Practical Pulmonary Pathology

A DIAGNOSTIC APPROACH

Elsevier CD-ROM license agreement

Practical Pulmonary Pathology

A DIAGNOSTIC APPROACH

Kevin O. Leslie MD
Consultant and Professor of Anatomic Pathology
Department of Laboratory Medicine and Pathology
Mayo Clinic Scottsdale
Scottsdale
Arizona
USA

Mark R. Wick MD
Professor of Pathology
Division of Surgical Pathology
University of Virginia Medical Center
Charlottesville
Virginia
USA

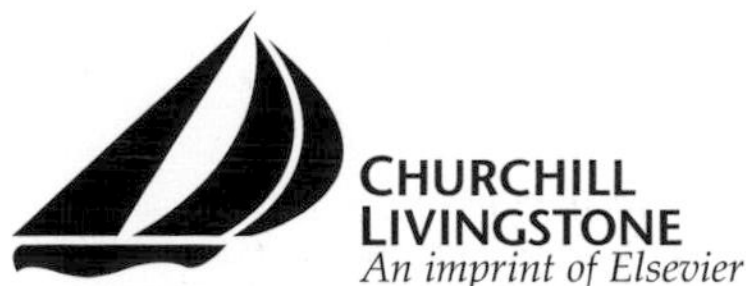

CHURCHILL LIVINGSTONE
An imprint of Elsevier

PHILADELPHIA EDINBURGH LONDON NEW YORK OXFORD ST LOUIS SYDNEY TORONTO 2005

CHURCHILL LIVINGSTONE
An imprint of Elsevier

First published 2005

ISBN 0443066310

British Library Cataloguing in Publication Data
A catalogue record for this book is available from the British Library

Library of Congress Cataloging in Publication Data
A catalog record for this book is available from the Library of Congress

Notice
Medical knowledge is constantly changing. Standard safety precautions must be followed, but as new research and clinical experience broaden our knowledge, changes in treatment and drug therapy may become necessary or appropriate. Readers are advised to check the most current product information provided by the manufacturer of each drug to be administered to verify the recommended dose, the method and duration of administration, and contraindications. It is the responsibility of the practitioner, relying on experience and knowledge of the patient, to determine dosages and the best treatment for each individual patient. Neither the Publisher nor the editors assumes any liability for any injury and/or damage to persons or property arising from this publication.

The Publisher

Last digit is the print number: 9 8 7 6 5 4 3 2

Commissioning Editor: Michael Houston
Project Development Manager: Belinda Kuhn
Project Manager: Alan Nicholson
Designer: Sarah Russell
Illustration Manager: Mick Ruddy

The publisher's policy is to use **paper manufactured from sustainable forests**

Printed in China

Contents

Contributors

Mattia Barbareschi MD, PhD
Associate Director
Department of Surgical Pathology
S. Chiara Hospital
Trento
ITALY

Kelly J. Butnor MD
Assistant Professor of Pathology
Department of Pathology
University of Vermont College of Medicine
Fletcher Allen Healthcare
Burlington, VT
USA

Lisa A. Cerilli MD
Pathologist
Health Partners Regional Laboratory
Richmond, VA
USA

Oi-Yee Cheung MD
Specialist Pathologist
Department of Pathology
Queen Elizabeth Hospital
Kowloon
HONG KONG

Andrew Churg MD
Professor of Pathology
Department of Pathology
University of British Columbia
Vancouver, BC
CANADA

Thomas V. Colby MD
Consultant and Professor of Anatomic Pathology
Department of Laboratory Medicine and Pathology
Mayo Clinic Scottsdale
Scottsdale, AZ
USA

Junya Fukuoka MD
Assistant Professor
Department of Pathology
Shiga University of Medical Science
Tsukinowa-cho, Seta, Otsu
JAPAN

Thomas E. Hartman MD
Consultant and Associate Professor of Radiology
Department of Radiology
Mayo Clinic Rochester
Rochester, MN
USA

Kirk D. Jones MD
Assistant Clinical Professor of Pathology
Department of Pathology
University of California
San Francisco, CA
USA

Andras Khoor MD
Consultant in Anatomic Pathology
Department of Pathology
Mayo Clinic Jacksonville
Jacksonville, FL
USA

Madeleine D. Kraus MD
Assistant Professor of Pathology
Department of Pathology
The University of Chicago Hospitals
Chicago, IL
USA

Kevin O. Leslie MD
Consultant and Professor of Anatomic Pathology
Department of Laboratory Medicine and Pathology
Mayo Clinic Scottsdale
Scottsdale, AZ
USA

Osamu Matsubara MD
National Defense Medical College
Department of Pathology
Tokoworaza
JAPAN

Stacey E. Mills MD
Professor of Pathology
Division of Surgical Pathology
University of Virginia Medical Center
Charlottesville, VA
USA

Cesar A. Moran MD
Professor of Pathology
Department of Pathology
MD Anderson Cancer Center
Houston, TX
USA

Stephen S. Raab MD
Professor of Pathology
Director of Cytology
Department of Pathology
University of Pittsburgh
Pittsburgh, PA
USA

Jon H. Ritter MD
Assistant Professor of Pathology
Department of Pathology
Washington University School of Medicine
St Louis, MO
USA

Victor L. Roggli MD
Professor of Pathology
Duke University Medical Center
Durham, NC
USA

Louis A. Rosati MD
Associate Pathologist
Banner Desert Medical Center
Department of Pathology
Mesa, AZ
USA

Charles D. Sturgis MD
Director of Cytopathology
Evanston Northwestern Healthcare
Assistant Professor of Pathology
Northwestern University Feinberg School of Medicine
Evanston, IL
USA

Victor F. Trastek MD
Professor of Surgery
Department of Thoracic Surgery
Mayo Clinic Scottsdale
Scottsdale, AZ
USA

William D. Travis MD
Professor of Pathology
Chairman
Department of Pulmonary and Mediastinal Pathology
Armed Forces Institute of Pathology
Washington DC
USA

Robert W. Viggiano MD
Consultant
Department of Pulmonary Medicine
Mayo Clinic Scottsdale
Scottsdale, AZ
USA

Mark R. Wick MD
Professor of Pathology
Division of Surgical Pathology
University of Virginia Medical Center
Charlottesville, VA
USA

Joanne L. Wright MD
Professor of Pathology
Department of Pathology
University of British Columbia
Vancouver, BC
CANADA

Samuel A. Yousem MD
Professor of Pathology
University of Pittsburgh Medical Center
Department of Pathology
Pittsburgh, PA
USA

Preface

A fundamental truth about medical textbooks is that they are often not read from beginning to end once the student of medicine has progressed beyond the basic medical school curriculum. In the *practice* of medicine, textbooks are more commonly used for learning about a disease or entity that we suspect a patient may have, based on history, physical findings and imaging/laboratory data gleaned from an initial screening evaluation. Such *disease-based* textbooks are much easier to use if you already have a good idea of where you need look for information on the patient's disease.

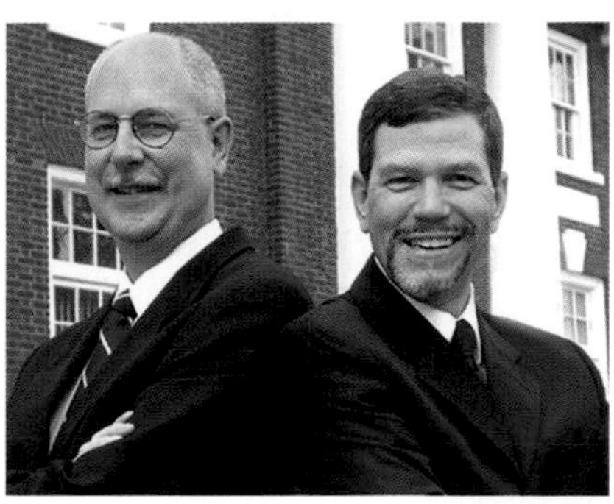

Today, medical textbooks continue to exist as a compendium of different subjects, each of which begins with an historical introduction and ends with treatment, expected clinical course, and prognosis. The subjects in this book are no different, but we have added this chapter as a visual index, based on patterns and findings in the biopsy specimen. We begin with the general pattern(s) of disease and then have added key morphologic findings that assist in focusing the reader to the appropriate section (or sections) in the book where similar findings are discussed. This approach is facilitated if we begin with a structural overlay that limits the patterns. We have found that six general patterns occur, and these are best appreciated at scanning magnification with the microscope. We could begin at an even lower "magnification" using the high-resolution computed tomogram (CT), and this is what our radiology colleagues commonly do as they assemble a differential diagnosis based on observed findings in this medium (see Ch. 3). In practice, the CT images may not be readily available to the pathologist, so we begin with a tissue section mounted on glass.

A basic knowledge of the two-dimensional structure of the lung is essential for accurately assessing patterns of disease. We assume that the reader is familiar with basic lung anatomy by the time a diagnostic problem is being evaluated in the patient care setting, but a brief review is always helpful (see Ch. 2.) An overview of the six patterns is presented in Box 1. Each pattern is further illustrated in the 12 pages that follow this introduction. Most of the patterns were devised to navigate the "diffuse lung diseases" commonly referred to as "interstitial lung diseases" or "ILD". Given the tumefactive nature of neoplasms, these are heavily represented in pattern 5 ("Nodules"), but some non-neoplastic diseases, such as sarcoidosis, nodular infections, Wegener's granulomatosis, and certain pneumoconioses, may also manifest as a nodular pattern. Rarely, neoplasms can present as diffuse "interstitial" lung disease clinically and radiologically.

Once the overriding or dominant pattern is recognized, the diagnostician is further aided by assessing the cellular composition and any other distinctive findings that accompany the pattern. In the case of a tumor forming a nodular mass, the presence of prominent spindled cells, or large granular cells, or clear cells provides a direction for creating a differential diagnosis. Within each pattern, we have attempted to use such qualifying elements to direct the reader to the appropriate chapter for further study, reasonably confident that the answer will lie within. For the unusual finding not identified in the list for a given pattern, the reader is directed to Appendix 1 where we have assembled a "visual encyclopedia" of distinctive findings and artifacts.

Naturally, overlap occurs between patterns and this too can be a useful guide to the correct diagnosis. For example, some infections are both *nodular* and have *airspace filling* (e.g. botyromycosis, aspiration pneumonia), while others are characterized by *acute lung injury* and diffuse *airspace filling* (e.g. pneumoccocal pneumonia, pneumocystis pneumonia.) In fact, some diffuse inflammatory conditions in the lung may manifest five of the six patterns, in different areas of the same biopsy (e.g. rheumatoid lung). Nevertheless, as more and more information is accrued from the biopsy, the differential diagnosis becomes more limited. In some cases, it may be necessary to include several possibilities in the final diagnosis, especially for the non-neoplastic diseases, where the effect of ancillary data not available at the time of diagnosis may be very large.

Kevin O Leslie
Mark R Wick
2004

Acknowledgments

This work is dedicated to my wife Peggy and our children Katie and Amy, whose support and tolerance over the years have made this work possible. I am also thankful for my good fortune in knowing Dr Tom Colby, long time friend, colleague, and mentor, and for the hundreds of pathologists and pulmonologists whose patients have provided me with insight and inspiration over the years.

Many thanks to Martha Cobb and Theresa Schwallier for providing invaluable assistance in manuscript preparation and to Drs. Joseph Collins, John English, Francesca Guddo, Felix Martinez, Harman Sekhon and Diana Ionescu for assistance in final proof review and for providing constructive criticism.

Kevin O Leslie, MD
Mayo Clinic Scottsdale

Many thanks are due to my children, Morgan and Robert, for allowing me to take time I would otherwise have spent with them to devote to finishing this work. Also, I am grateful to my colleagues in surgical pathology at the University of Virginia for their consistent encouragement and enthusiastic support of this project.

Mark R Wick, MD
University of Virginia Medical Center

Pattern-based approach to diagnosis

Pattern	Diseases to be considered
Acute lung injury	Diffuse alveolar damage (DAD) –infection –eosinophilic pneumonia –drug toxicity –certain systemic connective tissue diseases –diffuse alveolar hemorrhage –irradiation injury –idiopathic (acute interstitial pneumonia) Acute hypersensitivity pneumonitis Acute pneumoconiosis Acute aspiration pneumonia
Fibrosis	Usual interstitial pneumonia (UIP) Collagen vascular diseases Chronic eosinophilic pneumonia Chronic drug toxicity Chronic hypersensitivity pneumonitis Nonspecific interstitial pneumonia (NSIP) Sarcoidosis (advanced) Pneumoconioses Erdheim-Chester disease Hermansky-Pudlak syndrome
Chronic cellular infiltrates	Hypersensitivity pneumonitis Nonspecific interstitial pneumonia (NSIP) Systemic connective tissue diseases Certain chronic infections Certain drug toxicities Lymphocytic and lymphoid interstitial pneumonia Lymphomas and leukemias Lymphangitic carcinomatosis
Alveolar filling	Infections Airspace organization (organizing pneumonia) Diffuse alveolar hemorrhage Desquamative interstitial pneumonia (DIP) Respiratory bronchiolitis-associated ILD Alveolar proteinosis Dendriform (racemose) calcification Alveolar microlithiasis Mucostasis and mucinous tumors
Nodules	Primary and metastatic neoplasms Wegener granulomatosis Sarcoidosis/berylliosis Aspiration pneumonia Pulmonary Langerhans cell histiocytosis
Near normal biopsy	Chronic small airways disease Vasculopathic diseases Lymphangioleiomyomatosis (LAM)

PATTERN 1 **Acute lung injury**

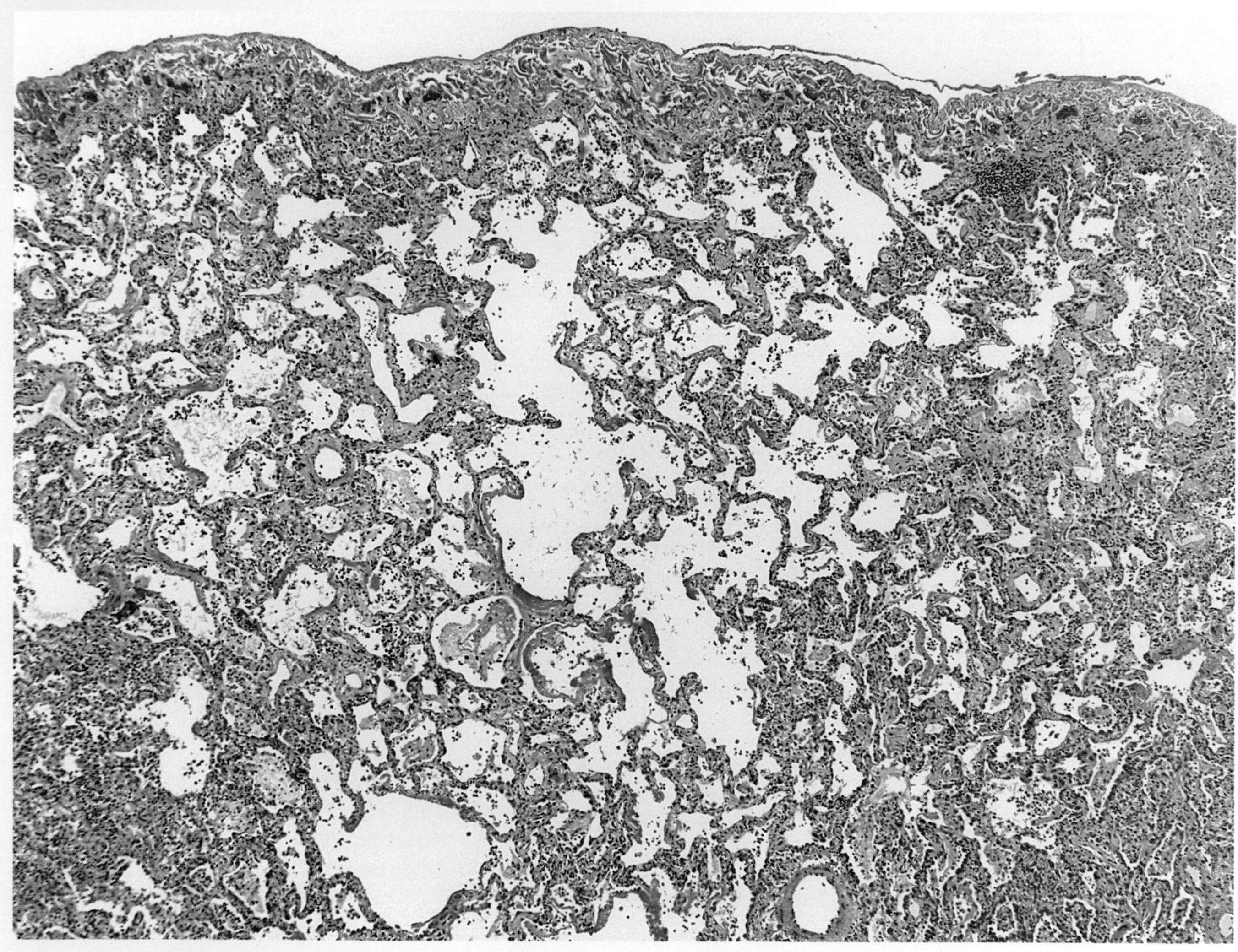

Elements of the pattern: The lung biopsy is *diffusely* involved by variable amounts of edema and fibrin accompanied by reactive type 2 cell hyperplasia. The dominance of non-cellular, protein-rich material imparts an overall red or pink appearance to the biopsy at scanning magnification (in routine hematoxylin-eosin stained sections.)

PATTERN 1 Acute lung injury

Additional findings	Diagnostic consideration	Chapter/page	
Hyaline membranes	Diffuse alveolar damage	(Ch 5:72,73; Ch 6:113)	■, ■
Necrosis in parenchyma	Infection	(Ch 5:75,91)	■
	Some tumors	(Ch 10:336,340,345; Ch 15:531,538)	■, ■
	Infarct	(Ch 6:153; Ch 10:365; Ch 17:604)	■, ■, ■
Necrosis in bronchioles	Infections	(Ch 5:78,82; Ch 6:125)	■, ■
	Acute aspiration	(Ch 8:277)	■
Fibrin in alveoli	Diffuse alveolar damage	(Ch 5:72)	■
	Drug toxicity	(Ch 5:72; Ch 7:218)	■, ■
	Connective tissue disease	(Ch 5:83)	■
	Infection	(Ch 4:59; Ch 5:75,81 Ch 6:109)	■, ■, ■
Eosinophils in alveoli	Eosinophilic lung diseases	(Ch 5:92; Ch 7:213)	■, ■
Siderophages in alveoli	Diffuse alveolar hemorrhage	(Ch 4:63; Ch 5:92; Ch 7:209; Ch 10:366)	■, ■, ■ ■
	Drug toxicity	(Ch 5:84; Ch 7:215)	■, ■
	Infarct	(Ch 10:365)	■
Fibrinous pleuritis	Connective tissue diseases	(Ch 5:83; Ch 7:204)	■, ■
	Eosinophilic pneumonia	(Ch 5:87)	■
	Pneumothorax	(Ch 7:238)	■
Neutrophils	Infections	(Ch 5:82)	■
	Capillaritis in diffuse alveolar hemorrhage	(Ch 10:336,355)	■,
Atypical cells	Acute lung injury	(Ch 5:92)	■
	Viral infections	(Ch 6:153)	■
	Leukemias	(Ch 15:531)	■
Fibrin + vacuolated macrophages	Drug toxicity	(Ch 5:84; Ch 7:215)	■, ■
	Connective tissue diseases	(Ch 5:83)	■

PATTERN 2 **Fibrosis**

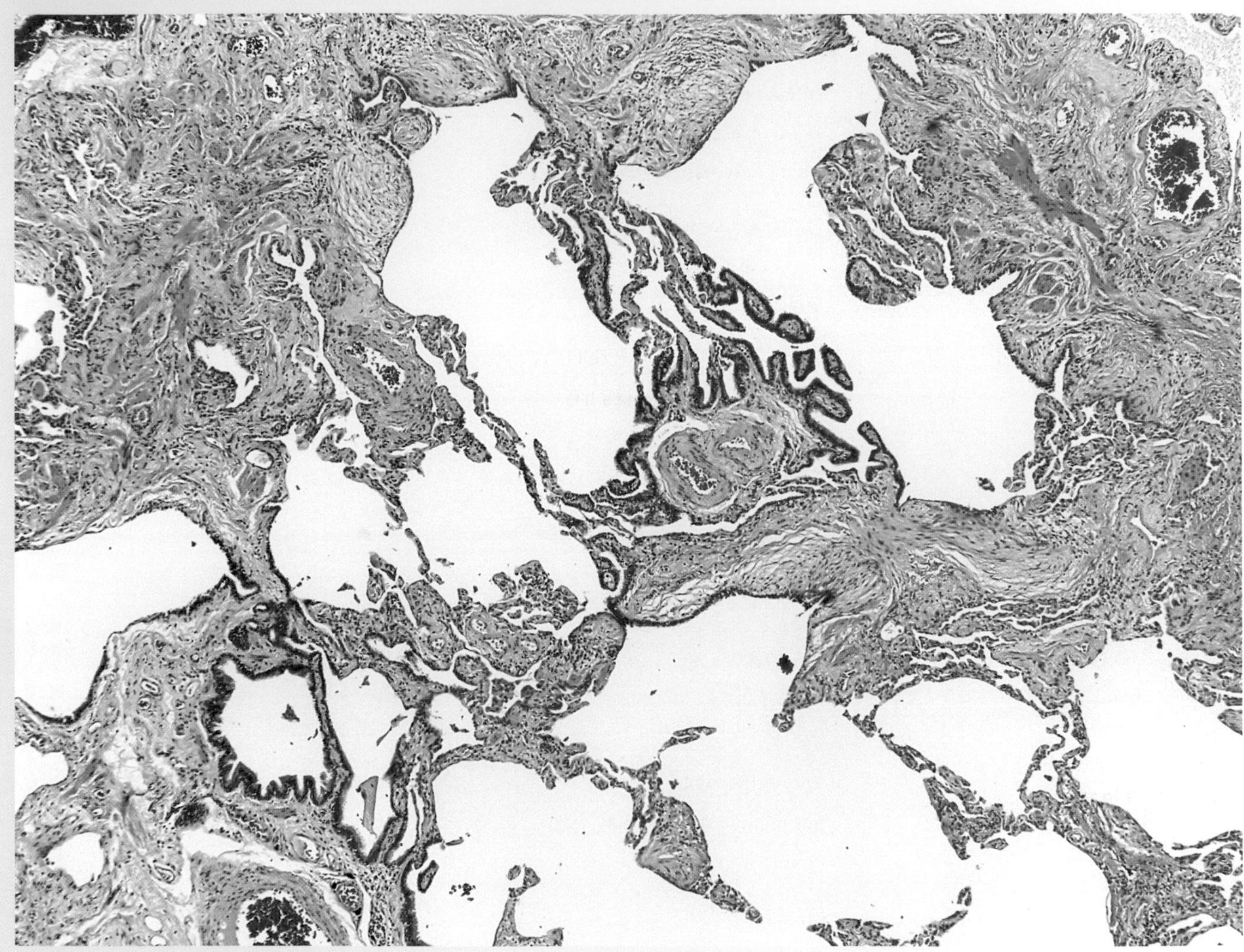

Elements of the pattern: The lung biopsy is involved by variable amounts of fibrosis. As in pattern 1, the biopsy tends to be more pink than blue at scanning magnification, as a result of collagen deposition (in routine hematoxylin-eosin stained sections.) Some fibrosis patterns are accompanied by chronic inflammation that may impart a blue tinge to the process, or even dark blue lymphoid aggregates.

PATTERN 2 **Fibrosis**

Additional findings	Diagnostic consideration	Chapter/page	
Hyaline membranes	Acute on chronic connective tissue disease	(Ch 7:204)	■
	Acute exacerbation of idiopathic pulmonary fibrosis (IPF)	(Ch 7:189)	■
Microscopic honeycombing	Usual interstitial pneumonia (UIP)	(Ch 7:185)	■
	Hypersensitivity pneumonitis	(Ch 7:228)	■
	Connective tissue disease	(Ch 7:203)	■
Prominent bronchiolization	Pulmonary Langerhans cell histiocytosis	(Ch 7:234)	■
	Respiratory bronchiolitis ILD	(Ch 7:196)	■
	Connective tissue diseases	(Ch 7:203)	■
	Chronic hypersensitivity pneumonitis	(Ch 7:228)	■
	Small airways disease	(Ch 8:265)	■
	Chronic aspiration	(Ch 8:289)	■
Uniform alveolar septal fibrosis	Connective tissue diseases	(Ch 7:191)	■
Peripheral lobular fibrosis	UIP/IPF	(Ch 7:185)	■
	Erdheim Chester disease	(Ch 7:238)	■
	Chronic eosinophilic pneumonia	(Ch 7:213)	■
Siderophages in alveoli	Chronic cardiac congestion	(Ch 7:201; Ch 9:323)	■, ■
	Chronic SLE with hemorrhage	(Ch 7:208; Ch 10:355)	■, ■
	Pneumoconiosis	(Ch 9:323)	■
	Pulmonary Langerhans cell histiocytosis	(Ch 7:234)	■
Fibrinous pleuritis	Connective tissue disease	(Ch 7:205)	■
	Eosinophilic pleuritis in pneumothorax	(Ch 7:238; Appendix:780)	■, ■
Prominent non-necrotizing granulomas	Sarcoidosis	(Ch 7:225)	■
Many vacuolated cells	Chronic obstruction	(Ch 7:233)	■
	Drug toxicity	(Ch 7:218)	■
	Hermansky-Pudlak syndrome	(Ch 7:243)	■
	Genetic storage diseases	(Ch 4:67)	■
Prominent chronic inflammation	Nonspecific interstitial pneumonia-fibrosis	(Ch 7:191)	■
	RA and other connective tissue disease	(Ch 7:203)	■
Bronchiolocentric scarring	Pulmonary Langerhans cell histocytosis	(Ch 7:234)	■
	Pneumoconiosis	(Ch 8:286; Ch 9:313)	■, ■
	Chronic Hypersensitivity	(Ch 7:228)	■
	Connective tissue diseases	(Ch 7:191)	■

PATTERN 3 Chronic cellular infiltrates

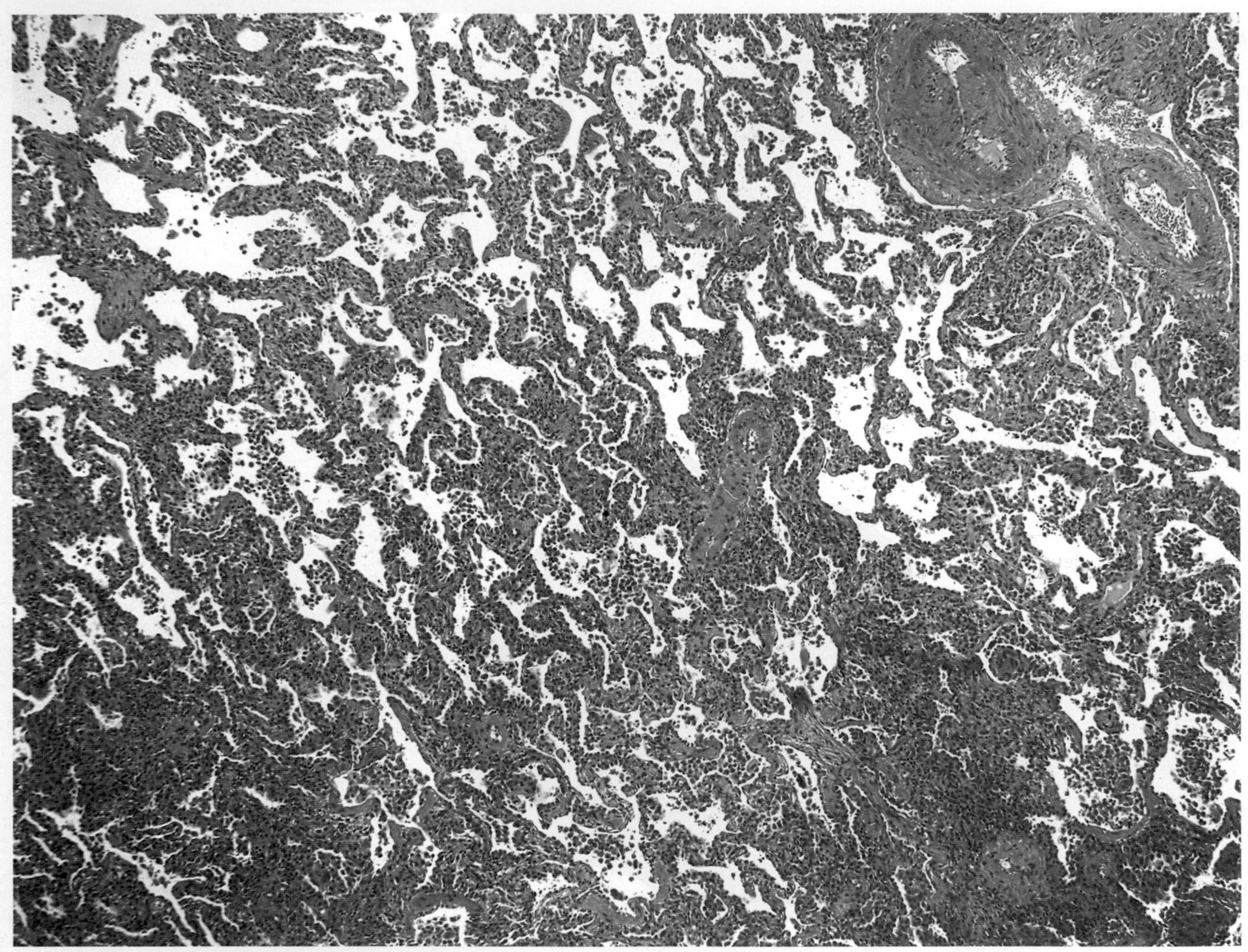

Elements of the pattern: The lung biopsy is involved by variable amounts of chronic inflammation and reactive type 2 cell hyperplasia. The dominance of mononuclear infiltrates may impart an overall blue appearance to the biopsy at scanning magnification (in routine hematoxylin-eosin stained sections.)

Additional findings	Diagnostic consideration	Chapter/page	
Hyaline membranes	"Acute on chronic" connective tissue disease	(Ch 7:204)	■
	Drug toxicity	(Ch 5:72,83)	■
	Diffuse alveolar hemorrhage	(Ch 5:83; Ch 7:208; Ch 10:372)	■, ■, ■
Necrosis in parenchyma	Viral and fungal infections	(Ch 5:79; Ch 6:116,131)	■, ■
	Aspiration	(Ch 6:112)	■
Necrosis in bronchioles	Viral infections	(Ch 5:75)	■
	Aspiration	(Ch 6:112)	■

(Continued)

PATTERN 3 Chronic cellular infiltrates

Additional findings	Diagnostic consideration	Chapter/page	
Poorly formed granulomas (Small and non-necrotizing)	Hypersensitivity pneumonitis	(Ch 7:228)	■
	Atypical mycobacterial infection	(Ch 6:126; Ch 8:275)	■, ■
	Lymphoid interstitial pneumonia	(Ch 4:64; Ch 7:201,212)	■, ■
	Drug toxicity	(Ch 7:218)	■
Well formed necrotizing granulomas	Infections	(Ch 6:123)	■
	Rare drug reactions	(Ch 7:215)	■
	Necrotizing sarcoidosis	(Ch 10:357)	■
Eosinophils in alveoli	Eosinophilic lung diseases	(Ch 7:213)	■
	Smoking-related diseases	(Ch 7:196)	■
Siderophages in alveoli	Diffuse alveolar hemorrhage	(Ch 10:366)	■
	Chronic passive congestion	(Ch 9:323)	■
	Drug toxicity	(Ch 10:355)	■
Fibrinous/chronic pleuritis	Connective tissue diseases	(Ch 7:194,205)	■
	Thoracic trauma/infection	(Ch 7:238)	■
	Pancreatitis-associated		
Patchy organizing pneumonia	Drug toxicity	(Ch 5:84; Ch 7:218)	■, ■
	Connective tissue diseases	(Ch 7:203)	■
	Infections	(Ch 6:112)	■
	Cryptogenic organizing pneumonia	(Ch 7:193)	■
	Diffuse alveolar hemorrhage	(Ch 10:354)	■
	Aspiration	(Ch 7:195)	■
Atypical cells*	Viral infections	(Ch 5:75; Ch 6:153)	■, ■
	Lymphangitic carcinoma	(Ch 7:249)	■
Multinucleated giant cells	Hard metal disease	(Ch 9:326)	■
	Mica pneumoconiosis	(Ch 9:318)	■
	Hypersensitivity pneumonitis	(Ch 7:228)	■
	IV drug abuse	(Ch 7:224)	■
	Drug toxicity	(Ch 7:218)	■
	Aspiration pneumonia	(Ch 7:195)	■
	Eosinophilic pneumonia	(Ch 7:213)	■
Dense mononuclear infiltration	Lymphomas	(Ch 8:273; Ch 10:347; Ch 15:529)	■, ■, ■
	Lymphoid interstitial pneumonia	(Ch 7:201)	■
	Connective tissue diseases	(Ch 7:212)	■
	Hypersensitivity pneumonitis	(Ch 7:228)	■
	Certain infections	(Ch 6:126; Ch 7:191)	■, ■
Lymphoid aggregates/germinal centers	Connective tissue diseases	(Ch 7:204)	■
	Diffuse lymphoid hyperplasia	(Ch 7:202)	■
	Lymphoid interstitial pneumonia	(Ch 7:201)	■
	Follicular bronchiolitis	(Ch 8:267)	■

PATTERN 4 **Alveolar filling**

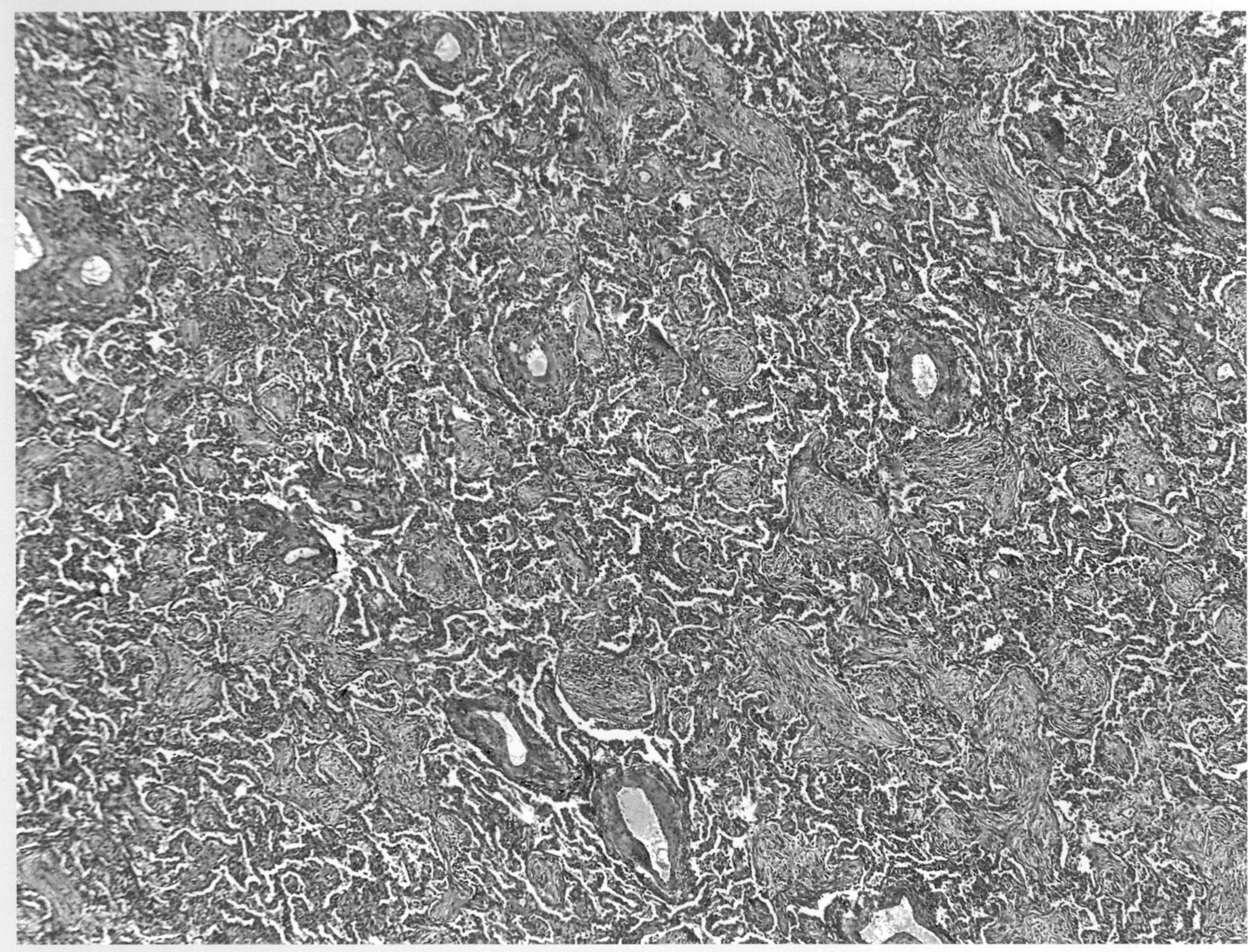

Elements of the pattern: The *dominant* finding is alveolar spaces filled with cells, or non-cellular elements.

PATTERN 4 Alveolar filling

Additional findings in airspaces	Diagnostic consideration	Chapter/page
Hyaline membranes and fibrin	Organizing diffuse alveolar damage	(Ch 5:72)
Necrosis and neutrophils	Bacterial infection	(Ch 5:82; Ch 6:109)
	Viral and fungal infection	(Ch 6:131,153)
Organizing pneumonia	Organizing infection	(Ch 6:109)
	Drug toxicity	(Ch 7:218)
	Cryptogenic organizing pneumonia	(Ch 7:193)
Fibrin and macrophages	Eosinophilic pneumonia post steroid	(Ch 7:213)
	Drug toxicity	(Ch 7:218)
	Connective tissue diseases	(Ch 7:212)
	Malakoplakia-like reaction	(Ch 6:122)
Eosinophils and macrophages	Eosinophilic lung diseases	(Ch 7:213)
Siderophages and fibrin	Diffuse alveolar hemorrhage	(Ch 10:354)
Mucin	Mucostasis in small airways disease	(Ch 8:283)
	Bronchioloalveolar carcinoma	(Ch 4:56; Ch 16:574)
	Cryptococcus infection	(Ch 6:136)
Bone/calcification	Dendriform calcification	(Ch 7:198)
	Metastatic calcification	(Appendix:784)
	Pulmonary alveolar microlithiasis	(Ch 7:246)
Atypical cells	Bronchioloalveolar carcinoma	(Ch 16:574)
	Herpesvirus infections	(Ch 5:79; Ch 6:158)
	Acute eosinophilic pneumonia	(Ch 5:87)
	Carcinomas and sarcomas	(Ch 14,16,17)
Proteinaceous exudates	Edema	(Ch 5:84; 6:116,155; Ch 7:190,209,248; Ch 12:403)
	Pulmonary alveolar proteinosis (PAP)	(Ch 7:247)
	PAP reactions	(Ch 7:248)
Multinucleated giant cells	Hard metal disease	(Ch 9:326)
	Eosinophilic pneumonia	(Ch 7:213)
	Wegener's granulomatosis	(Ch 10:337)
	Aspiration pneumonia	(Ch 7:195)
Polypoid mesenchymal bodies resembling chorionic villi	Bullous placental transmogrification	(Appendix:789)

PATTERN 5 **Nodules**

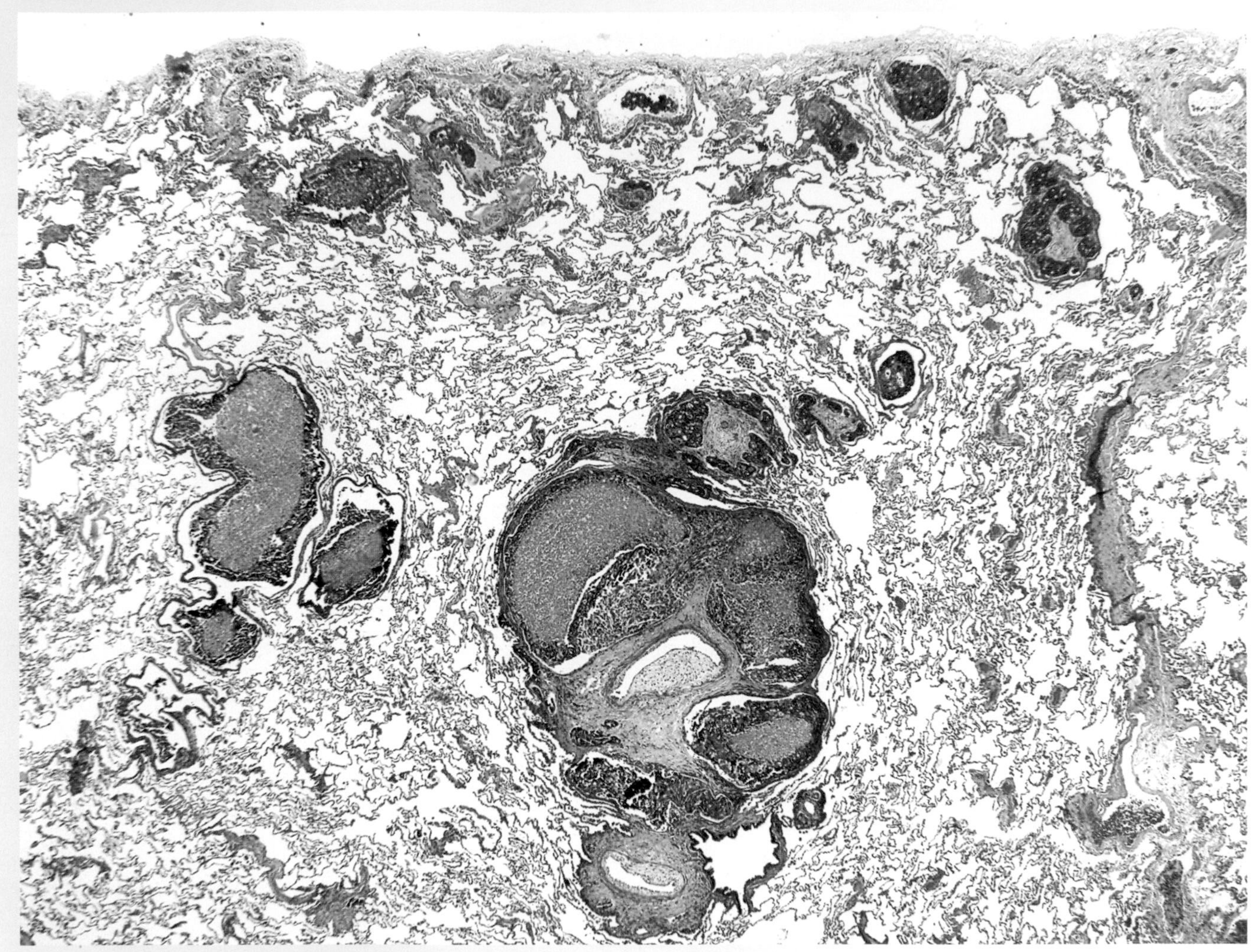

Elements of the pattern: Nodules of variable size and shape. An interface between the nodular lesion and more normal lung should be discernible. In the case of very large nodules encompassing the entire specimen, radiologic imaging can be used as part of the definition.

PATTERN 5 **Nodules**

Additional findings	Diagnostic consideration	Chapter/page	
Large lymphoid cells	Malignant lymphoma	(Ch 8:273; Ch 10:347; Ch 15:529)	■, ■, ■
Small lymphoid cells w/ germ ctrs	Lymphoid interstitial pneumonia	(Ch 7:201)	■
	MALT lymphoma, low grade	(Ch 8:272; Ch 15:527,529)	■, ■
	Follicular bronchiolitis	(Ch 7:204; Ch 8:267; Ch 10:345; Ch 15:524)	■, ■, ■, ■
	Diffuse lymphoid hyperplasia	(Ch 15:527)	■
	Intraparenchymal lymph node		
Giant multinucleated neoplastic cells	Sarcomatoid carcinoma	(Ch14:468)	■
	Large cell undifferentiated carcinoma	(Ch 13:444; Ch 16:579)	■, ■
	Primary and metastatic sarcomas	(Ch 14:475; Ch 17:623)	■, ■
	Metastatic pleomorphic carcinomas	(Ch 17:620)	■
	Primary or metastatic melanoma	(Ch 14:493; Ch 17:629)	■, ■
	Giant cell tumor (primary or metastatic)		
Small round blue neoplastic cells	Small cell undifferentiated carcinoma	(Ch 13:440)	■
	Malignant lymphoma	(Ch 15:527)	■
	Small cell squamous carcinoma	(Ch 16:566)	■
	Metastatic tumors		
	Ewing's sarcoma	(Ch 14:503)	■
	Primitive neuroectodermal tumor	(Ch 13:453; Ch 14:503)	■, ■
	Small cell osteosarcoma	(Ch 17:625)	■
	Neuroblastoma	(Ch 14:503; Ch 17:628)	■, ■
	Pleuropulmonary blastoma (with cysts)	(Ch 14:500,507)	■
Spindled or fusiform neoplastic cells	Primary sarcomatoid carcinoma	(Ch 14:468)	■
	Primary and metastatic sarcomas	(Ch 14:475; Ch 17:623)	■, ■
	Lymphangioleiomyomatosis (with cysts)	(Ch 3:43; Ch 7:239)	■, ■
	Inflammatory myofibroblastic tumor	(Ch 18:650; Ch 19:696)	■, ■
	Benign metastasizing leiomyoma	(Ch 19:683)	■
	Localized fibrous tumor	(Ch 19:704)	■
	Extraabdominal desmoid tumor	(Ch 14:468)	■
Large pink epithelioid neoplastic cells	Poorly differentiated primary carcinomas	(Ch 14:475; Ch 16:564; Ch 17:620)	■, ■, ■
	Large cell undifferentiated carcinoma	(Ch 13:444; Ch 16:579)	■, ■
	Metastatic carcinomas	(Ch 17:615–618,631)	■
	Metastatic sarcomas	(Ch 17:631)	■
	Epithelioid hemangioendothelioma	(Ch 14:481; Ch 19:723)	■, ■
	Melanoma (primary or metastatic)	(Ch 14:493; Ch 17:629)	■, ■

PATTERN 5 **Nodules** *(continued)*

Additional findings	Diagnostic consideration	Chapter/page	
Large clear epithelioid neoplastic cells	Primary adenocarcinoma	(Ch 16:565)	■
	Primary squamous carcinoma	(Ch 16:563)	■
	Large cell undifferentiated carcinoma	(Ch 16:580)	■
	Sugar tumor	(Ch 19:711)	■
	Perivascular epithelioid cell tumor (PEComa)	(Ch 19:690)	■
	Metastatic clear cell carcinoma	(Ch 17:612)	■
	Metastatic clear cell sarcoma	(Ch 17:620)	■
Large basophilic epithelial cells w/ peripheral pallisade	Large cell undifferentiated carcinoma	(Ch 16:579)	■
	Large cell neuroendocrine carcinoma	(Ch 13:444)	■
	Basaloid squamous carcinoma	(Ch 13:430; Ch 16:566)	■, ■
	Certain metastatic tumors	(Ch 17)	■
Glands or tubules- Malignant	Primary adenocarcinoma	(Ch 16:565)	■
	Metastatic adenocarcinoma	(Ch 17:611)	■
	Carcinoid tumor (primary or metastatic)	(Ch 13:434)	■
	Synovial sarcoma (primary or metastatic)	(Ch 17:622,642)	■
	Fetal-type primary adenocarcinoma	(Ch 16:570)	■
	Carcinosarcoma (primary or metastatic)	(Ch 14:466)	■
Glands or tubules- benign or mild atypia	Alveolar adenoma	(Ch 19:700)	■
	Adenoma of Type II cells	(Ch 16:576)	■
	Pulmonary sclerosing hemangioma	(Ch 19:700)	■
	Hamartoma	(Ch 18:648)	■
	Micronodular pneumocyte hyperplasia	(Ch 7:245; Ch 19:691)	■, ■
	Adenomatoid tumor	(Ch 19:693)	■
Malignant heterologous elements (cartilage, bone, skeletal muscle)	Carcinosarcoma	(Ch 14:466)	■
	Metastatic teratocarcinoma	(Ch 17:632; Ch 19:721)	■, ■
	Metastatic sarcoma	(Ch 17:623)	■
Distinct keratinization	Primary squamous cell carcinoma	(Ch 16:563)	■
	Squamous metaplasia of terminal airways	(Ch 5:77; Ch 18:660)	■, ■
	Basaloid squamous cell carcinoma	(Ch 13:430; Ch 15:566)	■, ■
	Adenosquamous carcinoma	(Ch 16:579)	■
	Metastatic squamous cell carcinoma	(Ch 17:604)	■

(Continued)

PATTERN 5 **Nodules**

Additional findings	Diagnostic consideration	Chapter/page	
Pigmented cells	Cellular phase of Langerhans cell histiocytosis	(Ch 7:234)	■
	Primary or metastatic melanoma	(Ch 14:493; Ch 17:629)	■, ■
	Melanotic carcinoid tumor		
	Metastatic angiosarcoma (hemosiderin)	(Ch 17:639)	■
Malignant w/Dominant Necrosis	Small cell undifferentiated carcinoma	(Ch 13:440)	■
	Sarcomatoid carcinoma (primary or metastatic)	(Ch 14:466)	■
	High-grade malignant lymphoma	(Ch 14:529)	■
Benign w/ necrosis	Necrotizing infections		
	Bacterial	(Ch 5:82; Ch 6:108)	■, ■
	Fungal	(Ch 6:131)	■
	Mycobacterial	(Ch 6:132)	■
	Viral	(Ch 6:153)	■
	Wegener granulomatosis	(Ch 10:337)	■
	Churg Strauss syndrome	(Ch 10:350)	■
	Lung infarct	(Ch 6:140; Ch 10:340)	■, ■
Benign w/dominant organizing pneumonia	Nodular organizing pneumonia	(Ch 6:112; Ch 7:193)	■, ■
	Aspiration pneumonia	(Ch 7:195)	■
Benign w/well formed granulomas	Granulomatous infection		
	Fungal	(Ch 6:131)	■
	Mycobacterial	(Ch 6:123)	■
	Bacterial (botyromycosis)	(Ch 6:109)	■
	Sarcoidosis/berylliosis	(Ch 7:225)	■
	Certain pneumoconioses	(Ch 9:320)	■
	Aspiration pneumonia	(Ch 7:195)	■
	Necrotizing sarcoidosis	(Ch 10:357)	■
Benign w/stellate airways centered lesions and variable fibrosis	Pulmonary Langerhans cell histiocytosis	(Ch 7:234)	■
	Certain inhalational injuries	(Ch 9:313)	■
	Pneumoconioses	(Ch 8:286; Ch 9:304,308,313)	■, ■

PATTERN 6 **Nearly normal lung**

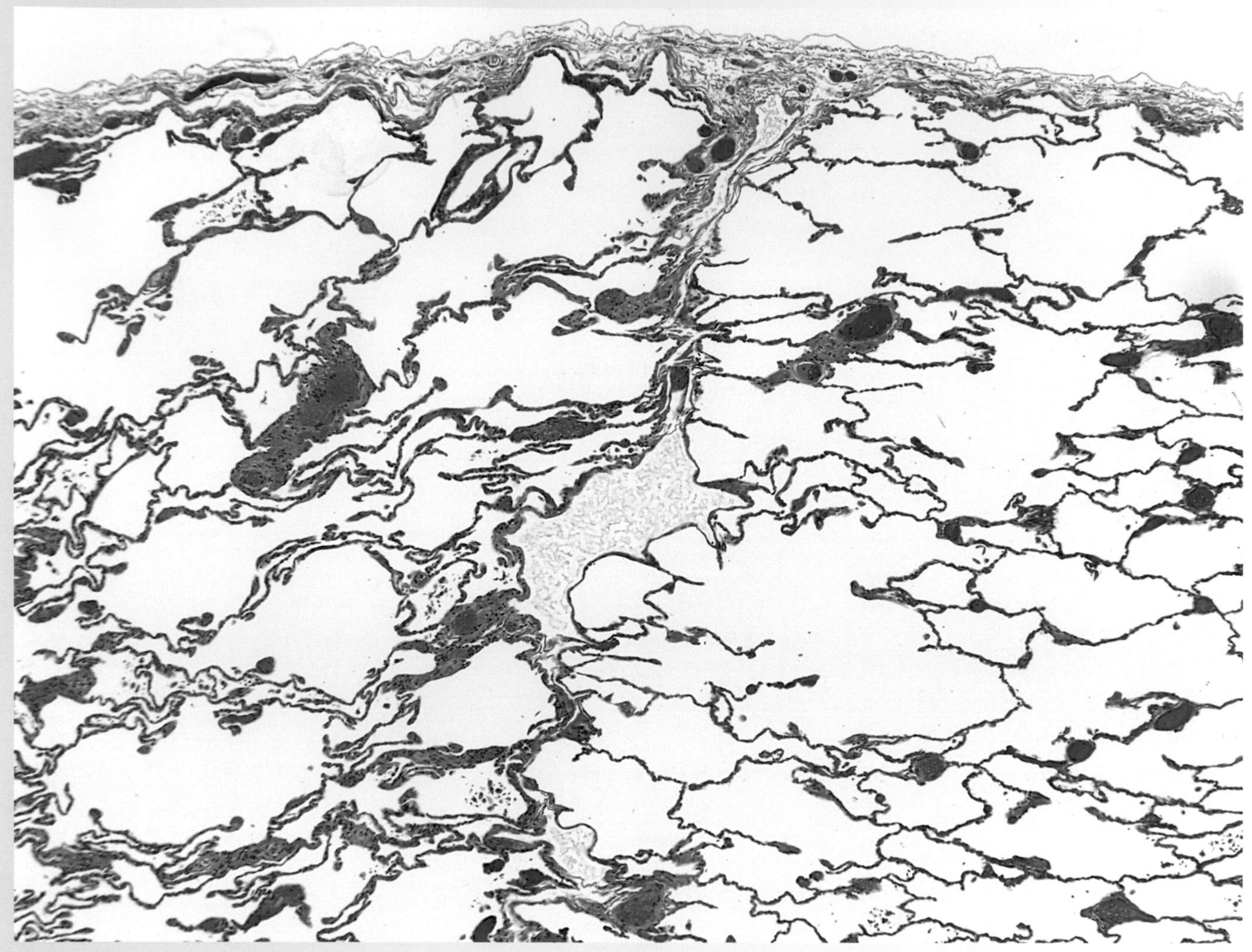

Elements of the pattern: The lung biopsy has little or no disease evident at scanning magnification.

PATTERN 6 Nearly normal lung

Additional findings	Diagnostic consideration	Chapter/page	
Thick pulmonary arteries	Pulmonary hypertension	(Ch 11:382)	■
	Chronic obstructive pulmonary disease	(Appendix:778)	■
Cysts	Lymphangioleiomyomatosis	(Ch 7:239)	■
	Pulmonary Langerhans cell histiocytosis	(Ch 7:234)	■
	Bullous emphysema	(Appendix:781)	■
Patchy Hyaline Membranes	Acute lung injury, early (may be subtle)	(Ch 5:72)	■
Airway scarring	Constrictive bronchiolitis (CB)	(Ch 8:284)	■
Bronchiolization (bronchiolar metaplasia)	Small airways disease +/- CB	(Ch 8:281)	■
Dilated bronchioles	Small airways disease +/- CB	(Ch 8:281)	■
Bronchioles absent or markedly decreased	Constrictive bronchiolitis	(Ch 8:284)	■
Prominent emphysema	Small airways disease +/- CB	(Ch 8:281)	■
Atypical cells	Lymphangitic and intravascular carcinoma	(Ch 7:249)	■

1

Lung anatomy

Kevin O Leslie   Mark R Wick

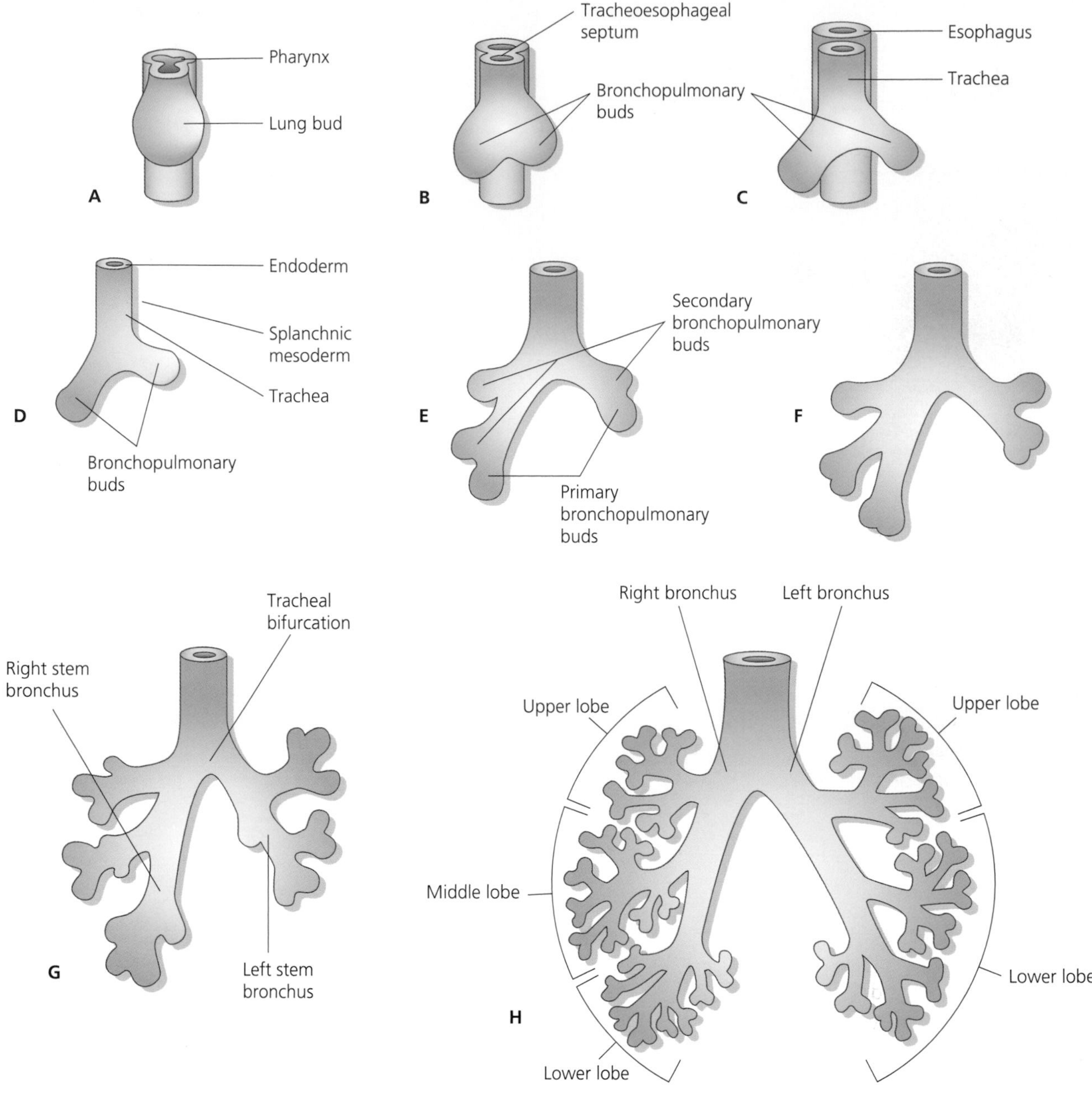

Fig. 1.1 Diagrammatic representation of the successive stages in the development of the bronchi and lungs: A–D, 4 weeks; E and F, 5 weeks; G, 6 weeks; H, 8 weeks. (Illustration courtesy of Moore[1] with permission.)

Development and gross anatomy

Airway development

During early embryogenesis (about day 21 post-fertilization), the lungs begin as a groove in the ventral floor of the foregut (Fig. 1.1) This foregut depression becomes a diverticulum of endoderm, surrounded by an amorphous condensation of splanchnic mesoderm that lengthens caudally in the midline, anterior to the esophagus. By the 4th week of gestation, two lung buds form as distal outpouchings.[1,2] A series of repetitive non-dichotomous branchings begins during week 5 and results in the formation of the primordial bronchial tree by the 8th week of gestation.

By 17 weeks, the rudimentary structure of the conducting airways has formed. This phase of lung development is referred to as the "pseudoglandular stage" because the fetal (postgestational week 7) lung is composed entirely of tubular elements that appear as circular gland-like structures in two-dimensional tissue

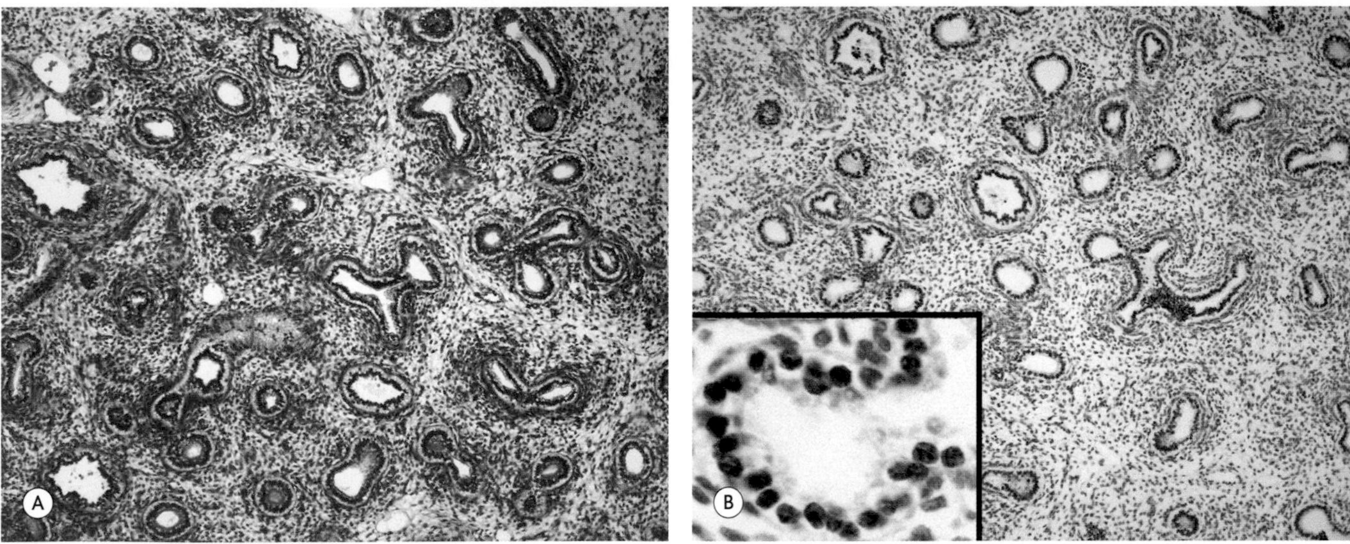

Fig. 1.2 In the early stage of lung development (A) the bronchi resemble tubular glands and are surrounded by undifferentiated mesenchyme. This stage is referred to as "pseudoglandular" because of this appearance (5–17 weeks gestation.) An immunohistochemical stain for thyroid transcription factor-1 (TTF-1, immunohistochemical stain, brown chromogen, hematoxylin counterstain) is positive in the nuclei of the immature airway cells (B).

sections (Fig. 1.2). The subsequent stages of development (*canalicular*, 13–25 weeks; *terminal sac*, 24 weeks to birth; and *alveolar*, late fetal to age 8–10 years) are dedicated to the formation of the essential units of respiration, the acini (Fig. 1.3).[1–5] The postnatal lung continues to accrue alveoli until about age 10 years (Fig. 1.4).

The pleura

Immediately after their formation, the lung buds grow into the medial walls of the pericardioperitoneal canals (splanchnic mesoderm) and in doing so become invested with a membrane that will be the visceral pleura (analogous to a fist being pushed into a balloon.) In this process, the lateral wall of the pericardioperitoneal canal becomes the parietal pleura, and the compressed space between becomes the pleural space (Fig. 1.5).

The lung lobes

By the end of gestation, five well-defined lung lobes are present, three on the right (upper, middle, and lower lobes) and two on the left (upper and lower lobes).[3,6,7] Each of the five primary lobar buds is invested with visceral pleura. Each lobe in turn is composed of one or more segments, resulting in a total of 10 segments per lung (Fig. 1.6). The presence of the heart leads to the formation of a rudimentary third lobe on the left side termed the lingula (more a part of the left upper lobe than an independent structure). In fact, the right middle lobe and lingula are analogous structures, given that each has an excessively long and narrow bronchus, predisposing these lobes to the pathologic effects of bronchial compression by adjacent lymph nodes or other masses. When this occurs, the chronic inflammatory changes that accrue in the respective lobe are referred to as "middle lobe syndrome."[8]

As gestation proceeds, airway branching continues to the level of the alveolar sacs, with a total of about 23 final subdivisions (20 of which occur proximal to the respiratory bronchioles). In successive order distally, the anatomic units formed are the lung segments, secondary and primary lobules (Fig. 1.7), and finally acini. With each successive division, the resulting airway branches are smaller than their predecessor, but each has a diameter greater than 50% of the airway parent. This phenomenon leads to a progressive increase in airway volume with each successive branching, and a significant reduction in airway resistance in more distal lung. The acinus consists of a central respiratory bronchiole that leads to an alveolar duct and terminates in an alveolar sac, comprised of many alveoli (Fig. 1.8).

Microscopic anatomy

The microscopic lung structure relevant to this chapter begins with the trachea and conducting airways and ends with the alveolar gas exchange units. This overview is intended to refresh the surgical pathologist's existing knowledge of the normal lung. For the reader interested

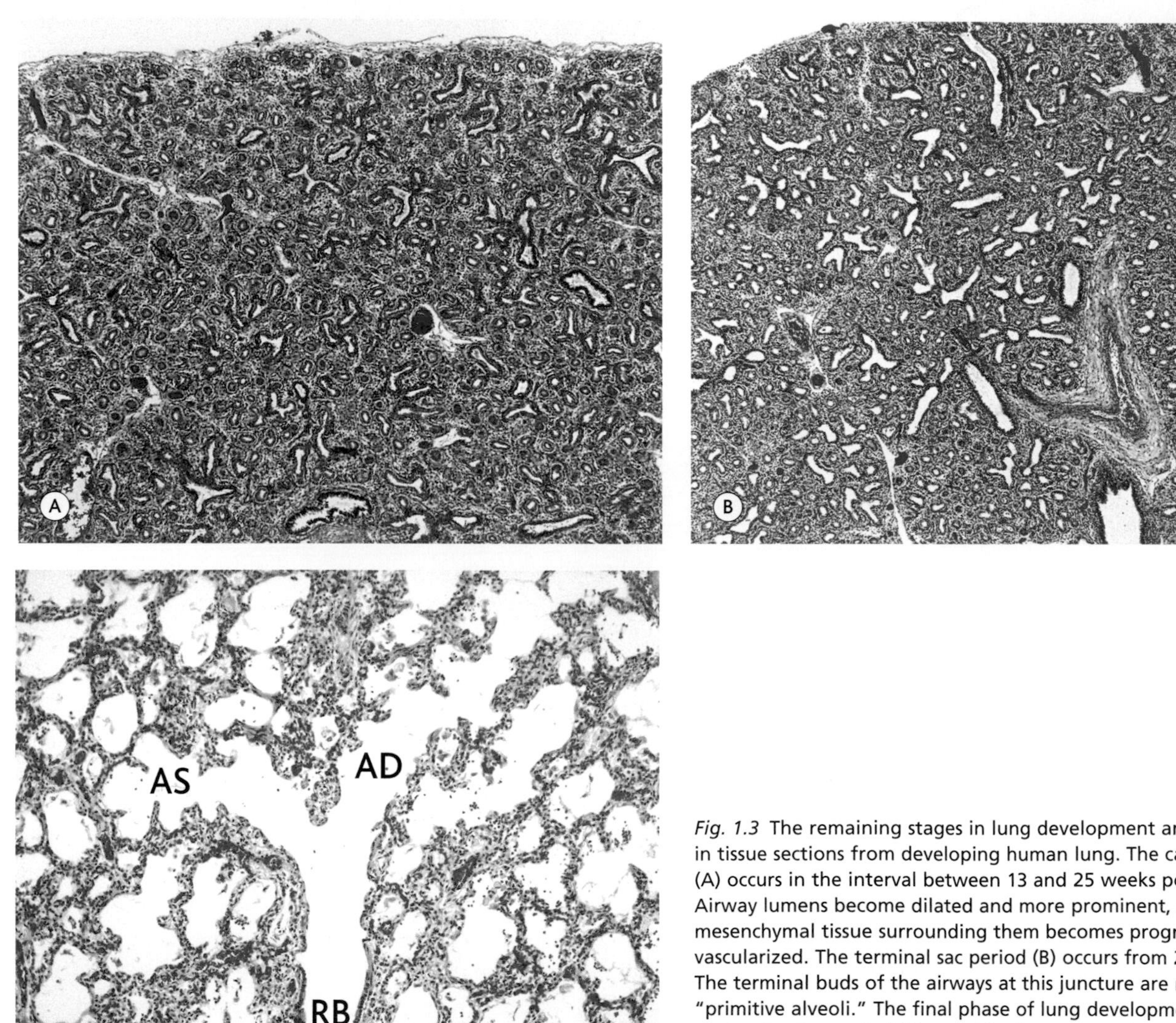

Fig. 1.3 The remaining stages in lung development are illustrated here in tissue sections from developing human lung. The canalicular period (A) occurs in the interval between 13 and 25 weeks postfertilization. Airway lumens become dilated and more prominent, and the mesenchymal tissue surrounding them becomes progressively vascularized. The terminal sac period (B) occurs from 24 weeks to birth. The terminal buds of the airways at this juncture are referred to as "primitive alveoli." The final phase of lung development is referred to as the alveolar period (C) and this phase crosses into childhood (late fetal to age 10 years). New alveoli continue to form well after birth. AD = alveolar duct; AS = alveolar sac; RB = respiratory bronchiole.

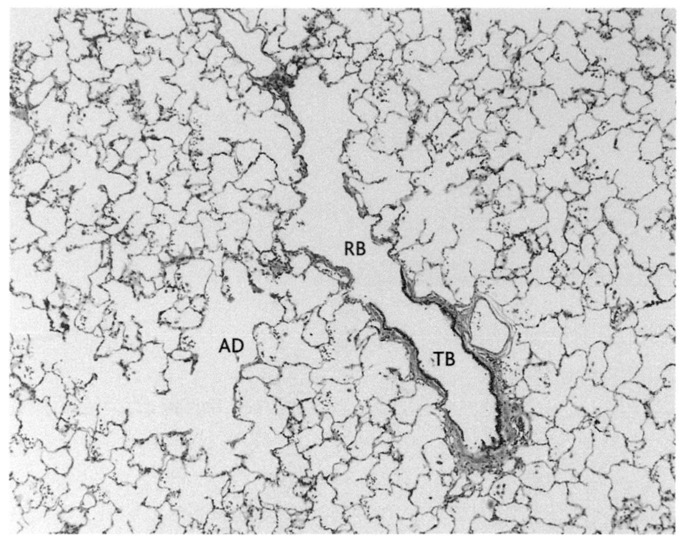

Fig. 1.4 The mature lung lobule consists of terminal bronchioles with their respective respiratory bronchioles, alveolar ducts, and alveolar sacs. Here the Y-shaped division of the terminal bronchiole into respiratory bronchioles and alveolar ducts can be seen in the lung of a child. TB = terminal bronchiole; RB = respiratory bronchiole; AD = alveolar duct.

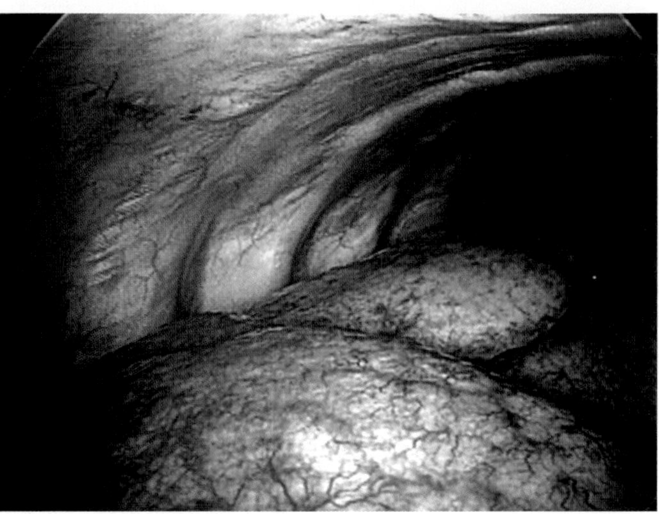

Fig. 1.5 The collapsed lung during thoracoscopic surgery demonstrates the visceral and parietal pleural surfaces.

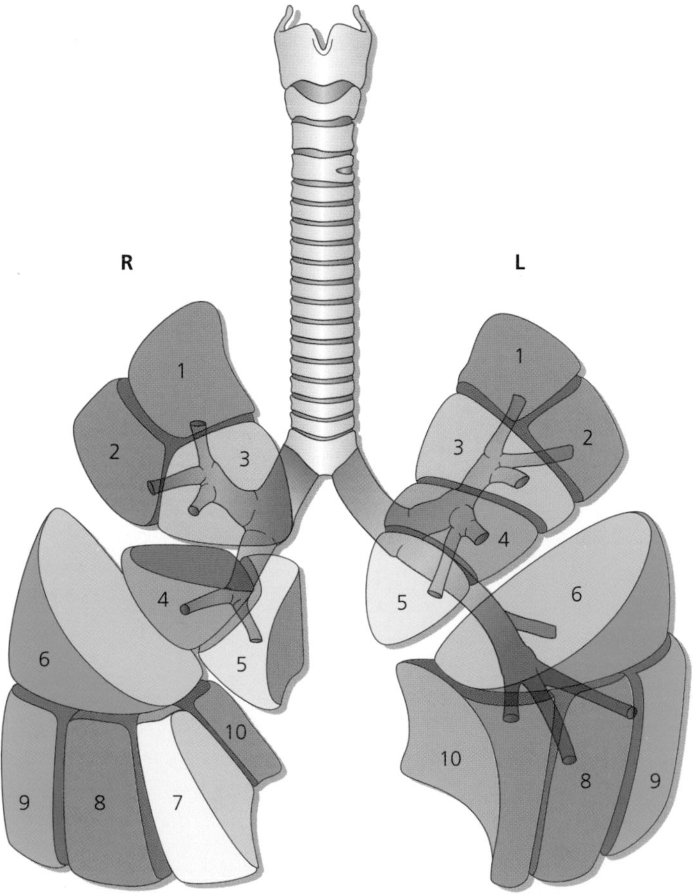

Fig. 1.6 Ten distinct segments are present in each lung. (Illustration courtesy of Nagaishi[4] with permission.)

in greater detail, the comprehensive and authoritative review of gross and microscopic lung anatomy by Nagaishi is recommended.[4]

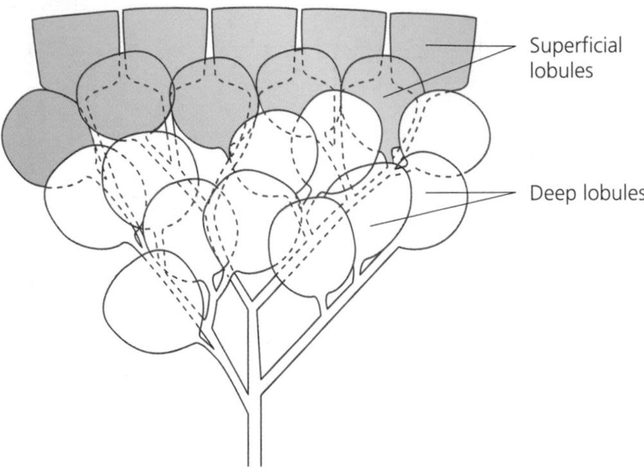

Fig. 1.7 The pulmonary lobules are configured into two layers that probably play important roles in the physical dynamics of respiration. The superficial layer is 3–4 cm thick. (Illustration courtesy of Nagaishi[4] with permission.)

The conducting airways

Each of the major divisions of the tracheobronchial tree (trachea, bronchi, bronchioles) has a specific role in lung function and this is reflected in their respective microscopic anatomy.

The trachea

The trachea is the gateway to the lung and is exposed to environmental factors in highest concentration. This rigid tube is designed for conducting gas, with rigid C-shaped cartilage rings that protect it from frontal injury and also prevent collapse during the negative changes in intrathoracic pressure that occur during respiration. The open side of the cartilage ring faces posteriorly, where the trachealis muscle completes the tracheal circumference. This arrangement allows the esophagus to abut the "soft" side of the trachea, down to the level of the carina. Respiratory epithelium (pseudostratified, ciliated, columnar-type), submucous glands, and smooth muscle combine to prepare inspired air for use in the lung by adding moisture and warmth (Fig. 1.9) while trapping dust particles and chemical vapor droplets before they can reach more delicate peripheral lung. For all these

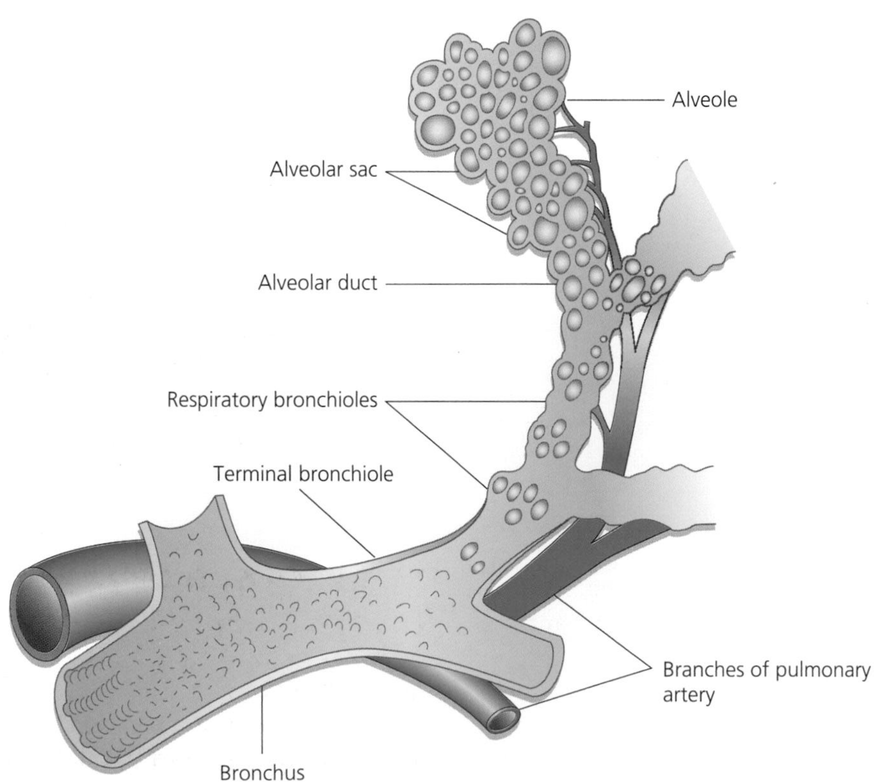

Fig. 1.8 This three-dimensional schematic diagram demonstrates the relationship between pulmonary artery and airway, and also illustrates the junction of a terminal bronchiole with the acinus. (Illustration courtesy of Nagaishi[4] with permission.)

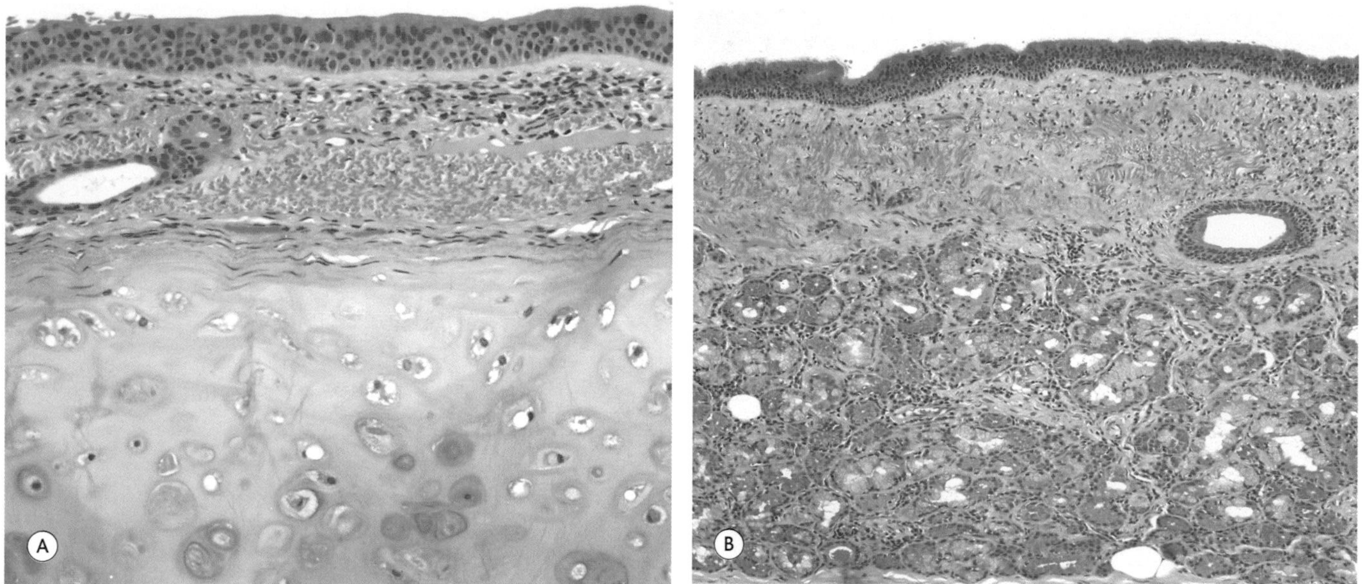

Fig. 1.9 (A) The tracheal mucosa is closely applied to the anterior cartilaginous portion with scant subepithelial tissue. (B) Posteriorly, cartilage is absent, tracheal glands are abundant, and muscle is prominent.

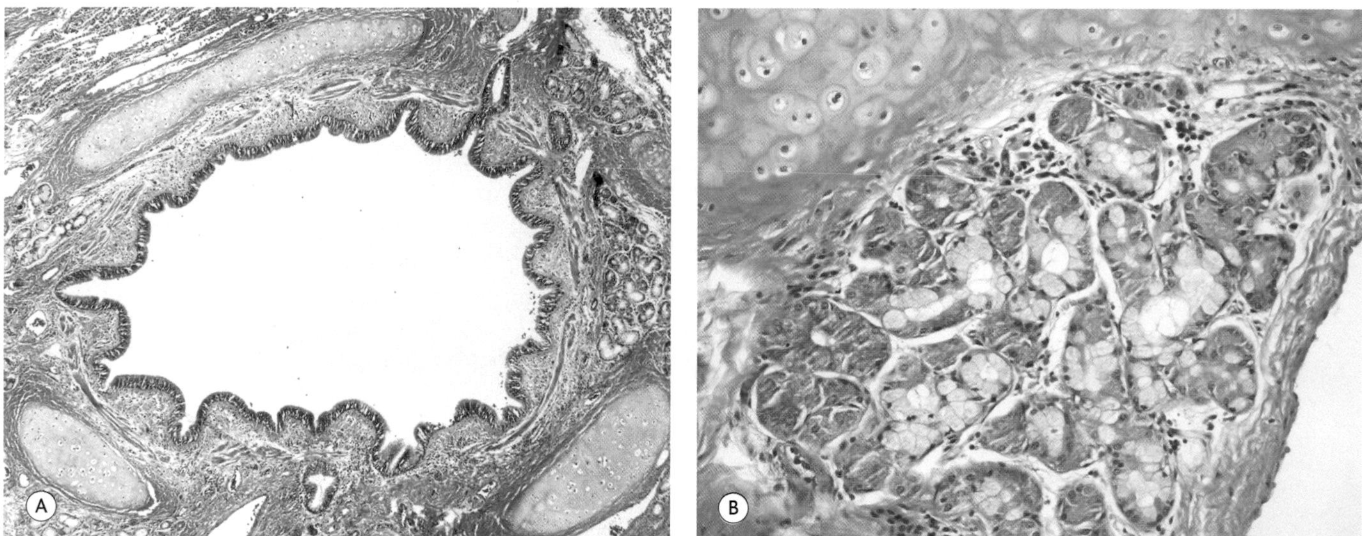

Fig. 1.10 A segmental bronchus in cross section (A) demonstrates the relationship of the structural elements of the cartilaginous airways. Discontinuous cartilage plates and a seromucus gland is evident (center right). (B) The relationship between serous and mucus glands in this structure is seen better at higher magnification.

reasons, when diseases affect the trachea the potential for impact on general respiratory function is significant.

The bronchi

The bronchi begin at the carina and extend into the substance of the lung. They are large conducting airways that have cartilage in their walls. Like the trachea, the cartilage of the main stem bronchi is C-shaped, but this configuration changes to that of puzzle piece-like plates once the bronchus enters the lung parenchyma. Within the substance of the lung, the cartilage plates decrease in density progressively as the bronchial diameter decreases, resulting in increasing area between individual plates. Mucus glands are positioned just beneath the surface epithelium and may be seen in endobronchial biopsies (Fig. 1.10). When inflamed, or distorted by crush artifact, they may simulate granulomas or tumor. These glands

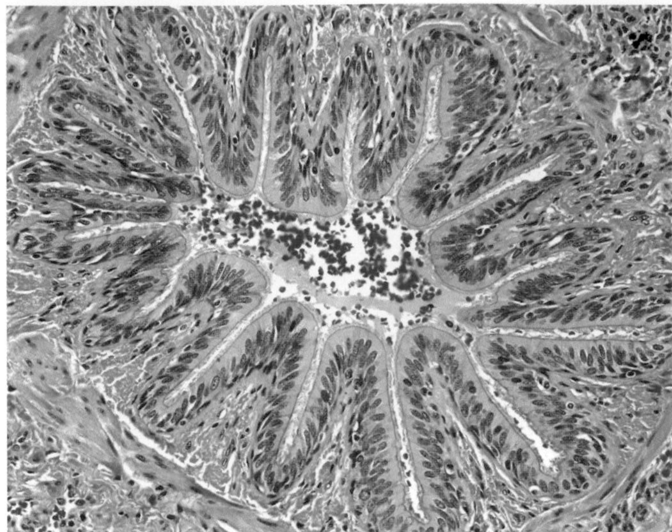

Fig. 1.11 The membranous airways (bronchioles) lack cartilage in their walls but rather have prominent smooth muscle. The mucosa is respiratory in type, with uniform delicate cilia.

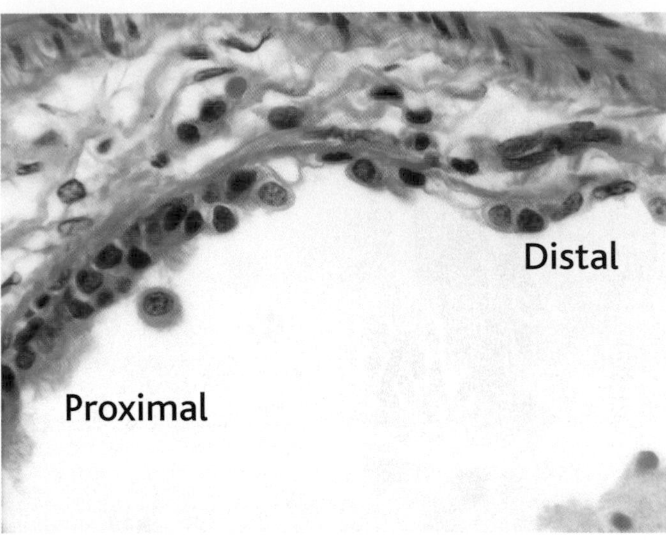

Fig. 1.13 The transition from respiratory columnar epithelium to flattened alveolar lining cells is rather abrupt with a recognized zone of cuboidal nonciliated cells present, although difficult to identify with consistency in lung sections.

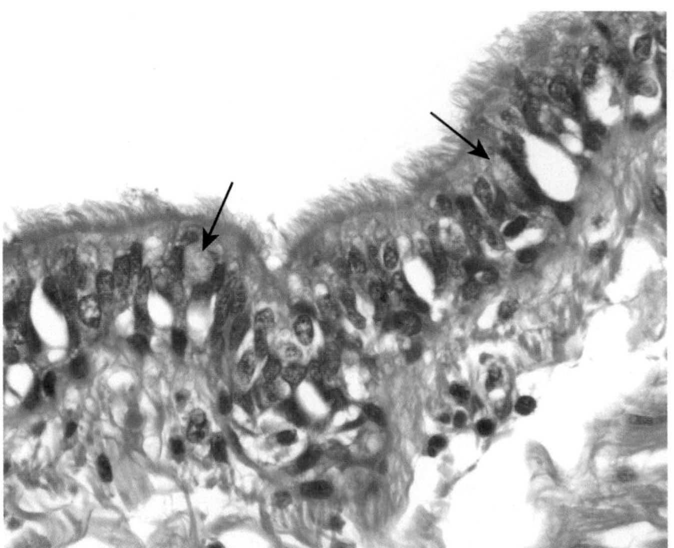

Fig. 1.12 The respiratory epithelium is columnar, pseudostratified, and ciliated. Scattered goblet cells can be seen interspersed between ciliated columnar cells (arrows), and the nuclei of the columnar cells are present at varying levels within the cell. The subepithelial region is loose areolar tissue and a basal lamina beneath the epithelium is easily recognizable, although not overly distinct or thickened.

connect to the airway lumen by a short duct. The bronchi divide and subdivide successively, becoming ever smaller on their way to the peripheral lung.

The bronchioles

The bronchioles are the final air conductors and by definition lack cartilage altogether (therefore sometimes referred to as "membranous") (Fig. 1.11). The bronchioles have no alveoli; these are acquired more distally in the pulmonary acinus. The terminal bronchiole is the smallest conducting airway without alveoli in its walls. There are about 30,000 terminal bronchioles in the lungs and each of these, in turn, directs air to approximately 10,000 alveoli. The cells that line the airways are columnar in shape and ciliated. Their nuclei are present at multiple levels in each cell, a phenomenon referred to as pseudostratification (Fig. 1.12).

Pseudostratified columnar epithelium is typically identifiable as far distal as the smallest terminal bronchioles, where the cells then rapidly become more cuboidal in shape and their nuclei more basally situated (Fig. 1.13). In the normal mucosa, mucus-secreting cells (goblet cells) are typically present in low numbers, and most often as individual units. It may be quite difficult to identify any goblet cells in the epithelium of small bronchioles. When these cells are numerous they may be distended with mucus and should suggest the presence of underlying airway disease (Fig. 1.14).

Airway mucosal neuroendocrine cells

Airway mucosal neuroendocrine cells typically present as single cells in the respiratory epithelium with clear cytoplasm (Fig. 1.15). Rarely, these cells may be present as groups, forming so-called *neuroepithelial bodies*. Immunohistochemical stains decorate these cells when addressed with antibodies directed against the common neuro-

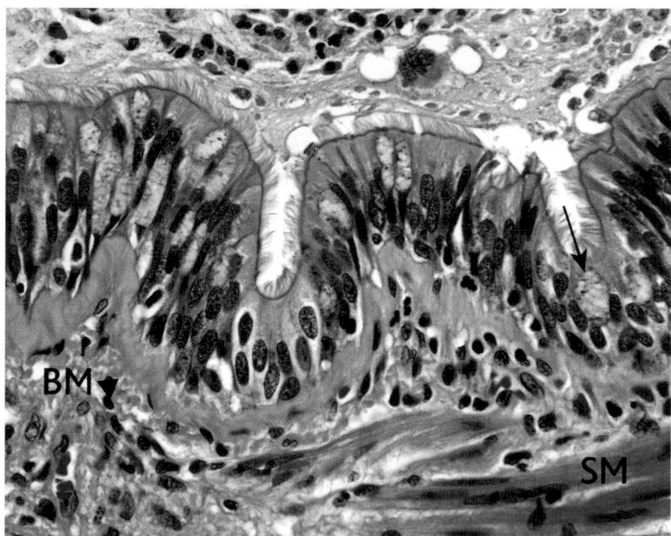

Fig. 1.14 Following irritation of the airway epithelium from any cause, goblet cell hyperplasia may occur (arrow on goblet cell). This phenomenon is typical in patients with asthma, as is prominent thickening of the basement membrane (BM, arrowhead) beneath the epithelium. SM = smooth muscle.

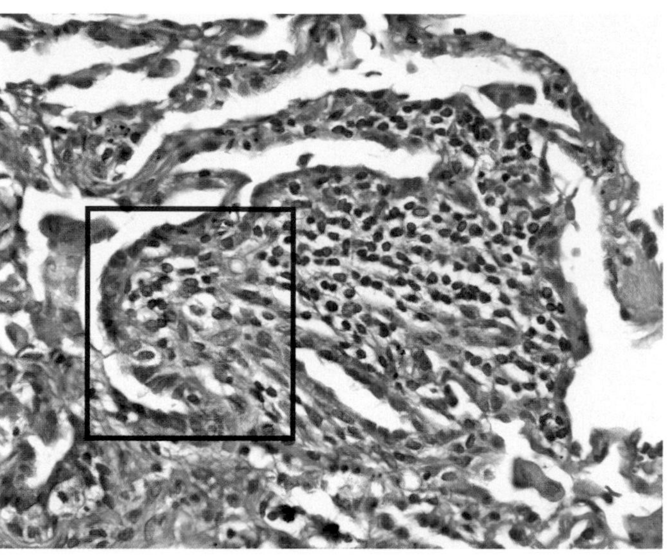

Fig. 1.16 The bronchus-associated lymphoid tissue (BALT) is uncommon in normal lungs but may be increased in smokers and in a number of other settings. These small aggregations of benign lymphoid cells are closely approximated to the airway epithelium (boxed area), typically with an intraepithelial component analogous to tonsillar epithelium.

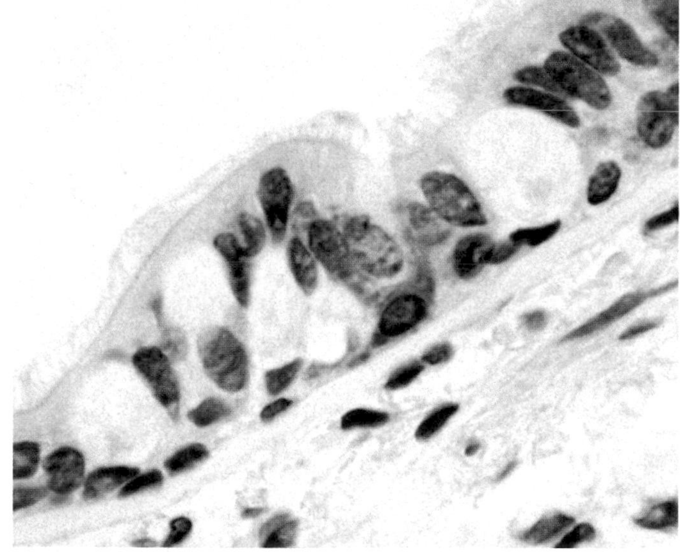

Fig. 1.15 Very sparse (and rare) neuroendocrine cells are present in the normal lung (immunohistochemical stain for synaptophysin with red chromogen, hematoxylin counterstain).

endocrine markers, chromogranin A and synaptophysin, as well as a number of more esoteric neuropeptides. The exact function of these cells is unknown. It has been suggested that lung neuroendocrine cells play a role in regulating ventilation–perfusion relationships, and may also be important in airway morphogenesis.[9]

Airway-associated lymphoid tissue

Airway-associated lymphoid tissue may be present in the normal lung, but it is very sparse, and typically occurs at the bifurcation points of the airways (Fig. 1.16). This lung lymphoid tissue is generally referred to as *bronchus-associated lymphoid tissue* (*BALT*), and is felt to be analogous to the mucosa-associated lymphoid tissue (MALT) of the gastrointestinal tract.[10] The strategic localization of BALT at airway divisions may be a consequence of exposure to inhaled antigens and other particles that are likely to impact these areas.[11] BALT foci are associated with specialized epithelial cells in the mucosa and the constituent lymphoid cells (mainly T lymphocytes) are admixed with macrophages and dendritic cells. The epithelial and dendritic cells of the BALT presumably play a role in the detection of inhaled allergens, viruses, and bacteria, such that BALT is considered to be a critical component of the lung's immune defense system. The bronchial BALT may become hyperplastic, with follicular germinal center formation. When this occurs, germinal centers may come to be sampled in bronchoscopic biopsies and pose a diagnostic challenge when crushed or cut in such a way that the follicular center lymphoid cells appear as a nodule or sheet in the specimen. BALT may also be important in diseases of immunologic origin that produce bronchiolitis, such as connective tissue diseases (e.g. Sjögren's syndrome and rheumatoid arthritis), as well as graft-versus-host disease

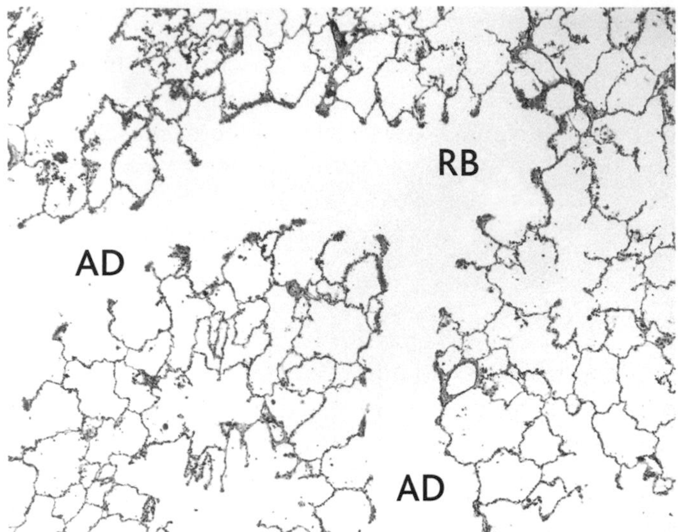

Fig. 1.17 A scanning magnification view of the acinus with a branched respiratory bronchiole (RB) leading into two primary alveolar ducts (AD), fully lined by alveoli.

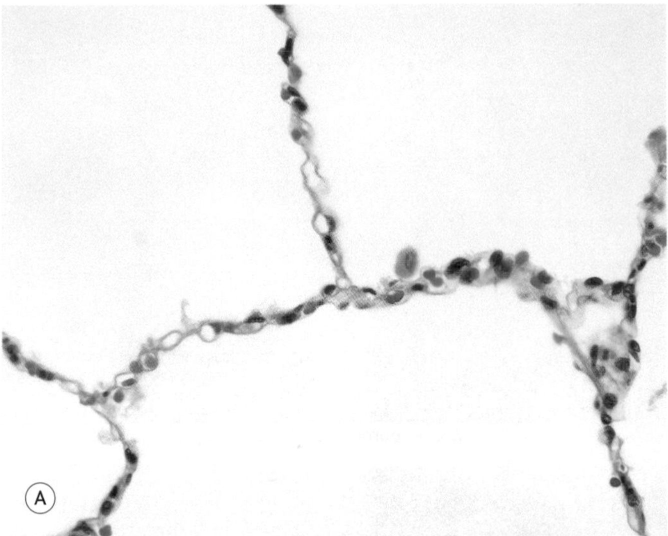

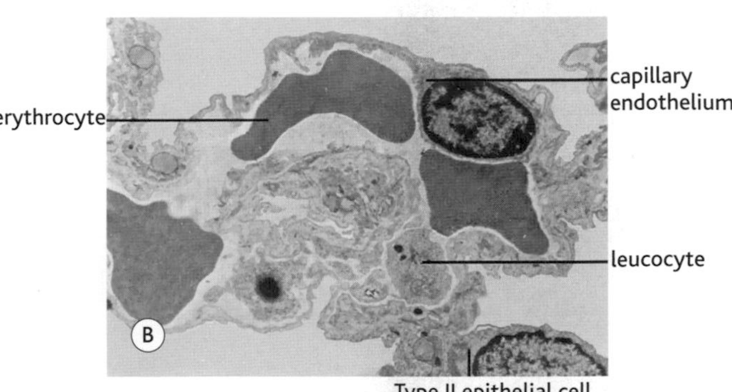

Fig. 1.18 High-magnification view of five adjacent alveoli with delicate alveolar walls. (A) Most of the visible nuclei in the normal alveolar wall belong to endothelial cells. (B) Electron microscopy emphasizes this point with a prominent endothelial cell nucleus adjacent to two red blood cells (RBCs). Note the extremely attenuated fusion of endothelial cytoplasm, basal laminae, and type I cell cytoplasm above these RBCs (not easily visible, even ultrastructurally). (Reproduced from Nagaishi[4] with permission.)

in organ transplantation, immunoglobulin deficiency states, and even inflammatory bowel disease.

Epithelial basement membrane

Epithelial basement membrane lies immediately beneath the airway epithelium and is routinely visible by association with an eosinophilic matrix of type III collagen. A fine layer of elastic tissue is present beneath the epithelial basement membrane. Collagen may come to separate this elastic tissue from the overlying basement membrane in airway injury associated with subepithelial fibrosis.

The smooth muscle of the airways

The smooth muscle of the airways is arranged in a complex spiral pattern. The *bronchovascular bundle* encompasses the airway, the accompanying pulmonary artery, a network of lymphatic channels, a common adventitia, and a sheath of loose connective tissue. The connective tissue of the bronchovascular bundle diminishes progressively in the smallest bronchioles of the lung.

The acinus

The acinus begins distal to the terminal bronchiole and is where most of the gas exchange occurs in the lungs. The acinus includes (in order proceeding distally) the *respiratory bronchioles (primary and secondary)*, the *alveolar ducts*, and the *alveolar sacs* (Fig. 1.17). Respiratory bronchioles have progressively more alveoli in their walls with successive distal generations. The last conducting structure, the alveolar duct, is entirely lined by alveoli. The alveolar ducts terminate in alveolar sacs, which are globular aggregations of adjacent alveoli. As the airways of the acinus branch and diminish in diameter progressively, a transition from cuboidal cells to flattened epithelium occurs abruptly.

The alveoli

Most of the alveolar surface that faces the inspired air is covered by extremely flat *type I epithelial cells* that are not easily seen with the light microscope. The thin and flattened nature of the type I epithelial cell is well-suited to gas exchange (Fig. 1.18). The *type II epithelial cells* are cuboidal in shape, and although they cover less surface

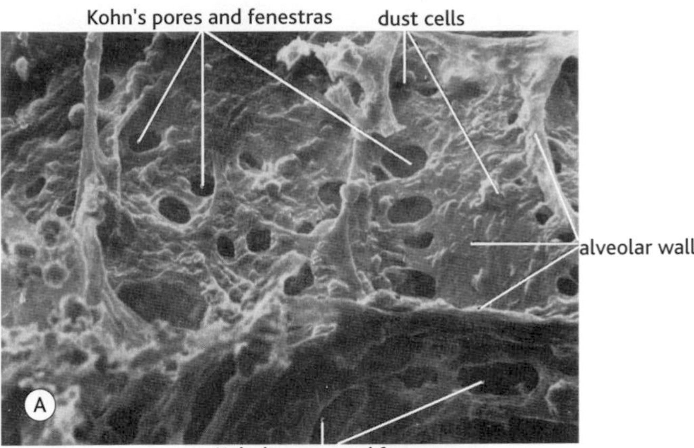

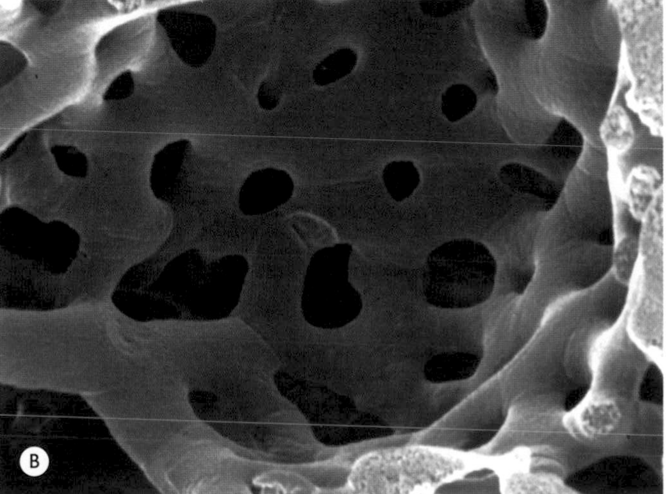

Fig. 1.19 A scanning electron micrograph (A) showing the internal aspect of the alveolus. The liberal communication between alveoli in adjacent alveolar sacs is made possible by the pores of Kohn. (This scanning electron micrograph of an adult human lung is reproduced from Nagaishi[4] with permission.) The capillary network of the alveolus (B) is demonstrated in this methacrylate vascular cast. (This scanning electron micrograph is courtesy of A Churg and J Wright.)

area, they are greater in total number than the type I cells. They are present at the angular junctions of alveolar walls (the alveolus being more like a geodesic dome than a sphere). The surface of the type II cell facing the alveolar airspace has microvilli that can sometimes be appreciated by light microscopy as slight roughening. Type II cells contain large numbers of organelles and are responsible for the production of surfactant, a substance that lowers surface tension and is essential for preventing alveolar collapse at low intra-alveolar pressures. Type II cells are the progenitor cells of the alveolar type I cells and, after an injury, divide and replace them. Type I and type II cells have tight junctions that present a physical barrier between the interstitial fluid and the alveolar air.

The alveolar walls

The alveolar walls are composed of a capillary net (Fig. 1.19), the extracellular matrix, and sparse cellular elements including mast cells, smooth muscle cells, pericytes, fibroblast-like cells, and occasional lymphocytes.[12] The mesenchymal cells of the interstitium have been the subject of considerable study. Unstimulated, they resemble fibroblasts and have few organelles. During the repair phase of an injury, actin and myosin appear in the cytoplasm, and they develop contractile properties that play an important role in lung repair.[13–15] *Capillary endothelial cells* within the acinus are joined by tight or semi-tight junctions. The semi-tight junctions exist to allow larger molecules to traverse the capillary wall.

Alveolar macrophages

Alveolar macrophages play an essential role as phagocytes and, under appropriate stimulation, secrete soluble factors that are an essential part of the lung's immunologic defense and response to injury. As mobile cellular elements, they are capable of removing engulfed particulates by migrating into the interstitium (and eventually, lymphatic channels) or ascending the mucociliary escalator of the airways.

The pulmonary arteries

The pulmonary arteries carry venous blood to the lungs for gas exchange with the inspired air in the alveolar spaces. The pulmonary circulation is a low-pressure system (mean systolic pressure = 14 mmHg) and one that is considerably shorter in length than the systemic circulation.[16,17] Nevertheless, a doubling of the resting blood flow to the lung results in only a small increase (about 5 mmHg) in pressure.

The pulmonary arteries arise from the conus arteriosus of the right ventricle of the heart and run in parallel with the airways within the lung.[18,19] The main trunk of the pulmonary artery bifurcates into right and left main trunks at the fourth thoracic vertebral body. These trunks follow the right and left main stem bronchi into their respective lung (Fig. 1.20). The diameter of the pulmonary artery and accompanying airway in cross section are roughly equal. The pulmonary arteries branch at a rate similar to the airways, but also have a second distinctive branching pattern identifiable in peripheral lung, with right-angle origins for branches having significantly smaller caliber (Fig. 1.21) designed to supply peribronchiolar alveoli. The pulmonary arteries are composed of three layers, the intima, the media, and the adventitia,

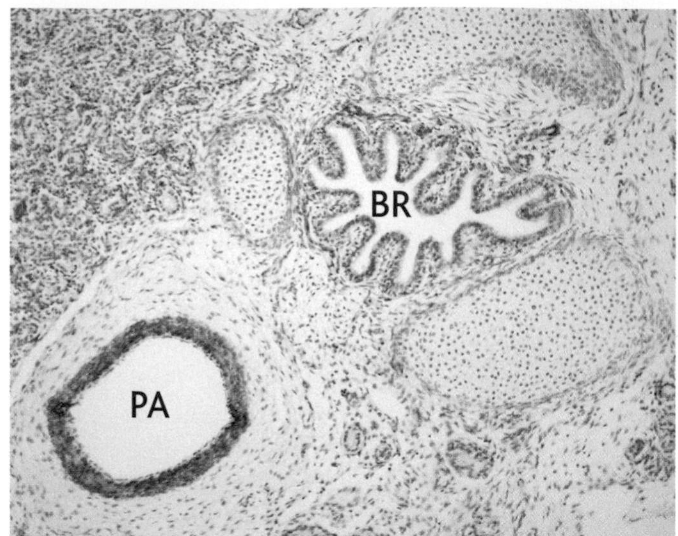

Fig. 1.20 This microscopic section of fetal lung shows the characteristic early relationship of pulmonary artery branches to bronchi (PA = pulmonary artery, BR = bronchus). The smooth muscle layers of each of these structures is outlined in brown. (Alpha smooth muscle actin (ASMA) immunohistochemical stain, brown chromogen, hematoxylin counterstain.)

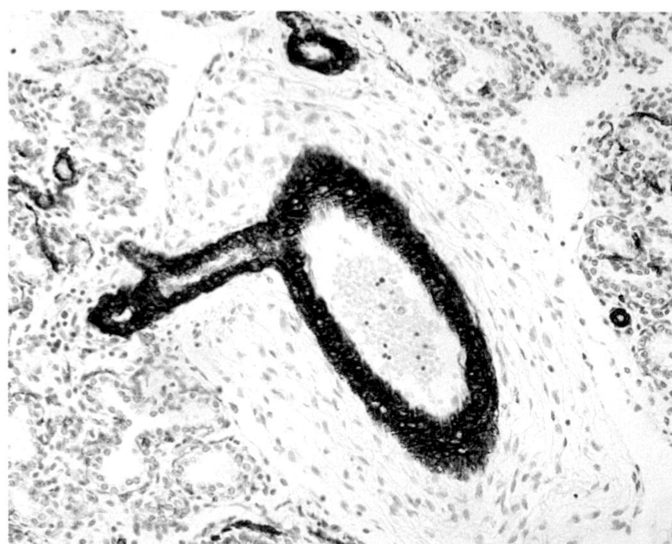

Fig. 1.21 The distinctive pattern of pulmonary artery branching in the lung parenchyma is nicely illustrated in this fetal lung stained with monoclonal antibody directed against alpha smooth muscle actin (ASMA immunohistochemical stain, brown chromogen, hematoxylin counterstain).

similar to systemic arteries; however, for arteries of the same diameter, systemic vessels have a significantly thicker muscular layer. In the adult, two or more elastic laminae are present in arteries larger than 1 mm in diameter. Arteries between 100 and 200 µm (0.1–0.2 mm) are muscular, and have internal and external elastic lamina

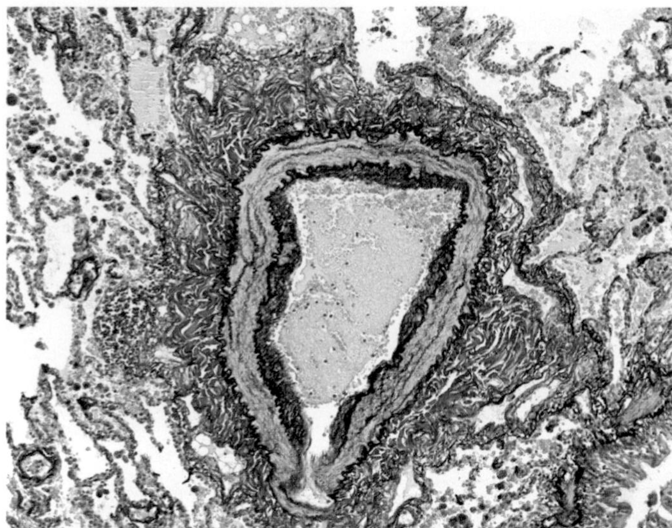

Fig. 1.22 Pulmonary artery in peripheral lung showing internal and external elastic lamina (elastic Van Gieson histochemical stain).

(Fig. 1.22). Smaller arteries may be muscular or non-muscular. The two elastic lamina appear fused in smaller arteries as a result of progressive attenuation of smooth muscle. Where muscle is absent, a single fragmented elastic lamina is all that separates the intima from the adventitia. In the adult, arterial muscle extends down to the level of the alveoli. The ratio of arterial wall thickness to external arterial diameter is often a useful marker for abnormality. Nondistended muscular arteries have a medial thickness that should represent about 5% of external arterial diameter.

The pulmonary veins

The pulmonary veins carry oxygenated blood back to the heart for systemic distribution. The large veins are present adjacent to the main arteries at the hilum, but the pulmonary veins within the lung parenchyma travel along a separate course within the interlobular septa, beginning on the venous side of the alveolar capillary bed. The intralobular pulmonary veins coalesce to form larger channels that join the interlobular septa at the periphery of the acinus (Fig. 1.23). The veins are indistinct structures in the lung and are often difficult to identify.[18,20] Most of the vascular structures identifiable at scanning magnification in tissue sections of lung are pulmonary arteries (with their adjacent airway). The most reliable method for locating a pulmonary vein in tissue sections is to find the junction of the pleura with an interlobular septum (Fig. 1.24). This is an important technique, since every lung biopsy for diffuse disease should be evaluated

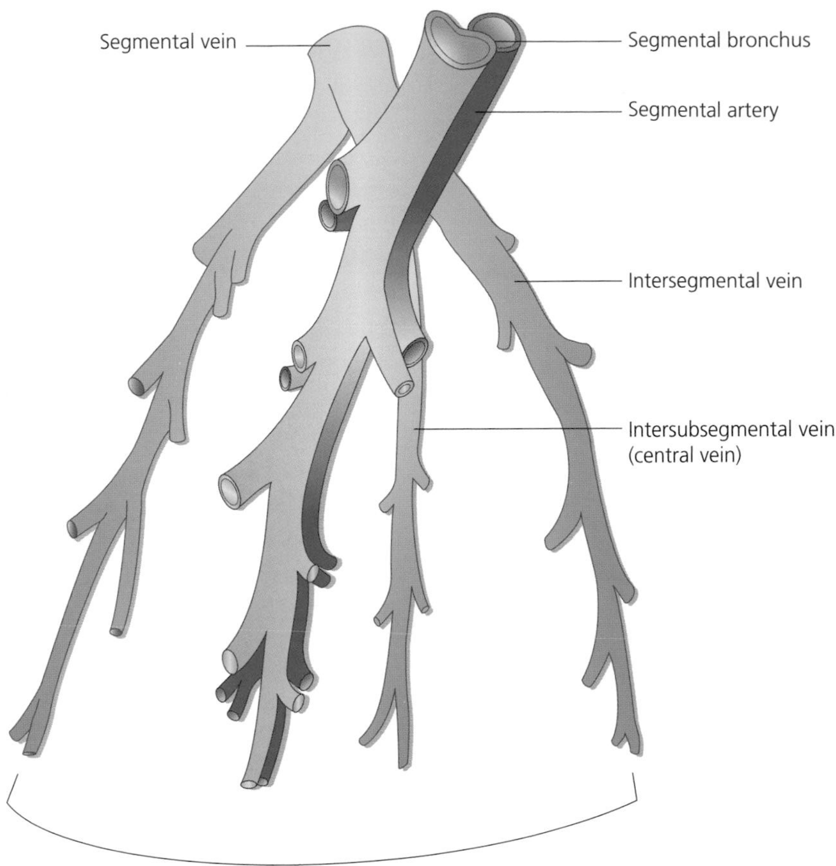

Fig. 1.23 The lobular relationship of pulmonary arteries and veins is illustrated in this simplified diagram. (Reproduced from Nagaishi[4] with permission.)

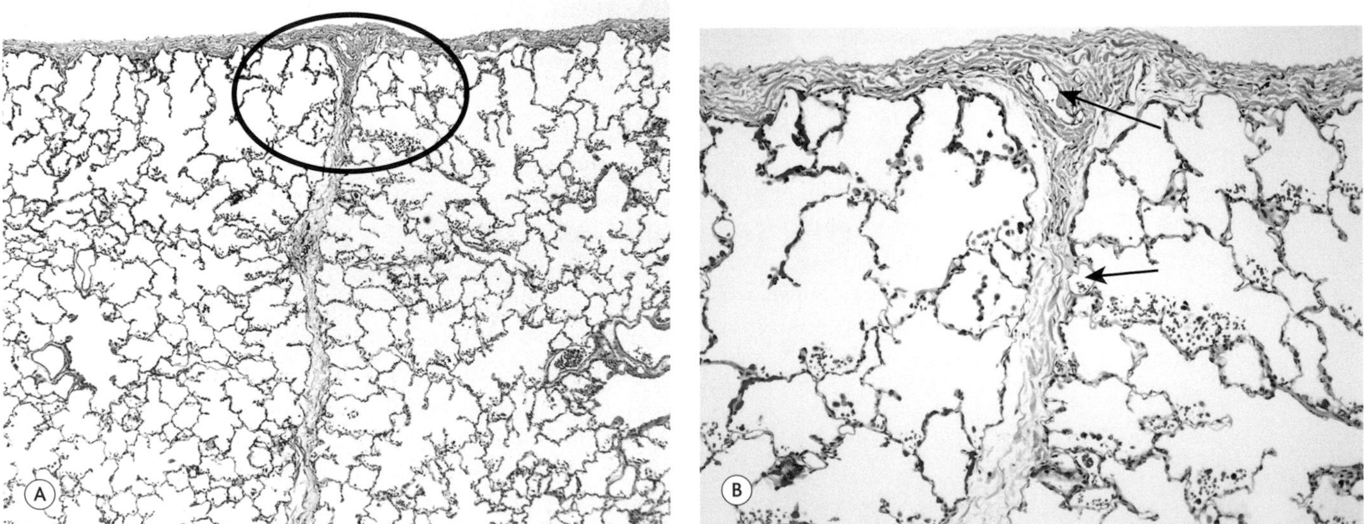

Fig. 1.24 (A) Study of the pulmonary veins and lymphatics is facilitated by finding junctions of pleura with interlobular septa. At higher magnification (B – oval area from A), the delicate vessels, with red blood cells (RBCs) in their lumen, are veins. The veins have slightly thicker walls than adjacent lymphatics. Large arrow = pleural vein; small arrow = peripheral lobular vein.

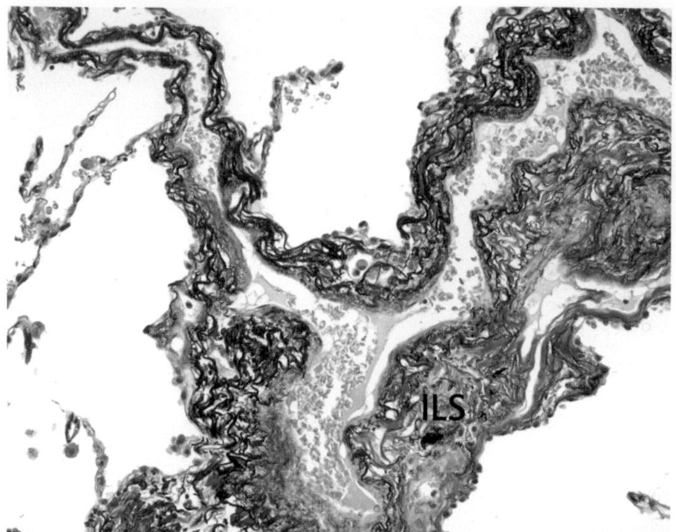

Fig. 1.25 A larger pulmonary vein stained for elastic tissue shows a single elastic lamina (elastic Van Gieson histochemical stain). ILS = interlobular septum.

systematically in search of pathologic alterations in each of the main compartments (airways, arteries, veins, acinar structures, and pleura). The veins have a single elastic lamina (Fig. 1.25) and sparse smooth muscle.

The bronchial arteries

The bronchial arteries supply arterial blood to the lung and arise most commonly from the descending aorta, although a number of anomalous origins are described. The bronchial arteries run parallel to the airways within the bronchovascular sheath where small branches supply capillary networks of the mucosa, airway smooth muscle, and adventitia.[20,21] The largest-diameter bronchial arteries can be seen in the adventitia of the airway. Submucosal branches are nearly imperceptible. On the venous side of the bronchial artery-supplied capillary net, bronchial veins within the lung eventually join pulmonary veins and return their blood to the left atrium.

The pulmonary lymphatics

The lymphatic vessels of the peripheral lung begin at the outer edge of the acinus, draining along interlobular septa to coalesce finally at the hilum.[22] A separate centriacinar system is present in the bronchovascular sheaths, beginning around the level of the respiratory bronchiole.[23] No lymphatics are present in the alveolar sacs, where it is believed that the interstitial space serves the purpose of extracellular fluid collection and drainage to more proximal regions. The lymphatic net of the pulmonary arteries extends further distally in the acinus than that associated with the terminal airways.[23] The lymphatic networks of the airways and pulmonary arteries anastomose freely during their course back to the hilum. The lymphatics (and veins) are also distributed over the surface of the lobes within the pleura. The relationship between airways, arteries, veins, and lymphatics is nicely illustrated by Okada[23] in Figure 1.26. When affected by certain diseases such as diffuse lymphangiomatosis (Fig. 1.27A) or lymphangiectasis (Fig. 1.27B) the distribution of the pulmonary lymphatics becomes much more apparent.

Other pulmonary lymphoid tissue

Lymphoid aggregates

Lymphoid aggregates are uncommon in the lung under normal circumstances. They have no capsule and are composed of B cells, T cells, and dendritic cells. Lymphoid aggregates increase in the lungs of cigarette smokers,[11,24] and may be present within interlobular septa, the pleura (Fig. 1.28), and in the subpleural connective tissue.[25] Lymphoid aggregates may be one of the sources for the condition known as *diffuse lymphoid hyperplasia*.

Dendritic cells

Dendritic cells are antigen-presenting cells that function in concert with T lymphocytes as part of acquired immunity. Dendritic cells occur in the epithelium and subepithelial tissue of the airways. They have a kidney-shaped nucleus that is eccentrically placed, and have prominent cytoplasmic protrusions. Dendritic cells strongly express the major histocompatibility complex (MHC) antigens.[26] A subpopulation of dendritic cells carry the Langerhans cell marker,[24] and contain Birbeck's granules in their cytoplasm on ultrastructural examination.[27] Langerhans cells are increased in the lungs of smokers, and can be identified by immunohistochemical techniques using antibodies directed against S100 protein and CD1a. The Langerhans cell is involved in the smoking-related disease known as pulmonary Langerhans cell histiocytosis (formerly known as pulmonary eosinophilic granuloma, or histiocytosis X).

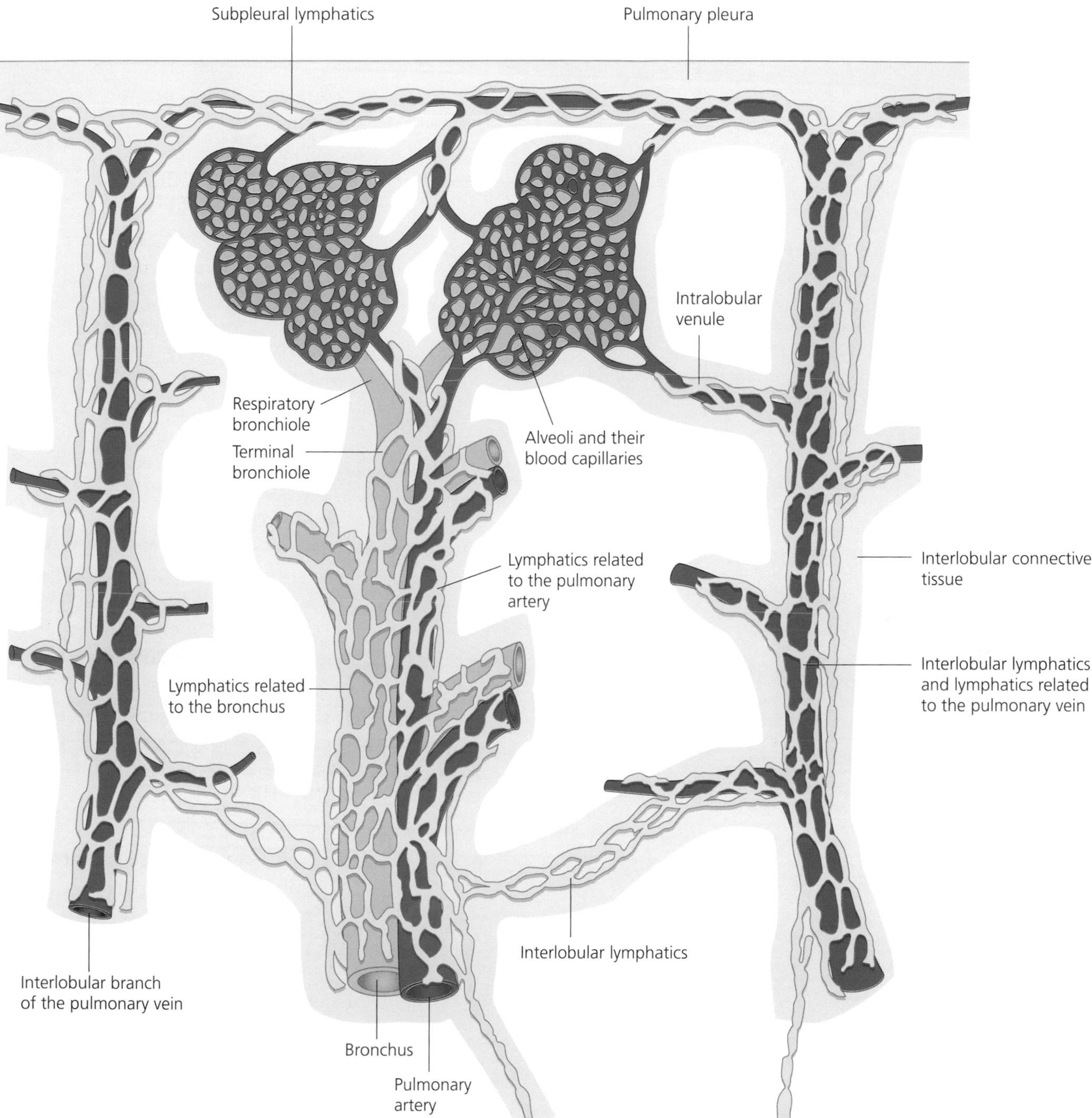

Fig. 1.26 Schematic illustration of the relationship between airways, pulmonary arteries, pulmonary veins, and lymphatics. (Illustration courtesy of Okada[23] with permission.)

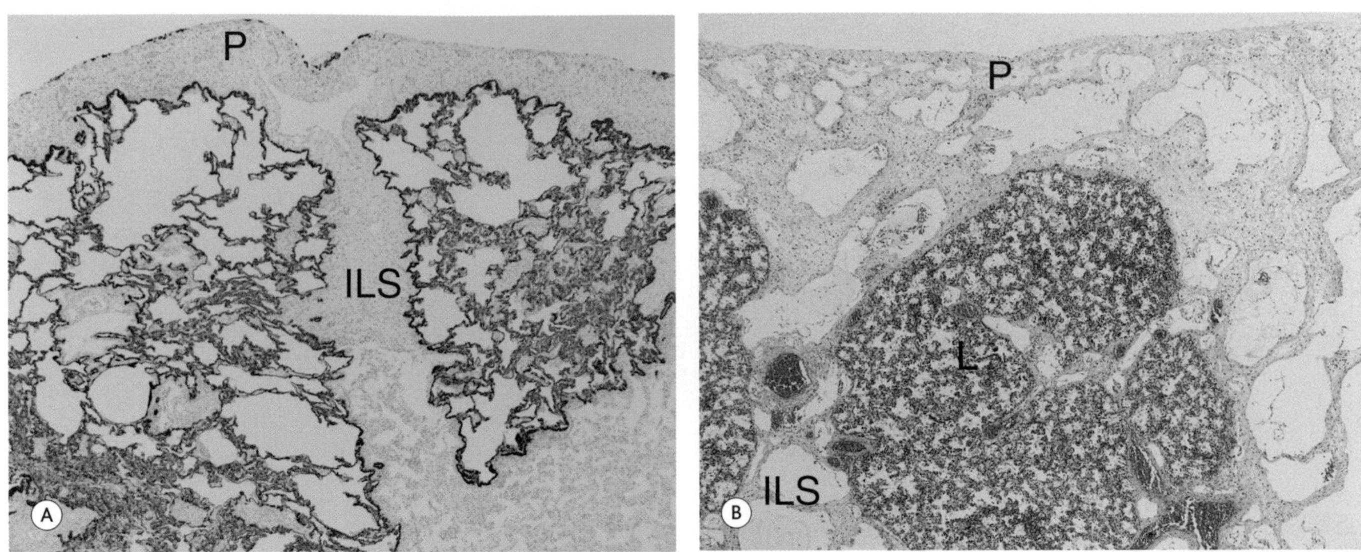

Fig. 1.27 (A) The pleural (P) and septal distribution (interlobular septum, ILS) of lymphatics is dramatically accentuated here in this example of the rare disorder of lymphatics known as diffuse pulmonary lymphangiomatosis. (B) Similar accentuation is produced by lymphangiectasis. L = lobule.

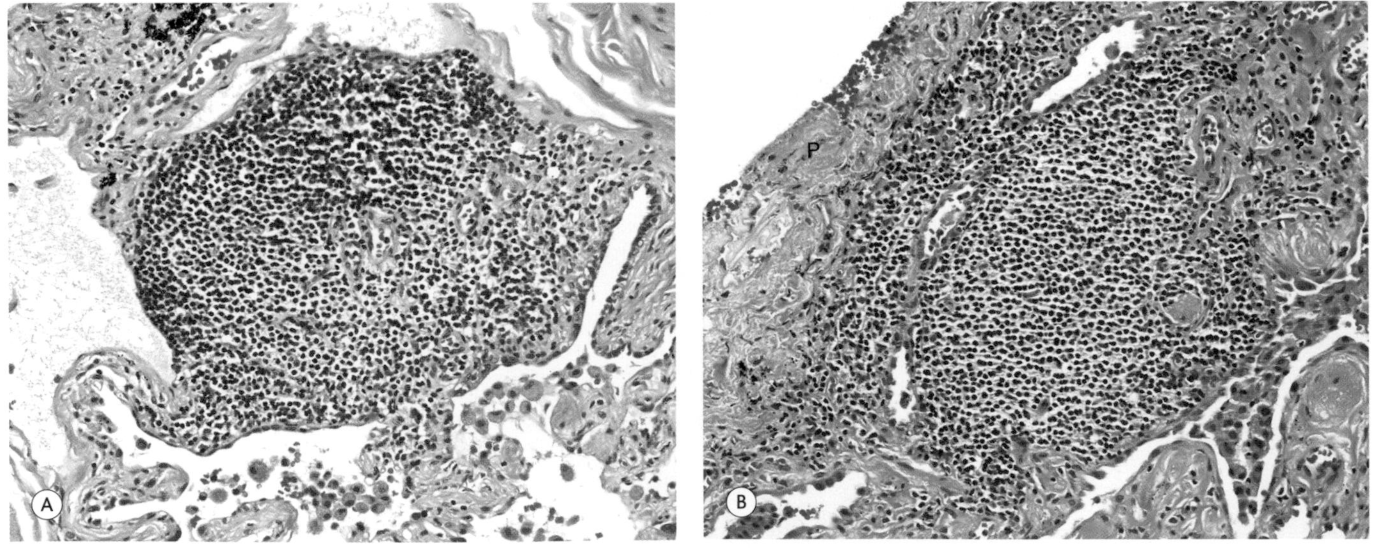

Fig. 1.28 Lymphoid aggregates in the lung may occur (A) along interlobular septa and (B) in the pleura (P). Germinal centers may be evident.

REFERENCES

1. Moore K: The developing human, 1st edn. 1973, WB Saunders, Philadelphia.
2. Langeman J: Medical embryology, 2nd edn. 1969, Williams and Wilkins, Baltimore.
3. Wells LJ, Boyden EA: The development of the bronchopulmonary segments in human embryos of horizons XVII to XIX. Am J Anat 1954; 95(2): 163–201.
4. Nagaishi C: Functional anatomy and histology of the lung, 1st edn. 1972, University Park Press, Baltimore.
5. Boyden EA: Development of the pulmonary airways. Minn Med 1971; 54(11): 894–897.
6. Boyden EA: Observations on the anatomy and development of the lungs. Lancet 1953; 73(12): 509–512.
7. Boyden EA: Observations on the history of the bronchopulmonary segments. Minn Med 1955; 38(9): 597–598.
8. Kwon KY, Myers JL, Swensen SJ, et al.: Middle lobe syndrome: a clinicopathological study of 21 patients. Hum Pathol 1995; 26(3): 302–307.
9. Aguayo S, Schuyler W, Murtagh J, et al.: Regulation of branching morphogenesis by bombesin-like peptides and neutral endopeptidase. Am J Respir Cell Mol Biol 1994; 10: 635–642.
10. Bienenstock J, Johnston N, Perey D: Bronchial lymphoid tissue I. Morphological characteristics. Lab Invest 1973; 28: 686–692.
11. Richmond I, Pritchard G, Ashcroft T, et al.: Bronchus associated lymphoid tissue (BALT) in human lung: its distribution in smokers and non-smokers. Thorax 1993; 48: 1130–1134.
12. Thurlbeck W. Chronic airflow obstruction. In: Pathology of the lung, 2nd edn, Churg A, Ed. 1995, Thieme Medical Publishers, New York, pp 739–825.
13. Fukuda Y, Ishizaki M, Masuda Y, et al.: The role of intraalveolar fibrosis in the process of pulmonary structural remodeling in patients with diffuse alveolar damage. Am J Pathol 1987; 126(1): 171–182.
14. Leslie K, King TE Jr, Low R: Smooth muscle actin is expressed by air space fibroblast-like cells in idiopathic pulmonary fibrosis and hypersensitivity pneumonitis. Chest 1991; 99(Suppl 3): 47S–48S.
15. Leslie KO, Mitchell J, Low R: Lung myofibroblasts. Cell Motil Cytoskeleton 1992; 22(2): 92–98.
16. Parker JC, Cave CB, Ardell JL, et al.: Vascular tree structure affects lung blood flow heterogeneity simulated in three dimensions. J Appl Physiol 1997; 83(4): 1370–1382.
17. Li CW, Cheng HD: A nonlinear fluid model for pulmonary blood circulation. J Biomech 1993; 26(6): 653–664.
18. Huang W, Yen RT, McLaurine M, et al.: Morphometry of the human pulmonary vasculature. J Appl Physiol 1996; 81(5): 2123–2133.
19. Hislop AA: Airway and blood vessel interaction during lung development. J Anat 2002; 201(4): 325–334.
20. Boyden EA: Human growth and development. Am J Anat 1971; 132(1): 1–3.
21. Boyden EA: The developing bronchial arteries in a fetus of the twelfth week. Am J Anat 1970; 129(3): 357–368.
22. Okada Y, Ito M, Nagaishi C: Anatomical study of the pulmonary lymphatics. Lymphology 1979; 12(3): 118–124.
23. Okada Y, Lymphatic system of the human lung, 1st edn. 1989, Kinpodo Publishing Co, Siga, Japan.
24. van Haarst J, de Wit H, Drexhage H, et al.: Distribution and immunophenotype of mononuclear phagocytes and dendritic cells in the human lung. Am J Respir Cell Mol Biol 1994; 10: 487–492.
25. Kradin R, Mark E: Benign lymphoid disorders of the lung, with a theory regarding their development. Hum Pathol 1983; 14: 857–867.
26. Van Voorhis W, Hair L, Steinman R, et al.: Human dendritic cells, enrichment and purification from peripheral blood. J Exp Med 1982; 155: 1172–1187.
27. Soler P, Moreau A, Basset F, et al.: Cigarette smoking-induced changes in the number and differentiated state of pulmonary dendritic/Langerhans cells. Am Rev Respir Dis 1989; 139: 1112–1117.

2

Optimal processing of diagnostic lung specimens

Kevin O Leslie   Robert W Viggiano   Victor F Trastek

Introduction

Optimal specimen handling is essential for the accurate interpretation of biopsies and cytologic preparations obtained in the course of evaluating the patient with lung disease.[1–9] The limited number of sampling techniques available can be divided into three general categories: specimen's obtained by bronchoscopy, specimens obtained by transthoracic needle core biopsy or aspiration, and specimens obtained by surgical wedge biopsy of peripheral lung through a transthoracic approach.[8, 10–13]

In this chapter we focus on the techniques and the specimens derived from them, with emphasis on how they should be managed in the laboratory. Once the sample is on target and of good quality, the addition of pertinent clinical data and radiologic information greatly increases the likelihood of a meaningful and accurate diagnosis.[13–15] Even when the differential diagnosis is simply "rule out malignancy", the effect of other information may be substantial, especially when the sample is of marginal quality or size. In the case of diffuse non-neoplastic lung diseases (often referred to as "interstitial lung diseases") a reasonable amount of clinical and radiologic information is essential for accurate interpretation. Without such information, even the experienced lung pathologist may need to resort to a purely descriptive diagnosis.[15]

In the pages that follow, the specimen characteristics and processing steps for the common lung samples taken in the course of clinical evaluation of pulmonary diseases are presented. Also, for each type of sample, the benefits and limitations are explored. Such a working knowledge of specimen handling for each procedure ensures the greatest likelihood of success in establishing a specific diagnosis and, in the end, a rational treatment plan. An overview of the sampling procedures and the specimens they generate is presented in Table 2.1.

Table 2.1 Diagnostic sampling techniques, the specimens generated by them, and the common analyses performed

Source	Specimens and common analyses performed
Sputum	Cytologic smears and centrifuge preparations. Fixed or air-dried, then stained for cytopathologic examination. Microbiological cultures performed as indicated
Bronchoscopy with:	
Washings	Cytologic smears and centrifuge preparations. Fixed or air-dried, then stained for cytopathologic examination. Microbiological cultures performed as indicated
Brushings	Cytologic smears and centrifuge preparations. Fixed or air-dried, then stained for cytopathologic examination. Microbiological cultures performed as indicated
(Endo) Bronchial biopsy	Forceps tissue biopsy, 2–3 mm in size. Fixed and processed for histopathologic examination. Microbiological cultures and other testing performed as indicated
Transbronchial biopsy	Forceps tissue biopsy, 2-3 mm in size. Processed for histopathologic examination. Microbiological cultures and other testing performed as indicated
Bronchoalveolar lavage (BAL)	Cytologic smears and centrifuge preparations. Fixed or air-dried, then stained for cytopathologic examination and biochemical analysis. Microbiological cultures and other testing performed as indicated
Transbronchial fine-needle aspiration	Cytologic smears and centrifuge preparations. Fixed or air-dried, then stained for cytopathologic examination. Microbiological cultures and other testing performed as indicated
Surgical "wedge" lung biopsy (either video-assisted or open)	3–5 cm peripheral lung tissue sample, including pleura and alveolar parenchyma. Specimens are fixed and processed for histopathologic examination. Microbiological cultures and specialized testing performed as indicated
Transthoracic needle core biopsy and aspiration	Core biopsy fragment(s), and cytologic smears/centrifuge preparations. Smears and cellular preparations can be fixed or air-dried, then stained for cytopathologic exam; special stains for organisms and other specialized techniques as indicated. Core tissue specimens are fixed and processed for histopathologic exam. Microbiological cultures and specialized assays performed as indicated
Thoracentesis	Cytologic centrifuge preparations. Fixed or air-dried, then stained for cytopathologic examination. Microbiological cultures, biochemical analysis, and specialized assays performed as indicated

Specimens obtained through the flexible bronchoscope

The flexible bronchoscope was introduced in the United States in the late 1960s, after successful use in Japan.[8] Despite several decades of experience with the rigid bronchoscope, the advent of the flexible bronchoscope (Fig. 2.1) allowed evaluation of the major conducting airways without general anesthesia and with less morbidity.[8,16] Furthermore, the flexible instrument has the advantage of providing better access to more distal and obliquely branched airways. The rigid bronchoscope still has major uses in certain settings, mainly where the device's larger bore is an advantage, but today pulmonary endoscopy is dominated by the flexible bronchoscope.

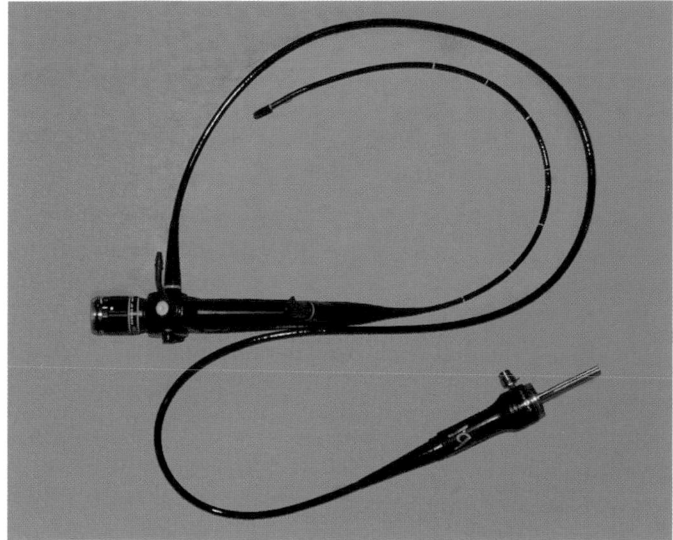

Fig. 2.1 **Bronchoscopy.** The modern flexible bronchoscope.

Endobronchial biopsies

Modern flexible bronchoscopes allow the operator to accurately visualize the structural integrity of the bronchial tree, and its mucosal surfaces, commonly as far distal as the sixth order-bronchi[17] (Fig. 2.2). Biopsy of visualized mucosal lesions is most commonly performed using cupped forceps (Fig. 2.3A) introduced through the flexible shaft of the bronchoscope.[8] With this technique, the airway mucosa, lamina propria and musculature are sampled with or without fragments of cartilage (Fig. 2.3B). The lymphovascular network of the peribronchial sheath is included, making it possible to identify metastatic disease when this is present in lymphatic or vascular

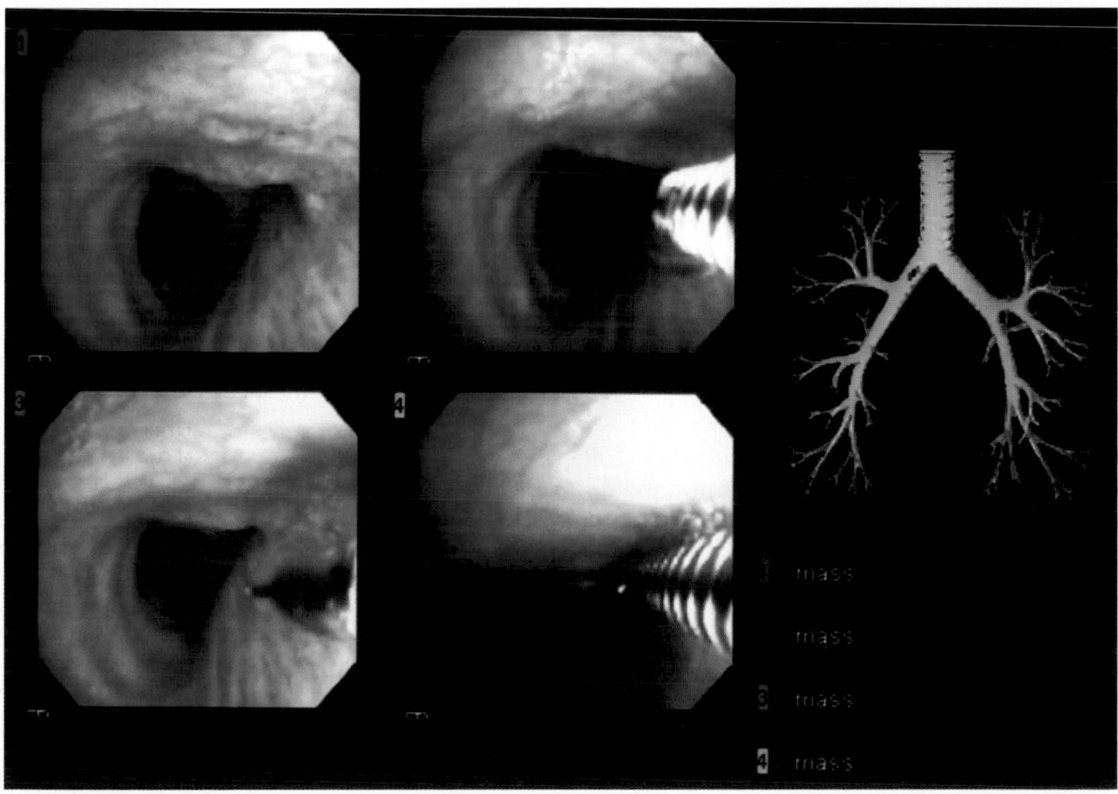

Fig. 2.2 **Bronchoscopy.** Endoscopic view of right mainstem bronchus with a needle biopsy device inserted (right upper and lower images and left lower image). Note the guide diagram (extreme right) with a red dot indicating the position of the bronchoscope tip.

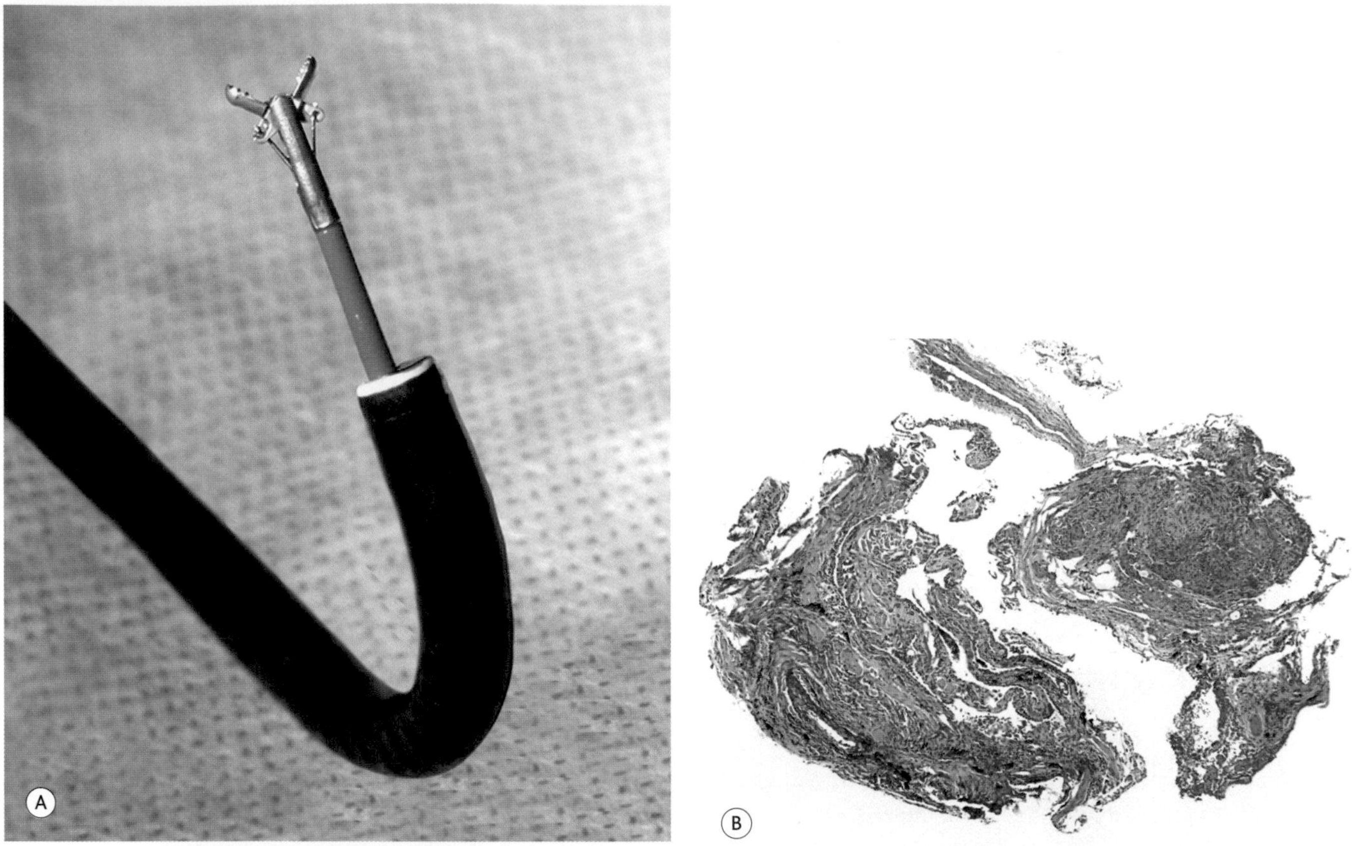

Fig. 2.3 **Bronchoscopic biopsy.** Cupped biopsy forceps (A) and bronchoscopic biopsy specimen (B). The airway epithelium, subepithelial tissue and muscle wall are typically present with variable cartilage.

channels. The closed forceps is extracted from the bronchoscope and the biopsy is dislodged from the cupped ends of the device and placed in fixative or other solution (see below). A sterile needle or fine-tipped forceps (Fig. 2.4) is useful for removing the delicate tissue specimen. The biopsies obtained in this way average 2–3 mm in size.

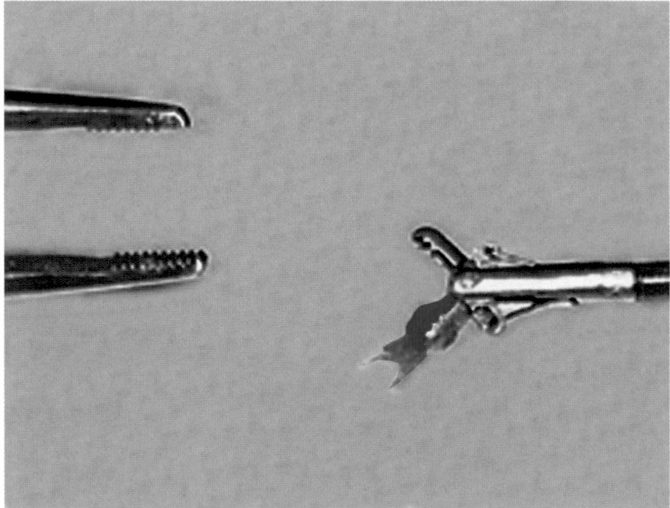

Fig. 2.4 **Bronchoscopic biopsy.** Removing the specimen from the device with fine-tipped forceps. Alternatively, a sterile needle can be used.

Specimens should be placed immediately into fixative solution or sterile transport medium. When these solutions are not available, specimens can be placed in a closed container on a sterile, saline-soaked, non-stick wound dressing pad and transferred to the laboratory for processing. Gauze or mesh pads are not appropriate for use, since the biopsy may become entwined in the mesh material, making extraction difficult, and tissue damage likely. As with all small biopsy specimens, caution must be exerted to avoid prolonged exposure to air, since drying artifact can make the specimen uninterpretable.

For tissue examination by light microscopy, the usual specimen fixation is accomplished using 10% neutral buffered formalin (4% formaldehyde solution). Biopsies should be submersed in fixative, with an optimal fixative-to-specimen volume ratio of at least 10:1. For reasons of safety and disposal cost, some laboratories have replaced their formalin solutions with special non-aldehyde fixatives, most of which use alcohol as the primary fixing agent. It is important to remember that all fixatives produce a certain degree of histologic artifact in tissues and cells, and that these artifacts can influence the accuracy

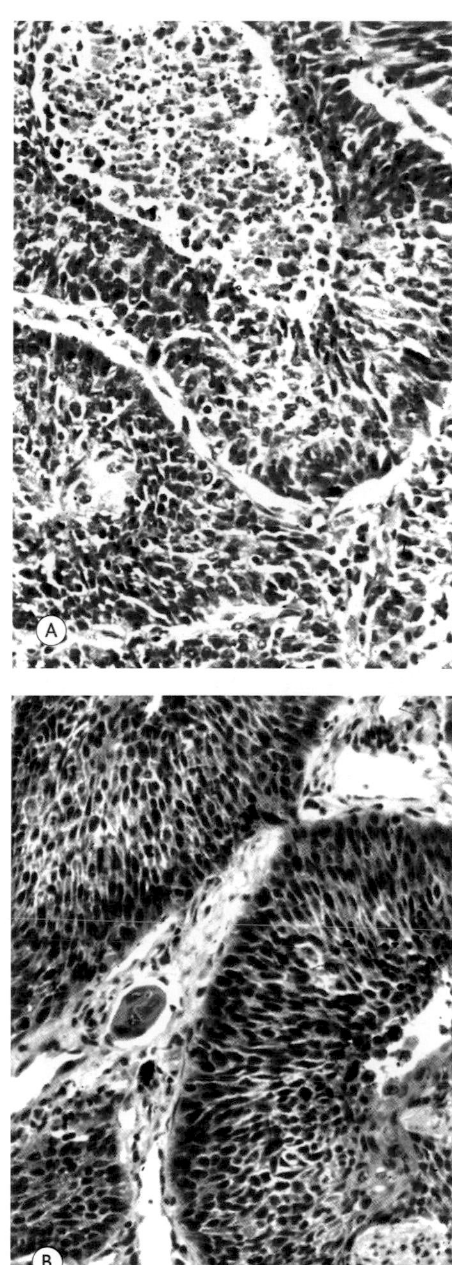

Fig. 2.5 **Artifacts produced by fixatives.** These can be appreciated in these two photos of the same tumor fixed in two different fixative solutions (A) formalin, (B) alcohol.

of the diagnosis (Fig. 2.5). For this reason, it is essential that the pathologist responsible for interpreting the specimen be consulted regarding the type of fixative to be used. Despite some hazards in handling and disposal, 10% neutral-buffered formalin remains the gold standard for lung biopsy fixation.

When transferring bronchoscopic biopsy specimens from carrier or fixative solutions into cassettes for paraffin embedment, a useful device is a polystyrene pipette with the tip cut off with scissors (Fig. 2.6). This pipetting device allows the operator to transfer delicate specimens without tearing or crushing. Transferring of these specimens using forceps is to be avoided.

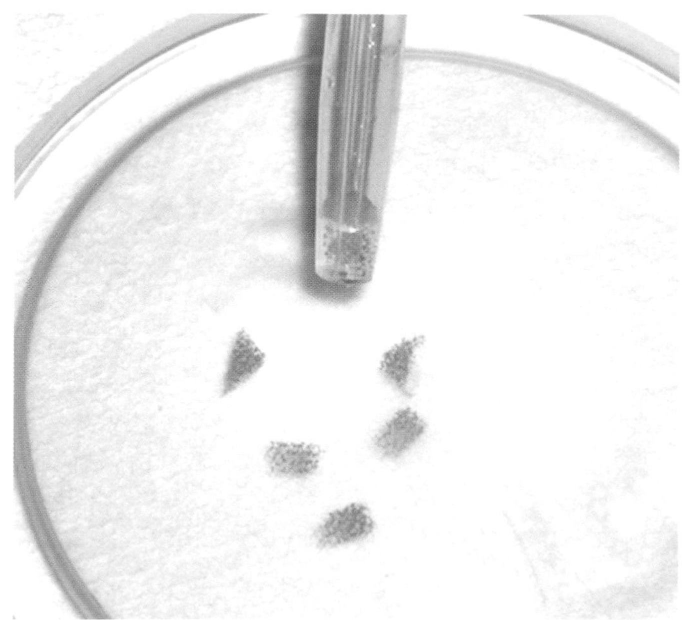

Fig. 2.6 **Transferring biopsy specimens.** Pipette transfer method. The pipette tip is cut off to provide a wider orifice.

When infection is a consideration, bronchoscopic biopsies can be transported directly to the microbiology laboratory for processing.[4,18,19] In most scenarios, biopsy samples are sent for both histopathologic evaluation and microbiological studies directly from the bronchoscopy suite or bedside. For both endobronchial and transbronchial biopsies, the optimal number of biopsies varies depending on the radiologic distribution of disease,[15,20–22] findings identified during bronchoscopy,[8,11,16] and other diagnostic considerations being entertained.[8,23,24] As a general guideline, if the patient is tolerating the procedure well, the greater the number of biopsies, the greater the likelihood of establishing a definitive diagnosis.[8,22,24]

Transbronchial biopsies

In contrast to the endobronchial biopsy, the transbronchial biopsy technique is intended to sample alveolar lung parenchyma beyond the cartilaginous bronchi.[8,16,17,25] This technique uses either crocodile-style forceps (Machida) or cupped forceps manipulated by the operator (Fig. 2.7). To obtain the biopsy, the forceps is advanced with the jaws closed into a distal airway until resistance is met. The forceps is retracted slightly and then advanced into more peripheral lung with the jaws open. The jaws are

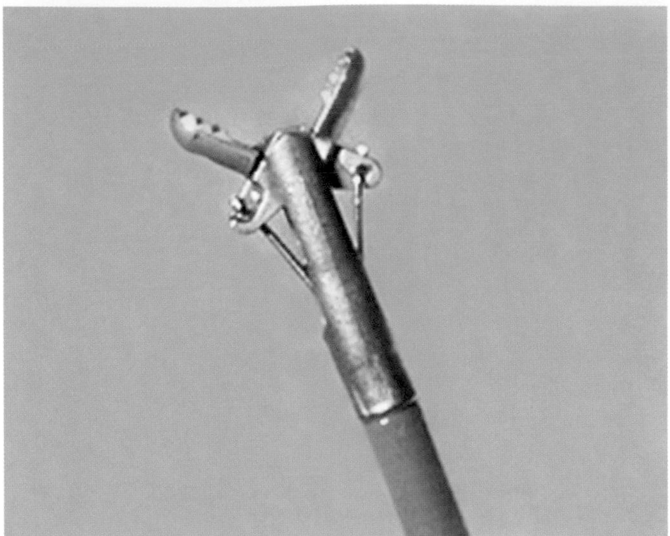

Fig. 2.7 **Transbronchial biopsy.** Cupped biopsy forceps with open jaws. This device is commonly used for transbronchial biopsies.

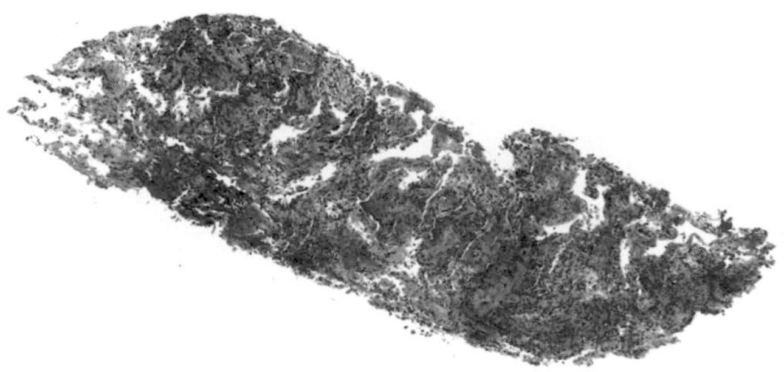

Fig. 2.8 **Transbronchial biopsy.** Low-magnification image of a typical transbronchial biopsy.

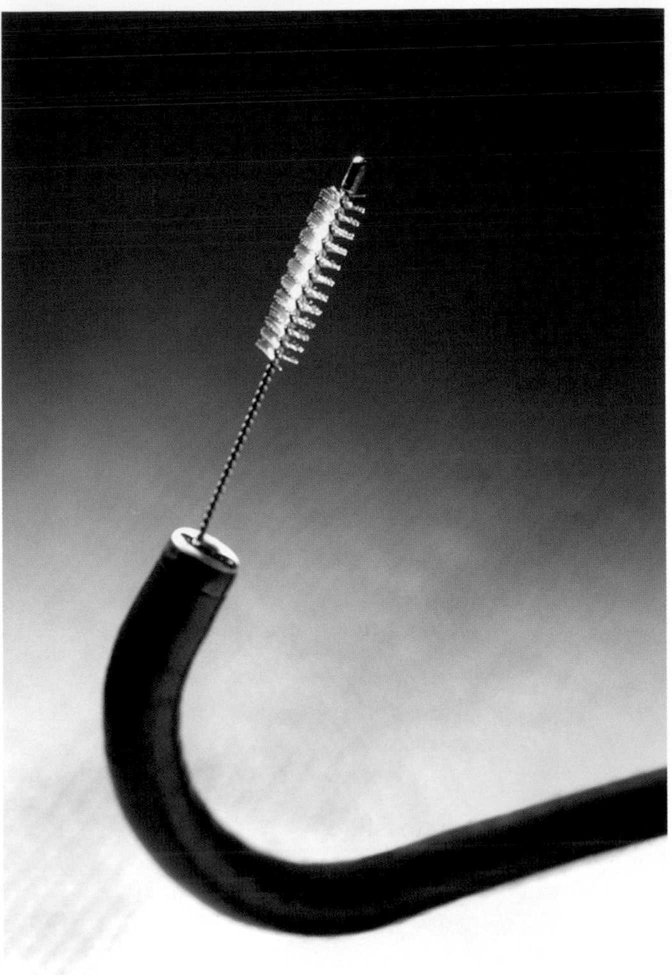

Fig. 2.9 **Bronchial brushing.** The conical bronchial bristle brush.

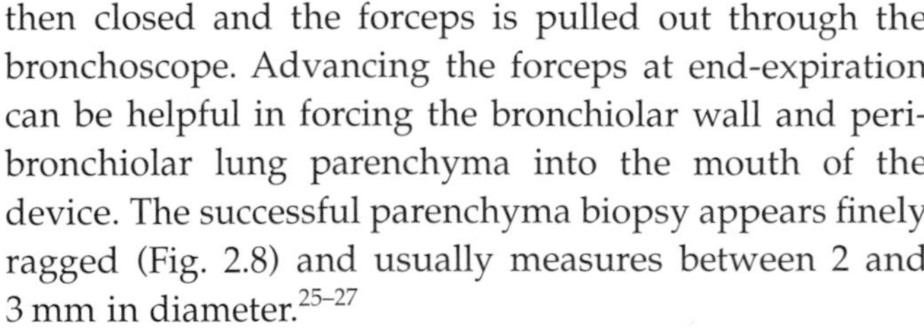

then closed and the forceps is pulled out through the bronchoscope. Advancing the forceps at end-expiration can be helpful in forcing the bronchiolar wall and peribronchiolar lung parenchyma into the mouth of the device. The successful parenchyma biopsy appears finely ragged (Fig. 2.8) and usually measures between 2 and 3 mm in diameter.[25–27]

As with endobronchial biopsies, the transbronchial biopsy is teased from the forceps with a sterile needle, and the same cautions are advisable to avoid damage during handling and transfer to fixative or other solution. The truncated pipette technique is also useful in this setting. Once processed, both types of biopsies should be serially sectioned for thorough microscopic evaluation.[2]

Bronchial brushings

Visualized lesions of the airway epithelium can be sampled for cytologic evaluation.[8,11,16] The technique involves the use of a conical bristle brush (Fig. 2.9). Under direct visualization the brush is agitated against the mucosal surface of the airway, forcing cells into the interstices of the brush (Fig. 2.10). The brush is removed from the bronchoscope and can be applied directly to glass slides. Cells and secretions smeared on slides can be subsequently fixed for cytologic evaluation using the Papanicolaou staining method, or air-dried for use with the Wright–Giemsa staining technique. Immediate fixation of slides is best accomplished with 95% alcohol by direct immersion immediately after smearing on the slide. Each fixation and staining technique produces characteristic artifacts and the use of one over the other depends on training and preference.

If slides are not available for smear preparations, the brush can be placed directly into a small vial of sterile saline, which is then shaken vigorously to dislodge cells into the fluid. This fluid sample of suspended cells is sent to the laboratory for millipore filtration or cytocentrifuge-

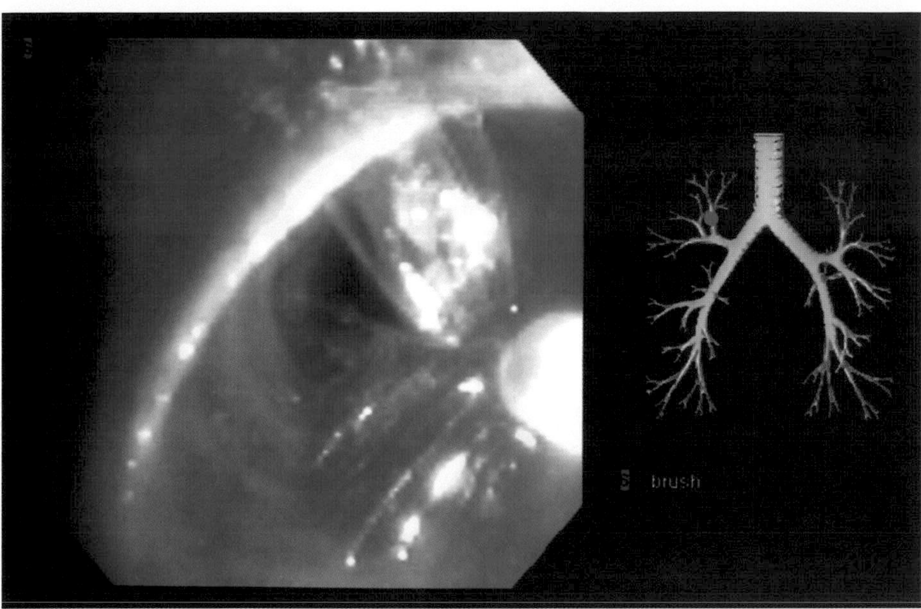

Fig. 2.10 **Bronchial brushing.** Application of the brush to the airway mucosa.

type application onto slides[8,11,16,28,29] analogous to the handling of washings and lavage specimens, discussed below.

Bronchial washings and bronchoalveolar lavage

Bronchial washings and bronchoalveolar lavage (BAL) specimens are less "lesion directed" sampling techniques, and rely on the presence of shed cells within the airways and peripheral alveolar spaces.[11,30–34] Bronchial washings are obtained by aspiration of sterile saline solution applied near the tip of the bronchoscope. They therefore consist of a rather concentrated cellular preparation of bronchial epithelial cells and macrophages with variable amounts of inflammatory cells and mucus. Because of the relatively small sample volume (similar to the bronchial brush sample, when this is placed into solution), a limited number of potential assays can be performed on the bronchial washing specimen. Cytologic examination and cultures are the most commonly ordered tests on these samples.

The BAL, by contrast, retrieves a large volume of saline that is injected into the airways (Fig. 2.11). This allows for sampling of a greater volume of lung parenchyma and airway luminal secretions. Cell density in the fluid is typically low and centrifuge or filter techniques are required for microscopic examination.

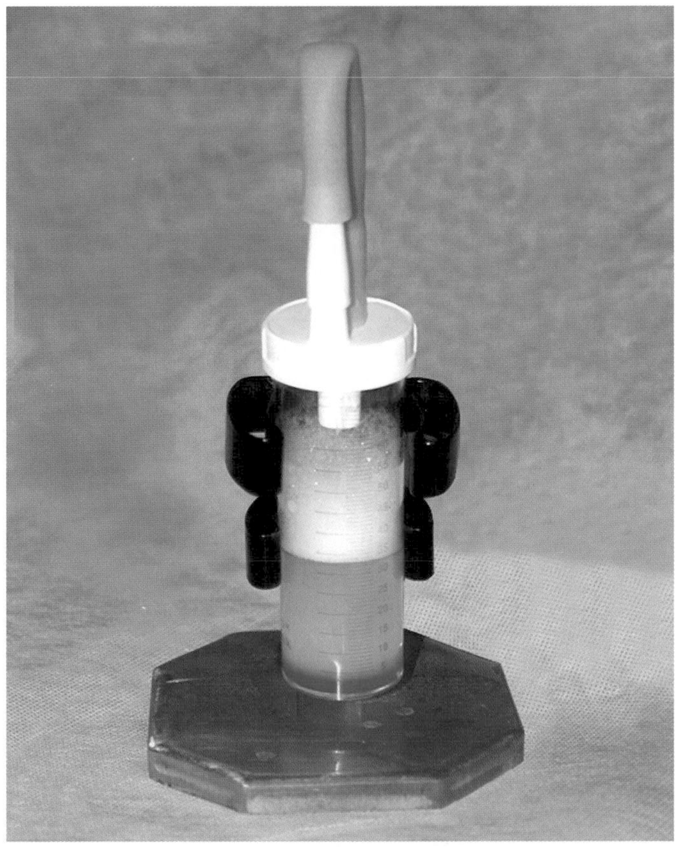

Fig. 2.11 **Bronchial washings.** These are obtained by aspiration of injected sterile saline solution.

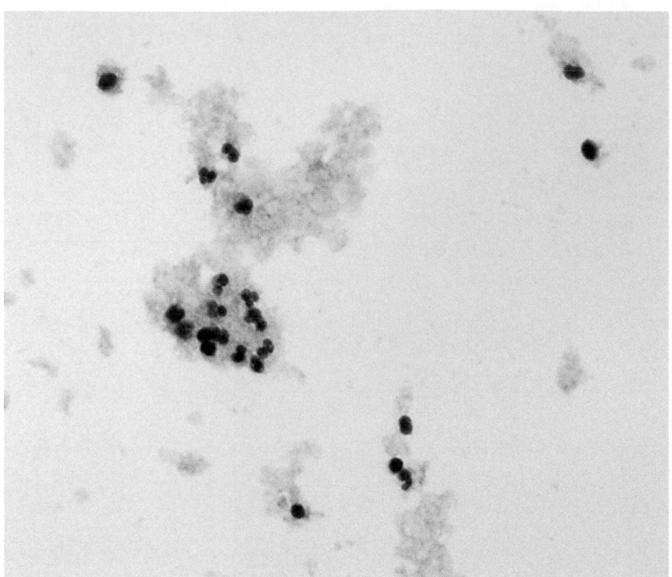

Fig. 2.12 **Bronchoalveolar lavage (BAL).** A BAL fluid with macrophages and neutrophils. (ThinPrep, Papanicolau stain, ×200 original magnification.)

The BAL technique is performed by instilling multiple aliquots of sterile saline (20–50 ml), followed by a variable dwell time and subsequent aspiration of this fluid into a flask or syringe at the bedside. The normal BAL fluid consists primarily of macrophages with a few inflammatory cells (Fig. 2.12).[33] A potential advantage of the BAL fluid is the ability to analyze non-cellular elements included, such as, surfactant content, serum proteins (albumin, immunoglobulins, enzymes, etc.) and mucus.[35,36] In current practice, the BAL technique is used primarily in the setting of the immunocompromised host for the diagnosis of infection.[35,37–40] However, as a research tool in the study of interstitial lung diseases, the BAL has been used extensively for quantitation of cellular components.[18,27,35,41–43]

In processing the BAL fluid, the operator must determine what types of analysis will be performed in advance. A typical sample might be divided into a number of aliquots, some of which would be sent to the cytopathology laboratory while others would be handled by the general laboratory (microbiology, chemistry, hematology). For cytopathologic evaluation, the bronchial washing smears and cytocentrifuge preparations can be air-dried for the Wright–Giemsa staining method. More commonly, in the United States, smears are fixed in an equal volume of either Saccomanno's fixative (2% Carbowax and 50% ethyl alcohol), or simply 50% (or greater) ethyl alcohol solution. These fixed smears are then stained using the Papanicolaou method or other staining techniques.

Transbronchial fine-needle aspiration

Transbronchial fine-needle aspiration (TBNA) was initially introduced by Wang and Terry in 1983[44] as a staging tool in the evaluation of patients with lung cancer. The use of TBNA has expanded considerably since that time[45–47] for the diagnosis of both central and peripheral lung lesions, even in the absence of endobronchial abnormalities.[47] The specimens generated by this technique are very small, sometimes no more than a drop or two, and when the target is solid tissue, these samples consist of thick cellular material. To prepare direct smear preparations for cytopathologic evaluation and rapid stains for organisms, the needle is removed from the syringe (or other aspiration device) and then reattached after air has been aspirated into the syringe. The air is then rapidly forced out through the needle tip, forcing the sample out of the needle hub and onto a slide. The slide is then either air-dried or immediately fixed, before staining. For microbiology cultures and fluid-based cytocentrifuge preparations, the needle is rinsed directly into culture or cytopathologic fixative medium, respectively.

Specimens obtained by transthoracic needle biopsy and aspiration

Thoracentesis specimens

Thoracentesis derives its greatest practical application in the evaluation of cells and noncellular elements in pleural effusions.[48–50] Like the BAL fluid, a number of specific analyses are typically performed. If collected after hours, the sterile thoracentesis fluid can be stored unfixed at 4 °C for processing the next day. The aliquoted thoracentesis fluid specimens are distributed to the appropriate laboratory for analysis (e.g. microbiology, chemistry, hematology). Chemical determinations of glucose, amylase, lactic dehydrogenase, and other analytes are compared with cellular composition determined by cytopathologic evaluation. The cytocentrifuge or millipore filter can also be evaluated cytopathologically for the presence of malignant neoplasm. Rapid stains for microorganisms can be performed as indicated.

Closed pleural biopsy

Available pleural needle biopsy devices include the Cope, Abrams, and True-Cut needles that produce a very small biopsy sample (Fig. 2.13). Inflammatory, infectious, and neoplastic diseases of the pleura can be diagnosed using these devices, despite the limitations of biopsy size

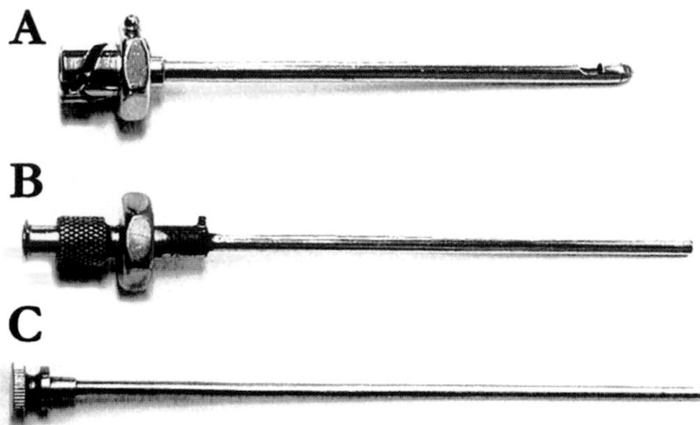

Fig. 2.13 **Pleural biopsy.** The Abrams pleural biopsy needle consists of an outer trocar with a blunt tip (A) and a side cutting port near the tip (right). The trocar is pulled across the parietal pleural edge, hooking this tissue into the side port. The inner cutting cannula (B) is then forced across the cutting port from within, following along a spiral guide path seen on the left end of the outer sheath. The stylet (C) keeps the needle channel closed during initial insertion into the pleural space, thereby avoiding the creation of a pneumothorax.

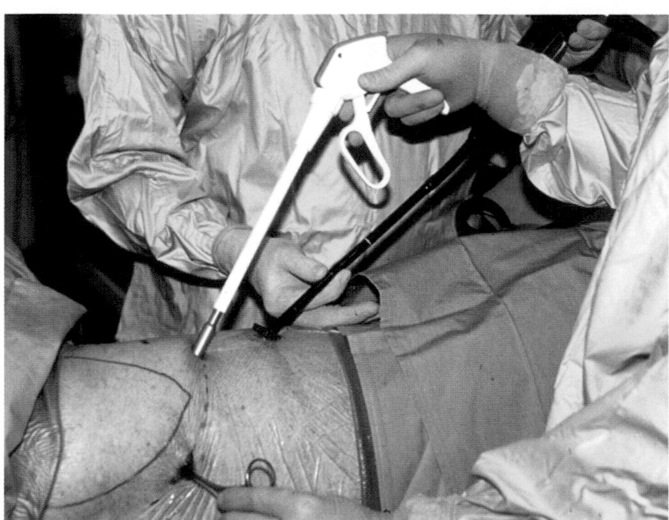

Fig. 2.14 **Video-assisted thoracoscopic surgery.** Three incisions are made for instruments: video scope (black), stapler (white), and manipulator device (bottom).

and somewhat randomness of sampling.[51] These small biopsy specimens should be handled in a fashion analogous to those obtained from bronchoscopic biopsy techniques (see above).

Transthoracic fine-needle aspiration and biopsy of the lung

In current practice, the use of transthoracic needle aspiration biopsy has become commonplace.[10,52–57] This technique is typically performed in the radiology department, since these biopsies are always performed under radiologic guidance. Samples are similar to those produced by transbronchial needle aspiration and should be handled accordingly (discussed previously). Assistance by a cytotechnologist during the procedure is a cost-effective benefit to ensure adequacy of specimen prior to termination of the procedure.[58] Recent advances in needle biopsy devices have allowed for better tissue samples and greater likelihood of accurate diagnosis.[59–62] If the technique generates a semi-liquid sample, this should be handled as described for transbronchial needle aspiration specimens. If a core of tissue is generated (typically 1 mm in diameter), this can be processed like other needle core biopsies received in surgical pathology. It is advisable to make 4–6 unstained sections at the time of initial sectioning in histology, in addition to those requested in advance for routine evaluation. Having these extra sections available saves time and avoids having to return to the tissue block (which can be a problem because block refacing wastes a certain amount of tissue) later when special stains may be necessary.

Specimens from thoracoscopy and thoracotomy

Surgical biopsy of lung parenchyma has become a relative gold standard for the evaluation and diagnosis of inflammatory lung disease in the United States.[63–69] In the early days of lung biopsy, open thoracotomy was the only available method. In the open biopsy procedure, the specimen is obtained through a limited thoracotomy, where exposure is gained to a reasonable amount of lung through an intercostal incision and retraction of the ribs. During the procedure, lung tissue is delivered into the incision and a wedge-shaped portion of lung with pleura is removed. A newer technique, becoming more widely available today, is the video-assisted thoracoscopic biopsy technique (VATS). With this procedure, smaller incisions are made and a thoracoscope with a video camera is introduced along with instruments. Figures 2.14–2.19 illustrate the technique.

Before any wedge lung biopsy procedure is performed, consultation between radiologist, chest physician, and thoracic surgeon is essential to ensure appropriate sampling and the identification of ideal locations for biopsies to be performed. For example, a single biopsy from the upper lobe in a patient with idiopathic pulmonary fibrosis may be futile, since the disease tends to involve the lower lobes predominantly. In the ideal scenario, the surgeon combines his best surgical judgment with the

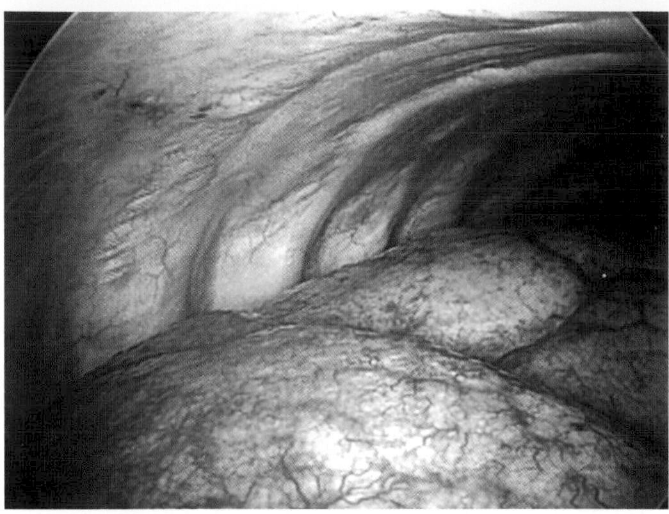

Fig. 2.15 **Video-assisted thoracoscopic surgery.** Videoscopic view of lung and parietal chest wall.

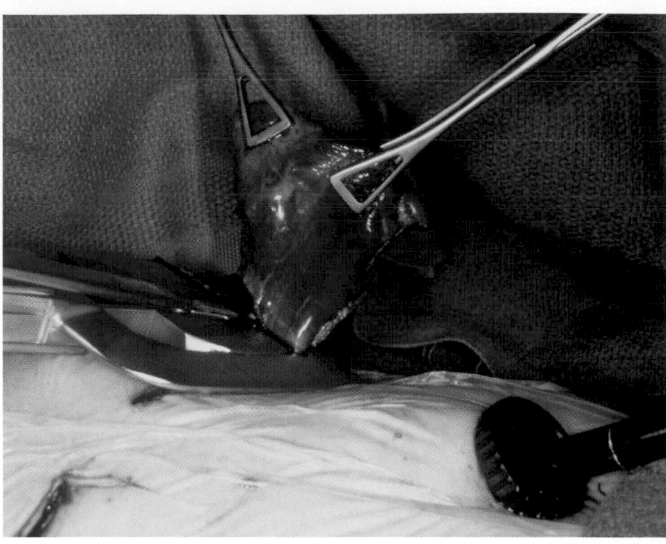

Fig. 2.17 **Video-assisted thoracoscopic surgery.** The stapled biopsy is extracted through one of the incisions.

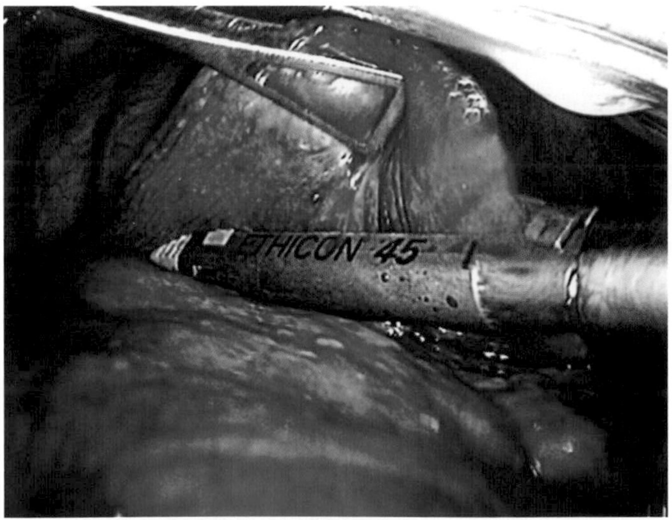

Fig. 2.16 **Video-assisted thoracoscopic surgery.** A selected portion of lung is held while the stapler isolates the biopsy from the surrounding lung. The double staple line produced allows safe surgical incision for removal.

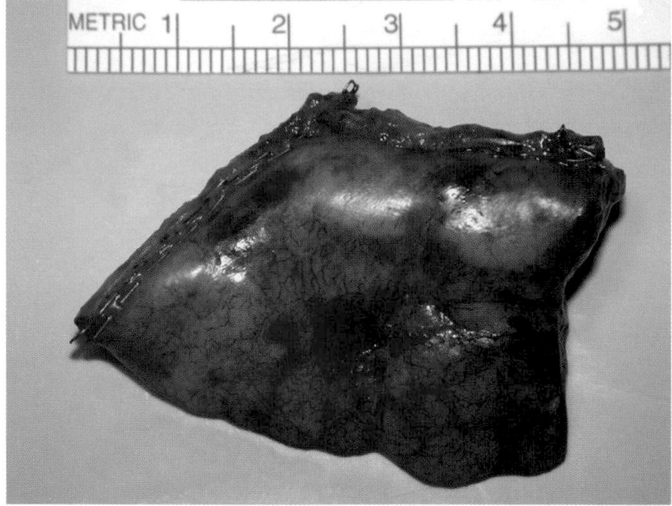

Fig. 2.18 **Optimal specimen size for surgical lung biopsies.** The surgical wedge biopsy should measure at least 3–5 cm in length and 3 cm in depth (from pleural surface to the stapled edge at mid-biopsy).

specific characteristics of the disease (if any) as identified on clinical and radiologic grounds.

With the VATS technique, more than one biopsy can be taken from widely separated areas. Such sampling is optimal for many diffuse inflammatory lung diseases.[70–72] Specimens measuring 2–3 cm can be easily obtained with little morbidity. The popularity of the VATS biopsy technique relates primarily to data suggesting faster patient recovery. Proponents claim shorter hospital stays with decreased morbidity as compared to open thoracotomy lung or pleural biopsy.[70,72–74] Unfortunately, no randomized studies have been performed to unequivocally support this position. We have found that the main differences between open thoracotomy and VATS biopsy procedures are more related to costs (higher for VATS) and specimen quality (slightly more artifacts for VATS biopsies). An indisputable benefit of the VATS procedure is greater accessibility to widely separated lung segments. On the question of where to biopsy, early reports discouraged using the lingula and middle lobe[75,76] for biopsy, arguing that these portions of lung tend to harbor non-representative and nonspecific inflammatory changes. More recent reports suggest that this is not the case.[5, 77]

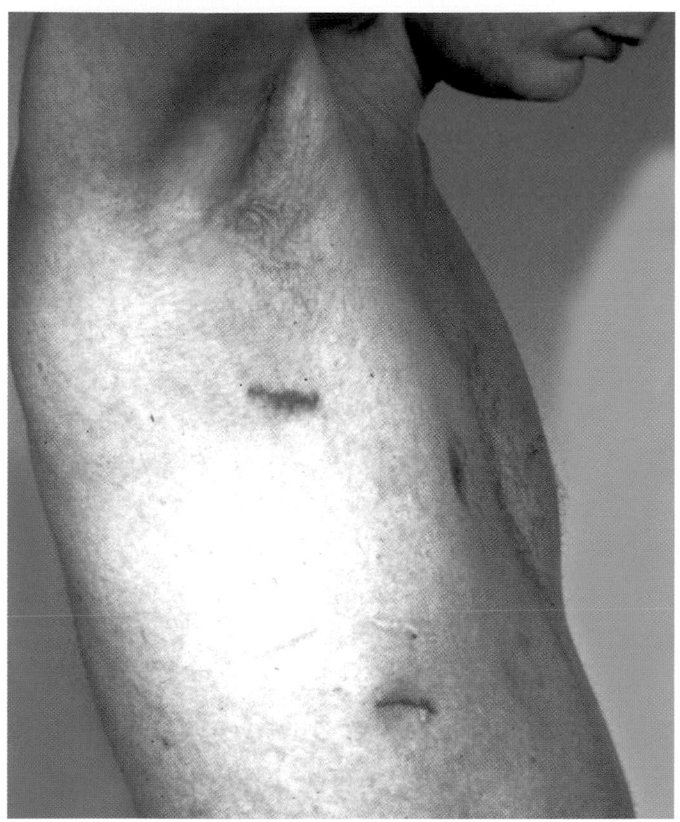

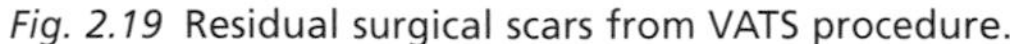

Fig. 2.19 Residual surgical scars from VATS procedure.

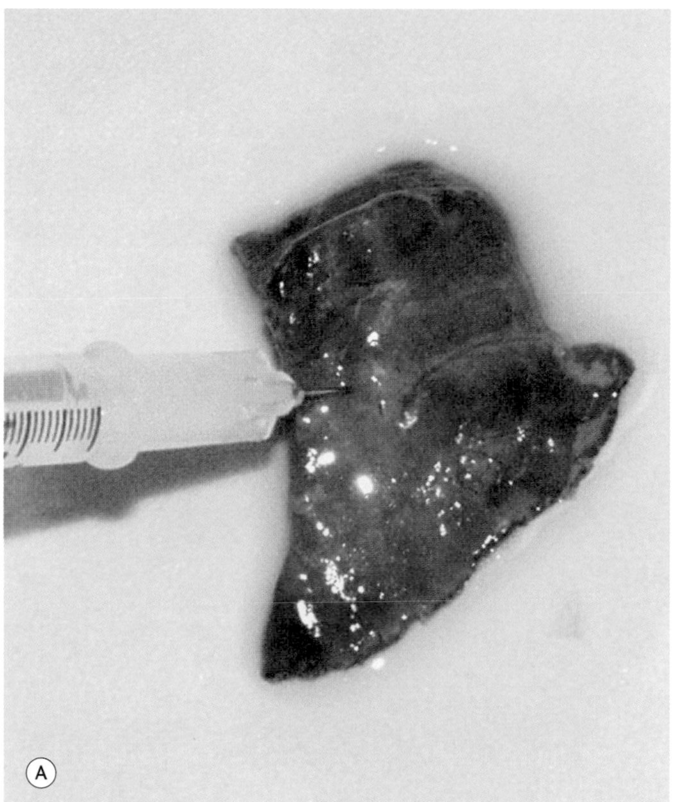

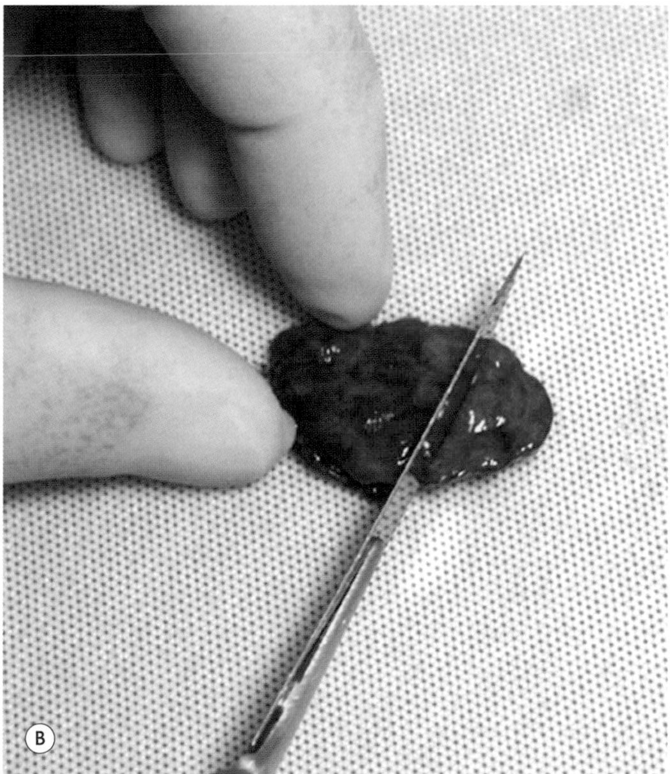

Fig. 2.20 **Handling the surgical wedge biopsy.** (A) tuberculin syringe (with 23–25 gauge needle) is useful for inflating lung wedge biopsies after the surgical staples have been removed. (B) Once inflated, submersion of the biopsy in fixative for an additional 30 minutes or more improves gross section quality and helps avoid damage to the specimen.

Processing of the wedge lung biopsy requires techniques different than those used in handling biopsies from other organs. Intraoperative consultation with immediate handling of the specimen is ideal, if only to guide appropriate specimen handling. If the wedge biopsy is to be divided for different types of analysis (e.g., microbiological cultures, electron microscopy, immunofluoresence studies, molecular studies) these portions can be removed before routine processing for morphologic assessment.

Performing frozen sections on air-filled lung tissue poses some special problems. Unfixed lung tissue is easily compressed, especially when attempts are made to slice it into thin sections unfixed (typically less than 5 mm). Severe compression may result in artifactual atelectasis, thereby compounding the difficulty of histopathologic assessment. The simplest and most reliable technique for frozen sections is to cut a 5–6mm slab from the biopsy using a fresh scalpel and freezing it without further preparation. For most lung diseases, the frozen sections generated this way are reasonably interpretable. Alternatively, some authors have recommended injecting the actual slab section (not the whole biopsy) with a stabilizing solution prior to freezing. To accomplish this, a dilute solution of embedding compound is gently infused

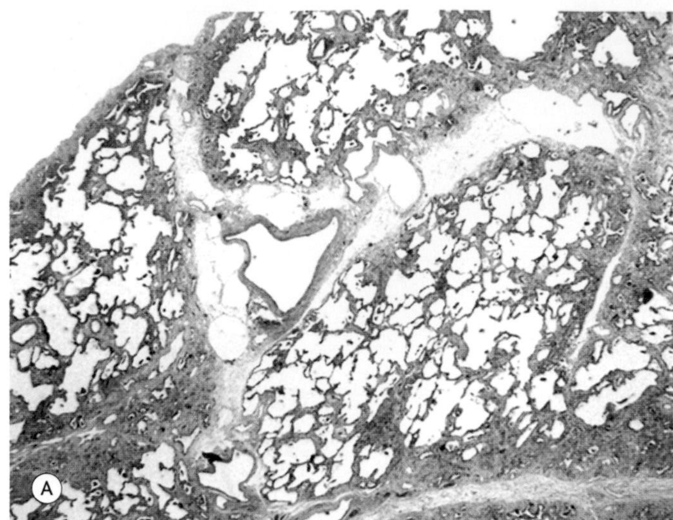

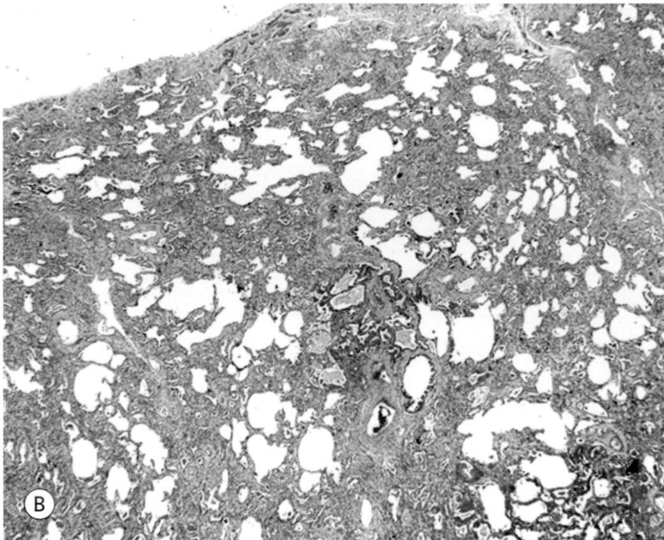

Fig. 2.21 **Inflation vs emersion fixation.** The wedge biopsy injection technique makes specimen sectioning easier, and allows the fixed specimen to more accurately reflect the normal lung histologic relationships in microscopic sections. The biopsy section in (A) was gently infused with fixative using a needle and syringe. The biopsy in (B) was emersion fixed after the staples were removed.

into the cut surface of the slab using a 21–23-gauge needle attached to a 5 ml syringe.

After frozen section consultation has been completed, the remainder of the specimen can be injected with 10% neutral-buffered formalin (or another fixative of choice). A number of methods have been recommended to accomplish this. First, the specimen can be vigorously shaken within a container of fixative. This action tends to distribute fixative within the lung parenchyma, but may not inflate atelectatic areas. Secondly, a small volume of carbonated water can be added to the fixative solution to assist in re-expansion of alveoli (no agitation required). Finally, the syringe inflation technique can be used and is the method we prefer (Fig. 2.20).[78] Here, a small needle (22–25 gauge) is attached to a 5 or 10 ml syringe filled with fixative. The needle is inserted through the open margin (after removal of the surgical staples) several times with gentle pressure, resulting in inflation of the specimen. Once inflation has been achieved, the specimen should be immersed in fixative for at least 30 minutes, before processing. Even a completely injected specimen will still only float just below the fixative surface, rather than sink to the bottom. After fixation, the specimen can be safely and easily sliced into 3–5 mm sections for final processing. While artifactual hyperinflation is a potential hazard with inflation, in practice this risk is overshadowed considerably by the benefits of adequately preserved and nicely separated alveolar walls within the specimen (Fig. 2.21).

Conclusions

Liberal communication between chest physician, radiologist, pathologist and thoracic surgeon is strongly advised before embarking on any lung biopsy procedure, especially those associated with procurement of wedge biopsies. Such a multidisciplinary approach is cost-effective and increases the likelihood of accurate results.

REFERENCES

1. Advanced laboratory methods in histology and pathology. Armed Forces Institute of Pathology, Washington, DC, 1994.
2. Nagata N, Hirano H, Takayama K, et al.: Step section preparation of transbronchial lung biopsy. Chest 1991; 100: 959–962.
3. Bonetti F, Chiodera F, Pea M, et al.: Transbronchial biopsy in lymphangiomyomatosis of the lung. HMB45 for diagnosis. Am J Surg Pathol 1993; 17: 1092–1102.
4. Chastre J, Fagon J, Soler P, et al.: Diagnosis of nosocomial bacterial pneumonia in intubated patients undergoing ventilation: comparison of the usefulness of bronchoalveolar lavage and the protected specimen brush. Am J Med 1988; 85: 499–506.
5. Miller R, Nelems B, Müller N, et al.: Lingular and right middle lobe biopsy in the assessment of diffuse lung disease. Ann Thorac Surg 1987; 44: 269–273.
6. Rosen P: Frozen section management of a lung biopsy for suspected Pneumocystis pneumonia. Am J Surg Pathol 1977; 1: 79–82.
7. Travis W, Borok Z, Roum J, et al.: Pulmonary Langerhans cell granulomatosis (histiocytosis X). A clinicopathologic study of 48 cases. Am J Surg Pathol 1993; 17: 971–986.
8. Zavala D: Diagnostic fiberoptic bronchoscopy: techniques and results of biopsy in 600 patients. Chest 1975; 68: 12–19.
9. Churg A: An inflation procedure for open-lung biopsies. Am J Surg Pathol 1983; 7: 69–71.
10. Yang P, Lee Y, Yu C, et al.: Ultrasonographically guided biopsy of thoracic tumors – a comparison of large-bore cutting biopsy with fine-needle aspiration. Cancer 1992; 69: 2553–2560.
11. Popp W, Rauscher H, Ritschka L, et al.: Diagnostic sensitivity of different techniques in the diagnosis of lung tumors with the flexible fiberoptic bronchoscope – comparison of brush biopsy, imprint cytology of forceps biopsy, and histology of forceps biopsy. Cancer 1991; 67: 72–75.
12. Burt ME, Flye W, Webber BL, et al.: Prospective evaluation of aspiration needle, cutting needle, transbronchial and open lung biopsy in patients with pulmonary infiltrates. Ann Thorac Surg 1981; 32: 146–153.

13. Leslie K, Lanza L, Helmers R, et al., Diagnostic sampling of lung tissues and cells. In: Medical management of pulmonary diseases, Davis G, Marcey T, Seward E, Eds. 1999, Marcel Dekker, New York, pp 213–220.
14. Leslie K, Colby T: Classification and pathology of diffuse interstitial lung disease. Semin Clin Immunol 1999; 1: 7–15.
15. Leslie K, Colby T, Swensen S: Anatomic distribution and histopathologic patterns in interstitial lung disease. In: Interstitial lung disease, Schwarz M, King TJ, Eds. 2002, BC Decker, Hamilton, pp 31–50.
16. Mitchell D, Emerson C, Collins J, et al.: Transbronchial lung biopsy with the fibreoptic bronchoscope: analysis of results in 433 patients. Br J Dis Chest 1981; 75: 258–262.
17. Kovnat DM, Rath GS, Anderson WM, et al.: Maximal extent of visualization of bronchial tree by flexible fiberoptic bronchoscopy. Am Rev Respir Dis 1974; 110(1): 88–90.
18. Haslam P, Turton C, Heard B, et al.: Bronchoalveolar lavage in pulmonary fibrosis: comparison of cells obtained with lung biopsy and clinical features. Thorax 1980; 35: 9–18.
19. Delvenne P, Arrese J, Thiry A, et al.: Detection of cytomegalovirus, Pneumocystis carinii, and aspergillus species in bronchoalveolar lavage fluid. A comparison of techniques. Am J Clin Pathol 1993; 100: 414–418.
20. Guinee DJ, Feuerstein I, Koss M, et al.: Pulmonary lymphangioleiomyomatosis. Diagnosis based on results of transbronchial biopsy and immunohistochemical studies and correlation with high-resolution computed tomography findings. Arch Pathol Lab Med 1994; 118: 846–849.
21. Colby TV, Swensen SJ: Anatomic distribution and histopathologic patterns in diffuse lung disease: correlation with HRCT. J Thorac Imaging 1996; 11(1): 1–26.
22. Popovich J, Kvale P, Eichenhorn M, et al.: Diagnostic accuracy of multiple biopsies from flexible fiberoptic bronchoscopy. A comparison of central versus peripheral carcinoma. Am Rev Respir Dis 1982; 125: 521–523.
23. Gilman M, Wang K: Transbronchial lung biopsy in sarcoidosis: an approach to determine the optimal number of biopsies. Am Rev Respir Dis 1980; 122: 721–724.
24. Flint A, Martinez F, Young M, et al.: Influence of sample number and biopsy site on the histologic diagnosis of diffuse lung disease. Ann Thorac Surg 1995; 60: 1605–1607.
25. Andersen H: Transbronchoscopic lung biopsy for diffuse pulmonary diseases. Results in 939 patients. Chest 1978; 73(5 Suppl): 734–736.
26. Cazzadori A, Di Perri G, Todeschini G, et al.: Transbronchial biopsy in the diagnosis of pulmonary infiltrates in immunocompromised patients. Chest 1995; 107(1): 101–106.
27. Guilinger R, Paradis I, Dauber J, et al.: The importance of bronchoscopy with transbronchial biopsy and bronchoalveolar lavage in the management of lung transplant recipients. Am J Respir Crit Care Med 1995; 152: 2037–2043.
28. Willcox M, Kervitsky A, Watters L, et al.: Quantification of cells recovered by bronchoalveolar lavage. Comparison of cytocentrifuge preparations with the filter method. Am Rev Respir Dis 1988; 138(1): 74–80.
29. Robb J, Melello C, Odom C: Comparison of Cyto-Shuttle and cytocentrifuge as processing methods for nongynecologic cytology specimens. Diagn Cytopathol 1996; 14(4): 305–309.
30. Poletti V, Romagna M, Allen K, et al.: Bronchoalveolar lavage in the diagnosis of disseminated lung tumors. Acta Cytol 1995; 39: 472–477.
31. Winterbauer R, Lammert J, Selland M, et al.: Bronchoalveolar lavage cell populations in the diagnosis of sarcoidosis. Chest 1993; 104: 352–361.
32. The BAL Cooperative Steering Committee. Bronchoalveolar lavage constituents in healthy individuals, idiopathic pulmonary fibrosis, and selected comparison groups. Am Rev Respir Dis 1990; 141: S169–202.
33. Merchant R, Schwartz D, Helmers R, et al.: Bronchoalveolar lavage cellularity – the distribution in normal volunteers. Am Rev Respir Dis 1992; 146: 448–453.
34. Cobben N, Jacobs J, Dieijen-Visser M, et al.: Diagnostic value of BAL fluid cellular profile and enzymes in infectious pulmonary disorders. Eur Respir J 1999; 14: 496–502.
35. American Thoracic Society Statement: Clinical role of bronchoalveolar lavage in adults with pulmonary disease. Am Rev Respir Dis 2001; 142: 481–486.
36. Reynolds HY, Fulmer JD, Kazmierowski JA, et al.: Analysis of cellular and protein content of broncho-alveolar lavage fluid from patients with idiopathic pulmonary fibrosis and chronic hypersensitivity pneumonitis. J Clin Invest 1977; 59(1): 165–175.
37. Abramson MJ, Stone CA, Holmes PW, et al.: The role of bronchoalveolar lavage in the diagnosis of suspected opportunistic pneumonia. Aust N Z J Med 1987; 17(4): 407–412.
38. Bye M, Bernstein L, Shah K, et al.: Diagnostic bronchoalveolar lavage in children with AIDS. Pediatr Pulmonol 1987; 3: 425–428.
39. Kahn FW, Jones JM: Diagnosing bacterial respiratory infection by bronchoalveolar lavage. J Infect Dis 1987; 155: 862–869.
40. Martin WJ, Smith TF, Sanderson DR, et al.: Role of bronchoalveolar lavage in the assessment of opportunistic pulmonary infections: utility and complications. Mayo Clin Proc 1987; 62: 549–557.
41. Goldstein RA, Rohatgi PK, Bergofsky EH, et al.: Clinical role of bronchoalveolar lavage in adults with pulmonary disease. Am Rev Respir Dis 1990; 142: 481–486.
42. Hunninghake GW, Gadek JE, Kawanami O, et al.: Inflammatory and immune processes in the human lung in health and disease: evaluation by bronchoalveolar lavage. Am J Pathol 1979; 97: 149–206.
43. Kvale PA: Bronchoscopic biopsies and bronchoalveolar lavage. Chest Surg Clin N Am 1996; 6(2): 205–222.
44. Wang K, Terry P: Transbronchial needle aspiration in the diagnosis and staging of bronchogenic carcinoma. Am Rev Respir Dis 1983; 127(3): 344–347.
45. Rosenthal D, Wallace J: Fine needle aspiration of pulmonary lesions via fiberoptic bronchoscopy. Acta Cytol 1984; 28: 203–210.
46. Wagner ED, Ramzy I, Greenberg SD, et al.: Transbronchial fine-needle aspiration. Reliability and limitations. Am J Clin Pathol 1989; 92: 36–41.
47. Mehta AC, Kavuru MS, Meeker DP, et al.: Transbronchial needle aspiration for histology specimens. Chest 1989; 96: 1228–1232.
48. Berquist TH, Bailey PB, Cortese DA, et al.: Transthoracic needle biopsy: accuracy and complications in relation to location and type of lesion. Mayo Clin Proc 1980; 55(8): 475–481.
49. Crosby JH, Hager B, Hoeg K: Transthoracic fine-needle aspiration. Experience in a cancer center. Cancer 1985; 56(10): 2504–2507.
50. Larscheid RC, Thorpe PE, Scott WJ: Percutaneous transthoracic needle aspiration biopsy: a comprehensive review of its current role in the diagnosis and treatment of lung tumors. Chest 1998; 114(3): 704–709.
51. Von Hoff DD, LiVolsi V: Diagnostic reliability of needle biopsy of the parietal pleura. A review of 272 biopsies. Am J Clin Pathol 1975; 64(2): 200–203.
52. Sanders C: Transthoracic needle aspiration. Clin Chest Med 1992; 13(1): 11–16.
53. Bocking A, Klose K, Kyll H, et al.: Cytologic versus histologic evaluation of needle biopsy of the lung, hilum and mediastinum-sensitivity, specificity and typing accuracy. Acta Cytol 1995; 39: 463–471.
54. Milman N: Percutaneous lung biopsy with semi-automatic, spring-driven fine needle – preliminary results in 13 patients. Respiration 1993; 60: 289–291.
55. Smyth R, Carty H, Thomas H, et al.: Diagnosis of interstitial lung disease by a percutaneous lung biopsy sample. Arch Dis Child 1994; 70: 143–144.
56. Lohela P, Tikkakoski T, Ammala K, et al.: Diagnosis of diffuse lung disease by cutting needle biopsy. Acta Radiol 1994; 35: 251–254.
57. Williams A, Santiago S, Lehrman S, et al.: Transcutaneous needle aspiration of solitary pulmonary masses: How many passes? Am Rev Respir Dis 1987; 136: 452–454.
58. Nasuti J, Gupta P, Baloch Z: Diagnostic value and cost-effectiveness of on-site evaluation of fine-needle aspiration specimens: Review of 5,688 cases. Diagn Cytopathol 2002; 27(1): 1–4.
59. Zavala DC, Bedell GN: Percutaneous lung biopsy with a cutting needle. An analysis of 40 cases and comparison with other biopsy techniques. Am Rev Respir Dis 1972; 106(2): 186–193.
60. Zavala DC: The diagnosis of pulmonary disease by nonthoracotomy techniques. Chest 1973; 64(1): 100–102.
61. Zavala DC, Rossi NP: Nonthoracotomy diagnostic techniques for pulmonary disease. Arch Surg 1973; 107(2): 152–154.
62. Zavala DC: Pulmonary biopsy. Adv Intern Med 1976; 21: 21–45.
63. Churg A, Wright JL: Nonneoplastic lung disease. Mod Pathol 1988; 1(1): 64–85.
64. Coren ME, Nicholson AG, Goldstraw P, et al.: Open lung biopsy for diffuse interstitial lung disease in children. Eur Respir J 1999; 14(4): 817–821.
65. Gaensler EA, Carrington CB: Open biopsy for chronic diffuse infiltrative lung disease: clinical, roentgenographic, and physiological correlations in 502 patients. Ann Thorac Surg 1980; 30(5): 411–426.

66. Krasna MJ, White CS, Aisner SC, et al.: The role of thoracoscopy in the diagnosis of interstitial lung disease. Ann Thorac Surg 1995; 59(2): 348–351.
67. Kramer MR, Berkman N, Mintz B, et al.: The role of open lung biopsy in the management and outcome of patients with diffuse lung disease. Ann Thorac Surg 1998; 65(1): 198–202.
68. Shah S, Tsang V, Goldstraw P: Open lung biopsy – a safe, reliable and accurate method for diagnosis in diffuse lung disease. Respiration 1992; 59: 243–246.
69. Wall C, Gaensler E, Carrington C, et al.: Comparison of transbronchial and open biopsies in chronic infiltrative lung disease. Am Rev Respir Dis 1981; 123: 280–285.
70. Bensard DD, McIntyre RC, Jr, Waring BJ, et al.: Comparison of video thoracoscopic lung biopsy to open lung biopsy in the diagnosis of interstitial lung disease. Chest 1993; 103(3): 765–770.
71. Molin LJ, Steinberg JB, Lanza LA: VATS increases costs in patients undergoing lung biopsy for interstitial lung disease. Ann Thorac Surg 1994; 58(6): 1595–1598.
72. Kadokura M, Colby TV, Myers JL, et al.: Pathologic comparison of video-assisted thoracic surgical lung biopsy with traditional open lung biopsy. J Thorac Cardiovasc Surg 1995; 109(3): 494–498.
73. Carnochan F, Walker W, Cameron E: Efficacy of video assisted thoracoscopic lung biopsy: an historical comparison with open lung biopsy. Thorax 1994; 49: 361–363.
74. Ravini M, Ferraro G, Barbieri B, et al.: Changing strategies of lung biopsies in diffuse lung diseases: the impact of video-assisted thoracoscopy. Eur Respir J 1998; 11: 99–103.
75. Newman S, Michel R, Wang N: Lingular lung biopsy: is it representative? Am Rev Respir Dis 1985; 132: 1084–1086.
76. Wetstein L: Sensitivity and specificity of lingular segmental biopsies of the lung. Chest 1986; 90: 383–386.
77. Temes RT, Joste NE, Allen NL, et al.: The lingula is an appropriate site for lung biopsy. Ann Thorac Surg 2000; 69(4): 1016–1018; discussion 1018–1019.
78. Churg A: An inflation procedure for open lung biopsies. Am J Surg Pathol 1983; 7(1): 69–71.

3

Basic pulmonary radiology

Thomas E Hartman

Introduction

The primary modalities available for imaging pulmonary parenchymal disease are the chest radiograph and chest computed tomography (CT). Other techniques – positron emission tomography (PET), magnetic resonance imaging (MRI), and ultrasound – have some usefulness in very specific situations but are not commonly applied to the initial evaluation of chest disease.

When evaluating lung parenchymal abnormalities, the *pattern*, the *distribution*, and the *chronicity* of the findings are the cornerstones upon which a workable differential diagnosis is built (Table 3.1). Some disease processes have imaging findings that are pathognomonic and allow the radiologist to offer a specific diagnosis with a high degree of confidence, but the majority of lung diseases do not have such a presentation. Fortunately, additional findings in the mediastinum, pleural space, abdomen, or chest wall, coupled with relevant clinical information, can be useful in further refining the differential diagnosis.

The *patterns* that are typically seen on the chest radiograph fall into three general categories:

- interstitial or linear opacities
- alveolar or confluent opacities
- nodular opacities.[1]

CT patterns are similar, but also include interlobular septal thickening, tree-in-bud pattern, and areas of ground glass attenuation.[2]

With regard to *distribution* of abnormalities on the chest X-ray, the primary distributions are central, peripheral, or diffuse (in the coronal plane). In the cephalocaudal plane there is also upper, mid, lower, or diffuse distribution.[1] CT shows distribution similar to the chest X-ray, but also includes a bronchovascular or perilymphatic distribution, a centrilobular or bronchiolocentric distribution, and a patchy or random distribution within the transaxial plane.[2] Sometimes abnormalities with a patchy distribution may have well-defined (geographic) borders and are referred to as having a "mosaic" pattern.

The initial approach to interpretation of the chest radiograph has long been based on the pattern of the abnormality that is visualized. Unfortunately, because there can be significant overlap between patterns, the distribution of abnormalities may prove more helpful in many cases. For example, some diseases may have an overlap in the pattern, but a distinctive distribution of abnormalities, while in other cases the pattern may be immediately recognizable and the distribution is a secondary consideration.

Finally, *chronicity* – determining whether an abnormality is acute or chronic – can help to narrow the differential diagnosis. This assessment requires obtaining any prior radiographs, or a history that strongly suggests an acute or a chronic process.

Differential diagnoses organized by distribution, pattern, and chronicity are now considered.

Distribution

Differential diagnoses based on distribution include: (1) upper lung diseases, (2) lower lung diseases, (3) peripheral diseases, and (4) central diseases.

Upper lung distribution

For diseases with upper lung distribution, "CHAPS" (Table 3.2) is a helpful mnemonic for remembering the elements in the differential diagnosis. Once an upper lung distribution has been recognized, the different patterns associated with the various diseases in the differential can be used to further narrow the diagnostic considerations. For example, bronchiectasis is the predominant finding in both cystic fibrosis[3,4] (Fig. 3.1) and allergic bronchopulmonary fungal disease (ABPFD),[5] whereas nodules can be seen with pulmonary Langerhans' cell histiocytosis,[6] silicosis,[7] and sarcoidosis.[8] However, if there

Table 3.1 Key evaluation parameters

Pattern		
Interstitial or linear opacities		Interlobular septal thickening (CT)
Alveolar or confluent opacities		Tree-in-bud pattern (CT)
Nodular opacities		Ground glass attenuation (CT)
Distribution		
Coronal plane	*Cephalocaudal plane*	
Central	Upper	Bronchovascular (CT)
Peripheral	Mid	Centrilobular (CT)
Diffuse	Lower	Patchy/random (CT)
	Diffuse	Mosaic pattern (CT)
Chronicity		
Prior films and/or clinical history		

Table 3.2 Chronic upper lung infiltrates on chest radiograph

Cystic fibrosis
Histiocytosis X (pulmonary Langerhans' cell histiocytosis)
Allergic bronchopulmonary aspergillosis
Pneumoconiosis (silicosis/coal workers' most common)
Sarcoidosis

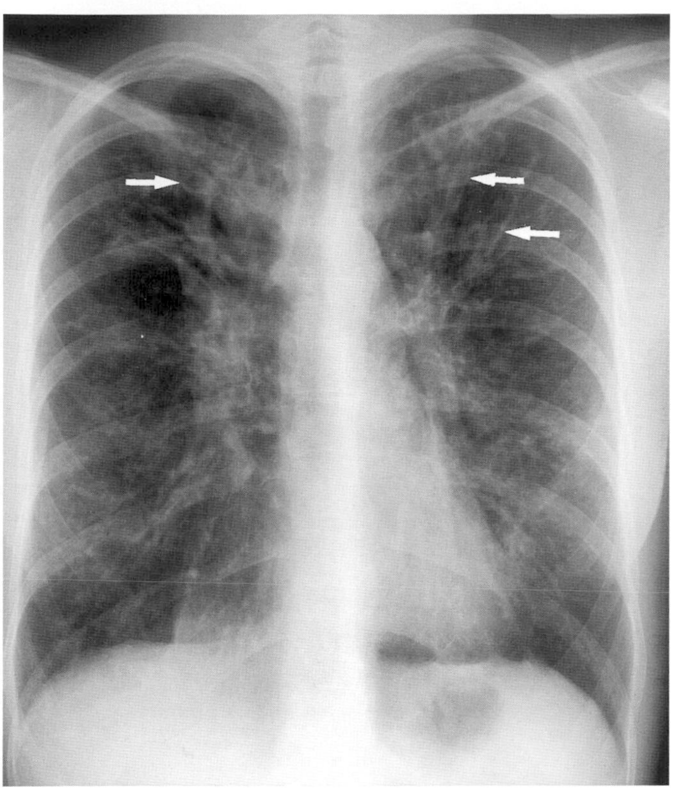

Fig. 3.1 PA chest radiograph from a 23-year-old woman with cystic fibrosis. Changes of bronchiectasis (arrows) are seen bilaterally. These are most marked in the upper lungs.

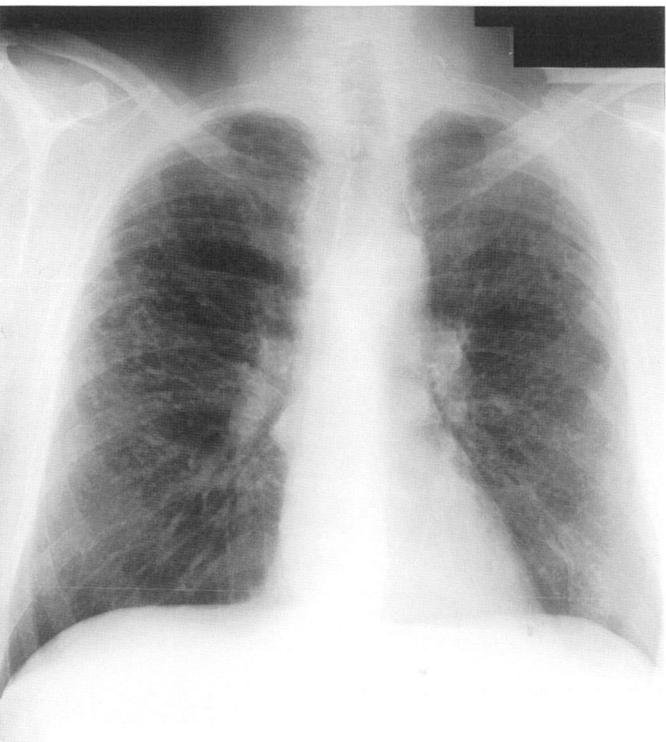

Fig. 3.2 PA chest radiograph of a 60-year-old man with silicosis. There are multiple small bilateral pulmonary nodules with a mid to upper lung predominance. There is also fullness of both hila compatible with adenopathy.

is significant adenopathy in addition to nodules, only silicosis (Fig. 3.2) and sarcoidosis should be considered.

Lower lung distribution

Diseases with this distribution include usual interstitial pneumonia (UIP), asbestosis, nonspecific interstitial pneumonia (NSIP), and organizing pneumonia (OP) patterns (previously referred to as "BOOP" patterns) (Table 3.3). Again, there is significant overlap between these patterns, but there are some findings that may allow the differential to be narrowed. If honeycombing is present, UIP is the most likely diagnosis.[9,10] If the predominant pattern is consolidation, organizing pneumonia pathology is most likely to be identified.[11] If pleural plaques are associated with the lower lung infiltrates, then asbestosis would be most likely[12] (Fig. 3.3).

Table 3.3 Chronic lower lung infiltrates on chest radiograph

Usual interstitial pneumonia
Asbestosis
Nonspecific interstitial pneumonia
Interstitial lung disease associated with collagen vascular diseases
Drug reactions
Chronic edema

Peripheral distribution

The primary diseases with a peripheral distribution are OP, eosinophilic pneumonia, and chronic hypersensitivity pneumonitis (Table 3.4). OP[11] and eosinophilic pneumonia[13] typically both present as consolidation and can occur in the upper or lower lungs. However, cryptogenic OP is more recognized as a lower lung disease and eosinophilic pneumonia is more recognized as an upper lung disease, especially in its chronic form (Fig. 3.4). Chronic hypersensitivity pneumonitis is more often a mid lung disease, but unlike eosinophilic pneumonia and OP, the predominant pattern is one of interstitial/irregular linear opacities[14] (Fig. 3.5). UIP, NSIP, and asbestosis can also have a peripheral distribution; however, a lower lung distribution is the predominant distribution for these diseases.

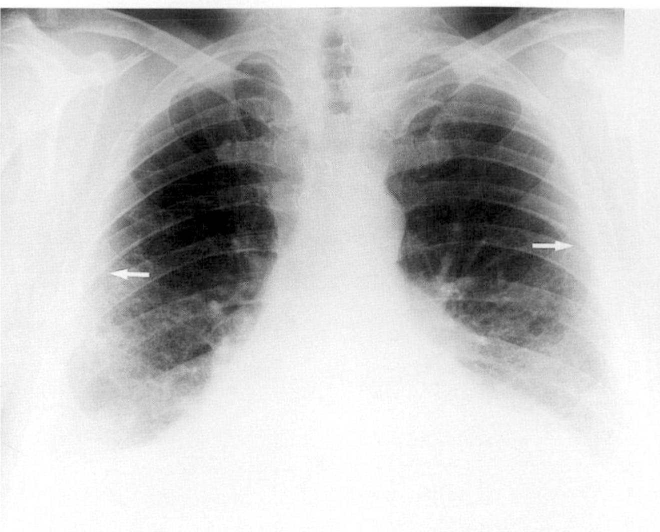

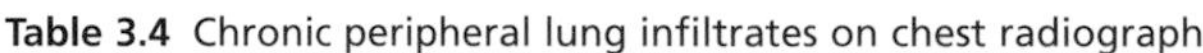

Fig. 3.3 PA chest radiograph of a 60-year-old man with asbestosis. There are bilateral interstitial infiltrates compatible with fibrosis. These have a basilar predominance. There are associated bilateral pleural plaques (arrows) which allow for a confident diagnosis of asbestosis.

Table 3.4 Chronic peripheral lung infiltrates on chest radiograph

Eosinophilic pneumonia (upper or lower lung zones)
Organizing pneumonia (OP) (lower lung zone dominant in cryptogenic form)
NSIP (lower lung zone)
UIP (lower lung zone)
Asbestosis (lower lung zone)

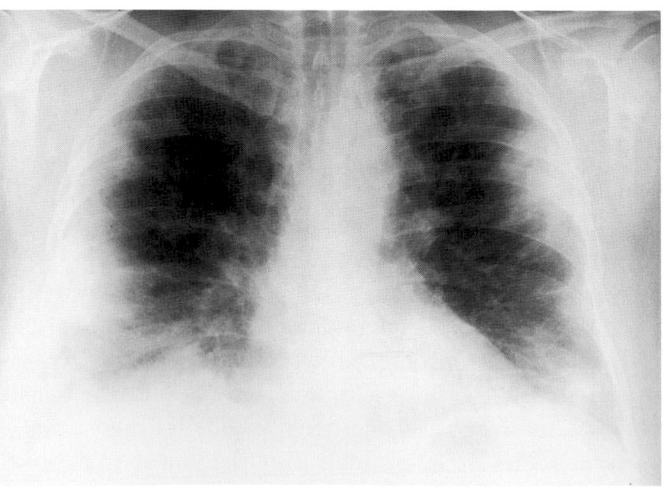

Fig. 3.4 PA chest radiograph of a 48-year-old woman with chronic eosinophilic pneumonia. There are bilateral areas of consolidation which have a peripheral distribution.

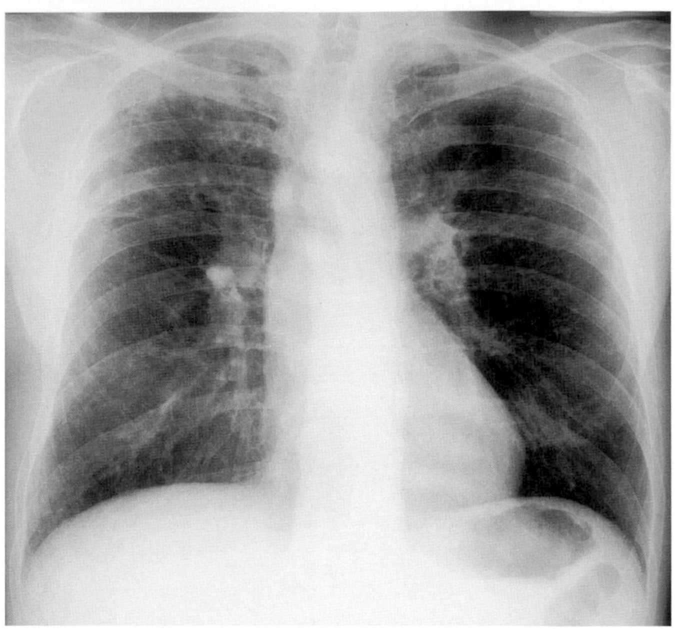

Fig. 3.5 PA chest radiograph of a 55-year-old man with chronic hypersensitivity pneumonitis. There are bilateral interstitial infiltrates with a predominantly upper lung and peripheral distribution.

Central distribution

Pulmonary edema in the setting of congestive heart failure (CHF) is the most common central abnormality, and is usually easily recognizable in the setting of cardiomegaly and pulmonary venous hypertension seen on the chest X-ray.[15] Non-cardiogenic pulmonary edema[15] and alveolar proteinosis[16] (Fig. 3.6) are other abnormalities with a primary central distribution (Table 3.5). Alveolar proteinosis differs from edema in that it is a chronic process. On CT, is it characterized by a "crazy paving" pattern[17] (Fig. 3.7). While a "crazy paving" pattern can be seen in other diseases, in the setting of a chronic infiltrate, it is virtually diagnostic of alveolar proteinosis.

Patterns

Alveolar pattern

The two main differentials for the alveolar pattern are based on whether the infiltrates are acute or chronic.

Acute

The main considerations for the acute alveolar pattern are blood, purulent exudates, edema, and aspiration. Within these general categories, more specific diseases can be defined. Causes of acute alveolar infiltrates resulting from blood include Goodpasture's syndrome[18]

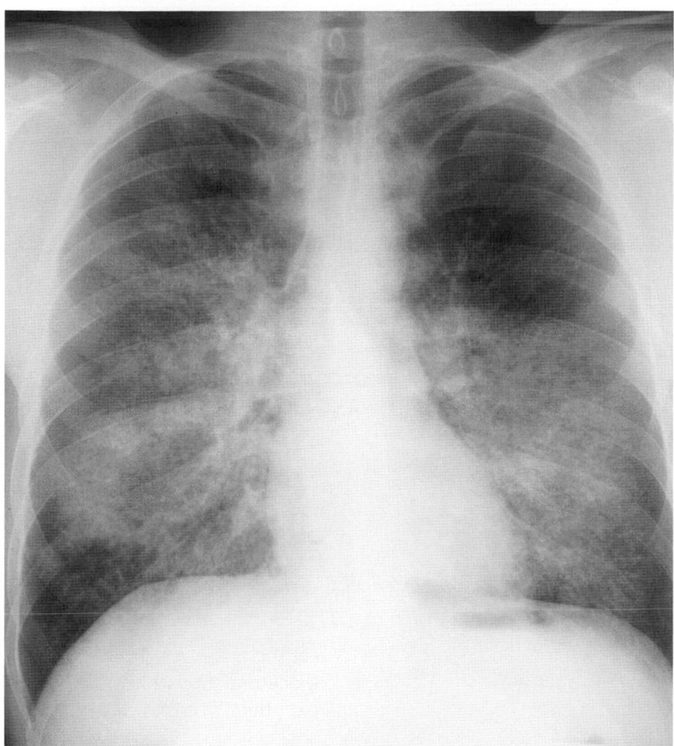

Fig. 3.6 PA chest radiograph of a 38-year-old man with an alveolar proteinosis. There are bilateral areas of consolidation which have a predominantly central/perihilar distribution. There is sparing of the apices and bases.

Table 3.5 Central lung infiltrates on chest radiograph

Pulmonary edema (CHF)
Pulmonary edema (non-cardiogenic)
Alveolar proteinosis (chronic)

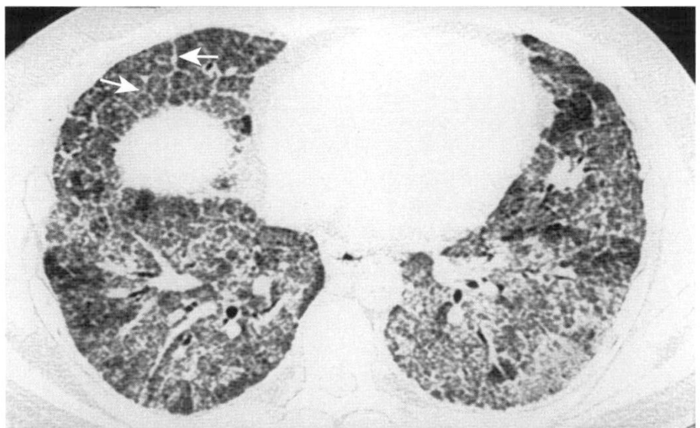

Fig. 3.7 High-resolution CT of a 32-year-old man with alveolar proteinosis. There are diffuse bilateral areas of ground glass attenuation. Within these areas there is a background of interlobular septal thickening (arrows). This combination has been called "crazy paving".

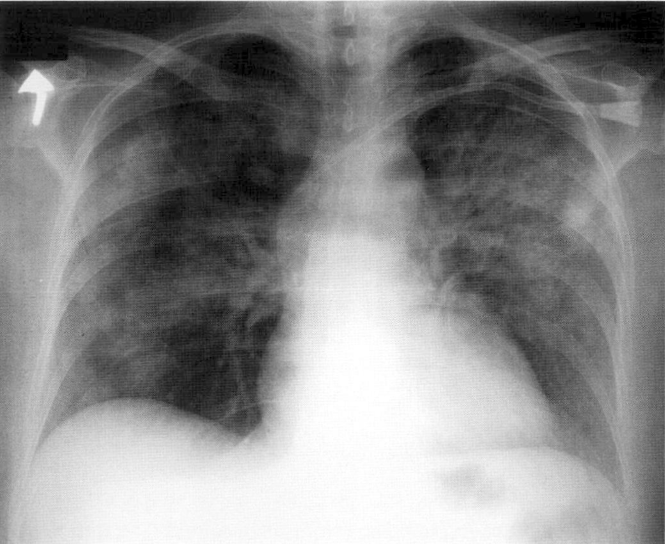

Fig. 3.8 Portable chest radiograph of a 35-year-old man with Goodpasture's syndrome. There are bilateral areas of consolidation in a predominantly perihilar distribution.

(Fig. 3.8), Wegener's granulomatosis,[19] systemic lupus erythematosus,[20] idiopathic pulmonary hemorrhage, disseminated intravascular coagulation (DIC), and trauma resulting in laceration or contusions. Less commonly, anticoagulants and low platelets can cause alveolar hemorrhage.

Causes of acute alveolar infiltrates resulting from purulent exudates (infection) depend on the status of the patient's immune system. Bacterial infections can be seen in both immunocompetent and immunocompromised patients. Immunocompetent patients typically will be at risk for bacterial, fungal, mycobacterial, and viral infections. Immunocompromised patients are at risk for all of these "usual" infections, plus a number of opportunistic infections, including pneumocystis pneumonia[21] (Fig. 3.9).

Acute edema may be cardiogenic or non-cardiogenic.[15] The non-cardiogenic differential can include volume overload, uremia, drug or transfusion reactions, neurogenic causes, and any causes of adult respiratory distress syndrome (ARDS).

Aspirations can include the aspiration of gastric contents,[22] smoke inhalation,[23] water in near-drowning situations,[24] and gas or hydrocarbon inhalation.[23]

Once alveolar infiltrates have been determined to be acute, the distribution of the infiltrates can be helpful in narrowing the differential further. Edema is most typically bilateral and symmetric with a perihilar or lower lung predominance.[15] Infections can be unilateral or bilateral. When bilateral, they tend to be patchy and asymmetric. Hemorrhage can either be localized or diffuse, while

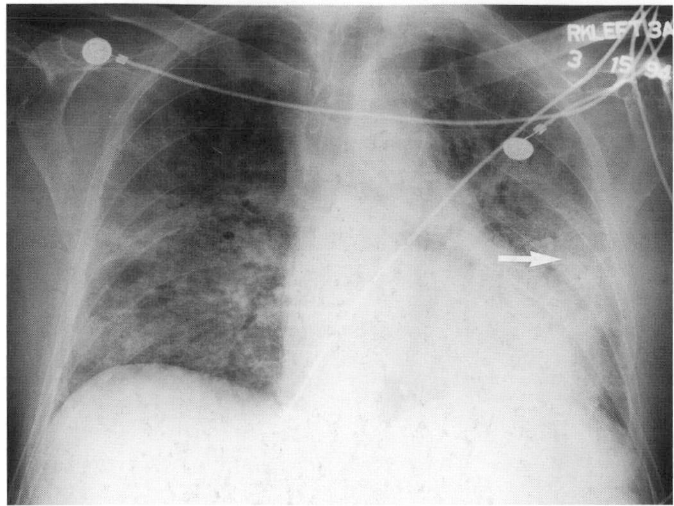

Fig. 3.9 Portable chest radiograph from a 52-year-old man with *Pneumocystis jiroveci* pneumonia. Bilateral pulmonary infiltrates are most prominent in the mid and lower lungs. These are predominantly airspace infiltrates with a more dense area of consolidation in the left lower lung (arrow).

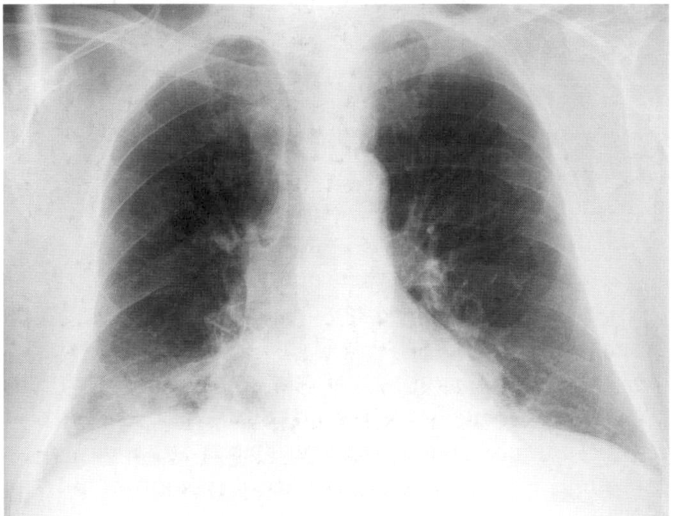

Fig. 3.10 PA chest radiograph of an 84-year-old man with mineral oil aspiration. There are bilateral areas of consolidation in the bases of the lower lobes.

aspiration typically presents in the dependent portions of the lungs[22] (Fig. 3.10).

Chronic

Chronic alveolar infiltrates include sarcoidosis, reactivation tuberculosis or fungal infections, bronchioloalveolar carcinoma, alveolar proteinosis, aspiration, lymphoma, and lipoid pneumonia.

Once alveolar infiltrates have been determined to be chronic, the distribution of the infiltrates can be helpful in narrowing the differential further. In sarcoidosis, the infiltrates typically have a perihilar or upper lung predominance[25] (Fig. 3.11). Reactivation tuberculosis (TB) also typically has an upper lung predominance, but in cases of TB, the apices are usually the predominant area of involvement.[26] Additionally, TB is often a unilateral process, whereas many of the other diseases are bilateral (Fig. 3.12). Alveolar proteinosis classically presents with perihilar alveolar infiltrates which spare the apices and bases[16] (see Fig. 3.6). Bronchioloalveolar carcinoma[27]and lymphoma[28] typically are solitary lesions but when multiple lesions are present they have a random distribution. Exogenous lipoid pneumonia is caused by aspiration of lipid and therefore like other aspirations occurs in the dependent portions of the lungs[29] (see Fig. 3.10).

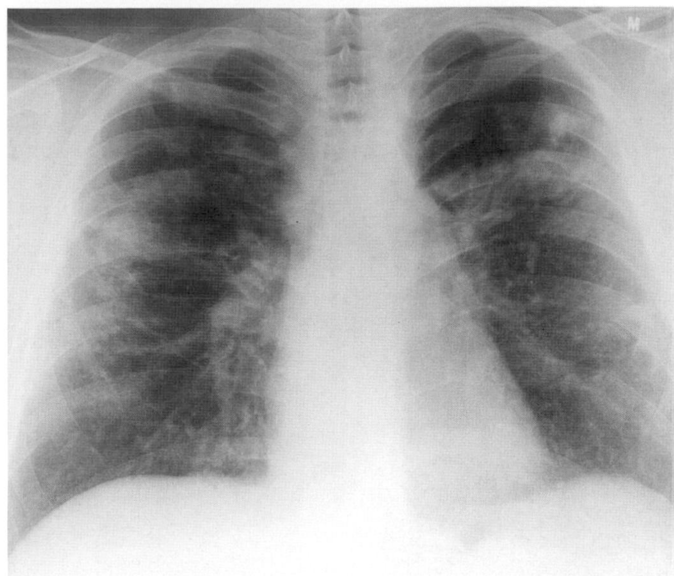

Fig. 3. 11 PA chest radiograph of a 33-year-old man with sarcoidosis. There are nodules and focal areas of consolidation bilaterally. These have a perihilar predominance.

Nodules

Nodule patterns that can be seen on the chest radiograph can be characterized as solitary, multiple, and cavitary. The diagnostic evaluation of solitary nodules as well as the differentials for multiple and cavitary nodules are discussed.

Solitary nodules

Radiologic evaluation of a solitary pulmonary nodule (SPN) has the primary function of differentiating benign from malignant lesions. There are certain imaging criteria on the chest radiograph or CT that can be used to evaluate the likelihood of a nodule being benign or malignant. The two primary criteria for the evaluation of

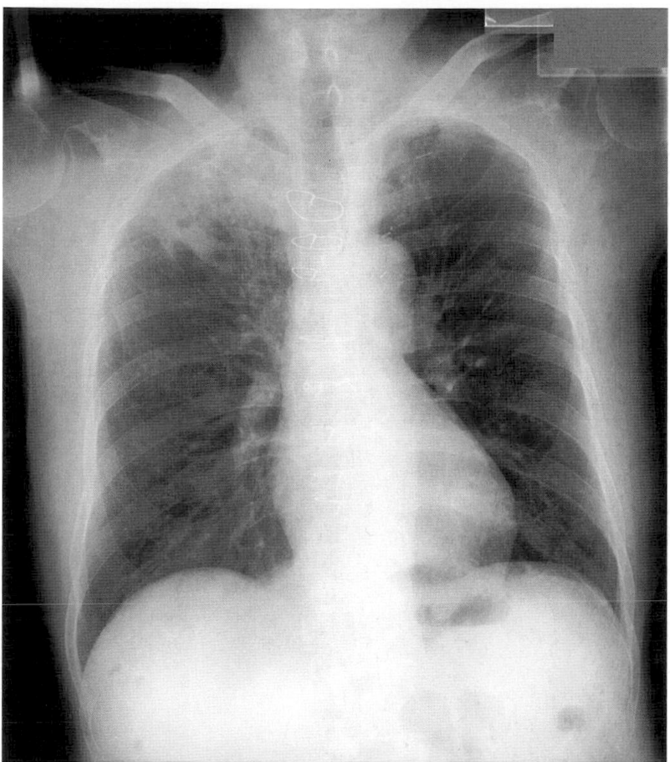

Fig. 3.12 PA chest radiograph of a 78-year-old man with recurrent tuberculosis infection. There is consolidation in the right apex. Note that this is a unilateral process which can allow a more confident suggestion of tuberculosis compared to the other causes of chronic alveolar infiltrates.

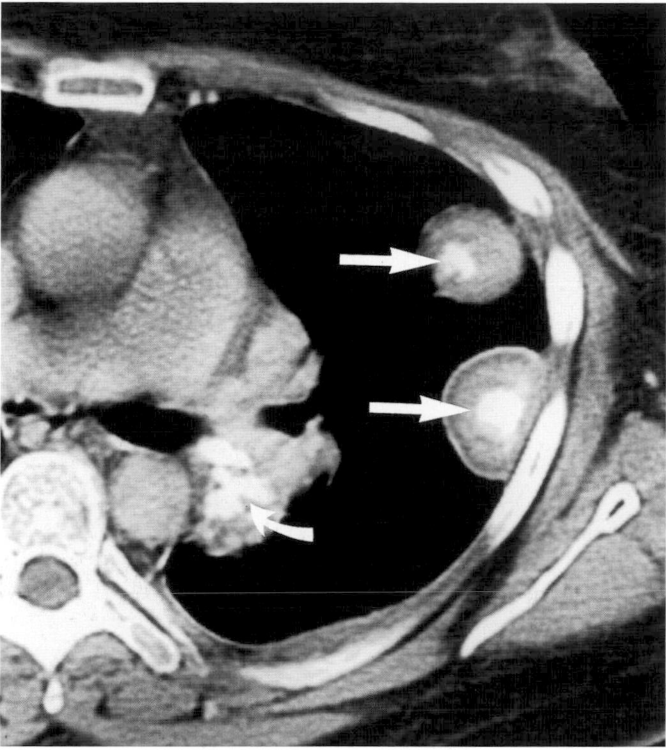

Fig. 3.13 CT scan of the chest in a 39-year-old woman with nodules in her left lung. Images through the two nodules in the left lung show areas of central calcification within both nodules (arrows). This allowed a confident diagnosis of benign calcified granulomas. Note also the calcified nodes in the left hilum (curved arrow).

SPNs are changes in the lesion over time and calcification within the nodule. Other criteria that may be helpful include the appearance of the margins of the lesion and the presence of satellite nodules.

Changes evident over time

Studies have shown that nodules that are unchanged over a 2-year period have a high incidence of benignity.[30,31] Therefore, the initial evaluation of an SPN should include an attempt to obtain older chest X-rays to assess whether there has been interval growth of the nodule. Growth, of itself, does not indicate malignancy, as benign nodules may grow. All things being equal, growth increases the likelihood that a nodule is malignant. An increase in nodule diameter of 26% equates to a doubling in volume of the nodule.[32]

Calcification

There are five types of calcification that can be seen within a pulmonary nodule. These include diffuse calcification, central calcification, lamellar calcification, chondroid (popcorn) calcification, and eccentric calcification.[32,33] Diffuse, central (Fig 3.13), lamellar, and chondroid calcification indicate a benign etiology. Chondroid calcification is not only a benign pattern of calcification but also indicates the specific diagnosis of a hamartoma. Eccentric calcification (Fig. 3.14) can be seen in benign lesions, and also in malignant lesions undergoing dystrophic calcification or engulfing a benign calcified lesion.

Margins

Nodule margins can be described as smooth, lobulated, irregular, or spiculated. The only margin characteristic that has significant predictive value is a spiculated margin (Fig. 3.15). A spiculated nodule has a predictive value for malignancy of approximately 90%.[34] Therefore, the presence of spiculation should prompt a more aggressive work-up of the pulmonary nodule.

The presence of a smooth border, however, does not necessarily indicate benignity, as up to 21% of malignant lesions can have smooth borders.[35] Therefore, nodules with smooth borders are indeterminate with regard to malignancy.

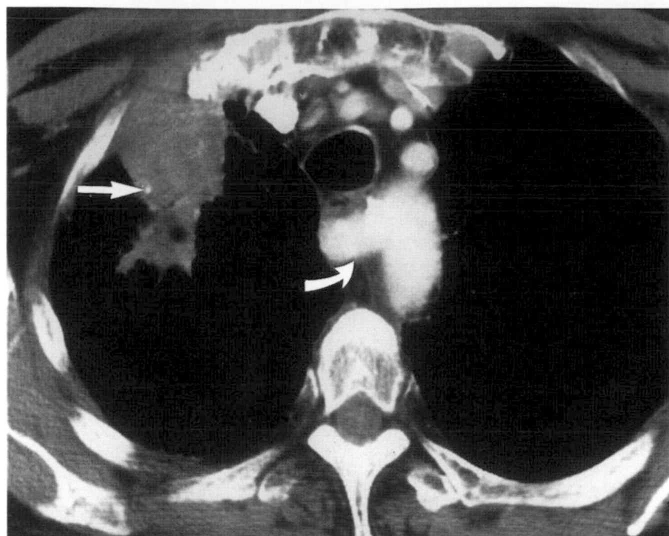

Fig. 3.14 CT scan of the chest in a 68-year-old man with actinomycoses. There is a large mass in the right upper lobe anteriorly. Within this mass there is a small area of eccentric calcification (arrow). This pattern of calcification is indeterminate and can be seen in either benign or malignant etiologies. Incidentally noted is an aberrant right subclavian artery passing posteriorly to the esophagus (curved arrow).

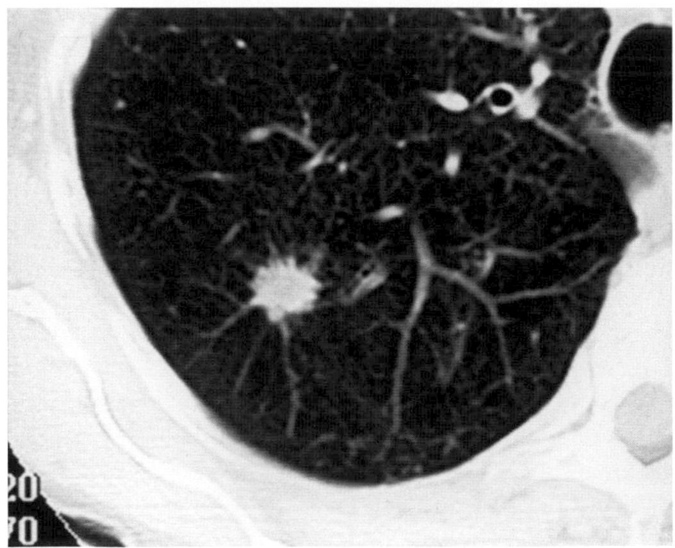

Fig. 3.15 CT scan of the chest in a 73-year-old woman with adenocarcinoma of the right lung. The nodule in the right upper lobe has spiculated margins which indicate an increased likelihood of malignancy.

Satellite nodules

Tiny nodules associated with a dominant pulmonary nodule are referred to as satellite nodules (Fig 3.16). The presence of satellite nodules indicates a high likelihood that the dominant nodule is benign, and a result of infection. The positive predictive value for benignity with satellite nodules is approximately 90%.[34]

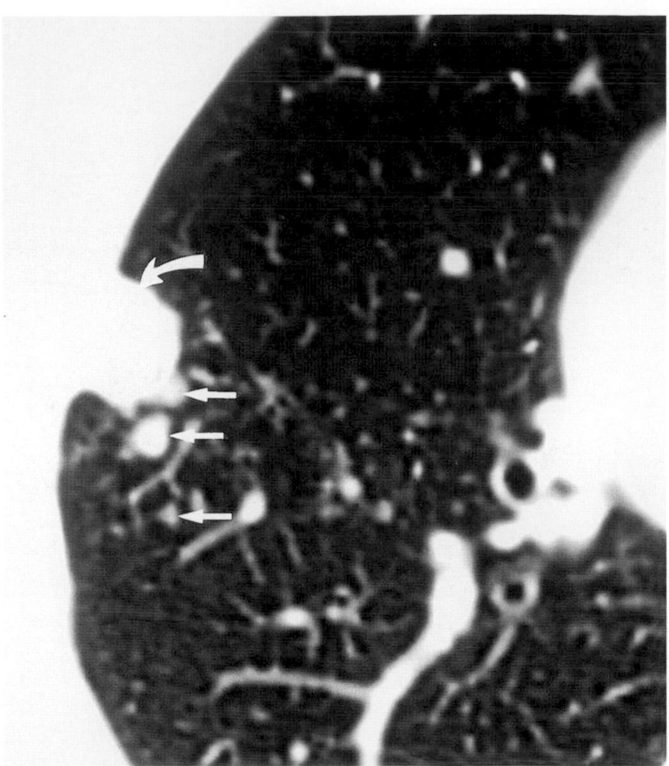

Fig. 3.16 A 75-year-old man with histoplasmosis. There are multiple satellite nodules (arrows) associated with the dominant nodule (curved arrow) in the right upper lobe. The presence of satellite nodules indicates an increased likelihood of benignity.

Computed tomography

While the chest radiograph is useful in the initial evaluation of solitary pulmonary nodules, CT can often provide additional information in the evaluation of SPNs. CT is more sensitive to the detection of calcification or fat within a pulmonary nodule. Therefore, nodules which are indeterminate on the chest X-ray can often be further characterized with CT. If CT shows a benign type of calcification, or fat within the nodule, further work-up will not be necessary.[35,36] The presence of fat on CT within a pulmonary nodule is virtually diagnostic of a hamartoma[37] (Fig. 3.17).

Nodule enhancement

CT with nodule enhancement is an additional test that can be performed to evaluate a pulmonary nodule. For a nodule enhancement study, contrast material is administered intravenously and the attenuation of the nodule is measured every 60 s for 4 min and compared with the attenuation measurement of the nodule taken

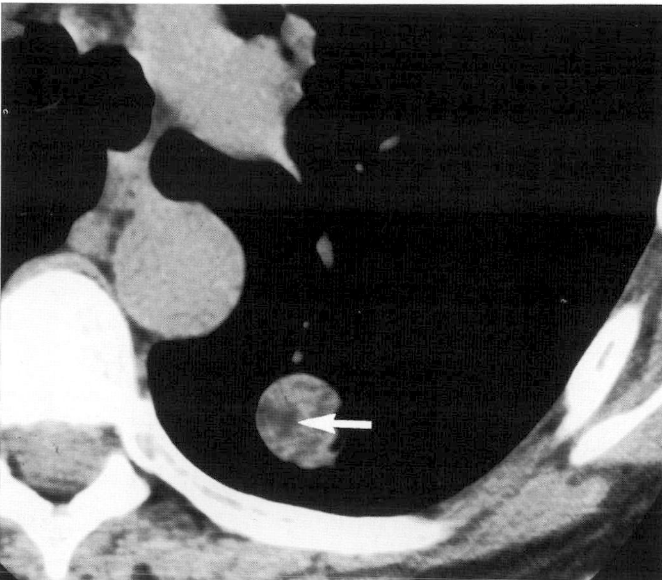

Fig. 3.17 CT scan of the chest in a 61-year-old woman with hamartoma. There are areas of fat attenuation (arrow) within the nodule in the superior segment of the left lower lobe. The presence of fat within a nodule is diagnostic of a hamartoma.

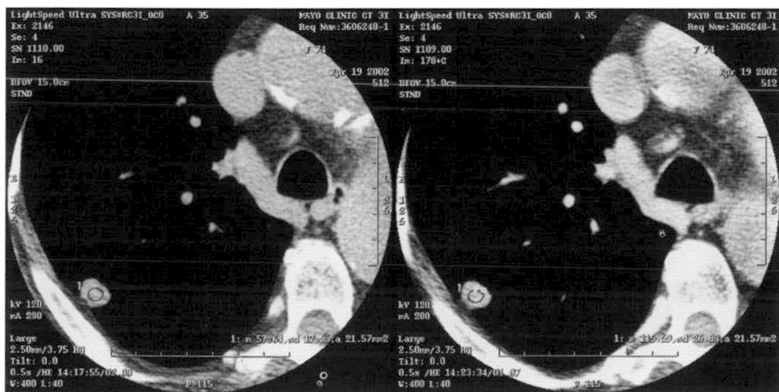

Fig. 3.18 CT scan of the chest in a 74-year-old woman with a pulmonary nodule in the right upper lobe posterolaterally. There is a pre-contrast image on the left and a 1-min post-contrast image on the right. The Hounsfield unit measurements from the region of interest on the pre-contrast is 58, while the Hounsfield unit measurements on the post-contrast scan is 116. Therefore, the nodule enhances 58 H, which would indicate a high likelihood of malignancy. At resection this was an adenosquamous carcinoma.

prior to the injection of contrast[38] (Fig 3.18). Nodule enhancement of less than 15 Hounsfield units is strongly predictive of benignity (positive predictive value for benignity of 99%). Nodule enhancement greater than 15 H indicates an increased risk of malignancy; however, only 58% of nodules with enhancement of greater than 15 H will be malignant.[39] Therefore, enhancing nodules, while more likely to be malignant, are still indeterminate. CT enhancement studies have some additional limitations. Nodules less than 8 mm in diameter, ground glass attenuation nodules, cavitary nodules, and nodules with central necrosis are not amenable to CT enhancement studies.[38,39]

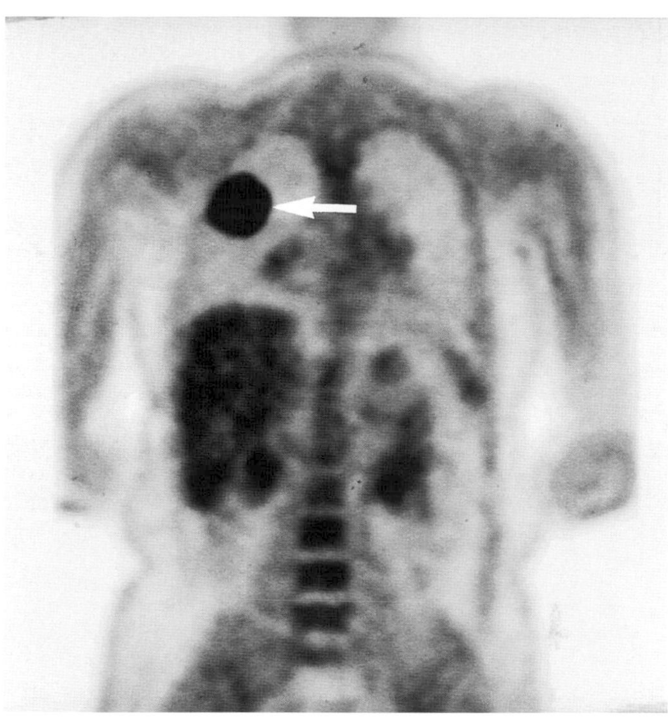

Fig. 3.19 PET scan of a 60-year-old woman with squamous cell carcinoma in the right upper lobe. There is intense increased FDG uptake in the right upper lobe nodule (arrow) compatible with malignancy.

Positron emission tomography

PET utilizes a glucose analog, FDG, labeled with a positron-emitting isotope. Increased glucose metabolism in malignant nodules results in increased uptake of FDG, permitting differentiation of benign and malignant nodules (Fig. 3.19). The sensitivity, specificity, and accuracy of PET in the diagnosis of benign nodules has been shown to be 90% or greater in several studies[40–42] The high specificity of PET for the diagnosis of benign lesions has important clinical utility in that lesions with low FDG uptake may be considered benign. However, there are instances with slow-growing malignancies such as bronchioloalveolar carcinoma[43] or well-differentiated tumors such as carcinoids[44] where false negatives can occur. Therefore, lesions that are FDG negative should be followed up to ensure that there is no interval growth. Another limitation is that PET typically has difficulty accurately evaluating lesions that are less than 10 mm in diameter.[40–42] Finally, PET can yield false positives in patients with active infectious or inflammatory processes such as tuberculosis and histoplasmosis.[45]

Table 3.6 Multiple small nodules on chest radiograph

Dust – organic – hypersensitivity pneumonitis – inorganic – silicosis /CWP
Eosinophilic granuloma (pulmonary Langerhans' cell histiocytosis)
Fungal infections
Tuberculosis
Sarcoidosis
Metastases

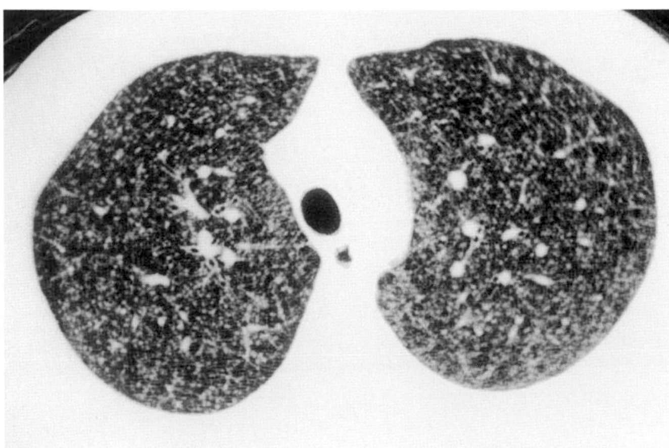

Fig. 3.20 CT scan of the chest in a 71-year-old man with miliary tuberculosis. There are innumerable tiny pulmonary nodules throughout both lungs.

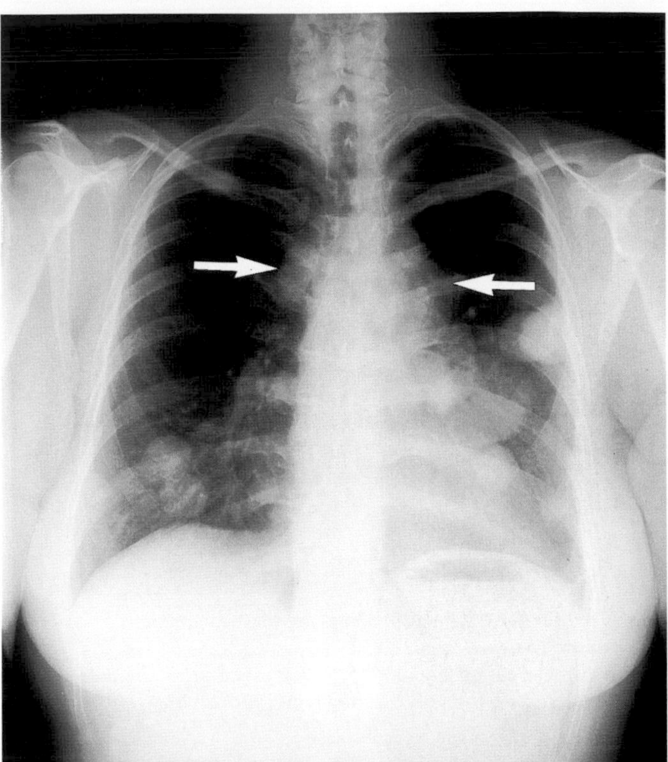

Fig. 3.21 PA chest radiograph of a 39-year-old woman with an old histoplasmosis infection. There are multiple bilateral pulmonary nodules as well as mediastinal adenopathy (arrows).

Multiple nodules

Multiple nodules also have a differential diagnosis based on size and distribution. It is useful to divide nodule size into small versus large. Smaller nodules (<5 mm) include miliary disease. However, the differential diagnosis does not change between nodules 3–5 mm in size and the <3 mm nodules which constitute miliary disease. A mnemonic which is helpful in this particular set of patients is DEFTS M (Table 3.6). D stands for dust and includes both organic causes, such as hypersensitivity pneumonitis in the subacute form,[46] and inorganic causes, such as silicosis[7] and coal workers'[47] pneumoconioses; E is for eosinophilic granuloma (pulmonary Langerhans' cell histiocytosis);[48] F is for fungal infections (histoplasmosis,[49] coccidioidomycosis,[50] cryptococcosis,[51] etc.); T is for tuberculosis and atypical mycobacterial infections[52] (Fig. 3.20); S is for sarcoidosis;[53] and M is for metastases.

Distribution can then be helpful in further narrowing the differential for multiple nodules. Sarcoidosis,[53] the pneumoconioses,[7, 47] and eosinophilic granuloma[48] have an upper lung predominance. Metastases typically have a lower lung predominance. When infections present as small nodules it is usually in the setting of disseminated disease and therefore such infections typically have a diffuse distribution.[49–52]

Nodules which are >5 mm would include all of the diseases discussed for nodules <5 mm (Fig. 3.21) except hypersensitivity pneumonitis. Additional diseases that could be considered for larger nodule sizes include Wegener's granulomatosis[54] and multiple arteriovenous malformations (AVMs).[55]

Cavitary nodules

Cavitary nodules invoke another differential list. The two main differential considerations for cavitary nodules include malignancy – either primary lung cancers or metastatic disease – and infections, particularily granulomatous infections.[49–51] Other lesions that may cavitate include infarction (septic emboli[56] or bland infarct), Wegener's granulomatosis[19] (Fig. 3.22), and rheumatoid nodules.[57] There are no features of cavitary nodules that allow confident differentiation of benign and malignant lesions. The most common source of cavitated lung metastases is primary squamous cell carcinoma of head and neck origin.

Chronic interstitial lung disease

Although there are over 120 diseases which can cause a chronic interstitial lung disease (CILD) pattern on the chest radiograph;[58] 14 of these diseases account for over 95% of the CILD that will typically be seen. It is in this category of diseases that high-resolution computed tomography (HRCT) has had the greatest impact. The common diseases and their characteristic HRCT findings are listed in Table 3.7.

UIP is the most common CILD seen. It is characterized by irregular linear opacities and honeycombing, with a subpleural and basilar predominance[10,59] (Fig. 3.23). Traction bronchiectasis is also commonly seen. Areas of ground glass attenuation can be seen, but are usually not

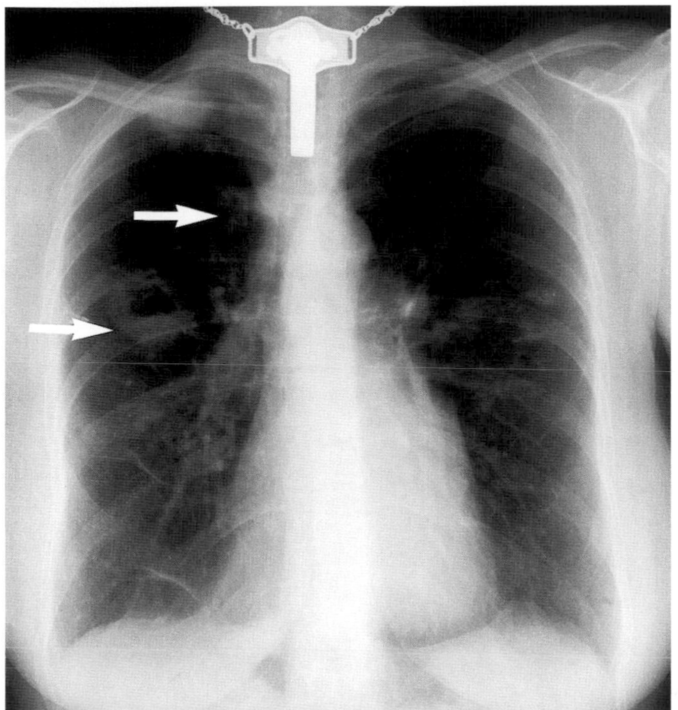

Fig. 3.22 PA chest radiograph of a 52-year-old woman with Wegener's granulomatosis. There are multiple bilateral pulmonary nodules, some of which are cavitated (arrows). A tracheostomy is in place below a subglottic stenosis, which is another finding which can be seen in association with Wegener's granulomatosis.

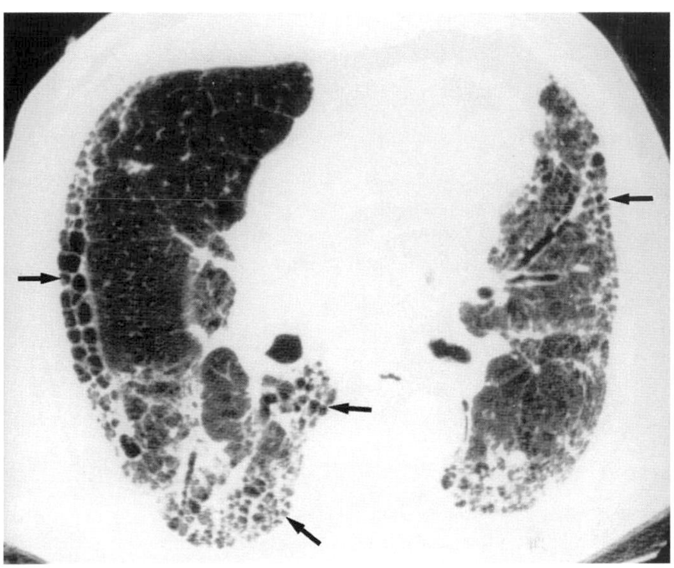

Fig. 3.23 High-resolution CT image through the lung basis of a 67-year-old man with usual interstitial pneumonia (UIP). The predominant finding is honeycombing in a subpleural distribution (arrows). This pattern of disease with a lower lung predominance is diagnostic of UIP.

Table 3.7 Diagnosis of chronic infiltrative lung disease with high-resolution computed tomography (HRCT)

Predominant pattern	Distribution	Diagnostic possibilities	Additional findings
Irregular lines with honeycombing	Subpleural, basilar	UIP	
		Asbestosis	Pleural plaques
	Subpleural, upper lung	Chronic HP	
Irregular lines without honeycombing	Subpleural, basilar	NSIP	Areas of ground glass attenuation
Nodules	Upper lung, perilymphatic	Sarcoidosis	
	Upper lung, posterior	Silicosis/CWP	
Areas of ground glass attenuation	Patchy, diffuse	Subacute HP	
	Subpleural, basilar	DIP, NSIP	
	Perihilar	Alveolar proteinosis	Interlobular septal thickening
Cysts	Upper lung, bases spared	Langerhans' cell histiocytosis	Nodules
	Diffuse, bases involved	LAM	
Nodular interlobular septal thickening	Basilar, symmetric or unilateral	Lymphangitic metastases	
Consolidation	Subpleural	Chronic eosinophilic pneumonia, OP	

CWP, coal workers' pneumoconioses; DIP, desquamative interstitial pneumonia; HP, hypersensitivity pneumonitis; LAM, lymphangioleiomyomatosis; NSIP, nonspecific interstitial pneumonia; OP, organizing pneumonia; UIP, usual interstitial pneumonia.

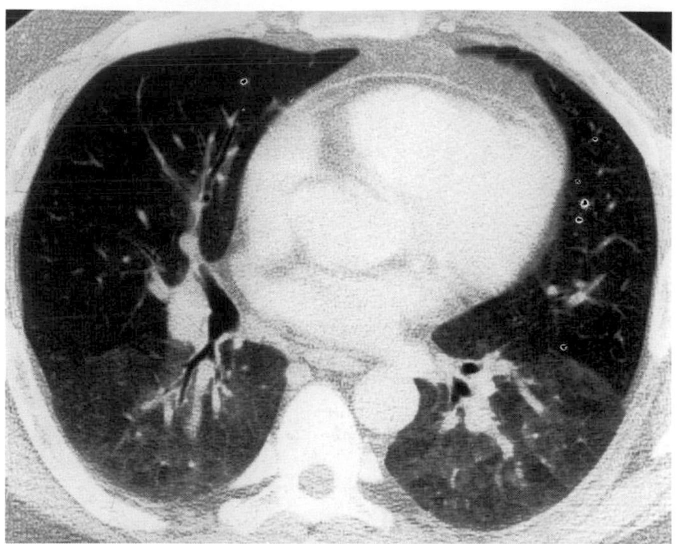

Fig. 3.24 High-resolution CT scan of the chest in a 73-year-old man with cellular NSIP. There are bilateral areas of ground glass attenuation which are most prominent in the posterior lungs. Although this is a nonspecific finding, at biopsy this was shown to be cellular NSIP.

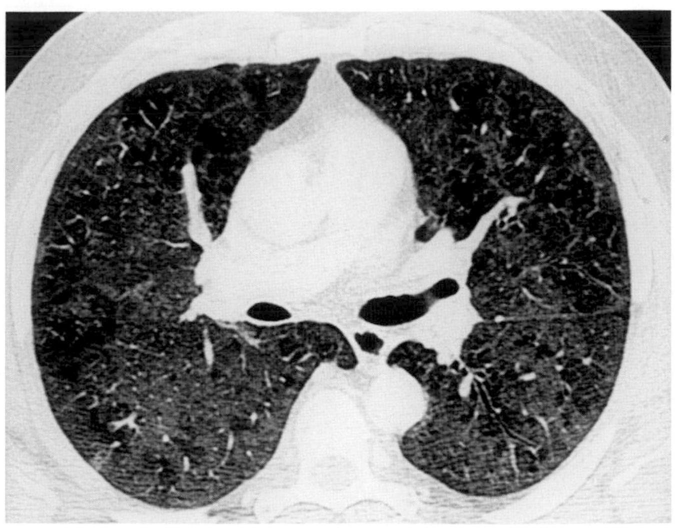

Fig. 3.26 High-resolution CT scan of a 50-year-old man with hypersensitivity pneumonitis. There are patchy areas of ground glass attenuation throughout both lungs with scattered areas of uninvolved lung bilaterally.

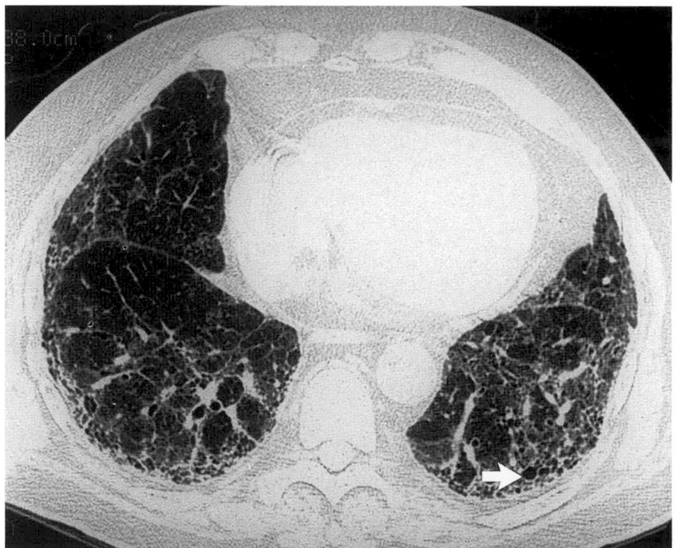

Fig. 3.25 High-resolution CT scan through the lower lungs of a 73-year-old man with fibrotic NSIP. The patient had associated rheumatoid arthritis. The predominant findings are course irregular linear opacities with a subpleural and basilar predominance. There is a small area of early honeycombing in the left lower lobe posteriorly (arrow). However, honeycombing is not the predominant finding and the lack of significant honeycombing favors NSIP over UIP. At biopsy this was shown to be the fibrotic form of NSIP.

a prominent feature and rarely occur in the absence of irregular linear opacities or honeycombing. If areas of ground glass attenuation are a prominent finding on HRCT, other diseases such as NSIP,[60] desquamative interstitial pneumonia (DIP),[61] and hypersensitivity pneumonitis[62] should be considered.

The key to the confident diagnosis of UIP on HRCT is the presence of honeycombing. If honeycombing in a subpleural and basilar distribution is a prominent finding, the diagnosis of UIP will be correct in over 95% of cases.[63] With the appropriate clinical findings, these HRCT findings can be used to obviate biopsy.

Cellular NSIP is characterized by areas of ground glass attenuation with a subpleural and basilar predominance[60,64] (Fig. 3.24). Fibrotic NSIP is characterized by irregular linear opacities with a basilar distribution.[65] However, unlike UIP, honeycombing is not a predominant finding in fibrotic NSIP (Fig. 3.25). There is often significant overlap of the findings in NSIP with the findings in DIP, and hypersensitivity pneumonitis. A smoking history may help in the differential between DIP and hypersensitivity pneumonitis, since DIP is unlikely in a nonsmoker,[66] whereas hypersensitivity pneumonitis is unlikely in a smoker.[67] In hypersensitivity pneumonitis, the areas of ground glass attenuation are typically more random with a geographic pattern[68,69] (Fig. 3.26). Small ground glass

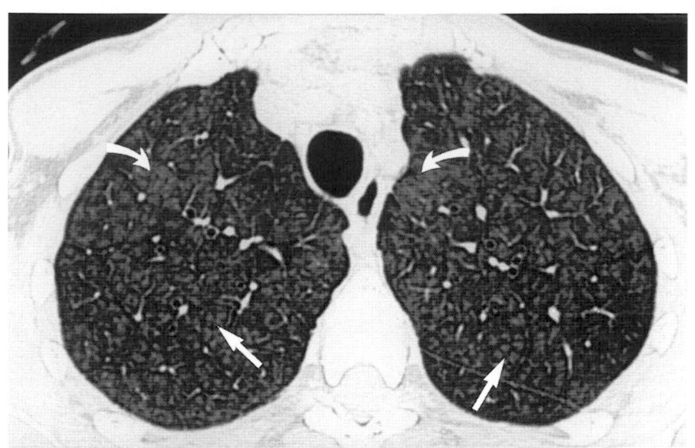

Fig. 3.27 High-resolution CT scan of a 54-year-old woman with hypersensitivity pneumonitis. There are ground glass attenuation centrilobular nodules bilaterally (arrows). There are also small areas of ground attenuation bilaterally (curved arrows).

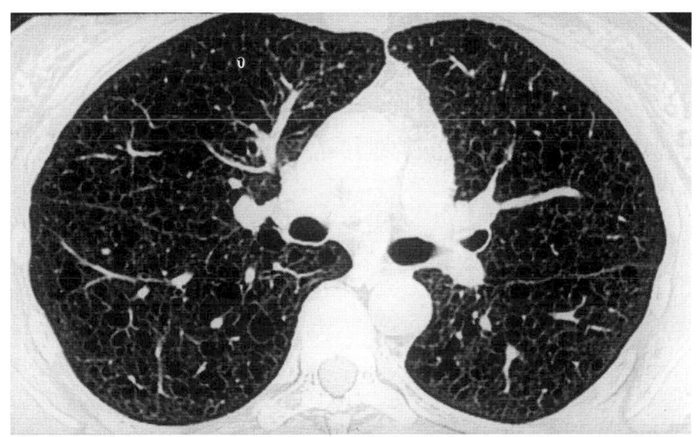

Fig. 3.28 High-resolution CT scan of a 52-year-old woman with lymphangioleiomyomatosis. There are multiple thin-walled cysts throughout both lungs. On lower images (not shown) these nodules could be seen to involve the lung bases. This pattern and diffuse distribution is diagnostic of LAM.

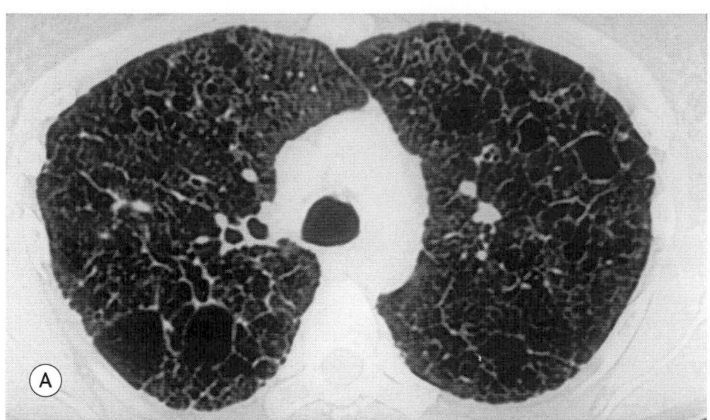

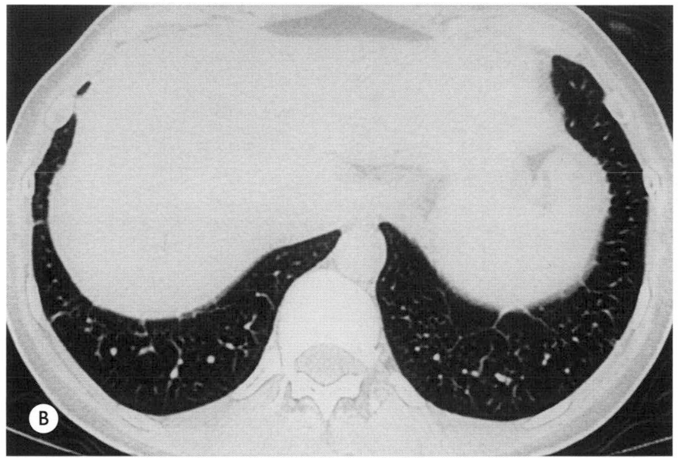

Fig. 3.29 High-resolution CT scans of a 45-year-old woman with pulmonary Langerhans' cell histiocytosis. (A) CT image through the upper lungs shows diffuse thin-walled cysts of varying sizes and shapes bilaterally. (B) CT image through the lung bases shows an absence of cysts. A pattern of cystic lung disease on high-resolution CT which spares the bases is diagnostic of pulmonary Langerhans' cell histiocytosis.

nodules with a centrilobular distribution are also typical of hypersensitivity pneumonitis[68,69] (Fig. 3.27), although NSIP may sometimes present with this pattern of abnormality.[65]

Lymphangioleiomyomatosis[59] (LAM) (Fig. 3.28) and pulmonary Langerhans' cell histiocytosis[70] (PLCH) (Fig. 3.29) are the CILDs that characteristically show cysts on HRCT. The distribution of the cysts allows confident differentiation of the two diseases.[63,71] LAM is a diffuse disease that has equivalent involvement of the apices and bases,[72,73] whereas PLCH typically spares the bases. If there is basilar involvement with PLCH, there is still relative sparing of the bases compared with the apices.[71] An additional finding that allows differentiation between

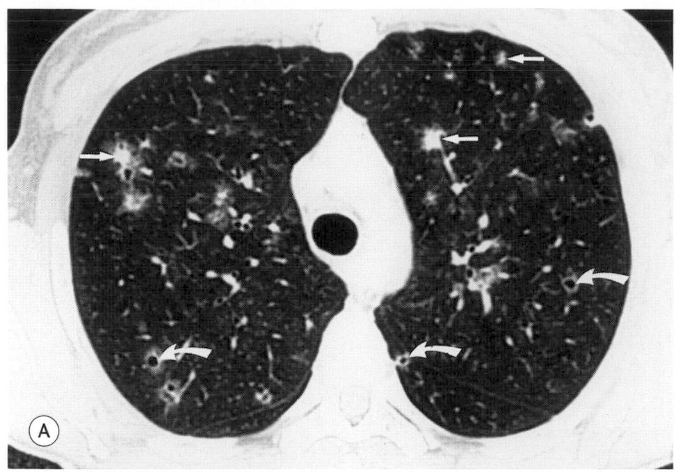

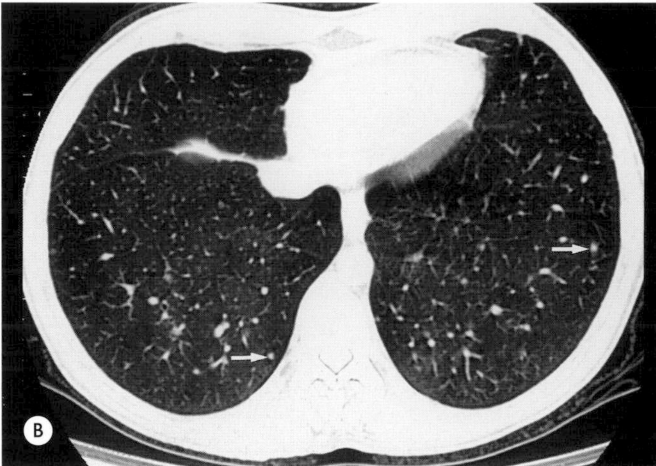

Fig. 3.30 High-resolution CT scans of a 33-year-old woman with pulmonary Langerhans' cell histiocytosis. (A) CT image through the upper lungs shows bilateral pulmonary nodules (arrows) as well as multiple bilateral cystic spaces (curved arrows). (B) CT image through the lower lungs shows only a few small nodules (arrows). The combination of nodules and cysts with relative sparing of the bases is diagnostic for pulmonary Langerhans' cell histiocytosis.

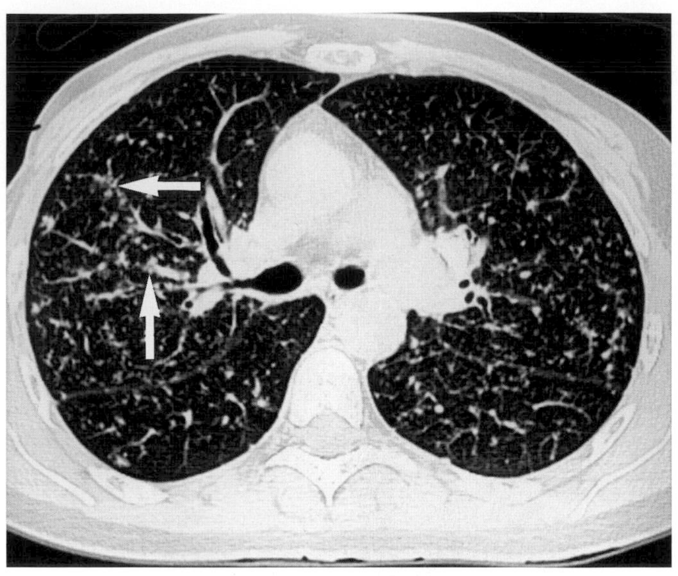

Fig. 3.31 High-resolution CT scan of the chest in a 44-year-old woman with sarcoidosis. There are bilateral pulmonary nodules with a perilymphatic/parabronchovascular distribution (arrows).

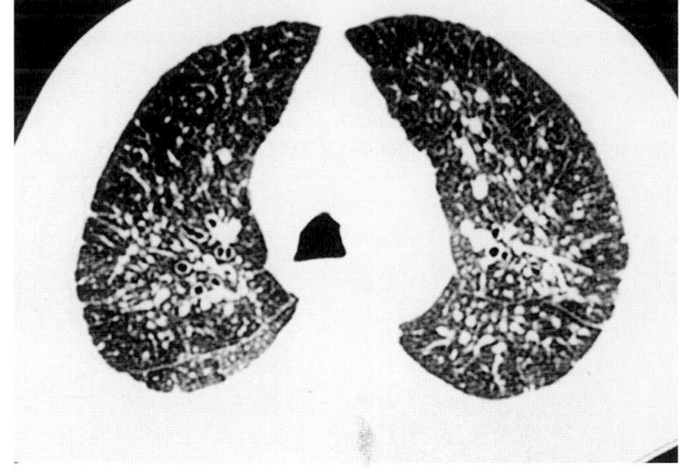

Fig. 3.32 High-resolution CT scan of a 68-year-old man with silicosis. The bilateral pulmonary nodules in silicosis have a random distribution. Note the difference in appearance compared to the sarcoidosis nodules in Fig. 3.30.

the two is the presence of nodules. PLCH will often have nodules and cysts present on HRCT[74, 75] (Fig. 3.30), particularly in the early stages of the disease, whereas nodules are rare in LAM.[72,73]

Nodules are the predominant finding in sarcoidosis and silicosis. Although both typically have a mid to upper lung predominance there is a distribution difference which will allow confident differentiation between the two. The nodules in sarcoidosis have a peribronchovascular/perilymphatic distribution[76,77] (Fig. 3.31), whereas the nodules in silicosis are randomly distributed[7,78] (Fig. 3.32).

Interlobular septal thickening is seen predominantly in the settings of pulmonary edema and lymphangitic metastases[79–81] (Fig. 3.33). In pulmonary edema, the interlobular septal thickening is smooth, whereas in lymphangitic metastases the interlobular septal thickening may be smooth or nodular.[79–81] Another potentially helpful feature is that lymphangitic metastases may be

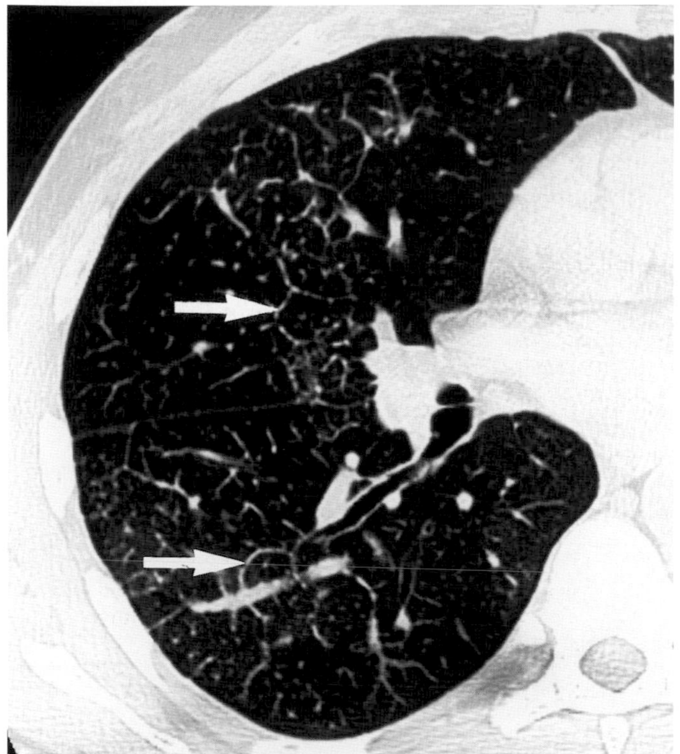

Fig. 3.33 High-resolution CT scan of a 55-year-old man with lymphangitic metastases from renal cell carcinoma. A CT image through the right lung shows areas of interlobular septal thickening (arrows). The polygonal shapes outlined by the interlobular septal thickening show the boundaries of the secondary pulmonary lobule.

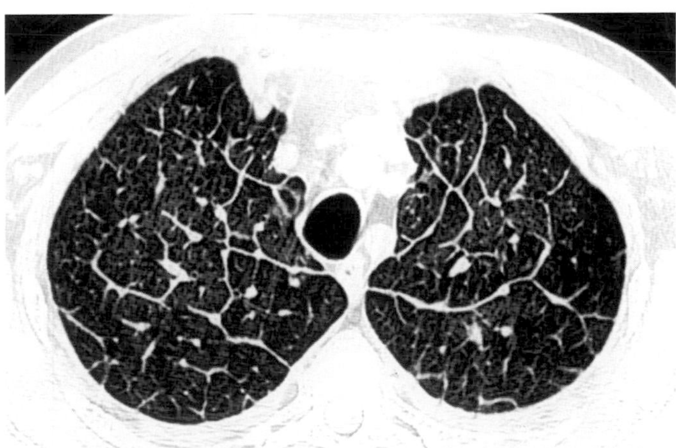

Fig. 3.34 High-resolution CT scan in a 71-year-old man with Erdheim–Chester disease. There is prominent smooth thickening of the intralobular septa in both lungs.

unilateral or asymmetric, whereas edema is typically bilateral and symmetric. Sarcoidosis can also present with some interlobular septal thickening; however, it is not typically a predominant finding. Other diseases which are predominantly characterized by interlobular septal thickening include Erdheim–Chester disease[82] involving the lungs (Fig. 3.34) and pulmonary veno-occlusive disease;[83] however, these are rare.

The tree-in-bud pattern seen on high-resolution CT consists of centrilobular nodules in association with branching centrilobular linear opacities, which when seen together resemble a budding tree branch. A tree-in-bud pattern is most commonly encountered with infectious etiologies,[84,85] although small airway diseases such as aspiration and panbronchiolitis[86] (Fig. 3.35) can also present with a tree-in-bud pattern.

Conclusion

When evaluating pulmonary parenchymal abnormalities the chest radiograph and CT are the primary modalities of choice. The pattern, distribution, and chronicity of findings helps to narrow the differential diagnosis.

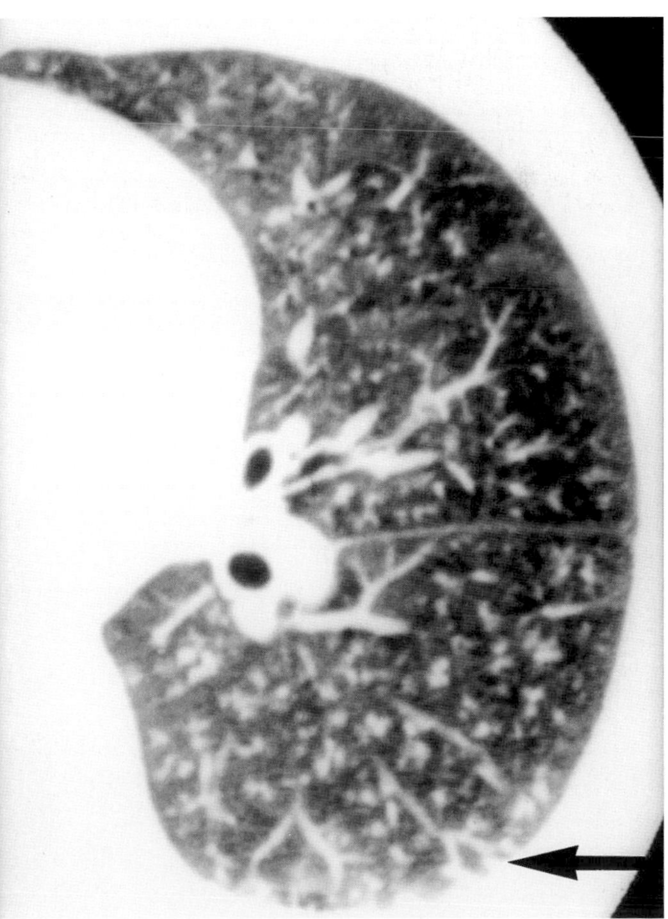

Fig. 3.35 High-resolution CT scan in a 32-year-old man with panbronchiolitis. There are numerous centrilobular nodules and branching opacities in the left lower lobe with an area of tree-in-bud pattern (arrow).

REFERENCES

1. Tuddenham WJ: Glossary of terms for thoracic radiology: recommendations of the Nomenclature Committee of the Fleischner Society. Am J Roentgenol 1984; 143: 509–517.
2. Austin JHM, Muller NL, Friedman PJ, et al.: Glossary of terms for CT of the lungs: recommendations of the nomenclature committee of the Fleischer Society. Radiology 1996; 200: 327–331.
3. Friedman PJ, Harwood IR, Ellenbogen PH: Pulmonary cystic fibrosis in the adult: early and late radiologic findings with pathologic correlation. AJR 1981; 136: 1131–1144.
4. Mitchell-Heggs P, Mearns M, Batten JC: Cystic fibrosis in adolescents and adults. QJM 1976; 179: 479–504.
5. Mintzer RA, Rogers LF, Kruglik GD, et al.: The spectrum of radiologic findings in allergic bronchopulmonary aspergillosis. Radiology 1978; 127: 301–307.
6. Lacronique J, Roth C, Battesti J-P, et al.: Chest radiological features of pulmonary histiocytosis X: a report based on 50 adult cases. Thorax 1982; 37: 104–109.
7. Bergin CJ, Muller NL, Vedall S, et al.: CT in silicosis: correlation with plain films and pulmonary function tests. AJR 1986; 146: 477–483.
8. DeRemee RA: The roentgenographic staging of sarcoidosis: historic and contemporary perspectives. Chest 1983; 83: 128–133.
9. Carrington CB, Gaensler EA, Coutu RE, et al.: Natural history and treated course of usual and desquamative interstitial pneumonia. N Engl J Med 1978; 298: 801–809.
10. Staples CA, Muller NL, Vedal S, et al.: Usual interstitial pneumonia correlation of CT with clinical, functional, and radiographic findings. Radiology 1987; 162: 377–381.
11. Muller NL, Guerry-Forces ML, Staples CA, et al.: Differential diagnosis of bronchiolitis obliterans with organizing pneumonia and usual interstitial pneumonia: clinical, functional, and radiologic findings. Radiology 1987; 162: 151–156.
12. Smith KW: Pulmonary disability in asbestos workers. AMA Arch Ind Health 1955; 12: 198.
13. Jederlinic PJ, Sicilian L, Gaensler EA: Chronic eosinophilic pneumonia: a report of 19 cases and a review of the literature. Medicine 1988; 67: 154–162.
14. Seal RME, Hapke EJ, Thomas GO, et al.: The pathology of acute and chronic stages of Farmer's Lung. Thorax 1968; 23: 469–489.
15. Milne EN, Pistolesi M, Miniati M, et al.: The radiologic distinction of cardiogenic and noncardiogenic edema. AJR 1985; 144: 879–894.
16. Wang BM, Stern EJ, Schmidt RA, et al.: Diagnosing pulmonary alveolar proteinosis: a review and an update. Chest 1997; 111: 460–466.
17. Murch CR, Carr DH: Computed tomography appearances of pulmonary alveolar proteinosis. Clin Radiol 1989; 40: 240–243.
18. Bowley NB, Steiner RE, Chin WS: The chest x-ray in antiglomerular basement membrane antibody disease (Goodpasture's syndrome). Clin Radiol 1979; 30: 419–429.
19. Cordier JF, Valeyre D, Guillevin L, et al.: Pulmonary Wegener's granulomatosis: a clinical and imaging study of 77 cases. Chest 1990; 97: 906–912.
20. Onomura K, Nakata H, Tanaka Y, et al.: Pulmonary hemorrhage in patients with systemic lupus erythematosus. J Thorac Imaging 1991; 6: 57–61.
21. Gamsu G, Hecht ST, Birnberg FA, et al.: *Pneumocystis carinii* pneumonia in homosexual men. AJR 1982; 139: 647–651.
22. Landay MJ, Christensen EE, Bynum LJ: Pulmonary manifestations of acute aspiration of gastric contents. AJR 1978; 131: 587–592.
23. Teixidor HS, Rubin E, Novick GS, et al.: Smoke inhalation: radiologic manifestations. Radiology 1983; 149: 383–387.
24. Rosenbaum HT, LTW, Fuller RH: Radiographic pulmonary changes in near drowning. Radiology 1964; 83: 306.
25. Kirks DR, McCormick VD, Greenspan RH: Pulmonary sarcoidosis: roentgenologic analysis of 150 patients. AJR 1979; 117: 777.
26. Krysl J, Korzeniewska-Kosela M, Muller NL, et al.: Radiologic features of pulmonary tuberculosis: an assessment of 188 cases. Can Assoc Radiol J 1994; 45: 101–107.
27. Hill CA: Bronchioloalveolar carcinoma: a review. Radiology 1984; 1984: 15–20.
28. Au V, Leung AN: Radiologic manifestations of lymphoma in the thorax. AJR 1997; 168: 93–98.
29. Kennedy JD, Costello P, Balikian JP, et al.: Exogenous lipoid pneumonia. AJR 1981; 136: 1145–1149.
30. Good CA, Wilson TW: The solitary circumscribed pulmonary nodule. JAMA 1958; 166: 210–215.
31. Hood RTJ, Good CA, Clagett OT, et al.: Solitary circumscribed lesions of the lung: study of 156 cases in which resection was performed. JAMA 1953; 152: 1185–1191.
32. Lillington GA, Caskey CE: Evaluation and management of solitary and multiple pulmonary nodules. Clin Chest Med 1993; 14: 111–119.
33. Midthun DE, Swensen SJ, Jett JR: Approach to the solitary pulmonary nodule. Mayo Clin Proc 1993; 68: 378–385.
34. Gurney JW: Determining the likelihood of malignancy in solitary pulmonary nodules with bayesian analysis. Radiology 1993; 186: 405–413.
35. Siegelman SS, Zerhouni EA, Leo FP, et al.: CT of the solitary pulmonary nodule. AJR 1980; 135: 1–13.
36. Zwirewich CV, Vedal S, Miller RR, et al.: Solitary pulmonary nodule: high resolution CT and radiologic/pathologic correlation. Radiology 1991; 179: 469–476.
37. Siegelman SS, Khouri NF, Scott WWJ, et al.: Pulmonary hamartoma: CT findings. Radiology 1986; 160: 313–317.
38. Swensen SJ, Brown LR, Colby TV, et al.: Lung nodule enhancement at CT: prospective findings. Radiology 1996; 201(2): 447–455
39. Swensen SJ, Vigianno RW, Midthun JE, et al.: Lung nodule enhancement at CT: multicenter study. Radiology 2000; 214: 73–80.
40. Patz EF, Lowe VJ, Hoffman JM, et al.: Focal pulmonary abnormalities: evaluation with F-18 fluorodeoxyglucose PET scanning. Radiology 1993; 188: 487–490.
41. Gupta NC, Frank AR, Dewan NA, et al.: Solitary pulmonary nodules: detection of malignancy with PET with 2-[F-18]-fluoro-2-deoxy-D-glucose. Radiology 1992; 184: 441–444.
42. Gupta NC, Maloof J, Gunel E: Probability of malignancy in solitary pulmonary nodules using fluorine-18-FDG and PET. J Nucl Med 1996; 37: 943–948.
43. Higashi K, Ueda Y, Seki H, et al.: Fluorine 18 FDG PET imaging in negative in bronchioloalveolar lung carcinoma. J Nucl Med 1998; 39: 1016–1020.
44. Erasmus JJ, McAdams HP, Patz EF, et al.: Evaluation of primary pulmonary carcinoid tumors using FDG PET. AJR 1998; 170: 1369–1373.
45. Lowe VJ, Fletcher JW, Gobar L: Prospective investigation of PET and lung nodules (PIOPILN). J Clin Oncol 1998; 16: 1075–1084.
46. Cook PG, Wells IP, McGavin CR: The distribution of pulmonary shadowing in farmer's lung. Clin Radiol 1988; 39: 21–27.
47. Crockcroft AE, Wagner JC, Seal EM, et al.: Irregular opacities in coal-workers' pneumoconiosis: correlation with pulmonary function and pathology. Ann Occup Hyg 1982; 26: 767.
48. Williams AW, Dunnington WG, Berte SJ: Pulmonary eosinophilic granulomas: a clinical and pathologic discussion. Ann Intern Med 1961; 54: 30.
49. Furcolow ML, Grayston JT: Occurrence of histoplasmosis in epidemics: etiologic studies. Am Rev Tuberc 1953; 68: 307.
50. Batra P: Pulmonary coccidioidomycosis. J Thorac Imag 1992; 7: 29–38.
51. Woodring JH, Ciporkin G, Lee C, et al.: Pulmonary cryptococcosis. Semin Roentgenol 1996; 1: 67–75.
52. Kwong JS, Carignan S, Kang EY, et al.: Miliary tuberculosis: diagnostic accuracy of chest radiography. Chest 1996; 110: 339–342.
53. McCloud TC, Epler GR, Gaensler EA, et al.: A radiographic classification for sarcoidosis: physiologic correlation. Invest Radiol 1982; 17: 129–138.
54. Aberle DR, Gamsu G, Lynch D: Thoracic manifestations of Wegener granulomatosis: diagnosis and course. Radiology 1990; 174: 703–709.
55. Gossage JR, Kanj G: Pulmonary arteriovenous malformations: a state of the art review. Am J Respir Crit Care Med 1998; 158(2): 643–661.
56. Huang RM, Naidich DP, Lubat E, et al.: Septic pulmonary emboli: CT-radiographic correlation. AJR 1989; 153: 41–45.
57. Sienewicz DJ, Martin JR, Moore S, et al.: Rheumatoid nodules in the lung. J Can Assoc Radiol 1962; 13: 73.
58. McCloud TC, Carrington CB, Gaensler EA: Diffuse infiltrative lung disease: a new scheme for description. Radiology 1983; 149: 353–363.
59. Muller NL, Miller RR: Computed tomography of chronic diffuse infiltrative lung disease: Part 1. Am Rev Respir Disease 1990; 142: 1206–1215.
60. MacDonald SLS, Rubens MB, Hansell DM, et al.: Nonspecific interstitial pneumonia and usual interstitial pneumonia: comparative appearances at and diagnostic accuracy of thin-section CT. Radiology 2001; 221(3): 600–605

61. Hartman TE, Primack SL, Swensen SJ, et al.: Desquamative interstitial pneumonia: thin section CT findings in 22 patients. Radiology 1993; 1993: 817–820.
62. Silver SF, Muller NL, Miller RR, et al.: Hypersensitivity pneumonitis: evaluation with CT. Radiology 1989; 173: 441–445.
63. Primack SL, Hartman TE, Hansell D, et al.: End-stage lung disease: CT findings in 61 patients. Radiology 1993; 189: 681–686.
64. Kim TS, Lee KS, Chung MP, et al.: Nonspecific interstitial pneumonia with fibrosis: high-resolution CT and pathologic findings. Am J Roentgenol 1998; 171: 1645–1650.
65. Hartman TE, Swensen SJ, Hansell D, et al.: Nonspecific interstitial pneumonia: variable appearance at high-resolution chest CT. Radiology 2000; 217: 701–705.
66. Heyneman L, Ward S, Lynch DA, et al.: Respiratory bronchiolitis, respiratory bronchiolitis-associated interstitial lung disease and desquamative interstitial pneumonia: different entities or part of the same spectrum of the same disease process? AJR 1999; 173: 1617–1622.
67. Warren CP: Extrinsic allergic alveolitis: a disease commoner in non-smokers. Thorax 1977; 32: 567–569.
68. Hansell DM, Moskovic E: High-resolution computed tomography in extrinsic allergic alveolitis. Clin Radiol 1991; 43: 8–12.
69. Matar LD, McAdams HP, Sporn TA: Hypersensitivity pneumonitis. AJR 2000; 174: 1061–1066.
70. Muller NL, Miller RR: Computed tomography of chronic diffuse infiltrative lung disease: Part 2. Am Rev Respir J 1990; 142: 1440–1448.
71. Bonelli FS, Hartman TE, Swensen SJ, et al.: Accuracy of high-resolution CT in diagnosing lung diseases. AJR 1998; 170: 1507–1512.
72. Muller NL, Chiles C, Kullnig P: Pulmonary lymphangiomyomatosis: correlation of CT with radiographic and functional findings. Radiology 1990; 175: 335–339.
73. Lenoir S, Grenier P, Brauner MW, et al.: Pulmonary lymphangiomyomatosis and tuberous sclerosis: comparison of radiographic and thin-section CT. Radiology 1990; 175: 329–334.
74. Moore AD, Godwin JD, Muller NL, et al.: Pulmonary histiocytosis X: comparison of radiographic and CT findings. Radiology 1989; 172: 249–254.
75. Brauner MW, Grenier P, Mouelhi MM, et al.: Pulmonary histocytosis X: evaluation with high-resolution CT. Radiology 1989; 172: 255.
76. Muller NL, Kullnig P, Miller RR: The CT findings of pulmonary sarcoidosis: analysis of 25 patients. AJR 1989; 152: 1179–1182.
77. Brauner MW, Grenier P, Mompoint D, et al.: Pulmonary sarcoidosis: evaluation with high-resolution CT. Radiology 1989; 172: 467–471.
78. Akira M, Higashihara T, Yokoyama K, et al.: Radiographic type p pneumoconiosis: high-resolution CT. Radiology 1989; 171: 117–123.
79. Stein MG, Mayo JR, Muller NL, et al.: Pulmonary lymphangitic spread of carcinoma: appearance on CT scans. Radiology 1987; 162: 371–375.
80. Munk PL, Muller NL, Miller RR, et al.: Pulmonary lymphangitic carcinomatosis: CT and pathologic findings. Radiology 1988; 166: 705–709.
81. Johkoh T, Ikezoe J, Tomiyama N, et al.: CT findings in lymphangitic carcinomatosis of the lung: correlation with histologic findings and pulmonary function tests. AJR 1992; 158: 1217–1222.
82. Wittenberg KH, Swensen SJ, Myers JL: Pulmonary involvement with Erdheim–Chester disease: radiographic and CT findings. AJR 2000; 174: 1327–1331.
83. Swensen SJ, Tashjiian JH, Myers JL, et al.: Pulmonary veno-occlusive disease: CT findings in eight patients. AJR 1996; 167: 937–940.
84. Muller NL, Miller RR: Diseases of the bronchioles: CT and histopathologic findings. Radiology 1995; 196: 3–12.
85. Gruden JF, Webb WR, Naidich DP, et al.: Multinodular disease: anatomic localization at thin-section CT-multi-reader evaluation of a simple algorithm. Radiology 1999; 210: 711–720.
86. Nishimura K, Kitaichi M, Izumi T, et al.: Diffuse parabronchiolitis: correlation of high-resolution CT and pathologic findings. Radiology 1992; 184: 779–785.

Developmental and pediatric lung disease

4

Kirk D Jones Thomas V Colby

Introduction

The diagnostic approach to the pediatric lung biopsy differs somewhat from that of the adult patient. Many of the usual questions that arise in adult pulmonary pathology are replaced by separate issues involving abnormal development, altered growth due to prematurity, or infections secondary to an immature immune system.[1] The spectrum of diseases observed in the pediatric lung biopsy differs from its adult counterpart and it is important to approach these biopsies with knowledge of lung development and anatomy. In addition, communication with the clinician, radiologist, and surgeon is essential, as one can usually build a tentative differential diagnosis based on clinical, radiologic, and intraoperative findings. This chapter covers the more common entities that the surgical pathologist may face when examining biopsies from pediatric patients.

Processing

Details on general processing of lung biopsy specimens are covered in Chapter 2. It should be emphasized that in both diffuse and localized disease of the pediatric lung, infection should always be considered. Consequently, a substantial portion (up to one-half) of the surgical lung biopsy should be sent for cultures if the surgeon has not done so already, directly from the operating room. Touch imprints of the biopsy cut surface can be performed and rapidly stained with silver stains for fungi or acid-fast stains for mycobacteria. All biopsies should have standard hematoxylin and eosin stains performed. Many cases of diffuse disease benefit from the addition of an elastic tissue stain for evaluating in the presence of vascular disease or small airway scarring. Stains for microorganisms, iron, and glycogen should be performed when indicated.

Cysts and masses

Many pediatric lung biopsies and resections are performed for localized abnormalities within the lungs, and these may be solid or cystic (Table 4.1). There are a number of clues that can be obtained from the history, the radiology, or the surgeon, and these can be helpful in making the correct diagnosis, even before biopsy slides have been reviewed. The location of the mass, the presence of cystic or solid areas, the vascular and bronchial supply, and the onset of symptoms can all be useful in narrowing the differential diagnosis.

Table 4.1 Intrathoracic cystic lesions in neonates and children

Bronchogenic cyst
Pulmonary sequestrations:
Intralobar sequestration
Extralobar sequestration
Foregut malformation
Congenital pulmonary airway malformations
Mediastinal cysts:
Esophageal cyst
Enteric cyst
Thymic cyst
Cystic teratoma
Pericardial cyst
Abscess
Cystic bronchiectasis
Post-infarction cyst
Acute or persistent interstitial emphysema
Peripheral cysts of pulmonary maldevelopment (Down syndrome)
Pleuropulmonary blastoma

Bronchogenic cysts

Bronchogenic cysts (or bronchial cysts) are developmental anomalies formed by abnormal budding of the tracheobronchial anlage of the primitive foregut in early development.[2,3] They are commonly found in the anterior mediastinum or along the tracheobronchial tree. Less often, they are found within the pulmonary parenchyma, within or below the diaphragm, or even within the pericardium.[4,5] Patients with bronchogenic cysts can present with infection or obstruction, although frequently these lesions are detected as an incidental radiologic finding.[3] The cyst is often unilocular and lined by a ciliated columnar epithelium. Many cysts communicate with the tracheobronchial tree. On occasion they may show focal or extensive squamous metaplasia, or mild chronic inflammation.

The differential diagnosis of the bronchogenic cyst includes esophageal duplication cyst for lesions occurring in the mediastinum and congenital pulmonary airway malformations (CPAM) for lesions occurring within the substance of the lung. The bronchogenic cyst typically has cartilaginous structures in its wall, and submucosal glands, similar to bronchi (Fig. 4.1). These structures may be sparse, but can help differentiate this lesion from the esophageal duplication cyst, which lacks these structures and has a double muscular layer in its wall. Both these entities can be lined by ciliated mucosa. The bronchogenic cyst lacks alveolar tissue, a feature that aids in its distinction from CPAM. On occasion, inflamed cysts within

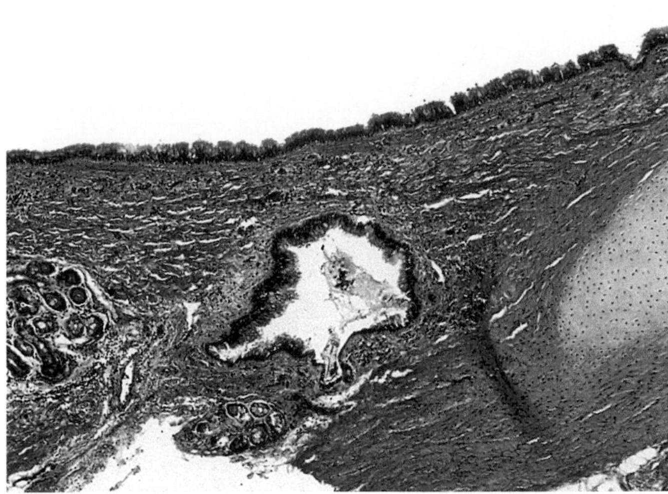

Fig. 4.1 **Bronchogenic cyst.** The wall of the bronchogenic cyst shows features similar to a normal bronchus, including submucosal glands (left and center) and cartilage (right).

Table 4.2 Pulmonary sequestrations compared

	Extralobar sequestration	Intralobar sequestration
Location	Outside pleura of lung	Within pleura of lung
		98% within lower lobe
Age at diagnosis	60% <6 months	50% >20 years
Arterial supply	Systemic (95%)	Systemic
Origin	Congenital anomaly	Mostly acquired
Histologic appearance	Normal lung	Inflamed, chronic pneumonia
	CPAM	Normal lung (rarely)
	Inflamed	

Source: modified from Stocker.[7]

the lung may be impossible to definitively diagnose. In these situations, the diagnosis of "inflamed intraparenchymal cyst" can be given with a differential diagnosis that includes abscess, CPAM, bronchogenic cyst, esophageal cyst, and intralobar sequestration. Radiologic and clinical features may help in further differentiating these entities.

Pulmonary sequestration

Pulmonary sequestration refers to the occurrence of lung tissue that does not communicate with the tracheobronchial tree and that typically has a systemic, rather than pulmonary, arterial supply.[6–9] Such lung tissue is therefore "sequestered" from the usual pulmonary airway and vascular connections. These lesions are further subdivided into an extralobar form, when they occur outside the visceral pleura of the lung, and an intralobar form, when they reside within the visceral pleura of the lung. Although they share common terminology, the two subtypes are most probably etiologically different (Table 4.2).[7] Extralobar sequestrations are congenital abnormalities, whereas most intralobar sequestrations are acquired lesions.

Extralobar sequestrations

Extralobar sequestrations (ELS) are thought to arise due to an abnormal budding from the tracheobronchial anlage. Lying outside the normal lung, these structures generally are completely surrounded by their own visceral pleura.[6–11] ELS are usually found in the lower thoracic cavity, but may be found above, within, or below the diaphragm. Grossly, they appear as irregularly ovoid portions of lung tissue surrounded by pleura. The key to the diagnosis of ELS is the identification of a systemic vascular supply. This finding plays trump over most others, since the ELS can have many different histologic appearances. The systemic artery can arise from a source above or below the diaphragm. Discussion with the surgeon and radiologist is often necessary in these cases, as it can be extremely difficult to definitively identify the artery in the gross specimen in the pathology laboratory.[12,13] The microscopic appearance can be varied (Fig. 4.2). In many cases, the tissue resembles nearly normal lung. When secondary infection occurs, various reactive changes can be seen, including type 2 pneumocyte hyperplasia, airway inflammation, and macrophage accumulation. Extralobar sequestrations may also have the histologic appearance of CPAM, and in some cases, both of these abnormalities may be at play.[7,10,11,14–17]

Intralobar sequestrations

Intralobar sequestrations (ILS) lie within the parenchyma of the lung. It was once thought that these malformations were congenital in origin but presented later in life. Today, it has been proposed that the majority of ILS are acquired lesions which arise as a result of obstruction of the bronchial tree and vascular supply to the affected segment of lung. It is hypothesized that concomitant secondary development of a systemic arterial supply occurs from hypertrophied pulmonary ligament arteries.[7] This hypothesis is consistent with the clinical observation

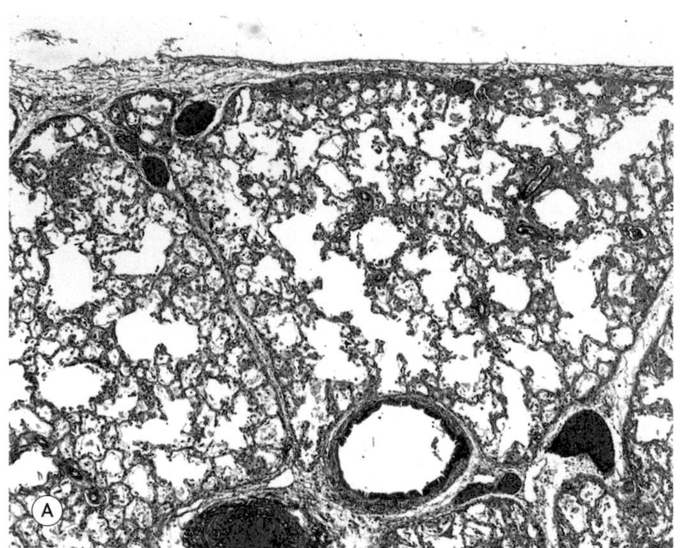

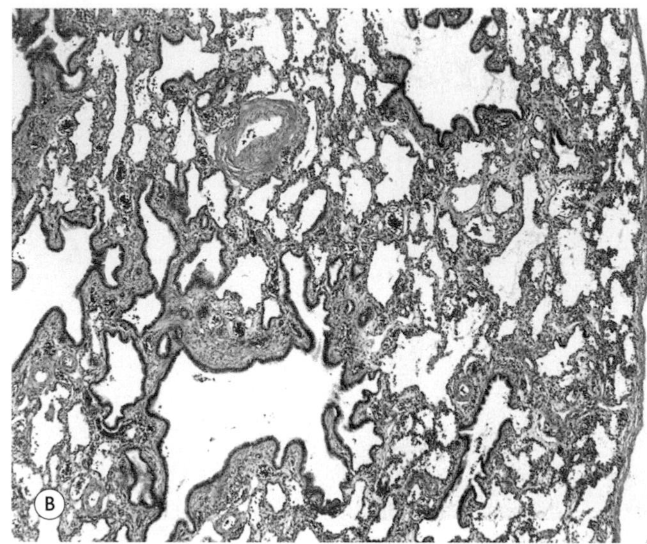

Fig. 4.2 **Extralobar sequestration.** Extralobar sequestrations can have various histologic appearances and may resemble (A) nearly normal lung or (B) congenital pulmonary airway malformations.

that most ILS occur in the medial areas of the lower lobes.[18] Radiologic studies can be extremely helpful in supporting the diagnosis.[19,20] Various modalities, including computed tomography (CT) and magnetic resonance imaging (MRI), will show a solid or cystic mass that lacks normal bronchovascular patterns. A systemic arterial supply may be confirmed radiologically or at the time of surgery. The gross and microscopic findings are markedly influenced by any accrued chronic inflammatory insults (usually secondary infections) endured by the sequestered lung tissue. The findings are usually similar in appearance to cases of localized bronchiectasis with recurrent infection. There is marked acute and chronic inflammation with fibrosis and cyst formation (Fig. 4.3). Occasional cases of intralobar sequestration can resemble nearly normal lung. In these cases, clinical and radiologic correlation is indispensable.

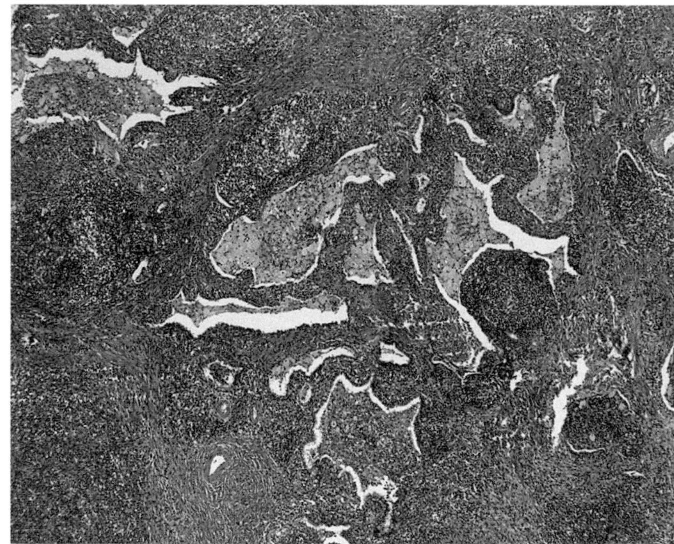

Fig. 4.3 **Intralobar sequestration.** Intralobar sequestrations frequently show evidence of chronic infection, including lymphoid hyperplasia, accumulation of foamy macrophages, and fibrosis.

Congenital pulmonary airway malformations

Congenital pulmonary airway malformations, historically referred to as congenital cystic adenomatoid malformations (CCAM), are masses of maldeveloped lung tissue that are classified according to their gross and microscopic appearance.[8,21–29] These lesions are identified most commonly in stillborn infants, or newborns with respiratory distress, but they can be first discovered in adolescence, and rarely in adults.[30] Stocker and colleagues proposed a classification scheme for CCAM which divided these malformations into three subtypes.[31] This was then expanded to five subtypes (type 0–4), with a subsequent change in the name from CCAM to CPAM.[32] The overriding concept of this subclassification is that, as one progresses from type 0 to type 4, the dominant findings move from malformed bronchi or large airways, to malformed bronchioles, and finally to malformed distal lung (alveolar) tissue. Type 0 is relatively rare and is composed of cartilaginous airways and loose mesenchyme. Type 0 CPAM has been termed acinar dysplasia.[33] Types 1–3 have a common general overall appearance of cystic spaces (distorted airways) with intervening structures more or less resembling alveoli (Figs 4.4, 4.5, and 4.6). The type 1 CPAM show larger cysts, having some bronchial

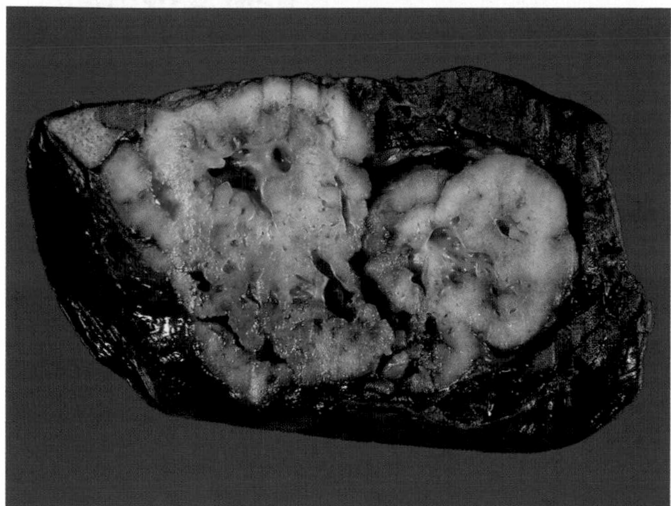

Fig. 4.4 **Congenital pulmonary airway malformation (CPAM).** Grossly, the CPAM shows a spongy mass of abnormal tissue with enclosed small cysts and adjacent darker atelectatic lung tissue.

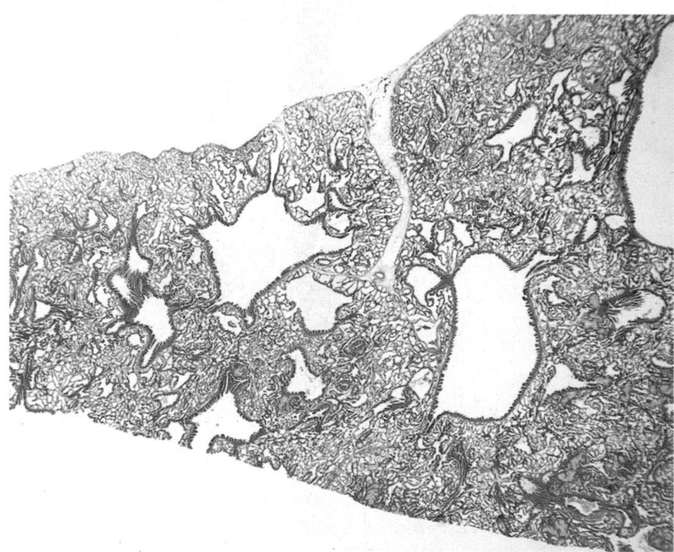

Fig. 4.5 **Congenital pulmonary airway malformation (CPAM).** The general architecture of the CPAM shows irregular dilated bronchiole-like spaces surrounded by alveoli-like structures.

differentiation in that they may contain a ciliated epithelial lining, papillary excrescences, mucinous type epithelium, or have cartilage in their walls. The type 2 CPAM show smaller cystic spaces that resemble ectatic irregular bronchioles, evenly separated from each other by alveolar structures. Striated muscle may be present in the stromal areas of type 2 CPAM. The type 3 CPAM are somewhat similar to type 2, but the majority of the tissue resembles immature lung in the early canalicular stage (16–28 weeks' gestation). Finally, type 4 CPAM are composed of large cysts with thin walls and a flattened epithelial lining somewhat resembling bullous emphysema.

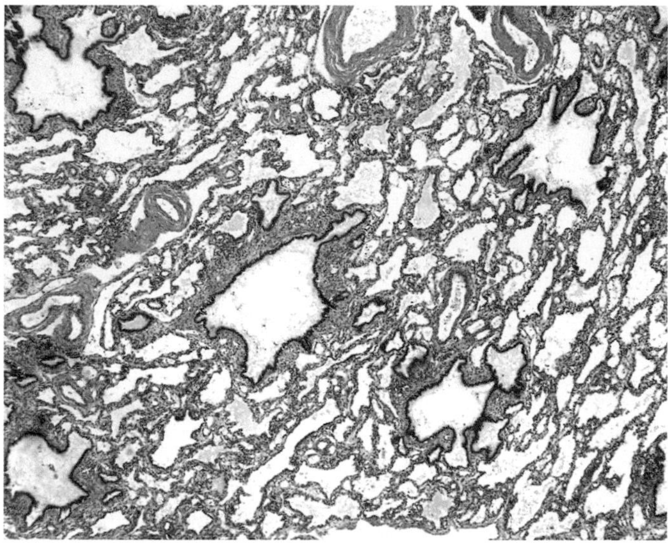

Fig. 4.6 **Congenital pulmonary airway malformation (CPAM).** This CPAM (type 2) shows numerous dilated evenly spaced bronchiole-like structures within a background of alveolar structures.

The traditional approach to these lesions has been to subclassify them, but this can be difficult, particularly in immature lungs.[23] In many cases, it is sufficient to render a diagnosis of CPAM without subclassification and to note the presence of mucinous cells and any specific types of mesenchymal tissue, such as skeletal muscle. The key to diagnosing the majority of these lesions is in the recognition of the general pattern of maldeveloped airways (which become cysts of varying size) surrounded by maldeveloped airspaces (which may closely resemble normal alveoli).

Although the prognosis in most cases is favorable following resection, there are reported cases of patients with a history of CPAM who have developed subsequent carcinomas.[34–40] Many of these lesions are mucinous bronchioloalveolar carcinomas, which has led to the proposal that the mucinous epithelium noted in CPAM type 1 is pre-neoplastic or even neoplastic (Fig. 4.7). Multifocal bilateral mucinous bronchioloalveolar carcinomas following incomplete resection of CPAM have been described in patients as young as 11 years.[36] The numbers of cases are too small to draw a conclusion; however, it is important to always note the presence of mucinous epithelium in CPAM, and also to comment on the completeness of resection for follow-up purposes.

An important disease to be distinguished from CPAM is pleuropulmonary blastoma (PPB).[41–45] This tumor can have a variety of gross appearances along a spectrum from completely solid to unilocular cystic forms. The cystic form can mimic both the type 1 and type 4 CPAM. In the case of type 4 CPAM, it is essential to verify the

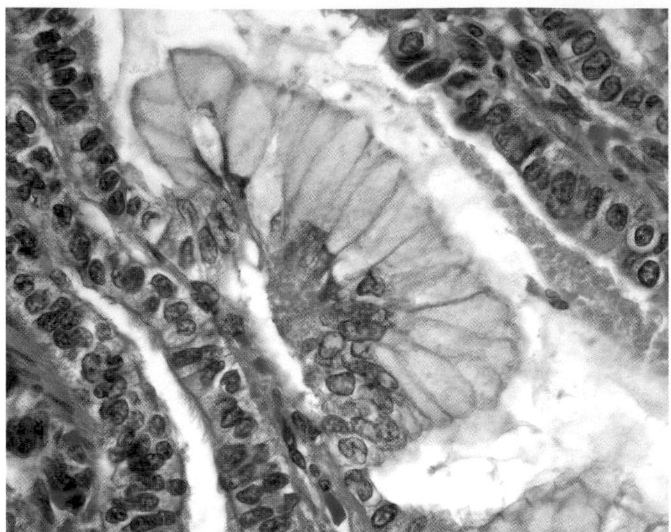

Fig. 4.7 **Congenital pulmonary airway malformation (CPAM).** An occasional finding in type 1 CPAM is well-differentiated mucinous epithelium that histologically resembles mucinous bronchioloalveolar carcinoma.

absence of the cambium layer of primitive rhabdomyoblasts in order to exclude PPB. Immunohistochemical staining for myogenin, desmin, and MyoD1 may be helpful in differentiating the cells of PPB from reactive fibroblastic proliferation or cellular mesenchyme in CPAM.

Interstitial pulmonary emphysema

Interstitial pulmonary emphysema results from the dissecting of air into the interstitial connective tissue of the lung. Rupture of alveoli or rents in the walls of airways are often responsible for this phenomenon.[8,46–49] Air accumulates in the interstitium along bronchovascular bundles and interlobular septa, and creates cystic spaces that may at first resemble tissue architecturally torn during sectioning. The usual clinical scenario is that of an infant receiving mechanical ventilation. In cases of infants less than 7 days old, the term acute interstitial pulmonary emphysema (AIPE) is generally employed, whereas in older patients, the term persistent interstitial pulmonary emphysema (PIPE) is used. Grossly, the process can involve both lungs diffusely or be localized to one or two lobes. Multiple small cysts can be seen to extend along interlobular septa. In the acute form of interstitial emphysema, the cysts tend to be rounded and are present around bronchovascular bundles. In persistent disease, the involved areas show multiple angulated cystic spaces that are frequently lined by multinucleated giant cells. The lesions of PIPE are distributed in the interstitium surrounding bronchovascular bundles and within interlobular septa (Fig. 4.8).

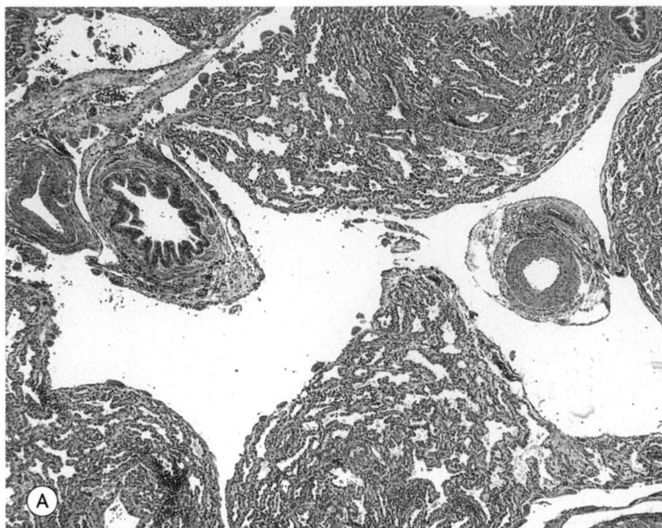

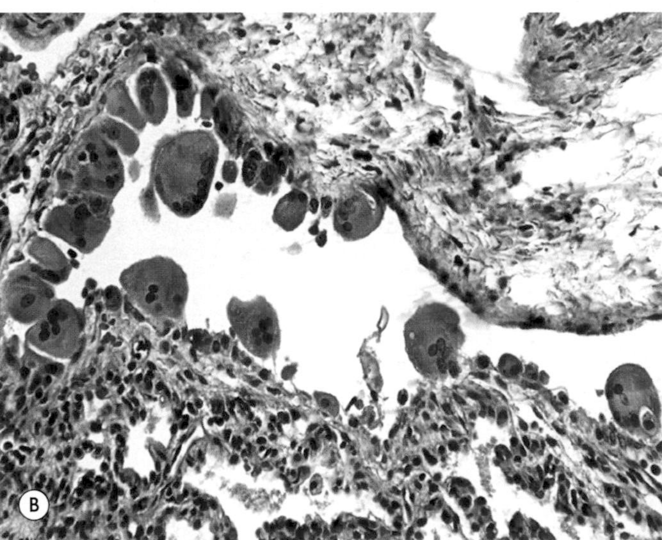

Fig. 4.8 **Persistent interstitial pulmonary emphysema (PIPE).** (A) In PIPE, angular cysts are formed from air dissecting from ruptured alveoli into the interstitium along bronchovascular bundles and interlobular septa. (B) Multinucleate giant cells line the cysts of PIPE.

Peripheral cysts secondary to lung maldevelopment

Hypoplastic lungs, and those damaged in the neonatal period, are susceptible to persistent alterations in lung growth. This maldevelopment frequently appears as alveolar enlargement, particularly in the subpleural areas and peripheral lobules. Cystic changes can occur in these cases, and microscopic examination reveals irregular airspace enlargement with fibrovascular walls lined by alveolar cells (Fig. 4.9). Several cases of peripheral cysts have been described in lungs of patients with Down syndrome.[50–55]

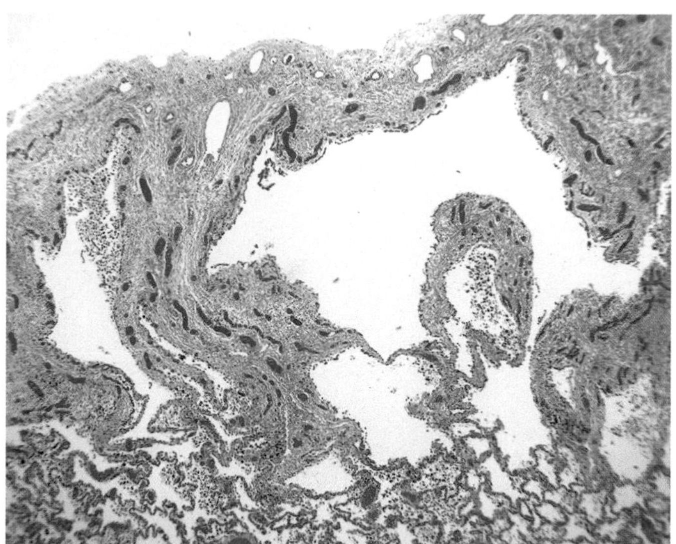

Fig. 4.9 **Down syndrome.** Peripheral cysts and alveolar simplification are a feature of lung maldevelopment in disorders such as Down syndrome.

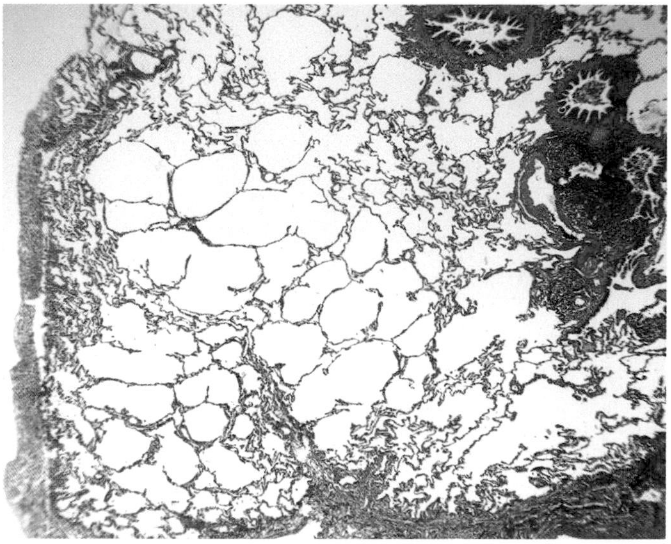

Fig. 4.10 **Infantile lobar overinflation.** Overinflation with alveolar distention is frequently secondary to obstruction from intrinsic or extrinsic sources.

Pulmonary hyperlucency

There are several conditions that will lead to the radiologic appearance of hyperlucency (Table 4.3). It is important to know that hyperlucency has led to the biopsy or lobectomy specimen, as these conditions can be extremely subtle when examined histologically, in the absence of such information. The clinical presentation can include shortness of breath, tachypnea, wheezing, and cough. The chest radiograph shows lobar enlargement with displacement of the mediastinum. The two most commonly occurring histologic patterns are congenital lobar emphysema (70%) and polyalveolar lobe (30%).

Table 4.3 Pathologic causes of radiologic hyperlucency in the lung

- Congenital lobar emphysema
  - Idiopathic
  - Bronchial stenosis or atresia
  - Small airway intrinsic disease
    - Post-infectious obliterative bronchiolitis
    - Meconium aspiration
    - Mucus plugging
    - Mucosal folds
  - Extrinsic compression by mass or abnormal vascular structure
- Polyalveolar lobe

Congenital lobar emphysema

Congenital lobar emphysema, or congenital lobar overinflation, occurs when there is overdistention of the normal alveolar parenchyma.[8,56] The etiology is variable, but is frequently a partial or complete obstruction of the bronchus supplying the affected lobe.[57] The obstruction can occur as a result of intrinsic factors such as congenital bronchial atresia, stenosis, or mucus plugging. Alternatively, congenital lobar emphysema can be extrinsic as a result of various vascular or neoplastic etiologies. Approximately half of the cases are idiopathic. The upper lobe is involved in nearly all cases. Lower lobe involvement is highly unusual except in acquired cases of lobar emphysema. The acquired cases tend to be observed in those patients who had prior hyaline membrane disease or bronchopulmonary dysplasia. These cases may arise secondary to trauma from tracheal suctioning during respiratory support.[58] On gross examination, the lobe is enlarged, but still maintains its basic shape. Alveoli and respiratory bronchioles may show dilatation histologically (Fig. 4.10). Occasionally, in both acquired or congenital forms, the source of obstruction is identified grossly or microscopically (Fig. 4.11).[59–61]

Polyalveolar lobe

Polyalveolar lobe occurs when there is an increase in the regional number of alveoli relative to the corresponding conducting airways and arteries.[62–64] Whereas the arteries and airways in these lungs are normal, the alveolar regions are enlarged by an increased number of nearly normal alveoli. The diagnosis can be made by radial–alveolar counts, which are performed by counting the number of alveoli transected by a line drawn from the respiratory bronchiole to the nearest acinar edge (pleura

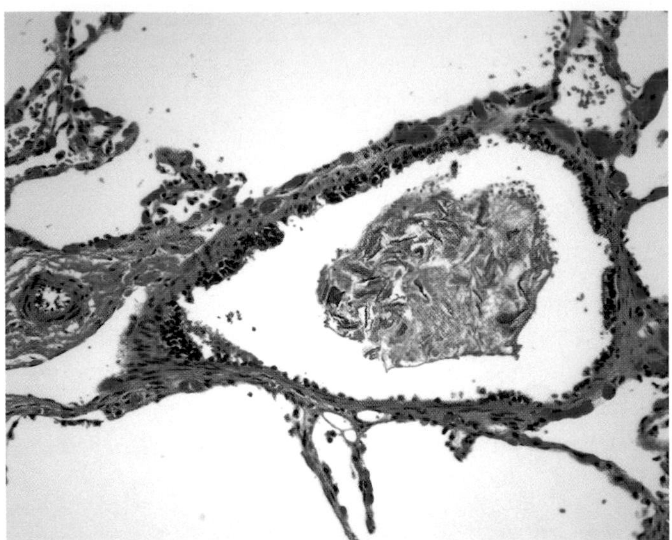

Fig. 4.11 Meconium aspiration is one of many small airway processes that can result in the dyspnea with hyperlucency due to congenital lobar overinflation.

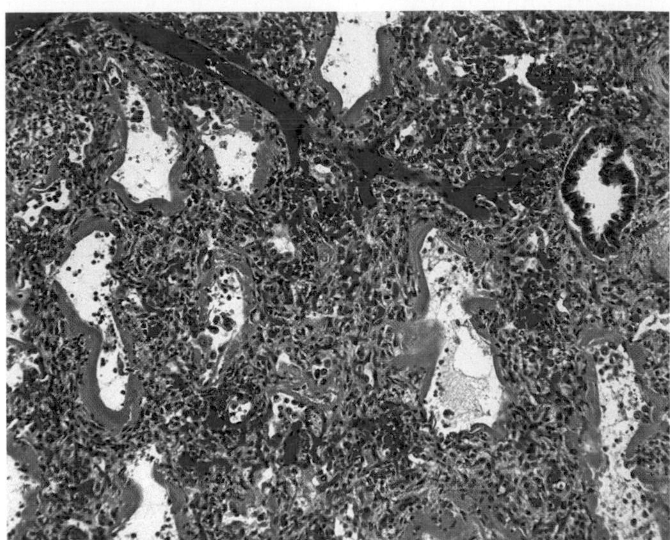

Fig. 4.13 **Hyaline membrane disease.** This case of hyaline membrane disease shows numerous hyaline membranes lining the alveolar ducts. Interstitial fibroblasts and congested alveolar capillaries thicken the alveolar septa.

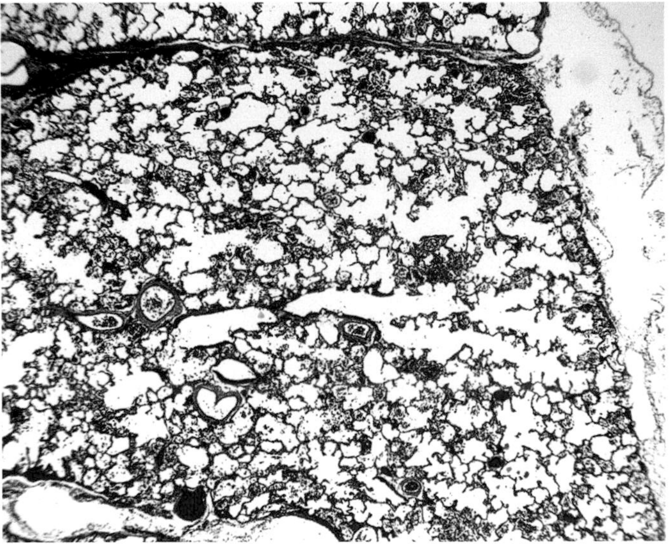

Fig. 4.12 **Polyalveolar lobe.** Polyalveolar lobe shows an increased number of alveoli within the affected region. Radial alveolar counts can be performed to determine increased values.

or septum).[65] The normal count varies with age but should be between 5 and 10 for infants, and 10 and 12 for young children. Radial–alveolar counts in polyalveolar lobe will be approximately two to three times that number (Fig. 4.12).

Hyaline membrane disease

Hyaline membrane disease is a form of acute lung injury seen in neonates and is the pathologic correlate of neonatal respiratory distress syndrome (RDS). Hyaline membrane disease arises as a result of surfactant deficiency.[66] Although surfactant granules can be observed in lung cells at 20 weeks' gestational age, surfactant is not produced in sufficient amounts until 34 weeks. Lack of surfactant can result either from prematurity, or from inadequate resorption of lung liquid at birth leading to a dilutional deficiency. Surfactant deficiency results in increased alveolar surface tension, with subsequent resistance to inflation and alveolar collapse. In this process, the alveoli become injured,[67] presumably as a result of shear stresses on the alveolar walls. Therefore, increases in either respiratory effort or mechanical ventilation pressures can increase the severity of the injury. This injury in turn leads to diffuse alveolar damage, which is similar in appearance to that observed in adult cases of acute respiratory distress syndrome.[68]

Grossly, the lungs are firm, red, and consolidated, without significant aeration. Microscopic examination reveals the presence of homogeneous lightly eosinophilic material closely adherent to the alveolar surface (Fig. 4.13). These hyaline membranes may look relatively uniform, but they are actually composed of a myriad of materials, including cytoplasm and nucleoplasm of dead cells, plasma transudate, and amniotic fluid. Hyaline membranes form within 3–4 hours of birth, and are well developed by 12–24 hours. An interesting finding in kernicteric infants with acute lung injury is the presence of yellow hyaline membranes secondary to bilirubin staining (Fig. 4.14).[69]

Cases of classical hyaline membrane disease (and subsequent bronchopulmonary dysplasia) have become relatively rare due to improvements in therapy, including surfactant replacement and advances in mechanical ventilation and oxygen therapy.[70] Of note, if numerous neutrophils or abundant fibrin accompany hyaline membranes, the possibility of acute infection or hemorrhage should be considered, as these are not usual components of hyaline membrane disease.

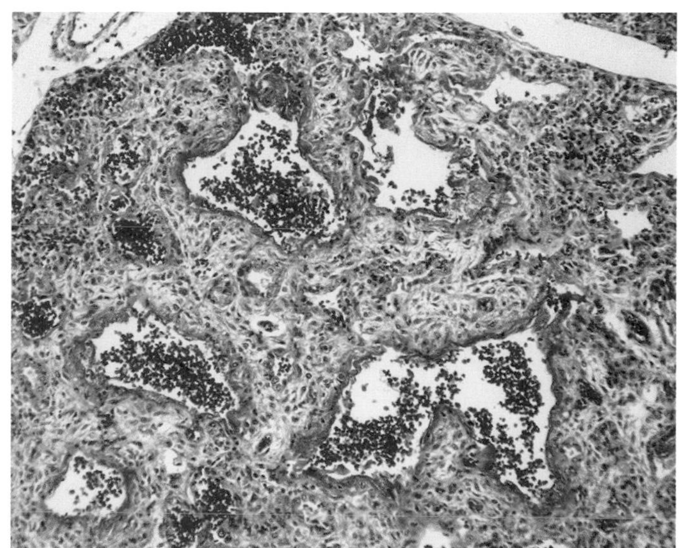

Fig. 4.14 **Hyaline membrane disease.** Yellow hyaline membranes may be observed in kernicteric infants with respiratory distress syndrome.

Bronchopulmonary dysplasia

Bronchopulmonary dysplasia (BPD) is a chronic lung disease that occurs in a proportion of children who require respiratory support in the neonatal period.[68,71,72] As the clinical treatment of prematurity has evolved, the pathologic appearance of this disease has changed.[70] The term was first used to describe patients with prior hyaline membrane disease who subsequently developed chronic lung disease.[73] These cases showed a variegated pattern on examination of the lung, with some lobules showing alveolar fibrosis and collapse, while adjacent lobules showed overdistention.[74–76] This appearance of the chronic disease was explained by observations in the pre-existing hyaline membrane disease. Early cases of hyaline membrane disease showed areas of necrotizing bronchiolitis with poor aeration of distal alveolar parenchyma. These areas were subsequently spared from the continuous alveolar insult related to oxygen therapy and mechanical ventilation. As the bronchioles and hyaline membranes healed, airway and interstitial fibroblast proliferation occurred (Fig. 4.15A). After fibrosis of the injured areas ensued, and healing of the bronchiole was complete, patchy fibrosis was evident in the affected regions, and nearly normal, overdistended alveoli were seen in the spared regions (Fig. 4.15B).

In current practice, neonates at risk for hyaline membrane disease are treated with respiratory support and surfactant replacement therapy. This strategy obviates the need for intense oxygen therapy and the mechanical stress that occurred historically. Nevertheless,

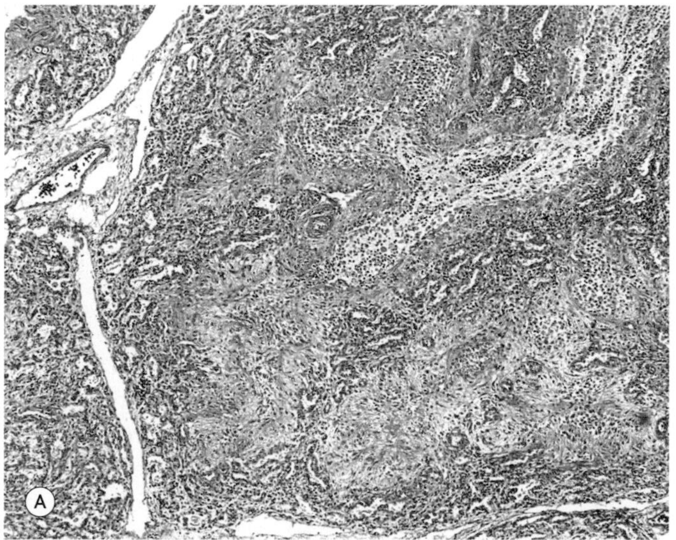

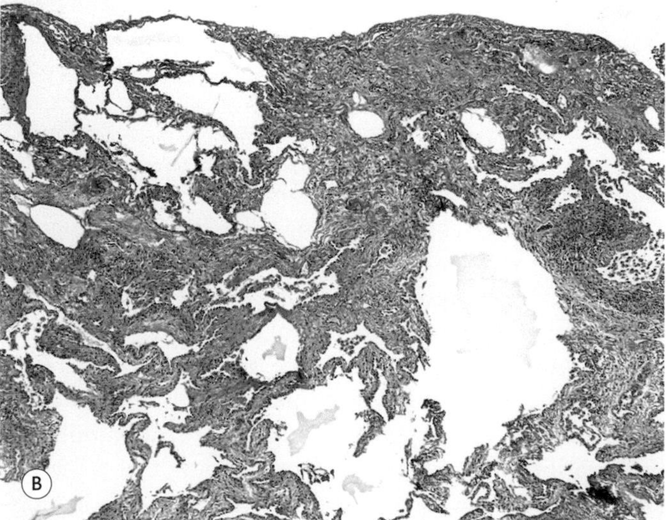

Fig. 4.15 **Organizing and chronic bronchopulmonary dysplasia (BPD).** In the organizing phase (A) one can see organization within alveolar ducts of a lobule. The surrounding alveoli are atelectatic. In chronic BPD (B) one may encounter patchy fibrosis and abnormally enlarged airspaces and differentiation from a chronic interstitial pneumonia would be difficult without the clinical history.

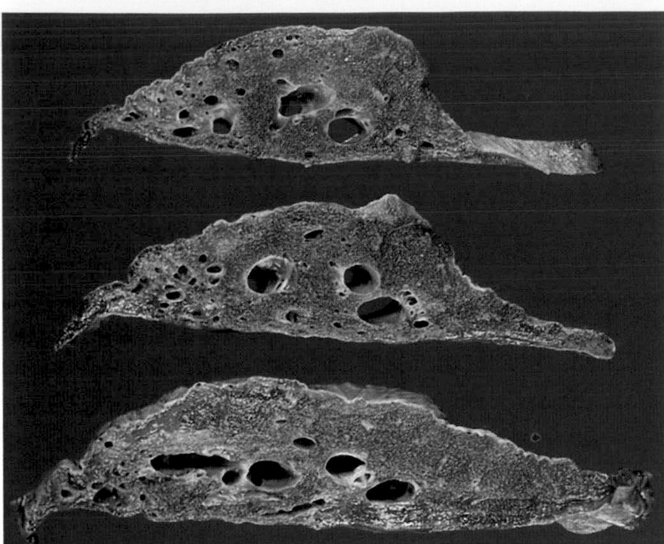

Fig. 4.16 **Arteriovenous malformation.** Multiple ectatic vessels may be seen grossly in arteriovenous malformations.

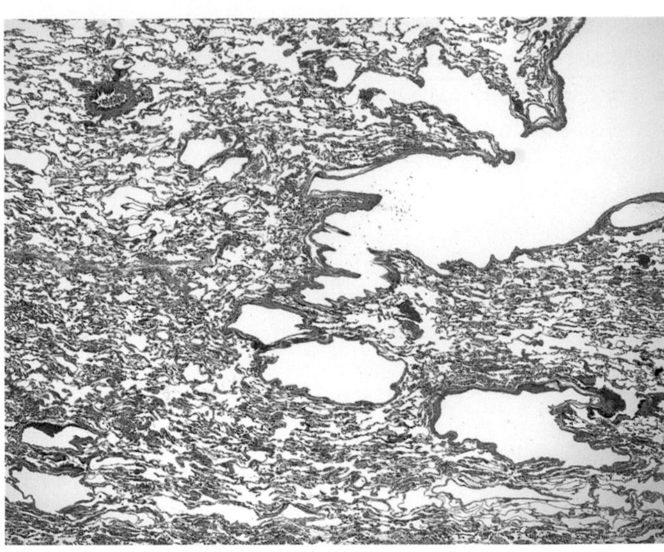

Fig. 4.17 Arteriovenous malformation. Scattered enlarged vessels are present in an abnormal distribution within the lung.

it is proposed that the lower levels of oxygen treatment in the current regimen result in a generalized uniform alveolar injury.[70] The injured alveoli continue to show maturation by thinning of their septa; however, there is a lack of additional subdivision and branching of the alveolar units of the lobule, thereby leading to an alveolar simplification.[70,72] This lack of normal maturation results in a decrease in the absolute numbers of alveoli. The alveolar walls may be of normal thickness or may be mildly fibrotic. As in polyalveolar lobe, radial alveolar counts can be used in BPD to assess the number of alveoli within lobules.[65,70]

Vascular abnormalities

Pulmonary arteriovenous malformations

Pulmonary arteriovenous malformations (PAVM) are defined as direct connections between branches of the pulmonary artery and pulmonary vein.[77] Common clinical symptoms are dyspnea, hemoptysis, palpitations, and chest pain. Pulmonary arteriovenous malformations are fairly rare in young children and infants, and tend to present in older children and adults. The diagnosis can be made on clinical and radiologic grounds, followed by pathologic confirmation. Grossly, the malformations can be single or multiple, and show ectatic vessels scattered amidst lung parenchyma (Fig. 4.16). Microscopic examination reveals dilated vessels and vascular tangles (Fig. 4.17). The vessels are ectatic and irregular, and are not always in their usual position adjacent to bronchioles (in the case of pulmonary arteries) or in the interlobular septa (in the case of pulmonary veins). Otolaryngologic examination is suggested in patients with PAVM to rule out Osler–Weber–Rendu disease, as approximately one-third of patients with single PAVM, and one-half of patients with multiple PAVM, will have this disease.[77,78] Rare cases of multiple small PAVM, occurring with polysplenia, have been described in young children with dyspnea.[79,80]

Congenital alveolar capillary dysplasia (misalignment of pulmonary veins)

Congenital alveolar capillary dysplasia is a disease characterized by a variety of diffuse pulmonary vascular abnormalities. The disease presents clinically soon after birth with profound respiratory distress.[81–83] The clinical picture is that of persistent pulmonary hypertension.[84–86] Histologic examination reveals thickened alveolar septa with a diminished number of alveolar capillaries. These alveolar capillaries tend to be abnormally located within the central portion of the septa rather than adjacent to the alveolar lumen (Fig. 4.18). The pulmonary arteries tend to show medial hypertrophy and the smaller branches continue to show complete or partial circumferential muscle, even as they extend into the walls of the alveoli. Additionally, there is misalignment of the pulmonary vessels, so the disease can be diagnosed by observing dilated pulmonary veins abnormally located adjacent to pulmonary arteries within bronchovascular sheaths

(Fig. 4.19). In some cases, the misalignment is partial, with several pulmonary veins lying in their normal location within interlobular septa.

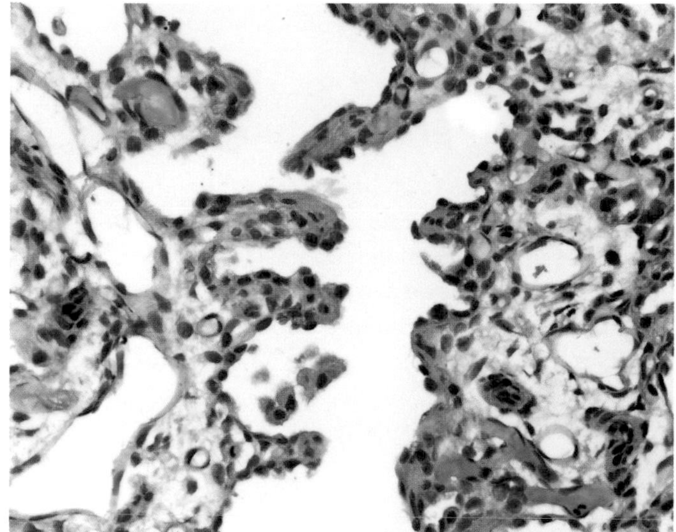

Fig. 4.18 **Alveolar capillary dysplasia.** Thickened alveolar septa contain capillaries that tend to be centrally located rather than abutting the alveolar lumina.

Congenital pulmonary lymphangiectasis

Congenital pulmonary lymphangiectasis is a disease of newborns that presents with dyspnea and cyanosis, and is uniformly lethal.[8,87–92] Panlobar diffuse ectasia of lymphatic channels is present (Fig. 4.20) along normal lymphatic routes (bronchovascular bundles, interlobular septa, and subpleural regions). Localized lymphangiectasis is occasionally observed in adults and children and is usually found as an incidental radiographic abnormality.[93,94] Chronic heart failure or pulmonary venous obstruction can lead to secondary lymphangiectasis, which has a similar histologic appearance.[95]

Diffuse pulmonary lymphangiomatosis

Diffuse pulmonary lymphangiomatosis is a rare disease, occurring in children or young adults, in which the normal lymphatic regions show an increased number of tangled lymphatic channels.[90,92,96,97] The patients generally present with dyspnea and occasionally with hemoptysis. Microscopic examination reveals increased numbers of anastomosing lymphatic channels with interspersed

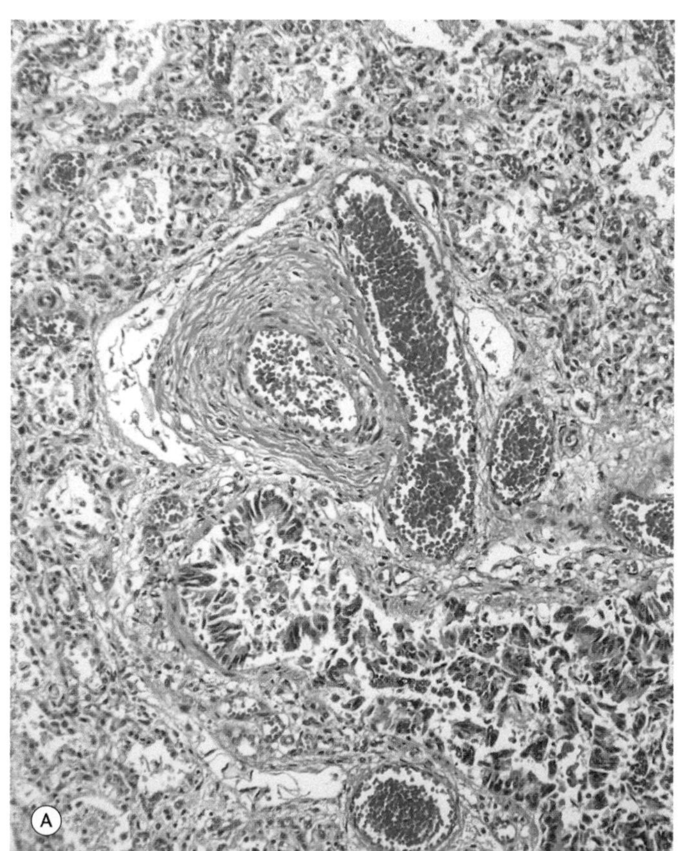

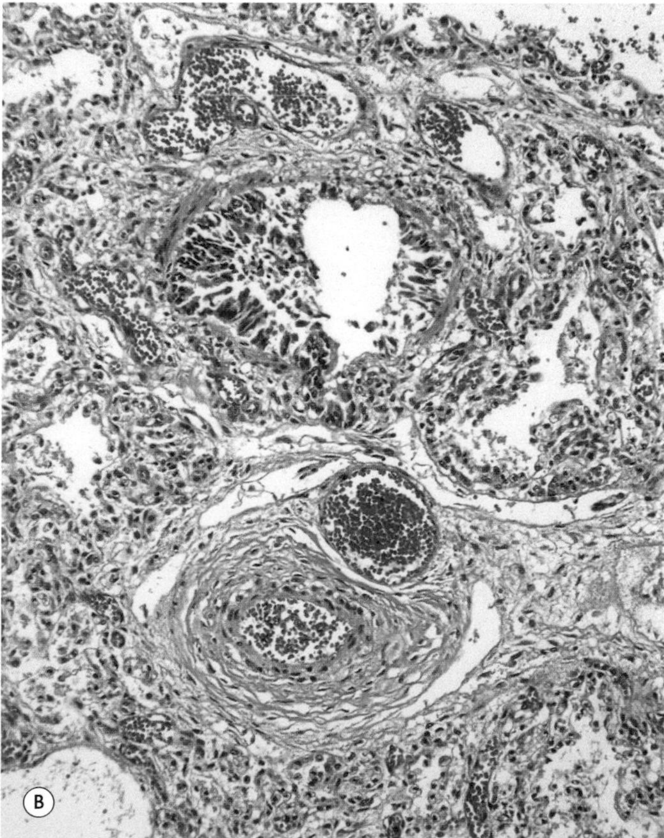

Fig. 4.19 **Alveolar capillary dysplasia.** (A,B) In this case of alveolar capillary dysplasia, congested pulmonary veins are located adjacent to thickened pulmonary arteries in the bronchovascular bundles.

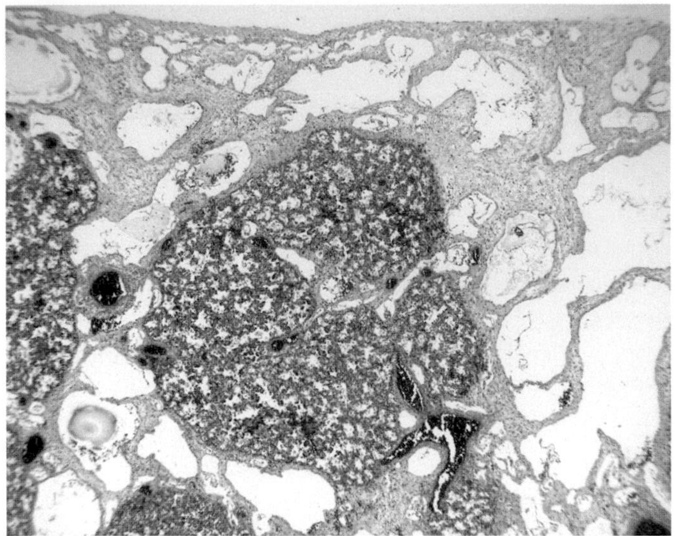

Fig. 4.20 **Lymphangiectasis.** In lymphangiectasis, dilated tortuous lymphatic vessels are present in the subpleural and septal regions.

fibroblasts, collagen, and small vessels distributed along the usual lymphatic routes of the lung. The lymphatics can be more easily observed by use of connective tissue stains, and immunohistochemical stains for keratin (to demonstrate these structures in negative relief), or CD31 (which stains the lymphatic endothelium) (Fig. 4.21).

Pediatric interstitial lung disease

Attempts to classify pediatric interstitial lung disease with the same categories used in adults can result in difficulties in classification, and misclassification.[1] Several of the patterns of diseases are similar between adults and children, but the underlying etiology and prognosis may be different in pediatric cases.[98–100] Some of the more common diseases in adults, such as usual interstitial pneumonia, may be virtually non-existent in children.[101]

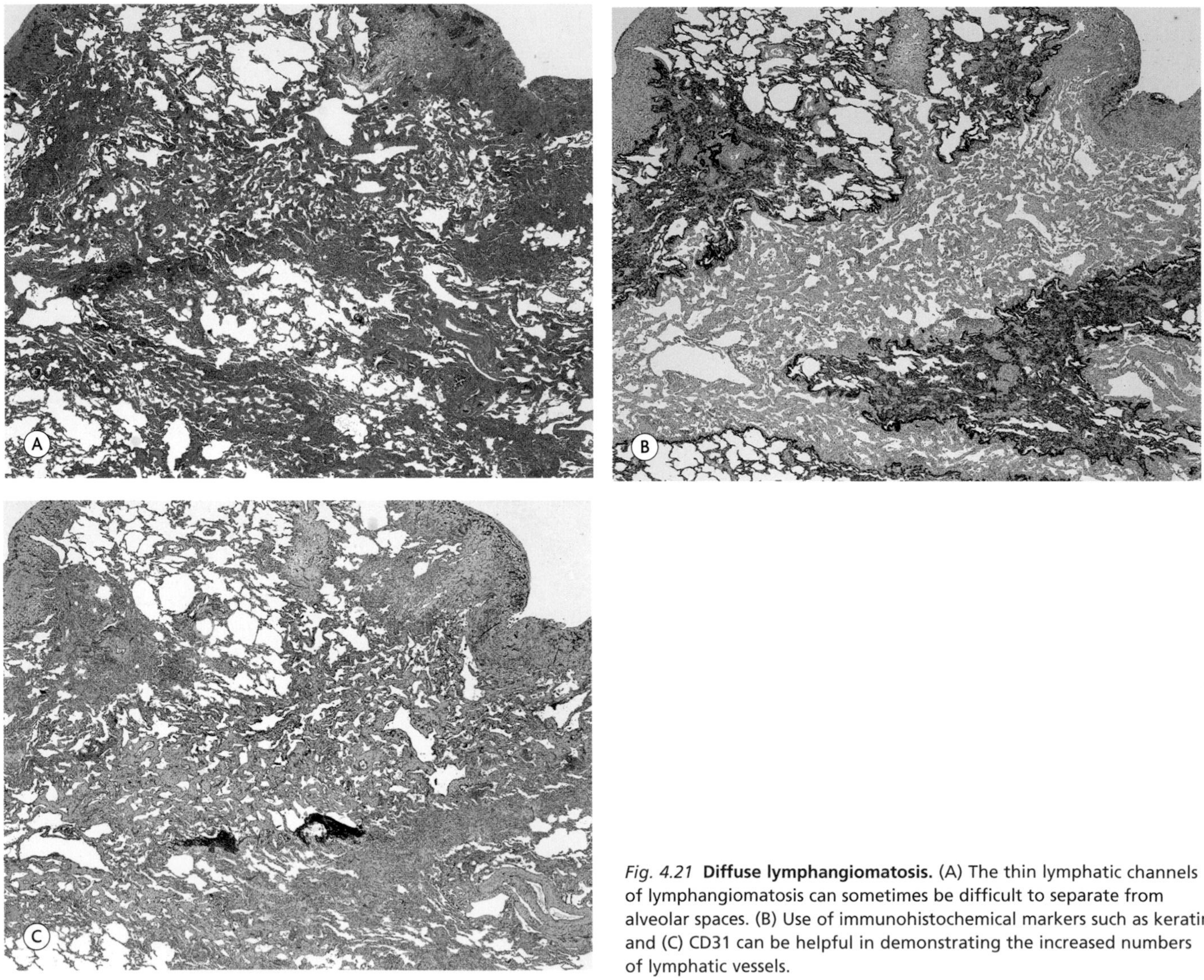

Fig. 4.21 **Diffuse lymphangiomatosis.** (A) The thin lymphatic channels of lymphangiomatosis can sometimes be difficult to separate from alveolar spaces. (B) Use of immunohistochemical markers such as keratin and (C) CD31 can be helpful in demonstrating the increased numbers of lymphatic vessels.

Table 4.4 Findings on biopsy in pediatric interstitial lung disease

Nonspecific interstitial pneumonitis
Infection (viral, mycoplasma, fungal, mycobacterial, bacterial, parasitic)
Lymphocytic interstitial pneumonitis
Follicular bronchiolitis
Desquamative interstitial pneumonitis
Pulmonary lymphatic disorders (e.g. lymphangiectasis)
Alveolar proteinosis
Metabolic storage diseases (e.g. Gaucher's disease)
Chronic pneumonitis of infancy
Pulmonary hemosiderosis
Veno-occlusive disease
Hypersensitivity pneumonitis
Aspiration pneumonia
Cardiovascular disease
Collagen vascular disease-related lung disease
Inflammatory bowel disease-related lung disease

Source: modified from Swensen et al.,[97] Coren et al.,[98] Fan et al.,[99] and Katzenstein and Myers.[101]

Recognition of patterns of interstitial disease remains as important in the diagnosis of pediatric diffuse lung disease as in adults[102] (Tables 4.4 and 4.5).

The subtypes of interstitial lung disease are described separately below but in practice precise characterization of an individual case may be difficult since there is overlap between many of the entities, such as nonspecific interstitial pneumonia (NSIP), cellular interstitial pneumonia, chronic pneumonitis of infancy, and desquamative interstitial pneumonia. Practically speaking, the most important diseases to recognize are the congenital diseases of metabolism or development, such as surfactant protein deficiency and alveolar capillary dysplasia.

Nonspecific interstitial pneumonia

The term "nonspecific interstitial pneumonia" is used to describe idiopathic pulmonary diseases that show a uniform expansion of the alveolar septa by inflammation, fibrosis, or both.[103] Whereas NSIP is the most commonly observed interstitial disease pattern in children,[98] it is important to consider other diseases first, such as surfactant abnormalities, infection, chronic pneumonia of infancy, cellular interstitial pneumonia of infancy, and hypersensitivity pneumonitis prior to making a diagnosis of NSIP.

Table 4.5 Histologic clues in interstitial lung disease

Histologic finding	Consider
Alveolar macrophages:	
Siderophages	Idiopathic pulmonary hemosiderosis Collagen vascular disease Alveolar hemorrhage Coagulopathy
Foamy (vacuolated) macrophages	Aspiration pneumonia Metabolic storage disorders Surfactant abnormalities Chronic pneumonitis of infancy Post-obstructive pneumonia
With eosinophils and fibrin	Eosinophilic pneumonia
Lightly pigmented or non-pigmented	Desquamative interstitial pneumonia Drug reaction
Granular proteinaceous material (distinct from that associated with *Pneumocystis* infection)	Pulmonary alveolar proteinosis Surfactant protein B deficiency Chronic pneumonitis of infancy (focal) Infection (especially viral)
Organizing pneumonia	Infection Collagen vascular disease Hypersensitivity pneumonitis Idiopathic
Alveolar septal thickening by lymphocytes:	
Bronchiolocentric	Hypersensitivity pneumonitis Infection Aspiration pneumonia Healing respiratory distress syndrome Cystic fibrosis Collagen vascular disease
Lymphocytic interstitial pneumonia/follicular bronchiolitis	Immune deficiency syndromes HIV infection Collagen vascular disease Infection
Alveolar septal thickening by fibrosis	Bronchopulmonary dysplasia Nonspecific interstitial pneumonia Cellular interstitial pneumonia of infancy Pulmonary interstitial glycogenosis Vascular/cardiogenic disease
Type 2 pneumocyte hyperplasia	Various organizing acute lung injuries Chronic pneumonitis of infancy
Alveolar septal thickening with prominent central vessels	Congenital alveolar capillary dysplasia

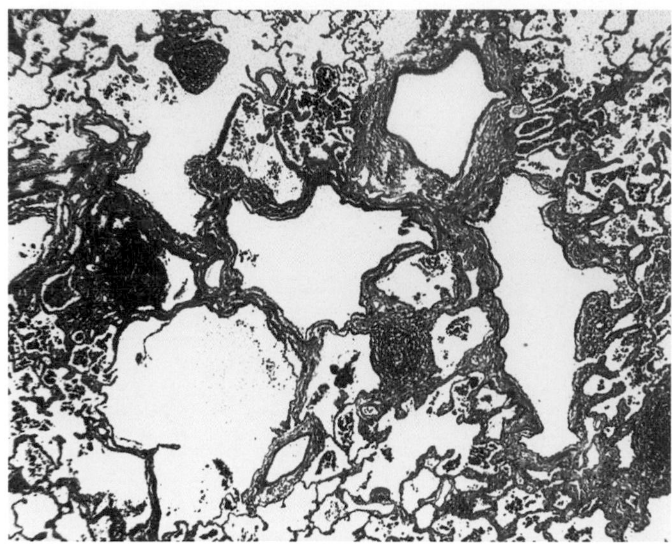

Fig. 4.22 **Follicular bronchiolitis.** In this case of juvenile rheumatoid arthritis, hemosiderin-filled macrophages are noted in airspaces, prominent lymphocyte follicles (follicular bronchiolitis) are present, and there is overinflation. Cystic changes were noted on CT scan.

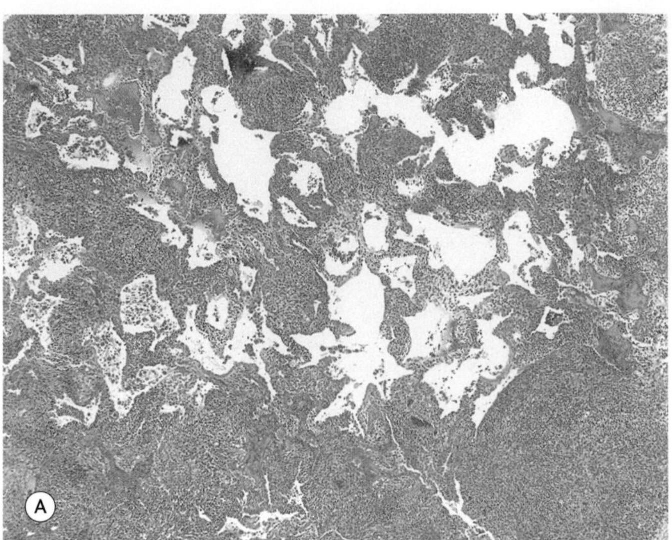

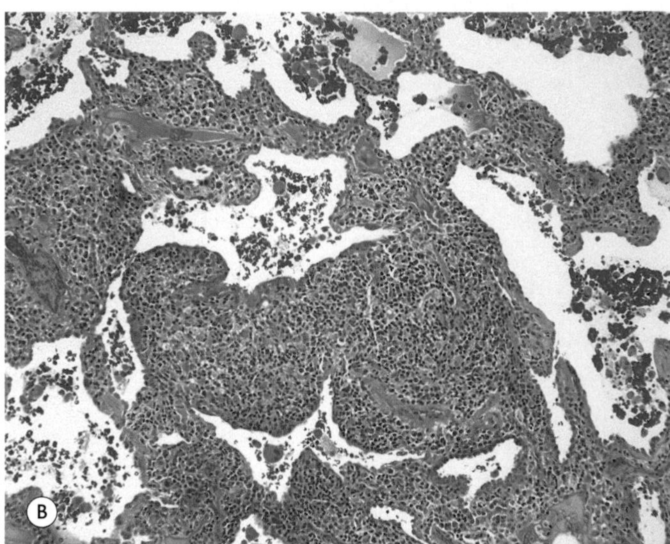

Fig. 4.23 **Congenital human immunodeficiency virus (HIV) infection.** (A,B) In this case of congenital HIV infection, numerous lymphocyte follicles are present and the interstitium is broadly expanded by a lymphocytic infiltrate.

Follicular bronchiolitis and lymphocytic interstitial pneumonia

Follicular bronchiolitis and lymphocytic interstitial pneumonia (LIP) that occurs in children is histologically identical to that observed in adults. The presence of lymphocyte aggregates with germinal centers surrounding bronchioles is characteristic of follicular bronchiolitis (Fig. 4.22), whereas a robust and diffuse lymphocytic interstitial infiltrate of the alveolar walls is the key finding in LIP (Fig. 4.23). These two patterns of lymphoid reaction can be observed in patients with immune deficiencies such as common variable immune deficiency or hypogammaglobulinemia,[102,104] collagen vascular diseases such as juvenile rheumatoid arthritis or Sjögren's syndrome,[102,105–107] and acquired, or maternal–fetal transmission of, human immune deficiency virus (HIV).[108–113]

Pulmonary alveolar proteinosis

Pulmonary alveolar proteinosis (PAP) is characterized by the accumulation of a granular appearing proteinaceous material within the alveolar spaces.[114] Several types of PAP can be identified and are subdivided into congenital forms, secondary forms, and acquired forms. Each has a characteristic clinical scenario and can be partially distinguished using clinical history. The three forms have similar histopathologic appearances; however, occasionally one can recognize viropathic changes or increased inflammation in secondary PAP (Fig. 4.24).

Congenital forms of pulmonary alveolar proteinosis are lethal diseases caused by defects in surfactant production and metabolism. Cases of congenital disease have been reported from mutations of the surfactant protein B gene and in genes related to secretion of surfactant proteins.[115–116a]

Secondary PAP is observed in infants with infections. The most common infections implicated are those caused by respiratory syncytial virus, cytomegalovirus, and parainfluenza virus. The patients are frequently immunosuppressed with severe combined immune deficiency syndrome, leukemia, or lysinuria.[117–120] These patients usually present with respiratory distress weeks to

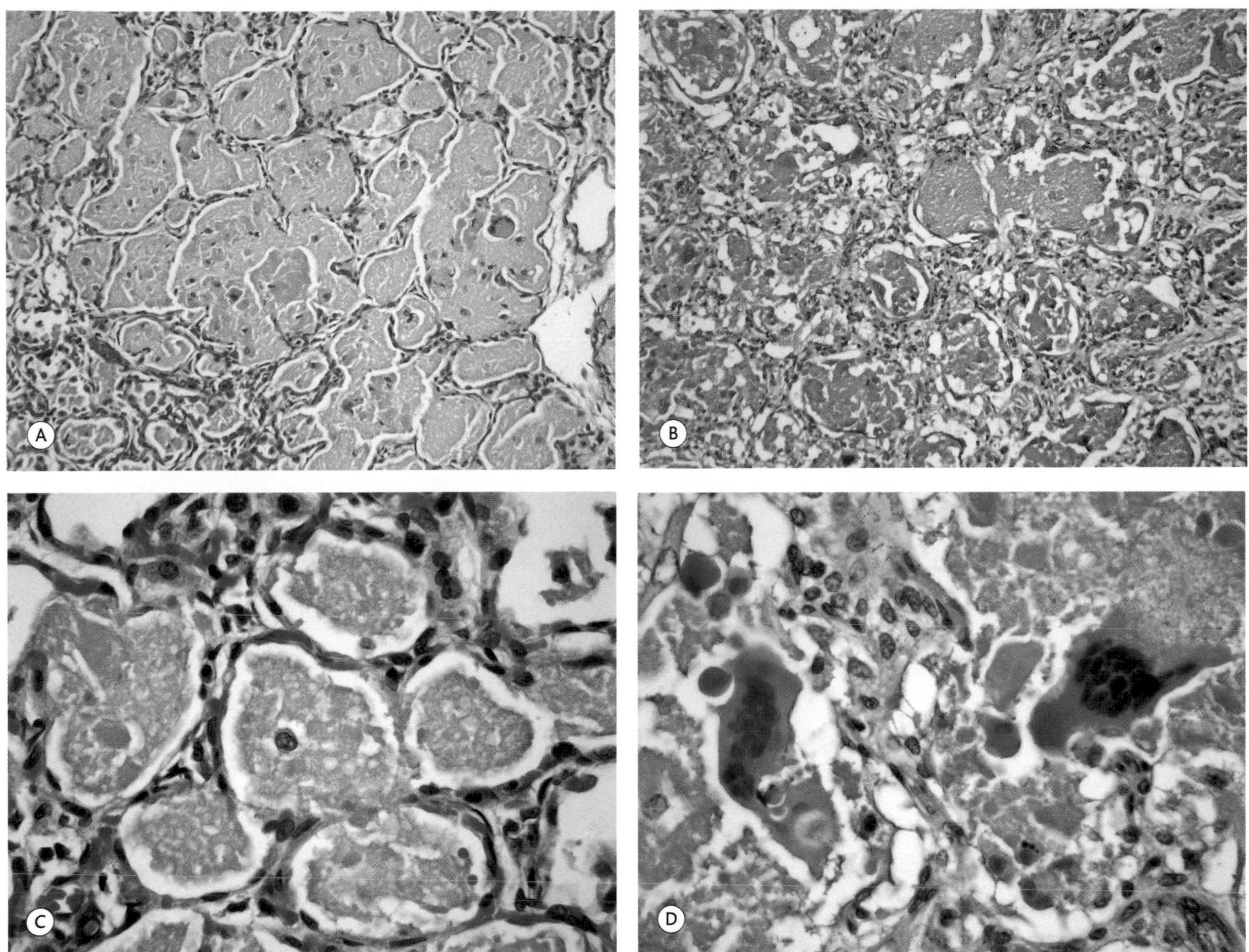

Fig. 4.24 **Pulmonary alveolar proteinosis.** Pulmonary alveolar proteinosis can result from (A,C) surfactant protein B deficiency or (B,D) in patients with immune deficiencies and superimposed infection.

months after delivery. The prognosis in this form of PAP is dependent upon clearance of the infection and management of any underlying disease.

Acquired PAP is unusual in infants and children, but can be observed in adolescents. Acquired PAP is felt to arise as a result of autoantibodies to granulocyte-macrophage colony-stimulating factor (GM-CSF), and is more common in adults.

Vascular disease as a cause of interstitial lung disease

Vascular diseases, especially those related to congenital heart defects, can mimic interstitial lung disease (ILD) clinically and radiologically.[99,100,121] While many of these cases are identified prior to biopsy, it is important to consider a vascular etiology when viewing a wedge biopsy in a patient being evaluated for ILD.

Chronic pneumonitis of infancy

Chronic pneumonitis of infancy is a diffuse interstitial lung disease that occurs in infants and young children. Katzenstein et al. described nine cases, aged 2 weeks to 11 months, at time of presentation.[122] Microscopically, the lungs showed alveolar septal thickening by myofibroblast-like spindle cells, and marked type 2 pneumocyte hyperplasia (Fig. 4.25). Inflammation and fibrosis were scant. Consolidation by airspace macrophages and proteinaceous material was a frequent finding. Subsequent cases have

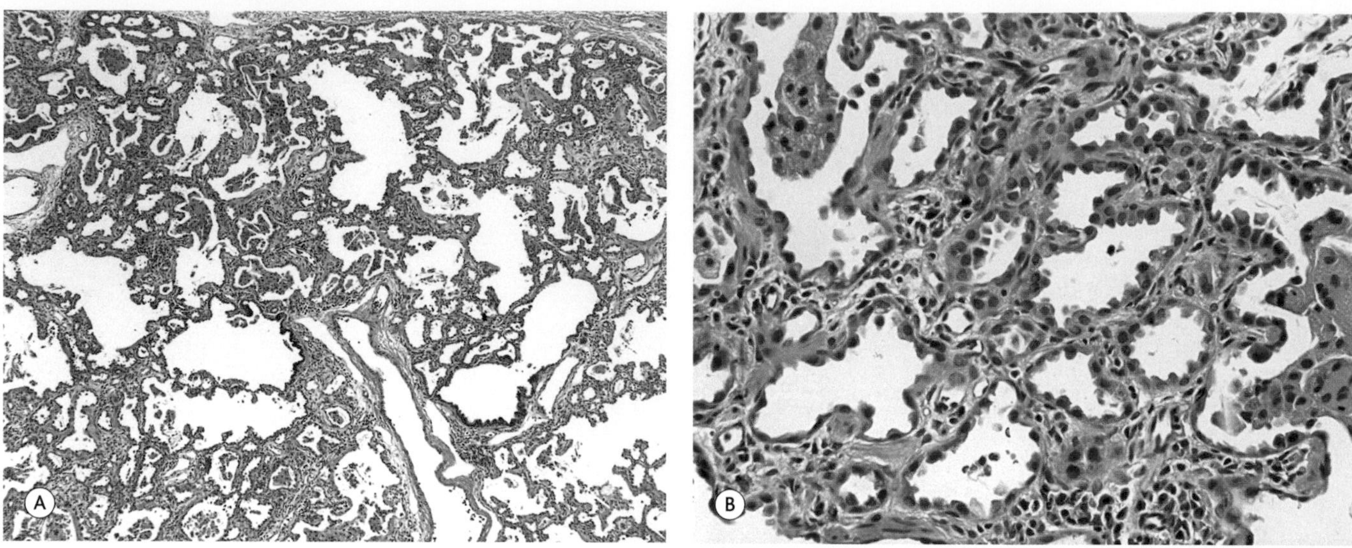

Fig. 4.25 **Chronic pneumonitis of infancy.** (A,B) Chronic pneumonitis of infancy shows thickening of alveolar septa by type 2 pneumocyte hyperplasia and a sparse inflammatory infiltrate. Airspace macrophages are noted, some with proteinaceous material and cholesterol clefts.

shown a poor prognosis, with the majority of affected infants developing chronic lung disease or dying of their disease. Some of these cases may be the result of defects or deficiencies of surfactant protein C.[123]

Infantile cellular interstitial pneumonitis (pulmonary interstitial glycogenosis)

Infantile cellular interstitial pneumonitis is a disease that occurs in infants from 1 day to approximately 1 month in age. The infants develop tachypnea and respiratory distress, and chest radiographs reveal bilateral interstitial infiltrates. Microscopic evaluation shows a uniform thickening of the alveolar septa due to infiltration by histiocytes, scattered lymphocytes, and spindle cells.[124] The spindle cells contain cytoplasmic glycogen granules demonstrable by their periodic acid–Schiff (PAS)-positive, diastase-digestible, staining characteristics.[125] The term "pulmonary interstitial glycogenosis" has been proposed in light of this feature. Although these patients sometimes require ventilatory support, they tend to show good recovery from their disease over the course of weeks and have normal development following resolution. The key to diagnosis is the uniform thickening of the alveolar septa by cells with glycogen-rich cytoplasm (Fig. 4.26).

Extrinsic allergic alveolitis (hypersensitivity pneumonitis)

Extrinsic allergic alveolitis (EAA) can occur in children, and it is histologically similar to that seen in adults with this disorder. The patient generally presents with exercise intolerance and cough. Although the list of antigens in adult EAA is relatively broad, in children, the vast majority of cases involve either bird antigens (70%) or molds (15%).[126,127] Histologically, there is a diffuse interstitial lymphocytic infiltrate with bronchiolocentric accentuation and scattered poorly formed granulomas. The airspaces may show consolidation, with macrophages or organizing pneumonia.

Desquamative interstitial pneumonia

Desquamative interstitial pneumonia (DIP) in adults is generally a smoking-related illness resulting in filling of the alveoli with lightly pigmented macrophages. There are cases of DIP which occur in early childhood that have shown stabilization with systemic corticosteroid treatment.[98,102] There are several diseases that can result in DIP-like reactions, including chronic pneumonitis of infancy, various viral infections, aspiration, and alveolar proteinosis. Therefore, when findings suggest DIP in infants and young children, consideration should be given to these diseases.

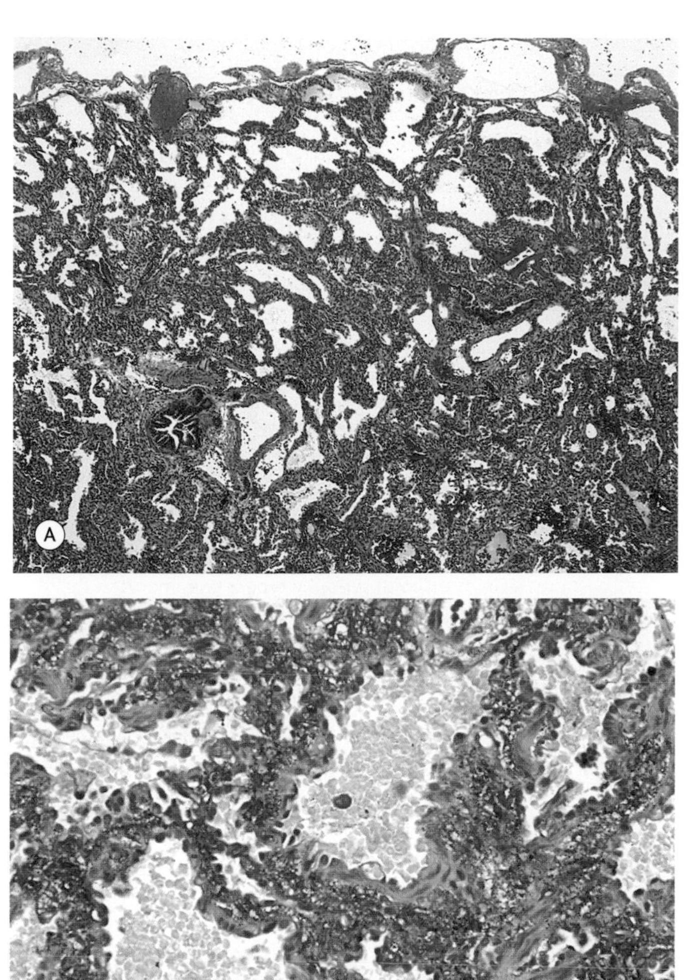

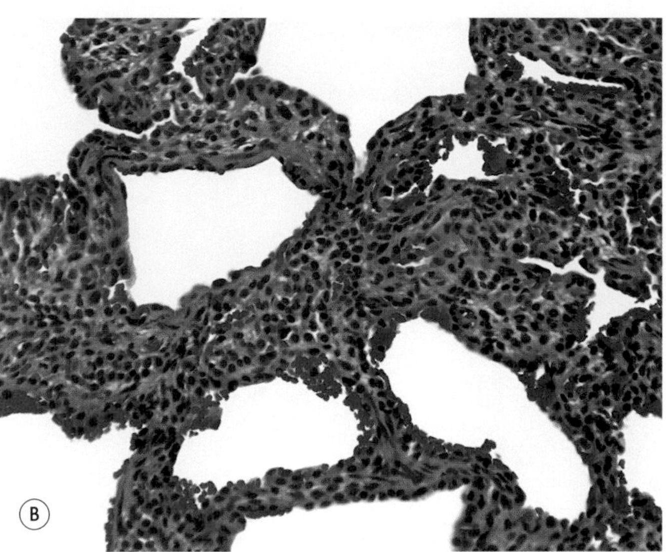

Fig. 4.26 **Cellular interstitial pneumonitis of infancy/pulmonary interstitial glycogenosis.** (A,B) In cellular interstitial pneumonitis of infancy, the alveolar septa are thickened by numerous round and spindle cells. (C) A periodic acid–Schiff (PAS) stain highlights the presence of cytoplasmic glycogen in these cells.

Aspiration injury

Children with abnormal swallowing function, or gastroesophageal reflux, may aspirate food or gastric fluids into the lung, resulting in aspiration injury. The histologic features of aspiration are variable. Chronic airway irritation can result in follicular bronchiolitis or organizing pneumonia with granulation tissue plugs occurring within airway lumina. In severe chronic cases, bronchiectasis can occur.[128] Accumulation of intra-alveolar foamy macrophages is occasionally observed. Diagnosis using oil red O stains for lipophages on bronchioalveolar lavage specimens has been suggested. Although this method is relatively sensitive, it is not very specific, since many other diseases including storage diseases can result in increased lipophages.[129] Aspirated food particles may be observed and may have a granulomatous reaction surrounding them.[130] An interesting but unusual interaction has been described in infants who aspirate fat or oils and who develop coincident infection by rapid-growing mycobacteria. The

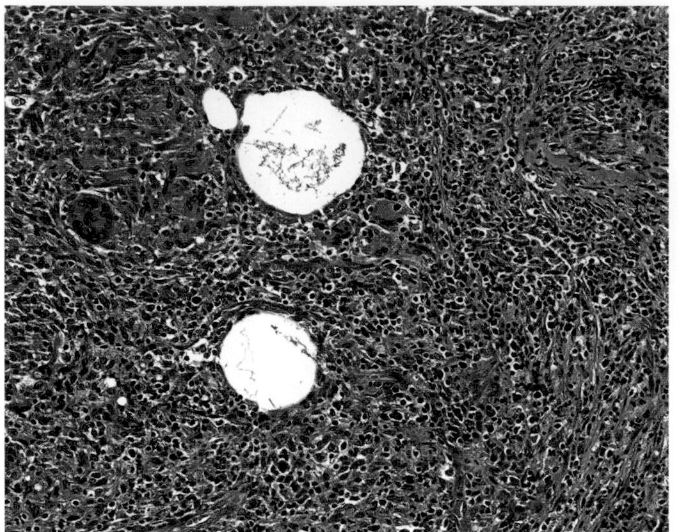

Fig. 4.27 **Aspiration pneumonia with mycobacterial infection.** The interaction of aspirated lipid and rapid-growing mycobacteria create an unusual lipoid granulomatous pneumonia with vacuoles surrounded by neutrophils and a histiocytic reaction with multinucleate giant cells. Stains for acid-fast bacilli reveal clusters of organisms within the vacuoles.

result is a lipoid pneumonia with granulomas.[131] Acid-fast bacteria can be demonstrated within the lipid droplets in such cases (Fig. 4.27).

Eosinophilic pneumonia

Eosinophilic pneumonia has a similar appearance in children as it does in adults. The causes are also similar, with many cases being secondary to drug reactions, parasite infections, or systemic diseases.[132] Many cases are idiopathic. The histologic triad of eosinophils, macrophages, and fibrin filling the alveolar spaces is usually easily appreciated in acute eosinophilic pneumonia.

REFERENCES

1. Fan LL, Langston C: Pediatric interstitial lung disease: children are not small adults. Am J Respir Crit Care Med 2002; 165(11): 1466–1467.
2. Aktogu S, Yuncu G, Halilcolar H, et al.: Bronchogenic cysts: clinicopathological presentation and treatment. Eur Respir J 1996; 9(10): 2017–2021.
3. Cioffi U, Bonavina L, De Simone M, et al.: Presentation and surgical management of bronchogenic and esophageal duplication cysts in adults. Chest 1998; 113(6): 1492–1496.
4. Coselli MP, de Ipolyi P, Bloss RS, et al.: Bronchogenic cysts above and below the diaphragm: report of eight cases. Ann Thorac Surg 1987; 44(5): 491–494.
5. Kanemitsu Y, Nakayama H, Asamura H, et al.: Clinical features and management of bronchogenic cysts: report of 17 cases. Surg Today 1999; 29(11): 1201–1205.
6. Louie HW, Martin SM, Mulder DG: Pulmonary sequestration: 17-year experience at UCLA. Am Surg 1993; 59(12): 801–805.
7. Stocker JT: Sequestrations of the lung. Semin Diagn Pathol 1986; 3(2): 106–121.
8. Stocker JT, Drake RM, Madewell JE: Cystic and congenital lung disease in the newborn. Perspect Pediatr Pathol 1978; 4: 93–154.
9. Stocker JT, Kagan-Hallet K: Extralobar pulmonary sequestration: analysis of 15 cases. Am J Clin Pathol 1979; 72(6): 917–925.
10. Aulicino MR, Reis ED, Dolgin SE, et al.: Intra-abdominal pulmonary sequestration exhibiting congenital cystic adenomatoid malformation. Report of a case and review of the literature. Arch Pathol Lab Med 1994; 118(10): 1034–1037.
11. Morad NA, al-Malki T, e-Tahir M: Intra-abdominal pulmonary sequestration: diagnostic difficulties. Pathology 1997; 29(2): 218–220.
12. Chan YF, Oldfield R, Vogel S, et al.: Pulmonary sequestration presenting as a prenatally detected suprarenal lesion in a neonate. J Pediatr Surg 2000; 35(9): 1367–1369.
13. Rosado-de-Christenson ML, Frazier AA, Stocker JT, et al.: From the archives of the AFIP. Extralobar sequestration: radiologic–pathologic correlation. Radiographics 1993; 13(2): 425–441.
14. Zangwill BC, Stocker JT: Congenital cystic adenomatoid malformation within an extralobar pulmonary sequestration. Pediatr Pathol 1993; 13(3): 309–315.
15. Conran RM, Stocker JT: Extralobar sequestration with frequently associated congenital cystic adenomatoid malformation, type 2: report of 50 cases. Pediatr Dev Pathol 1999; 2(5): 454–463.
16. Cass DL, Crombleholme TM, Howell LJ, et al.: Cystic lung lesions with systemic arterial blood supply: a hybrid of congenital cystic adenomatoid malformation and bronchopulmonary sequestration. J Pediatr Surg 1997; 32(7): 986–990.
17. Fraggetta F, Cacciaguerra S, Nash R, et al.: Intra-abdominal pulmonary sequestration associated with congenital cystic adenomatoid malformation of the lung: just an unusual combination of rare pathologies? Pathol Res Pract 1998; 194(3): 209–211.
18. Frazier AA, Rosado-De-Christenson ML, Stocker JT, et al.: Intralobar sequestration: radiologic–pathologic correlation. Radiographics 1997; 17(3): 725–745.
19. Zylak CJ, Eyler WR, Spizarny DL, et al.: Developmental lung anomalies in the adult: radiologic–pathologic correlation. Radiographics 2002; 22(Spec No): S25–43.
20. Au VW, Chan JK, Chan FL: Pulmonary sequestration diagnosed by contrast enhanced three-dimensional MR angiography. Br J Radiol 1999; 72(859): 709–711.
21. Bale PM: Congenital cystic malformation of the lung. A form of congenital bronchiolar ("adenomatoid") malformation. Am J Clin Pathol 1979; 71(4): 411–420.
22. Benning TL, Godwin JD, Roggli VL, et al.: Cartilaginous variant of congenital adenomatoid malformation of the lung. Chest 1987; 92(3): 514–516.
23. Cha I, Adzick NS, Harrison MR, et al.: Fetal congenital cystic adenomatoid malformations of the lung: a clinicopathologic study of eleven cases. Am J Surg Pathol 1997; 21(5): 537–544.
24. Cloutier MM, Schaeffer DA, Hight D: Congenital cystic adenomatoid malformation. Chest 1993; 103(3): 761–764.
25. Luck SR, Reynolds M, Raffensperger JG: Congenital bronchopulmonary malformations. Curr Probl Surg 1986; 23(4): 245–314.
26. Miller RK, Sieber WK, Yunis EJ: Congenital adenomatoid malformation of the lung. A report of 17 cases and review of the literature. Pathol Annu 1980; 15(Pt 1): 387–402.
27. Moerman P, Fryns JP, Vandenberghe K, et al.: Pathogenesis of congenital cystic adenomatoid malformation of the lung. Histopathology 1992; 21(4): 315–321.
28. Nakamura Y: Pulmonary disorders in infants. Acta Pathol Jpn 1993; 43(7–8): 347–359.
29. Rosado-de-Christenson ML, Stocker JT: Congenital cystic adenomatoid malformation. Radiographics 1991; 11(5): 865–886.
30. Avitabile AM, Greco MA, Hulnick DH, et al.: Congenital cystic adenomatoid malformation of the lung in adults. Am J Surg Pathol 1984; 8(3): 193–202.
31. Stocker JT, Madewell JE, Drake RM: Congenital cystic adenomatoid malformation of the lung. Classification and morphologic spectrum. Hum Pathol 1977; 8(2): 155–171.
32. Stocker JT: Congenital and developmental diseases. In: Pulmonary pathology, Hammar SP, Ed. 1994, Springer-Verlag, New York, pp 155–190.

33. Rutledge JC, Jensen P: Acinar dysplasia: a new form of pulmonary maldevelopment. Hum Pathol 1986; 17(12): 1290–1293.
34. Sheffield EA, Addis BJ, Corrin B, et al.: Epithelial hyperplasia and malignant change in congenital lung cysts. J Clin Pathol 1987; 40(6): 612–614.
35. Benjamin DR, Cahill JL: Bronchioloalveolar carcinoma of the lung and congenital cystic adenomatoid malformation. Am J Clin Pathol 1991; 95(6): 889–892.
36. Kaslovsky RA, Purdy S, Dangman BC, et al.: Bronchioloalveolar carcinoma in a child with congenital cystic adenomatoid malformation. Chest 1997; 112(2): 548–551.
37. Usui Y, Takabe K, Takayama S, et al.: Minute squamous cell carcinoma arising in the wall of a congenital lung cyst. Chest 1991; 99(1): 235–236.
38. Ribet ME, Copin MC, Soots JG, et al.: Bronchioloalveolar carcinoma and congenital cystic adenomatoid malformation. Ann Thorac Surg 1995; 60(4): 1126–1128.
39. Ota H, Langston C, Honda T, et al.: Histochemical analysis of mucus cells of congenital adenomatoid malformation of the lung: insights into the carcinogenesis of pulmonary adenocarcinoma expressing gastric mucins. Am J Clin Pathol 1998; 110(4): 450–455.
40. Granata C, Gambini C, Balducci T, et al.: Bronchioloalveolar carcinoma arising in congenital cystic adenomatoid malformation in a child: a case report and review on malignancies originating in congenital cystic adenomatoid malformation. Pediatr Pulmonol 1998; 25(1): 62–66.
41. Federici S, Domenichelli V, Tani G, et al.: Pleuropulmonary blastoma in congenital cystic adenomatoid malformation: report of a case. Eur J Pediatr Surg 2001; 11(3): 196–199.
41a. MacSweeney F, Papagiannopoulos K, Goldstraw P, et al.: An assessment of the expanded classification of congenital cystic adenomatoid malformations and their relationship to malignant transformation. Am J Surg Pathol 2003; 27(8): 1139–1146.
42. Dehner LP: Pleuropulmonary blastoma is THE pulmonary blastoma of childhood. Semin Diagn Pathol 1994; 11(2): 144–151.
42a. Langston C: New concepts in the pathology of congenital lung malformations. Semin Pediatr Surg 2003; 12(1); 17–37.
43. Manivel JC, Priest JR, Watterson J, et al.: Pleuropulmonary blastoma. The so-called pulmonary blastoma of childhood. Cancer 1988; 62(8): 1516–1526.
44. Merriman TE, Beasley SW, Chow CW, et al.: A rare tumor masquerading as an empyema: pleuropulmonary blastoma. Pediatr Pulmonol 1996; 22(6): 408–411.
45. Indolfi P, Casale F, Carli M, et al.: Pleuropulmonary blastoma: management and prognosis of 11 cases. Cancer 2000; 89(6): 1396–1401.
46. Yao JL, Fasano M, Morotti R, et al.: Demonstration of communication between alveolus and interstitium in persistent interstitial pulmonary emphysema: case report. Pediatr Dev Pathol 1999; 2(5): 484–487.
47. Zimmermann H: Progressive interstitial pulmonary lobar emphysema. Eur J Pediatr 1982; 138(3): 258–262.
48. Stocker JT, Madewell JE: Persistent interstitial pulmonary emphysema: another complication of the respiratory distress syndrome. Pediatrics 1977; 59(6): 847–857.
49. Brewer LL, Moskowitz PS, Carrington CB, et al.: Pneumatosis pulmonalis: a complication of the idiopathic respiratory distress syndrome. Am J Pathol 1979; 95(1): 171–190.
50. Cooney TP, Thurlbeck WM: Pulmonary hypoplasia in Down's syndrome. N Engl J Med 1982; 307(19): 1170–1173.
51. Cooney TP, Wentworth PJ, Thurlbeck WM: Diminished radial count is found only postnatally in Down's syndrome. Pediatr Pulmonol 1988; 5(4): 204–209.
52. Gonzalez OR, Gomez IG, Recalde AL, et al.: Postnatal development of the cystic lung lesion of Down syndrome: suggestion that the cause is reduced formation of peripheral air spaces. Pediatr Pathol 1991; 11(4): 623–633.
53. Gyves-Ray K, Kirchner S, Stein S, et al.: Cystic lung disease in Down syndrome. Pediatr Radiol 1994; 24(2): 137–138.
54. Schloo BL, Vawter GF, Reid LM: Down syndrome: patterns of disturbed lung growth. Hum Pathol 1991; 22(9): 919–923.
55. Tyrrell VJ, Asher MI, Chan Y: Subpleural lung cysts in Down's syndrome. Pediatr Pulmonol 1999; 28(2): 145–148.
56. Hislop A, Reid L: New pathological findings in emphysema of childhood. 2. Overinflation of a normal lobe. Thorax 1971; 26(2): 190–194.
57. Stanger P, Lucas RV Jr, Edwards JE: Anatomic factors causing respiratory distress in acyanotic congenital cardiac disease. Special reference to bronchial obstruction. Pediatrics 1969; 43(5): 760–769.
58. Miller KE, Edwards DK, Hilton S, et al.: Acquired lobar emphysema in premature infants with bronchopulmonary dysplasia: an iatrogenic disease? Radiology 1981; 138(3): 589–592.
59. Newman B, Yunis E: Lobar emphysema associated with respiratory syncytial virus pneumonia. Pediatr Radiol 1995; 25(8): 646–648.
60. Nathan L, Leveno KJ, Carmody TJ 3rd, et al.: Meconium: a 1990s perspective on an old obstetric hazard. Obstet Gynecol 1994; 83(3): 329–332.
61. Swaminathan S, Quinn J, Stabile MW, et al.: Long-term pulmonary sequelae of meconium aspiration syndrome. J Pediatr 1989; 114(3): 356–361.
62. Hislop A, Reid L: New pathological findings in emphysema of childhood. 1. Polyalveolar lobe with emphysema. Thorax 1970; 25(6): 682–690.
63. Tapper D, Schuster S, McBride J, et al.: Polyalveolar lobe: anatomic and physiologic parameters and their relationship to congenital lobar emphysema. J Pediatr Surg 1980; 15(6): 931–937.
64. Munnell ER, Lambird PA, Austin RL: Polyalveolar lobe causing lobar emphysema of infancy. Ann Thorac Surg 1973; 16(6): 624–628.
65. Emery JL, Mithal A: The number of alveoli in the terminal respiratory unit of man during late intrauterine life and childhood. Arch Dis Child 1960; 35: 544–557.
66. Farrell PM, Avery ME: Hyaline membrane disease. Am Rev Respir Dis 1975; 111(5): 657–688.
67. Ikegami M, Jacobs H, Jobe A: Surfactant function in respiratory distress syndrome. J Pediatr 1983; 102(3): 443–447.
68. O'Brodovich HM, Mellins RB: Bronchopulmonary dysplasia. Unresolved neonatal acute lung injury. Am Rev Respir Dis 1985; 132(3): 694–709.
69. Morgenstern B, Klionsky B, Doshi N: Yellow hyaline membrane disease. Identification of the pigment and bilirubin binding. Lab Invest 1981; 44(6): 514–518.
70. Husain AN, Siddiqui NH, Stocker JT: Pathology of arrested acinar development in postsurfactant bronchopulmonary dysplasia. Hum Pathol 1998; 29(7): 710–717.
71. Nickerson BG: Bronchopulmonary dysplasia. Chronic pulmonary disease following neonatal respiratory failure. Chest 1985; 87(4): 528–535.
72. Jobe AH, Bancalari E: Bronchopulmonary dysplasia. Am J Respir Crit Care Med 2001; 163(7): 1723–1729.
73. Northway WH Jr, Rosan RC, Porter DY: Pulmonary disease following respirator therapy of hyaline-membrane disease. Bronchopulmonary dysplasia. N Engl J Med 1967; 276(7): 357–368.
74. Northway WH Jr: Bronchopulmonary dysplasia: then and now. Arch Dis Child 1990; 65(10 Spec No): 1076–1081.
75. Stocker JT: Pathologic features of long-standing "healed" bronchopulmonary dysplasia: a study of 28 3- to 40-month-old infants. Hum Pathol 1986; 17(9): 943–961.
76. Northway WH Jr, Moss RB, Carlisle KB, et al.: Late pulmonary sequelae of bronchopulmonary dysplasia. N Engl J Med 1990; 323(26): 1793–1799.
77. Burke CM, Safai C, Nelson DP, et al.: Pulmonary arteriovenous malformations: a critical update. Am Rev Respir Dis 1986; 134(2): 334–339.
78. child with hereditary hemorrhagic telangiectasia (Osler–Weber–Rendu disease). Pediatr Pulmonol 1992; 13(2): 124–127.
79. Kapur S, Rome J, Chandra RS: Diffuse pulmonary arteriovenous malformation in a child with polysplenia syndrome. Pediatr Pathol Lab Med 1995; 15(3): 463–468.
80. Papagiannis J, Kanter RJ, Effman EL, et al.: Polysplenia with pulmonary arteriovenous malformations. Pediatr Cardiol 1993; 14(2): 127–129.
81. Wagenvoort CA: Misalignment of lung vessels: a syndrome causing persistent neonatal pulmonary hypertension. Hum Pathol 1986; 17(7): 727–730.
82. Janney CG, Askin FB, Kuhn C 3rd: Congenital alveolar capillary dysplasia – an unusual cause of respiratory distress in the newborn. Am J Clin Pathol 1981; 76(5): 722–727.
83. Langston C: Misalignment of pulmonary veins and alveolar capillary dysplasia. Pediatr Pathol 1991; 11(1): 163–170.
84. Tibballs J, Chow CW: Incidence of alveolar capillary dysplasia in severe idiopathic persistent pulmonary hypertension of the newborn. J Paediatr Child Health 2002; 38(4): 397–400.

85. Alameh J, Bachiri A, Devisme L, et al.: Alveolar capillary dysplasia: a cause of persistent pulmonary hypertension of the newborn. Eur J Pediatr 2002; 161(5): 262–266.
86. Haraida S, Lochbuhler H, Heger A, et al.: Congenital alveolar capillary dysplasia: rare cause of persistent pulmonary hypertension. Pediatr Pathol Lab Med 1997; 17(6): 959–975.
87. Scully RE, Mark EJ, McNeely WF, McNeely BU, Eds: Case records of the Massachusetts General Hospital. Weekly clinicopathological exercises. Case 13-1992. A full-term newborn boy with chronic respiratory distress. N Engl J Med 1992; 326(13): 875–884.
88. Noonan JA, Walters LR, Reeves JT: Congenital pulmonary lymphangiectasis. Am J Dis Child 1970; 120(4): 314–319.
89. Hunter WS, Becroft DM: Congenital pulmonary lymphangiectasis associated with pleural effusions. Arch Dis Child 1984; 59(3): 278–279.
90. Hilliard RI, McKendry JB, Phillips MJ: Congenital abnormalities of the lymphatic system: a new clinical classification. Pediatrics 1990; 86(6): 988–994.
91. Brown M, Pysher T, Coffin CM: Lymphangioma and congenital pulmonary lymphangiectasis: a histologic, immunohistochemical, and clinicopathologic comparison. Mod Pathol 1999; 12(6): 569–575.
92. Faul JL, Berry GJ, Colby TV, et al.: Thoracic lymphangiomas, lymphangiectasis, lymphangiomatosis, and lymphatic dysplasia syndrome. Am J Respir Crit Care Med 2000; 161(3 Pt 1): 1037–1046.
93. Wagenaar SS, Swierenga J, Wagenvoort CA: Late presentation of primary pulmonary lymphangiectasis. Thorax 1978; 33(6): 791–795.
94. Verlaat CW, Peters HM, Semmekrot BA, et al.: Congenital pulmonary lymphangiectasis presenting as a unilateral hyperlucent lung. Eur J Pediatr 1994; 153(3): 202–205.
95. France NE, Brown RJ: Congenital pulmonary lymphangiectasis. Report of 11 examples with special reference to cardiovascular findings. Arch Dis Child 1971; 46(248): 528–532.
96. Tazelaar HD, Kerr D, Yousem SA, et al.: Diffuse pulmonary lymphangiomatosis. Hum Pathol 1993; 24(12): 1313–1322.
97. Swensen SJ, Hartman TE, Mayo JR, et al.: Diffuse pulmonary lymphangiomatosis: CT findings. J Comput Assist Tomogr 1995; 19(3): 348–352.
98. Coren ME, Nicholson AG, Goldstraw P, et al.: Open lung biopsy for diffuse interstitial lung disease in children. Eur Respir J 1999; 14(4): 817–821.
99. Fan LL, Mullen AL, Brugman SM, et al.: Clinical spectrum of chronic interstitial lung disease in children. J Pediatr 1992; 121(6): 867–872.
100. Fan LL, Langston C: Chronic interstitial lung disease in children. Pediatr Pulmonol 1993; 16(3): 184–196.
101. Katzenstein AL, Myers JL: Idiopathic pulmonary fibrosis: clinical relevance of pathologic classification. Am J Respir Crit Care Med 1998; 157(4 Pt 1): 1301–1315.
102. Nicholson AG, Kim H, Corrin B, et al.: The value of classifying interstitial pneumonitis in childhood according to defined histological patterns. Histopathology 1998; 33(3): 203–211.
103. Katzenstein AL, Fiorelli RF: Nonspecific interstitial pneumonia/fibrosis. Histologic features and clinical significance. Am J Surg Pathol 1994; 18(2): 136–147.
104. Yousem SA, Colby TV, Carrington CB: Follicular bronchitis/bronchiolitis. Hum Pathol 1985; 16(7): 700–706.
105. Athreya BH, Doughty RA, Bookspan M, et al.: Pulmonary manifestations of juvenile rheumatoid arthritis. A report of eight cases and review. Clin Chest Med 1980; 1(3): 361–374.
106. Uziel Y, Hen B, Cordoba M, et al.: Lymphocytic interstitial pneumonitis preceding polyarticular juvenile rheumatoid arthritis. Clin Exp Rheumatol 1998; 16(5): 617–619.
107. Lovell D, Lindsley C, Langston C: Lymphoid interstitial pneumonia in juvenile rheumatoid arthritis. J Pediatr 1984; 105(6): 947–950.
108. Grieco MH, Chinoy-Acharya P: Lymphocytic interstitial pneumonia associated with the acquired immune deficiency syndrome. Am Rev Respir Dis 1985; 131(6): 952–955.
109. Kornstein MJ, Pietra GG, Hoxie JA, et al.: The pathology and treatment of interstitial pneumonitis in two infants with AIDS. Am Rev Respir Dis 1986; 133(6): 1196–1198.
110. Teirstein AS, Rosen MJ: Lymphocytic interstitial pneumonia. Clin Chest Med 1988; 9(3): 467–471.
111. Pitt J: Lymphocytic interstitial pneumonia. Pediatr Clin North Am 1991; 38(1): 89–95.
112. Marchevsky A, Rosen MJ, Chrystal G, et al.: Pulmonary complications of the acquired immunodeficiency syndrome: a clinicopathologic study of 70 cases. Hum Pathol 1985; 16(7): 659–670.
113. Rubinstein A, Morecki R, Silverman B, et al.: Pulmonary disease in children with acquired immune deficiency syndrome and AIDS-related complex. J Pediatr 1986; 108(4): 498–503.
114. Rosen SH, Castleman B, Liebow AA: Pulmonary alveolar proteinosis. N Engl J Med 1958; 258(23): 1123–1142.
115. Nogee LM, de Mello DE, Dehner LP, et al.: Brief report: deficiency of pulmonary surfactant protein B in congenital alveolar proteinosis. N Engl J Med 1993; 328(6): 406–410.
115a. Shulenin S, Nogee LM, Annilo T, et al.: ABCA3 gene mutations in newborns with fatal surfactant deficiency. N Engl J Med, 2004; 350(13): 1296–1303.
116. Nogee LM, Garnier G, Dietz HC, et al.: A mutation in the surfactant protein B gene responsible for fatal neonatal respiratory disease in multiple kindreds. J Clin Invest 1994; 93(4): 1860–1863.
116a. Tryka AF, Wert SE, Mazursky JE, et al.: Absence of lamellar bodies with accumulation of dense bodies characterizes a novel form of congenital surfactant defect. Pediatr Dev Pathol, 2000; 3(4): 335–345.
117. Bedrossian CW, Luna MA, Conklin RH, et al.: Alveolar proteinosis as a consequence of immunosuppression. A hypothesis based on clinical and pathologic observations. Hum Pathol 1980; 11(5 suppl): 527–535.
118. Nachajon RV, Rutstein RM, Rudy BJ, et al.: Pulmonary alveolar proteinosis in an HIV-infected child. Pediatr Pulmonol 1997; 24(4): 292–295.
119. Samuels MP, Warner JO: Pulmonary alveolar lipoproteinosis complicating juvenile dermatomyositis. Thorax 1988; 43(11): 939–940.
120. Parto K, Svedstrom E, Majurin ML, et al.: Pulmonary manifestations in lysinuric protein intolerance. Chest 1993; 104(4): 1176–1182.
121. Sondheimer HM, Lung MC, Brugman SM, et al.: Pulmonary vascular disorders masquerading as interstitial lung disease. Pediatr Pulmonol 1995; 20(5): 284–288.
122. Katzenstein AL, Gordon LP, Oliphant M, et al.: Chronic pneumonitis of infancy. A unique form of interstitial lung disease occurring in early childhood. Am J Surg Pathol 1995; 19(4): 439–447.
123. Nogee LM, Dunbar AE 3rd, Wert SE, et al.: A mutation in the surfactant protein C gene associated with familial interstitial lung disease. N Engl J Med 2001; 344(8): 573–579.
124. Schroeder SA, Shannon DC, Mark EJ: Cellular interstitial pneumonitis in infants. A clinicopathologic study. Chest 1992; 101(4): 1065–1069.
125. Canakis AM, Cutz E, Manson D, et al.: Pulmonary interstitial glycogenosis: a new variant of neonatal interstitial lung disease. Am J Respir Crit Care Med 2002; 165(11): 1557–1565.
126. Fan LL: Hypersensitivity pneumonitis in children. Curr Opin Pediatr 2002; 14(3): 323–326.
127. Yee WF, Castile RG, Cooper A, et al.: Diagnosing bird fancier's disease in children. Pediatrics 1990; 85(5): 848–852.
128. Annobil SH, Morad NA, Kameswaran M, et al.: Bronchiectasis due to lipid aspiration in childhood: clinical and pathological correlates. Ann Trop Paediatr 1996; 16(1): 19–25.
129. Colombo JL, Hallberg TK: Recurrent aspiration in children: lipid-laden alveolar macrophage quantitation. Pediatr Pulmonol 1987; 3(2): 86–89.
130. Gadol CL, Joshi VV, Lee EY: Bronchiolar obstruction associated with repeated aspiration of vegetable material in two children with cerebral palsy. Pediatr Pulmonol 1987; 3(6): 437–439.
131. Annobil SH, Benjamin B, Kameswaran M, et al.: Lipoid pneumonia in children following aspiration of animal fat (ghee). Ann Trop Paediatr 1991; 11(1): 87–94.
132. Oermann CM, Panesar KS, Langston C, et al.: Pulmonary infiltrates with eosinophilia syndromes in children. J Pediatr 2000; 136(3): 351–358.

Acute lung injury

Oi-Yee Cheung Kevin O Leslie

5

Introduction

A wide variety of insults can produce acute lung damage, inclusive of those that injure the lungs directly. Early terms for diffuse acute lung injury occurring indirectly in the setting of overwhelming non-thoracic trauma accompanied by hypovolemia were "shock lung", "postperfusion lung", "traumatic wet lung", and "congestive atelectasis".[1,2]

In 1967, Ashbaugh and coworkers formally described a syndrome in which patients developed severe respiratory distress of acute onset following an identifiable injury. Patients developed dyspnea, reduced lung compliance, diffuse chest radiographic infiltrates, and hypoxemia refractory to supplementary oxygen.[3] Today this sequence of clinical events is referred to as the adult respiratory distress syndrome (ARDS). The clinical course is rapid and the mortality rate is high, with more than half of patients affected dying of respiratory failure within days to weeks.[2,4,5]

The American–European Consensus Conference (AECC) formally defined ARDS in 1994 by the following criteria: acute onset; bilateral chest radiographic infiltrates; hypoxemia regardless of the positive end-expiratory pressure oxygen concentration; an arterial partial pressure of oxygen to inspired oxygen fraction ratio less than 200; and no evidence of left atrial hypertension.[6] The AECC also agreed that ARDS represents the most severe form in a spectrum of disease encompassed under the general term "acute lung injury" (ALI).

The histologic counterpart of ARDS is distinctive and referred to as diffuse alveolar damage (DAD). Diffuse alveolar damage is the most extreme manifestation of lung injury and can occur as a result of a large number of direct injuries to the lungs (e.g. infection). In this chapter, our discussion is centered on DAD and less severe manifestations of ALI. Some authors have considered organizing pneumonia to be a form of ALI, but we and others believe that organization is a subacute phenomenon with a more protracted clinical course (several days to weeks). Subacute organizing pneumonia of unknown etiology (previously known as idiopathic bronchiolitis obliterans organizing pneumonia)[7] will be discussed with the chronic diffuse diseases (see Ch. 7).

Diffuse alveolar damage: the morphologic prototype of acute lung injury

The causes of acute lung injury are numerous (Table 5.1). The lung reacts to various types of insults in similar ways, regardless of the etiology. The resultant endothelial and alveolar epithelial cell injury is attended by fluid and cellular exudation. Subsequent reparative fibroblastic proliferation is accompanied by type II pneumocyte hyperplasia.[4,8] The microscopic appearance depends on the time interval between the insult and biopsy, and on the severity and extent of the injury.[2] Diffuse alveolar damage is the usual pathologic manifestation of ARDS and is the best-characterized prototype of acute lung injury. From studies of ARDS, the pathologic changes appear to proceed consistently through discrete but

Table 5.1 Causes of diffuse alveolar damage

Idiopathic Acute interstitial pneumonia (Hamman–Rich syndrome) **Infection** Any infection in the immunosuppressed patient, especially *Pneumocystis carinii* Viral infection: adenovirus, influenza, herpes, CMV, hanta virus, etc. Legionella Mycoplasma/chlamydia Rickettsiae **Drugs** Chemotherapeutic drugs Busulfan, bleomycin, methotrexate, azathioprine, BCNU, cytoxan, melphalan, mitomycin Amiodarone Gold Nitrofurantoin Hexamethonium Placidyl Penicillamine **Collagen vascular disease** Systemic lupus erythematosus Rheumatoid arthritis Polymyositis/dermatomyositis Scleroderma Mixed connective disease **Pulmonary hemorrhage syndrome and vasculitis** Goodpasture's syndrome Microscopic polyangiitis Polyarteritis nodosa Wegener's granulomatosis Vasculitis associated with collagen vascular disease **Ingestants** Paraquat Kerosene Denatured rapeseed oil	**Inhalants** Oxygen Amitrole-containing herbicide Ammonia and bleach mixture Chlorine gas Hydrogen sulfide Mercury vapor Nitric acid fume Nitrogen dioxide Paint remover Smoke Smoke bomb Sulfur dioxide War gases **Shock** Traumatic Hemorrhage Neurogenic Cardiogenic **Sepsis** **Radiation** **Others** Acute massive aspiration Acute pancreatitis Burn Cardiopulmonary bypass Heat High altitude Intravenous administration of contrast material Leukemic cell lysis Molar pregnancy Near-drowning Peritoneal-venous shunt Post lymphangiography Toxic shock syndrome Transfusion therapy Uremia Venous air embolism

Source: From Katzenstein and Askin's *Surgical Pathology of Non-neoplastic Lung Disease*, with modifications.

overlapping phases (Fig. 5.1) – an early exudative (acute) phase (Fig. 5.2A,B), a subacute proliferative (organizing) phase (Fig. 5.2C), and a late fibrotic phase (Fig. 5.3).[2,4,5,7,9] The exudative phase is most prominent in the first week of injury. The earliest changes include interstitial and intra-alveolar edema with varying amounts of hemorrhage and fibrin deposition (Fig. 5.4). Hyaline membranes (Fig. 5.5), the histologic hallmark of the exudative phase of ARDS, are most prominent from 3 to 7 days after injury. Mild interstitial mononuclear inflammatory infiltrates (Fig. 5.6) and fibrin thrombi in small pulmonary arteries (Fig. 5.7) are also seen. Type II pneumocyte hyperplasia (Fig. 5.8) begins by the end of this phase and persists through the proliferative phase. The reactive type II pneumocytes may have marked nuclear atypia and mitotic figures may be numerous (Fig. 5.9). The proliferative phase begins 1 week after the injury and is characterized by fibroblastic proliferation, mainly within the interstitium, but also focally in the alveolar spaces (Fig. 5.10). The fibrosis consists of loose aggregates of fibroblasts admixed with scattered inflammatory cells (Fig. 5.11); collagen deposition is minimal. Reactive type II pneumocytes persist. Immature squamous metaplasia may occur (Fig. 5.12) in and around terminal bronchioles. The degree of cytologic atypia in this squamous epithelium can be so severe as to mimic malignancy (Fig. 5.13). The hyaline membranes are mostly resorbed by the late proliferative stage but a few remnants may remain along alveolar septa. Some cases of DAD resolve completely with little residual morphologic effects, but in other cases, fibrosis may progress to extensive structural remodeling and honeycomb lung. As might be expected, a recent outcomes review of 109 survivors of ARDS revealed persistent functional disability 1 year after discharge from intensive care.[10]

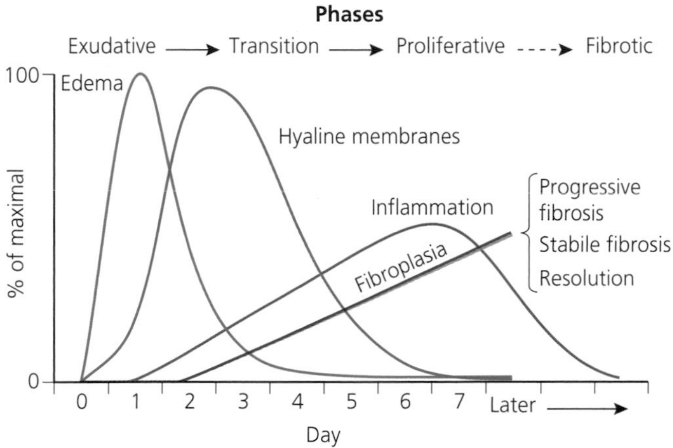

Fig. 5.1 **ARDS timeline.** The phases of ARDS are reproducible and reflect the global mechanisms of wound repair (exudation, proliferation, fibrogenesis). In experimental ARDS the exact time of injury is known and all of the lung proceeds through the phases at the same time. In a patient who develops DAD from any cause, the acute lung injury may begin in different areas at different times, so a biopsy specimen may have injury at varying phases in this sequence. (Modified after Katzenstein.[5])

It should be noted that, by definition, ARDS has a known inciting event. The above description is based on a model of ARDS due to oxygen toxicity, where the evolution of pathologic abnormalities can be studied over a defined time period.[2,5] In practice, lung biopsies are most often performed in patients without a known etiology or specific onset of injury. Moreover, some causes of ALI produce injury over a protracted period of time, or may injure the lung in a repetitive fashion (e.g.

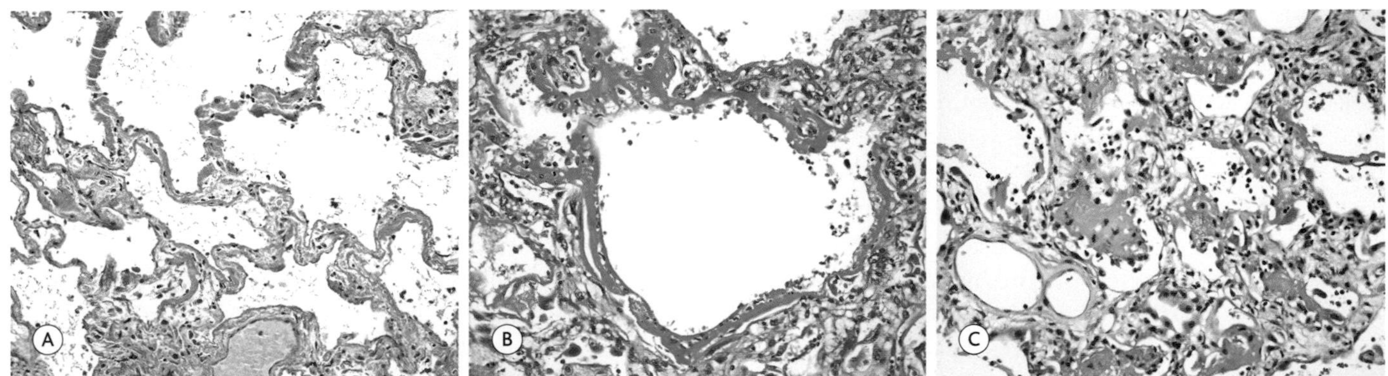

Fig. 5.2 **ARDS – exudative and proliferative phases.** (A) The early exudative phase of ARDS with some edema, cellular debris, and early hyaline membrane formation evolves to (B) well-defined hyaline membranes. Note here the increased cellularity in the interstitium, with some spindled fibroblast-like cells evident. (C) Organization of hyaline membranes occurs in the early proliferative phase. There is increased airspace cellularity at this stage.

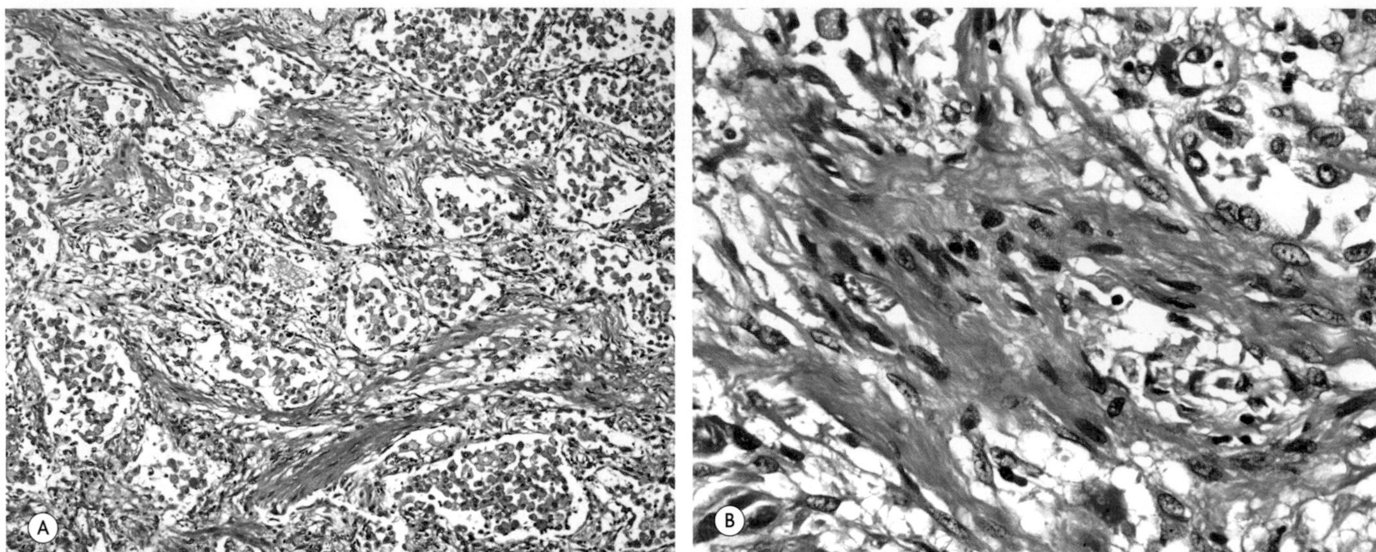

Fig. 5.3 **ARDS – late proliferative and fibrosis stages.** (A) The cellular late proliferative phase of ARDS may evolve to (B) fibrosis, with cellular fibroblastic proliferation and collagen deposition.

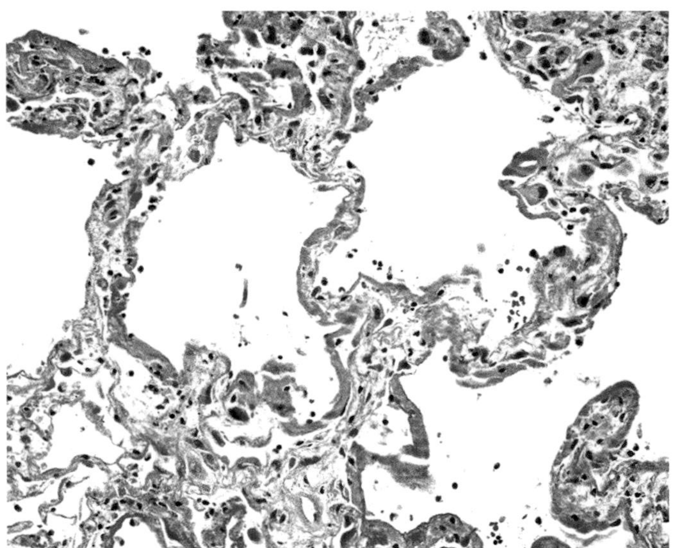

Fig. 5.4 **ARDS – early exudative phase.** Mild interstitial edema with hyaline membranes outlining alveolar spaces are characteristic findings.

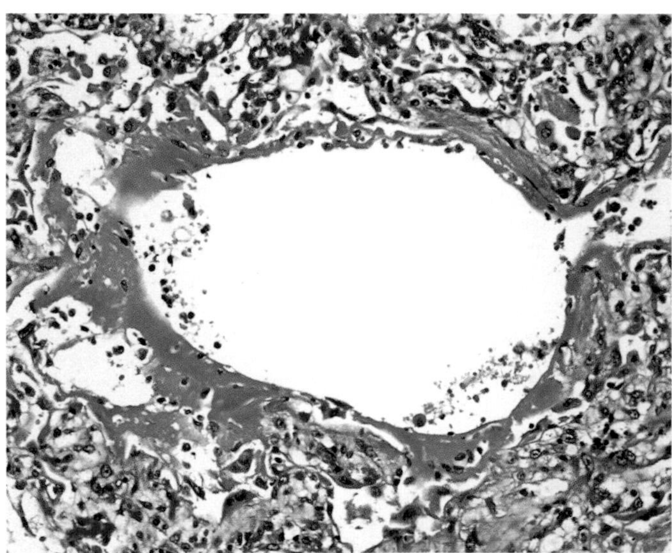

Fig. 5.5 **ARDS – hyaline membranes.** Proteinaceous alveolar exudates accumulate along the periphery of alveoli, closely adherent to alveolar wall–airspace interface.

drug toxicity). In these circumstances, the pathology does not necessarily progress sequentially through the defined stages as in ARDS, so both acute and organizing phases may be encountered in the same biopsy specimen. The basic histopathologic elements of ALI are presented in Table 5.2.

Acute fibrinous and organizing pneumonia (AFOP) is a recently recognized histopathologic pattern of acute lung injury with a similar clinical presentation to that of classical DAD, both in terms of potential etiologies as well as outcome. It differs from DAD in that hyaline membranes are absent. The dominant feature is intra-alveolar fibrin "balls" or aggregates. The distribution of these is typically patchy. Organizing pneumonia in the form of luminal loose fibroblastic tissue is present surrounding the fibrin. The alvolar septa adjacent to

Table 5.2 Defining features of acute lung injury

Interstitial (alveolar septal) edema
Fibroblastic proliferation in alveolar septa
Alveolar edema
Alveolar fibrin and cellular debris, +/- hyaline membranes
Reactive type II pneumocytes

areas of fibrin deposition show a variety of changes similar to that of DAD, such as septal edema, type II pneumocyte hyperplasia and acute and chronic inflammatory infiltrates. The intervening lung shows minimal histological changes. AFOP may represent a fibrinous variant of DAD.[10a]

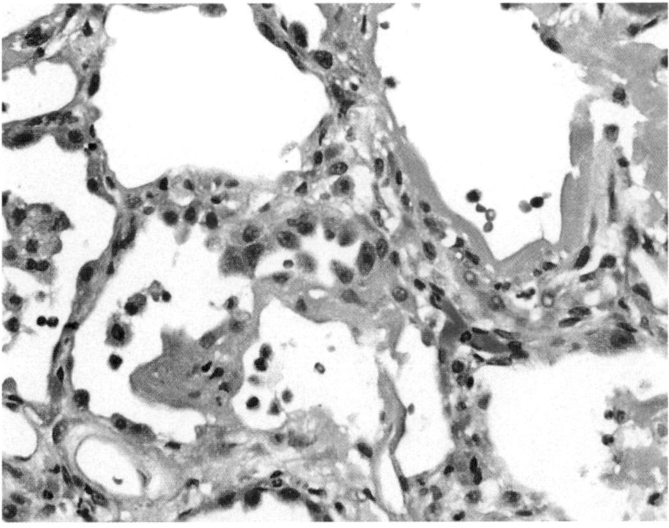

Fig. 5.6 **ARDS – mild interstitial inflammation.** In ARDS, the inciting event is frequently extrathoracic and lung injury is therefore superimposed on normal pre-existing structure.

Specific causes of acute lung injury

Infection

Infection is one of the most common causes of acute lung injury. Among infectious organisms, viruses most consistently produce DAD.[2,5] Occasionally, fungi (e.g. *Pneumocystis*), and bacteria (e.g. *Legionella*) can also present as DAD. Some of the organisms that are well known as causing acute lung injury histology are discussed here.

Viral infection

Influenza is a common cause of viral pneumonia. The pathology ranges from mild organizing acute lung injury (resembling organizing pneumonia) in non-fatal cases, to severe DAD with necrotizing tracheobronchitis (Fig. 5.14) in fatal cases.[11,12] Specific viral cytopathic effects are not identifiable by light microscopy. Ultrastructurally, intranuclear fibrillary inclusions have been found in epithelial and endothelial cells.[13]

Measles virus produces a mild pneumonia in the normal host, but can cause serious pneumonia in immunocompromised children. Pathologic features include interstitial pneumonia, bronchitis/bronchiolitis, and DAD.[14] The characteristic histology is the presence of multinucleated giant cells (Fig. 5.15A) with characteristic eosinophilic intranuclear and intracytoplasmic in-

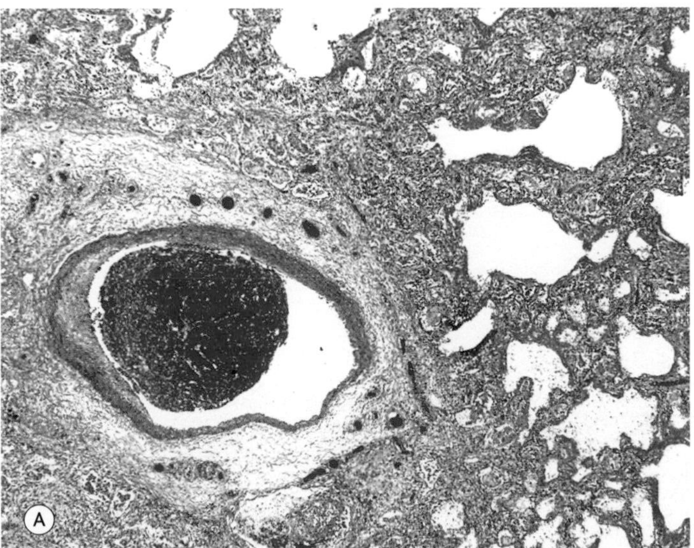

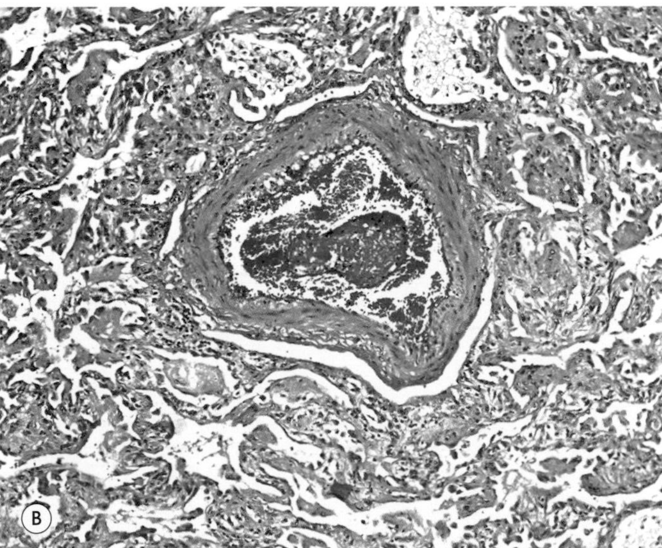

Fig. 5.7 **ARDS – fibrin thrombi in arteries.** Acute lung injury results in local conditions that lead to arterial thrombosis. Thrombi in varying stages of organization may be seen (larger pulmonary artery in A, smaller pulmonary artery in B).

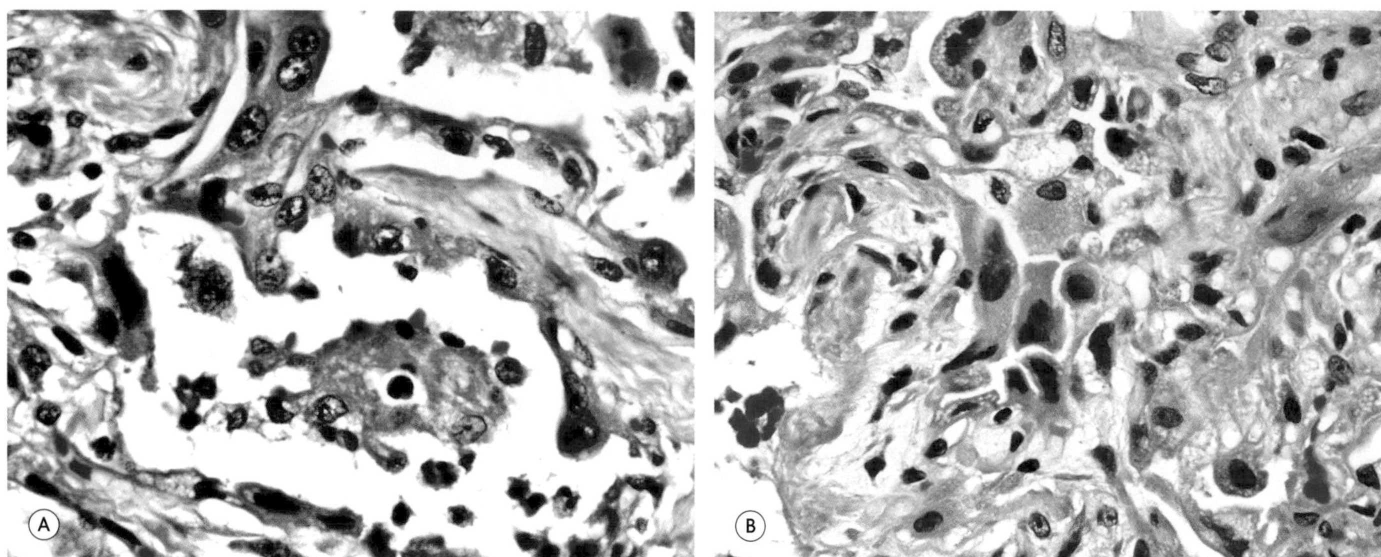

Fig. 5.8 **ARDS – type II cell hyperplasia.** Cuboidal type II cells are nearly always prominent in the late exudative phase and throughout the proliferative phase of ARDS. These hyperchromatic and enlarged epithelial cells repopulate the damaged type I cell lining of the alveolar spaces. Depending on the mechanism of injury, atypia of regenerating type II cells may be mild, moderate, or severe: (A) prominent type II cells having a "hobnail" appearance, simulating viropathic change: (B) brightly eosinophilic type II cells aggregated at the center of a collapsed alveolus. Considerable structural remodeling may take place following ARDS, as these atelectatic spaces fuse to form consolidated areas of lung parenchyma at the microscopic level.

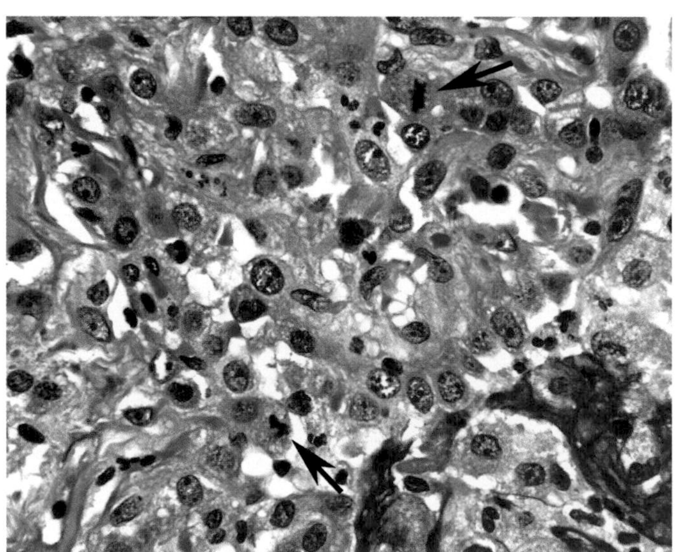

Fig. 5.9 **ARDS – mitotic figures in type II cells.** Mitotic activity can be quite brisk in all forms of acute lung injury (mitotic figures at arrows).

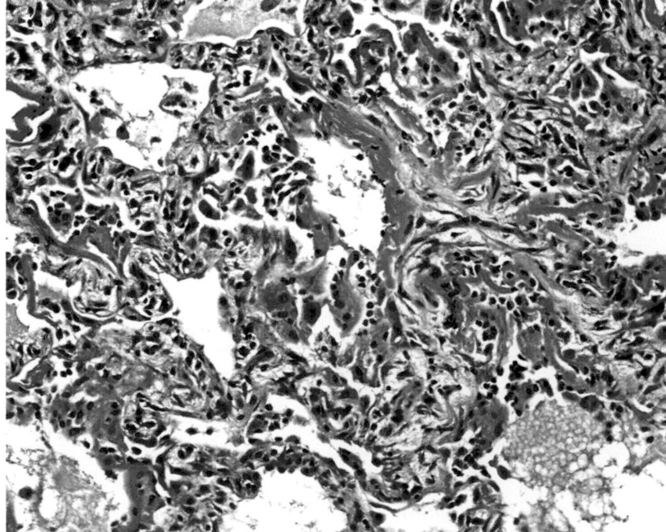

Fig. 5.10 **ARDS – fibroblastic proliferation.** Fibroblastic proliferation occurs to variable degree in both the interstitium and within airspaces in the proliferative and early fibrotic phases of ARDS.

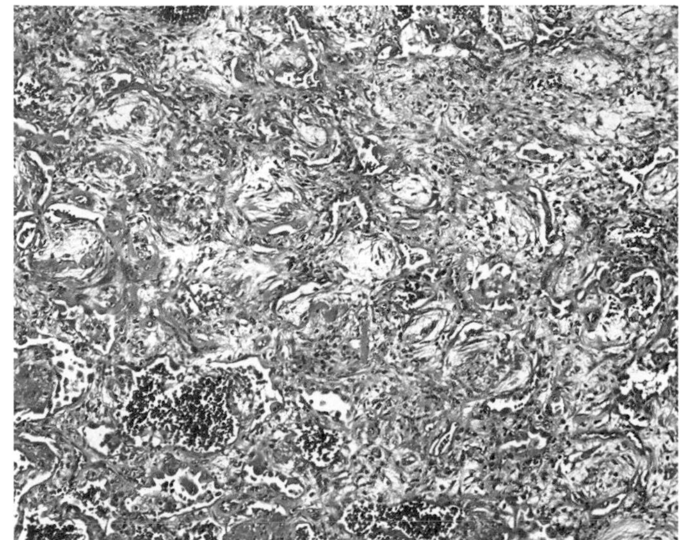

Fig. 5.11 **ARDS – airspace organization.** Organizing pneumonia-like airspace organization can be quite prominent in the late proliferative phase of ARDS.

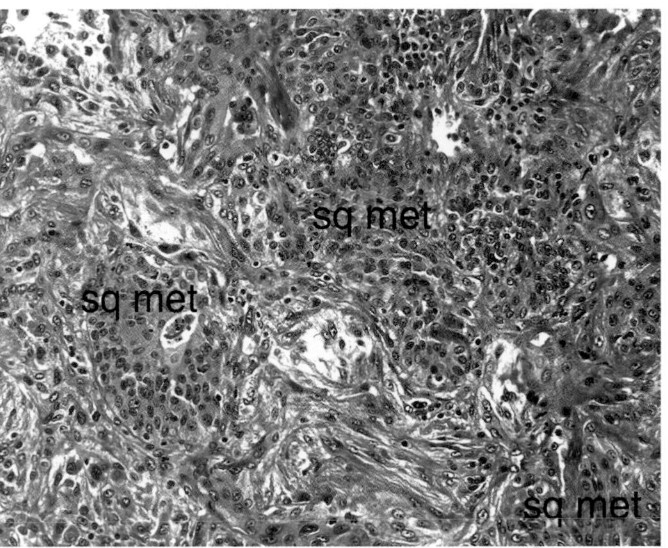

Fig. 5.13 **ARDS – squamous metaplasia.** A high magnification image of a case of ARDS with prominent squamous metaplasia (sq met). In some instances squamous metaplasia may be so prominent as to suggest neoplasm.

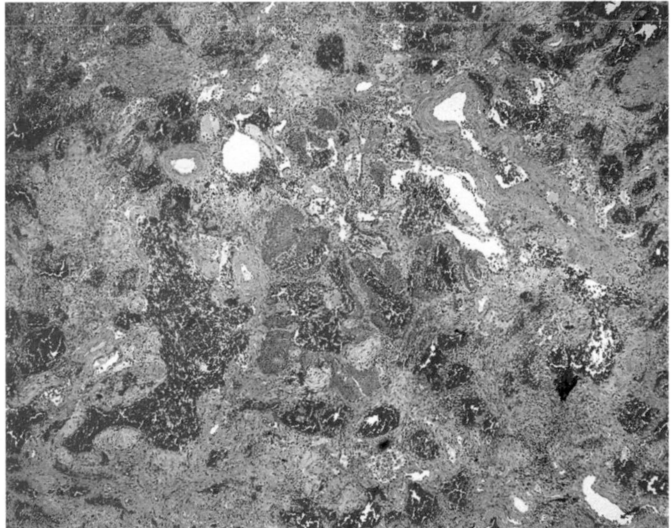

Fig. 5.12 **ARDS – squamous metaplasia.** Squamous metaplasia of terminal airways may occur as a subacute proliferative event in ARDS and other forms of diffuse alveolar damage. The nested squamous epithelium is often nodular, appearing at scanning magnification by virtue of patchy terminal airway involvement.

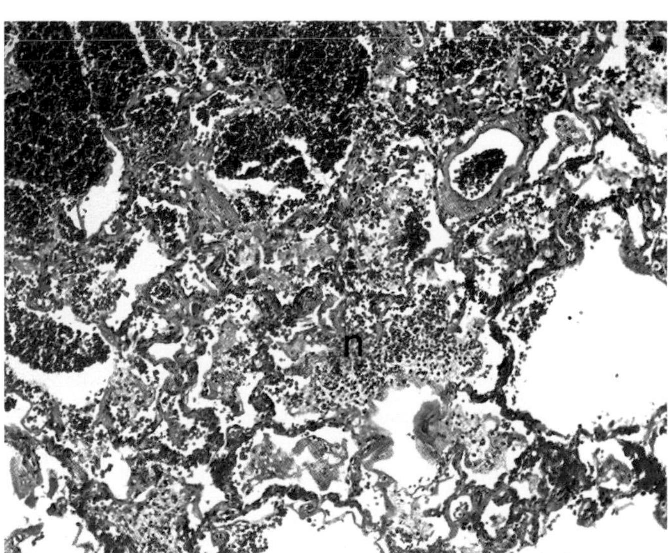

Fig. 5.14 **DAD – influenza pneumonia.** Influenza pneumonia produces a fibrinous and focally neutrophilic diffuse alveolar damage. Note the sparse neutrophils present in an airspace (n), and abundant blood in this case of influenza pneumonia. No specific inclusions are produced by the influenza viruses.

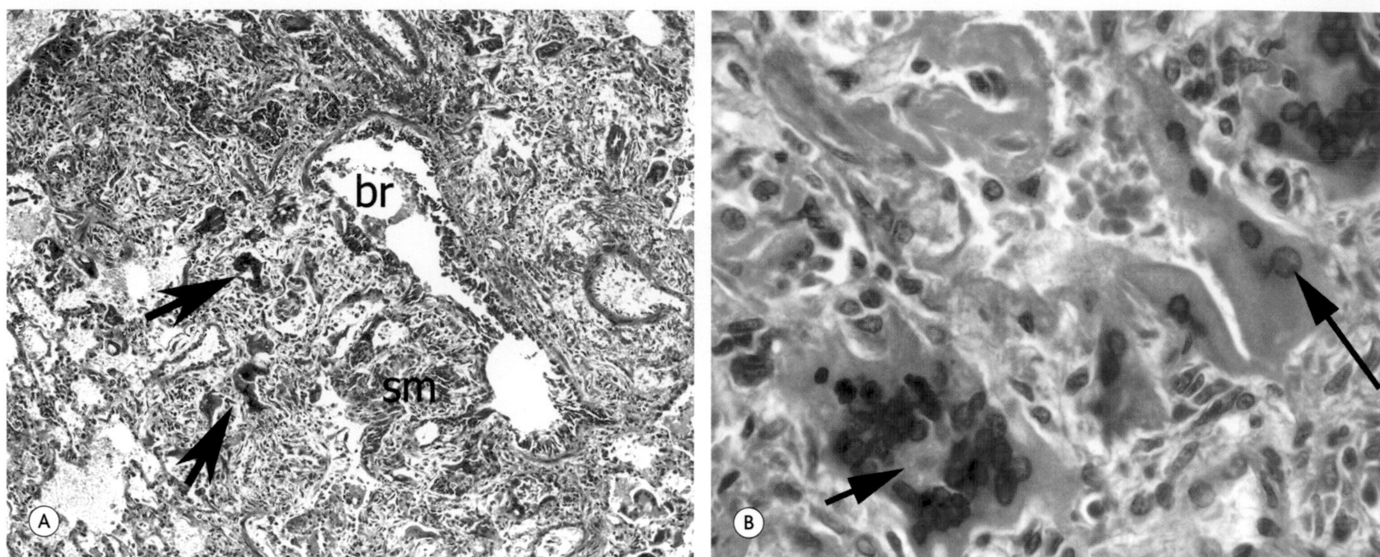

Fig. 5.15 **DAD – measles pneumonia.** (A) A terminal airway (br) in a case of acute measles pneumonia with diffuse alveolar damage. Squamous metaplasia of the airway is also present (sm). The arrows denote multinucleated giant cells, present here in a bronchiolocentric distribution. (B) The characteristic multinucleated giant cells of measles pneumonia. Note the glassy intranuclear inclusions (long arrow) and occasional eosinophilic cytoplasmic inclusions (short arrow).

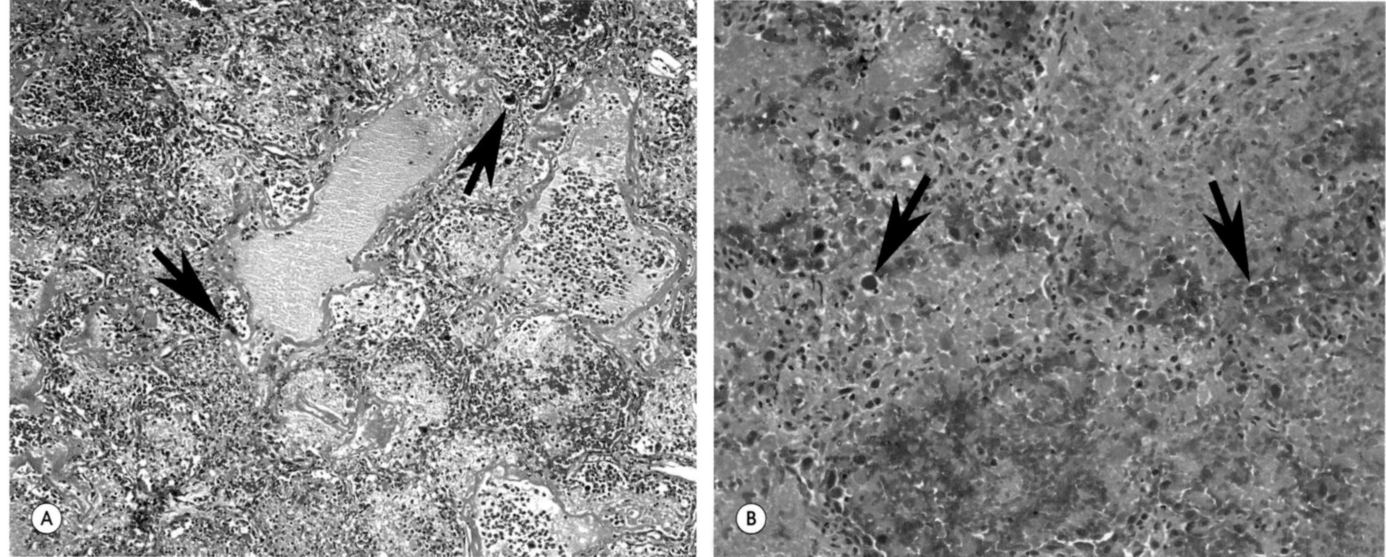

Fig. 5.16 **DAD – adenovirus pneumonia.** Adenovirus produces necrotizing bronchitis/bronchiolitis and this is especially prominent in the setting of diffuse alveolar damage caused by this infection. The "smudge cells" of adenovirus infection can be seen at scanning magnification (A; arrows) in this case of DAD produced by adenovirus pneumonia. (B) Smudge cells at higher magnification (arrows).

clusions.[14–18] These cells are found in the alveolar spaces and within alveolar septa (Fig. 5.15B). Viral inclusions are seen ultrastructurally as tightly packed tubules.[18]

Adenovirus is an important cause of lower respiratory tract disease in children,[19,20] although adults (particularly those who are immunocompromised)[21] and military recruits are also occasionally affected.[22] The lung shows necrotizing bronchitis/bronchiolitis accompanied by DAD. The pathologic changes are more severe in bronchi, bronchioles, and peribronchiolar regions (Fig. 5.16A). Two types of inclusions can be observed in lung epithelial cells. An eosinophilic intranuclear inclusion with a halo is usually less conspicuous than the more readily identifiable "smudge cells" (Fig. 5.16B). These latter cells are larger than normal, entirely basophilic, and have no defined inclusion or halo by light microscopy.[19] Ultrastructurally, smudge cell inclusions are represented by arrays of hexagonal particles.[23]

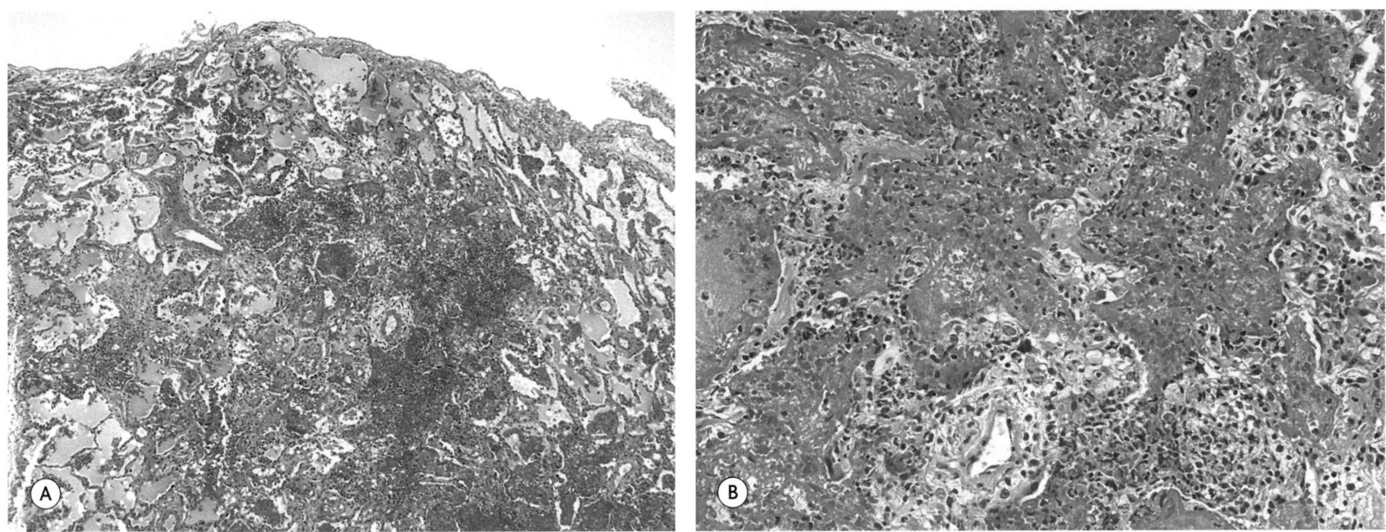

Fig. 5.17 **DAD – Herpes simplex pneumonia.** The Herpesviridae produce nodular necrotizing pneumonia (see Chapter 6). (A) The nodular appearance of herpes simplex pneumonia is evident with zonal areas of hemorrhage and necrosis. (B) A higher magnification view of the hemorrhagic and necrotizing pneumonia produced by herpes simplex.

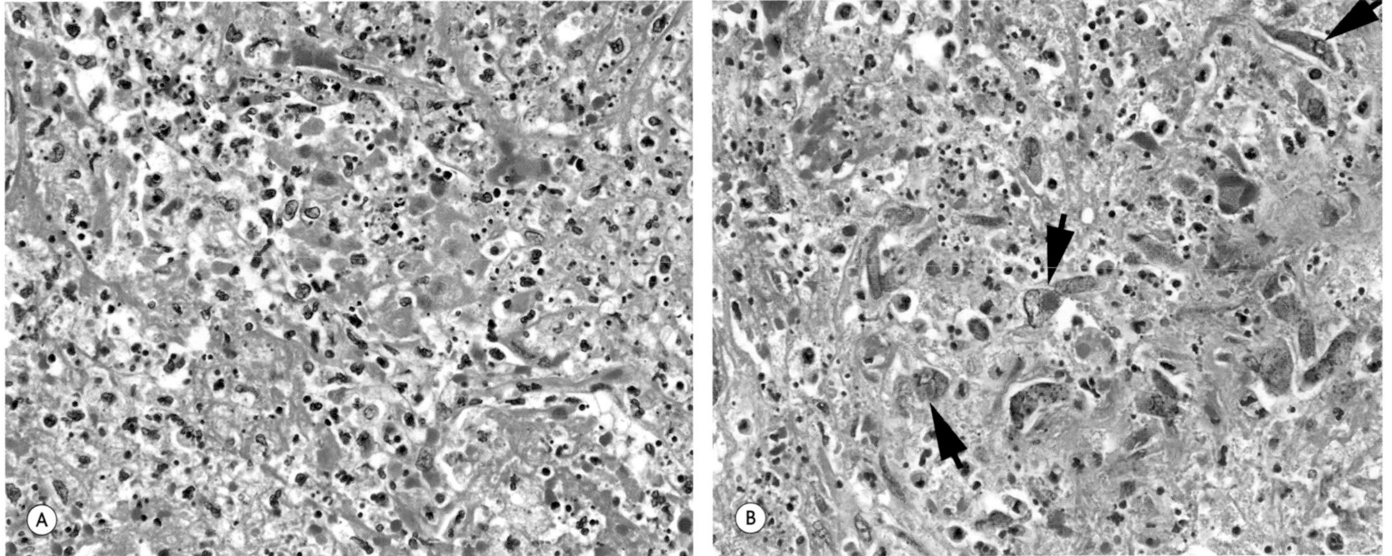

Fig. 5.18 **Herpes simplex pneumonia – inclusions.** (A) Diffuse alveolar damage caused by herpes pneumonia. (B) The viral cytopathic effects of herpes pneumonia, where the classic Cowdry A intranuclear inclusions (short arrows) are usually easy to find, compared to the basophilic, smudged or ground-glass, nuclear inclusion (Cowdry B).

Herpes simplex virus is mainly a cause of respiratory infection in the immunocompromised host. There are two patterns of infection: airway spread that results in necrotizing tracheobronchitis (Fig. 5.17), and blood-borne dissemination that produces miliary necrotic parenchymal nodules. DAD and hemorrhage can occur in both forms.[24,25] Characteristic inclusions may be seen in bronchial and alveolar epithelial cells (Fig. 5.18). The more obvious is an intranuclear eosinophilic inclusion surrounded by clear halo (Cowdry A) and the other is represented by a basophilic to amphophilic ground glass nucleus (Cowdry B). Rounded viral particles with double membranes are seen under the electron microscope.[24,25]

Varicella-zoster virus predominantly affects children and is the cause of chickenpox.[26] Pulmonary complications rarely occur in children with normal immunity (less than 1%). However, 15% of adults with chickenpox develop pneumonia, and both immunocompetent and immuno-compromised individuals are equally affected.[22,26] The histopathology of varicella pneumonia (Fig. 5.19) is

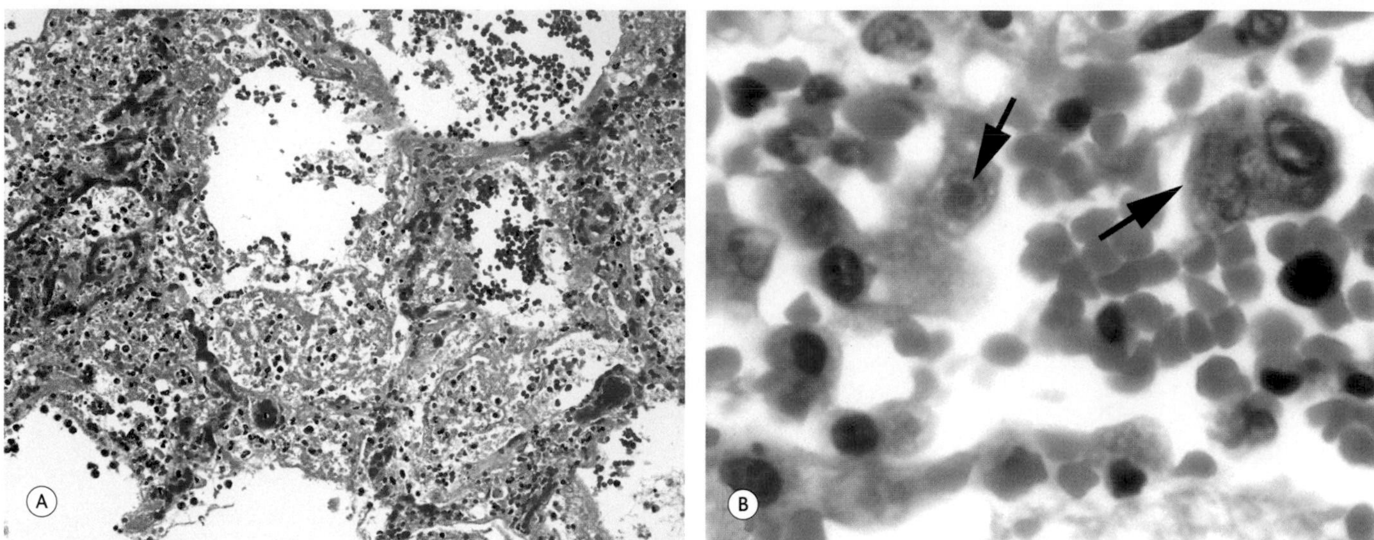

Fig. 5.19 **DAD – varicella-zoster.** The inclusions are similar to those produced by herpes simplex. (A) A fibrinous diffuse alveolar damage with neutrophils in airspaces in a case of chickenpox pneumonia. (B) The rare intranuclear eosinophilic inclusions identifiable in this infection (arrows).

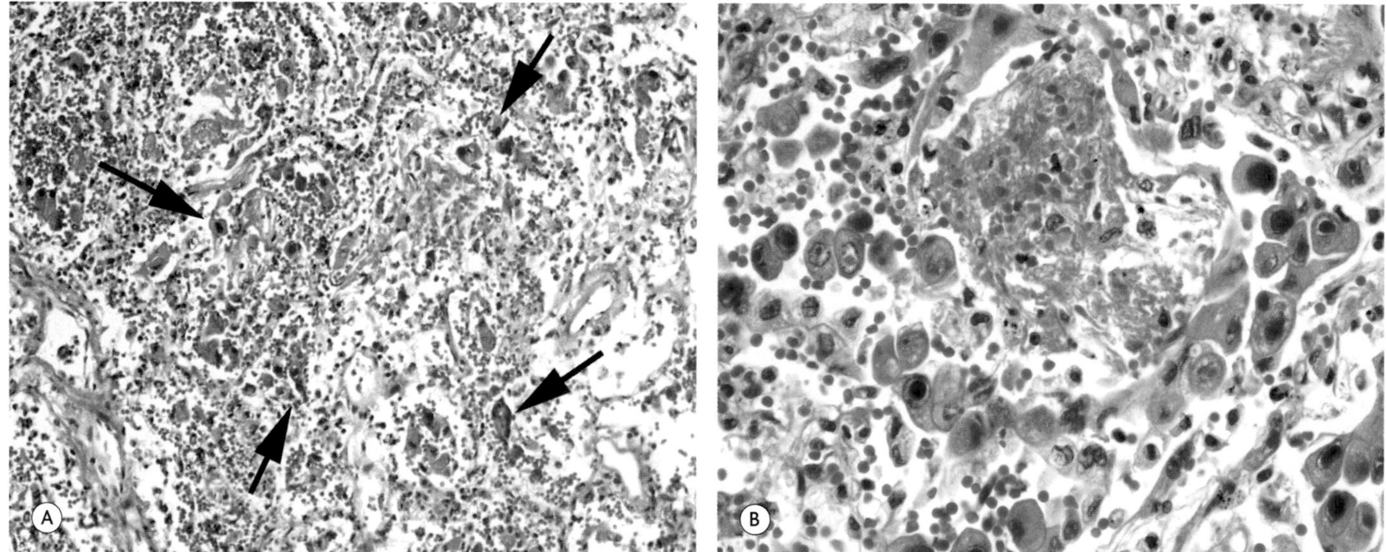

Fig. 5.20 **DAD – CMV pneumonia.** Diffuse alveolar damage produced by CMV infection can be quite dramatic in the immunocompromised host. (A) DAD with numerous CMV cells evident at scanning magnification (arrows). (B) These CMV infected cells at higher magnification, with their prominent intranuclear inclusions evident.

similar to that of herpes simplex. While identical intranuclear inclusions are reported to occur,[22,26] these can be considerably more difficult to identify in chickenpox pneumonia.

Cytomegalovirus is an important cause of symptomatic pneumonia in the immunocompromised host, especially those who have received bone marrow or solid organ transplants, and those with HIV infection.[27–29] The pathology varies from little or no inflammatory response to hemorrhagic nodules with necrosis (Fig. 5.20A) and DAD.[27] The diagnostic feature is seen in endothelial cells, macrophages and epithelial cells and consists of cellular enlargement, a prominent intranuclear inclusion and an intracytoplasmic basophilic inclusion (Fig. 5.20B).[27]

Hantavirus is a rare cause of ALI.[30–32] The infection produces alveolar edema, hyaline membranes, and atypical interstitial mononuclear inflammatory infiltrates (Fig. 5.21).[30–32] Spherical membrane-bound viral particles have been found in the cytoplasm of endothelial cells by electron microscopy.

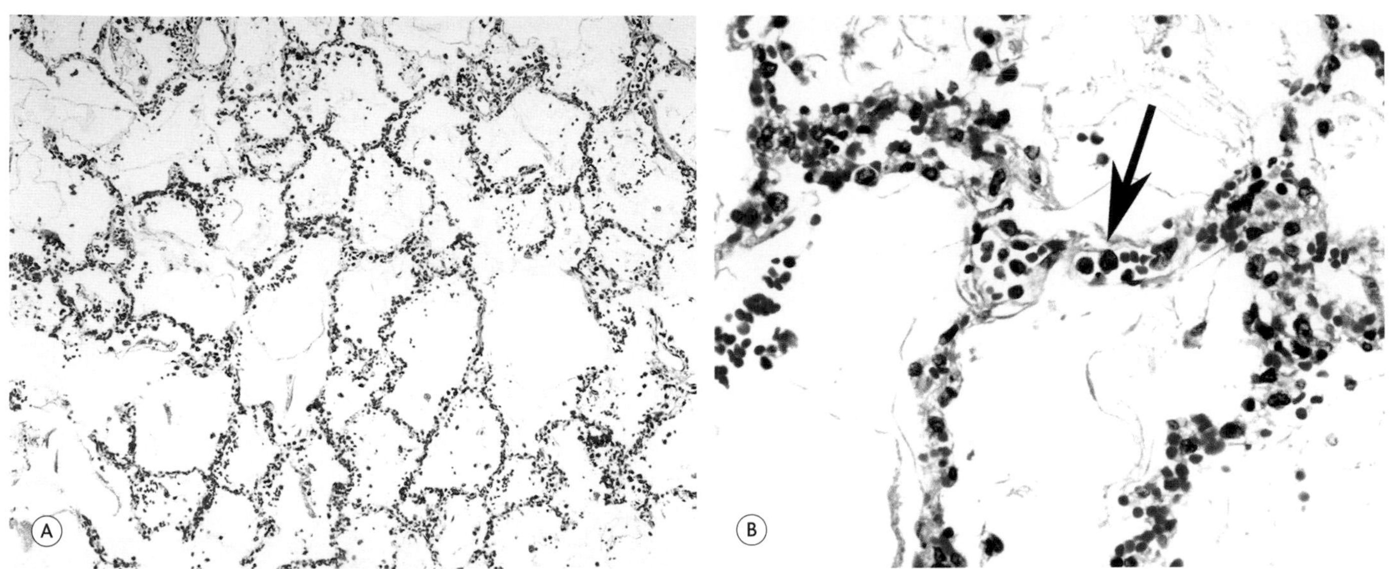

Fig. 5.21 **DAD – Hantavirus pneumonia.** Hantavirus pneumonia is characterized by alveolar edema, hyaline membranes (A), and scattered atypical interstitial mononuclear cells (B, arrow).

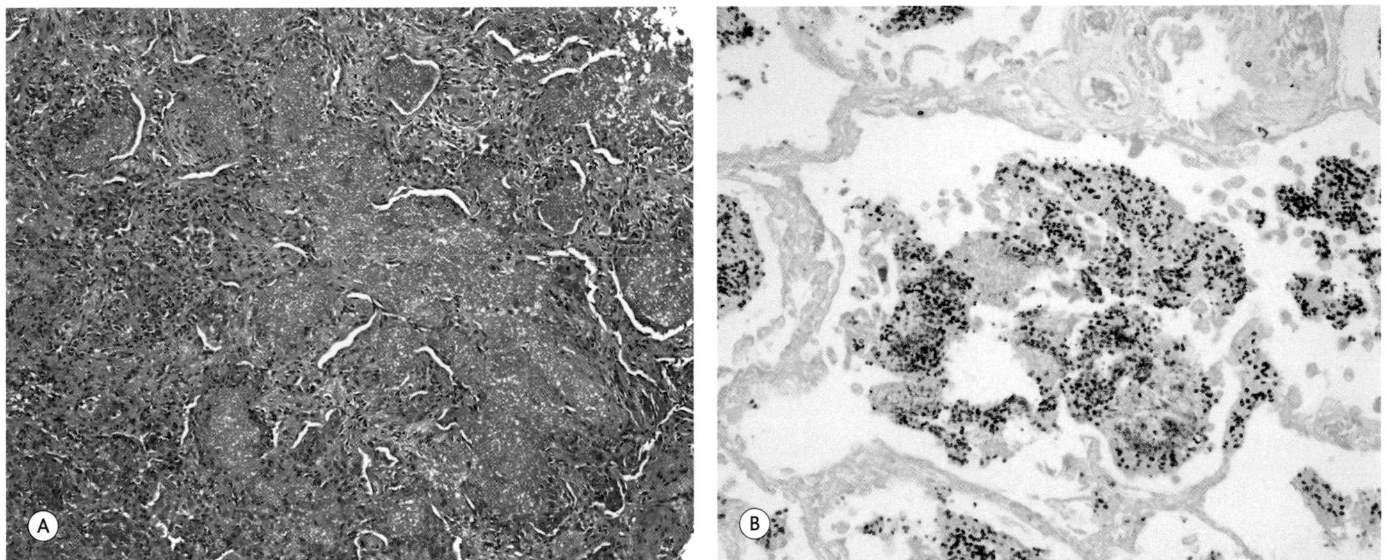

Fig. 5.22 **DAD – pneumocystis pneumonia.** (A) The characteristic frothy "alveolar casts" of pneumocystis pneumonia in the profoundly immunocompromised host (classically AIDS in HIV infection). Numerous silver-stained organisms are evident within these eosinophilic exudates (B, methenamine silver stain).

Fungal infection

Pneumocystis jiroveci (previously known as *Pneumocystis carinii*) is the most common fungus to cause DAD.[33–35] The histology of pneumocystis infection in the setting of profound immunodeficiency is that of frothy intra-alveolar exudates (Fig. 5.22A) (so-called "alveolar casts"), with many organisms (Fig. 5.22B).[34,35] However, in the mildly immunocompromised patient this feature is not observed or may be subtle. In such individuals several "atypical" manifestations are described.[33,35,36] DAD is the most dramatic of these atypical presentations (Fig. 5.23A), with the organisms present within hyaline membranes (Fig. 5.23B) and in isolated intra-alveolar fibrin deposits.[36] The Grocott's methenamine silver method (GMS) is routinely used to stain the organisms, which typically occur in small groups and clusters (Figs 5.22B and 5.23B).[33,35,36]

Bacterial infection

Common bacterial pneumonias rarely cause DAD; however, this lung injury pattern has been described in legionnaires' disease, *Mycoplasma* pneumonia, and *Rickettsia* infection.[37–41]

Legionella is a fastidious Gram-negative bacillus that causes acute respiratory infection in elderly and immunodeficient individuals.[37,38,41] The histopathology is that of a pyogenic necrotizing bronchopneumonia (Fig. 5.24A) that affects the respiratory bronchioles, alveolar ducts, and adjacent alveolar spaces. DAD commonly occurs.[37,38,41] The rod-shaped organisms (Fig. 5.24B) can be identified by Dieterle silver stain.[41]

It should be noted that in immunocompromised patients, any type of infection can cause DAD, with pneumocystis pneumonia being the most common.[18] For

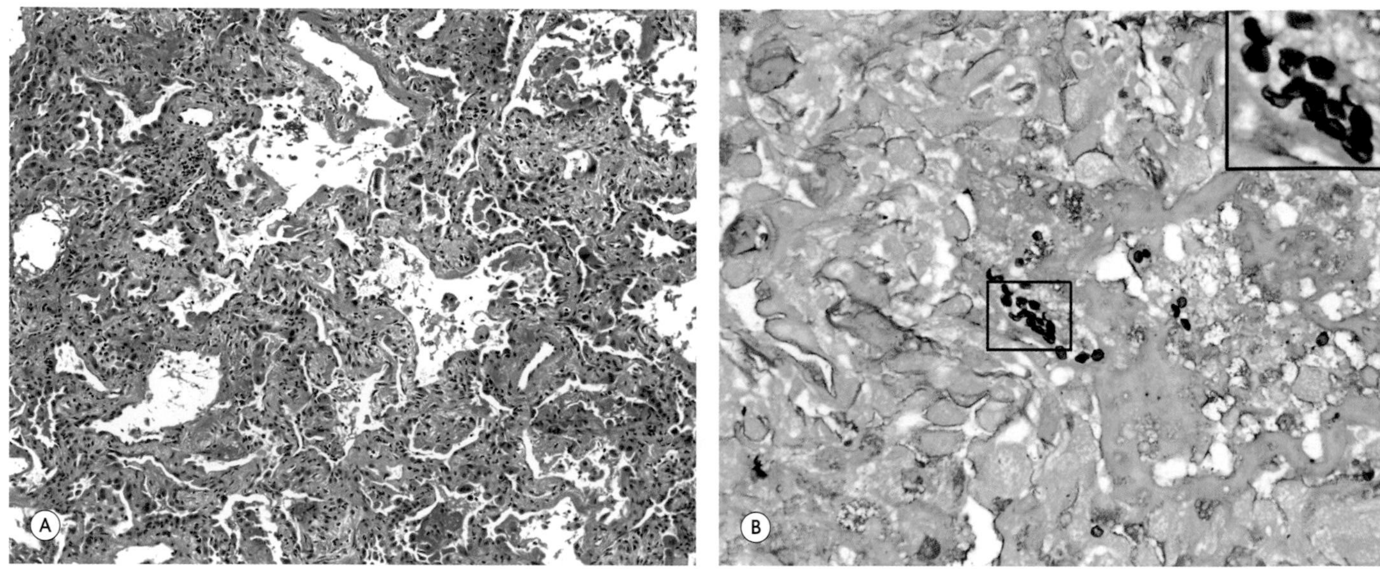

Fig. 5.23 **DAD – pneumocystis pneumonia.** (A) In patients less severely immunocompromised, diffuse alveolar damage may occur, with few organisms identifiable by silver stains (B, methenamine silver stain). A colony of pneumocystis is shown in the inset (upper right corner).

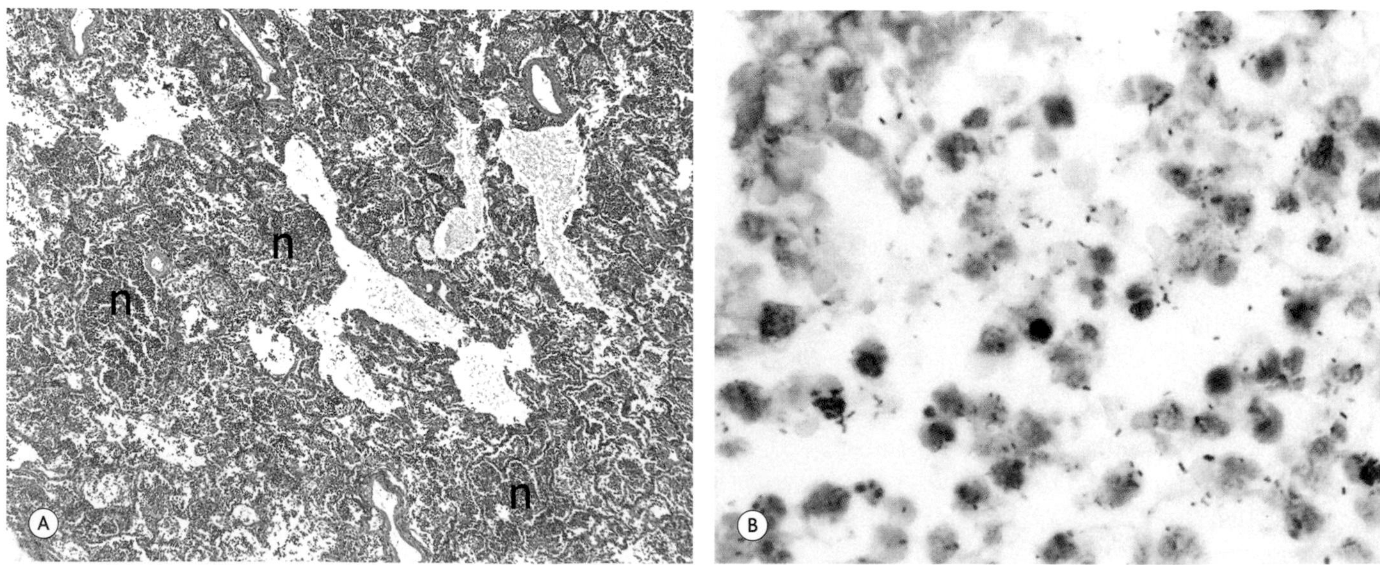

Fig. 5.24 **DAD – *Legionella* pneumonia.** (A) The diffuse alveolar damage caused by *Legionella* infection is prominently neutrophilic (n). Within these areas, a silver stain shows numerous rod-shaped stained organisms (B, Dieterle silver method).

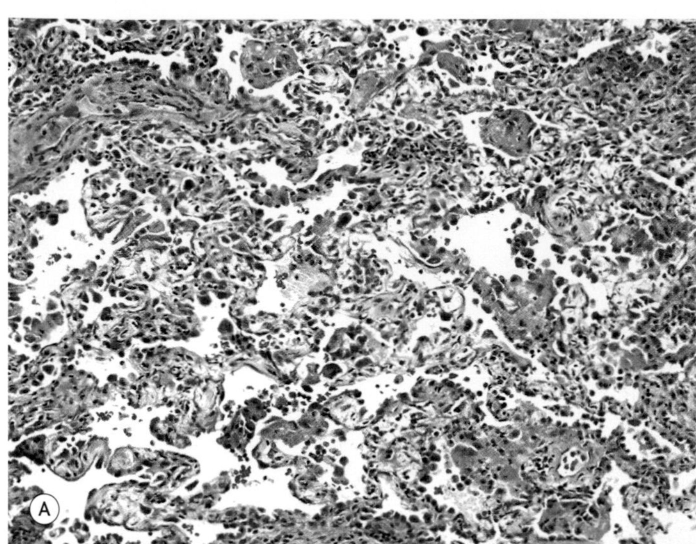

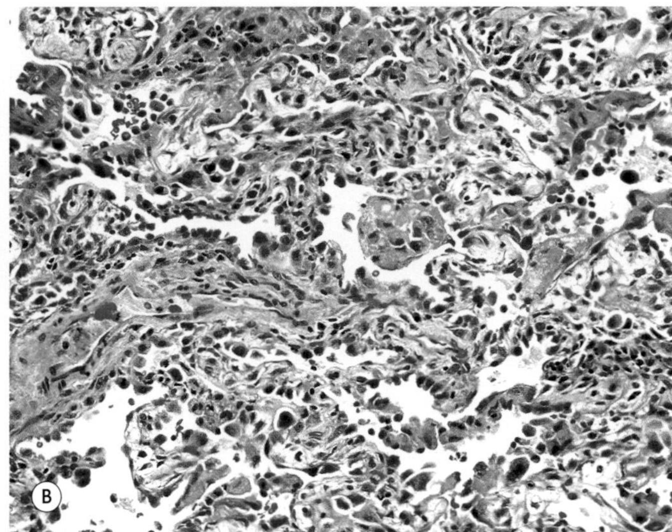

Fig. 5.25 **DAD in SLE.** The diffuse alveolar damage associated with lupus may be quite hemorrhagic and associated with a "pneumonitis". Note the increased mononuclear cells within the alveolar interstitium in both A and B. Sometimes the alveolar hemorrhage of SLE may overlap with diffuse alveolar damage on morphologic grounds.

this reason, it is essential to perform special stains (AFB, GMS, Warthin–Starry, etc.) on every lung biopsy with DAD.

Collagen vascular diseases

Systemic collagen vascular disorders are a well-known cause of diffuse lung disease.[42–49] In some cases, lung involvement may be the first manifestation of the systemic disease, even without identifiable serologic evidence.[47] Acute lung injury has been reported to occur in the following collagen vascular diseases.

Systemic lupus erythematosus

Pulmonary manifestations in systemic lupus erythematosus (SLE) may present as pleural disease, acute or chronic diffuse inflammatory lung disease, airway disease and/or vascular disease (vasculitis and thromboembolic lesions). Acute lupus pneumonitis (ALP) is a form of fulminant interstitial disease (Fig. 5.25A) with a high mortality rate.[42] Patients present with severe dyspnea, tachypnea, fever, and arterial hypoxemia. ALP represents the first manifestation of SLE in about 50% of individuals affected.[42,48] The most common pathology of this acute disease is DAD. Alveolar hemorrhage, with capillaritis and small vessel vasculitis (Fig. 5.25B), and pulmonary edema, are also observed.[42,47,50] Immunofluorescence studies demonstrate immune complexes in lung parenchyma and both immune complexes and tubuloreticular inclusions may be seen ultrastructurally.[47,48,50]

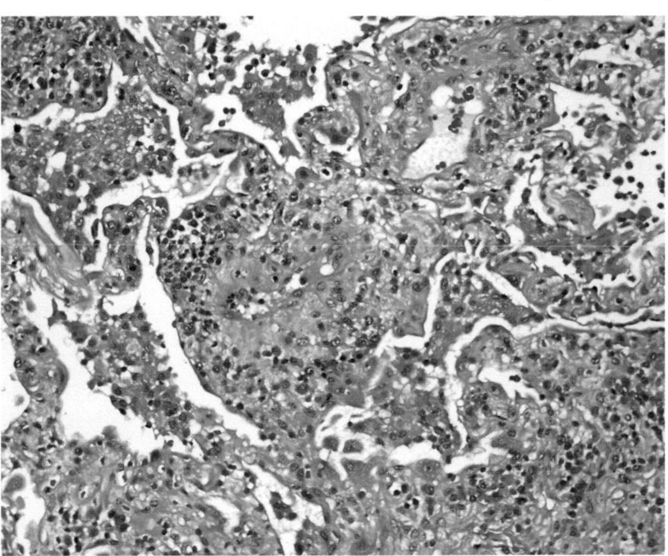

Fig. 5.26 **DAD in RA.** When diffuse alveolar damage occurs in rheumatoid arthritis, sometimes hints at more chronic disease may be present, with lymphoplasmacellular infiltrates, chronic bronchiolitis, and chronic pleuritis. Here, a perivascular lymphoplasmacellular infiltrate is evident with surrounding airspace fibrin and macrophages.

Rheumatoid arthritis

A significant percentage of patients with rheumatoid arthritis (RA) have lung disease.[43,44,51–54] There are many different morphologic patterns of lung disease in RA,[44,47,49] with the rheumatoid nodule being the most specific. Acute lung injury has been reported (Fig. 5.26); it is referred to as acute interstitial pneumonia (AIP) in some publications[55] and DAD in others.[44]

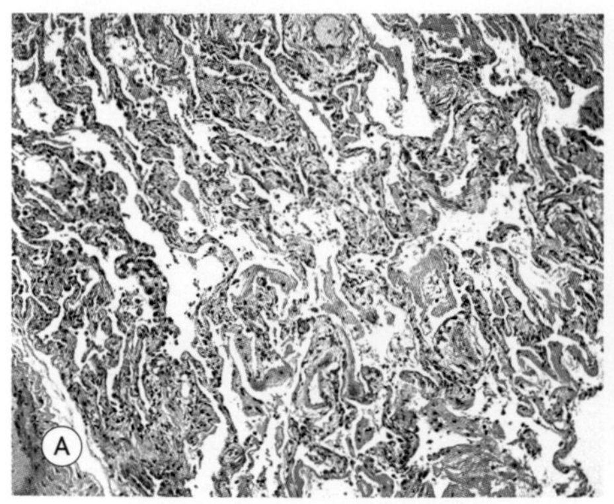

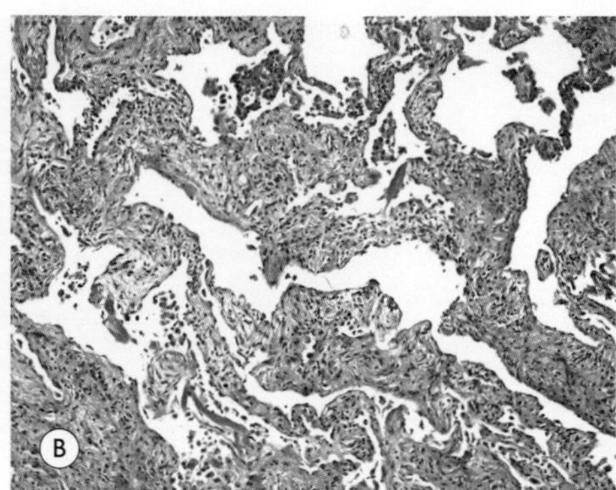

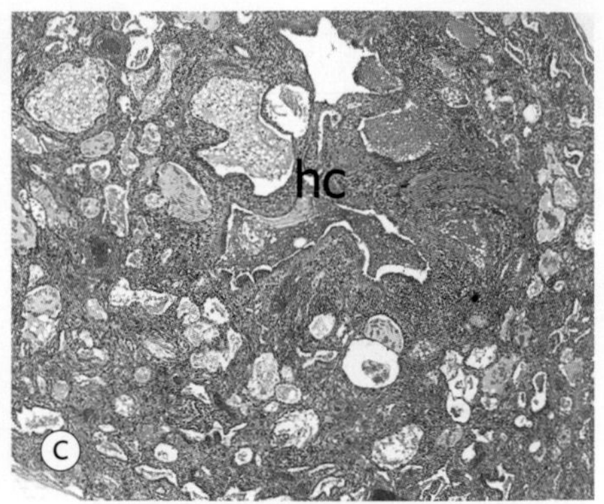

Fig. 5.27 **DAD in PM/DM.** All of the systemic connective tissue diseases can manifest acute, subacute, and chronic lung disease. Three examples of diffuse lung disease accompanying polymyositis/dermatomyositis are presented. (A) DAD occurring in PM/DM; (B) a subacute organizing pneumonia with an interstitial mononuclear infiltrate (NSIP-like – see Chapter 7); and (C) a UIP-like pattern of lung fibrosis with microscopic honeycomb remodeling (hc).

Polymyositis/dermatomyositis

This systemic connective tissue disorder is well known to be associated with interstitial lung disease.[45,46] Three main clinical presentations include:

1. acute fulminant respiratory distress, resembling Hamman–Rich syndrome
2. slowly progressive dyspnea
3. an asymptomatic form, with abnormal radiologic findings and pulmonary function studies.[49]

Three major patterns of histopathology have been observed, including DAD (Fig. 5.27A), organizing pneumonia (Fig. 5.27B), and chronic fibrosis (Fig. 5.27C) (UIP pattern).[56] The rapidly progressive clinical presentation shows DAD histology on lung biopsy and carries the worst prognosis.[46]

Scleroderma and mixed connective disease diffuse alveolar damage

In scleroderma and mixed connective disease, DAD has been reported to occur.[47,57] Many patients with collagen vascular disease receive drug therapy during the course of their illness. A large number of drugs (including cytotoxic agents used for immunosuppression) are known to cause DAD. Also, as a desired result of therapy, patients may be immunosuppressed, making the exclusion of infection a high priority in the case of acute clinical lung disease.

Drug effect

Drugs can produce a wide range of lung manifestations and the causative agents are numerous.[58–71] The spectrum of drug-induced lung disease runs the entire gamut, from DAD to fibrosis. Between these two extremes, subacute clinical manifestations occur, including organizing pneumonia, chronic interstitial pneumonia, eosinophilic pneumonia, obliterative bronchiolitis, pulmonary hemorrhage, pulmonary edema, pulmonary hypertension, veno-occlusive disease, and granulomatous interstitial pneumonia.[68,72,73]

DAD is a common and dramatic manifestation of pulmonary drug toxicity.[68] Many drugs are known to cause DAD.[72] A few of the more common ones are discussed below.

Chemotherapeutic agents

DAD is frequently caused by cytotoxic drugs and the commonly implicated ones include bleomycin (Fig. 5.28), busulfan (Fig. 5.29), and carmustine.[5,68,72] Patients usually present with dyspnea, cough, and diffuse pulmonary infiltrates.[74–78] The histology is most commonly represented by nonspecific acute lung injury with hyaline membranes, but some changes may be present to at least suggest a causative agent. For example, the presence of acute lung injury with associated atypical type II pneumocytes with markedly enlarged pleomorphic nuclei[79] and prominent nucleoli (Fig. 5.29) are characteristic for busulfan-induced pulmonary toxicity, and ultrastructural intranuclear tubular structures have been found in type II pneumocytes associated with busulfan and bleomycin.[79–82] In most cases, the possibility that a drug is the cause of DAD can only be inferred from the clinical history. The differential diagnosis typically includes other treatment-related injury or complication of therapy (e.g. concomitant irradiation or infection). For example, oxygen therapy is a well-recognized cause of DAD (Fig. 5.30), and also may

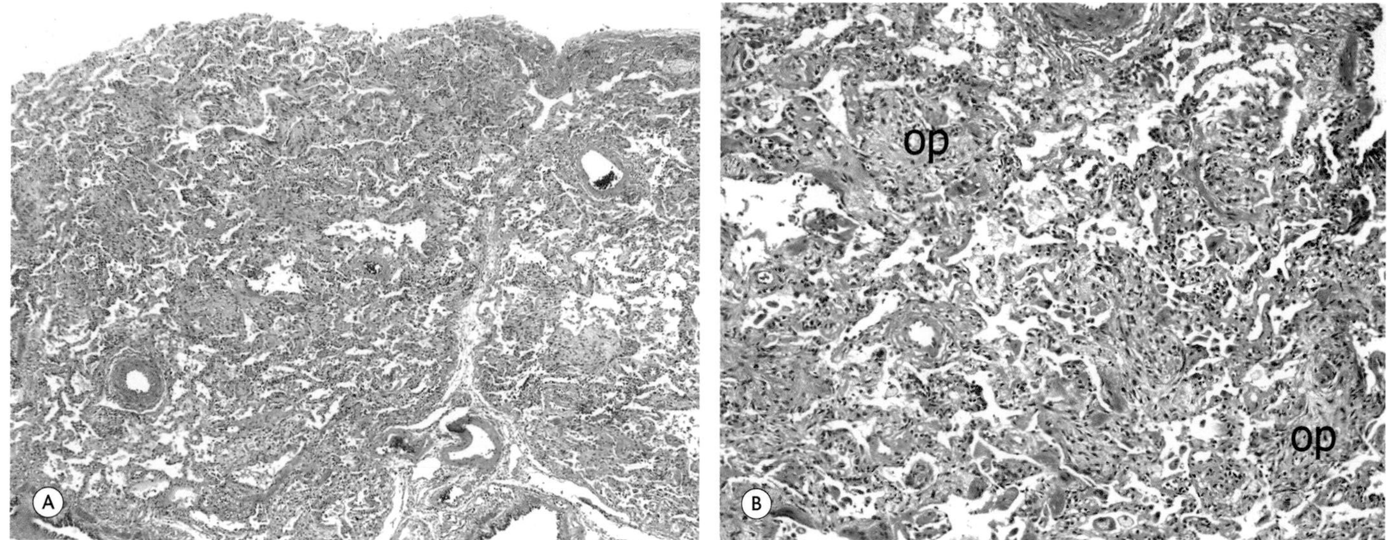

Fig. 5.28 **DAD – bleomycin toxicity.** Bleomycin produces a characteristic lung injury in experimental animal models. (A) In humans, DAD may occur often typified by (B) the presence of reactive type II cells and organizing pneumonia (op).

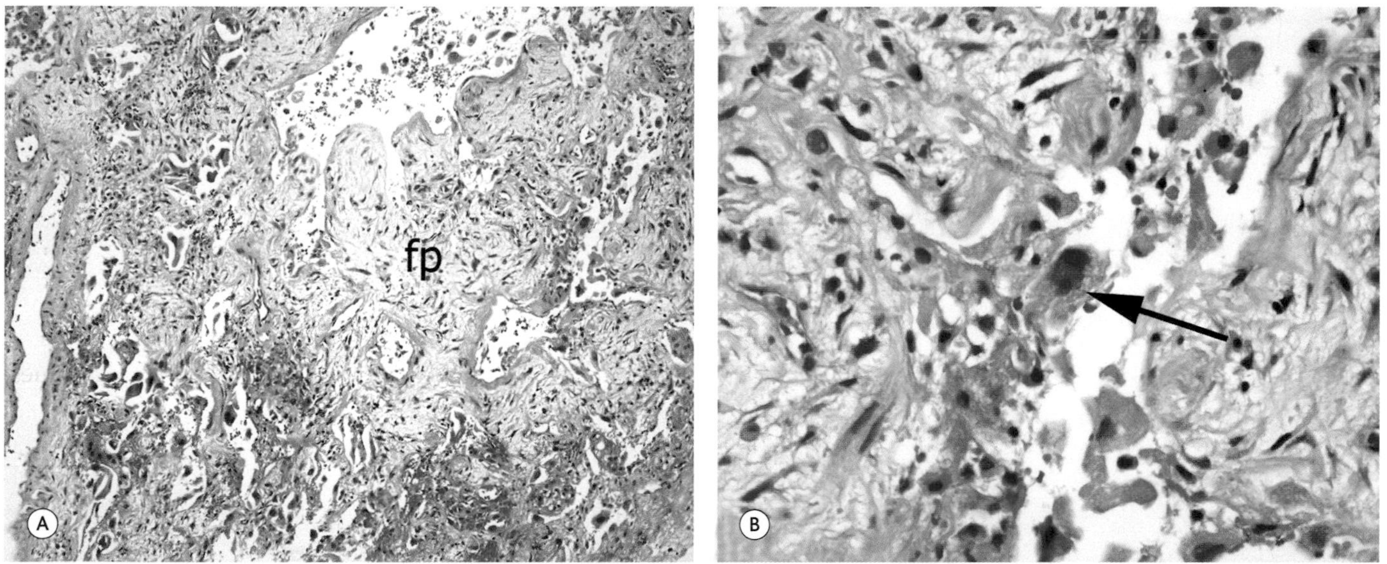

Fig. 5.29 **DAD – busulfan toxicity.** (A,B) Busulfan can produce DAD characterized by the presence of prominently atypical type II cells. In this case, prominent interstitial organization with edematous fibroblastic proliferation is seen (fp) and hyaline membranes are evident. Reactive type II cells (B) may appear alarmingly atypical (arrow).

exacerbate bleomycin-induced lung injury.[83] Methotrexate (Fig. 5.31) is another commonly used cytotoxic drug that can cause acute and organizing DAD.[84] Methotrexate also produces other distinctive patterns, such as granulomatous interstitial pneumonia (see Ch. 7), which is seldom seen in association with other commonly used chemotherapeutic agents. To complicate matters further, methotrexate is also used in the treatment of rheumatoid arthritis, a disease known to independently produce DAD as one of its pulmonary manifestations.[47,52]

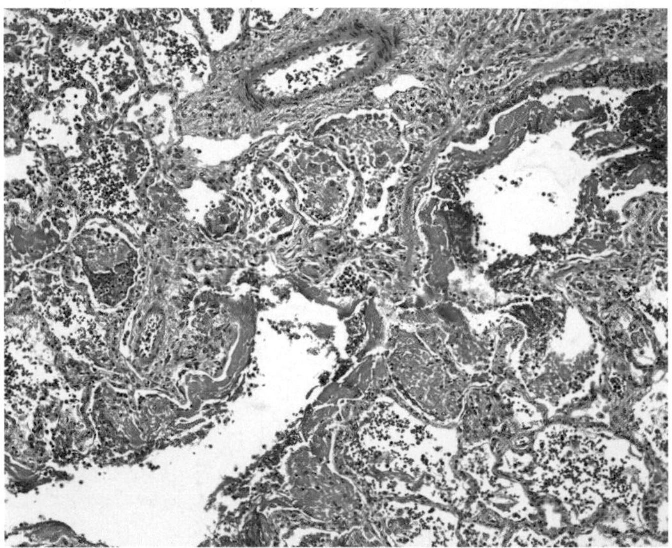

Fig. 5.30 **DAD – oxygen toxicity.** Classic oxygen toxicity causes DAD and necrosis of terminal airway epithelium as illustrated in this photomicrograph.

Amiodarone

This highly effective anti-arrhythmic drug is increasingly recognized as a cause of pulmonary toxicity.[67,85–89]

Because patients taking amiodarone have known cardiac disease, they often present with a complicated clinical picture, with several superimposed processes potentially affecting the lungs in various ways. Clinical and radiologic considerations typically include congestive heart failure, pulmonary emboli, and acute lung injury due to other causes.[67,89]

Distinctive features may be present on chest CT scans (see Ch. 3).[67] The lung biopsy commonly shows acute and organizing lung injury (Fig. 5.32A). Other patterns include chronic interstitial pneumonitis with fibrosis, and organizing pneumonia.[87] Characteristically, type II pneumocytes and alveolar macrophages show finely vacuolated cytoplasm in response to amiodarone therapy (Fig. 5.32B), but these changes alone are not evidence of toxicity since they may also be seen in patients taking amiodarone who do not have clinical lung toxicity.[85–88]

Anti-inflammatory drugs

Methotrexate and gold, common therapies for patients with rheumatoid arthritis, are most frequently implicated in lung toxicity. Methotrexate has been discussed earlier

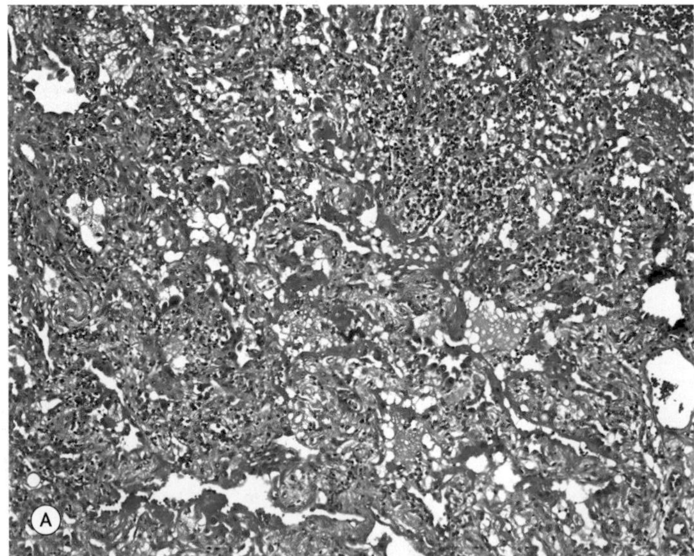

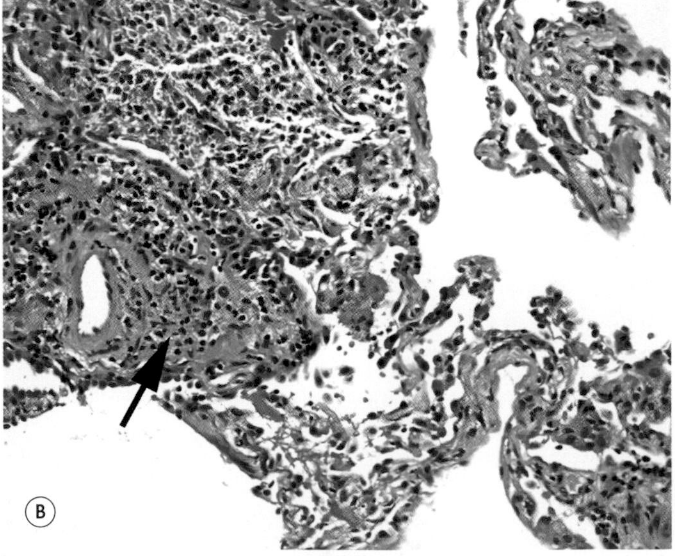

Fig. 5.31 **DAD – methotrexate toxicity.** (A,B) Methotrexate produces small poorly formed granulomas in subacute and chronic manifestations of lung toxicity. Early aggregations of macrophages may be seen resembling poorly formed granulomas in cases where diffuse alveolar damage is the manifestation of injury, but these are not required for the diagnosis (B; arrow).

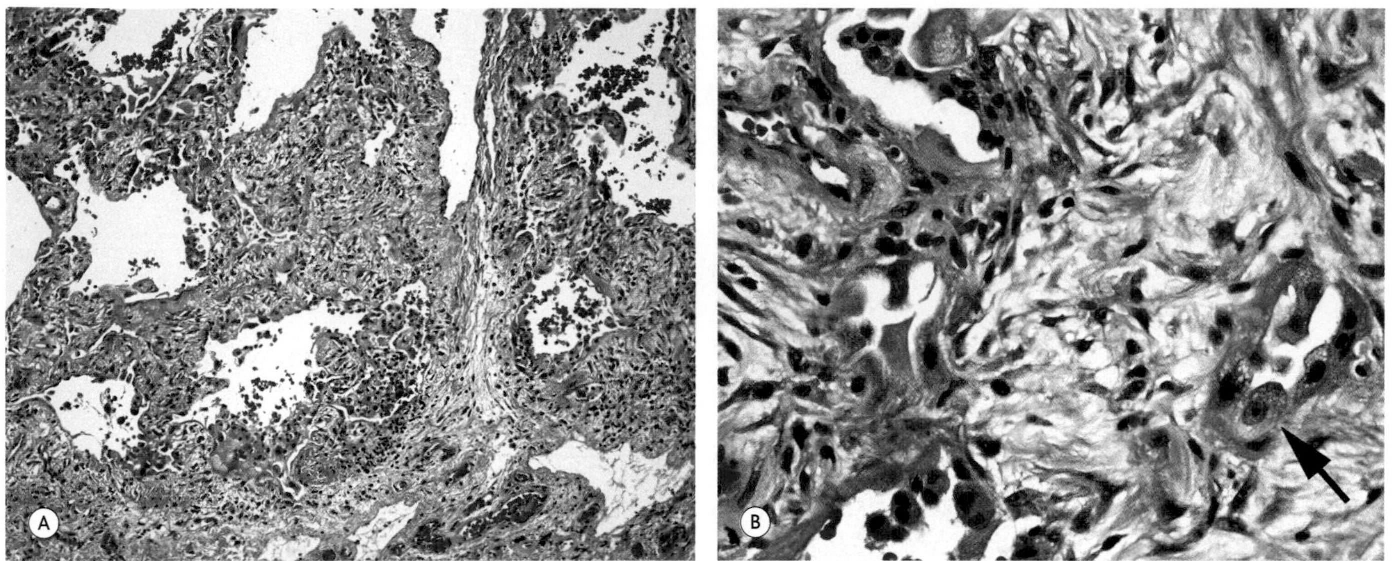

Fig. 5.32 **DAD – amiodarone toxicity.** Amiodarone can produce acute, subacute, and chronic lung toxicity. (A) A scanning magnification image of DAD, resulting from amiodarone toxicity. (B) The finely vacuolated macrophages and type II cells are clearly evident (arrow).

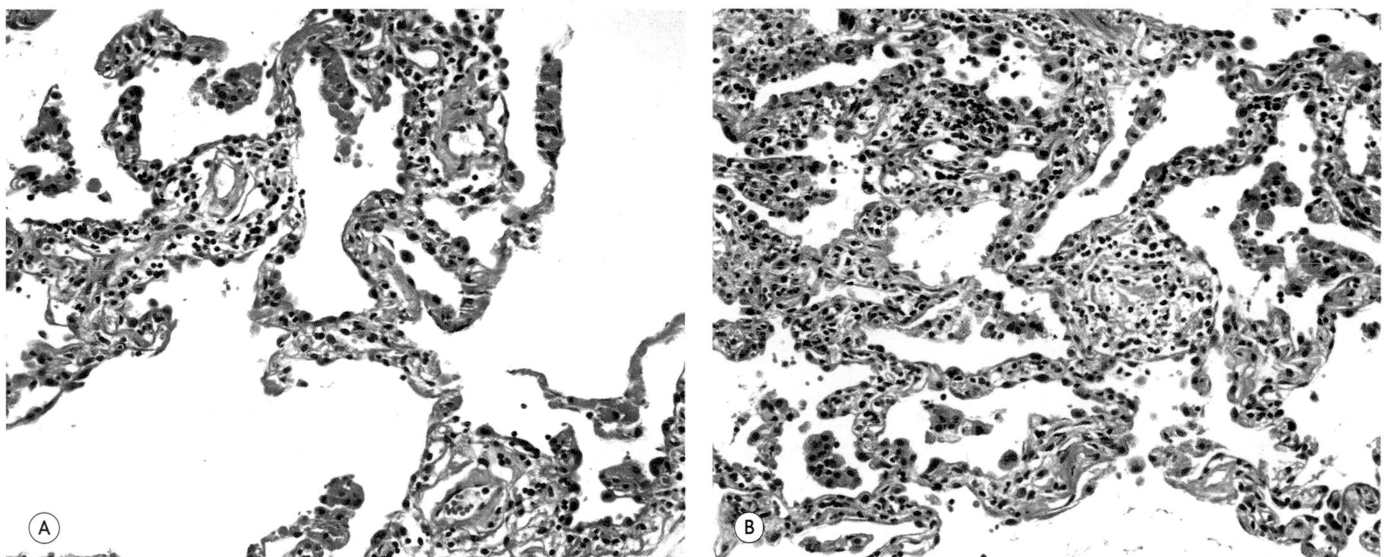

Fig. 5.33 **DAD – gold therapy toxicity.** (A) Gold therapy for rheumatoid arthritis may produce diffuse alveolar damage with hyaline membranes. (B) A chronic or subacute cellular inflammatory process is also described.

in this chapter. Organizing DAD (Fig. 5.33) and chronic interstitial pneumonia are commonly described pulmonary manifestations of "gold toxicity".[64,66,90]

Acute eosinophilic pneumonia

Acute eosinophilic pneumonia (AEP) was first described in 1989[91] and is characterized by acute respiratory failure, fever of days to weeks duration, diffuse pulmonary infiltrates radiologically, and eosinophilia in bronchoalveolar lavage (BAL) fluid or lung biopsy specimens in the absence of infection, atopy, and asthma.[92] Peripheral eosinophilia is frequently described, but is not a consistent finding at initial presentation.[93,94] Acute eosinophilic pneumonia is easily confused with acute interstitial pneumonia (AIP), because both present as acute respiratory distress without an obvious underlying cause.[92]

Histologically, the disease is characterized by acute and organizing lung injury showing classical features (Fig. 5.34) of:

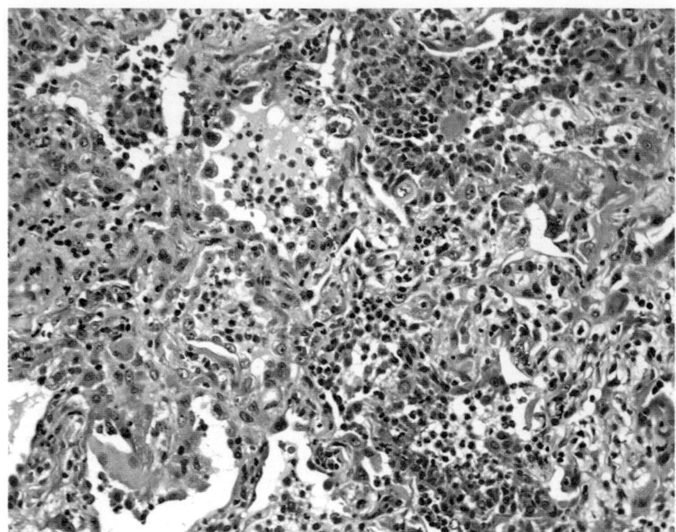

Fig. 5.34 **AEP.** The histopathologic findings seen in eosinophilic pneumonia are well known to most pathologists. The combination of reactive type II cell hyperplasia, airspace fibrin, eosinophilic airspace macrophages, and scattered eosinophils all combine to produce a characteristic picture.

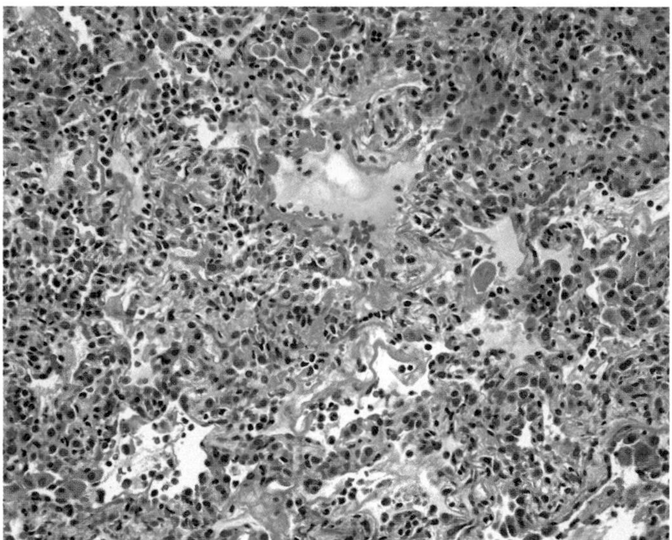

Fig. 5.35 **DAD with AEP – hyaline membranes.** Hyaline membranes may occur in the acute lung injury associated with eosinophilic pneumonia. This is an important occurrence to be aware of so as not to exclude eosinophilic pneumonia from the differential diagnosis of DAD with hyaline membranes.

- alveolar septal edema
- eosinophilic airspace macrophages
- tissue and airspace eosinophils in varying numbers, and
- marked reactive atypia of alveolar type II cells.

Intra-alveolar fibroblastic proliferation (patchy organizing pneumonia) and inflammatory cells are present to variable degree. Hyaline membranes and organizing intra-alveolar fibrin may be present (Fig. 5.35). The most significant feature is the presence of interstitial and alveolar eosinophils. Infiltration of small blood vessels by eosinophils also may be seen. It is important to distinguish AEP from other causes of DAD, because patients typically benefit from systemic corticosteroid treatment with prompt recovery. However, before initiating immunosuppressive therapy, infection should be rigorously excluded by culture and special stains, since parasitic and fungal infections can also manifest as tissue eosinophilia.

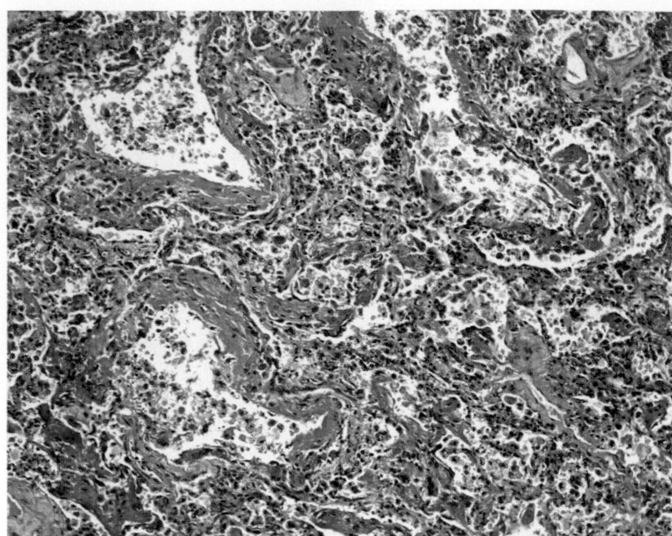

Fig. 5.36 **AIP.** Idiopathic acute interstitial pneumonia (AIP) may take the form of every morphologic manifestation of ARDS, depending on the timing of the biopsy relative to the onset of symptoms. Here, a classic DAD with hyaline membranes of variable cellularity is presented (mid-proliferative phase). Interstitial fibroblastic proliferation may be more or less prominent from case to case and should not serve as a qualifying morphologic finding for the diagnosis. AIP is nothing more than diffuse alveolar damage of unknown causation.

Acute interstitial pneumonia

Acute interstitial pneumonia, also commonly referred to as the Hamman–Rich syndrome, is a fulminant lung disease of unknown etiology occurring in previously healthy patients.[95–97] Patients usually report a prodromal illness simulating viral infection of the upper respiratory tract, followed by rapidly progressive respiratory failure. Mortality is high, with death occurring weeks or months after the acute onset.[95, 97] The classical histopathology is acute and organizing DAD,[95, 97] with septal edema and hyaline membranes in the early phase, and septal fibroblastic proliferation with reactive type II pneumocytes prominent in the organizing phase. In practice, a combination of acute and organizing changes (Fig. 5.36)

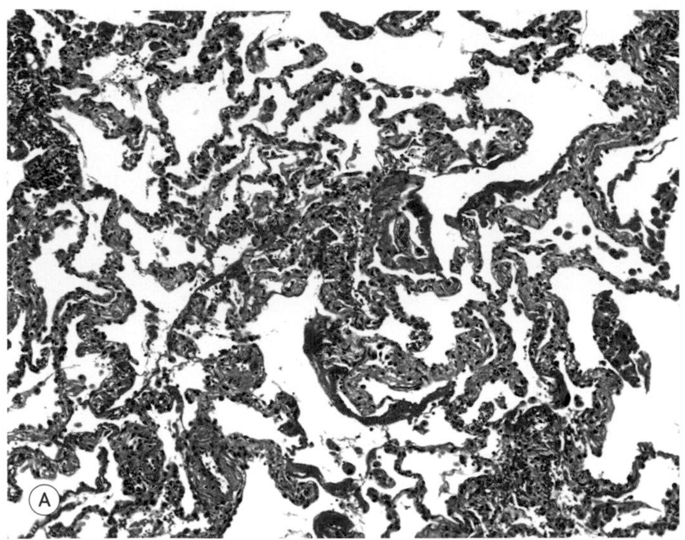

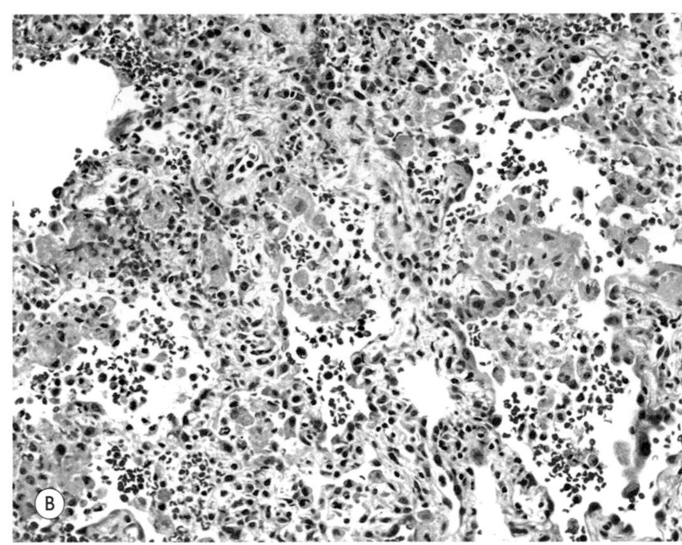

Fig. 5.37 **DAD in Goodpasture's syndrome.** (A) Goodpasture's syndrome characteristically produces alveolar hemorrhage, but acute lung injury with hyaline membranes can occur. Another example of DAD in Goodpasture's syndrome is presented in B. Here, greater interstitial fibroblast proliferation is evident, along with more numerous airspace macrophages.

are often seen in the lung at the time of biopsy.[98] Varying degrees of airspace organization, mononuclear inflammatory infiltrates, thrombi in small pulmonary arteries and reparative peribronchiolar squamous metaplasia are also seen in most cases.

Since AIP is idiopathic, potential causes of acute lung injury must be excluded before making this diagnosis. The differential diagnosis includes infection, collagen vascular disease, acute exacerbation of usual interstitial pneumonia, drug effect, and other causes of DAD.[98] Most cases of DAD are not AIP, and detailed clinical information, radiologic findings (localized versus diffuse disease), serologic data, and microbiological results will often resolve a specific etiology. Special stains applied to tissue sections or cytologic preparations (AFB, GMS, Warthin–Starry, etc.) are also essential to rule out infectious organisms in this setting.

Immunologically mediated pulmonary hemorrhage and vasculitis

So-called pulmonary hemorrhage syndromes may show acute lung injury,[99] in addition to alveolar hemorrhage and hemosiderin-laden macrophages. In some patients, DAD may be the dominant pathology.[100] In the study by Lombard et al. on patients with Goodpasture's syndrome, all showed acute lung injury that varied from focal to diffuse lung involvement.[100] Histopathologically, typical acute and organizing DAD was present, showing widened and edematous alveolar septa, fibroblastic proliferation, reactive type II pneumocytes and, rarely, even hyaline membranes (Fig. 5.37A). Alveolar hemorrhage was present in all cases, focally or diffusely. Capillaritis, an important finding indicating true alveolar hemorrhage,[99] was seen, evidenced by marked septal neutrophilic infiltration. Capillaritis was absent in one case for which DAD was the dominant histopathology.

Microscopic polyangiitis can present as an acute interstitial pneumonia both clinically and pathologically. These patients have vasculitis as the known cause of acute lung injury.[101] Alveolar hemorrhage with arteritis, capillaritis, and venulitis may be seen in some of these cases.[101]

Polyarteritis nodosa and vasculitis associated with systemic connective tissue disease (notably systemic lupus erythematosus and rheumatoid arthritis), can also show acute lung injury with alveolar hemorrhage as the dominant pathologic finding.[47,102]

Radiation pneumonitis

Radiation can produce both acute and chronic damage to the lung, causing acute radiation pneumonitis and chronic progressive fibrosis, respectively.[103] The effect is dependent on the dosage and total time of irradiation and the volume irradiated. Concomitant chemotherapy and infections, which by themselves are causes of DAD, may potentiate the effect of radiation injury.[5,69,104,105]

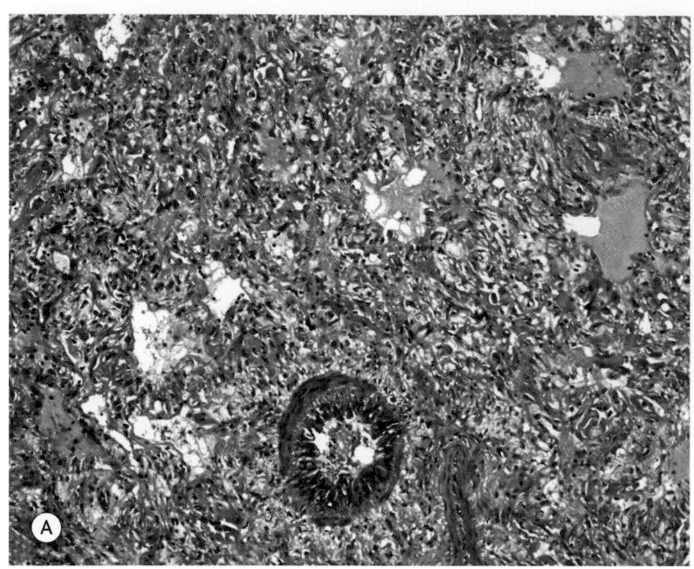

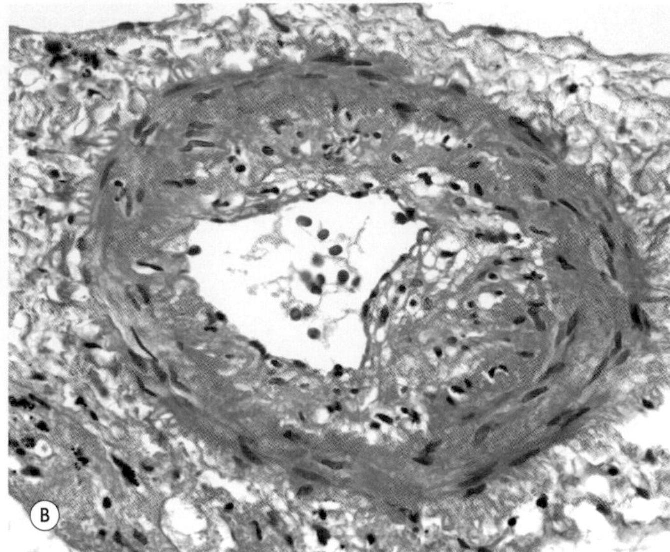

Fig. 5.38 **DAD – radiation injury.** (A) Radiation injury to the lung can produce DAD with striking reactive type II cell hyperplasia. In (B) foamy macrophages in the wall of a pulmonary artery following radiation pneumonitis can be seen.

Acute radiation pneumonitis occurs 1–2 months after radiation therapy.[5,105] Clinical features include dyspnea, cough, pleuritic pain, fever, and chest infiltrates. The lung biopsy shows acute and organizing DAD.[103,105] Markedly atypical type II pneumocytes with enlarged hyperchromatic nuclei and vacuolated cytoplasm are a hallmark of the disease (Fig. 5.38A) and increased numbers of alveolar macrophages are seen. Foamy cells are present in the intima and media of pulmonary blood vessels in some cases, and thrombosis (Fig. 5.38B), with or without transmural fibrinoid necrosis, is common.[69,106–108]

Disease presenting as classical ARDS

By definition, ARDS must be associated with an identifiable inciting event. The histopathology is classical DAD. The histologic changes should be consistent with those expected for the time interval from the onset of clinical disease (see below). In many cases, the ARDS may be caused by a combination of factors, each potentiating the other.[4] For illustration purposes, a few thoroughly studied causes are discussed here.

Oxygen toxicity and inhalants

Oxygen is a well-known cause of ARDS and a useful model for all types of DAD.[4,109,110] Oxygen toxicity is also important in that oxygen is widely used in the care of patients, often in the setting of other injuries that can potentially cause ARDS, e.g. sepsis, shock, trauma. Exposure to high concentrations of oxygen for prolonged periods can lead to characteristic pulmonary damage. In 1958, Pratt first noted pulmonary changes due to high concentrations of inspired oxygen.[111] In 1967, Nash et al. described the sequential pathologic changes of this injury,[109] later re-emphasized by Pratt.[110] In neonates receiving oxygen for hyaline membrane disease, bronchopulmonary dysplasia was reported to occur.[112] As might be expected, the features of hyaline membrane disease in neonates and oxygen-induced DAD in adults are indistinguishable (see Fig. 5.30). Other inhalants such as chlorine gas, mercury vapor, high concentrations of carbon dioxide, and nitrogen mustard have all been reported to cause ARDS.[2,4,5]

Shock and trauma

Massive extrapulmonary trauma and shock first became recognized as causes of unexplained respiratory failure during the wars of the second half of the 20th century. A variety of names were assigned to this war-time condition, including shock lung, congestive atelectasis, traumatic wet lung, Da Nang lung, respiratory insufficiency syndrome, post-traumatic pulmonary insufficiency, and progressive pulmonary consolidation.[2] It became clear that shock of any cause (e.g. hypovolaemia due to hemorrhage, cardiogenic shock, sepsis), could cause ARDS and

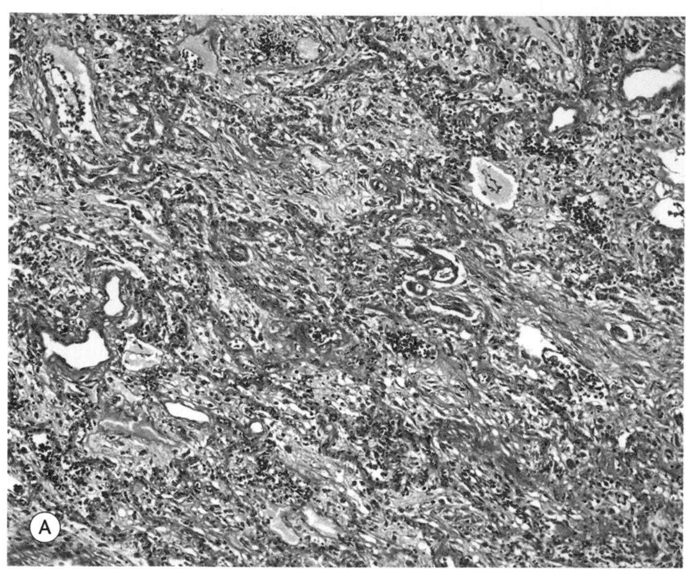

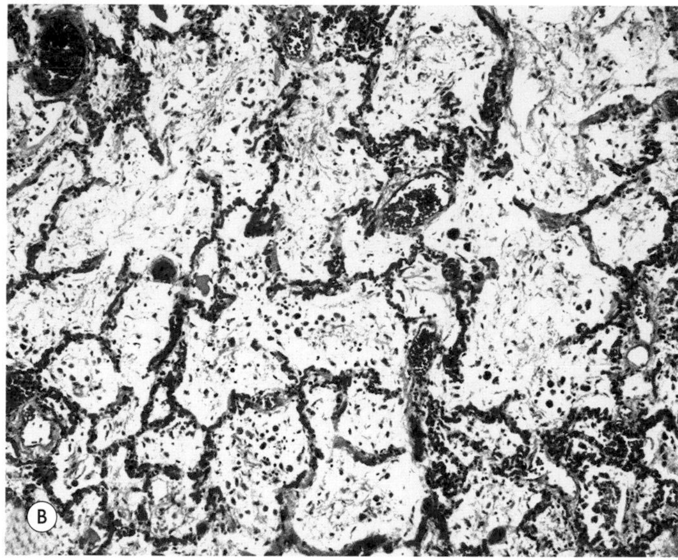

Fig. 5.39 **DAD – paraquat poisoning.** Paraquat produces a dramatic and characteristic pattern of lung injury with (A) prominent airspace fibroplasia and (B) eventual fibrosis with collagen deposition in a loose pattern.

in most cases, a number of factors come into play. Patients typically develop dyspnea of rapid onset accompanied by diffuse chest infiltrates several hours to days after an episode of shock. Once ARDS begins, the mortality rate is high.[1,2,113]

Ingested toxins

Paraquat is a potent herbicide which causes hydrogen peroxide and superoxide free radicals to be released causing damage to cell membranes.[114–116] Oropharyngitis is the initial symptom of poisoning, followed by impaired renal and liver function. About 5 days later, patients develop ARDS. The histopathology in most cases is one of organizing DAD (Fig. 5.39). The diagnosis is confirmed by tissue analysis for paraquat, which can be performed even on autopsy specimens. Other ingested toxins (e.g. kerosene, rapeseed oil) have also been reported to cause ARDS.[5]

Additional features in the differential diagnosis of acute lung injury

Acute lung injury is a pathologic pattern and by itself is nonspecific. The following additional features often help narrow the possible etiologies.

Presence of hyaline membranes

The most commonly encountered etiologies include: infection, collagen vascular disease, drug toxicity, and an idiopathic form (i.e. acute interstitial pneumonia).[2,5]

Presence of neutrophils

The presence of neutrophils in lung alveolar spaces should always raise the possibility of infection.[105,117] For example, legionnaires' disease characteristically shows acute bronchopneumonia with DAD.[41]

Presence of frothy exudates

The presence of frothy exudates in alveolar spaces is a classical feature of pneumocystis pneumonia. However, this feature is not always present. In some cases, especially in mildly immunocompromised patients, DAD may be the only finding.[36]

Presence of necrosis

Among the infectious causes of DAD, viral infection figures prominently. Influenza, herpes simplex, varicella-zoster and adenovirus are well known to produce DAD,[19,21,24–26] and all of these viral infections are typically accompanied by necrosis. *Legionella* and *Pneumocystis* infection can also produce ALI with necrosis.[36,41,118]

Presence of eosinophils

Acute and organizing diffuse alveolar damage with prominent interstitial and alveolar eosinophils is characteristic of acute eosinophilic pneumonia.[92] However, if the patient has been treated with steroid prior to biopsy, there may be very few eosinophils left and the diagnosis may be difficult or impossible.

Presence of siderophages and capillaritis

Hemosiderin-laden macrophages with or without capillaritis in the setting of acute lung injury should raise consideration for immunologically mediated pulmonary hemorrhage.[99] Care must be taken not to interpret the pigmented macrophages seen in the lungs of cigarette smokers as evidence of hemorrhage.[119] The hemosiderin in macrophages related to true hemorrhage in the lung (from any cause) is globular, often slightly refractile, and golden-brown in color.[47,99–101]

Presence of atypical cells

Viral infections often produce cytopathic effects, including intracellular inclusions (see Chapter 6). Examples of intracellular inclusions are the Cowdry A and B inclusions seen in herpes infection, cytomegaly with intranuclear and intracytoplasmic inclusions of cytomegalovirus, the multinucleated giant cells of measles and respiratory syncytial virus, and the smudged cells of adenovirus infection.[23,27,28,120,121] Chemotherapeutic drugs such as busulfan and bleomycin are often associated with markedly atypical type II pneumocytes that may have enlarged pleomorphic nuclei and prominent nucleoli.[80,81] Markedly atypical type II pneumocytes that may simulate viropathic effect are also seen in radiation pneumonitis.[69,107,108]

Presence of foamy cells

Alveolar lining cells with vacuolated cytoplasm accompanied by intra-alveolar foamy macrophages are characteristic features seen in patients taking amiodarone, and amiodarone toxicity may produce acute lung injury changes.[85–87,89] In some cases of radiation pneumonitis, foam cells are seen in the intima and media of blood vessels.[69,108]

Presence of advanced interstitial fibrosis

Clinical idiopathic pulmonary fibrosis (IPF) has usual interstitial pneumonia on pathologic examination (see Ch. 7) with advanced lung remodeling. Interestingly, IPF undergoes episodic exacerbation, and on occasion such exacerbation may be overwhelming and produce DAD.[122] It is prudent to examine lung biopsy sections for the presence of dense fibrosis with structural remodeling (microscopic honeycombing) in cases of DAD to identify the rare case of IPF that presents for the first time as an acute episode of exacerbation.

Clinicopathologic correlation

Because the morphologic manifestations of acute diffuse lung disease may be relatively stereotypic, clinicopathologic correlation is often helpful in arriving at a specific etiology. A summary of the more important history and laboratory data pertinent to this correlation is presented in Table 5.3.

One of the first questions to be addressed is whether or not a known inciting event was identified clinically (i.e. Is this ARDS?). Next, the results of any sampling procedures to identify infection should be checked, along with special stains applied to the tissue sections, to exclude infection. Finally, data regarding related disease, such as infection, autoimmune disease, underlying lung disease, are needed. For example, if the patient is immunosuppressed, infection should always lead the differential diagnosis. Keep in mind that patients with certain diseases may be taking medications that may cause DAD (e.g. cardiac arrhythmia and amiodarone). Moreover, laboratory studies may reveal antibodies related to connective tissue disease (ANA, RF, Jo-1, Scl-70, anti-fibrillarin, anti-Mpp 10, SS-A, SS-B, etc.).

Table 5.3 Essential information for determining etiology

Immune status
Acuity of onset
Radiologic distribution and character of abnormalities
History of inciting event (e.g. shock)
History of lung disease (e.g. usual interstitial pneumonia with current acute exacerbation)
History of systemic disease (e.g. connective tissue disease, heart disease)
History of medication use or drug abuse
History of other recent treatment (e.g. radiotherapy for malignancy)
Serology – sedimentation rate, autoimmune antibodies (e.g. ANA, RF, ANCA)
Results of microbiology studies

Regarding the pathologist's role and responsibility, every biopsy case of acute lung injury should have special stains performed for organisms (at a minimum, methenamine silver and acid-fast stains). Additional stains (auramine–rhodamine, Dieterle, Warthin–Starry, immunohistochemical stains for specific organisms and molecular probes) should be done as necessary.

REFERENCES

1. Petty T: 41st Aspen Lung Conference: overview. Chest 1999; 116: 1S–2S.
2. Tomashefski J, Jr: Pulmonary pathology of acute respiratory distress syndrome. Clin Chest Med 2000; 21(3): 435–466.
3. Ashbaugh D, Bigelow D, Petty T, et al.: Acute respiratory distress in adults. Lancet 1967; 2: 319–323.
4. Katzenstein A, Bloor C, Liebow A: Diffuse alveolar damage – the role of oxygen, shock and related factors. Am J Pathol 1976; 85: 209–228.
5. Katzenstein A: Acute lung injury patterns: diffuse alveolar damage and bronchiolitis obliterans – organizing pneumonia. In: Surgical pathology of non-neoplastic lung disease, Katzenstein A, Askin F, Eds. 1997, WB Saunders, Philadelphia.
6. Bernard G, Artigas A, Briham K, et al.: The American–European Consensus Conference on ARDS. Definitions, mechanisms, relevant outcomes, and clinical trial coordination. Am J Respir Crit Care Med 1994; 149: 818–824.
7. Wright J: Adult respiratory distress syndrome. In: Pathology of the lung, Thurlbeck W, Churg A, Eds. 1995, Thieme, New York.
8. Bellingan G: The pulmonary physician in critical care 6: the pathogenesis of ALI/ARDS. Thorax 2002; 57: 540–546.
9. Colby T, Lombard C, Yousem S, et al.: Atlas of pulmonary surgical pathology. 1991, WB Saunders, Philadelphia.
10. Herridge MS, Cheung AM, Tansey CM, et al.: One-year outcomes in survivors of the acute respiratory distress syndrome. N Engl J Med 2003; 348(8): 683–693.

10a. Beasley MB, Franks TJ, Galvin JR, et al: Acute Fibrinous and organizing Pneumonia: A histologic pattern of lung injury and possible variant of diffuse alveolar damage. Arch Pathol Lab Med 2002; 126: 1064–1070.

11. Oseasohn R, Adelson L, Kaji M: Clinicopathology study of 33 fatal cases of Asian influenza. N Engl J Med 1959; 260: 509–518.
12. Yeldandi A, Colby T: Pathologic features of lung biopsy specimens from influenza pneumonia cases. Hum Pathol 1994; 25: 47–53.
13. Tamura H, Aronson B: Intranuclear fibrillary inclusions in influenza pneumonia. Pathol Lab Med 1978; 102: 252–257.
14. Sobonya RE, Hiller FC, Pingleton W, et al.: Fatal measles (rubeola) pneumonia in adults. Arch Pathol Lab Med 1978; 102: 366–371.
15. Enders JF, McCarthy K, Mitus A, et al.: Isolation of measles virus at autopsy in cases of giant-cell pneumonia without rash. N Engl J Med 1959; 261: 875–881.
16. Mitus A, Enders JF, Craig JM, et al.: Persistence of measles virus and depression of antibody formation in patients with giant-cell pneumonia after measles. N Engl J Med 1959; 261: 882–889.
17. Haram K, Jacobsen J: Measles and its relationship to giant cell pneumonia (Hecht pneumonia). Acta Pathol Microbiol Immunol Scand [A] 1973; 81: 761–769.
18. Katzenstein A, Infection I. Unusual pneumonias. In: Surgical pathology of non-neoplastic lung disease, Katzenstein A, Askin F, Eds. 1997, WB Saunders, Philadelphia.
19. Becroft D: Histopathology of fatal adenovirus infection of the respiratory tract in young children. J Clin Pathol 1967; 20: 561–569.
20. Becroft D: Bronchiolitis obliterans, bronchiectasis and other sequelae of adenovirus type 21 infection in young children. J Clin Pathol 1971; 24: 72–79.
21. Zahradnik J, Spencer M, Porter D: Adenovirus infection in the immunocompromised patient. Am J Med 1980; 68: 725–732.
22. Miller R: Viral infections of the respiratory tract. In: Pathology of the lung, 2nd edn, Thurlbeck W, Churg A, Eds. 1995, Thieme Medical Publishers, New York, pp 195–222.
23. Abbondanzo S, English C, Kagan E, et al.: Fatal adenovirus pneumonia in a newborn identified by electron microscopy and in-situ hybridization. Arch Pathol Lab Med 1989; 113: 1349–1353.
24. Ramsey P, Fife K, Hackman RC, et al.: Herpes simplex virus pneumonia: clinical, virologic, and pathologic features in 20 patients. Ann Intern Med 1982; 97: 813–820.
25. Graham B, Snell JJ: Herpes simplex virus infection of the adult lower respiratory tract. Medicine (Baltimore) 1983; 62: 384–393.
26. Pugh RN, Omar RI, Hossain MM: Varicella infection and pneumonia among adults. Int J Infect Dis 1998; 2(4): 205–210.
27. Craighead J: Cytomegalovirus pulmonary disease. Pathobiol Annu 1975; 5: 197–220.
28. Beschorner W, Hutchins G, Burns W, et al.: Cytomegalovirus pneumonia in bone marrow transplant recipients: miliary and diffuse patterns. Am Rev Respir Dis 1980; 122: 107–114.
29. Winston D, Ho W, Champlin R: Cytomegalovirus after allogenic bone marrow transplantation. Rev Infect Dis 1992; 12(suppl): S776–792.
30. Colby TV, Zaki SR, Feddersen RM, et al.: Hantavirus pulmonary syndrome is distinguishable from acute interstitial pneumonia. Arch Pathol Lab Med 2000; 124(10): 1463–1466.
31. Duchin J, Koster F, Peters C, et al.: Hantavirus pulmonary syndrome. A clinical description of 17 patients with a newly recognized disease. N Engl J Med 1994; 330: 949–955.
32. Nolte K, Feddersen R, Foucar K, et al.: Hantavirus pulmonary syndrome in the United States. A new pathological description of a disease caused by a new agent. Hum Pathol 1995; 26: 110–120.
33. Weber W, Askin F, Dehner L: Lung biopsy in *Pneumocystis carinii* pneumonia. A histopathologic study of typical and atypical features. Am J Clin Pathol 1977; 67: 11–19.
34. Ognibene F, Shelhamer J, Gill V, et al.: The diagnosis of *Pneumocystis carinii* pneumonia in patients with the acquired immunodeficiency syndrome using subsegmental bronchoalveolar lavage. Am Rev Respir Dis 1984; 129: 929–932.
35. Grimes M, LaPook J, Bar MH, et al.: Disseminated *Pneumocystis carinii* infection in a patient with acquired immunodeficiency syndrome. Hum Pathol 1987; 18: 307–308.
36. Askin F, Katzenstein A: Pneumocystis infection masquerading as diffuse alveolar damage: a potential source of diagnostic error. Chest 1979; 4: 420–422.
37. Blackmon J, Hicklin M, Chandler F: Legionnaires' disease. Pathological and historical aspects of a new disease. Arch Pathol Lab Med 1978; 102: 337–343.
38. Lattimen G, Rachman R, Scarlato M: Legionnaires' disease pneumonia: histopathologic features and comparison with microbial and chemical pneumonias. Ann Clin Lab Sci 1979; 9: 353–361.
39. Rollin S, Colby T, Clayton F: Open lung biopsy in *Mycoplasma pneumoniae* pneumonia. Arch Pathol Lab Med 1986; 110: 34–41.
40. Torres A, de Celis M, Roisin R, et al.: Adult respiratory distress syndrome in Q fever. Eur J Respir Dis 1987; 70: 322–325.
41. Winn WJ, Myerowitz R: The pathology of the *Legionella* pneumonias. A review of 74 cases and the literature. Hum Pathol 1981; 12: 401–422.
42. Matthay R, Schwanz M, Petty T, et al.: Pulmonary manifestations of systemic lupus erythematosus: review of twelve cases of acute lupus pneumonitis. Medicine 1974; 54: 397–409.
43. Hunninghake G, Fauci A: Pulmonary involvement in the collagen vascular diseases. Am Rev Respir Dis 1979; 119: 471–503.
44. Yousem S, Colby T, Carrington C: Lung biopsy in rheumatoid arthritis. Am Rev Respir Dis 1985; 131: 770–777.
45. Lakhanpal S, Lie J, Conn D, et al.: Pulmonary disease in polymyositis/dermatomyositis: a clinicopathological analysis of 65 autopsy cases. Ann Rheum Dis 1987; 46: 23–29.
46. Tazelaar H, Viggiano R, Pickersgill J, et al.: Interstitial lung disease in polymyositis and dermatomyositis. Clinical features and prognosis as correlated with histologic findings. Am Rev Respir Dis 1990; 141: 727–733.
47. Colby T: Pulmonary pathology in patients with systemic autoimmune disease. Clin Chest Med 1998; 19: 587–612.
48. Quismorio Jr F, Cheema G: Interstitial lung disease in systemic lupus erythematosus. Curr Opin Pulm Med 2000; 6: 424–429.
49. Lamblin C, Bergoin C, Saelens T, et al.: Interstitial lung disease in collagen vascular disease. Eur Respir J 2001; 18(Suppl 32): 69s–80s.
50. Myers J, Katzenstein A: Microangiitis in lupus-induced pulmonary hemorrhage. Am J Clin Pathol 1986; 85: 552–556.
51. Walker W, Wright V: Pulmonary lesions and rheumatoid arthritis. Medicine (Baltimore) 1968; 47: 501–515.

52. Laitinen O, Nissila M, Salorinne Y, et al.: Pulmonary involvement in patients with rheumatoid arthritis. Scand J Respir Dis 1975; 56: 297–304.
53. Hakala M, Paakko P, Huhti E, et al.: Open lung biopsy of patients with rheumatoid arthritis. Clin Rheumatol 1990; 9(4): 452–460.
54. Gochuico BR: Potential pathogenesis and clinical aspects of pulmonary fibrosis associated with rheumatoid arthritis. Am J Med Sci 2001; 321(1): 83–88.
55. Pratt D, Schwartz M, May J, et al.: Rapidly fatal pulmonary fibrosis: the accelerated variation of interstitial pneumonitis. Thorax 1979; 34: 587–593.
56. Douglas WW, Tazelaar HD, Hartman TE, et al.: Polymyositis–dermatomyositis-associated interstitial lung disease. Am J Respir Crit Care Med 2001; 164(7): 1182–1185.
57. Muir T, Tazelaar H, Colby T, et al.: Organizing diffuse alveolar damage associated with progressive systemic sclerosis. Mayo Clin Proc 1997; 72: 639–642.
58. Clarysse A, Cathey W, Cartwright G, et al.: Pulmonary disease complicating intermittent therapy with methotrexate. JAMA 1969; 209: 1861–1864.
59. Bone R, Wolfe J, Sobonya R, et al.: Desquamative interstitial pneumonia following chronic nitrofurantoin therapy. Chest 1976; 69(2): 296–297.
60. Kruban Z: Pulmonary changes induced by amphophilic drugs. Environ Health Perspect 1976; 16: 111–115.
61. Samuels M, Johnson D, Holoye P, et al.: Large-dose bleomycin therapy and pulmonary toxicity. A possible role of prior radiotherapy. JAMA 1976; 235: 1117–1120.
62. Kilburn K: Pulmonary disease induced by drugs. In: Pulmonary diseases and disorders, Fishman AP, Ed. 1980, McGraw-Hill, New York, pp 707–724.
63. Williams T, Eidus L, Thomas P: Fibrosing alveolitis, bronchiolitis obliterans and sulfalazine therapy. Chest 1982; 81: 766–768.
64. Schapira D, Nahir M, Scharf Y: Pulmonary injury induced by gold salts treatment. Med Interne 1985; 23(4): 259–263.
65. Yousem S, Lifson J, Colby T: Chemotherapy-induced eosinophilic pneumonia. Relation to bleomycin. Chest 1985; 88(1): 103–106.
66. Slingerland R, Hoogsteden H, Adriaansen H, et al.: Gold-induced pneumonitis. Respiration 1987; 52(3): 232–236.
67. Rosenow E 3rd, Myers J, Swensen S, et al.: Drug-induced pulmonary disease. An update. Chest 1992; 102: 239–250.
68. Rossi S, Eramus J, McAdams H, et al.: Pulmonary drug toxicity: radiologic and pathologic manifestations. Radiographics 2000; 20(5): 1245–1259.
69. Abid S, Malhotra V, Perry M: Radiation-induced and chemotherapy-induced pulmonary injury. Curr Opin Oncol 2001; 13(4): 242–248.
70. Fassas A, Gojo I, Rapoport A, et al.: Pulmonary toxicity syndrome following CDEP (cyclophosphamide, dexamethasone, etoposide, cisplatin) chemotherapy. Bone Marrow Transplant 2001; 28(4): 399–403.
71. Erasmus J, McAdams H, Rossi S: Drug-induced lung injury. Semin Roentgenol 2002; 37(1): 72–81.
72. Myers J: Pathology of drug-induced lung disease. In: Surgical pathology of non-neoplastic lung disease, Katzenstein A, Askin F, Eds. 1997, WB Saunders, Philadelphia.
73. Cleverley J, Screaton N, Hiorus M, et al.: Drug-induced lung disease: high-resolution CT and histological findings. Clin Radiol 2002; 57: 292–299.
74. Cooper J, Jr., White D, Mathay R: Drug-induced pulmonary disease (Parts 1 and 2). Am Rev Respir Dis 1986; 133: 321–338, 488–502.
75. Limper AH, Rosenow EC 3rd: Drug-induced interstitial lung disease. Curr Opin Pulm Med 1996; 2(5): 396–404.
76. Copper JA Jr.: Drug-induced lung disease. Adv Intern Med 1997; 42: 231–268.
77. Camus PH, Foucher P, Bonniaud PH, et al.: Drug-induced infiltrative lung disease. Eur Respir J Suppl 2001; 32: 93s–100s.
78. Ozkan M, Dweik RA, Ahmad M: Drug-induced lung disease. Cleve Clin J Med 2001; 68(9): 782–785, 89–95.
79. Littler W, Kay J, Haselton P, et al.: Busulphan lung. Thorax 1969; 24(6): 639–655.
80. Koss l, Melamed M, Mayer K: The effect of bulsufan on human epithelia. Am J Clin Pathol 1965; 44: 385–397.
81. Feingold M, Koss L: Effect of long-term administration of bulsufan. Arch Intern Med 1969; 124: 66–71.
82. Gyorkey F, Gyorkey P, Sinkovies J: Origin and significance of intranuclear tubular inclusions in type II pulmonary alveolar epithelial cells of patients with bleomycin and bulsufan toxicity. Ultrastruc Pathol 1980; 1: 211– 221.
83. Ingrassia T 3rd, Ryu J, Trastek V, et al.: Oxygen-exacerbated bleomycin pulmonary toxicity. Mayo Clin Proc 1991; 66: 173–178.
84. Imokawa S, Colby T, Leslie K, et al.: Methotrexate pneumonitis: review of the literature and histopathological findings in nine patients. Eur Respir J 2000; 15: 373–381.
85. Dean P, Groshart K, Potterfield JG, et al.: Amiodarone-associated pulmonary toxicity: a clinical and pathologic study of eleven cases. Am J Clin Pathol 1987; 87: 7–13.
86. Kennedy JI, Myers JL, Plumb VJ, et al.: Amiodarone pulmonary toxicity. Clinical, radiologic, and pathologic correlations. Arch Intern Med 1987; 147(1): 50–55.
87. Myers JL, Kennedy JI, Plumb VJ: Amiodarone lung: pathologic findings in clinically toxic patients. Hum Pathol 1987; 18(4): 349–354.
88. Martin W 2nd, Rosenow E 3rd: Amiodarone pulmonary toxicity. Recognition and pathogenesis (Part I). Chest 1988; 93: 1067–1075.
89. Donaldson L, Grant I, Naysmith M, et al.: Acute amiodarone-induced lung toxicity. Intens Care Med 1998; 24(6): 626–630.
90. Blancas R, Moreno J, Martin F, et al.: Alveolar-interstitial pneumopathy after gold-salts compounds administration, requiring mechanical ventilation. Intens Care Med 1998; 24(10): 1110–1112.
91. Allen J, Pacht E, Gadek J, et al.: Acute eosinophilic pneumonia as a reversible cause of noninfectious respiratory failure. N Engl J Med 1989; 321: 569–574.
92. Tazelaar H, Linz L, Colby T, et al.: Acute eosinophilic pneumonia: histopathologic findings in nine patients. Am J Respir Crit Care Med 1997; 155: 296–302.
93. Hayakawa H, Sato A, Toyoshima M: A clinical study of idiopathic eosinophilic pneumonia. Chest 1994; 105: 1462–1466.
94. Pope-Harman A, Davis W, Allen E, et al.: Acute eosinophilic pneumonia: a review of 12 cases. Chest 1994; 106: 156s.
95. Hamman L, Rich A: Acute diffuse interstitial fibrosis of the lungs. Bull Johns Hopkins Hosp 1944; 74: 177–212.
96. Katzenstein A, Myers J, Mazur M: Acute interstitial pneumonia. A clinicopathologic, ultrastructural, and cell kinetic study. Am J Surg Pathol 1986; 10: 256–267.
97. Olson J, Colby T, Elliott C: Hamman–Rich syndrome revisited. Mayo Clin Proc 1990; 65: 1538–1548.
98. Bouros D, Nicholson A, Polychronopoulos V, et al.: Acute interstitial pneumonia. Eur Respir J 2000; 15: 412–418.
99. Colby T, Fukuoka J, Ewaskow S, et al.: Pathologic approach to pulmonary hemorrhage. Ann Diagn Pathol 2001; 5: 309–319.
100. Lombard C, Colby T, Elliott C: Surgical pathology of the lung in anti-basement membrane antibody-associated Goodpastures syndrome. Hum Pathol 1989; 20: 445–451.
101. Akikusa B, Kondo Y, Irabu N, et al.: Six cases of microscopic polyarteritis exhibiting acute interstitial pneumonia. Pathol Int 1995; 45: 580–588.
102. Matsumoto T, Homma S, Okada M, et al.: The lung in polyarteritis nodosa: a pathologic study of 10 cases. Hum Pathol 1993; 24: 717–724.
103. Fajardo L, Berthrong M: Radiation injury in surgical pathology. Part I. Am J Surg Pathol 1978; 2: 159–199.
104. Einhorn L, Krause M, Hornback N, et al.: Enhanced pulmonary toxicity with bleomycin and radiotherapy in oat cell lung cancer. Cancer 1976; 37: 2414–2416.
105. Flint A, Colby T, Diffuse alveolar damage. In: Surgical pathology of diffuse infiltrative lung disease. 1987, Grune and Stratton, Orlando.
106. Gross N: Pulmonary effects of radiation therapy. Ann Intern Med 1977; 86: 81–92.
107. Fajardo L, Pathology of radiation injury. Masson monographs in diagnostic pathology, No. 6, Sternberg SS, series Ed. Masson Publishing, New York, 1982.
108. Coggle J, Lambert B, Moores S: Radiation effects in the lung. Environ Health Perspect 1986; 70: 261–291.
109. Nash G, Blennerhassett J, Pontoppidan H: Pulmonary lesions associated with oxygen therapy and artificial ventilation. N Engl J Med 1967; 276: 368–374.
110. Pratt P: Pathology of pulmonary oxygen toxicity. Am Rev Respir Dis 1974; suppl 110: 51–57.
111. Pratt P: Pulmonary capillary proliferation induced by oxygen. Am J Pathol 1958; 34: 1033–1050.
112. Northway W Jr , Rosan R, Porter D: Pulmonary disease following

respirator therapy of hyaline-membrane disease: bronchopulmonary dysplasia. N Engl J Med 1967; 276: 357–368.
113. Milberg J, Davis D, Steinberg K, et al.: Improved survival of patients with acute respiratory distress syndrome (ARDS): 1983–1993. JAMA 1995; 273(4): 306–309.
114. Anderson C: Paraquat and the lung. Australas Radiol 1970; 14: 409–411.
115. Dearden L, Fairshter R, McRae D, et al.: Pulmonary ultrastructure of the late aspects of human paraquat poisoning. Am J Pathol 1978; 93: 667–680.
116. Fairshter R: Paraquat poisoning an update. West J Med 1978; 128: 56–58.
117. Chian CF, Chang FY: Acute respiratory distress syndrome in Mycoplasma pneumonia: a case report and review. J Microbiol Immunol Infect 1999; 32(1): 52–56.
118. Weber W, Akin F, Dehner L: Lung biopsy in *Pneumocystis carinii* pneumonia: a histolopathologic study of typical and atypical features. Am J Clin Pathol 1977; 67: 11–19.
119. Yousem S, Colby T, Gaensler E: Respiratory bronchiolitis-associated interstitial lung disease and its relationship to desquamative interstitial pneumonia. Mayo Clin Proc 1989; 64: 1373–1380.
120. Everard M, Milner A: The respiratory syncitial virus and its role in acute bronchiolitis. Eur J Pediatr 1992; 151(9): 638–651.
121. Ebsen M, Anhenn O, Roder C, et al.: Morphology of adenovirus type-3 infection of human respiratory epithelial cells in vitro. Virchows Arch 2002; 440(5): 512–518.
122. Knodoh Y, Taniguchi H, Kawabata Y, et al.: Acute exacerbation in idiopathic pulmonary fibrosis: analysis of clinical and pathologic findings in three cases. Chest 1993; 103: 1808–1812.

Lung infections

Louis A Rosati Kevin O Leslie

6

Introduction

Lower respiratory tract infections are the leading causes of morbidity and mortality worldwide.[1] Included in this category are bronchitis/bronchiolitis, community acquired and nosocomial pneumonias, and pneumonias in the immunocompromised host. However, only a relatively small percentage of these infections come to the attention of the surgical pathologist. More often than not, if a diagnosis of pneumonia is made in pathology, it occurs in the microbiology laboratory. Nevertheless, the surgical pathologist sometimes plays a pivotal role by identifying an organism that fails detection by microbiologic techniques[2] (Table 6.1). Culture diagnosis is not always possible; the organism may not reproduce in culture, a culture may not have been requested, or the culture technique may have failed for one of various technical reasons. Even when culture is successful, the timeframe for diagnostic purposes may not be clinically useful, or the culture result, in the absence of a tissue response, may not permit distinction of pathogens from innocent bystanders, be they colonizers or contaminants. For all of these reasons, the biopsied pulmonary infection is often one that has eluded standard microbiologic techniques, has failed empirical therapy, or requires morphologic analysis for clarification of a critical differential diagnosis. In these situations, the diagnostic pathologist is indispensible.[3,4] Moreover, the immediate reporting of a frozen section, or the use of new tissue processing systems (which permit the preparation of a paraffin block in about an hour), can positively impact patient management by rapid, same day, reporting of results from a biopsy.[5]

Diagnostic tools and strategies

The history of pathology is intertwined with the discovery of pathogenic bacteria and the development of the science of microbiology.[6] Today, pathologists and microbiologists approach the diagnosis of infectious disease with techniques and methods that share some similarities, but have important differences.[7] The surgical pathologist or cytopathologist grounded in clinical microbiology is able to apply the tools of both disciplines, listed in Tables 6.2A and 6.2B, and achieve a diagnosis by correlating the data from histopathology or cytopathology with microbiology. Unfortunately, the diagnostic work-up and reporting in surgical or cytopathology and microbiology typically run in parallel, often without one group knowing the findings of the other. An interdisciplinary approach that is based on mutual understanding and

Table 6.1 Role of the diagnostic pathologist

Rapid diagnosis: frozen section; cytologic smears; rapid tissue process
Identify unculturable pathogens
Establish diagnosis when cultures negative
Evaluate pathogenic significance of culture isolate
Define "new" infectious diseases
Exclude infectious etiology; detect co-morbid process
Intraoperative triage of limited biopsy tissue
Clinicopathologic and microbiologic correlation

Source: modified from Watts and Chandler.[4]

Table 6.2A Diagnostic tools of the pathologist

Activity	Objective
Pre/intra/postoperative consultation	Information exchange and strategies
Gross examination	Tissue handling and triage
Histopathologic examination	Organism morphology; cytopathic effect; host response
Histochemical stains	Detection and morphologic detail
Immunohistochemical stains	Detection of organisms; confirmation of genus/species
Electron microscopy	Selective use for virus, fungi, parasite, & bacteria
Molecular techniques (ISH; PCR)	Sensitive & specific detection & identification of nonculturable organisms; stain negative cases
Report	Clinicopathologic & microbiologic correlation

ISH = in-situ hybridization; PCR = polymerase chain reaction.

Table 6.2B Diagnostic tools of the microbiologist

Activity	Objective
Pre/intra/postoperative consultation	Information exchange and strategies
Direct visualization (smears & imprints)	Rapid detection
Culture	Identify genus & species; susceptibility studies
Antigen detection	Rapid identification
Serology	Specific antibody response
Molecular techniques	Sensitive & specific detection and identification
Report	Traditional vs interpretive format

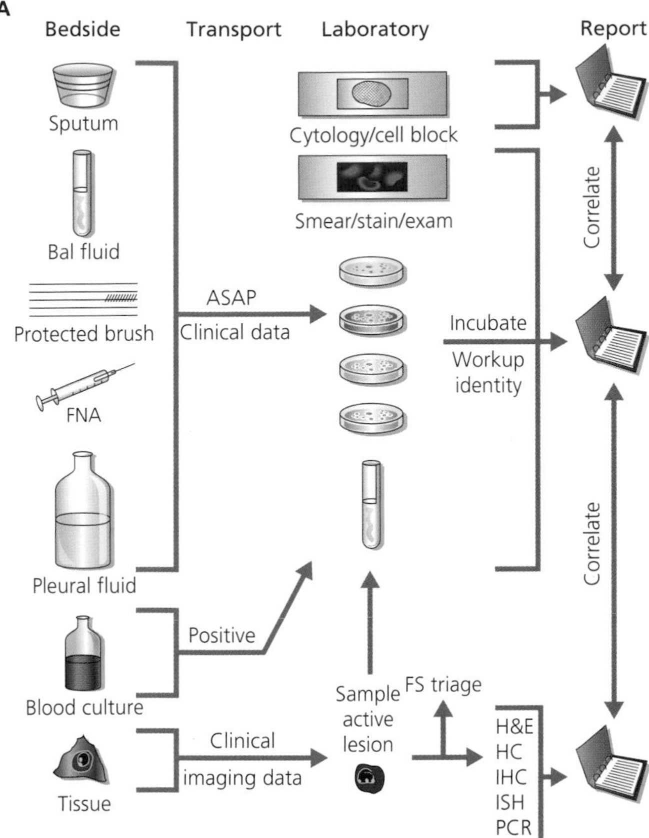

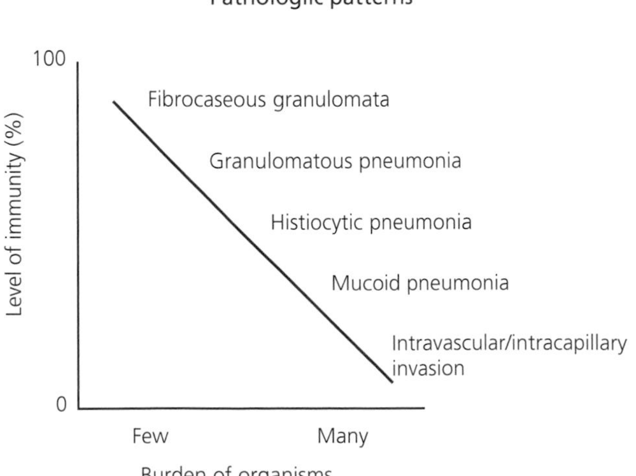

Fig. 6.1 (A) Laboratory work-up and reporting of respiratory tract infection through correlative database inquiry. (B) Pathologic patterns: level of immunity and organism burden – cryptococcosis. In cryptococcal pneumonia, patients with normal and near normal immunity form granulomas with few organisms. Immunocompromised patients have histiocytic infiltrates or mucoid pneumonia with little or no inflammatory reaction and many organisms. (Based on data from Mark EJ: N Engl J Med 2002; 347: 523.)

communication would seem to be a logical, if not ideal, scenario for optimal clinical management.[8] Such an integrated morphologic and microbiologic approach is presented schematically in Fig. 6.1A and should be achievable by correlative database enquiry using contemporary laboratory information systems.

Because the distinction of one organism's genus or species from another can have important prognostic and therapeutic implications, correlation of the histopathologic findings with the results of culture is essential. To accomplish this, foresight in obtaining and properly handling tissue for culture is vital.[9] The correlation of the morphologic and microbiologic data can be facilitated in the surgical pathology report by appending a comment that seeks to enhance the morphologic diagnosis by suggesting a specific etiology, differential diagnosis, or additional work-up with culture, serology, or molecular studies. In certain situations, it is also appropriate to include the preliminary results of microbiology stains and cultures, and to correlate this information with the morphologic findings whenever possible.

Knowledge of the clinical setting

Clinical data such as any known risk factors, age, and the immune status of the patient are most important, as these parameters typically influence the spectrum of morphologic changes and the type and burden of etiologic agents.[10–15] Also, because the degree of immunosuppression influences the burden of organisms, the effort required to identify them is different. For example, organisms are less often found in lung tissues from patients with normal or near-normal immunity. In this setting, cultures, serologic studies and epidemiologic data must be relied upon to provide the diagnosis.[16] By contrast, the HIV-infected patient with acquired immune deficiency and atypical mycobacterial infection, manifest poorly formed granulomas or histiocytic infiltrates with an overabundance of organisms identified by tissue stains. *Pneumocystis* organisms may be easily identified in AIDS patients who manifest diffuse alveolar damage accompanied by abundant, foamy alveolar casts but when immunosuppression is less severe (such as that produced by corticosteroids administered for arthritis), the morphologic features can be less typical, and the organisms sparse. The relationship between the level of immunity, burden of organisms, and patterns of disease is illustrated for cryptococcosis (Fig. 6.1B).

In the immunocompromised host, one must also consider a broader differential diagnosis. In addition to infection, pulmonary involvement by any underlying

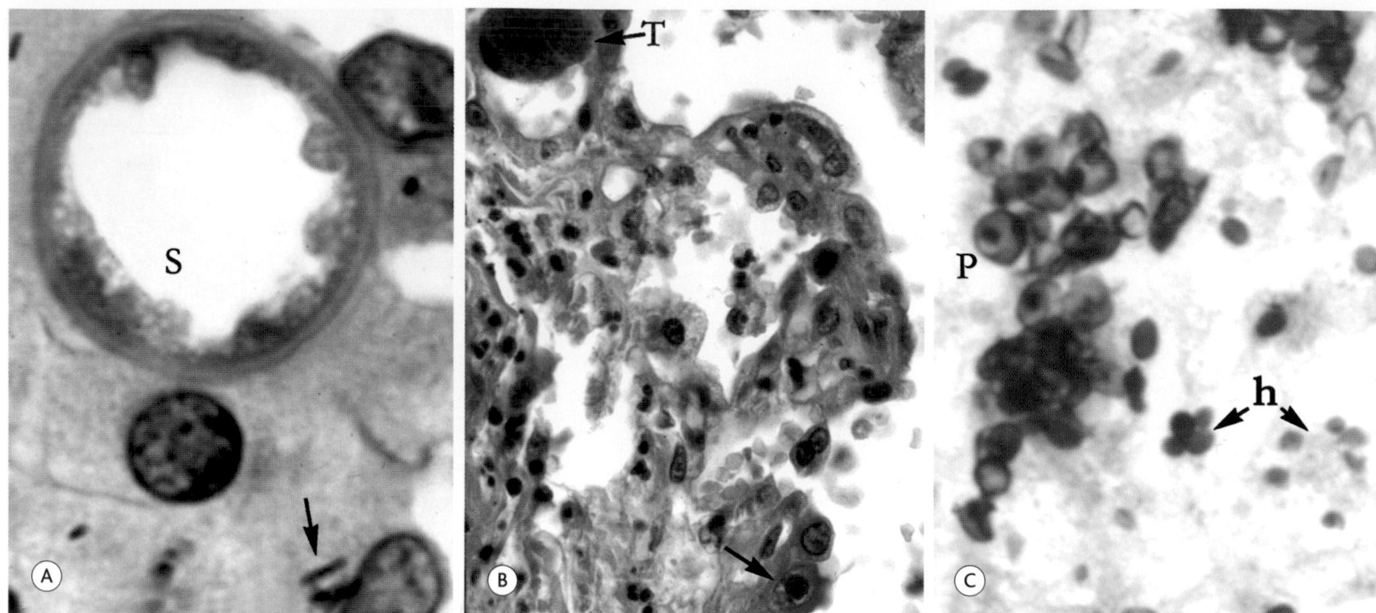

Fig. 6.2 **Dual infections.** (A) Spherule of *Coccidioides* (S) and *Mycobacterium avium* complex (MAC) acid-fast bacilli (M) (Ziehl–Neelsen/H&E); (B) *Toxoplasma* pseudocysts (T) and cytomegalovirus (B) infected alveolar lining cell (arrow; H&E); (C) Clusters of *Pneumocystis* cysts (P) in the midst of *Histoplasma capsulatum* yeast cells (H) (GMS).

disease, drug-induced and treatment-related disease, noninfectious interstitial pneumonias, malignancy, and new pulmonary diseases unrelated to the patient's immunocompromised state, such as aspiration, heart failure, pulmonary emboli, and other disorders come into consideration. Furthermore, iatrogenic immunosuppression in the transplant patient poses additional unique challenges such as the question of rejection, graft vs host disease and Epstein–Barr virus-associated lymphoproliferative disorders. Importantly, because multiple different morphologic patterns of injury and infections can occur in the immunosuppressed patient, when one organism is found, careful search for another is always warranted (Fig. 6.2).

Pattern recognition

Knowledge of the radiographic pattern of the lesion (e.g. localized, diffuse, bilateral) also helps to narrow the differential diagnosis.[17] Review of the imaging studies with the radiologist can be very useful in arriving at a diagnosis. Correlating these data with the clinical history and the histopathologic pattern of lung injury allows the pathologist to reduce the number of diagnostic possibilities (Fig. 6.3). The histopathologic patterns are finite and these typically correlate with a particular group of organisms (Table 6.3).

Useful tissue stains in lung infection

Many diagnostic pathologists have a general aversion to the use of special stains for identifying organisms in tissue sections based on less than optimal specificity and sensitivity and the technical difficulty of performing some of these (especially silver impregnation methods, such as the Dieterle, Steiner, and Warthin–Starry stains). Nevertheless, several histochemical stains are quite useful in detecting bacteria, mycobacteria, and fungi in tissue sections. A list of these is presented in Table 6.4. These stains can be applied as part of an algorithmic strategy, especially in the immunocompromised patient, regardless of history.[2]

For example, when bacteria are being sought, some would prefer to begin with the tissue Gram stain (e.g. Brown & Hopps and Brown & Brenn) (Fig. 6.4), but silver impregnation techniques (e.g. Warthin–Starry) are more

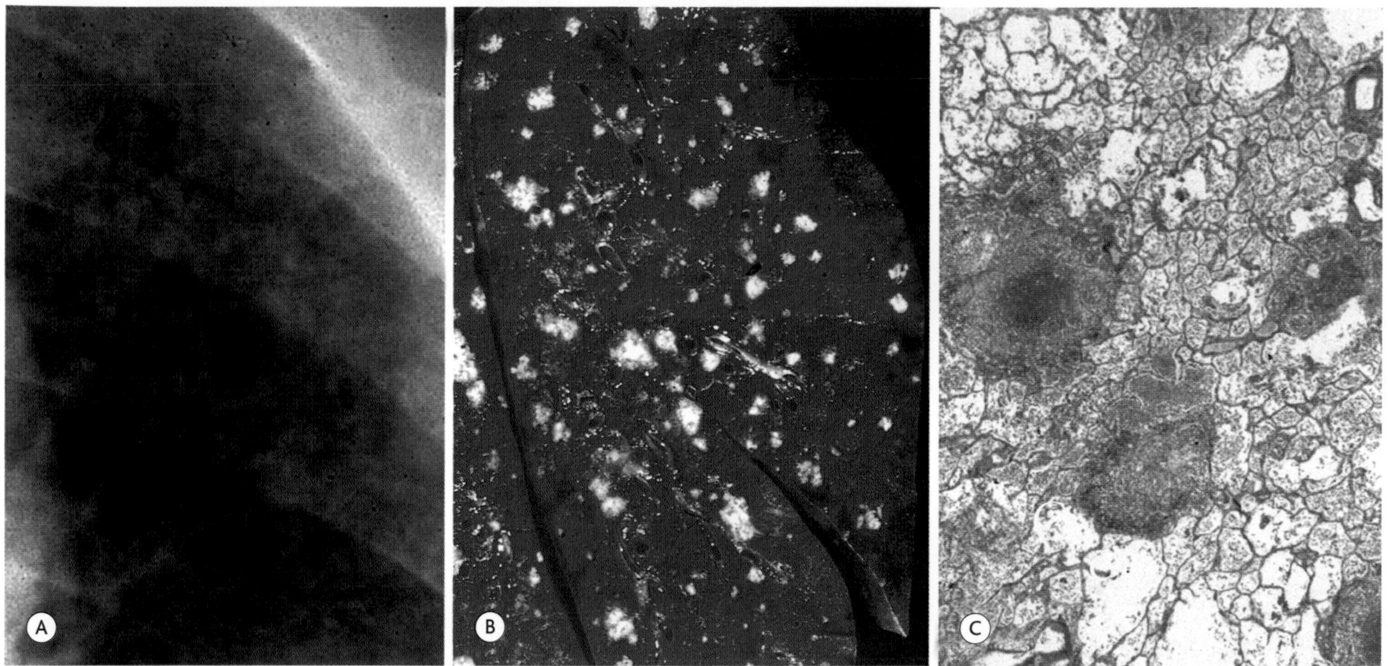

Fig. 6.3 **The miliary pattern (tuberculosis).** (A) Chest X-ray; close-up view of miliary infiltrate. (B) Gross cut surface of pulmonary parenchyma with miliary nodules. (C) Histopathology of miliary necrotizing granulomas (H&E).

sensitive and a good starting point for approaching a suspected bacterial infection. By coating the bacteria with metallic silver, the bacterial silhouettes are enhanced (Fig. 6.5) and become more visible.[2] Other stains (e.g. Giemsa) will sometimes detect bacteria that do not stain well with more conventional stains (Fig. 6.6).

The Grocott's methenamine silver (GMS) stain (Fig. 6.7), or one of its rapid variants, is the best stain for most fungi in tissue, and also stains *Actinomycetes*, *Nocardia*, *Pneumocystis* (cysts), free-living soil amoeba, algal cells, the spores of certain microsporidia, and the cytoplasmic inclusions of cytomegalovirus (CMV).[18]

Most mycobacteria stain well with the Ziehl–Neelsen procedure (Fig. 6.8) but the auramine–rhodamine fluorescent procedure is superior in terms of sensitivity (Fig. 6.9). *Nocardia* spp., *Legionella micdadei*, and *Rhodococcus equi* are weakly or partially acid-fast, and modified acid-fast stains such as the Fite–Farraco procedure are more satisfactory for these organisms. Some mycobacterial species, such as *M. avium* complex, are also PAS-positive, GMS-positive, and weakly Gram-positive.

Finally, for completeness, it can be said that for most protozoa and helminths, as well as viral inclusions, a good-quality hematoxylin and eosin (H&E) stained section suffices; in fact, a good H&E stained section alone is diagnostic for many infectious diseases. It can often detect and distinguish even bacterial cocci and bacilli when the burden of organisms is high (Fig. 6.10).

Immunologic and molecular techniques

The application of ancillary studies, such as immunohistochemistry, in-situ hybridization[19] (Fig. 6.11) or nucleic acid amplification technology, such as the polymerase chain reaction method (PCR), can provide a specific etiologic diagnosis in certain cases, and are the techniques that have the best chance for diagnosing infections caused by fastidious species that are difficult or impossible to culture from any sample, including formalin-fixed, paraffin-embedded tissues. Since the introduction of the original PCR method in the 1980s, a number of modifications have been made. Non-PCR DNA amplification methods and methods based not on the amplification of the DNA target per se but on amplification of the signal or probe have also been introduced.[20] Among the newly emergent technologies is rapid-cycle "real time" PCR, an especially powerful advancement that is significantly more sensitive than

Table 6.3 Pathologic patterns and agents of pulmonary infection

Pattern	Most common agents
Airway disease	
– Bronchitis/bronchiolitis	Virus; bacteria; mycoplasma
– Bronchiectasis	Bacteria; mycobacteria
Acute exudative pneumonia	
– Purulent (neutrophilic)	Bacteria
Lobular (bronchopneumonia)	Bacteria
Confluent (lobar pneumonia)	Bacteria
With granules	Botryomycosis; actinomycosis
– Eosinophilic	Parasites
– Foamy alveolar cast	Pneumocystis
– Acute diffuse/localized alveolar damage	Virus; polymicrobial
Chronic pneumonia	
– Fibroinflammatory	Bacteria
– Organizing diffuse/localized alveolar damage	Virus
– Eosinophilic	Parasite
– Histiocytic	Mycobacteria
Interstitial pneumonia	
– Perivascular lymphoid	Virus; atypical agents
– Eosinophilic	Parasite
– Granulomatous	Mycobacteria
Nodules	
– Large	
Necrotizing	Fungal; mycobacteria
Granulomatous	Fungal; mycobacteria
Fibrocaseous	Fungal; mycobacteria
Calcified	Fungal; mycobacteria
– Miliary	
Necrotizing	Viral; mycobacteria; fungi
Granulomatous	Fungi
Cavities and cysts	Fungi; mycobacteria
Intravascular/infarct	Fungi
Spindle cell pseudotumor	Mycobacteria
Minimal ("ID") reaction	Polymicrobial

Table 6.4 Useful tissue stains in lung infection

Gram stains:
- Brown & Brenn
- Brown & Hopps

Silver stains:
- Warthin–Starry
- Steiner
- Dieterle

Fungal stains:
- Gomori methenamine silver (GMS)
- Periodic acid schiff (PAS)

Mycobacterial stains
- Ziehl–Neelsen (heat)
- Kinyoun (cold)
- Auromine O (fluorochrome)
- Fite–Ferraco (peanut or mineral oil)

Others:
- Giemsa; DiffQuik
- Mucicarmine
- Modified trichrome (Weber)
- Fontana–Masson
- Chemofluorescent (optical brighteners)
- Immunofluorescent antibodies
- Immunohistochemistry

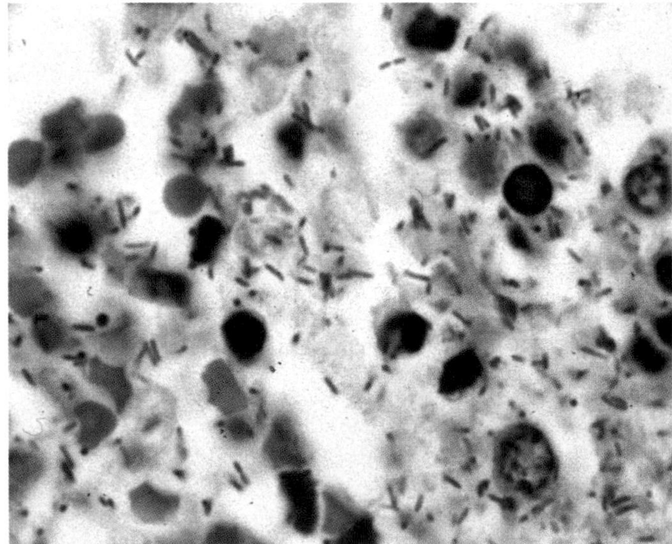

Fig. 6.4 Gram-negative bacilli (*Escherichia coli*) in alveolar exudate (Brown & Hopps stain).

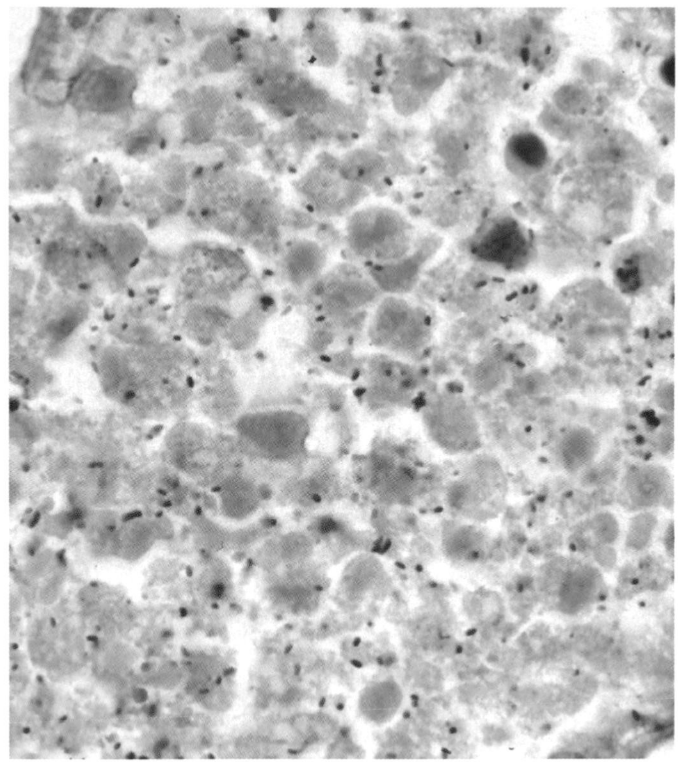

Fig. 6.5 Black (silver-coated) bacilli (*Legionella pneumophilia*) in alveolar exudate (Dieterle stain).

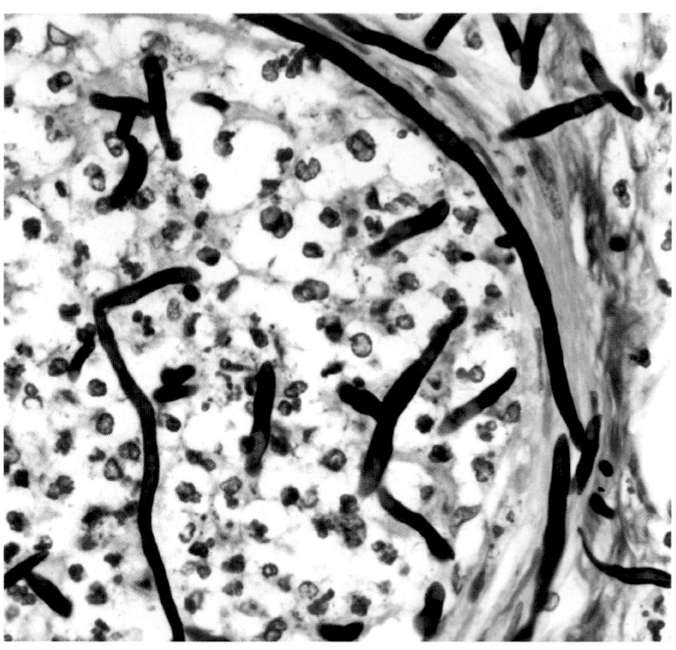

Fig. 6.7 **Angioinvasive *Aspergillus* sp. (GMS).** (Courtesy of Dr Francis Chandler, Augusta, GA.)

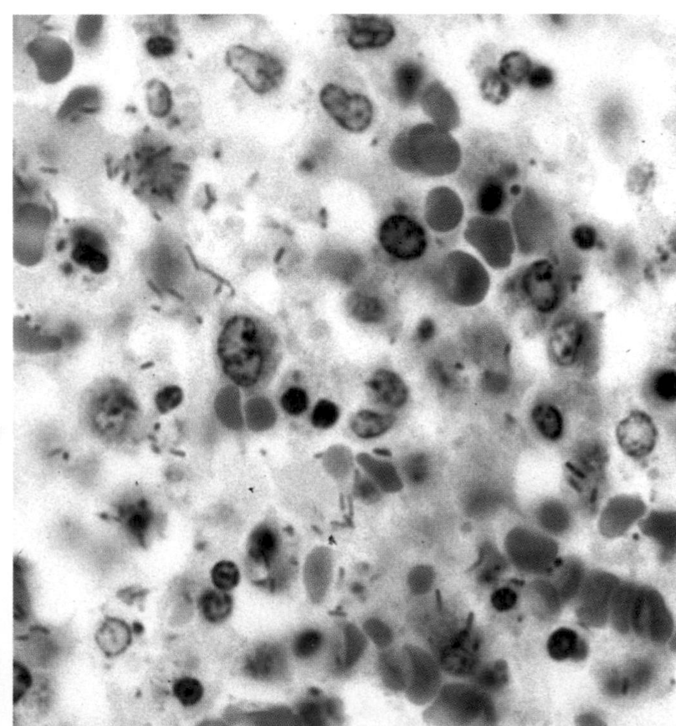

Fig. 6.6 Bacillary organisms in alveolar exudates (Giemsa stain).

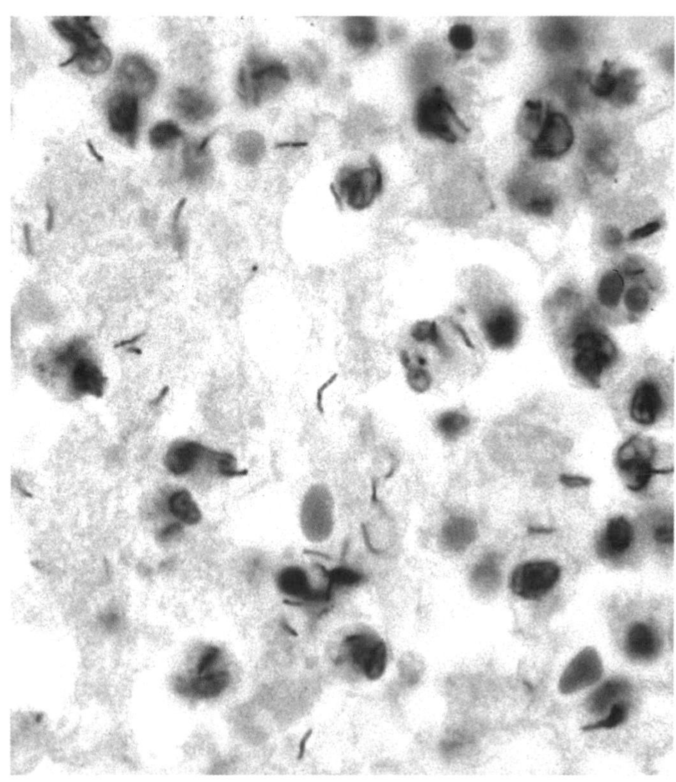

Fig. 6.8 **Acid-fast bacilli (*M. tuberculosis*).** Ziehl–Neelsen stain.

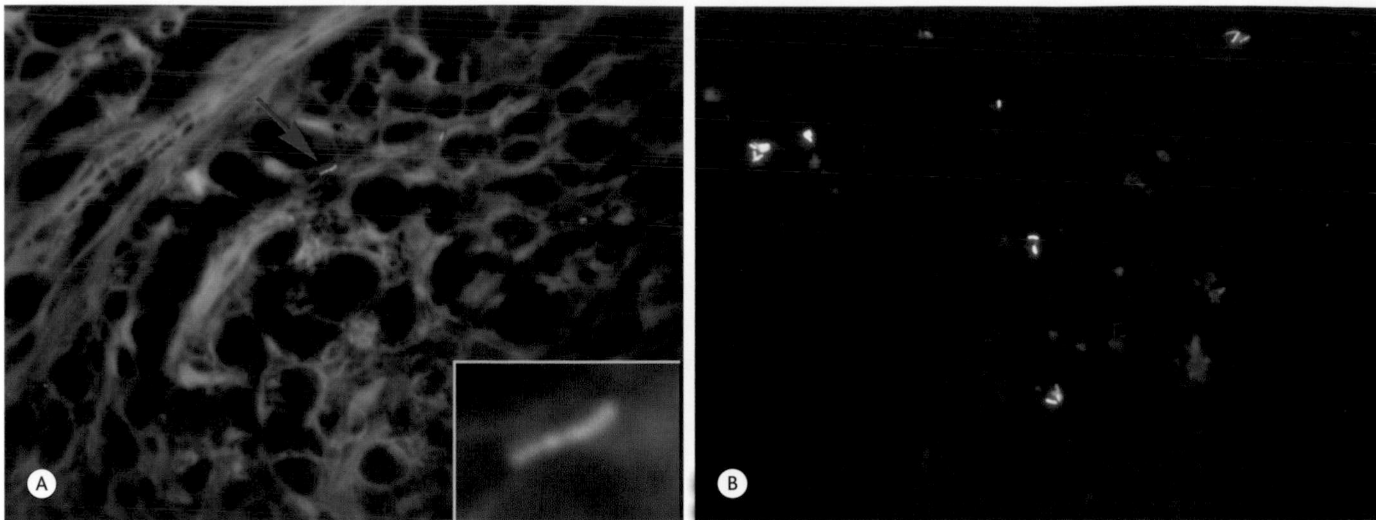

Fig. 6.9 **Fluorescent bacillary organisms (*M. tuberculosis*).** (A) Tissue section with two bacilli. Note beaded character in close-up view (inset). Auromine–rhodamine stain. (B) Fluorescent bacillary organisms at low-scanning power.

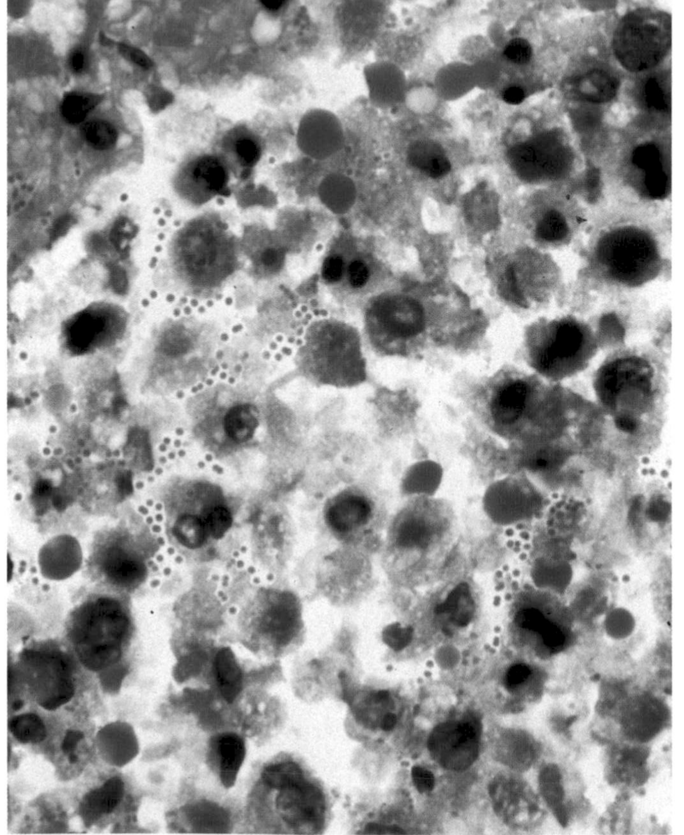

Fig. 6.10 Streptococci in necrotizing pneumonia. H&E stain.

Fig. 6.11 **Blastomyces dermatitidis.** In-situ hybridization. (Courtesy of Ricardo Lloyd, M.D., Rochester, MN.)

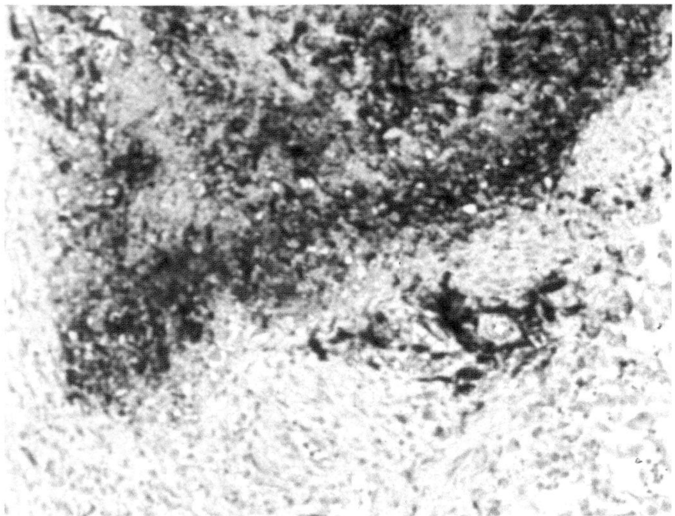

Fig. 6.12 Herpes simplex necrotizing pneumonitis (immunohistochemistry).

Table 6.5 Limitations of diagnostic tools

Morphology
Histopathology: inflammatory pattern nonspecific, atypical or absent; organisms not visualized or nonspecific morphology, e.g. "Aspergillus-like"; unexpected or unfamiliar site
Special stains/IHC/molecular techniques: sensitivity and specificity issues; misinterpretation, e.g. aberrant forms, artifacts, non-microbial mimics; limited reagents, false-negative and false-positive results
Cytopathology: limitations similar to histopathology
Microbiology
Direct visualization: sensitivity & specificity.
Culture/identifications: Normal flora or pathogens? Colonization or asymptomatic shedding vs invasion; difficult, dangerous, or slow to grow; treated; fixed, contaminated tissue; too small or nonrepresentative
Serology: single sample; no early response or lack of response; nondiagnostic for highly prevalent/persistent microbe; cross reaction; acute vs chronic; false-positive IgM tests

culture. In time, it will find a place in laboratories of all sizes, and dramatically impact the speed and accuracy of microbiologic testing practice for all types of microorganisms.[21]

Immunohistochemical reagents for microbiological detection are becoming increasingly available and provide added power to determining specific diagnoses on formalin-fixed paraffin-embedded tissue[22] (Fig. 6.12). Although these techniques provide the diagnostic equivalence of culture confirmation, they are not without limitations, and considerations of sensitivity, specificity, and accuracy must be applied if diagnostic pitfalls are to be avoided.

Limiting factors

Needless to say, the diagnostic tools employed by both pathologists and microbiologists have their limitations, in terms of sensitivity and specificity.[7,18] Some of these are listed in Table 6.5. Culture alone cannot distinguish contamination from colonization, or in the case of viruses, asymptomatic shedding from true infection. However, if a surgical biopsy is available, correlation of the histopathologic features can help assign an etiologic role to an agent recovered in culture. The host inflammatory pattern and morphologic features of an organism can be characteristic for certain types of infections, but often the organism's morphology alone is not sufficiently accurate for a diagnosis at the genus or species level. Furthermore, the classic histopathologic findings for a given infection may be incomplete or lacking, making specific morphologic diagnosis possible for relatively few organisms. For example, etiologic diagnosis is straightforward when large spherules with endospores characteristic of *Coccidioides* spp. are present, when small budding yeasts of *Histoplasma capsulatum* are seen or yeasts with large mucoid capsules of *Cryptococcus neoformans* are identified. However, atypical forms of these organisms can be misleading.[23] Similarly, hyphal morphology is helpful when it is characteristic of a specific genus or group but there are many look-alikes (Fig. 6.13) that require separation by searching for subtle differences under high magnification or oil immersion, or reliance on special techniques and culture.[24]

Certain viruses may have characteristic inclusions in tissue, but there are notable pitfalls. For example, eosinophilic intranuclear inclusions of adenovirus may resemble the early inclusions in herpes simplex virus or CMV, especially when the typical smudged cellular forms of adenovirus are absent. Simulators of viral cytopathic effect, such as macronucleoli, optically clear nuclei, and intranuclear cytoplasmic invaginations occur commonly in pathology and can be problematic (Fig. 6.14).

Pseudomicrobic artifacts also exist for bacteria and fungi on routine and special stains. These include fragmented reticulin fibers, pigments, calcium deposits, Hamazaki–Wesenberg (yellow-brown) yeast-like bodies (Fig. 6.15), pollen grains, and even lymphoglandular bodies.[25] For all of the above reasons, the pathologist must maintain a high threshold for diagnosing organisms

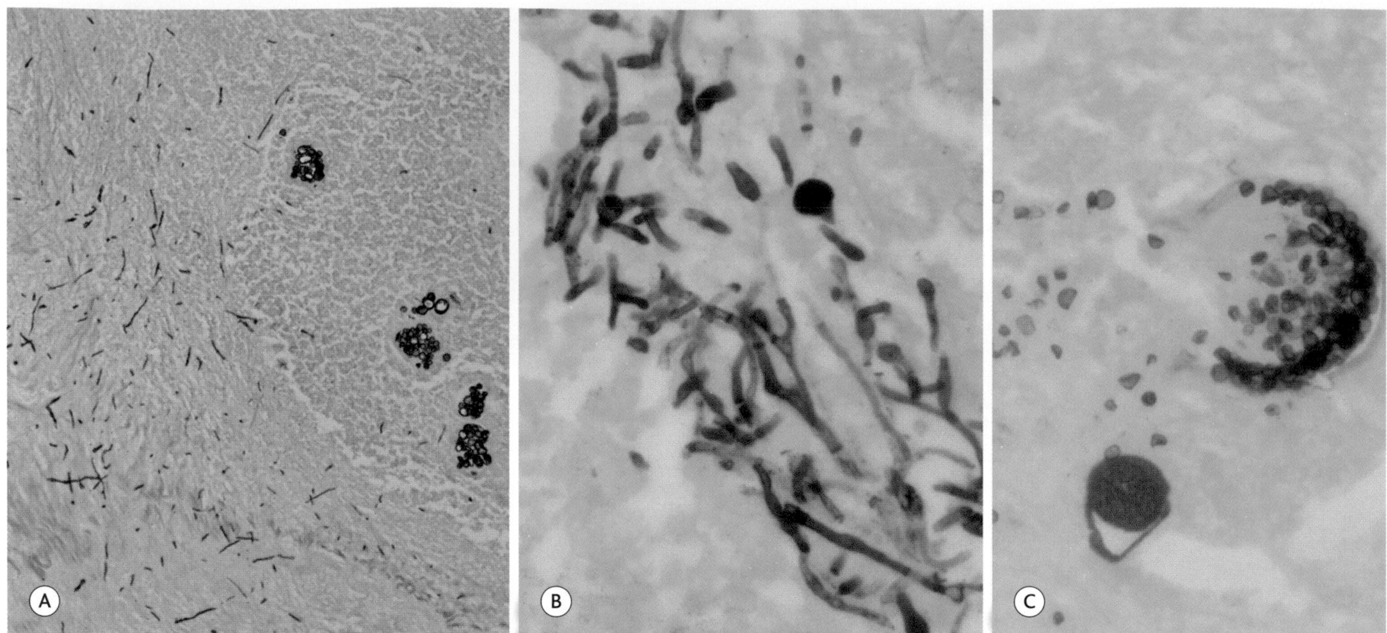

Fig. 6.13 *Coccidioides immitis*, biphasic features vs other species. Culture grew *C. immitis* and *Fusarium* spp. (A) Spherules and mycelia. (B) Mycelia. (C) Ruptured spherule with endospores (GMS stain).

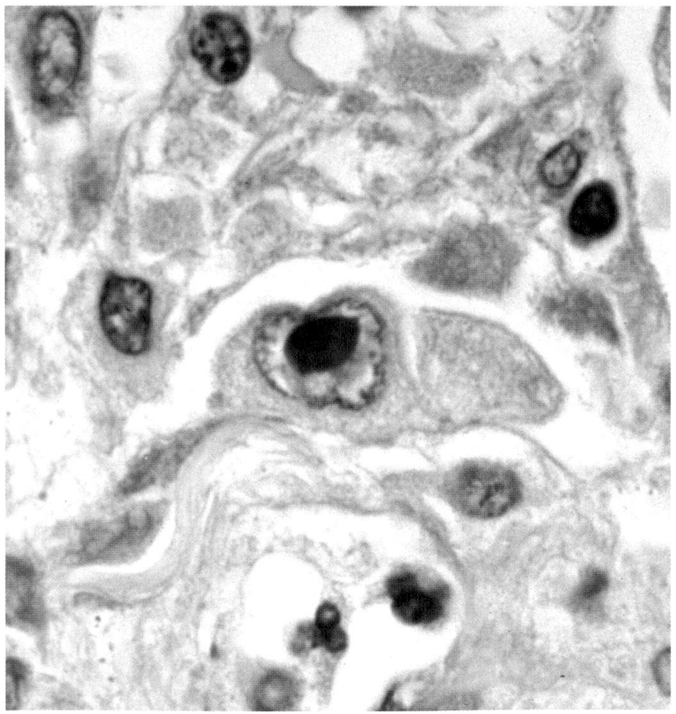

Fig. 6.14 Macronucleolus mimicking a viral inclusion in an alveolar lining cell (H&E stain).

on morphologic grounds. If there is any question, repeating special stains liberally on deeper levels and/or different blocks is advisable.

There are times when the clinical suspicion of an infectious disease cannot be confirmed by the pathologist or microbiologist, despite a thorough microscopic evaluation and culture of the tissue. The histologic features for infection may be lacking, and all stains and molecular techniques may prove negative. Still, this negative information is useful, since the clinical findings may actually reflect a noninfectious disease: e.g. a pulmonary infiltrate in an immunocompromised patient may have a noninfectious etiology, such as a drug reaction, lymphangitic neoplasm or graft versus host disease.

The role of cytopathology in lung infection

A wide variety of infectious diseases of the lung, including bacterial, mycobacterial, fungal, viral, and parasitic, can be diagnosed through exfoliative or fine-needle aspiration cytologic techniques.[26–28] Fine-needle aspiration is an especially powerful tool, compared to exfoliative cytology of respiratory secretions (sputa, bronchial washings, brushings, and bronchoalveolar lavage). Exfoliative cytology is often limited due to problems associated with distinguishing colonizing organisms in the airways from true pathogens. Nonetheless, these diagnostic techniques are complementary, and have been used in recent years to evaluate pneumonias and pulmonary nodules in both normal hosts and immunocompromised patients.

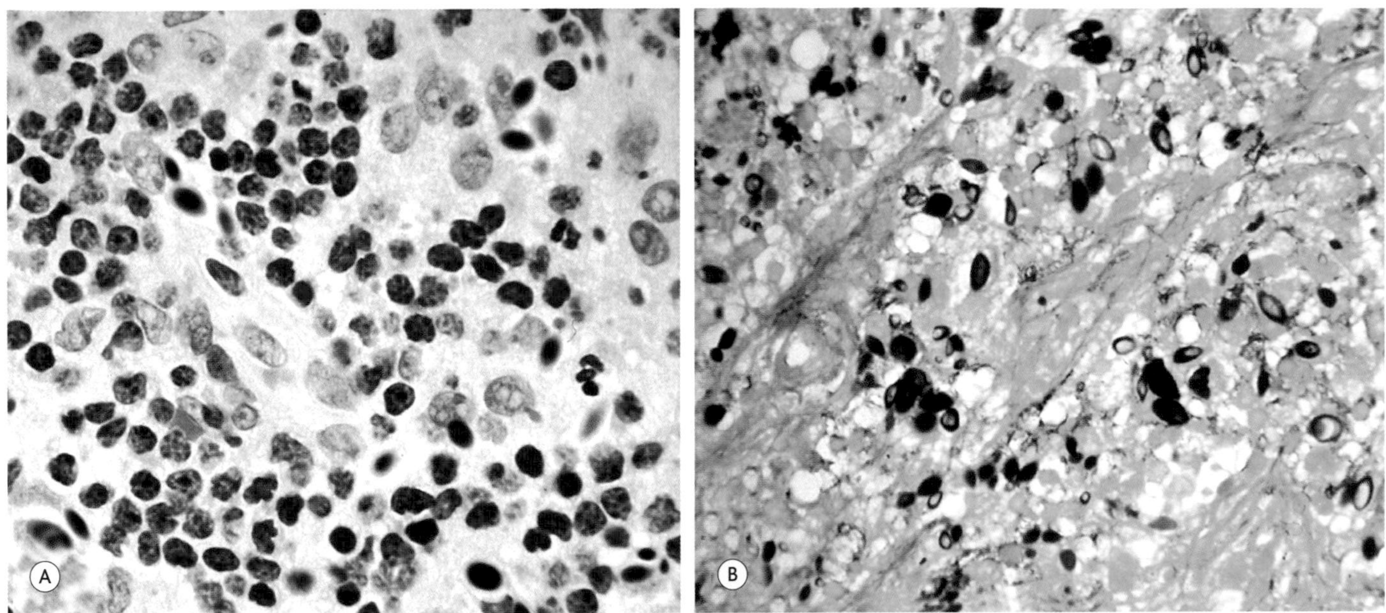

Fig. 6.15 **Yellow-brown Hamazaki–Wesenberg bodies.** (A) H&E stain. (B) GMS stain.

Mass-like infiltrates are often the target of aspiration biopsy needles where suspicion or exclusion of an infectious process ranks high in the differential diagnosis. Besides the morphologic features of the microorganism, important cytologic clues to the diagnosis include the accompanying cellular response and the presence and character of any necrotic debris present, as outlined in Table 6.6. Although nonspecific, such features can suggest certain possibilities to the cytopathologist and assist the microbiology laboratory in triaging the specimen.[29] To this end, the presence of a cytopathologist, microscope, and staining setup during the aspiration process can be useful. The cytopathologist can correlate the clinical setting, radiographic features, and clues from the gross character of the aspirate (color, consistency, odor, etc.), thereby assisting in narrowing the diagnostic possibilities and avoiding false-positive and false-negative diagnoses.[30] Also, immediate evaluation of smears by rapid stain allows the cytopathologist to either make or suggest a specific diagnosis, similar to a frozen section prepared during intraoperative consultation. Smears can be prepared for special stains, needle rinses can be made for culture and other ancillary studies, and additional aspirations may be encouraged for these purposes. Special stains for bacteria, mycobacteria, and fungi should be performed whenever the character of the aspirate and the clinical setting indicate they might be potentially useful. They may not be routinely warranted in all categories of patients, particularly in the non-immunosuppressed host.

Some interventionalists prefer to provide only a needle core biopsy in lieu of an aspirate for a variety of reasons. These two techniques can be viewed as complementary; whereas needle core biopsies work well for neoplasms and many granulomas, the aspirate is often superior for many types of infections, especially

Table 6.6 Fine-needle aspirate (FNA) patterns of pulmonary infectious diseases

Patterns	Possible etiology
Acute purulent inflammation/abscess	Bacteria Fungi
Granuloma pattern (epithelioid cells with/ without necrosis)	
– Caseous/necrotizing	Fungi
– Suppurative	Mycobacteria
– Epithelial	Bacteria
– Mixed	Parasite
Foamy alveolar cast (FAC) pattern	*P. Jiroveci*
Histiocytic	Mycobacterial Bacteria Fungi
Chronic inflammation (lymphocyte & plasma cell)	Virus Any other
Null/id reaction	Virus Any other

bacterial abcesses. Sometimes a rapid and specific etiologic diagnosis is possible at the bedside, based on the microscopic features of the organism itself. However, when the organism is not readily apparent or its features are inconclusive, the microbiology laboratory can be invaluable for its role in isolation and identification.

Summary

The successful treatment of pulmonary infections depends on the accuracy of the etiologic diagnosis. In turn, this requires collecting the best specimens, transporting them to the anatomic and microbiology sections of the laboratory under optimum conditions, and processing them with techniques appropriate for the spectrum of possible etiologies. An interdisciplinary approach enhances this process. Therefore, it behooves pathologists, clinicians, and microbiologists to communicate frequently and to understand the strengths and weaknesses of their respective disciplines. Joint strategies can be developed for the approach to certain types of suspected infections, helping foster the development of laboratory "foresight" in surgical colleagues and medical consultants. As methods of diagnosis, strategies for treatment, and prophylaxis change, the pathologist must remain vigilant to a changing spectrum of etiologic agents and tissue injury patterns. Laboratories with a standard protocol in place are optimally positioned to choose the appropriate combination of diagnostic methods (morphologic, culture, immunologic, molecular) that will provide an accurate etiologic diagnosis. An example of such an operational protocol is presented in Table 6.7.

Table 6.7 Work-up of pulmonary infections

Preop/intraop consult
- Inquiry regarding:
  History
  Risk factors; immune status
  Radiographic pattern
- Advise regarding:
  How & what to collect
  What culture & tests to order
  Devices, transport media & containers
  Fixatives for morphologic study

Written protocol
- Handling tissue for cultures
- Special stains & ancillary tests
- Logistics
- Requisition – designed to communicate

Morphologic examination
- Inflammatory pattern
- Persistence & repeat studies
- Oil immersion, if necessary
- High threshold for positive
- Consider multiple pathogens

Report
- Presumptive vs definitive diagnosis; correlate with culture; other studies
- Comment:
  Clinicopathologic/ microbiologic correlation
  Differential diagnosis
  Ancillary tests
  Suggestions for further work-up

Bacterial pneumonias

The surgical pathologist rarely receives biopsy specimens from patients with community-acquired or nosocomial pneumonias. Most are suspected clinically by symptoms, physical and radiographic findings; some are confirmed immediately by Gram stains or later by culture performed on respiratory secretions in the microbiology laboratory. Sometimes, serologic studies prove diagnostic. However, even when conventional microbiologic approaches are utilized, about 50% of bacterial pneumonias remain undiagnosed.[31–33] Patients with mild disease are often not tested, but simply treated empirically with antibiotic regimens. By contrast, patients with severe disease, whether immunocompromised or not, often become candidates for invasive procedures.

Etiologic agents

Bacterial pneumonia may be classified according to a number of parameters, including pathogenesis, epidemiology, anatomic pattern, clinical course, and organism type (Table 6.8)[34] Using bacterial type as a starting point allows the pathologist to correlate anatomic and histopathologic patterns of lung injury with categories of etiologic agents.

Pyogenic bacteria

The pyogenic bacteria most commonly associated with community-acquired pneumonias include *Streptococcus pneumoniae*, *Haemophilus influenzae*, and *Moraxella catarrhalis*.[33] Others, such as *Legionella* spp., *Chlamydia pneumoniae* and *Mycoplasma pneumoniae* (often referred to

Table 6.8 Classification of bacterial pneumonia

Pathogenesis:
- Primary
  Exogenous
  Endogenous
- Secondary

Epidemiology:
- Community acquired
- Nosocomial

Anatomic type:
- Lobular
- Lobar

Clinical course:
- Acute
- Chronic

Bacterial type:
- Pyogenic species
- Atypical agents
- Granule/filamentous group

as the "atypical" group) are clinically important but controversy exists with regard to the relative frequency that these organisms are etiologically responsible. Although community-acquired pneumonia is considered to be fundamentally different in children and adults, severe or complicated pneumonias in both of these age groups have similar etiologies.[35] The enteric Gram-negative bacilli cause relatively few community-acquired pneumonias, whereas they account for most of the nosocomial pneumonias, along with *Pseudomonas* spp., *Acinetobacter* spp. *Staphylococcus aureus*, and anaerobes.[36–37a] Most nosocomial pneumonias result from aspiration of these bacterial species that colonize the oropharynx of hospitalized patients; they are often polymicrobial. Any of the bacterial organisms listed (including mixtures with fungi and viruses) can cause pneumonia in immunocompromised patients.[14,38]

Atypical pneumonia agents

The atypical pneumonia agents are those which do not commonly produce lobar consolidation. Although this potentially implicates a wide variety of bacterial, viral, and protozoal pathogens, a selective list by convention includes *Mycoplasma pneumoniae*, *Legionella* spp., *Chlamydia* spp., *Bordetella* spp., and *Coxiella burnetii*.[39]

Filamentous/granule group

The filamentous/granule group refers to those bacteria that form long, thin, branching filaments in tissues, such as the *Actinomyces* spp. (anaerobic actinomycete) or *Nocardia* spp. (aerobic actinomycete).[40] Botryomycosis is caused by nonfilamentous bacteria, especially *Staphylococcus aureus*, or Gram-negative bacilli, such as *Pseudomonas aeruginosa* and *Escherichia coli*, which form organized aggregates referred to as grains or granules.[41]

Table 6.9 Patterns of bacterial lung injury

Patterns of bacterial lung injury
Bronchitis/bronchiolitis
Acute exudative pneumonia
Lobular (bronchopneumonia)
Confluent (lobar pneumonia)
With granules
Fibroinflammatory and/or organizing pneumonia
Interstitial pneumonia
Nodular/necrotizing lesions
Miliary lesions
Abscess

Histopathologic patterns

Bacterial lung injury patterns will vary based on the virulence of the organism and the host's response. These patterns are further modulated by therapeutic or immunologic factors. While some of the patterns presented in Table 6.9 are characteristic, none are diagnostic. Overlap and mixed patterns occur.[42]

Acute exudative pneumonia

Acute exudative pneumonia is caused by pyogenic bacteria, such as the streptococcal species, which typically produce a neutrophil-rich intra-alveolar exudate with variable amounts of fibrin and red cells. Pathologists recognize this constellation of findings as acute lobular pneumonia (Fig. 6.16) and this usually correlates with patchy segmental infiltrates on X-ray.[43–45]

With increasing organism virulence and disease severity, lobular exudates may become confluent (lobar pneumonia). In milder cases, the disease may be limited to the airways (bronchitis/bronchiolitis), with a mixed cellular infiltrate of mononuclear cells and neutrophils (Fig. 6.17).

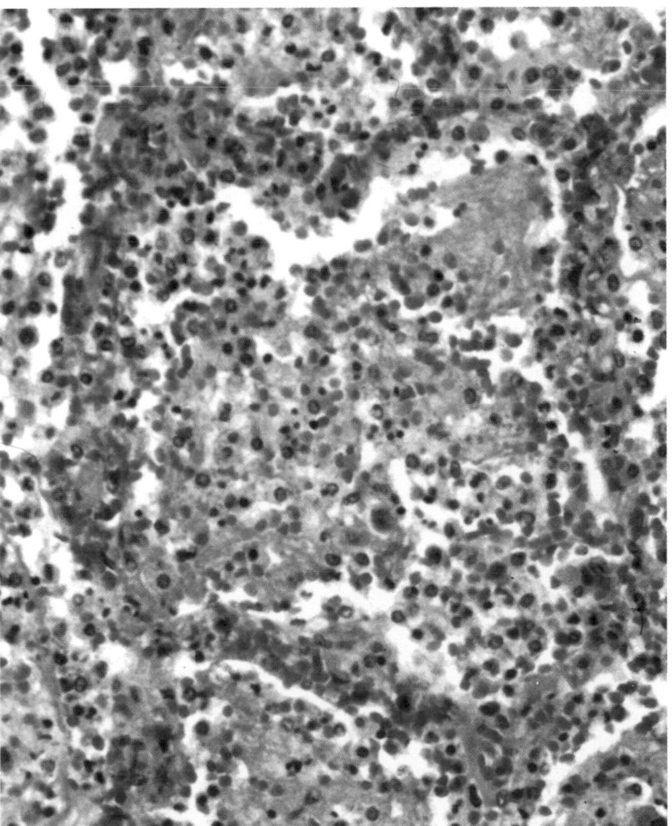

Fig. 6.16 Alveoli filled with fibrinopurulent exudate with variable hemorrhage (H&E stain).

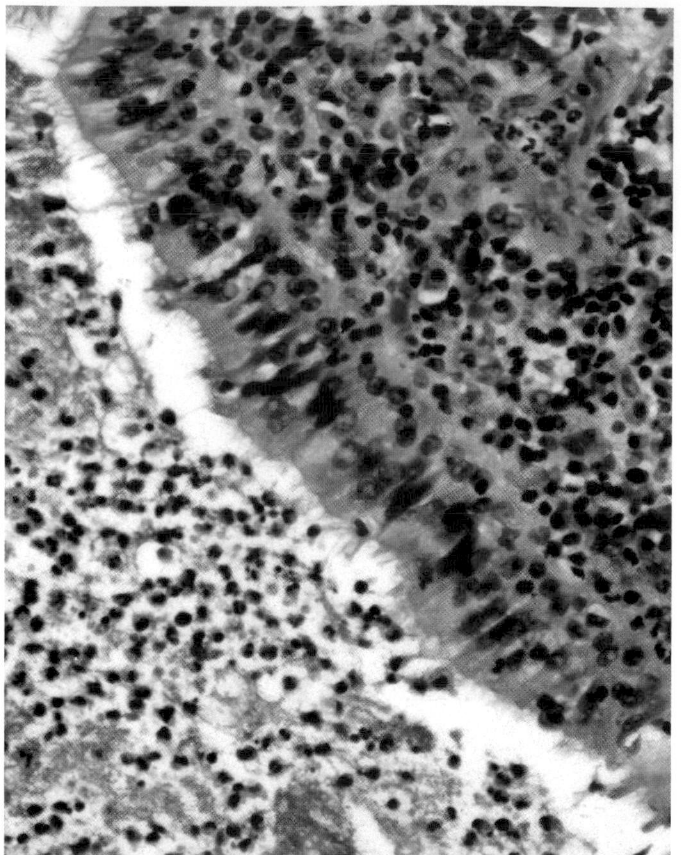

Fig. 6.17 Bronchiolitis with intraluminal exudate (H&E stain).

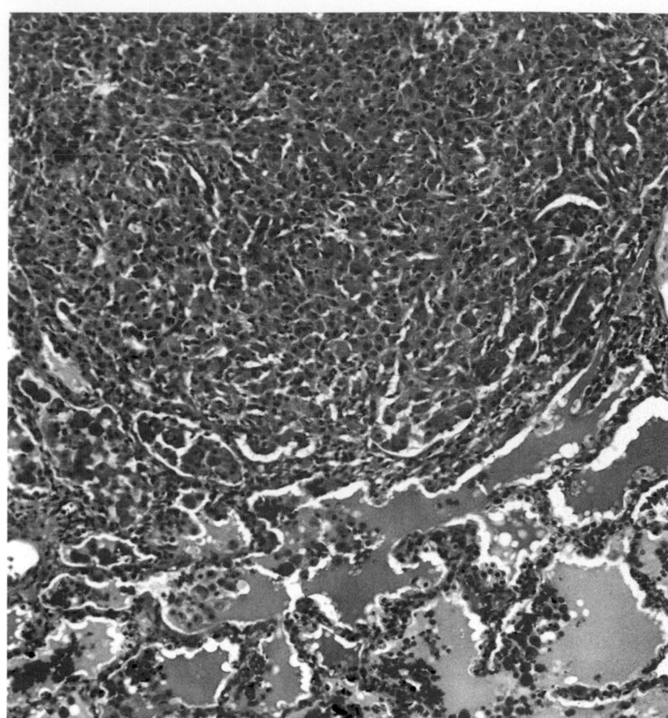

Fig. 6.18 Nodular histiocytic infiltrate in rhodococcal pneumonia (H&E stain).

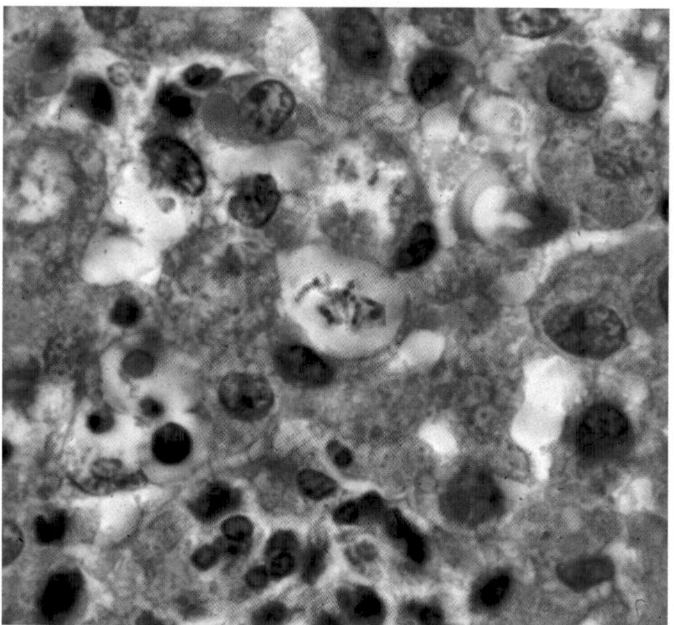

Fig. 6.19 *Rhodococcus equi* bacilli in macrophage (H&E stain).

Nodular infiltrates with or without necrotizing features

Nodular infiltrates with or without necrotizing features (Fig. 6.18) are characteristic of certain species, such as *Rhodococcus equi* (Fig. 6.19).[46] Necrotizing pneumonias may also be produced by pyogenic bacteria such as *Staphlococcus aureus*, *Streptococcus pyogenes* and the Gram-negative bacilli, *Klebsiella*, *Acinetobacter*, *Pseudomonas*, and *Burkholderia* spp. Histopathologic patterns of injury in these cases likely reflect the route of infection, the virulence of the particular species and the immune status of the patient.

Miliary lesions

Miliary lesions (Fig. 6.20) suggest pneumonia secondary to hematogenous spread (septicemia), but are also characteristic of certain organisms, such as *Nocardia* and the anaerobic actionomycetes.

Lung abscess

The lung abscess is usually a polymicrobic mixture of aerobic and anaerobic bacteria,[47] most often secondary to aspiration (Fig. 6.21). *Actinomyces* spp. (Fig. 6.22) and *Nocardia* spp. may also manifest this pattern, as can certain pyogenic bacteria, such as *Staphylococcus aureus*, and the other organisms listed above for necrotizing pneumonias. In the setting of aspiration, in addition to

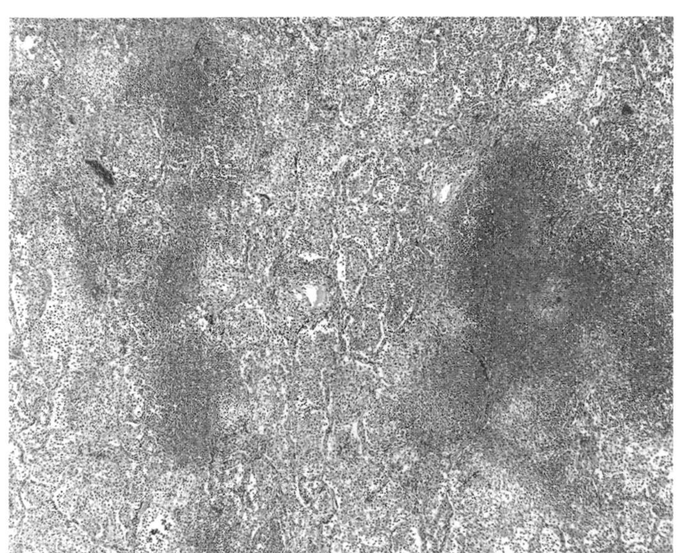

Fig. 6.20 Necrotizing pneumonia, miliary pattern (H&E stain).

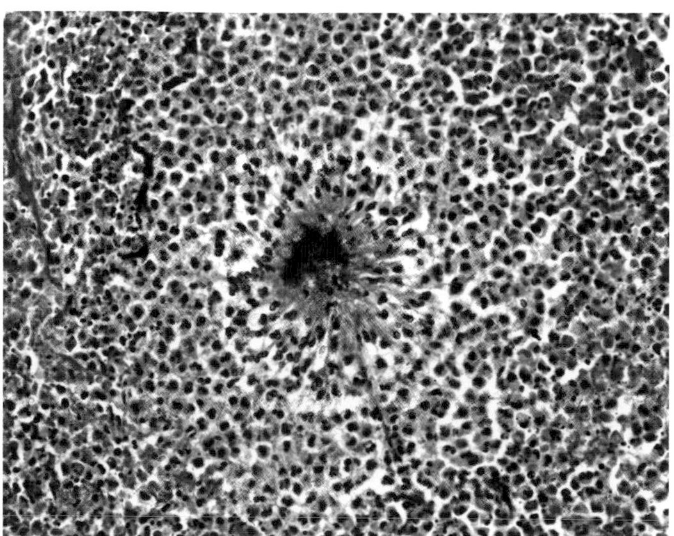

Fig. 6.22 Lung abscess with sulfer granule of actinomycosis in purulent exudate (H&E stain).

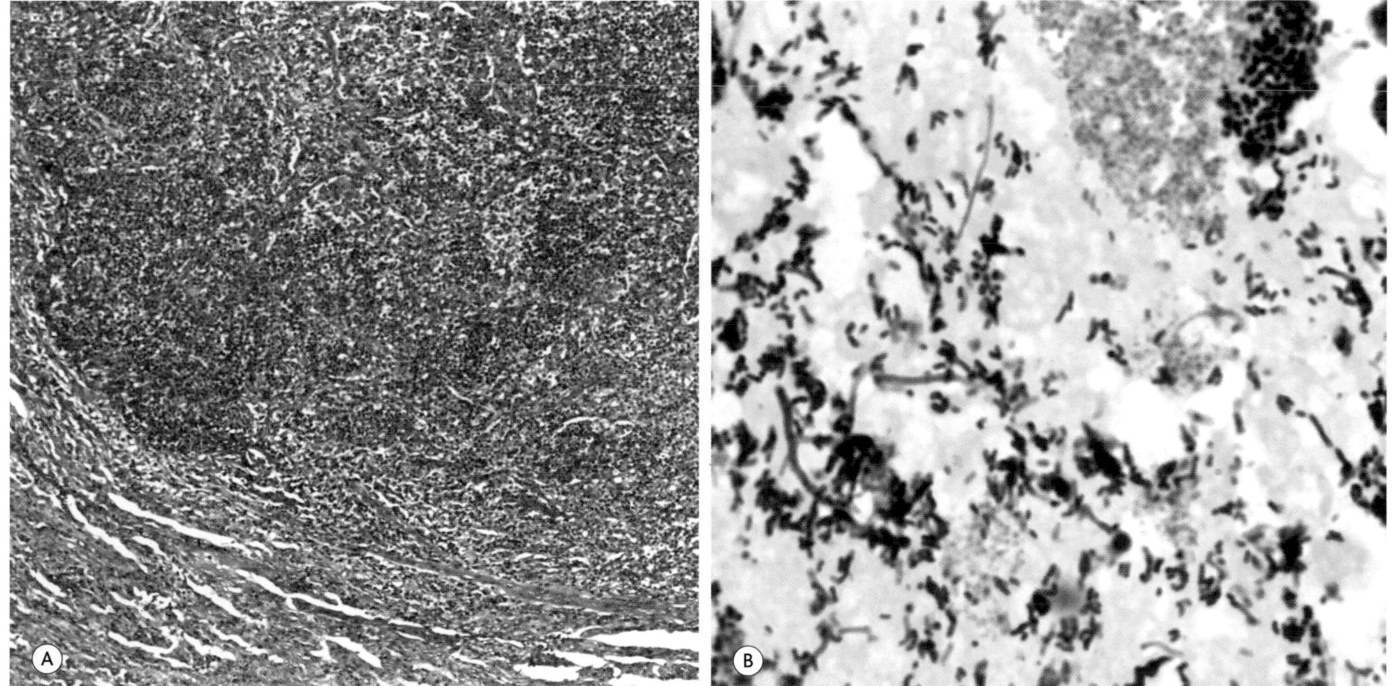

Fig. 6.21 (A) Lung abscess with suppurative inflammation (H&E stain). (B) Lung abscess with polymicrobial bacterial population (Gram stain).

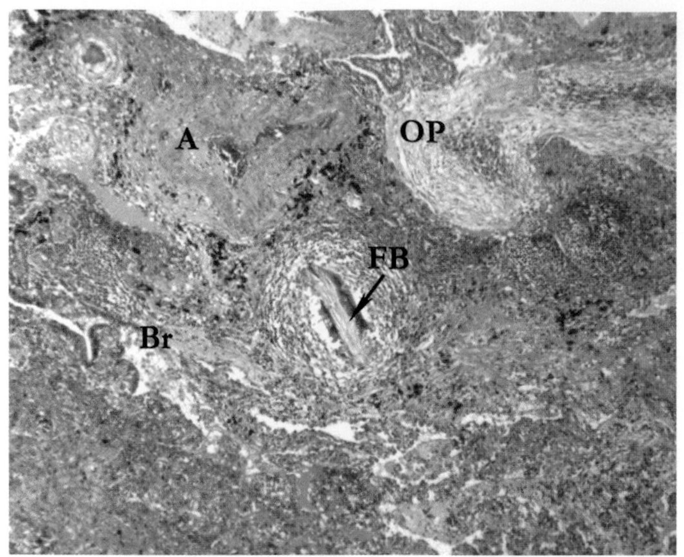

Fig. 6.23 **Aspiration pneumonia.** Giant cells surround vegetable matter (FB) in purulent exudates, organizing pneumonia (OP), bronchiolitis (BR), artery (A).

abscess, lung injury can take the form of bronchiolitis, lobular pneumonia, necrotizing pneumonia, lipoid pneumonia, empyema, or various combinations of these patterns. Granulomatous foci (Fig. 6.23) with foreign material and giant cells may also be seen.[45]

Chronic bacterial pneumonias

Chronic bacterial pneumonias (Fig. 6.24) can produce a nonspecific fibroinflammatory process, with lymphoplasmacytic infiltrates, macrophages, and/or organization with fascicles of fibroblasts in alveolar ducts and alveolar spaces.[48,49] Eventually, if not resorbed, these may become areas of fibrosis or scar. Such scarring is often associated with localized interlobular septal and pleural thickening (Fig. 6.25) that may serve as clues to the diagnosis of chronic infection.

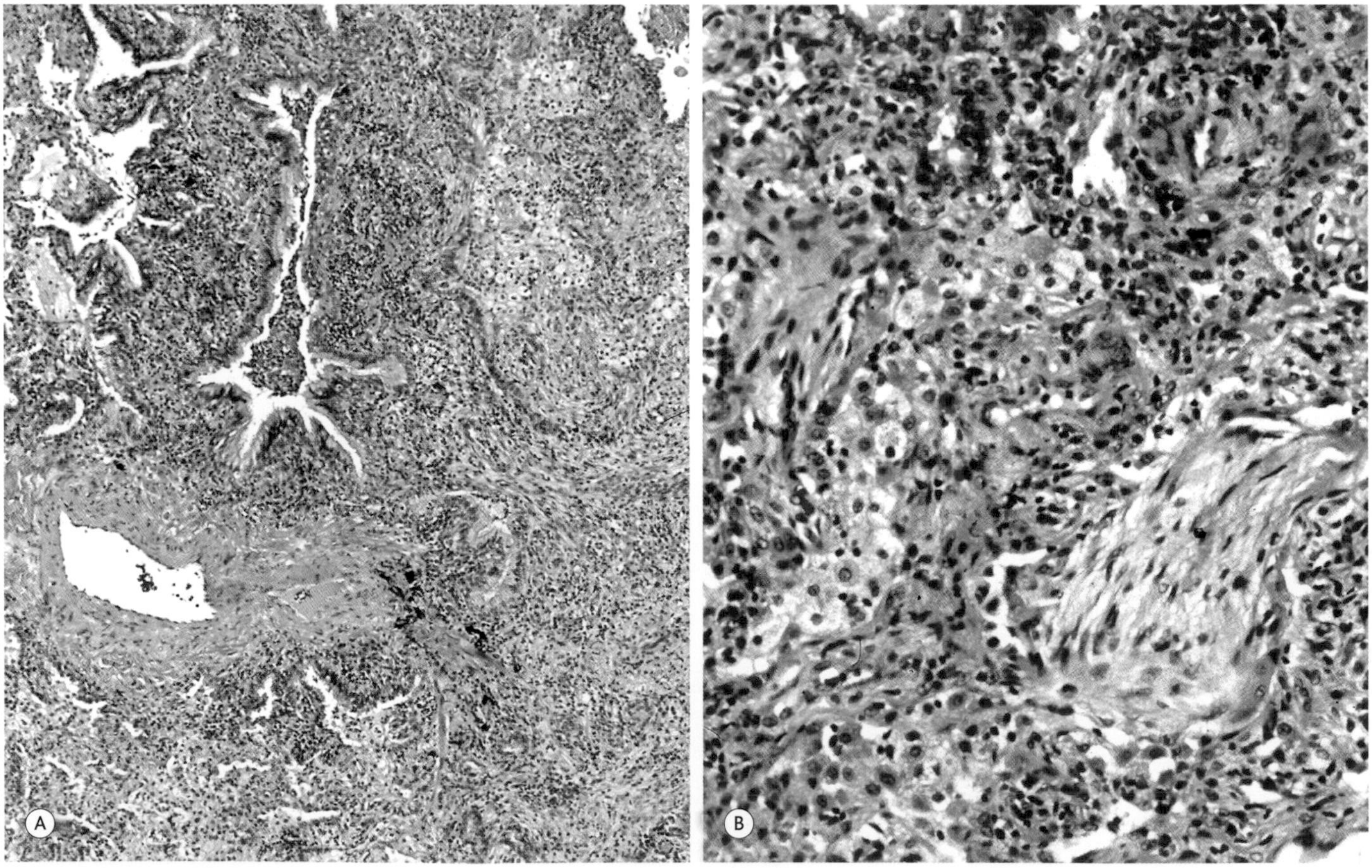

Fig. 6.24 **Chronic pneumonia.** (A) Lymphoplasmacytic infiltrate. (B) Fascicles of fibroblasts in alveolar ducts and spaces (H&E stain).

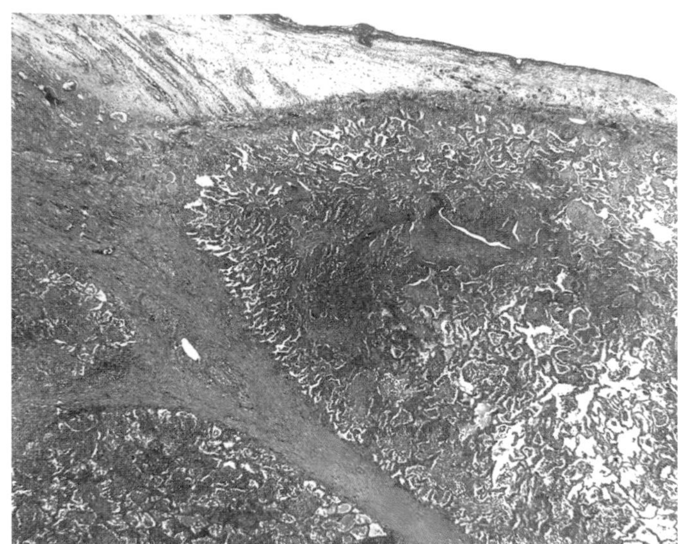

Fig. 6.25 Chronic pneumonia with thickened interlobular septum (H&E stain).

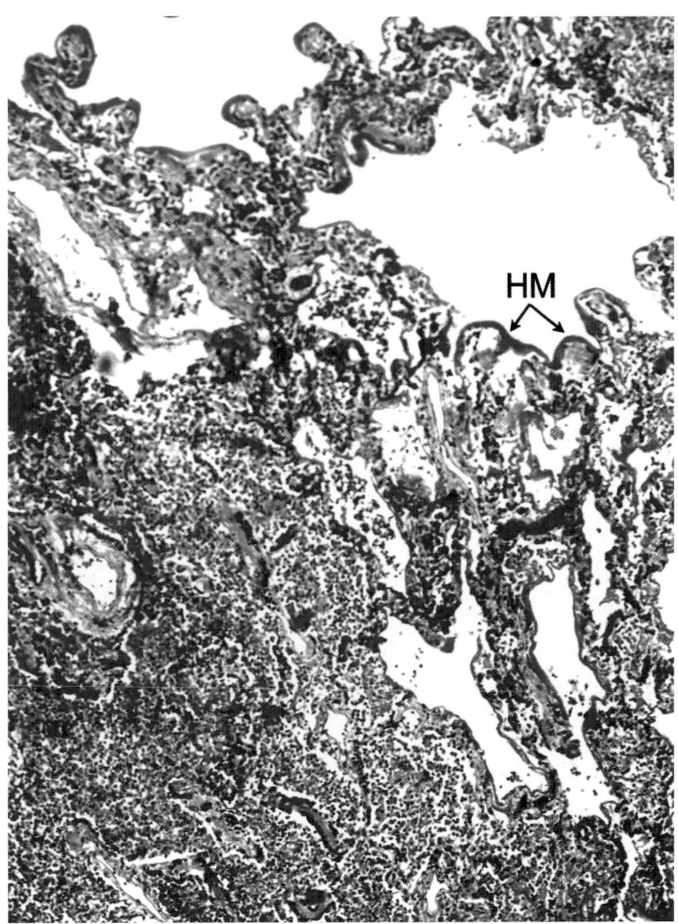

Fig. 6.26 Bacterial pneumonia with hyaline membranes (HM) at periphery (H&E stain).

Diffuse alveolar damage

Diffuse alveolar damage may coexist with any of the necroinflammatory patterns described. Acute diffuse alveolar damage is accompanied by hyaline membranes (Fig. 6.26), whereas the organizing form is attended by airspace fibroplasia.

Atypical pneumonias

The atypical pneumonias include the well-described cases due to *Legionella* spp. and the less well-described cases caused by other organisms comprising the atypical group. *Legionella* spp. typically cause an acute fibrinopurulent lobular pneumonia[43] (Fig. 6.27A). *Legionella* bacilli can often be identified in silver impregnation-stained sections (Fig. 6.27B) or recovered in culture, but newer diagnostic methods, such as real-time PCR and in-situ hybridization (Fig. 6.28), can also be applied when standard approaches fail.[50] The pathologic findings of the other members of the atypical group (i.e. *Chlamydia*; *Mycoplasma*) are not well characterized, mainly because these pneumonias are rarely biopsied. The few well-documented cases of *Mycoplasma*, *Chlamydia*, and *Coxiella* infections that have been described in the literature resemble viral bronchitis or bronchiolitis with mixed inflammatory infiltrates in airway walls and in the adjacent interstitium (Fig. 6.29).[51] There is relative sparing of the peribronchiolar alveolar spaces; although patchy organized fibrinous exudates are seen in some cases, and complications may superimpose additional findings.

Grains and granules

The grains and granules formed by the actinomycetes, and bacteria of botryomycosis may have a uniform tinctorial hue but, more often, these have a hematoxylinophilic core and an outer investment of eosinophilic material known as the Splendore–Hoepplei phenomenon (Fig. 6.30). *Actinomyces* spp. form similar granules, and both they and the bacteria of botryomycosis are typically found in the midst of purulent exudates.[40] The *Nocardia* spp. may aggregate in colonies simulating granules, but with a much looser texture (Fig. 6.31) and more monochromatic tinctorial properties.[52] Rarely, these colonies may be identical in appearance to the grains or granules of botryomycosis or actinomycosis in H&E sections.

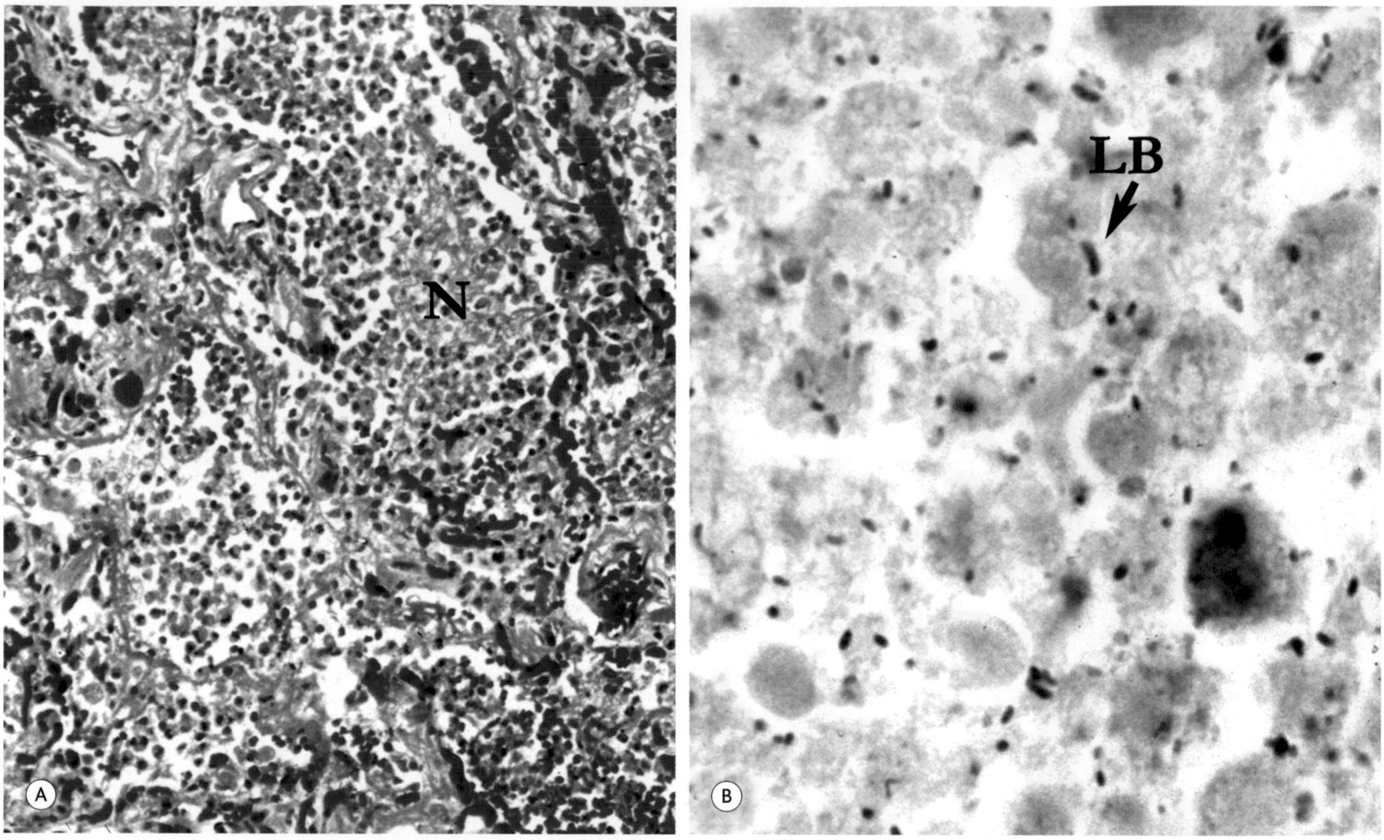

Fig. 6.27 (A) Legionnaires' disease with intra-alveolar necroinflammatory exudates (N) and hemorrhage (H&E stain). (B) Enhanced silhouette of Legionnaires' bacilli (LB) in alveolar exudate with silver impregnation stain (Dieterle stain).

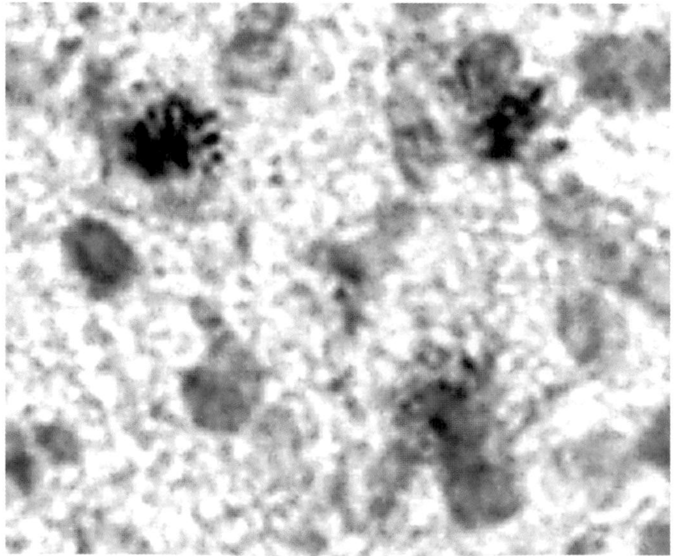

Fig. 6.28 **Legionnaires' disease.** Detection of organisms by in-situ hybridization (Courtesy of Ricardo Lloyd, M.D., Rochester, MN.)

Bacterial agents of bioterrorism

The use of microbial pathogens as agents of bioterrorism requires that pathologists become familiar with the histopathologic features they produce. In this context, respiratory disease caused by the inhalation of *Bacillus anthracis*, *Yersinia pestis*, and *Francisella tularensis* are pertinent to this section.

Bacillus anthracis

In 1877, Robert Koch's conclusive demonstration that *Bacillus anthracis* was the etiologic agent of anthrax revolutionized medicine by linking microbial cause and effect for the first time.[6] Set against its historic importance to medicine, the recent use of anthrax as a bioterrorist agent is sadly tragic. Inhalational anthrax causes a severe hemorrhagic mediastinitis.[53–57] This, and the toxemia (*B. anthracis* produces an exotoxin with three potent components: protective antigen, lethal factor, and edema factor) from the ensuing massive bacteremia, severely compromises pulmonary function and leads to death in 40% or more of the cases. Pleural effusion may be present

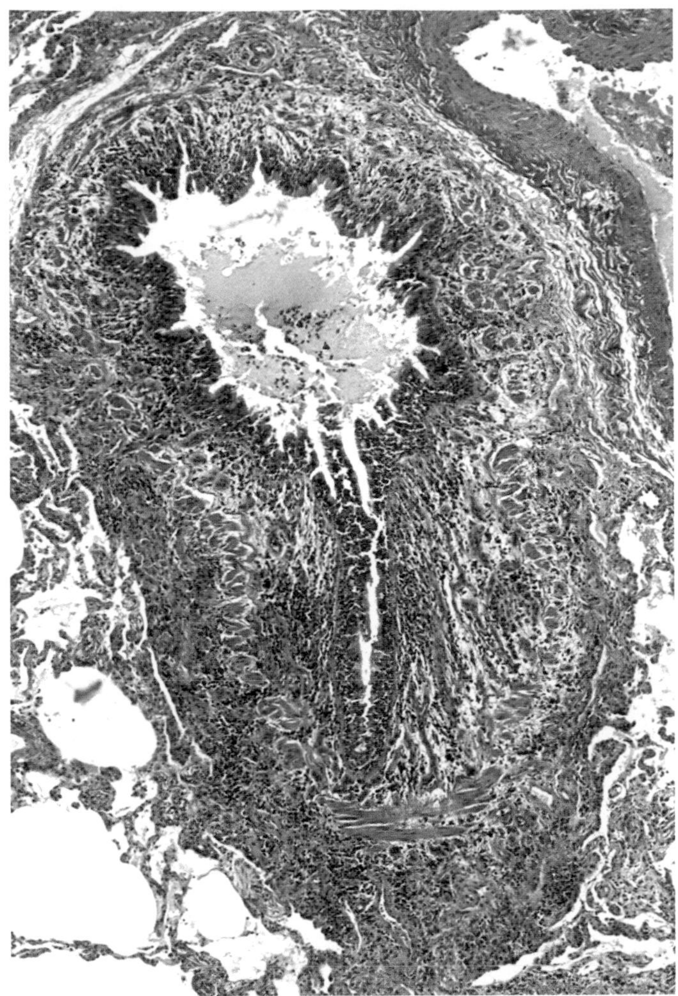

Fig. 6.29 **Mycoplasma pneumonia.** Bronchiolitis with patchy infiltrates in peribronchial interstitium (H&E stain).

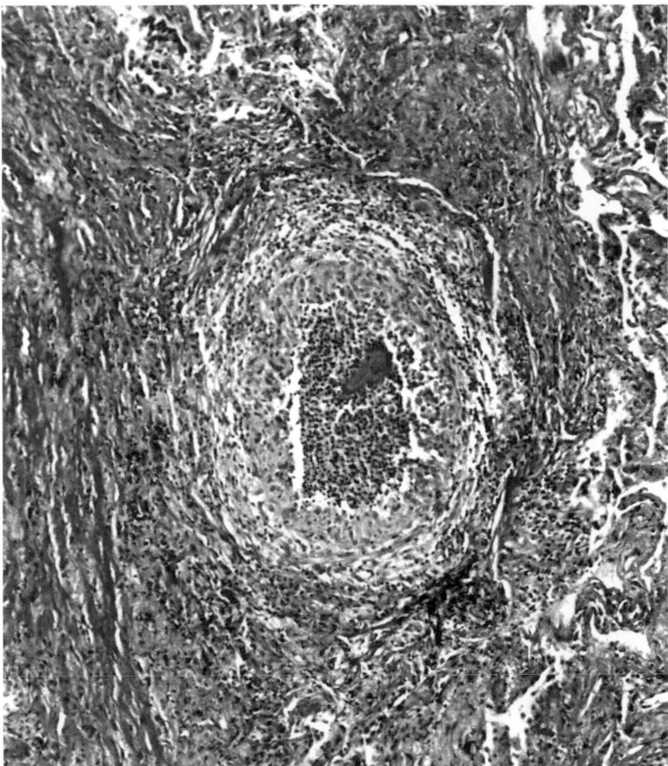

Fig. 6.30 Botryomycosis granule with hematoxylinophilic core and eosinophilic investment known as Splendore–Hoepplei effect (H&E stain).

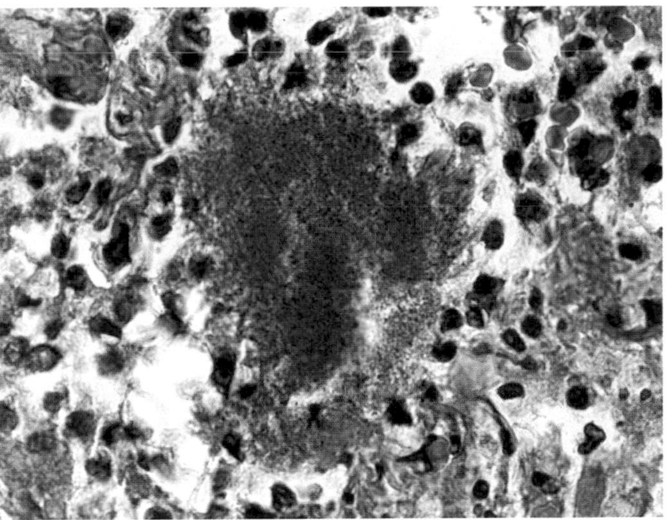

Fig. 6.31 Loose-textured aggregate of *Nocardia* filamentous bacteria surrounded by neutrophils (H&E stain).

but pneumonia is generally minor and secondary. In those patients in whom pulmonary parenchymal changes are found, the alveolar spaces contain a serosanguinous fluid with minimal fibrin deposits, some mononuclear cells but few if any neutrophils.[56] Large Gram-positive bacilli (some may appear partially Gram-negative), without spores, pervade the alveolar septal vessels with a few in the alveolar spaces. This gradient suggests a hematogenous rather than an airway acquisition. Hemorrhagic mediastinitis in a previously healthy adult is essentially pathognomonic of inhalational anthrax. The lymph node parenchyma is generally teeming with intact and fragmented Gram-positive bacilli which can be identified as *B. anthracis* by immunohistochemistry.[56,57] Cultures of blood and pleural fluid, if available, are likely to be the earliest positive diagnostic tests.[55] Sputum studies are much less useful.

Yersinia pestis

Primary pneumonic plague follows inhalation of *Yersinia pestis* bacilli in a potential bioterrorist scenario.[58] The infection begins as bronchiolitis and alveolitis that progresses to a lobular and eventual lobar consolidation. The histopathologic features evolve over time, beginning

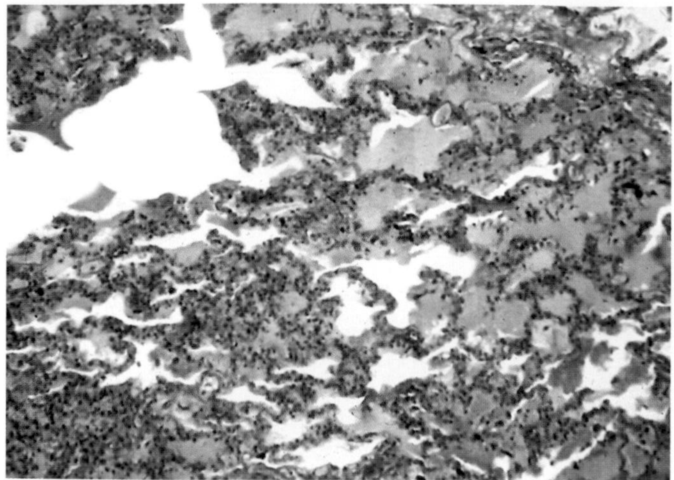

Fig. 6.32 **Plague pneumonia.** Early phase with edema, fibrin, and sparse inflammatory cells (H&E stain).

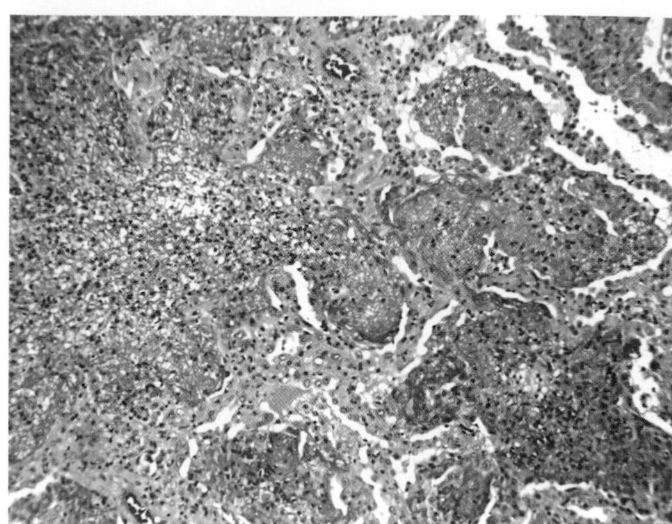

Fig. 6.34 **Tularemia.** Fibrinous lobular pneumonia phase (H&E stain).

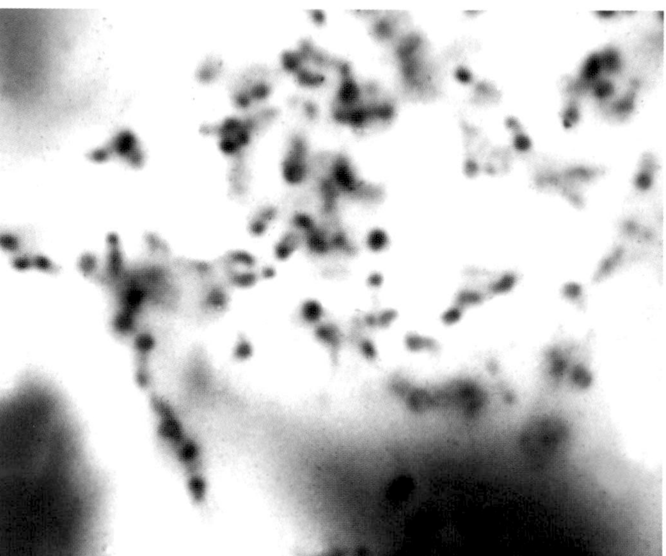

Fig. 6.33 Yersinia pestis bacilli in alveolar space (H&E stain).

with a serosanguinous intra-alveolar fluid accumulation with variable fibrin deposits (Fig. 6.32), progressing through a fibrinopurulent phase, and culminating in a necrotizing lesion.[59] Myriad bacilli in the intra-alveolar exudates with significantly fewer organisms in the interstitium (a characteristic of primary pneumonia) is one of several pulmonary and extrapulmonary features used to distinguish primary from secondary pneumonic plague.[60] These bacilli may be obvious in H&E-stained sections (Fig. 6.33) and are generally better visualized with Giemsa than Gram stains. Immunohistochemistry provides a rapid and specific diagnosis.[61] In contrast to inhalational anthrax, sputum Gram stain and culture are useful tests that are likely to be positive at clinical presentation. Also, because sepsis is an integral component of the pneumonia, it is important to collect blood cultures.

Francisella tularensis

Inhalation of *Francisella tularensis* bacilli, following a bioterrorist aerosol release, is generally expected to result in a slowly progressing pneumonia, with a lower case fatality rate than either inhalational anthrax or plague.[62] Initially, a hemorrhagic and ulcerative bronchiolitis is followed by a fibrinous lobular pneumonia with many macrophages but relatively few neutrophils (Fig. 6.34). Necrosis then supervenes and evolves into a granulomatous reaction. The small, Gram-negative coccobacillary organisms are difficult to identify in a tissue Gram stain and require silvering techniques (Steiner; Dieterle; Warthin–Starry) to enhance their silhouette.[63] Specific fluorescent antibody tests for formalin-fixed tissue and immunohistochemistry are also available through public health laboratories. In the microbiology laboratory, Gram stains and cultures of respiratory secretions are useful for diagnosis, but blood cultures are not often positive. Antigen detection and molecular techniques, such as PCR, can be used to identify *F. tularensis*. Serologic tests are available but should not be expected to provide timely information in an outbreak situation.[62]

Cytopathology

The stereotypic cellular response to pyogenic bacteria is acute inflammation, characterized by variable numbers

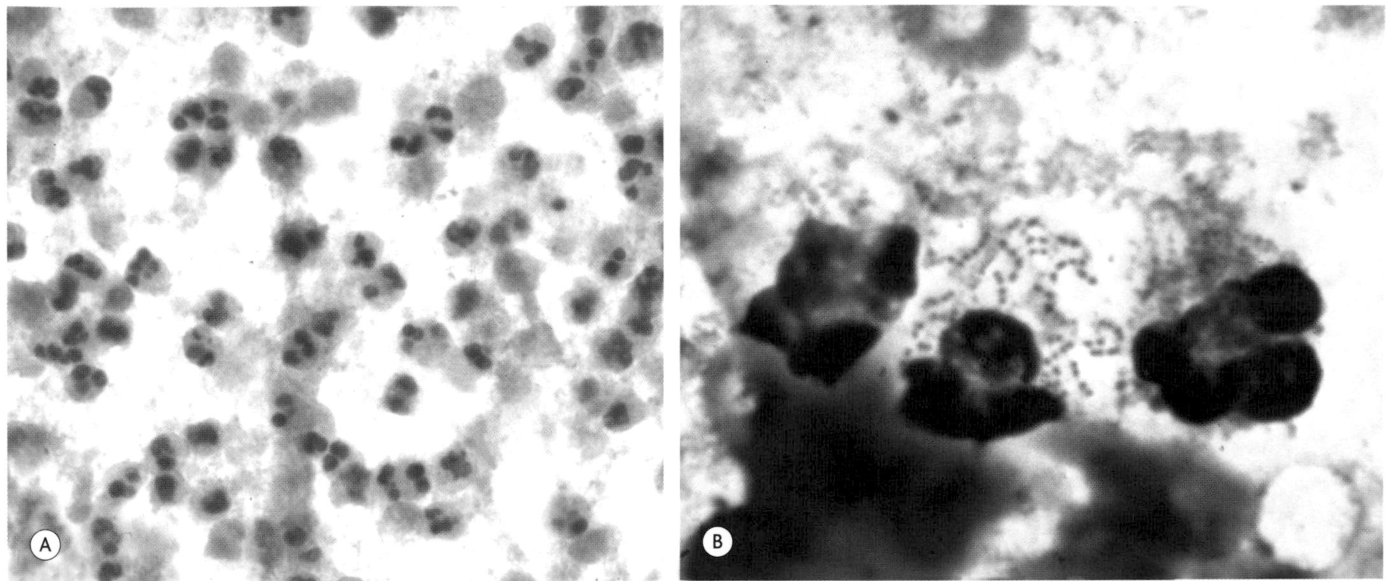

Fig. 6.35 (A) Purulent exudate of nodular pulmonary infiltrate; fine-needle aspirate (alcohol-fixed H&E stain). (B) Streptococci (viridans group) in cytoplasm of neutrophil; fine-needle aspirate (Diff-Quik).

of neutrophils. Bacteria may be visualized in various stained preparations made from respiratory tract secretions and washings using the Papanicolaou and Diff-Quik methods.[26] The clinical significance is rather limited in these specimens due to the potential contamination by oral flora and the problem of distinguishing colonization from infection. However, when the upper respiratory tract can be bypassed, either through transtracheal or transthoracic needle aspiration, the presence of bacteria becomes much more significant, especially when sheets of neutrophils and/or necroinflammatory debris are present (Fig. 6.35A), as would be the case with a typical lobar or lobular consolidation, lung abscess, or other complex pneumonia.[32,64,65] In this context, transthoracic needle aspiration can establish the etiologic diagnosis of community and nosocomial pneumonias in both children and adults when coupled with contemporary microbiologic methods.[37,66] Proponents consider it an underutilized technique whose potential benefits, in experienced hands, outweigh its modest risks.

Many types of bacilli and cocci can be seen within and around neutrophils on Diff-Quik stained smears (Fig. 6.35B) A smear can also be prepared for Gram stain and the aspirate needle rinsed in nonbacteriostatic sterile saline or nutrient broths for culture. The size (length and width), shape of organisms, and the Gram reaction allow rough categorization of organisms into groups such as enteric type bacilli, pseudomonads, fusiform anaerobic type bacilli, tiny coccobacillary types suggestive of the hemophilus/bacteroides group (Fig. 6.36) or Gram-positive cocci.[67] Branching filamentous forms suggest actinomycetes or *Nocardia* spp. (Fig. 6.37), with the latter distinguished by their being partially acid fast.[68] Needless to say, care must be exercised in the staining laboratory to prevent contamination of staining solutions, as this can be a cause of false-positive results.

While most aspirated cavitary lung lesions with the abscess pattern are the result of infection, the differential diagnosis includes a necrotic neoplasm (particularly squamous cell carcinoma), Wegener's granulomatosis, and nonbacterial infections associated with suppurative granulomas due to fungi and mycobacteria.

Microbiology

Contemporary techniques for the laboratory diagnosis of bacterial pneumonia are listed in Table 6.10.[69,70] The traditional morphologic and culture-based approach to microbiologic diagnosis is gradually shifting to molecular methods, but the routine application of these procedures is the hope for the near future.

The work-up of respiratory secretions such as sputum in the microbiology laboratory may or may not be indicated based on the clinical and immunologic status of the patient. Certainly, the value of this work-up for community-acquired pneumonias has been questioned for some time and the guidelines from two specialty societies (the American Thoracic Society and the

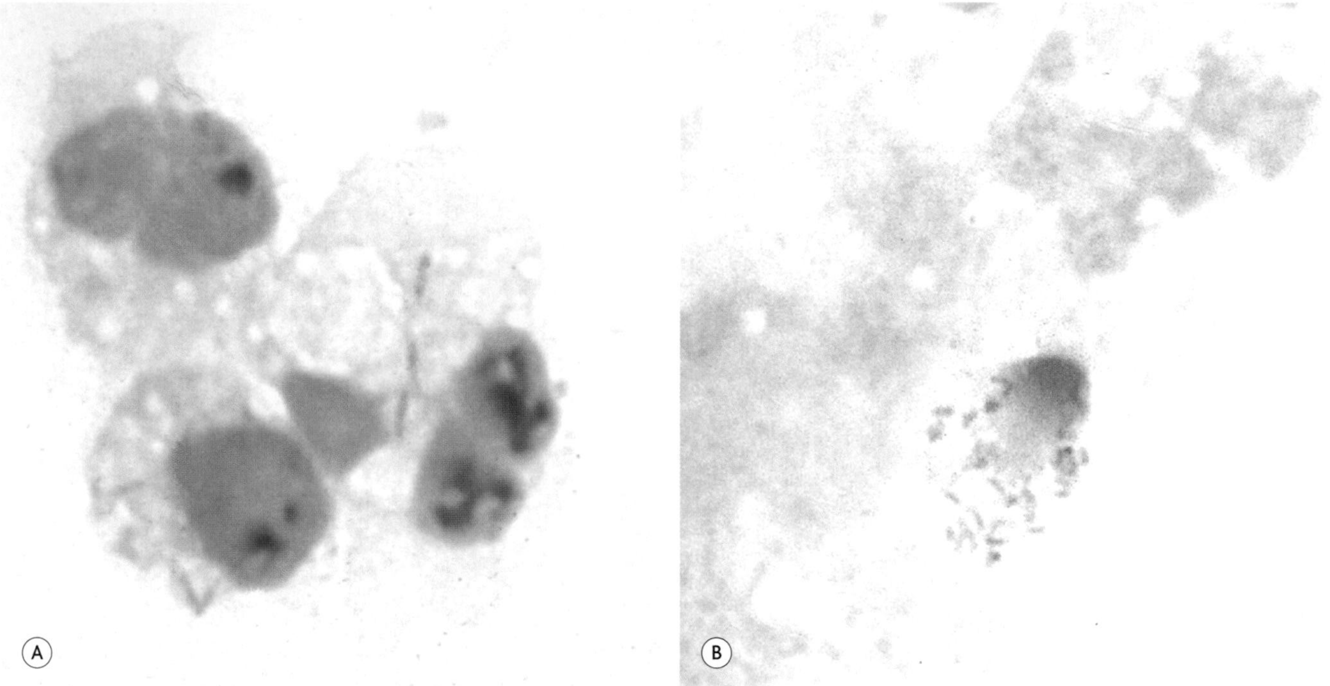

Fig. 6.36 (A) Fusiform bacteria (*Fusobacterium* sp.) in cytoplasm of neutrophil; fine-needle aspirate (Gram stain). (B) Coccobacilli (*Haemophilus influenzae*) in cytoplasm of leukocyte; fine-needle aspirate (Gram stain).

Table 6.10 Laboratory diagnosis of bacterial pneumonia

Direct detection of organisms:
– Gram; other stains of respiratory secretions and fluids
– Direct fluorescent antibody stain
– Histopathology & cytopathology
– Immunohistochemistry
Antigen detection:
– *Legionella pneumophila* [LP1] and *Streptococcus pneumoniae*
Culture:
– Conventional media for usual pyogenic bacteria
– Special media for fastidious/atypical agents
Serology
Molecular methods:
– In-situ hybridization
– DNA amplification

Infectious Disease Society of America) differ in this regard.[71–73] However, when a carefully collected specimen and well-prepared Gram stain reveals one or two predominant bacterial morphotypes (Fig. 6.38), especially in the presence of neutrophils and few or no squamous cells, a presumptive diagnosis can be offered and correlated with whatever grows on culture plates. Conversely, the presence of a mixed bacterial population, especially in the absence of inflammation and/or with many squamous cells is nondiagnostic, potentially misleading and raises doubts about the validity of culture results. However, pneumonia in the hospitalized, and especially the immunocompromised patient, requires an aggressive strategy to collect a good sputum sample for Gram stain and culture. If this attempt is unsatisfactory or nondiagnostic, then invasive techniques beginning with fiberoptic bronchocopy and bronchoalveolar lavage with protected catheters, for quatitative culture, can be considered.[74] The anaerobic pulmonary infection, typically a lung abscess, can also be approached in this way or with trans-thoracic needle aspiration.[47]

Gram stains of tissue sections from bronchoscopic or surgical biopsies, as well as cytologic samples of respiratory secretions, are also notoriously insensitive and nonspecific. Nevertheless, as with sputum, the presence of a predominant bacterial morphotype in a distinctive necroinflammatory background carries diagnostic weight when correlated with whatever data are available clinically and in the microbiology laboratory. It is again worth cautioning that tissues, like smears, are prone to false-positive results if care is not exercised in the laboratory to prevent contamination of staining solutions.

In those cases where bacteria are visible on H&E stained sections, the Gram stain is especially helpful in confirming a presumptive etiology. For example, pairs and short or long chains of Gram-positive cocci in a

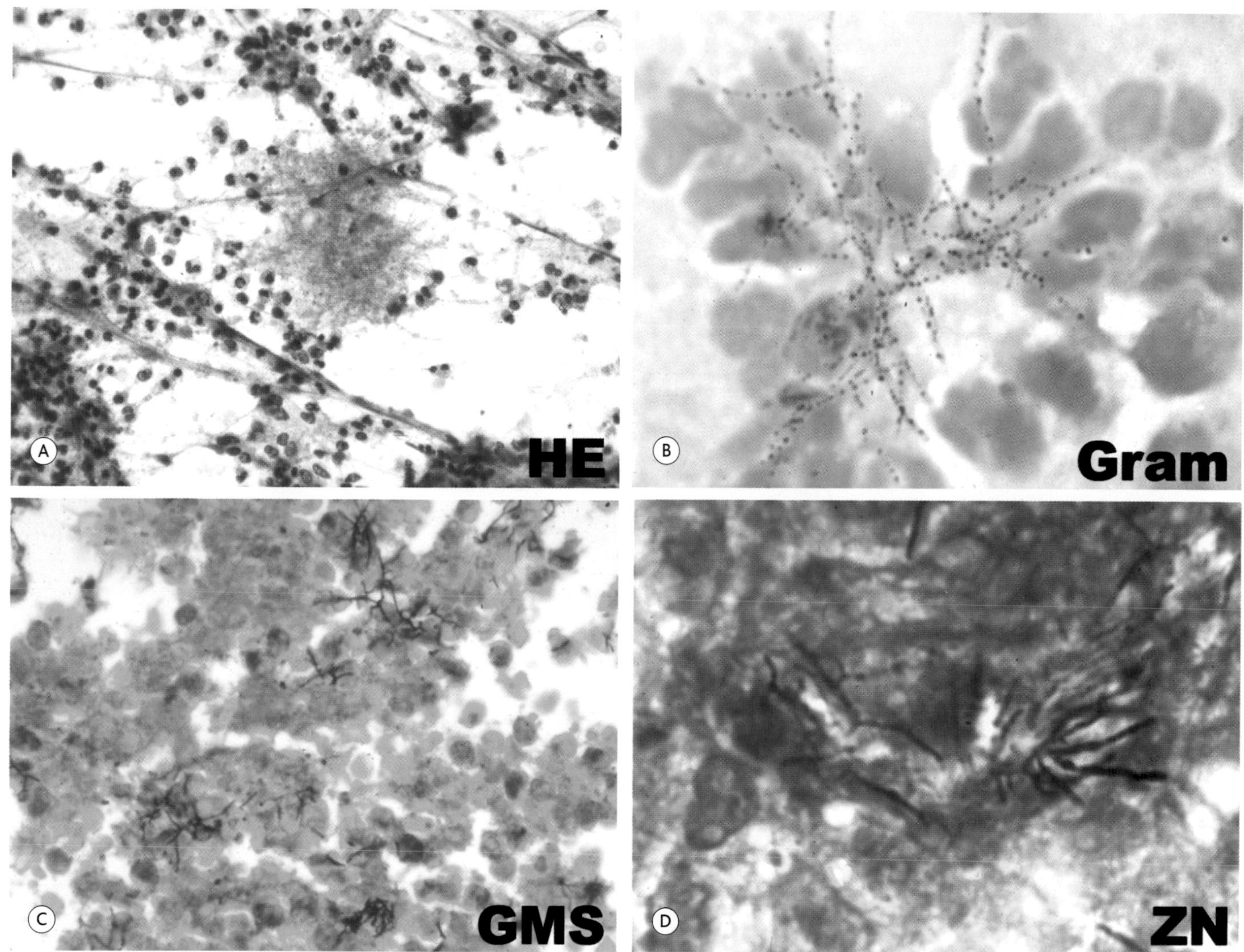

Fig. 6.37 ***Nocardia.*** (A) Loose, feathery cluster of bacilli in purulent exudate; fine needle aspirate (alcohol-fixed H&E). (B) Gram stain; (C) GMS stain; (D) Ziehl–Neelsen stain.

necroinflammatory background suggest a streptococcal pneumonia, whereas numerous slender Gram-negative bacilli investing and infiltrating blood vessels are characteristic of a pseudomonas pneumonia (Fig. 6.39). Other types of Gram-negative pneumonias (Fig. 6.40) can also be confirmed with well-prepared Gram stains.[49] In the case of an abscess, mixtures of Gram-positive cocci and Gram-negative bacilli in tissue, as illustrated in Fig. 6.21, are a useful finding, and are helpful in supporting a diagnosis of an anaerobic infection.

When organisms are sparse, other stains such as Giemsa or silver impregnation may highlight the organisms in the exudates (Fig. 6.41). The Gram stain is also useful for evaluating infections with granules and allows differentiation of the agents of botryomycosis (the Gram-positive cocci or Gram-negative bacilli) from the filamentous *Actinomyces* spp. (Fig. 6.42). The methenamine silver stain is the best procedure for detecting *Nocardia* spp. and the modified Ziehl–Neelsen allows for differentiation of *Nocardia* spp. (positive) from the anaerobic *Actinomyces* (negative).

Commercially available immunohistochemical reagents exist for relatively few bacterial species. Immunohistochemistry is available for the potential bioterrorist agents discussed in this chapter through the Centers for Disease Control and Prevention (CDC, Atlanta, Georgia). It is expected that commercial reagents will become increasingly available for the common etiologic agents in the near future.[22]

Culture media that will allow recovery of common bacterial species causing pneumonia from various types of respiratory secretions, washings, brushings, aspirates,

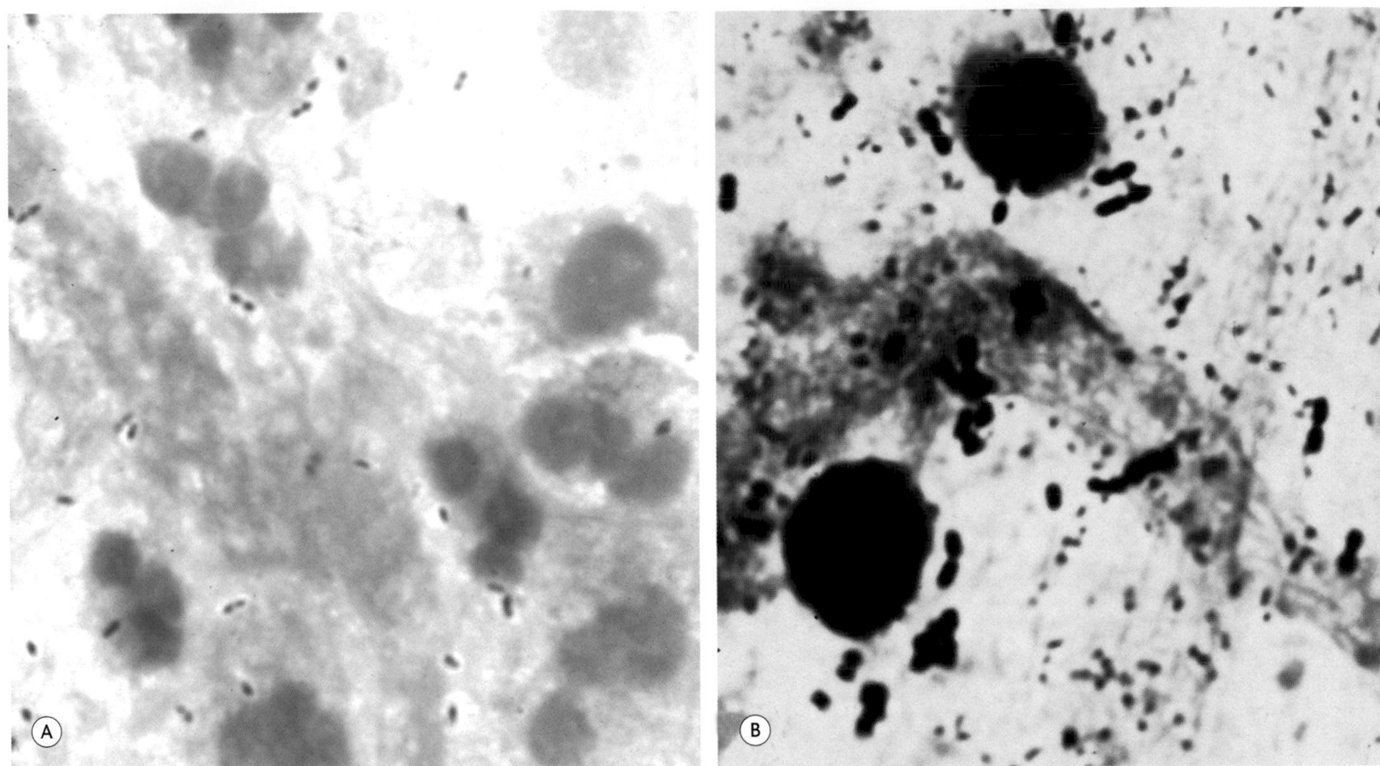

Fig. 6.38 **Sputum Gram stain.** (A) Gram-positive diplococci (*Streptococcus pneumoniae*) with neutrophils, but no squamous cells. (B) Gram-positive diplococci (*S. pneumoniae*) and Gram-negative coccobacili (*Haemophilus influenzae*).

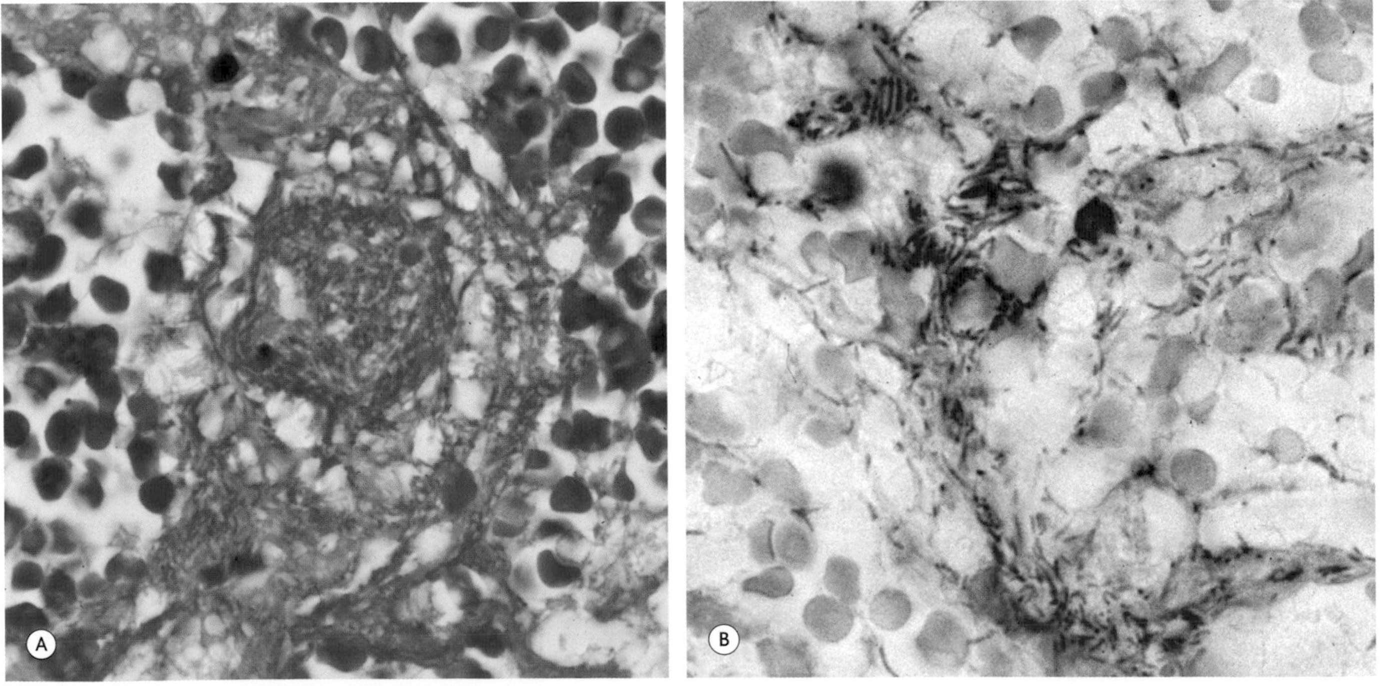

Fig. 6.39 (A) The slender Gram-negative bacilli are nicely demonstrated on Gram stain. (B) *Pseudomonas aeruginosa* bacilli investing interstitial vessels (Brown & Hopps stain).

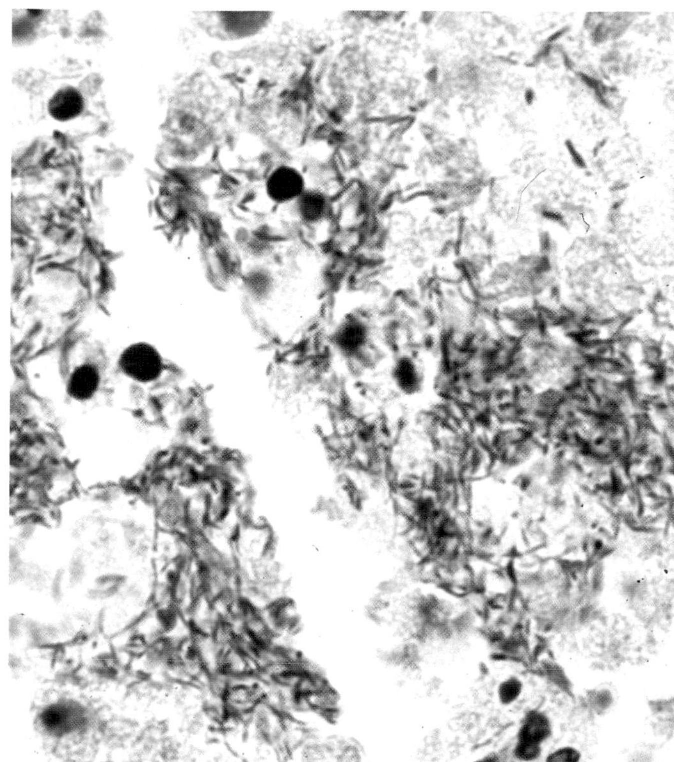

Fig. 6.40 *Berkholderia cepacia* bacilli (Brown & Hopps stain).

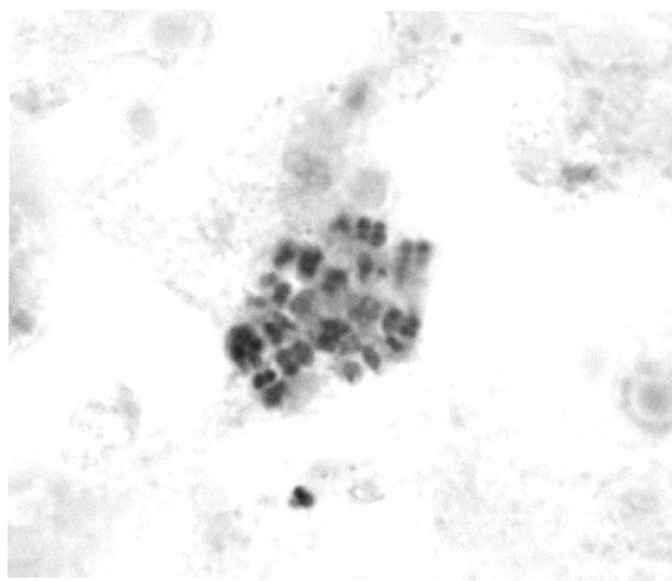

Fig. 6.41 Bacterial tetrads in alveolar exudate (Giemsa stain).

and tissues include sheep blood agar, chocolate agar, and MacConkey agar. These media will also support growth of *B. anthracis* and *Y. pestis*. Buffered charcoal yeast extract (BYE) agar is the primary medium for *Legionella* spp. Because *Legionella* spp. survive poorly in respiratory

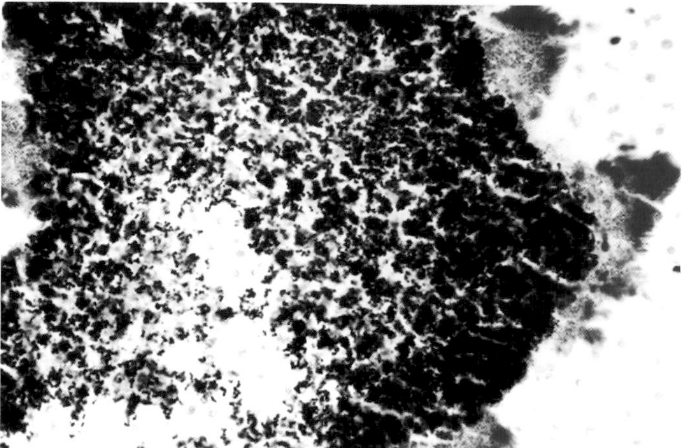

Fig. 6.42 **Botryomycosis.** Cluster of Gram-positive cocci (*Staphylococcus aureus*) invested by Gram-negative staining Splendore–Hoeppli material (Brown & Brenn stain). (Courtesy of Dr. Francis Chandler, Augusta, GA.)

secretions, rapid transport and immediate plating is essential for recovery. BYE is also a good "all purpose" medium for other fastidious species including *F. tularensis*. However, *F. tularensis* grows best in cysteine-enriched media.[75]

In addition to respiratory samples, blood cultures can be performed in patients sick enough to suspect bacteremias, and pleural fluid culture can be employed when effusions are present. Positive cultures of these normally sterile fluids circumvent the interpretive problems associated with bacterial growth in sputum samples.

The actinomycetes are best isolated from invasive specimens such as needle aspirates, transbronchial and surgical wedge biopsies. The laboratory should be alerted to search for these agents because special consideration must be given to culture set-up and incubation conditions. The actinomycetes responsible for actinomycosis require anaerobic media and atmosphere as well as prolonged incubation. *Nocardia*, an aerobic actinomycete, grows well on most nonselective media but requires extended incubation. Colonial morphology, Gram and acid-fast stains and a few biochemical tests generally suffice to identify these organisms at the genus level. However, genotyping rather than phenotypic characteristics are required to identify newly emergent species.[76]

In general, the laboratory diagnosis of pneumonia caused by most of the atypical agents is difficult because systems are not routinely available or are costly, cumbersome, or unsafe. For the atypical agents (*Mycoplasma*, *Chlamydia* and *Coxiella* spp.), serology has been the method of choice for diagnosis.[39,77] Classic cold agglutinin and complement fixation tests for these agents have largely been replaced by enzyme immunoassay and microimmunofluorescence. Serology is also useful for tularemia, because of the difficulty in culturing the fastidious bacterium.

Legionella pneumonia is a common form of severe pneumonia not readily diagnosed for a number of reasons, including lack of its clinical consideration and the organism's fastidiousness.[78] In the microbiology laboratory, the direct fluorescent antibody test and culture on buffered charcoal yeast extract agar have been the mainstays of diagnosis. Culture is considered the diagnostic gold standard but is only 60% sensitive. Serology is available for most of the *L. pneumophilia* serotypes, which account for 90% of the pneumonia cases; however, the need to collect paired sera weeks apart limits its usefulness for the acutely ill patient. Antigen detection in urine has become commercially available and, because the need to collect acute and convalesent sera is obviated, it has become a frequently used diagnostic test.[78] Its advantage lies in its potential to effect early treatment decisions through rapid diagnosis. Its disadvantage lies in the fact that it only detects patients infected with *L. pneumophila* serogroup 1 (LP1), the most prevalent species and serotype, but none of the non-LP1 serotypes, or cases due to other *Legionella* spp.[79,80]

The use of molecular diagnostic tools (in-situ hybridization and nucleic acid amplification by PCR or other methods) to detect these agents has been reported.[50,81,82] The recent introduction of real-time PCR appears promising as a highly sensitive, specific, and rapid diagnostic technique that will likely find routine clinical application. It provides a platform for the simultaneous amplification and detection of target DNA in a single tube through the use of one of several types of fluorescence resonance energy transfer (FRET) fluorescent probe quencher techniques or melting curve analysis. Furthermore, it obviates the concern for amplicon contamination in the laboratory.[83] The development of a multiplex assay, to detect multiple agents in a single reaction, would seem to be an ideal pursuit for the laboratory diagnosis of the atypical pneumonia agents.[84]

Differential diagnosis

The key morphologic and microbiologic features of the bacterial pneumonias are summarized in Table 6.11. The presence of purulent exudates or significant numbers of neutrophils in biopsy or cytologic samples should always trigger a search for bacterial infection. However, since lung biopsies are usually performed late in the time course of an evolving infiltrate, after many procedures have been performed and bacteria have been excluded or treated with antibiotics, neutrophilic exudates may not signify bacterial infection unless accompanied by necrosis, as in an abscess. Instead, consideration should be given to one of several non-infectious acute inflammatory diseases, with an immunologic basis, that can mimic bacterial infection. Some of these include Wegener's granulomatosis, Goodpasture's syndrome, systemic lupus erythematosus, and microscopic polyangiitis, all conditions that can produce acute inflammation centered

Table 6.11 Bacterial pneumonia synopsis

Pyogenic bacteria	
Surgical pathology:	Acute purulent inflammation with/without necrosis; organization; diffuse alveolar damage may be present, most often non-specific. Some pathogens characteristic, e.g. pseudomonas (perivascular bacillary pattern); *Rhodococcus* (histiocytic/malakoplakia pattern). Acute phase resolves or progresses to chronic organizing pneumonia.
Cytopathology:	Acute inflammation with/without visible bacteria on Diff-Quik stained smear
Microbiology:	Gram stain reactivity and morphology (visual detection requires heavy bacterial burden; 10^6/g tissue). Culture sterile lung tissue on standard nonselective and selective media (blood; chocolate; MacConkey agars); anaerobic broth and agars for abscesses. Urinary antigen for *S. pneumoniae*
Atypical pneumonia agents	
Surgical pathology:	*Legionella* pneumonia – fibrinopurulent with bacilli visible in silver stained (Dieterle; Warthin–Starry) sections. DAD often present. *Chlamydia* and *Mycoplasma* – polymorphous bronchiolar and interstitial infiltrate
Cytopathology:	Acute inflammation with bacilli stained with silver or by immunofluorescence (*Legionella* pneumonia).
Microbiology:	DFA for *L. pneumophilia* serotypes. Culture on selective (BCYE) agar for *Legionella*; urinary antigen for *Legionella*. Serology and/or PCR for *Mycoplasma* and *Chlamydia*
Filamentous–granule group	
Surgical pathology:	Granules or loose filamentous aggregates in purulent exudate with abscess formation and poorly formed granulomas in some cases
Cytopathology:	Filamentous tangles or aggregates or granules with neutrophils and/or necroinflammatory background
Microbiology:	Gram-positive branching filaments; *Nocardia* (aerobic actinomycete) and *Actinomyces* (anaerobic actinomycete). *Nocardia* partially acid-fast and GMS-positive. Gram-positive cocci or Gram-negative bacilli (botryomycosis). Culture on standard nonselective media and selective (BCYE) media; anaerobic broths and media for *Actinomyces*

on alveolar septal blood vessels ("capillaritis"). On occasion, capillaritis can result in airspace accumulation of neutrophils, further raising concern for bronchopneumonia. Centrally necrotic or cavitary neoplasms of various types may mimic abscesses grossly and microscopically, and exceptionally well-differentiated adenocarcinomas containing glands filled with detritus may mimic inflammatory and bacterial diseases. Suppurative granulomas can have a bacterial, mycobacterial, or fungal etiology. Even the miliary necroinflammatory lesion typical of bacterial infection can be produced by viruses, some fungi, and even protozoa (e.g. *Toxoplasma gondii*).

Mycobacterial infection

The surgical pathologist encounters mycobacterial infections in lung biopsies when standard clinical diagnostic approaches to pulmonary infiltrates are unsuccessful and the lesions persist or progress. In this scenario, an invasive procedure such as transbronchial biopsy, transthoracic needle biopsy, and surgical lung biopsy are often a last resort. In recent years, delays in diagnosis of mycobacterial infection have markedly decreased, thanks in part to recommendations from the CDC for improving laboratory turnaround time, and the response of the diagnostics industry with better methods and technology. However, given the fact that direct AFB (acid-fast bacilli) smears of respiratory specimens are negative in at least half the cases,[85] and many mycobacterial species are fastidious and slow growing, the biopsy may be the first suggestion of a mycobacterial infection. The biopsy can also define the organism's relationship to any lesion, or the host response. This is important when evaluating the significance of a culture result, because while an isolate of *Mycobacterium tuberculosis* is always taken seriously, a single isolate of a non-tuberculous mycobacterium from the respiratory tract does not necessarily implicate it as the cause of disease.[86]

Etiologic agents

Mycobacteria can be categorized into two clinically relevant groups: *Mycobacterium tuberculosis* complex (MTC) and the non-tuberculous mycobacteria (NTM). MTC includes the subspecies *M. tuberculosis*, *M. bovis*, *M. africanum*, and *M microti*. The latter three species produce tuberculosis in some areas of the world but in the United States the incidence is very low.

Mycobacterium tuberculosis

Mycobacterium tuberculosis is the most virulent mycobacterial species and an unequivocal pathogen. It is responsible for more deaths worldwide than any single microbe and is the etiologic agent of tuberculosis worldwide in its various forms, which are listed in Table 6.12. Primary tuberculosis occurs in patients without previous exposure or loss of acquired immunity. Progressive primary tuberculosis occurs in patients with inadequate acquired immunity, i.e. impaired cellular immunity. Post-primary tuberculosis, also referred to as secondary or reinfection/reactivation tuberculosis, occurs in patients with previous immunity to the organism.[87,88] Many clinical experts consider that most cases of active tuberculosis in adults with normal immunity arise from reactivation of latent infection (post-primary tuberculosis), whereas reinfection with a new strain derived from the environment (primary or post-primary tuberculosis) can occur in the immunocompromised patient. However, DNA fingerprinting methods (genotyping) have challenged this dogma by showing that exogenous reinfection accounts for a significant percentage of cases in some areas of the world.[88a]Miliary tuberculosis and extrapulmonary disease can occur with any of these forms.[87,89] Primary tuberculosis is usually a mild illness that often is not clinically recognized. However, the bacillemia that occurs during its development can seed extrapulmonary organs and set the stage for subsequent reactivation. About 5% of patients pass through latency to post-primary disease within 2 years of primary infection and another 5% do so later in their lives.[90]

The non-tuberculous mycobacteria

The NTM include more than 90 species, many of which have been identified during the past decade.[91,91a] However, relatively few cause pulmonary disease.[86] These organisms are acquired from the environment where they are ubiquitous. In contrast to *M. tuberculosis*, the NTM are

Table 6.12 Classification of tuberculosis

Primary tuberculosis: – Exogenous first infection – Exogenous reinfection
Progressive primary tuberculosis
Postprimary tuberculosis: – Endogenous reactivation – Exogenous infection in BCG vaccinated – Exogenous superinfection

Source: from Allen,[87] Table 13-1, p 233 with permission.

not spread from person to person. In most instances, patients who develop infection with the NTM have chronic lung disease and other risk factors, such as AIDS, alcoholism, or diabetes. There are increasing reports of NTM infections in non-immunocompromised patients.[16,92] *Mycobacterium avium* complex (MAC), followed by *M. kansasii*, are the most frequent isolates in all settings. Among a growing list of species causing lung disease are *M. abscessus*, *M. fortuitum*, *M. szulgai*, *M. simiae*, *M. xenopi*, *M. malmoense*, *M. celatum*, *M. asiaticum*, and *M. shimodii*. These latter species manifest marked geographic variability with respect to prevalence and severity. It is noteworthy, however, that since 1985, there have been more MAC isolates than *M. tuberculosis* in the USA.[86]

The histopathologic patterns produced by mycobacteria are listed in Table 6.13. The radiographic, gross, and microscopic patterns of mycobacterial disease reflect the virulence of the various mycobacterial species, as well as the patients' prior exposure and immune status.[93]

Table 6.13 Patterns of mycobacterial lung injury

Patterns
Large nodules with or without cavities: – Well-formed granuloma – Poorly formed granuloma – Suppurative granuloma – Histiocytic aggregates
Miliary nodules
Calcified nodules
Granulomatous interstitial pneumonitis
Bronchitis/bronchiectasis
Spindle cell pseudotumors

Primary tuberculosis

Mycobacterium tuberculosis occurs typically in the best aerated lung regions (anterior segments of the upper lobes, lingula and middle lobe, or basal segments of the lower lobes).[86a] The disease passes through progressive phases of exudation, recruitment of macrophages and T lymphocytes, and granuloma formation followed by repair with granulation tissue, fibrosis, and mineralization.[88] Macrophage-laden bacilli also travel to the hilar lymph nodes, where the phases are repeated. This combination of events produces the classic Ghon complex, consisting of a peripheral 1–2 cm lung nodule and an enlarged, sometimes calcified, hilar lymph node. In both locations, the histopathologic hallmark is a necrotizing granuloma (Fig. 6.43) composed of epithelioid cells with variable numbers of Langhans' giant cells, a peripheral investment of lymphocytes, and a central zone of caseation necrosis.[87] A spectrum of lesions may be seen, from the tuberculoid "hard" granuloma without necrosis and rare organisms, to the multibacillary necrotic lesion with scant epithelioid cells.[94] In a minority of patients the lesions enlarge and progress due to increased necrosis and/or liquefaction.

The complications of tuberculosis are listed in Table 6.14 and illustrated in Fig. 6.46. These include extension into blood vessels with miliary (Fig. 6.44) or systemic

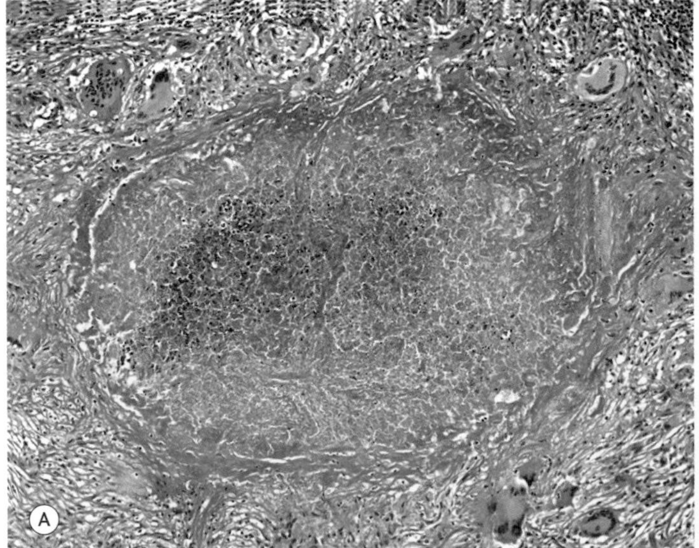

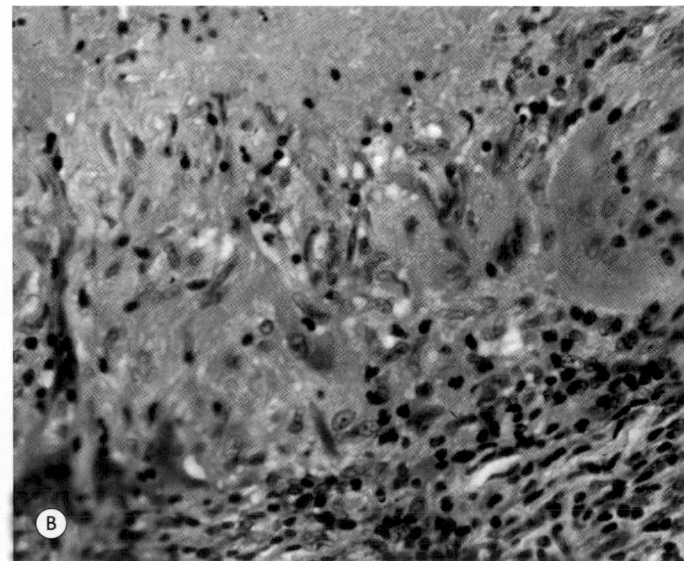

Fig. 6.43 (A) Tuberculoid granuloma with central zone of caseation necrosis surrounded by epithelioid cells, giant cells, and outer investment of lymphocytes. (B) Palisade of epithelioid histiocytes in giant cells at edge of necrotic zone (H&E stain).

dissemination, lymphatic drainage into the pleura with granulomatous pleuritis and effusions, or involvement of bronchi with bronchocentric granulomatous lesions (Fig. 6.45) or tuberculous bronchopneumonia. Granulomas may also encroach upon blood vessels, mimicking a "granulomatous" vasculitis.

Post-primary tuberculosis

Post-primary tuberculosis, the most common form in adults, typically involves the apices of the upper lobes, producing granulomatous lesions with greater caseation, often with cavities and variable degrees of fibrosis and retraction of the parenchyma.[89] Extension to other lobes, hilar, or mediastinal lymph nodes and miliary spread through the lungs and to extrapulmonary sites can also complicate this form of disease. Other presentation patterns include acute and organizing diffuse alveolar damage with advanced or miliary disease, acute tuberculous bronchopneumonia, and the solitary pulmonary nodule (tuberculoma). An endobronchial form may mimic a neoplasm and is also noteworthy for extensive necrosis and often large numbers of bacilli.[95] Because characteristic granulomatous morphology may not be visible around the necrotic material, stains for mycobacteria should be considered in cases of necrotic endobronchial samples.

Table 6.14 Complications of tuberculosis

Miliary tuberculosis
Granulomatous pleuritis and effusions
Tuberculous bronchopneumonia
Extrapulmonary dissemination to: - Meninges - Kidney - Bone - Other

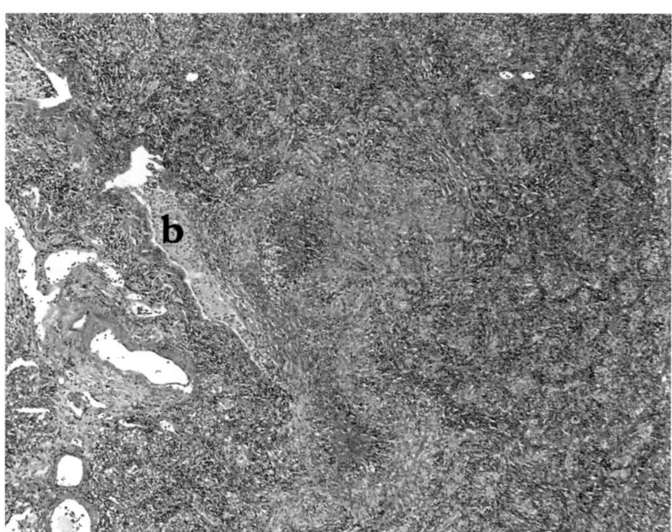

Fig. 6.45 Bronchocentric granuloma (b).

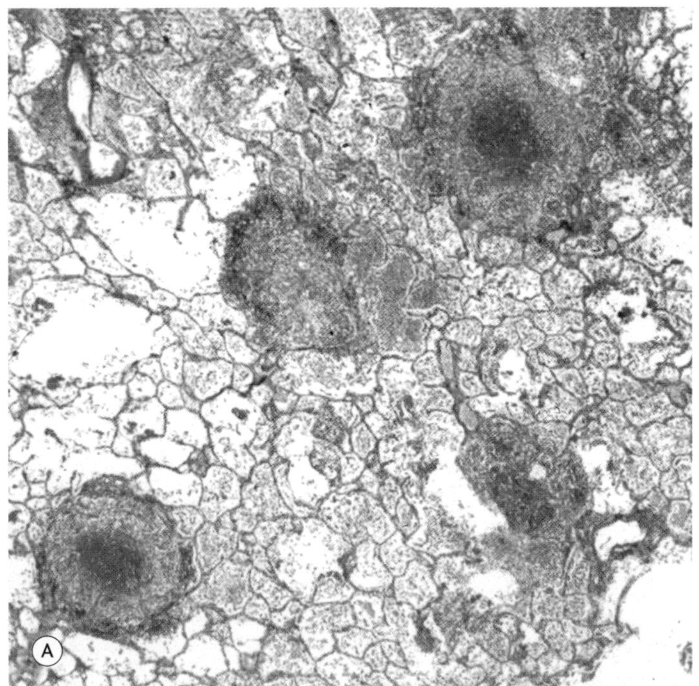

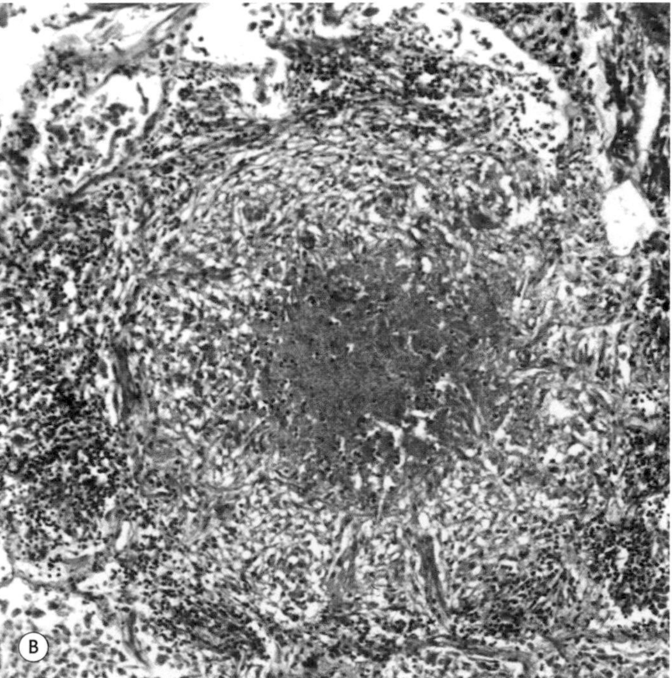

Fig. 6.44 **Miliary tuberculosis.** (A) Miliary pattern. (B) Epithelioid granulomas with necrotic central zones (H&E stain).

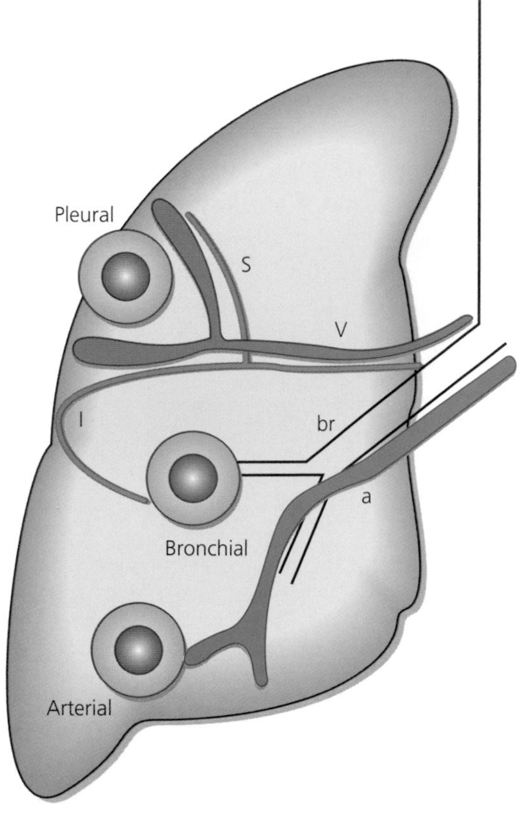

Fig. 6.46 **Complications of tuberculosis.** Invasion of arteries (a) with miliary spread; bronchi (br) with tuberculous bronchopneumonia; lymphatics (l) with granulomatous pleuritis and effusions. Invasion of septal (S) veins (V) leads to extrapulmonary dissemination.

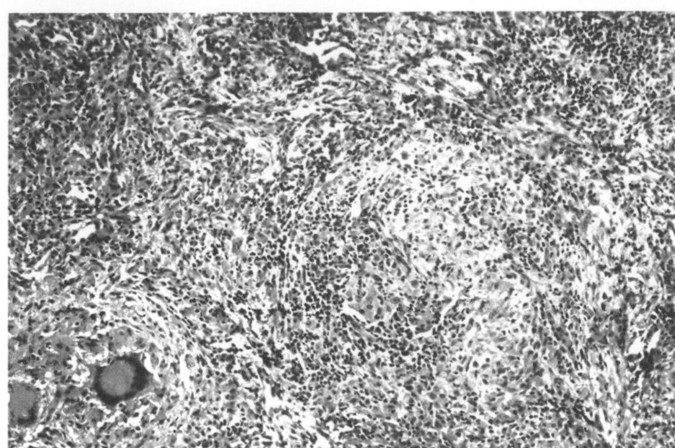

Fig. 6.47 **Non-necrotizing granuloma.** *Mycobacterium avium* complex (MAC) (H&E stain).

Non-tuberculous mycobacterial infections

Non-tuberculous mycobacterial infections may be similar to *M. tuberculosis*, but there are differences. For example, the NTM do not cause the same sequence of primary/post-primary disease, and dissemination does not occur except in the immunocompromised patient. *M. kansasii* is more virulent than MAC, and its histopathology is more like that produced by M. tuberculosis.[96]

Mycobacterium avium complex produces a variety of syndromes.[97] In primary infection, upper lobe thin-walled cavities may be seen. Histologically, a spectrum of granulomatous inflammation occurs, including loosely formed and well-defined granulomas that generally have less tendency to necrose (Fig. 6.47). Multiple confluent granulomas can mimic sarcoidosis. Organisms are usually sparse and more difficult to find in the immunocompetent individual.

In the HIV-infected patient, the disease is more commonly centered in the gastrointestinal tract, which is considered to be the portal of entry. Pulmonary disease usually signifies dissemination or colonization.[98] Well-formed tuberculoid granulomas may be found at involved sites, but in general, poorly-formed granulomas without lymphocyte cuffing, or clusters of macrophages alone typify MAC infection in these patients. Plump, finely vacuolated macrophages (pseudo-Gaucher's cells) containing abundant phagocytosed intracytoplasmic bacilli are a distinctive finding in this clinical setting (Fig. 6.48).

Mycobacterium avium complex can also colonize pre-existing cavitary lung disease from any cause, including old tuberculous cavities, which, interestingly, may also be occupied by fungus balls of *Aspergillus* or other fungal genera. *Mycobacterium avium* complex can also colonize bronchiectatic lung, presumably because of decreased mucociliary clearance. Here, the fundamental histopathology is granulomatous inflammation centered in the airway walls (Fig. 6.49). Another rather indolent airway-centered process produced by MAC in otherwise healthy adults has been referred to as Lady Windermere's syndrome. Typically, elderly females without apparent risk factors develop multiple pulmonary nodules with preferential involvement of the middle lobe and lingula. Biopsy shows bronchiectasis and chronic bronchiolitis with granulomatous features. This constellation of clinical, radiographic, gross, and microscopic findings has been recognized as one of the patterns of middle lobe syndrome.[99] Recently, MAC has been cultured from the lungs of adults who use hot tubs. So called "hot tub lung" is associated with a miliary bronchiolocentric and interstitial pattern (Fig. 6.50A) similar to that produced by hypersensitivity pneumonitis.[16] Importantly, in our experience, the computed tomographic (CT) appearance

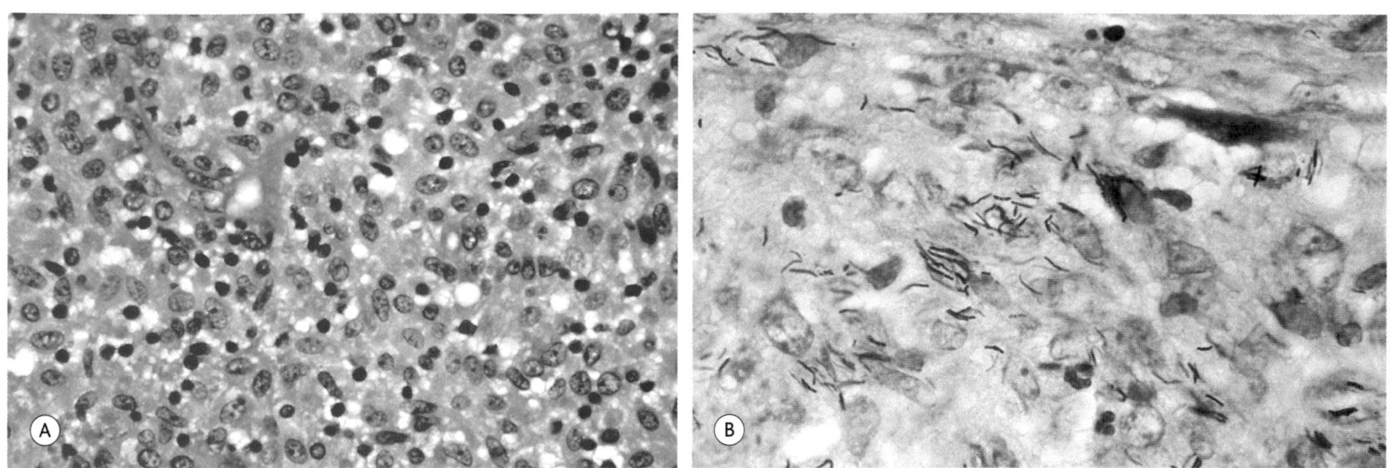

Fig. 6.48 (A) Clusters of macrophages. *Mycobacterium avium* complex (MAC) infection in patient with AIDS (H&E stain). (B) Numerous acid-fast bacilli (MAC) in histiocytic infiltrate (Ziehl–Neelsen stain).

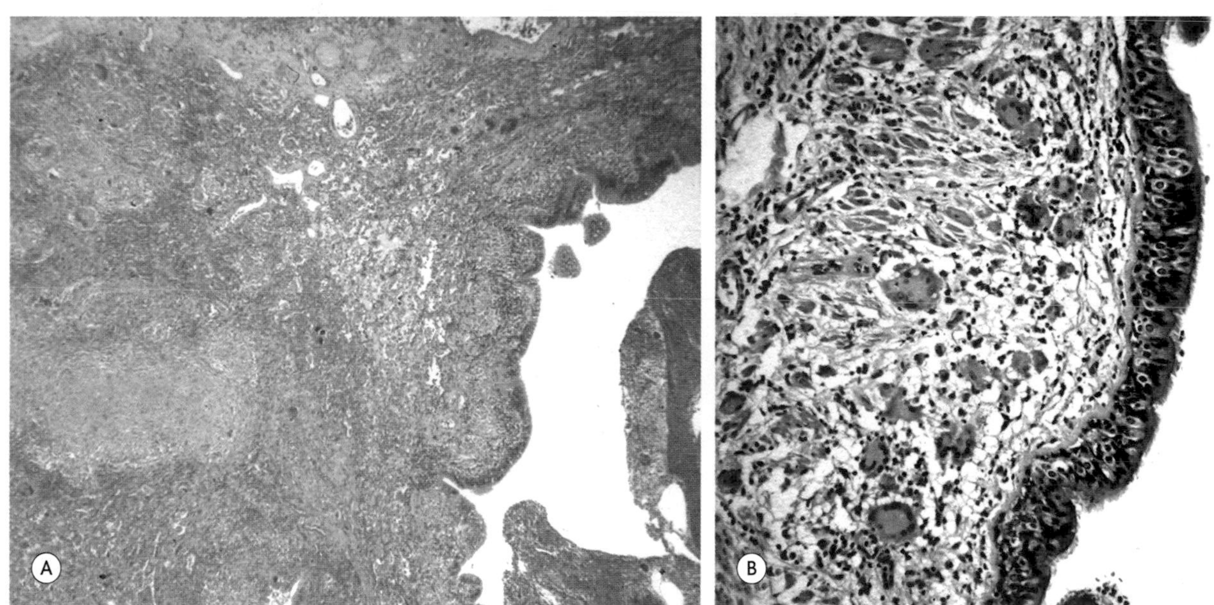

Fig. 6.49 **Middle lobe syndrome.** (A) Bronchiectasis with peribronchial granulomas (MAC). (B) Airway mucosa with granuloma (H&E stain).

can also be indistinguishable from that associated with hypersensitivity pneumonitis (Fig. 6.50B). Organisms are difficult to find in these cases but can sometimes be recovered in cultures. Whether this condition is an infection, a hypersensitivity reaction, or a hybrid of both conditions is unresolved at this time.

Another rare morphologic manifestation of mycobacterial infection is the so-called spindle cell pseudotumor (Fig. 6.51) which may occur in lung, skin, lymph nodes, and a number of other sites in immunocompromised patients.[100] The etiologic agents are usually NTM (MAC and *M. kansasii*), but *M. tuberculosis* has also been identified in some cases.

Certain species of rapidly growing mycobacteria (RGM) are capable of producing pulmonary disease, albeit infrequently.[101] *Mycobacterium abscessus* is the leading RGM recovered from the lung. It produces chronic lung infection that has a striking clinical and pathologic similarity to MAC infections, including the propensity to involve the lungs of patients with

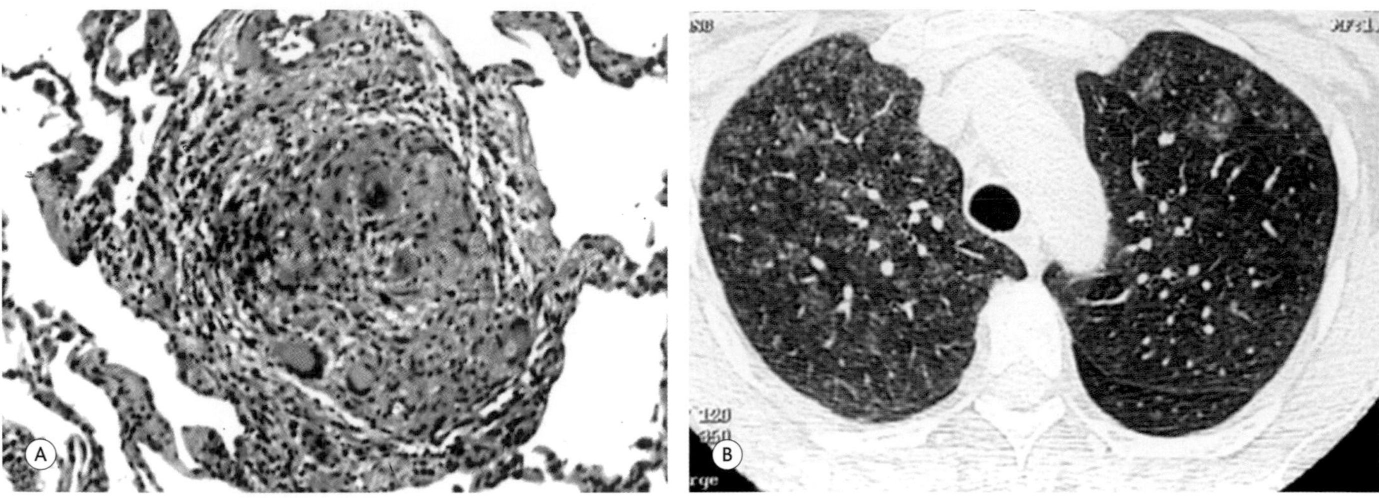

Fig. 6.50 (A) Non-necrotizing granuloma (hot tub lung) (H&E stain). (B) CT image of hot tub lung resembling hypersensitivity pneumonitis.

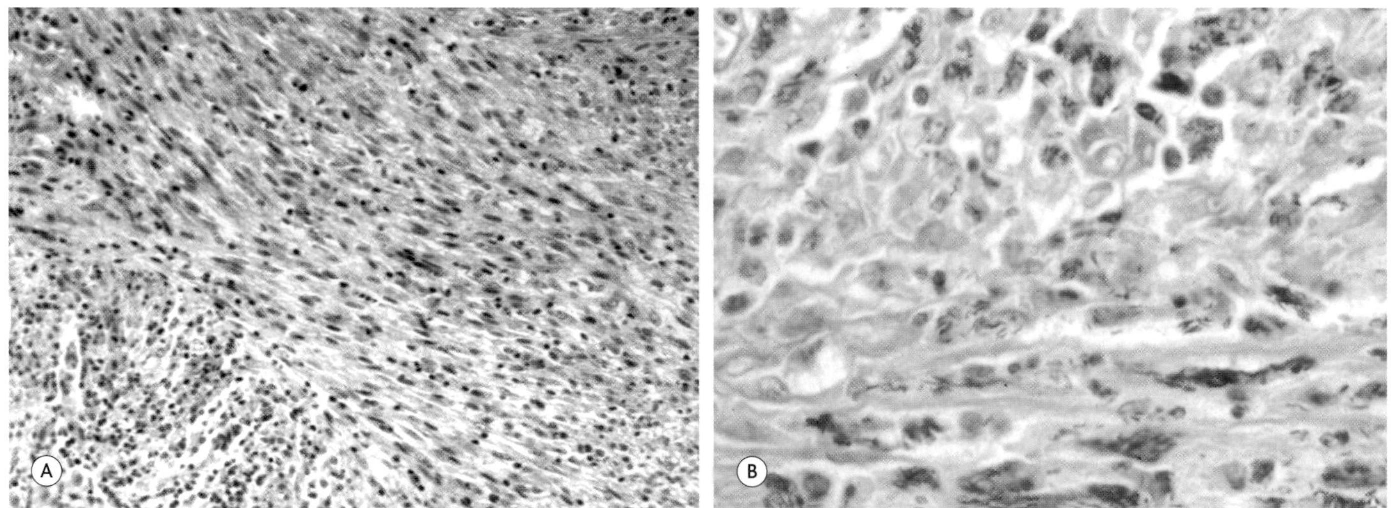

Fig. 6.51 **Spindle-cell pseudotumor.** (A) The fascicles of fibroblasts with scattered lymphocytes (H&E stain). (B) Myriad acid-fast bacilli (Ziehl-Neelsen stain).

bronchiectasis. *Mycobacterium fortuitum* is recovered less often, usually in the setting of chronic aspiration. *Mycobacterium smegmatis* has been recovered in cases of pneumonia associated with inhalation or aspiration of lipid-containing medicines, foods, and oils.

Cytopathology

Fine-needle aspiration biopsy has been successfully utilized to diagnose both tuberculous pulmonary lesions and NTM infections.[102] The finding of finely granular amorphous necrotic debris associated with aggregates of epithelioid histiocytes (with or without multinucleated giant cells) (Fig. 6.52) is suggestive of a mycobacterial or fungal infection.[103] In this setting, necrotic cancers must be excluded by a thorough search for atypical cells.

Special stains for acid-fast bacilli can be applied to aspirate smears but culture of the aspirate is more likely to yield the etiologic agent when bacilli are sparse. Also, culture is still necessary for species identification and, if necessary, antimicrobial susceptibility testing. Epithelioid granulomas manifest a similar cellular pattern, but the granular necrotic debris is absent. Another pattern that may be seen, particularly in the immunocompromised patient, is a pure histiocytic or macrophage reaction with few or no epithelioid or multinucleated giant cells or necrotic debris. Numerous bacilli may be present in the distended cytoplasm of histiocytes and in the

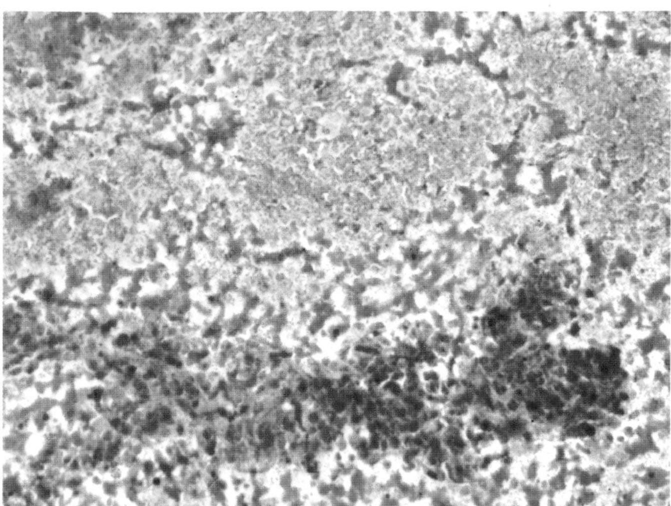

Fig. 6.52 **Necrotizing granuloma (Mycobacterium kansasii).** Sheets of epithelioid cells in a background of granular necroinflammatory debris; fine-needle aspirate (Diff-Quik stain).

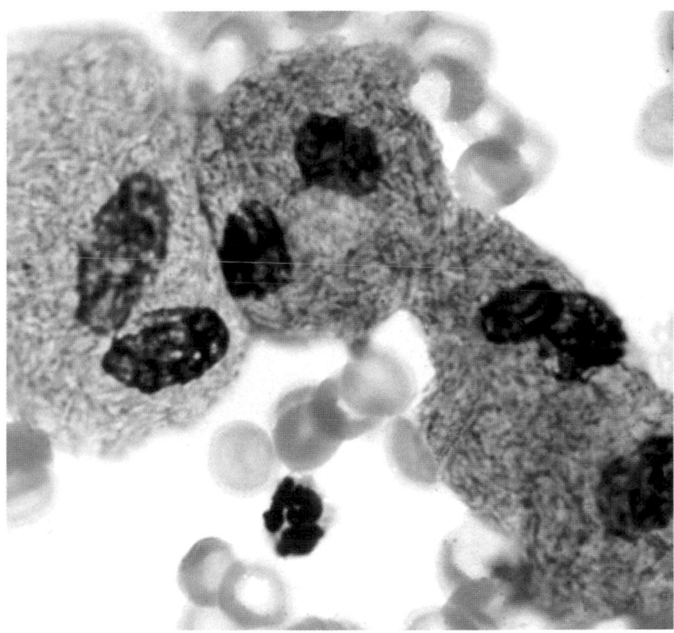

Fig. 6.53 Pseudo-Gaucher histiocytes filled with myriad mycobacteria as negative images; fine-needle aspirate (Diff-Quik stain).

extracellular background. In air-dried (Diff-Quik) and alcohol-fixed (H&E or Papanicolaou stained) smears, the bacilli may be recognized as negative images (Fig. 6.53).

Microbiology

The traditional and some of the newer molecular approaches to the laboratory diagnosis of mycobacterial lung infection are outlined in Table 6.15.

Table 6.15 Laboratory diagnosis of mycobacterial lung infection

Direct detection of organisms:
- Ziehl–Neelsen; Kinyoun acid-fast stains
- Auramine O fluorescent stain
- Histopathology and cytopathology
- Immunohistochemistry

Culture:
- Conventional solid and broth media
- Radiometric liquid media system
- Nonradiometric (fluorescent; colorimetric) liquid media systems

Molecular methods:
- In-situ hybridization
- DNA amplification

The mycobacterium is a slender but slightly curved bacillus, 4 μm in length, often with a beaded appearance; the length, curvature, and beadedness is sometimes accentuated in *M. kansasii*.[104] In tissue sections or on smears, the Ziehl–Neelsen acid-fast stain or auramine–rhodamine fluorescent stains are most often recommended for best visualization. Organisms are most often found in the central necrotic zone of the granulomas or the lining of cavities. Sections from two tissue blocks may be required to find organisms, but some cases require more sections as well as perseverance in examination under oil immersion. Bacilli are rarely found in histiocytes and granulomas without necrosis, except in immunocompromised patients where they may be visible in pseudo-Gaucher's cells on H&E stained sections, or as ghosted outlines with Giemsa-type stains. Dead bacilli lose their acid-fast character but may sometimes be identified with GMS. A commercial immunohistochemical reagent for mycobacteria is now available but is effective only in cases that are positive by traditional acid-fast stains.[22] The differentiation of mycobacterial species in Ziehl–Neelsen-positive, formalin-fixed sections, has also been achieved by in-situ hybridization techniques with specific nucleic acid probes.[105] PCR amplification and identification is likely to be the most sensitive technique for those cases that are suspected to harbor mycobacteria but are negative by acid-fast staining.[106] This technique may also be useful in cases that lack the characteristic granulomatous pattern of inflammation.[107]

Conventional wisdom states that culture is more sensitive than direct examination; however, the literature clearly documents cases where acid-fast stains on tissue biopsies succeeded where cultures of tissue have failed, an outcome that speaks to the virtue of perseverance in the face of compelling histopathology.[108] Furthermore, tissue culture is prone to sampling error unless more than one site is sampled.[109] Specimens may also be smear-positive and culture-negative in patients whose disease has been treated. When only a rare bacillus is found, a high threshold must be maintained and artifactual "pseudo" acid-fast bacilli excluded. As a general rule, a cutoff value of three organisms for a positive result seems prudent. False-positive smears can also result from contamination with local tap water that may harbor mycobacteria.

Traditional solid media (Lowenstein–Jensen, Petragani, and Middlebrook agars) have given way to liquid media (radiometric and nonradiometric) as the first-line systems. Liquid media have demonstrated increased recovery of mycobacteria and decreased time to detection. They also facilitate rapid and accurate susceptibility testing.[85,110] Some of these liquid systems are manual with visual inspection, whereas others are fully automated and continuously monitored. Most laboratories back up liquid systems with conventional media, because no system, at this time, is capable of identifying all isolates. Commercially available nucleic acid probes which hybridize to the mycobacterial RNA have largely replaced traditional biochemical testing, and have significantly shortened the time to identification of *M. tuberculosis* and selected NTM.[111] The less-frequently isolated species of NTM, for which probes are not available, are usually referred to reference or state laboratories, where identification is accomplished either by biochemical testing, cell wall analysis using chromatographic techniques, or genotypic sequencing.[91]

The rapid differentiation of *M. tuberculosis* from NTM is most important clinically, as the latter are much less infectious. In this context, molecular techniques have decreased the time to detection and identification of mycobacteria to less than 3 weeks in most instances. Direct nucleic acid amplification (NAA) testing of clinical specimens using commercially available polymerase chain reaction (PCR) or transcription-mediated amplification (TMA) methods can reduce detection and identification times to less than 8 hours.[109] Immunochromatographic techniques based on the detection of secreted mycobacterial proteins have the potential to reduce these times even further.[112] Although faster, the overall accuracy of NAA is higher than that of smears but less than that of culture.[111] In fact, no single test at this time has sufficient sensitivity and specificity to stand alone, and a combination of available techniques, depending on the clinical and economic setting, may be the best overall strategy.[113,114]

Interpretation of a culture isolate can sometimes be difficult. The presence of *M. tuberculosis* is always significant. *Mycobacterium kansasii* is an important pathogen, and its isolation is usually also significant, although it may represent colonization. The significance of other non-tuberculous mycobacterial isolates is variable, depending on whether there is clinical and radiographic evidence of disease. It is in this setting that histopathology plays an important role. *Mycobacterium avium* complex can be isolated from the respiratory tract of otherwise healthy adults, as well as HIV-infected patients with no clinical or radiographic evidence of disease. The American Thoracic Society has proposed diagnostic criteria which require that certain clinical, radiographic, and laboratory parameters be met in order to prove pathogenicity.[86] The laboratory criteria include three positive respiratory specimens within a year (two positive cultures and one positive smear, or three positive cultures) or a single positive bronchial wash with moderate to heavy growth, or a 4+ AFB smear. A tissue biopsy with appropriate histopathology and a positive culture or positive tissue acid-fast stain is also considered diagnostic.

Differential diagnosis

The key morphologic and microbiologic features of mycobacterial lung infections are summarized in Table 6.16. Mycobacteria produce a wide spectrum of

Table 6.16 Mycobacterial pneumonia synopsis

M. tuberculosis	
Surgical pathology:	Various patterns reflect immune status and complications: Necrotizing (tuberculoid) granuloma; granulomatous pneumonia; miliary granulomas; tuberculous (caseous) bronchopneumonia; pleural fibrosis and granulomas; endobronchial necrosis.
Cytopathology:	Epithelioid cells and necroinflammatory debris. Acid-fast bacilli detected with Ziehl–Neelsen or auramine O stains of cellblock sections, more sensitive than smears
Microbiology:	Acid-fast bacilli detected with Ziehl–Neelsen; Kinyoun stains or fluorescent bacilli with auramine O stain. Culture on Lowenstein–Jensen and Middlebrook selective and nonselective agar and/or liquid media systems. DNA probes or NAA for identification
Non-tuberculous mycobacteria (NTM; MOTT)	
Surgical pathology:	Granulomas generally with less necrosis; often epithelioid only. Unusual patterns, e.g. pseudo-Gaucher and spindle cell proliferation in immunocompromised patients
Cytopathology:	Epithelioid cells; pseudo-Gaucher or spindle cells with little or no necrosis. Negative images in Diff-Quik, confirmed as acid-fast bacilli with Ziehl–Neelsen. Organisms sparse, except in immunocompromised patient
Microbiology:	See *M. tuberculosis*

Table 6.17 Common fungal pathogens in the lung

Dimorphic fungi (mycelia at 25–30° C; yeast at 37° C): – *Blastomyces dermatitidis* – *Coccidioides immitis* – *Histoplasma capsulatum* – *Paracoccidioides braziliensis* – *Sporothrix schenckii* – *Penicillium marneffei*
Yeast: – *Cryptococcus neoformans* – *Candida* spp.
Hyaline (non-pigmented) molds: – *Aspergillus* spp. – *Zygomycetes* spp.
Phaeoid (pigmented; dematiaceous) molds: – *Bipolaris* spp.; *Alternaria*; *Curvularia* – *Pseudoallescheria boydii/Scedosporium apiospermum*
Miscellaneous: – Pneumocystis jiroveci

inflammatory patterns, both granulomatous and non-granulomatous. While the potential differential diagnosis is long, in practical terms, major considerations are fungal infections, sarcoidosis, Wegener's granulomatosis, and bacterial infections that produce suppurative granulomas, such as *Nocardia*, *Actinomyces*, *Brucella*, and *Francisella* spp. Generally, the use of special stains and cultures will resolve most diagnostic dilemmas. Wegener's granulomatosis (see Chapter 10) can usually be excluded, based on the lack of the characteristic tinctorial properties of the necrosis in the granulomas, the presence of granulomas without necrosis, and the absence of vasculitis or capillaritis. Sarcoidosis can be a difficult exclusion when necrosis is absent or sparse in a mycobacterial infection. Radiographic evidence of bilateral hilar adenopathy and other systemic findings of sarcoidosis often resolve the issue.

Fungal pneumonias

The pathologist examining tissue sections containing fungal forms is in a unique position to provide at least a provisional diagnosis at the group or genus level, and to make a judgment as to the significance of the organism in terms of its invasiveness or presence as a saprophobe or allergen. Indeed, often the most effective diagnostic strategy available is the rapid identification of fungi in tissue sections or cytologic samples.[26,115] This is especially important when opportunistic infection is being considered in the immunocompromised patient. However, optimal performance also requires knowing when the morphologic features of a fungal organism are insufficient to permit group or genus level diagnosis, and when integration of microbiologic data and histopathologic findings is required.

Table 6.18 Patterns of fungal lung injury

Large nodules: – Non-necrotizing granulomas – Necrotizing granulomas – Suppurative granulomas – Poorly formed granulomas
Cavitary lesions
Miliary nodules
Acute bronchopneumonia
Airway disease
Intravascular/infarct
Diffuse alveolar damage, acute and organizing
Foamy alveolar casts

Etiologic agents

Nearly 70,000 fungi are known, and about 100 have been recovered from respiratory infections.[116] Fortunately, only a small number are implicated as pathogenic on a consistent basis, and these are listed in Table 6.17.

Patterns of fungal lung injury

Inflammatory patterns that suggest the presence of a fungal infection are listed in Table 6.18. As is the case for other categories of etiologic agents, there are no absolutely characteristic or diagnostic patterns. Overlap is common and atypical reactions occur, ranging from overwhelming diffuse alveolar damage to little or no reaction in the immunocompromised patient. Detection of the etiologic agent in tissue by microscopic examination, ancillary tests, or culture confers specificity and significance to the listed patterns. Large spherules with endospores characteristic of *Coccidioides immitis* or yeast with large mucoid capsules of *Cryptococcus neoformans* can be diagnostic. However, atypical forms of these organisms can be misleading and challenging. For example, in aerated cavities or in the setting of bronchopleural fistula, *Coccidioides* spp. may produce branching septate and moniliform hyphae or immature morula-like spherules mimicking other fungi (e.g. hyaline molds and *Blastomyces dermatitidis*).[23] Similarly, *C. neoformans*, *Histoplasma capsulatum*, and *Sporothrix schenckii* have been reported to produce hyphae or pseudohyphae in tissue, while acapsular *C. neoformans* may mimic other yeasts or *Pneumocystis* organisms.[117]

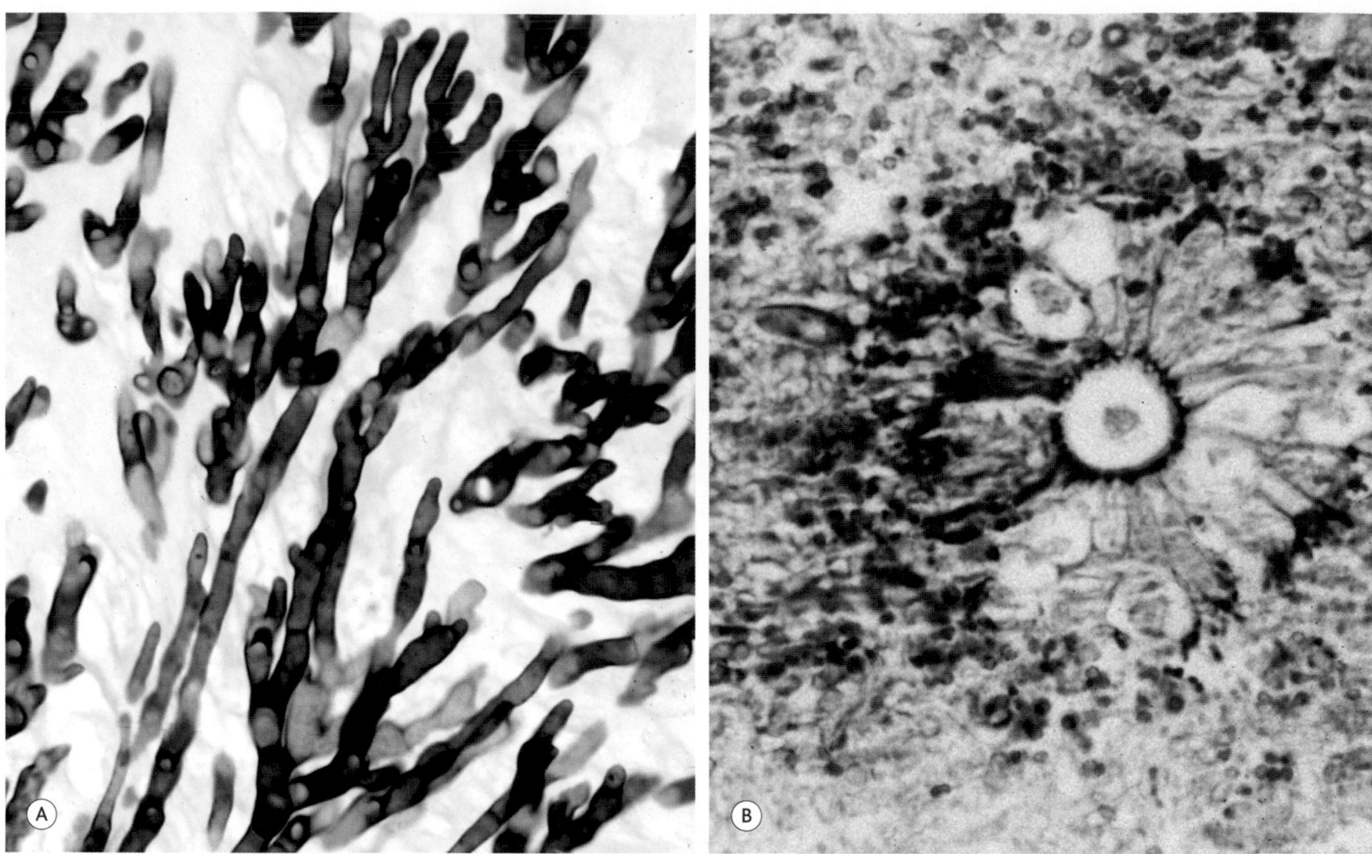

Fig. 6.54 ***Aspergillus*** **sp.** (A) Septate mycelia with 45° angle branching (GMS stain). (B) Fruiting body (conidiophore with sterigmata and conidia) (GMS stain).

Mycelial morphology is helpful when it is characteristic of a specific genus or group. For example, broad, sparsely septate, nonparallel, twisted or irregular diameter, thin-wall mycelia, with variable wide-angle branching, characterize *Zygomycetes;* whereas progressively proliferating, regularly septate, 45° angle, dichotomously branching mycelia with parallel walls are typical of *Aspergillus* spp. (Fig. 6.54). In the case of *Aspergillus*, it is important to remember that only the presence of a fruiting body (conidiophore with sterigmata and conidia) permits diagnosis at the genus level; and there are many *Aspergillus* look-alikes in tissue, such as *Fusarium, Paecilomyces, Acremonium, Bipolaris, Pseudoallescheria boydii* and its asexual anamorph, *Scedosporium apiospermum.*[117] Sometimes careful examination of tissue with special stains under high magnification or oil emersion will reveal clues, such as in-situ sporulation, allowing a more definitive diagnosis.[24] However, these clues are often subtle, even for experienced microscopists, and it is important to defer to culture, immunohistologic, or molecular techniques whenever possible.[118] Typical morphologic injury patterns and related etiologic agents are briefly highlighted below. The references should be consulted for further details.

Blastomycosis

This chronic granulomatous and suppurative infection is essentially a North American disease with a particularly high prevalence in the State of Mississippi. It may be found in patients with normal immunity as well as in those immunocompromised by diseases and therapy.[119] Although some *Blastomyces dermatitidis* infections are asymptomatic, blastomycosis can be quite diverse clinically, presenting as a mild to severe pneumonia, adult respiratory distress syndrome, or tumor. The disease almost always begins in the lungs, although skin and bone are other common sites of involvement. In the lung, pathologic substrates include focal or diffuse infiltrates, rare lobar consolidation, miliary nodules, solitary nodules, and acute or organizing diffuse alveolar damage (Table 6.19).[120–122]

Necrotizing granulomas, especially the suppurative type are characteristic (Fig. 6.55A), but non-necrotizing granulomas may be found as well.

Few to numerous, refractile, double-contoured wall, multinucleated yeast cells (8–15 µm range up to 30 µm) with broad-based budding are characteristic (Fig. 6.55B) but large forms can mimic small *Coccidioides* spherules;[123] smaller forms ("microforms") may also be found which can mimic *Cryptococcus neoformans*.[120]

Coccidioidomycosis

Endemic in the Lower Sonoran Life Zone of the southwestern USA, the soil fungus *Coccidioides immitis* and the newly recognized species *C. posadasii*[124] may be encountered outside the endemic area as a result of fomite transmission of arthroconidia (e.g. Asian textile workers handling imported Arizona cotton) or in travelers who have returned from an endemic area. Most primary pulmonary infections are asymptomatic. The spectrum of pulmonary pathology in patients with clinically apparent disease, outlined in Table 6.20, ranges from upper and lower airway involvement, solitary parenchymal nodules, acute pneumonia, eosinophilic pneumonia, chronic progressive disease with cavitary nodules, bronchopleural fistula, empyema, and even miliary and systemic dissemination.[125–127] Granulomas are characteristic and may occur with or without necrosis. Intact spherules induce fibrocaseous granulomas (Fig. 6.56A), whereas ruptured spherules may incite suppurative and BCG-like granulomatous reactions (Fig. 6.56B).[125]

Table 6.19 Patterns of pulmonary blastomycosis

Patterns
Acute pneumonia:
– Lobular
– Lobar
Diffuse alveolar damage
Miliary nodule
Solitary nodule

Table 6.20 Patterns of coccidioidal respiratory tract disease

Patterns
Airway disease:
– Pharyngeal granuloma
– Laryngeal granuloma
– Tracheobronchial granuloma
Pulmonary parenchymal disease:
– Acute pneumonia
– Eosinophilic pneumonia
– Chronic progressive infection
Fibrocavitary lesions
Bronchopleural fistula; empyema
– Solitary pulmonary nodule
– Disseminated disease
Miliary
Extrapulmonary

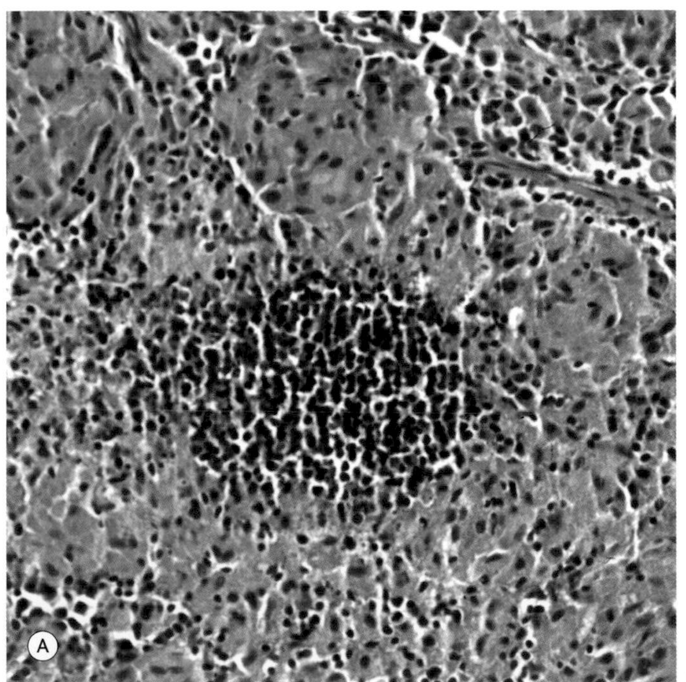

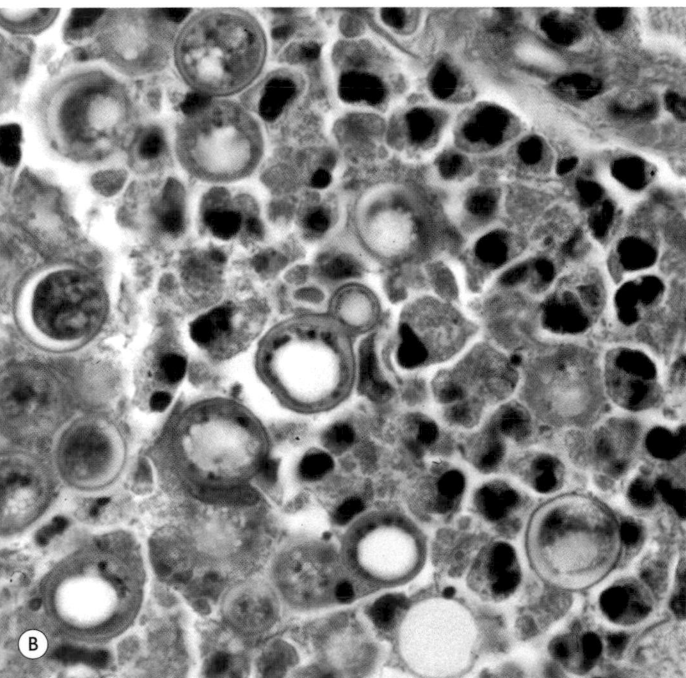

Fig. 6.55 **Blastomycosis.** (A) The suppurative granuloma is characteristic (H&E stain). (B) Double-contoured wall yeast with broad-based budding (H&E stain).

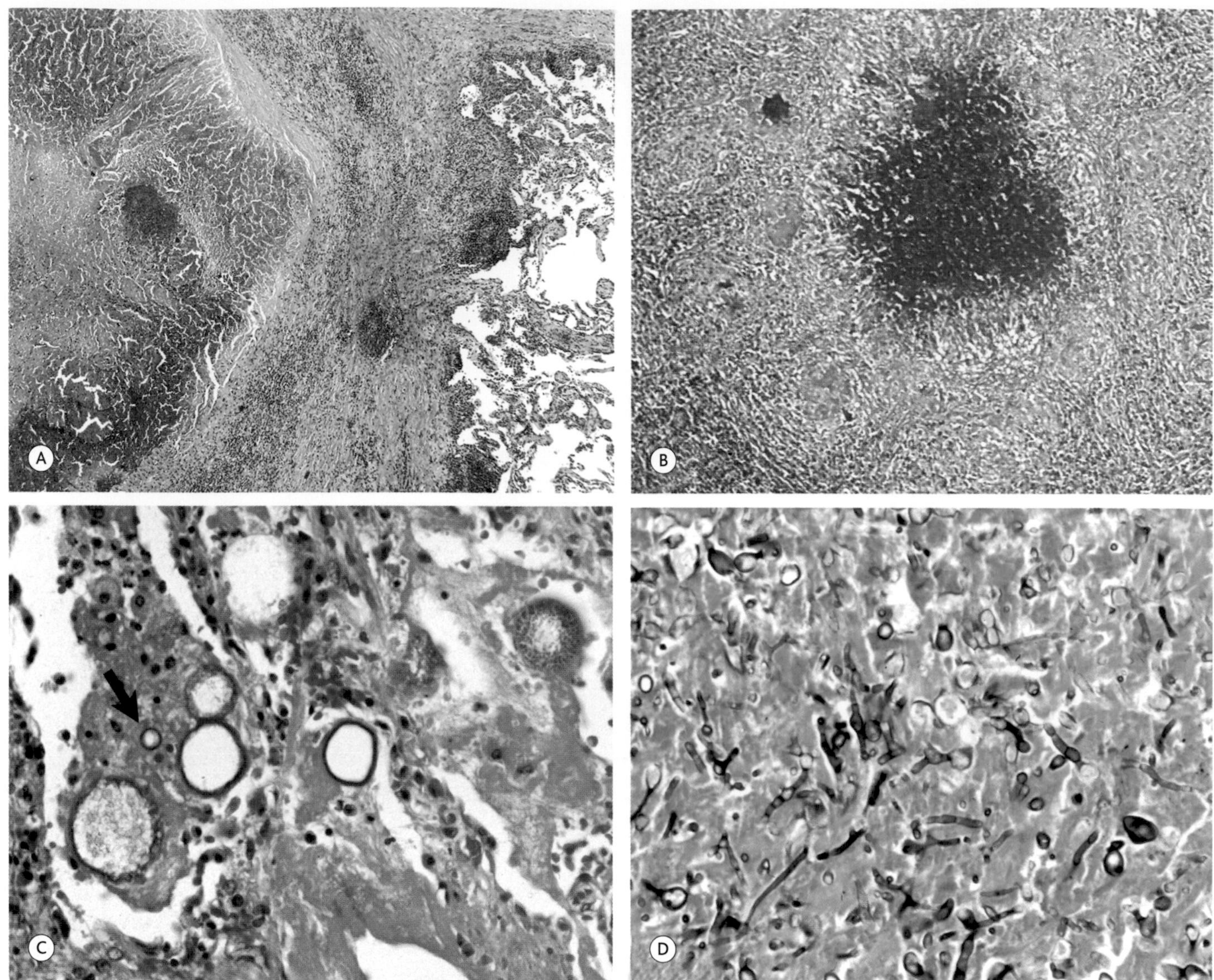

Fig. 6.56 **Coccidioidomycosis.** (A) Fibrocaseous granuloma (H&E stain). (B) BCG-like granuloma (H&E stain). (C) Coccidioides immitis, small (arrow) and large spherules with/without endospores (H&E stain). (D) Biphasic pattern with mycelia and spore-like swellings (GMS stain).

The large mature spherule (up to 40–60 μm) has a thick refractile wall lined by or filled with endospores and is the key to the diagnosis (Fig. 6.56C). This finding allows the distinction of coccidioidomycosis from other fungi such as blastomycosis and histoplasmosis, which produce similar histopathologic reaction patterns. In aerated cavities or the setting of bronchopleural fistula, mycelia resembling various hyaline molds may be seen with or without a variety of mature and immature spherules (Fig. 6.56D; see also Fig. 6.13). Look-alikes include large variant *B. dermatitidis*, adiaspiromycosis, pollen grains, and pulses (legume seeds).

Histoplasmosis

This most common pulmonary fungal infection worldwide is endemic in the Ohio and Mississippi river valleys of North America and is the most common endemic mycosis in AIDS.[128] The clinical forms of *Histoplasma capsulatum* infection, outlined in Table 6.21, include primary acute, chronic latent and progressive, disseminated, and mediastinal sclerosing and lymphadenopathy types.[34,129] The pathologic correlates involve a spectrum of histopathology, from an exudative to a granulomatous process, influenced by such factors as the fungal burden and the immune status of the patient. In patients with normal defenses, necrotizing and non-necrotizing granulomas, including sarcoid-like lesions, occur as large solitary lesions, miliary nodules (Fig. 6.57A), cavitary lesions, and laminated fibrous solitary nodules. In patients with impaired immunity, striking macrophage response with numerous intracellular yeasts is a characteristic pattern (Fig. 6.57B). The exudative lesion resembles acute lobular pneumonia with fibrinopurulent exudates.[130]

Histoplasma capsulatum are yeast (2–5 μm), with narrow-based unequal budding (Fig. 6.57C). They may be seen on H&E stained sections, and, when numerous, appear as small refractile ovoid structures within macrophages. Yeasts typically occur in clusters, but may be rare or very localized in old granulomas. A search for budding organisms in these situations may prove futile. Sometimes, yeasts may have dark staining foci, resembling *Pneumocystis* organisms. Also, some yeast cells may be surrounded by a clear space and may be mistaken for *Cryptococcus*.[34] Other look-alikes include *Candida* spp., *Penicillium marneffei*, capsule-deficient cryptococci, intracellular *Blastomyces dermatidis* and Hamazaki–Wesenberg bodies.

Table 6.21 Clinical forms of pulmonary histoplasmosis

Benign, self limited
Acute: - Acute respiratory distress syndrome - Acute self-limited, upper lobe (in smokers with emphysema)
Chronic: - Asymptomatic pulmonary nodule +/- calcification (histoplasmoma) - Progressive (chronic cavitary) pulmonary
Progressive disseminated
Mediastinal: - Lymphadenopathy - Middle lobe syndrome - Fibrosis

Source: from Travis et al.,[34] Table 12-6, with permission.

Paracoccidioidomycosis (South American blastomycosis)

Seven clinical forms occur, but rarely cause lung infections in North America. The histopathology resembles other mycoses and can be exudative or granulomatous. *Paracoccidioides braziliensis* appears as a large spherical yeast (10–60 μm) with multiple buds attached by narrow necks ("steering wheel" or "ship's wheel").[131] When budding is sparse, look-alikes include *H. capsulatum* with small intracellular forms, *B. dermatitides*, and capsule-deficient *Cryptococcus* for medium-size forms, and *Coccidioides immitis* or *C. posadasii* for large forms.

Sporotrichosis

Infection by *Sporothrix schenckii* is usually confined to the skin, subcutaneum, and lymphatic pathways, but the organism can disseminate to the lungs. Rarely, *S. schenckii* is a primary pulmonary pathogen. The organism can produce cavitary disease in the form of a single lesion.

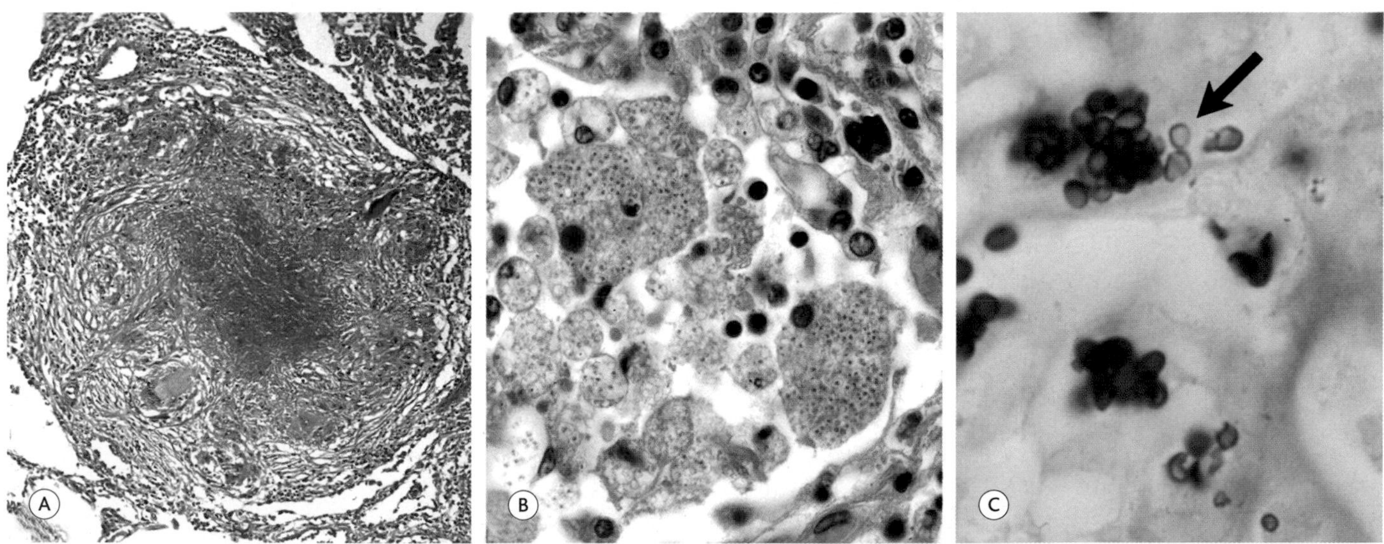

Fig. 6.57 **Histoplasmosis.** (A) Miliary nodule with central zone of necrosis invested by epithelioid histiocytes, multinucleated giant cells, and outer collarette of lymphocytes. (B) Myriad *Histoplasma capsulatum* yeast cells in macrophages. (C) Clusters of *H. capsulatum* yeast cells in macrophages. Note narrow-based budding (arrow; GMS stain).

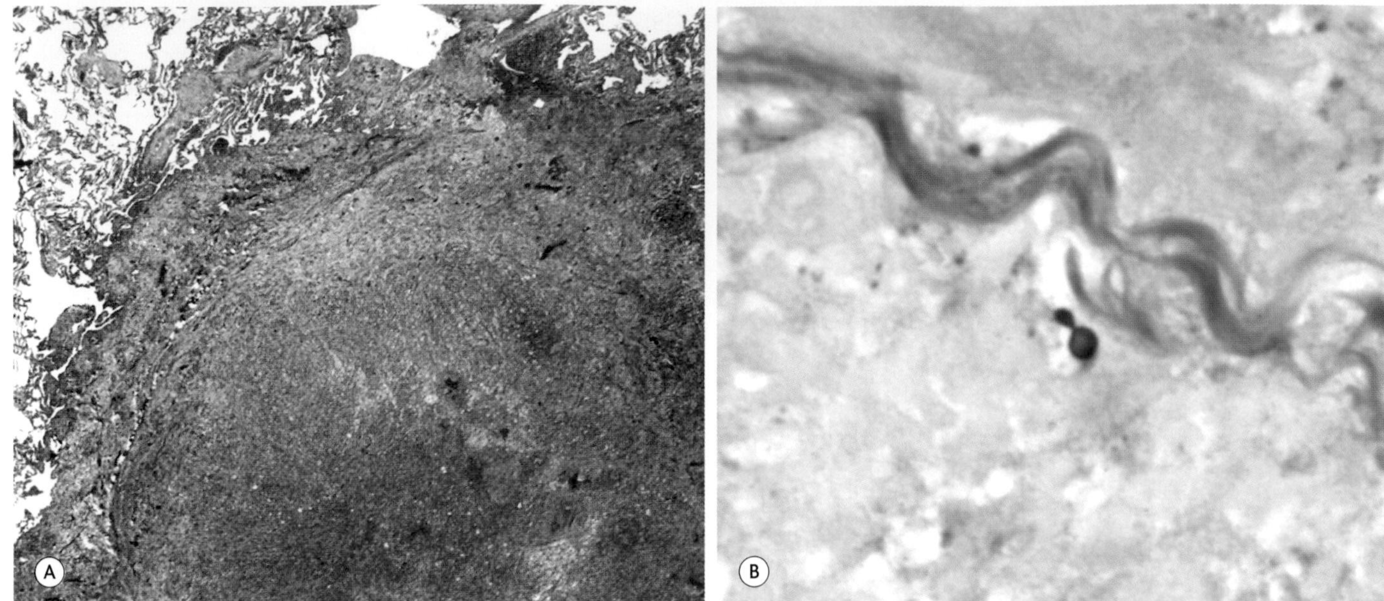

Fig. 6.58 **Sporotrichosis.** (A) Cavitary granuloma presenting as a solitary pulmonary nodule (H&E stain). (B) A rare, oval, narrow, budding yeast (GMS stain).

Infection may be bilateral and apical, progressive and destructive or may be identified clinically as a solitary pulmonary nodule. Microscopically, caseous and suppurative type granulomas (Fig. 6.58A) occur, with variable numbers of round to oval, small (2–3 μm) narrow budding yeast (Fig. 6.58B) or cigar-shaped forms.[132] Non-necrotizing granulomas also occur. Asteroid bodies are an important clue, especially when organisms are sparse, as is often the case. Look-alikes include *H. capsulatum*, acapsular *Cryptococcus*, *Candida* spp., and Hamazaki–Wesenberg bodies.

Penicilliosis

Southeast Asia is the endemic setting of the unique dimorphic fungus *Penicillium marneffei*. The disease it produces is not seen in North America except in travelers, especially immunocompromised hosts. It is one of the commonest opportunistic infections in AIDS patients in Southeast Asia and a significant clue to the presence of AIDS in that area. The respiratory tract is the portal of entry, with pulmonary infiltrates and disseminated disease, especially to skin. Microscopically, alveolar macrophages stuffed with spherical to oval yeast-like cells (2.5–5 μm) are seen, each with a single transverse septum; short hyphal forms and elongated, curved "sausage" forms may be formed in necrotic and cavitary lesions.[133,134] The septum distinguishes it from its look-alike, *H. capsulatum*.

Table 6.22 Patterns of cryptococcal lung disease (in order of decreasing immunity)

Fibrocaseous granuloma
Granulomatous pneumonia
Histiocytic pneumonia
Mucoid pneumonia
Intracapillary cryptococcosis

Source: from Mark EJ,[135] with permission.

Cryptococcosis

Cryptococcus neoformans is a ubiquitous, facultative, intracellular organism whose pathogenicity in the lung largely depends on the patient's immune status, as illustrated earlier in Fig. 6.1 and listed in Table 6.22. In the normal host, a substantial proportion of patients are asymptomatic and the remainder have characteristic respiratory symptoms associated with infiltrates or nodules. Immunocompromised patients are almost invariably symptomatic and often have signs of disseminated disease. Pulmonary injury patterns include single or multiple nodules, segmental or diffuse infiltrates, cavitary lesions, and miliary nodules. Microscopically, patients with intact immune systems manifest

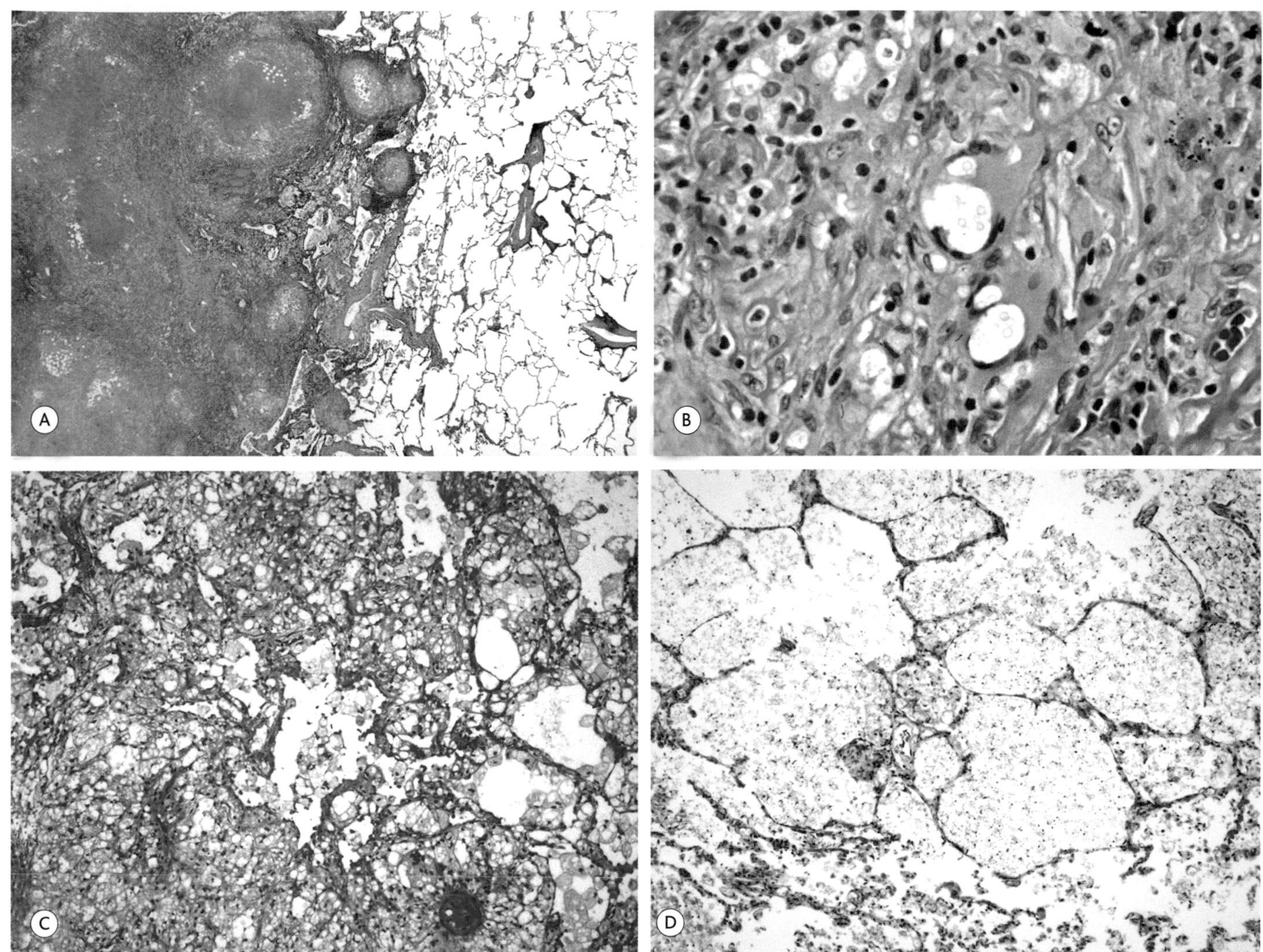

Fig. 6.59 **Cryptococcosis.** (A) Solitary pulmonary nodule with small satellite granulomas (H&E stain). (B) Granulomatous pneumonia with clusters of pale staining yeast in clear spaces surrounded by histiocytes and multinucleated giant cells (H&E stain). (C) Histiocytic pneumonia. (D) Mucoid pneumonia with no inflammatory cell reaction.

fibrocaseous granulomas (Fig. 6.59A) or granulomatous pneumonia (Fig. 6.59B), whereas immunocompromised patients are more likely to have histiocytic (Fig. 6.59 C) or mucoid infiltrates without inflammation (Fig. 6.59 D). The lungs of patients with the most severe immunodeficiency may contain myriad yeasts in the alveolar septal capillaries (Fig. 6.60), with little if any intra-alveolar reaction.[135] However, the intracapillary form may be associated with mucoid pneumonia.[136] The distinctive manifestation of mucoid pneumonia (Fig. 6.61A) can be confirmed with mucin stains such as alcian blue (Fig. 6.61B).

The organisms are round, budding yeast forms (4–7 µm, range from 2 to 15 µm). In H&E stained sections pale gray to light blue, pleomorphic yeast-like cells can simulate artifact surrounded by clear space. They often occur in clusters and can be found within giant cells, as illustrated in Fig 6.59B.[136] Mucicarmine stains the capsule, as shown in Fig. 6.60A, but capsule-deficient forms occur (Fig. 6.60B) and their pleomorphic appearance can be confused with other yeast forms, including *H. capsulatum*, *B. dermatitidis*, *S. schenckii* and *Pneumocystis* spp.

Candidiasis

Candida spp. are yeasts that can produce pseudohyphae, and are the most common invasive fungal organisms in humans. Primary *Candida* pneumonia is rare outside of the setting of an immunocompromised patient in the intensive care unit.[34] In general, *Candida albicans* is the most frequently isolated of the more than 80 known species. Among the several other medically important species, *C. glabrata* (formerly *Torulopsis glabrata*) is now

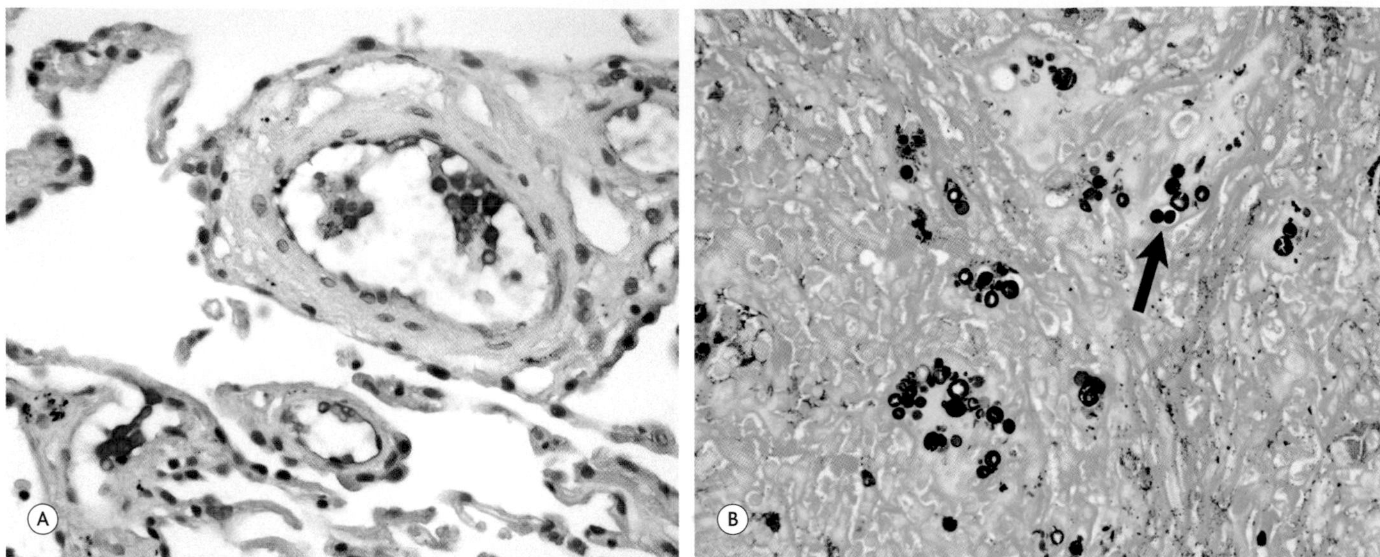

Fig. 6.60 (A) Intravascular *Cryptococcus*. Yeast cells with stained capsules (mucicarmine stain). (B) Capsule-deficient *Cryptococcus* (GMS stain).

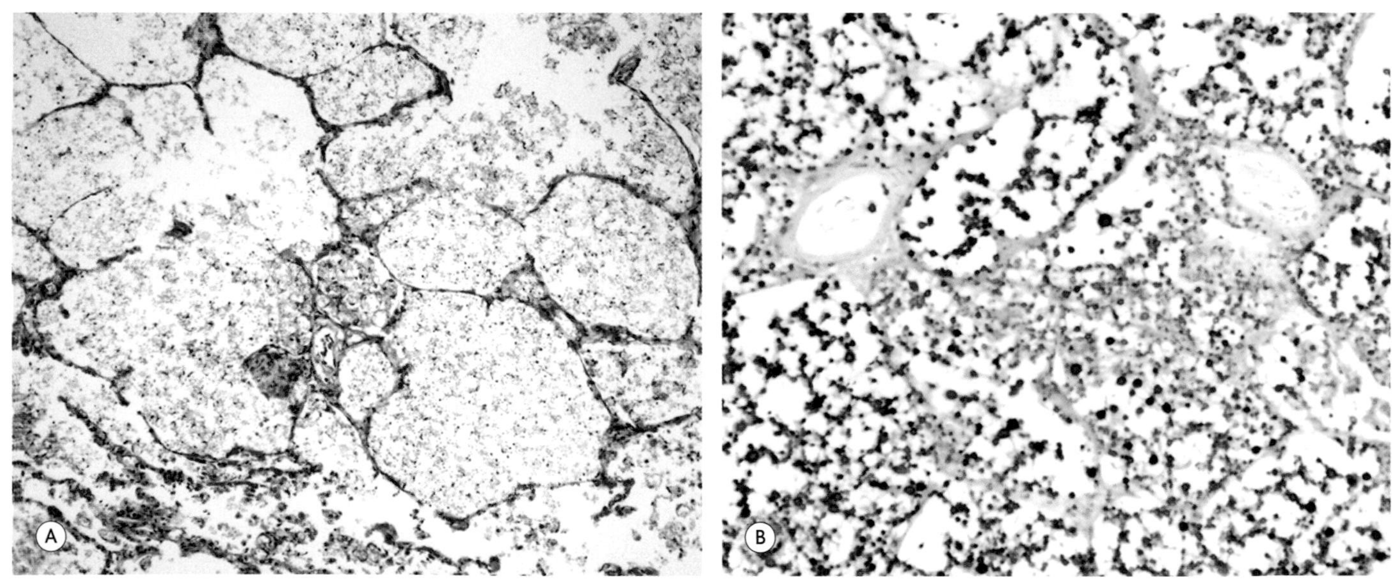

Fig. 6.61 **Cryptococcal mucoid pneumonia.** (A) Myriad blue-gray yeast in mucoid matrix (H&E stain); (B) Alcian blue mucin stain accentuates the mucoid matrix.

the second most common yeast species isolated from clinical specimens. It only produces yeast in tissue (compared to other species which may manifest yeast and pseudohyphae). Whereas primary *Candida* pneumonia is rather uncommon, pulmonary disease can occur secondary to hematogenous dissemination or aspiration from the oropharynx. When bloodborne, miliary nodules with a necroinflammatory center and a hemorrhagic rim reflect an intravascular distribution of fungi. In the case of aspiration, the organisms may be found in the airways associated with a pattern of bronchopneumonia[137] (Fig. 6.62A) or, much less commonly, a bronchocentric granulomatosis pattern.

In tissue sections, oval budding yeast-like cells (blastoconidia) 2–6 µm in diameter may appear with pseudohyphae, which constrict at points of budding,

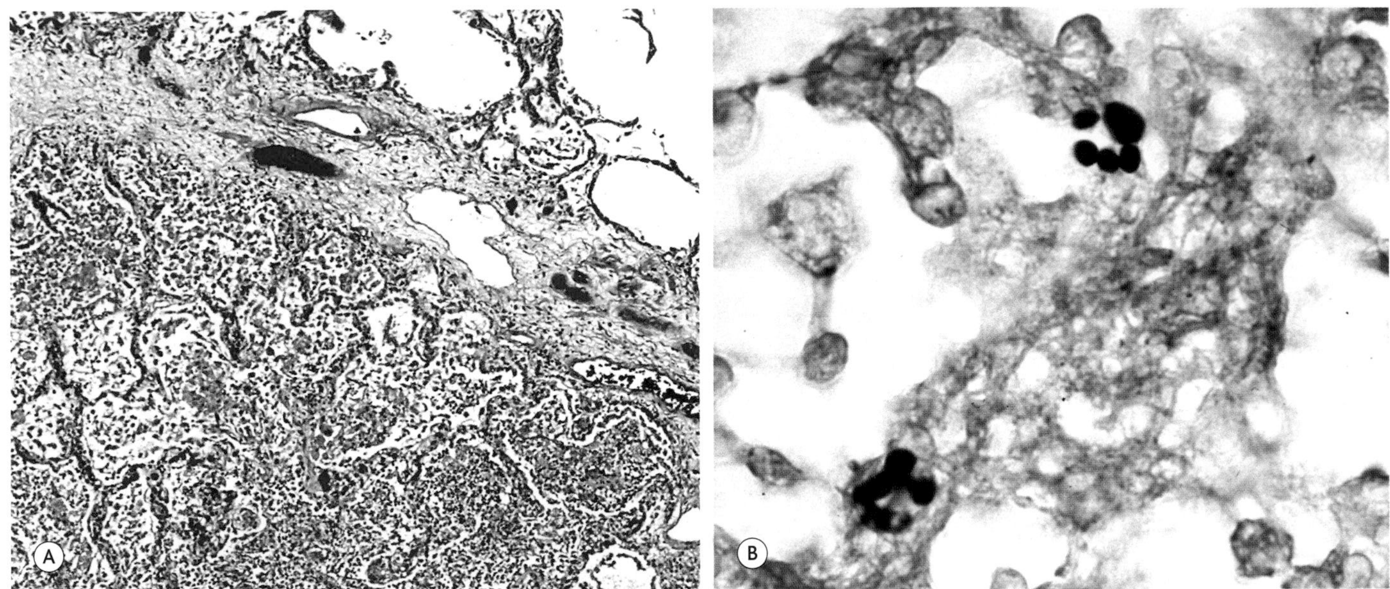

Fig. 6.62 (A) *Candida* bronchopneumonia. (B) *Candida* yeast cells – blastoconidia (GMS stain).

creating the impression of bulging rather than parallel walls (Fig. 6.62B). The pseudohyphae branch at acute angles and their width can overlap with the true hyphae of *Aspergillus*, from which they must be distinguished.

Rarely, giant blastoconidia ("chlamydaspore-like") have been identified in tissue where they may be potentially confused with *Cryptococcus*, *Blastomyces*, and *Paracoccidioides* spp.[138] Other look-alikes include *Histoplasma capsulatum*, *Trichosporon beigeli*, and *Malassesia furfur*, depending on whether pseudohyphae or yeast forms alone are present. They can be distinguished from *Histoplasma* by their extracellular location and Gram stain positivity. *Trichosporon beigeli* tends to be somewhat larger and more pleomorphic. Malasseziasis is clinically associated with parenteral nutrition, Intralipid, and indwelling catheters. Pulmonary lesions include pneumonia, mycotic thromboemboli, infarcts, and vasculitis. *Malassesia furfur* may be found in small arteries, where they appear as small, 2–5 µm yeast-like cells. They form distinctive unipolar broad-based buds but no pseudohyphae.[34]

Aspergillosis

Worldwide, species of *Aspergillus* are the most common invasive molds. They are the second most common fungal pathogens after *Candida* spp., but in contrast to *Candida*, are more commonly isolated from the lung. There are several species, but *A. fumigatus* is the one most often seen in the clinical laboratory and most often isolated from the lungs of immunocompromised patients.[139] Respiratory aspergillosis can be classified into a colonizing or saprophytic form (intrabronchial and preexisting cavity-fungus ball) (Fig. 6.63A); hypersensitivity forms (allergic bronchopulmonary aspergillosis, including mucoid impaction of bronchi and hypersensitivity pneumonitis) (Fig. 6.63B); and invasive disease (minimally invasive/chronic necrotizing or angioinvasive/disseminated), as outlined in Table 6.23.[34,139–141] Invasive disease tends to occur in the immunocompromised patient and typically is angiocentric, with intravascular

Table 6.23 Patterns of pulmonary aspergillosis

Patterns
Colonization:
– Fungus ball
Hypersensitivity reaction:
– Allergic bronchopulmonary aspergillosis
– Eosinophilic pneumonia
– Mucoid impaction
– Bronchocentric granulomatosis
– Hypersensitivity pneumonitis
Invasive:
– Acute invasive aspergillosis
– Necrotizing pseudomembranous tracheobronchitis
– Chronic necrotizing pneumonia
– Bronchopleural fistula
– Empyema

Source: from Travis et al.,[34] Table 12-10, with permission.

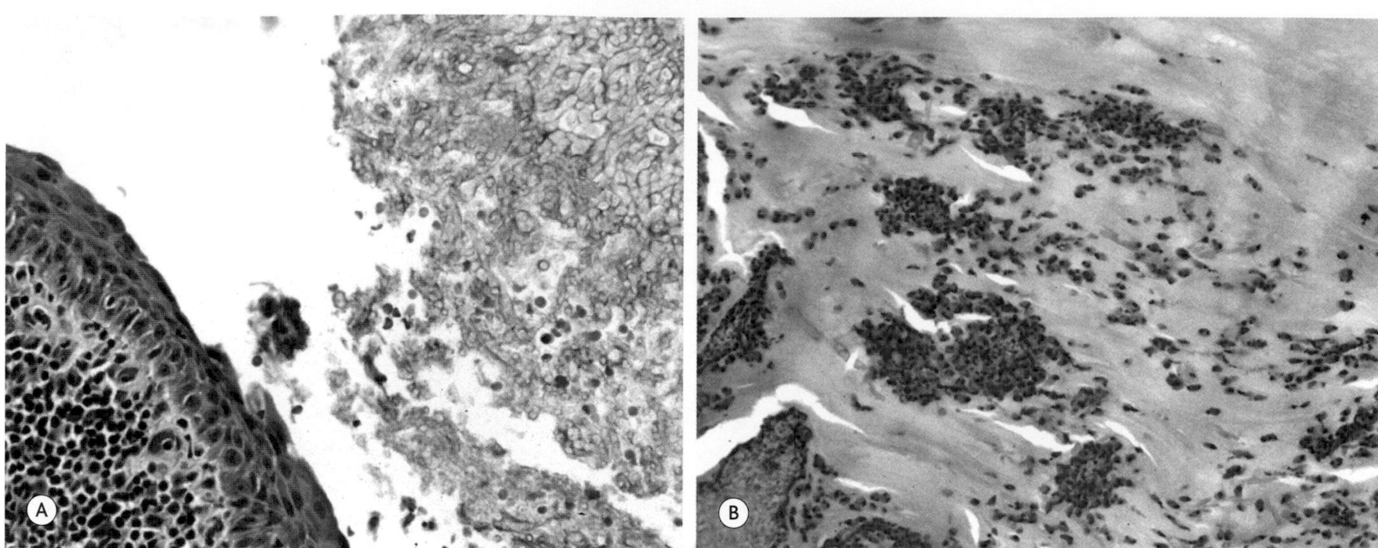

Fig. 6.63 (A) Aspergillosis fungus ball (H&E stain). (B) Allergic bronchopulmonary aspergillosis. Intraluminal allergic mucin with laminated clusters of eosinophils in inspissated basophilic mucin with scattered Charcot–Leyden crystals (H&E stain).

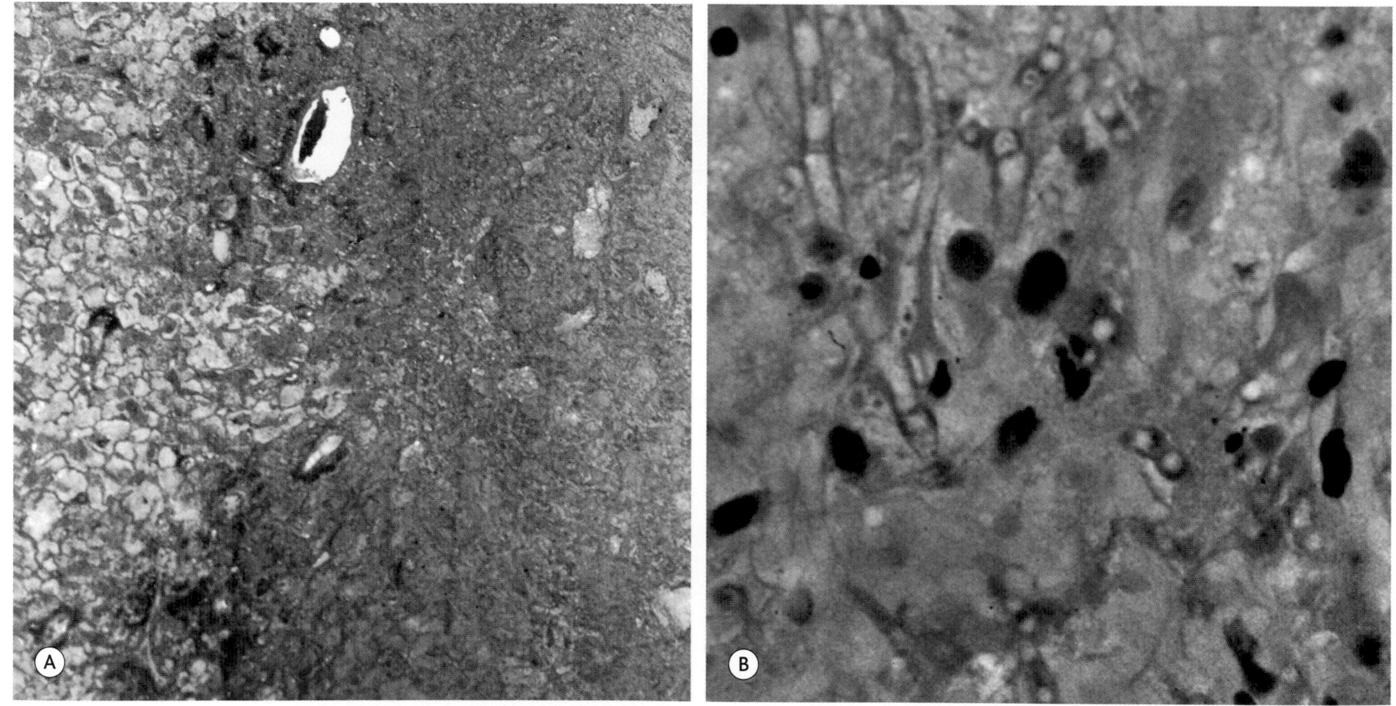

Fig. 6.64 **Invasive aspergillosis.** (A) Hemorrhagic infarct (H&E stain). (B) 45° angle branching septate hyphae.

spread producing hemorrhagic infarcts (Fig. 6.64A). Some cases defy categorization, are unique, e.g. bronchocentric (Fig. 6.65A) and miliary patterns (Fig. 6.65B), or are hybrids of infection and hypersensitivity.[142]

Microscopically, septate hyphae, dichotomatously branched at a 45° angle, have uniform, consistent width (3–6 μm) without constrictions at points of septation, as previously illustrated in Fig. 6.54. When numerous, as in some angioinvasive lesions and fungus balls, these features can be readily appreciated in H&E stained sections (Fig. 6.64B). Fruiting heads, previously illustrated in Fig. 6.54B, are sometimes formed in cavities. Oxalate

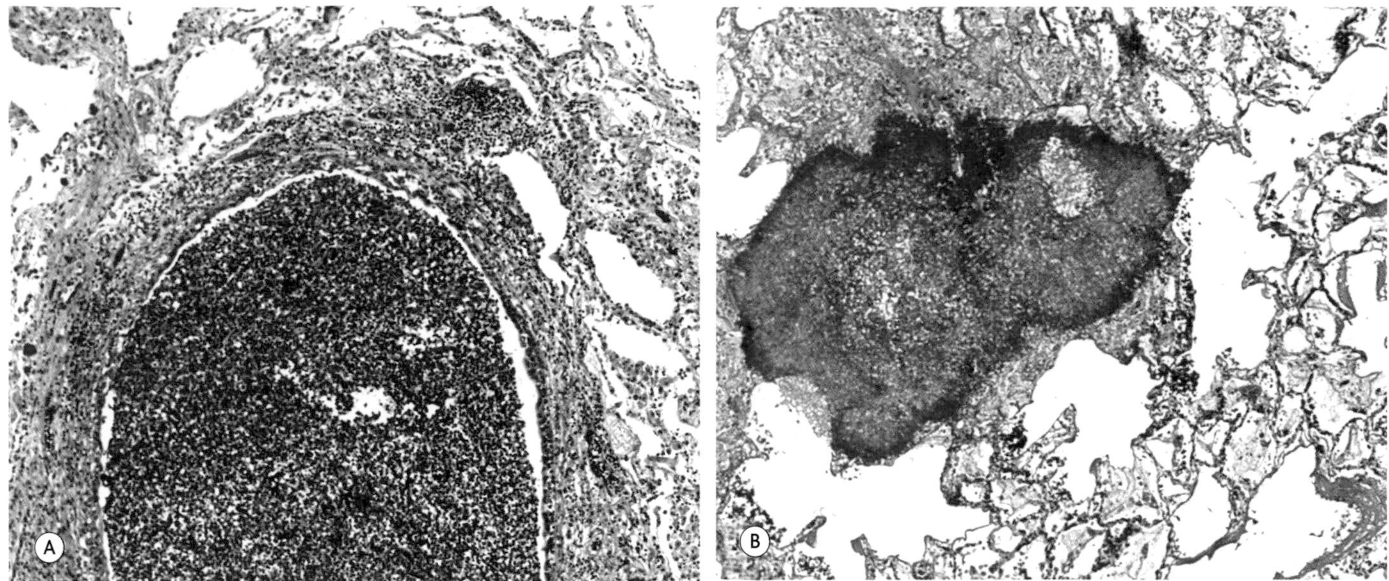

Fig. 6.65 **Bronchiolocentric and miliary aspergillosis.** (A) Bronchiole expanded and filled with purulent exudate (H&E stain). (B) Miliary pattern. Expanding colony of organisms with hyaline membranes at periphery.

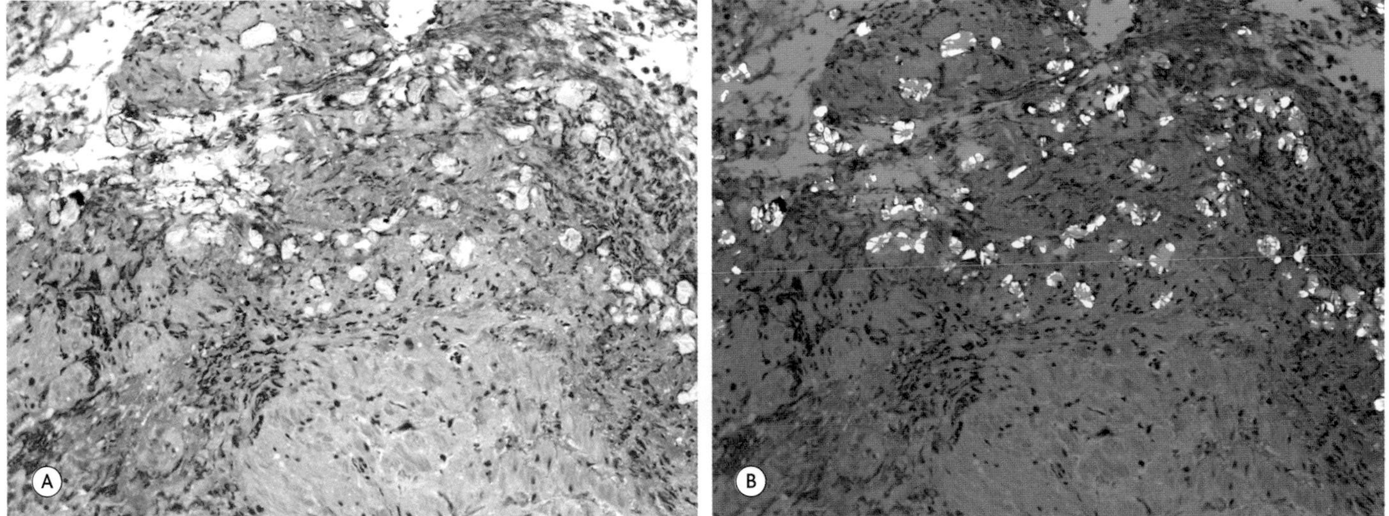

Fig. 6.66 (A) Pale yellow oxalate crystal sheaths in necroinflammatory debris (H&E stain). (B) Birefringent oxylates under polarized light.

crystals, visible in plane-polarized light (Fig. 6.66), are an important clue to *Aspergillus* infection when hyphae cannot be identified.

Look-alikes include various hyaline molds such as *Zygomycete* and *Candida* spp., as well as *Pseudoallescheria boydii*.[143] Another look-alike is *Fusarium* spp. Fusariosis is an emerging mycosis in the immunocompromised host and the second most common opportunist after *Aspergillus* spp. in immunosuppresed patients with hematologic malignancies.[144] The clinical and pathological features in the lung and at sites of dissemination mimic those of aspergillosis and the mycelia are essentially indistinguishable. Isolation in culture, immunohistochemistry, or molecular techniques such as in-situ hybridization or PCR are required for definitive diagnosis.

Zygomycosis

The taxonomic organization of the fungal phylum *Zygomycota*, includes the class *Zygomycetes*, which is subdivided into two orders: *Mucorales* and *Entomophthorales*. These orders contain the agents of human zygomycosis.[145]

The order *Mucorales* includes the genera *Absidia*, *Apophysomyces*, *Rhizopus*, *Rhizomucor*, and *Mucor* from which the often taxonomically incorrect term 'mucormycosis' is derived. In fact, most infections are due to *Rhizopus* and *Absidia* spp.[146] The *Zygomycete* spp. share clinical and pathologic features with invasive *Aspergillus* spp., being angiotropic and capable of inducing hemorrhagic infarcts with sparse inflammation.

Clinical syndromes produced by these fungi include rhinocerebral, pulmonary, cutaneous, gastrointestinal, and neonatal infections. Hematopoietic malignancies and diabetes mellitus with acidosis underlie most cases of pulmonary infection. Table 6.24 lists a broad spectrum of pulmonary disease that includes solitary or multiple and bilateral nodular lesions, segmental or lobar consolidation, cavitary lesions, fistulas, infarcts (Fig. 6.67); direct extension into mediastinal, thoracic soft tissue, chest wall and diaphragm; chronic tracheal and endobronchial infection; and fungus ball similar to aspergilloma.[147] An endobronchial syndrome with a propensity to erode blood vessels has also been described, sometimes resulting in fatal hemoptysis.[148]

Table 6.24 Patterns of pulmonary zygomycosis

Acute lobular or lobar pneumonia
Nodules
Cavities
Endobronchial mass
Fistulas
Infarcts
Thoracic soft tissue/mediastinum
Fungus ball

Hyphae, are broad (6–25 μm), thin-walled, and pauciseptate (Fig. 6.68A). They display considerable variation in width, with twisted, non-parallel contours and random wide-angle branching, nearing 90 degrees.[149] They also have a tendency to fragment more commonly than *Aspergillus* spp., which tend to retain their elongate sweeping profiles. Additional features include variability in tinctorial staining in H&E sections, ranging from basophilia to eosinophilia. Weakly stained hyphae are especially prone to occur in frozen sections, and they often have a bubbly or vacuolated appearance.[146] In addition to being angiotropic, they are neurotropic.[149] In lesions exposed to air, the hyphae may form ovoid or spherical thick-walled chlamydoconidia, within or at the terminal ends[150] (Fig. 6.68B) Look-alikes at the lower width range include *Aspergillus* and other *Aspergillus*-like hyaline molds. The pseudohyphae of *Candida* spp. sometimes can be closely simulated.

Phaeohyphomycosis

A few genera of dematiacious molds produce infections like those of *Aspergillus*, including allergic broncho-pulmonary disease (Fig. 6.69A) and bronchocentric granulomatosis patterns.[151,152] These include *Bipolaris*, *Exserohilum*, *Xylohypha*, *Alternaria*, *Curvularia*, and the

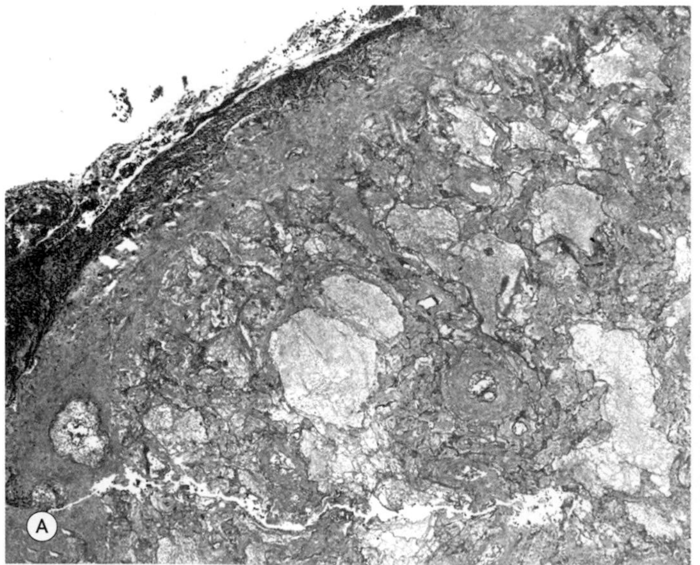

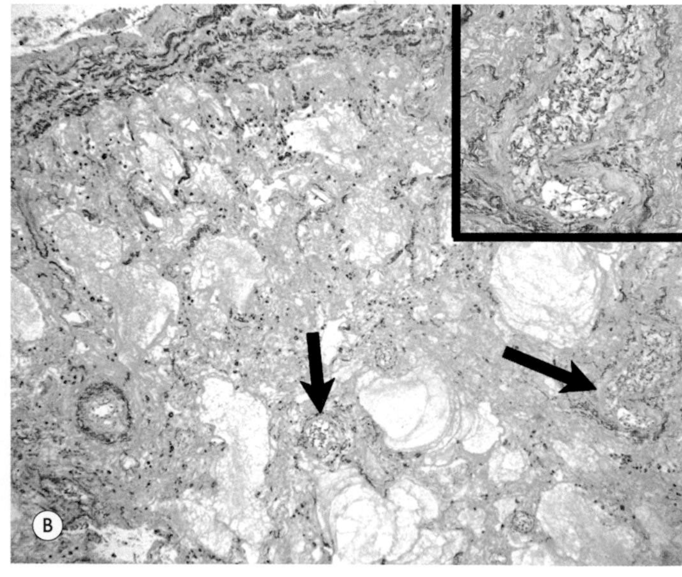

Fig. 6.67 **Zygomycosis.** (A) Nodular infarct (H&E stain). (B) Intravascular organisms. Vessel at right arrow is shown at high magnification (inset; GMS stain).

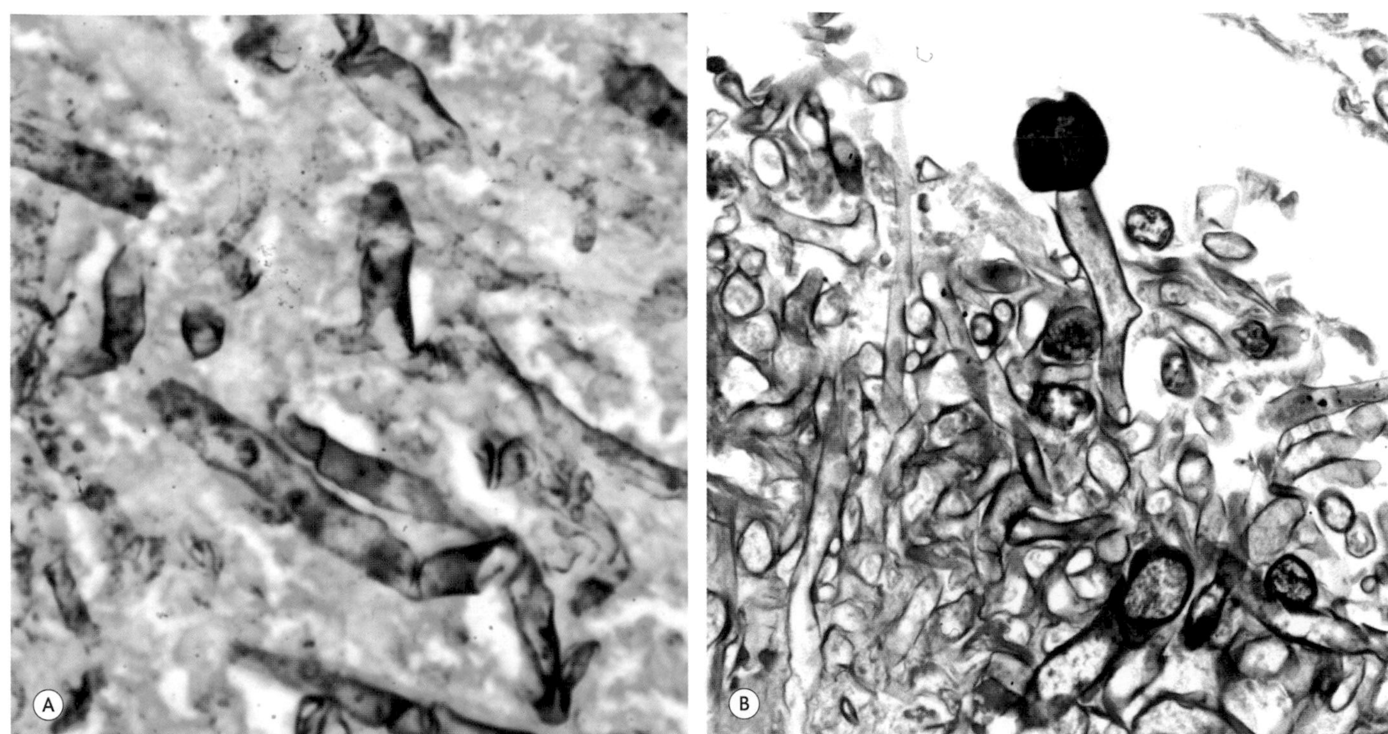

Fig. 6.68 **Zygomycosis.** (A) Twisted pauciseptate, broad mycelia characteristic of zygomycetes (GMS stain). (B) Endobronchial zygomycosis with chlamydospores (H&E stain).

species *Pseudoallescheria boydii.*[116] In the allergic mucin or other deposits of necroinflammatory debris, the phaeoid (dark brown to black pigmented) hyphae (2–6 μm) are generally sparse but can resemble *Aspergillus* and other hyaline molds, especially when lightly or non-pigmented. Typically, only small mycelial fragments, which may be mistaken for artifacts, are seen, sometimes with terminal swellings resembling chlamydoconidia (Fig. 6.69B). The dematiacious agents of subcutaneous forms of chromoblastomycosis appear as pigmented muriform cells in granulomas and do not form mycelia; rarely they are encountered in the lung. *Pseudoallescheria boydii*, another *Aspergillus* look-alike, usually has a more ragged, disorganized and dense clustered pattern of mycelia.

Pneumocystosis

The face of pneumocystis pneumonia continues to change. Once considered to be a protozoan, *Pneumocystis carinii* is now classified as a fungus and the species infecting humans has been renamed *P. jiroveci.*[153] Once a disease primarily of malnourished children and occasionally occurring in the setting of treatment for childhood leukemia, today infection is identified most commonly in patients with defective immunity, especially AIDS, or those on immunosuppressive therapies for hematopoietic malignancies, organ transplants, and collagen-vascular diseases. With the success of contemporary therapy for AIDS, the pathologist is now more likely to encounter the disease in the latter group of patients in whom it is apt to be more subtle.[154] The classic pattern during the HIV epidemic was the foamy alveolar cast (Fig. 6.70) with moderate to numerous organisms, type 2 pneumocyte hyperplasia, and a scant to moderate interstitial lymphoplasmacytic infiltrate.[155]

In recent years, a number of atypical and unusual patterns have been described that are potentially misleading.[34,156] These are listed in Table 6.25. *Pneumocystis jiroveci* can mimic any lung injury pattern, including acute diffuse alveolar damage with hyaline membranes (Fig. 6.71) and minimal or no foamy exudates, to an organizing phase with sparse organisms. There is also a spectrum of granulomatous infection, both non-necrotizing and necrotizing, that may overlap morphologically with mycobacterial or other fungal infections

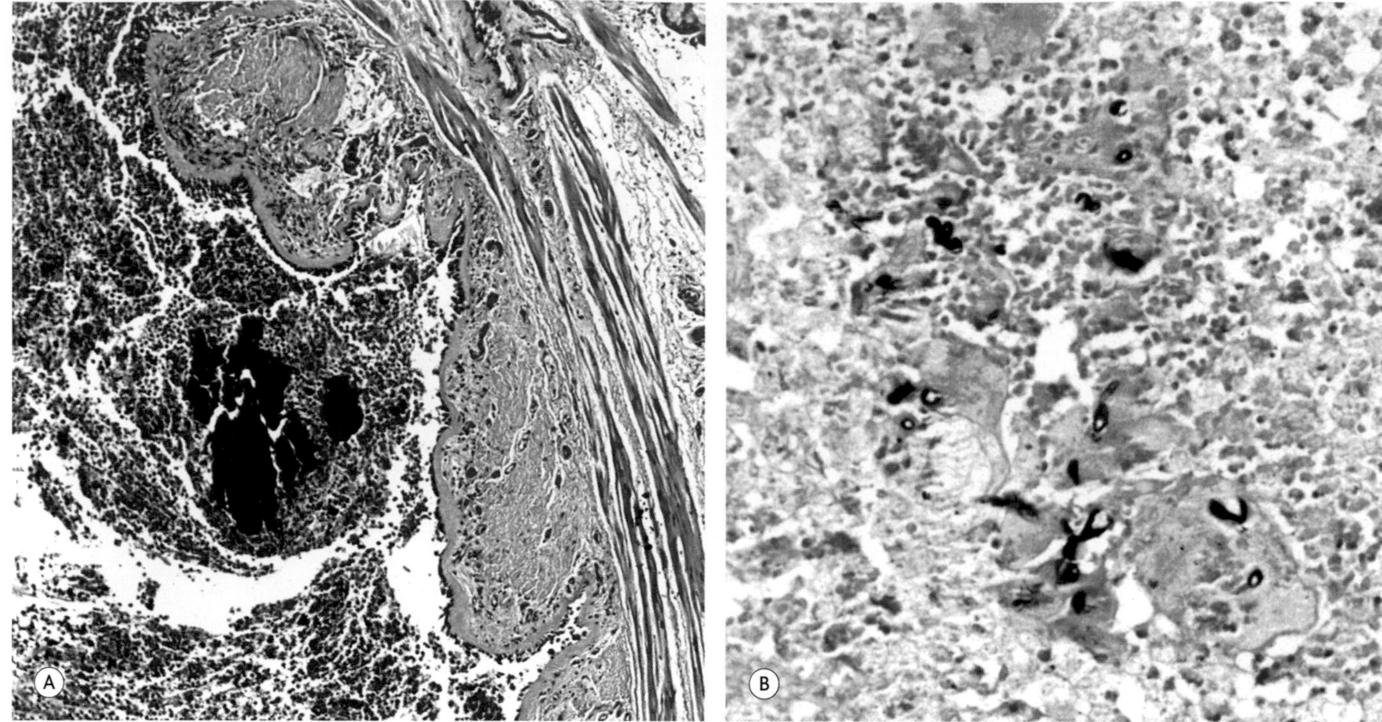

Fig. 6.69 **Allergic bronchopulmonary fungal disease.** (A) Ectatic bronchus with thick eosinophilic basement membrane and intraluminal necroinflammatory debris (H&E stain). (B) Mycelial fragments of *Bipolaris* sp. (GMS stain).

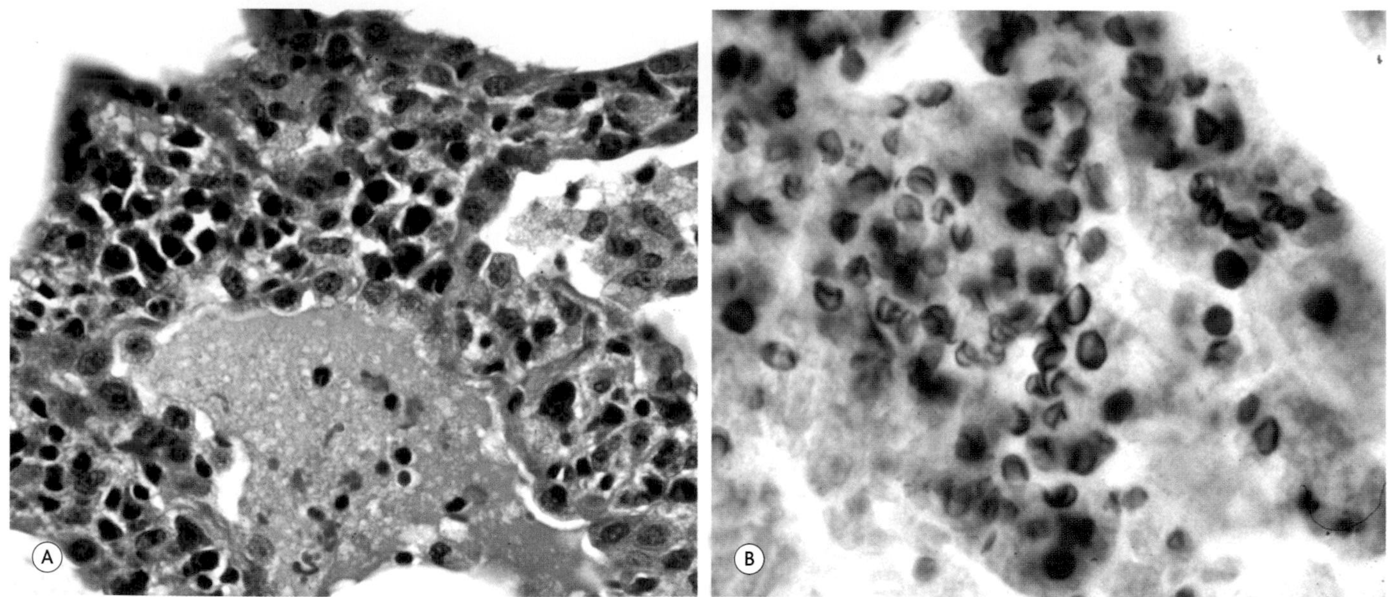

Fig. 6.70 **Pneumocystis pneumonia.** (A) Lymphoplasmacytic interstitial infiltrate and intraalveolar foamy alveolar cast (H&E stain). (B) Numerous yeast-like cells of *Pneumocystis jiroveci* in varying shapes (GMS stain).

(especially histoplasmosis) (Fig. 6.72). Cavitary disease, solitary pulmonary nodules that may be relatively fibrotic, cysts, and dystrophic calcification are also described.[157,158]

Microscopically, three life stages of the organisms are still referred to as sporozoites, trophozoites, and cysts. The cyst is the most commonly recognized form and, when stained with GMS, are oval (4–7 μm) yeast-like cells with collapsed, helmet, and crescentic forms. The intracystic dot or paired-comma structures are important keys to distinguish *P. jiroveci* cysts from look-alikes such as *Histoplasma*, acapsular *Cryptococcus*, *Candida* spp., and overstained red blood cells. Sporozoites and trophozoites are seen to best advantage in touch imprints and cytologic preparations of respiratory samples.

Table 6.25 Patterns of pulmonary pneumocystis infection

Foamy alveolar cast
Diffuse alveolar damage
Id reaction (minimal change)
Granulomas
Miliary disease
Vascular invasion/vasculitis/infarct
Lymphoid interstitial pneumonia
Cavities & cysts
Subpleural blebs & bullae
Microcalcification

Cytopathology

Many of the fungal pathogens involving the respiratory tract can be detected by cytologic techniques in sputa, bronchial washings and brushings, bronchoalveolar lavage (BAL), and needle aspirates.[27] The aspirates and other samples can also be submitted for culture and ancillary studies.[159] The four most common yeast forms – *Cryptococcus neoformans*, *Coccidioides immitis* or *posadasii*, *Histoplama capsulatum*, and *Blastomyces dermatitidis* – must be distinguished from each other, and *P. jiroveci* can also enter the differential diagnosis.[26]

Morphologic features of these organisms are often better visualized in cytologic preparations than in tissue sections, usually permitting a rapid and definitive diagnosis on routinely stained smears (Papanicolaou, Diff-Quik, and H&E). More specific fungal stains, GMS, Gridley, and Fontana–Masson, can often be held in reserve.

The inflammatory background that may be observed in needle aspirates of fungal infections are listed in Table 6.6. Amorphous granular debris, and epithelioid cells characterize many necrotizing granulomas. Typically, a background of neutrophils is seen when suppurative granulomas are aspirated. Histoplasma infections may manifest an epithelioid or phagocytic cell population. Cryptococcal infections can be similar or have little or no accompanying inflammation in the immunocompromised patient.

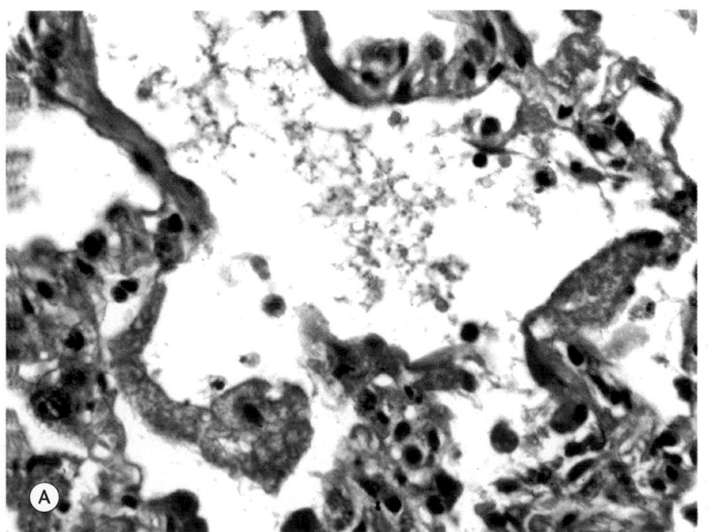

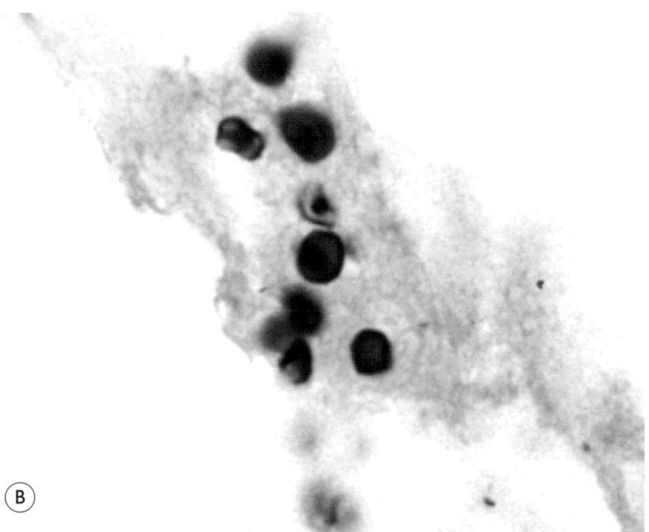

Fig. 6.71 **Pneumocystis pneumonia.** (A) Diffuse alveolar damage pattern with hyaline membranes (H&E stain). (B) Cysts in hyaline membrane (GMS stain).

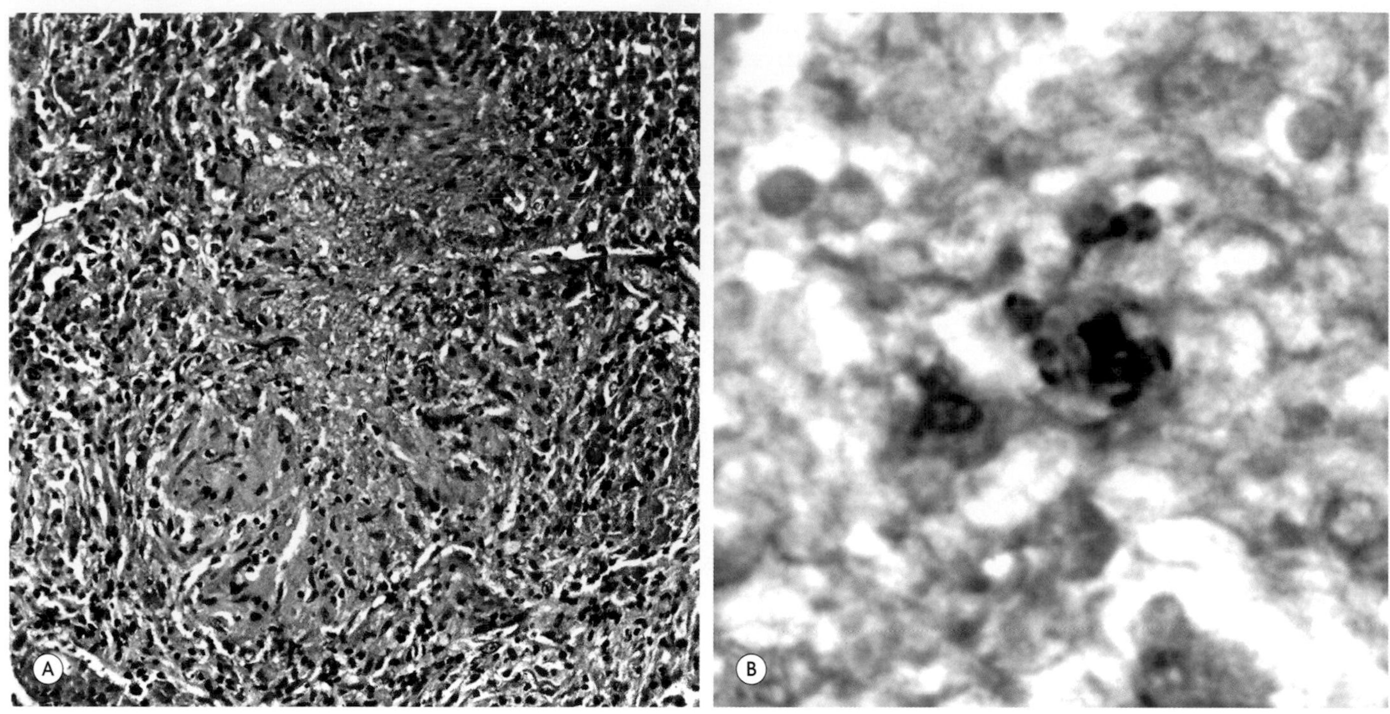

Fig. 6.72 **Pneumocystis pneumonia.** (A) Miliary granuloma with central necrosis (H&E stain). (B) Sparse organisms in granuloma (GMS stain).

Table 6.26 Morphologic features of selective yeast forms

	Small			Intermediate		Large
Feature	*Candida*	*Pneumocystis*	*Histoplasma*	*Cryptococcus*	*Blastomyces*	*Coccidioides*
Size (μm)	3–4	5–8	2–5	5–15	8–20	20–200
Shape	Oval	Pleomorphic	Oval	Pleomorphic	Round	Round
Budding	None	None	Narrow-based	Narrow-based	Broad-based	None
Wall thickness	Thin	Thin	Thin	Thin	Thick	Thick
Hyphae/ pseudohyphae	Common; characteristic	Absent	Rare	Rare	Rare	Occasional
Other features	Single and chains	Intracystic body Trophozoite forms	Intracellular Refractile	Mucicarmine + capsule Acapsular forms	Double contour wall	Endospores & immature spherules

Source: modified from Chandler and Watts.[117]

Cytology of common yeast forms

Morphologic features of some of the more common yeast forms that the pathologist encounters in cytologic material are presented in Table 6.26.

Cryptococcus neoformans are single budding yeast with narrow, pinched-off base about 4–7 μm, but ranging from 2 to 15 μm. In needle aspirates, the mucoid capsule investing the yeast imparts a "spare tire" appearance (Fig. 6.73).

Blastomyces dermatitidis are refractile, double-contoured, and range from 8 to 15 μm with broad-based budding (Fig. 6.74).

An internal amorphous mass can be appreciated in some stained preparations. Smaller or larger yeast cells can be mistaken for *C. neoformans* and *C. immitis*, respectively.

Coccidioidies immitis/posadasii spherules manifest a variety of sizes and shapes, from large spherules packed with endospores (Fig. 6.75A) to empty collapsed spheres

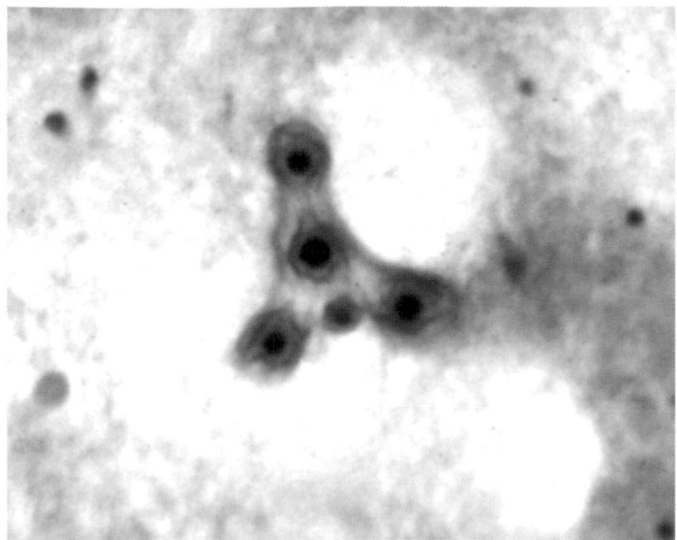

Fig. 6.73 ***Cryptococcus neoformans.*** Clusters of yeast cells resembling "spare tires" invested by capsule in sparse inflammatory background; fine-needle aspirate (alcohol-fixed H&E stain).

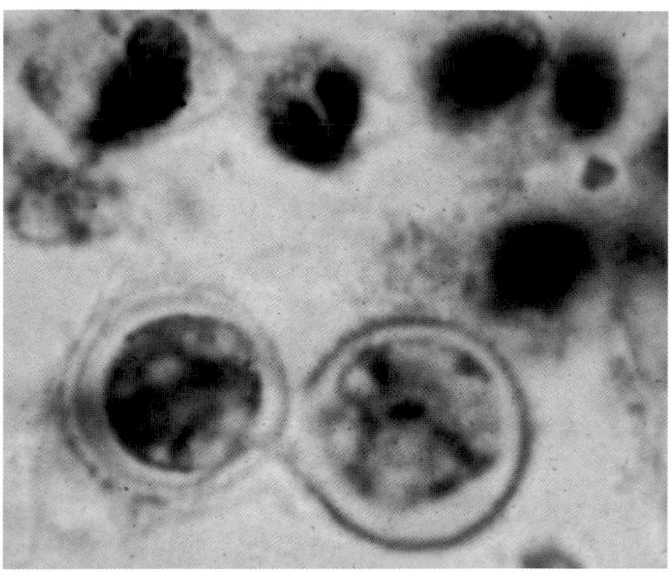

Fig. 6.74 ***Blastomyces dermatitidis.*** Double-contoured yeast with broad-based budding; bronchoalveolar lavage (alcohol-fixed Papanicolaou stain).

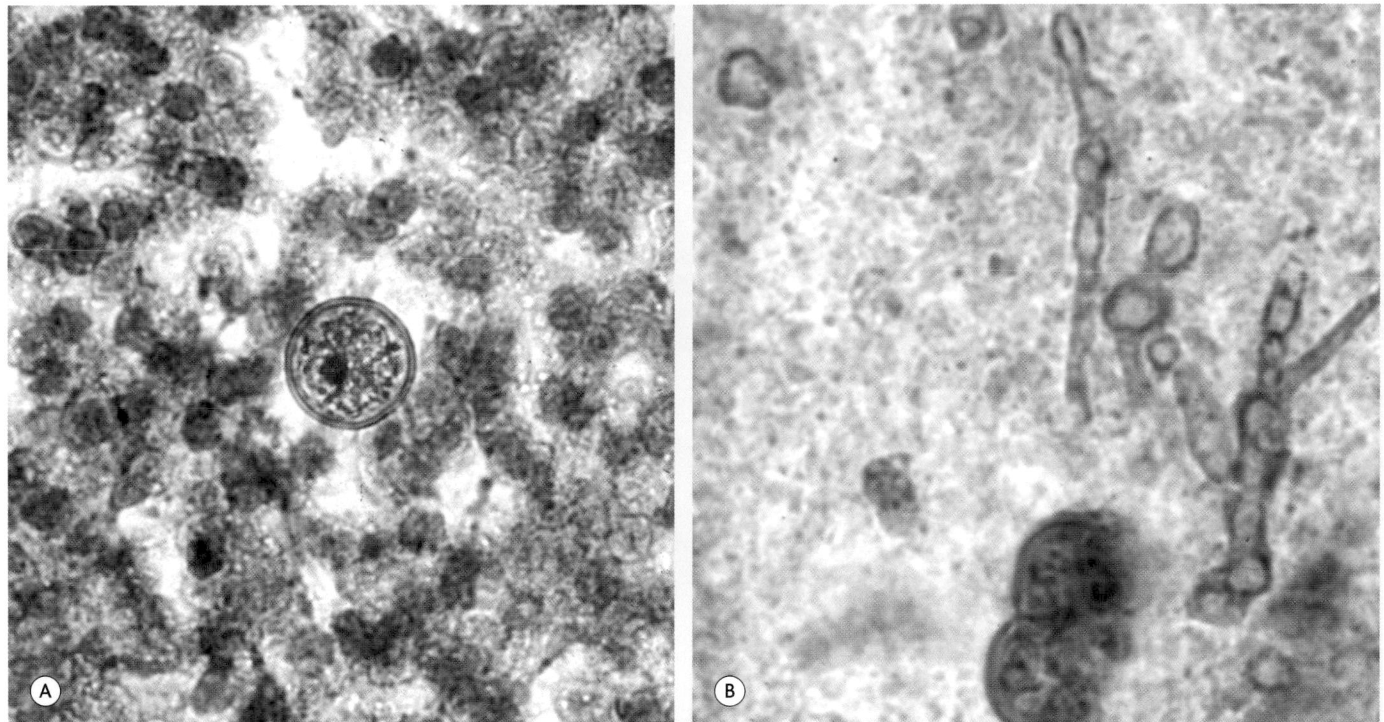

Fig. 6.75 ***Coccidioides* sp.** (A) Negative staining spherule in suppurative inflammatory background; fine-needle aspirate (alcohol-fixed H&E stain). (B) Ruptured spherules and mycelia with arthrospores in granular necrotic background. Fine-needle aspirate (alcohol-fixed H&E stain).

and small immature spherules.[160] The latter may overlap with *Blastomyces* and other yeasts. Mycelial forms of *Coccidioides* spp., with arthrospores, may be found in aspirates of cavitary nodules exposed to air (Fig. 6.75B).

Histoplasma capsulatum yeast cells are small (2–5 μm) and stain poorly in routine smears, but can be suspected by their dot-like refractile appearance in the cytoplasm of macrophages. In Diff-Quik stained smears, the characteristic purple polarized yeast forms are discernable and they are outlined entirely in GMS stained smears (Fig. 6.76).

Pneumocystis jiroveci's most characteristic cytologic presentation in exfoliative samples and aspirates is the foamy alveolar cast, which varies from eosinophilic to basophilic and is highly characteristic (Fig. 6.77A). These organisms rarely occur singly. The GMS stain outlines the characteristic cysts (Fig. 6.77B).

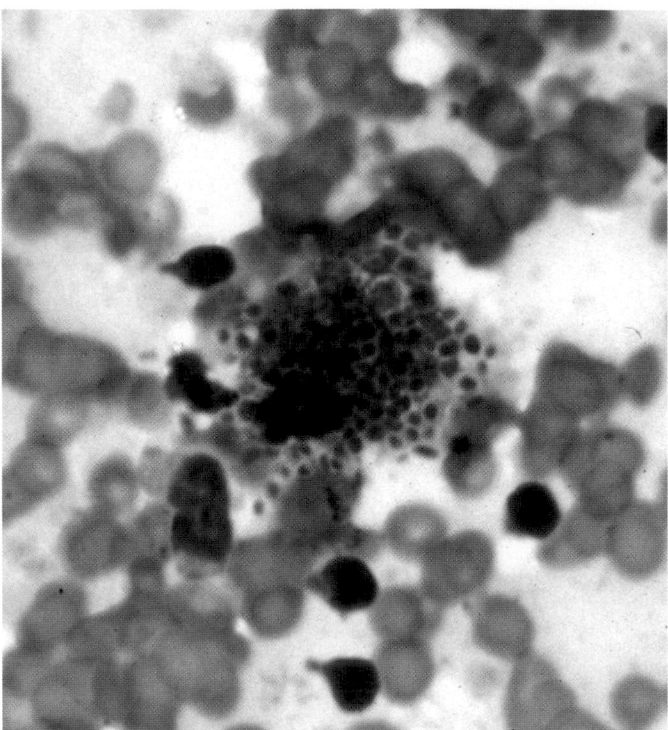

Fig. 6.76 **Histoplasma capsulatum.** Clusters of purple polarized yeast cells; fine-needle aspirate (Diff-Quik stain).

Cytology of common mycelial forms

The cytopathologist's most frequent challenge is the interpretation of mycelial forms in exfoliated material, especially the distinction between *Aspergillus* look-alikes, *Zygomycetes*, and *Candida* hyphae. The morphologic features of some of the more common agents are compared in Table 6.27.

Candida spp. may present in different forms, including unicellular yeasts (blastoconidia), chains of budding blastoconidia referred to as pseudohyphae, elongated hyphal appendages called germ tubes, and true hyphae with septa. They are easily diagnosed when both yeasts and pseudohyphae are present. However, interpretation of their significance is difficult in all except transthoracic needle aspirates, where the presence of any mycelial structure, particularly in the setting of mass-like and cavitary infiltrates, provides strong morphologic evidence of infection.

Aspergillus spp. are characterized by septate mycelia that branch at angles approaching 45° (Fig. 6.78). *Aspergillus* hyphae lack constrictions at points of septation. However, *Aspergillus* organisms cannot be differentiated from one of their mimics by morphology alone, unless accompanied by a fruiting body. A recently described, rapid in-situ hybridization technique specific for *Aspergillus* spp. can be performed on pulmonary cytospin specimens, as well as tissue.[161] The recent availability of a commercial immunohistochemical

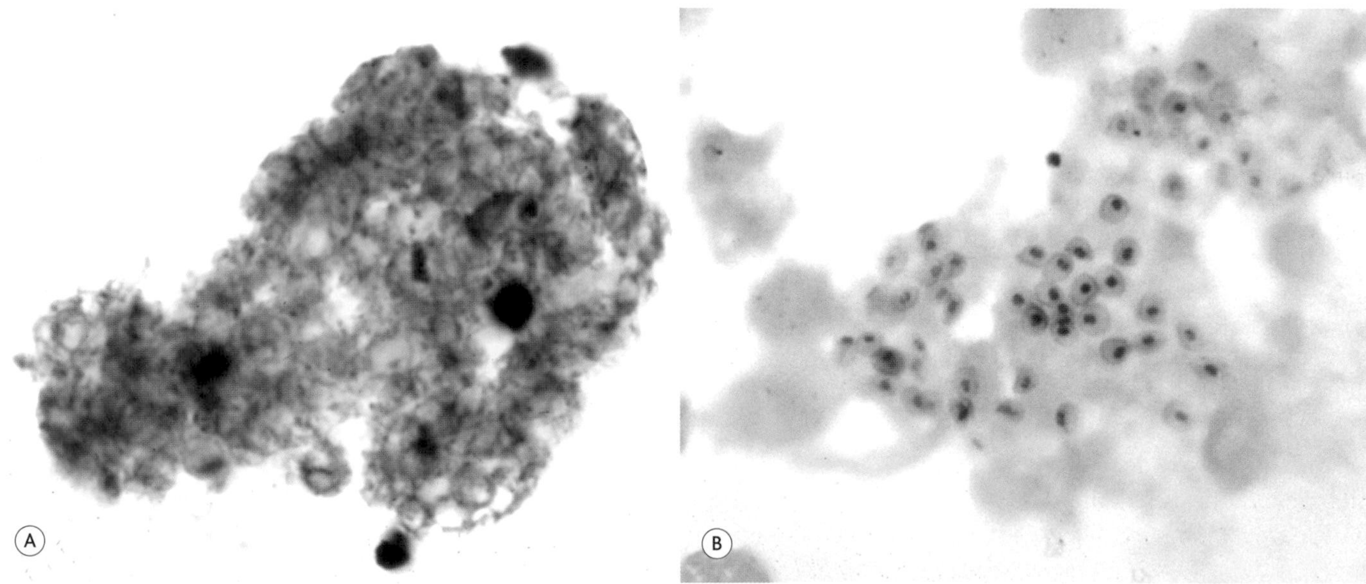

Fig. 6.77 ***Pneumocystis jiroveci.*** (A) Foamy alveolar cast. Bronchial washing (Thin Prep, Papanicolaou stain). (B) Cysts with intracystic dot (bronchial washing/Thin Prep, GMS stain).

Table 6.27 Morphologic features of selected fungal mycelia

	Aspergillus	*Bipolaris*	*Zygomycetes*	*P. boydii*	*Fusarium*
Width (μm)	3–6	2–6	5–20	2–5	3–8
Contour	Parallel	Parallel	Irregular	Parallel	Parallel
Branching	Dichotomous	Haphazard	Wide angle	Haphazard	90° angle
Branch orientation	Parallel	Random	Random	Random	Random
Septation	Frequent	Frequent	Infrequent	Frequent	Frequent
Phaeoid (brown)	No	Yes	No	Usually not	No
Angioinvasive	Yes	No	Yes	Yes	Yes
Other features	Fruiting body; oxalate crystals sometime	Chlamydoconidia sometimes. One of many dematiacious genera	Rarely Chlamydoconidia	***Aspergillus*** "look-alikes"	***Aspergillus*** "look-alikes"

Source: modified from Chandler and Watts.[117]

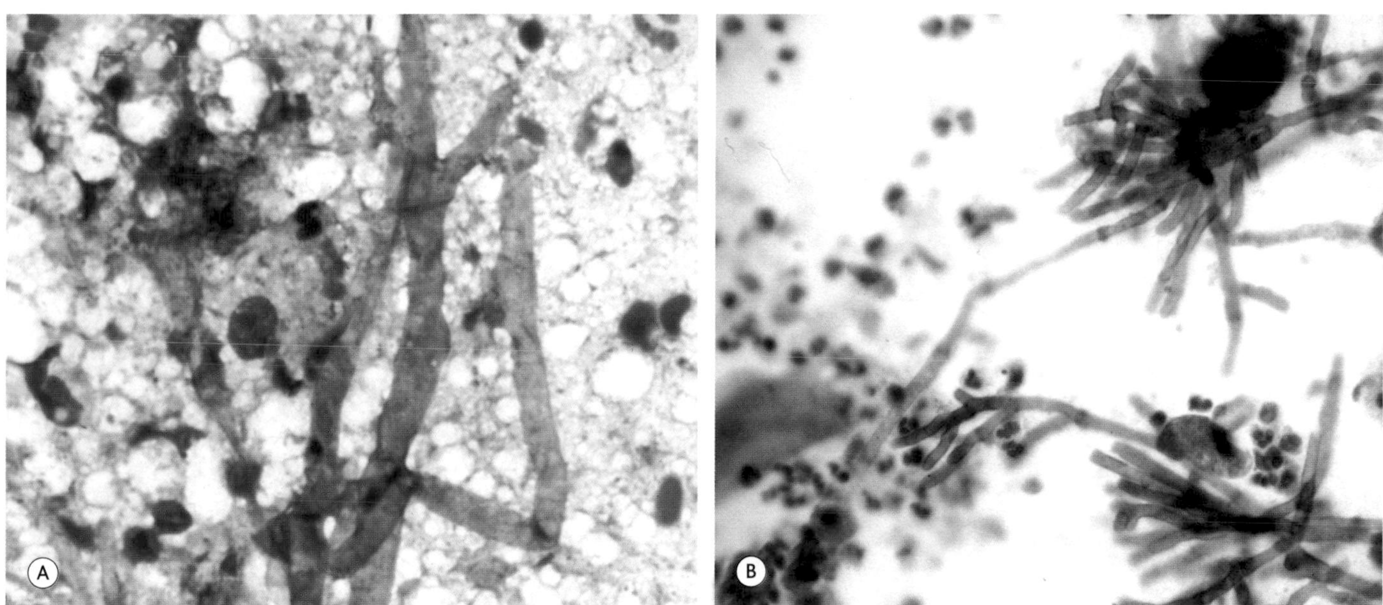

Fig. 6.78 ***Aspergillus* sp.** (A) Twisted sparsely septate mycelia. Difficult to differentiate from mimics, including *Zygomycetes*; fine-needle aspirate (Diff-Quik stain). (B) Characteristic mycelia (bronchial washing, Papanicolaou stain).

reagent may also prove to be an aid to a specific cytodiagnosis.[170a] An additional advantage is that this technique could assist in sorting out this otherwise difficult differential diagnosis.

Zygomycetes mycelia are distinguished from *Aspergillus* and *Candida* forms by their often broader width and their pleomorphic, twisted ribbon-like, pauciseptate features. It must be noted, however, that in aspirates of aspergilloma, the mycelia may also have a twisted appearance, as illustrated in Fig. 6.78A.

In fungal infections, in general, a potential pitfall in the evaluation of cytopathologic samples (both exfoliative and needle aspirates), is the confounding presence of atypical reactive squamous cells and type 2 pneumocytes which can mimic neoplasms.[30] Furthermore, pathologists interpreting lung biopsies, especially transbronchial biopsies, should always attempt to correlate their findings with samples that may have been collected for cytology or microbiology. This is especially advisable because etiologic agents that escape detection in tissue, such as *Pneumocystis*, *Aspergillus*, and cytomegalovirus, may be found in the washings or lavage specimens.[162]

Microbiology

Complimentary laboratory methods are often required for diagnosis of fungal infection, and these are listed in Table 28.[116]

Under the microscope, many fungi are readily apparent in H&E stained sections, where they appear colorless (negative staining) or phaeoid (naturally pigmented). The Grocott's methenamine silver stain (GMS) is the best histologic stain for demonstrating fungi when they are sparse or not visible on H&E sections. However, some fungi, notably the *Zygomycetes*, may stain poorly with GMS. The GMS can be counterstained with H&E, allowing co-evaluation of the host inflammatory response. The Fontana–Masson stain has been used to detect melanin in *C. neoformans* and phaeoid fungi, but many *Aspergillus* spp. and some *Zygomycetes* will also stain with this reagent.[163] The PAS stain can be useful in select circumstances, and histochemical stains for mucin (alcian blue or mucicarmine) are useful for *C. neoformans* infections. The PAS and mucin stains can also be counterstained with GMS or Fontana–Masson to simultaneously highlight cell walls and capsules of *Cryptococcus*.

It is important to remember that not everything that stains with the silver methods is a fungus, and care must be taken to distinguish organisms from pseudomicrobes, such as overstained red cells, white blood cell nuclei, reticulin and elastic fibers, calcium deposits, and even Hamazaki–Wesenberg bodies.[25]

In the microbiology laboratory, the age-old technique of direct light microscopic visualization of fluids, exudates, and tissue homogenates treated with potassium hydroxide (KOH prep) is being replaced by chemofluorescent cotton brightening agents (such as calcofluor white). Fluorescence microscopy with these reagents can detect a wide variety of fungi in wet mounts as well as frozen sections and paraffin-embedded tissue.[164,165]

The time-honored laboratory techniques for the identification of fungi (gross colonial and microscopic morphology after isolation on fungal media followed by biochemical testing) may be the principal means to an etiologic diagnosis. For deep tissues, including the lung and other sterile sites, the Emmons modification of Saboraud glucose agar with choramphenicol is recommended by many mycologists.[166] Additional use of enriched media such as brain-heart infusion agar can improve recovery of *C. neoformans*, *B. dermatitidis*, and *H. capsulatum*. Selective media containing cyclohexamide are not recommended for normally sterile sites, as they are potentially inhibitory for yeasts, such as *Cryptococcus* and *Candida* spp. and molds, such as *Aspergillus* and *Zygomycetes* species.

Table 6.28 Laboratory diagnosis of fungal pneumonia

Direct detection of organisms: – Chemofluorescent stains – Direct fluorescent antibody stain – Histopathology and cytopathology – Immunohistochemistry
Antigen detection: – (Histoplasmosis & cryptococcosis)
Culture: – Emmons modified Sabouraud agar – Brain heart infusion agar – Special and selective media
Serology
Molecular methods: – In-situ hybridization – DNA amplification

The interpretation of a positive fungal culture must be made in the clinical context. In the absence of proof of tissue invasion, or compelling ancillary data, the interpretation of laboratory results requires considerable judgment. This is because many fungi are ubiquitous in the environment, and most fungal isolates from nonsterile respiratory samples do not represent disease unless there are also significant risk factors such as human immunodeficiency virus infection, organ transplant, or immunocompromising drug therapy.[167]

For most of the dimorphic fungi, hyphae to yeast conversion studies have given way to commercially available nucleic acid probes for rapid specific identification. Procurement of tissue for culture prior to formalin fixation is important whenever fungal infections are suspected. The tissue sample should be kept moist using sterile, nonbacteriostatic saline or Ringer's solution. Specimens are minced, but not ground, before plating.

The value of bringing multiple, often complimentary, laboratory methods to bear on inconclusive morphologic findings cannot be overemphasized. In this context, while culture has been considered the most reliable method for definitive diagnosis, and histopathology often the fastest, the greatest yield results from combining histopathology with traditional culture and one or more of the newer molecular methods.[168] Culture may fail to yield an isolate even in the face of positive microscopic findings. In fact, the yield from tissue, needle aspirates, BAL, and bronchial washings is quite low for molds and other fungi for reasons that are not entirely clear.[169] Immunofluorescence using specific monoclonal antibodies can achieve rapid and specific diagnosis in selected infections, especially when tissue has not been submitted for culture. Antibodies directed against the antigens of *Aspergillus* spp. and selected other fungi have been described but, except for Aspergillus species, most are not yet commercially available. For the problematic case, the mycology section of the Center for Disease Control and Prevention (CDC; Atlanta, Georgia) can provide assistance. Immunohistochemical identification of fungi can be accomplished fairly easily for those species for which reagents are commercially available.[22,170,170a]

Molecular techniques, including in-situ hybridization and amplification technologies such as PCR, are other powerful tools that can provide rapid, accurate diagnosis for yeasts and molds which may be present in small numbers or manifest overlapping histologic features with one another.[165,171–173] A few laboratories (including the CDC) are performing such assays. Quantitative real-time PCR on blood, body fluids, and other samples holds promise for relatively rapid, definitive diagnosis when routine methods of isolation and identification fail in critical situations.[174]

Serologic tests can support a morphologic diagnosis when positive titers are present, but effective serodiagnosis of systemic fungal infections is not available for most fungi.[175] Unfortunately, an antibody response does not necessarily correlate with invasive disease; and an antibody response may be lacking for various reasons. False-positive results due to cross reactions, and false-negative results for a variety of reasons plague many of these assays. Some of the most accurate serologic tests (sensitivity and specificity) for fungal infections are those for histoplasmosis and coccidioidomycosis, yet tests for both have limitations that must be recognized when interpreting results.[176,177]

The detection of macromolecular antigens shed into various body fluids requires a relatively large microbial burden, which tends to limit sensitivity for most fungal infections, except histoplasmosis and crytococcosis.[168] For these two fungi, useful antigen detection techniques are available for serum, urine, cerebrospinal, and BAL fluids. They are especially sensitive in patients with defective immunity.[159,176] In patients with pneumonia and normal immunity, however, these tests may be positive in lavage fluid but negative in urine unless the disease has disseminated. Recently, an enzyme immunoassay for galactomannan antigen has been approved by the FDA for use in diagnosis and monitoring invasive aspergillus infections.[176a] A real-time PCR method for this purpose has also been reported.[176b]

Differential diagnosis

The key morphologic and mycologic features of the fungal pneumonias are summarized in Table 6.29. When H&E and GMS stains fail to detect or clearly identify fungal elements in a suspected fungal infection, the use of ancillary procedures may provide the specific diagnosis. Sometimes, if tissue or other patient specimens have been submitted for culture, the answer may lie in the mycology section of the microbiology laboratory, as many species begin to grow in a matter of days. When fungi are not readily identified by any of these techniques or strategies, other granulomatous infections should be considered, especially mycobacterial; uncommon bacterial (e.g. tularemia and brucellosis) and parasitic infections. Non-infectious necrotizing and non-necrotizing granulomatous disorders also enter the differential. These include Wegener's granulomatosis, idiopathic bronchocentric granulomatosis, aspiration, sarcoidosis,

Table 6.29 Fungal pneumonia synopsis

Blastomycosis	
Surgical pathology:	Suppurative granuloma most characteristic; also, tuberculoid (necrotizing) types. Round, thick (double contoured) wall yeast with broad-based budding
Cytopathology:	Neutrophils and epithelioid cells with characteristic refractile yeast cell with double-contoured wall and broad-based budding
Microbiology:	Characteristic yeast in wet mount, KOH and calcofluor stained smear. Culture sterile lung tissue on nonselective fungal media (e.g. Emmons modified Sabouraud) and enriched media (e.g. brain-heart infusion). Add selective media for bronchial/transbronchial samples. Colonies produce oval conidia on terminal ends of conidiophore at right angle to mycelium. Confirm with DNA probe. Serology not useful.
Coccidioidomycosis	
Surgical pathology:	Fibrocaseous granuloma. Large intact and/or ruptured spherules, full, partially or completely empty of endospores. Mycelial forms in aerated cavities and fistula may be only or predominant form.
Cytopathology:	Necroinflammatory debris with epithelioid histiocytes. Intact, viable, colorless spherules with variable number of endospores and/or ruptured degenerating forms with stained wall vary in size from large mature to small immature types.
Microbiology:	Characteristic mature spherules in wet mount, KOH and calcofluor smear. Culture of sterile lung tissue on nonselective fungal media yields mycelia with characteristic arthroconidia. Confirm with DNA probe. Serologic diagnosis with tests for IgG and IgM antibodies by immunodiffusion, EIA; complement fixation for titers

Table 6.29 Fungal pneumonia synopsis—cont'd

Histoplasmosis	
Surgical pathology:	Macrophage reaction and/or granulomas, based on immunity, including miliary and solitary pulmonary, variably-hyalinized nodule. Small, thin-wall, oval yeast with narrow-based buds, often refractile
Cytopathology:	Macrophage and epithelioid cells with characteristic yeast cell, often intracellular, stained purple with Diff-Quik; black with GMS
Microbiology:	Rarely detected by direct examination of most clinical specimens. Culture sterile lung tissue on nonselective and enriched fungal media produces tuberculate macroconidia. Confirm with DNA probe. Antigen detection by EIA available for BAL fluid, CSF, serum, and urine.
Paracoccidioidomycosis	
Surgical pathology:	Exudative or granulomatous lesion with large, globose yeast cell with multiple buds
Cytopathology:	Suppurative or granulomatous reaction with characteristic yeast cell
Microbiology:	Direct detection in wet mount, KOH and calcofluor smear. Culture sterile lung tissue on standard nonselective fungal media. Serology by immunodiffusion, EIA; complement fixation for titer
Sporotrichosis	
Surgical pathology:	Necrotizing granuloma, often cavitary with small, usually round, sometimes cigar-shape yeast with sparse, narrow buds
Cytopathology:	Suppurative or necrotizing granuloma pattern. Yeast cells generally sparse or absent
Microbiology:	Rarely detected by direct examination of most clinical specimens. Culture of sterile lung tissue on nonselective fungal media yield thin, hyphae bearing conidia in a rosette pattern. Converts to a yeast phase at 37°C on blood agar. No serology
Penicilliosis	
Surgical pathology:	Alveolar macrophages stuffed with yeast cells resemble ***Histoplasma*** spp., but with septum reflecting binary fission, not budding reproduction
Cytopathology:	Macrophage with intracellular characteristic yeast forms
Microbiology:	Culture of sterile lung tissue on nonselective fungal media yields a mold with a red pigment evident as culture ages. Erect conidiophores sometimes branched with metulae bearing one or several phialides with long, loose chains of oval conidia. New urinary antigen test
Cryptococcosis	
Surgical pathology:	Granulomas, histiocytic infiltrate, or mucoid pneumonia, based on immunity with pale, round, budding pleomorphic yeast cells, often in clusters. Mucoid capsules usually; acapsular types sometimes
Cytopathology:	Yeast cell with mucoid capsular halos resemble "spare tire." Combination of mucicarmine and GMS or Fontanna–Masson outlines capsule and cell wall. Background of epithelioid cells or necroinflammatory debris may be sparse or absent
Microbiology:	Oval to lemon-shaped calcofluor positive yeast cell with capsule in India ink stained touch imprint. Culture on nonselective fungal media yields mucoid yeast-type colonies. No pseudohyphae; germ tube negative. Dark brown pigment on birdseed (Niger) agar. Confirm with biochemical tests. Antigen detection test (latex agglutination or EIA) on serum, BAL, CSF, and needle aspirates
Candidiasis	
Surgical pathology:	Miliary necroinflammatory lesions or bronchopneumonia with small, oval, budding yeasts with or without pseudohyphae. *C. glabrata* yeast only
Cytopathology:	Yeasts and/or pseudohyphae in a necroinflammatory background
Microbiology:	Budding yeast and pseudohyphae in wet mounts, KOH and calcofluor stained smears. Cultures on selective and nonselective fungal media yield creamy tan to white yeast-type colonies. Identification by germ tube production, carbohydrate assimilation, and cornmeal agar morphology.
Aspergillosis	
Surgical pathology:	Various forms include saprophytic (fungus ball), allergic (ABPA and mucoid impaction, hypersensitivity pneumonitis) and invasive disease, varying from minimal chronic necrotizing to extensive pneumonia. Angiotrophic with necrotizing infarcts; also hybrid forms of disease. Septate, dichotomous, 45° angle mycelia; oxalate crystals. Presence of fruiting body is genus specific
Cytopathology:	Tangled clusters of septate mycelia in a necroinflammatory background. May appear sparsely septate and twisted, mimicking *Zygomycetes* in aspirates, more typical morphology in exfoliative specimens
Microbiology:	Calcofluor and GMS stain positive mycelia. Culture of sterile lung tissue on nonselective fungal media produces mold-type colonies in a range of colors. Species differentiation by conidial and conidiophore morphology Antigen detection (galactomannan) by EIA in blood for invasive infection.
Zygomycosis	
Surgical pathology:	Nodular lesions, lobar consolidations, cavitary lesions, fungus ball, and airway infections tend to be necrotizing and ischemic secondary to angio-invasive characteristic. Broad pauciseptate mycelia with 90° angle branching; often twisted ribbon morphology
Cytopathology:	Pauciseptate mycelia often with twisted ribbon morphology in a necroinflammatory background
Microbiology:	Calcofluor and GMS stain positive mycelia. Rapidly growing cottony colonies on most nonselective fungal media, but "controlled baiting" with bread sometimes necessary. Identification based on presence and locations of rhizoids, shape of sporangia, presence of columnella, and shape of sporangiospores

Table 6.29 Fungal pneumonia synopsis—cont'd

Phaeohyphomycosis	
Surgical pathology:	Allergic bronchopulmonary fungal disease similar to ***Aspergillus***
Cytopathology:	Similar to allergic bronchopulmonary aspergillosis pattern, i.e. "allergic mucin" with eosinophils, Charcot–Leiden crystals in inspissated mucus. Fungal mycelial fragments sparse or absent
Microbiology:	Dematiaceous (phaeoid) dark brown to black colonies on nonselective fungal media. Identified by shape and cross walls of multicelled, pigmented conidia
Pneumocystosis	
Surgical pathology:	Pneumonia with foamy alveolar cast is classic; other patterns include diffuse alveolar damage, granulomatous lesions, and minimal changes. Variable numbers of cysts noted in GMS stained sections
Cytopathology:	Foamy alveolar cast with characteristic cysts outlined by GMS
Microbiology:	Classified as a fungus and renamed *P. jiroveci*, but cannot be cultured. Detection with fluorescent monoclonal antibody or GMS stained smears

Table 6.30 Viral pathogens of the lung

RNA viruses	DNA viruses
Influenza	Adenovirus
Parainfluenza	Herpes simplex
Respiratory syncytial virus	Varicella-zoster
Human metapneumovirus	Cytomegalovirus
Measles	Epstein–Barr virus
Hantavirus	
Coronavirus	

Table 6.31 Patterns of viral lung injury

Diffuse alveolar damage
Bronchitis and bronchiolitis
Diffuse interstitial pneumonia
Perivascular lymphoid infiltrates
Miliary small nodules
Airspace organization (BOOP pattern)
Calcified nodules

rheumatoid nodules, pyoderma gangrenosum-like lung lesions in inflammatory bowel disease patients, and Churg-Strauss syndrome.

Viral pneumonia

Viruses cause more infections than all other types of microorganisms combined, and involve the respiratory tract more commonly than other organ systems.[178] Fortunately, the lung diseases produced by viruses are usually mild and self-limited. Nevertheless, viruses cause major public health illnesses and account for many of the new and emerging diseases in today's headlines. At times, viruses are also capable of producing serious and life-threatening infections that come to the attention of pathologists in both immunocompromised patients and young healthy individuals.[179] The viruses that commonly infect the lung are presented in Table 6.30.

The conventional respiratory viruses (influenza, parainfluenza, respiratory syncytial virus, and adenovirus) cause outbreaks of respiratory illness in the general population each year. In infants, the elderly, and in those patients with chronic diseases, they can cause serious pneumonias. Pneumonia in the immunocompromised host is usually attributed to the herpesviruses (herpes simplex and cytomegalovirus). Less appreciated, is the fact that the conventional respiratory viruses are frequent causes of respiratory illness in these patients, and that these infections result in high rates of morbidity and mortality.[180] Pneumonia due to measles, Hantavirus, and Epstein–Barr virus (EBV) are uncommon but with the exception of EBV, they have distinctive pathologic findings. Other viruses, not listed in the table, such as the picornavirus group (Rhinovirus and Enterovirus) and human metapneumovirus can also cause pneumonia, especially in the immunocompromised patient.

Patterns of lung injury

The respiratory tract viruses have a tendency to target specific regions of the tracheobronchial tree and lungs, producing characteristic clinical syndromes. However, sufficient overlap clinically, radiographically, and pathologically often limits a strict anatomic classification. The gross/radiographic and histopathologic patterns of injury at scanning magnification, as listed in Table 6.31, can sometimes be useful in narrowing the search for a specific etiologic agent.

The histopathologic diagnosis of viral infection is impossible without characteristic "cytopathic effect (CPE)". This term has traditionally been used by

Table 6.32 Pulmonary viral cytopathic effect (CPE)

Virus	Intranuclear	Intracytoplasmic	Inclusion characteristics
Herpes simplex; varicella zoster	+	–	Early ground glass; later eosinophilic (Cowdry A type) multinucleated cells
Adenovirus	+	–	Early eosinophilic (Cowdry A); later basophilic smudged nucleus
Cytomegalovirus	+	+	Cytomegaly with large "owl eye" amphophilic (Cowdry A) nuclear & multiple smaller basophilic (GMS+) cytoplasmic type
Respiratory syncytial virus	–	+	Eosinophilic smooth, small, often indistinct. Multinucleated syncytia in some cases
Measles	+	+	Eosinophilic nuclear (Cowdry A) in multinucleated cells. Cytoplasmic type – eosinophilic & pleomorphic
Parainfluenza	–	+	Rarely observed, pleomorphic, eosinophilic. Multinucleated syncytia rarely
Influenza	–	–	No inclusions or other distinctive CPE

virologists to describe cellular changes in unstained cell culture monolayers by light microscopy,[181,182] but it can be applied to all virus-associated nuclear and cytoplasmic alterations seen on H&E stained slides or highlighted by immunohistochemical staining. Diffuse alveolar damage, often with bronchiolitis, is the most typical pattern of viral lung injury. However, as we have shown in previous sections, diffuse alveolar damage also occurs in bacterial, mycobacterial, and fungal pneumonias, so a careful search for specific viral CPE becomes important in this setting. For the surgical pathologist, CPE manifests mainly as the viral inclusion present in the nucleus and/or cytoplasm of an infected cell. Viral inclusions confer diagnostic specificity to the pathologic pattern of injury in which they are found, and for the common respiratory tract viruses, the features are presented in Table 6.32. Finally, it is worth mentioning that most clinically significant viral pneumonias that have CPE also show necrosis somewhere in the biopsy.

Influenza viruses

Influenza viruses are the most pathogenic of the respiratory viruses and predispose patients most commonly to secondary bacterial pneumonia. These viruses also account for the greatest public health burden. Annually, they cause epidemic outbreaks of respiratory disease that are often associated with considerable morbidity; periodically, they produce pandemics with high mortality. These viruses target the ciliated epithelium of the tracheobronchial tree, producing a spectrum of changes that vary depending on the stage of the disease (early vs late), outcome (fatal vs nonfatal) and the presence or absence of secondary bacterial pneumonia. These changes include necrotizing bronchitis and bronchiolitis with or without superimposed diffuse alveolar damage of exudative and/or organizing type (Fig. 6.79). Fibrinous lung injury with organization, lacking hyaline membranes, can also occur.[183] Epithelial damage to the airway provides a nidus for the bacterial pneumonias (*Haemophilus influenzae, Staphylococcus aureus, Streptococcus pneumoniae*) that account for much of the morbidity and mortality of influenza. Since these viruses produce no characteristic cellular inclusions, etiologic diagnosis is not possible by morphology alone, and requires antigen detection by immunofluorescence, immunohistochemistry, in-situ hybridization, or culture.[184]

Parainfluenza virus

Parainfluenza virus comprises four serotypes (I–IV) that typically target the upper respiratory tract, classically in the form of croup.[185] Some cases involve distal airways, similar to respiratory syncytial virus and influenza, but are milder, with less morbidity and requiring fewer hospitalizations. A few documented cases have been described with a diffuse alveolar damage pattern or an interstitial pneumonitis with giant cells, the latter resembling those of measles and respiratory syncytial virus infection. The giant cells of parainfluenza tend to be larger and with more intracytoplasmic inclusions.[34] Parainfluenza virus is a potential opportunist in the immunocompromised host.

Respiratory syncytial virus

Respiratory syncytial virus (RSV) causes annual outbreaks of bronchiolitis and pneumonia in infants that are especially severe during the first year of life, and in those of low birth weight or with cardiopulmonary disease.[185] Primarily considered a childhood virus, RSV has more recently been recognized as the etiologic agent

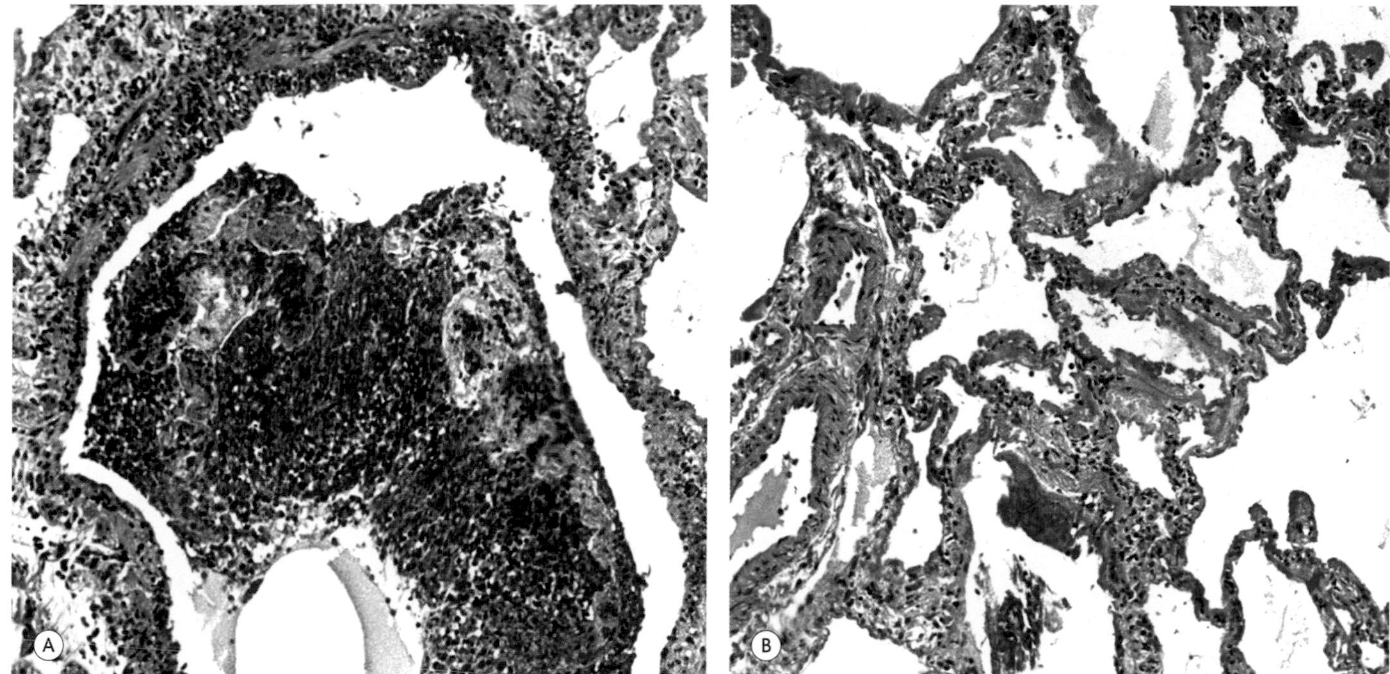

Fig. 6.79 **Influenza.** (A) Bronchiolitis with intraluminal necroinflammatory debris. (B) Acute diffuse alveolar damage pattern with hyaline membranes (H&E stain).

of community-acquired pneumonia in adults with chronic lung disease requiring hospitalization.[186,187] Also, RSV is often an unsuspected opportunistic pathogen in immunocompromised patients.[180,188] RSV targets the epithelium of the distal airway, producing bronchiolitis with disorganization of the epithelium and sloughing[189] (Fig. 6.80A). Diffuse alveolar damage may be seen in immunocompromised hosts. Giant cells (syncytia), similar to the cytopathic changes seen in cell culture, may be present in alveolar ducts and airspaces around bronchiolitis (Fig. 6.80B). Eosinophilic inclusions in cytoplasm may be seen in tissues and cytology specimens from immunosuppressed patients; however, these are difficult to confirm as diagnostic of RSV without immunohistochemistry. Human metapneumovirus is a newly isolated and described RNA virus that infects children and adults. It is a significant cause of respiratory disease in the first year of life and produces a spectrum of disease similar to RSV.[189a]

Measles virus

Measles virus causes a childhood viral exanthem, which, unlike varicella (chickenpox), leads to complications that are common and serious. Measles pneumonia accounts for the vast majority of measles-related deaths and most of these are a consequence of secondary bacterial pneumonia. Primary viral pneumonia occurs, but is uncommon, even in immunocompromised hosts. Microscopically, bronchial and bronchiolar epithelial degeneration and reactive hyperplasia with squamous metaplasia is typically accompanied by peribronchial inflammation. Diffuse alveolar damage may occur. Characteristic giant cells show distinctive intranuclear eosinophilic inclusions surrounded by halos (Fig. 6.81).[189] Minute intracytoplasmic eosinophilic inclusions precede the development of the intranuclear inclusions and are often difficult to identify. Pneumonia with giant cells should always suggest measles, but similar changes can be seen in RSV and parainfluenza pneumonia.[189] Hard metal pneumoconiosis (giant cell interstitial pneumonia) is in the differential diagnosis, but the overall appearance of hard metal disease is one of a chronic disease with some fibrosis, and few if any acute changes.

Hantavirus

Hantavirus produces a rapidly evolving cardiopulmonary syndrome with a high mortality rate. It first came to public attention as an emerging infection following an outbreak in the southwestern United States in 1993 that was causally linked to a previously unrecognized hantavirus. All members of this genera are zoonotic and found in rodents around the world. The specific type responsible for the cardiopulmonary syndrome, designated Sin Nombre (without a name), is present in rodent feces and is acquired from the environment through inhalation. It produces florid pulmonary edema with

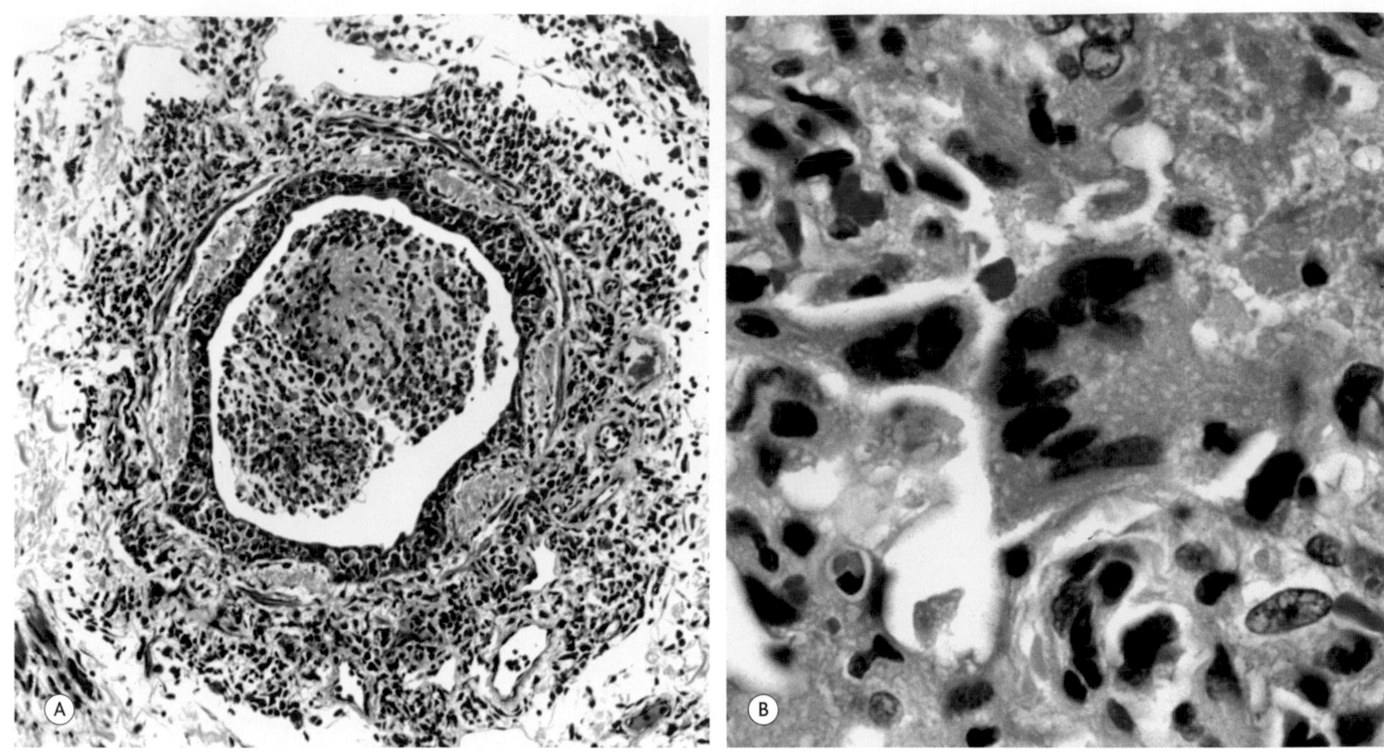

Fig. 6.80 **Respiratory syncytial virus.** (A) Bronchiolitis with intraluminal sloughing (H&E stain). (B) Bronchiolitis with giant cell syncytia (H&E stain).

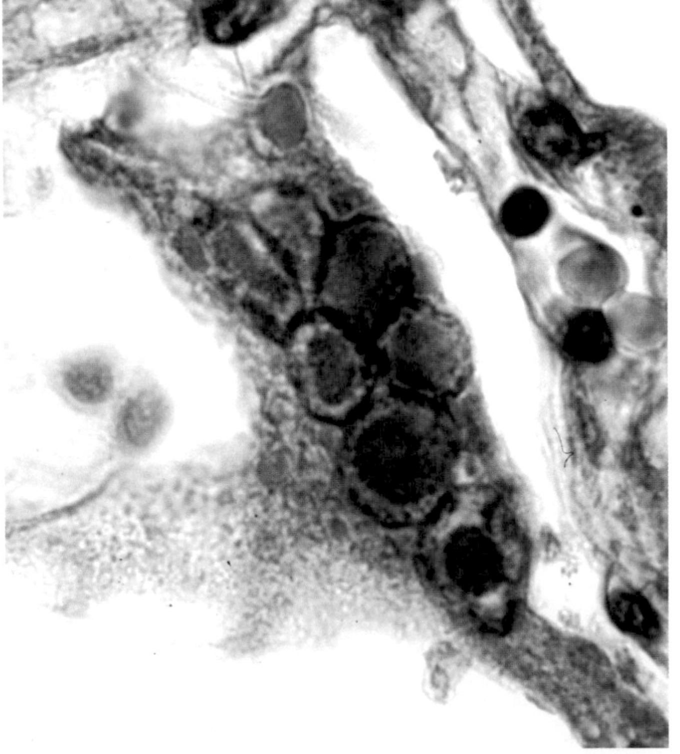

Fig. 6.81 Measles virus pneumonia with characteristic red intranuclear inclusions in giant cell (H&E stain).

pleural effusions, variable fibrin deposits, and focal wispy hyaline membranes[190] (Fig. 6.82A). Immunoblast-like cells are present in vascular spaces and in the peripheral blood (Fig. 6.82B). Morphologic diagnosis is presumptive, since hantaviral antigen in endothelial cells, detected by immunohistochemistry, is required for definitive diagnosis.[191] In the appropriate clinical setting, clues to the diagnosis can sometimes be found in a constellation of morphologic findings on a peripheral blood smear, and confirmation can be achieved serologically by detection of hantavirus-specific IgM antibodies, or by detection of hantaviral RNA by PCR in peripheral blood leukocytes.[192,193]

Coronaviruses

Coronaviruses are ubiquitous RNA viruses known to cause disease in many animals. In humans, they are responsible for the majority of common colds, along with the rhinoviruses. In certain epidemiologic situations, they can cause pneumonia in children, in frail elderly individuals and in immunocompromised adults.[194,195]

In November 2002, an atypical pneumonia appeared in China, and was subsequently labeled severe acute

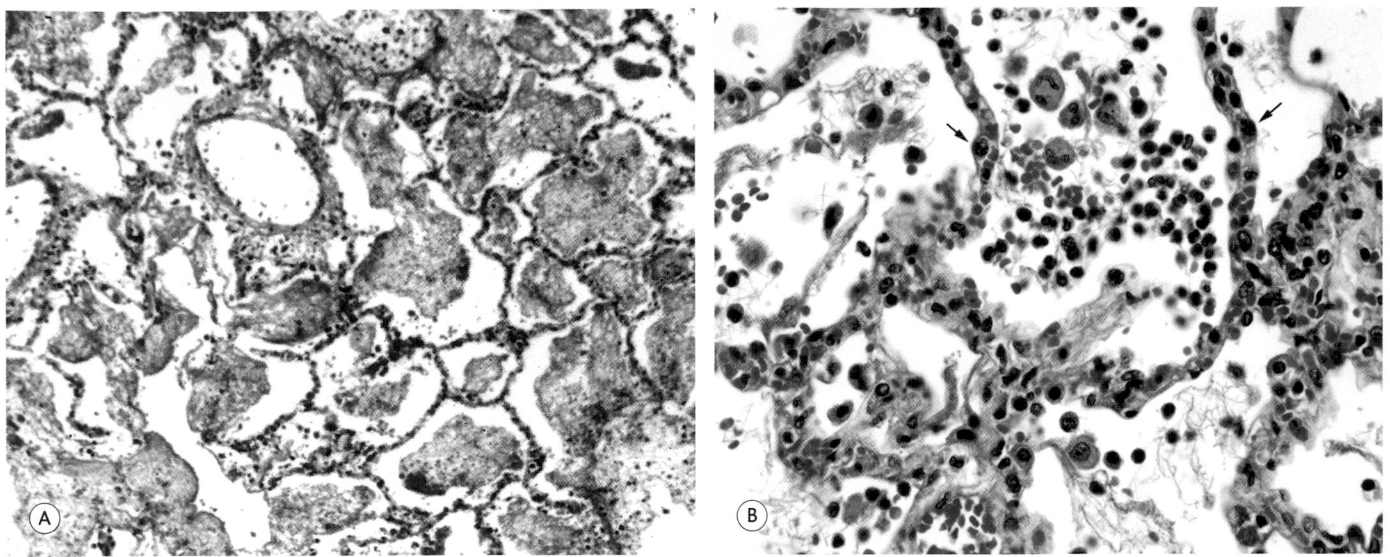

Fig. 6.82 **Hantavirus.** (A) Pulmonary edema with fibrin deposits (H&E stain). (B) Immunoblast-like cells in alveolar capillaries at arrows (H&E stain)

respiratory syndrome (SARS). The disease became an alarming global health problem in the space of a few months,[196] and was linked (Koch's postulates were fulfilled) by tissue culture isolation, electron microscopy, and molecular analysis to an emergent novel coronavirus, proposed as the "Urbani strain of SARS-associated coronavirus".[197]

Clinically, the disease ranges from a non-hypoxemic febrile respiratory disease (with minimal symptoms in some patients) to one of severe pulmonary dysfunction, manifesting as adult respiratory distress syndrome and terminating in death for approximately 5% of the patients affected.[198] In the reported cases, chest X-rays on presentation were either normal or showed unilateral, predominantly peripheral areas of consolidation, which progressed to bilateral, patchy consolidation, the degree and extent of which correlated with the development of respiratory failure. In patients who presented with normal X-rays, CT scans often revealed bilateral ground glass consolidation resembling bronchiloitis obliterans with organizing pneumonia (cryptogenic organizing pneumonia). Laboratory abnormalities in some, but not all, patients included leukopenia with lymphopenia and thrombocytopenia. The partial thromboplastin time and D-dimer levels were increased. Biochemical abnormalities included elevated lactate dehydrogenase, alanine aminotransferase, and creatinine levels. Lymphopenia and elevated LDH were helpful clues, but the clinical, radiographic, and laboratory features, while characteristic, were not distinguishable from those of patients with pneumonia caused by other viruses, bacteria, and various atypical agents.

Histopathologic findings in lung biopsies and autopsy tissues revealed acute lung injury (diffuse alveolar damage) in various stages of organization.[199] In milder cases seen in lung biopsy specimens, relatively scant intra-alveolar fibrin deposits with some congestion and edema were present (Fig. 6.83). However, the spectrum of findings included hyaline membrane formation, interstitial lymphocytic infiltrates, desquamation of alveolar pneumocytes, and areas undergoing organization of the acute phase injury. In some patients, multinucleated syncytial cells reminiscent of the cytopathic effect seen in influenza, respiratory syncytial virus, and measles virus infections were noted. Viral inclusions were not identified and immunohistochemical studies failed to reveal viral antigen. It was speculated that the antigen may have been cleared by the time the tissues were obtained for study, or that possibly the histopathology reflected a response to the secondary effects of inflammatory cytokines or other factors induced by the virus. Nonetheless, although no direct involvement in the pathologic process was documented, the isolation of a unique coronavirus (Fig. 6.84) from lung tissue, implicated it as the etiologic agent of the disease. More recently the SARS viral signal has been detected in alveolar type II pneumocytes by in-situ hybridization.[199a]

Adenovirus

Adenovirus comprises several genera and multiple serotypes which cause infections of the upper and lower respiratory tract, conjunctiva, and gut. Respiratory tract infections are most common, and can be especially severe in neonates and children, as well as in adults who are

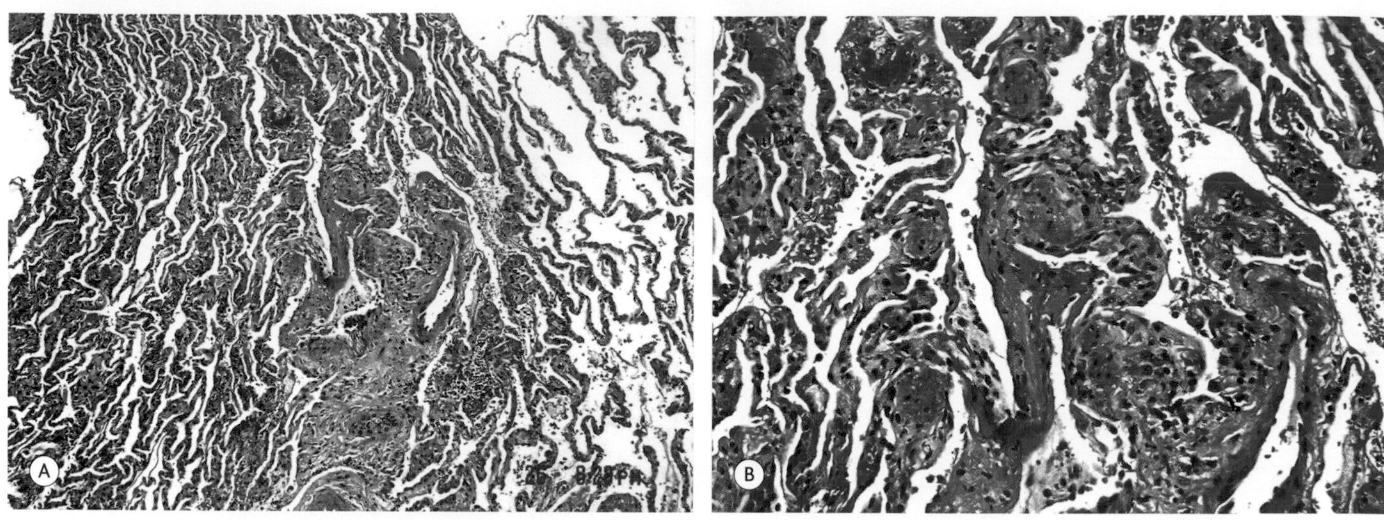

Fig. 6.83 **Coronavirus pneumonia (SARS).** (A,B) Acute fibrinous lung injury. (Courtesy of Dr. Oi-Yee Cheung, Queen Elizabeth Hospital, Hong Kong, China.)

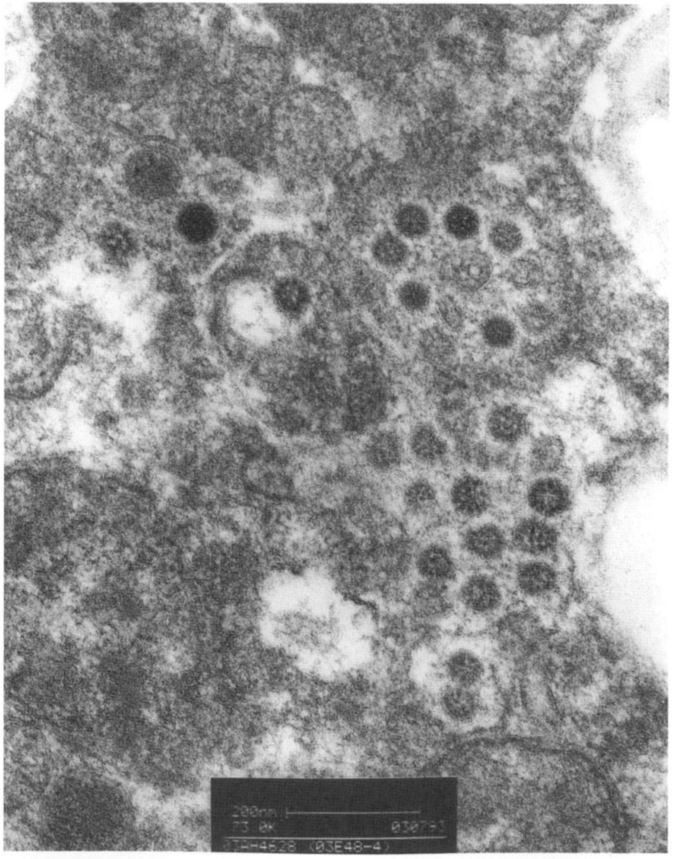

Fig. 6.84 Coronavirus infected cell; electron photomicrograph. (Courtesy of Dr. Oi-Yee Cheung, Queen Elizabeth Hospital, Hong Kong, China.)

immunocompomised. In the lung, they produce two patterns of lung injury – diffuse alveolar damage with or without necrotizing bronchiolitis, and pneumonitis with "dirty" or karyorrhectic necrosis (Fig. 6.85).[200] These patterns may coexist in some cases. Two types of adenoviral CPE may be seen. The pneumonia may be accompanied by extensive intraalveolar hemorrhage due to adenoviral endothelial damage.[200a] Initially an eosinophilic (Cowdry A) intranuclear inclusion occurs surrounded by a halo with marginated chromatin, similar to herpes simplex virus (Fig. 6.86A). This later enlarges and becomes more basophilic, obliterating the nuclear membrane, and producing the characteristic "smudge cell"[189] (Fig. 6.86B).

Herpes simplex viruses

Herpes simplex viruses (HSV), types I and II, have had traditional assigned roles as etiologic agents of mucocutaneous disease of the head and neck (I) and genitalia (II). However, there is considerable crossover with both types isolated from patients with disease at either site. Tracheobronchitis and pneumonia due to these viruses are rare in healthy adults with intact immune systems. They occur primarily in patients with underlying pulmonary disease and in association with inhalational and intubational trauma. They also occur in neonates and in patients who are immunosuppressed or

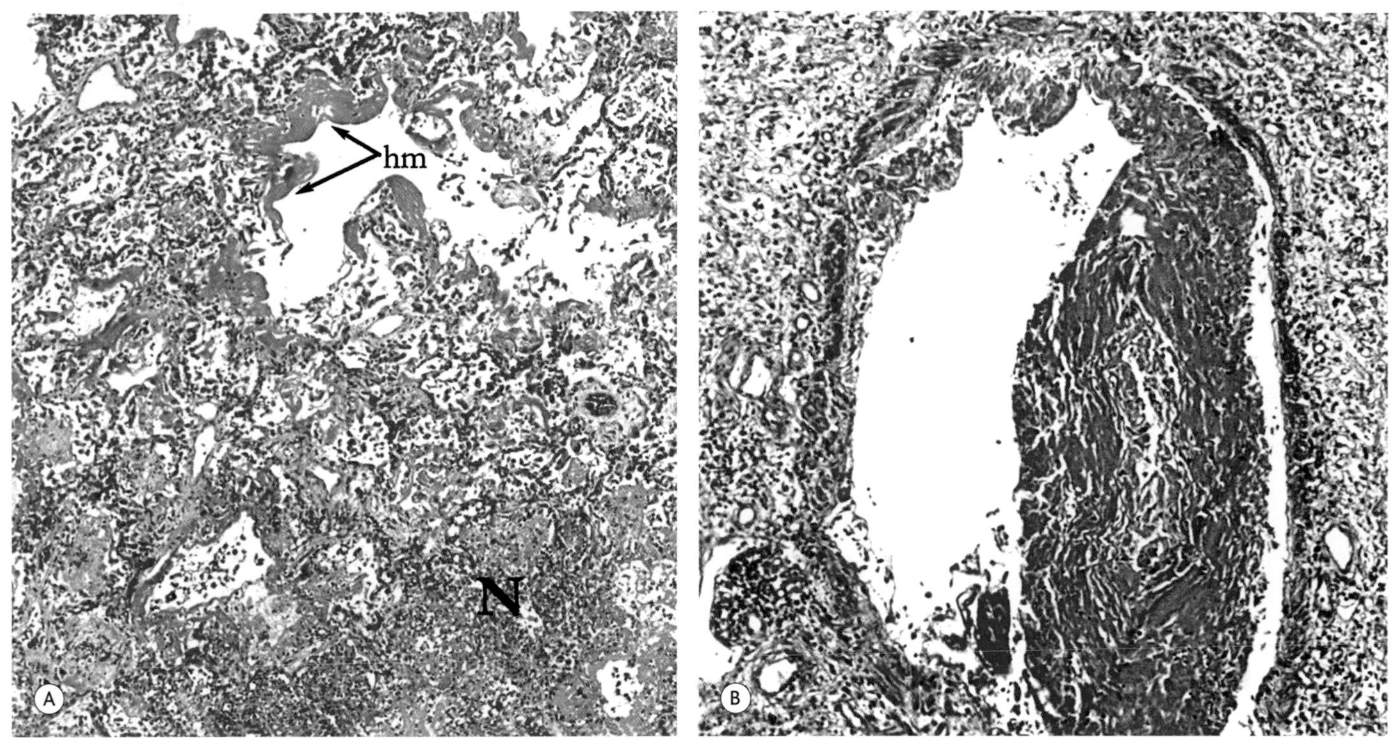

Fig. 6.85 **Adenoviral pneumonia.** (A) Necrosis (N) and diffuse alveolar damage (hm). (B) Nectrotizing bronchiolitis.

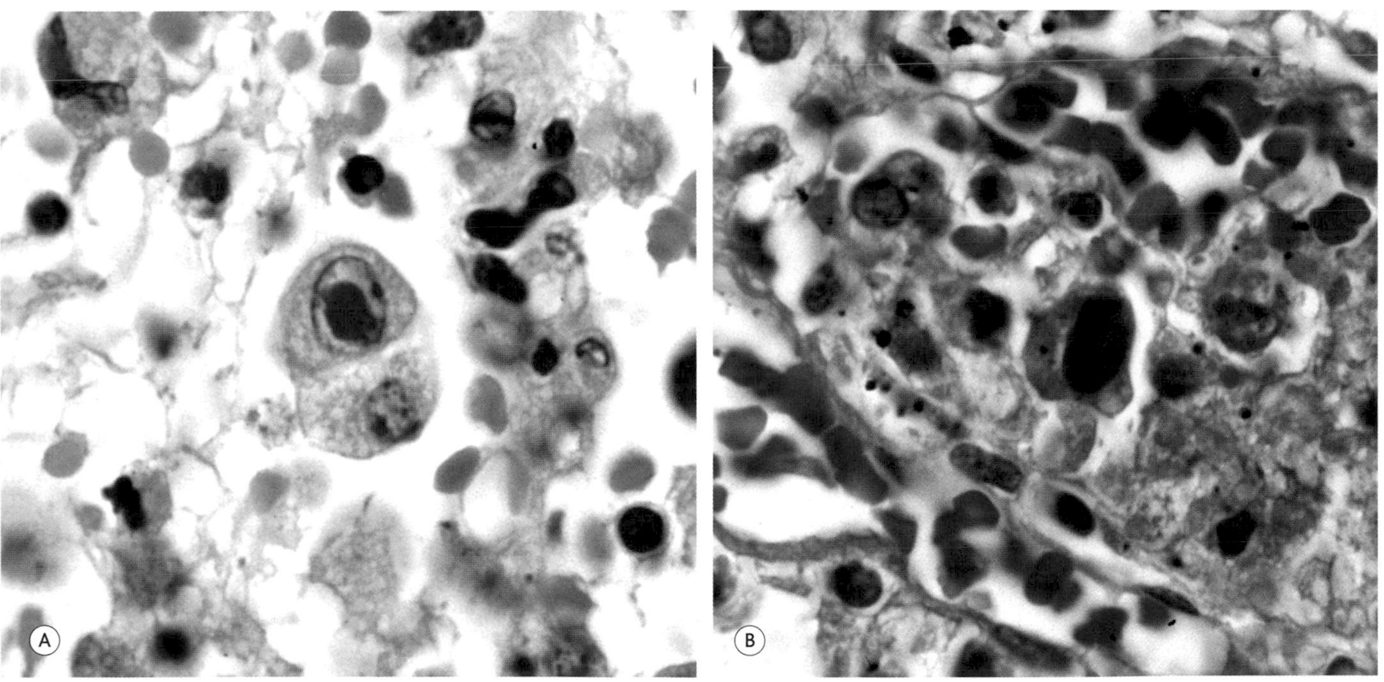

Fig. 6.86 **Adenovirus.** (A) Cowdry A intranuclear inclusions (H&E stain). (B) Smudged cell (H&E stain).

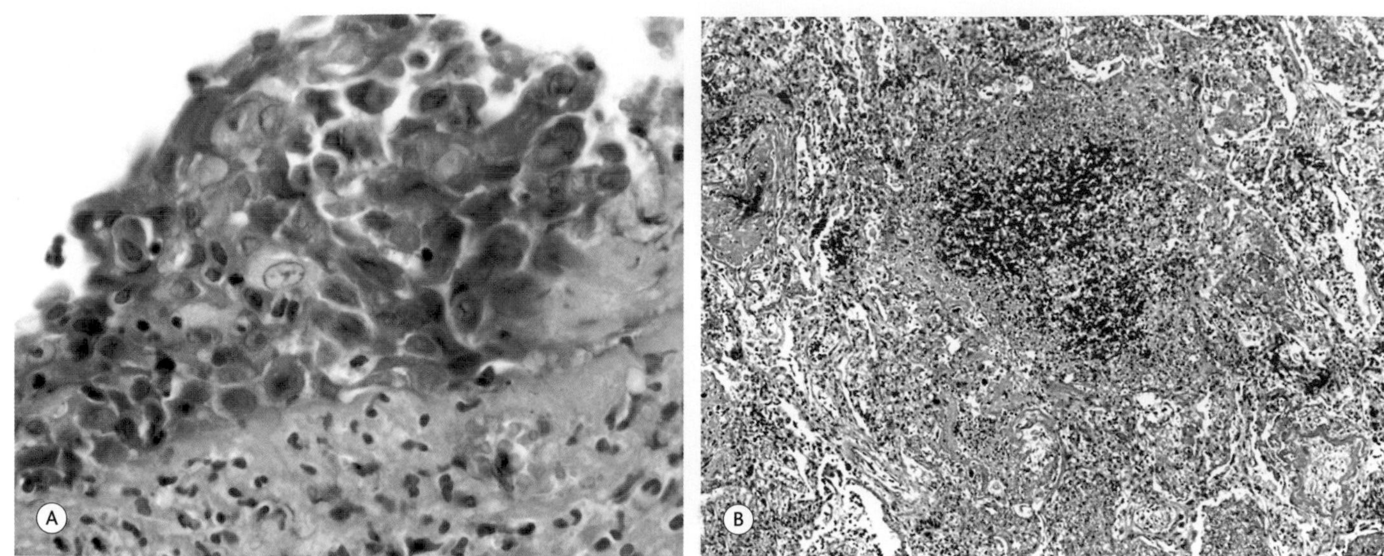

Fig. 6.87 **Herpes simplex viral pneumonia.** (A) Tracheobronchitis. Note cells with ground glass inclusion. (B) Miliary nodular pattern of hemorrhagic necrosis (H&E stain).

compromised by various chronic diseases. Characteristic lesions include tracheobronchitis (Fig. 6.87A) with ulcers and hemorrhagic diffuse alveolar damage. Necrosis in a miliary small, or rarely large, nodular pattern is a helpful clue and the best location to identify CPE (Fig. 6.87B).[45] Like adenovirus, HSV also has two types of CPE: initially a "ground glass" amphophilic intranuclear inclusion (Cowdry B) appears with marginated chromatin. Later, a single eosinophilic (Cowdry A) inclusion (Fig. 6.88) surrounded by a halo, similar to adenovirus, develops.[189] In the absence of smudge cells, HSV and adenoviral infections can look identical. Fortunately, immunohistochemistry or in-situ hybridization can resolve this differential diagnosis.

Varicella-zoster virus

Varicella-zoster (V-Z) virus produces considerable morbiditiy in the newborn, adult, and immunocompromised host, both in its primary form (varicella), and in its reactivated form (zoster). Varicella pneumonia is rarely observed in otherwise healthy children but is a major complication of adult varicella. However, in those adults without underlying diseases and normal immunity, the course is generally mild and self-limited. In contrast, high mortality rates occur among immunosuppressed patients. Microscopically, miliary, small, nodular foci of necrosis associated with interstitial pneumonitis, edema, fibrin deposits, or patchy hyaline membranes may be seen (Fig. 6.89A). HSV-like intranuclear inclusions are present, but may be sparse and difficult to identify. A miliary pattern of calcified nodules (Fig. 6.89B) may be seen in the healed phase.[189]

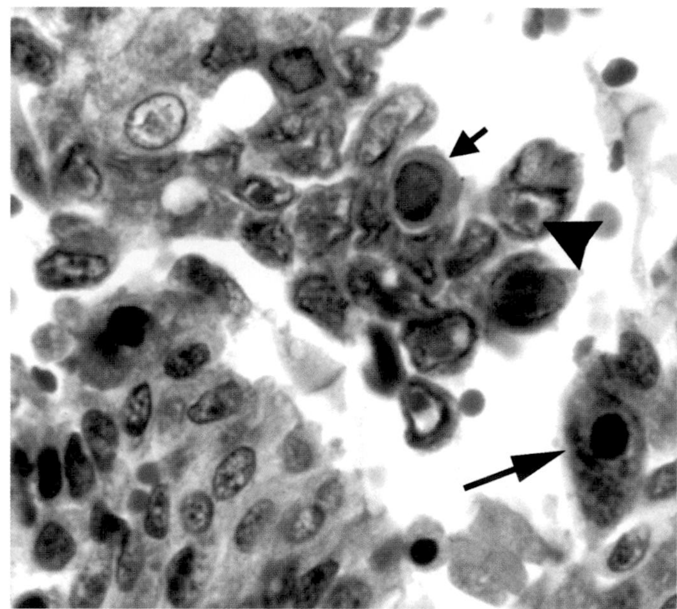

Fig. 6.88 **Herpes simplex viral pneumonia.** Note two types of CPE: Cowdry A ground glass type and Cowdry B eosinophilic inclusion. Compare to CMV intranuclear inclusion at long arrow (H&E stain).

Cytomegalovirus

Cytomegalovirus (CMV) infections are acquired throughout life. This virus can cause considerable morbidity and mortality in the neonate but infection is generally

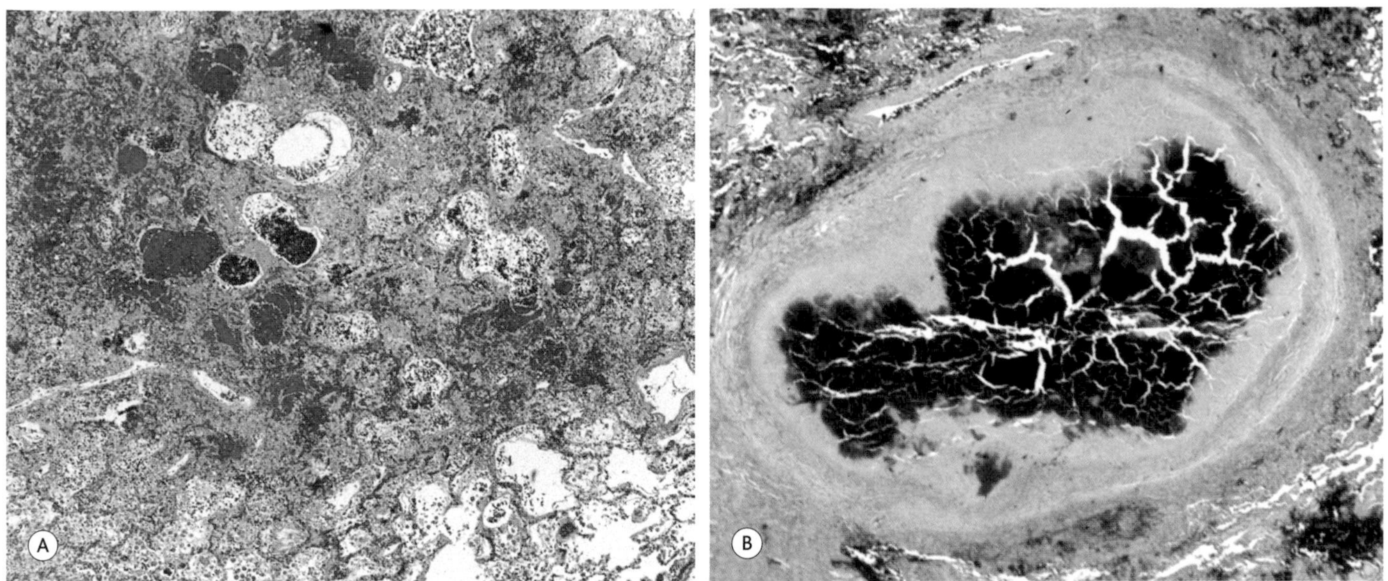

Fig. 6.89 **Varicella pneumonia.** (A) A hemorrhagic miliary nodule (H&E stain). (B) Late phase with calcified nodules (H&E stain).

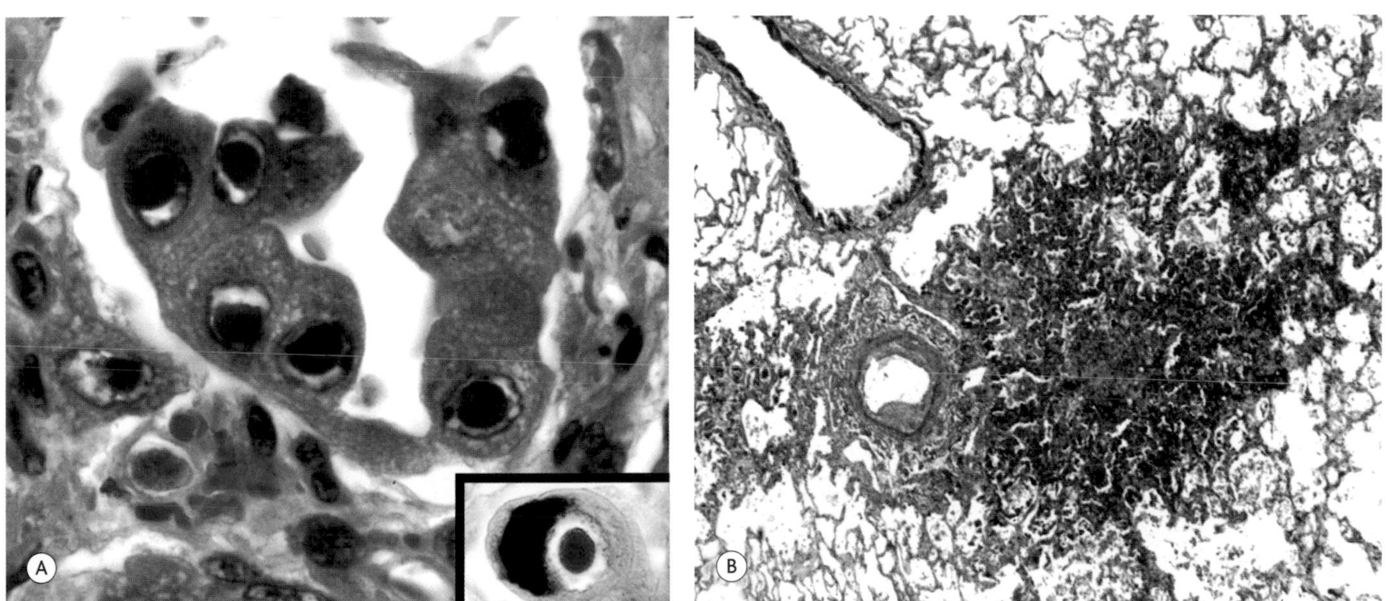

Fig. 6.90 **CMV pneumonia.** (A) Multiple characteristic intranuclear and intracytoplasmic inclusions in alveolar lining cells (H&E stain). Note GMS positive staining of inclusions (inset) (Courtesy of Dr. Francis Chandler, Augusta, GA.) (B) Miliary nodule pattern of CMV pneumonia (H&E stain).

asymptomatic in older healthy children and adults. Like other herpesviruses, primary infection is followed by latency, which persists until immune deficiency or immunosuppressive therapy causes it to reactivate and disseminate. CMV has therefore become one of the most common opportunists in patients with AIDS and those who receive organ transplants. In these settings, CMV can produce a variety of patterns, including "minimal changes," where only scattered alveolar lining cells with typical viropathic changes are seen. The CPE of CMV produces cytomegalic cells with large, round to oval, smooth "owl eye" eosinophilic to basophilic intranuclear inclusions surrounded by a clear halo (Fig. 6.90A).

Later, multiple eosinophilic cytoplasmic inclusions develop that may be positive with PAS and GMS stains (see inset, Fig. 6.87A). The more numerous the cytomegalic cells, the greater the clinical significance. Miliary, small nodules with central hemorrhage surrounded by necrotic alveolar walls (Fig. 6.90B) is another characteristic pattern which suggests viral infection.[45] Interstitial pneumonitis is the least common pattern of CMV infection. Ulcers may be seen in the trachea and bronchi, but occur less often than in herpetic infections, as shown in Fig. 6.88. In CMV pneumonias, look for other pathogens, typically *P. jiroveci* (Fig. 6.91), but bacteria, fungi, protozoa, as well as other viruses are possible.[201]

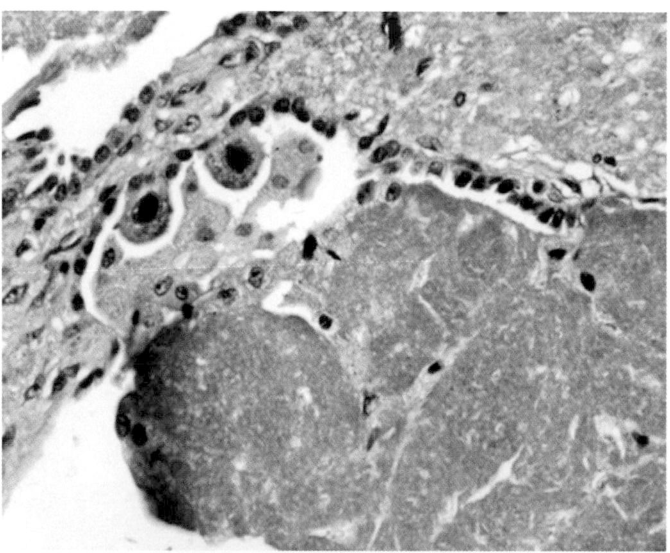

Fig. 6.91 CMV-infected alveolar lining cells associated with the foamy alveolar casts of *P. jiroveci* (H&E stain).

Epstein–Barr virus

Epstein–Barr virus (EBV) infections are usually acquired in childhood and are generally asymptomatic. The pathologist most often encounters this virus in the lung in the context of pulmonary lymphomas or in other EBV-associated lymphoproliferative disorders that can occur in transplant patients and other immunocompromised individuals. However, the most common symptomatic primary EBV infection is infectious mononucleosis. Most of these patients recover uneventfully but a few develop one or more complications. Pneumonitis is one of them, albeit rare and not well-characterized. The few reports describing pathology indicate a nonspecific lymphocytic interstitial pneumonitis that may be bronchiolocentric (Fig. 6.92).[202,203] There is no CPE, and while serologic studies can be supportive of a clinicopathologic diagnosis, etiologic proof of EBV infection requires demonstration of the virus in lymphoid cells by in-situ hybridization for EBV-encoded RNA-1 (EBER-1).

Cytopathology

The cytologic features of viral infections in the respiratory tract are most likely to be found in exfoliative specimens, such as bronchial washings and bronchoalveolar lavages, rather than needle aspirates, although viral diagnosis has been achieved with this technique.[204,205] This is because viral infections are less likely to produce radiographic mass-like infiltrates, which are the most common targets of needle biopsy procedures. Herpes

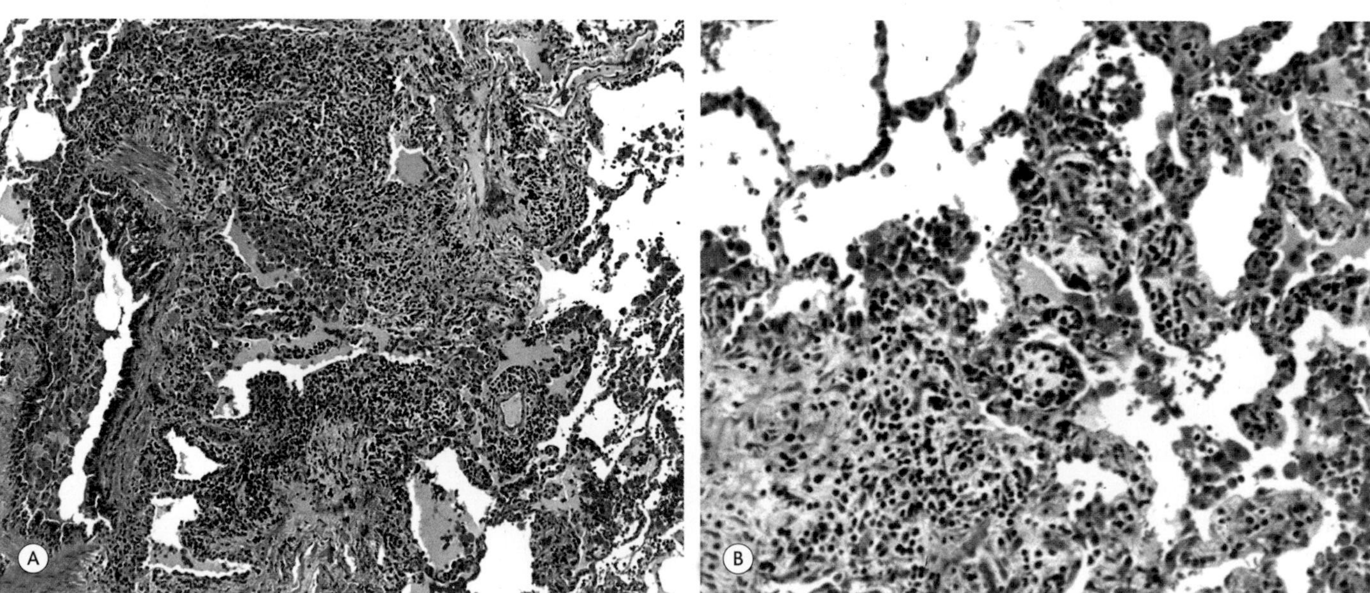

Fig. 6.92 **EBV pneumonitis.** (A) Nonspecific cellular interstitial pneumonitis (H&E stain). (B) Patchy interstitial infiltrate (H&E stain).

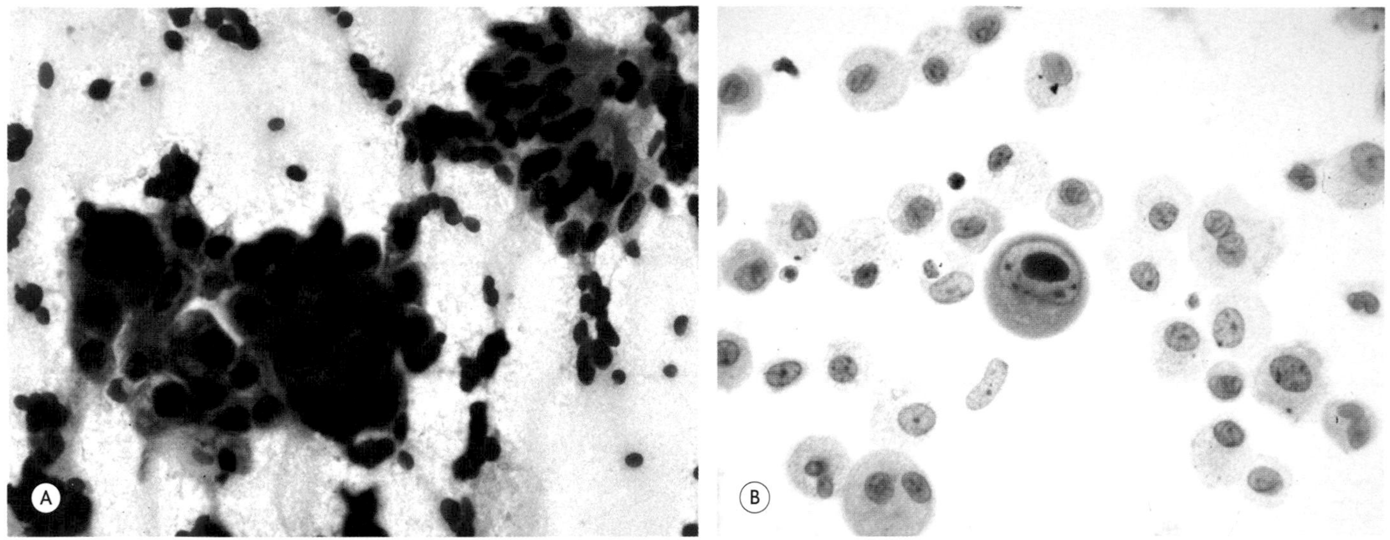

Fig. 6.93 **CMV pneumonitis; characteristic cytopathic effect.** (A) Fine-needle aspirate (H&E stain). (B) Bronchoalveolar lavage specimen.

simplex, cytomegalovirus (Fig. 6.93), and adenovirus are the most commonly identified viral pathogens in respiratory cytologic specimens, but varicella virus, parainfluenza virus, respiratory syncytial virus, and measles virus have also been detected.

Characteristic CPE produced by these viruses, is often better appreciated in cytologic smears rather than in tissue sections, which may in fact be negative. Therefore, review of any cytology sample taken at the time of biopsy can be valuable. Other less-specific changes may be found. These include ciliocytophoria (free cilia complexes with terminal bars) and cytologic atypia mimicking cancer.[27]

Table 6.33 Laboratory diagnosis of viral pneumonia

Direct detection of organisms: – Histopathology and cytopathology for CPE – Immunohistochemistry – Electron microscopy
Antigen detection: – Direct immunofluorescence – Enzyme immunoassay
Culture: – Conventional roller tube – Shell vial
Serology
Molecular methods: – In-situ hybridization – DNA amplification

Microbiology

Diagnostic virology is the newest of the microbiology and infectious disease specialties to have benefited from the technologic revolution in laboratory medicine. Rapid and accurate diagnosis can often be achieved today using practical, convenient laboratory methods that employ reliable, commercially-available mammalian cells, media, and reagent systems.[179,206,207] This has allowed many rural and small urban hospital laboratories to provide timely viral diagnostic services not possible a short time ago. Soon, it is predicted, self-contained, rapid-cycle real-time PCR will account for the majority of viral assays in laboratories of all sizes.[21] As a result, the pathologist who suspects a viral infection will increasingly have a variety of tools to achieve an etiologic diagnosis when morphologic manifestations are suggestive of viral infection.

The basic approaches to laboratory diagnosis are listed in Table 6.33. Characteristic cytopathic effects of various respiratory viruses, including intranuclear and intracytoplasmic inclusions, are summarized in Table 6.32. In questionable cases, confirmation by immunohistochemistry (Fig. 6.94A) in-situ hybridization (Fig. 6.94B), or electron microscopy may be helpful.[208,209]

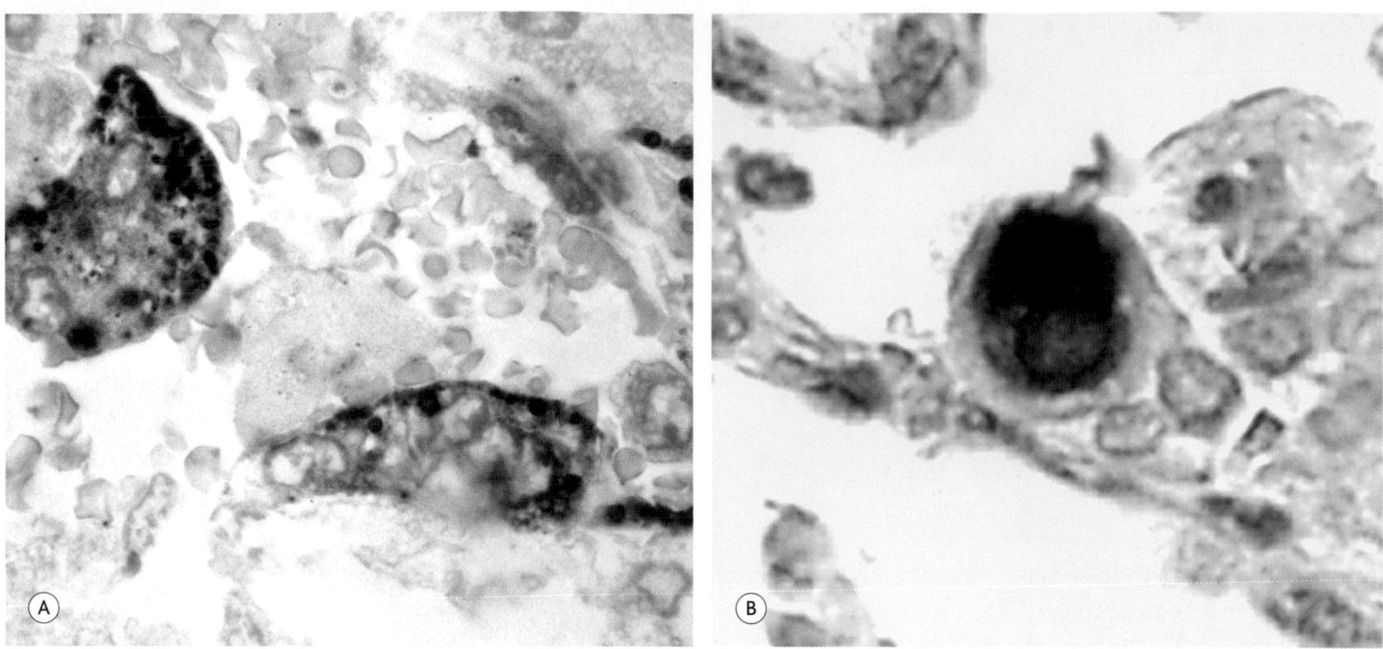

Fig. 6.94 (A) RSV cytoplasmic inclusions detected by immunohistochemistry. (B) CMV-infected cell with cytoplasmic inclusions detected by in-situ hybridization. (Courtesy of RV Lloyd, M.D., Rochester, MN.)

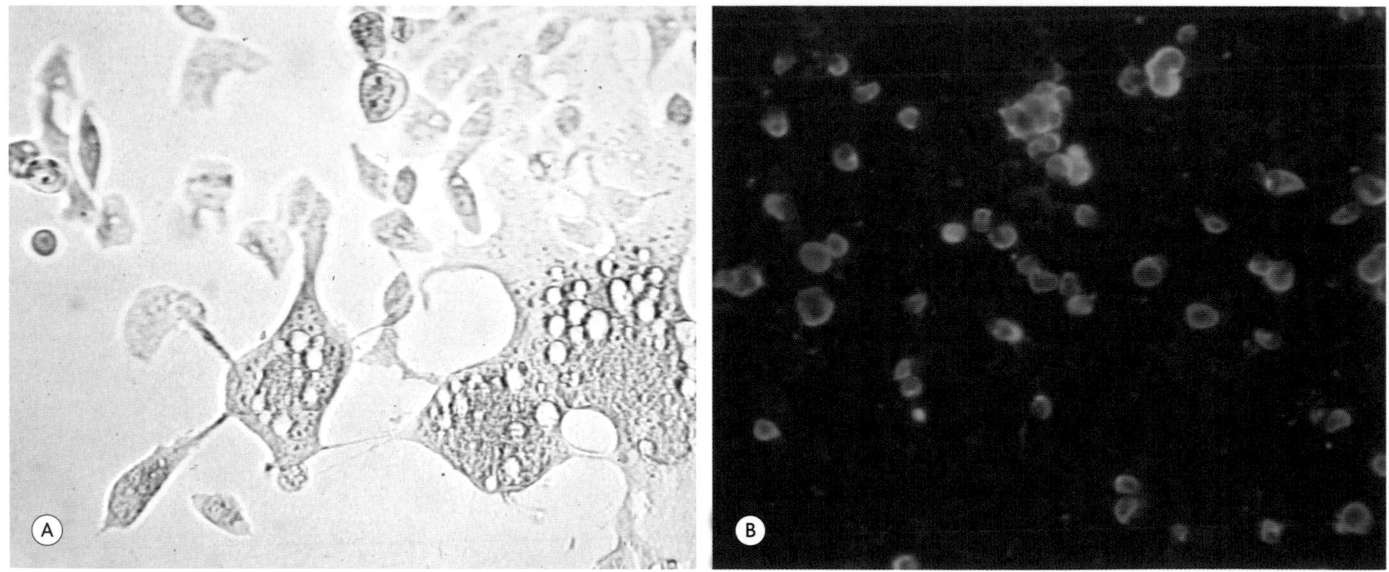

Fig. 6.95 (A) RSV cytopathic effect in tissue culture. (B) RSV antigen in nasopharyngeal swab specimen detected by direct immunofluorescence.

In the microbiology laboratory, the diagnosis of viral respiratory infections is based primarily on antigen detection and culture (Fig. 6.95). Direct antigen detection in clinical specimens collected by nasopharyngeal swabs, nasal washings and aspirates, or bronchoalveolar lavage (but not sputum or throat swabs) are performed utilizing monoclonal antibodies by either immunofluorescence microscopy or enzyme immunoassay. By utilizing a single reagent containing the monoclonal antibodies against several viruses and dual flurochromes, the common respiratory viruses can be rapidly screened by direct immunofluoresence. Positive specimens can then be tested with individual reagents to determine the specific etiologic agent, while negative specimens can be submitted for culture.[210] Enzyme immunoassay includes methods that offer speed and convenience at the point of care. However, they are less sensitive than standard virologic methods, which still must be used to test negative specimens. Direct detection can also be accomplished in cellular samples, including tissue, by in-situ hybridization or amplification techniques such as PCR. For RNA viruses, PCR employs a reverse transcriptase step. PCR multiplex techniques permit simultaneous detection of multiple viruses (as do cultures) or alternatively a virus and a different type of pathogen, e.g. CMV and *Toxoplasma gondii*.[211,212] These assays, at the present, are more technically demanding than culture and antigen detection by immunofluorescence or enzyme immunoassay, but are more sensitive. For the present at least, isolation still remains useful for many respiratory viral infections and antigen detection methods offer the speed and immediacy of reporting that many molecular methods lack.

Traditional viral cultures in tubes with various types of cell monolayers are currently performed with greater sensitivity and turnaround time using the shell vial technique. This technique employs centrifugation of clinical specimen suspensions onto coverslipped cell monolayers, followed by brief incubation (1–2 days) and antigen detection.[206] It is important therefore to preserve a portion of tissue from a bronchial/transbronchial biopsy or thoracotomy specimen in viral transport medium, especially in the immunocompromised patient, who may not have had bronchoalveolar lavage fluid submitted for culture.

Viral serology has been used commonly for diagnosis but may be the least-sensitive approach. A positive serodiagnosis, typically based on a four-fold rise in titer between acute and convalescent sera, is not very useful in the acutely ill patient; antigen detection or culture of respiratory tract specimens is much preferred. However, a serologic strategy, utilizing a panel of antigens in an immunofluorescence or enzyme immunoassays format on a single specimen is useful for suspected EBV infections.[213]

A beneficial case can also be made for CMV serology for assessment of the antibody status of organ donors and recipients for predicting the risk of post-transplant CMV disease. Tests for the detection of actual disease in these transplant patients, when tissue is not available or findings are inconclusive, includes the p65 antigenemia assay on peripheral blood leukocytes and amplification of CMV DNA in various peripheral blood compartments (plasma, whole blood, and leukocytes).[214] These assays may eventually replace culture of bronchoalveolar lavage fluid for surveillance of CMV infection in these patients.[215]

Differential diagnosis

The key morphologic and microbiologic features of the viral pneumonias are summarized in Table 6.34. In the absence of CPE, diffuse alveolar damage and other patterns of lung injury are not diagnostic of viral infection. Diffuse alveolar damage is a nonspecific response to many types of infection, including bacterial, mycobacterial, fungal, and protozoal, all of which must be considered in the differential diagnosis. In addition, other noninfectious causes include reactions to drugs, radiation, toxic inhalants, and shock of any type. Occasionally, CPE may not be diagnostic: for example, the early inclusions of adenovirus, herpes simplex, and cytomegalovirus may be quite similar. In most cases, immunohistochemistry or molecular techniques can resolve the diagnostic dilemma. Mimics of CPE, which must be distinguished, include macronuclei in both reactive processes and occult neoplastic infiltrates, and intranuclear cytoplasmic invaginations, which can occur in a variety of cells. Cytoplasmic viral inclusions can also be simulated by aggregated altered protein and particulate matter.

Parasitic infections

It is estimated that about 300 species of helminth worms and 70 species of protozoa have been acquired by humans during our short history on Earth.[216] Most of these are rare, but about 90 are relatively common and some of them have been found in the lung. A world made smaller by globalization and travel to endemic areas, and the appearance of emerging and re-emerging parasitic pathogens in immunocompromised patients, guarantee that pathologists will be increasingly challenged by diagnostic problems associated with these organisms.[217] Nevertheless, pulmonary parasitic infections are relatively rare and continue to be exotic diseases for surgical and cytopathologists in the United States.

Several parasite species migrate through the lungs as part of their normal life cycle, but few preferentially infect the human lung.[218] Most are aberrant pulmonary localizations in the human host, where they become lost in transit or are part of a secondary disseminated infection from another organ system, often in the setting of compromised immunity. The etiologic list in Table 6.35 is selective, based on the more commonly cited pulmonary incidences. The reader is encouraged to consult the references for a more comprehensive compilation.

Table 6.34 Viral pneumonia synopsis

Influenza	
Surgical pathology:	Diffuse alveolar damage, bronchitis, and bronchiolitis. Secondary acute purulent pneumonia. Antigen detection by immunofluorescence, immunohistochemistry, or in-situ hybridization
Cytopathology:	Nonspecific changes may include reactive-type pneumocytes; ciliocytophoria
Microbiology:	Antigen detection by DFA or EIA. Culture on primary monkey kidney cells, noncytopathic. Detection by hemadsorption
Respiratory syncytial virus	
Surgical pathology:	Bronchiolitis with lumen detritus; may be associated with syncytial giant cells. Diffuse alveolar damage in immunocompromised hosts. Confirm with immunohistochemistry
Cytopathology:	Giant cell syncytia characteristic, but often not seen. Eosinophilic inclusions may be seen in bronchial epithelial cells in immunocompromised patients; rarely in normal hosts. Rarely diagnosed by cytology alone
Microbiology:	Antigen detection by DFA and EIA usually more sensitive than culture. Cultures on continuous epithelial cell lines (Hep-2) and primary monkey kidney yield characteristic syncytial cytopathic effect
Measles	
Surgical pathology:	Bronchitis, bronchiolitis, diffuse alveolar damage with giant cells containing Cowdry A inclusions and small cytoplasmic inclusions
Cytopathology:	Eosinophilic intranuclear and cytoplasmic inclusions. Rarely diagnosed by cytology
Microbiology:	Antigen detection by DFA and EIA. Culture on primary monkey kidney produces spindle cell or multinucleated CPE. Serology (measles-specific IgM) available
Hantavirus	
Surgical pathology:	Pulmonary edema pattern with variable fibrin deposits. Immunoblast-like cells in vascular spaces. Confirm by immunohistochemistry
Cytopathology:	Noncytopathic
Microbiology:	Serology – hantavirus-specific IgM or detection of specific RNA by PCR in peripheral blood leukocytes
Coronavirus (SARS–cov)	
Surgical pathology:	Acute and/or organizing DAD varies according to duration. Coronavirus particles by electron microscopy
Cytopathology:	Cytopathic in veno EG cells; giant cell syncytial in lung
Microbiology:	Culture on veno EG cells. Conventional RT–PCR or real-time PCR serology available – IFA; ELISA.
Adenovirus	
Surgical pathology:	Diffuse alveolar damage with or without necrotizing bronchiolitis and/or pneumonitis with necrosis and karyorrhexis
Cytopathology:	Early Cowdry A intranuclear inclusions, later smudge cell. Reactive and reparative type atypia in background
Microbiology:	Antigen detection by EIA and DFA. Culture on continuous epithelial cell lines produces characteristic grape-like clustered cytopathic effect
Herpesvirus	
Surgical pathology:	Tracheobronchitis; diffuse alveolar damage; miliary necroinflammatory lesions
Cytopathology:	Ground glass (Cowdry B) intranuclear inclusions; later Cowdry A inclusions in multinucleated cells, often resemble "seeds in a pomegranate" on Pap, H&E, and Diff-Quik stained smears. Background reactive and reparative atypia
Microbiology:	Antigen detection by immunofluorescence. Culture on diploid fibroblasts produces characteristic cytopathic effect, sometimes within 24 hours. Serology less useful
Varicella-zoster	
Surgical pathology:	Miliary necroinflammatory lesions; calcified nodules in healed phase
Cytopathology:	Intranuclear Cowdry A inclusions sparse and less well defined than herpes simplex
Microbiology:	Antigen detection by immunofluorescence. Culture on human embryonic lung or vero cells produce CPE more slowly than herpes viruses (3–7 days). Serology available
Cytomegalovirus	
Surgical pathology:	Minimal changes with scattered cytomegalic cells; miliary necroinflammatory lesions; interstitial pneumonitis
Cytopathology:	Large "owl eye" Cowdry A inclusions with halo; cytoplasmic inclusions stained with GMs
Microbiology:	Culture on human diploid fibroblasts produces characteristic CPE slowly in traditional tube cultures, but more rapidly by shell vial technique. p65 antigenemia assay and PCR. Selective application of serology useful
Epstein–Barr virus	
Surgical pathology:	Polymorphous lymphoid interstitial pneumonitis. Confirm by in-situ hybridization
Cytopathology:	Noncytopathic
Microbiology:	No routine culture; diagnosis by serology with panel of antibodies (EA; IgG and IgM VCA; EBNA)

Patterns of lung injury

When parasites, in the form of adult worms, larvae, or eggs, invade or become deposited in lung tissue, they usually provoke an intense inflammatory reaction with neutrophils, eosinophils, and various mononuclear cells. One or more of the patterns listed in Table 6.36 may be identified. When the predominant site of involvement is the bronchial mucosa, a bronchitis and bronchiolitis pattern is observed; when they become impacted in pulmonary arteries, a nodular angiocentric pattern is observed, although it may be overshadowed by thrombosis and infarction. Some parasites invade the alveolar parenchyma, resulting in a pattern of miliary small nodules or pneumonitis. Naturally, none of these patterns are consistently present and combinations of patterns may be seen. In some cases, an acute Loeffler's-like eosinophilic pneumonia may reflect an allergic reaction to the transient passage of larvae through the pulmonary vasculature.

Table 6.35 Some common parasitic lung pathogens

Protozoa:
- *Toxoplasma gondii*
- *Entamoeba histolytica*
- Cryptosporidia
- Microsporidia

Metazoa (helminths):
- Nematodes
  Dirofilaria immitis
  Strongyloides stercoralis
- Cestodes
  Echinococcus spp.
- Trematodes
  Paragonimus spp.
  Schistosoma spp.

Table 6.36 Patterns of parasitic lung injury

Eosinophilic pneumonia
Large nodule(s)
Miliary small nodules
Bronchitis and bronchiolitis
Abscess, cavities, and cysts
Intravascular reaction

The various patterns, although nondiagnostic, can be suggestive of a parasitic infection, particularly when they incorporate a heavy eosinophilic infiltrate or granulomatous component. The challenge for the pathologist is the identification of a parasite, distinguishing it from artifact or foreign body, and classifying it as precisely as possible based on its size and unique morphologic features. Once suggestive morphologic features are present, the patient's travel history can help to further narrow the differential diagnosis. Of interest, a common "parasite" encountered in practice is not a parasite at all but aspirated vegetable material simulating the complex structure of an organism.[219]

Toxoplasmosis

Toxoplasma gondii is an obligate, intracellular protozoan and a common opportunist in patients with AIDS, the disease underlying most cases of toxoplasmosis seen in recent years. The brain and retina are most commonly involved in these patients but pulmonary lesions may also be present in cases of disseminated disease. These often take the form of miliary small nodules with fibrinous exudates, which may progress to a confluent fibrinopurulent pneumonia.[220] Free forms (crescent-shaped tachyzoites) and cysts may be identified (Fig. 6.96). Pseudocysts packed with tachyzoites can be distinguished from true cysts with bradyzoites, the latter staining with PAS and GMS.[221]

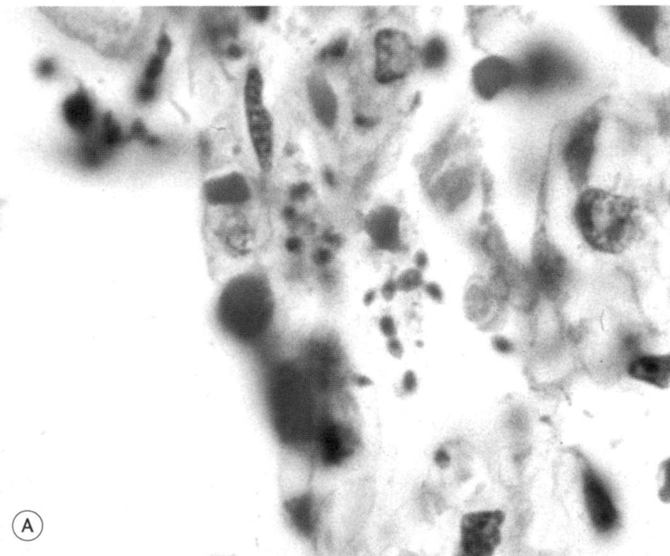

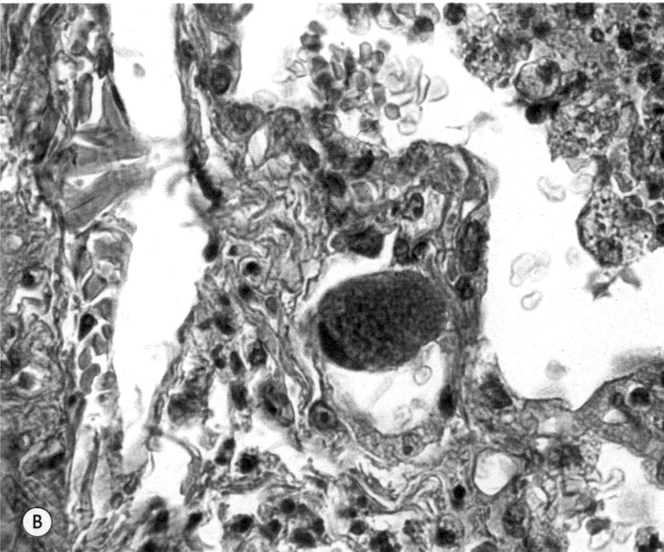

Fig. 6.96 **Toxoplasmosis.** (A) Tachyzoites. (B) Pseudocysts packed with tachyzoites (H&E stain).

Amoebiasis

Amoebic dysentery becomes invasive in a small percentage of patients. When the trophozoites of *Entamoeba histolytica* leave the gut, they most commonly travel to the liver. From the liver, either by direct extension, or rarely by hematogenous spread, the lungs may become involved. In this scenario, abscesses composed of liquefactive debris with few polys (in contrast to bacterial abscess), usually form in the right lower lobe.[222,223] Trophozoites can be best seen at the margin of viable tissue (Fig. 6.97). They resemble histiocytes, but are usually larger with a lower nucleo-cytoplasmic ratio. A tiny central karyosome within a round nucleus having vesicular chromatin is characteristic.[224,225] Bronchial fistula and empyema can occur as complications; amoebae may be found in sputum and pleural fluid, respectively, in these situations. Free-living amoebic species (*Acanthamoeba, Balamuthia, Naegleria*) have the central nervous system as their principal focus of infection. However, disseminated disease, including lung infection (Fig. 6.98) may occur in certain epidemiologic situations, especially in immunocompromised patients.[226]

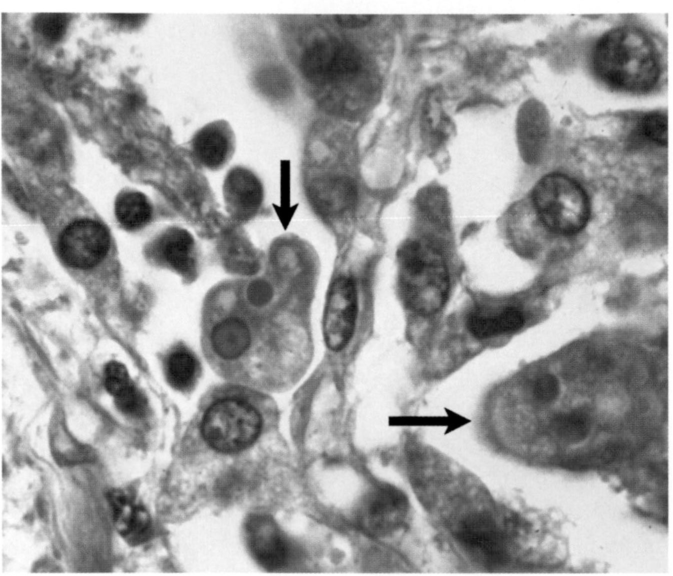

Fig. 6.97 **Amoebic trophozoite in lung tissue.** Note delicate marginal nuclear chromatin with small central karyosome and small red blood cell in cytoplasm. (Courtesy of Ronald Neafi, AFIP, Washington DC.)

Cryptosporidiosis

Ten species of the intracellular coccidian protozoa are currently recognized, but one of them, *Cryposporidium parvum*, causes most human infections.[227] Clinically, this organism may have three major manifestations: asymptomatic shedding; acute watery diarrhea that lasts for about 2 weeks; and persistent diarrhea that lasts several weeks. Patients with AIDS have a wider spectrum of disease severity and duration that includes a fulminant cholera-like illness.[227] AIDS patients are also most likely to manifest extraintestinal disease. In the lung, the organism targets the epithelium of the airways just as it does the surface epithelium of the gut and biliary tract.[228] In H&E sections, cryptosporidia appear as small, 4–6 μm, round to oval, protrusions from the cell surface. Electron

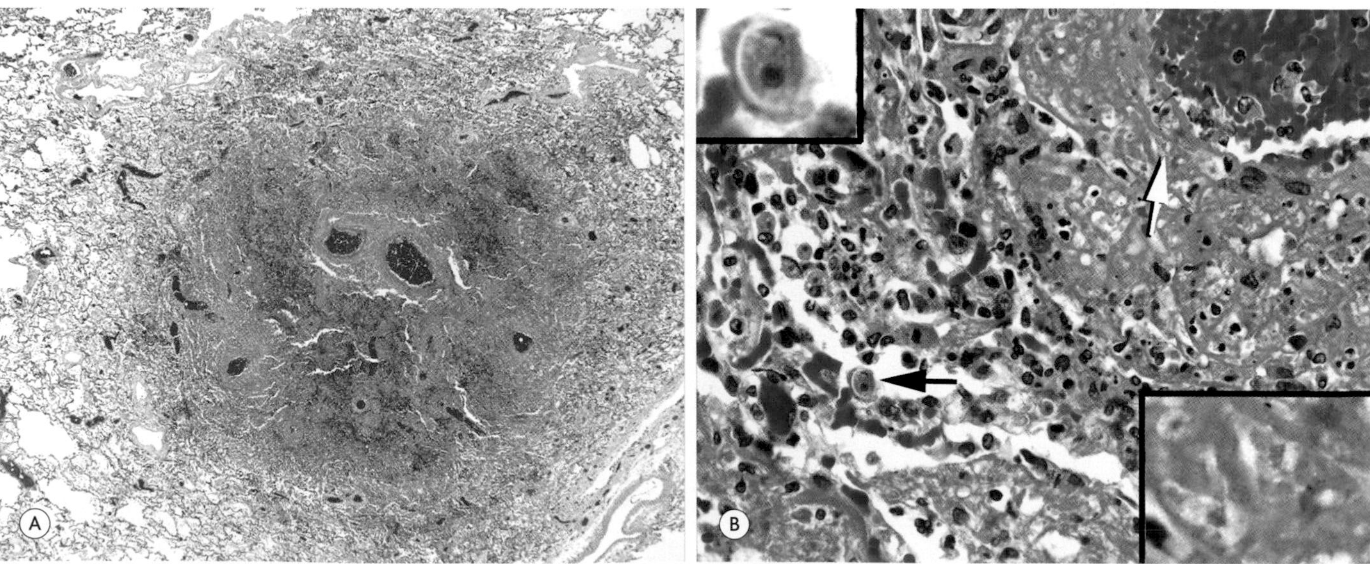

Fig. 6.98 **Free-living amoeba in lung tissue.** (A) Necroinflammatory nodule. (B) Incysted form, black arrow and left upper inset; trophozoite, white arrow and lower right inset (H&E stain).

microscopy reveals that they are intracellular but extracytoplasmic. In addition to H&E, they stain with Giemsa, PAS, GMS, and acid-fast stains. A mild to moderate chronic inflammatory cell infiltrate is usually present in the submucosa. Recognition of this disease in AIDS patients can be challenging because the findings may be subtle and coexistent pneumonias caused by other pathogens can divert the pathologist's attention.

Microsporidiosis

The microsporidia are obligate intracellular, spore-forming protozoa. There are more that 140 genera and 1200 species, but only seven genera, and a few species have been confirmed as human pathogens.[229] They are opportunists that have recently emerged in severely immunocompromised patients, especially AIDS and transplant recipients. They are found less often in people with intact immunity. Clinically, they primarily cause chronic diarrhea and cholangitis. In the lung, they cause bronchitis and/or bronchiolitis, usually in patients who also have intestinal infection and/or disease in other sites, especially the biliary tract.[230] The pathologic findings are centered on the airways and these show a mixed inflammatory cell infiltrate of mononuclear and polymorphonuclear leukocytes.[231] The organisms are found within vacuoles in the apical portion of epithelial cells lining the airways. They appear as very small (1.0–1.5 µm) basophilic dots, whose recognition depends on organism load. However, even when heavy, the findings can be subtle. Also, as with cryptosporidiosis, their presence is often overlooked or obscured by coexistent pneumonias. Special stains such as modified trichrome, Warthin–Starry-type silver, and Gram stains are more sensitive and specific, especially when used in combination.[232]

Dirofilariasis

The zoonosis caused by *Dirofilaria immitis*, a parasite of dogs and other mammals, is transmitted by mosquitos and black flies to humans. Larvae injected by these insect vectors, migrate from the subcutaneum into veins and travel to the heart, where they die before maturing into adult worms. They are then washed into the lungs by the pulmonary arterial blood flow, where they form the nidus of a thrombus. An infarct follows, which typically presents as an asymptomatic solitary pulmonary nodule ("coin lesion") in the lung periphery. Microscopically, the nodule resembles a typical infarct with a core of coagulation necrosis, but also with degenerated worm fragments in the remnant of an arteriole (Fig. 6.99). A peripheral investment of chronic granulation tissue forms an interface with the alveolated parenchyma. Step sections and trichrome stains may be needed when H&E sections do not show the parasite.[233]

Strongyloidiasis

This infection is most often found in patients or travelers in the tropics, but endemic foci are present in the southeastern United States. Rabitiform larvae of the nematode *Strongyloides stercoralis*, after hatching from ingested eggs, invade the small intestinal mucosa. At this site occult infection may remain asymptomatic for years. Dissemination typically follows debilitation brought on by immunocompromising diseases and therapies. When this occurs, filariform larvae leave the gut and travel through the pulmonary vasculature. When they penetrate alveoli (Fig. 6.100), they provoke hemorrhage and inflammation.[234] Loeffler's syndrome, eosinophilic pneumonia, and abscesses may develop. When migration is interrupted, filariform larvae may metamorphose in situ to adult worms, which can produce eggs and rabitiform larvae. Larvae identified in the sputum indicate hyperinfection.[235] Disseminated strongyloidiasis is but one example of an infection that may become manifest, particularly in immunocompromised patients, years after emigration from or travel to an endemic area harboring pathogens considered unusual or exotic by pathologists in the United States.

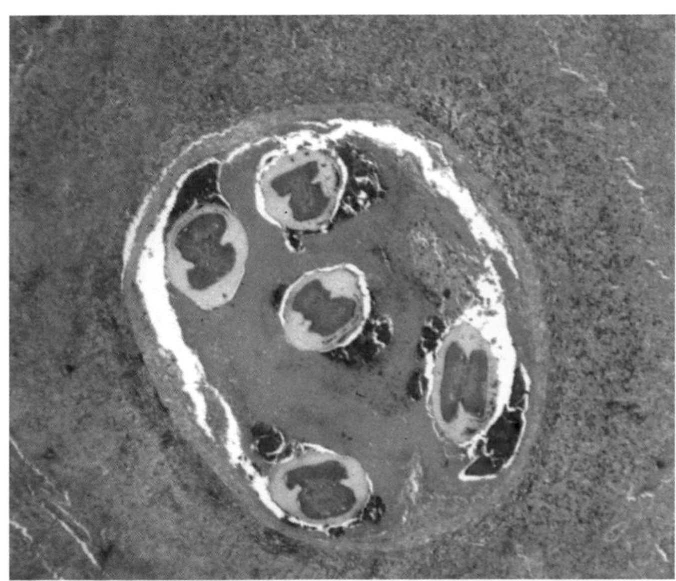

Fig. 6.99 Dirofilarial nodule with worm remnants in organizing thrombosed vessel (H&E stain).

Echinococcosis

This zoonosis occurs wherever sheep, dogs, or other canidae and man live in close contact. Ingested eggs of this tapeworm hatch in the gut, releasing oncospheres, which invade the mucosa, enter the circulation, and travel to various sites where they develop into hydatid cysts. In the lung, unilocular slow-growing cysts are produced by *Echinococcus granulosus*.[236] *Echinococcus multilocularis* proliferates by budding, producing an alveolar pattern of microvesicles.[225] The cyst of *E. granulosus* has a trilayered membrane (Fig. 6.101A) with an outer fibrous, middle-laminated hyaline, and inner germinal layer that gives rise to brood capsules containing infective protoscolices with hooklets and suckers (Fig. 6.101B). The layers usually become separated in tissue, with the outer fibrous layer containing chronic inflammatory cells forming an interface with the alveolated parenchyma. Cysts that rupture into bronchi may be expectorated as debris with protoscolices or portions of the cyst wall. Abscesses and granulomas may also form in the lung, pleura, and chest wall.[237]

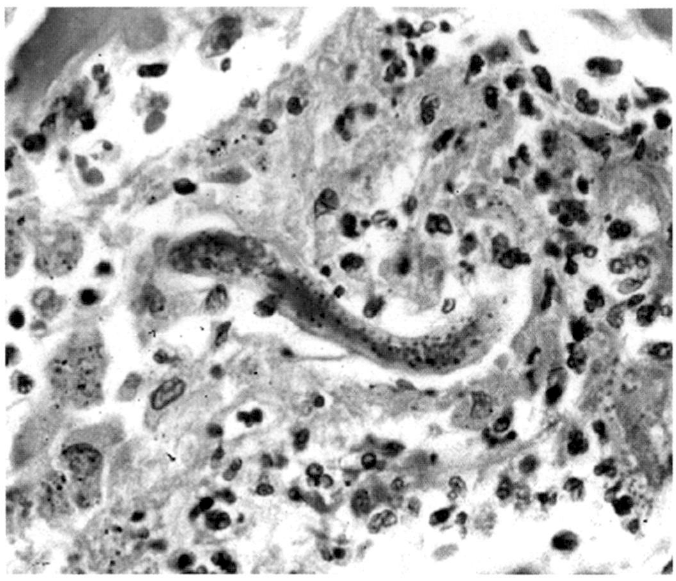

Fig. 6.100 Filariform larvae of *Strongyloides stercoralis* penetrating into alveolar space with associated inflammation (H&E stain).

Paragonimoniasis

This infection is acquired by the ingestion of freshwater crabs or crayfish infected with the metacercarial larva of *Paragonimus* spp. Most cases worldwide are due *to P. westermani,* but several other species exist in Asia, Africa, and South and North America. In the United States, infections due to *P. kellicotti* have been reported.[238] The disease manifestations are related to the migratory route and the inflammatory response these hermaphroditic flukes stimulate as they enter lung parenchyma and

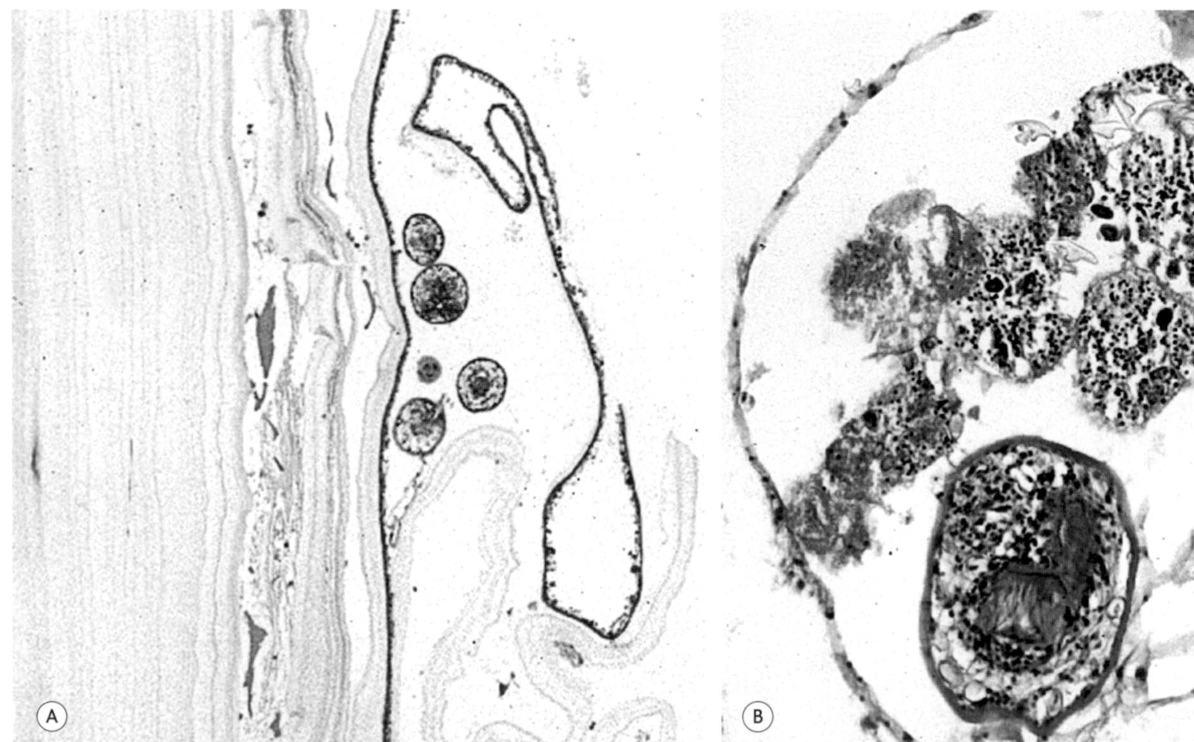

Fig. 6.101 ***Echinococcus granulosus.*** (A) Cyst with trilayered membrane (H&E stain). (B) Brood capsules (H&E stain).

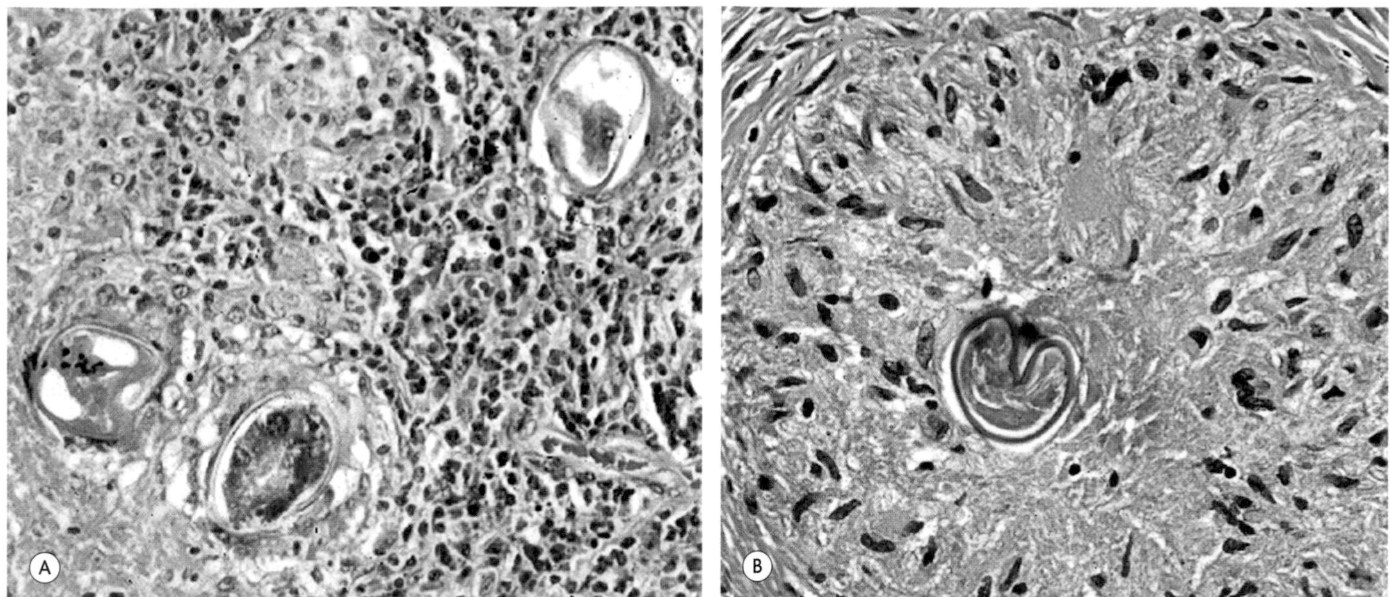

Fig. 6.102 (A) *Paragonimus westermani* with yellowish refractile eggs in eosinophil-rich exudates (H&E stain); (B) Distorted egg (*Paragonimus kellicotti*) in granuloma (H&E stain).

travel to sites near larger bronchioles or bronchi. Typically, an eosinophil-rich inflammatory reaction surrounds them and this reaction may condense to form a fibrous pseudocyst or capsule containing worms, exudate, and debris (Fig. 6.102A). Cysts rupturing into bronchioles may result in eggs, blood, and inflammatory cells being coughed up in the sputum. Alternatively, eggs may become embedded in parenchyma, producing nodular granulomatous lesions (Fig. 6.102B) that progress to scars.[239] The eggs are yellowish, ovoid, operculated, and 75–110 µm × 45–60 µm in size. The opercula unfortunately are not easily seen in tissue; however, the eggs are birefringent under polarized light, which helps to distinguish them from non-birefringent schistosome eggs.[218]

Schistosomiasis

The public health burden of this parasitic infection is enormous, affecting as it does, 200 million people in 74 countries while continuing to expand its geographic range.[240] The life cycle and disease manifestations of the three major *Shistosoma* spp. (*S. mansoni*, *S haematobium*, and *S. japonicum*) involve eggs, snail intermediate hosts, and free swimming cercaria, which penetrate the skin of susceptible animals and man and develop into adult worms. The male and female worms eventually come to reside in various human venous plexuses, depending on the species, where egg deposition occurs. Pulmonary disease is almost always secondary to severe hepatic involvement with portal hypertension. In this setting, the eggs of *S. mansoni*, and rarely *S. japonicum* or *S. haematobium*, may be shunted through portosystemic collateral veins to the lungs. The eggs lodge in arterioles, provoking a characteristic granulomatous endarteritis with pulmonary symptoms and radiographic infiltrates.[241,242] When the endarteritis is accompanied by angiomatoid changes, the lesion is considered pathognomonic of pulmonary schistosomiasis.[218] Eggs are typically surrounded by epithelioid cells and collagen (Fig. 6.103). Most schistosome eggs lack birefringence and are larger than paragonimus eggs, with which they share a superficial resemblance. Acute larval pneumonitis and a Loeffler-like eosinophilic pneumonia may occur as a manifestation of acute schistosomiasis.[240,243] Adult schistosomes may rarely be found in pulmonary blood vessels.

Cytopathology

The cytologic literature contains many reports of the successful identification of parasites in pulmonary infections recovered by exfoliative (sputum, bronchial washing, brushing, broncholveolar lavage, pleural fluid) and needle aspiration techniques. Some of these are listed

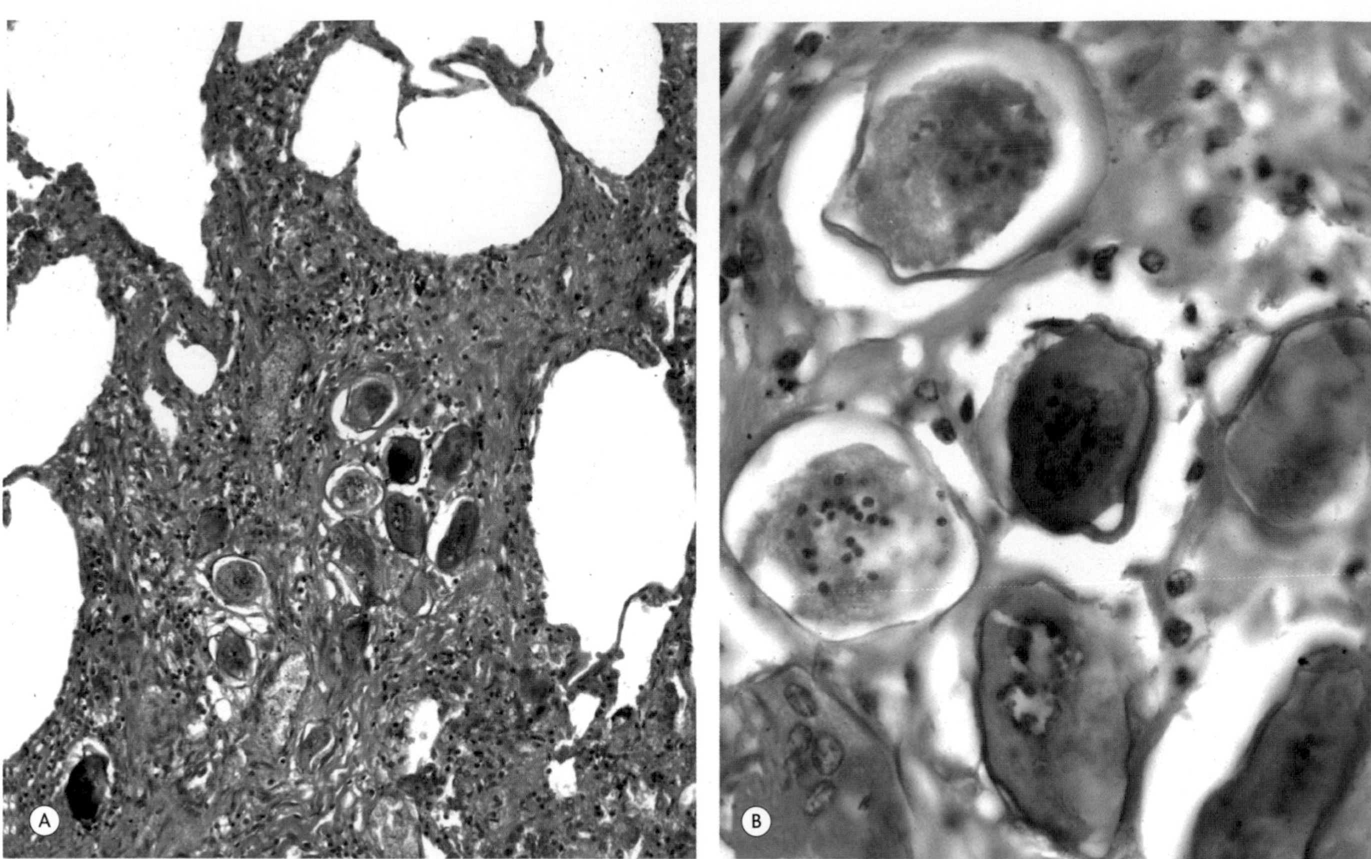

Fig. 6.103 (A) Schistosome eggs in lung parenchyma. (B) Schistosome eggs (*S. japonicum*) (H&E stain). (Courtesy of Ronald Neafi, AFIP, Washington DC.)

in Table 6.37.[237,238,244–259] Cited commonly in textbooks and reviews is the occurrence of *Strongyloides stercoralis* larvae in expectorated sputum or bronchial washings of patients with hyperinfections (Fig. 6.104). Also common, are reports of echinococcus protoscolices and hooklets in needle aspirates from patients with pleuropulmonary disease.[26,27] Although large-bore and cutting needle biopsies have traditionally been contraindicated in the setting of potential echinococcus infections, reports of successful fine-needle aspirates, without untoward reactions, suggests that this is a relatively safe procedure in which the benefits outweigh the risks.[245]

Cytology is a sensitive and often preferred method to diagnose cryptosporidiosis, microsporidiosis, and other respiratory tract infections in the immunocompromised host, as it has the advantage of being less invasive. Specimens such as bronchial washings and BAL fluids can be prepared by high-speed centrifugation followed by standard smear preparation, cytocentrifugation or ThinPrep technology. A battery of special stains, including Gram, modified trichrome, Giemsa, GMS, acid-fast, chemofluorescent, and immunofluorescent, depending on reagent availability, can then be applied to detect cryptosporidial oocysts, microsporidial spores, or other etiologic agents.

The morphologic features of many of the organisms cited above are usually better defined in cytologic prepartions than in tissue biopsies, provided that there is little obscuring background debris and that cytotechnique and staining have been well-performed. Pseudoparasites such as vegetable matter, textile fibers, pollens, red cell

Table 6.37 Parasites reported in respiratory cytology specimens

Toxoplasma
Amoeba
Trichomonas
Cryptosporidia
Microsporidia
Leishmania
Paragonimus
Echinococcus
Strongyloides
Schistosoma
Dirofilaria
Microfilaria

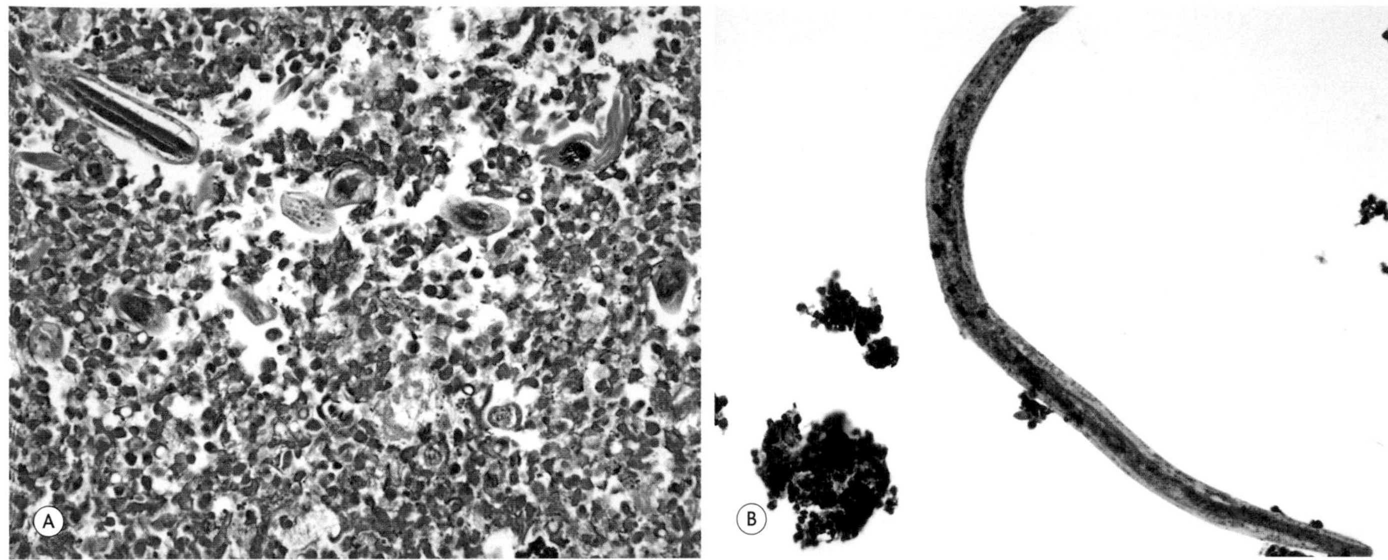

Fig. 6.104 ***Strongyloides stercoralis* larvae in bronchial washing.** (A) ThinPrep smear. (B) Larval fragments in cell block.

ghosts, and other extraneous matter must be recognized and excluded. Thus, as for all of the various categories of microorganisms cited in this chapter, cytopathology adds synergy to surgical pathologic and microbiologic methods.

Microbiology

The laboratory diagnosis of parasitic disease depends on the collection of appropriate specimens, which in turn requires appropriate clinical evaluation. For example, just as stool examination is the most efficient means of diagnosing most intestinal protozoa and helminths, respiratory specimens (e.g. sputum, bronchial washes, bronchoalveolar lavages, and touch imprints of lung biopsies) can provide a specific etiologic diagnosis when pulmonary infections are suspected.[217] As is the case for cytologic samples, these specimens often reveal the characteristic microanatomic features of parasite larvae and eggs that usually cannot be easily seen when they are embedded in tissue. Moreover, the identification of organisms in respiratory specimens is diagnostic of pulmonary infection, whereas the presence of the organism in the feces of a patient suspected of having pulmonary disease provides only presumptive evidence.

Serodiagnosis with immunologic and molecular methods can be useful when parasites are located deep within tissue, such as the lung, and not easily accessible to biopsy or cytologic sampling.[260] Serodiagnosis of parasitic diseases has been plagued by tests with low sensitivity and specificity, mainly as a result of the complex composition of parasitic antigens and the occurrence of frequent cross reactions.[217] However, in recent years, there have been significant refinements in antigenic preparations and improvements in technology, resulting in assays with greater predictive value. The newer tests employ enzyme immunoassay and immunoblot methodology. Many test kits are commercially available and diagnostic services are provided by the Center for Disease Control and Prevention and other reference laboratories.[261] Among protozoal infections, serology is especially useful for the diagnosis of toxoplasmosis. Several commercial kits are available for IgG and IgM antibodies; however, false-negative results can be seen in immunocompromised patients and positive results must be interpreted with caution, especially when the index of suspicion is low.[262] Real-time PCR has been successfully used for the diagnosis of toxoplasmosis in the immunocompromised patient.[262a] Antibody determinations also have value in cases of pulmonary and other tissue invasive forms of amebiasis, as compared to antigen detection methods that are more useful for noninvasive amoebic intestinal diseases. For the cryptosporidia, the new immunofluorescent tests and enzyme immunoassays that have been developed for intestinal infections may have application in respiratory infections. Similar tests are not available for the microsporidia and diagnosis for these organisms continues to rely on direct staining techniques at this time. For the helminths, serodiagnosis is possible for *Echinococcus*, *Paragonimus*, *Strongyloides*, and *Schistosoma* spp., utilizing enzyme immunoassay methods that have fair sensitivity and

Table 6.38 Parasitic pneumonia synopsis

Toxoplasmosis	
Surgical pathology:	Miliary small necroinflammatory nodules with fibrin; fibrinous pneumonia
Cytopathology:	Crescent-shaped tachyzoites, pseudocysts, and true cysts.
Microbiology:	Serologic diagnosis by IFA or EIA. Identification of tachyzoites or pseudocyst in tissue
Amebiasis	
Surgical pathology:	Lung abscess
Cytopathology:	Trophozoite in necroinflammatory debris resembles histiocytes. Confirm with immunohistochemistry
Microbiology:	Identification of trophozoite characteristics. Serologic methods positive in most cases of extraintestinal disease. DNA probes
Cryptosporidiosis	
Surgical pathology:	Bronchitis and/or bronchiolitis with cryptosporidia seen on H&E sections as small, round protrusions along the epithelial surface of the mucosa
Cytopathology:	Red oocysts in smears prepared from bronchial washes and BAL fluid stained with modified acid-fast stains
Microbiology:	Findings on direct examination of specimens similar to cytology. Immunofluorescence and enzyme immunoassay developed for intestinal infection
Microsporidiosis	
Surgical pathology:	Bronchitis and/or bronchiolitis. Small basophilic dots in vacuoles may be visible in H&E sections when burden of organism is heavy; highlighted with Gram and modified trichrome stains; toluidine blue stain plastic sections; electron microscopy
Cytopathology:	Characteristic pink capsule-shaped spores with dark band in modified trichrome stained preparations of BAL fluid. Giemsa, Gram, and chemofluorescent stains also useful
Microbiology:	Findings on direct examination of fluids similar to cytology. Culture in research setting by special arrangement. Molecular methods
Dirofilariasis	
Surgical pathology:	Solitary pulmonary nodule with infarct pattern and worm fragments
Cytopathology:	Intact or fragmented worm in necroinflammatory debris
Microbiology:	Identification of characteristic round worm in tissues. Serology not useful
Strongyloidiasis	
Surgical pathology:	Eosinophilic pneumonia, abscess, Loeffler's syndrome with filariform larvae
Cytopathology:	Filariform larvae in sputum indicates hyperinfection
Microbiology:	Primary diagnostic stage in stool is rhabitiform larvae; filariform larvae may be seen in sputum and lung tissue. Eggs resemble hookworm eggs, but rarely seen
Echinococcosis	
Surgical pathology:	Trilayered cyst with brood capsules containing protoscolices. Fibrous wall forms interface with lung parenchyma; sometimes abscess and granulomas
Cytopathology:	Protoscolices with sucker and hooklets or detached hooklets in granular background debris
Microbiology:	Identification of hooklets and protoscolices in needle aspirates, pleural fluid, and sputum. Serology available
Paragonimoniasis	
Surgical pathology:	Eosinophilic pneumonia. Fibrous pseudocysts containing worms and necroinflammatory debris. Egg granulomas
Cytopathology:	Yellow ovoid birefringent eggs with flattened operculum
Microbiology:	Identification of characteristic egg in sputum or tissue. Serology available
Schistosomiasis	
Surgical pathology:	Granulomatous endarteritis; eggs in epithelioid granulomas
Cytopathology:	Characteristic nonbirefringent, nonoperculated eggs. Presence and position of spine determines species
Microbiology:	Embryonated eggs may be present in feces or urine; not sputum. Serology available

specificity.[261] The available tests for *Dirofilaria* suffer from poor sensitivity and specificity and are not clinically useful at this time.

Differential diagnosis

The key morphologic and microbiologic features of the selected parasitic lung infections are summarized in Table 6.38. In the absence of eggs, larvae, worms, or trophozoa, the various inflammatory patterns must be distinguished from that of other infections and various non-infectious diseases due to toxins, drugs, and such entities as the Churg–Strauss and hypereosinophilic syndromes.[263] Eosinophilic pneumonia, especially, has a varied etiology that includes parasitic infections.[264] False-positive morphologic diagnoses of parasitic infections may be caused by objects resembling parasites,[219,265] such as lentil grains in aspiration pneumonia, pollen grains, and Liesegang rings. These ring-like structures can simulate various types of nematodes.[266] Careful attention to the microanatomy of an apparent foreign body and comparison to parasites illustrated in atlases can often resolve diagnostic dilemmas. Some cases, however, may require referral to pathologists with specialized training and experience in parasitic diseases.

REFERENCES

1. Fauci AS: Infectious diseases: considerations for the 21st century. Clin Infect Dis 2001; 32: 675–685.
2. Chandler F: Approaches to the pathologic diagnosis of infectious diseases. In: Pathology of infectious disease, Connor D, Chandler FW, Schwartz DA, Manz HJ, Lack EE, Eds. 1997, Appleton & Lange, Stamford, CT, pp 3–7.
3. Watts JC: Surgical pathology and the diagnosis of infectious disease. Am J Clin Pathol, 1994; 102: 711–712.
4. Watts JC, Chandler FW: The surgical pathologists role in the diagnosis of infectious disease. J Histotechnol 1995; 18: 191–193.
5. Morales A, et al.: Continuous-specimen-flow, high-throughput, 1-hour tissue processing. Arch Pathol Lab Med 2002; 126: 583–590.
6. Rosati L: The microbe, creator of the pathologist: an interrelated history of pathology, microbiology and infectious disease. Ann Diagn Pathol 2001; 5: 184–189.
7. Woods GL: Role of the clinical microbiologist in the tissue diagnosis of infectious disease. In: Special course. Contemporary diagnostic pathology of infectious diseases. 1996. United States and Canadian Academy of Pathology. Washington, DC.
8. Procop GW, Wilson MR: Infectious disease pathology. Clin Infect Dis 2001; 32: 1589–1601.
9. Braunstein H: The value of microbiologic culture of tissue samples in surgical pathology. Mod Pathol 1989; 2: 217–221.
10. Travis WD: Surgical pathology of pulmonary infections. Semin Thorac Cardiovasc Surg 1995; 7: 81–95.
11. Colby TV, Weiss RL: Current concepts in the surgical pathology of pulmonary infections. Am J Surg Path 1987; 11: 25–37.
12. Dunn DL: Diagnosis and treatment of opportunistic infections in immunocompromised patients. Am Surg 2000; 66: 117–125.
13. Levine SJ: An approach to the diagnosis of pulmonary infections in immunocompromised patients. Semin Respir Infect 1992; 7: 81–95.
14. Dichter JR, Levine SJ, Shellhammer: Approach to the immunocompromised host with pulmonary symptoms. Hematol Oncol Clin North Am 1993; 7: 887–912.
15. Wilson WR, Cockerill FR, Rosenow AC: Pulmonary disease in the immunocompromised host. Mayo Clin Proc 1985; 60: 610–631.
16. Khoor A, Leslie KO, Tazelar HD: Diffuse pulmonary disease caused by nontuberculous mycobacteria in nonimmunocompromised people. Am J Clin Pathol 2001; 115: 755–762.
17. Colby TV, Swanson SJ: Anatomic distribution and histopathologic patterns in diffuse lung disease:correlation with HRCT. J Thoracic Imag 1996; 11: 1–26.
18. Woods GL, Walker DH: Detection of infection or infectious agents by use of cytologic and histologic stains. Clin Micro Rev 1996; 9: 382–404.
19. Mantone KT, Park C: In situ hybridization with oligonucleotide probes: application to infectious agent detection. In: Advances in pathology. 1996, Mosby-Year Book, London, pp 329–357.
20. Wolk D, Mitchell S, Patel R: Principles of molecular microbiology testing methods. Infect Dis Clin N Am 2001; 15: 1157–1204.
21. Cockerill F, Smith T: Rapid-cycle real-time PCR: a revolution for clinical microbiology. ASM News 2002; 68: 77–83.
22. Cartun RW: Use of immunohistochemistry in the surgical pathology laboratory for the diagnosis of infectious disease. Pathol Case Rev 1999; 4: 260–265.
23. Kaufman L, Valero G, Padhye AA: Misleading manifestations of *Coccidioides immitis* in vivo. J Clin Microbiol 1998; 36: 3721–3723.
24. Liu K, Howell DN, Perfect JR: Morphologic criteria for the identification of species of fusarium, paecilomyces and acremonium by histopathology. Am J Clin Pathol, 1998; 109: 45–48.
25. Gorelkin L, Chandler F: Pseudomicrobes: some potential diagnostic pitfalls in the histopathologic assessment of inflammatory lesions. Human Path 1988; 19: 954–959.
26. Powers CN: Diagnosis of infectious disease: a cytopathologists perspective. Clin Micro Rev 1998; 11: 341–365.
27. Johnston WW, Elson CE: Respiratory tract. In: Comprehensive cytopathology, Bibbo M, Ed. 1991, WB Saunders: Philadelphia, pp 340–352.
28. DeMay RM: A micromiscellany. In: The art and science of cytopathology. Exfoliative cytology, DeMay RM, Ed. 1996, ASCP Press, Chicago, pp 53–58.
29. Silverman JF, Gay RM: Fine-needle aspiration and surgical pathology of infectious lesions: morphologic features and the role of the clinical microbiology laboratory for rapid diagnosis. Clin Lab Med 1995; 15: 251–278.
30. Crapanzano JP, Zakowski MF: Diagnostic dilemmas in pulmonary cytology. Cancer (Cyopathology), 2001; 93(6): 364–375.
31. Fang G, Fine M, Orloff J: New and emerging etiologies for community-acquired pneumonia with implications for therapy. Medicine 1990; 69: 307–316.
32. Ruiz-Gonzalez A, Falquera M. Nogues A: Is *Streptococcus pneumoniae* the leading cause of pneumonia of unknown etiology? A microbiologic study of lung aspirates in consecutive patients with community acquired pneumonia. Am J Med 1999; 106: 385–390.
33. Reimer LG: Community-acquired bacterial pneumonia. Semin Respir Infect 2000; 15: 95–100.
34. Travis WD, Colby TV, Koss MN: Lung infections. In: Non-neoplastic disorders of the lower respiratory tract. Atlas of non tumor pathology, King DW, Ed., Vol. 2. 2002, American Registry of Pathology Washington, DC, pp 539–728.
35. McIntosh K: Community-acquired pneumonia in children. N Engl J Med 2002; 346: 429–436.
36. Pennigton JE: Hospital acquired pneumonia. In Respiratory infections. Diagnosis and management, Pennington JE, Ed. 1994, Raven Press, New York, pp 207–227.

37a. Bonifacio SL, Kitterman JA, Ursell PC: Pseudomonas pneumonia in infants. An autopsy study. Human Pathol 2003; 34: 929–938.

37. Mayer J: Laboratory diagnosis of nosocomial pneumonia. Semin Respir Infect 2000; 15: 119–131.
38. Baselski V, Mason K: Pneumonia in the immunocompromised host: the role of bronchoscopy and newer diagnostic techniques. Semin Respir Infect 2000; 15: 144–161.
39. Hindizeh M, Carroll KC: Laboratory diagnosis of atypical pneumonia. Semin Respir Infect 2000; 15: 101–113.
40. Chandler F, Connor D: Actinomycosis. In: Pathology of infectious disease, Chandler F, Connor D, Schwartz D, Eds. 1997, Appleton & Lange, Stamford, CT, pp 391–396.
41. de Montpreville VT, Nashashibi N, Dulmet EM: Actinomycosis and other bronchopulmonary infections with bacterial granules. Ann Diagn Pathol 1999; 3: p. 67–74.
42. Kuhn C: Bacterial infections. In: Pathology of the lung, Thurlbeck W, Churg AM, Eds. 1995, Thieme Medical Publishers: New York, pp 267–302.
43. Winn WC, Chandler FC: Bacterial infections. In: Pulmonary pathology, D. DH and H. SP, Eds. 1994, Springer-Verlag, New York. pp 255–330.
44. Hazelton PS: Pulmonary bacterial infection: in Spencer's pathology of the lung, Hazelton PS, Ed. 1996, McGraw Hill, New York, pp 189–256.
45. Colby TV, Lombard CM, Sousen SA: Atlas of pulmonary pathology. 1991, WB Saunders, Philadelphia.
46. Kwon KY, Colby TV: *Rhodococcus equi* pneumonia and pulmonary malakoplakia in acquired immunodeficiency syndrome. Arch Pathol Lab Med 1994; 118: 744–748.
47. Verma P: Laboratory diagnosis of anaerobic pleuropulmonary infections. Semin Respir Infect 2000; 15: 114–118.
48. Corley DE, Winderbaust RH: Infectious diseases that result in slowly resolving chronic pneumonia. Semin Respir Infect 1993; 8: 3-13.
49. Belchis DA, Simpson E, Colby TV: Histopathologic features of *Burkholderia cepacia* pneumonia in patients without cystic fibrosis. Mod Pathol 2000; 13: 369–372.
50. Hayden RT, Uhl JR, Hopkins MK: Direct detection of *Legionella* species from bronchoalveolar lavage and open biopsy specimens: comparison of light cycler PCR, insitu hybridization, direct immunoflorescence, antigen detection and culture. J Clin Microbiol 2001; 39: 2618–2626.

51. Rolands S, Colby TV, Clayton F: Open lung biopsy in *Mycoplasma pneumoniae* pneumonia. Arch Pathol Lab Med 1986: 110: 34–41.
52. Oddo D, Gonzales S: Actinomycosis and nocardiosis: a morphologic study of 17 cases. Pathol Res Pract 1986; 181: 320–326.
53. Bush L, Abrams BH, Beal A: Index case of inhalational anthrax due to bioterrorism in the United States. N Engl J Med 2001; 345: 1607–1610.
54. Borio L, Frank D, Mani V: Death due to bioterrorism-related inhalational anthrax. JAMA 2001; 286: 2554–2560.
55. Ingelsby T, Dennis DT, Henderson DA: Anthrax as a biologic weapon. JAMA 1999; 281: 1735–1746.
56. Grinberg L, Abramova FA, Yampolska OV: Quantitative pathology of inhalational anthrax I: quantitative microscopic findings. Mod Pathol 2001; 14: 482–495
57. Barakat L, Quentzel LA, Jerigan DL: Fatal inhalational anthrax in a 94-year-old Connecticut woman. JAMA 2002; 287: 863–868.
58. Ingelsby T, Dennis DT, Henderson DA: Plague as a biological weapon. JAMA 2000; 283: 2281–2291.
59. Smith J, Reisner B: Plague. In: Pathology of infectious disease, Connor DH, et al., Eds. 1997, Appleton & Lange, Stamford, CT, pp 729–738.
60. Dennis D, Meier F (eds): Plague. Pathology of emerging infection, Horsburgh CR, Nelson A, Eds. 1997, ASM Press, Washington, DC, pp 21–45.
61. Guarner J, Wun-Ju S, Greer P: Immunohistochemical detection of *Yersinia pestis* in formalin-fixed, paraffin-embedded tissue. Am J Clin Pathol 2002; 117: 205–209.
62. Dennis D, Ingelsby TV, Henderson DA: Tularemia as a biologic weapon. JAMA 2001; 285: 2763–2773.
63. Geyer S, Burkey A, Chandler F: Tularemia. Pathology of infectious disease, Connor D, Chandler FW, Schwartz DA, Manz HJ, Lack EE, Eds. 1997, Appleton & Lange, Stamford, CT, pp 869–873.
64. Grinan NP, Lucerna FM, Romero JV: Yield of percutaneous needle aspiration in lung abcess. Chest 1990; 97: 69–74.
65. Yang PC, Luk KT, Lee YC: Lung abscess: US-guided transthoracic aspiration. Radiology 1991; 180: 171–175.
66. Vuori-Holopainen E, Salo E, Saxon H: Etiological diagnosis of childhood pneumonia by use of transthoracic needle aspiration and modern microbiologic methods. Clin Infect Dis 2002; 34: 583–590.
67. Bartlett RC: Medical microbiology: how far to go – how fast to go in 1982. In: Significance of medical microbiology in the care of patients, Lorian V, Ed. 1982, Williams and Wilkins: Baltimore, pp 12–44.
68. Busmanis I, Harvey M, Hellyar A: Nocardiosis diagnosed by FNA: a case report. Diagn Cytopathol 1995; 12: 56–58.
69. Saubolle M, McKeller P: Laboratory diagnosis of community-acquired lower respiratory tract infection. Infect Dis Clin N Am 2001; 15: 1025–1045.
70. Carroll KC: Laboratory diagnosis of lower respiratory tract infections: controversy and conundrums. J Clin Microbiol 2002; 40: 3115–3120.
71. Barrett-Connor E: The nonvalue of sputum culture in the diagnosis of pneumococcal pneumonia. Am Rev Resp Dis 1970; 103: 845–848.
72. Society AT: Guidelines for the initial management of adults with community-acquired pneumonia: diagnosis, assessment of severity and initial antimicrobial therapy. Am Rev Resp Dis 1993; 148: 1418–1426.
73. Bartlett J, Brieman JG, Mandell IA: Community-acquired pneumonia in adults: guidelines for management. Clin Infect Dis 1998; 26: 811–838.
74. Danes C, Gonzales-Martin J, Pumarola T: Pulmonary infiltrates in immunosuppressed patients: analysis of a diagnostic protocol. J Clin Microbiol 2002; 40: 2134–2140.
75. Ellis J, Broun JM, Steigerwalt AG: Tularemia. Clin Micro Rev 2002; 15: 631–646.
76. Conville P, et al.: *Nocardia veterana* as a pathogen in North American patients. J Clin Microbiol 2003; 41: 2560–2568.
77. Petitjean J, Vabret A, Gourin VS: Evaluation of four commercial immunoglobulin G (IgG) and IgM-specific enzyme immunoassays for the diagnosis of *Mycoplasma pneumoniae* infections. J Clin Microbiol 2002; 40: 165–171.
78. Fields B, Benson R, Besser R: *Legionella* and Legionaires' disease: 25 years of investigation. Clin Micro Rev 2002; 15: 506–526.
79. Muder R, Yu V: Infection due to *Legionella* species other than *L. pneumophila*. Clin Infect Dis 2002; 35: 990–998.
80. Benin A, Benson R, Besser R: Trends in Legionnaires disease, 1980–1998: declining mortality and new patterns of diagnosis. Clin Infect Dis 2002; 35: 1039–1046.
81. Waring AL, Tanga A, Hulse CK: Development of a genomics-based PCR assay for detection of mycoplasma pneumonias in a large outbreak in New York State. J Clin Microbiol 2001; 39: 1385–1390.
82. Reischl U, et al.: Direct detection and differentiation of *Legionella* spp. and *Legionella pneumophilia* in clinical specimens by dual-color real-time PCR and melting curve analysis. J Clin Microbiol 2002; 40: 3814–3417.
83. Krafft A, Kulesh D: Applying molecular biologic techniques to detection biologic agents. Clin Lab Med 2001; 21: 631–660.
84. Wittwer C, Hermann M, Gundry C: Real time multiplex assays. Methods 2001; 25: 430–442.
85. Gardiner DF, Beavis KG: Laboratory diagnosis of mycobacterial infections. Semin Respir Infect 2000; 15: 132–143.
86. American Thoracic Society: Diagnosis and treatment of disease caused by nontuberculous mycobacteria. Am J Crit Care Med 1997; 156: S1–25.
86a. Van Dyke P, Van Hoenacker FM, Van den Brande P, De Schepper AM: Imaging of pulmonary tuberculosis. Eur Radiol 2003; 13: 1771–1785.
87. Allen EA: Tuberculosis and other mycobacterial infections of the lung. In: Pathology of the lung, Thurlbeck WM, Churg AM, Eds. 1995, Thieme Medical Publisher, New York, pp 229–265.
88. Hruban RH, Hutchin GM: Mycobacterial infections. In: Pulmonary pathology, Dail DH, Hammer SP, Eds. 1994, Springer-Verlag, New York, pp 331–350.
88a. Barnes PF, Cave D: Molecular epidemiology of tuberculosis. N Engl J Med 2003; 12: 1149–1156.
89. Lack EE, Connor CH: Tuberculosis. In: Pathology of infectious disease, Connor DH, et al., Eds. 1997, Appleton & Lange, Stamford, CT, pp 857–868.
90. Small PM, Fujiwara PI: Management of tuberculosis in the United States. N Engl J Med 2001; 345: 189–200.
91. Tortoli E: Impact of genotypic studies on mycobacterial taxonomy: the new mycobacteria of the 1990s. Clin Micro Rev 2003; 16: 319–354.
91a. Primm TP, Lucero CA, Falkinham JO: Health impacts of environmental myobacteria. Clin Micro Rev. 2004; 17: 98–106.
92. Prince DS, Damster B, Gribetz A: Infection with *Mycobacterium avium* complex in patients without predisposing conditions. N Engl J Med 1989; 321: 863–868.
93. Marchevesky A, Damster B, Gribetz A: The spectrum of pathology of nontuberculous mycobacterial infection in open-lung biopsy specimens. Am J Clin Pathol 1982; 78: 755–700.
94. Tang Y, Procop GW, Zeng X: Histologic parameters predictive of mycobacterial infection. Am J Clin Pathol 1998; 109: 321–324.
95. Hoheisel G, Chan BKM, Chan CHS: Endobronchial tuberculosis: diagnosotic features and theraputic outcome. Respir Med 1994; 88: 593–597.
96. Bloch KC, Zwerling L, Pletcher MJ: Incidence and clinical implications of isolation of *Mycobacterium kansasii*: result of a five-year population based study. Ann Intern Med 1998; 129: 698–704.
97. Rotterdam H: *Mycobacterium avium* complex infection. Pathology of Infectious Disease, Connor DH, et al., Eds. 1997, Appleton & Lange, Stamford, CT.
98. Horsburgh CR: *Mycobacterium avium* complex infection in the acquired immunodeficiency syndrome. N Engl J Med 1991; 324: 332–338.
99. Kwon K, Meyers J, Swensen S: Middle lobe syndrome. a clinicopathologic study of 21 patients. Human Path 1995; 26: 302–307.
100. Sekosan M, Cleto M, Senseng C: Spindle cell pseudotumors in the lungs due to *Mycobacterium tuberculosis* in a transplant patient. Am J Surg Path 1994; 18:1065–1068.
101. Brown-Elliott B, Wallace R: Clinical and taxonomic status of pathogenic nonpigmented or late-pigmenting rapidly growing mycobacteria. Clin Micro Rev 2002; 15: 716–746.
102. Das DK: Fine needle aspiration cytology in the diagnosis of tuberculous lesions. Lab Med 2000; 31: 625–632.
103. Dalgren SE, Eastrom P: Aspiration cytology in the diagnosis of pulmonary tuberculosis. Scand J Respir Dis 1972; 53: 196–201.
104. Smith M, Molina CP, Schnadig VJ: Pathologic features of *Mycobacterium kansasii* infection in patients with acquired immunodeficiency syndrome. Arch Pathol Lab Med 2003; 127: 554–560.
105. Zerbi P, Schoonau A, Bonetto S: Amplified in situ hybridization with peptide nucleic acid probes for differentiation of *Mycobacterium tuberculosis* complex and nontuberculous mycobacterium species on

formalin-fixed, paraffin-embedded archival biopsy and autopsy samples. Am J Clin Pathol 2001; 116: 770–775.

106. Hardman WJ, Benian GM, Howard T: Rapid detection of mycobacteria in inflammatory necrotizing granulomas from formalin-fixed, paraffin-embedded tissues by PCR in clinically high risk patients with acid-fast and culture negative tissue biopsies. Am J Clin Pathol 1996; 106: 384–389.
107. Park D, Kim JX, Choi KU: Comparison of polymerase chain reaction with histopathologic features for diagnosis of tuberculosis in formalin-fixed, paraffin-embedded histologic specimens. Arch Pathol Lab Med 2003; 2003: 326–330.
108. Renshaw AA: The relative sensitivity of special stains and culture in open lung biopsies. Am J Clin Pathol 1994; 102: 736–740.
109. O'Sullivan C, Miller DM, Schneider PS: Evaluation of Gen-Probe amplified *Mycobacterium tuberculosis* direct test by using respiratory and nonrespiratory specimens in a tertiary care laboratory. J Clin Microbiol 2002; 40: 1723–1727.
110. Bemer P, Palicova F, Rush-Gerdes S: Multicenter evaluation of fully automated BACTEC mycobacteria growth indicator tube 960 system for susceptibility testing of *Mycobacterium tuberculosis*. J Clin Microbiol 2002; 40: 150–154.
111. Woods GL: Molecular techniques in mycobacterial detection. Arch Pathol Lab Med 2001; 125: 122–126.
112. Hasegawa N, Miura T, Ishii K: New simple and rapid test for culture confirmation of *Mycobacterium tuberculosis* complex: a multicenter study. J Clin Microbiol 2002; 40: 908–912.
113. Al Zahrani K, Al Jahdali H, Poirer L: Accuracy and utility of commercially available amplification and serologic tests for the diagnosis of mimimal pulmonary tuberculosis. Am J Respir Crit Care Med 2000; 162: 1323–1329.
114. Schluger NW: Changing approaches to the diagnosis of tuberculosis. Am J Respir Crit Care Med 2001; 164: 2020–2024.
115. Sobonya RE: Fungal disease, including allergic bronchopulmonary aspergillosis, 2nd edn. Pathology of the lung, Thurlbeck WM, Churg AM, Eds. 1995, Thieme Medical Publisher, New York, pp 303–331.
116. Saubolle M: Fungal pneumonias. Semin Respir Infect 2000; 15: 162–177.
117. Chandler F, Watts JC: Pathologic diagnosis of fungus infections. 1987, ASCP Press, Chicago.
118. Watts JC, Chandler F: Morphologic identification of mycelial pathogens in tissue sections. a caveat. Am J Clin Pathol 1998; 109: 1–2.
119. Lemos LB, Baliga M, Guo M: Blastomycosis: the great pretender can also be an opportunist. Initial clinical diagnosis and underlying disease in 123 patients. Ann Diagn Pathol 2002; 6: 194–203.
120. Chandler FC: Blastomycosis. In: Pathology of infectious diseases, Connor D, Chandler FW, Schwartz DA, Manz HJ, Lack EE, Eds. 1997, Appleton & Lange, Stamford, CT, pp 943–951.
121. Lemos LB, Balugh M, Go M: Acute respiratory distress syndrome and blastomycosis. Presentation of nine cases and review of the literature. Ann Diagn Pathol 2001; 5: 1–9.
122. Lemos LB, Go M, Balugh M: Blastomycosis: organ involvement and etiologic diagnosis. A review of 123 patients from Mississipppi. Ann Diagn Pathol 2000; 4: 391–406.
123. Hussain Z, Martin A, Youngberg GA: *Blastomyces dermatitidis* with large yeast forms. Arch Pathol Lab Med 2001; 125: 663–664.
124. Fisher M, Koenig TJ, White JW: Molecular and phenotypic description of *Coccidioides posadasii* sp nov., previously recognized as the non-California population of *Coccidioides immitis*. Mycologia 2002; 94: 73–84.
125. Pappagianis D, Chandler FC: *Coccidioidomycosis*. In: Pathology of infectious diseases, Connor D, Chandler FW, Schwartz DA, Manz HJ, Lack EE, Eds. 1997, Appleton & Lange, Stamford, CT, pp 977–987.
126. DiTomasso JP, Angel NM, Roe JD: Bronchoscopic diagnosis of pulmonary coccidioidomycosis. Diagn Infect Dis 1994; 18: 83–87.
127. Polesky A, Kirsch CM, Snyder LS: Airway coccidioidomycosis. Clin Infect Dis 1999; 28: 1273–1280.
128. Wheat J: Endemic mycoses in AIDS: a clinical review. Clin Micro Rev 1995; 8: 146–159.
129. Goodwin RA, Shapiro JL, Thurman GH: Disseminated histoplasmosis. Medicine 1980; 59: 1–33.
130. Chandler FC, Watts JC: *Histoplasmosis capsulati*. In: Pathology of infectious diseases, Connor D, Chandler FW, Schwartz DA, Manz HJ, Lack EE, Eds. 1997, Appleton & Lange, Stamford, CT, pp 1007–1015.
131. Londero AT, Chandler FW: Paracoccidioidomycosis. In: Pathology of infectious diseases, Connor D, Chandler FW, Schwartz DA, Manz HJ, Lack EE, Eds. 1997, Appleton & Lange, Stamford, CT, pp 1045–1053.
132. England DM, Hochholzer L: Primary pulmonary sporotrichosis. Am J Surg Path 1985; 9: 193–204.
133. Deng Z, Connor DH: Progressive disseminated penicilliosis caused by *Penicillium marneffei*: report of eight cases and differentiation of the causative organism from *Histoplasma capsulatum*. Am J Clin Pathol 1985; 84: 323–327.
134. McGinnis MR, Chandler FC: *Penicilliosis marneffei*. In: Pathology of infectious diseases, Connor D, Chandler FW, Schwartz DA, Manz HJ, Lack EE, Eds. 1997, Appleton & Lange, Stamford, CT, pp 1055–1058.
135. Mark EJ: Case records of the Massachusetts General Hospital. N Engl J Med 2002; 347: 518–524.
136. Menefee J, Hutchins GM: Pulmonary cryptococcosis. Human Path 1985; 16: 121–128.
137. Luna MA: Candidiasis. In: Pathology of infectious diseases, Connor D, Chandler FW, Schwartz DA, Manz HJ, Lack EE, Eds. 1997, Appleton & Lange, Stamford, CT, pp 953–964.
138. Alasio T, Lento P, Bottone E: Giant blastoconidia of *Candida albicans*. Arch Pathol Lab Med 2003; 127: 868–871.
139. Latge J: *Aspergillus fumigatus* and aspergillosis. Clin Micro Rev 1999; 12: 310–350.
140. Bosken CH, Meyers JL. Greenberger PA: Pathologic features of allergic bronchopulmonary aspergillosis. Am J Surg Path 1988; 12: 216–222.
141. Yousem SA: The histopathologic spectrum of chronic necrotizing forms of pulmonary aspergillosis. Human Path 1997; 28: 650–656.
142. Scully RE, Mank EJ, McNeeley WJ: Case records of the Massachusetts General Hospital, Case 24-2001. N Engl J Med 2001; 345: 443–449.
143. Tadros TS, et al.: Pathology of hyalohyphomycosis caused by *Scedosporium apiospermum* (*Pseudoallescheria boydii*): an emerging mycosis. Human Path 1998; 29: 1266–1272.
144. Boutati E, Anaissie E: Fusarium, a significant emerging pathogen in patients with hematologic malignancy: ten years experience at a cancer center and implications for management. Blood 1997; 90: 999–1008.
145. Guarro J, Gene J: Developments in fungal taxonomy. Clin Micro Rev 1999; 12: 454–500.
146. Ribes J, Vanover-Sams C, Baker D: Zygomycetes in human disease. Clin Micro Rev 2000; 13: 236–301.
147. Irwin R, Rinaldi M, Walsh T: *Zygomycosis* of the respiratory tract. In: Fungal diseases of the lung, 3rd edn, Sarosi S, Davies S, Ed. 2000, Lippincott, Williams & Wilkins, Philadelphia, pp 163–185.
148. Hanson LA, Prakash UBS, Colby TV: Pulmonary complications in diabetes mellitus. Mayo Clin Proc 1989; 64: 791–799.
149. Frater JL, Hall GS, Procop GW: Histologic features of zygomycosis. Emphasis on perineural invasion and fungal morphology. Arch Pathol Lab Med 2001; 125: 375–378.
150. Kimura M: Chlamydoconidia formation in zygomycosis due to *Rhizopus* species. Arch Pathol Lab Med 1998; 122: 1120–1122.
151. Lake FR, Froudist JH, McAleer R: Allergic bronchopulmonary fungal disease caused by *Bipolaris* and *Curvularia*. Aust NZ Med 1991; 21: 871–874.
152. Travis WD, Kwon-Chung KJ, Kleiner DE: Unusual aspects of allergic bronchpulmonary fungal disease: a report of two cases due to *Curvularia* organisms associated with allergic fungal sinusitis. Human Path 1991; 22: 1240–1248.
153. Stringer J, Beard CB, Miller RF: A new name (*Pneumocystis jiroveci*) for pneumocystis from hemans. Emerg Infect Dis 2002; 8(9): 891–896.
154. Zahar J, Pattaluga S, Lipschik GY: *Pneumocystis carinii* pneumonia in critically ill patients with malignancy. Clin Infect Dis 2002; 35: 929–934.
155. Schliep TC: *Pneumocystis pneumonia*. Semin Respir Infect 1999; 14: 333–343.
156. Travis WD, et al.: Atypical pathologic manifestations of *Pneumocystis carinii* in the acquired immunodeficiency syndrome. Am J Surg Path 1990; 14: 615–625.
157. Hartz JW, Geisinger RK, Schalryj M (Cherl): Granulomatous pneumocystosis presenting as a solitary pulmonary nodule. Arch Pathol Lab Med 1985; 106: 466–469.
158. Couples JB, Blackie SP, Roe JD: Granulomatous *Pneumocystis carinii* pneumonia mimicking tuberculosis. Arch Pathol Lab Med 1989; 113: 1281–1284.
159. Liaw Y, Yang PC, Yu C: Direct determination of cryptococcal antigen

in transthoracic needle aspirate for diagnosis of pulmonary cryptococcosis. J Clin Microbiol 1995; 53: 1588–1591.
160. Raab SS, Silverman JF, Zimmerman KG: Fine needle aspiration biopsy of pulmonary coccidioidomycosis: spectrum of cytologic findings in 73 patients. Am J Clin Pathol 1993; 99: 582–587.
161. Zimmerman RL, Montone KT, Fogt F: Ultra fast identification of *Aspergillus* species in pulmonary cytology specimens by in situ hybridization. Int J Mol Med 2000; 5: 427–429.
162. Aubry M, Frasier R: The role of bronchial biopsy and washings in the diagnosis of allergic bronchopulmonary aspergillosis. Mod Pathol 1998; 11: 607–610.
163. Kimura M, McGinnis MR: Fontana–Masson stained tissue from culture-proven mycoses. Arch Pathol Lab Med 1998; 122: 1107–1111.
164. Monheit J, Cowan D, Moore D: Rapid detection of fungi in tissues using calcofluor white and fluorescence microscopy. Arch Pathol Lab Med 1984; 108: 616–619.
165. Bialek R, Ernst F, Dietz K: Comparison of staining methods and a nested PCR assay to detect *Histoplasma capsulatum* in tissue sections. Am J Clin Pathol 2002; 117: 597–603.
166. Rosner E, Reiss E, Warren NG: Evaluation of the status of laboratory practices and the need for continuing education in medical mycology. Am J Clin Pathol 2002; 118: 278–286.
167. Perfect JR, Cox GM, Lee JY: The impact of culture isolation of *Aspergillus* species: a hospital-based survey of aspergillosis. Clin Infect Dis 2001; 33: 1824–1833.
168. Yeo S, Wong B: Current status of nonculture methods for diagnosis of invasive fungal infections. Clin Micro Rev 2002; 15: 465–484.
169. Tarrand J, Lichterfeld M, Warraich I: Diagnosis of invasive septate mold infections. Am J Clin Pathol 2003; 119: 854–858.
170. Moskowitz L, Ganjei P, Ziegels-Weissman J: Immunohistologic identification of fungi in systemic and cutaneous mycoses. Arch Pathol Lab Med 1986; 110: 433–436.
170a. Choi JK, Mauger J, McGowan KL: Immunohistochemical detection of aspergillus species in pediatric tissue samples. Am J Clin 2004; 121: 18–25.
171. Hayden RT, Roberts CD, Lloyd RV: In situ hybridization for the identification of yeastlike organism in tissue section. Diagn Molec Pathol 2001; 10: 15–23.
172. Sandhu GS, Kline BC, Stockman L: Molecular probes for diagnosis of fungal infections. J Clin Microbiol 1995; 33: 2913–2919.
173. Lindsley, MD, Hurst SF, Iqbal NJ: Rapid identification of dimorphic and yeast-like fungal pathogens using specific DNA probes. J Clin Microbiol 2001; 39: 3505–3511.
174. Pham A, Tarrand JJ, May GS: Diagnosis of invasive mold infection by real-time quantitative PCR. Am J Clin Pathol 2003; 119: 38–44.
175. Wheat LJ: Serologic diagnosis of fungal disease. In: Fungal disease of the lung, Sarosi G, Davies S, Eds. 2000, Lippincott, Williams & Wilkins: Philadelphia, pp 17–29.
176. Wheat J: Laboratory diagnosis of histoplasmosis. Semin Respir Infect 2001; 16: 141–148.
176a. Kwak EJ, Husain S, Obman A et al.: Efficacy of galactomannan antigen in the platelia aspergillus enzyme immunoassay for diagnosis of invasive aspergillosis in liver transplant patients . J Clin Microbiol 2004; 42: 435–438.
176b. Challier S, Boyer S, Abachin E, et al.: Development of a serum-based Taqman real-time PCK assay for diagnosis of invasive aspergillosis. J Clin microbiol 2004; 42: 844–846.
177. Pappagianis D, Zimmer BL: Serology of coccidioidomycosis. Clin Micro Rev 1990; 3: 247–268.
178. Treanor J: Respiratory infections. In: Clinical virology, Richman DD, Whitley RJ, Hayden RT, Eds. 1997, Churchhill-Livingstone, New York, pp 5–34.
179. Storch GA: Diagnostic virology. Clin Infect Dis 2000; 31: 739–751.
180. Rabella N, Rodriquez P, Labeaga R: Conventional respiratory viruses recovered from immunocompromised patients: clinical considerations. Clin Infect Dis 1999; 28: 1043–1048.
181. Malherbe HH, Strickland-Cholmley M: Viral cytopathology. 1980, CRC Press, Boca Raton, FL.
182. Fields BN, Knipe DM: Virology. 1990, Raven Press, New York.
183. Anjuna V, Colby TV: Pathologic features of lung biopsy specimens from influenza pneumonia cases. Human Path 1994; 25: 47–53.
184. Guarner J, Wem-Ja S, Dawson J: Immunohistochemical and in situ hybridization studies of influenza A infection in human lungs. Am J Clin Pathol 2000; 114: 227–233.
185. Hall CB: Respiratory syncytial virus and parainfluenza virus. N Engl J Med 2001; 344: 1917–1928.
186. Falsey A, Formica M, Walsh E: Diagnosis of respiratory syncytial virus infection: comparison of reverse transcription-PCR to viral culture and serology in adults with respiratory infection. J Clin Microbiol 2002; 40: 817–820.
187. Griffin M, Coffey CS, Meezil KM: Winter viruses. Influenza and respiratory syncytial virus-related morbidity in chronic lung disease. Arch Intern Med 2002; 162: 1229–1236.
188. Krinzman S, Basgoz N, Kardin R: Respiratory syncytial virus-associated infections in adults and adult recipients of solid organ transplants. J Heart Lung Transplant 1998; 17: 202–210.
189. Miller R: Viral infections of the respiratory tract. In: Pathology of the lung, Thurlbeck W, Churg AM, Eds. 1995, Thieme Medical Publishers: New York, pp 195–222.
189a. Williams JV, Harris PA, Tollefson BA et al.: Human metapneumovirus and lower respiratory tract disease in otherwise healthy infants and children. N Engl J Med 2004; 350: 443–450.
190. Nolte KB, Fedderman RM, Foucar K: Hantavirus pulmonary syndrome in the United States: a pathologic description of a disease caused by a new agent. Human Path 1995; 26: 110–120.
191. Colby TV, Zaki SR, Fedderman RM: Hantavirus pulmonary syndrome is distinguishable from acute interstitial pneumonia. Arch Pathol Lab Med 2000; 14: 1463–1466.
192. Koster F, Foucar K, Hjelle B: Rapid presumptive diagnosis of hantavirus cardiopulmonary syndrome by peripheral blood smear review. Am J Clin Pathol 2001; 116: 665–672.
193. Peters C, Khan A: Hantavirus pulmonary syndrome: the new American hemorrhagic fever. Clin Infect Dis 2002; 34: 1224–1231.
194. MacIntosh K: Coronaviruses. In: Clinical virology, R. DD, W. RJ, and H. FG, Eds. 1997, Churchhill-Livingstone, New York, pp 1123–1130.
195. Falsey A, Walch E, Hayden F: Rhinovirus and Coronavirus infection-associated hospitalization among older adults. J Infect Dis 2002; 185: 1338–1341.
196. Wenzel R, Edmund M: Managing SARS amidst uncertainty. N Engl J Med 2003; 348: 1947–1950.
197. Ksiazek T, Erdman M, Goldsmith C: A novel coronavirus associated with severe acute respiratory syndrome. N Engl J Med 2003; 348: 1953–1966.
198. Booth C, Marukas L, Tomlinson G: Clinical features and short-term outcomes of 144 patients with SARS in the greater Toronto area. JAMA 2003; 289: 2801–2809.
199. Lee N, Hui D, Leu A: A major outbreak of severe acute respiratory syndrome in Hong Kong. N Engl J Med 2003; 348: 1986–1994.
199a. Chow K-C. Hsiao C-H, Lin T-Y et al.: Detection of severe acute respiratory syndrome-associated coronavirus in pneumocytes of the lung. Am J Clin Pathol 2004; 121(4): 574–580.
200. Ohori NP, Michaels MG, Jaffee R: Adenovirus pneumonia in lung transplant recipients. Human Path 1995; 26: 1073–1079.
200a. Pham TT, Burchette JL, Hale LP: Fatal disseminated adenovirus infection in immunocompromised patients. Am J Clin Pathol. 2003; 120: 575–583.
201. Landry ML: Multiple viral infections in the immunocompromised host: recognition and interpretation. Clin Diagn Virol 1994; 2: 313–321.
202. Schooley R, Carey RW, Miller G: Chronic Epstein–Barr virus infection associated with fever and interstitial pneumonitis. Ann Intern Med 1986; 104: 636–643.
203. Wick M, Woronzoff-Dashkoff K, McGlennen R: The molecular characterization of fatal infectious mononucleosis. Am J Clin Pathol 2002; 117: 582–588.
204. Buchanan AJ, Gupta RK: Cytomegalovirus infection of the lung. Cytomorphologic diagnosis by fine needle aspiration cytology. Diagn Cytopathol 1986; 2: 341–342.
205. Feldman P, Covell J: Fine needle aspiration cytology and its clinical applications: breast and lung. 1985, American Society of Clinical Pathology, Chicago.
206. Leland DS, Immanuel D: Laboratory diagnosis of viral infections of the lung. Semin Respir Infect 1995; 10: 189–198.
207. Barenfanger J, Drake C, Leon N: Clinical and financial benefits of rapid detection of respiratory viruses: an outcome study. J Clin Microbiol 2000; 38: 2824–2828.
208. Montone KT, Park C: In situ hybridization with oligonucleotide probes: applications to infectious agent detection. 1996, Mosby Year Book, St Louis, pp 329–357.

209. Payne C: Electron microscopy in the diagnosis of infectious diseases. In: Pathology of infectious diseases, Connor D, Chandler FW, Schwartz DA, Manz HJ, Lack EE, Eds. 1997, Appleton & Lange, Stamford, CT, pp 9–34.
210. Murphy P, Roberts Z, Waner J: Differential diagnosis of influenza A virus, influenza B virus and respiratory syncytial virus by direct immunofluoresence using mixtures of monoclonal antibodies of different isotypes. J Clin Microbiol 1996; 34: 1798–2000.
211. Liolios T, Jenney D, Spelman T: Comparison of multiplex reverse transcriptase-PCR-enzyme hybridization assay with conventional cell culture and immunofluorescence for the detection of seven viral respiratory pathogens. J Clin Microbiol 2001; 39: 2779–2783.
212. Hindizeh M, Hillyard DR, Carroll KC: Evaluation of the Prodesse Hexaplex multiplex PCR assay for direct detection of seventeen respiratory viruses in clinical specimens. Am J Clin Pathol 2001; 116: 218–224.
213. Rea T, Ashley RL, Russo JE: A systemic study of Epstein–Barr virus serologic assays following acute infection. Am J Clin Pathol 2002; 117: 156–161.
214. Razonable R, Paya C, Smith T: Role of the laboratory in diagnosis and management of cytomegalovirus infection in hematopoietic stem cell and solid-organ transplant recipients. J Clin Microbiol 2002; 40: 746–752.
215. Weinberg A, Schissel D, Giller R: Molecular methods for cytomegalovirus surveillance in bone marrow transplant recipients. J Clin Microbiol 2002; 40: 4203–4306.
216. Cox F: History of human parasitology. Clin Micro Rev 2002; 15: 595–612.
217. Fritsche TR, Smith JW: Medical parasitology. In: Clinical diagnosis and management by laboratory methods, Henry JB, Ed. 2001, WB Saunders, Philadelphia.
218. Baird JK, Neafie RC, Marty AM: Parasitic infections. In: Pulmonary pathology, Dail DH, Hammer ST, Eds. 1994, Springer-Verlag, New York.
219. Ali A, Hoda SA: Vegetable matter in histology sections may simulate pathogenic microrganisms. Abst 1127 USCAP Annual Meeting. Mod Pathol 2002; 15: 272A.
220. Nash G, Kerschmann RL, Herndier B: The pathologic manifestations of pulmonary toxoplasmosis in the acquired immune-deficiency syndrome. Human Path 1994; 25: 652–658.
221. Frenkel JK: Toxoplasmosis. In: Pathology of infectious diseases, Connor DH, Chandler FC, Schwartz DA, Eds. 1997, Appleton & Lange, Stamford, CT, pp 1270–1271.
222. Lyche KD, Jensen WA: Pleuropulmonary amoebiasis. Semin Respir Infect 1997; 12: 106–112.
223. Wilson ES: Pleuropulmonary amebiasis. Am J Roentgenol Radium Ther Nucl Med 1971; 111(3): 518–524.
224. Ash LR, Orihel TC: Atlas of human parasitology, 4th edn. 1997, ASCP Press, Chicago.
225. Sun T: Parasitic disorders. Pathology, diagnosis and management, 2nd edn. 1999, Williams and Wilkins, Baltimore.
226. Marciano-Cabral F, Cabral G: *Acathamoeba* spp as agents of disease in humans. Clin Micro Rev 2003; 16: 273–307.
227. Chen X, Keithly JS, Paya CV: Cryptosporidiosis. N Engl J Med 2002; 346: 1729–1731.
228. Pearl M, Villanueva TG, Kaufman D: Respiratory cryptosporidiosis in the acquired immune deficiency syndrome. JAMA 1984; 252: 1290–1301.
229. Garcia L: Laboratory identification of the microsporidia. J Clin Microbiol 2002; 40: 1892–1901.
230. Weber R, Bryan RT, Schwartz DA: Human microsporidial infections. Clin Micro Rev 1994; 7: 426–461.
231. Schwartz D, Visvesvara G, Leitch G.: Pathology of symptomatic microsporidial (*Encephalitozoon hellem*) bronchiolitis in acquired immunodeficiency syndrome: a new respiratory pathogen diagnosed from lung, biopsy, bronchoalveolar lavage, sputum and tissue culture. Human Path 1993; 24 937–943.
232. Lamps L, Bonner MP, Vnencak-Jones CL: Optimal screening and diagnosis of microspoidia in tissue sections. A comparison of polarization, special stains and molecular techniques. Am J Clin Pathol 1998; 109: 404–410.
233. Flieder DB, Moran CA: Pulmonary dirofilariasis: a clinicopathologic study of 41 lesions in 39 patients. Human Path 1999; 30: 251–256.
234. Byard RW, Bourne AJ, Matthews N: Pulmonary strongyloidiasis in a child diagnosed on open lung biopsy. Surg Pathol 1993; 5: 55–61.
235. Upadhyay D, Corbridge T, Jain M: Pulmonary hyperinfection syndrome with *Strongyloides stercoralis*. Am J Med 2001; 111: 167–179.
236. Baden L, Elliott D: Case 4-2003: a 42 year-old woman with cough, fever and abnormalities on thoracoabdominal computed tomography. N Engl J Med 2003; 348: 447–455.
237. Redington AE, Russell SG, Ladhani S: Pulmonary echinococcosis with chest wall involvement in a patient with no apparent risk factors. J Infect 2001; 42: 285–288.
238. Procop GW, Marty AM, Scheck DW: North American paragonimiasis. a case report. Acta Cytol 2000; 44: 75–80.
239. Sinniah B: Paragonimiasis. In: Pathology of infectious diseases, Connor DH, Chandler FC, Schwartz DA, Eds. 1997, Appleton & Lange, Stamford, CT, pp 1527–1530.
240. Ross G, Bartley PB, Sleigh AC: Schistosomiasis. N Engl J Med 2002; 346: 1212–1220.
241. Bethem EP, Schettino GD, Carvalho CR: Pulmonary schistosomiasis. Curr Opin Pulm Med 1997; 3: 361–365.
242. Schwarrtz E, Rozenman J, Perlman M: Pulmonary manifestations of early schistosome infection among nonimmune travelers. Am J Med 2000; 9: 718–722.
243. Cooke GS, L. A., Gleeson FV: Acute pulmonary schistosomiasis in travelers returning from Lake Malawi, sub-Saharan Africa. Clin Infect Dis 1999; 29: 836–839.
244. Singh A, Singh X, Sharma VK: Diagnosis of hydatid disease of abdomen and thorax by ultrasound guided fine needle aspiration cytology. Indian J Pathol Microbiol 1999; 42: 155–156.
245. Handa U, Mohan H, Ahal S: Cytodiagnosis of hydatid cyst disease presenting with Horner' syndrome. Acta Cytol 2001; 45: 784–788.
246. Brown RW, Clarke RJ, Denham I: Pulmonary paragonimiasis in a immigrant from Laos. Med J Australia 1983; 2: 688–689.
247. Abdulla MA, Hombal SM, al-Juwaiser A: Detection of *Schistosoma mansoni* in bronchalveolar lavage fluid. A case report. Acta Cytol 1999; 43: 856–858.
248. Kramer MR, Gregg PA, Goldstein M: Disseminated strongyloidiasis in AIDS and non-AIDS immunocompromised hosts: diagnosis by sputum and bronchoalveolar lavage. South Med J 1990; 83: 1226–1229.
249. Kapila K, Verma K: Cytologic detection of parasitic disorders. Acta Cytol 1982; 26: 359–362.
250. Marsan C, Marais MH, Sollet JP: Disseminated strongyloidiasis: a case report. Cytopathol 1993; 4: 123–126.
251. Didier ES, Rogers LB, Orenstein JM: Chacterization of *Encephalitozoan (septata) intestinalis* isolates cultured from nasal mucosa and bronchoalveolar lavage fluids of two AIDS patients. J Eukar Microbiol 1996; 43: 34–43.
252. Weber R, Kaster H, Keller R: Pulmonary and intestinal microsporidiosis in a patient with the acquired immunodeficiency syndrome. Am Rev Resp Dis 1992; 146: 1603–1605.
253. Ro JY, Tsakalakis PJ, White VA: Pulmonary dirofilariasis: the great imitator of primary or metastatic lung cancer. A clinicopathologic analysis of seven cases and a review of the literature. Human Path 1989; 20: 69–76.
254. Akagogi E, Ishibashi O, Mitsui K: Pulmonary dirofilariasis cytologically mimicking lung cancer. A case report. Acta Cytol 1993; 531–534.
255. Nicholson CP, Allen MS, Trastek VF: *Dirofilaria immitis*: a rare increasing cause of pulmonary nodules. Mayo Clin Proc 1992; 67: 646–650.
256. Jokipii L, Salmela K, Saha H: Leishmaniasis diagnosed from bronchalveolar lavage. Scan J Infect Dis 1992; 24: 677–781.
257. Wheeler RR, Bardales RH, North PE: Toxoplasma pneumonia: diagnosis by bronchoalveolar lavage. Diagn Cytopathol 1994; 11: 52–55.
258. Radosavljevic-Asie G, Jovanovic D, Tuckovic M: Trichomonas in pleural effusion. Europe Respir J 1994; 7: 1906–1908.
259. Newsome AL, Curtis FT, Culbertson CG: Identification of Acanthamoeba in bronchoalveolar lavage specimens. Diagn Cytopathol 1992; 8: 231–234.
260. Wilson MR, Schantz P, Pieniazk N: Diagnosis of parasitic infection: immunologic and molecular methods. In: Manual of clinical microbiology, Murry PR, Baron EJ, Pfaller MA, Eds. 1995, ASM Press, Washington, DC.
261. Maddison SE: Serodiagnosis of parasitic disease. Clin Micro Rev 1991; 4: 457–469.

262. Wilson MR, Remington JS, Clavet C: Evaluation of six commercial kits for detection of human immunoglobulin M antibodies to *Toxoplasma gondii*. J Clin Microbiol 1997; 35: 3112–3115.
262a. Remington JS, Thulliez P, Montoya JC: Recent developments for diagnosis of toxoplasmosis. J Clin Microbiol 2004; 42: 941–945.
263. Churg AM: Recent advances in the diagnosis of Churg–Strauss syndrome. Mod Pathol 2001; 14: 1284–1293.
264. Allen JM, Davis DB: Eosinophilic lung diseases. Am J Respir Crit Care Med 1994; 150: 1423–1438.
265. Burgers JA, Sluiters JA, deJong DW: Pseudoparasitic pneumonia after bone marrow transplantation. Neth J Med 2001; 59: 170–176.
266. Thuur SM, Nelson AM, Gibson FB et al.: Liesegang rings in tissue. How to distinguish Liesegang rings from the giant kidney worm. Dioctophyma renale. Am J Surg Pathol. 1987; 11(8): 598–605.

7 Chronic diffuse lung diseases

Junya Fukuoka Kevin O Leslie

Introduction

The diffuse lung diseases (DLDs) include a spectrum of primarily non-neoplastic conditions that all share the common property of diffusely involving the lung parenchyma.[1–9] The term "interstitial lung disease" or "ILD" is often used to describe these conditions, but we prefer the term "diffuse lung disease" as a better general descriptor, and a less restrictive implication of the exact microanatomical compartment involved.

This chapter focuses on the subacute and chronic forms of DLD (acute DLD is discussed in Ch. 5), and includes diseases that typically evolve over weeks, months, and/or years. Patients with DLD share a number of clinical and radiologic manifestations, including:

1. shortness of breath (dyspnea)
2. diffuse abnormalities in lung mechanics and gas transfer (pulmonary function)
3. diffuse abnormalities on chest radiographs and computed tomographic (CT) scans of the chest.

An overview of DLDs from the pathologist's perspective is presented in Table 7.1. We will restrict our focus in this chapter to a limited number of predominantly inflammatory diseases that come to biopsy relatively frequently (Table 7.2). Our emphasis is on the histopathologic patterns of these diseases as observed through the microscope. These patterns help narrow the differential diagnosis and often allow for a definitive diagnosis when coupled with clinical and radiologic data.

The DLDs have in common the accumulation of inflammatory and immune effector cells in the lung interstitium as their main histopathologic finding. The interstitium of the lung is the compartment that exists between the basement membrane of lung epithelial cells (the lining cells of the airways and alveoli in direct contact with inspired air) and that of adjacent blood vessels. There is a general misconception that the lung interstitium is confined to the "space" that exists within the alveolar walls. In fact, this compartment extends as a continuum from the alveolar septa to the pleura.

Unlike neoplasms that may have distinctive or even unique morphologic features, the DLDs are distinguished from one another by:

1. location involved (anatomical compartment or structure)
2. distribution (focal or diffuse)
3. cellular composition (acute, chronic, histiocytic, etc.) of the inflammatory reaction.[7–9]

Coupled with these, is the mechanism by which repair is taking place (organizing or not) and the age of the reparative process.[10]

Transbronchial and surgical wedge biopsy interpretation in the DLD patient is complicated by several factors. First, these diseases involve the interstitium, but they are frequently attended by reactive changes in the surrounding alveolar spaces and associated terminal airways. Such reactive changes can be quite impressive,

Table 7.1 Inclusive overview of the chronic diffuse lung diseases (DLDs)

1. Idiopathic interstitial pneumonias (UIP, NSIP, COP, RBILD/DIP, LIP)
2. Chronic manifestations of the systemic collagen vascular diseases
3. Eosinophilic lung disease (chronic eosinophilic pneumonia)
4. Chronic drug reactions
5. Interstitial diseases with granulomas (some infections, sarcoidosis, hypersensitivity pneumonitis, berylliosis)
6. Diffuse alveolar hemorrhage
7. Pneumoconioses
8. Pulmonary hypertension and related disorders
9. Miscellaneous diseases (Langerhans cell histiocytosis, lymphangioleiomyomatosis, pulmonary alveolar proteinosis, amyloidosis, pulmonary alveolar microlithiasis, Erdheim–Chester disease, Hermansky–Pudlak syndrome)
10. Malignant neoplasms (carcinomatosis, malignant lymphomas, metastatic sarcomas)

COP = cryptogenic organizing pneumonia; DIP = desquamative interstitial pneumonia; LIP = lymphoid interstitial pneumonia; NSIP = nonspecific interstitial pneumonia; RBILD = respiratory bronchiolitis interstitial lung disease; UIP = usual interstitial pneumonia.

Table 7.2 Diffuse lung diseases presented in this chapter

1. Idiopathic interstitial pneumonias (UIP, NSIP, COP, RBILD/DIP, LIP)
2. Chronic manifestations of systemic collagen vascular disease
3. Eosinophilic lung disease (chronic eosinophilic pneumonia)
4. Chronic drug reactions
5. Interstitial diseases with granulomas (some infections, sarcoidosis, hypersensitivity pneumonitis, berylliosis)
6. Miscellaneous diseases (Langerhans cell histiocytosis, lymphangioleiomyomatosis, pulmonary alveolar proteinosis, amyloidosis, Erdheim–Chester disease, Hermansky–Pudlak syndrome)
7. Malignant neoplasms (lymphangitic carcinomatosis)

COP = cryptogenic organizing pneumonia; DIP = desquamative interstitial pneumonia; LIP = lymphoid interstitial pneumonia; NSIP = nonspecific interstitial pneumonia; RBILD = respiratory bronchiolitis interstitial lung disease; UIP = usual interstitial pneumonia.

and commonly distract the observer from recognizing the interstitial nature of the process. Secondly, the inherent variability and natural history of inflammatory diseases pose problems, wherein early phases of a disease may differ in appearance from later phases, and the intensity of a reaction may vary from individual to individual. Thirdly, more than one inflammatory disease can involve the lung simultaneously, adding further complexity to the morphologic picture. Finally, and perhaps most importantly, these predominantly medical diseases cannot be diagnosed accurately without some clinical and radiologic correlation.

Despite extensive clinical and experimental research efforts over the past several decades, the etiology and pathogenesis of most DLDs remains unknown. In certain DLDs, a specific exposure can be identified (for example, hypersensitivity pneumonitis or toxic reaction to a drug), while in others a systemic autoimmune disease may be present (for example, rheumatoid arthritis manifesting in the lung). When no associated exposure or underlying condition is identified, a DLD is considered to be "idiopathic."

Like most human organs, the lung has a limited repertoire of responses to injury of any type, and most of these responses are nonspecific. Without guidelines for interpretation and appropriate nomenclature, the surgical pathologist may experience difficulty in coming to a clinically meaningful diagnosis for the DLD patient. Additionally, since the lung biopsy for DLD is always a limited sampling, the pathologist and clinician must work cooperatively in establishing a differential diagnosis based on the clinical presentation, laboratory data, and radiologic findings. A purely descriptive pathologic diagnosis (for example "chronic lung fibrosis"), without clinical or radiologic correlation, or a focused differential diagnosis, is of marginal use in the contemporary practice of pulmonary medicine. In this chapter, we will present the essential clinical, radiologic and histopathologic elements of the chronic DLD, and provide the reader with specific terminology for use in diagnosing these diseases, wherever possible.

One of the most important chronic lung diseases in pulmonary medicine today is one known clinically as "idiopathic pulmonary fibrosis" or "IPF." This most devastating of the chronic DLDs is often the diagnosis of exclusion from a clinical perspective, and one against which all other chronic lung diseases are judged. The reason for this is that IPF is a disease that progresses despite therapy and rivals many cancers in causing death, often within 3 years of the diagnosis.[4] As emphasized in a recent joint consensus statement of the American Thoracic Society (ATS) and the European Respiratory Society (ERS), the pathologic manifestation of IPF in the lung is "usual interstitial pneumonia" (UIP).[4] UIP was a term introduced by Liebow, in reference to one of five forms of "idiopathic interstitial pneumonia."[2] In Liebow's words, UIP represented "chronic lung fibrosis of the common or usual type," a seemingly broad category of chronic lung disease.[2]

As we explore the chronic DLD, it seems most appropriate to begin with UIP, recognizing that our current concept of this disease is more restrictive than perhaps was initially intended.[4] The pathologist who is able to recognize the subtle but distinctive features of UIP, and confidently distinguish it from other DLDs, is well on the way to mastering the art of pulmonary pathology.

The idiopathic interstitial pneumonias

Liebow's initial classification of the idiopathic interstitial pneumonias (IIPs) is presented for historical purposes in Table 7.3.[2] In the years following the introduction of this classification scheme, new information led to the modification or elimination of certain of these idiopathic interstitial pneumonias, and the addition of others not previously included (Table 7.4).[11,12] We have learned since Liebow's time that desquamative interstitial pneumonia (DIP), initially thought to be an early manifestation of UIP,[13] is in fact a smoking-related disease in the majority of cases, and one that most often affects adults.[14,15] We also have come to realize that giant cell interstitial

Table 7.3 Liebow classification of the idiopathic interstitial pneumonias

Usual interstitial pneumonia (UIP)
Desquamative interstitial pneumonia (DIP)
Bronchiolitis obliterans interstitial pneumonia (BIP)
Lymphoid interstitial pneumonia (LIP)
Giant cell interstitial pneumonia (GIP)

Source: from Liebow and Carrington.[2]

Table 7.4 Katzenstein classification of idiopathic interstitial pneumonias

Usual interstitial pneumonia (UIP)
Desquamative interstitial pneumonia (DIP)
Respiratory bronchiolitis interstitial lung disease (RBILD)
Acute interstitial pneumonia (AIP)
Nonspecific interstitial pneumonia (NSIP)

Source: from Katzenstein and Askin,[1] Table 3-1, p 49, with permission.

pneumonia (GIP) was actually a manifestation of cobalt exposure, as a pneumonoconiosis in "hard metal disease" (see Ch. 8, pneumoconiosis).[16] Finally, it became apparent that many early cases of lymphoid interstitial pneumonia (LIP) evolved into lymphoproliferative disease, and likely were not "inflammatory" diseases in the true sense of the word.[17–19]

Based on this evolution in our understanding, a modification to Liebow's original classification of the IIPs was proposed by Katzenstein.[11,12] This included the major categories of UIP and DIP, but coupled DIP with "respiratory bronchiolitis-associated interstitial lung disease" (RBILD), and acknowledged the strong relationship of these diseases to cigarette smoking. Katzenstein also proposed a new category of "acute interstitial pneumonia" (AIP),[20] as an entity separate from UIP, a distinction that Liebow did not make in his initial classification. Finally, Katzenstein created a new category to encompass a group of inflammatory diseases that differed in appearance from UIP, DIP, or AIP. The term "nonspecific interstitial pneumonia" (NSIP) was proposed for this "new" pattern.[21] In our experience, the majority of idiopathic interstitial pneumonias can be classified using this scheme. We would add "idiopathic (or cryptogenic) organizing pneumonia" (previously known as idiopathic bronchiolitis obliterans organizing pneumonia, or BOOP) to this classification as well, as did a recent international workshop on the classification of the IIPs.[4] That workshop maintained LIP in the classification (Table 7.5), acknowledging that when diffuse interstitial lymphoplasmacellular infiltration is present, and non-neoplastic, most observers would consider such a pattern to be a manifestation of NSIP. Importantly, the consensus panel felt that NSIP should be included in the IIPs as a provisional category, until additional data accrue.[4]

The IIPs are classically defined as diffuse pulmonary diseases that involve two or more lobes of the lung and, in most patients, they are bilateral in distribution. Some localized lesions (such as infection, atelectasis, or tumor) may mimic the IIPs in a biopsy specimen. It is safe to say that if a disease process is confined to the biopsy area sampled, it is unlikely to be an IIP. AIP is an acute form of IIP and is discussed in detail in Chapter 5. A comparison of the histopathologic findings in each of the IIPs is presented in Table 7.6.

Table 7.5 2002 International consensus classification of idiopathic interstitial pneumonias

Pathologic pattern	Clinical–radiologic–pathologic diagnosis
Usual interstitial pneumonia	Idiopathic pulmonary fibrosis/cryptogenic fibrosing alveolitis
Nonspecific interstitial pneumonia	Nonspecific interstitial pneumonia *(provisional)*
Respiratory bronchiolitis	Respiratory bronchiolitis interstitial lung disease
Desquamative interstitial pneumonia	Desquamative interstitial pneumonia
Organizing pneumonia	Cryptogenic organizing pneumonia
Diffuse alveolar damage	Acute interstitial pneumonia
Lymphoid interstitial pneumonia	Lymphoid interstitial pneumonia

Source: from Travis et al.,[4] p 281, Table 2, with permission.

Table 7.6 Contrasting pathologic features of the idiopathic interstitial pneumonias

Features	NSIP	UIP	DIP	AIP	LIP	COP
Temporal appearance	Uniform	Variegated	Uniform	Uniform	Uniform	Uniform
Interstitial inflammation	Prominent	Scant	Scant	Scant	Prominent	Scant
Interstitial fibrosis (collagen)	Var, diffuse	Patchy	Var, diffuse	No	Some cases	No
Interstitial fibrosis (fibroblasts)	Occas, diffuse	No	No	Yes, diffuse	No	No
OP pattern	Occas, focal	Occas, focal	No	Occas, focal	No	Prominent
Fibroblast foci	Occas, focal	Typical	No	No	No	No
Honeycomb areas	Rare	Typical	No	No	Sometimes	No
Intra-alveolar macrophages	Occas, patchy	Occas, focal	Yes, diffuse	No	Occas, Patchy	No
Hyaline membranes	No	No	No	Yes, focal	No	No
Granulomas	No	No	No	No	Focal, poorly formed	No

NSIP = nonspecific interstitial pneumonia; DIP = desquamative interstitial pneumonia; UIP = usual interstitial pneumonia; AIP = acute interstitial pneumonia; LIP= lymphocytic interstitial pneumonia; COP = cryptogenic organizing pneumonia; Occas = occasional; Var = variable.
Source: from Katzenstein and Fiorelli[367] and Travis et al.[6]

Usual interstitial pneumonia

Pulmonary pathologists have debated for years what is and what is not UIP. To many, UIP is a relatively non-specific pattern of chronic lung injury with fibrosis and "honeycomb" remodeling (see below). Today, we know that not all lung diseases with fibrosis behave similarly and in particular do not run the aggressive course expected for clinical "idiopathic pulmonary fibrosis."[4] The most honest answer may be that clinical and radiologic IPF has UIP pathologic changes, but that a "UIP pattern" of parenchymal fibrosis with remodeling seen in biopsy specimens may not necessarily correlate with clinical and radiologic IPF. Fortunately, not all lung diseases that produce scarring fit the pattern now defined as UIP.[4] Asbestosis,[22–24] chronic hypersensitivity pneumonitis,[25–27] systemic collagen vascular diseases,[28–31] and even some chronic toxic drug reactions[32] can all produce lung fibrosis. In the 30 years following Liebow's introduction of UIP as an "idiopathic" interstitial disease, pathologists often used the term "UIP" in a variety of non-idiopathic settings (e.g. "UIP from asbestosis"). If we define UIP as simply any form of lung fibrosis, then applying UIP as a synonym for fibrosis is perfectly reasonable. On the other hand, if UIP is a distinctive pathologic entity that corresponds to a clinical disease (IPF), then UIP should have identifiable features that afford its status as a unique disease process. That there is a continued misconception of UIP is underscored by our clinical colleagues, who tell us that many UIP diagnoses that they receive on their patients do not correspond to clinical IPF in presentation, response to therapy, or expected prognosis.

If we examine the subset of DLD that corresponds to clinical and radiologic IPF, we find a disease that is not overtly inflammatory, but one with a clear tendency to produce fibrosis. Moreover, the fibrosis seen in the lungs of IPF patients has a relatively reproducible pattern and distribution. Through such a focused analysis, we can begin to see the subtle differences that exist between the UIP of IPF and the fibrosis that may occur in other lung diseases, most of which have an identifiable cause, etiologic agent, or associated systemic disease process.

Clinical presentation

The incidence of UIP varies between males and females, with males predominating. The disease may have a prevalence in the United States as high as 55,000,[33] and roughly two-thirds of patients are over the age of 60.[34, 35] For this reason, lung biopsies from patients less than 50 years of age should be diagnosed with caution, and preferably with the addition of expert consultation. Symptoms typically progress insidiously for months to years prior to diagnosis. The onset of a non-productive cough and slowly progressive dyspnea is characteristic. Dry inspiratory crackles (so-called "Velcro" crackles) are detected at the lung bases on chest auscultation in more than 80% of patients at presentation.[35] Clubbing of the digits is seen in 25–50% of patients at presentation. Fever is rare and its presence should suggest an alternate diagnosis, as should a significantly elevated erythrocyte sedimentation rate (greater than 100 mm/h). Serologic studies may be mildly elevated (ANA or rheumatoid factor) but when significant elevation is present, a systemic connective tissue disease should be strongly considered. Also, patients who present with clinical features of UIP/IPF and later develop a defined collagen vascular disease might require their disease to be reclassified.[4]

Radiologic findings

On plain chest radiography, the presence of peripheral reticular opacities involving the lung bases is a characteristic finding.[36] When present, these are usually bilateral and often asymmetrical. Lung volumes are typically decreased at presentation, except when there is severe upper lobe (centriacinar) emphysema.[37] Importantly, a normal chest radiograph does not exclude the diagnosis.[38] Confluent alveolar opacities are rare and, if present, suggest an alternate diagnosis or a comorbid process. Computed tomograms (CTs), preferably of the high-resolution type (scan sections of 1 mm or less), commonly show patchy, predominately peripheral (subpleural), reticular abnormalities involving the lung bases bilaterally.[39] Some asymmetry is expected between right and left lungs, and skip areas with better-preserved lung immediately adjacent are typical (so-called radiologic heterogeneity.) The earliest findings may be quite subtle, with delicate peripherally accentuated pleural-based reticular opacities in the lower lung zones (Fig. 7.1). Ground glass opacities are not typical, and if present, should be limited in extent.[40–42] Subpleural cysts ranging from a few millimeters in diameter to a centimeter or more (radiologic "honeycombing") increase in prominence as the disease advances (Fig. 7.2). In areas of more severe involvement there is often traction bronchiectasis. Diagnostic accuracy for IPF on high-resolution CT (HRCT) scan by trained observers is in the range of 90% when typical findings are present (high specificity); however, approximately one-third of UIP patients will be missed by relying on HRCT diagnosis alone (low sensitivity).[27,43]

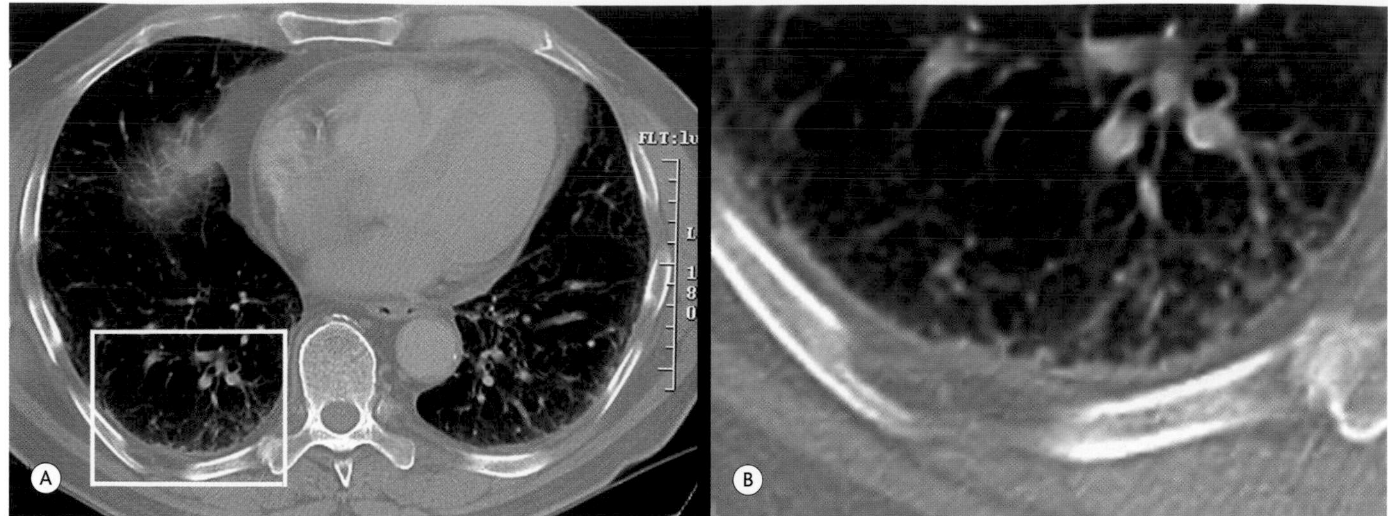

Fig. 7.1 **Usual interstitial pneumonia (UIP).** (A) This CT scan shows the early subtle findings in UIP, with delicate pleural-based reticular opacities in the lower lung zones and a few small honeycomb cysts (B–boxed area from A).

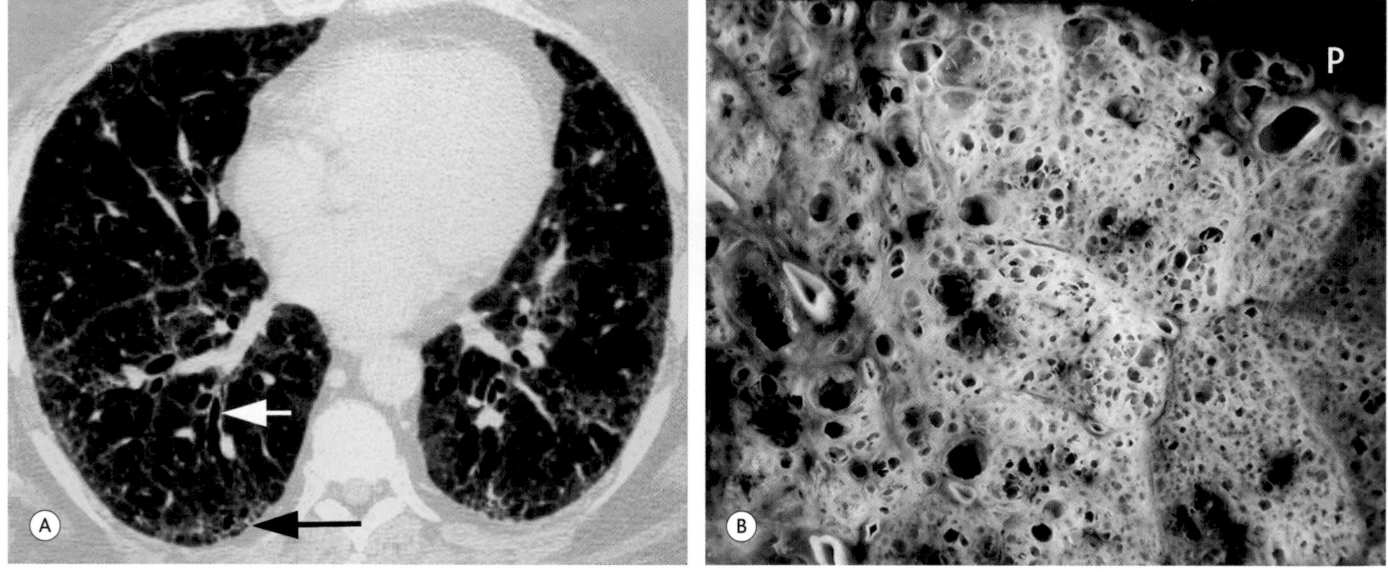

Fig. 7.2 **Usual interstitial pneumonia (UIP).** (A) Another CT example with characteristic changes of UIP, with subpleural cysts (black arrow) and traction bronchiectasis (white arrow). The gross lung specimen in UIP (B) shows subpleural (P) cysts ranging from a few millimeters in diameter to a centimeter or more (radiologic "honeycombing"), that increase in prominence as the disease advances.

Pathologic findings

UIP cannot be diagnosed with the bronchoscopic or transbronchial biopsy specimen. Surgically derived wedge lung biopsies (3–5 cm in length by 2–3 cm in breadth), from video-assisted thoracoscopic surgery (VATS) or open thoracotomy, are the appropriate specimen for diagnosis (see Ch. 2 for additional details on the lung biopsy). Occasionally, UIP will be evident in lobectomy and pneumonectomy specimens performed for other diseases. UIP is a process that involves the periphery of the lung lobule and these areas are not sampled adequately in even the most ambitious transbronchial biopsy scenario (where many large fragments of alveolar parenchyma may be present, but these are mainly derived from the central portion of the lung lobules). More than one biopsy site should be sampled, and preferably a biopsy sample should be obtained from all lobes in the hemithorax chosen for surgical intervention. If only two areas can be sampled, mid lung and lower lung are preferable to upper and mid lung, and biopsies taken from the lower lobe should be taken above the most advanced areas of fibrosis.

The characteristic histopathologic findings of UIP have been referred to as "temporally heterogeneous,"[36,44–47] a term and concept that is often misunderstood by many surgical pathologists and pulmonologists. The observed findings are quite reproducible and specific in our experience. An expanded description of "temporal heterogeneity" is that of abrupt transitions in the biopsy, from dense (old) remodeled lung parenchyma to normal alveolar walls toward the center of the lobule (new or yet to be involved lung). This transition occurs through patchy areas of lung injury evidenced by the "fibroblast" or "fibroblastic" focus (Fig. 7.3). The remodeled lung is present mainly beneath the pleura and at the periphery of the secondary lobule, adjacent to interlobular septa (Fig. 7.4). When UIP is recognizable as a distinct pathologic entity, the pleural fibrosis contains smooth muscle proliferation in disorganized fascicles (Fig. 7.5) and foci

Fig. 7.3 **Usual interstitial pneumonia (UIP).** The histopathologic "temporal heterogeneity" of UIP is characterized by abrupt transitions in the biopsy, from dense remodeled lung parenchyma ("old" injury, evident in the right side of this image) to normal alveolar walls ("new" or not yet involved lung, center and left side of this image) at the center of the lobule. This transition occurs through patchy areas of lung injury evidenced by the "fibroblast" or "fibroblastic" focus (ff.).

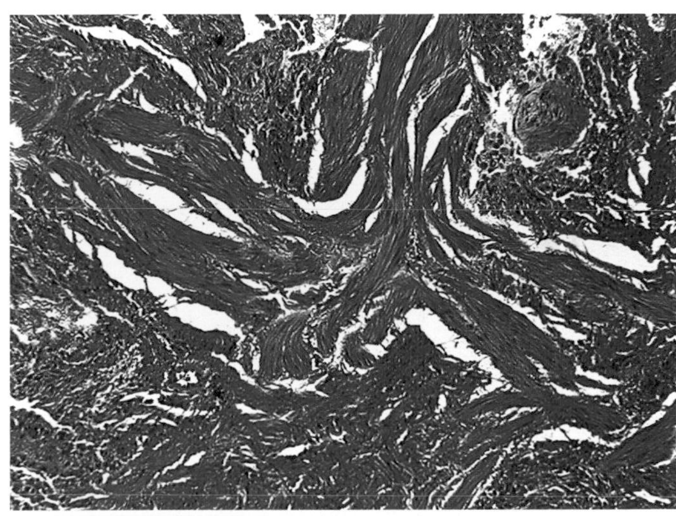

Fig. 7.5 **Usual interstitial pneumonia (UIP).** When UIP is recognizable as a distinct pathologic entity, the subpleural fibrous tissue contains smooth muscle proliferation, seen here as large disorganized fascicles.

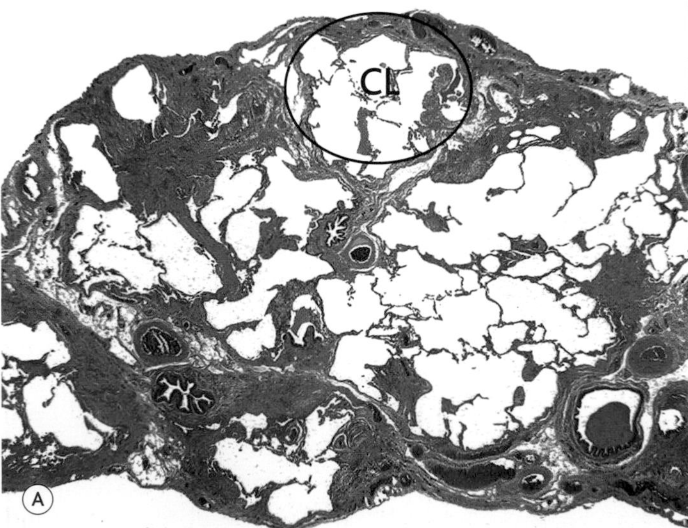

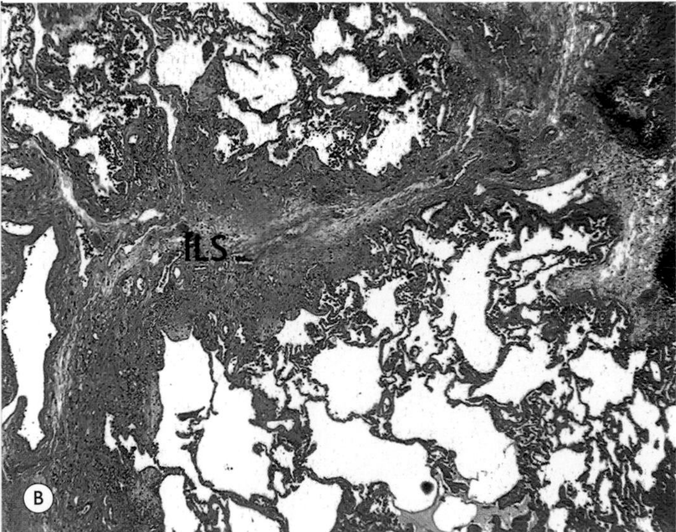

Fig. 7.4 **Usual interstitial pneumonia (UIP).** (A) The remodeled lung is present mainly beneath the pleura and at the periphery of the secondary lobule, adjacent to interlobular septa. A slightly shrunken lobule is circled at upper center (CL = center of lobule). (B) An interlobular septum (ILS) widened by fibrosis, with less involved lung lobules above and below center.

of microscopic honeycombing (Fig. 7.6). Microscopic honeycombing probably represents one of the early manifestations of the gross honeycomb cysts seen in the end stage of UIP. The radiologist's use of the term "honeycombing" corresponds to much larger cysts (in the range of 0.5–3 cm or larger) as a localized manifestation of advanced lung remodeling (Fig. 7.7). Microscopic honeycomb cysts are considerably smaller (in the range of 1–3 mm) and are typically present subpleurally (Fig. 7.8). The cysts are lined by columnar ciliated epithelium and typically are filled with mucus, with variable amounts of acute inflammation and

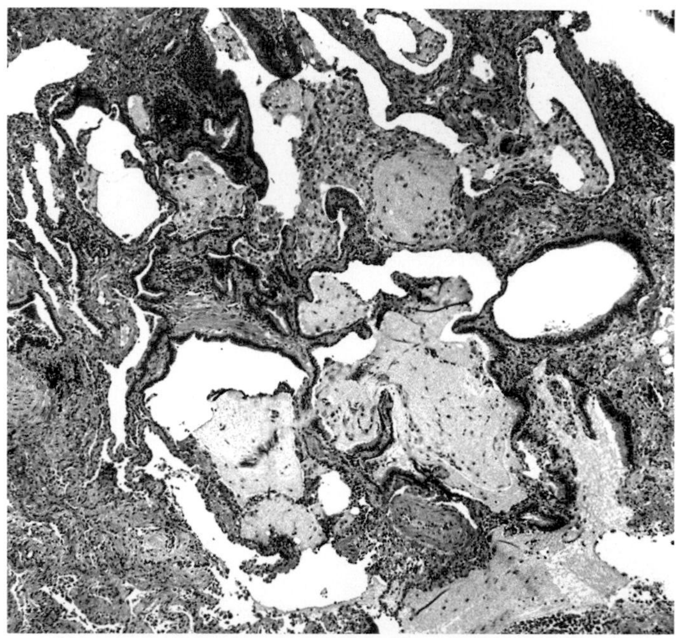

Fig. 7.6 **Usual interstitial pneumonia (UIP).** Even in patients with "early" disease radiologically, foci of microscopic honeycombing are typically present. To distinguish bronchiolar metaplasia from microscopic honeycombing, noting the location of the lesion is often helpful, as microscopic honeycombing is present more peripherally in lobules and associated with dense scar, while bronchiolar metaplasia is a phenomenon that develops at the center of lobules, in association with respiratory bronchioles.

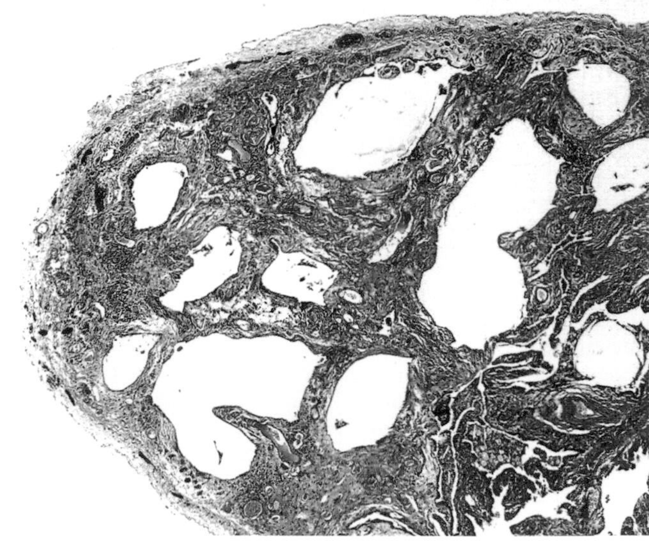

Fig. 7.8 **Usual interstitial pneumonia (UIP).** Microscopic honeycomb cysts are considerably smaller (in the range of 1–3 mm) than those identified radiologically.

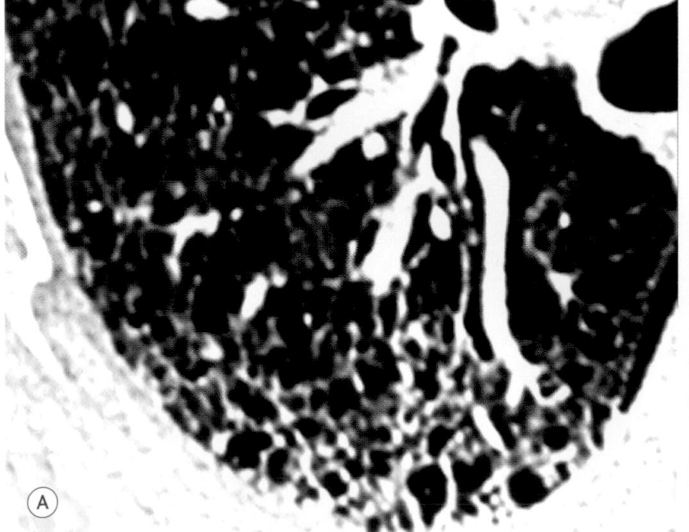

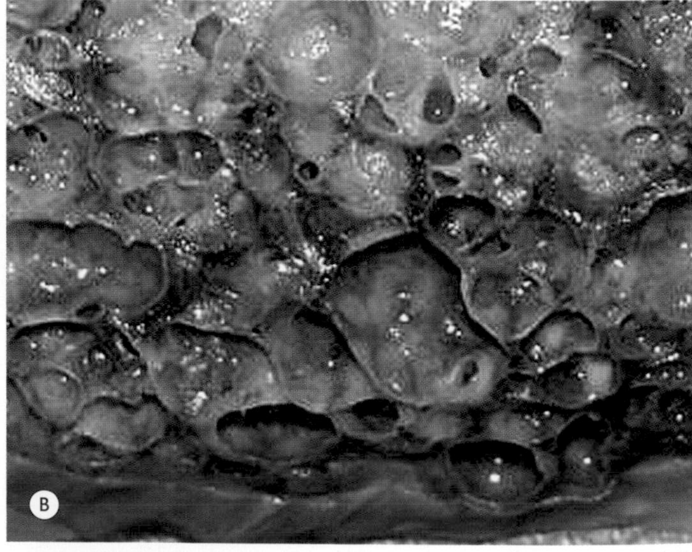

Fig. 7.7 **Usual interstitial pneumonia (UIP).** The radiologist's use of the term "honeycombing" corresponds to much larger cysts (in the range of 0.5–3 cm or larger) as a localized manifestation of advanced lung remodeling. (A) Here a patient with advanced UIP has many peripheral honeycomb cysts and traction bronchiectasis. (B) The gross lung shows dramatic confluent cyst formation.

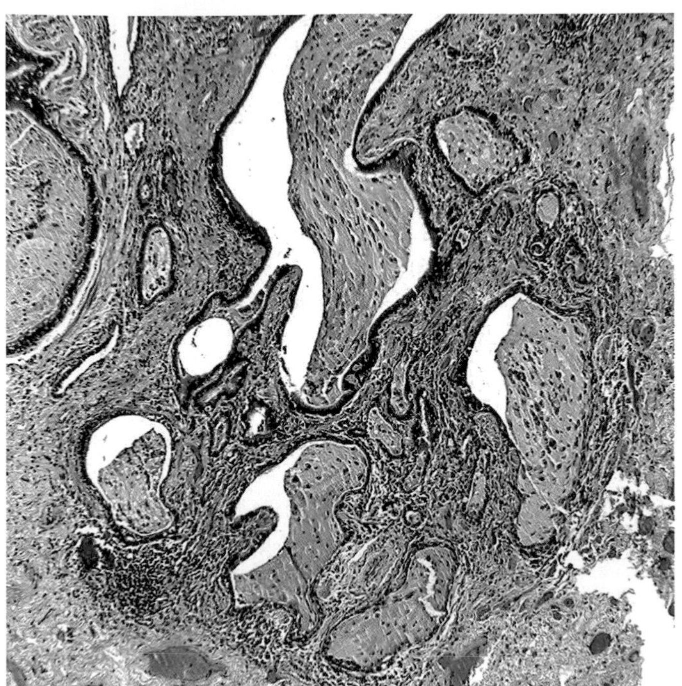

Fig. 7.9 **Usual interstitial pneumonia (UIP).** Microscopic honeycomb cysts are lined by columnar ciliated epithelium and typically are filled with mucus, with variable amounts of acute inflammation and inflammatory debris. When dense chronic inflammation is present in UIP, it is most often seen around microscopic honeycombing.

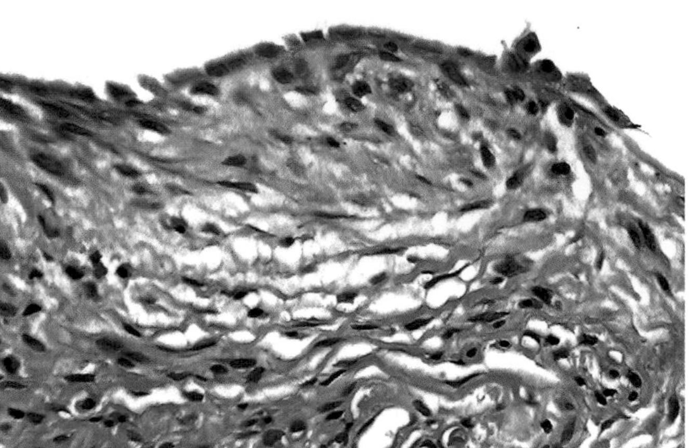

Fig. 7.10 **Usual interstitial pneumonia (UIP).** The fibroblastic foci of UIP are patchy and present immediately beneath reactive-appearing cuboidal alveolar lining epithelium (type II cell hyperplasia). The fibroblastic proliferation bulges toward the airspace, but does not appear to make a polypoid structure.

inflammatory debris (Fig. 7.9). When dense chronic inflammation is present in UIP, it is seen around these localized inflammatory lesions.

Exactly how honeycomb cysts (gross or microscopic) form is unclear, but it is possible that they represent centrilobular airways, trapped in the fibrous remodeling, that are then pulled to the periphery of the lobule. In support of this concept, lobules with foci of microscopic honeycombing often lack a visible central airway, and tractional emphysema is nearly always present. This hypothesis would also explain the presence of smooth muscle fascicles in subpleural fibrosis, and might be more tenable than the hypothesis that this muscle forms by fibroblast metaplasia.

Between the two "temporal" extremes of "old" peripheral fibrosis and uninvolved lung present centrally in the lobule is the presumed active zone of injury in UIP, evidenced by a crescent-shaped bulge of immature fibroblasts (technically "myofibroblasts") and ground substance (see Fig. 7.3). This lesion is known as the "fibroblastic focus" and typically is not extensive in the biopsy. Some investigators have postulated that an increased number of these foci in a given UIP patient's biopsy is associated with a worse prognosis, and that a relative lack of fibroblastic foci may be an explanation for the better prognosis observed for patients with lung fibrosis related to systemic collagen vascular diseases.[48]

UIP is not an overtly inflammatory condition in the absence of so-called "acute exacerbation" (see below). This is not to imply that fibrosis occurs "mysteriously" in the disease. Some form of injury is occurring in UIP but it seems to be subtle, and is probably focused on the alveolar epithelium and its basement membrane. The fibroblastic foci of UIP appear immediately beneath reactive-appearing alveolar lining epithelium, where they obscure the epithelial basement membrane and bulge into the adjacent airspace (Fig. 7.10), as though they were aborted "Masson polyps" of the type seen in organizing pneumonia (see Cryptogenic organizing pneumonia section). Further evidence that UIP/IPF is an inflammatory disease is the presence of reactive type II cells proliferation at the transition from areas of fibroblastic foci to relatively normal alveolar walls. Conceptually, the subtle inflammatory disease of UIP burns through the lung like a smoldering fire, leaving fibrosis, smooth muscle proliferation, microscopic honeycombing, and fibrosis in its path.

Acute exacerbation

Liebow conceived of UIP as a chronic lung disease resulting from repeated subclinical episodes of "diffuse alveolar damage" (DAD).[2] In support of this hypothesis, episodic deterioration is typical in IPF patients.[35] However, in some patients with IPF, clinical deterioration is abrupt and overwhelming. This large-scale manifestation of otherwise focal and episodic injury has been referred

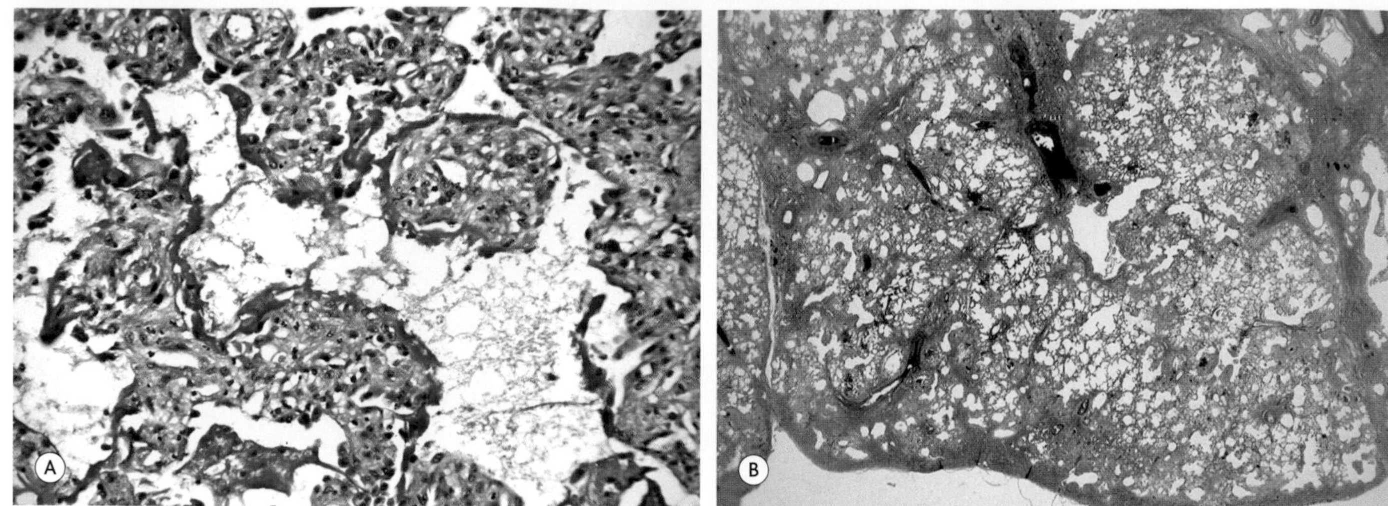

Fig. 7.11 **Usual interstitial pneumonia (UIP).** *Acute exacerbation* of idiopathic pulmonary fibrosis (IPF) has mixed histopathologic changes, typically with diffuse alveolar damage (A) superimposed on a background of older fibrosis and microscopic honeycombing of UIP. The background disease may be highlighted with the trichrome stain (B) that shows peripherally accentuated perilobular fibrosis. These two images are taken from the same biopsy section.

to as "acute exacerbation" and corresponds to overwhelming diffuse alveolar damage, possibly related to immunologic exacerbation of the underlying disease process or undetected infection.[49] Such exacerbation of IPF has mixed histopathologic changes, since the background older fibrosis with microscopic honeycombing of UIP is often overshadowed by diffuse acute lung injury with variable "organizing pneumonia" and even hyaline membranes (Fig. 7.11). In a group of three patients reported by Kondoh and coworkers, all showed some degree of improvement in the short-term, following high-dose corticosteroid therapy. Several authors have proposed such acute exacerbation as the terminal episode in many patients with IPF, even though respiratory failure has always been presumed to be a slower evolution than that implied by "acute exacerbation."[5] Based on a recent large randomized, double-blind, placebo-controlled trial of recombinant interferon gamma in IPF, approximately 15% of patients with UIP experience overwhelming acute exacerbation during the course of their disease, and this is often the fatal event for those affected (GIPF-001 clinical trial data[123]).

Differential diagnosis

The differential diagnosis for the UIP pattern includes a number of diseases that produce lung fibrosis. When this is a diffuse bilateral process, the main entities in the differential diagnosis are listed in Table 7.7.

Table 7.7 The many potential causes of lung fibrosis, with or without honeycomb remodeling

1. Idiopathic pulmonary fibrosis (idiopathic usual interstitial pneumonia)
2. Desquamative interstitial pneumonia (DIP)
3. Lymphocytic interstitial pneumonia
4. Systemic collagen vascular disease
5. Certain drug reactions
6. Pneumoconioses (asbestosis, berylliosis, silicosis, hard metal pneumoconiosis, others)
7. Sarcoidosis
8. Pulmonary Langerhans cell histiocytosis (histiocytosis X)
9. Chronic granulomatous infections
10. Chronic aspiration
11. Chronic hypersensitivity pneumonitis
12. Organized chronic eosinophilic pneumonia
13. Organized, and organizing, diffuse alveolar damage
14. Chronic interstitial pulmonary edema/passive congestion
15. Radiation (chronic)
16. Healed infectious pneumonias and other inflammatory processes
17. Nonspecific interstitial pneumonia/fibrosis (NSIP/F)
18. Hermansky–Pudlak syndrome (oculocutaneous albinism with platelet dysfunction)

Clinical course

The most common causes of death in patients with IPF are summarized in Table 7.8. As defined clinically, IPF has a median survival of less than 3 years.[50] At present, no effective therapy has been established for IPF, but newer therapies are on the horizon, using human recombinant cytokines, agents antagonistic to the effects of transforming

Table 7.8 Cause of death in 543 patients with UIP/IPF (1–7 year follow-up)

60% died in the follow-up period
Respiratory failure = 38.7%
Infection = 6.5%
Lung cancer = 10.4%
Pulmonary embolism = 3.4%
Heart failure = 14.4%
Ischemic heart disease = 9.5%
Other = 17.1% (including pneumothorax, corticosteroid-induced metabolic side-effects and myopathy, and therapy-related immunosuppression)

IPF = idiopathic pulmonary fibrosis; UIP = usual interstitial pneumonia.
Source: from Panos et al.[5]

growth factor β (TGF-β), and antifibrotic agents (e.g. interferon γ-1b, TGF-β antagonists, perfenidone).

Essential requirements for accurate diagnosis

For pulmonary physicians, a pathologic diagnosis of UIP implies clinical idiopathic pulmonary fibrosis and as such should never be made in the absence of clinical and radiologic correlation. The gravity of the prognosis and lack of current available therapy strongly support this notion.[35] If the pathologic findings are compelling for the "UIP pattern," it is reasonable to use a descriptive diagnosis, such as that presented in Table 7.9. This approach provides an opportunity for further correlation by clinical colleagues and radiologists in solidifying the diagnosis.

Table 7.9 Sample diagnosis in a case where the UIP histologic pattern is seen in a surgical lung biopsy

Diagnosis: Fibrosing interstitial pneumonia with microscopic honeycombing and peripheral smooth muscle prominence. Fibroblast focus activity is [*high/intermediate/low*].

Comment: ***The histopathologic changes identified are characteristic of those seen in patients with clinical idiopathic pulmonary fibrosis (IPF).*** *Radiologic and clinical correlation is required for a definitive diagnosis.*

Criteria for the UIP pattern
Chronic fibrosing interstitial pneumonia with:
- Patchy involvement
- Architectural loss
- Mainly peripheral zones of chronic scarring with honeycomb change
- Marked smooth muscle metaplasia/hyperplasia
- Typical peripheral lobular and paraseptal accentuation
- Centrilobular sparing is an expected finding
- Fibroblastic foci are present at the junction of fibrosis with normal lung
- Interstitial inflammation is usually mild and focal (typically around areas of microscopic honeycombing)
- Pleuritis is uncommon unless there has been a pneumothorax

Nonspecific interstitial pneumonia

For many years after Liebow's classification of the idiopathic interstitial pneumonias was widely adopted, a number of diffuse inflammatory lung diseases were identified that did not fit well within this classification scheme. A number of terms were applied to such diffuse lung diseases, including "unclassified" or "unclassifiable" interstitial pneumonia.[51] In 1994 the term "non-specific interstitial pneumonia (NSIP)" was proposed by Katzenstein and Fiorelli, who described a group of 64 patients who presented with diffuse lung disease and a chief complaint of dyspnea, usually present for several months prior to evaluation.[21] Radiologic studies showed bilateral interstitial infiltrates with variable consolidation. Importantly, the 64 patients in this study had a significantly better prognosis than that observed for patients with UIP.

Katzenstein and Fiorelli recognized that the constellation of histologic patterns seen in NSIP did not represent one disease and, in follow-up, found that these patients often had hypersensitivity, resolving infection, or systemic collagen vascular disease, among other occurrences. Subsequently, Nagai and coworkers studied a group of patients with nonspecific interstitial pneumonia and rigorously excluded possible etiologies. The reported survival in this "idiopathic NSIP" was 90% at 5 years.[52] Thus, when used in the true idiopathic context, the term "NSIP" may actually be useful if it consistently implies an interstitial chronic inflammatory disease of unknown etiology, with an expected good response to therapy and excellent survival. If, on the other hand, the term is applied indiscriminately, as a substitute for any unrecognized DLD pathologically, consistent clinical behavior will be impossible to predict and the clinician will be no better off than before subjecting the patient to the biopsy procedure.

Clinical presentation

Some general statements can be made regarding the clinical presentation in NSIP, recognizing that most of the available data have been derived from studies where a heterogeneous group of disorders was represented. Patients with NSIP histopathology in lung biopsies (i.e. an "NSIP pattern") tend to be younger than patients with UIP[52–54] and the NSIP pattern can occur in children.[21] As with many of the chronic diffuse lung diseases, symptoms appear gradually. Shortness of breath, cough, fatigue, and weight loss are the most commonly reported complaints. Fever and digital clubbing have been reported but are uncommon.[21,53]

Radiologic findings

Most chest X-ray abnormalities are confined to the lower lung zones in NSIP and tend to be bilateral and symmetrical.[55] Less than 40% of the lung volume is typically involved. Patchy parenchymal (alveolar) opacification is a commonly reported abnormality[55] but reticular (interstitial) changes have also been identified.[21] HRCT findings are variable and nonspecific.[56] Ground glass attenuation is common, followed less frequently by irregular linear opacities, patchy honeycombing, and nodular opacities.[56] As one might anticipate, most of the described findings in NSIP overlap with those of other DLD, such as hypersensitivity pneumonitis and cryptogenic organizing pneumonia.

Pathologic findings

Katzenstein and Fiorelli emphasized that the histopathology of NSIP was temporally "uniform" (Fig. 7.12), in contrast to the UIP pattern where variable zones of older fibrosis, more active fibroplasia, and normal lung all coexist in the same biopsy specimen (*temporal heterogeneity*).

As initially defined, the inflammatory process in NSIP is diffuse and uniform, mainly involving the alveolar walls (Fig. 7.13) and variably affecting the bronchovascular sheaths (Fig. 7.14) and pleura (Fig. 7.15).[21] In some patients, infiltrates are predominantly peribronchial, while in others germinal centers may be seen along with chronic pleuritis. When airspace organization (the organizing pneumonia pattern) is present, it is not uniformly distributed (Fig. 7.16) as might occur in organizing infectious pneumonia.[21] When fibrosis occurs in NSIP, it is usually mild and preserves lung structure (Fig. 7.17), generally without microscopic honeycombing.[21]

Whether or not NSIP is a new "interstitial lung disease," or simply a wastebasket category of diseases with some overlapping features, remains to be resolved. Caution is advised in using this term for any lung disease with interstitial inflammation, just as it is imprudent to diagnose all fibrosing lung diseases as UIP.

Differential diagnosis

The main entities in the differential diagnosis of the NSIP pattern include hypersensitivity pneumonitis, systemic collagen vascular diseases manifesting in the lung, resolving infection, and low-grade lymphoproliferative disease masquerading as LIP (see below). Cellular NSIP and LIP may be difficult to distinguish from each other on histopathologic grounds so they might be considered synonyms from the pathologist's perspective, once lymphoproliferative disease has been reasonably excluded.

Clinical course

The purely "cellular" form of NSIP seems to be a disease with a good prognosis, compared with UIP and AIP.

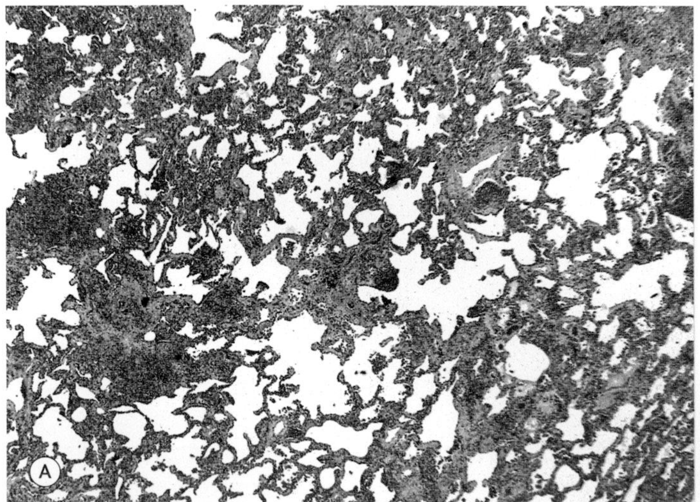

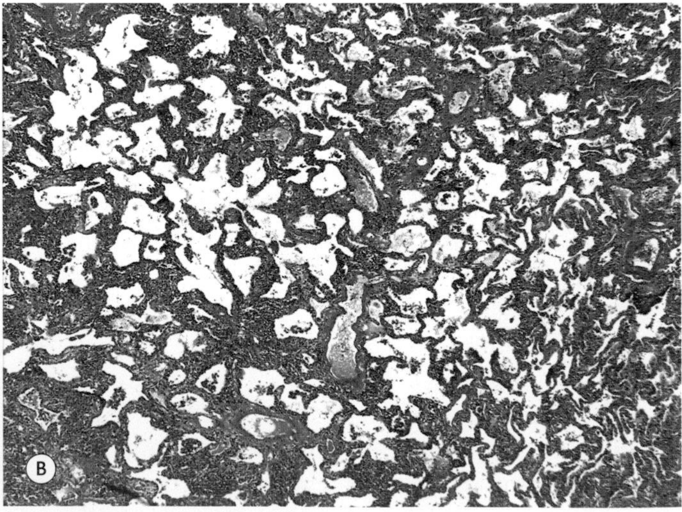

Fig. 7.12 **Nonspecific interstitial pneumonia (NSIP).** The histopathology of NSIP is temporally "uniform," in contrast to the temporal *heterogeneity* of the UIP pattern. Two examples are shown here: (A) small lymphoid aggregates can be appreciated at scanning magnification; (B) the process is uniform and may be associated with interstitial widening and some interstitial fibrosis.

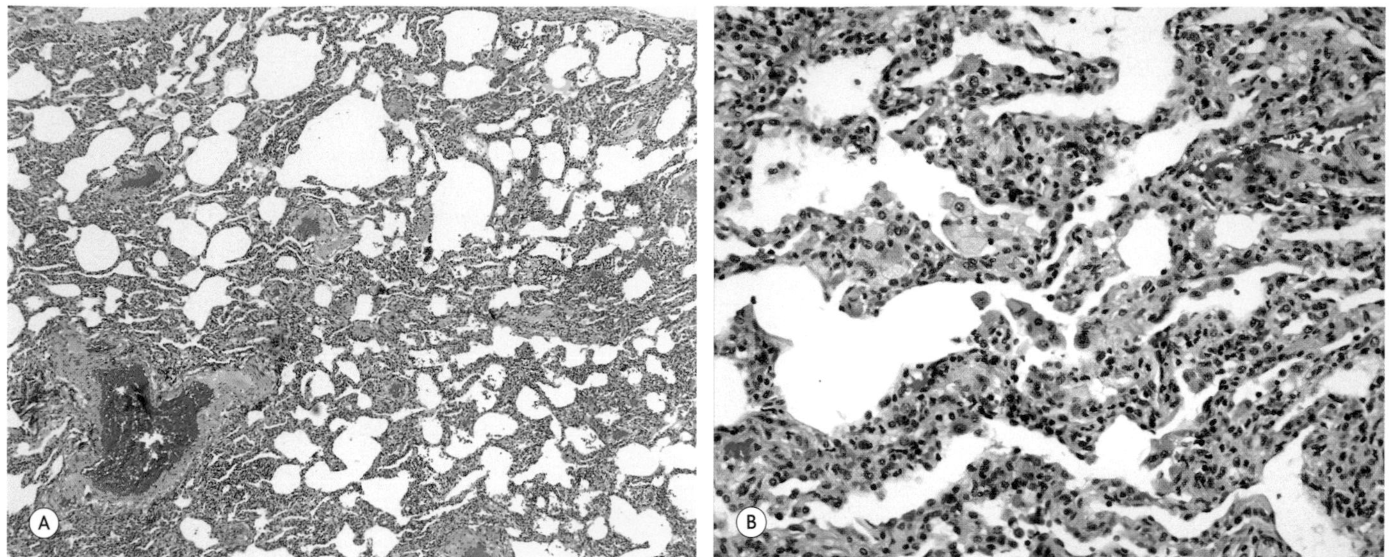

Fig. 7.13 **Nonspecific interstitial pneumonia (NSIP).** (A) The chronic inflammatory infiltration in NSIP is diffuse and relatively uniform, mainly involving the alveolar walls. (B) Lymphocytes and plasma cells are the dominant cells.

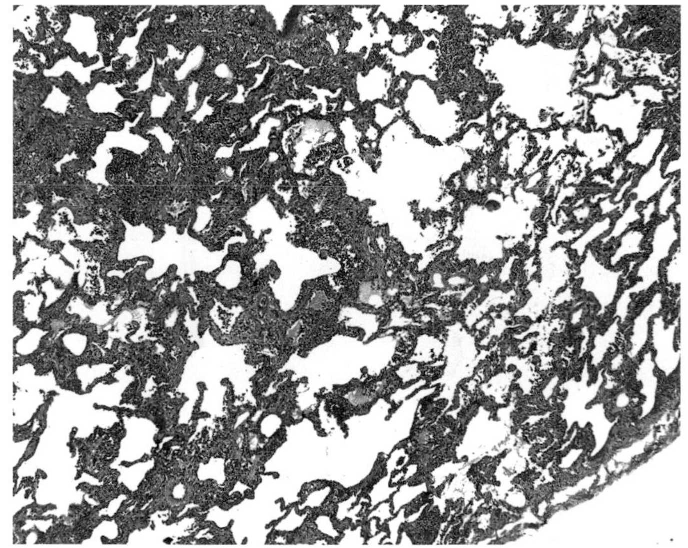

Fig. 7.14 **Nonspecific interstitial pneumonia (NSIP).** There is variable widening of alveolar walls by chronic inflammation, with little if any spared alveolar parenchyma in the biopsy. Bronchovascular sheaths are also typically involved by inflammatory cells, to variable degree.

When fibrosis and honeycombing are added as modifiers to NSIP, 5- and 10-year survivals change significantly for the worse.[52, 57] This observation suggests that fibrotic forms of NSIP may be within the spectrum of other fibrosing lung diseases, such as the UIP of IPF, and certain systemic connective tissue diseases that manifest in the lung with fibrosis.

Cryptogenic organizing pneumonia

Airspace organization is an extremely common manifestation of lung injury and can be seen following a wide variety of insults: from organizing lung infection to bacterial pneumonia (Table 7.10). For this reason, the organizing pneumonia pattern in the lung biopsy is the least specific and perhaps the most misunderstood.

It is well known that lung repair following a wide spectrum of injuries frequently evolves through a phase of airspace organization. When organization is diffuse, involving the entire surgical biopsy, organizing pneumonia (or "diffuse airspace organization") is an appropriate terminology. When no etiology can be identified for an organizing pneumonia pattern, the term cryptogenic organizing pneumonia (COP) has been proposed (also referred to as idiopathic bronchiolitis obliterans organizing pneumonia).[4,58,59]

The term "bronchiolitis obliterans organizing pneumonia" (BOOP), as an idiopathic disease, was first proposed by Davison and coworkers,[58] and later by Epler and coworkers[59], to define a group of patients who had a specific clinical disease course and who had lung biopsies with variable amounts of airspace organization (organizing pneumonia pattern) of unexplained etiology.[59] The clinical-pathologic entity of idiopathic BOOP is now referred to as "cryptogenic organizing pneumonia."[4] The importance of recognizing the pattern of organizing pneumonia in the clinical context defined relates to therapy and prognosis. Patients with clinical COP respond

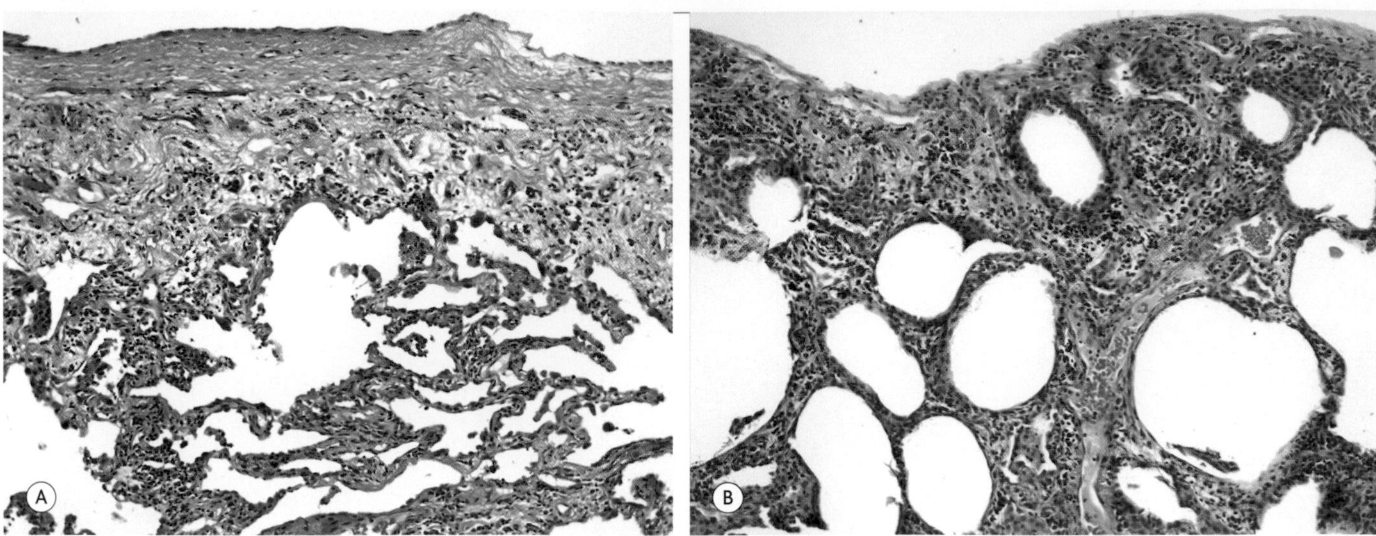

Fig. 7.15 **Nonspecific interstitial pneumonia (NSIP).** Pleuritis is very common in NSIP (A,B), emphasizing the strong association between the NSIP pattern in biopsy and the presence of known, or evolving, systemic collagen vascular disease.

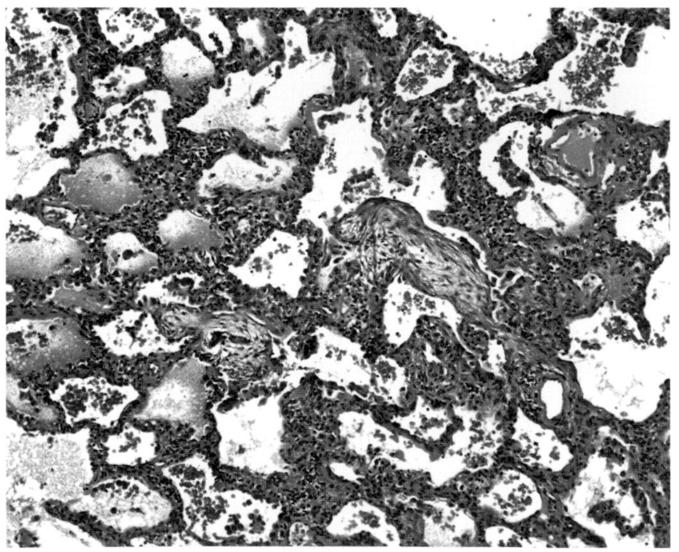

Fig. 7.16 **Nonspecific interstitial pneumonia (NSIP).** When airspace organization (organizing pneumonia pattern) is seen (center), it is not diffusely or uniformly distributed, as might occur in organizing infectious pneumonia.

well to systemic corticosteroid administration, and pulmonologists expect a good prognosis when this diagnosis is implied. When a pathologist uses the term "BOOP" to refer to any occurrence of organizing pneumonia in a biopsy, the clinician may misunderstand and assume "idiopathic BOOP." For example, the "BOOP" pattern might be seen in a disease with abundant fibrosis. In this setting, the prognosis may be guarded.[60]

Clinical presentation

The typical presentation, as described by Epler et al. for the original idiopathic "BOOP," is that of a patient who presents several weeks after an episode of clinical symptoms suggesting upper respiratory tract infection.[59] The mean age at onset is 55 years and the majority of patients are non-smokers.[61,62] Slowly increasing symptoms of cough (sometimes productive) and dyspnea are typically present, often resulting in a surgical lung biopsy within 3 months of disease onset. Weight loss, night sweats, chills, intermittent fever, and myalgias are common. Mild to moderate restrictive pulmonary function studies are identified in the majority of patients.[62–64] Hemoptysis and wheezing are typically absent. There is often a marked increase in the erythrocyte sedimentation rate (ESR). Digital clubbing is not a feature of the disease.

Radiologic findings

Chest radiograph and CT scan show a number of abnormal findings, none of which are specific for one disease. Patchy airspace consolidation (loss of visible structure underlying opacification) is the most consistent finding and is present in 90% of cases.[65,66] Air bronchograms can be seen in areas of consolidation. Ground glass attenuation accompanies consolidation in more than half of the patients. The disease involves the lower lung zones more often then the upper lung zones.[67] Small nodular opacities can be seen in 10–50% of patients.[68]

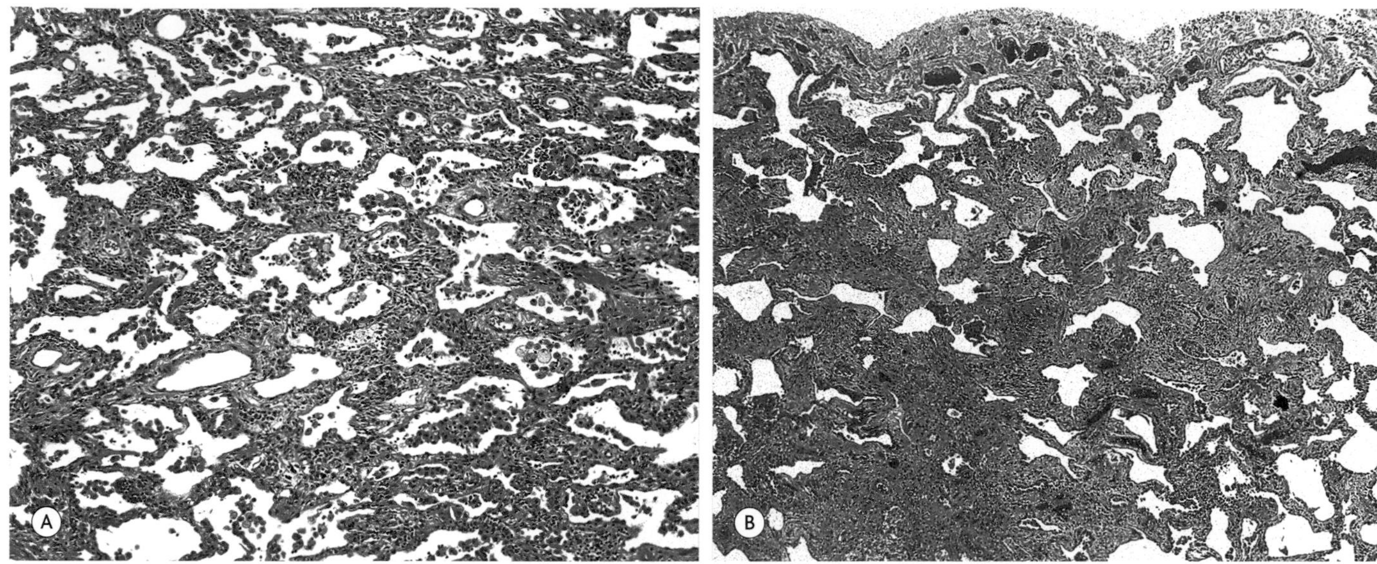

Fig. 7.17 **Nonspecific interstitial pneumonia (NSIP).** When fibrosis occurs in NSIP (so-called "fibrotic NSIP"), it is usually mild to moderate in amount and preserves lung structure, generally without microscopic honeycombing, or heterogeneity (i.e. normal lung adjacent to advanced fibrosis). (A) Low magnification of one example; (B) a higher magnification of another case.

Table 7.10 Causes of the organizing pneumonia pattern

Causes
Organizing infections
Organizing diffuse alveolar damage
Drug and toxic reactions
Collagen vascular diseases
Hypersensitivity pneumonitis
Chronic eosinophilic pneumonia
Airway diseases (bronchitis and emphysema, bronchiectasis, cystic fibrosis, aspiration pneumonia, and chronic bronchiolitis) complicated by infection
Airway obstruction
Peripheral reaction around abscesses, infarcts, Wegener granulomatosis, and others
Idiopathic (likely immunologic) lung disease (cryptogenic organizing pneumonia)

Source: from Leslie et al.,[3] p 40, with permission.

In a small percentage of patients large nodules may be seen,[68] and rarely reticulonodular infiltrates occur.[64] It is speculated that this latter finding identifies a subset of COP that may not respond to therapy. Opacities may be recurrent and/or migratory.[69–71] Lung volumes are typically normal in most patients and pleural effusions rarely occur.[65,66,72]

Pathologic findings

The organizing pneumonia (OP) pattern is characterized by variably dense airspace aggregates of loose fibroblasts in ground substance (immature collagen matrix) (Fig. 7.18). This alveolar filling process can be seen to extend into or from terminal bronchioles (Fig. 7.19). In COP the lung architecture is typically preserved, and lymphocytes, plasma cells, and histiocytes are present to variable degree within the interstitium (Fig. 7.20).[59,73,74] Fibrin may be seen focally in association with airspace organization (Fig. 7.21). Alveolar macrophage accumulation may be present, attesting to some degree of airway obstruction.[59,73,74] When airspace organization is confluent and diffuse in the biopsy, COP is less likely to be the accurate diagnosis. Interstitial fibrosis and honeycomb lung remodeling are not components of the cryptogenic (idiopathic) form of OP.[59,73,74]

Treatment and prognosis

The expected response to systemic corticosteroid therapy for COP is excellent.[59,69,75] Therapy generally requires extended tapering, sometimes for more than a year, because relapses occur in some patients whose corticosteroid therapy is tapered too soon.[59,69,75]

Differential diagnosis

As mentioned above, the differential diagnosis for the organizing pneumonia histopathologic pattern is too

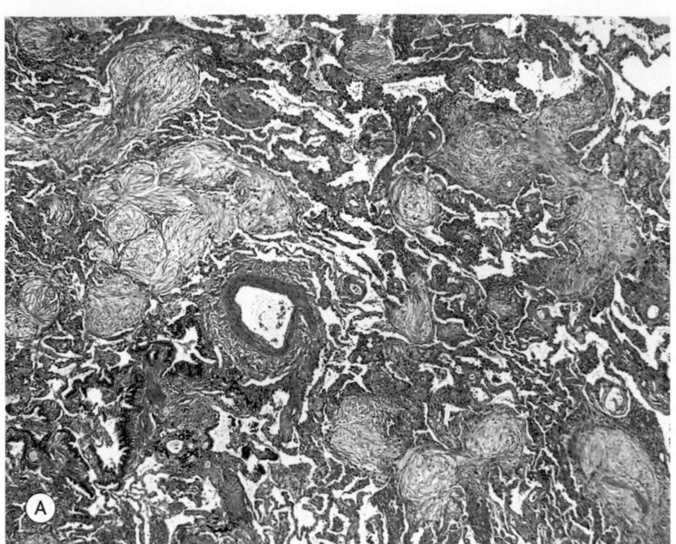

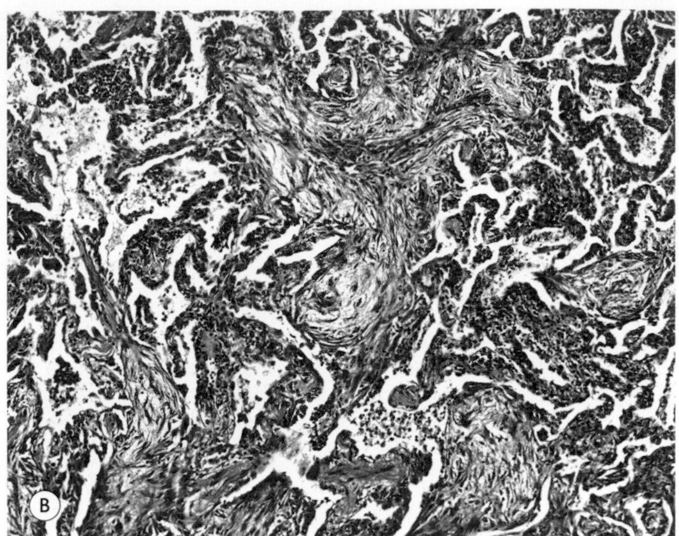

Fig. 7.18 **Organizing pneumonia (OP) pattern.** The OP pattern is characterized by variably dense airspace aggregates of loose fibroblasts present within ground substance (immature collagen associated with an acellular pale/basophilic matrix). (A) Scanning magnification, showing slight nodularity of the process. (B) Higher magnification, showing growth of loose granulation tissue within terminal airways and adjacent alveolar spaces.

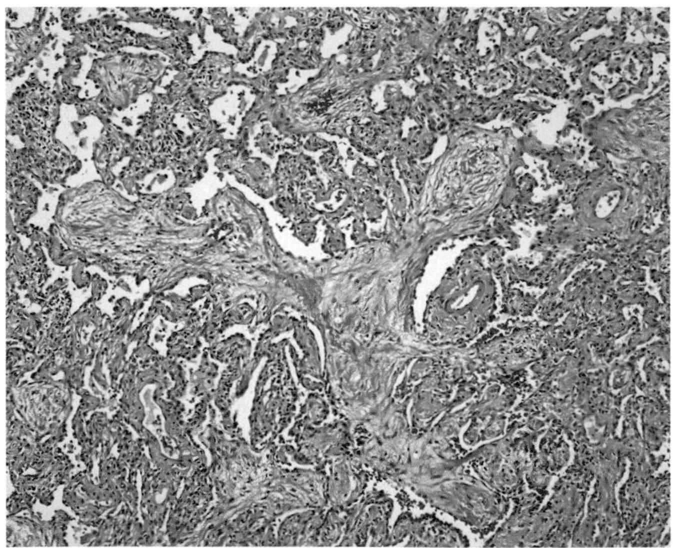

Fig. 7.19 **Organizing pneumonia pattern.** A branching tongue of fibroblastic proliferation can be seen to extend into, or from, an alveolar duct. Note the mild inflammatory interstitial infiltrate in surrounding alveolar walls.

broad to have any clinical meaning. In general, it is fair to say that the presence of the OP pattern is much more commonly associated with slowly organizing infection, systemic connective tissue diseases, hypersensitivity pneumonitis, and idiosyncratic reaction to drug or medication, rather than a "cryptogenic" disease. Rarely, airspace organization may ossify and produce so-called "racemose" or "dendriform" ossification (Fig. 7.22).

Clinical course

In the case of cryptogenic organizing pneumonia, patients typically experience an excellent response to systemic corticosteroid therapy.

Respiratory bronchiolitis-associated interstitial lung disease

Respiratory bronchiolitis (RB) is a histopathologic lesion of the small airways that occurs commonly in cigarette smokers.[76] In some smokers, an exuberant form of RB occurs as a clinical and radiologic manifestation of diffuse "interstitial" lung disease. This DLD manifestation of RB has been referred to as respiratory bronchiolitis-associated interstitial lung disease (RBILD).[77] RB, RBILD, and desquamative interstitial pneumonia (DIP) have been proposed as existing along a continuum in smokers,[78] with RB on the asymptomatic end of a spectrum that culminates in DIP. Whether RB, RBILD, and DIP are truly manifestations of a single disease process remains to be proven. Certainly all three have some histopathologic elements in common, but the two main clinical manifestations in the spectrum (RBILD and DIP) also differ in a number of ways clinically and radiologically.

Clinical presentation

Patients with RBILD are typically a decade younger than those with DIP and present in early midlife, with a mean

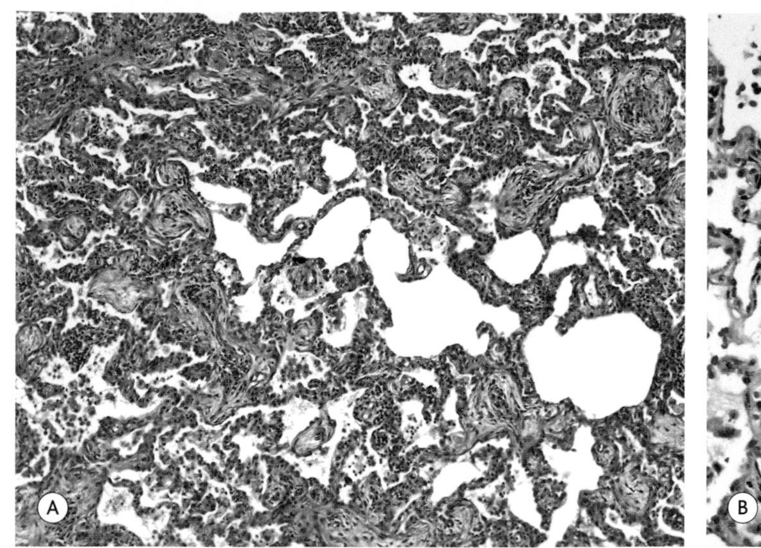

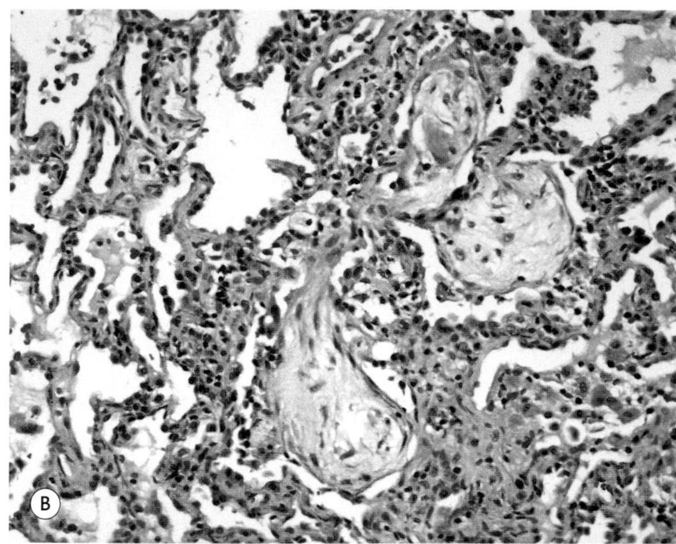

Fig. 7.20 **Organizing pneumonia pattern.** In cryptogenic organizing pneumonia (COP) the lung architecture is typically preserved. Lymphocytes, plasma cells, and histiocytes are present to variable degree within the interstitium. (A) Note the very patchy organization here. (B) The prototypic appearance of COP, with patchy organization and mild interstitial pneumonia, is evident here.

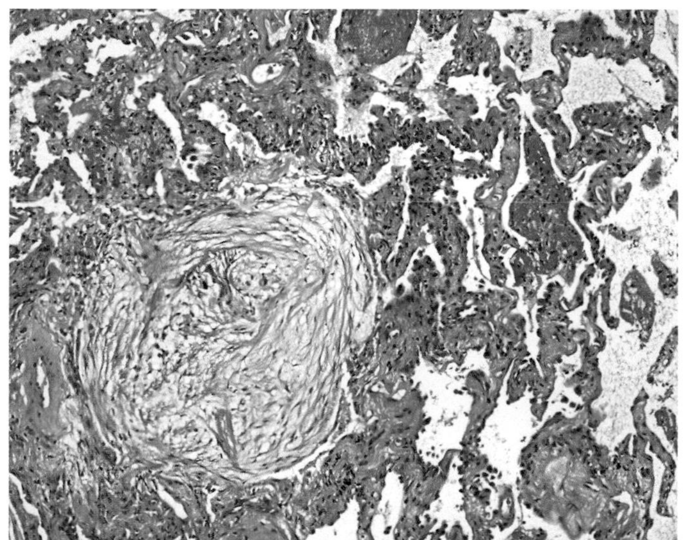

Fig. 7.21 **Organizing pneumonia pattern.** Fibrin (center right) may be seen focally in association with airspace organization (center left) in cryptogenic organizing pneumonia (COP).

age of 36 years in two studies.[77,79] A relationship between smoking pack-years and onset of diseases suggests a dose-related effect, with a threshold in the vicinity of 30 pack-years. There tends to be a gender predilection in favor of men,[78,80] but the sexes were equally affected in one study.[79] Mild symptoms of breathlessness and cough are the most common initial complaints.[77,79] Clubbing of the digits is unusual in RBILD.[79,81,82] Pulmonary function abnormalities parallel the mild clinical symptoms and may show evidence of both obstruction and restriction, with mild reduction in the diffusing capacity.[80]

Radiologic findings

The chest X-ray appearance of RBILD reflects the presence of disease focused on the airways, mainly with thickening of airway walls.[78] Ground glass opacity is seen in more than 50% of chest radiographs in RBILD. On CT scans, ground glass opacities and centrilobular nodules are typical findings.[78]

Pathologic findings

Respiratory bronchiolitis is a common reaction in the lungs of cigarette smokers and its presence alone does not imply the diffuse lung disease manifestation.[82] Moreover, even when the histopathology is diffuse and distinctive in the biopsy specimen, clinical correlation is required for accurate diagnosis. For example, a patient with a lung mass, resected and found to be a bronchogenic carcinoma, may have extensive RB in surrounding lung parenchyma. In the absence of a clinically and radiologically defined DLD, a diagnosis of RBILD would be inappropriate.

The essential morphologic constituents of respiratory bronchiolitis (RB) are (1) scant inflammation around the

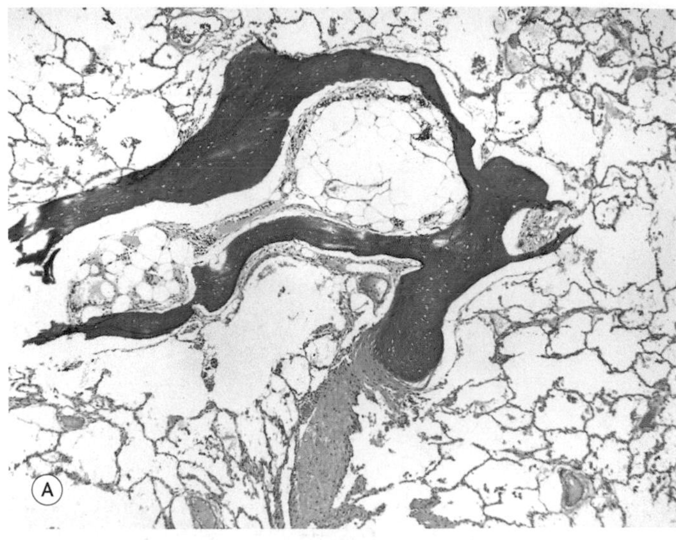

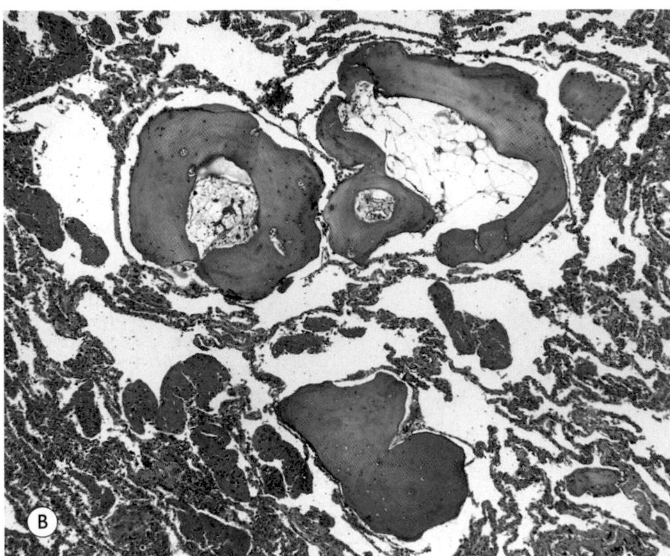

Fig. 7.22 **Racemose (dendriform) alveolar calcification.** Rarely, airspace organization may ossify and produce so-called "racemose" or "dendriform" ossification (A,B).

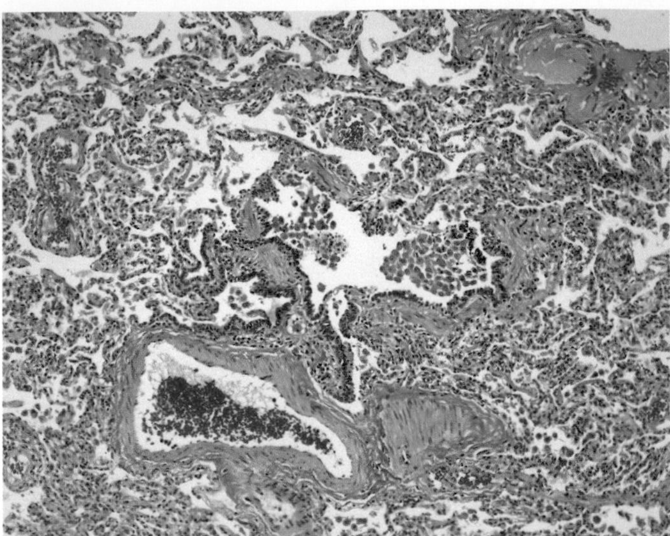

Fig. 7.23 **Respiratory bronchiolitis (RB).** Respiratory bronchiolitis is characterized by the presence of scant inflammation around the terminal airways.

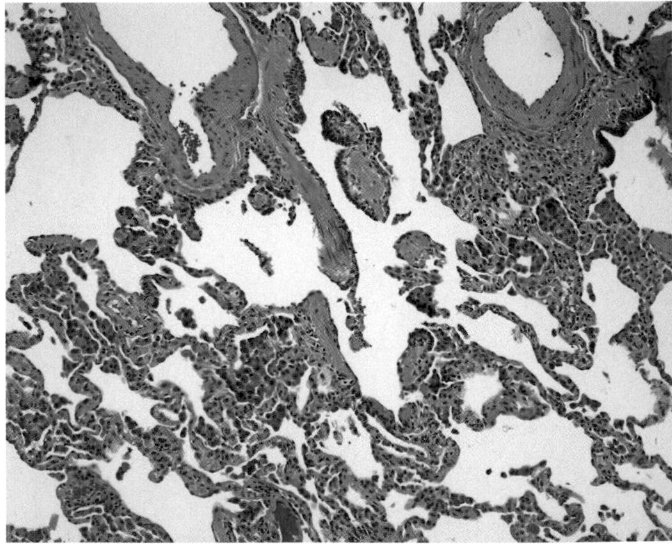

Fig. 7.24 **Respiratory bronchiolitis (RB).** Metaplastic bronchiolar epithelium extends out from terminal airways to involve alveolar ducts.

terminal airways (Fig. 7.23), (2) metaplastic bronchiolar epithelium extending out from terminal airways to involve alveolar ducts (Fig. 7.24), and (3) variable numbers of lightly pigmented, dusty brown, airspace macrophages, which are seen within bronchiolar lumens and in immediate surrounding alveoli (Fig. 7.25). Scant peribronchiolar fibrosis may be present and this may extend to involve contiguous alveolar walls (Fig. 7.26).

Differential diagnosis

Respiratory bronchiolitis may be confused on occasion with bronchiolitis of other etiology. When bronchiolar metaplasia is a prominent component, distinction from other small airways disease (SAD), such as idiopathic constrictive bronchiolitis, may be difficult. Patients with idiopathic constrictive bronchiolitis in surgical biopsies tend to have more severe pulmonary function abnormalities than those patients with RB or RBILD (see Ch. 8 for a discussion of SAD).

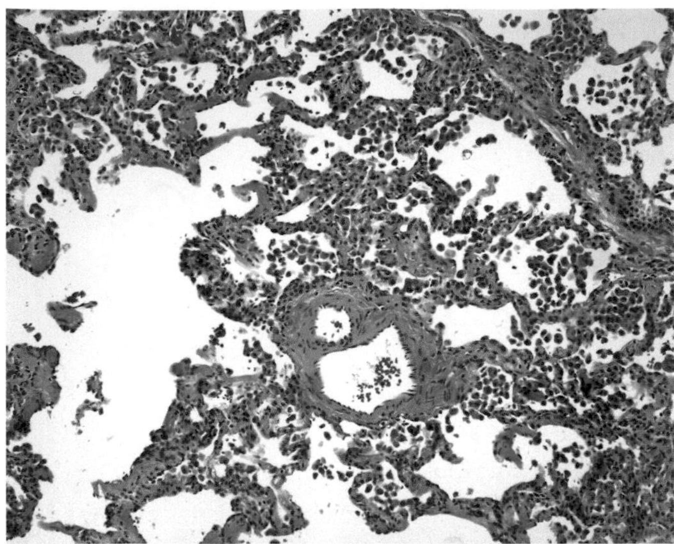

Fig. 7.25 **Respiratory bronchiolitis (RB).** Variable numbers of lightly pigmented (dusty brown) airspace macrophages are seen within bronchiolar lumens and in immediate surrounding alveoli.

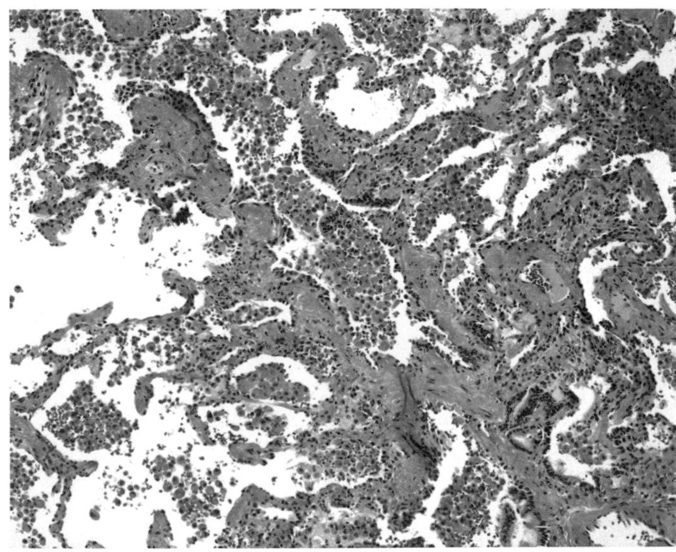

Fig. 7.26 **Respiratory bronchiolitis (RB).** Scant peribronchiolar fibrosis may be present and this may extend to involve contiguous alveolar walls, with or without prominent smooth muscle bundles.

Clinical course

RBILD has an excellent prognosis. When patients are mildly symptomatic, improvement has been reported with smoking cessation alone.

Desquamative interstitial pneumonia

Leibow[2] proposed the term "desquamative interstitial pneumonia" for a diffuse lung disease that occurred in patients who were typically a decade or more younger than those who developed UIP. The disease often presented in mid-adulthood and most patients were cigarette smokers.[83] Liebow also believed that the "desquamated" cells that filled the airspaces in DIP were epithelial cells. Today we know that the airspace cells of Liebow's DIP are actually macrophages, and that DIP is not a credible precursor lesion for UIP, as was proposed by some authorities.

Our current concept of DIP overlaps with that of RBILD, with both being considered components of the "smoking-related diffuse lung diseases" (see pulmonary Langerhans cell histiocytosis below). Whether DIP occurs as a separate disease in non-smoking adolescents remains debatable, but is unlikely. Another debate is centered on whether a form of UIP coexists with DIP as a "hybrid" entity. Those who still believe that DIP is a precursor lesion to UIP embrace instances where this association is suggested in surgical lung biopsies, as proof of concept. The counter-argument is that smokers accumulate alveolar macrophages in areas of lung fibrosis, and since the majority of patients with UIP are current or ex-smokers, some of these patients will have prominent smokers-type macrophages coexistent with UIP.

Clinical presentation

As currently defined, DIP is a very rare smoking-related lung disease. Patients with DIP are typically older than those with RBILD[78] and roughly a decade younger than those with UIP.[82,83] Most patients with DIP are cigarette smokers and men are more frequently affected than women. Like UIP, the clinical presentation is dominated by insidious onset of dyspnea and dry cough over several weeks or months.[82,84] Digital clubbing is present in 50% of patients with DIP, a finding in sharp contrast to RBILD. The symptoms of DIP are usually more pronounced and more severe than those of RBILD,[78] and supported by pulmonary function testing showing mild restriction and moderate reductions in diffusing capacity.[84]

Radiologic findings

The plain film of the chest may be normal in 3–22% of patients with DIP. When abnormalities are present, patchy areas of ground glass opacification are dominant. The lung bases and periphery are most commonly affected.[78,85,86] On CT scans, ground glass opacification is universally present, mostly in a bibasilar distribution.[85] Linear and reticular opacities may accompany ground glass opacities at the bases but tend to be quite limited in extent. Focal areas of peripheral honeycombing may be

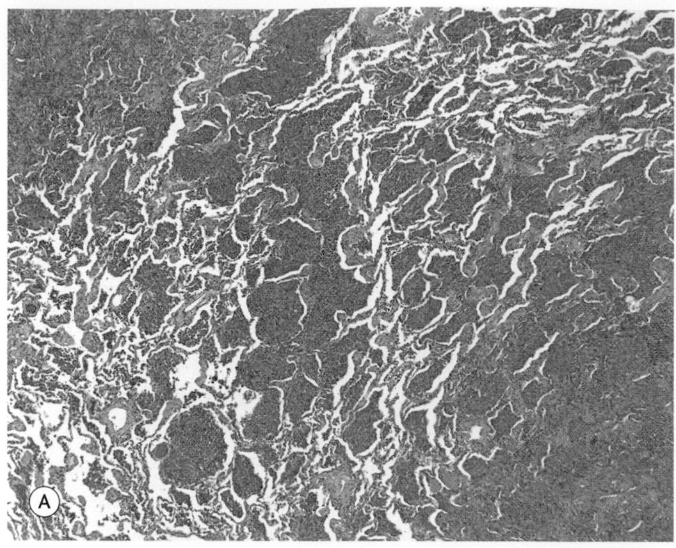

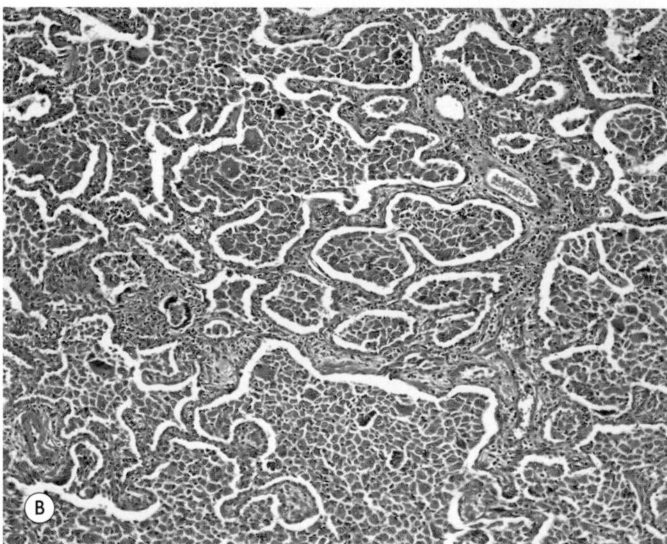

Fig. 7.27 **Desquamative interstitial pneumonia (DIP).** (A) DIP is often a scanning magnification diagnosis. (B) The surgical lung biopsy has an eosinophilic appearance due to the presence of eosinophilic macrophages uniformly filling airspaces.

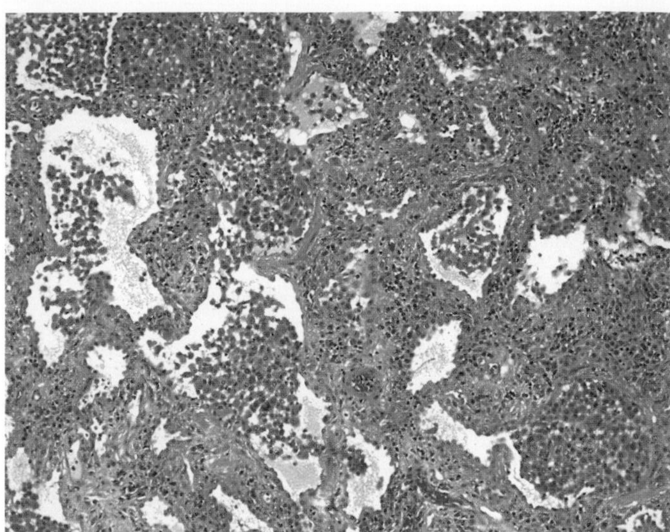

Fig. 7.28 **Desquamative interstitial pneumonia (DIP).** Variable thickening of alveolar walls by fibrous tissue is the rule in DIP and this is typically uniform in appearance. The expected presence of some alveolar wall fibrosis often makes the distinction of DIP from fibrotic forms of NSIP in heavy smokers the main issue, especially since the prognosis may be quite different between the two diseases.

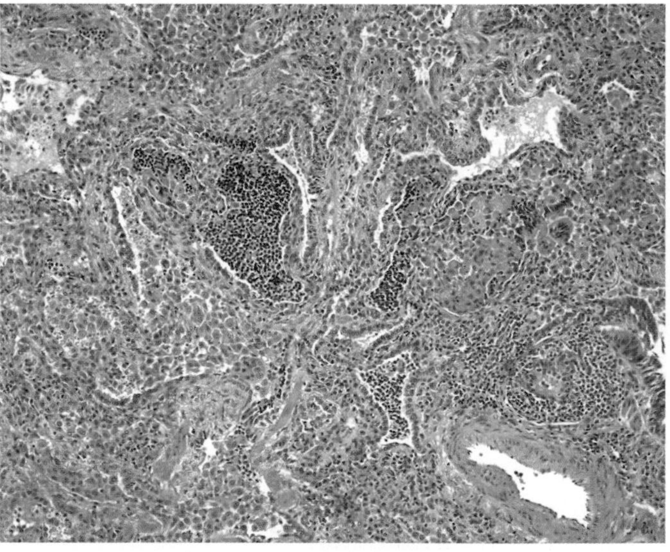

Fig. 7.29 **Desquamative interstitial pneumonia (DIP).** When chronic inflammation is evident in DIP at scanning magnification, it is centrilobular and associated with respiratory bronchioles.

identified in as many as one-third of patients[85] but, when prominent and associated with more pronounced reticular opacification, should raise a differential diagnosis to include other chronic fibrosing lung disorders (e.g. UIP).

Pathologic findings

On scanning magnification, the surgical lung biopsy in DIP has an eosinophilic appearance due to the presence of eosinophilic macrophages uniformly filling airspaces (Fig. 7.27).[14,79] Mild interstitial thickening by fibrous tissue is the rule and this is uniform in appearance (Fig. 7.28). When chronic inflammation is evident at scanning magnification, it is centrilobular and associated with respiratory bronchioles (Fig. 7.29). Scant numbers of plasma cells and rare eosinophils may be seen within slightly thickened alveolar walls at high magnification (Fig. 7.30).

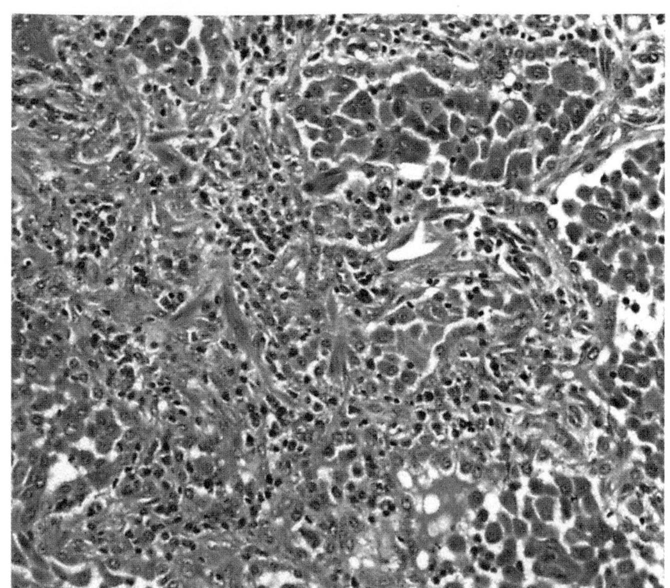

Fig. 7.30 **Desquamative interstitial pneumonia (DIP).** Scant numbers of plasma cells and rare eosinophils may be seen within slightly thickened alveolar walls at high magnification.

Differential diagnosis

Distinguishing DIP from RBILD is probably a useless exercise for pathologists, and inclusion of these two smoking-related diseases together as a diagnostic entity seems reasonable in the absence of clinical and radiologic data. Eosinophilic lung disease can simulate the low-magnification appearance of DIP, as can chronic passive congestion, pulmonary hemorrhage syndromes, giant cell interstitial pneumonia in hard metal disease, and pulmonary Langerhans cell histiocytosis (pulmonary histiocytosis X) when a prominent "DIP reaction" is identified. Progression to end-stage fibrotic lung disease is atypical and should raise consideration of another diagnosis, or comorbid disease.

Clinical course

Like RBILD, the prognosis for patients with DIP tends to be good, with an estimated 10-year survival of 70%.[84] Smoking cessation and corticosteroid therapy have proven effective.[83]

Lymphoid interstitial pneumonia

Lymphoid interstitial pneumonia (original LIP) was conceived as a chronic cellular interstitial pneumonia with distinctive histopathologic features, quite different in cellular composition and form than Liebow's other IIPs (e.g. UIP, BIP, DIP, and GIP).[2] LIP became controversial because many of the patients who were classified by Liebow and others as LIP, evolved into (or were indolent forms of) low-grade lymphoproliferative disease involving the lung.[87–89] It is now generally acknowledged that the accrual of dense lymphoid tissue in the lung carries strong implications for lymphoproliferative disease, especially small B-cell lymphomas of extranodal marginal zone type (so-called lymphomas of the mucosa-associated lymphoid tissue, or MALT).[87–90] Lymphoid interstitial pneumonia, as currently defined, is included as an entity in this chapter because a recent international consensus panel chose to keep LIP as a form of idiopathic interstitial pneumonia,[4] partly for historical reasons, all the while recognizing that many pulmonary pathologists would classify the described histopathologic findings of "idiopathic LIP," as a cellular form of "NSIP."

Clinical presentation

The clinical manifestations of the rare idiopathic form of the "LIP pattern" are not well studied but seem to be similar to those of other subacute/chronic diffuse lung diseases. Women are more commonly affected than men and patients are typically between 40 and 50 years of age.[91] Slowly progressive breathlessness is commonly present, with or without non-productive cough, and the disease may evolve over months to years.

In the classic description of LIP, systemic symptoms such as weight loss, pleuritic pain, arthralgias, adenopathy, and fever were reported, depending on any associated systemic condition.[91–93] Bibasilar crackles, cyanosis, and clubbing may be seen. Immunoglobulin abnormalities in serum are present in some patients.[94,95] More commonly, the LIP pattern is associated with a systemic condition that dominates the clinical presentation and clinical course (e.g. Sjögren's syndrome, pernicious anemia, hypogammaglobulinemia).

Radiologic findings

The published radiologic features of idiopathic LIP seem to describe more than one pattern of disease.[96] Bibasilar reticular opacities are the most frequent abnormality observed.[96,97] There may be mixed alveolar and interstitial infiltrates, cysts, honeycombing, and changes suggesting pulmonary hypertension late in the disease.[98,99] Nodular patterns can also occur.[100] Pleural effusion is rare and if present should increase concern for low-grade malignant lymphoma.

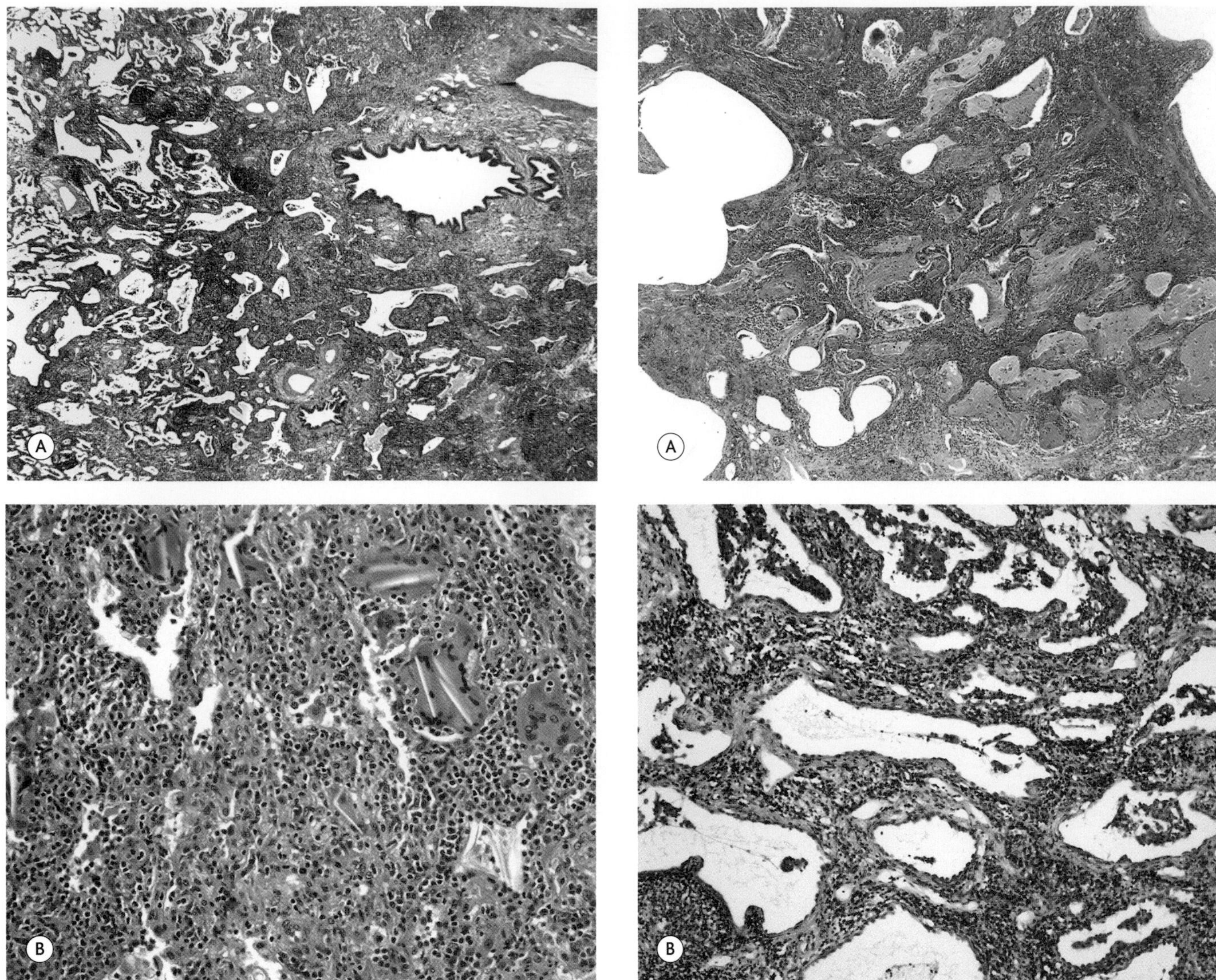

Fig. 7.31 **Lymphoid interstitial pneumonia (LIP).** (A) The histopathology of the LIP pattern is characterized by the presence of a dense and diffuse alveolar septal infiltrate made up of lymphocytes, plasma cells, plasmacytoid cells, and histiocytes. (B) Multinucleated giant cells and small non-necrotizing granulomas are commonly present.

Fig. 7.32 **Lymphoid interstitial pneumonia (LIP).** (A) Microscopic honeycomb cystic remodeling, with some interstitial fibrosis (B), can also be components of idiopathic LIP.

Pathologic findings

The histopathology of the LIP pattern is characterized by the presence of a dense and diffuse alveolar septal infiltrate made up of lymphocytes, plasma cells, plasmacytoid cells, and histiocytes (Fig. 7.31). This definition helps exclude diseases with less intense cellular interstitial infiltrates such as certain hypersensitivity reactions and systemic connective tissue diseases. Multinucleated giant cells and/or small ill-defined granulomas in the interstitium have been described in the idiopathic form of LIP, but should always raise concern for hypersensitivity pneumonitis, atypical mycobacterial infections, and certain drug reactions. Microscopic honeycomb cystic remodeling, with some interstitial fibrosis (Fig. 7.32), can also be a part of idiopathic LIP. Germinal centers may be present to a variable extent along airways and lymphatic routes (Fig. 7.33). When these are prominent, the term "diffuse lymphoid hyperplasia" has been used as a preferable term. When the idiopathic form of the LIP pattern (as currently defined) is identified, immunophenotyping and gene rearrangement studies typically show an absence of clonality.[101] When nodular lymphoid hyperplasia is prominent around bronchioles, typically

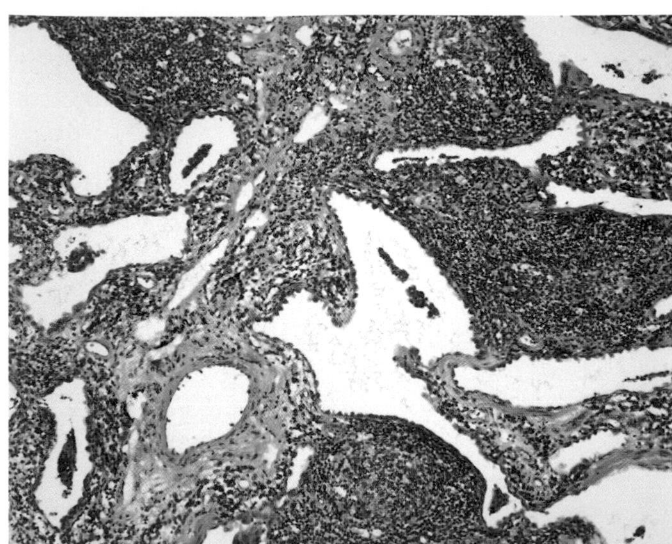

Fig. 7.33 **Lymphoid interstitial pneumonia (LIP).** Germinal centers may be present to a variable extent along airways and lymphatic routes. When these are prominent, the term "diffuse lymphoid hyperplasia" has been used as a preferable term to LIP.

accompanied by an interstitial infiltrate, Sjögren syndrome should be rigorously investigated as a potential etiology.

Differential diagnosis

The LIP pattern is most consistently seen when systemic collagen vascular diseases manifest in the lung.[91,102,103] The LIP pattern may also be seen in the setting of bone marrow transplantation[104] and frequently occurs in both children and adults with congenital or acquired immunodeficiency syndromes,[105] and in the setting of adult HIV infection, including vertical transmission infection from mother to child.[102,106–109]

Much of what has been written about the pathology of LIP is similar to that written about the pathologic pattern of NSIP. If LIP and cellular NSIP can be distinguished microscopically, it is usually on the basis of the intensity of the lymphoid infiltrate. Naturally, in this setting, gene rearrangement studies are important in distinguishing idiopathic LIP from low-grade lymphoproliferative disease (see Ch. 15 for further discussion). Once the pattern is established, it is useful to suggest the potential systemic conditions that may be associated with this pattern (Table 7.11) in a comment section of the surgical pathology report.

Table 7.11 Systemic conditions associated with the lymphoid interstitial pneumonia (LIP) histopathologic pattern

- Certain infections (e.g. *Pneumocystis jiroveci* pneumonia, Epstein–Barr virus, HIV infection)
- Connective tissue diseases (Sjögren's syndrome, rheumatoid arthritis, systemic lupus erythematosus)
- Immune deficiency diseases (HIV infection, heritable immunodeficiency syndromes)
- Autoimmune diseases (Hashimoto's thyroiditis, myasthenia gravis, pernicious anemia)
- Drug- or toxin-related lung injury

Clinical course

The clinical outcome and response to therapy for patients with the LIP pattern depend largely on the presence of systemic disease. In the idiopathic form, an accurate prognosis has not been forthcoming. In symptomatic patients, corticosteroid administration may result in significant benefit[91] and further supports the notion that LIP is an immunologic disease process in most instances, rather than a neoplastic one. When honeycomb cysts, clubbing, or cor pulmonale are present, the prognosis is less favorable, with as many as one-third of patients succumbing to the disease.[91,100] Infection is a common complication, especially when LIP is associated with dysproteinemia.[91,92,110]

Chronic manifestations of systemic collagen vascular diseases

Systemic collagen vascular diseases (CVDs) play an extremely important role in the DLD. It is estimated that DLD in CVDs is responsible for 1600 deaths annually in the United States, a figure that corresponds to roughly 25% of all DLD deaths and 2% of deaths from all respiratory causes.[111] Not suprisingly, most interstitial pneumonia patterns raise collagen vascular disease as an etiology in the differential diagnosis. On the other hand, certain CVDs are associated with reasonably reproducible findings in the lung. Table 7.12 lists the different patterns of inflammatory lung disease that have been described as lung manifestations of the known connective tissue diseases. The five CVDs that are more commonly associated with DLD are:

1. rheumatoid arthritis
2. progressive systemic sclerosis
3. systemic lupus erythematosus
4. polymyositis/dermatomyositis
5. Sjögren's syndrome.

In this chapter we will restrict our focus to the more chronic manifestations of these diseases. Acute lung manifestations of the CVDs are presented in Chapter 5.

Table 7.12 Lung manifestations of the collagen vascular diseases

	RA	SLE	PSS	DM/PM	MCTD	SS	AS
Pleural inflammation, fibrosis, effusions	X	X	X	X	X	X	X
Airway disease:							
– Inflammation (bronchiolitis)	X	X		X	X	X	
– Constrictive bronchiolitis	X				X		
– Bronchiectasis	X				X		
– Follicular bronchiolitis	X	X			X	X	
Interstitial disease:							
– Acute (DAD), with or without hemorrhage	X	X	X	X	X		
– Subacute/organizing (OP pattern)	X	X	X	X	X	X	
– Subacute cellular	X	X	X	X	X	X	
– Chronic cellular and fibrotic	X	X	X	X	X	X	
– Eosinophilic infiltrates	X				X		
– Granulomatous interstitial pneumonia	X	X			X		
Vascular diseases; hypertension/vasculitis	X	X	X	X	X	X	
Parenchymal nodules	X						
Apical fibrobullous disease	X		X		X		
Lymphoid proliferation (reactive, neoplastic)	X		X		X		

RA = rheumatoid arthritis; SLE = systemic lupus erythematosus; PSS = progressive systemic sclerosis; DM/PM = polymyositis/dermatomyositis; MCTD = mixed connective tissue disease; SS = Sjögren's syndrome; AS = ankylosing spondylitis; OP = organizing pneumonia; DAD = diffuse alveolar damage.
Source: adapted from Colby et al.[368] and Travis et al.[6]

Rheumatoid arthritis

Rheumatoid arthritis (RA) is a chronic systemic disease that produces symmetrical arthritis, and occurs more commonly in women then men. DLD was not recognized as a manifestation of RA until 1948,[112] possibly because lung manifestations of the disease are difficult to recognize on purely clinical grounds. Today, with the advent of pulmonary function testing, bronchoalveolar lavage, and computed tomograms, significant lung disease is seen in 14% of patients who meet the American Rheumatism Association criteria for RA, and subclinical disease is seen in as many as 44%.[113] Interestingly, men are three times as likely to develop DLD with RA than are women.[28] Clinically significant DLD in RA is associated with increased morbidity and mortality.[28]

Clinical presentation

Diffuse lung disease in RA typically occurs in patients with diagnosed disease, but rarely, DLD may precede articular manifestations.[114,115] The clinical presentation is dominated by shortness of breath and cough. Adults are more commonly affected than children,[116] and despite a higher incidence of RA in women, men with long-standing rheumatoid disease and subcutaneous nodules seem to develop lung manifestations more often.[114] Physical examination may reveal bibasilar inspiratory crackles, digital clubbing, and evidence of cor pulmonale, the latter occurring when pulmonary hypertension arises as a result of hypoxic vasoconstriction.[28,114] When fibrosis and honeycomb remodeling accompany diffuse lung disease in RA, UIP enters into the differential diagnosis. Such patients are often younger than those with idiopathic UIP. Cigarette smoking has been reported as an independent predictor of lung disease in RA.[117]

Radiologic findings

Several radiologic manifestations are described in RA, including reticular opacities with or without honeycombing, airway-associated abnormalities (bronchiectasis, nodules, centrilobular branching lines), and parenchymal opacities.[118] When ground glass infiltrates and reticular opacities are present, there is a predilection for involving the bases and lung periphery. HRCT findings include ground glass attenuation with mixed alveolar and interstitial infiltrates. As lung disease advances, dense reticular and nodular opacities appear, and honeycomb lung may be seen in late stages of the disease.[118,119]

Pathologic findings

Despite the seemingly nonspecific nature of the described pathologic manifestations of RA, a few key elements emerge on review of many well-documented cases of RA-DLD. Chronic inflammation, in the form of lymphocyte aggregates and germinal centers, is typical, although not

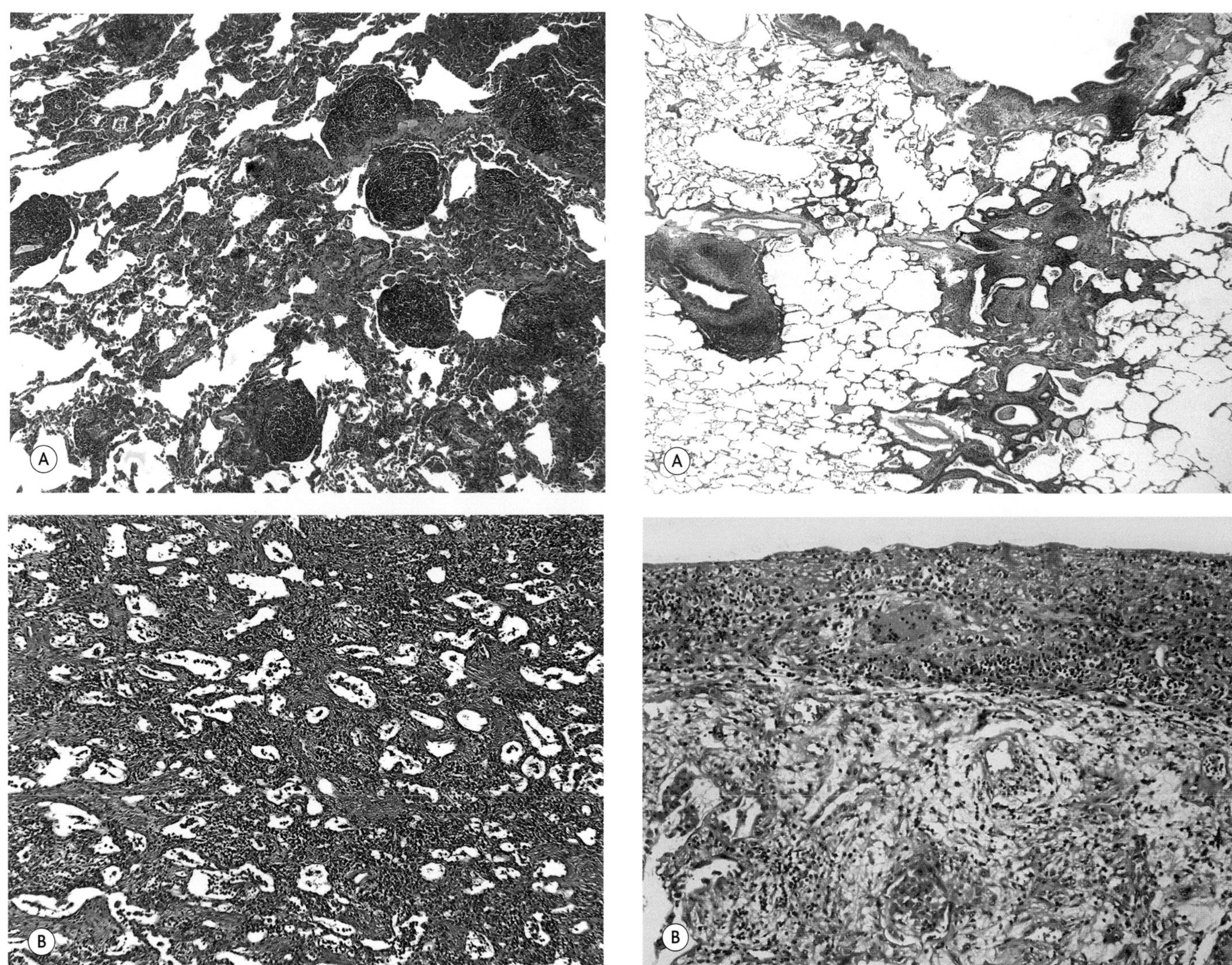

Fig. 7.34 **Rheumatoid arthritis (RA) lung disease.** (A) Chronic inflammation typically occurs in RA lung as lymphoid aggregates and follicular lymphoid germinal centers. (B) A variably cellular chronic interstitial infiltrate rich in plasma cells and lymphocytes is typical.

Fig. 7.35 **Rheumatoid arthritis (RA) lung disease.** Most of the lymphoid aggregations in RA (A) are present around the terminal airways ("follicular bronchiolitis" when lymphoid germinal centers are prominent) but lymphoid follicles may also be present in the pleura. In fact, the presence of chronic pleuritis (B) should always raise RA in the differential diagnosis.

unique (Fig. 7.34) Most of the lymphoid aggregations are present around the terminal airways ("follicular bronchiolitis" when lymphoid germinal centers are prominent) (Fig. 7.35), but lymphoid follicles may also be present in the pleura. In fact, the presence of chronic pleuritis should always raise RA in the differential diagnosis. Areas of subacute lung injury, attended by reactive type II cells and airspace organization (Fig. 7.36), can be seen with cellular interstitial pneumonia (Fig. 7.37) and variable interstitial fibrosis (Fig. 7.38). This combination of subacute and chronic inflammatory reactions haphazardly involving the same lung biopsy, including the pleura, should raise consideration for RA lung disease. Importantly, this spectrum of disease in the same biopsy specimen differs from that seen in UIP by not being present as an orderly transition from inactive fibrosis to normal lung (temporal heterogeneity). Vasculitis (including capillaritis) and even pulmonary hemorrhage have been described as manifestations of RA lung. When silicosis occurs with rheumatoid arthritis, the resulting disease is referred to as "Caplan's syndrome." Rheumatoid nodules can occur in the lung and pleura, and must be distinguished from granulomatous infection or Wegener's granulomatosis. Intrapulmonary lymph

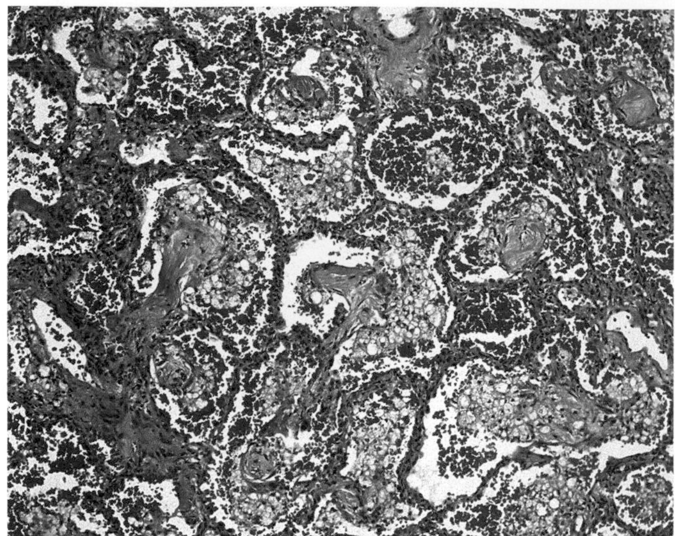

Fig. 7.36 **Rheumatoid arthritis (RA) lung disease.** Areas of subacute lung injury, attended by reactive type II cells and airspace organization, can be seen (here with fresh hemorrhage, probably related to the procedure).

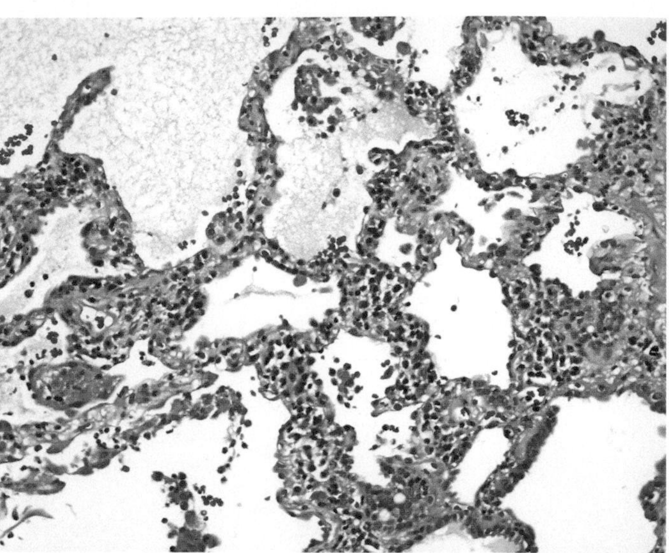

Fig. 7.37 **Rheumatoid arthritis (RA) lung disease.** The cellular interstitial pneumonia of RA may be attended by diffuse reactive type II cell hyperplasia, but is not particularly diagnostic absent of other more characteristic findings of RA (lymphoid germinal centers, follicular bronchiolitis, pleuritis, rheumatoid nodules).

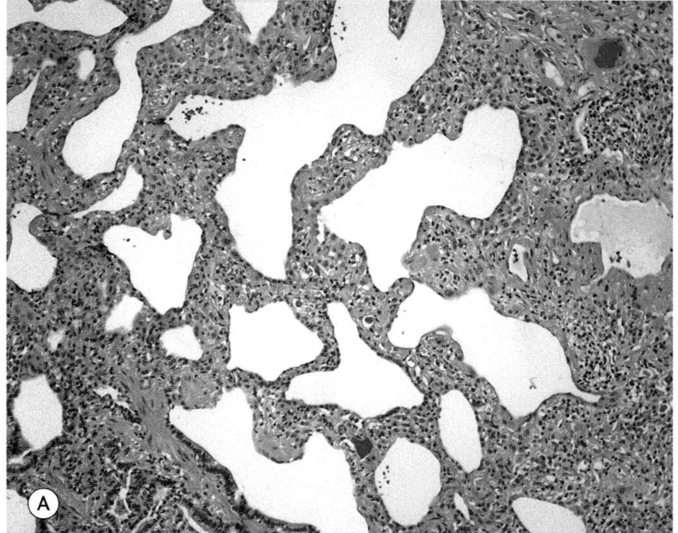

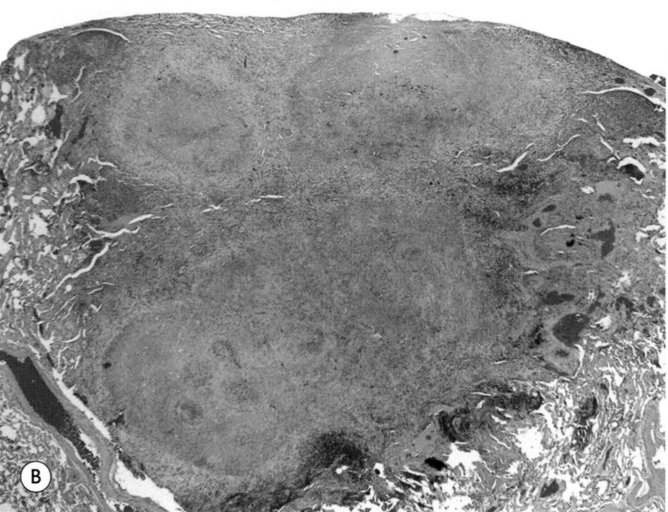

Fig. 7.38 **Rheumatoid arthritis (RA) lung disease.** Variable interstitial fibrosis (A) is typical and often resembles the fibrotic form of NSIP. Typical rheumatoid nodules may occur in RA lung (B) and must be distinguished from infection and Wegener's granulomatosis.

nodes may become prominent in rheumatoid arthritis and typically show reactive lymphoid hyperplasia when subjected to biopsy.

Differential diagnosis

RA lung manifestations are frequently confused with the idiopathic interstitial pneumonias (COP, NSIP, or even UIP), especially when the lung disease precedes the systemic disease. When patients with rheumatoid arthritis develop pulmonary symptoms, biopsies are usually performed only when superimposed lung infection or drug reaction is suspected clinically. Surgical lung biopsy in this context can be extremely difficult to interpret, given significant overlap in the morphologic patterns of drug reactions, low-grade infection, and the systemic collagen vascular disease itself.

Clinical course

As with other connective tissue diseases, therapeutic strategies in RA have focused on immunosuppression.[28] The development of pulmonary fibrosis has a significant negative impact on survival.[115,117,120]

Progressive systemic sclerosis

Progressive systemic sclerosis (PSS) is a relatively rare systemic autoimmune disease with cutaneous manifestations (dermal sclerosis) frequently accompanied by Raynaud's phenomenon. Pulmonary involvement (mainly DLD) occurs more commonly in patients with PSS than any other connective tissue disease,[121,122] with lung disease ranking fourth in frequency (after skin, peripheral vascular disease, and esophageal manifestations) in the disease. As in patients with RA, lung involvement in PSS is associated with increased morbidity and mortality.[122]

Clinical presentation

Chronic exertional dyspnea is the most common presentation, followed in frequency by chronic cough. Bibasilar inspiratory "crackles" are present in two-thirds of patients.[28,122] Digital clubbing may be present, but is uncommon. Pulmonary fibrosis and cor pulmonale may eventually occur.[124] Like other CVDs, lung involvement can precede the development of diagnostic systemic manifestations.[122,125]

Radiologic findings

Bibasilar interstitial infiltrates with relative sparing of the upper lung zones are typical radiologic features.[126,127] Loss of lung volume, honeycomb cysts, and findings consistent with pulmonary hypertension may also occur. Mixed reticular and nodular infiltrates are common.[126,127] Pleural effusion and/or pleural thickening may occur as minor findings.

Pathologic findings

Of all the CVD manifestations in lung, those produced by PSS are perhaps the most characteristic. The interstitial fibrosis of PSS is paucicellular and diffuse, with preservation of underlying lung architecture (Fig. 7.39). This distinctive "collagenization" of the lung interstitium has been confused with the pattern of lung fibrosis seen in idiopathic UIP.[124] The lack of "temporal heterogeneity" (see UIP above) is a useful finding and helps exclude UIP (of idiopathic pulmonary fibrosis) from the differential diagnosis. Pulmonary hypertensive changes (Fig. 7.40) may be present and deserve careful attention, since this is a major cause of mortality in scleroderma patients with lung disease.[128] As patients with PSS can also develop esophageal motility problems, subclinical chronic aspiration should be carefully excluded as a comorbid disease process.[129,130]

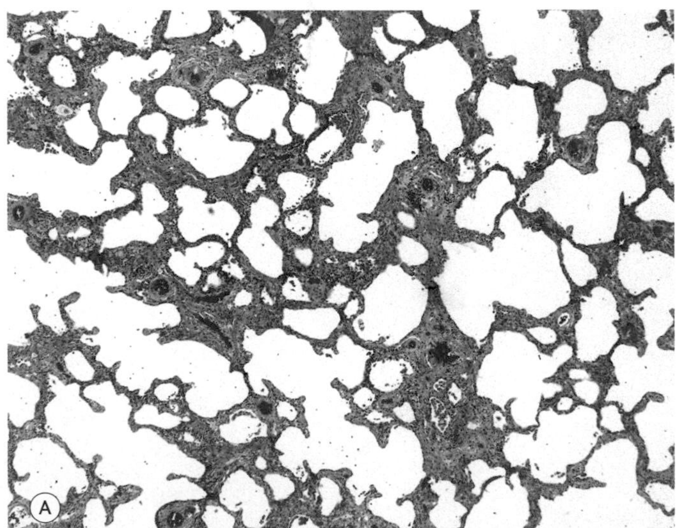

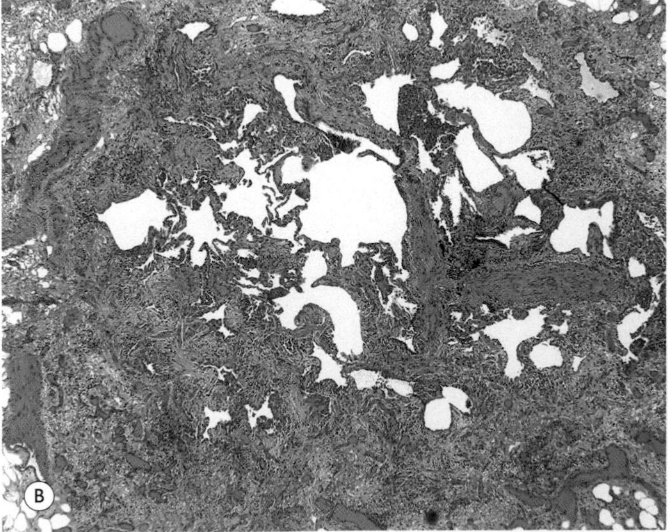

Fig. 7.39 **Progressive systemic sclerosis (PSS).** (A) The interstitial fibrosis of PSS is typically paucicellular and diffuse, with preservation of underlying lung architecture. (B) When fibrosis is more advanced, distinction from UIP (of idiopathic pulmonary fibrosis) may be difficult on morphologic grounds.

Clinical course

The mean survival for patients with scleroderma is 12 years from the time of diagnosis, and pulmonary disease has emerged as the major cause of death.[131] Pulmonary function status at presentation is a reasonable predictor of survival, and high-dose immunosuppressive therapy seems to benefit those patients with severe manifestations.[132]

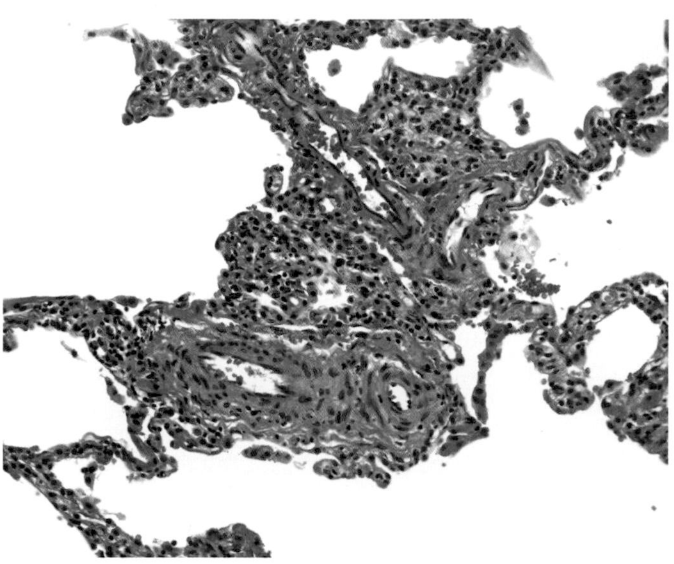

Fig. 7.40 **Progressive systemic sclerosis (PSS).** Pulmonary hypertensive changes may be present and deserve careful attention, since this is a major cause of mortality in scleroderma patients with lung disease.

Systemic lupus erythematosus

Systemic lupus erythematosus (SLE) is a chronic systemic autoimmune disease characterized by arthropathy, mucocutaneous manifestations, renal disease, and serositis.[133] The lung can be the major site of involvement in SLE, ranging from acute lupus pneumonitis, at one end of the spectrum, to fibrotic forms of "NSIP," at the other.[134–136] Acute lung injury and pulmonary hemorrhage are more commonly associated with SLE than with other systemic connective tissue diseases,[136,137] but hemoptysis only occurs in little more than half of the affected patients.[138,139]

Clinical presentation

SLE rivals PSS as the leader in pleuropulmonary manifestations in CVD.[134,140–142] The spectrum of lung disease in SLE is quite broad[135–137,143] and includes pleuritis (Fig. 7.41), acute lupus pneumonitis (Fig. 7.42), nonspecific interstitial pneumonia (NSIP) with fibrosis (Fig. 7.43), and diffuse alveolar hemorrhage (Fig. 7.44). Constrictive small airway disease, pulmonary arterial hypertension, and pulmonary embolism can also occur as rare manifestations. Patients with lung disease often have a high serum antinuclear antibody (ANA) or rheumatoid factor (RF) titer.

Radiologic findings

The radiologic findings are similar to those seen in other connective tissue diseases, with variable ground glass

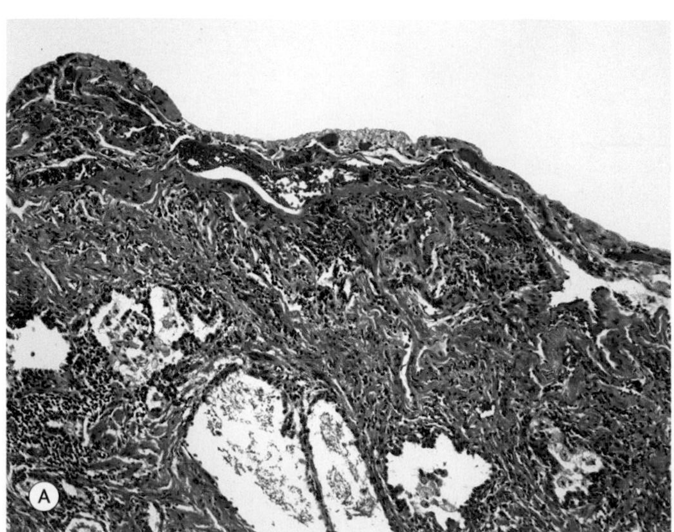

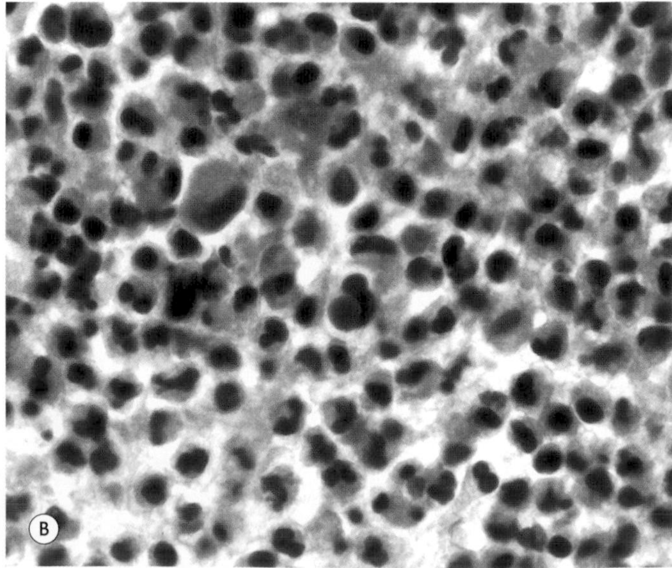

Fig. 7.41 **Systemic lupus erythematosus (SLE).** The spectrum of lung disease in SLE is quite broad and includes (A) pleuritis, sometimes accompanied by so-called LE bodies (B – center).

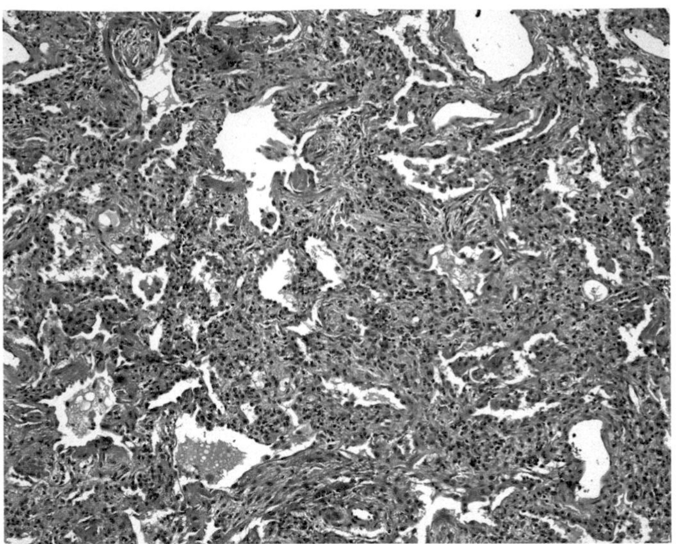

Fig. 7.42 **Systemic lupus erythematosus (SLE).** Acute lupus pneumonitis (ALP) is the most dramatic manifestation of SLE lung disease and is a form of acute lung injury.

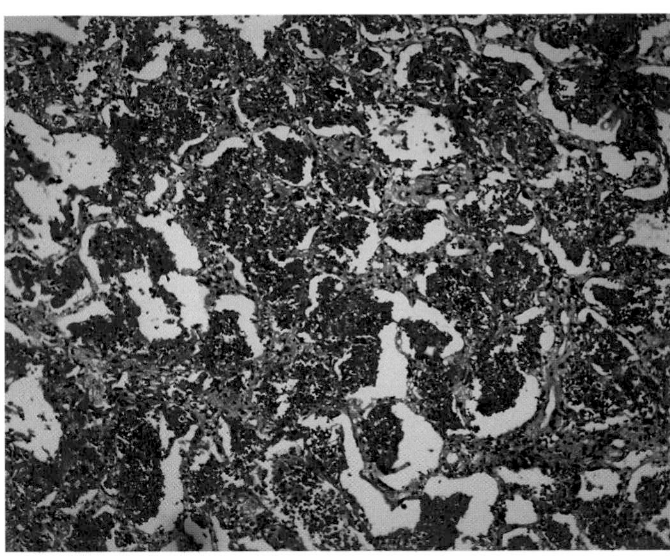

Fig. 7.44 **Systemic lupus erythematosus (SLE).** Diffuse alveolar hemorrhage may occur in SLE, often without hemoptysis. Here, prominent airspace fibrin and blood are accompanied by siderophages and marked reactive type II cell hyperplasia. An interstitial pneumonia is also evident in the widened alveolar walls.

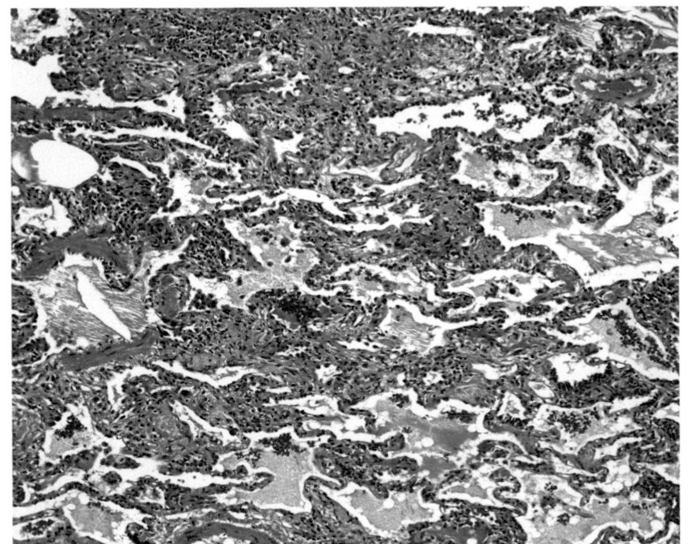

Fig. 7.43 **Systemic lupus erythematosus (SLE).** The second most common manifestation of SLE lung disease is "NSIP pattern" cellular interstitial pneumonia with variable interstitial fibrosis.

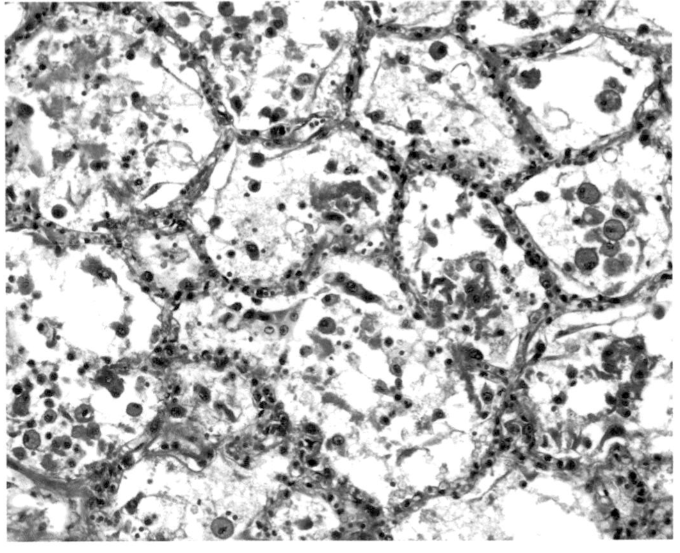

Fig. 7.45 **Systemic lupus erythematosus (SLE).** At high magnification the acute lung injury of acute lupus pneumonitis (ALP) is characterized by alveolitis with variable interstitial inflammation and edema.

attenuation, pleural thickening, pleural and pericardial effusions, and linear parenchymal opacities.[136,144–147] Acute pneumonitis can produce more extensive changes but rarely may show a normal chest radiograph and HRCT.[148]

Pathologic findings

Two general categories of pulmonary disease are described in SLE. The first is acute lupus pneumonitis (ALP). ALP is characterized by alveolitis with variable interstitial inflammation and edema (Figs. 7.42 and 7.45). Siderophages and capillaritis occur to variable degree (Fig. 7.46). Pleuritis is commonly present. The second category of disease is cellular interstitial pneumonia (lymphocytes and plasma cells) with variable interstitial fibrosis (Fig. 7.47). This latter nonspecific interstitial pneumonia, or "NSIP" pattern, is associated with a better prognosis than ALP. When pulmonary hemorrhage occurs, the prognosis may be adversely affected.[149]

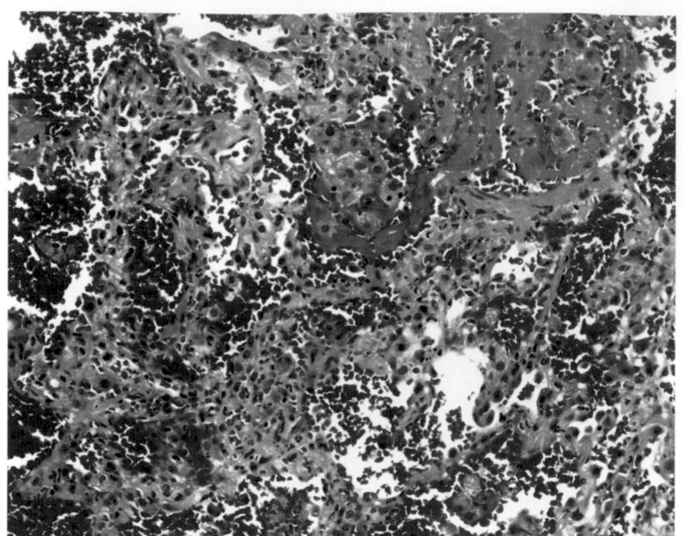

Fig. 7.46 **Systemic lupus erythematosus (SLE).** Siderophages and capillaritis may be present in the diffuse alveolar hemorrhage of SLE.

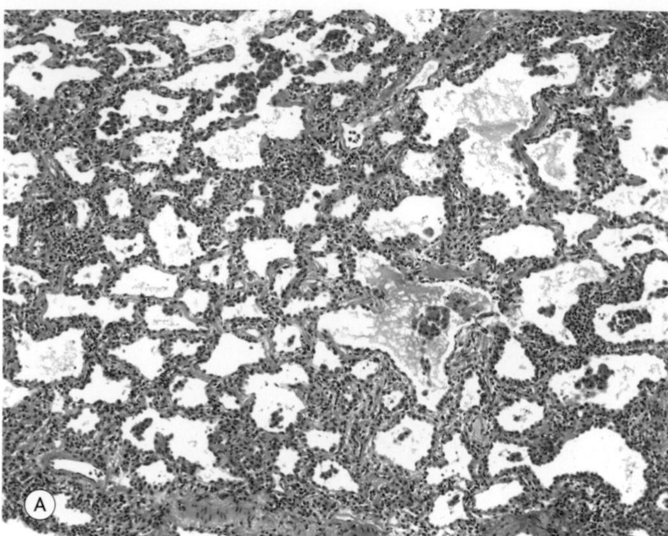

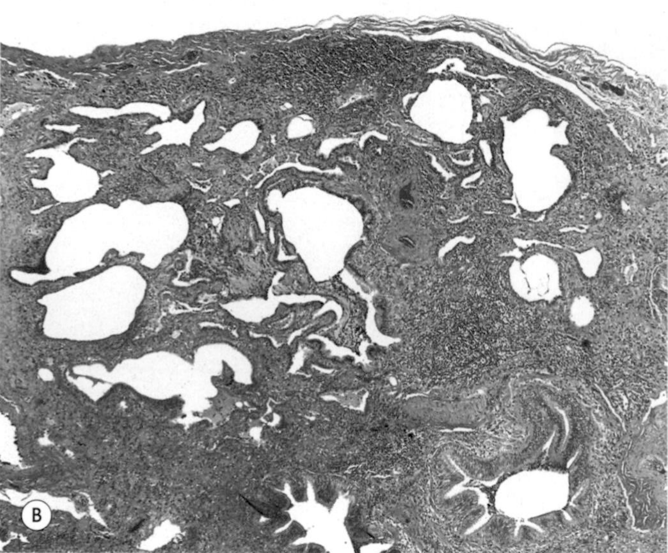

Fig. 7.47 **Systemic lupus erythematosus (SLE).** The cellular interstitial pneumonia of SLE lung is often accompanied by subacute lung injury with reactive type II cells and variable amounts of airspace fibrin (A). Some diffuse fibrosis is typically present in the nonspecific interstitial pneumonia (NSIP) manifestation of lupus, but advanced pulmonary fibrosis (B) may occur in SLE, here with chronic pleuritis.

Clinical course

Systemic corticosteroid therapy may be effective in SLE-associated lung disease, although sometimes the addition of a cytotoxic agent (e.g. cyclophosphamide, azathioprine) may be required.[150] Acute lupus pneumonitis has a reported high mortality rate in some series.[141] More chronic forms of diffuse lung disease in SLE have a relatively good prognosis and response to therapy.[151]

Polymyositis/dermatomyositis (PM/DM)

Polymyositis/dermatomyositis (PM/DM) are inflammatory disorders of the dermis and skeletal muscle. Five groups of primary or secondary disease are recognized, including childhood forms and overlap syndromes.[152,153] Pulmonary complications in PM/DM occur less commonly than in other systemic connective tissue diseases but, in a percentage of patients, the pulmonary manifestations can be quite dramatic.[154]

Clinical presentation

While most patients with PM/DM develop lung manifestations after the clinical diagnosis has been established, on occasion lung disease can precede the clinical and serologic diagnosis by months or even years.[155] Onset of pulmonary symptoms may occur at any age, with a mean occurrence in the sixth decade.[121,155,156] Women are more commonly affected than men. Digital clubbing is rare. In contrast to most other systemic connective tissue diseases (with the exception of SLE), patients with PM/DM can present with acute lung disease, typically manifesting as rapidly progressive diffuse alveolar damage.[154,156] Importantly, acute aspiration pneumonitis secondary to underlying respiratory muscle weakness, or bronchopneumonia occurring after immunosuppressive therapy, is each more common in PM/DM than is chronic diffuse lung disease.[157,158]

Radiologic findings

As with other CVDs manifesting in the lung, radiologic abnormalities predominately affect the lung bases.[156]

Ikezoe and colleagues reviewed the HRCT findings in 23 of 25 patients with PM/DM who had HRCT abnormalities.[159] They identified ground glass opacities in 92%, linear opacities in 92%, irregular interfaces in 88%, airspace consolidation in 52%, parenchymal micronodules in 28%, and honeycombing in 16%. The most dramatic radiologic finding associated with PM/DM is the rapid onset of airspace consolidation associated with the development of diffuse alveolar damage.[155,156]

Pathologic findings

The most frequent lung manifestation of PM/DM is a cellular interstitial pneumonia (Fig. 7.48) with some fibrosis,[155,156] indistinguishable from "nonspecific interstitial pneumonia" (see "The idiopathic interstitial pneumonias" section). The next most common pattern is diffuse alveolar damage (Fig. 7.49). The fibrosis associated with PM/DM is distinguishable from that of idiopathic UIP based on a relative lack of peripheral accentuation (Fig. 7.50) and absence of the typical transitions from

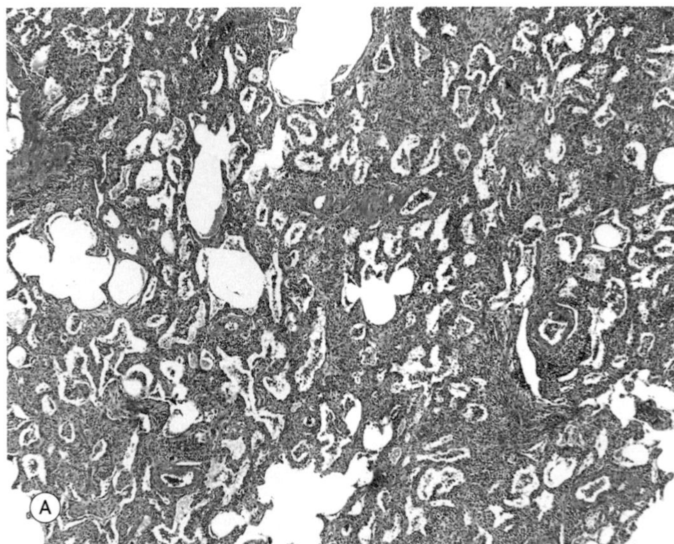

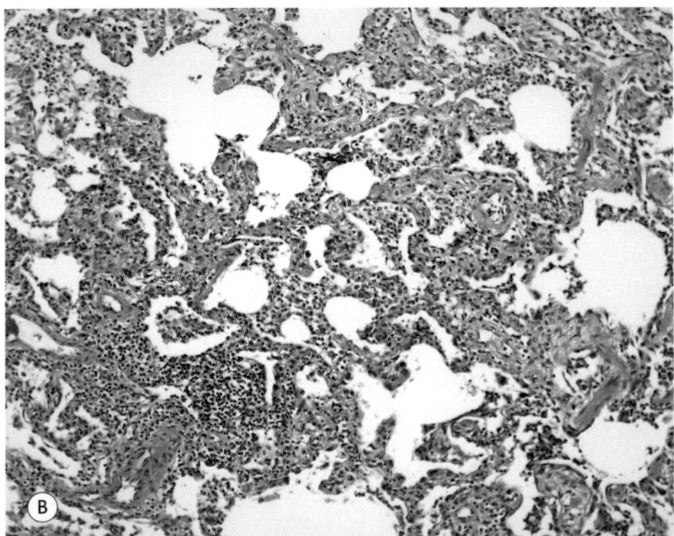

Fig. 7.48 **Polymyositis/dermatomyositis (PD/DM).** The most frequent lung manifestation of PM/DM is a cellular interstitial pneumonia (A,B) with some fibrosis, indistinguishable from cellular or fibrotic forms of "nonspecific interstitial pneumonia."

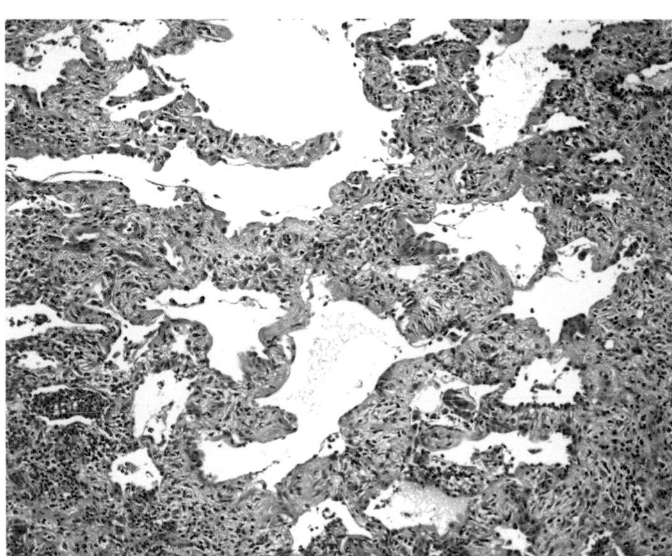

Fig. 7.49 **Polymyositis/dermatomyositis (PD/DM).** The diffuse alveolar damage (DAD) manifestation of PM/DM may precede the systemic and serologic manifestations of the disease by a year or more. Note the prominent hyaline membranes. Without an explanation for this acute lung disease, idiopathic "acute interstitial pneumonia" may be the clinical diagnosis until the systemic disease manifests itself.

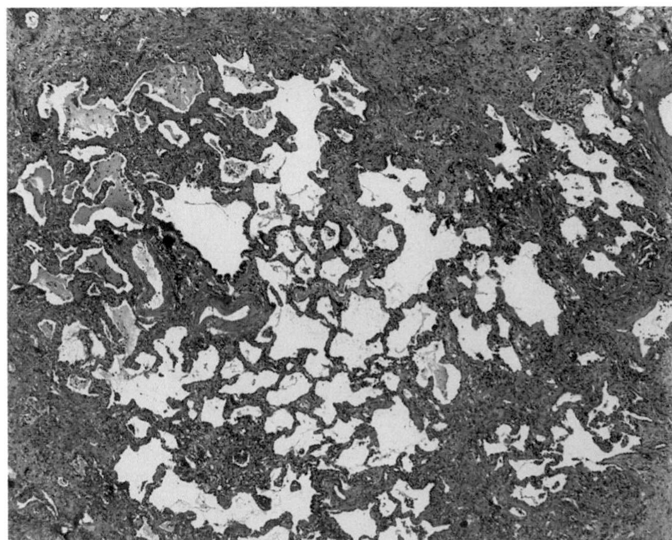

Fig. 7.50 **Polymyositis/dermatomyositis (PD/DM).** The fibrosis associated with PM/DM may be indistinguishable from that of idiopathic UIP in limited samples. In general, there is a relative lack of peripheral accentuation and absence of the typical transitions from older lung fibrosis to normal lung through fibroblastic foci.

older lung fibrosis to normal lung through fibroblastic foci. Pleuritis, inflammatory small airways disease, and pulmonary hypertension are unusual findings and their occurrence should suggest a manifestation of some other connective tissue disease.

Sjögren's syndrome

Sjögren's syndrome (SS) is an immune-mediated exocrinopathy characterized by lymphocytic infiltration of the salivary glands, with resulting dry mouth and dry eyes.[160] Lung involvement is common, and is similar to that of other collagen vascular diseases manifesting in the lung.[93,161,162] SS can occur as a primary connective tissue disease or as a complication associated with other connective tissue diseases (the occurrence is about equally divided).[160] Whether a primary or secondary form, the consistent pathologic manifestation is that of lymphoid accumulation in an airway-centered distribution, and the NSIP/LIP pattern of cellular interstitial pneumonia.

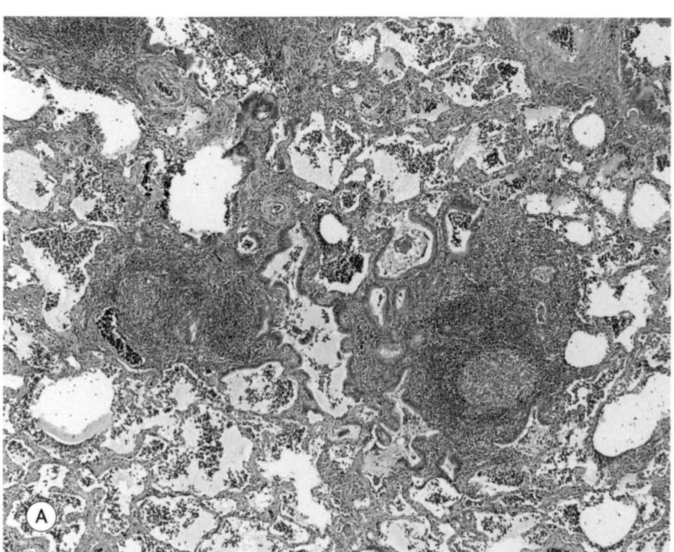

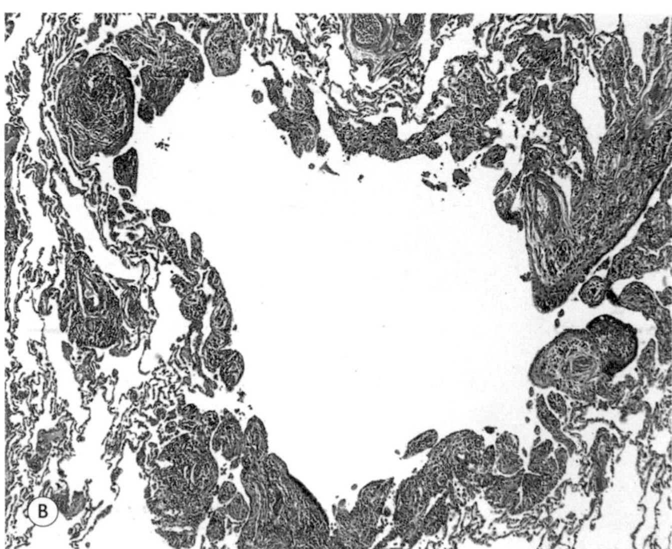

Fig. 7.51 **Sjögren's syndrome (SS).** The histologic spectrum of pulmonary SS includes bronchiolitis as the dominant and consistent feature (A). Cysts may occur in SS and be seen both radiologically and in surgical biopsy specimens (B).

Clinical presentation

Women are more commonly affected with lung disease in SS than men and the most frequent presenting complaint is cough and dyspnea.[93,161] A positive rheumatoid factor and ANA are expected findings, as well as positive reactions to extractable nuclear antigens (anti-SSA, anti-SSB).[163] These latter serologic tests are specific for the primary form of the disease.[164]

Radiologic findings

Mixed alveolar and interstitial infiltrates are characteristic in SS and they usually have a finely reticular or nodular pattern.[162,165] The occurrence of pleural effusion or hilar/mediastinal adenopathy in SS should raise concern for lymphoma.[166]

Pathologic findings

The histologic spectrum of pulmonary SS includes bronchiolitis (Fig. 7.51) with or without airspace organization, follicular lymphoid hyperplasia along airways (Fig. 7.52), diffuse NSIP or LIP pattern interstitial inflam-

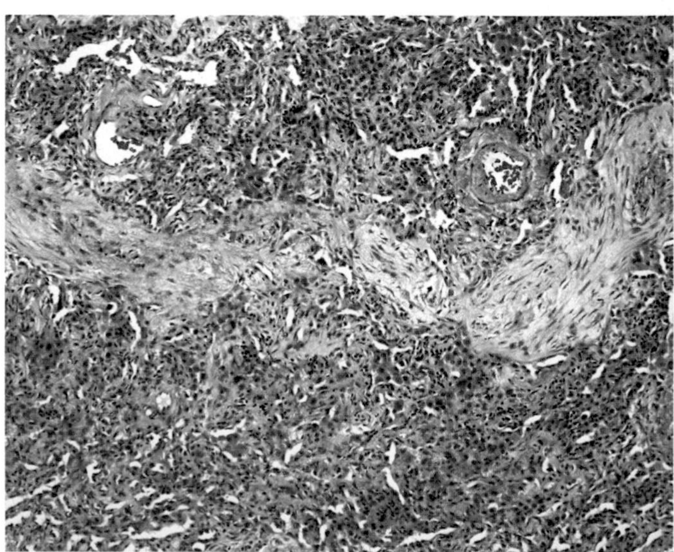

Fig. 7.52 **Sjögren's syndrome (SS).** Terminal airway and alveolar space organization commonly accompany the bronchiolitis and cellular interstitial pneumonia of SS.

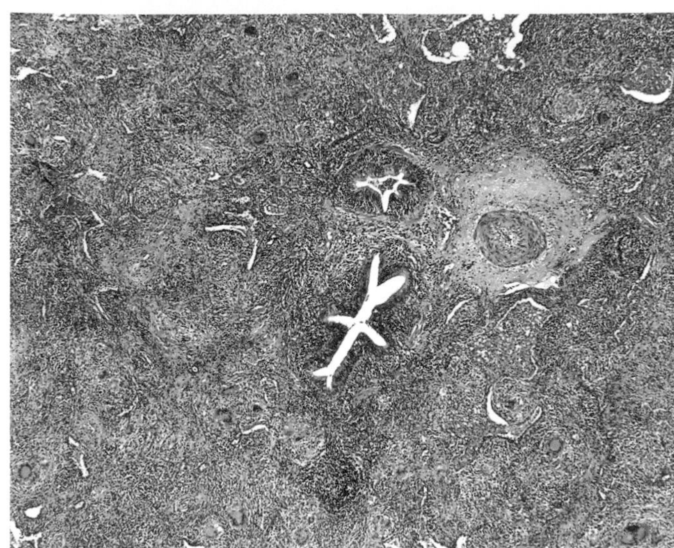

Fig. 7.53 **Sjögren's syndrome (SS).** Nonspecific interstitial pneumonia (NSIP) or lymphoid interstitial pneumonia (LIP) pattern interstitial inflammation in SS lung must be distinguished from low-grade lymphoproliferative disease when lymphocytes are dense and dominant. Note the numerous multinucleated giant cells and poorly formed granulomas here. Prominent arteriopathic changes with marked adventitial fibrosis can be seen in the pulmonary artery at center right.

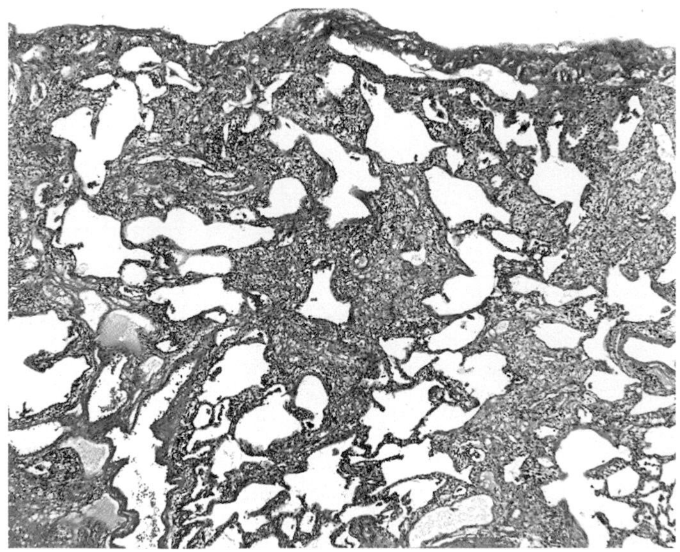

Fig. 7.54 **Sjögren's syndrome (SS).** Advanced interstitial fibrosis occurs rarely in SS lung disease, and may raise concern for an inflammatory version of usual interstitial pneumonia (UIP). Note the absence of transitions to normal lung and absence of peripheral accentuation here.

mation (Fig. 7.53), and, rarely, interstitial fibrosis (Fig. 7.54), the latter raising concern for an inflammatory version of UIP. Small, non-necrotizing granulomas, resembling those of hypersensitivity pneumonitis, are frequently identified in the interstitium (Fig. 7.55). In some cases, more

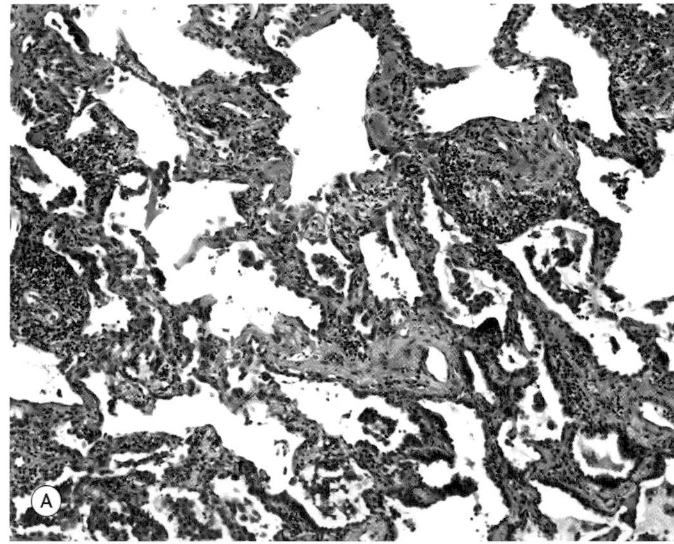

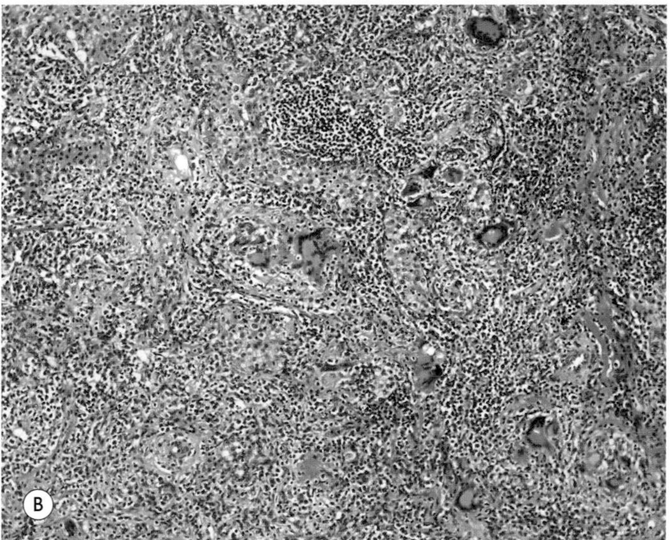

Fig. 7.55 **Sjögren's syndrome (SS).** (A) Small, non-necrotizing granulomas, resembling those of hypersensitivity pneumonitis, are frequently identified in the interstitium in the lymphoid interstitial pneumonia pattern (LIP) of SS. (B) Sometimes the granulomas are more diffusely present, raising infection and aspiration pneumonia high in the differential diagnosis.

prominent granulomatous inflammation can be seen, especially in association with the LIP pattern of cellular infiltration. Patients with SS are at risk for lymphoid hyperplasia and lymphoproliferative diseases and this should be kept in mind in evaluating the lung biopsy in this setting.

Diffuse eosinophilic lung disease

Several different conditions have been described in which the airspaces of the lungs contain a large number of eosinophils.[167,168] An etiologic and clinical classification of

Table 7.13 Etiologic and clinical classification of eosinophilic pneumonia

Idiopathic (unknown cause)
- Chronic eosinophilic pneumonia
- Acute eosinophilic pneumonia
- Simple eosinophilic pneumonia (Loffler's)
- Incidental eosinophilic pneumonia

Secondary eosinophilic pneumonia
- Infection:
  - Parasitic
    - Tropical eosinophilic pneumonia
    - *Ascaris lumbricoides, Toxicara canis, Filaria*
    - *Dirofilaria*
    - Fungal
    - *Aspergillus*
- Drug-induced:
  - Antibiotics
  - Cytotoxic drugs
  - Anti-inflammatory agents
  - L-tryptophan
- Immunologic or systemic diseases:
  - Allergic bronchopulmonary fungal disease
  - Asthma
  - Collagen vascular disease
  - Churg–Strauss syndrome
  - HIV infection
  - Malignancy
  - Hypereosinophilic syndrome

Source: from Travis et al.,[6] p 161, with permission.

the eosinophilic lung diseases is presented in Table 7.13. When disease manifests over many weeks to months, the term "chronic eosinophilic pneumonia" has been applied, even though the pathologic findings in biopsy specimens may not reflect this chronicity with fibrosis.

Clinical features

Patients with the "chronic" form of eosinophilic pneumonia often manifest a typical clinical syndrome and radiographic appearance.[169] The condition frequently affects middle-aged women, and asthma is present in about one-quarter of the cases. Nasal symptoms occur in about one-third of affected individuals. The disease typically presents with severe systemic effects, including fever, sweats, weight loss, cough and dyspnea. Peripheral blood eosinophilia can often be identified, but this may be transient or in some cases absent.

Radiologic findings

Bilateral subpleural airspace consolidation with poorly defined margins is seen on chest radiographs, most commonly present at the apices and in the axillary region. The infiltrates may disappear spontaneously and recur in the same position, or elsewhere (so-called "migratory" infiltrates). In the most extreme cases, the infiltrates are densest in the periphery of the lung and spare the central region. This phenomenon has been referred to as the "photographic negative of pulmonary edema."[169] Computed tomographic scans detect the peripheral location of infiltrates even when this distribution is not apparent on the chest radiograph.[170] Once the characteristic presentation is recognized, corticosteroid administration can lead to dramatic improvement and may even be used as a diagnostic test. Atypical presentations occur, so that surgical wedge biopsy may be required to establish the diagnosis.

Pathologic findings

The histologic features are similar to those of the acute form and it has been said that the distinction must rely on the clinical course rather than the constellation of morphologic findings. Alveolar spaces are filled with eosinophils and plump eosinophilic macrophages (Fig. 7.56) and there is an associated mild interstitial pneumonia. Type II hyperplasia is characteristic (Fig. 7.57), and fibrin is often present in the airspaces (Fig. 7.58). Angiitis of small vessels may be seen and patchy airspace and alveolar duct organization may be present. A vaguely granulomatous accumulation of dense macrophages may be seen within the alveolar spaces (Fig. 7.59), sometimes accompanied by multinucleated giant cells whose nuclei and cytoplasm closely resembles that of adjacent macrophages (Fig. 7.60). Chronicity may be suggested by the presence of variable interstitial fibrosis.

Differential diagnosis

When airspace organization is prominent, the organizing pneumonia pattern differential diagnosis must be considered (see Table 7.10). An overlap syndrome between cryptogenic organizing pneumonia and eosinophilic pneumonia with subacute clinical course has been proposed, and it is interesting that both conditions are expected to have a favorable response to systemic corticosteroid administration. When corticosteroids have been administered before biopsy, eosinophils may be absent or inconspicuous in lung sections. In such cases, the differential diagnosis may include granulomatous disease if the dense histiocytic response and multinucleated giant cells dominate the picture. When fibrin is prominent in the setting of pretreatment with corticosteroids, acute lung injury may enter the pathologic differential diagnosis. Some patients with long-standing symptoms may have fibrosis on biopsy. In these individuals consideration for a fibrosing lung disease may enter the differential diagnosis.

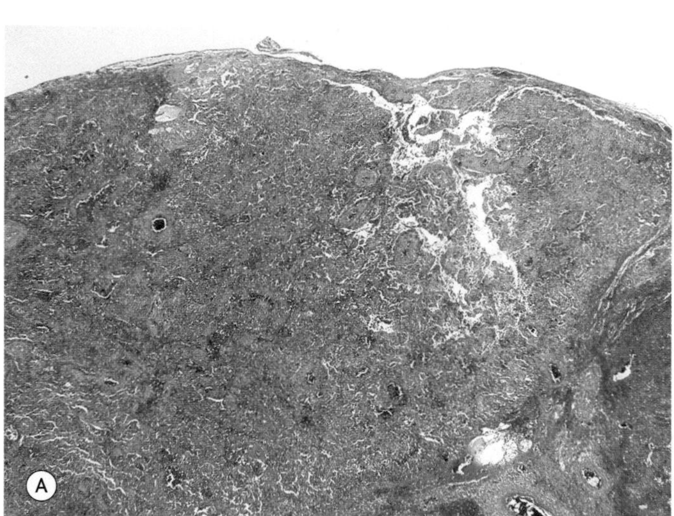

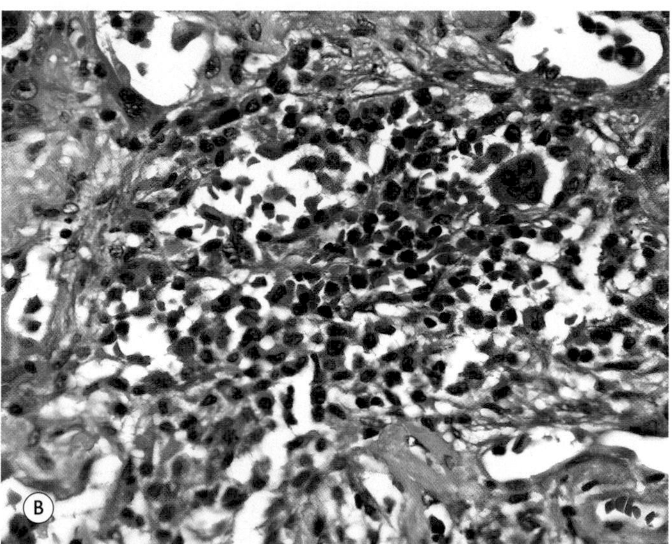

Fig. 7.56 **Eosinophilic pneumonia.** In acute eosinophilic pneumonia, the alveolar spaces are diffusely filled with eosinophils and plump eosinophilic macrophages (A) and there may be an associated mild interstitial pneumonia. (B) Eosinophilic microabscesses may be present.

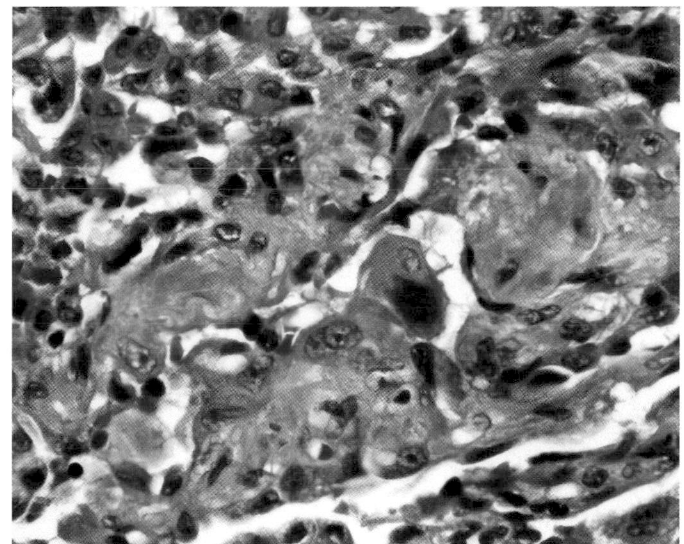

Fig. 7.57 **Eosinophilic pneumonia.** Highly atypical type II hyperplasia is characteristic in acute eosinophilic pneumonia (AEP), often raising concern for viral cytopathic changes.

Clinical course

The clinical course is somewhat dependent on the underlying cause of the eosinophilic pneumonia but, in general, most affected individuals will benefit from high-dose corticosteroid therapy (although the speed of recovery may not be as rapid for those cases with other than acute onset eosinophilic pneumonia). As in all cases of eosinophilic pneumonia, it is always worthwhile to suggest the possibility of Churg–Strauss syndrome (see Ch. 10), since the pulmonary manifestations of that systemic vasculitic disease in the lung are most commonly those of eosinophilic pneumonia.

Drug-associated diffuse lung disease

An increasing number of medications have been implicated in chronic diffuse lung disease.[171,172] Three distinct forms are recognized:[173]

1. drug-mediated chronic diffuse lung disease
2. acute lung injury associated with drug administration
3. vascular diseases produced by medications.[174]

The latter two conditions are dealt with in other chapters (see Chs 5 and 10).

The accurate recognition of drug-induced diffuse lung disease is a major challenge in lung pathology because most of the histologic changes identified are nonspecific (Table 7.14) and simulate other causes of diffuse lung disease.[175] Moreover, many affected patients have underlying diseases for which a drug has been administered, and some of these diseases also have pulmonary manifestations. The diagnosis of a drug-mediated diffuse lung disease requires careful exclusion of other causes.[176] A clear onset of pulmonary symptoms in association with drug administration, and reduction of symptoms on cessation of the drug, may not be easily discernable. Clinical information regarding specific drug type, dose, and timing of administration relative to onset of symptoms are all essential components for accurate diagnosis.

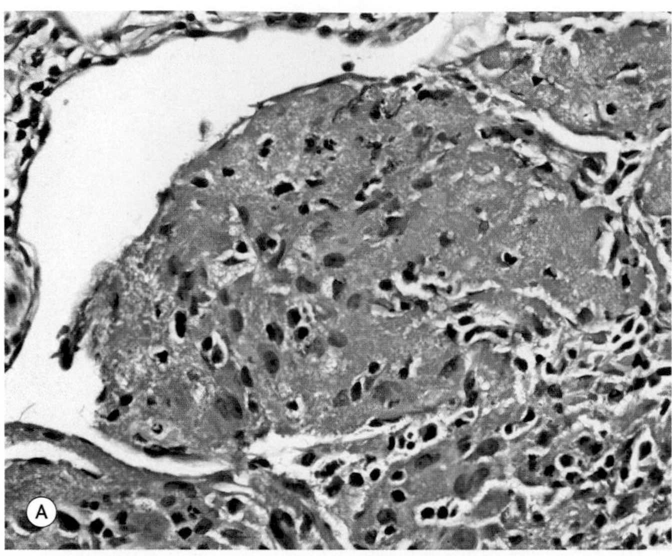

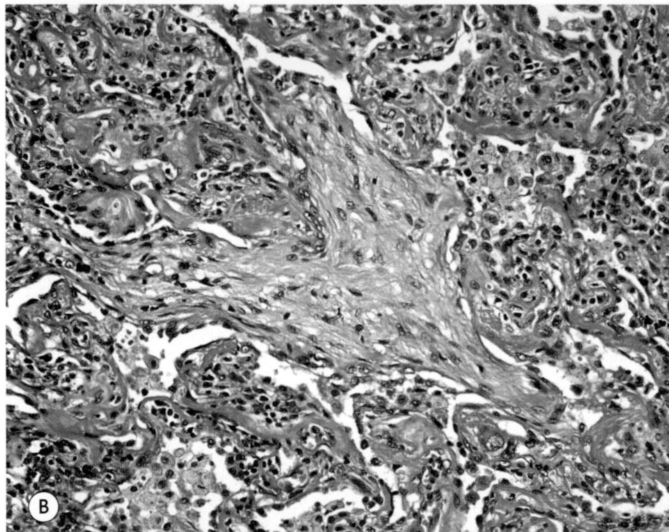

Fig. 7.58 **Eosinophilic pneumonia.** (A) Fibrinous airspace exudates are commonly present, typically with admixed eosinophils, as seen here. (B) Organizing pneumonia pattern repair may also occur.

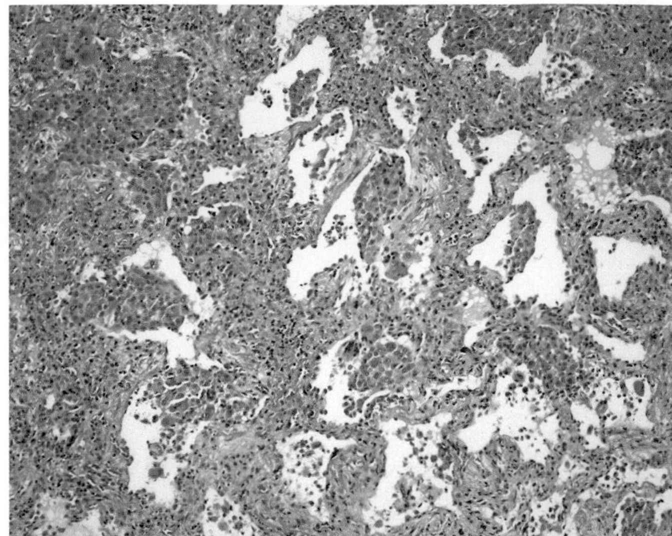

Fig. 7.59 **Eosinophilic pneumonia.** A vaguely granulomatous accumulation of dense macrophages may be seen within the alveolar spaces, sometimes accompanied by plump multinucleated macrophages.

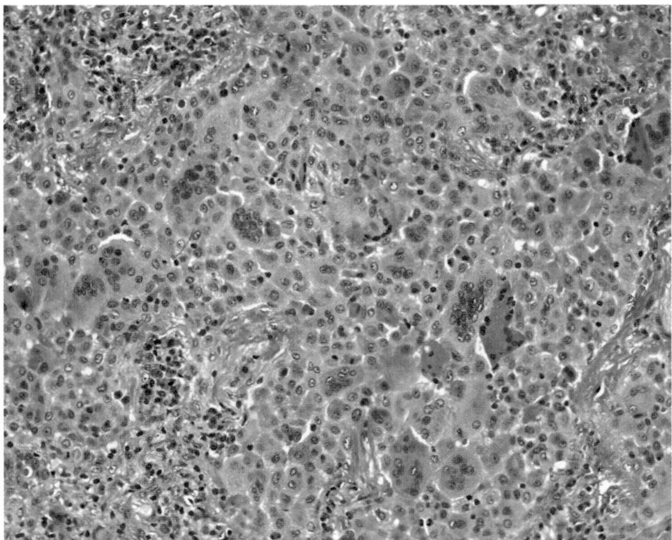

Fig. 7.60 **Eosinophilic pneumonia.** The multinucleated giant cells of eosinophilic pneumonia have nuclei and cytoplasm that closely resembles that of adjacent alveolar macrophages, but occasionally they may be more brightly eosinophilic.

Table 7.14 Pulmonary reactions and associated drugs

Drugs	FIP	CIP	OP	EDM	DAD	EOS	AH	BO	PVOD	Gran
Amiodarone	+	++	+	++	+	+	++			
β blockers	+	++	+			+				
Bleomycin	++	++	+	++	+	+			+	
Busulfan	+				+			+	+	
Carmustine (BCNU)	+	++		++	+				+	
Cocaine					+	+	+			+
Cyclophosphamide	+		+	++	+		+			
Ergots	+	++	+							
Etoposide		++			+					
Gefitinib (Iressa)					+					
G(M)-CSF		++		++	+	+				
Heroin		++		++			+			
Hexamethonium	+		+		+					
Hydrochlorothiazide		++		++	+	+				
L-tryptophan		+				+				
Lomustine (CCNU)	+				+					
Methotrexate	++	++	+	+	+	+		+		+
Minocycline			+	++		+				
Mitomycin C	+	++		++	+		++		+	
Nitrofurantoin	+	++	+	++	+	+	++			+
Penicillamine		+	+		+	+	++	+		
Phenytoin		+	+			+	++			
Procarbazine		+			+	+				+
Prozac		+								
Sulfasalazine	+	++		++	+	+				
Zinostatin					+				+	

FIP = fibrosing interstitial pneumonia, including UIP and fibrosing NSIP pattern; CIP = cellular interstitial pneumonia, including cellular NSIP and LIP pattern; OP = organizing pneumonia; EDM = edema; DAD = diffuse alveolar damage; EOS = tissue eosinophilia; AH = alveolar hemorrhage; BO = bronchiolitis obliterans; PVOD = pulmonary veno-occlusive disease; Gran = granulomatous inflammation; G(M)-CSF = granulocyte (macrophage) colony-stimulating factor.
Source: amiodarone,[191,369,370] β-blockers,[371–373] bleomycin,[206,74,375] busulfan,[205,376,377] carmustine (BCNU),[201,375,378] cocaine,[379,380] cyclophosphamide,[381–384] ergolines,[385] etoposide,[386] Gefitinib,[387] heroin,[388,389] hexamethonium,[390–392] hydrochlothiazide,[393–395] L-tryptophan,[396,397] lomustine (CCNU),[398] methotrexate,[175,180] minocycline,[399, 400] mitomycin C,[401,402] nitrofurantoin,[403–406] penicillamine,[407–409] phenytoin,[410, 411] procarbazine,[412–414] Prozac (fluoxetine),[415] sulfasalazine,[416] zinostatin.[417]

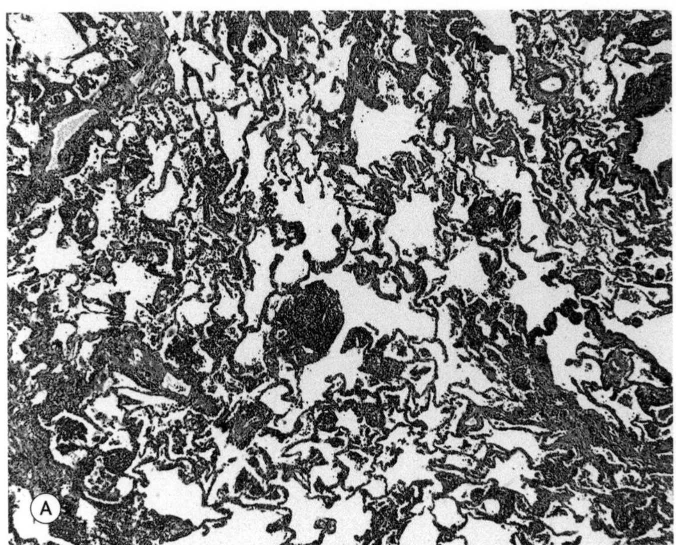

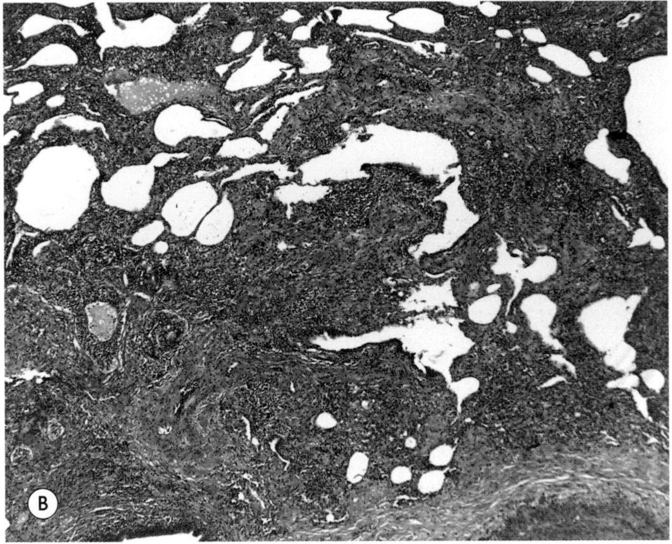

Fig. 7.61 **Methotrexate (MTX).** In MTX toxicity, nonspecific interstitial inflammation (A) and fibrosis (B) are common findings, and scattered lymphoid aggregates may be seen. When the latter are prominent, and accompanied by bronchiolitis, concern for exacerbation of an underlying connective tissue disease being treated comes into the differential diagnosis (e.g. rheumatoid arthritis).

General pathologic findings

Most of the inflammatory changes in the lung related to drug toxicity are nonspecific. More often than not, a mixture of both acute and chronic disease is apparent and can be a clue to the diagnosis of drug-mediated injury.[175] In chronic drug toxicity, lung fibrosis may occur, sometimes with honeycomb remodeling. In such cases, UIP may be simulated. Tissue eosinophilia can occur in drug reactions and some drugs are associated with the production in the lung of small, poorly formed granulomas,

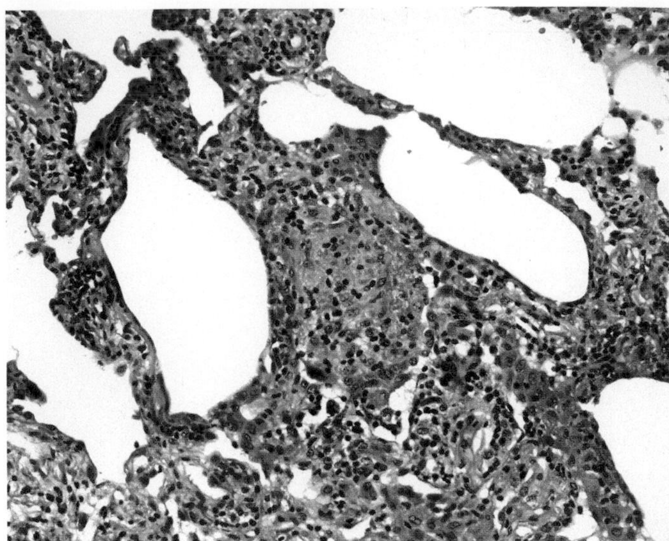

Fig. 7.62 **Methotrexate (MTX).** The presence of giant cells and scattered small non-necrotizing granulomas (center) are the only relatively specific markers for MTX, in comparison to other drugs.

simulating infection, hypersensitivity, or even Sjögren's syndrome.[171]

General treatment and prognosis

Most patients with drug-mediated diffuse lung disease have a favorable prognosis when the implicated drug is withdrawn. Once fibrosis has occurred, changes may be stable, with little improvement. Systemic corticosteroid therapy may be added when symptoms are severe.

Specific drugs associated with diffuse lung diseases

Methotrexate

Methotrexate (MTX) lung toxicity is predominately a manifestation seen in women taking the drug.[177,178] Because MTX is used in the treatment of a variety of disorders (e.g. rheumatoid arthritis, some leukemias, some visceral cancers), these tend to be the associated underlying diseases that must be considered in the differential diagnosis for the lung manifestations identified. Interstitial inflammation and fibrosis (Fig. 7.61) are common findings in the surgical lung biopsy.[179–181] The presence of giant cells and small non-necrotizing granulomas (Fig. 7.62) are the only relatively specific markers for MTX, in comparison to other drugs.[180] Type II pneumocyte

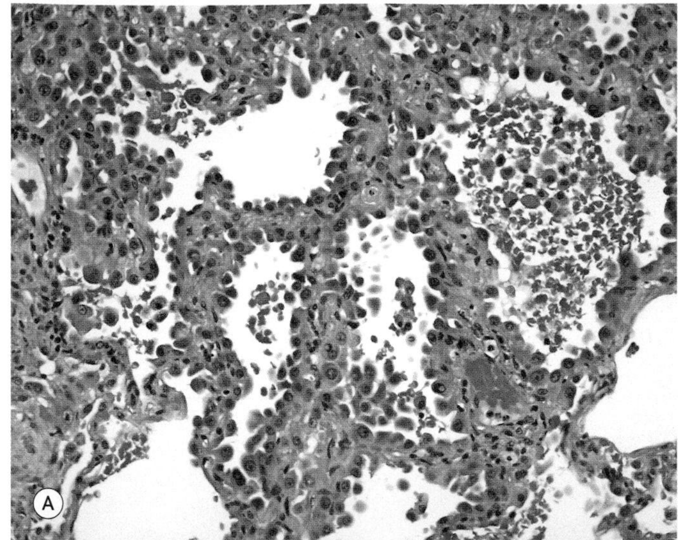

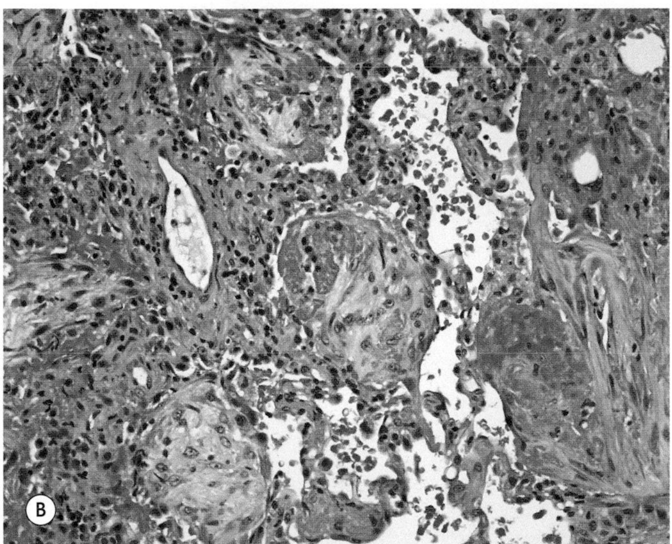

Fig. 7.63 **Methotrexate (MTX).** (A) Type II pneumocyte hyperplasia and (B) variable acute lung injury with airspace organization, with or without tissue eosinophilia, can be seen.

hyperplasia and tissue eosinophilia can be seen (Fig. 7.63). Hyaline membranes are rarely identified.[180]

Amiodarone

Amiodarone is the drug of choice for certain refractory cardiac arrhythmias. Pulmonary toxicity has been reported in 5–10% of patients taking this medication. Older patients are more likely to develop lung disease. The clinical onset is characterized by slowly progressive dyspnea and dry cough, occurring within months of initiating therapy. About one-third of patients manifest an acute fibrile illness mimicking infectious pneumonia.[182–185] HRCT scans show diffuse infiltrates, combined with basal/

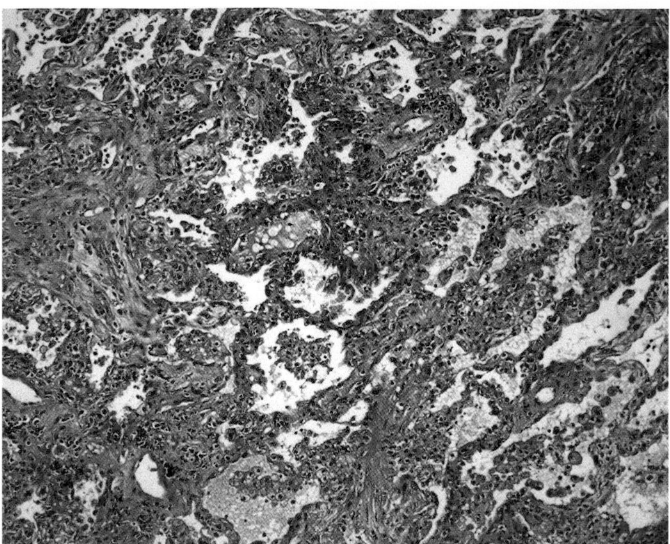

Fig. 7.64 **Amiodarone.** The most common pathologic change seen in amiodarone toxicity is a cellular interstitial pneumonia associated with prominent intra-alveolar macrophages whose cytoplasm shows fine vacuolation.

peripheral high attenuation opacities, and nonspecific infiltrates.[186,187] The most common pathologic manifestation is a cellular interstitial pneumonia (Fig. 7.64) associated with prominent intra-alveolar macrophages whose cytoplasm shows fine vacuolation.[182,188–190] This vacuolation also can be seen in reactive type II pneumocytes (Fig. 7.65) and published reports have described the presence of characteristic lamellar cytoplasmic inclusions ultrastructurally.[191] Unfortunately, these cytoplasmic changes are an expected manifestation of the drug, so that the mere presence of this change is not sufficient to warrant a diagnosis of amiodarone toxicity.[188] Pleural inflammation and pleural effusion have been reported.[192] Some patients with amiodarone toxicity can develop an organizing pneumonia (Fig. 7.66) pattern (OP pattern) or even diffuse alveolar damage.[188,193,194] The majority of patients who develop pulmonary toxicity related to amiodarone will recover once the drug is discontinued.[182,183,188–190]

BCNU (carmustine)

BCNU is the treatment of choice for patients with certain brain tumors and is used in some combination chemotherapy regimens. Acute and organizing diffuse alveolar damage is the most common manifestation in acute BCNU pulmonary toxicity.[195–198] Delayed lung toxicity has been described in survivors of childhood brain tumors who received BCNU, with lung changes appearing 8–20 years after cessation of treatment.[195,199–201] The histiologic features of BCNU toxicity can be

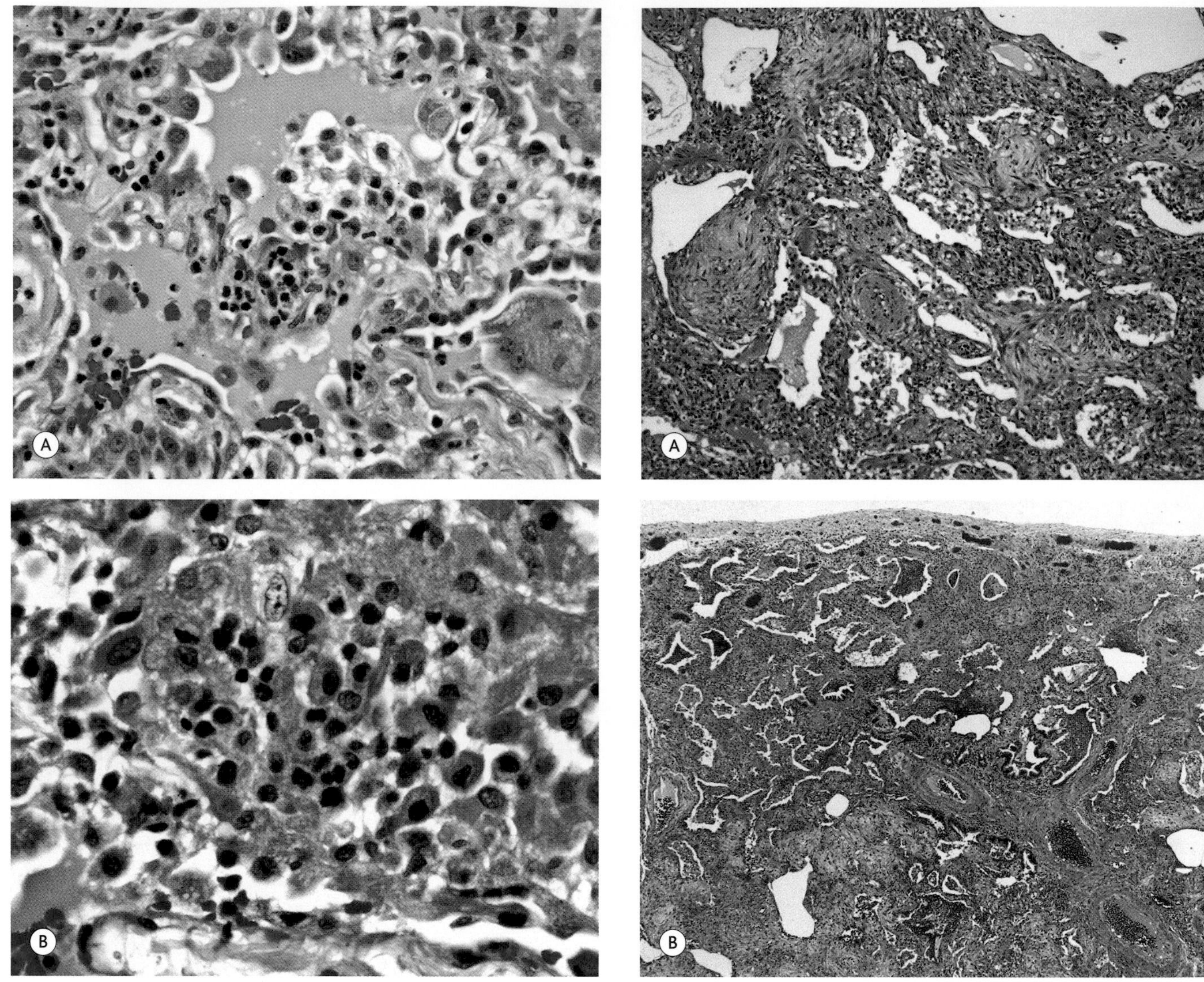

Fig. 7.65 **Amiodarone.** (A,B) Amiodarone effect also can be seen in reactive type II pneumocytes. Published reports have described the presence of characteristic lamellar cytoplasmic inclusions ultrastructurally. Unfortunately, these cytoplasmic and ultrastructural changes are expected manifestations of the drug, so that the mere presence of this change is not sufficient to warrant a diagnosis of amiodarone toxicity.

Fig. 7.66 **Amiodarone.** (A) Some patients with amiodarone toxicity develop an organizing pneumonia pattern (OP pattern), producing a mass effect on thoracic imaging studies. (B) Rarely, chronic toxicity may result in advanced lung fibrosis.

generally grouped within the NSIP pattern (Fig. 7.67) and, in children, fibrosis develops in the upper lung zones, with peripheral accentuation.[200,201] In adults, this upper lobe distribution is uncommon. Pleural disease can accompany pulmonary abnormalities in some patients.

Busulfan

Busulfan is an alkylating agent that has been used in the treatment of chronic myelogenous leukemia. Pulmonary toxicity has been reported to occur in 4% of patients,[202–204] most commonly as acute lung injury . Unfortunately, the prognosis for patients who develop busulfan-induced acute lung disease is poor. Rarely, patients with busulfan toxicity develop chronic diffuse lung disease (Fig. 7.68).[205]

Bleomycin

Bleomycin is a chemotherapeutic agent used in the treatment of lymphomas, epidermoid carcinomas, and malignant testicular tumors. Lung toxicity appears to be dose related, but irradiation or oxygen therapy may

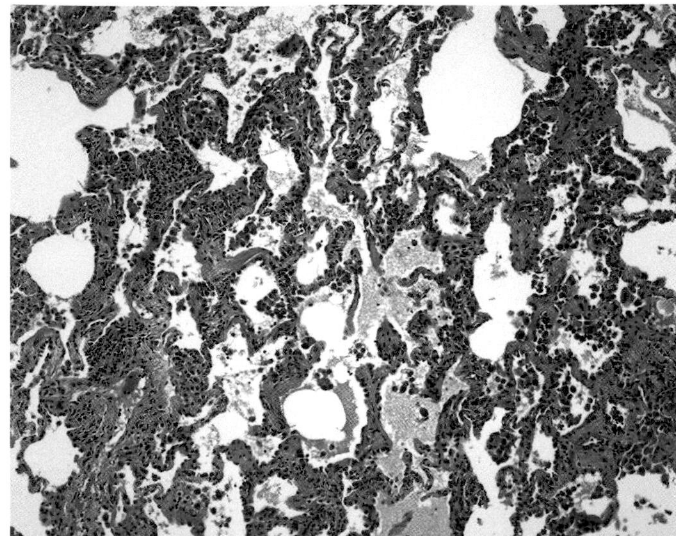

Fig. 7.67 **BCNU.** The histologic features of BCNU toxicity are those of a nonspecific cellular interstitial pneumonia with variable interstitial fibrosis.

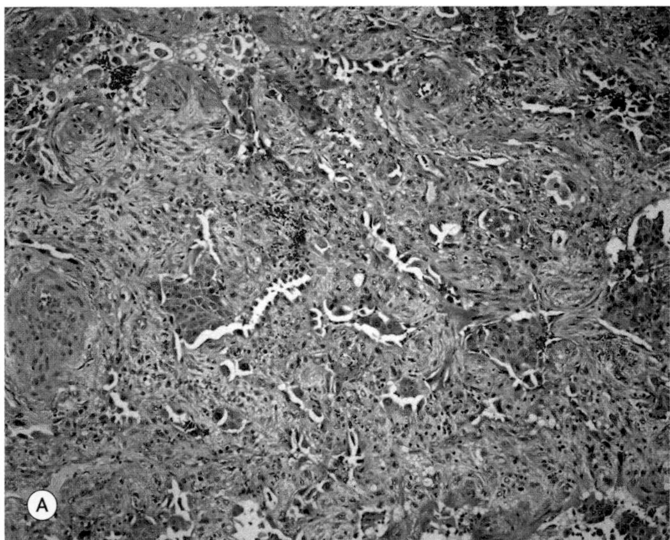

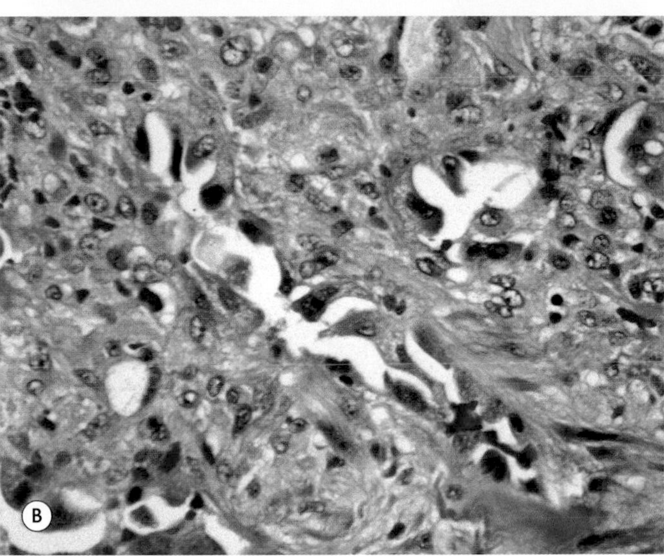

Fig. 7.68 **Busulfan.** (A,B) The prognosis for patients who develop busulfan-induced acute lung disease is poor. In the subacute form of injury, airspace organization is often accompanied by marked atypia of reactive type II cells.

predispose the lung to injury.[206–209] The typical clinical presentation begins with dry cough, progressing to breathlessness. Chest imaging reveals areas of nodular consolidation and/or diffuse reticulation.[210] In experimental models, the initial site of injury seems to be the venous endothelial cell, followed by necrosis of type I cells with consequent fibroplasia.[211–214] In humans, toxicity results in acute lung injury with airspace organization in the early phase and fibrosis as a late consequence (Fig. 7.69).

Illicit drug abuse

Many of the described pulmonary manifestations of illicit drug use (Table 7.15) are related to infections derived from the use of contaminated needles, or comorbidity related to the use of non-injected substances (typically sniffed or inhaled).[215] For a minority of substance abusers, intravenous injection of solubilized analgesic tablets is the drug of choice. Today, the presence of perivascular talc particles usually indicates a residual injury from another time in the patient's life, because tablet manufacturing today uses microcrystalline cellulose compounds as binding and filling agents, rather than talc as was the practice many years ago. Today, when intravenous drug use occurs by injection of crushed analgesic tablets, microcrystalline cellulose is the commonly identified injurious particle in the lung parenchyma. The physical characteristics and histochemical staining reactions of this material are different than those of talc, and these may be useful distinguishing features on occasion.[216]

Injected particles generally average 10–15 µm[216–218] in diameter, in contrast to inhaled substances where particle sizes tend to be smaller, usually less than 5 µm (use the red blood cells for size comparison). The most commonly used fillers historically have included talc, microcrystalline cellulose, and cornstarch. Cornstarch appears as a spherical structure with a Maltese cross pattern

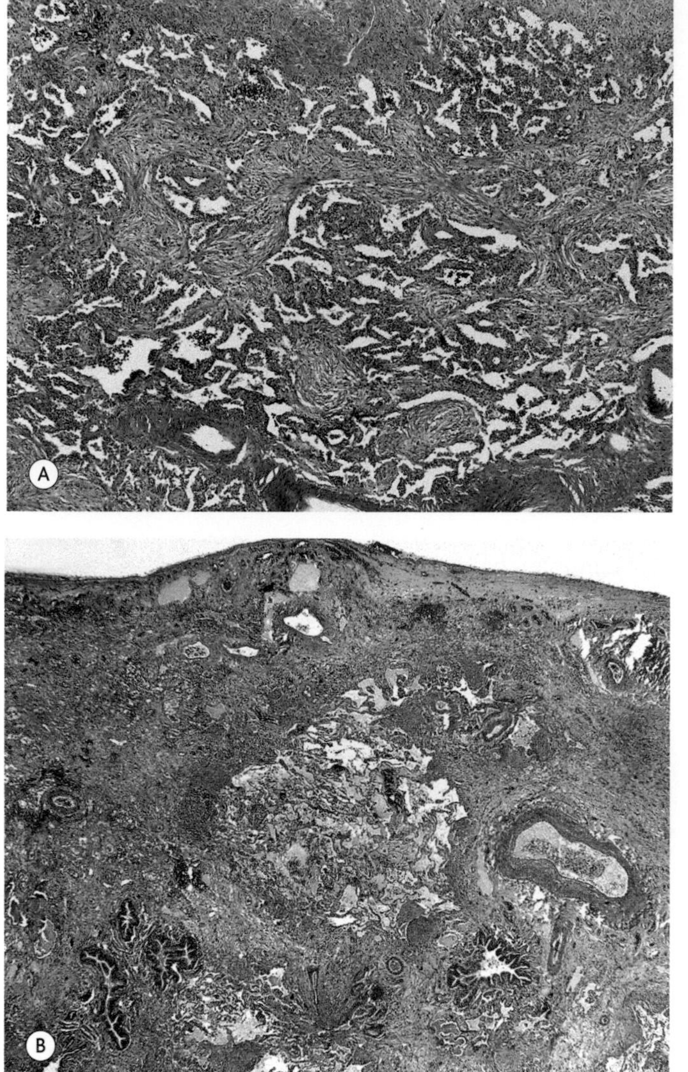

Fig. 7.69 **Bleomycin.** (A) Bleomycin toxicity may produce acute lung injury with airspace organization in the early phase and (B) fibrosis resembling that of usual interstitial pneumonia (UIP) as a late consequence.

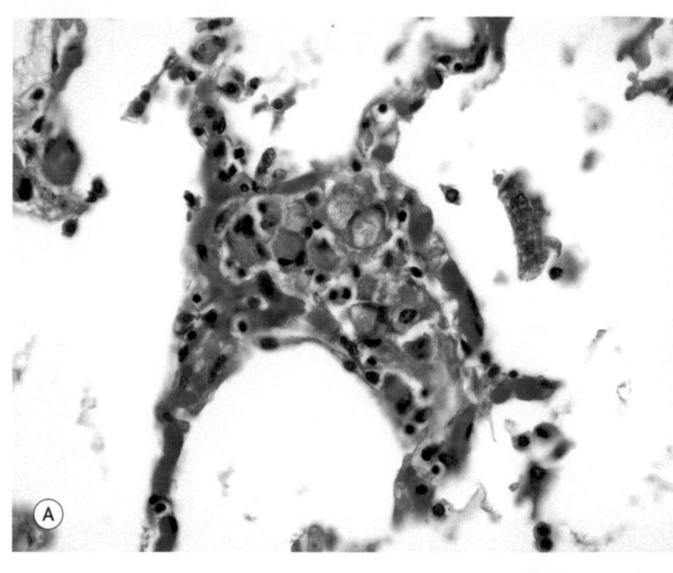

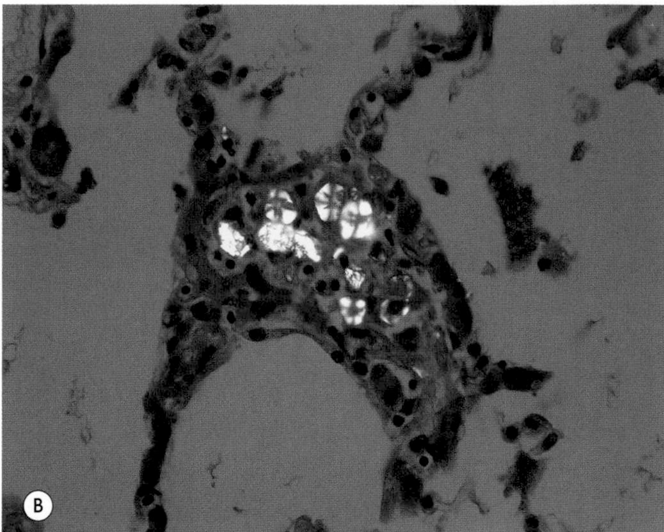

Fig. 7.70 **Intravenous (IV) drug – talc.** (A) This patient with IV talcosis has small clusters of multinucleated histiocytes containing irregular plate-like crystals that are strongly birefringent under full polarization. (B) Talc particles may be slightly yellow on routine hematoxylin and eosin staining in partially polarized light (single filter).

Table 7.15 The pulmonary complications of intravenous drug abuse

Infections (including HIV) and infection-related diseases: – Pneumonia – Abscesses – Mycotic aneurysms – Septic emboli
Adult respiratory distress syndrome
Pulmonary hypertension
Interstitial fibrosis with interstitial lung disease
Massive fibrosis
Emphysema

under plane-polarized light. Talc appears as irregular, plate-like crystals that are strongly birefringent (Fig. 7.70), and may be slightly yellow on routine hematoxylin and eosin staining when a single polarizing filter is in place. Microcrystalline cellulose particles appear as elongated crystalline structures (Fig. 7.71) that may stain positively using digested PAS, methenamine silver and Congo red stains. The reaction in the lung is generally interstitial and perivascular (Fig. 7.72) rather than intra-alveolar. Intravenous foreign material rarely may become encrusted with iron (ferruginated).

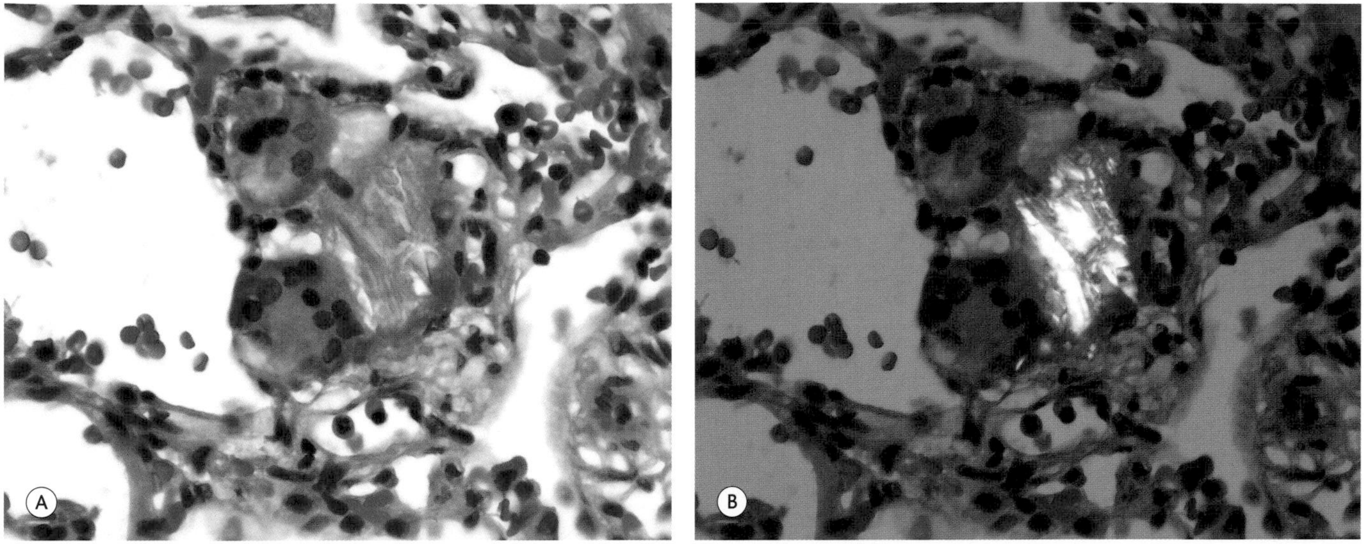

Fig. 7.71 **Intravenous (IV) drug – microcrystalline cellulose.** (A) Microcrystalline cellulose particles appear as elongated crystalline structures in the cytoplasm of foreign body giant cells in the perivascular interstitium. (B) These are strongly birefringent in polarized light.

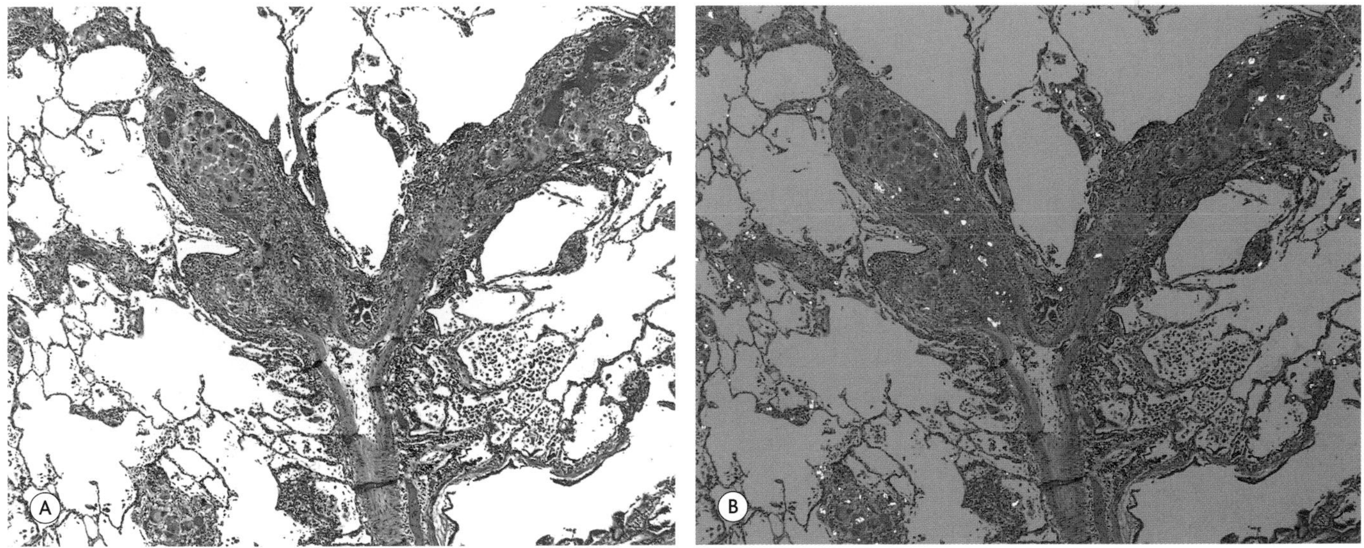

Fig. 7.72 **Intravenous (IV) drug – microcrystalline cellulose.** (A) The reaction in the lung is generally interstitial and perivascular rather than intra-alveolar. (B) The extent of intravenous foreign material may be better appreciated using polarizing filters.

Pathologic findings

As the intravenous material becomes lodged in the pulmonary microvasculature, a perivascular interstitial foreign body-type granulomatous reaction is produced (Fig. 7.73) that may be associated with prominent vascular changes (including pulmonary hypertension/ thrombotic lesions, etc.),[219] as well as interstitial fibrosis (Fig. 7.74) that may be focal or diffuse and sometimes massive.[220] Among the pathologic manifestations presented in Table 7.16, pulmonary hypertension is the most common, while emphysema is quite uncommon. Emphysema associated with intravenous drug abuse is typically of the panacinar type (similar to alpha-1-antitrypsin deficiency) and has been most frequently associated with methylphenidate (Ritalin) abuse.[221] In contrast to smoking-associated emphysema, the radiologic changes seen in Ritalin lung are more severe in the lower lobes. Bulla may be present. In one report it was suggested that the presence of basilar pulmonary emphysema should always alert the radiologist to the possibility of intravenous drug abuse.[221] The pathogenesis

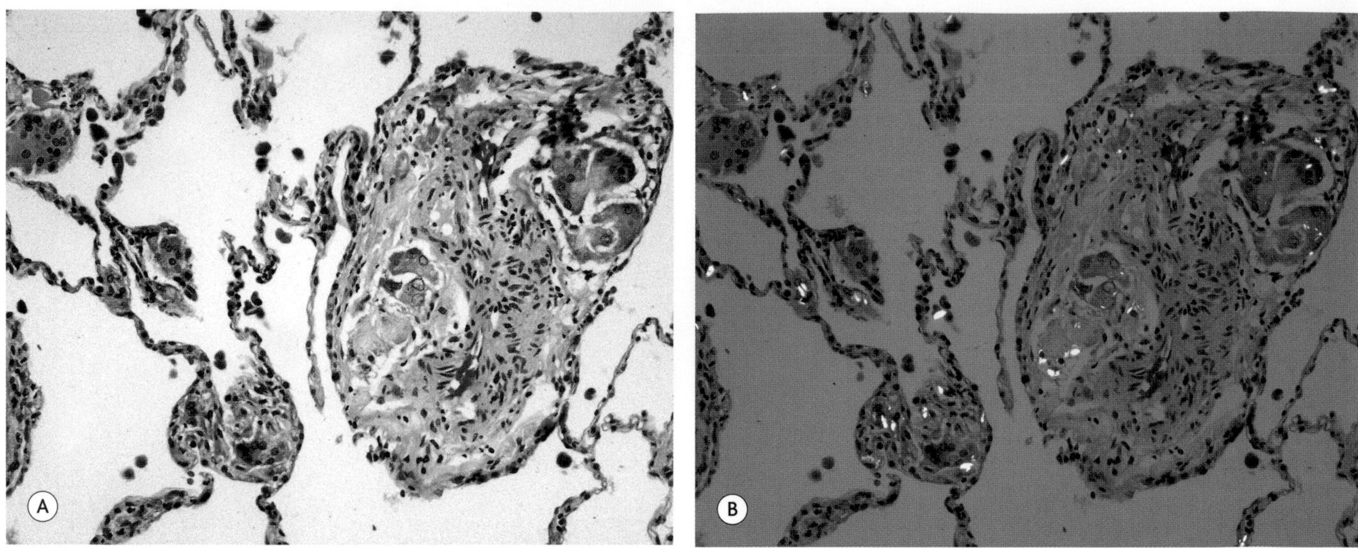

Fig. 7.73 **Intravenous (IV) drug.** (A, B – polarized light) A perivascular interstitial foreign body-type granulomatous reaction is produced that may be associated with prominent vascular changes as illustrated here.

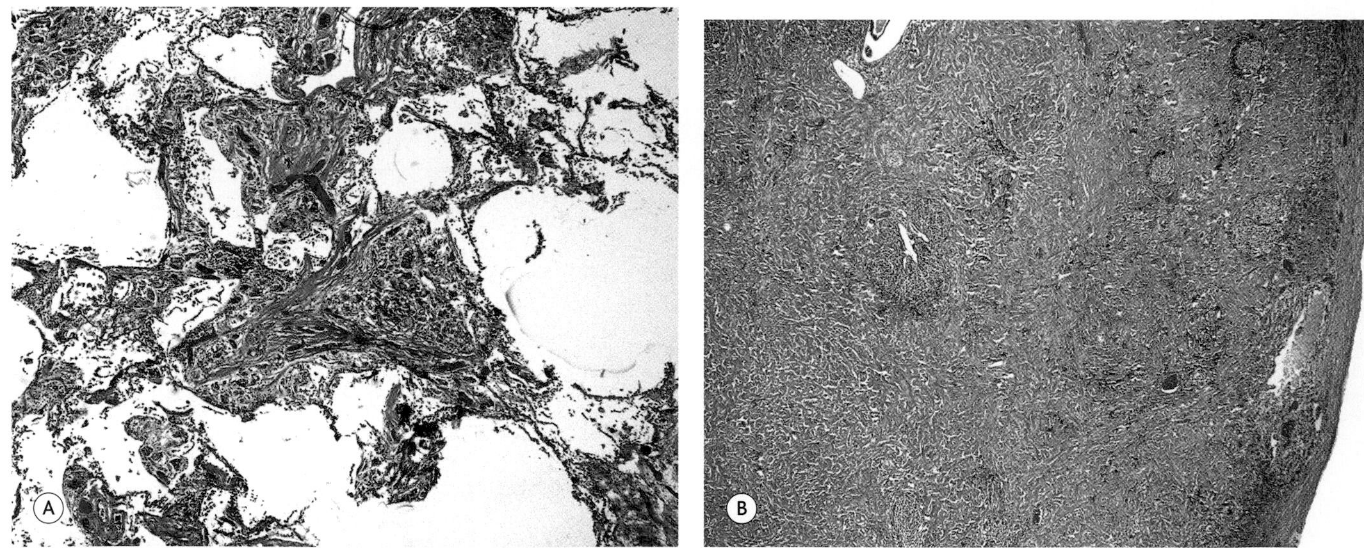

Fig. 7.74 **Intravenous (IV) drug.** One complication of IV drug abuse is (A) lung fibrosis, and (B) sometimes this can be massive.

Table 7.16 Pathologic lesions and clinical syndromes related to intravenous drug use

Pathologic lesions	Clinical syndromes
Vascular, perivascular and interstitial foreign body granulomas with:	
Pulmonary arterial hypertension – with thrombotic lesions – without thrombotic lesions	Pulmonary hypertension (may cause sudden death)
Interstitial fibrosis	Interstitial lung disease
Massive fibrosis	Complicated "pneumoconiosis" (tends to be bilateral and involves mid and upper lung zones)
Panacinar emphysema	Emphysema/chronic airflow obstruction

Table 7.17 Granulomatous interstitial pneumonias

Granulomas commonly encountered	Granulomas infrequently encountered or inconsistent
Sarcoidosis/ berylliosis	Bronchiectasis/bronchiolitis with secondary granulomatous infection
Infections: Mycobacteria, fungi, pneumocystis, actinomyces, nocardia, others	Some pneumoconioses Drug reactions
Hypersensitivity pneumonitis	Collagen vascular diseases (e.g. Sjögren's syndrome)
	Intravenous talcosis
	Vasculitis:* – Wegener's granulomatosis – Churg–Strauss syndrome
	Bronchocentric granulomatosis
	Eosinophilic pneumonia
	Foreign body granulomas (aspiration pneumonia)
	Immunoglobulin deficiency
	Lymphoid interstitial pneumonia/diffuse lymphoid hyperlasia
	Giant cell interstitial pneumonia/ hard metal lung disease
	Diffuse neoplastic involvement of the lungs (lymphoma, leukemia, others)
	Inflammatory bowel disease (Crohn's disease)
	Incidental granulomas
	Unclassifiable

*Vasculitis syndromes rarely present as diffuse granulomatous lung disease.
Source: adapted from Cheung et al.[7]

of panlobular emphysema associated with intravenous drug abuse is unknown. Some of the postulated mechanisms include synergism with cigarette smoke, direct toxic effects of the drug, and induced intravascular leukocyte sequestration causing proteolytic pulmonary injury.

Because the foreign material remains in the lung, there may be progression of the clinical and pathologic lesions after discontinuation of intravenous drug abuse. Recurrence of the changes of intravenous drug abuse have been described rarely in transplanted lung tissue, although this appears to be a consequence of resumed intravenous drug abuse.[222]

Diffuse lung diseases with granulomas

Granulomas occur in the lung in a variety of infectious and non-infectious diseases (Table 7.17).[7] Infectious diseases with granulomas are discussed in Chapter 6. While non-infectious granulomas can occur diffusely in the lungs in certain drug reactions, and in Sjögren's syndrome, the relatively specific disease entities of sarcoidosis, berylliosis, and hypersensitivity pneumonitis are presented here separately because of their distinctive clinical, radiologic, and histopathologic presentations.

Sarcoidosis

Clinical presentation

Sarcoidosis is a systemic disease of uncertain etiology, with frequent lung manifestations.[223–227] Lung disease is usually mild, accompanied by variable degrees of shortness of breath, chest pain, and cough.[227] As many as two-thirds of patients are asymptomatic.[228,229] Sarcoidosis is predominately a disease of young adults but has been described in patients of all ages. [230–232] Sarcoidosis can have an acute, subacute, or chronic presentation in the lung. In symptomatic patients, restrictive defects and decreased diffusing capacity are commonly described. Serum angiotensin-converting enzyme (ACE) is elevated in 30–80% of patients. ACE has also been detected within granulomas, bronchial alveolar lavage fluid, tears, and even cerebrospinal fluid in these patients. Unfortunately, ACE levels can be elevated in a variety of disorders, including infectious granulomatous diseases, lymphoma, hepatitis, and diabetes.[228] The Kveim test[233] is relatively specific for sarcoidosis, employing an injected antigenic serum derived from human sarcoid granuloma extracts, but the test is not widely used today,[227] given the widespread use of bronchoscopic biopsy in confirming the diagnosis in patients suspected of having the disease on clinical and radiologic grounds.

Radiologic findings

The clinical staging of sarcoidosis is based on chest radiographic findings. Five stages of pulmonary sarcoidosis are described, corresponding to extent of disease. Stages I and II disease are most common, with only 15% of patients presenting with parenchymal infiltrates alone.[227,228] When sarcoidosis involves the lung parenchyma, the disease is upper lobe predominant.[227] CT scans are usually not necessary for the diagnosis, but

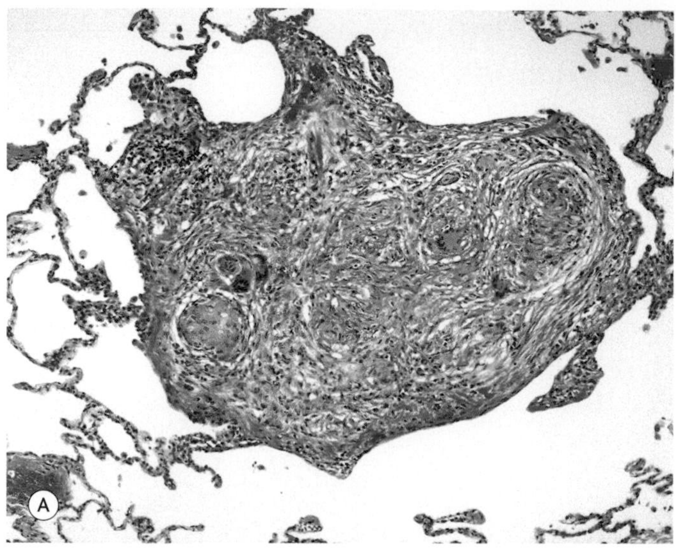

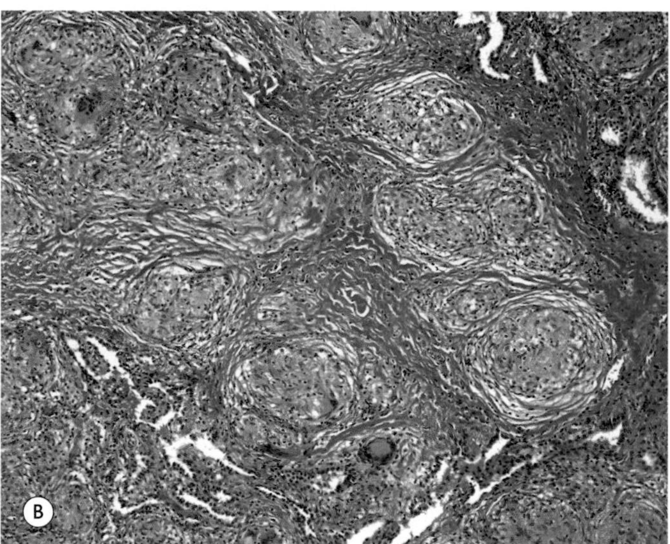

Fig. 7.75 **Sarcoidosis.** (A) The characteristic pathologic lesion of pulmonary sarcoidosis is the non-necrotizing (immune) granuloma, (B) typically occurring within sclerotic fibrosis.

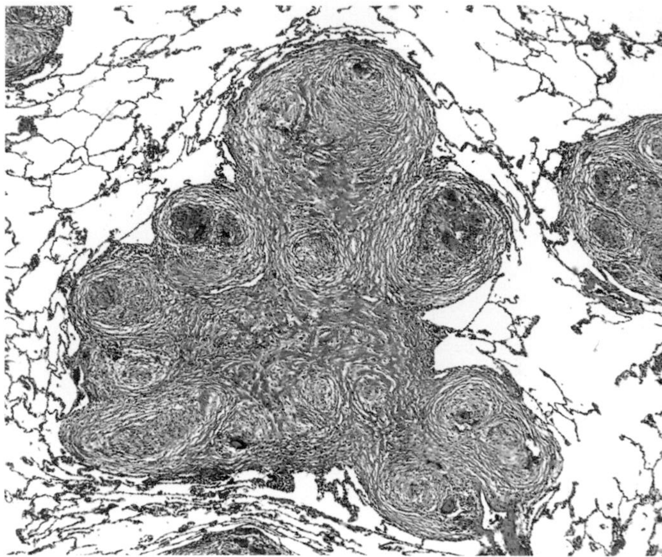

Fig. 7.76 **Sarcoidosis.** In sarcoidosis, small granulomas have a tendency to coalesce and form larger nodular lesions, all embedded in refractile eosinophilic collagen.

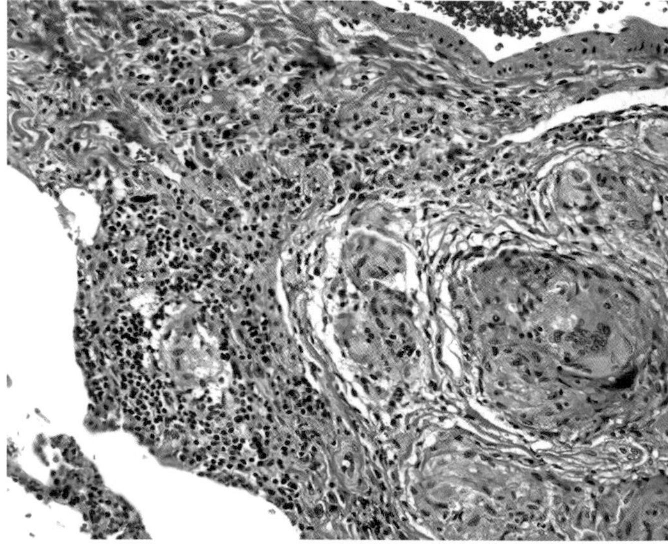

Fig. 7.77 **Sarcoidosis.** A variable (but rarely intense) rim of lymphocytic inflammation is typically seen at the periphery of confluent granulomas.

do show reticulonodular opacities following lymphatic routes, with or without alveolar infiltrates.[228,234–236] Bullae formation with honeycombing can occur in advanced disease, sometimes associated with progressive lung fibrosis.[237,238] A peculiar form of sarcoidosis with rapid onset of symptoms and a diffuse alveolar filling pattern on CT scans has been referred to as "alveolar sarcoidosis."[239] The pathologic manifestations of this form of the disease are distinctive only for the large number of small interstitial granulomas present throughout the lung parenchyma.

Pathologic findings

The characteristic pathologic lesion of pulmonary sarcoidosis is the non-necrotizing (immune) granuloma, typically occurring within sclerotic fibrosis (Fig. 7.75). In sarcoidosis, small granulomas have a tendency to coalesce and form larger nodular lesions, all embedded in refractile eosinophilic collagen (Fig. 7.76). A rim of lymphocytic inflammation is typically seen at the periphery of these confluent nodules (Fig. 7.77). Granulomas are distributed along lymphatic routes in the pleura, the intralobular

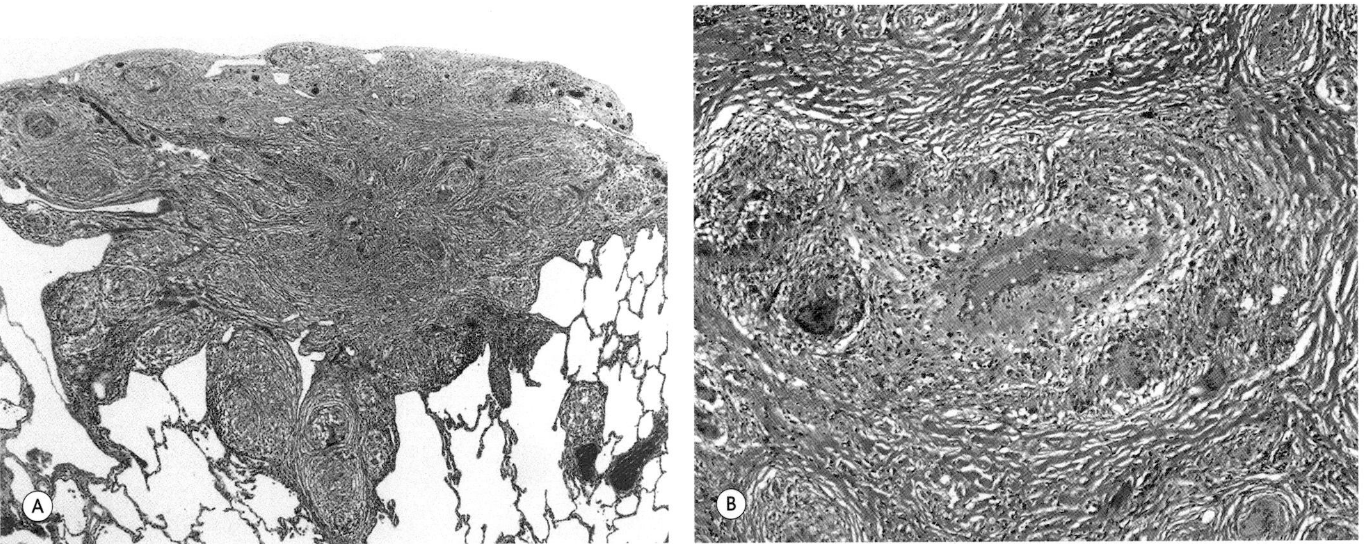

Fig. 7.78 **Sarcoidosis.** (A) Granulomas are distributed along lymphatic routes in the pleura, the intralobular septa, and along the bronchovascular bundles. This image is diagnostic of sarcoidosis, but berylliosis should always be included as a diagnostic possibility. (B) Perivascular granulomas embedded in sclerosis are commonly seen. Despite this potential for vasocentric growth, pulmonary hypertension is an uncommon complication in sarcoidosis.

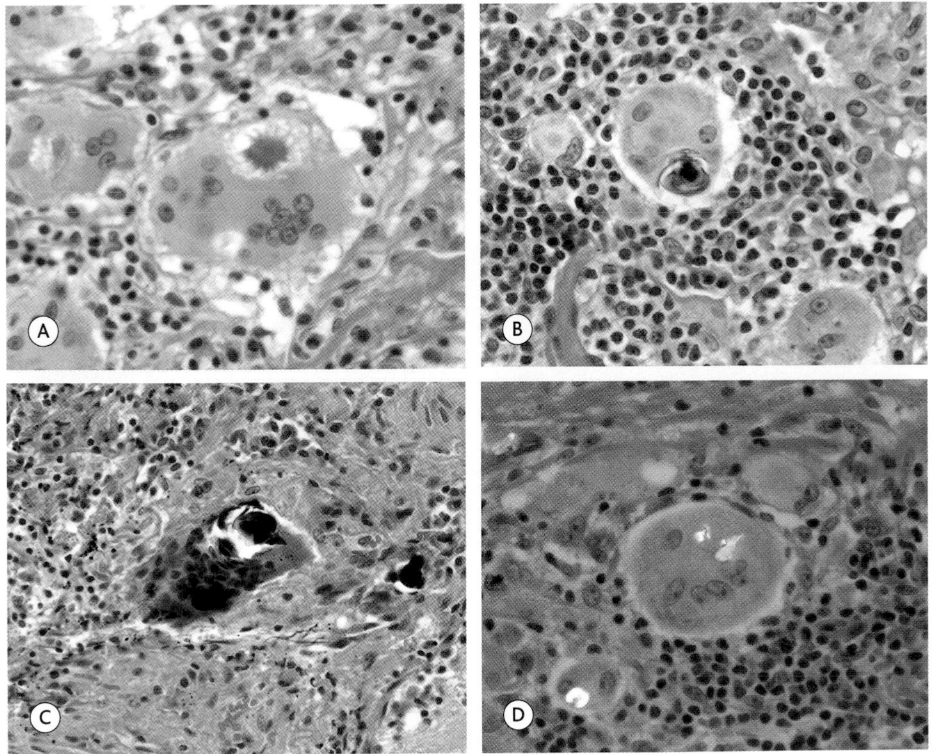

Fig. 7.79 **Sarcoidosis.** Multinucleated giant cells are characteristically present in the disease, often accompanied by a variety of distinctive (but not specific) cytoplasmic inclusions: (A) upper left, asteroid body; (B) upper right, Schaumann (conchoidal) body; (C) lower left, Schaumann bodies; (D) lower right, Schaumann body in polarized light.

septa, and along the bronchovascular bundles (Fig. 7.78). Multinucleated giant cells are characteristically present in the disease, often accompanied by a variety of distinctive cytoplasmic inclusions (e.g. Schaumann bodies, asteroid bodies, etc.) (Fig. 7.79). A mild inflammatory interstitial infiltrate is said to occur occasionally in pulmonary sarcoidosis, but in practice this is rarely seen. In bronchoscopic or transbronchial biopsies, granulomas

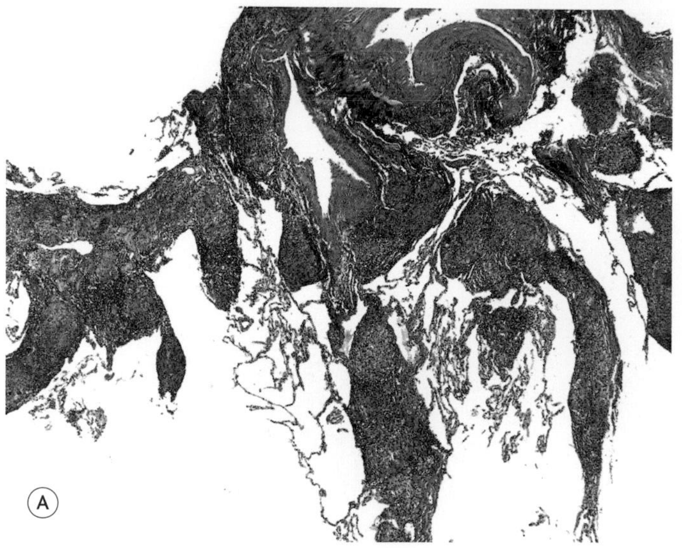

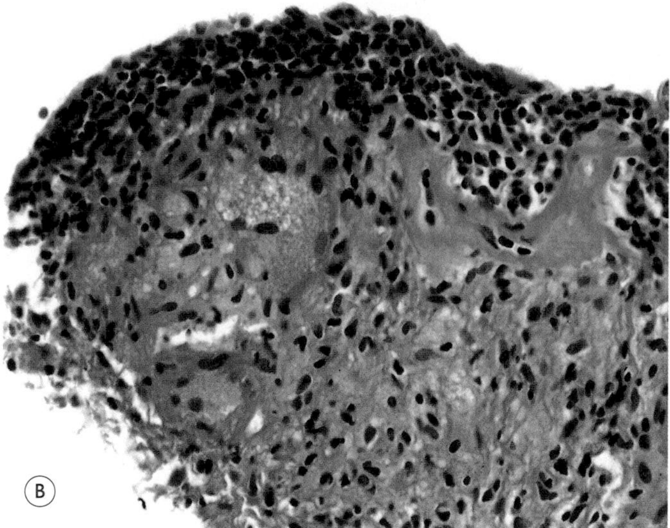

Fig. 7.80 **Sarcoidosis.** (A) In bronchoscopic or transbronchial biopsies, granulomas may be quite dramatic, but (B) sometimes they are more subtle, present typically in the immediate subepithelial region of the airway.

typically occur in the submucosa (Fig. 7.80). Gilman and coworkers showed that the chance of obtaining a positive result in patients with sarcoidosis increased to 90% when four biopsy specimens were obtained.[240] When five to six biopsies were obtained, the probability rose to 100% for patients with stage II and III disease. Special stains for organisms (acid-fast stains and silver stains) should be routinely performed when granulomas are identified in lung biopsies, to exclude infection, even in the absence of necrosis. In a retrospective study performed by Hsu et al., positive microbiological cultures were identified in 11% of biopsies in which granulomas were present despite negative special stains on tissue sections.[241] In the culture-positive cases, clinical and radiographic findings were judged to be of low or intermediate suspicion for sarcoidosis. As one might expect, necrosis in granulomas was more frequently associated with culture-positive cases.

Differential diagnosis

Granulomatous infection leads the differential diagnosis for sarcoidosis and is the diagnosis of exclusion. The granulomas of hypersensitivity pneumonitis are vague and poorly formed. Aspiration pneumonia can be associated with granuloma formation, but these tend to resemble foreign body-type granulomas with characteristic multinucleated giant cells, often containing foreign (partially digested food, primarily) material.

Chronic berylliosis

Beryllium, derived from the mineral beryl, is the etiologic agent for berylliosis.[242–244] The disease occurs after inhalation of this metal or its salts.[245] Exposure to beryllium occurs today mainly as an occupational lung disease, particularly in the computer manufacturing and aerospace engineering fields.[246,247](For additional discussion see Ch. 9) Acute berylliosis occurs after heavy exposure and is thankfully rare today given strict industrial exposure regulations and aggressive surveillance in this setting. When acute berylliosis occurs, the pathologic findings are those of diffuse alveolar damage (DAD). The chronic form of berylliosis is indistinguishable from sarcoidosis on histopathologic grounds.[242–244] Like sarcoidosis, chronic berylliosis produces variable fibrosis and distinct granulomas with giant cells (Fig. 7.81). Chronic berylliosis may produce large centrally hyalinized nodules (Fig. 7.82), which can simulate resolved lesions of histoplasmosis. When granulomas are less prominent, chronic berylliosis may also simulate hypersensitivity pneumonitis histopathologically (Fig. 7.83).

Hypersensitivity pneumonitis (extrinsic allergic alveolitis)

Environmental antigens (typically "organic" protein antigens) are known to produce characteristic inflammatory reactions in the lung in certain predisposed individuals.[248–251] The classic descriptions of "farmer's lung," resulting from exposure to thermophilic actinomyces in hay; and "bird fancier's lung," resulting from inhalation from avian antigens are examples of hypersensitivity pneumonitis (HSP). Similar reactions can occur to

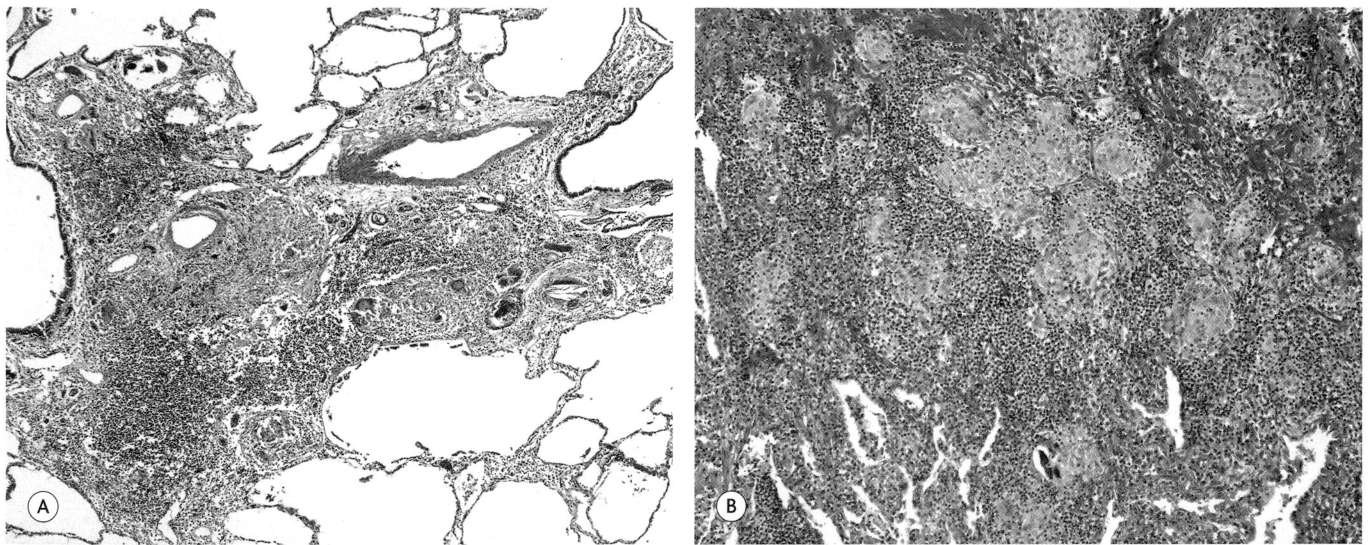

Fig. 7.81 **Berylliosis.** Like sarcoidosis, chronic berylliosis produces (A) variable fibrosis and (B) distinct granulomas with giant cells. There may be a suggestion of more lymphocytic inflammation, but this is not sufficiently reliable to be useful diagnostically.

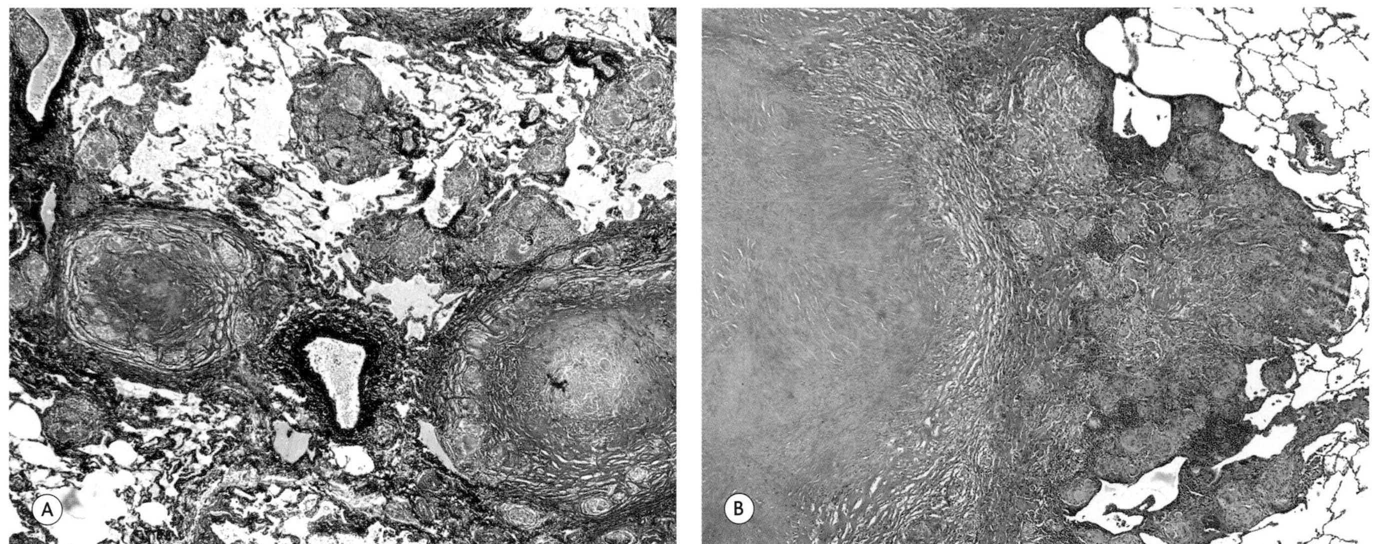

Fig. 7.82 **Berylliosis.** (A,B) Chronic berylliosis may produce large centrally hyalinized nodules, which can simulate resolved lesions of histoplasmosis.

ingested antigens associated with some medications, but, in general usage, HSP refers to disease occurring as a result of inhalation exposure. The more common antigens implicated in HSP are presented in Table 7.18.

Clinical presentation

The disease can occur as acute and chronic forms. The acute form occurs within hours of inhalational exposure to antigen. Affected individuals experience malaise, dyspnea, and dry cough, sometimes associated with fever and chills. The symptom complex raises a differential diagnosis including viral infection. Recurrence of symptoms and signs follows subsequent exposure episodes.[252] Cigarette smoking seems to reduce the risk of developing hypersensitivity, although the mechanism for this protective action is unknown.[253]

The chronic form of HSP probably results from lower levels of antigen exposure over time, presumably accompanied by more subtle symptoms that may not allow the patient to associate the symptom with a specific exposure.[252, 254] Unfortunately, the chronic form of HSP may be progressive and can lead to death from end-stage lung fibrosis.[252,254] As in the acute phase, chronic malaise and varying degrees of breathlessness on exertion occur, sometimes accompanied by weight loss. Several excellent reviews of hypersensitivity pneumonitis are available.[250–252,254–256]

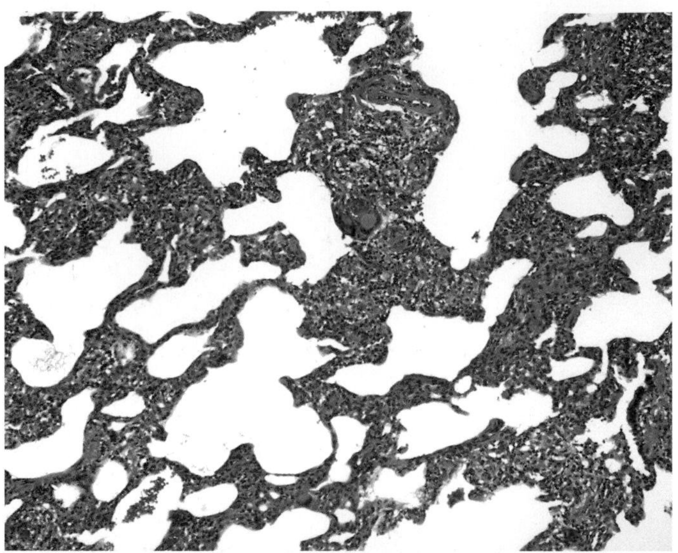

Fig. 7.83 **Berylliosis.** When granulomas are less prominent, as illustrated in this case of berylliosis, hypersensitivity pneumonitis may enter the differential diagnosis.

Radiologic findings

In acute HSP, a diffuse ground glass appearance is seen on CT scans of the chest, sometimes accompanied by fine nodules.[257] In subacute disease, abnormalities tend to be confined to the upper half or two-thirds of the lung. In more chronic forms, small nodules, variable ground glass change, and irregular linear opacities may be seen, most often in the middle lung zones (with relative sparing of the apices and bases) or without a specific zonal predilection.[26] The presence of irregular linear opacities correlates with the presence of lung fibrosis.[252,256,257] In very late stage chronic HSP, honeycomb remodeling may be identified radiologically, mimicking usual interstitial pneumonia.[26,27] Interestingly, the CT appearance of subacute hypersensitivity pneumonitis may be indistinguishable from low-grade atypical mycobacterial infection that occurs in the immunocompetent host, as a result of bioaerosol exposure to non-tuberculous mycobacteria[258,259] (so called "hot tub lung" – see Ch. 6).

Pathologic findings

The histopathologic features of HSP are typically those of a chronic inflammatory interstitial pneumonia associated with bronchiolitis, and small, indistinct, non-necrotizing

Table 7.18 Causes of hypersensitivity pneumonitis (extrinsic allergic alveolitis)

Antigen	Source	Disease
Thermophilic bacteria		
Micropolyspora faeni	Moldy hay	Farmer's lung
Thermoactinomyces vulgaris	Moldy compost	Mushroom worker's disease
Thermoactinomyces saccharii	Moldy sugar cane	Bagassosis
Thermoactinomyces vulgaris	Air conditioners, humidifers	Air conditioner lung/humidifier lung
Thermoactinomyces candidus	Air conditioners, humidifers	Air conditioner lung/humidifier lung
Molds		
Cryptostroma corticale	Moldy maple bark	Maple bark stripper's disease
Aspergillus clavatus	Moldy barley	Malt worker's lung
Graphium spp.	Moldy wood dust	Sequoiosis
Pullularia spp.	Moldy wood dust	Sequoiosis
Trichosporon cutaneum	Home environment	Summer-type hypersensitivity pneumonitis (Japan)
Other bacteria		
Bacillus subtilis	Water	Detergent worker's lung
Bacillus cereus	Water	Humidifier lung
Bacterial products	Cotton	Byssinosis
Amoebi	Water	Humidifier lung
Insect products	Grain	Wheat weevil disease
Chemicals		
Trimellitic anhydride (TMA)	Plastics, rubber manufacturing	Chemical worker's lung
Methylene diisocyanate (MDI)	Plastics, rubber manufacturing	Chemical worker's lung
Toluene diisocyanate (TDI)	Plastics, rubber manufacturing	Chemical worker's lung
Pyromellitic dianhydride (PMDA)	Epoxy resin	

Source: from Katzenstein and Askin,[1] p 139, with permission.

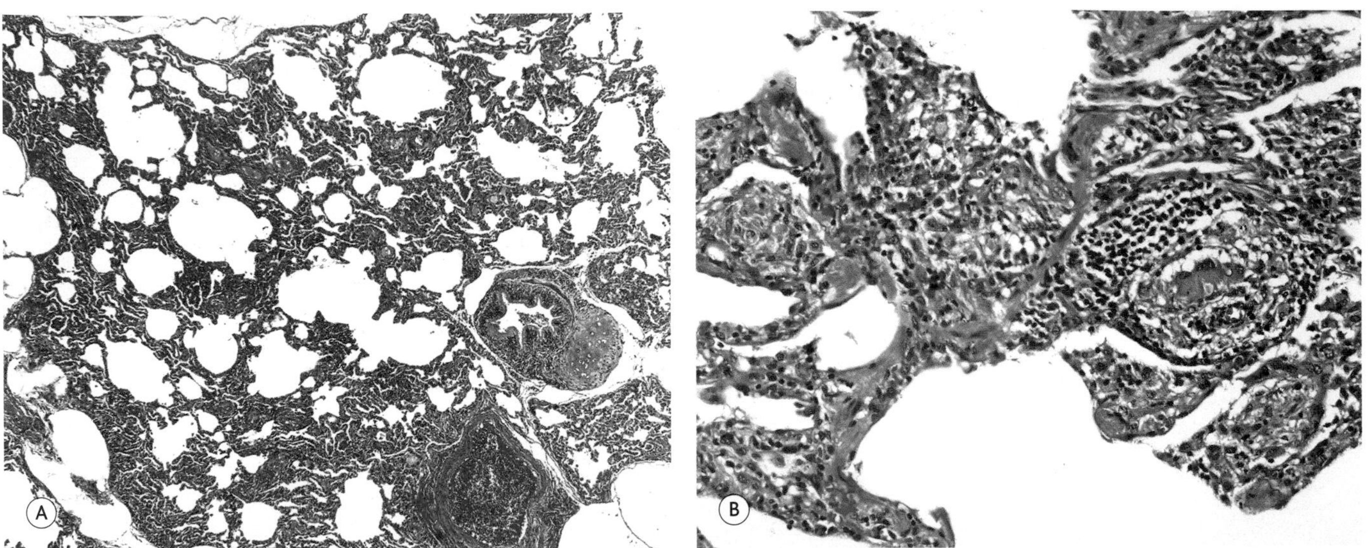

Fig. 7.84 **Hypersensitivity pneumonitis (HSP).** HSP produces a chronic inflammatory interstitial pneumonia associated with (A) bronchiolitis and (B) small, indistinct, non-necrotizing *interstitial* granulomas.

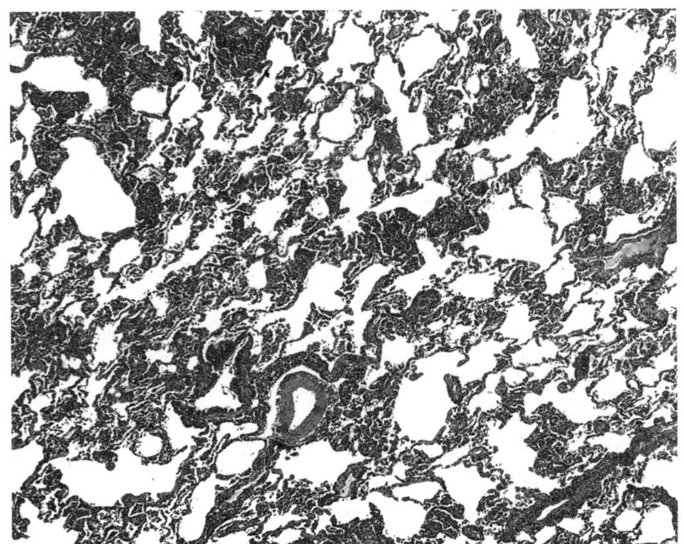

Fig. 7.85 **Hypersensitivity pneumonitis (HSP).** At low magnification, the surgical lung biopsy shows a moderately dense interstitial infiltrate, causing slight widening of the alveolar walls.

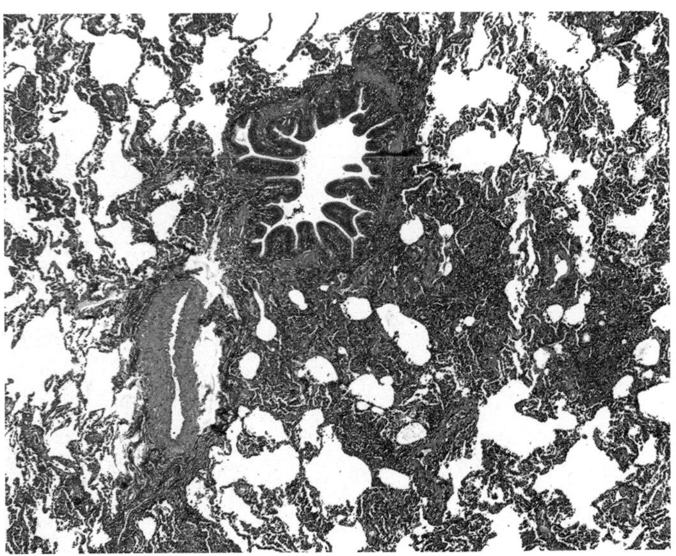

Fig. 7.86 **Hypersensitivity pneumonitis (HSP).** A bronchiolocentric distribution may be evident, either by the presence of a terminal bronchiole or by some degree of nodularity to the infiltrates at low magnification.

interstitial granulomas (Fig. 7.84).[248,260,261] In early reports of "farmer's lung," acute inflammation and vasculitis were also observed.[262] The histopathology of HSP raises a differential diagnosis that includes other cellular interstitial pneumonias, such as nonspecific interstitial pneumonia (NSIP). At low magnification, the surgical lung biopsy shows a moderately dense interstitial infiltrate, comprised of plasma cells and small lymphocytes, causing slight widening of the alveolar walls (Fig. 7.85). A bronchiolocentric distribution may be evident, either by the presence of a terminal bronchiole or by some degree of nodularity to the infiltrates at low magnification (Fig. 7.86). The interstitial "granulomas" of hypersensitivity pneumonitis are sufficiently vague in

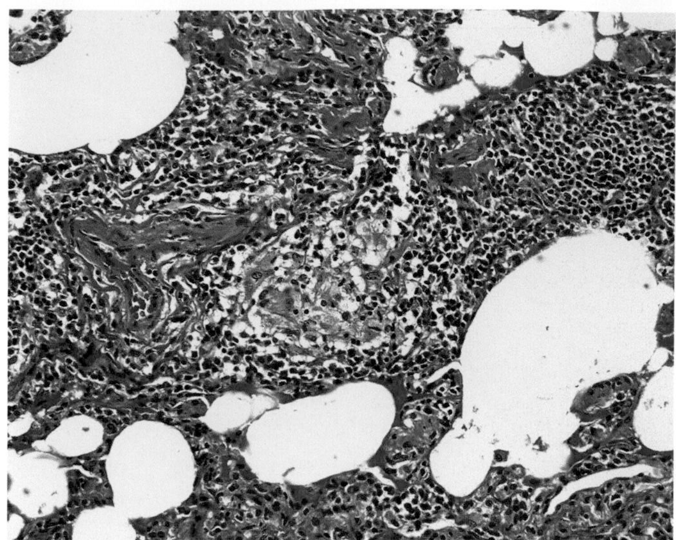

Fig. 7.87 **Hypersensitivity pneumonitis (HSP).** The interstitial "granulomas" of hypersensitivity pneumonitis are sufficiently vague in their appearance as to escape notice in many cases. Prominent, well-formed granulomas are not a typical manifestation of the disease.

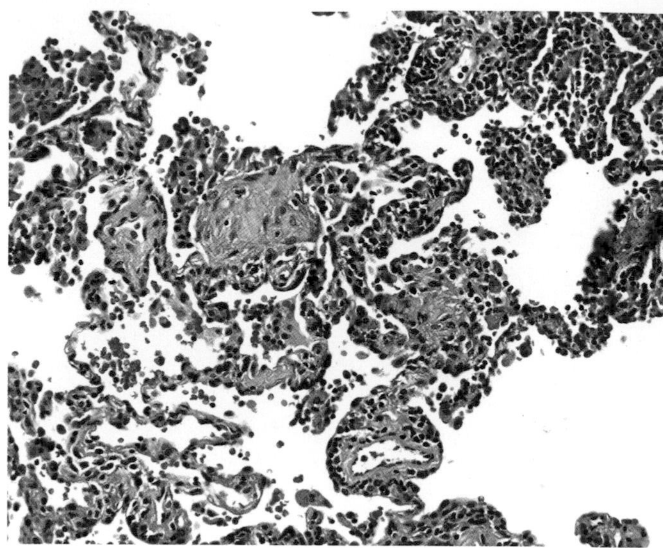

Fig. 7.89 **Hypersensitivity pneumonitis (HSP).** Patchy airspace organization can be seen in as many as 60% of patients with hypersensitivity pneumonitis.

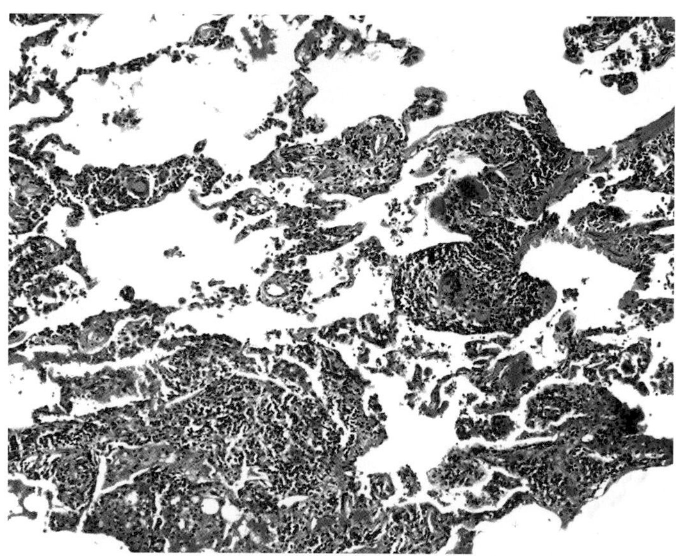

Fig. 7.88 **Hypersensitivity pneumonitis (HSP).** Multinucleated giant cells may also be seen in the interstitium and are a helpful feature at low magnification in drawing the eye to closer examination.

their appearance (Fig. 7.87) as to escape notice in many cases. Multinucleated giant cells (Fig. 7.88) may be seen in the interstitium at scanning magnification and are a helpful feature in drawing the eye to closer examination of the interstitium for epithelioid histiocytes in small aggregates. Necrosis is not a component of the granulomatous reaction in hypersensitivity pneumonitis.

Airspace organization (Fig. 7.89) with immature fibroblast and matrix (organizing pneumonia pattern) can be seen in as many as 60% of patients with hypersensitivity pneumonitis,[260] but in general this is not confluent organization, as is seen in organizing pneumonia of infectious etiology. Rather, small tufted patches of organization can be seen scattered throughout the lung biopsy. Some degree of bronchiolitis is expected in HSP, and this is characterized by aggregates of lymphocytes and plasma cells surrounding terminal airways (Fig. 7.90) A mild perivascular lymphoid accumulation is typically present in hypersensitivity pneumonitis, but prominent germinal centers or dense lymphoplasmacellular infiltration along lymphatic routes is not typical and should raise concern for lymphoproliferative disease (which on occasion can simulate the cellular phase of chronic hypersensitivity pneumonitis). In the chronic form of hypersensitivity, dense fibrosis with microscopic honeycombing can be seen (Fig. 7.91). Refractile oxalate crystals in giant cells may be sufficiently prominent to suggest aspiration pneumonia or even pneumoconiosis (Fig. 7.92).

Clinical course

The clinical course of HSP varies with the intensity and chronicity of exposure.[252,262,263] If an offending antigen cannot be identified in the patient's environment, the prognosis is guarded, since patients may not respond to corticosteroid therapy in the continued presence of the

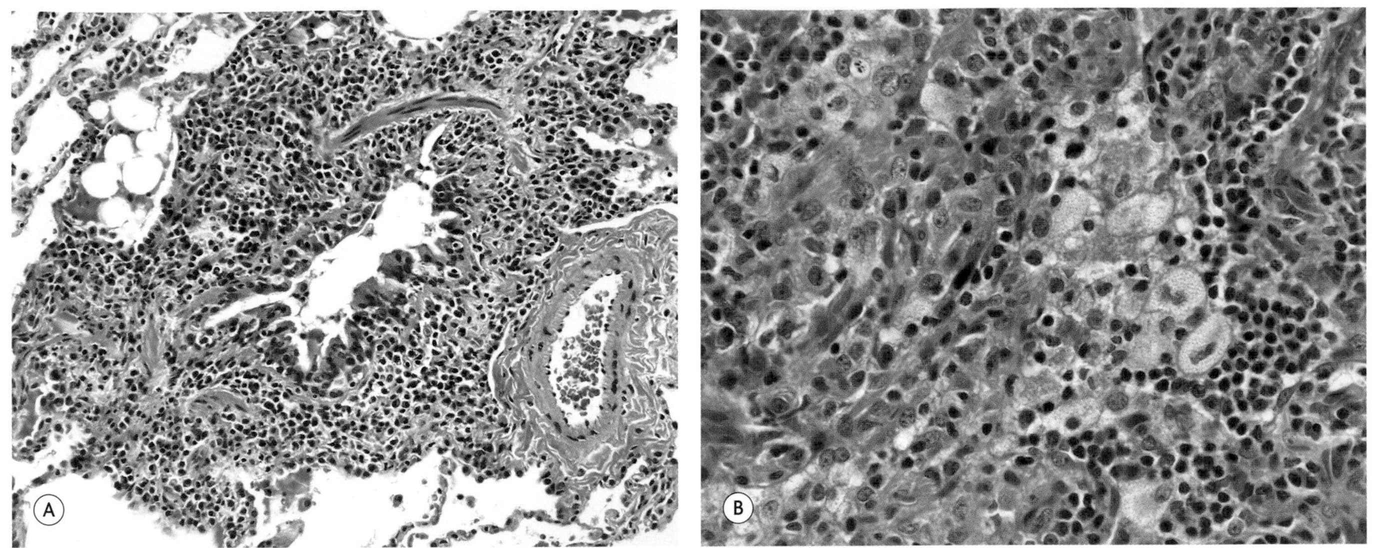

Fig. 7.90 **Hypersensitivity pneumonitis (HSP).** (A) Bronchiolitis is expected in HSP, manifested here as aggregates of lymphocytes and plasma cells surrounding a terminal airway. (B) Presumably, as a consequence of bronchiolitis and some degree of obstruction, prominently vacuolated macrophages may be present in a bronchiolocentric distribution.

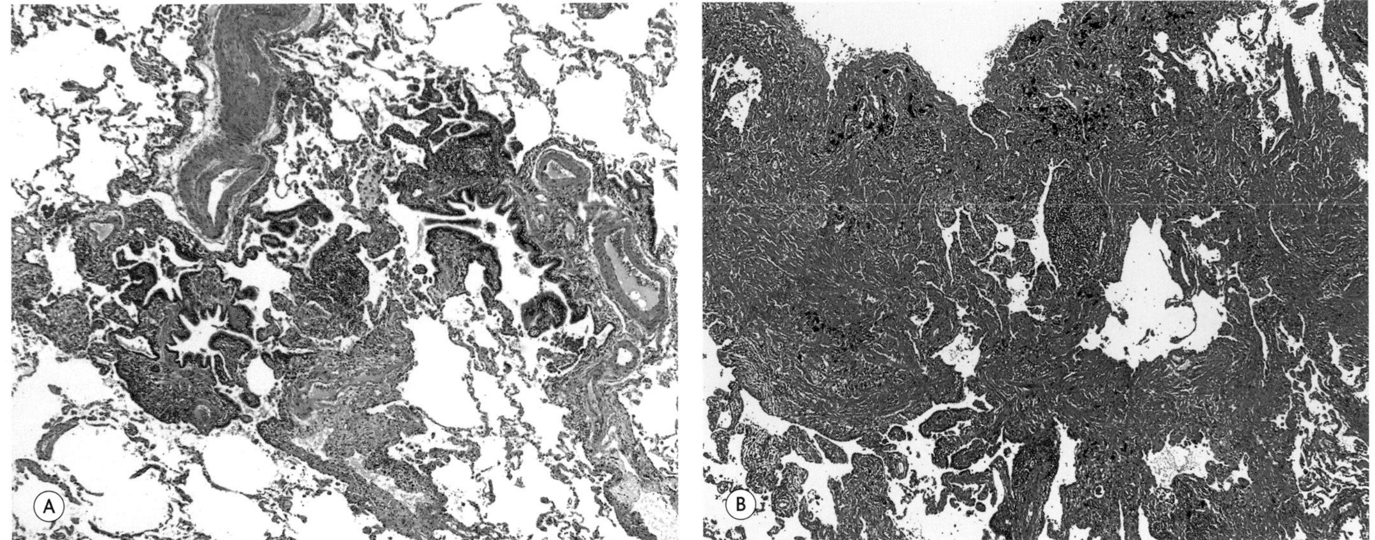

Fig. 7.91 **Hypersensitivity pneumonitis (HSP).** (A) In chronic hypersensitivity pneumonitis, prominent bronchiolization (Lambertosis) attests to chronic airway injury from inhaled antigen. (B) Dense fibrosis with microscopic honeycombing resembling usual interstitial pneumonia (UIP) may also be seen.

offending antigen.[264–268] Once lung fibrosis occurs, immunosuppressive therapy may be of little benefit, especially if there is ongoing exposure to antigen.[268]

Differential diagnosis

Cellular interstitial pneumonias with or without small non-necrotizing granulomas can be a component of drug reactions and low-grade infections (especially that produced by atypical mycobacterial species). Whether true hypersensitivity pneumonitis can occur to ingested drug or medication is controversial. Early sarcoidosis is in the differential diagnosis, but the more characteristic "tuberculoid" granulomas of sarcoidosis and presence of sclerotic matrix surrounding granulomas is helpful in differentiating this disease from HSP. Also, interstitial inflammation can be seen in sarcoidosis, but it is exceedingly mild, if it occurs at all. As mentioned earlier,

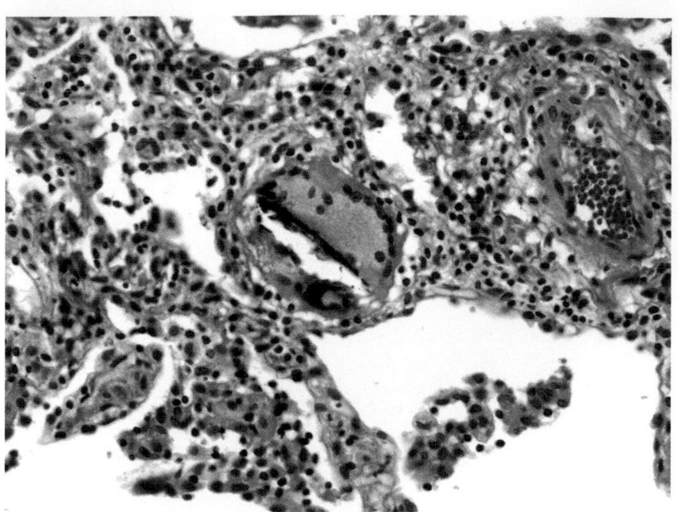

Fig. 7.92 **Hypersensitivity pneumonitis (HSP).** Refractile oxalate crystals in giant cells may be sufficiently prominent to suggest aspiration pneumonia or even pneumoconiosis.

when lymphoplasmacellular infiltrates are dense or confluent, LIP or low-grade malignant lymphoma of MALT enters the differential diagnosis. In the latter situation, immunohistochemical stains for lymphoid antigens (CD3 and CD20) may be helpful in demonstrating a predominance of CD20 positive B lymphocytes, a finding that should raise serious consideration for malignant lymphoma.

Miscellaneous diffuse lung diseases

Pulmonary Langerhans cell histiocytosis

The concept of smoking-related ILD has been presented earlier with RBILD and DIP. Here we focus on pulmonary Langerhans cell histiocytosis (PLCH), another important consequence of smoking, and a lung disease previously referred to as pulmonary eosinophilic granuloma or pulmonary histiocytosis X. PLCH is considered to be a reactive proliferative disease of Langerhans cells,[269,270] in contrast to extrapulmonary forms of Langerhans cell histiocytosis that are felt to be neoplastic.[271] A compelling association with cigarette smoking has led to the general acceptance of this lung disorder as a smoking-related disease.[15,272] A comprehensive up-to-date review of the pathobiology of PLCH can be found in a recent publication by Vassallo et al.[270] Although PLCH is unrelated to the systemic diseases of Langerhans cells (eosinophilic granuloma, Letterer–Siwi disease, Hand–Schüller–Christian disease), when systemic eosinophilic granuloma involves the lung it is said to be indistinguishable from the cellular phase of PLCH on histopathologic grounds.[273]

Two distinctive pathologic manifestations of PLCH occur: a cellular form and a fibrotic form. The natural history of PLCH suggests that the early lesions of PLCH are cellular, with many Langerhans cells and tissue eosinophils, while older lesions are predominately fibrotic. Such a natural progression may occur continuously in the same patient, with "younger" cellular lesions admixed with "older" ones. In most surgical biopsies, one form of the disease seems to predominate.[270] Often, the fibrotic lesions of the disease are not recognized as such because of the paucity or absence of Langerhans cells, and the proliferative lesions are typically mistaken for neoplasm.

Clinical presentation

The true incidence and prevalence of PLCH is unknown. Most patients are between 20 and 50 years of age at the onset of symptoms and women may be more commonly affected than men.[270,272,274] Chronic cough and dyspnea are typical presenting complaints; however, a significant percentage of patients are asymptomatic. Rarely, hemoptysis or pneumothorax can occur.

Radiologic findings

PLCH is a disease of the upper lung zones. Small nodules and cysts are present to varying degree on plain films of the chest.[274–277] The nodules range in size from 0.2 to 1 cm. When fibrosis occurs, it is best seen on HRCT and appears as reticular opacities.[276,278] When significant fibrosis occurs in PLCH, the disease may simulate idiopathic pulmonary fibrosis.[274,275,278]

Pathologic findings

Proliferative (cellular) phase

At scanning magnification, the nodules of PLCH have a stellate appearance and are centered on the small airways (Fig. 7.93) Cysts are formed at the periphery of nodules by traction on surrounding alveolar walls or the central terminal airway, resulting in variably sized spaces, typically lacking distinctive lining cells (Fig. 7.94). Stellate cellular nodules may be as large as 1.5 cm,[273] and confluence of nodules affecting adjacent airways may impart a serpentine outline to the lesions (Fig. 7.95). Based on a recent three-dimensional reconstruction study, the lesions of PLCH seem to form a sheath around the small airways exclusively, and extend proximally and distally in a continuous fashion.[279] In many cases, a rim of

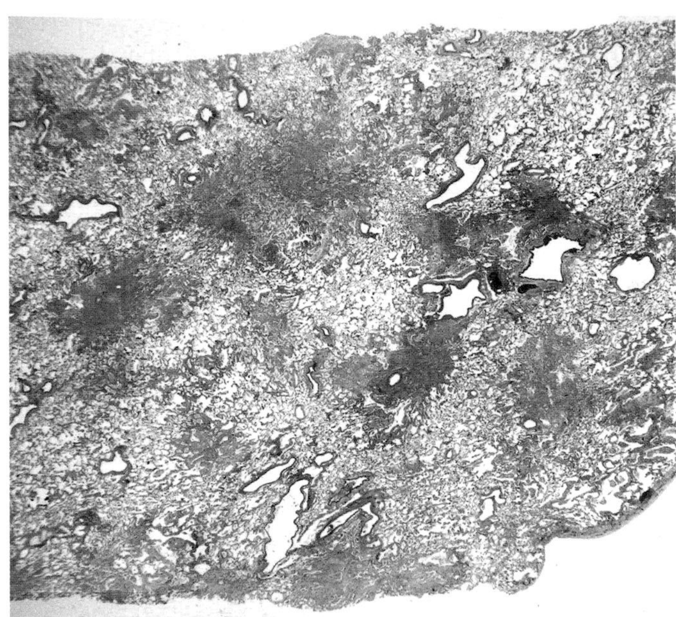

Fig. 7.93 **Pulmonary Langerhans cell histiocytosis (PLCH).** At scanning magnification, the nodules of PLCH have a stellate appearance and are centered on the small airways.

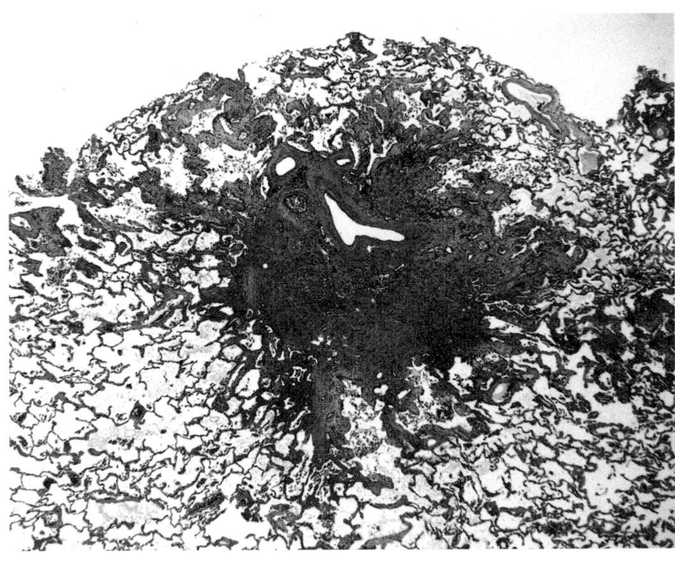

Fig. 7.95 **Pulmonary Langerhans cell histiocytosis (PLCH).** Stellate cellular nodules of PLCH may be as large as 1.5 cm.

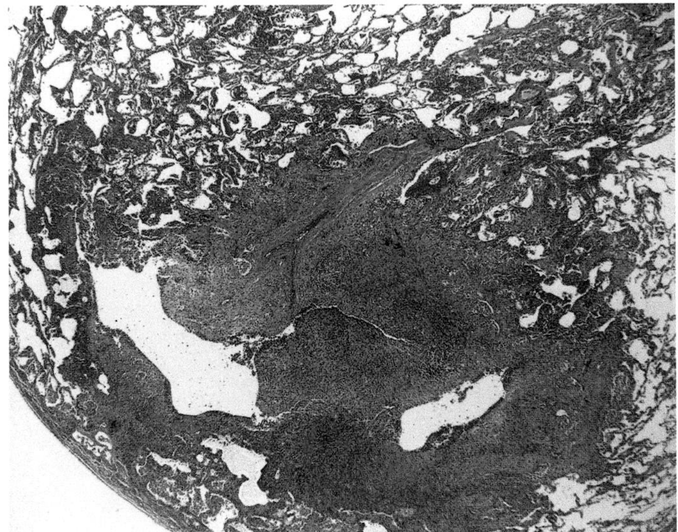

Fig. 7.94 **Pulmonary Langerhans cell histiocytosis (PLCH).** The cysts in PLCH are formed by traction on surrounding alveolar walls or the central terminal airway, resulting in variably sized spaces, typically lacking distinctive lining cells.

brown-pigmented macrophages ("smoker's macrophages") is present in and around the nodules (Fig. 7.96). Eosinophils in variable numbers occupy the next innermost layer of the nodules (Fig. 7.97) and this is the location where aggregated Langerhans cells are most easily found in the thickened interstitium (Fig. 7.98). The Langerhans cells have a pale basophilic nucleus with characteristic sharp nuclear infoldings, imparting a "crumpled tissue paper" nuclear contour (Fig. 7.99). The cytoplasm of the Langerhans cell is granular and mildly eosinophilic, with indistinct margins. In these cellular lesions of PLCH, immunohistochemical stains for S100 protein and CD1a can be used to highlight the presence of Langerhans cells (Fig. 7.100) but in most instances the morphology of the lesions is sufficiently compelling that a definitive diagnosis can be established without the aid of special stains. In some cases, patchy interstitial and airspace organization (Fig. 7.101) may be present, and typically there is respiratory bronchiolitis. Other smoking-related lung changes may be present, adding further complexity to the morphologic picture (e.g. DIP/RBILD, small airways disease with mucostasis, areas of bronchiolization, etc.).

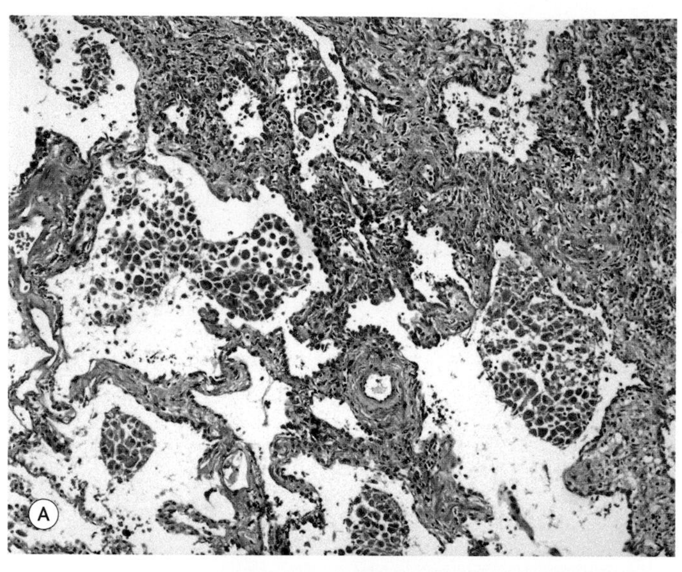

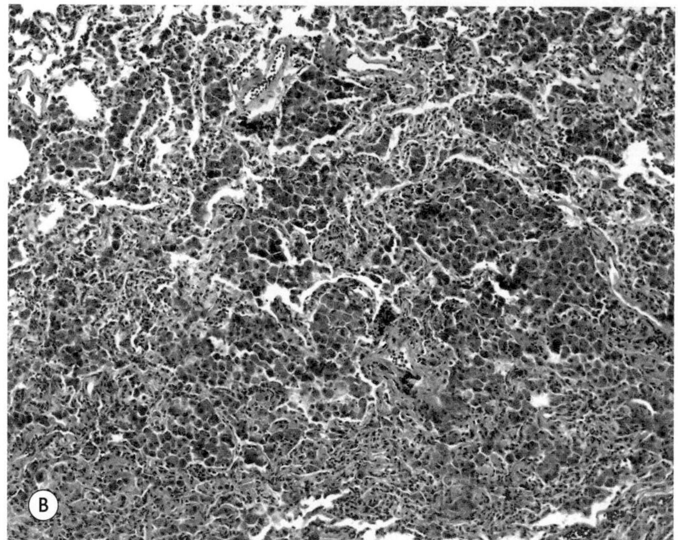

Fig. 7.96 **Pulmonary Langerhans cell histiocytosis (PLCH).** (A,B) In many cases, a rim of brown-pigmented macrophages ("smoker's macrophages") is present within and around the nodules.

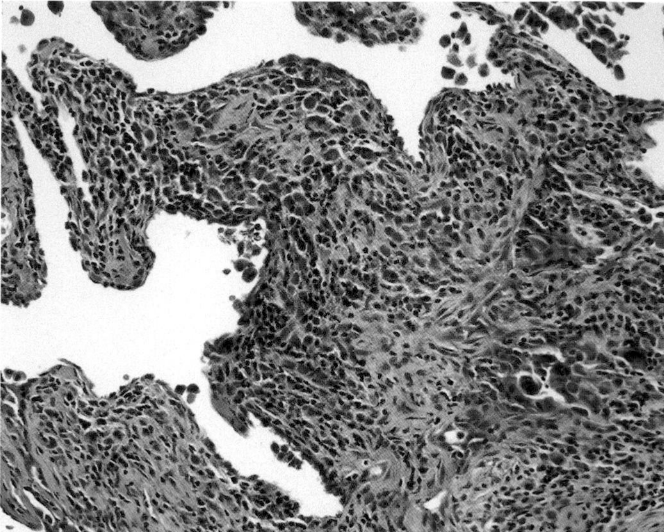

Fig. 7.97 **Pulmonary Langerhans cell histiocytosis (PLCH).** Eosinophils in variable numbers occupy the next innermost layer of the nodules.

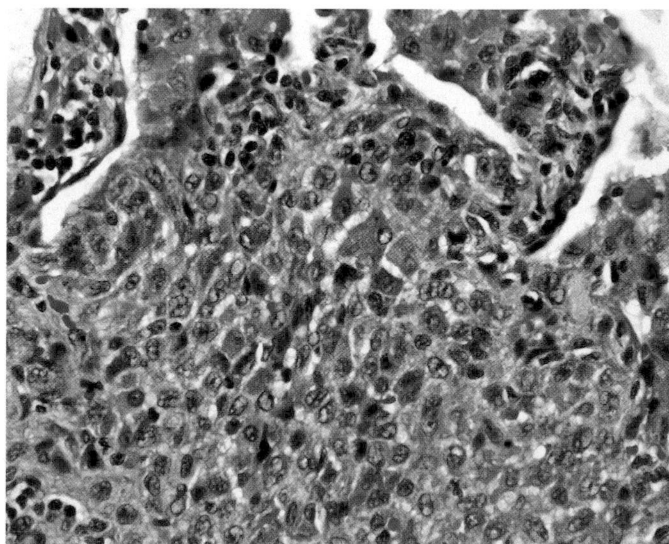

Fig. 7.98 **Pulmonary Langerhans cell histiocytosis (PLCH).** Aggregated Langerhans cells are most easily found in the thickened interstitium of the stellate ramifications of the lesions.

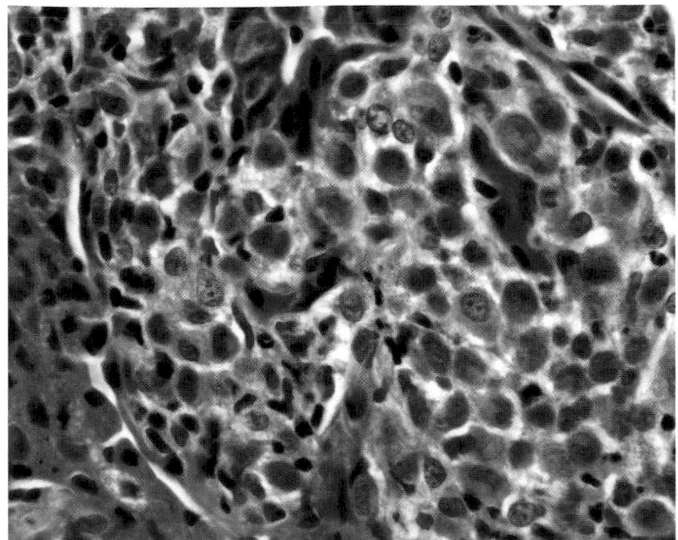

Fig. 7.99 **Pulmonary Langerhans cell histiocytosis (PLCH).** The Langerhans cells have a pale nucleus with characteristic sharp nuclear infoldings, imparting a "crumpled tissue paper" outline. The cytoplasm of the Langerhans cell is variably eosinophilic and indistinct.

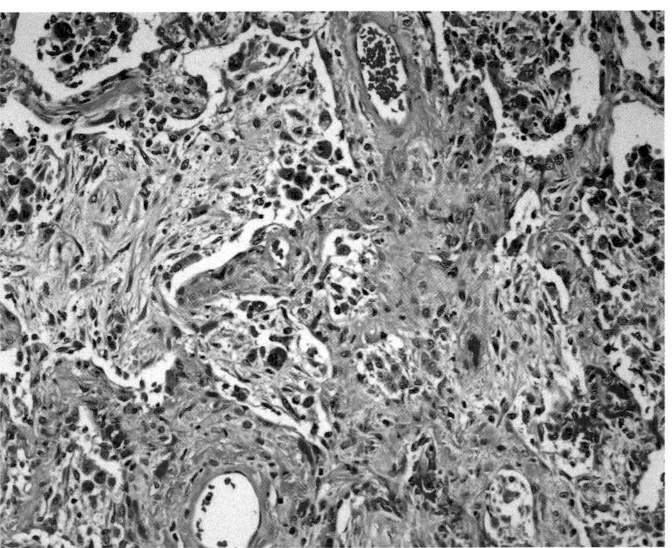

Fig. 7.101 **Pulmonary Langerhans cell histiocytosis (PLCH).** In some cases, patchy airspace organization may be present, but it is not a particularly characteristic feature of the disease.

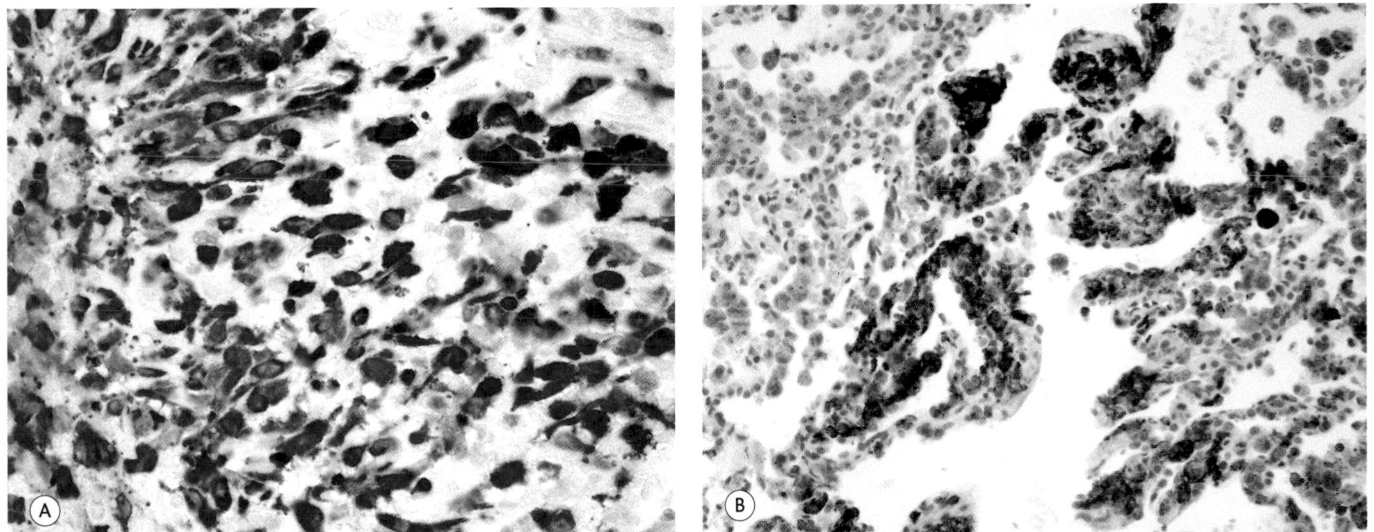

Fig. 7.100 **Pulmonary Langerhans cell histiocytosis (PLCH).** In the cellular lesions of PLCH, (A) immunohistochemical stains for S100 protein and CD1a (B) can be used to highlight the presence of Langerhans cells. In most cases, the morphology of the lesions is sufficiently compelling that a definitive diagnosis can be established without the aid of special stains.

Fibrotic lesions

As the lesions of PLCH "age," Langerhans cells become progressively depleted and overshadowed by fibrosis (Fig. 7.102). The mechanism for this transformation is unknown. In some patients, only residual stellate parenchymal scars are found and pulmonary function may be significantly compromised (analogous to constrictive bronchiolitis). Lung function and radiologic studies may suggest a diffuse lung disease, but the biopsy may have only stellate fibrotic lesions centered on the terminal airways, without an identifiable interstitial inflammatory disease. Another scenario in which such scars can be seen is in portions of lung removed for other reasons (e.g. bronchogenic carcinoma). Presumably these "footprints" of prior PLCH are incidental findings and do not necessarily imply active disease elsewhere in the lung.

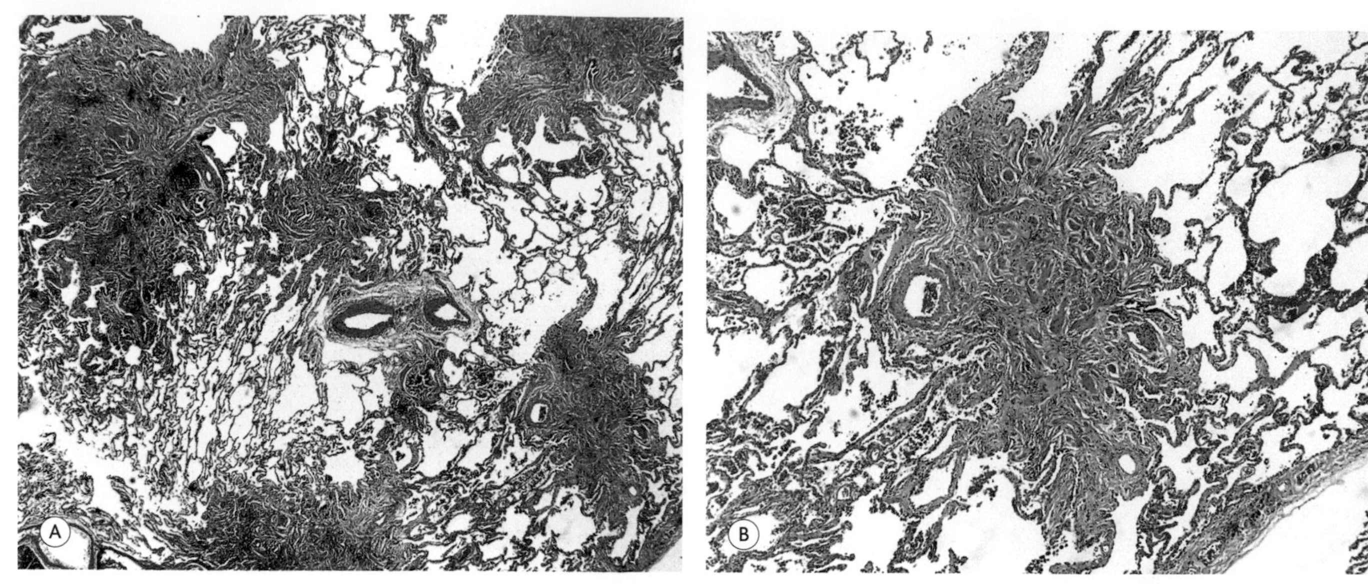

Fig. 7.102 **Pulmonary Langerhans cell histiocytosis (PLCH).** (A) As the lesions of PLCH "age," they become progressively fibrotic, and (B) Langerhans cells become depleted and overshadowed by fibrosis.

Differential diagnosis

Nodular infections and neoplasm are commonly in the differential diagnosis radiologically, the latter especially in the setting of a young woman with known breast carcinoma, being screened for metastatic disease to the lungs. Pathologically, the proliferative lesions may be mistaken for neoplasm as well, but careful attention to the layered or zonal composition of the nodules and the distinctive morphology of the Langerhans cells will typically bring the diagnosis of PLCH to the forefront. When cysts are prominent, lymphangioleiomyomatosis (LAM) enters the differential (see below). In this setting, immunohistochemical stains may be useful in establishing the correct diagnosis (S100 protein immunoreactivity in Langerhans cells, versus HMB45 and actin in LAM cells). Other nodular lung diseases are occasionally confused with PLCH, including Wegener's granulomatosis, Hodgkin's disease, and certain metastatic low-grade sarcomas. When fibrotic lesions are dominant, usual interstitial pneumonia (clinical idiopathic pulmonary fibrosis), and other fibrosing lung disorders may be suggested. The stellate appearance of the PLCH lesion, the tendency for lesions to spare the pleura and immediate subpleural lung, and the association of scars with the airways may be helpful distinguishing features. Rarely, pneumothorax (from any cause) can produce subpleural fibrosis with sheets of tissue eosinophils (so-called reactive eosinophilic pleuritis.)[280,281] Such lesions are not usually confused with PLCH but on occasion may be the only identified pathologic change in a biopsy following pneumothorax (sometimes performed during surgical intervention for the pneumothorax), raising concern of under-sampled or "upstream" PLCH. Radiologic correlation may be very helpful in this setting.

Clinical course

Smoking cessation is the most effective therapy and is the treatment of choice.[270] Immunosuppression with corticosteroids, with or without the addition of a cytotoxic agent, has met with variable success. In larger reviews, the median survival is 12 years[270,282] with 5- and 10-year survival of 70% and 60%, respectively. The most frequent cause of death is related to respiratory complications associated with neoplasms of hematologic, pulmonary, and/or other organs. A worse survival is observed for patients with poor respiratory function at diagnosis.[270]

Erdheim–Chester disease

Erdheim–Chester disease (ECD) is a rare non-familial systemic histiocytosis affecting middle-aged adults without gender predilection.[283–285] The disease is characterized by xanthogranulomatous infiltration of the long tubular bones, resulting in symmetrical osteosclerosis.[283,286–289] Extraskeletal involvement is relatively common, occurring in about half of those affected. Of the

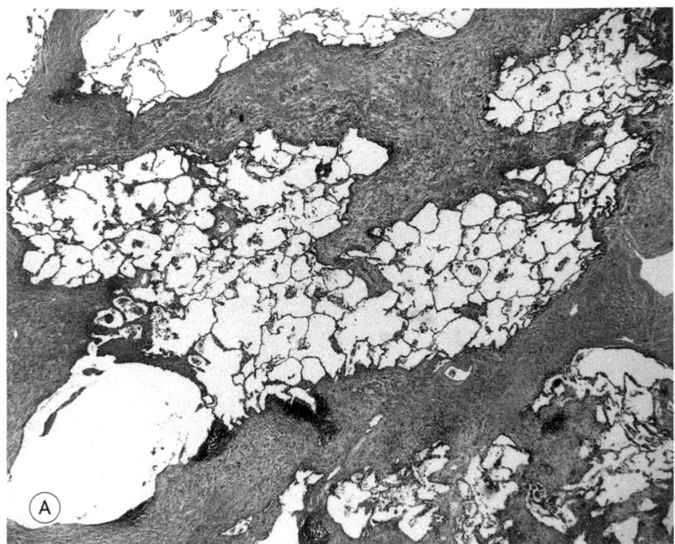

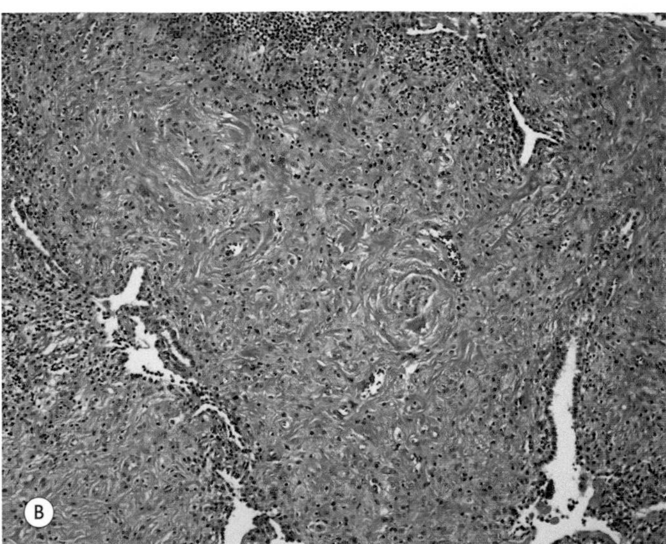

Fig. 7.103 **Erdheim–Chester disease (ECD).** (A) In surgical wedge lung biopsies or resected lung lobes, a distinctive pattern of pleural and septal fibrosis is evident, with a distinctive lymphatic distribution. (B) Admixed lymphoid aggregates are typical. The interface with surrounding lung is generally abrupt.

reported extraskeletal sites involved, the pituitary area, skin, orbit, pericardium, and retroperitoneum are most often involved.

Clinical presentation

Pulmonary involvement occurs in about one-third of patients and is associated with significant morbidity and mortality.[283,290–294] Progressive breathlessness is the typical presentation.

Radiologic findings

Computed tomograms reveal thickening of the visceral pleura, thickened interlobular septa, fine reticular and centrilobular opacities, and ground glass attenuation.[293]

Pathologic findings

In surgical wedge lung biopsies, a distinctive interstitial infiltrate is observed,[292] consisting of xanthomatous histiocytes, lymphocytes, and scattered Touton-type giant cells. Prominent fibrosis is present in a characteristic subpleural and lymphatic distribution (Fig. 7.103). Using immunohistochemistry, the cells of ECD (Fig. 7.104) express histiocytic markers (CD68 and factor XIIIa), but typically lack CD1a immunoreactivity. S100 protein immunoreactivity occurs in a subset of patients.

Differential diagnosis

The differential diagnosis includes advanced lung fibrosis associated with pulmonary Langerhans cell histiocytosis, and the exceedingly rare lung occurrence of Rosai–Dorfman disease (sinus histiocytosis with massive lymphadenopathy). In advanced PLCH, the fibrosis tends to be more confluent, and particularily bronchiolocentric, with blunt stellate-shaped scars. In Rosai–Dorfman disease (discussed further in chapter 18) the histiocytic nature of the process is often overshadowed by the inflammatory component (Fig. 7.105).

Clinical course

Patients with pulmonary involvement by ECD typically follow a progressive downhill course with respiratory compromise and death. The disease is unresponsive to therapy.

Lymphangioleiomyomatosis

Lymphangioleiomyomatosis (LAM) is a rare chronic lung disease characterized by the presence of cysts accompanied by bundles of distinctive smooth muscle cells.[295–301] LAM is a disease of women and has a distinctive relationship to the genetic disorder known as the tuberous sclerosis complex (TSC).[302,303] Recent experimental data have demonstrated loss of heterozygosity of chromosomes 9p and 16p, and mutation in the tuberous sclerosis complex gene (TSC2) in LAM, suggesting that LAM is a neoplastic disease.[304–306] Nevertheless, debate continues as to whether or not LAM is a true neoplasm or a hyperplasia of genetically aberrant cells. LAM was considered to be a disease

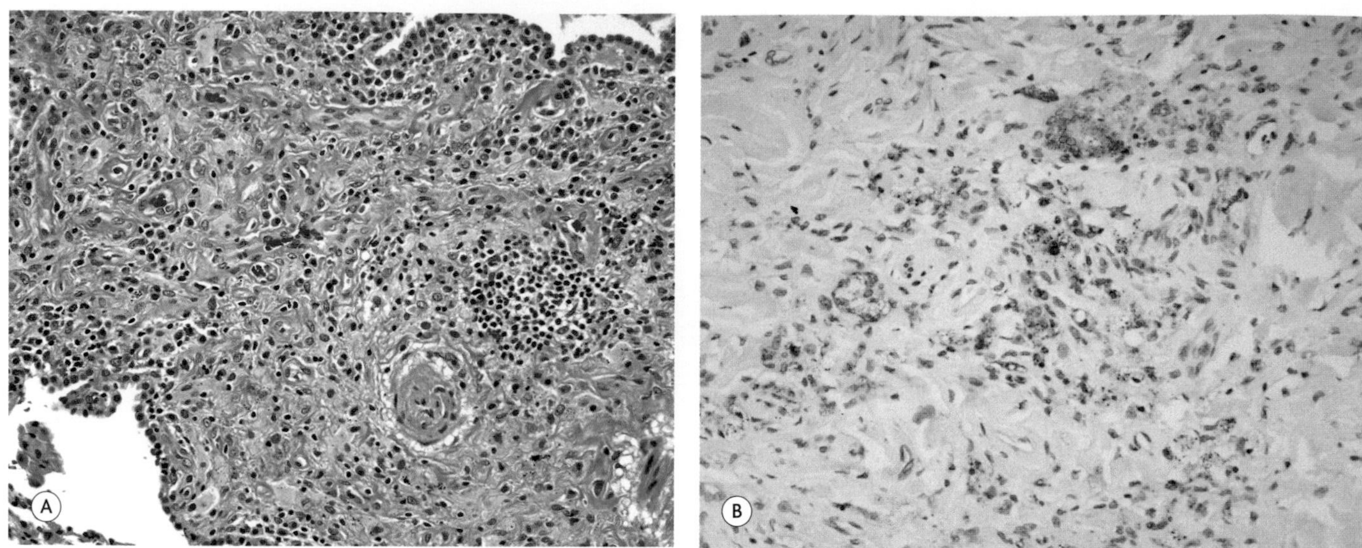

Fig. 7.104 **Erdheim–Chester disease (ECD).** (A) At closer inspection, the fibrosis of ECD contains xanthomatous histiocytes, lymphocytes, and scattered Touton-type giant cells. (B) These latter giant cells, and other histiocytes in the infiltrate, can be highlighted with immunohistochemical stains for CD68 and factor XIIIa.

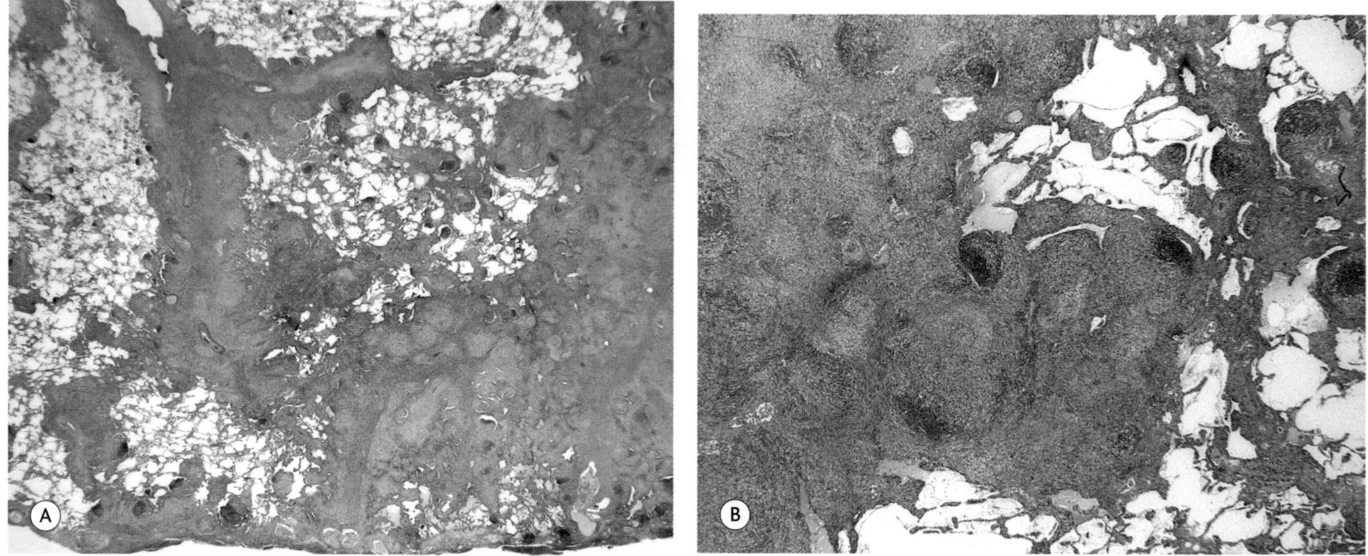

Fig. 7.105 **Rosai–Dorfman disease.** (A) Nodular expansion of interlobular septa, pleura and bronchovascular sheaths is apparent at low magnification. The mixed inflammatory composition of the process becomes more evident at higher magnification.

unique to women, but rare cases of LAM in males have been reported,[307,308] and we have seen an additional case in consultation (unpublished data) in a phenotypic male with TSC. LAM is discussed in this chapter because the disease typically presents as a chronic diffuse lung process clinically and radiologically.

Clinical presentation

LAM occurs most frequently in women of childbearing age, with a peak incidence in the fourth decade of life.[295,299,309] Two forms of the disease occur, one sporadically, and the other in association with the genetic marker for TSC. In both forms of the disease, extrathoracic (especially renal) angiomyolipomas commonly occur.[310–315] Of note, the rare males reported to have LAM also had TSC.[307,308] LAM is often asymptomatic in its early stage and many affected individuals are identified based on chest radiographs performed for other reasons. The most common clinical complaint is shortness of breath.[295,299,300] Pneumothorax occurs and pleurocentesis may reveal a chylous effusion.

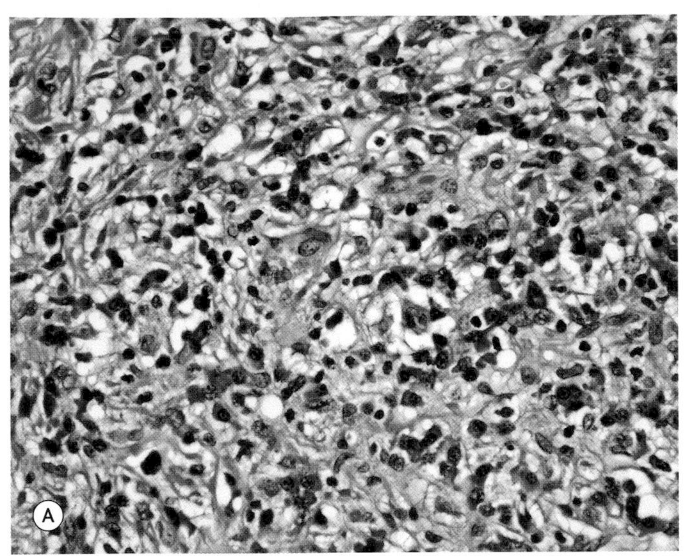

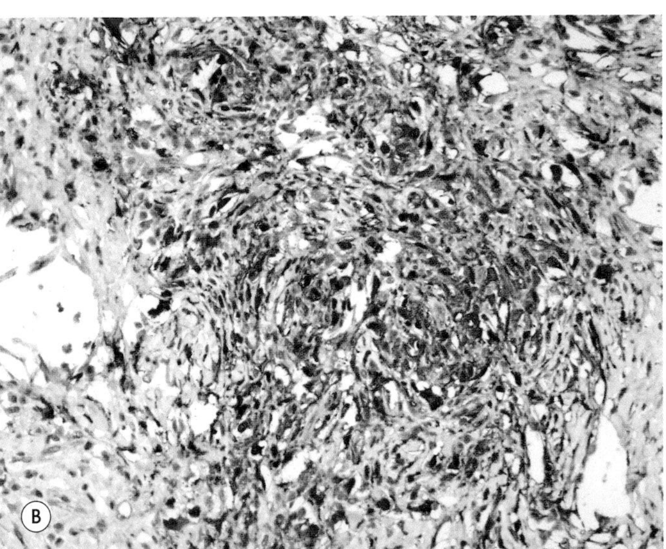

Fig. 7.106 **Rosai–Dorfman disease.** (A) In Rosai–Dorfman disease, the histiocytic nature of the process is often overshadowed by the inflammatory component. (B) An S100 protein stain may be very useful in establishing the diagnosis. Emperipolesis, the typical finding in the more common lymph node manifestation of the disease, may be difficult to appreciate on routine hematoxylin and eosin (H&E) stained sections of lung tissue.

Radiologic features

Plain films of the chest may be interpreted as normal,[316] but in the presence of pneumothorax, air or fluid may be present in the pleural space. Small nodules and cysts may be detected and typically are present diffusely in the lungs, in contrast to the upper lobe distribution of lesions in PLCH. CT scans show diagnostic changes with small nodules and thin-walled cysts throughout both lungs.[316–321]

Pathologic features

LAM lesions may be difficult to appreciate at scanning magnification, particularly in cases where smooth muscle lesions are sparse or of small size (Fig. 7.107). In most cases, thin-walled cysts are easily visible (Fig. 7.108) and useful for searching out diagnostic smooth muscle bundles at higher magnification (Fig. 7.109). The smooth muscle of LAM is distinctive (Fig. 7.110). The LAM cell is fusiform and plump. The nucleus is larger than that of other smooth muscle cells in the lung (Fig. 7.111) and the nuclear/cytoplasmic ratio is typically higher. Smooth muscle bundles may be small or attenuated at the periphery of cysts (Fig. 7.112), or quite cellular and prominent (Fig. 7.113).

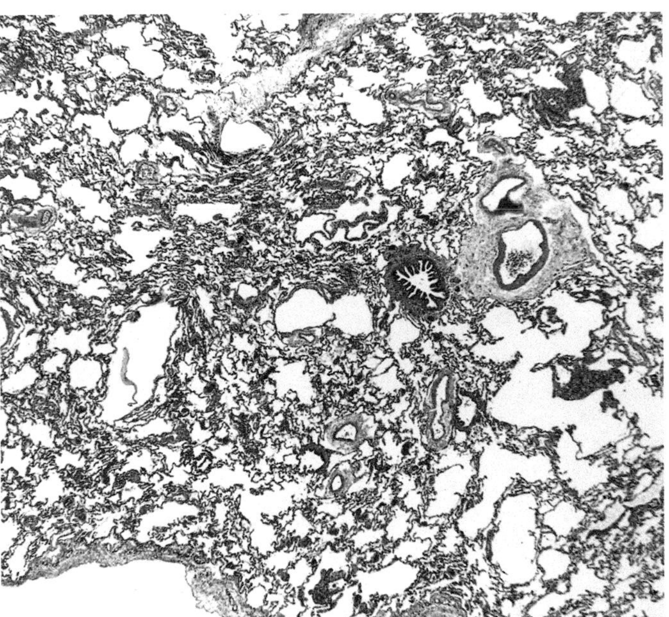

Fig. 7.107 **Lymphangioleiomyomatosis (LAM).** LAM lesions may be difficult to appreciate at scanning magnification, particularly in cases where smooth muscle lesions are sparse or of small size.

Differential diagnosis

The differential diagnosis of LAM includes alveolar duct smooth muscle hyperplasia, pulmonary Langerhans cell histiocytosis, metastatic low-grade sarcomas in the lung, and cystic terminal airways in small airways disease (SAD), especially when these diseases occur in the setting of pneumothorax.

Clinical course

No effective therapy has emerged for LAM. In spite of this, antihormonal therapy[322–325] has been the mainstay of

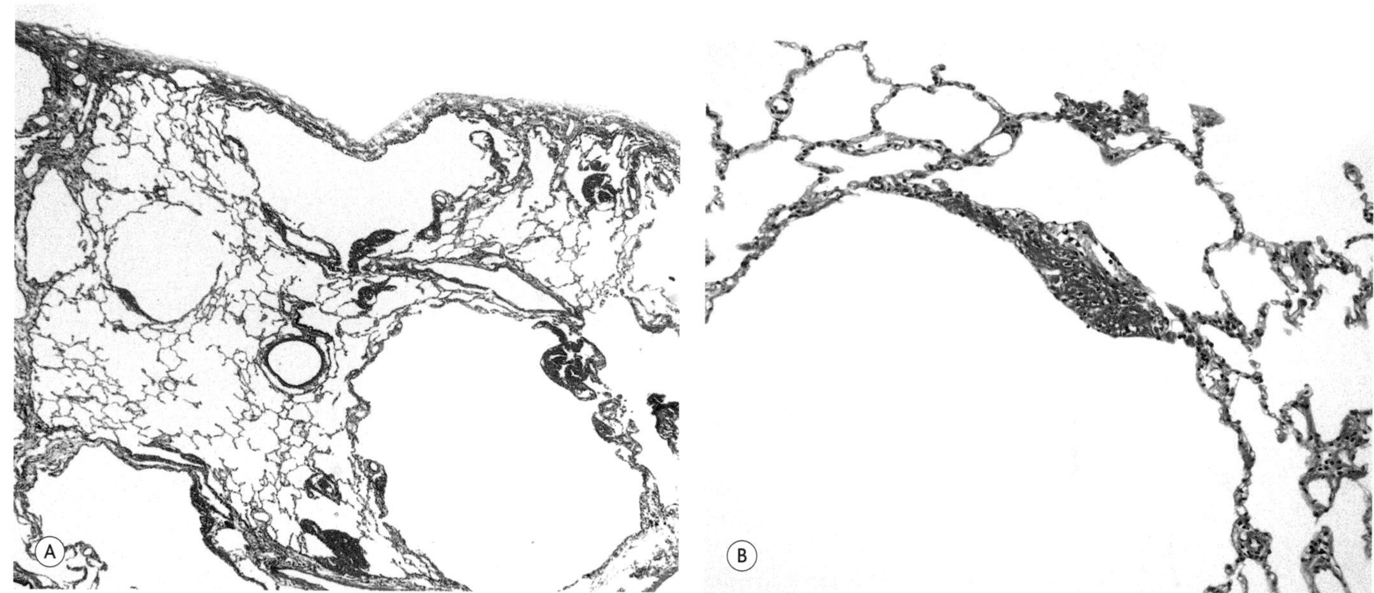

Fig. 7.108 **Lymphangioleiomyomatosis (LAM).** (A) In most cases, thin-walled cysts are easily visible and (B) useful for searching out the characteristic smooth muscle of LAM.

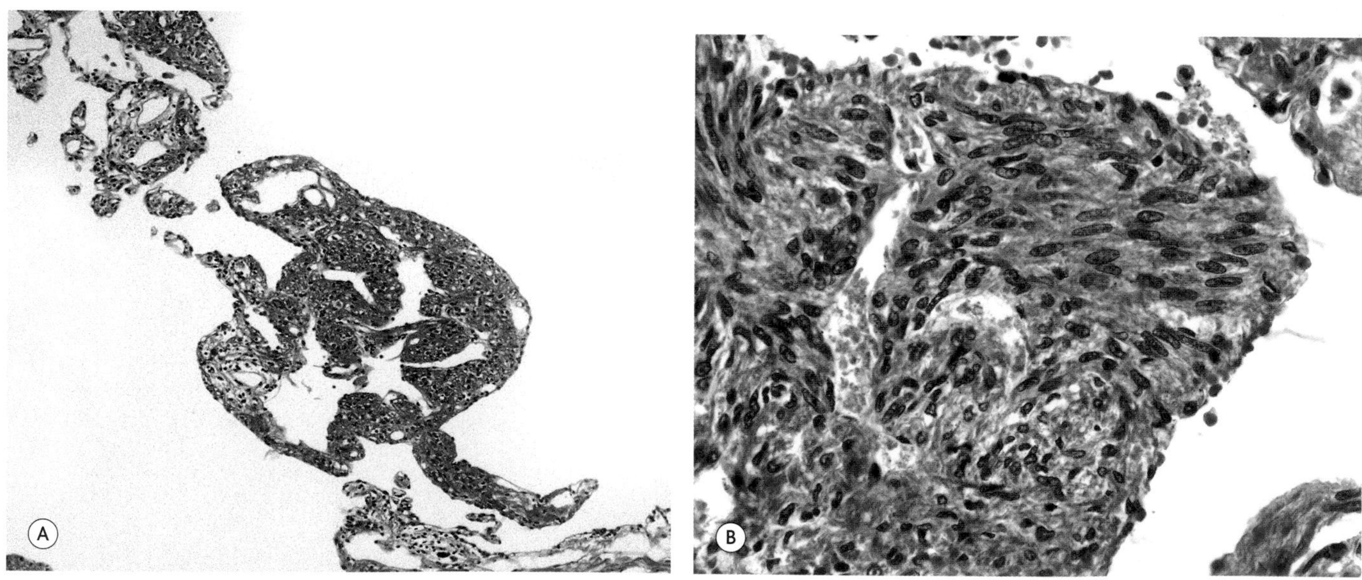

Fig. 7.109 **Lymphangioleiomyomatosis (LAM).** (A,B) The smooth muscle of LAM more resembles a low-grade neoplasm than any normally occurring smooth muscle.

treatment, given the presence of estrogen and progesterone receptors in the abnormal smooth muscle cells in this disease.[300,324,326,327] Lung transplantation may be considered as a last resort.[328] Recurrence of LAM in transplanted lung is reported to occur.[329] The median survival is in the range of 10 years, with an early subset of deaths occurring within the first 5 years of diagnosis.[330,331]

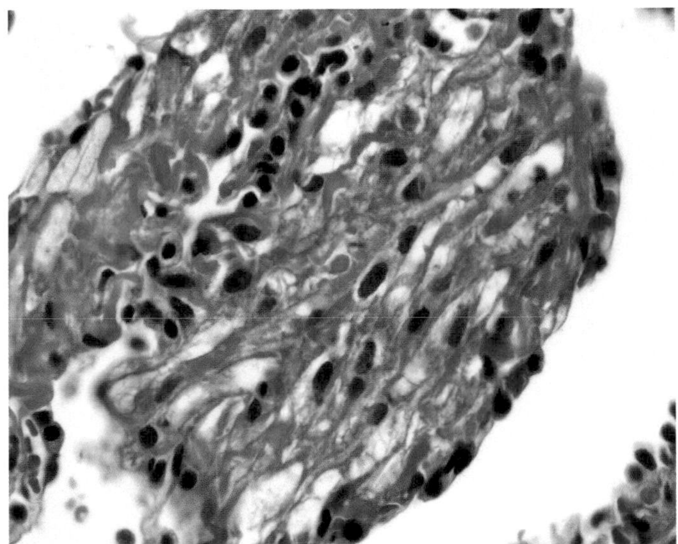

Fig. 7.110 **Lymphangioleiomyomatosis (LAM).** The smooth muscle cells of LAM are distinctive. The LAM cell is fusiform and plump, with irregular pale vacuoles in its cytoplasm.

Hermansky–Pudlak syndrome

The Hermansky–Pudlak syndrome (HPS) encompasses a group of autosomal recessive inherited genetic disorders that share oculocutaneous albinism, platelet storage pool deficiency, and variable tissue lipofuscinosis.[332–334] The most common form of HPS arises from a 16 base pair duplication in the HPS1 gene at exon 15 on the long arm of chromosome 10 (10q23).[335] This form is referred to as HPS1 and is associated with progressive, lethal pulmonary fibrosis. HPS1 affects between 400 and 500 individuals in northwest Puerto Rico.[336,337] Pulmonary fibrosis typically begins in the fourth decade and results in death from respiratory failure within 1–6 years of onset.[338] A granulomatous colitis may also occur in HPS patients.

Radiologic findings

Avila and coworkers[339] reviewed chest radiographs and CT scans from 67 patients with HPS1. CT scans with minimal abnormalities had normal corresponding chest radiographs. When abnormalities were present on radiographs, these consisted of diffuse reticulonodular interstitial infiltrates, perihilar fibrosis, and pleural thickening. HRCT findings included peribronchovascular thickening, ground glass opacification, and septal thickening. Increasing severity of these changes, as assessed using a fibrosis scoring system, were inversely correlated with forced vital capacity (FVC).

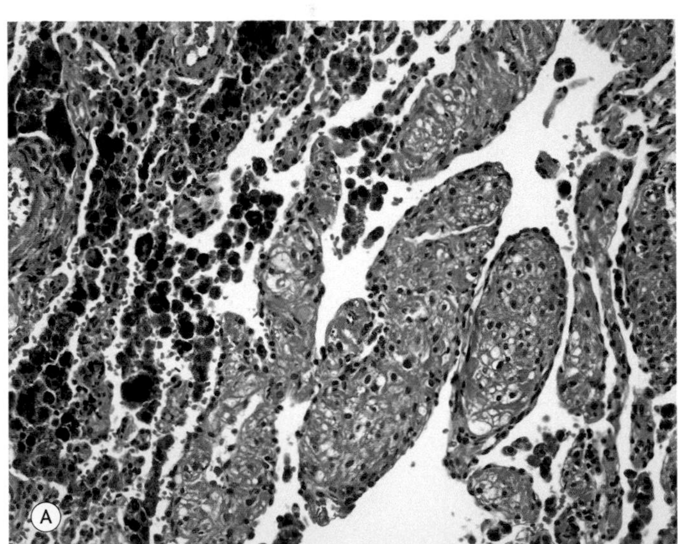

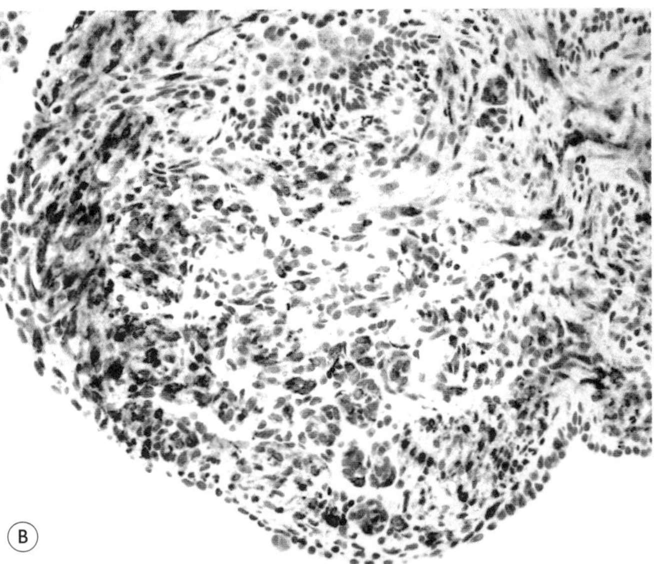

Fig. 7.111 **Lymphangioleiomyomatosis (LAM).** (A) The nucleus of the LAM smooth muscle cell is larger than that of other smooth muscle cells in the lung, and the nuclear/cytoplasmic ratio is typically higher. (B) In this example, hemosiderosis is present in adjacent alveolar spaces. Immunohistochemical stains for HMB45 are very helpful in establishing the correct diagnosis.

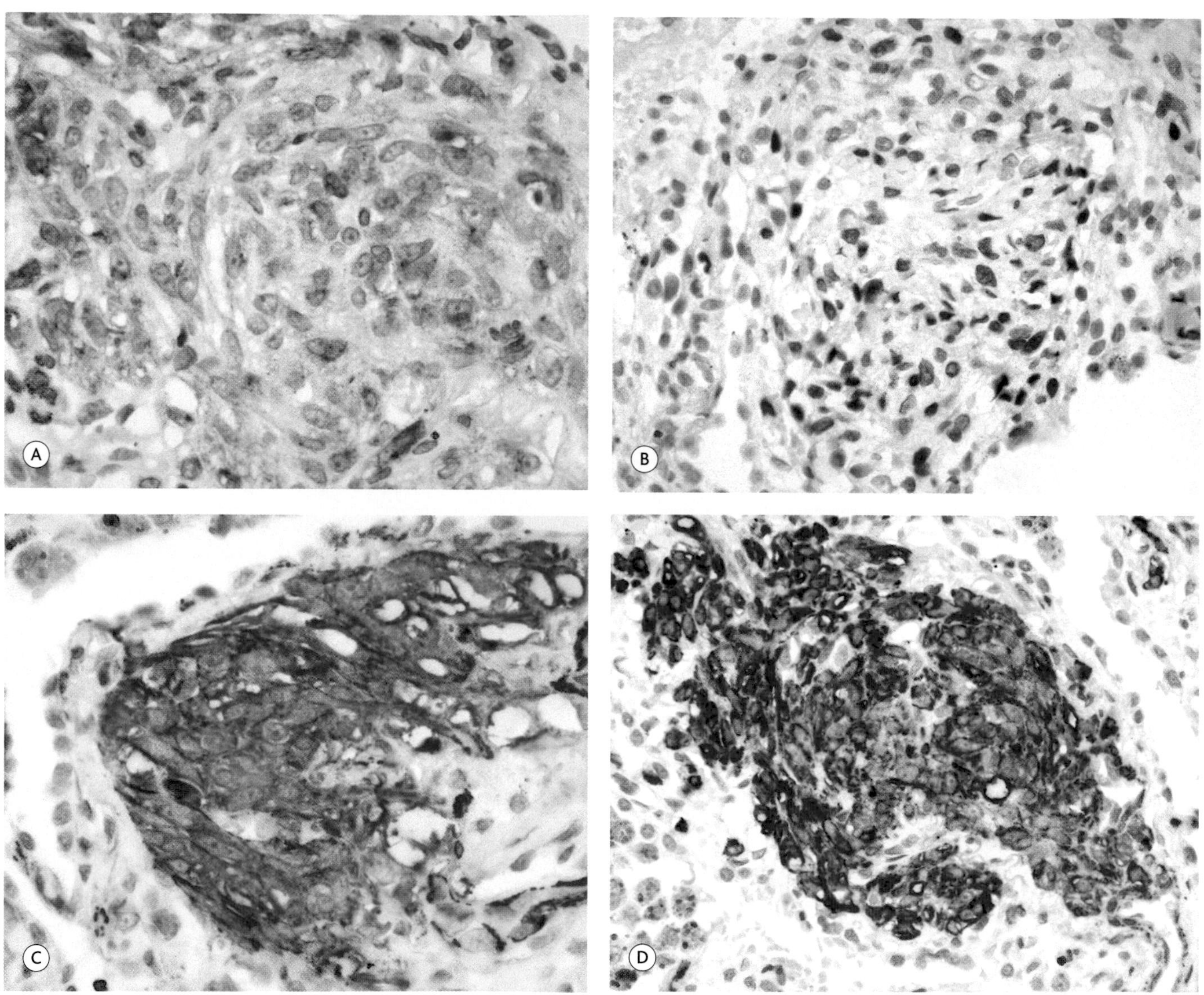

Fig. 7.112 **Lymphangioleiomyomatosis (LAM).** (A) Other positive stains in LAM smooth muscle include MelanA/MART-1, (B) estrogen receptor, (C) smooth muscle actin, and (D) desmin.

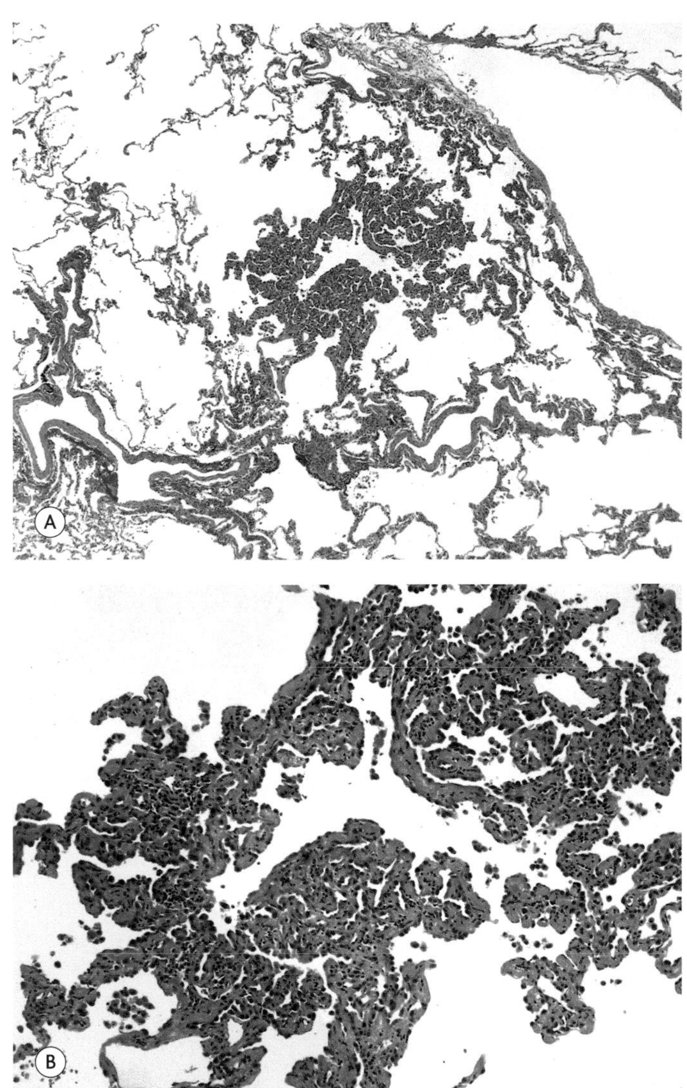

Fig. 7.113 **Lymphangioleiomyomatosis (LAM).** (A) Another distinctive lesion that may be seen in association with LAM, especially in those patients who also have tuberous sclerosis complex (TSC), is micronodular pneumocyte hyperplasia (MNPH). (B) MNPH lesions are epithelial and probably represent a hamartomatous proliferation. The cells of MNPH do not stain with antibodies directed against HMB45 or MelanA/MART-1 but, rather, stain with cytokeratin and surfactant apoprotein antibodies.

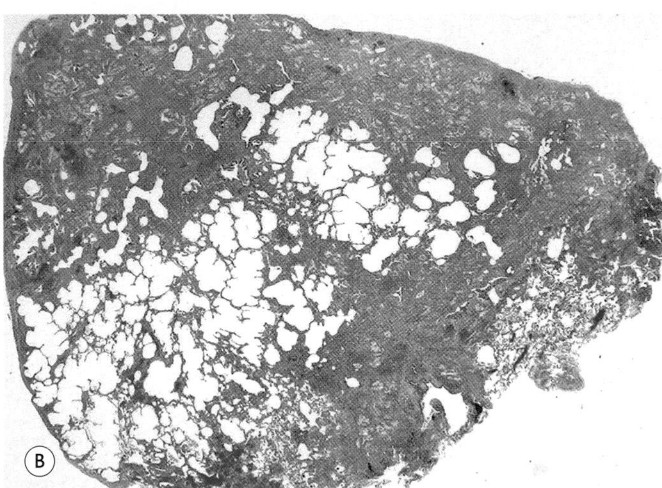

Fig. 7.114 **Hermansky–Pudlak syndrome.** (A) This genetic disease produces lethal lung fibrosis in affected individuals. The CT scan findings are dramatic and characterized by diffuse reticular opacities. (B) Tissue sections show advanced lung remodeling with fibrosis, typically without an easily characterized distribution.

Pathologic findings

Surgical biopsies and autopsy lungs from five patients with HPS were studied by Nakatani et al.[340] They described alveolar septal thickening (Fig. 7.114) associated with prominent clear vacuolated type II pneumocytes (Fig. 7.115), patchy zones of fibrosis with an apparent bronchiolocentric distribution, some evidence of constrictive bronchiolitis, and haphazard microscopic honeycombing without a consistent peripheral lobular or subpleural distribution. Numerous giant lamellar bodies were present in the macrophages and type II cells on ultrastructural examination, and the phospholipid material in the vacuoles was weakly positive with antibodies directed against surfactant apoprotein by immunohistochemistry.

Clinical course

No effective therapy has been identified for HPS patients with lung fibrosis, but newer antifibrotic therapies are being explored.[341]

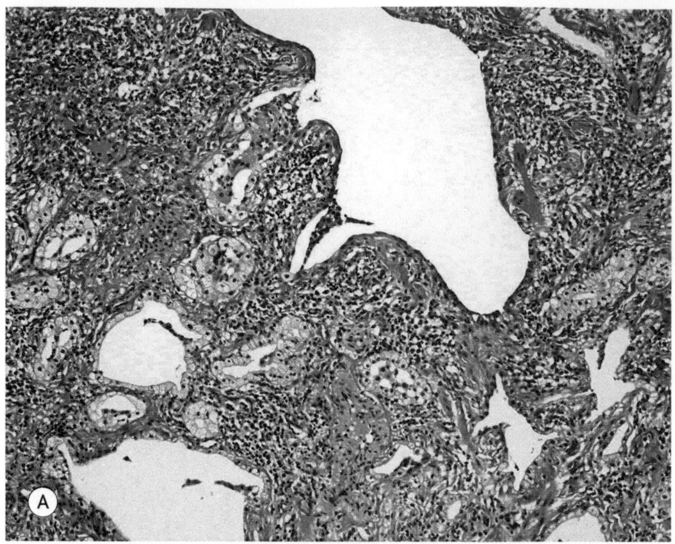

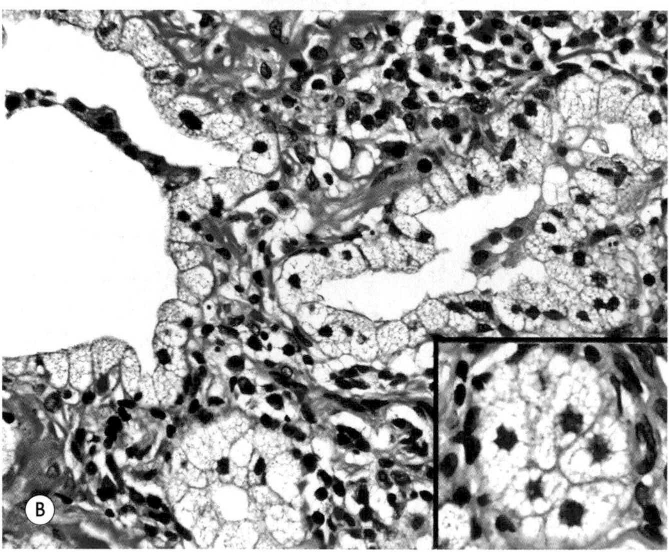

Fig. 7.115 **Hermansky–Pudlak syndrome.** (A,B) At higher magnification, prominent clear vacuolated type II pneumocytes, patchy zones of fibrosis with an apparent bronchiolocentric distribution, and some evidence of constrictive bronchiolitis are seen.

Pulmonary alveolar microlithiasis

Pulmonary alveolar microlithiasis (PAM) is a rare but distinctive autosomal recessive heritable lung disease with approximately 300 cases reported in the literature.[342–346] A significant number of cases identified are familial (siblings); however, PAM occurring in both a parent and a child is uncommon. The exact incidence of the disease is unknown, but in a 46-year period, the Mayo Clinic identified only eight cases.[344] Patients are typically diagnosed in the fourth decade of life, but the disease has an age range from childhood to 80.[344] There appears to be an increased incidence in individuals of Turkish descent and a recent report described a Turkish family with six affected members.[347]

Clinical presentation

Most cases are diagnosed in adult life, but the disease can manifest at any age.[343–345] It is hypothesized that the condition results from a congenital metabolic disorder, resulting in slow progressive disease during life. The most common presentation is that of an asymptomatic patient. Some patients may experience varying degrees of dyspnea, and death has been reported to occur following accelerated respiratory failure. Affected patients typically exhibit a restrictive pulmonary function defect,[343] but this is generally mild when compared with the dramatic appearance of the chest radiograph, especially in young patients. Associated nephrolithiasis and pleural calcification have been reported.[348]

Radiologic findings

The chest radiograph is almost immediately diagnostic, with sand-like micronodular opacities present throughout both lungs diffusely. The lower lung zones tend to be more opacified than the upper lobes. The chest radiograph may remain static for many years.[343–345] HRCT scans reveal intra-alveolar microcalcifications bilaterally, with increased concentration of microliths along bronchovascular bundles, interlobular fissures, and in the subpleural lung parenchyma.[349,350]

Pathologic findings

Grossly, the lungs are firm, gritty, and rigidly maintain their shape before fixation. On microscopic examination, the airspaces contain innumerable tiny calcified bodies that are concentrically laminated and have radial striations (Fig. 7.116) These microliths are composed of calcium and phosphorus, in concentrations similar to bone.[345] Magnesium and iron are typically present in small amounts. Microliths may be as large as 1 mm or more, but most often they are uniform and in the range of 250 µm in diameter. Rarely, they may be present within the alveolar walls, often accompanied by some degree of interstitial thickening and chronic inflammation (Fig. 7.117).

Differential diagnosis

The differential diagnosis includes corpora amylacea, and alveolar calcification from any cause. The microliths of PAM can be distinguished from incidental corpora amylacea by the larger size of the former and the lack of calcification in the latter. Also, corpora amylacea typically

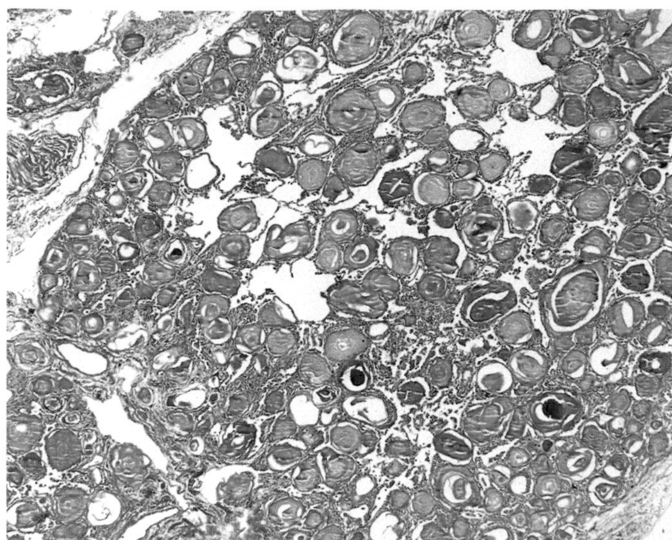

Fig. 7.116 **Pulmonary alveolar microlithiasis.** The airspaces contain innumerable tiny calcified bodies that are concentrically laminated and have radial striations.

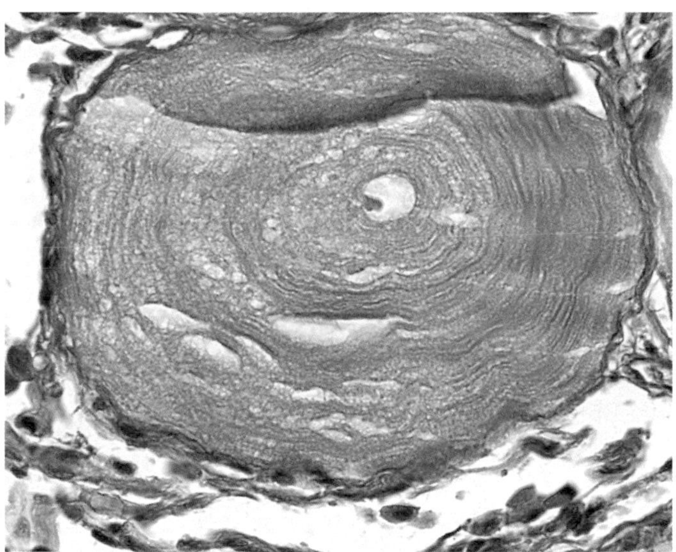

Fig. 7.117 **Pulmonary alveolar microlithiasis.** Rarely, they may be present within the alveolar walls, often accompanied by some degree of interstitial thickening and chronic inflammation.

have a small black pigment core, while the microliths of PAM lack this feature. The sheer number of alveolar microliths in PAM distinguish this condition from other forms of lung calcification.

Clinical course

The majority of patients with PAM survive many years with little disease progression. There is no current therapy for the symptomatic patient.

Pulmonary alveolar proteinosis

Pulmonary alveolar proteinosis (PAP) is a diffuse lung process of unknown etiology characterized by the presence of alveolar spaces filled with amorphous eosinophilic material. PAP is often multilobar, bilateral, and of subacute or chronic onset. Other subacute or chronic DLDs that have an alveolar component are in the differential diagnosis of PAP (e.g. cryptogenic organizing pneumonia, RBILD/DIP, LIP, and NSIP).

Clinical presentation

The disease occurs commonly as a primary idiopathic form, but may also be seen as a secondary phenomenon in the settings of occupational disease (especially dust-related), drug-induced injury, hematologic diseases, and in many settings of immunodeficiency.[351–355] The disease is commonly associated with exposure to crystalline material and silica, although other substances have also been implicated.[352,356] The idiopathic form is the most common presentation, where there is a male predominance and an age range of 30–50 years. The usual presenting symptom is insidious dyspnea, sometimes with cough.[355–357] Experimental data from knock-out mice used in the study of granulocyte-monocyte colony-stimulating factor (GM-CSF) have implicated deficiency of this cytokine as one potential etiology for the disease.[355,358]

Radiologic findings

Chest radiographs show extensive bilateral airspace consolidation, involving mainly the perihilar regions, and often the symptoms belie the severe radiographic abnormalities. CT demonstrates what appears to be smooth thickening of lobular septa that is not seen on the chest radiograph. The thickening of lobular septa within areas of ground glass attenuation is characteristic of alveolar proteinosis on CT and is referred to as the "crazy paving pattern."[359] The areas of ground glass attenuation and consolidation are often sharply demarcated from the surrounding normal lung without an apparent anatomic reason.

Pathologic findings

Pulmonary alveolar proteinosis (alveolar lipoproteinosis) is characterized by an intra-alveolar accumulation of lipid-rich eosinophilic material.[351] PAP presumably occurs as a result of overproduction of surfactant by type II cells, impaired clearance of surfactant by alveolar macrophages, or a combination of these mechanisms. The gross lung shows firm yellow-white nodules, some as large as 2 cm in diameter. Microscopically, the scanning magnification appearance is distinctive, if not diagnostic. Pink granular material fills the airspaces, sometimes with a rim of retraction that separates the alveolar wall slightly from the exudate (Fig. 7.118). Closer inspection of this material shows embedded clumps of dense globular material and cholesterol clefts (Fig. 7.119). The periodic acid–Schiff (PAS) stain may be useful in demonstrating a diastase-resistant, positive reaction in the proteinaceous material of PAP. By immunohistochemistry this material is immunoreactive, with antibodies directed against surfactant. There may be few other associated changes in the lung biopsy, although patients with long-standing disease may develop some interstitial fibrosis and chronic inflammation. More dramatic inflammatory changes should suggest comorbid disease, such as infection. For example, *Nocardia* infection is known to be associated with PAP. PAP can be patchy in the lungs and even in biopsy specimens, so a high index of suspicion is required, coupled with good clinical and radiologic data.

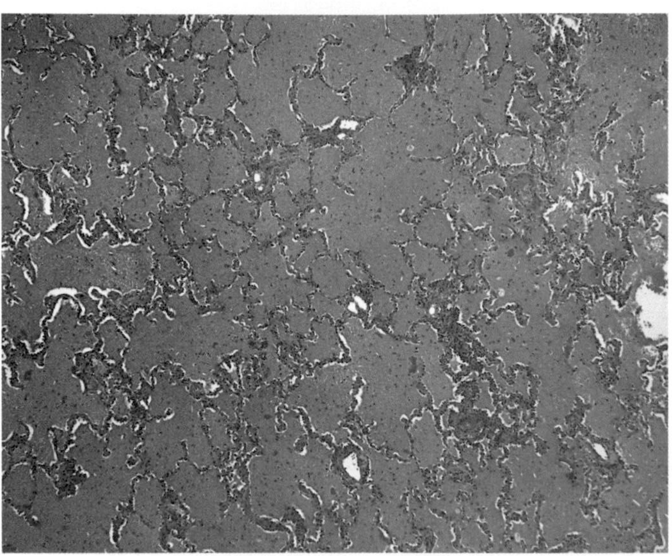

Fig. 7.118 **Pulmonary alveolar proteinosis (PAP).** The nearly diagnostic appearance of PAP at scanning magnification demonstrates pink granular material filling the airspaces, sometimes with a rim of retraction that separates the alveolar wall slightly from the exudate.

Differential diagnosis

The differential diagnosis includes pulmonary edema and pneumocystis pneumonia. Pulmonary edema lacks the globular material and cellular debris seen in PAP. Pneumocystis pneumonia can be distinguished from PAP by a more dramatic clinical presentation, exudates that appear finely vacuolated or foamy, and background lung with significantly more inflammatory changes.

Clinical course

Despite significant radiologic abnormalities, the disease may be unusually silent, producing little if any clinical manifestations in the absence of superimposed infection. When patients have severe dyspnea and hypoxemia, treatment can be accomplished using one or more sessions of whole lung lavage, which usually induces remission and excellent long-term survival.[360]

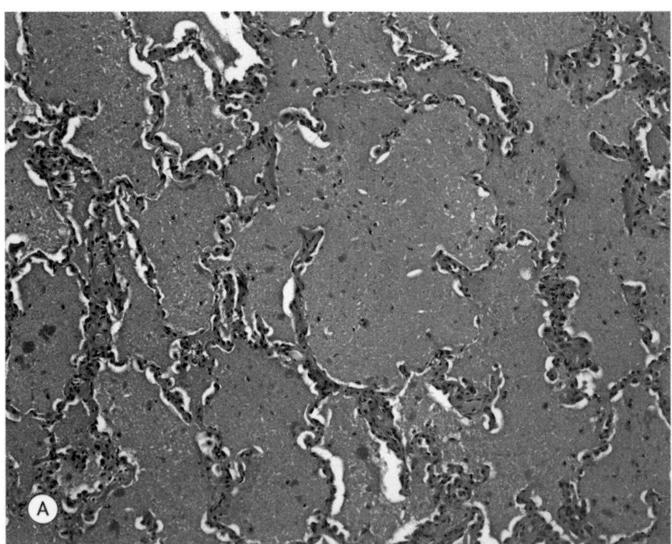

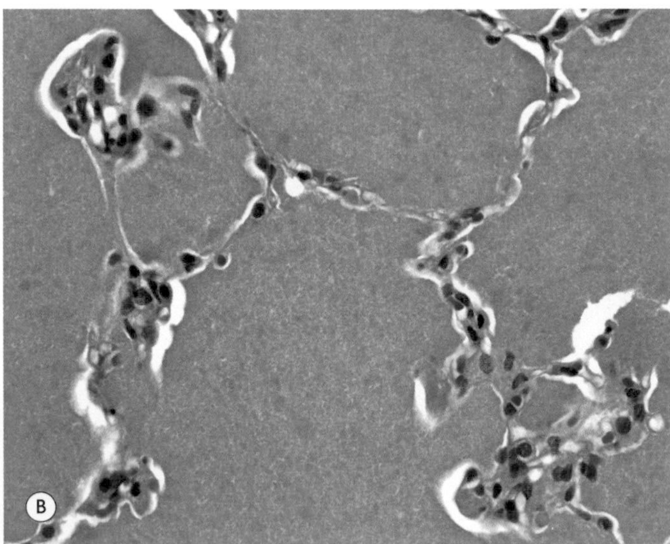

Fig. 7.119 **Pulmonary alveolar proteinosis (PAP).** (A) Closer inspection of this material shows embedded clumps of dense globular material and cholesterol clefts. (B) The clumps may be variably prominent: in this example they are less distinct.

Lymphangitic carcinomatosis

Metastatic carcinoma involving the lung primarily within lymphatics is known as pulmonary lymphangitic carcinomatosis (lymphangitis carcinomatosa). The tumor type is most often adenocarcinoma and the phenomenon accounts for as much as 8% of all metastases to the lung. The most common sites of origin are breast, lung, and stomach, although primary disease in pancreas, ovary, kidney, and uterine cervix can also spread to the lungs in this manner.[361,362] The published reports on the subject are found predominately in the radiology literature.[361–364]

Clinical presentation

Patients often present with insidious onset of dyspnea, frequently accompanied by an irritating non-productive cough.

Radiologic findings

On plain chest films, the changes are often subtle and nonspecific. In one study, the correct diagnosis was only made in 20 of 87 of cases (23%) and 50% of films were interpreted as normal.[365] Abnormalities include linear opacities, horizontal linear lines abutting the pleura, mostly in the lower lobes (Kerley B lines), subpleural edema, and, commonly, hilar and mediastinal lymph node enlargement.[363] By contrast, the HRCT findings are highly characteristic and accurately reflect the macroscopic abnormalities in this disease. Because the major lymphatic vessels in the lung are located in the pleura, interlobular septa, and bronchovascular bundles, the abnormalities are found primarily in this distribution, thickening and accentuating these structures. HRCT scanning shows irregular thickening of the bronchovascular bundles and lobular septa, giving them a beaded appearance.[362,364]

Pathologic findings

Small aggregates of tumor cells are present within lymphatic channels of the bronchovascular sheath and pleura (Fig. 7.120). Because the lymphatics of the bronchi are involved in this process, lymphangitic carcinoma is one of the few diffuse lung diseases that can be diagnosed definitively by bronchial or transbronchial biopsy (Fig. 7.121).[366] Variable amounts of tumor may be present throughout the lung, involving the interstitium of the alveolar walls, the airspaces themselves, and the lumens of small muscular pulmonary arteries. This latter finding (microangiopathic obliterative endarteritis) may be the origin of the edema, inflammation, and interstitial fibrosis that frequently accompanies the disease, and probably accounts for the clinical and radiologic impression of non-neoplastic diffuse lung disease.[361,363]

The pathogenesis of lymphangitic carcinoma is unknown. Seeding of the lung lymphatics from retrograde spread of microvascular tumor emboli has been postulated and supported by observations of intravascular tumor present in other organs at autopsy from patients so affected.[361,363]

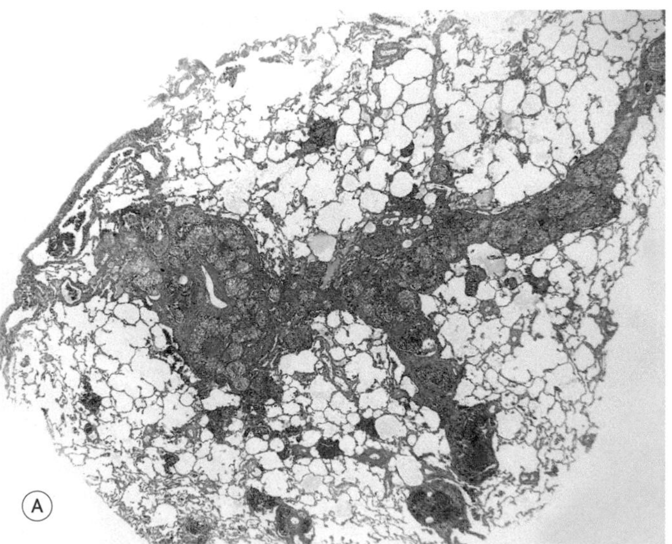

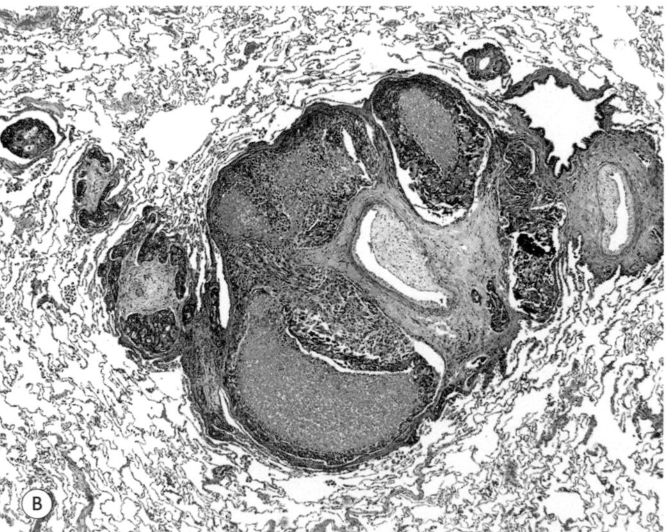

Fig. 7.120 **Lymphangitic carcinomatosis.** Few lung disease are as dramatic (or as devastating to those affected) than lymphangitic carcinomatosis. The characteristic distribution of the disease is demonstrated in (A) where the peribronchial and septal lymphatics are filled by metastatic tumor. Bronchovascular sheath lymphatics are overwhelmed by tumor in (B).

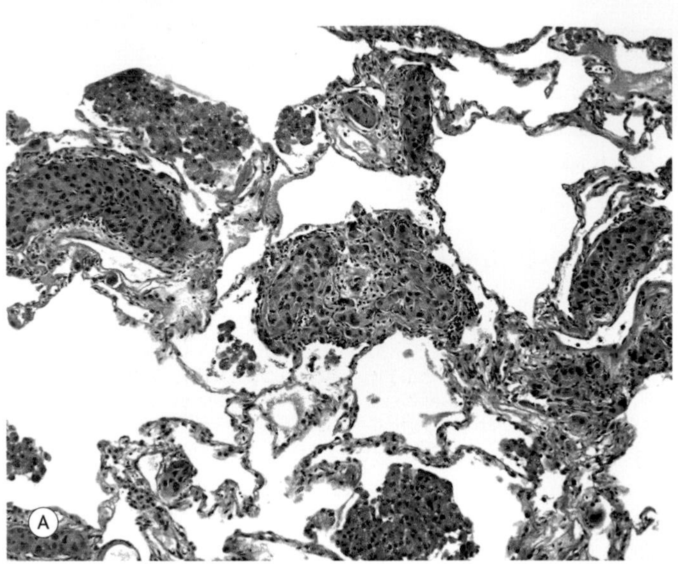

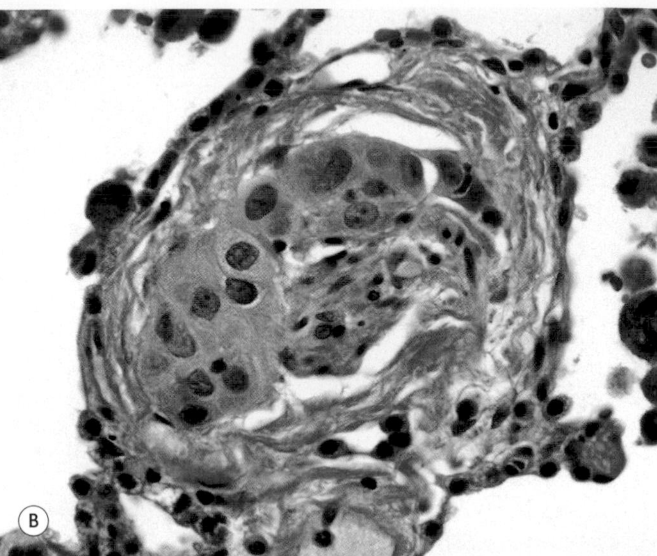

Fig. 7.121 **Lymphangitic carcinomatosis.** (A) At times the disease may be more subtle and present as an interstitial infiltrate in lung biopsies. (B) Lymphangitic carcinoma is one of the few diffuse lung diseases that can be diagnosed definitively by bronchial or transbronchial biopsy.

Differential diagnosis

Lesions that may mimic lymphangitic carcinoma include intravascular lymphoma, thromboembolic disease, and foreign material from intravenous injection.

Clinical course

The prognosis is grim, with most patients dying before 6 months. Rarely, long-term survivors are reported.[361]

REFERENCES

1. Katzenstein A-L, Askin F: Surgical pathology of non-neoplastic lung disease, 3rd edn. 1997, WB Saunders, Philadelphia.
2. Liebow A, Carrington C: The interstitial pneumonias. In: Frontiers of pulmonary radiology pathophysiologic, roentgenographic and radioisotopic considerations, Simon M, Potchen E, LeMay M, Eds. 1969, Grune & Stratton, Orlando, Florida, pp 109–141.
3. Leslie K, Colby T, Swenson S: Anatomic distribution and histopathologic patterns of interstitial lung disease. In: Interstitial lung disease, Schwarz MI, King TE, Eds. 2003, BC Decker, Hamilton, pp 31–53.
4. Travis W, King TJ, Bateman E, et al.: American Thoracic Society/European Respiratory Society international multidisciplinary consensus classification of the idiopathic interstitial pneumonias. Am Rev Respir Crit Care Med 2002; 165: 227–304.
5. Panos RJ, Mortenson RL, Niccoli SA, et al.: Clinical deterioration in patients with idiopathic pulmonary fibrosis: causes and assessment. Am J Med 1990; 88(4): 396–404.
6. Travis W, Colby T, Koss M, et al.: Non-neoplastic disorders of the lower respiratory tract. In: Atlas of nontumor pathology, Vol. 2, King D, Ed. American Registry of Pathology, Armed Forces Institute of Pathology, Washington, DC, 2002, p 939.
7. Cheung O, Muhm J, Helmers R, et al.: Surgical pathology of granulomatous interstitial pneumonia. Ann Diagn Pathol 2003; 7: 127–138.
8. Colby T, Carrington C: Interstitial lung disease. In: Pathology of the lung, 2nd edn, Thurlbeck W, Churg A, Eds. 1995, Thieme Medical Publishers, New York, pp 589–737.
9. Colby TV: Surgical pathology of non-neoplastic lung disease. Mod Pathol 2000; 13(3): 343–358.
10. Leslie KO, Mitchell J, Low R: Lung myofibroblasts. Cell Motil Cytoskeleton 1992; 22(2): 92–98.
11. Katzenstein AL: Idiopathic interstitial pneumonia: classification and diagnosis. Monogr Pathol 1993; 36: 1–31.
12. Katzenstein AL, Myers JL: Nonspecific interstitial pneumonia and the other idiopathic interstitial pneumonias: classification and diagnostic criteria. Am J Surg Pathol 2000; 24(1): 1–3.
13. Crystal R, Fulmer J, Roberts W, et al.: Idiopathic pulmonary fibrosis. Clinical histologic, radiographic, physiologic, scintigraphic, cytologic and biochemical aspects. Ann Intern Med 1976; 85: 769–788.
14. Carrington CB, Gaensler EA, Coutu RE, et al.: Usual and desquamative interstitial pneumonia. Chest 1976; 69(Suppl 2): 261–263.
15. Aubry MC, Wright JL, Myers JL: The pathology of smoking-related lung diseases. Clin Chest Med 2000; 21(1): 11–35, vii.
16. Ohori NP, Sciurba FC, Owens GR, et al.: Giant-cell interstitial pneumonia and hard-metal pneumoconiosis. A clinicopathologic study of four cases and review of the literature. Am J Surg Pathol 1989; 13(7): 581–587.
17. Banerjee D, Ahmad D: Malignant lymphoma complicating lymphocytic interstitial pneumonia: a monoclonal B-cell neoplasm arising in a polyclonal lymphoproliferative disorder. Hum Pathol 1982; 13(8): 780–782.
18. Herbert A, Walters MT, Cawley MI, et al.: Lymphocytic interstitial pneumonia identified as lymphoma of mucosa associated lymphoid tissue. J Pathol 1985; 146(2): 129–138.
19. Schuurman HJ, Gooszen HC, Tan IW, et al.: Low-grade lymphoma of immature T-cell phenotype in a case of lymphocytic interstitial pneumonia and Sjögren's syndrome. Histopathology 1987; 11(11): 1193–1204.
20. Katzenstein A, Myers J, Mazur M: Acute interstitial pneumonia: a clinicopathologic, ultrastructural, and cell kinetic study. Am J Surg Pathol 1986; 10: 256–267.
21. Katzenstein AL, Fiorelli RF: Nonspecific interstitial pneumonia/fibrosis. Histologic features and clinical significance. Am J Surg Pathol 1994; 18(2): 136–147.
22. Gough J: Differential diagnosis in the pathology of asbestosis. Ann NY Acad Sci 1965; 132: 368–372.
23. Gadek J, Hunninghake G, Schoenberger C, et al.: Pulmonary asbestosis and idiopathic pulmonary fibrosis: pathogenetic parallels. Chest 1981; 80(Suppl 1): 63–64.
24. Yamamoto S: Histopathological features of pulmonary asbestosis with particular emphasis on the comparison with those of usual interstitial pneumonia. Osaka City Med J 1997; 43(2): 225–242.

25. Leslie K, King TE Jr, Low R: Smooth muscle actin is expressed by air space fibroblast-like cells in idiopathic pulmonary fibrosis and hypersensitivity pneumonitis. Chest 1991; 99(Suppl 3): 47S–48S.
26. Adler B, Padley S, Müller N, et al.: Chronic hypersensitivity pneumonitis: high resolution CT and radiographic features in 16 patients. Radiology 1992; 185: 91–95.
27. Lynch DA, Newell JD, Logan PM, et al.: Can CT distinguish hypersensitivity pneumonitis from idiopathic pulmonary fibrosis? AJR Am J Roentgenol 1995; 165(4): 807–811.
28. Hunninghake G, Fauci A: Pulmonary involvement in the collagen vascular diseases. Am Rev Respir Dis 1979; 119: 471–503.
29. Colby T: Pathology of the lung in collagen vascular diseases. In: The lung in rheumatic diseases, Lenfant C, Ed. 1990, Marcel Dekker, New York, pp 145–178.
30. DeSpain JD, Swinfard RW: Collagen vascular disease. Dermatol Clin 1992; 10(1): 1–18.
31. Lamblin C, Bergoin C, Saelens T, et al.: Interstitial lung diseases in collagen vascular diseases. Eur Respir J Suppl 2001; 32: 69s–80s.
32. Rossi SE, Erasmus JJ, McAdams HP, et al.: Pulmonary drug toxicity: radiologic and pathologic manifestations. Radiographics 2000; 20(5): 1245–1259.
33. Weycker D, Oster G, Edelsberg J, et al.: Economic costs of idiopathic pulmonary fibrosis. Chest 2002; 122(Suppl 4): 150.
34. Coultas DB: Epidemiology of idiopathic pulmonary fibrosis. Semin Respir Med 1993; 14: 181–196.
35. American Thoracic Society/European Respiratory Society International Multidisciplinary Consensus Classification of the Idiopathic Interstitial Pneumonias: This joint statement of the American Thoracic Society (ATS), and the European Respiratory Society (ERS) was adopted by the ATS board of directors, June 2001 and by the ERS Executive Committee, June 2001. Am J Respir Crit Care Med 2002; 165(2): 277–304.
36. Guerry-Force M, Müller N, Wright J, et al.: A comparison of bronchiolitis obliterans with organizing pneumonia, usual interstitial pneumonia and small airways disease. Am Rev Respir Dis 1987; 135(3): 705–712.
37. Staples C, Müller N, Vedal S, et al.: Usual interstitial pneumonia: correlations of CT with clinical, functional and radiologic findings. Radiology 1987; 162: 377–381.
38. Epler G, McLoud T, Gaensler E, et al.: Normal chest roentgenograms in chronic diffuse inflitrative lung disease. N Engl J Med 1978; 298: 934–939.
39. Akira M, Sakatani M, Ueda E: Idiopathic pulmonary fibrosis: progression of honeycombing at thin-section CT. Radiology 1993; 189(3): 687–691.
40. Nishimura K, Itoh H: High-resolution computed tomographic features of bronchiolitis obliterans organizing pneumonia. Chest 1992; 102: 26S–31S.
41. Lynch DA: Ground glass attenuation on CT in patients with idiopathic pulmonary fibrosis. Chest 1996; 110(2): 312–313.
42. Kazerooni EA, Martinez FJ, Flint A, et al.: Thin-section CT obtained at 10-mm increments versus limited three-level thin-section CT for idiopathic pulmonary fibrosis: correlation with pathologic scoring. AJR Am J Roentgenol 1997; 169(4): 977–983.
43. Hunninghake GW, Zimmerman MB, Schwartz DA, et al.: Utility of a lung biopsy for the diagnosis of idiopathic pulmonary fibrosis. Am J Respir Crit Care Med 2001; 164(2): 193–196.
44. Katzenstein A, Myers J, Prophet W, et al.: Bronchiolitis obliterans and usual interstitial pneumonia. A comparative clinicopathologic study. Am J Surg Pathol 1986; 10: 373–376.
45. Lee JS, Gong G, Song KS, et al.: Usual interstitial pneumonia: relationship between disease activity and the progression of honeycombing at thin-section computed tomography. J Thorac Imaging 1998; 13(3): 199–203.
46. Myers JL: NSIP, UIP, and the ABCs of idiopathic interstitial pneumonias. Eur Respir J 1998; 12(5): 1003–1004.
47. Nagao T, Nagai S, Kitaichi M, et al.: Usual interstitial pneumonia: idiopathic pulmonary fibrosis versus collagen vascular diseases. Respiration 2001; 68(2): 151–159.
48. Flaherty KR, Colby TV, Travis WD, et al.: Fibroblastic foci in usual interstitial pneumonia: idiopathic versus collagen vascular disease. Am J Respir Crit Care Med 2003; 167(10): 1410–1415.
49. Kondoh Y, Taniguchi H, Kawabata Y, et al.: Acute exacerbation in idiopathic pulmonary fibrosis. Analysis of clinical and pathologic findings in three cases. Chest 1993; 103(6): 1808–1812.
50. Bjoraker JA, Ryu JH, Edwin MK, et al.: Prognostic significance of histopathologic subsets in idiopathic pulmonary fibrosis. Am J Respir Crit Care Med 1998; 157(1): 199–203.
51. Kitaichi M: Pathologic features and the classification of interstitial pneumonia of unknown etiology. Bull Chest Dis Res Inst Kyoto Univ 1990; 23(1–2): 1–18.
52. Nagai S, Kitaichi M, Itoh H, et al.: Idiopathic nonspecific interstitial pneumonia/fibrosis: comparison with idiopathic pulmonary fibrosis and BOOP. Eur Respir J 1998; 12(5): 1010–1019.
53. Cottin V, Donsbeck AV, Revel D, et al.: Nonspecific interstitial pneumonia. Individualization of a clinicopathologic entity in a series of 12 patients. Am J Respir Crit Care Med 1998; 158(4): 1286–1293.
54. Daniil ZD, Gilchrist FC, Nicholson AG, et al.: A histologic pattern of nonspecific interstitial pneumonia is associated with a better prognosis than usual interstitial pneumonia in patients with cryptogenic fibrosing alveolitis. Am J Respir Crit Care Med 1999; 160(3): 899–905.
55. Park JS, Lee KS, Kim JS, et al.: Nonspecific interstitial pneumonia with fibrosis: radiographic and CT findings in seven patients. Radiology 1995; 195(3): 645–648.
56. Hartman TE, Swensen SJ, Hansell DM, et al.: Nonspecific interstitial pneumonia: variable appearance at high-resolution chest CT. Radiology 2000; 217(3): 701–705.
57. Travis WD, Matsui K, Moss J, et al.: Idiopathic nonspecific interstitial pneumonia: prognostic significance of cellular and fibrosing patterns: survival comparison with usual interstitial pneumonia and desquamative interstitial pneumonia. Am J Surg Pathol 2000; 24(1): 19–33.
58. Davison A, Heard B, McAllister W, et al.: Cryptogenic organizing pneumonia. Q J Med 1983; 207: 382–394.
59. Epler GR, Colby TV, McLoud TC, et al.: Bronchiolitis obliterans organizing pneumonia. N Engl J Med 1985; 312(3): 152–158.
60. Yousem SA, Lohr RH, Colby TV: Idiopathic bronchiolitis obliterans organizing pneumonia/cryptogenic organizing pneumonia with unfavorable outcome: pathologic predictors. Mod Pathol 1997; 10(9): 864–871.
61. Izumi T, Nagai S, Nishimura K, et al.: [BALF cell findings in patients with BOOP, particularly in comparison with UIP]. Nihon Kyobu Shikkan Gakkai Zasshi 1989; 27(4): 474–480.
62. King TJ, Mortensen R: Cryptogenic organizing pneumonitis. Chest 1992; 102: 8S–13S.
63. Muller NL, Guerry-Force ML, Staples CA, et al.: Differential diagnosis of bronchiolitis obliterans with organizing pneumonia and usual interstitial pneumonia: clinical, functional, and radiologic findings. Radiology 1987; 162(1 Pt 1): 151–156.
64. Cordier J, Loire R, Brune J: Idiopathic bronchiolitis obliterans organizing pneumonia: definition of clinical profiles in a series of 16 patients. Chest 1989; 96: 999–1004.
65. Muller NL, Staples CA, Miller RR: Bronchiolitis obliterans organizing pneumonia: CT features in 14 patients. AJR Am J Roentgenol 1990; 154(5): 983–987.
66. Lee K, Kullnig P, Hartman T, et al.: Cryptogenic organizing pneumonia. CT findings in 43 patients. AJR Am J Roentgenol 1994; 162(3): 543–546.
67. Preidler KW, Szolar DM, Moelleken S, et al.: Distribution pattern of computed tomography findings in patients with bronchiolitis obliterans organizing pneumonia. Invest Radiol 1996; 31(5): 251–255.
68. Akira M, Yamamoto S, Sakatani M: Bronchiolitis obliterans organizing pneumonia manifesting as multiple large nodules or masses. AJR Am J Roentgenol 1998; 170(2): 291–295.
69. Izumi T, Kitaichi M, Nishimura K, et al.: Bronchiolitis obliterans organizing pneumonia. Clinical features and differential diagnosis. Chest 1992; 102(3): 715–719.
70. Reich J, Scott D: Levitating lung lesions due to bronchiolitis obliterans organizing pneumonia. Chest 1993; 103(2): 623–624.
71. King TE Jr: BOOP: an important cause of migratory pulmonary infiltrates? Eur Respir J 1995; 8(2): 193–195.
72. Bouchardy L, Kuhlman J, Ball W, et al.: CT findings in bronchiolitis obliterans organizing pneumonia (BOOP) with radiographic, clinical, and histologic correlation. J Comput Assist Tomogr 1993; 17: 352–357.
73. Colby TV: Pathologic aspects of bronchiolitis obliterans organizing pneumonia. Chest 1992; 102(Suppl 1): 38S–43S.
74. Kitaichi M: Bronchiolitis obliterans organizing pneumonia (BOOP). In: Basic and clinical aspect of pulmonary fibrosis, Takishima T, Ed. 1994, CRC Press, Boca Raton, FL, pp 463–488.

75. Cordier JF: Cryptogenic organizing pneumonitis. Bronchiolitis obliterans organizing pneumonia. Clin Chest Med 1993; 14(4): 677–692.
76. Niewoehner D, Kleinerman J, Rice D: Pathologic changes in the peripheral airways in young cigarette smokers. N Engl J Med 1974; 291: 755–758.
77. Myers J, Veal C, Shin M, et al.: Respiratory bronchiolitis causing interstitial lung disease. A clinicopathologic study of six cases. Am Rev Respir Dis 1987; 135: 880–884.
78. Heyneman LE, Ward S, Lynch DA, et al.: Respiratory bronchiolitis, respiratory bronchiolitis-associated interstitial lung disease, and desquamative interstitial pneumonia: different entities or part of the spectrum of the same disease process? AJR Am J Roentgenol 1999; 173(6): 1617–1622.
79. Yousem SA, Colby TV, Gaensler EA: Respiratory bronchiolitis-associated interstitial lung disease and its relationship to desquamative interstitial pneumonia. Mayo Clin Proc 1989; 64(11): 1373–1380.
80. Myers JL, Veal CF Jr, Shin MS, et al.: Respiratory bronchiolitis causing interstitial lung disease. A clinicopathologic study of six cases. Am Rev Respir Dis 1987; 135(4): 880–884.
81. King TE Jr.: Respiratory bronchiolitis-associated interstitial lung disease. Clin Chest Med 1993; 14(4): 693–698.
82. Moon J, du Bois RM, Colby TV, et al.: Clinical significance of respiratory bronchiolitis on open lung biopsy and its relationship to smoking related interstitial lung disease. Thorax 1999; 54(11): 1009–1014.
83. Carrington C, Gaensler E, Coutu R, et al.: Natural history and treated course of usual and desquamative interstitial pneumonia. N Engl J Med 1978; 298(15): 801–809.
84. Katzenstein AL, Myers JL: Idiopathic pulmonary fibrosis: clinical relevance of pathologic classification. Am J Respir Crit Care Med 1998; 157(4 Pt 1): 1301–1315.
85. Hartman TE, Primack SL, Swensen SJ, et al.: Desquamative interstitial pneumonia: thin-section CT findings in 22 patients. Radiology 1993; 187(3): 787–790.
86. Gruden JF, Webb WR: CT findings in a proved case of respiratory bronchiolitis. AJR Am J Roentgenol 1993; 161(1): 44–46.
87. Nicholson AG, Wotherspoon AC, Diss TC, et al.: Pulmonary B-cell non-Hodgkin's lymphomas. The value of immunohistochemistry and gene analysis in diagnosis. Histopathology 1995; 26(5): 395–403.
88. Nicholson AG, Wotherspoon AC, Diss TC, et al.: Reactive pulmonary lymphoid disorders. Histopathology 1995; 26(5): 405–412.
89. Nicholson AG, Wotherspoon AC, Jones AL, et al.: Pulmonary B-cell non-Hodgkin's lymphoma associated with autoimmune disorders: a clinicopathological review of six cases. Eur Respir J 1996; 9(10): 2022–2025.
90. Koss MN: Pulmonary lymphoproliferative disorders. Monogr Pathol 1993; 18(36): 145–194.
91. Strimlan C, Rosenow EI, Weiland L, et al.: Lymphocytic interstitial pneumonitis. Review of 13 cases. Ann Intern Med 1978; 88: 616–621.
92. Liebow A, Carrington C: Diffuse pulmonary lymphoreticular infiltrations associated with dysproteinemia. Med Clin North Am 1973; 57: 809–843.
93. Strimlan CV, Rosenow EC 3rd, Divertie MB, et al.: Pulmonary manifestations of Sjögren's syndrome. Chest 1976; 70(3): 354–361.
94. DeCoteau WE, Tourville D, Ambrus JL, et al.: Lymphoid interstitial pneumonia and autoerythrocyte sensitization syndrome. A case with deposition of immunoglobulins on the alveolar basement membrane. Arch Intern Med 1974; 134(3): 519–522.
95. Kurusu Y, Yamashita J, Ogawa M: Detection of circulating tumor cells by reverse transcriptase-polymerase chain reaction in patients with resectable non-small-cell lung cancer. Surgery 1999; 126(5): 820–826.
96. Julsrud PR, Brown LR, Li CY, et al.: Pulmonary processes of mature-appearing lymphocytes: pseudolymphoma, well-differentiated lymphocytic lymphoma, and lymphocytic interstitial pneumonitis. Radiology 1978; 127(2): 289–296.
97. Schwarz MI: A man with dyspnea, productive cough, and chest radiograph showing hyperinflation and a diffuse nodular pattern. Chest 1998; 113(4): 1123–1124.
98. Macfarlane A, Davies D: Diffuse lymphoid interstitial pneumonia. Thorax 1973; 28(6): 768–776.
99. Strimlan C, Rosenow E, Weiland L, et al.: Lymphocytic interstitial pneumonitis. Ann Intern Med 1978; 88: 616–621.
100. Johkoh T, Muller NL, Pickford HA, et al.: Lymphocytic interstitial pneumonia: thin-section CT findings in 22 patients. Radiology 1999; 212(2): 567–572.
101. Julsrud P, Brown L, Li CY, Rosenow EC 3rd, Crowe JK: Pulmonary processes of mature-appearing lymphocytes: pseudolymphoma, well-differentiated lymphocytic lymphoma, and lymphocytic interstitial pneumonitis. Radiology 1978; 127: 289–296.
102. Kradin RL, Mark EJ: Benign lymphoid disorders of the lung, with a theory regarding their development. Hum Pathol 1983; 14(10): 857–867.
103. Strimlan CV: Pulmonary function in patients with primary Sjögren's syndrome. Ann Rheum Dis 2001; 60(4): 429.
104. Palmas A, Tefferi A, Myers JL, et al.: Late-onset noninfectious pulmonary complications after allogeneic bone marrow transplantation. Br J Haematol 1998; 100(4): 680–687.
105. Grieco M, Chinoy-Acharya P: Lymphoid interstitial pneumonia associated with the acquired immune deficiency syndrome. Am Rev Respir Dis 1985; 131: 952–955.
106. Berdon WE, Mellins RB, Abramson SJ, et al.: Pediatric HIV infection in its second decade – the changing pattern of lung involvement. Clinical, plain film, and computed tomographic findings. Radiol Clin North Am 1993; 31(3): 453–463.
107. Couderc LJ, Clauvel JP, Caubarrere I: Lung limited lymphocytic proliferation in human immunodeficiency virus (HIV) infection. Respir Med 1993; 87(7): 559.
108. Ikeogu MO, Wolf B, Mathe S: Pulmonary manifestations in HIV seropositivity and malnutrition in Zimbabwe. Arch Dis Child 1997; 76(2): 124–128.
109. Khare MD, Sharland M: Pulmonary manifestations of pediatric HIV infection. Indian J Pediatr 1999; 66(6): 895–904.
110. Church JA: Lymphoid interstitial pneumonia and rheumatoid arthritis. J Pediatr 1985; 107(3): 485.
111. Black L, Katz S: Respiratory disease: task force report on problems, research approaches, needs. 1977, National Heart and Lung Institute, Bethesda, Maryland.
112. Ellman P, Ball RE: "Rheumatoid disease" with joint and pulmonary manifestations. BMJ 1948; 2: 816–820.
113. Gabbay E, Tarala R, Will R, et al.: Interstitial lung disease in recent onset rheumatoid arthritis. Am J Respir Crit Care Med 1997; 156(2 Pt 1): 528–535.
114. Anaya JM, Diethelm L, Ortiz LA, et al.: Pulmonary involvement in rheumatoid arthritis. Semin Arthritis Rheum 1995; 24(4): 242–254.
115. Hakala M: Poor prognosis in patients with rheumatoid arthritis hospitalized for interstitial lung fibrosis. Chest 1988; 93(1): 114–118.
116. Athreya BH, Doughty RA, Bookspan M, et al.: Pulmonary manifestations of juvenile rheumatoid arthritis. A report of eight cases and review. Clin Chest Med 1980; 1(3): 361–374.
117. Saag KG, Kolluri S, Koehnke RK, et al.: Rheumatoid arthritis lung disease. Determinants of radiographic and physiologic abnormalities. Arthritis Rheum 1996; 39(10): 1711–1719.
118. Akira M, Sakatani M, Hara H: Thin-section CT findings in rheumatoid arthritis-associated lung disease: CT patterns and their courses. J Comput Assist Tomogr 1999; 23(6): 941–948.
119. Remy-Jardin M, Remy J, Cortet B, et al.: Lung changes in rheumatoid arthritis: CT findings. Radiology 1994; 193(2): 375–382.
120. Laitinen O, Nissila M, Salorinne Y, et al.: Pulmonary involvement in patients with rheumatoid arthritis. Scand J Respir Dis 1975; 56: 297–304.
121. Schwarz MI, Matthay RA, Sahn SA, et al.: Interstitial lung disease in polymyositis and dermatomyositis: analysis of six cases and review of the literature. Medicine (Baltimore) 1976; 55(1): 89–104.
122. Cheema GS, Quismorio FP Jr: Interstitial lung disease in systemic sclerosis. Curr Opin Pulm Med 2001; 7(5): 283–290.
123. Raghu G, Brown KK, Bradford WZ, et al.; Idiopathic Pulmonary Fibrosis Study Group: a placebo-controlled trial of interferon gamma-1b in patients with idiopathic pulmonary fibrosis. N Engl J Med 2004; 350(2): 125–133.
124. Bouros D, Wells AU, Nicholson AG, et al.: Histopathologic subsets of fibrosing alveolitis in patients with systemic sclerosis and their relationship to outcome. Am J Respir Crit Care Med 2002; 165(12): 1581–1586.
125. Kim DS, Yoo B, Lee JS, et al.: The major histopathologic pattern of pulmonary fibrosis in scleroderma is nonspecific interstitial pneumonia. Sarcoidosis Vasc Diffuse Lung Dis 2002; 19(2): 121–127.

126. Kim EA, Johkoh T, Lee KS, et al.: Interstitial pneumonia in progressive systemic sclerosis: serial high-resolution CT findings with functional correlation. J Comput Assist Tomogr 2001; 25(5): 757–763.
127. Cozzi F, Chiesura-Corona M, Rizzi M, et al.: [Lung fibrosis quantified by HRCT in scleroderma patients with different disease forms and ANA specificities]. Reumatismo 2001; 53(1): 55–62.
128. Yamane K, Ihn H, Asano Y, et al.: Clinical and laboratory features of scleroderma patients with pulmonary hypertension. Rheumatology (Oxford) 2000; 39(11): 1269–1271.
129. Johnson DA, Drane WE, Curran J, et al.: Pulmonary disease in progressive systemic sclerosis. A complication of gastroesophageal reflux and occult aspiration? Arch Intern Med 1989; 149(3): 589–593.
130. Montesi A, Pesaresi A, Cavalli ML, et al.: Oropharyngeal and esophageal function in scleroderma. Dysphagia 1991; 6(4): 219–223.
131. Mayes MD: Scleroderma epidemiology. Rheum Dis Clin North Am 2003; 29(2): 239–254.
132. McSweeney PA, Nash RA, Sullivan KM, et al.: High-dose immunosuppressive therapy for severe systemic sclerosis: initial outcomes. Blood 2002; 100(5): 1602–1610.
133. Dubois E, Tufanelli, DL: Clinical manifestations of systemic lupus erythematosus. JAMA 1964; 190: 104–111.
134. Eisenberg H, Dubois E, Sherwin R, et al.: Diffuse interstitial lung disease in systemic lupus erythematosus. Ann Intern Med 1973; 79: 37–45.
135. Gammon R, Bridges T, Al-Nezir H, et al.: Bronchiolitis obliterans organizing pneumonia associated with systemic lupus erythematosus. Chest 1992; 102: 1171–1174.
136. Cheema GS, Quismorio FP Jr: Interstitial lung disease in systemic lupus erythematosus. Curr Opin Pulm Med 2000; 6(5): 424–429.
137. Myers JL, Katzenstein AA: Microangiitis in lupus-induced pulmonary hemorrhage. Am J Clin Pathol 1986; 85(5): 552–556.
138. Chang MY, Fang JT, Chen YC, et al.: Diffuse alveolar hemorrhage in systemic lupus erythematosus: a single center retrospective study in Taiwan. Ren Fail 2002; 24(6): 791–802.
139. Santos-Ocampo AS, Mandell BF, Fessler BJ: Alveolar hemorrhage in systemic lupus erythematosus: presentation and management. Chest 2000; 118(4): 1083–1090.
140. Murin S, Wiedemann HP, Matthay RA: Pulmonary manifestations of systemic lupus erythematosus. Clin Chest Med 1998; 19(4): 641–665, viii.
141. Matthay R, Schwarz M, Petty T, et al.: Pulmonary manifestations of systemic lupus erythematosus: review of twelve cases with acute lupus pneumonitis. Medicine 1974; 54: 397–409.
142. Kim JS, Lee KS, Koh EM, et al.: Thoracic involvement of systemic lupus erythematosus: clinical, pathologic, and radiologic findings. J Comput Assist Tomogr 2000; 24(1): 9–18.
143. Hughson MD, He Z, Henegar J, et al.: Alveolar hemorrhage and renal microangiopathy in systemic lupus erythematosus. Arch Pathol Lab Med 2001; 125(4): 475–483.
144. Bankier AA, Kiener HP, Wiesmayr MN, et al.: Discrete lung involvement in systemic lupus erythematosus: CT assessment. Radiology 1995; 196(3): 835–840.
145. Fenlon HM, Doran M, Sant SM, et al.: High-resolution chest CT in systemic lupus erythematosus. AJR Am J Roentgenol 1996; 166(2): 301–307.
146. Sant SM, Doran M, Fenelon HM, et al.: Pleuropulmonary abnormalities in patients with systemic lupus erythematosus: assessment with high resolution computed tomography, chest radiography and pulmonary function tests. Clin Exp Rheumatol 1997; 15(5): 507–513.
147. Ooi GC, Ngan H, Peh WC, et al.: Systemic lupus erythematosus patients with respiratory symptoms: the value of HRCT. Clin Radiol 1997; 52(10): 775–781.
148. Susanto I, Peters JI: Acute lupus pneumonitis with normal chest radiograph. Chest 1997; 111(6): 1781–1783.
149. Zamora MR, Warner ML, Tuder R, et al.: Diffuse alveolar hemorrhage and systemic lupus erythematosus. Clinical presentation, histology, survival, and outcome. Medicine (Baltimore) 1997; 76(3): 192–202.
150. Urman JD, Rothfield NF: Corticosteroid treatment in systemic lupus erythematosus. Survival studies. JAMA 1977; 238(21): 2272–2276.
151. Rosner S, Ginzler EM, Diamond HS, et al.: A multicenter study of outcome in systemic lupus erythematosus. II. Causes of death. Arthritis Rheum 1982; 25(6): 612–617.
152. Bohan A, Peter JB, Bowman RL, et al.: Computer-assisted analysis of 153 patients with polymyositis and dermatomyositis. Medicine (Baltimore) 1977; 56(4): 255–286.
153. Bohan A: History and classification of polymyositis and dermatomyositis. Clin Dermatol 1988; 6(2): 3–8.
154. Nobutoh T, Kohda M, Doi Y, et al.: An autopsy case of dermatomyositis with rapidly progressive diffuse alveolar damage. J Dermatol 1998; 25(1): 32–36.
155. Tazelaar HD, Viggiano RW, Pickersgill J, et al.: Interstitial lung disease in polymyositis and dermatomyositis. Clinical features and prognosis as correlated with histologic findings. Am Rev Respir Dis 1990; 141(3): 727–733.
156. Douglas WW, Tazelaar HD, Hartman TE, et al.: Polymyositis-dermatomyositis-associated interstitial lung disease. Am J Respir Crit Care Med 2001; 164(7): 1182–1185.
157. Hepper N, Ferguson, RH, Howard, FM: Three types of pulmonary involvement in polymyositis. Med Clin North Am 1964; 48: 1031–1042.
158. Benbassat J, Gefel D, Larholt K, et al.: Prognostic factors in polymyositis/dermatomyositis. A computer-assisted analysis of ninety-two cases. Arthritis Rheum 1985; 28(3): 249–255.
159. Ikezoe J, Johkoh T, Kohno N, et al.: High-resolution CT findings of lung disease in patients with polymyositis and dermatomyositis. J Thorac Imaging 1996; 11(4): 250–259.
160. Whaley K, Alspaugh, MA: Sjögren's syndrome. In: Textbook of rheumatology, Kelley WN, Harris ED, Ruddy S, Sledge CB, Eds. 1985, WB Saunders, Philadelphia, p 956.
161. Baruch HH, Firooznia H, Sackler JP, et al.: Pulmonary disorders associated with Sjögren's syndrome. Rev Interam Radiol 1977; 2(2): 77–81.
162. Franquet T, Gimenez A, Monill JM, et al.: Primary Sjögren's syndrome and associated lung disease: CT findings in 50 patients. AJR Am J Roentgenol 1997; 169(3): 655–658.
163. Deheinzelin D, Capelozzi VL, Kairalla RA, et al.: Interstitial lung disease in primary Sjögren's syndrome. Clinical–pathological evaluation and response to treatment. Am J Respir Crit Care Med 1996; 154(3 Pt 1): 794–799.
164. Reveille JD, Wilson RW, Provost TT, et al.: Primary Sjögren's syndrome and other autoimmune diseases in families. Prevalence and immunogenetic studies in six kindreds. Ann Intern Med 1984; 101(6): 748–756.
165. Meyer CA, Pina JS, Taillon D, et al.: Inspiratory and expiratory high-resolution CT findings in a patient with Sjögren's syndrome and cystic lung disease. AJR Am J Roentgenol 1997; 168(1): 101–103.
166. Hansen LA, Prakash UB, Colby TV: Pulmonary lymphoma in Sjögren's syndrome. Mayo Clin Proc 1989; 64(8): 920–931.
167. Carrington C, Addington W, Goff A, et al.: Chronic eosinophilic pneumonia. N Engl J Med 1969; 280: 787–798.
168. Liebow A, Carrington C: The eosinophilic pneumonias. Medicine (Baltimore) 1969; 48: 251–285.
169. Gaensler E, Carrington C: Peripheral opacities in chronic eosinophilic pneumonia. The photographic negative of pulmonary edema. AJR 1977; 128: 1–13.
170. Mayo J, Müller N, Road J, et al.: Chronic eosinophilic pneumonia: CT findings in six cases. AJR 1989; 153: 727–730.
171. Copper JA Jr: Drug-induced lung disease. Adv Intern Med 1997; 42: 231–268.
172. Camus PH, Foucher P, Bonniaud PH, et al.: Drug-induced infiltrative lung disease. Eur Respir J Suppl 2001; 32: 93s–100s.
173. Ozkan M, Dweik RA, Ahmad M: Drug-induced lung disease. Cleve Clin J Med 2001; 68(9): 782–785, 89–95.
174. Cuellar ML: Drug-induced vasculitis. Curr Rheumatol Rep 2002; 4(1): 55–59.
175. Myers JL: Pathology of drug-induced lung disease. In: Katzenstein and Askin's surgical pathology of non-neoplastic lung disease, Katzenstein AL, Ed. 1997, WB Saunders, Philadelphia, pp 81–111.
176. Zitnik RJ, Matthay RA: Drug-induced lung disease. In: Interstitial lung disease, Schwartz MI, King TE, Eds. 1998, BC Decker, London, pp 423–449.
177. Sostman HD, Matthay RA, Putman CE, et al.: Methotrexate-induced pneumonitis. Medicine (Baltimore) 1976; 55(5): 371–388.
178. Goodman TA, Polisson RP: Methotrexate: adverse reactions and major toxicities. Rheum Dis Clin North Am 1994; 20(2): 513–528.
179. Bedrossian CW, Miller WC, Luna MA: Methotrexate-induced diffuse interstitial pulmonary fibrosis. South Med J 1979; 72(3): 313–318.

180. Imokawa S, Colby TV, Leslie KO, et al.: Methotrexate pneumonitis: review of the literature and histopathological findings in nine patients. Eur Respir J 2000; 15(2): 373–381.
181. Zisman DA, McCune WJ, Tino G, et al.: Drug-induced pneumonitis: the role of methotrexate. Sarcoidosis Vasc Diffuse Lung Dis 2001; 18(3): 243–252.
182. Kennedy JI, Myers JL, Plumb VJ, et al.: Amiodarone pulmonary toxicity. Clinical, radiologic, and pathologic correlations. Arch Intern Med 1987; 147(1): 50–55.
183. Dusman RE, Stanton MS, Miles WM, et al.: Clinical features of amiodarone-induced pulmonary toxicity. Circulation 1990; 82(1): 51–59.
184. Weinberg BA, Miles WM, Klein LS, et al.: Five-year follow-up of 589 patients treated with amiodarone. Am Heart J 1993; 125(1): 109–120.
185. Fraire AE, Guntupalli KK, Greenberg SD, et al.: Amiodarone pulmonary toxicity: a multidisciplinary review of current status. South Med J 1993; 86(1): 67–77.
186. Nicholson AA, Hayward C: The value of computed tomography in the diagnosis of amiodarone-induced pulmonary toxicity. Clin Radiol 1989; 40(6): 564–567.
187. Kuhlman JE, Teigen C, Ren H, et al.: Amiodarone pulmonary toxicity: CT findings in symptomatic patients. Radiology 1990; 177(1): 121–125.
188. Myers JL, Kennedy JI, Plumb VJ: Amiodarone lung: pathologic findings in clinically toxic patients. Hum Pathol 1987; 18(4): 349–354.
189. Martin WJ 2nd, Rosenow EC 3rd: Amiodarone pulmonary toxicity. Recognition and pathogenesis (Part I). Chest 1988; 93(5): 1067–1075.
190. Martin WJ 2nd, Rosenow EC 3rd: Amiodarone pulmonary toxicity. Recognition and pathogenesis (Part 2). Chest 1988; 93(6): 1242–1248.
191. Liu FL, Cohen RD, Downar E, et al.: Amiodarone pulmonary toxicity: functional and ultrastructural evaluation. Thorax 1986; 41(2): 100–105.
192. Gonzalez-Rothi RJ, Hannan SE, Hood CI, et al.: Amiodarone pulmonary toxicity presenting as bilateral exudative pleural effusions. Chest 1987; 92(1): 179–182.
193. Wood DL, Osborn MJ, Rooke J, et al.: Amiodarone pulmonary toxicity: report of two cases associated with rapidly progressive fatal adult respiratory distress syndrome after pulmonary angiography. Mayo Clin Proc 1985; 60(9): 601–603.
194. Van Mieghem W, Coolen L, Malysse I, et al.: Amiodarone and the development of ARDS after lung surgery. Chest 1994; 105(6): 1642–1645.
195. Durant JR, Norgard MJ, Murad TM, et al.: Pulmonary toxicity associated with bischloroethylnitrosourea (BCNU). Ann Intern Med 1979; 90(2): 191–194.
196. Lieberman A, Ruoff M, Estey E, et al.: Irreversible pulmonary toxicity after single course of BCNU. Am J Med Sci 1980; 279(1): 53–56.
197. Litam JP, Dail DH, Spitzer G, et al.: Early pulmonary toxicity after administration of high-dose BCNU. Cancer Treat Rep 1981; 65(1–2): 39–44.
198. Cao TM, Negrin RS, Stockerl-Goldstein KE, et al.: Pulmonary toxicity syndrome in breast cancer patients undergoing BCNU-containing high-dose chemotherapy and autologous hematopoietic cell transplantation. Biol Blood Marrow Transplant 2000; 6(4): 387–394.
199. Holoye PY, Jenkins DE, Greenberg SD: Pulmonary toxicity in long-term administration of BCNU. Cancer Treat Rep 1976; 60(11): 1691–1694.
200. O'Driscoll BR, Hasleton PS, Taylor PM, et al.: Active lung fibrosis up to 17 years after chemotherapy with carmustine (BCNU) in childhood. N Engl J Med 1990; 323(6): 378–382.
201. Hasleton PS, O'Driscoll BR, Lynch P, et al.: Late BCNU lung: a light and ultrastructural study on the delayed effect of BCNU on the lung parenchyma. J Pathol 1991; 164(1): 31–36.
202. Littler W, Kay J, Haselton P, et al.: Busulphan lung. Thorax 1969; 24(6): 639–655.
203. Cooper JA Jr, White DA, Matthay RA: Drug-induced pulmonary disease. Part 1: Cytotoxic drugs. Am Rev Respir Dis 1986; 133(2): 321–340.
204. Kreisman H, Wolkove N: Pulmonary toxicity of antineoplastic therapy. Semin Oncol 1992; 19(5): 508–520.
205. Feingold ML, Koss LG: Effects of long-term administration of busulfan. Report of a patient with generalized nuclear abnormalities, carcinoma of vulva, and pulmonary fibrosis. Arch Intern Med 1969; 124(1): 66–71.
206. Iacovino JR, Leitner J, Abbas AK, et al.: Fatal pulmonary reaction from low doses of bleomycin. An idiosyncratic tissue response. JAMA 1976; 235(12): 1253–1255.
207. Holoye P, Luna M, MacKay B, et al.: Bleomycin hypersensitivity pneumonitis. Ann Intern Med 1978; 8: 47–49.
208. Hay JG, Haslam PL, Dewar A, et al.: Development of acute lung injury after the combination of intravenous bleomycin and exposure to hyperoxia in rats. Thorax 1987; 42(5): 374–382.
209. Borzone G, Moreno R, Urrea R, et al.: Bleomycin-induced chronic lung damage does not resemble human idiopathic pulmonary fibrosis. Am J Respir Crit Care Med 2001; 163(7): 1648–1653.
210. Lien HH, Brodahl U, Telhaug R, et al.: Pulmonary changes at computed tomography in patients with testicular carcinoma treated with cis-platinum, vinblastine and bleomycin. Acta Radiol Diagn (Stockh) 1985; 26(5): 507–510.
211. Adler KB, Callahan LM, Evans JN: Cellular alterations in the alveolar wall in bleomycin-induced pulmonary fibrosis in rats. An ultrastructural morphometric study. Am Rev Respir Dis 1986; 133(6): 1043–1048.
212. Lazo JS: Bleomycin. Cancer Chemother Biol Response Modif 1999; 18: 39–45.
213. Bowler RP, Nicks M, Warnick K, et al.: Role of extracellular superoxide dismutase in bleomycin-induced pulmonary fibrosis. Am J Physiol Lung Cell Mol Physiol 2002; 282(4): L719–726.
214. Taatjes DJ, Leslie KO, von Turkovich M, et al.: Alveolocapillary remodeling in bleomycin-induced rat lung injury: interpretation from lectin-binding studies. Prog Histochem Cytochem 1991; 23(1–4): 194–199.
215. Stern W, Subbarao K: Pulmonary complications of drug addiction. Semin Roentgenol 1983; 28: 183–197.
216. Abraham J, Brambilla C: Particle size for differentiation between inhalation and injection pulmonary talcosis. Environ Res 1980; 21(1): 94–96.
217. Abraham JL: Identification and quantitative analysis of tissue particulate burden. Ann NY Acad Sci 1984; 428: 60–67.
218. Abraham JL, Burnett BR, Hunt A: Development and use of a pneumoconiosis database of human pulmonary inorganic particulate burden in over 400 lungs. Scanning Microsc 1991; 5(1): 95–104; discussion 5–8.
219. Tomashefski J, Hirsch C: The pulmonary vascular lesions of intravenous drug abuse. Hum Pathol 1980; 11: 133–145.
220. Crouch E, Churg A: Progressive massive fibrosis of the lung secondary to intravenous injection of talc: a pathologic and mineralogical analysis. Am J Clin Pathol 1983; 80: 520–526.
221. Stern E, Frank M, Schmutz J, et al.: Panlobular pulmonary emphysema caused by IV injection of methylphenidate (Ritalin): findings on chest radiographs and CT scans. AJR 1994; 162: 555–560.
222. Cook RC, Fradet G, English JC, et al.: Recurrence of intravenous talc granulomatosis following single lung transplantation. Can Respir J 1998; 5(6): 511–514.
223. Judd PA, Finnegan P, Curran RC: Pulmonary sarcoidosis: a clinicopathological study. J Pathol 1975; 115: 191–198.
224. Saltini C, Crystal RG: Pulmonary sarcoidosis: pathogenesis, staging and therapy. Int Arch Allergy Appl Immunol 1985; 76(Suppl 1): 92–100.
225. Lynch JP 3rd, Kazerooni EA, Gay SE: Pulmonary sarcoidosis. Clin Chest Med 1997; 18(4): 755–785.
226. Muller-Quernheim J: Sarcoidosis: immunopathogenetic concepts and their clinical application. Eur Respir J 1998; 12(3): 716–738.
227. Hunninghake GW, Costabel U, Ando M, et al.: ATS/ERS/WASOG statement on sarcoidosis. American Thoracic Society/European Respiratory Society/World Association of Sarcoidosis and other Granulomatous Disorders. Sarcoidosis Vasc Diffuse Lung Dis 1999; 16(2): 149–173.
228. Moller DR: Systemic sarcoidosis. In: Fishman's pulmonary diseases and disorders, Fishman AP, Elias, JA, Fishman JA, et al., Eds. 1997, McGraw-Hill, New York, pp 1055–1068.
229. Stirling RG, Cullinan P, Du Bois RM: Sarcoidosis. In: Interstitial lung disease, Schwartz MI, King, TE, Eds. 1998, BC Decker, London, pp 279–322.
230. Milman N, Selroos O: Pulmonary sarcoidosis in the Nordic countries 1950–1982. Epidemiology and clinical picture. Sarcoidosis 1990; 7(1): 50–57.
231. Milman N, Selroos O: Pulmonary sarcoidosis in the Nordic countries 1950–1982. II. Course and prognosis. Sarcoidosis 1990; 7(2): 113–118.

232. Sartwell PE, Edwards LB: Epidemiology of sarcoidosis in the U.S. Navy. Am J Epidemiol 1974; 99(4): 250–257.
233. Teirstein AS: Kveim antigen: what does it tell us about causation of sarcoidosis? Semin Respir Infect 1998; 13(3): 206–211.
234. Lynch D, Webb W, Gamsu G, et al.: Computed tomography in pulmonary sarcoidosis. J Comput Assist Tomogr 1989; 13: 405–410.
235. Kuhlman JE, Fishman EK, Hamper UM, et al.: The computed tomographic spectrum of thoracic sarcoidosis. Radiographics 1989; 9(3): 449–466.
236. Muller NL, Kullnig P, Miller RR: The CT findings of pulmonary sarcoidosis: analysis of 25 patients. AJR Am J Roentgenol 1989; 152(6): 1179–1182.
237. Padley SP, Padhani AR, Nicholson A, et al.: Pulmonary sarcoidosis mimicking cryptogenic fibrosing alveolitis on CT. Clin Radiol 1996; 51(11): 807–810.
238. Abehsera M, Valeyre D, Grenier P, et al.: Sarcoidosis with pulmonary fibrosis: CT patterns and correlation with pulmonary function. AJR Am J Roentgenol 2000; 174(6): 1751–1757.
239. Battesti J, Saumon G, Valeyre D, et al.: Pulmonary sarcoidosis with an alveolar radiographic pattern. Thorax 1982; 37: 448–452.
240. Gilman MJ, Wang KP: Transbronchial lung biopsy in sarcoidosis. An approach to determine the optimal number of biopsies. Am Rev Respir Dis 1980; 122(5): 721–724.
241. Hsu RM, Connors AF Jr, Tomashefski JF Jr: Histologic, microbiologic, and clinical correlates of the diagnosis of sarcoidosis by transbronchial biopsy. Arch Pathol Lab Med 1996; 120(4): 364–368.
242. Freiman D, Hardy H: Beryllium disease: the relation of pulmonary pathology to clinical course and prognosis based on a study of 130 cases from the U.S. Beryllium Case Registry. Hum Pathol 1970; 1: 25–44.
243. Matilla A, Galera H, Pascual E, et al.: Chronic berylliosis. Br J Dis Chest 1973; 67: 308–314.
244. Aronchik J, Rossman M, Miller W: Chronic beryllium disease: diagnosis, radiographic findings, and correlation with pulmonary function tests. Radiology 1987; 163: 677–678.
245. Kriebel D, Brain JD, Sprince NL, et al.: The pulmonary toxicity of beryllium. Am Rev Respir Dis 1988; 137(2): 464–473.
246. Kriebel D, Sprince NL, Eisen EA, et al.: Pulmonary function in beryllium workers: assessment of exposure. Br J Ind Med 1988; 45(2): 83–92.
247. Kriebel D, Sprince NL, Eisen EA, et al.: Beryllium exposure and pulmonary function: a cross sectional study of beryllium workers. Br J Ind Med 1988; 45(3): 167–173.
248. Kawanami O, Basset F, Barrios R, et al.: Hypersensitivity pneumonitis in man: light and electron microscopic studies of 18 lung biopsies. Am J Pathol 1983; 110: 275–289.
249. Salvaggio J, Karr R: Hypersensitivity pneumonitis: state of the art. Chest 1979; 75(Suppl 2): 270–274.
250. Wild LG, Lopez M: Hypersensitivity pneumonitis: a comprehensive review. J Investig Allergol Clin Immunol 2001; 11(1): 3–15.
251. Bourke SJ, Dalphin JC, Boyd G, et al.: Hypersensitivity pneumonitis: current concepts. Eur Respir J Suppl 2001; 32: 81s–92s.
252. Selman M: Hypersensitivity pneumonitis. In: Interstitial lung disease, Schwartz MI, King TE, Eds. 1998, BC Decker, London, pp 393–422.
253. Murin S, Bilello KS, Matthay R: Other smoking-affected pulmonary diseases. Clin Chest Med 2000; 21(1): 121–137, ix.
254. Patel AM, Ryu JH, Reed CE: Hypersensitivity pneumonitis: current concepts and future questions. J Allergy Clin Immunol 2001; 108(5): 661–670.
255. Ando M, Suga M: Hypersensitivity pneumonitis. Curr Opin Pulm Med 1997; 3(5): 391–395.
256. Glazer C, Rose C, Lynch D: Clinical and radiologic manifestations of hypersensitivity pneumonitis. J Thorac Imaging 2002; 17(4): 261–272.
257. Cook PG, Wells IP, McGavin CR: The distribution of pulmonary shadowing in farmer's lung. Clin Radiol 1988; 39(1): 21–27.
258. Khoor A, Leslie KO, Tazelaar HD, et al.: Diffuse pulmonary disease caused by nontuberculous mycobacteria in immunocompetent people (hot tub lung). Am J Clin Pathol 2001; 115(5): 755–762.
259. Pham R, Vydareny K, Gal A: High-resolution computed tomography appearance of pulmonary *Mycobacterium avium* complex infection after exposure to hot tub: case of hot-tub lung. J Thorac Imaging 2003; 18(1): 48–52.
260. Coleman A, Colby TV: Histologic diagnosis of extrinsic allergic alveolitis. Am J Surg Pathol 1988; 12(7): 514–518.
261. Colby T, Coleman A: Histologic differential diagnosis of extrinsic allergic alveolitis. Prog Surg Pathol 1989; 10: 11–26.
262. Seal RM, Hapke EJ, Thomas GO, et al.: The pathology of the acute and chronic stages of farmer's lung. Thorax 1968; 23(5): 469–489.
263. Barbee RA, Callies Q, Dickie HA, et al.: The long-term prognosis in farmer's lung. Am Rev Respir Dis 1968; 97(2): 223–231.
264. Kokkarinen J, Tukiainen H, Seppa A, et al.: Hypersensitivity pneumonitis due to native birds in a bird ringer. Chest 1994; 106(4): 1269–1271.
265. Kokkarinen J, Tukiainen H, Terho EO: Mortality due to farmer's lung in Finland. Chest 1994; 106(2): 509–512.
266. Kokkarinen JI, Tukiainen HO, Terho EO: Effect of corticosteroid treatment on the recovery of pulmonary function in farmer's lung. Am Rev Respir Dis 1992; 145(1): 3–5.
267. Sansores R, Salas J, Chapela R, et al.: Clubbing in hypersensitivity pneumonitis. Its prevalence and possible prognostic role. Arch Intern Med 1990; 150(9): 1849–1851.
268. Perez-Padilla R, Gaxiola M, Salas J, et al.: Bronchiolitis in chronic pigeon breeder's disease. Morphologic evidence of a spectrum of small airway lesions in hypersensitivity pneumonitis induced by avian antigens. Chest 1996; 110(2): 371–377.
269. Brabencova E, Tazi A, Lorenzato M, et al.: Langerhans cells in Langerhans cell granulomatosis are not actively proliferating cells. Am J Pathol 1998; 152(5): 1143–1149.
270. Vassallo R, Ryu JH, Colby TV, et al.: Pulmonary Langerhans'-cell histiocytosis. N Engl J Med 2000; 342(26): 1969–1978.
271. Willman CL, Busque L, Griffith BB, et al.: Langerhans'-cell histiocytosis (histiocytosis X) – a clonal proliferative disease. N Engl J Med 1994; 331(3): 154–160.
272. Travis WD, Borok Z, Roum JH, et al.: Pulmonary Langerhans cell granulomatosis (histiocytosis X). A clinicopathologic study of 48 cases. Am J Surg Pathol 1993; 17(10): 971–986.
273. Colby TV, Lombard C: Histiocytosis X in the lung. Hum Pathol 1983; 14(10): 847–856.
274. Friedman PJ, Liebow AA, Sokoloff J: Eosinophilic granuloma of lung. Clinical aspects of primary histiocytosis in the adult. Medicine (Baltimore) 1981; 60(6): 385–396.
275. Lacronique J, Roth C, Battesti JP, et al.: Chest radiological features of pulmonary histiocytosis X: a report based on 50 adult cases. Thorax 1982; 37(2): 104–109.
276. Moore AD, Godwin JD, Muller NL, et al.: Pulmonary histiocytosis X: comparison of radiographic and CT findings. Radiology 1989; 172(1): 249–254.
277. Kulwiec EL, Lynch DA, Aguayo SM, et al.: Imaging of pulmonary histiocytosis X. Radiographics 1992; 12(3): 515–526.
278. Brauner MW, Grenier P, Tijani K, et al.: Pulmonary Langerhans cell histiocytosis: evolution of lesions on CT scans. Radiology 1997; 204(2): 497–502.
279. Kambouchner M, Basset F, Marchal J, et al.: Three dimensional characterization of pathologic lesions in pulmonary Langerhans cell histiocytosis. Am J Respir Crit Care Med 2002; 166(11): 1419–1421.
280. McDonnell TJ, Crouch EC, Gonzalez JG: Reactive eosinophilic pleuritis. A sequela of pneumothorax in pulmonary eosinophilic granuloma. Am J Clin Pathol 1989; 91(1): 107–111.
281. Askin F, McCann B, Kuhn C: Reactive eosinophilic pleuritis: a lesion to be distinguished from pulmonary eosinophilic granuloma. Arch Pathol Lab Med 1977; 101: 187–192.
282. Delobbe A, Durieu J, Duhamel A, et al.: Determinants of survival in pulmonary Langerhans' cell granulomatosis (histiocytosis X). Groupe d'Etude en Pathologie Interstitielle de la Societe de Pathologie Thoracique du Nord. Eur Respir J 1996; 9(10): 2002–2006.
283. Veyssier-Belot C, Cacoub P, Caparros-Lefebvre D, et al.: Erdheim–Chester disease. Clinical and radiologic characteristics of 59 cases. Medicine (Baltimore) 1996; 75(3): 157–169.
284. Devouassoux G, Lantuejoul S, Chatelain P, et al.: Erdheim–Chester disease: a primary macrophage cell disorder. Am J Respir Crit Care Med 1998; 157(2): 650–653.
285. Bisceglia M, Cammisa M, Suster S, et al.: Erdheim–Chester disease: clinical and pathologic spectrum of four cases from the Arkadi M. Rywlin slide seminars. Adv Anat Pathol 2003; 10(3): 160–171.
286. Bancroft LW, Berquist TH: Erdheim–Chester disease: radiographic findings in five patients. Skeletal Radiol 1998; 27(3): 127–132.

287. Breuil V, Brocq O, Pellegrino C, et al.: Erdheim–Chester disease: typical radiological bone features for a rare xanthogranulomatosis. Ann Rheum Dis 2002; 61(3): 199–200.
288. Gottlieb R, Chen A: MR findings of Erdheim–Chester disease. J Comput Assist Tomogr 2002; 26(2): 257–261.
289. Olmos JM, Canga A, Velero C, et al.: Imaging of Erdheim–Chester disease. J Bone Miner Res 2002; 17(3): 381–383.
290. Kambouchner M, Colby TV, Domenge C, et al.: Erdheim–Chester disease with prominent pulmonary involvement associated with eosinophilic granuloma of mandibular bone. Histopathology 1997; 30(4): 353–358.
291. Egan AJ, Boardman LA, Tazelaar HD, et al.: Erdheim–Chester disease: clinical, radiologic, and histopathologic findings in five patients with interstitial lung disease. Am J Surg Pathol 1999; 23(1): 17–26.
292. Rush WL, Andriko JA, Galateau-Salle F, et al.: Pulmonary pathology of Erdheim–Chester disease. Mod Pathol 2000; 13(7): 747–754.
293. Wittenberg KH, Swensen SJ, Myers JL: Pulmonary involvement with Erdheim–Chester disease: radiographic and CT findings. AJR Am J Roentgenol 2000; 174(5): 1327–1331.
294. Shamburek RD, Brewer HB Jr, Gochuico BR: Erdheim–Chester disease: a rare multisystem histiocytic disorder associated with interstitial lung disease. Am J Med Sci 2001; 321(1): 66–75.
295. Taylor JR, Ryu J, Colby TV, et al.: Lymphangioleiomyomatosis. Clinical course in 32 patients. N Engl J Med 1990; 323(18): 1254–1260.
296. Kitaichi M, Nishimura K, Itoh H, et al.: Pulmonary lymphangioleiomyomatosis: a report of 46 patients including a clinicopathologic study of prognostic factors. Am J Respir Crit Care Med 1995; 151(2 Pt 1): 527–533.
297. Kalassian KG, Doyle R, Kao P, et al.: Lymphangioleiomyomatosis: new insights. Am J Respir Crit Care Med 1997; 155(4): 1183–1186.
298. Athavale A, Chhajed P, Singhal P, et al.: Pulmonary lymphangioleiomyomatosis. J Assoc Physicians India 1999; 47(6): 649–650.
299. Urban T, Lazor R, Lacronique J, et al.: Pulmonary lymphangioleiomyomatosis. A study of 69 patients. Groupe d'Etudes et de Recherche sur les Maladies "Orphelines" Pulmonaires (GERM"O"P). Medicine (Baltimore) 1999; 78(5): 321–337.
300. Chu SC, Horiba K, Usuki J, et al.: Comprehensive evaluation of 35 patients with lymphangioleiomyomatosis. Chest 1999; 115(4): 1041–1052.
301. Kelly J, Moss J: Lymphangioleiomyomatosis. Am J Med Sci 2001; 321(1): 17–25.
302. Capron F, Ameille J, Leclerc P, et al.: Pulmonary lymphangioleiomyomatosis and Bourneville's tuberous sclerosis with pulmonary involvement: the same disease? Cancer 1983; 52(5): 851–855.
303. Costello LC, Hartman TE, Ryu JH: High frequency of pulmonary lymphangioleiomyomatosis in women with tuberous sclerosis complex. Mayo Clin Proc 2000; 75(6): 591–594.
304. Sato T, Seyama K, Fujii H, et al.: Mutation analysis of the TSC1 and 7TC2 genes in Japanese patients with pulmonary lymphangioleiomyomatosis. J Hum Genet 2002; 47(1): 20–28.
305. Yu J, Astrinidis A, Henske EP: Chromosome 16 loss of heterozygosity in tuberous sclerosis and sporadic lymphangiomyomatosis. Am J Respir Crit Care Med 2001; 164(8 Pt 1): 1537–1540.
306. Carsillo T, Astrinidis A, Henske EP: Mutations in the tuberous sclerosis complex gene TSC2 are a cause of sporadic pulmonary lymphangioleiomyomatosis. Proc Natl Acad Sci USA 2000; 97(11): 6085–6090.
307. Kang HW, Kim CJ, Kang SK, et al.: Pulmonary lymphangioleiomyomatosis in a male. J Korean Med Sci 1991; 6(1): 83–85.
308. Aubry MC, Myers JL, Ryu JH, et al.: Pulmonary lymphangioleiomyomatosis in a man. Am J Respir Crit Care Med 2000; 162(2 Pt 1): 749–752.
309. Corrin B, Liebow AA, Friedman PJ: Pulmonary lymphangiomyomatosis. A review. Am J Pathol 1975; 79(2): 348–382.
310. Lack EE, Dolan MF, Finisio J, et al.: Pulmonary and extrapulmonary lymphangioleiomyomatosis. Report of a case with bilateral renal angiomyolipomas, multifocal lymphangioleiomyomatosis, and a glial polyp of the endocervix. Am J Surg Pathol 1986; 10(9): 650–657.
311. Uzzo RG, Libby DM, Vaughan ED Jr, et al.: Coexisting lymphangioleiomyomatosis and bilateral angiomyolipomas in a patient with tuberous sclerosis. J Urol 1994; 151(6): 1612–1615.
312. Bernstein SM, Newell JD Jr, Adamczyk D, et al.: How common are renal angiomyolipomas in patients with pulmonary lymphangiomyomatosis? Am J Respir Crit Care Med 1995; 152(6 Pt 1): 2138–2143.
313. Maziak DE, Kesten S, Rappaport DC, et al.: Extrathoracic angiomyolipomas in lymphangioleiomyomatosis. Eur Respir J 1996; 9(3): 402–405.
314. Neumann HP, Schwarzkopf G, Henske EP: Renal angiomyolipomas, cysts, and cancer in tuberous sclerosis complex. Semin Pediatr Neurol 1998; 5(4): 269–275.
315. Tuzel E, Kirkali Z, Mungan U, et al.: Giant angiomyolipoma associated with marked pulmonary lesions suggesting lymphangioleiomyomatosis in a patient with tuberous sclerosis. Int Urol Nephrol 2000; 32(2): 219–222.
316. Muller NL, Chiles C, Kullnig P: Pulmonary lymphangiomyomatosis: correlation of CT with radiographic and functional findings. Radiology 1990; 175(2): 335–339.
317. Rappaport DC, Weisbrod GL, Herman SJ, et al.: Pulmonary lymphangioleiomyomatosis: high-resolution CT findings in four cases. AJR Am J Roentgenol 1989; 152(5): 961–964.
318. Templeton PA, McLoud TC, Muller NL, et al.: Pulmonary lymphangioleiomyomatosis: CT and pathologic findings. J Comput Assist Tomogr 1989; 13(1): 54–57.
319. Sherrier RH, Chiles C, Roggli V: Pulmonary lymphangioleiomyomatosis: CT findings. AJR Am J Roentgenol 1989; 153(5): 937–940.
320. Templeton P, McLoud T, Müller N, et al.: Pulmonary lymphangioleiomyomatosis: CT and pathologic findings. J Comput Assist Tomogr 1989; 13: 54–57.
321. Kirchner J, Stein A, Viel K, et al.: Pulmonary lymphangioleiomyomatosis: high-resolution CT findings. Eur Radiol 1999; 9(1): 49–54.
322. Shen A, Iseman MD, Waldron JA, et al.: Exacerbation of pulmonary lymphangioleiomyomatosis by exogenous estrogens. Chest 1987; 91(5): 782–785.
323. Eliasson AH, Phillips YY, Tenholder MF: Treatment of lymphangioleiomyomatosis. A meta-analysis. Chest 1989; 96(6): 1352–1355.
324. Ohori NP, Yousem SA, Sonmez-Alpan E, et al.: Estrogen and progesterone receptors in lymphangioleiomyomatosis, epithelioid hemangioendothelioma, and sclerosing hemangioma of the lung. Am J Clin Pathol 1991; 96(4): 529–535.
325. Rajjoub S, Blatt MW, Ritterspach J: Response to treatment with progesterone in a patient with pulmonary lymphangioleiomyomatosis. W V Med J 1995; 91(7): 322–323.
326. Colley MH, Geppert E, Franklin WA: Immunohistochemical detection of steroid receptors in a case of pulmonary lymphangioleiomyomatosis. Am J Surg Pathol 1989; 13(9): 803–807.
327. Berger U, Khaghani A, Pomerance A, et al.: Pulmonary lymphangioleiomyomatosis and steroid receptors. An immunocytochemical study. Am J Clin Pathol 1990; 93(5): 609–614.
328. Boehler A, Speich R, Russi EW, et al.: Lung transplantation for lymphangioleiomyomatosis. N Engl J Med 1996; 335(17): 1275–1280.
329. Bittmann I, Dose TB, Muller C, et al.: Lymphangioleiomyomatosis: recurrence after single lung transplantation. Hum Pathol 1997; 28(12): 1420–1423.
330. Schiavina M, Fabiani A, Cornia B, et al.: Lymphangioleiomyomatosis: clinical course. Monaldi Arch Chest Dis 1994; 49(1): 6–14.
331. Seyama K, Kira S, Takahashi H, et al.: Longitudinal follow-up study of 11 patients with pulmonary lymphangioleiomyomatosis: diverse clinical courses of LAM allow some patients to be treated without anti-hormone therapy. Respirology 2001; 6(4): 331–340.
332. Davies BH, Tuddenham EG: Familial pulmonary fibrosis associated with oculocutaneous albinism and platelet function defect. A new syndrome. Q J Med 1976; 45(178): 219–232.
333. DePinho RA, Kaplan KL: The Hermansky–Pudlak syndrome. Report of three cases and review of pathophysiology and management considerations. Medicine (Baltimore) 1985; 64(3): 192–202.
334. Dimson O, Drolet BA, Esterly NB: Hermansky–Pudlak syndrome. Pediatr Dermatol 1999; 16(6): 475–477.
335. Huizing M, Gahl WA: Disorders of vesicles of lysosomal lineage: the Hermansky–Pudlak syndromes. Curr Mol Med 2002; 2(5): 451–467.
336. Anikster Y, Huizing M, White J, et al.: Mutation of a new gene causes a unique form of Hermansky–Pudlak syndrome in a genetic isolate of central Puerto Rico. Nat Genet 2001; 28(4): 376–380.

337. Hermos CR, Huizing M, Kaiser-Kupfer MI, et al.: Hermansky–Pudlak syndrome type 1: gene organization, novel mutations, and clinical-molecular review of non-Puerto Rican cases. Hum Mutat 2002; 20(6): 482.
338. Okano A, Sato A, Chida K, et al.: [Pulmonary interstitial pneumonia in association with Hermansky–Pudlak syndrome]. Nihon Kyobu Shikkan Gakkai Zasshi 1991; 29(12): 1596–1602.
339. Avila NA, Brantly M, Premkumar A, et al.: Hermansky–Pudlak syndrome: radiography and CT of the chest compared with pulmonary function tests and genetic studies. AJR Am J Roentgenol 2002; 179(4): 887–892.
340. Nakatani Y, Nakamura N, Sano J, et al.: Interstitial pneumonia in Hermansky–Pudlak syndrome: significance of florid foamy swelling/degeneration (giant lamellar body degeneration) of type-2 pneumocytes. Virchows Arch 2000; 437(3): 304–313.
341. Gahl WA, Brantly M, Troendle J, et al.: Effect of pirfenidone on the pulmonary fibrosis of Hermansky–Pudlak syndrome. Mol Genet Metab 2002; 76(3): 234–242.
342. Sosman M, Dodd G, Jones W, et al.: The familial occurrence of pulmonary alveolar microlithiasis. AJR 1957; 77: 947–952.
343. Fuleihan F, Abboud R, Balikian J, et al.: Pulmonary alveolar microlithiasis: lung function in five cases. Thorax 1969; 24: 84–90.
344. Prakash UB, Barham SS, Rosenow EC 3rd, et al.: Pulmonary alveolar microlithiasis. A review including ultrastructural and pulmonary function studies. Mayo Clin Proc 1983; 58(5): 290–300.
345. Moran CA, Hochholzer L, Hasleton PS, et al.: Pulmonary alveolar microlithiasis. A clinicopathologic and chemical analysis of seven cases. Arch Pathol Lab Med 1997; 121(6): 607–611.
346. Castellana G, Gentile M, Castellana R, Fiorente P, Lamorgese V: Pulmonary alveolar microlithiasis: clinical features, evolution of the phenotype, and review of the literature. Am J Med Genet 2002; 111(2): 220–224.
347. Senyigit A, Yaramis A, Gurkan F, et al.: Pulmonary alveolar microlithiasis: a rare familial inheritance with report of six cases in a family. Contribution of six new cases to the number of case reports in Turkey. Respiration 2001; 68(2): 204–209.
348. Pant K, Shah A, Mathur R, et al.: Pulmonary alveolar microlithiasis with pleural calcification and nephrolithiasis. Chest 1990; 98: 245–246.
349. Schmidt H, Lorcher U, Kitz R, et al.: Pulmonary alveolar microlithiasis in children. Pediatr Radiol 1996; 26(1): 33–36.
350. Chang Y, Yang P, Luh K, et al.: High-resolution computed tomography of pulmonary alveolar microlithiasis. J Formos Med Assoc 1999; 98(6): 440–443.
351. Singh G, Katyal S, Bedrossian C, et al.: Pulmonary alveolar proteinosis; staining for surfactant apoprotein in alveolar proteinosis and in conditions simulating it. Chest 1983; 83: 82–86.
352. Miller R, Churg A, Hutcheon M, et al.: Pulmonary alveolar proteinosis and aluminum dust exposure. Am Rev Respir Dis 1984; 130: 312–315.
353. Bedrossian C, Luna M, Conklin R, et al.: Alveolar proteinosis as a consequence of immunosuppression. A hypothesis based on clinical and pathologic observations. Hum Pathol 1980; Suppl 11: 527–535.
354. Wang Y, Xia J, Wang QW: Clinical report on 62 cases of acute dimethyl sulfate intoxication. Am J Ind Med 1988; 13(4): 455–462.
355. Seymour J, Presneill J: Pulmonary alveolar proteinosis: progress in the first 44 years. Am J Respir Crit Care Med 2002; 166(2): 215–235.
356. Shah P, Hansell D, Lawson P, et al.: Pulmonary alveolar proteinosis: clinical aspects and current concepts in pathogenesis. Thorax 2000; 55: 67–77.
357. Davidson J, MacLeod W: Pulmonary alveolar proteinosis. Br J Dis Chest 1969; 63: 13–16.
358. Carraway M, Piantadosi C, Wright J: Alveolar proteinosis: a disease of mice and men. Am J Physiol Lung Cell Mol Physiol 2001; 280(3): L377–L78.
359. Godwin JD, Muller NL, Takasugi JE: Pulmonary alveolar proteinosis: CT findings. Radiology 1988; 169(3): 609–613.
360. Claypool W, Roger R, Matuschak G: Update on the clinical diagnosis, management, and pathogenesis of pulmonary alveolar proteinosis (phospholipidosis). Chest 1984; 85: 550–558.
361. Heitzman ER: The lung: radiologic-pathologic correlations, 2nd edn. 1984, CV Mosby, St Louis.
362. Munk P, Müller N, Miller R, et al.: Pulmonary lymphangitic carcinomatosis: CT and pathologic findings. Radiology 1988; 166: 705–709.
363. Janower M, Blennerhassett J: Lymphangitic spread of metastatic cancer to the lung. A radiologic-pathologic classification. Radiology 1971; 101: 267–273.
364. Stein M, Mayo J, Müller N, et al.: Pulmonary lymphangitic spread of carcinoma: appearance on CT scans. Radiology 1987; 162: 371–375.
365. Goldsmith S, Bailey H, Callahan E, et al.: Pulmonary metastases from breast carcinoma. Surgery 1967; 94: 483–488.
366. Wall C, Gaensler E, Carrington C, et al.: Comparison of transbronchial and open biopsies in chronic infiltrative lung disease. Am Rev Respir Dis 1981; 123: 280–285.
367. Katzenstein A, Fiorelli R: Nonspecific interstitial pneumonia/fibrosis: histologic features and clinical significance. Am J Surg Pathol 1994; 18: 136–147.
368. Colby TV, Lombard C, Yousem S, et al.: Atlas of pulmonary surgical pathology. In: Atlases in diagnostic surgical pathology, 1st Vol, Bordin G, Ed. 1991, WB Saunders, Philadelphia, p 380.
369. Kennedy JI, Myers JL, Plumb VJ, et al.: Amiodarone pulmonary toxicity. Clinical, radiologic, and pathologic correlations. Arch Intern Med 1987; 147(1): 50–55.
370. Olivieri D, Pesci A, Bertorelli G: Eosinophilic alveolitis in immunologic interstitial lung disorders. Lung 1990; 168(Suppl): 964–973.
371. Musk AW, Pollard JA: Pindolol and pulmonary fibrosis. Br Med J 1979; 2(6190): 581–582.
372. Levy MB, Fink JN, Guzzetta PA: Nadolol and hypersensitivity pneumonitis. Ann Intern Med 1986; 105(5): 806–807.
373. Camus P, Lombard JN, Perrichon M, et al.: Bronchiolitis obliterans organising pneumonia in patients taking acebutolol or amiodarone. Thorax 1989; 44(9): 711–715.
374. Luna MA, Bedrossian CW, Lichtiger B, et al.: Interstitial pneumonitis associated with bleomycin therapy. Am J Clin Pathol 1972; 58(5): 501–510.
375. Lombard CM, Churg A, Winokur S: Pulmonary veno-occlusive disease following therapy for malignant neoplasms. Chest 1987; 92(5): 871–876.
376. Littler WA, Kay JM, Hasleton PS, et al.: Busulphan lung. Thorax 1969; 24(6): 639–655.
377. Hasleton PS: Busulphan lung: histopathology. Thorax 1970; 25(2): 257.
378. Mitsudo SM, Greenwald ES, Banerji B, et al.: BCNU (1,3-bis-(2-chloroethyl)-1-nitrosurea) lung. Drug-induced pulmonary changes. Cancer 1984; 54(4): 751–755.
379. Forrester JM, Steele AW, Waldron JA, et al.: Crack lung: an acute pulmonary syndrome with a spectrum of clinical and histopathologic findings. Am Rev Respir Dis 1990; 142(2): 462–467.
380. Murray RJ, Albin RJ, Mergner W, et al.: Diffuse alveolar hemorrhage temporally related to cocaine smoking. Chest 1988; 93(2): 427–429.
381. Abdel Karim FW, Ayash RE, Allam C, et al.: Pulmonary fibrosis after prolonged treatment with low-dose cyclophosphamide. A case report. Oncology 1983; 40(3): 174–176.
382. Patel AR, Shah PC, Rhee HL, et al.: Cyclophosphamide therapy and interstitial pulmonary fibrosis. Cancer 1976; 38(4): 1542–1549.
383. Spector JI, Zimbler H, Ross JS: Early-onset cyclophosphamide-induced interstitial pneumonitis. JAMA 1979; 242(26): 2852–2854.
384. Slavin RE, Millan JC, Mullins GM: Pathology of high dose intermittent cyclophosphamide therapy. Hum Pathol 1975; 6(6): 693–709.
385. Pfitzenmeyer P, Foucher P, Dennewald G, et al.: Pleuropulmonary changes induced by ergoline drugs. Eur Respir J 1996; 9(5): 1013–1019.
386. Gurjal A, An T, Valdivieso M, et al.: Etoposide-induced pulmonary toxicity. Lung Cancer 1999; 26(2): 109–112.
387. Inoue A, Saijo Y, Maemondo M, et al.: Severe acute interstitial pneumonia and gefitinib. Lancet 2003; 361(9352): 137–139.
388. Warnock ML, Ghahremani GG, Rattenborg C, et al.: Pulmonary complication of heroin intoxication. Aspiration pneumonia and diffuse bronchiectasis. JAMA 1972; 219(8): 1051–1053.
389. Karne S, D'Ambrosio C, Einarsson O, et al.: Hypersensitivity pneumonitis induced by intranasal heroin use. Am J Med 1999; 107(4): 392–395.
390. Stableforth DE: Chronic lung disease. Pulmonary fibrosis. Br J Hosp Med 1979; 22(2): 128, 32–35.
391. Petersen AG, Dodge M, Helwig FC: Pulmonary changes associated with hexamethonium therapy. Arch Intern Med 1959; 103: 285–288.
392. Perry HM Jr, O'Neal RM, Thomas WA: Pulmonary disease following chronic chemical ganglionic blockade. Am J Med 1957; 22: 37–50.

393. Beaudry C, Laplante L: Severe allergic pneumonitis from hydrochlorothiazide. Ann Intern Med 1973; 78(2): 251–253.
394. Kaufman A, Montilla E, Helfgott M, et al.: Pneumonitis and hydrochlorothiazide. Ann Intern Med 1973; 79(2): 282–283.
395. Dorn MR, Walker BK: Noncardiogenic pulmonary edema associated with hydrochlorothiazide therapy. Chest 1981; 79(4): 482–483.
396. Travis WD, Kalafer ME, Robin HS, et al.: Hypersensitivity pneumonitis and pulmonary vasculitis with eosinophilia in a patient taking an L-tryptophan preparation. Ann Intern Med 1990; 112(4): 301–303.
397. Catton CK, Elmer JC, Whitehouse AC, et al.: Pulmonary involvement in the eosinophilia-myalgia syndrome. Chest 1991; 99(2): 327–329.
398. Cordonnier C, Vernant JP, Mital P, et al.: Pulmonary fibrosis subsequent to high doses of CCNU for chronic myeloid leukemia. Cancer 1983; 51(10): 1814–1818.
399. Bentur L, Bar-Kana Y, Livni E, et al.: Severe minocycline-induced eosinophilic pneumonia: extrapulmonary manifestations and the use of in vitro immunoassays. Ann Pharmacother 1997; 31(6): 733–735.
400. Piperno D, Donne C, Loire R, et al.: Bronchiolitis obliterans organizing pneumonia associated with minocycline therapy: a possible cause. Eur Respir J 1995; 8(6): 1018–1020.
401. Waldhorn RE, Tsou E, Smith FP, et al.: Pulmonary veno-occlusive disease associated with microangiopathic hemolytic anemia and chemotherapy of gastric adenocarcinoma. Med Pediatr Oncol 1984; 12(6): 394–396.
402. Fielding JW, Crocker J, Stockley RA, et al.: Interstitial fibrosis in a patient treated with 5-fluorouracil and mitomycin C. Br Med J 1979; 2(6189): 551–552.
403. Israel KS, Brashear RE, Sharma HM, et al.: Pulmonary fibrosis and nitrofurantoin. Am Rev Respir Dis 1973; 108(2): 353–356.
404. Geller M, Dickie HA, Kass DA, et al.: The histopathology of acute nitrofurantoin-associated penumonitis. Ann Allergy 1976; 37(4): 275–279.
405. Carrington CB, Addington WW, Goff AM et al.: Chronic eosinophilic pneumonia. N Engl J Med 1969; 280(15): 787–798.
406. Magee F, Wright JL, Chan N, et al.: Two unusual pathological reactions to nitrofurantoin: case reports. Histopathology 1986; 10(7): 701–706.
407. Epler GR, Snider GL, Gaensler EA, et al.: Bronchiolitis and bronchitis in connective tissue disease. A possible relationship to the use of penicillamine. JAMA 1979; 242(6): 528–532.
408. Sternlieb I, Bennett B, Scheinberg IH: D-penicillamine induced Goodpasture's syndrome in Wilson's disease. Ann Intern Med 1975; 82(5): 673–676.
409. Davies D, Jones JK: Pulmonary eosinophilia caused by penicillamine. Thorax 1980; 35(12): 957–958.
410. Chamberlain DW, Hyland RH, Ross DJ: Diphenylhydantoin-induced lymphocytic interstitial pneumonia. Chest 1986; 90(3): 458–460.
411. Michael JR, Rudin ML: Acute pulmonary disease caused by phenytoin. Ann Intern Med 1981; 95(4): 452–454.
412. Dohner VA, Ward HP, Standord RE: Alveolitis during procarbazine, vincristine and cyclophosphamide therapy. Chest 1972; 62(5): 636–639.
413. Farney RJ, Morris AH, Armstrong JD, et al.: Diffuse pulmonary disease after therapy with nitrogen mustard, vincristine, procarbazine, and prednisone. Am Rev Respir Dis 1977; 115(1): 135–145.
414. Horton LW, Chappell AG, Powell DE: Diffuse interstitial pulmonary fibrosis complicating Hodgkin's disease. Br J Dis Chest 1977; 71(1): 44–48.
415. Gonzalez-Rothi RJ, Zander DS, Ros PR: Fluoxetine hydrochloride (Prozac)-induced pulmonary disease. Chest 1995; 107(6): 1763–1765.
416. Parry SD, Barbatzas C, Peel ET, et al.: Sulphasalazine and lung toxicity. Eur Respir J 2002; 19(4): 756–764.
417. Calvo DB 3rd, Legha SS, McKelvey EM, et al.: Zinostatin-related pulmonary toxicity. Cancer Treat Rep 1981; 65(1–2): 165–167.

8

Pathology of the large and small airways

Mattia Barbareschi   Kevin O Leslie

The conducting airways

The trachea and conducing airways play a vital role in lung function. The diseases that affect these structures are commonly related to inhalation exposure, but may also arise from developmental anomalies and systemic diseases (Table 8.1). In this chapter we will begin with the trachea and proceed distally to the bronchi and bronchioles. Our focus remains centered on those diseases and conditions that are likely to come to the attention of the surgical pathologist. We begin with descriptions of individual lesions of the trachea and conducting airways along with the different diseases where these lesions may be encountered. In a separate section we will describe a few of the more specific clinicopathologic entities classically associated with disease of the airways, such as asthma, chronic obstructive pulmonary disease (COPD), and emphysema.

Table 8.1 Non-neoplastic diseases of the trachea and bronchi

Asthma
Bronchitis: Infectious Irritant Collagen vascular disease Miscellaneous inflammatory diseases
Bronchiectasis
Bronchocentric granulomatosis
Mucoid impaction of the bronchi
Allergic bronchopulmonary fungal disease
Plastic bronchitis
Tracheobronchomegaly
Congenital bronchial cartilage deficiency
Relapsing polychondritis
Broncholithiasis, bronchostenosis
Miscellaneous conditions (tracheobronchial amyloid, tracheomalacia, tracheobronchopathia osteochrondroplastica)

The trachea

The pathology of the trachea can be subdivided into intrinsic and extrinsic diseases. Diseases intrinsic and unique to the trachea are few and include congenital and metabolic diseases primarily. Most of the non-neoplastic diseases recognized in the trachea also involve the larynx and/or the conducting airways. We will discuss and illustrate three of these – tracheal amyloid, tracheobronchomalacia, and tracheobronchopathia osteochondroplastica – since each may be encountered in bronchoscopic biopsy specimens.

Tracheal amyloid

Tracheobronchial amyloidosis is an idiopathic disease characterized by amyloid deposition, often throughout the tracheobronchial tree but sometimes restricted to the trachea.[1] Approximately 100 patients have been reported in the literature. Tracheobronchial amyloidosis most frequently produces dyspnea, wheezing (sometimes misdiagnosed as asthma), recurrent pneumonia, and atelectasis, which are believed to be sequelae of the narrowed airways. Pulmonary function tests usually show fixed obstruction. Pathologically, amyloid deposits usually occur in the submucosa and may involve the entire tracheal or bronchial wall with irregular masses or sheets (Fig. 8.1). Amyloid may be accompanied by multinucleated giant cells; calcification and ossification are frequent (Fig. 8.2).[1–4] When amyloid is identified in bronchoscopic biopsy specimens, this is typically an organ-limited manifestation, similar to nodular parenchymal amyloid. Of the three major types of amyloid (AL, AA, and transthyretin), tracheobronchial amyloid is most commonly of the AL type. The prognosis is poor, as almost one-third of patients die within 7–12 years of diagnosis.[1] Therapy is limited to debulking procedures for localized lesions, although there are suggestions that radiation therapy may provide more definitive treatment.[5–8]

Tracheobronchomalacia

Tracheobronchomalacia (soft or collapsing trachea/bronchi) is a disease of the airway wall, that may affect children but also occurs in adults.[9] In children, the disease is most often related to prematurity and prolonged mechanical ventilation. In most affected individuals, the disease is self-limited.[10,11] In adults, it is seen in the middle aged and elderly, and is a progressive condition. Tracheobronchomalacia may be related to *relapsing polychondritis*, a systemic disease affecting the cartilaginous tissue in several organs, including the airways.[9,12–14] Pathologically, the tracheal wall becomes soft as a result of inflammatory destruction of the cartilage (Fig. 8.3). Over time, the cartilage becomes replaced by inflammation, accompanied by vascular proliferation and fibrous tissue.

Tracheobronchopathia osteochondroplastica

This rare lung disease is characterized by the presence of cartilaginous and/or osseous submucosal nodules that

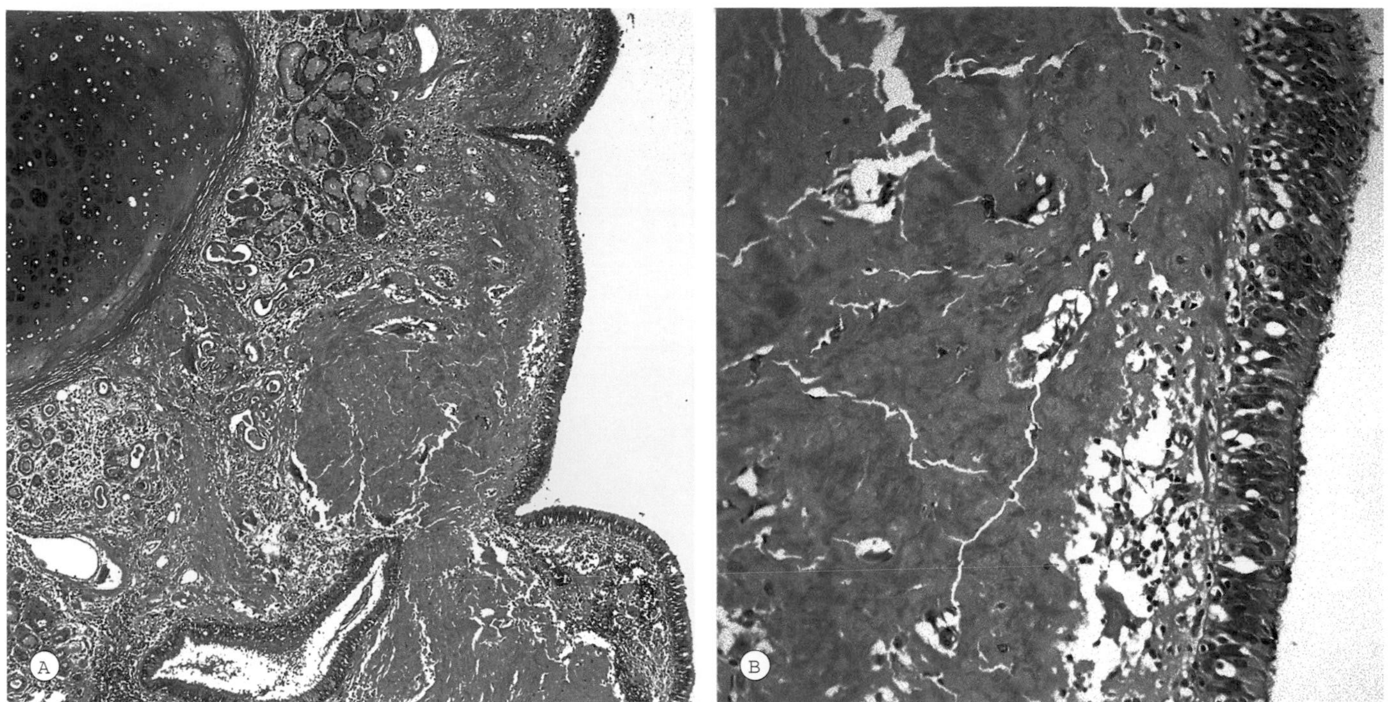

Fig. 8.1 **Tracheal amyloid.** (A) A low-power magnification view shows the tracheal wall with diffuse amyloid deposition. (B) At higher magnification the amyloid is present just below the respiratory epithelium.

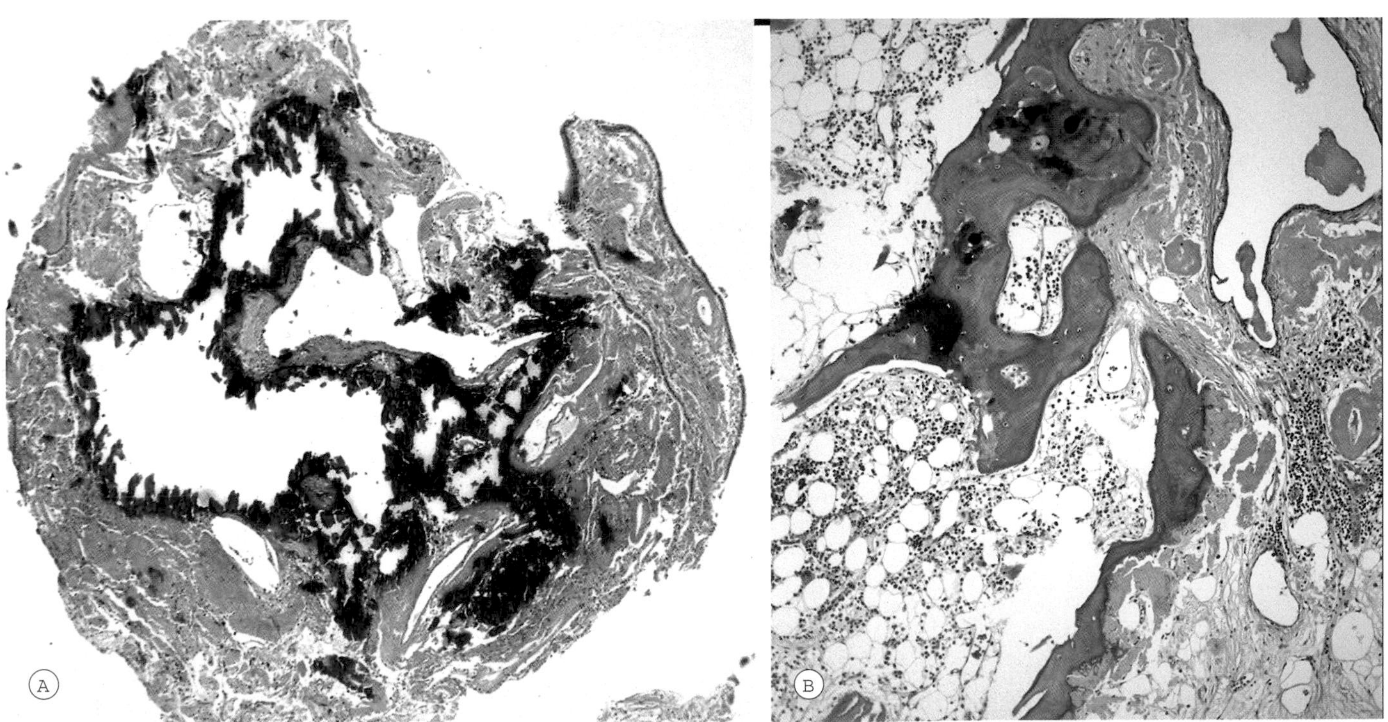

Fig. 8.2 **Tracheal amyloid.** (A) Tracheal biopsy, showing an example where the amyloid is diffusely calcified. (B) Osseous metaplasia can occur in tracheal amyloid.

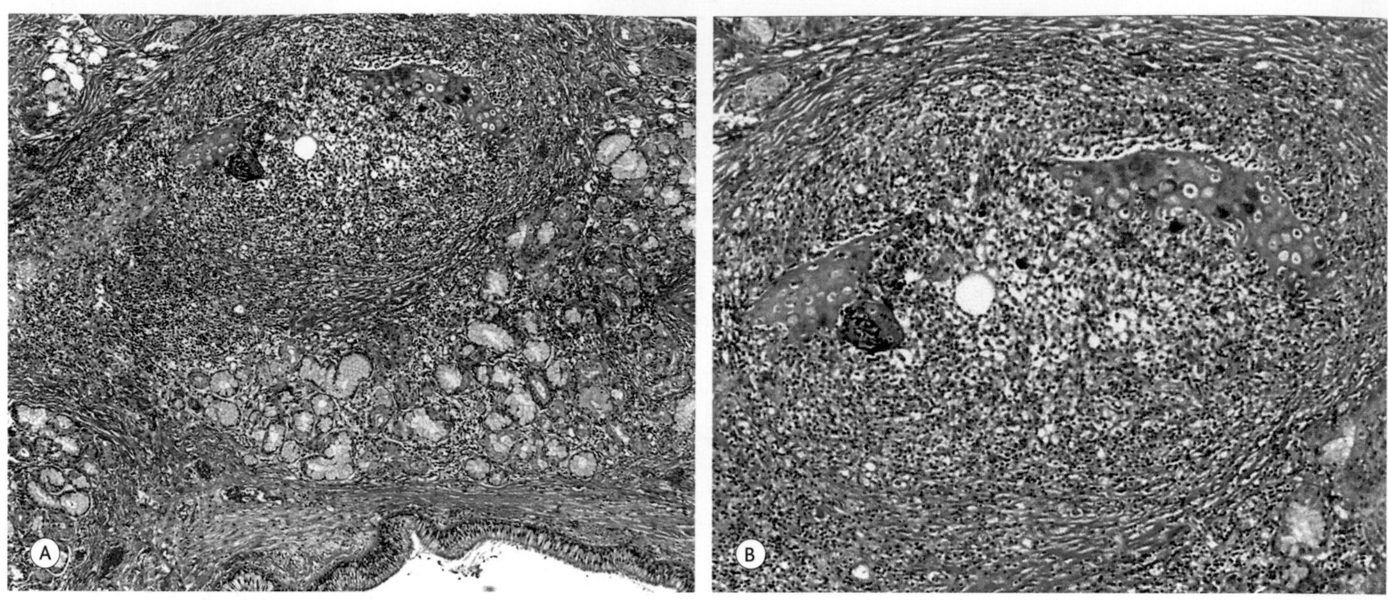

Fig. 8.3 **Tracheal chondritis.** (A) The cartilage of the tracheal wall is surrounded and replaced by inflammatory, vascular, and fibrous tissue. A higher magnification of the cartilage destruction in this process is presented in B (from A, upper-center).

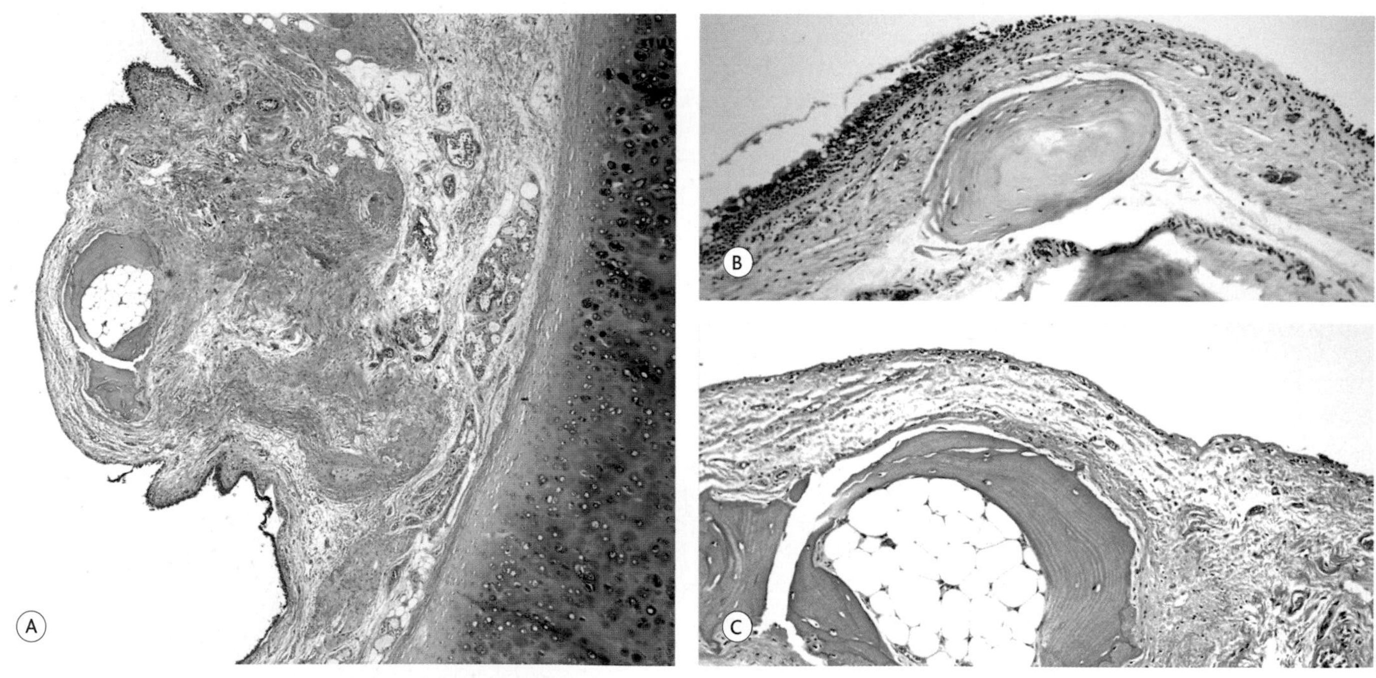

Fig. 8.4 **Tracheobronchopathia osteochondroplastica.** (A) The panoramic view shows a nodular protrusion into the tracheal lumen, composed of fibrous tissue and mature bone. (C) An area from the same nodule is shown at higher magnification. (B) An example from a different patient, showing osseous metaplasia.

bulge into the lumen of the trachea and bronchi (Fig. 8.4), sparing the posterior membranous portion.[15–17] The etiology and pathogenesis are unknown. The disease affects adults more commonly than children and there is a male gender predilection. Most cases are asymptomatic and are most often diagnosed incidentally during intubation or bronchoscopy. A minority of patients may experience cough, dyspnea, and hemoptysis. When the cartilaginous or ossified lesions of tracheobronchopathia osteochondroplastica are seen in bronchoscopic biopsies, the differential diagnosis includes ossified amyloid deposits. Other conditions associated with endoluminal nodular lesions include endobronchial sarcoidosis, endobronchial granulomatous infections, papillomatosis, and tracheobronchial calcinosis.[16,17]

The bronchi

The conducting airways begin at the carina and extend distally in the lung to the level of the noncartilaginous bronchioles. While many diffuse lung diseases may involve the large airways secondarily, there are some primary diseases that will be presented here. Asthma-associated diseases, typically observed in the large airways, are discussed in the final section of this chapter. Cystic fibrosis and ciliary disorders will not be discussed here as detailed expositions can be found in other sources.[18–20]

Bronchitis

Infectious and inflammatory conditions of the large airways are particularly relevant to the surgical pathologist and cytopathologist, given the prominence of inflammatory manifestations seen in biopsies obtained through the bronchoscope (endobronchial and transbronchial biopsies). In practice, the presence of acute and/or chronic inflammation in endobronchial biopsies, where bronchial mucosa and muscle or cartilage are evident, demand a descriptive diagnosis (Fig. 8.5). It is best to avoid the use of the term "chronic bronchitis" in reference to such inflammatory changes involving respiratory mucosa since they carry a clinical implication regarding the diffuse nature of the disease and specific clinical manifestations. When bronchitis occurs as a direct result of respiratory infection, necrosis of the mucosa may be present (acute necrotizing bronchitis). In the post-infection period, residual chronic inflammatory changes may be the dominant findings. Unfortunately, the list of possible etiologies for the presence of chronic inflammation in bronchial mucosa is quite long (Table 8.2) and sufficiently diverse as to not be useful in narrowing the clinical differential diagnosis. For this reason, a careful search for other more specific findings is always in order and these are worth mentioning as a list of pertinent negative findings (vasculitis, granulomas, necrosis, tumor, etc.).

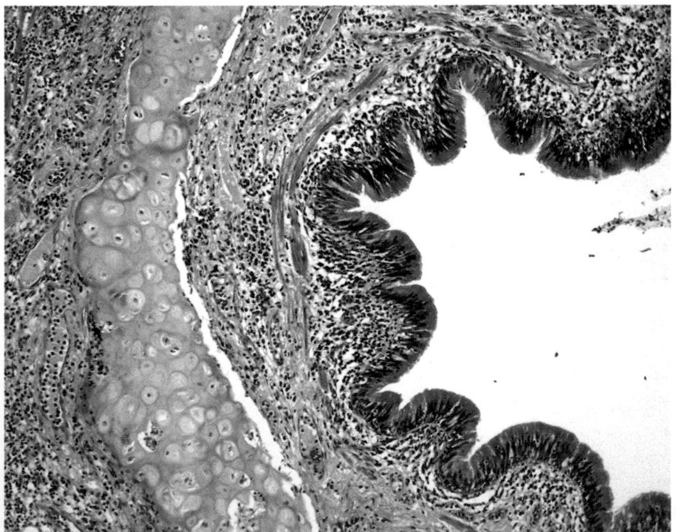

Fig. 8.5 **Bronchitis.** The bronchial wall shows a chronic inflammatory infiltrate in the subepithelial connective tissue and surrounding cartilage.

Bronchiectasis

Bronchiectasis is a worldwide problem, less prominent in the United States possibly as a consequence of liberal antibiotic use in childhood infections. In specific conditions, such as cystic fibrosis, bronchiectasis may dominate the pulmonary pathology. Bronchiectasis is defined as a permanent dilatation of the cartilaginous airways (bronchi), often attended by acute and chronic inflammation. Conceptually, bronchiectasis can be considered the end result of any number of conditions that damage the airway wall and result in weakening over time and dilatation. Primary causes are most commonly related to inherited abnormalities (ciliary dysfunction, abnormal mucus production), whereas secondary causes are numerous. Bronchiectasis in the living patient is a radiologic diagnosis, having distinctive features in resected lungs, lobes and, rarely, in surgical biopsies.

The proposed historical classification of bronchiectasis divided the process into:

- saccular type, characterized by progressive dilatation of the bronchi from central to peripheral
- varicose type, where combined dilatation and constriction dominate the picture without a consistent pattern

Table 8.2 Possible causes of chronic inflammation in bronchoscopic biopsies

Clinical chronic bronchitis
Post-infectious
Hypersensitivity reactions
Allergic bronchopulmonary fungal disease
Bronchiectasis
Reaction at the periphery of a tumor, abscess, or infection
MALT lymphoma
Follicular bronchiolitis
Drug reactions
Toxic inhalation

MALT = mucosa-associated lymphoid tissue.

- cylindrical type, where uniform dilatation is evident, primarily as a manifestation of loss of normal tapering.

Such a classification has come under intense scrutiny with the advent of high-resolution computed tomography (HRCT) scanning, where the airways can be better defined in three-dimensional space, through computer-enhanced reconstruction.

Clinical presentation

Presenting symptoms include cough, production of purulent sputum, fever, shortness of breath, and, occasionally, hemoptysis. No age or sex predilection occurs and the disease tends to run a course of recurrent exacerbation, sometime with superimposed infection. In a review of multiple published series of bronchiectasis between 1935 and 1981, Barker and Bardana[21] found a significant proportion of idiopathic cases (as much as 30% according to Nicotra et al.[22]) Among recognizable causes of bronchiectasis are infections, primary ciliary dyskinesia, immunodeficiency, cystic fibrosis, rheumatoid arthritis, and inflammatory bowel disease.[23] An intriguing implication of *Helicobacter pylori* in the pathogeneses has been raised in some studies.[24,25]

Findings in bronchoscopy

Inflammatory changes in biopsies obtained with the bronchoscope correlate poorly with the presence or absence of bronchiectasis. Nevertheless, such biopsies may be useful for ancillary laboratory studies (such as ultrastructural studies in search of ciliary abnormalities).

Radiologic findings

On plain films of the chest, classic parallel linear opacities (referred to as "tram tracks") correspond to thickened bronchial walls, whereas tubular opacities reflect mucus-filled bronchi. Today, most cases of bronchiectasis are diagnosed by HRCT scans.[26] Overall, the sensitivity of HRCT in detecting bronchiectasis is quite high.[27,28] The HRCT findings in bronchiectasis are presented in Table 8.3.

Pathologic findings

The gross findings in bronchiectasis have been well described from autopsy studies.[29] For the surgical pathologist, acute and chronic inflammatory changes dominate the biopsy picture. The presence of necrotic debris and mucus in airways may be a sign of coexistent bronchiectasis, but, in most instances, the surgical lung biopsy findings only reflect "downstream" secondary manifestations of obstruction or infection occurring more proximally. Lymphoid hyperplasia surrounding the large airways may occur in bronchiectasis and bronchoscopically derived biopsies may sample such hyperplastic lymphoid tissue, raising concern for tumor on occasion (especially when a portion of a germinal center dominates the small biopsy specimen) (Fig. 8.6). Caution is always advisable in these settings to avoid the overdiagnosis of lymphoproliferative disease. Also, the necrotic granular debris that may accompany bronchiectasis may be sampled in bronchoscopic biopsies, thereby raising concern for necrotic neoplasm or abscess. Again, a broad differential diagnosis is the best approach here to avoid confusion and possible misdirection of clinical management.

Table 8.3 High-resolution computed tomography findings in bronchiectasis

- Lack of bronchial tapering
- Presence of visible bronchi within 1 cm of the costal pleura
- Visible bronchial lumens abutting mediastinal pleura, bronchi as horizontally disposed parallel lines (tram tracks)
- Bronchial diameter exceeding adjacent pulmonary artery diameter ("signet ring sign")
- Irregular bronchial dilatation
- Clustered thin-walled cystic spaces with or without air-fluid levels

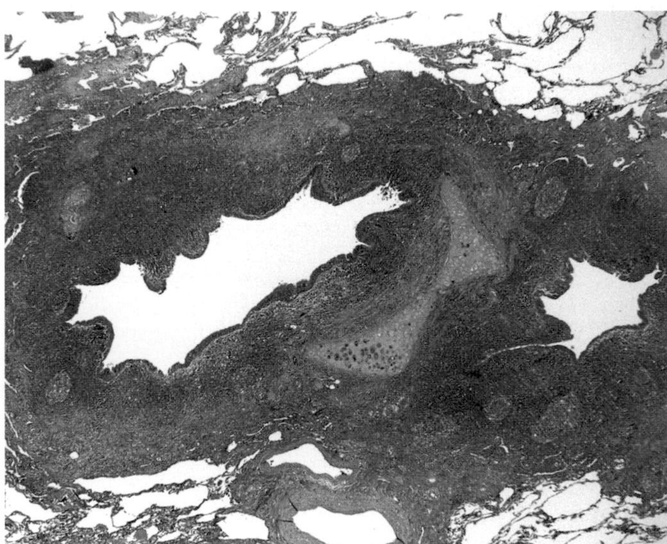

Fig. 8.6 **Bronchiectasis.** The lumen of the bronchus is dilated and there is prominent chronic inflammation in the bronchial wall.

Middle lobe syndrome

Middle lobe syndrome is discussed here because the disease is fundamentally one of chronic large airway obstruction with secondary bronchiectasis, bronchitis, and bronchiolitis-associated parenchymal changes that

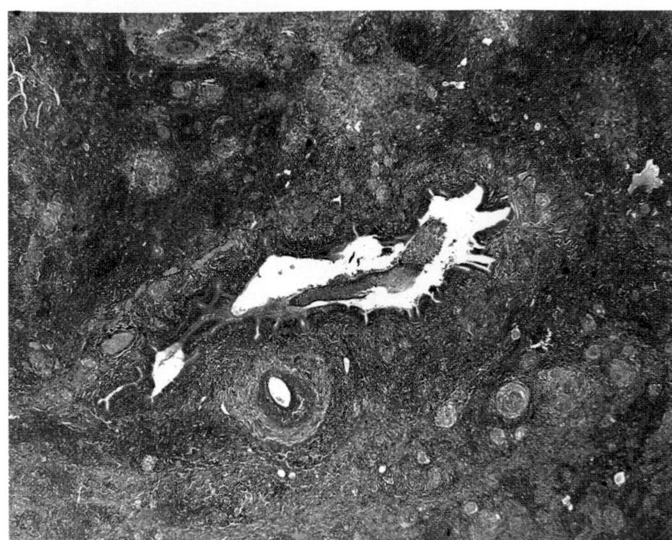

Fig. 8.7 **Middle lobe syndrome.** The bronchial wall shows prominent lymphoid infiltration, with many germinal centers.

arise as additional downstream effects of these airway abnormalities.

The concept of right middle lobe syndrome was highlighted in studies of children with chronic failure to thrive and right middle lobe abnormalities on chest radiographs. The hypothesis proposed was based on the notion that lymphoid hyperplasia occurring around the right middle lobe bronchus produced compression and narrowing of the bronchial lumen. Also, the position of the middle lobe (and the lingula of the left lung) relative to the remainder of the lung and tracheal bronchial tree makes it susceptible to subacute obstruction and secondary chronic inflammatory changes in the lobe (long narrow bronchus). In practice, the disease occurs more frequently in adults, often without an identifiable obstructing lesion,[30] and this population is dominated by middle-aged or elderly women (so-called Lady Windemere's syndrome).[31,32]

Radiographic findings

Consolidation of the right middle lobe, or lingula, attended by bronchiectasis, is typical.[30]

Pathologic findings

In surgical lung biopsies of the right middle lobe or lingula, advanced remodeling, granulomatous inflammation, extensive inflammatory infiltrates, and mucostasis, when present together, should always raise middle lobe syndrome as a possibility (Fig. 8.7). Colonization by atypical mycobacterial species may occur and acid-fast organisms may be identified in granulomas.[31] It has been suggested that atypical mycobacterial species actually participate in the early stages of the disease process but this notion is based mainly on circumstantial evidence. A number of inflammatory changes are observed in middle lobe syndrome and these are listed in Table 8.4.[33]

Table 8.4 Pathologic findings in middle lobe syndrome

- Bronchiectasis
- Follicular bronchiolitis
- Organizing pneumonia
- Bronchial lithiasis
- Atelectasis
- Granulomas (mainly due to *Mycobacterium avium-intracellulare*)
- Abscesses
- Hemosiderosis
- Interstitial fibrosis and honeycomb changes
- Pleural fibrosis

Source: modified from Kwon et al.[30]

Treatment

Removal of any obstructing lesions, whether neoplasm or other, in early stages of the disease process may avoid surgical resection.[32]

The small airways (bronchioles and alveolar ducts)

The small airways of the lung include the small bronchi, with a diameter less than 2–3 mm, and the membranous bronchioles (terminal and respiratory bronchioles). Terminal bronchioles (TB) have a diameter of less than 1 mm and are just proximal to the respiratory bronchioles (RB), the first airways that have alveoli budding from their walls. The TB are located in the center of the pulmonary lobule and, like all conducting airways, are always accompanied by a pulmonary artery branch (Fig. 8.8). In cross-sectional views, their respective diameters are approximately equal (Fig. 8.9A). The lumen of the TB is uniform in longitudinal histologic sections, but minor variations in size can be seen (Fig. 8.9B).

It is said that the small airways are the "Achilles heel" of the lung, as they play an important role in air distribution and flow, but lack the rigid structure of the bronchi to protect them from collapse during exhalation, especially when affected by disease. The small airways can be affected secondarily by inflammatory diseases that involve primarily the bronchi and/or the alveoli, or by primary diseases that selectively involve these delicate anatomic structures.

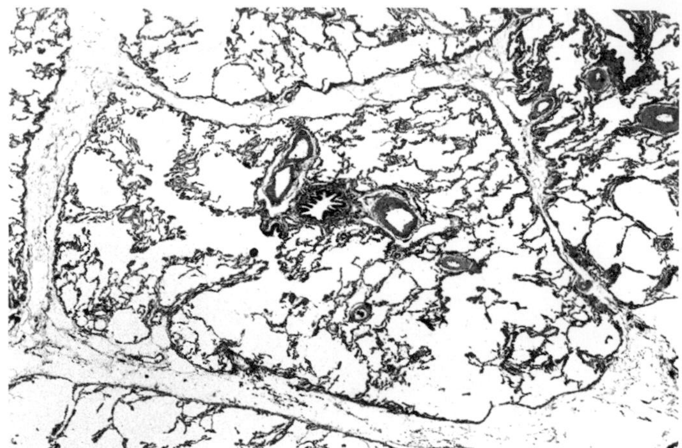

Fig. 8.8 **Normal lobule.** A near-normal pulmonary lobule, whose outlines are enhanced in this patient by a slight degree of edema of the septa. In the middle of the lobule is the bronchiole along with the adjacent pulmonary artery. Note that the diameter of the terminal bronchiole, seen here in cross section, is very similar to that of the nearby arteries.

Patients are rarely subjected to lung biopsy with a preoperative diagnosis of "small airways disease." The reasons for this are legion, but mainly result from the small airways being relatively "silent" clinically and radiologically. In addition, some of the small airways lesions are quite subtle histologically and, at first glance, may be overlooked.[34,35] Here, we will present the elemental histopathologic lesions of the small airways observable in lung biopsies and relate them to the main diseases/patterns where they can be encountered. We will also briefly overview some general histologic patterns of lesions or specific diseases that may involve the small airways. It is important to recognize that the elementary lesions rarely occur in isolation, and are frequently combined together.

It is the rare lung biopsy that does not show some degree of histopathologic alteration in the small airways. Critical to the evaluation of such changes is the knowl-

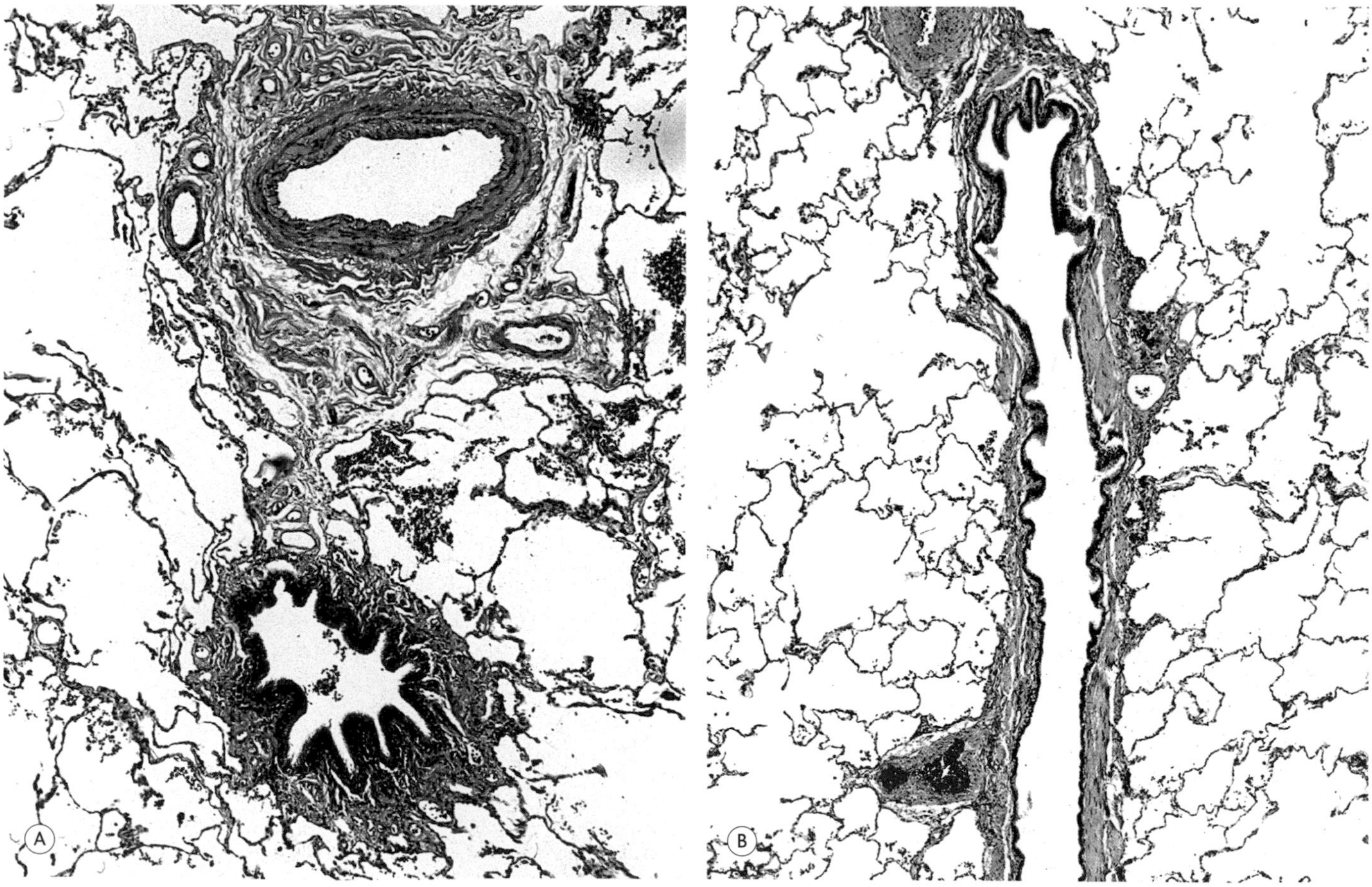

Fig. 8.9 **Terminal bronchiole.** (A) A cross section of a terminal bronchiole and adjacent artery. The normal terminal bronchiole has a thin wall and an open lumen. The wall is composed of a variably enfolded mucosa, showing a columnar to cuboidal epithelium with ciliated columnar cells and Clara cells. In longitudinal sections, the lumen of the normal bronchiole is regular and there is little tortuosity evident. (B) This bronchiole is cut lengthwise, its major axis is relatively straight, and the lumen has a relatively constant diameter.

Table 8.5 High-resolution computed abnormalities tomography of the small airways

Radiologic finding	Pathologic pattern
Centrilobular nodularity	Cellular bronchiolitis Follicular bronchiolitis Respiratory bronchiolitis
Peribronchial nodules	Follicular bronchiolitis
Tree in bud pattern	Cellular bronchiolitis Panbronchiolitis
Diffuse or geographic air-trapping Mosaic pattern	Constrictive bronchiolitis
Bronchioloectasis, bronchiectasis	Panbronchiolitis
Patchy ground-glass attenuation	Respiratory bronchiolitis
Ground-glass opacity	Follicular bronchiolitis

Source: modified from Lynch.[125]

edge of the clinical manifestations, the radiologic distribution of disease (whether localized, or bilateral and diffuse), and the patient's cigarette smoking history. Attempts to predict clinical disease based on isolated abnormalities of the small airways, as viewed through the microscope, can be exquisitely unrewarding. A high-resolution computed tomography scan may provide valuable information regarding the possible pathologic pattern of disease, as shown in Table 8.5.

What follows is a compilation of the specific elementary pathologic changes in the small airways that can be identified histopathologically, along with the lists of conditions that should be considered when each is encountered. It is always important to realize that many of these lesions are part of a dynamic process, where one single causative agent may produce distinct pathologic features at different times in the natural history of the disease. In addition, the same clinicopathologic condition may result in a variety of pathologic changes in the small airways. In other words, frequently, there may be no direct relationship between a clinicopathologic condition and a specific histopathologic lesion in the small airways.

Inflammatory bronchiolitis

Inflammatory bronchiolitis, also known as cellular bronchiolitis, is a generic term that includes acute bronchiolitis, chronic bronchiolitis, and combined forms with variable amounts of both. All forms may be associated with bronchiolar fibrosis.[34] It is important to emphasize that both acute and chronic forms of bronchiolitis may have significant overlap, with one form typically being dominant. Diseases of the airways rarely have histopathologic findings sufficiently specific to point to a single etiology or a specific disease in the absence of some characteristic finding (e.g. viral inclusions, aspirated foreign material). When confronted with isolated inflammatory changes in the small airways, it is important to invoke a differential diagnosis to stimulate clinicopathologic correlation, and thereby help to narrow considerations in the clinical differential diagnosis.

Acute bronchiolitis

Florid acute bronchiolitis is characterized by predominately acute inflammation of the small airways, with variable epithelial sloughing. Extension of acute inflammation into surrounding peribronchiolar parenchyma is typical (Fig. 8.10). Very often, acute bronchiolitis is associated with some degree of chronic inflammatory infiltration, as described below. Conditions associated with relatively pure acute bronchiolitis include the early phase of certain infections (most of which also produce epithelial necrosis).[36,37] A careful search for viral inclusions is especially relevant in this scenario. Acute fume or toxic gas inhalation can also produce acute small airways injury, with few if any chronic changes. Loose connective tissue polyps may be present as a consequence of basement membrane disruption with fibroblastic migration into the airway lumens from subepithelial regions (so-called Masson polyps). Acute aspiration can manifest occasionally as acute bronchiolitis (most commonly seen at autopsy when aspiration may be part of the terminal event). Acute bronchiolitis can be an uncommon manifestation of Wegener's granulomatosis.[38]

Acute and chronic bronchiolitis

Acute and chronic inflammation of the small airways (Fig. 8.11) is one of the most common manifestations of "cellular bronchiolitis."[39] This inflammatory process is frequently associated with other bronchiolocentric manifestations, including intraluminal polyp formation, constriction and obliteration, and lymphoid follicles within the peribronchiolar sheath (follicular bronchiolitis).

When acute and chronic bronchiolitis are the primary manifestation in the lung biopsy, clinical manifestations may be accompanied by completely obstructive, completely restrictive, or a mixture of obstructive and restrictive pulmonary physiology. High-resolution computed tomography scans may show a predominantly nodular pattern, although reticulonodular infiltrates are more commonly observed. Table 8.6 lists the most frequent diseases associated with acute and chronic bronchiolitis.

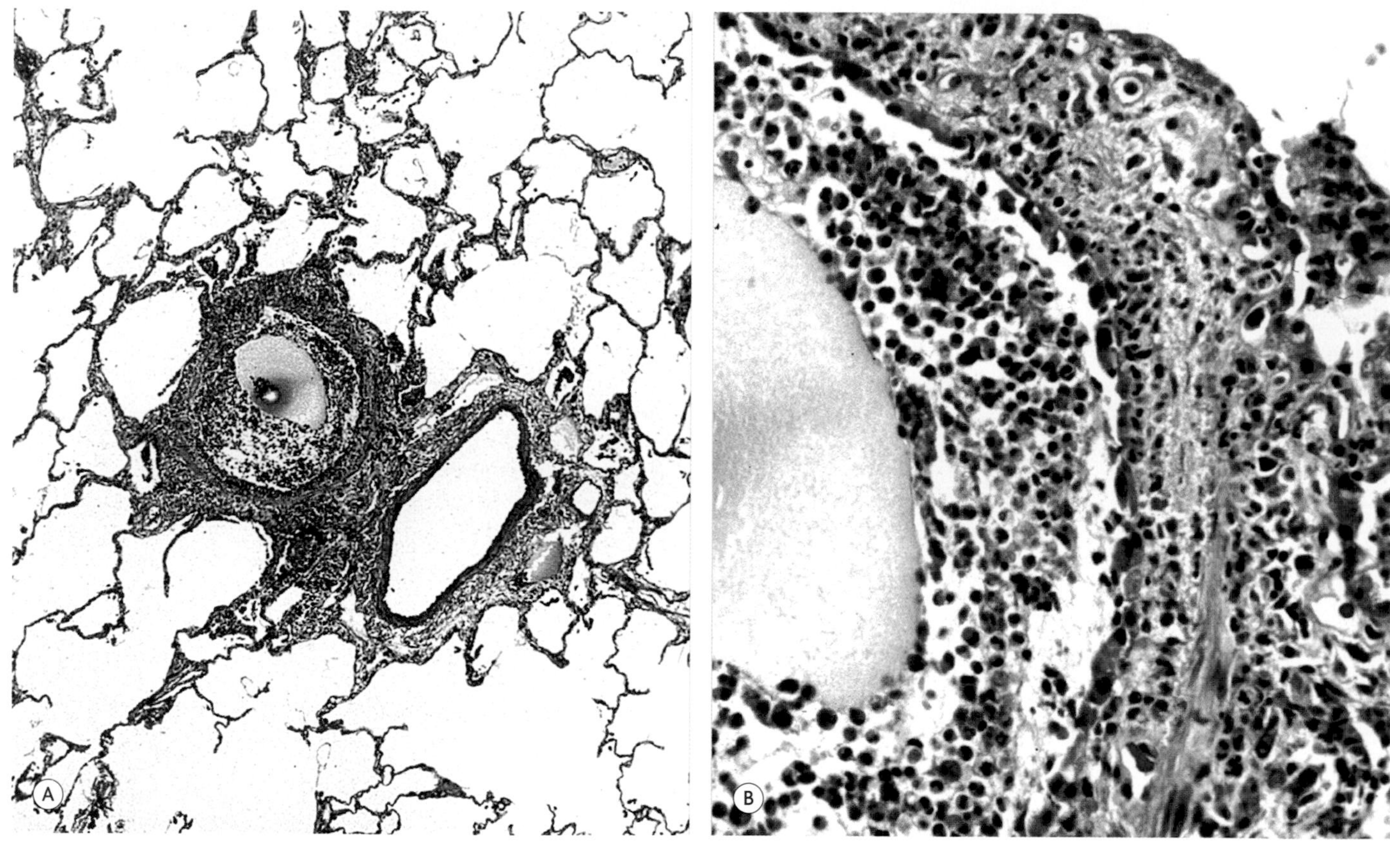

Fig. 8.10 **Acute bronchiolitis.** (A) A bronchovascular bundle with the small artery and the respiratory bronchiole. There is increased cellularity of the bronchiolar wall and many neutrophils are present within its lumen, accompanied by some acellular exudate. The surrounding lung parenchyma is uninvolved by the disease. (B) At higher magnification, the bronchiolar wall shows a cellular infiltrate composed of neutrophils, which expand the adventitial connective tissue and the subepithelial tissue (note by comparison the normal bronchiole in Fig. 8.9A, where epithelial cells are almost in direct contact with the underlying muscular layer of the airway). Rare individual epithelial cells are necrotic and are sloughed into the lumen.

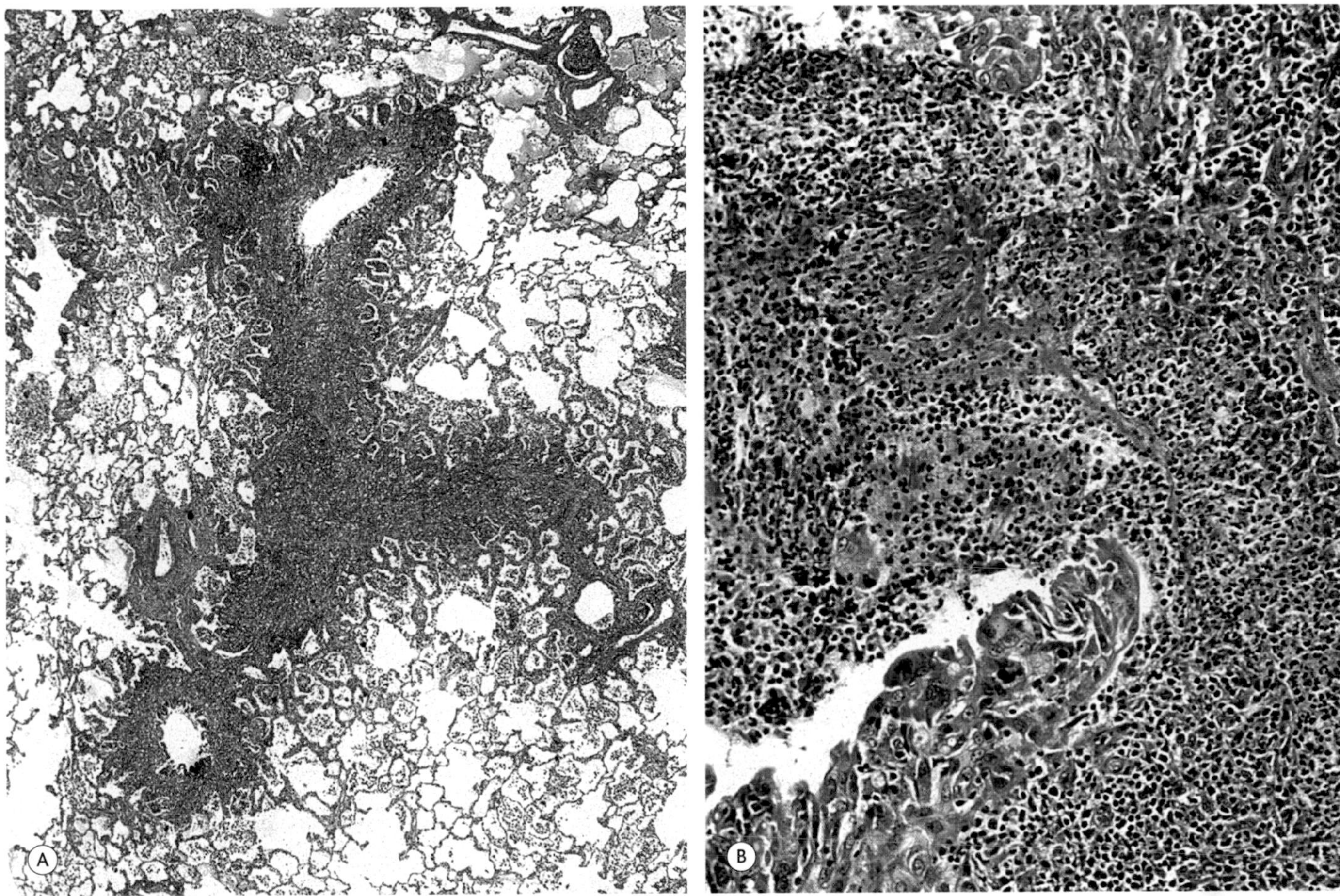

Fig. 8.11 **Acute and chronic bronchitis/bronchiolitis.** At low magnification (A) a definite peribronchiolar lesion is seen that also involves the adjacent lung parenchyma. (B) The cellular infiltrate is composed of neutrophils and lymphocytes. This image is from a case of bronchiolocentric Wegener's granulomatosis.

Table 8.6 Diseases and conditions associated with acute and chronic bronchiolitis

Infections
Allergic reactions
Collagen vascular diseases
Bronchocentric granulomatosis
Allergic bronchopulmonary fungal disease
Distal to bronchiectasis
Associated with inflammatory bowel disease
Aspiration pneumonia
Graft versus host disease
Wegener's granulomatosis
Idiopathic forms

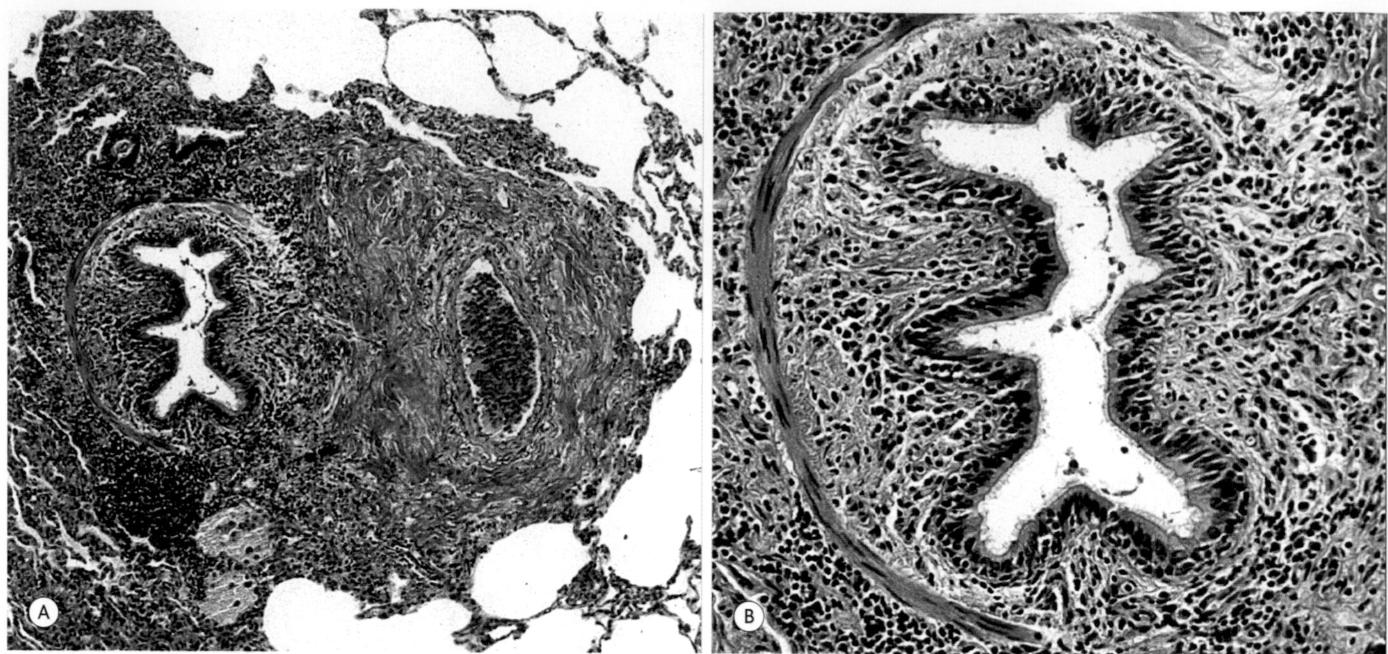

Fig. 8.12 **Chronic bronchiolitis.** (A) The bronchiole shows an inflammatory reaction that expands the subepithelial connective tissue, whereas the actual diameter of the airway is similar to that of the adjacent artery. (B) At higher magnification the chronic inflamatory infiltrate can be seen to fill the subepithelial area and also extends across the muscular wall to involve the bronchovascular sheath. This patient had a severe restrictive ventilatory defect.

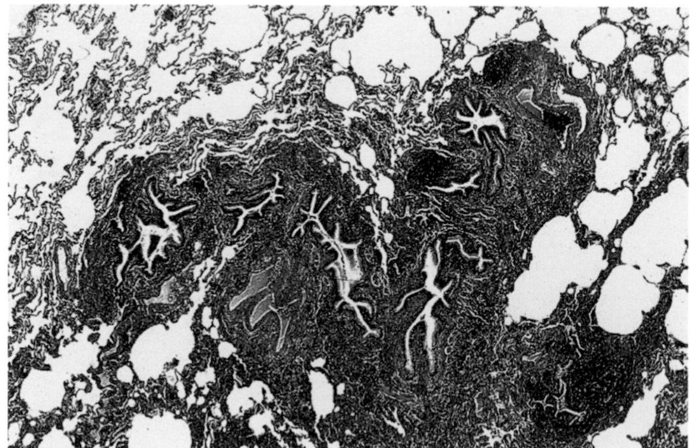

Fig. 8.13 **Chronic bronchiolitis:** Effects on the structure of the terminal bronchioles. The image shows a longitudinal section of a terminal bronchiole along with the adjacent artery. The airway is surrounded by a prominent lymphocytic infiltrate and shows distortion of the lumen, with variable stricture and dilatation. This case is from a patient with a severe restrictive ventilatory defect. The irregular shape of this bronchiole is best appreciated in comparison with the normal bronchiole shown in Fig. 8.9B.

Chronic bronchiolitis

Chronic inflammation within and surrounding the walls of small airways (Figs 8.12 and 8.13) can be seen in several conditions (Table 8.7). Chronic bronchiolitis can occur with or without lymphoid follicles and/or some degree of fibrosis. *Follicular bronchiolitis* is a specific subtype of chronic bronchiolitis, characterized by the presence of lymphoid follicles with well-formed germinal centers surrounding the bronchiolar walls, sometimes with lymphocytes migrating in the respiratory epithelium, either singly or in small clusters (Figs 8.14–8.16). Follicular bronchiolitis may be seen in several connective tissue diseases.[40–42] In cases with severe lymphoid infiltrates, especially if lymphoepithelial lesions are prominent, one should always consider the possibility of a lung lymphoma, most of which are low-grade B cell lymphomas of extranodal marginal zone type, arising from the mucosa-associated lymphoid tissue (MALT) (Fig. 8.17).[43–45] Low-grade lymphomas of the lung typically follow a very indolent course.[46] Follicular bronchiolitis may also be seen in some occupational exposure settings, such as nylon flock workers.[47–50]

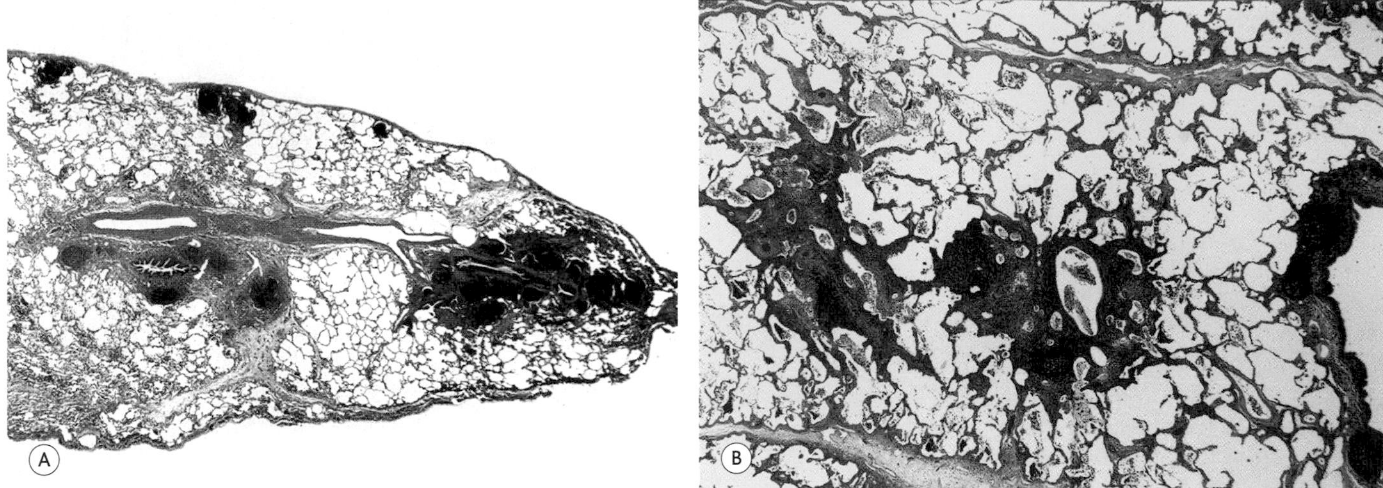

Fig. 8.14 **Follicular bronchiolitis.** The low-magnification view (A) shows the characteristic bronchiolocentric lymphoid infiltrate of follicular bronchiolitis in a biopsy from a patient with Sjögren's syndrome. (B) Lymphoid follicles with germinal centers are readily apparent and associated with bronchiolar injury (B-center). Follicular bronchiolitis may have a number of causes, including collagen vascular disease (as in the present case), cystic fibrosis, ciliary defects, immunodeficiency syndromes, or may be secondary to bronchiectasis, prior infection, or aspiration.

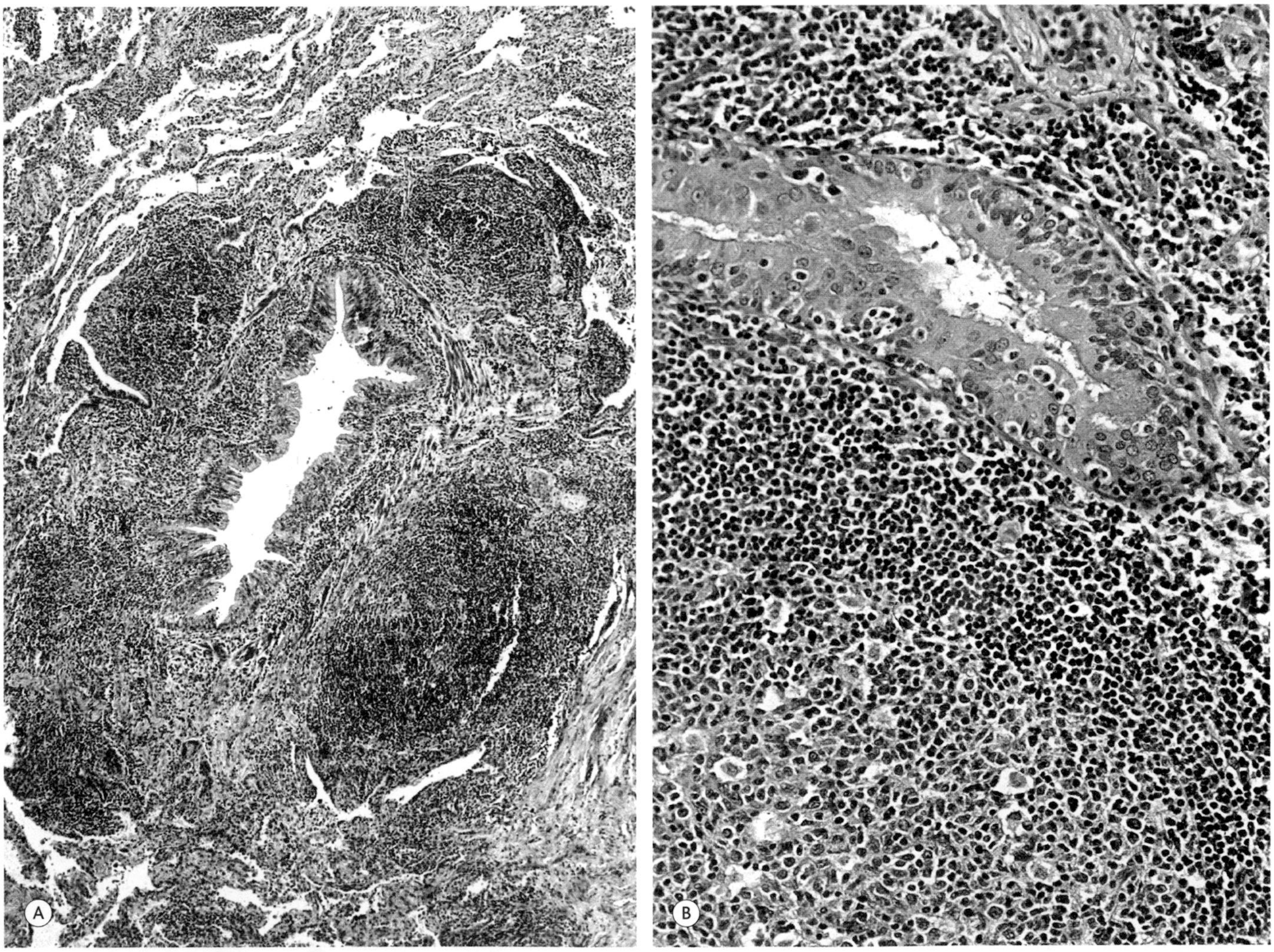

Fig. 8.15 **Follicular bronchiolitis.** (A) The terminal bronchiole is surrounded by a prominent inflammatory infiltrate with lymphoid follicles having well-formed germinal centers. The inflammatory process involves both the subepithelial layer and the adventitial tissue. (B) The subepithelial layer has a diffuse lymphoid infiltrate composed of mature small lymphocytes, which may show a tendency toward intraepithelial migration, simulating the lymphoepithelial lesions seen in low-grade lymphomas of the MALT/BALT tissue. (From a patient with bronchiectasis in the setting of a middle lobe syndrome.)

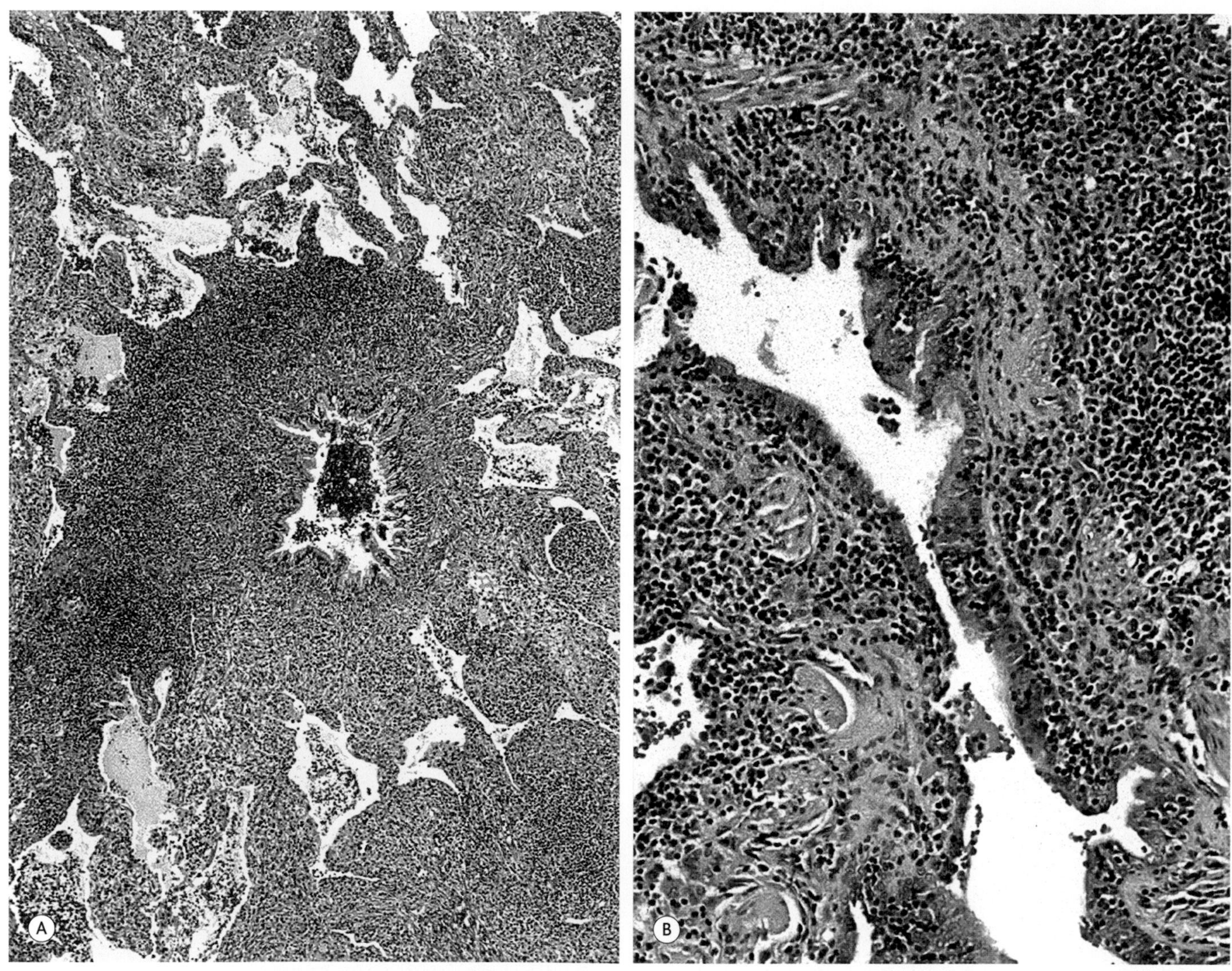

Fig. 8.16 **Follicular bronchiolitis.** (A) This respiratory bronchiole is surrounded by several lymphoid follicles. (B) The lymphoid tissue expands the bronchiolar wall, and many mononuclear cells are seen between the epithelial cell layer and the *muscularis propria*. (From a patient with IgA deficiency.)

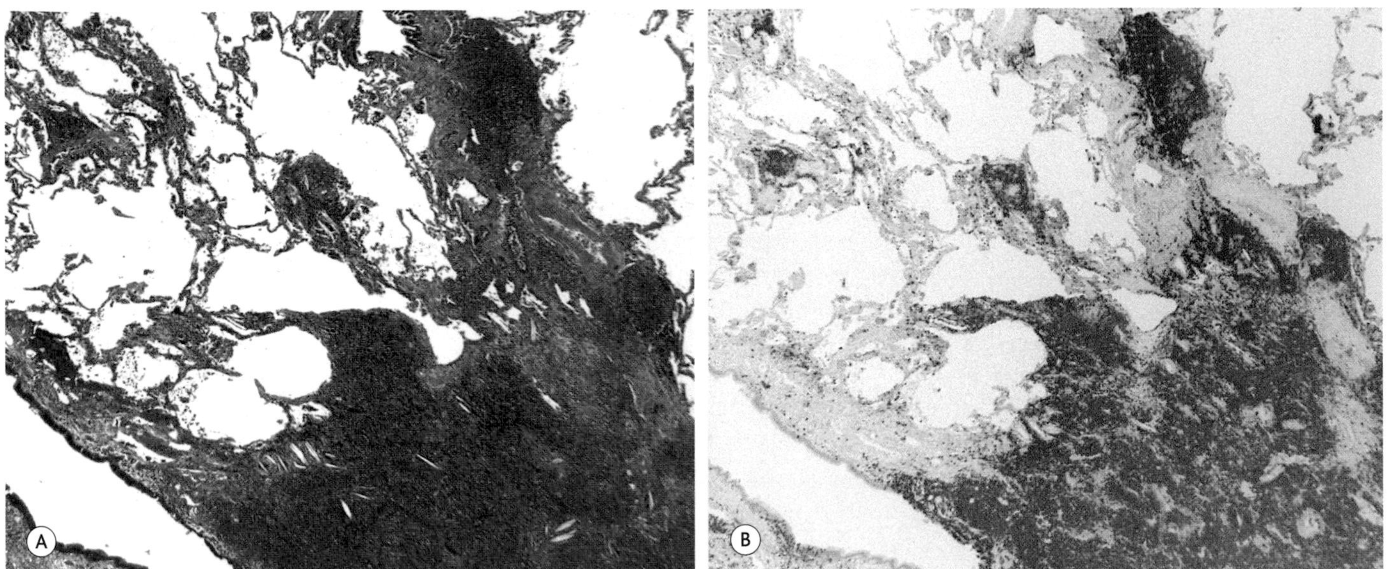

Fig. 8.17 **Low-grade lymphoma of the bronchus-associated lymphoid tissue (BALT).** This lymphoma, the bronchial counterpart of gastric MALToma, is a marginal zone lymphoma that originated from the BALT lymphoid tissue. (A) The present case shows a dense and homogeneous cellular infiltrate composed predominantly of small lymphocytes, which extends along the bronchiolar wall. (B) A CD20 immunostain highlights the diffuse and monomorphous spread of small B lymphocytes.

Table 8.7 Chronic inflammation of the small airways

Bronchiectasis (especially in airways distal to markedly dilated airways)
Collagen vascular diseases
Small airway disease in asthma
Graft versus host disease
Lymphoproliferative diseases (especially-low grade MALT lymphomas)
Respiratory bronchiolitis
Chronic aspiration pneumonia
Associated with inflammatory bowel disease
Nylon flock-associated interstitial lung disease
As a minor component of a localized inflammatory reaction (i.e. in right middle lobe syndrome)
Idiopathic forms

MALT = mucosa-associated lymphoid tissue.

Granulomatous bronchiolitis

Isolated granulomatous bronchiolitis is unusual. Sarcoidosis is the leading consideration in the differential diagnosis in the absence of necrosis (Fig. 8.18). On the other hand, when necrosis is present, granulomas are usually present in the surrounding lung parenchyma as well, and herald the strong possibility of infection (especially infection caused by mycobacteria and fungi (Fig. 8.19).[51] Necrotizing granulomatous bronchiolitis may also be seen in the setting of chronic necrotizing forms of pulmonary aspergillosis.[52] However, even in the absence of necrosis, infection should still remain high in the differential diagnosis. Non-necrotizing granulomatous bronchiolitis can be seen in association with inflammatory bowel disease, such as Crohn's disease, sometimes accompanied by microabscesses.[53] Non-necrotizing peribronchiolar granulomas are also seen in the majority of patients with hypersensitivity pneumonitis (Fig. 8.20) and aspiration pneumonia.[39] When isolated peribronchiolar multinucleated giant cells are the major finding, one should consider Wegener's granulomatosis (Fig. 8.21), aspiration pneumonia (Figs 8.22 and 8.23) and hard metal (cobalt) pneumoconiosis (so-called giant cell interstitial pneumonia).

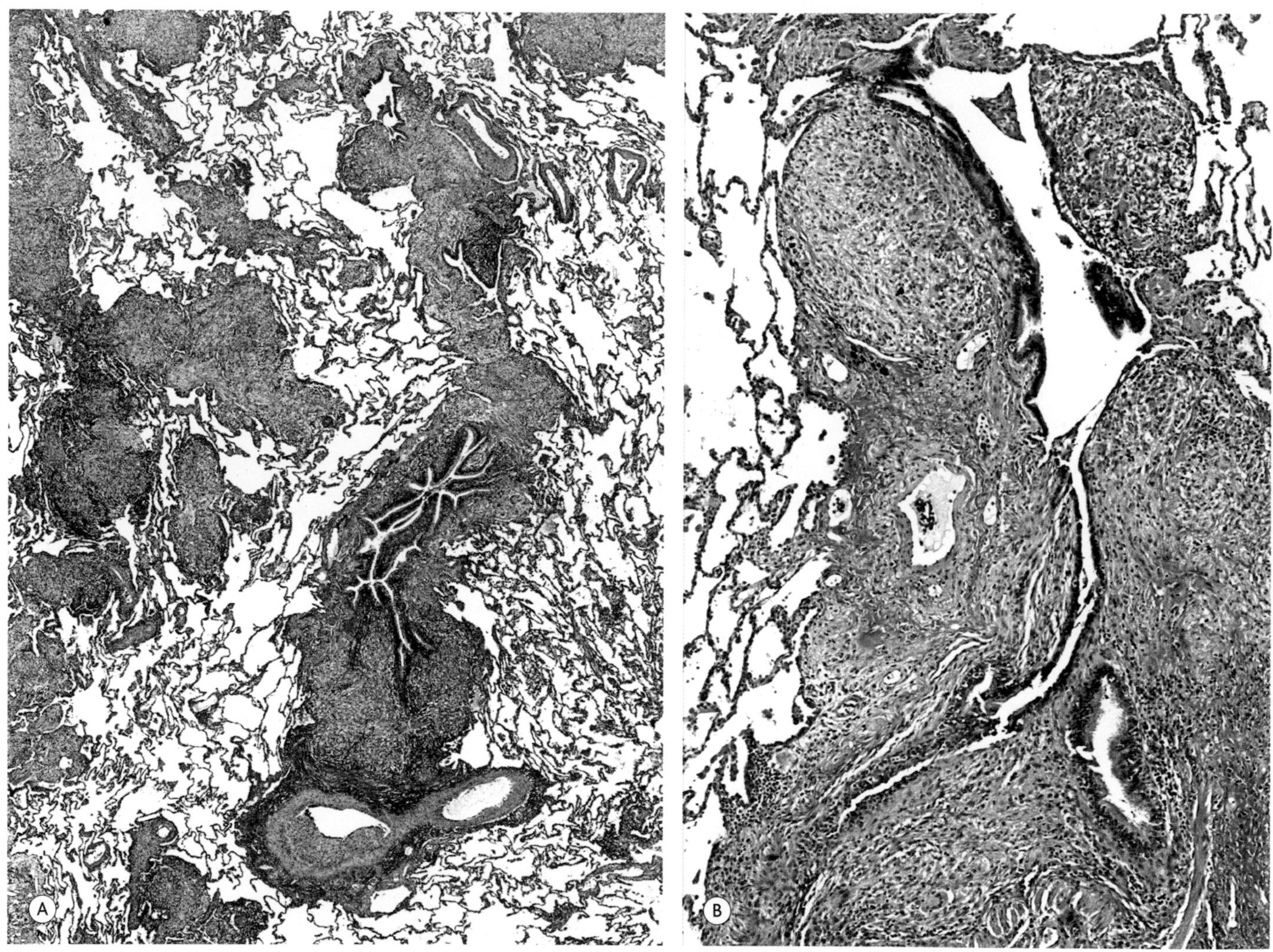

Fig. 8.18 **Sarcoidosis.** At scanning magnification (A), the serpiginous outline of the bronchovascular bundle is accentuated by pale pink granulomas, collagen, and scant chronic inflammation. (B) The bronchiole shows the typical granulomas and sclerotic background matrix of sarcoidosis, which involves the airway wall and impinges on the adjacent arterial wall. The granulomas are well formed, with a definite fibrous demarcation, and show a tendency toward coalescence. Inflammatory cells are scant and the whole process has an eosinophilic appearance, which is clearly different from the lesions seen in granulomatous bronchiolitis due to infection (see Fig. 8.19 for comparison).

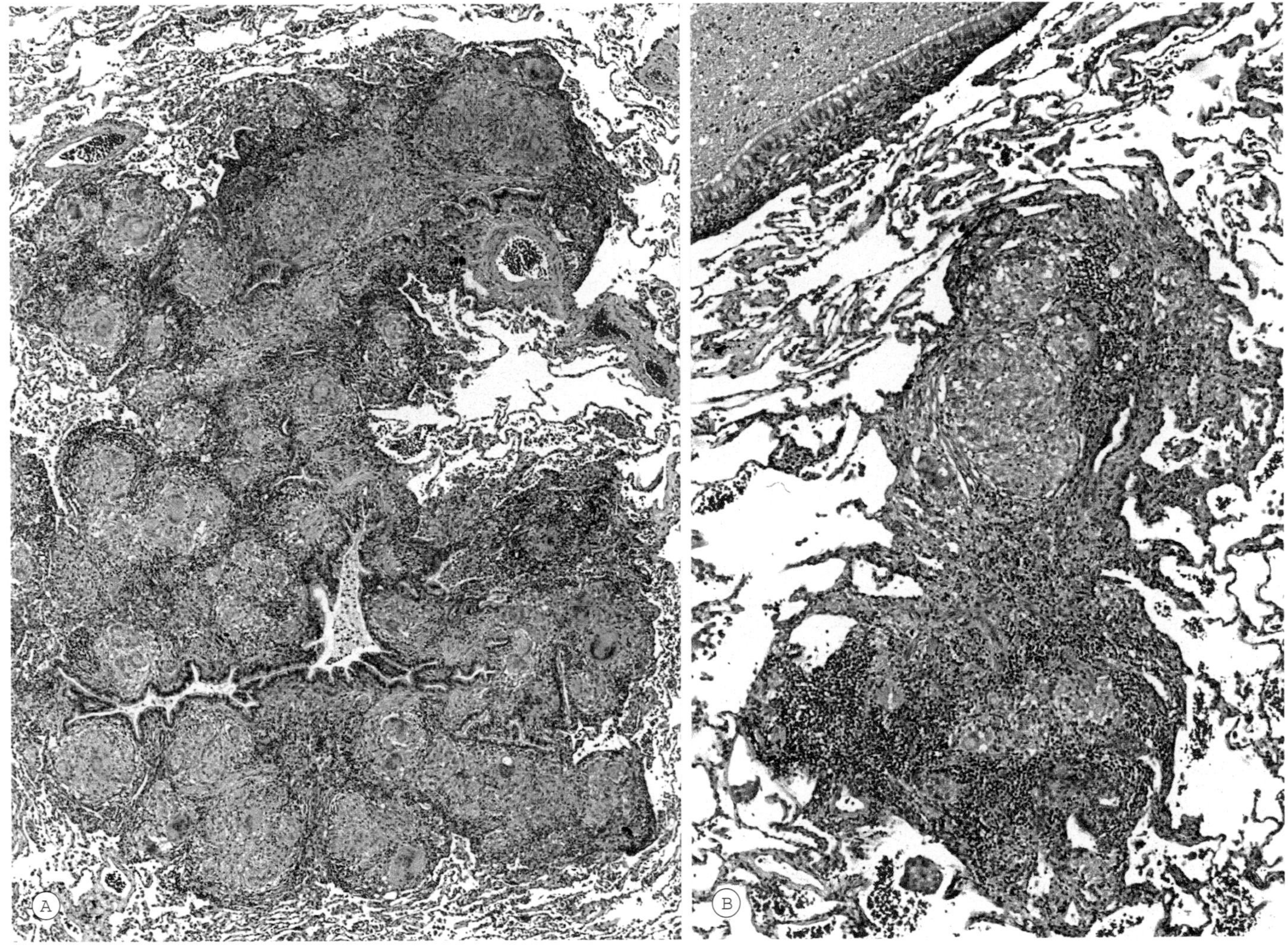

Fig. 8.19 **Granulomatous bronchiolitis due to infection.** (A) A granulomatous bronchiolitis in *Mycobacterium tuberculosis* infection: granulomas are abundant and have distinct giant cells. (B) A case of *Mycobacterium avium* complex (MAC) infection, with non-necrotizing granulomas centered on the bronchioles (note the dilated bronchiole in the left upper corner). The small granulomas are usually solitary with a cuff of lymphocytes, and involve respiratory and terminal bronchioles. These lesions are frequently seen in association with a predisposing factor (e.g. bronchiectasis) or in healthy patients exposed to a contaminated environment (such as that seen in hot tub use). The inflammatory process surrounding the granulomas is greater than that associated with sarcoidosis. On the other hand, MAC granulomas are much better organized than those seen in hypersensitivity pneumonitis, where "granulomas" tend to be nothing more than loose clusters of interstitial epithelioid histiocytes and giant cells.

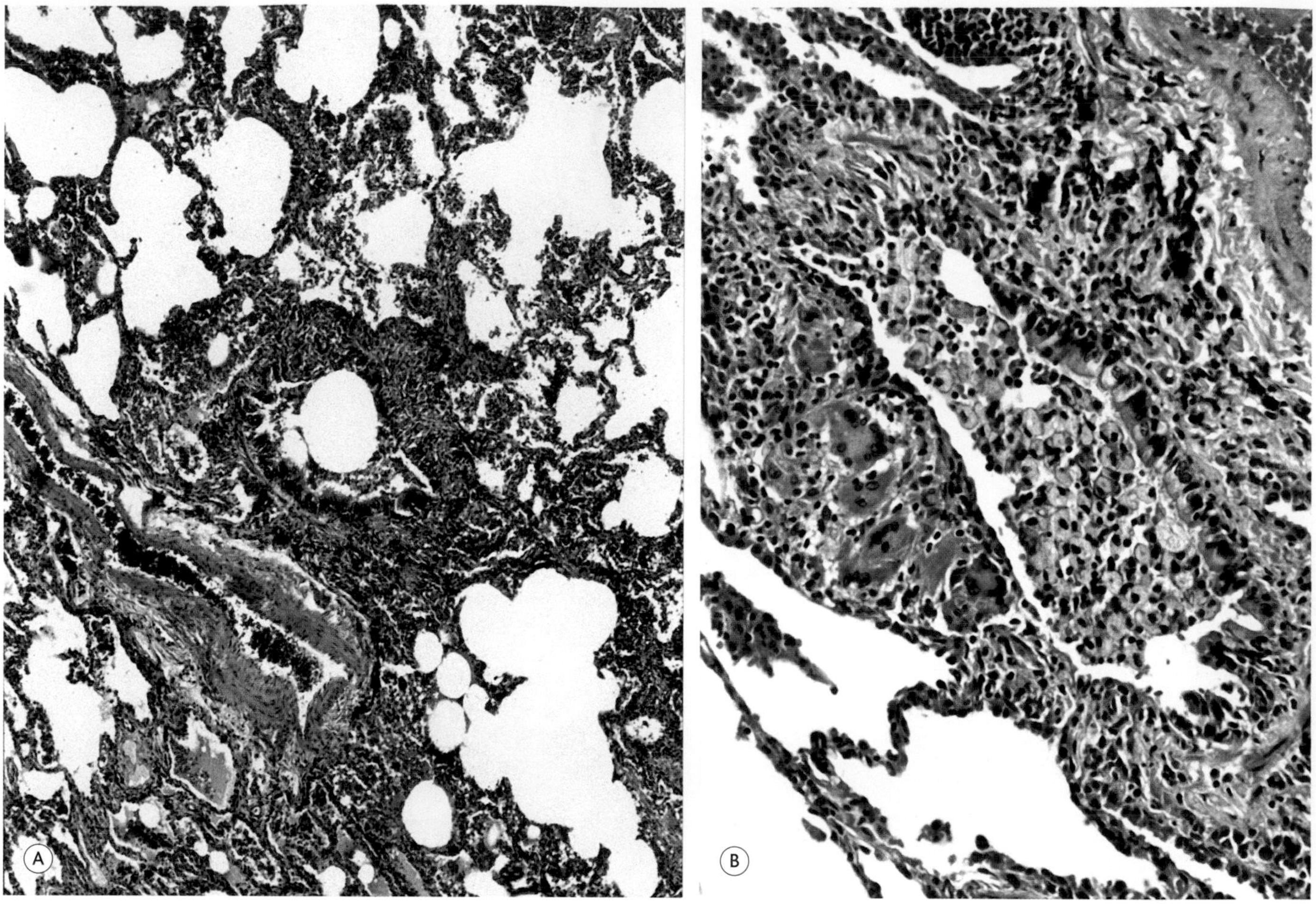

Fig. 8.20 **Hypersensitivity pneumonitis.** (A) A bronchiolocentric cellular infiltrate is typically present, accompanied by (B) an ill-defined granulomatous reaction in the interstitium focally, and sometimes adjacent to the bronchioles. This patient had a hypersensitivity reaction after using a polyurethane spray indoors.

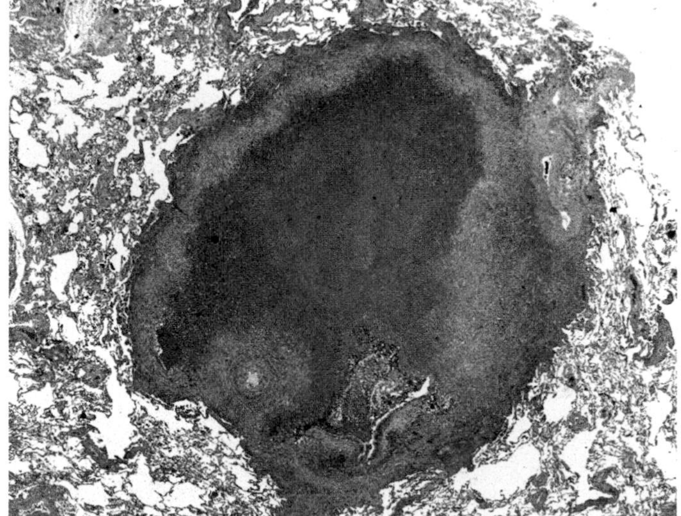

Fig. 8.21 **Bronchiolocentric granulomas in Wegener's granulomatosis.** This lung biopsy shows a granulomatous reaction, with central necrosis, involving a small airway. Note the typical basophilic appearance of the necrosis.

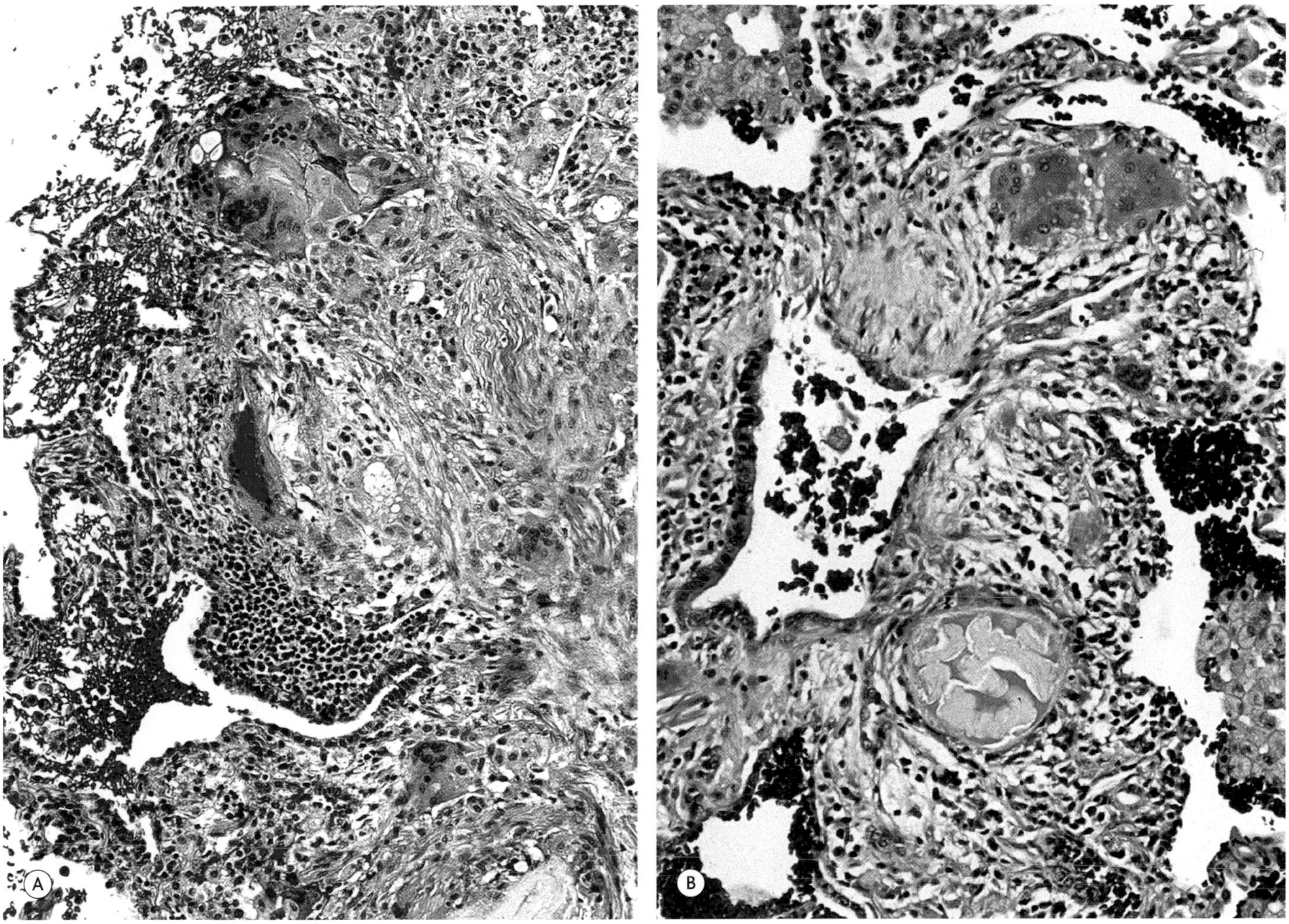

Fig. 8.22 **Aspiration bronchiolitis.** This biopsy is from a patient who suffered from gastroesophageal reflux disease (GERD): he developed the sudden onset of pneumonia, which did not resolve, and underwent lung biopsy 4 weeks later. (A) The pattern is one of non-necrotizing granulomatous bronchiolitis with many giant cells, (B) some of which surround typical aspirated starch grains.

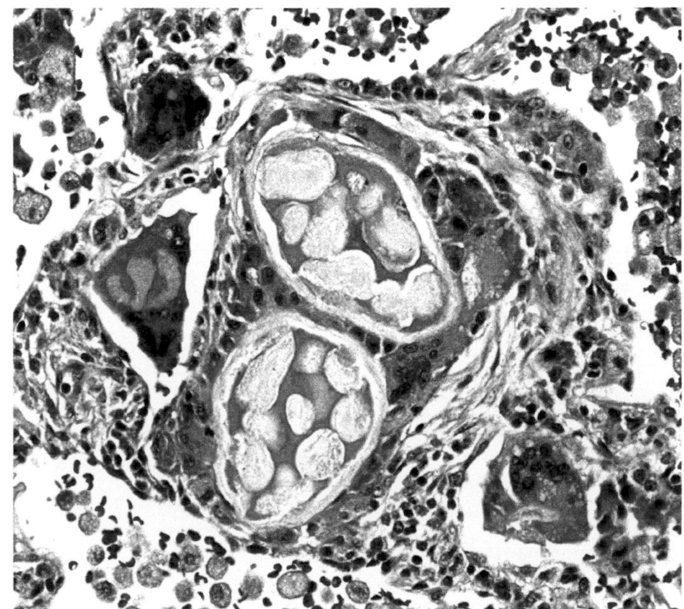

Fig. 8.23 **Aspiration bronchiolitis.** Typical starch grains surrounded by foreign body-type giant cells.

Table 8.8 Causes of bronchiolar necrosis (mucosal necrosis, epithelial sloughing, and variable acute inflammation)

Infections (especially viral infections and certain bronchocentric fungal infections)
Toxic fume exposure
Bronchocentric granulomatosis
Wegener's granulomatosis

Bronchiolar necrosis

Complete mucosal necrosis with epithelial sloughing and variable acute inflammation is typical of a limited number of lung diseases, mainly those of infectious origin (Table 8.8). In the presence of bronchiolar necrosis, a careful search for viropathic changes or micro-organisms (bacterial and fungal) should be undertaken (Figs 8.24–8.26). When the process is intensely suppurative

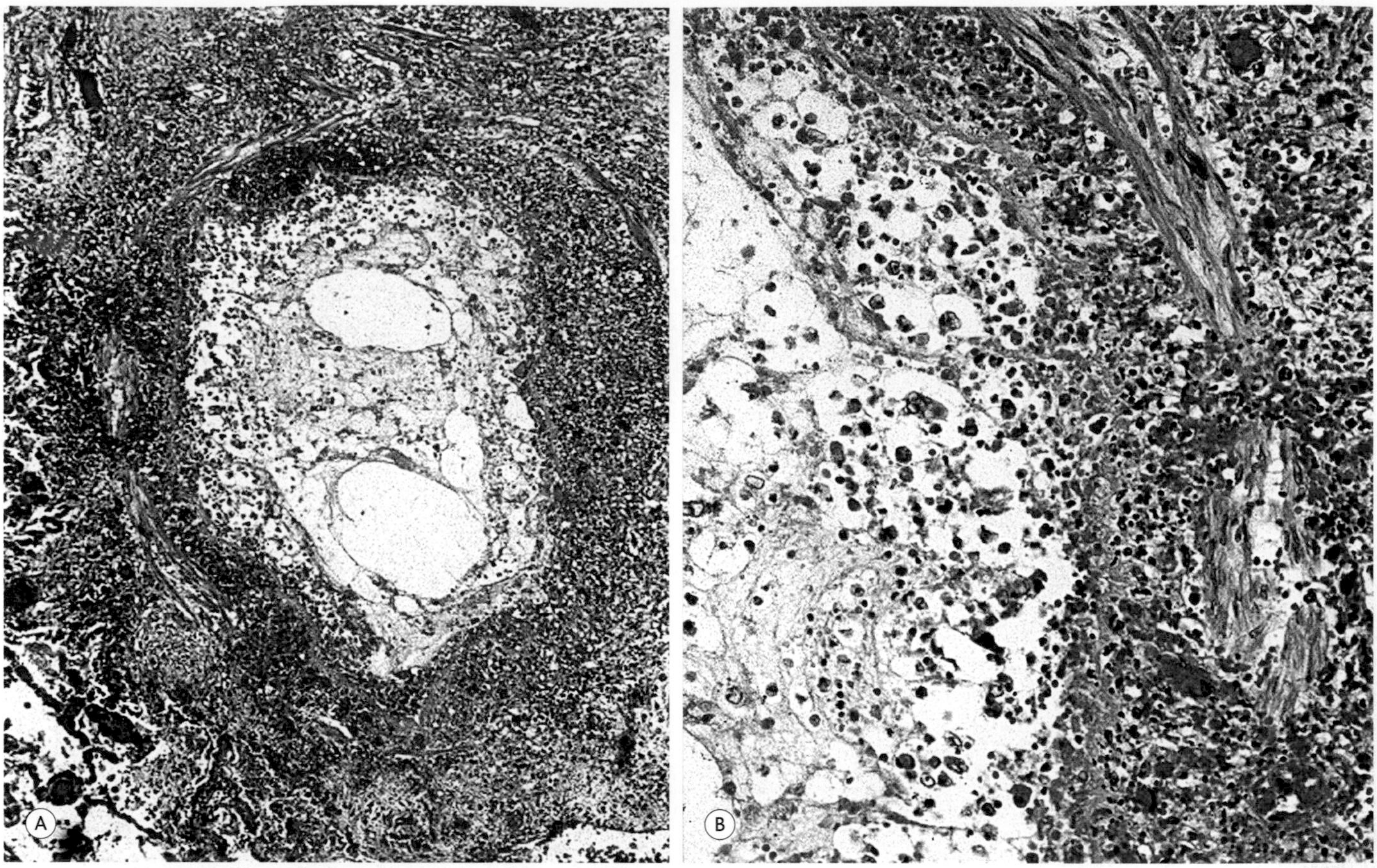

Fig. 8.24 **Herpetic necrotizing bronchiolitis.** (A) An acute necrotizing inflammatory process involves the entire bronchiolar wall with involvement of surrounding alveolar septa. (B) The lumen of the bronchiole contains exudate, red blood cells, and single epithelial cells.

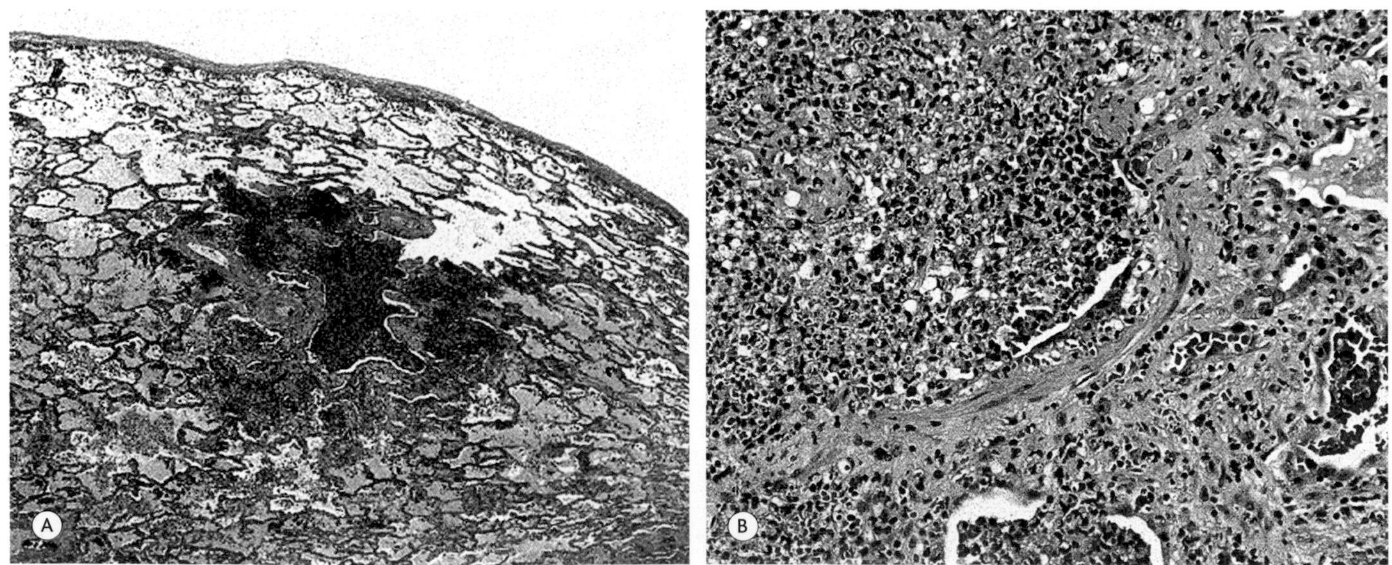

Fig. 8.25 **Adenovirus necrotizing acute bronchiolitis.** This biopsy is from a renal transplant patient receiving immunosuppressive therapy. The lung biopsy shows a bronchiolocentric acute inflammatory process characterized by prominent epithelial necrosis. (A) The lumen of the bronchiole has been obliterated. (B) At higher magnification one can appreciate the presence of the muscular layer, whereas the epithelial layer is almost completely destroyed. Adenovirus was cultured from the biopsy specimen.

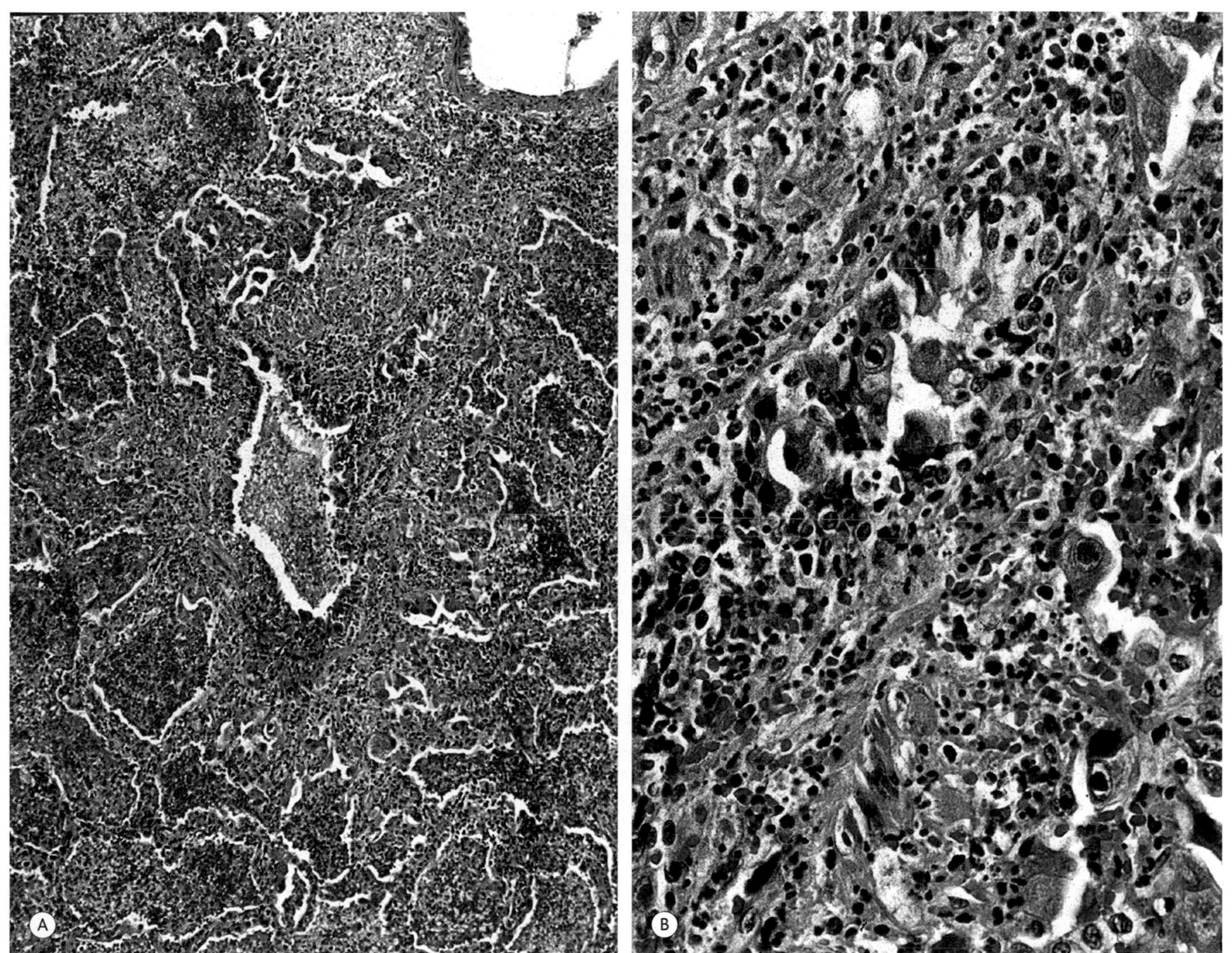

Fig. 8.26 **Cytomegalovirus bronchiolitis.** (A) The bronchiole shows an acute inflammatory necrotizing process. (B) Viral inclusions are seen at higher magnification.

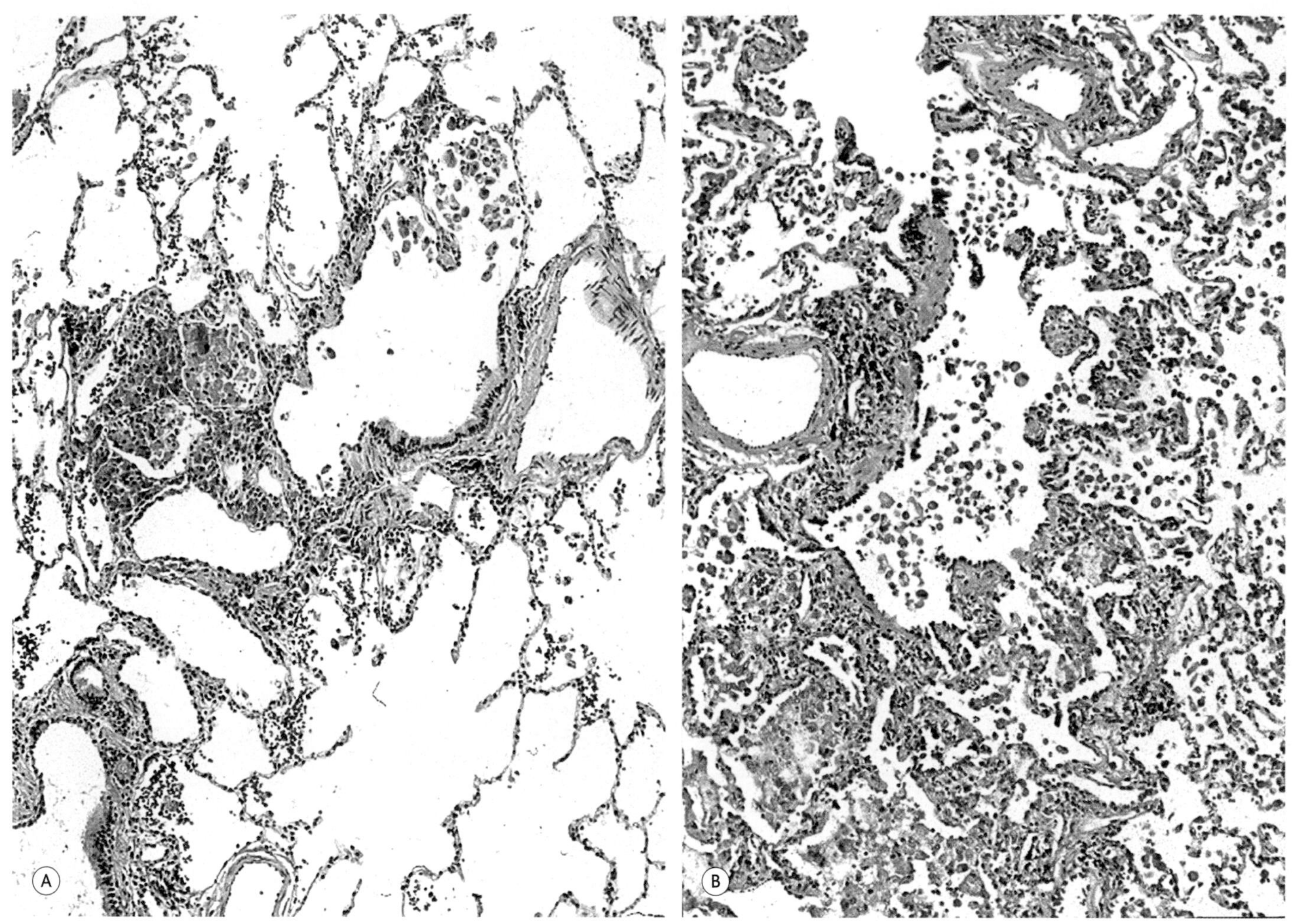

Fig. 8.27 **Respiratory bronchiolitis.** These two bronchioles represent different patterns with distortion and inflammation in so-called "smokers bronchiolitis." (A) The bronchiole is dilated, mildly distorted, and there is prominent filling of the alveolar spaces by finely granular and pigmented macrophages. (B) The bronchiolar wall shows mild thickening with chronic inflammation, along with "smoker's macrophages" in the lumen.

with large nodular foci of necrosis, consideration should be given to the possibility of pyoderma gangrenosum lesions in the lung associated with inflammatory bowel disease (e.g. ulcerative colitis)[54,55] or occurring de novo without IBD.[56–60]

Respiratory (smoker's) bronchiolitis

Respiratory bronchiolitis is a very special marker for smoking-related lung injury and is extremely common in lung biopsies and surgical specimens (by virtue of cigarette smoking being a cause of, or associated with, many lung diseases).[61–65] The histopathologic lesion is characterized by mild inflammation of the respiratory bronchiole with variable extension of inflammation into the surrounding alveolar walls. The peribronchiolar alveoli contain variable numbers of lightly pigmented macrophages (smoker's macrophages) that give the lesion its characteristic appearance (Figs 8.27 and 8.28). On occasion, respiratory bronchiolitis can be sufficiently extensive to produce clinical and radiologic manifestations of diffuse interstitial lung disease, so-called respiratory bronchiolitis-associated interstitial lung disease, or RBILD (see Ch. 7). Desquamative interstitial pneumonia is also a consideration when this occurs. Respiratory bronchiolitis is very commonly seen with Langerhans cell histiocytosis (pulmonary eosinophilic granuloma).[61,62,64]

When respiratory bronchiolitis is the sole pathologic finding in a smoker, a careful search for another disease process is in order, since mild respiratory bronchiolitis alone is unlikely to produce sufficient clinical and radiographic findings to warrant lung biopsy.[66] Conversely, in a lifelong non-smoker, changes resembling respiratory

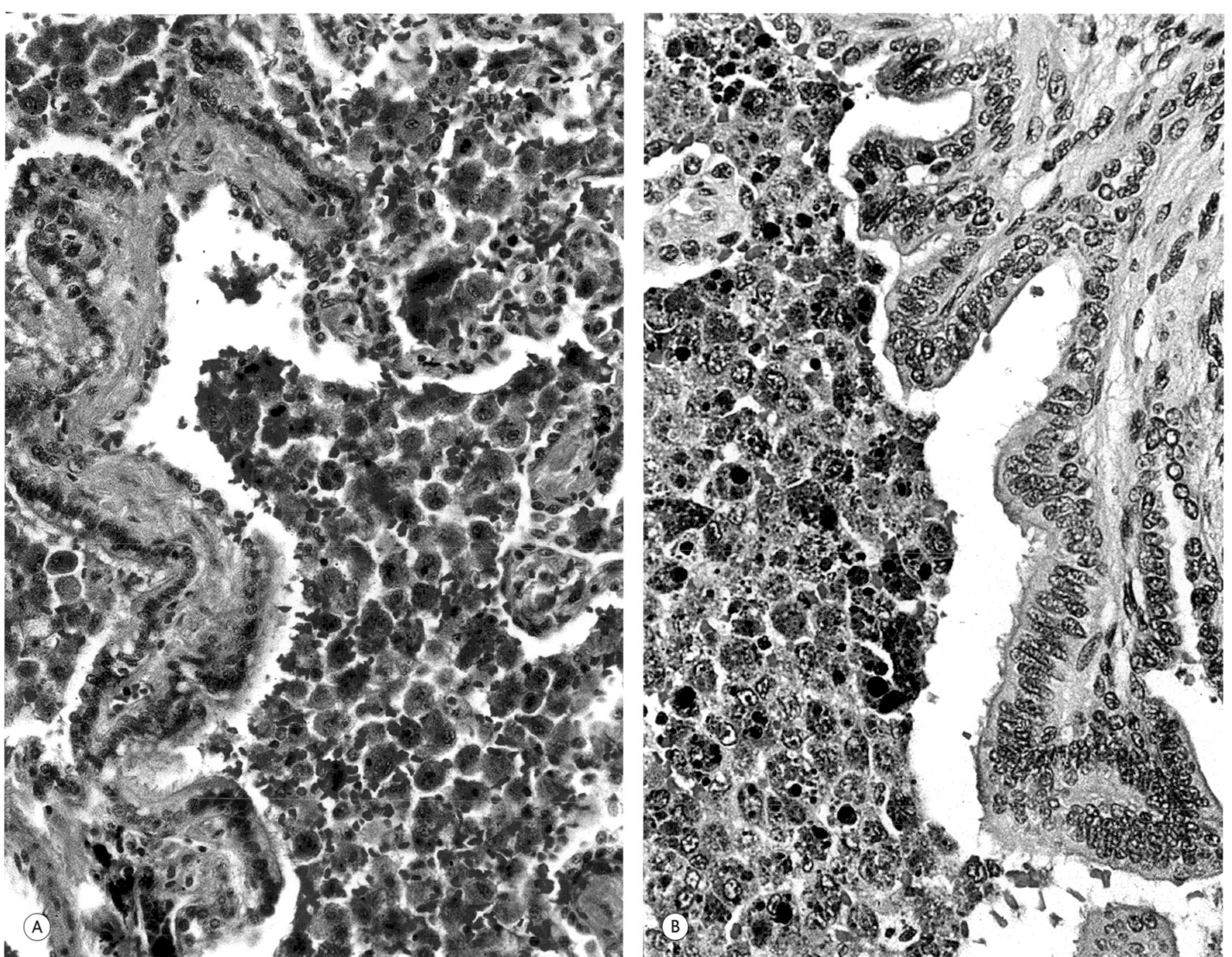

Fig. 8.28 **Respiratory bronchiolitis.** (A) Alveolar macrophages with fine, gold-brown, cytoplasmic pigment accumulate in the respiratory bronchiole, alveolar ducts, and peribronchiolar alveoli. (B) On the right, by comparison, the heavily pigmented macrophages seen in hemorrhage syndromes. In pulmonary hemorrhage, the hemosiderin pigment granules are more abundant and more coarse.

bronchiolitis usually indicate significant small airways pathology and some of these patients may have profound clinical symptoms with significant hypoxia and manifestations on CT scan suggesting interstitial lung disease. Trichrome and elastic tissue stains may be useful in better defining the small airways pathology in the biopsy, such as excessive peribronchiolar fibrosis and obliterative scars. In this situation, high-resolution inspiratory and expiratory CT scans may provide additional radiologic evidence to support the small airways as the primary focus of the lung disease (see Constrictive bronchiolitis, below).

Bronchiolar metaplasia (lambertosis)

Bronchiolar metaplasia is a pathologic process where bronchiolar epithelial cells extend beyond the respiratory bronchioles along alveolar septa, replacing the normal alveolar lining cells (Fig. 8.29). This lesion is often described as "lambertosis," as it is hypothesized that the metaplastic epithelium derives from the canals of Lambert that normally directly connect non-respiratory bronchioles to adjacent alveoli. Lambertosis can be seen in a number of pathologic entities, including COPD and constrictive

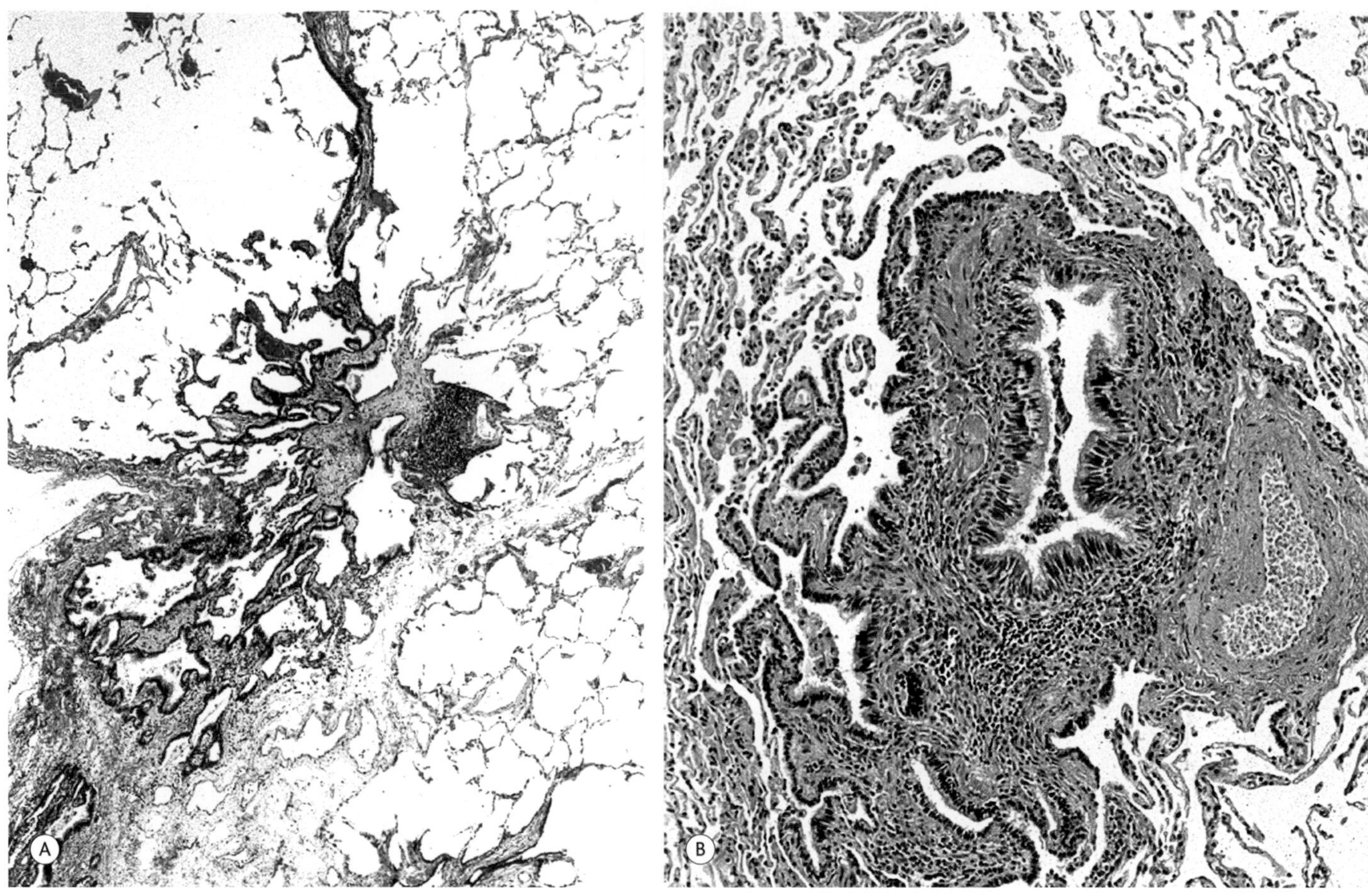

Fig. 8.29 **Bronchiolar metaplasia (so-called lambertosis).** (A) Proliferation of cuboidal epithelial cells, extending from alveolar ducts into proximal lobular acini along the alveolar septa is a common finding in smokers and may be considered as a reactive/reparative process involving chronic injury to the terminal and respiratory bronchiole. (B) At higher magnification, the bronchiolocentric nature is easily appreciated. This image is from a patient who was a heavy smoker.

bronchiolitis among others. In most cases the lesion is felt to be postinflammatory in origin and therefore could potentially be seen as a consequence of any number of inflammatory diseases involving the small airways. No specific cause is identified in some patients and the disease may be an idiopathic manifestation of an unidentified remote injury to the small airways. When this is the case, the disease may manifest clinically as an interstitial lung disease with restrictive physiology. The histopathology of bronchiolar metaplasia is that of variable extension of columnar, sometimes ciliated, epithelium, out beyond the alveolar ducts to involve alveolar walls. When the lesions are exuberant, they may appear as nodules measuring 2–5 mm in diameter. These lesions must be distinguished from microscopic honeycombing, atypical adenomatous hyperplasia,[67–70] and the micronodular pneumocyte hyperplasia of tuberous sclerosis complex.[71]

When prominent bronchiolar metaplasia is identified, along with some other significant pathology (e.g. in association with a lobectomy for carcinoma), the exact significance of this process relative to the patient's clinical manifestations is unclear. In our experience, bronchiolar metaplasia in the setting of smoking-related lung disease may or may not have a clinical or radiologic correlation. Conversely, such changes in a non-smoker are always significant. Diseases associated with prominent bronchiolar metaplasia are listed in Table 8.9.

Table 8.9 Diseases associated with bronchiolar metaplasia (lambertosis)

Healed bronchiolitis (from any cause)
Chronic hypersensitivity pneumonitis (extrinsic allergic alveolitis)
Distal to bronchiectasis (from any cause)
As a component of constrictive bronchiolitis

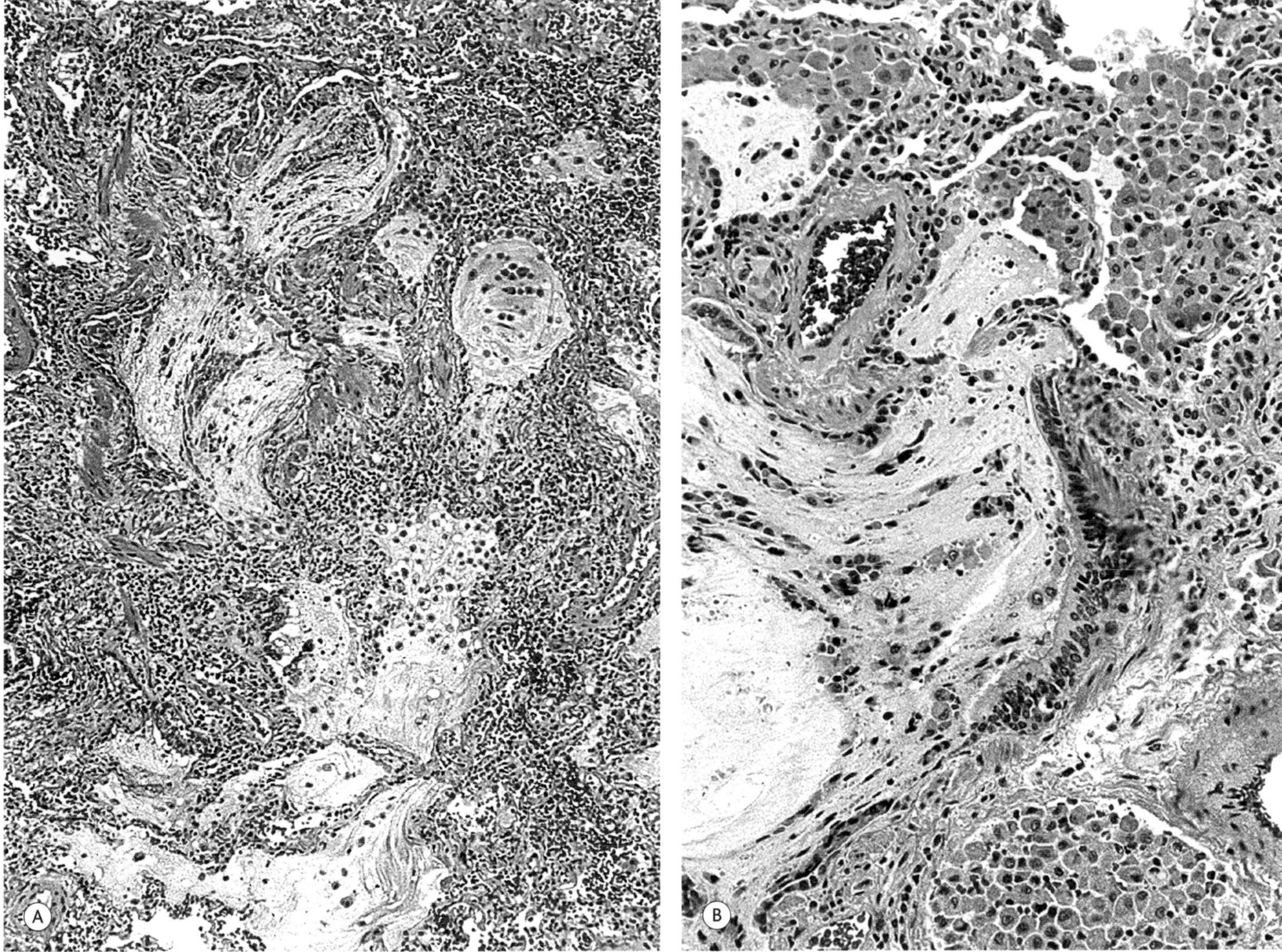

Fig. 8.30 **Mucostasis in respiratory bronchiolitis.** (A) The respiratory bronchioles and alveolar ducts are filled with mucinous material. (B) Extension of free mucus into peribronchiolar alveoli is seen and many smokers' type macrophages with dusty brown pigment are visible (B, center right).

Mucostasis

Mucostasis (also referred to as mucus stasis) is defined as visible amphophilic mucin within dilated terminal airways or in surrounding alveolar ducts and alveolar spaces (Fig. 8.30).[39,72] Mucostasis is a common finding in cigarette smokers, and can occur in a number of other settings, as detailed in Table 8.10.

When mucus extrusion into alveolar spaces is extensive, a careful search for bronchioloalveolar carcinoma (BAC) is in order, especially in the absence of another specific pathologic entity in the biopsy. Correlation with imaging studies may be helpful in excluding BAC.

Table 8.10 Diseases associated with mucostasis

COPD
Respiratory bronchiolitis
Asthma
Mucoid impaction/allergic pulmonary fungal disease
Constrictive bronchiolitis
Distal to bronchiectasis
As part of a localized inflammatory reaction (e.g. middle lobe syndrome)
Bronchioloalveolar carcinoma

COPD = chronic obstructive pulmonary disease.

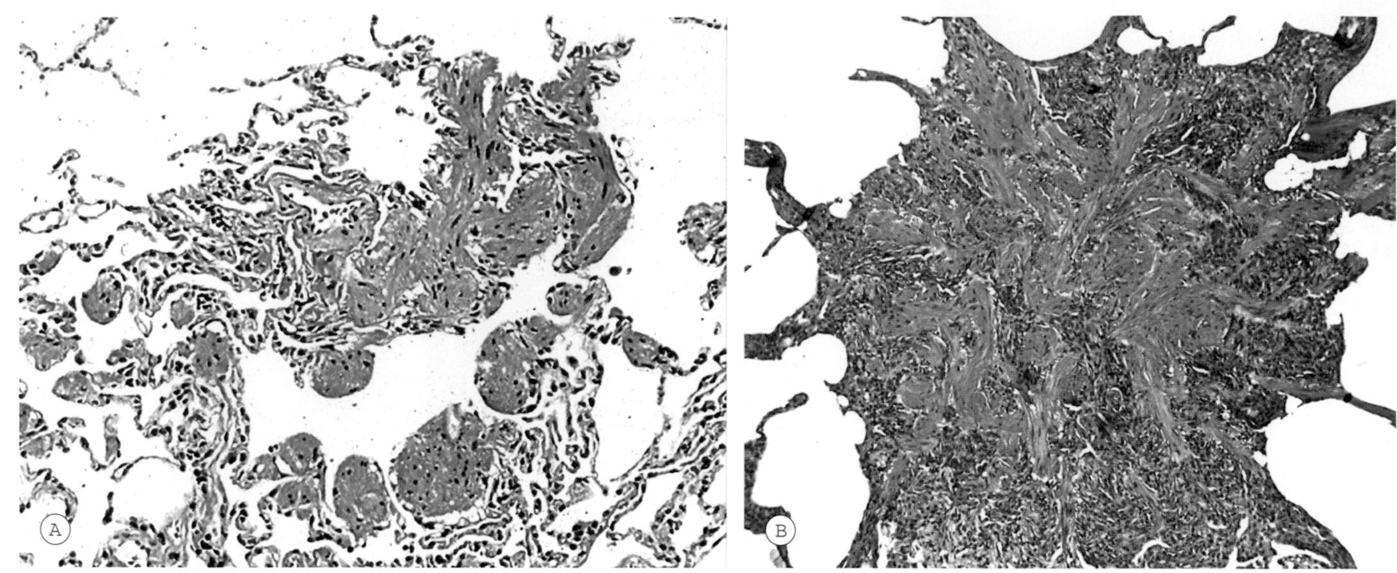

Fig. 8.31 **Smooth muscle hyperplasia.** (A) This terminal bronchiole is from a patient with previous history of radiation therapy and presents an irregular lumen with an excessively thick smooth muscle layer. (B) A typical "smoker's nodule," characterized by radial fascicles of smooth muscle present in a centrilobular distribution.

Table 8.11 Diseases associated with airway smooth muscle hyperplasia

Asthma
As a component of constrictive bronchiolitis
Associated with fibrosing lung diseases
As part of a localized inflammatory process
As a focal incidental finding
As a component of generalized bronchiolar scarring and peribronchiolar metaplasia
Aguayo–Miller disease (neuroendocrine cell hyperplasia with occlusive bronchiolar fibrosis)

Bronchiolar smooth muscle hyperplasia

Generalized thickening of the smooth muscle around conducting airways and alveolar ducts can be seen in a number of inflammatory lung diseases (Fig. 8.31A). Sometimes smooth muscle nodules formed of haphazard fascicles can be seen in smokers and are of unknown clinical relevance (Fig. 8.31B). Smooth muscle associated with subpleural fibrosis is common in usual interstitial pneumonia (UIP) as well. The diseases associated with smooth muscle hyperplasia are listed in Table 8.11.

Constrictive bronchiolitis and bronchiolitis obliterans with intraluminal Masson polyps

The term bronchiolitis obliterans is an historical term derived from *bronchiolitis obliterans fibrosa*, where the terminal airways are filled with Masson-type fibroblastic polyps.[73–75] However, the term bronchiolitis obliterans has also been used to describe other specific clinicopathologic situations. For example, a form of idiopathic interstitial lung disease characterized by numerous Masson-type fibroblastic polyps in the terminal airways and in surrounding alveoli was termed idiopathic bronchiolitis obliterans organizing pneumonia or BOOP[73,75] (now termed cryptogenic organizing pneumonia, COP). An entirely different clinical and pathologic condition with variable constriction and obliteration of the small airways has also been referred to by this term (also called "obliterative bronchiolitis").[76,77] We believe that the term "bronchiolitis obliterans" should be used only to describe the airway injury of chronic lung transplant rejection, where it has now become entrenched (so-called bronchiolitis obliterans syndrome, or BOS).[78–83] We also feel that the original description of intraluminal bronchiolar fibroblastic polyps occurring as part of many lung repair reactions should be referred to as "organizing pneumonia pattern" (OP), or simply "airspace organization".

We use the term "constrictive bronchiolitis" to describe the small airways disease in which variable narrowing or obliteration of the small airways occurs in the non lung transplant patient, often without an identified etiology (but sometimes with the conditions in Table 8.12).[34,84–88] It is useful to consider constrictive bronchiolitis in the same way hepatopathologists describe ductal loss or "ductopenia" in some liver diseases. Affected bronchioles may show lesions of different ages and the injury is not

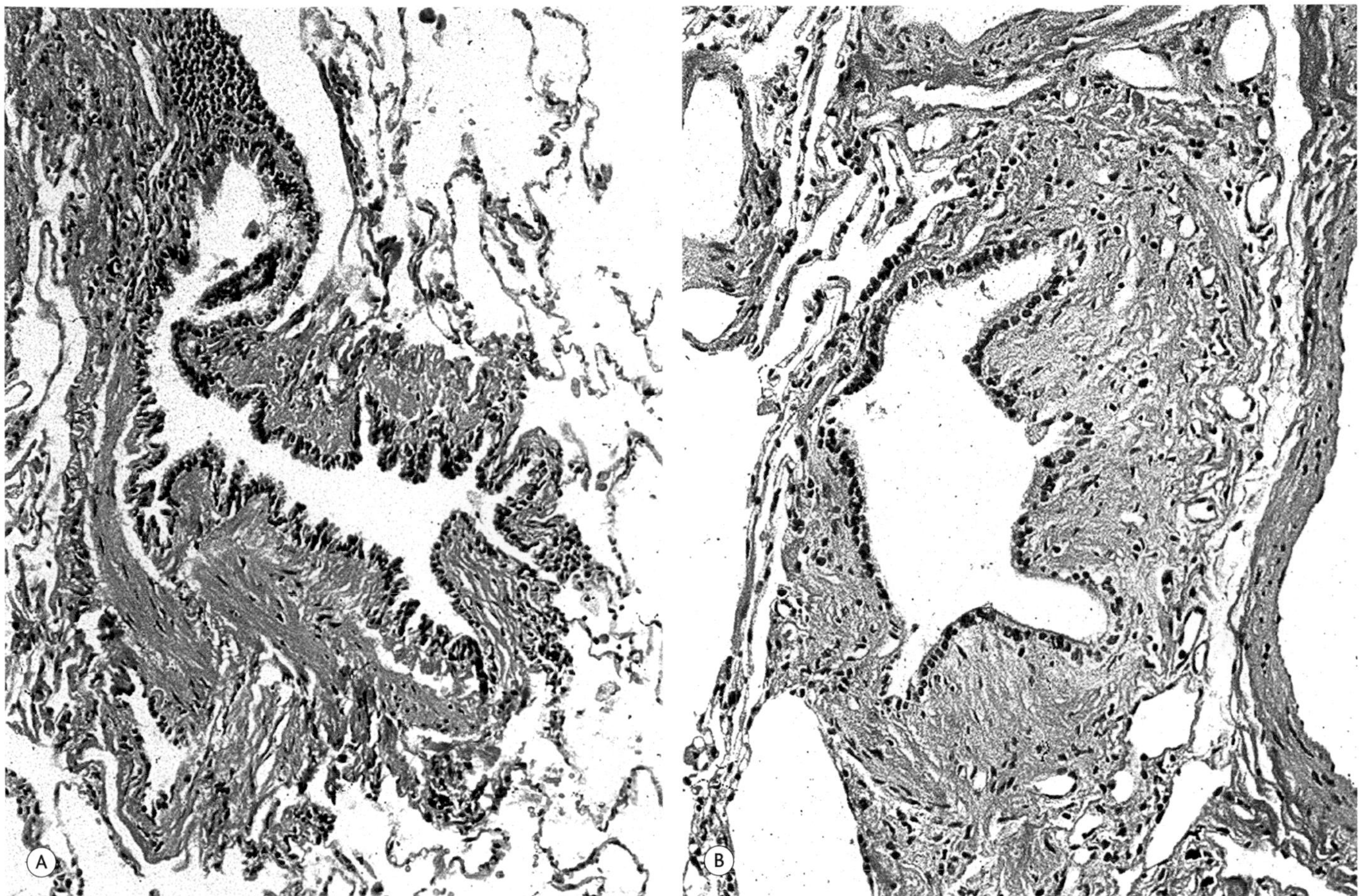

Fig. 8.32 **Idiopathic constrictive bronchiolitis.** (A) The wall of this bronchiole is thick and fibrotic without much associated inflammatory changes. The luminal profiles may be highly variable, here (B) slightly dilated and tortuous, despite abundant mural fibrosis.

uniform throughout the biopsy (or presumably the lung as a whole.) A number of mechanisms have been proposed in the lung transplantation setting, where the earliest stage is characterized by eccentric subepithelial fibrosis with scattered admixed chronic inflammatory cells. Concentric fibrosis then progresses over time until the lumen becomes markedly narrowed, or entirely obliterated. In other instances, the lumen may be initially occluded by loose fibrous tissue, presumably as a manifestation of active repair following an injury to the airway epithelium and basal lamina. Some authors have distinguished these latter lesions as more typical of bronchiolitis obliterans – asserting that the outer dimensions of the bronchiole remains stable (i.e. not necessarily constricted).

Given the limited repertoire of airway repair after injury, it is probably best to think of constrictive and obliterative forms of bronchiolitis simply as a representation of a later evolution of the repair process, whereas organizing intraluminal polyps (bronchiolitis obliterans fibrosa) are a more subacute manifestation of injury. Why some injuries resolve with little permanent structural abnormalities, whereas others result in persistent damage, is unknown. In an analogy with alveolar injury, a good example is pneumoccocal pneumonia, which results in extensive fibroplasia in the organizing (grey hepatization) phase. Complete structural recovery is the rule, with minimal permanent alterations. However, other infectious pneumonias (such as Gram-negative bacterial pneumonia) may resolve with advanced lung damage and permanent structural remodeling. Examples of the spectrum of constrictive airway injury are presented in Figs 8.32–8.34.

Bronchiolar fibrosis

Increased fibrous tissue beneath the epithelium of the small airways or around the airways, as an expansion of the adventitia, may be seen with or without smooth

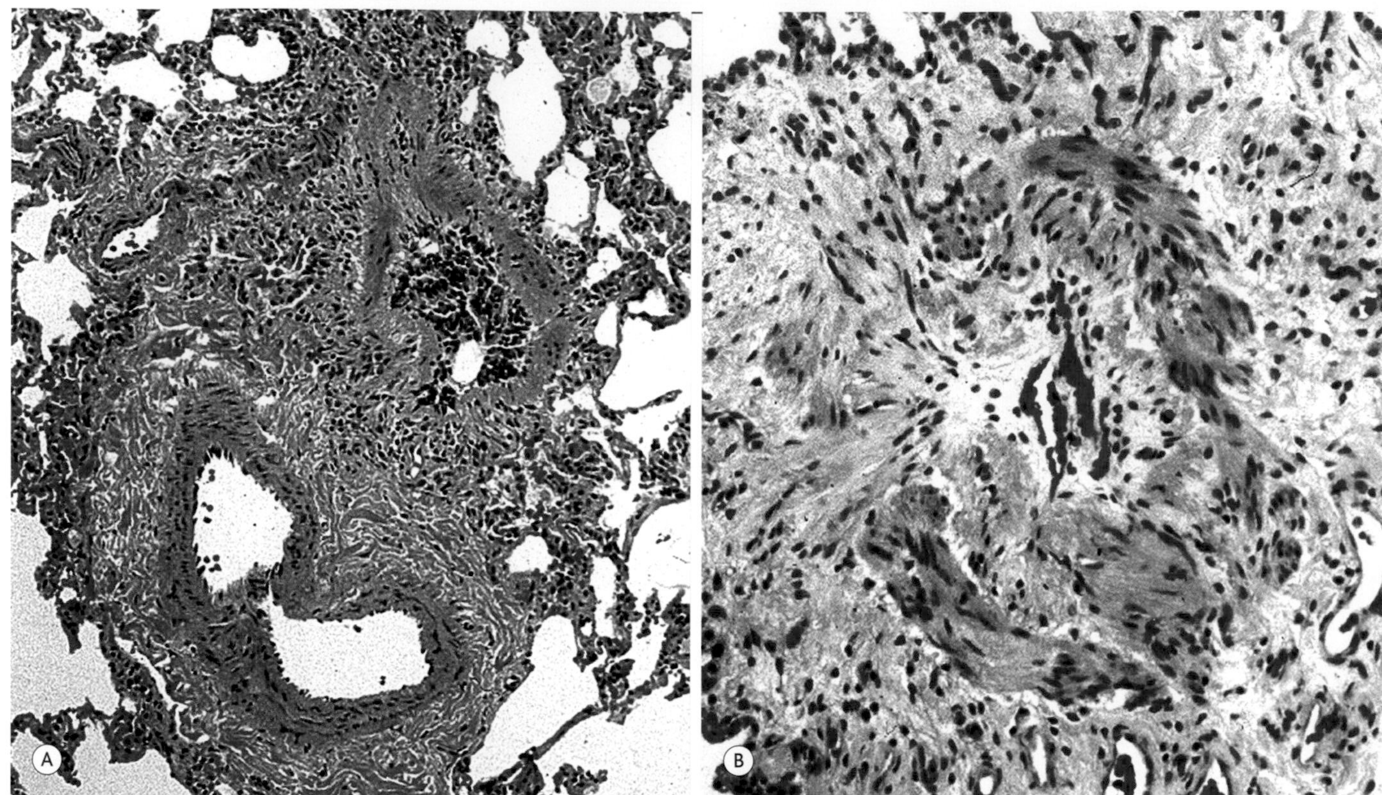

Fig. 8.33 **Constrictive bronchiolitis.** (A) From a child, following a viral infection: the lumen of the bronchiole is small, the walls are fibrotic, and the epithelial cells are sloughed into the lumen. (B) From a patient who developed obstructive lung disease after having had an acute pneumonia due to mycoplasma infection. The bronchiole is almost completely obliterated by fibrous tissue. The epithelial cells are lost, while the muscularis propria is still preserved.

muscle hyperplasia and bronchiolar metaplasia. The presence of subepithelial fibrosis in the small airways is almost a universal finding in heavy cigarette smokers and the significance of this change is often difficult to reconcile with a clinical or radiographic manifestation. Bronchiolar fibrosis, in the non-smoker, could be a component of several conditions, including pathophysiologically defined constrictive bronchiolitis (discussed above), that in turn may be related to one or more of the potential etiologies listed in Table 8.12. It is worth noting that the pathologic findings of constrictive bronchiolitis may be quite subtle. When no other explanation for a patient's significant hypoxia or "interstitial lung disease" on radiographic studies can be identified in the biopsy, trichrome and elastic tissue stains may be helpful in the identification of small airways obliteration.

Organizing pneumonia pattern with intraluminal polyps

The formation of intraluminal fibroblastic polyps in the small airways is almost always associated with significant inflammatory changes in the airway wall and surrounding lung parenchyma. The terms "bronchiolitis obliterans organizing pneumonia" or "organizing pneumonia" have been used in these settings. On occasions, such intraluminal polyps may be the predominant finding,[89] such as in very acute fume inhalation (Figs 8.35 and 8.36). Intraluminal fibroblastic polyps can be seen in many lung disorders, as detailed in Table 8.13.

Terminal airway fibrosis with dust deposition (pneumoconiosis-associated small airways disease)

Variable dust deposition around airways, accompanied by fibrosis, can be seen commonly in smokers. Under polarized light, small refractile silicate (aluminum and magnesium silicates typically) particles may be identified within areas of pigment deposition, either as a consequence of lifelong dust exposure in the older patient, or as a common finding in cigarette smoking. When "dust nodules" are numerous and prominent (typically over 1 cm in diameter), consideration for a pneumoconiosis

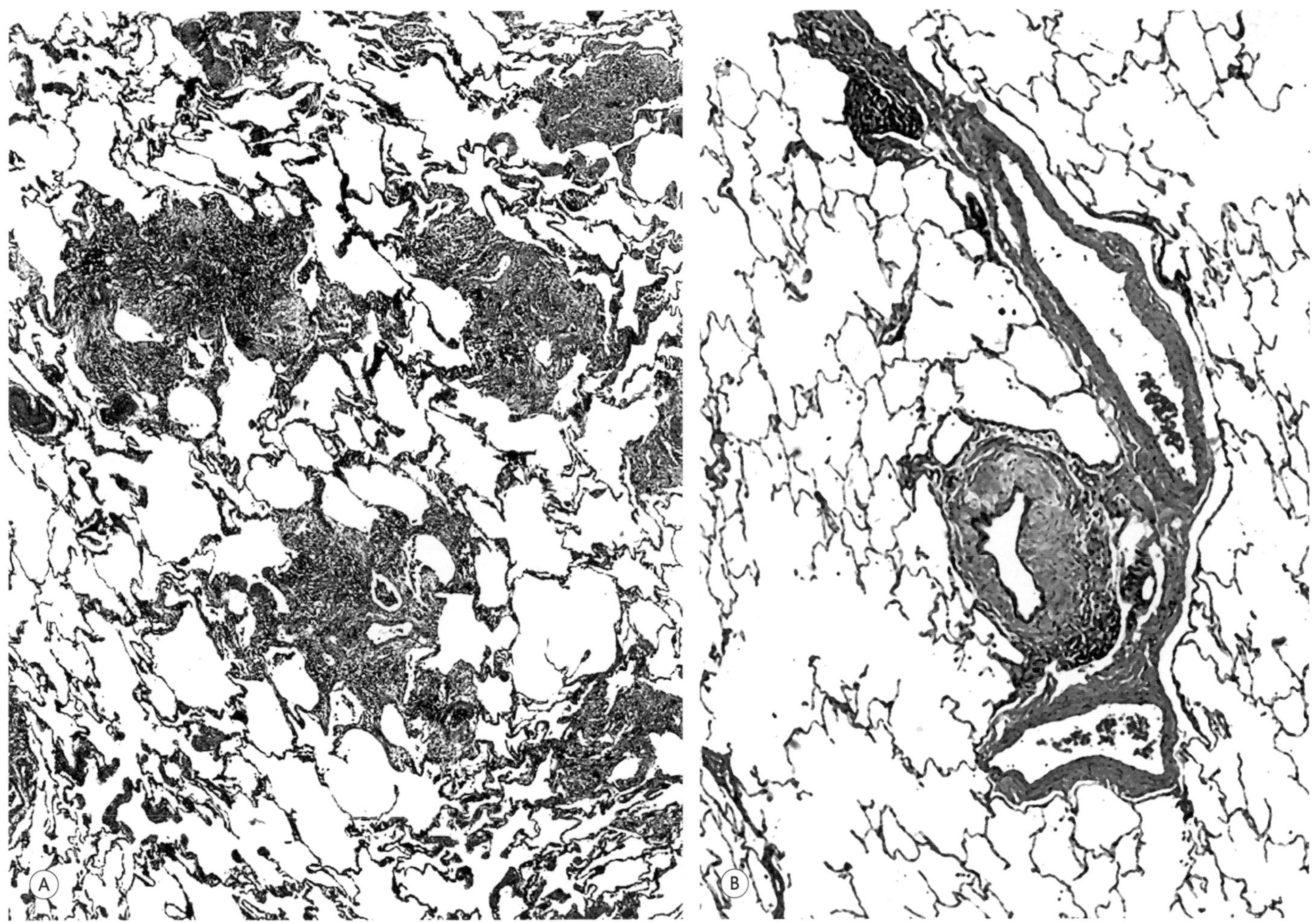

Fig. 8.34 **Constrictive bronchiolitis associated with inflammatory bowel disease.** (A) Low-magnification image showing bronchiolocentric lesions, characterized by fibrosis and a chronic inflammatory infiltrate with almost complete destruction of the terminal bronchioles. (B) A higher-magnification image from another patient shows changes that are quite subtle. There is no inflammation in the bronchiolar wall, but the diameter of the airway is smaller than that of the artery, and the subepithelial connective tissue is dense and fibrotic.

Table 8.12 Known causes of constrictive bronchiolitis

Infection:
Respiratory syncytial virus
Cytomegalovirus
Adenovirus
Influenza virus
Parainfluenza virus
Varicella
Mycoplasma
Fumes
Toxins
Systemic connective tissue disease
Drugs
Transplant associated (lung)
Idiopathic

Source: data from Colby and Leslie[39] and King.[126]

enters into the differential diagnosis. Fibrosis often accompanies such nodules.

Small airways associated with specific mineral dust exposure such as that produced by asbestos, aluminum oxide, iron oxide, silicates, and coal, for example, is referred to as "pneumoconiosis-associated small airways disease."[77] Pneumoconiosis-associated small airways injury is frequently only minimally inflammatory (Figs 8.37 and 8.38). The alveolar duct walls are thickened by fibrous tissue and dust deposition is seen in association with the small airways. Clinical and radiographic correlation are essential before making a pathologic diagnosis of clinically significant pneumoconiosis (see Ch. 9). When hemosiderin is present along with alveolar duct fibrosis and other pigment deposition, a careful search for asbestos bodies is in order. In this setting, iron stains (Prussian blue) may be helpful for

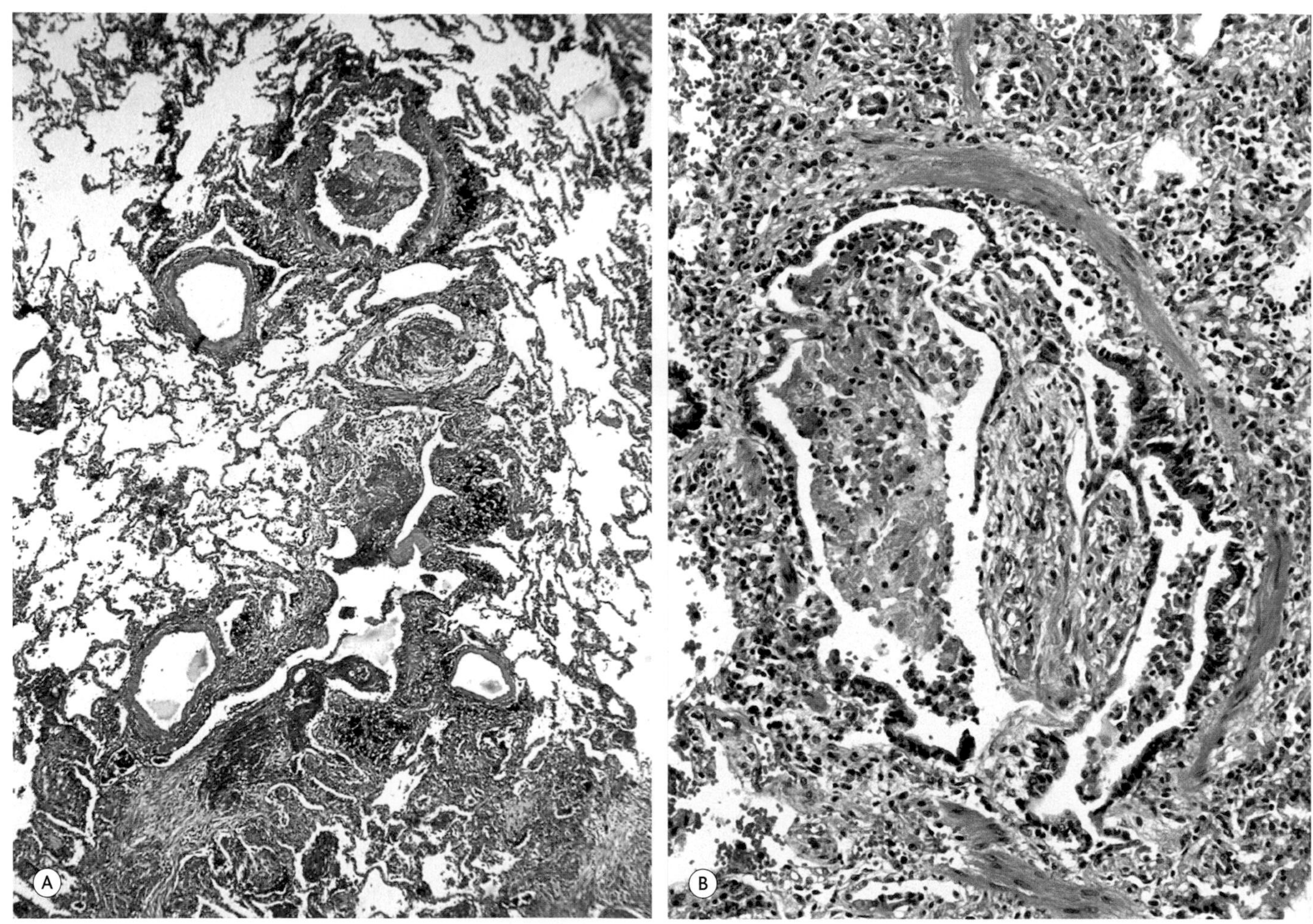

Fig. 8.35 **Organizing pneumonia with Masson polyps and fibrin (bronchiolitis obliterans).** These images are from a silo filler's lung biopsy. The patient developed an acute illness and died 3 days after this biopsy, despite steroid therapy. (A) The bronchioles are filled with polypoid formations, (B) some of which are partially fibroblastic and partially fibrinous, while others are purely fibroblastic and show an investing epithelial layer.

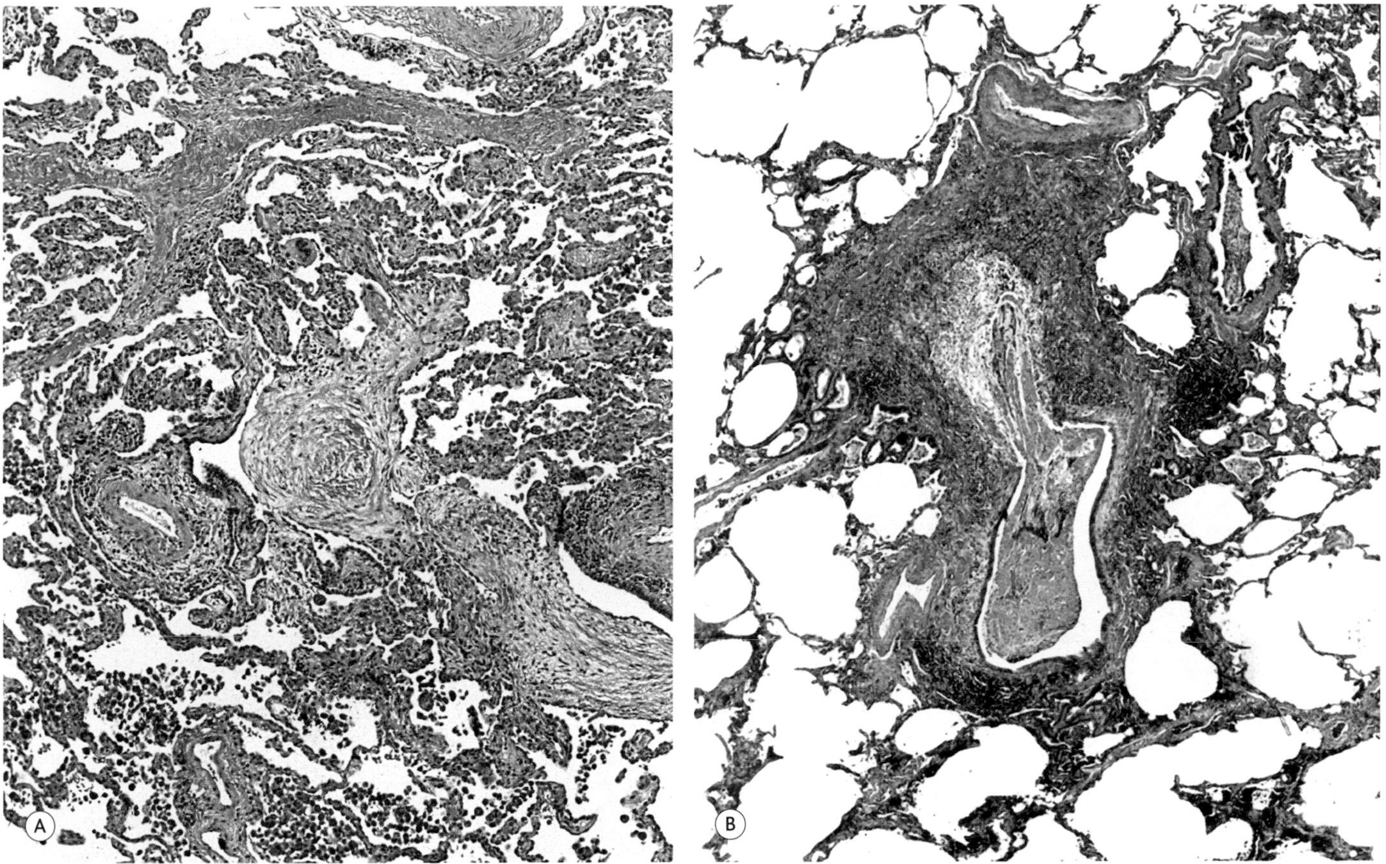

Fig. 8.36 **Organizing pneumonia with Masson polyps and fibrin (bronchiolitis obliterans).** (A) A polyp extending along the terminal airway in a patient with Wegener's granulomatosis. (B) A bronchiole in a patient with rheumatoid arthritis shows luminal polypoid myofibroblastic proliferation, accompanied by a peribronchiolar lymphoid infiltrate.

Table 8.13 Conditions associated with the organizing pneumonia/ BOOP pattern

As a phase of diffuse alveolar damage
Result of infection
Distal to bronchial obstruction
With aspiration pneumonia
Following certain drug reactions and toxic exposures
In association with systemic connective tissue disease
In hypersensitivity pneumonitis
In eosinophilic pneumonia
As a consequance of chronic bronchiolitis or diffuse panbronchiolitis
As an idiopathic process, usually associated with mild interstitial pneumonia
As a nonspecific reaction in other inflammatory lung diseases as in, for example, Wegener's granulomatosis, abscesses, necrosis, in tumors, and infarcts
In lung transplants with graft verus host disease

Source: modified from Travis et al.[18]

identifying foci of iron deposition, thereby attracting the pathologist's attention to areas where asbestos bodies (ferruginous bodies) are more likely to be identified (Fig. 8.38B).

Dilated and irregular bronchiolar shapes

Variations in the shape and other distortions of the terminal airways can be seen as a secondary phenomenon in many inflammatory airway diseases and is a common finding in smokers. A useful method for assessing such changes is to search for terminal airways that are present in cross section such that the diameter of the airway and of the adjacent artery can be compared. In this setting, the diameters should be equal. When considerable bronchiolar distortion is present, thin-walled dilated airways may greatly exceed the pulmonary artery diameter or, alternatively, may be significantly smaller. Such variable saccular, or varicose, dilatation and constriction is common in chronic small airway diseases that result in fibrosis.

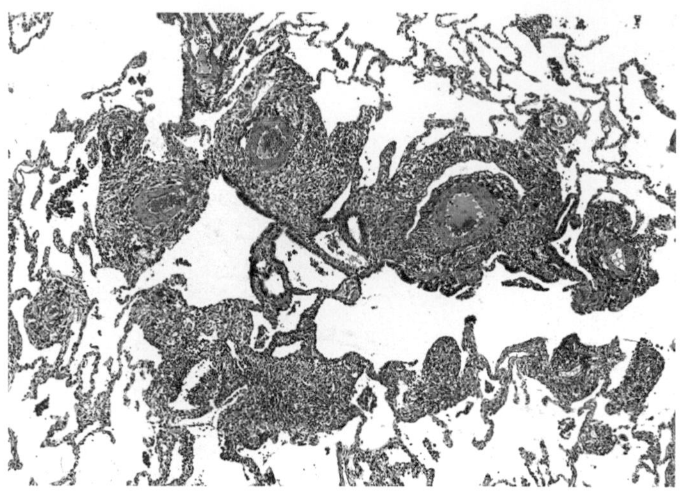

Fig. 8.37 **Silicatosis.** This biopsy from a pottery factory worker shows the wall of a thickened and distorted respiratory bronchiole. The majority of cells in the wall are histiocytes. On polarized light there are many needle-shaped, birefringent silicate crystals present.

Bronchiolocentric nodules

A number of diseases may produce nodular lesions centered on the small airways (bronchiolocentric nodules).[34] The diseases that can produce such bronchocentric nodules include primarily inflammatory lesions (e.g. panbronchiolitis[90]), inflammatory and fibrotic lesions (e.g. pulmonary Langerhans cell histiocytosis[91,92]) (Fig. 8.39), and miscellaneous disease processes (e.g. multiple carcinoid tumorlets with or without constrictive bronchiolitis,[93,94] and lymphangitic tumor, including malignant lymphoma).

Clinicopathologic entities with prominent airway manifestations

Defined clinical diseases with distinctive inflammatory reaction patterns in the airways are few. In this section we

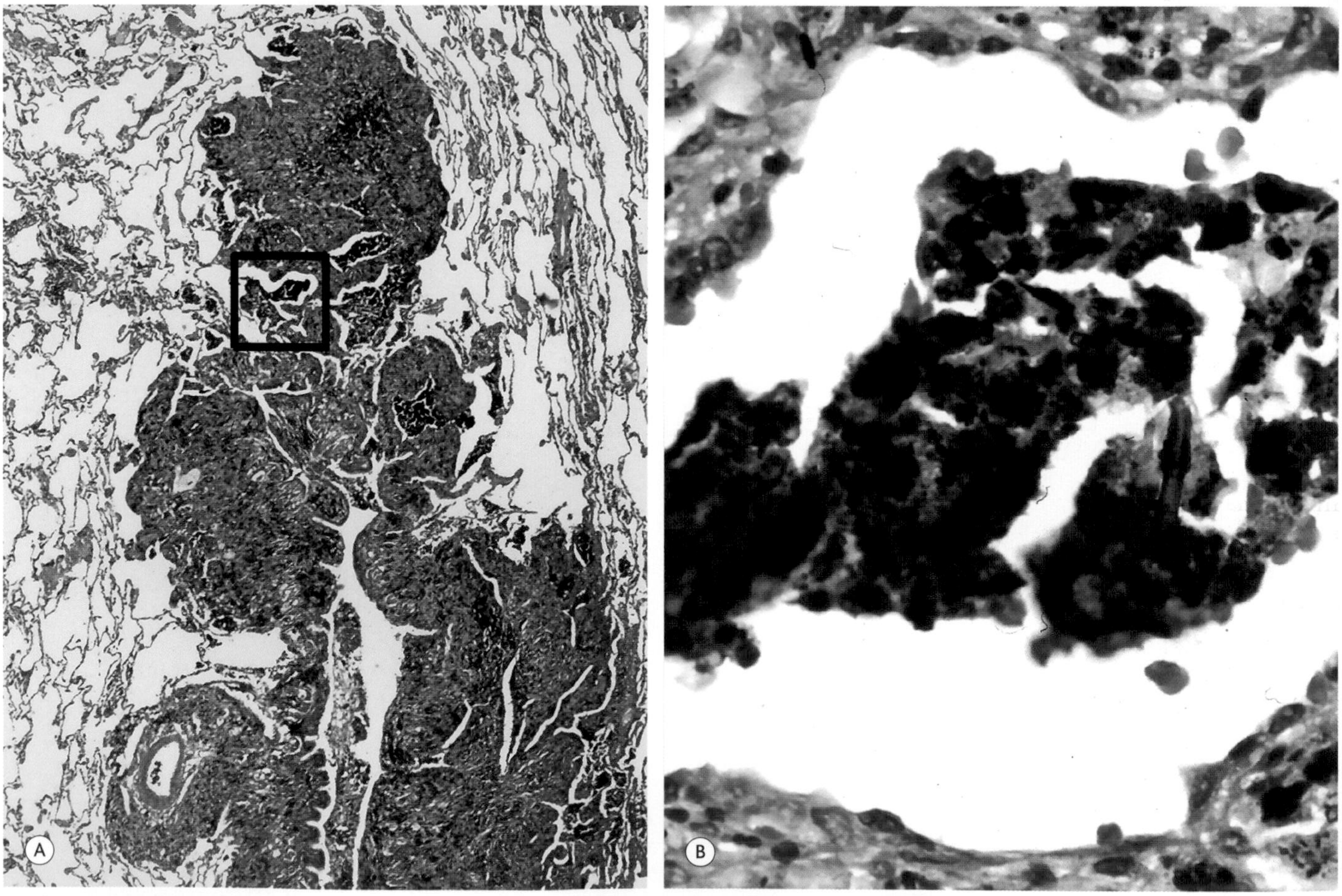

Fig. 8.38 **Mixed dust pneumoconiosis.** (A) At low magnification the bronchiole and accompanying artery are surrounded by densely pigmented fibrous tissue, which distorts the normal architecture of the bundle. (B) The histiocytic cells within the fibrous tissue contain abundant black pigment and the lumen of the bronchiole contains densely pigmented cells, most of which contain hemosiderin, and occasionally, ferruginous bodies.

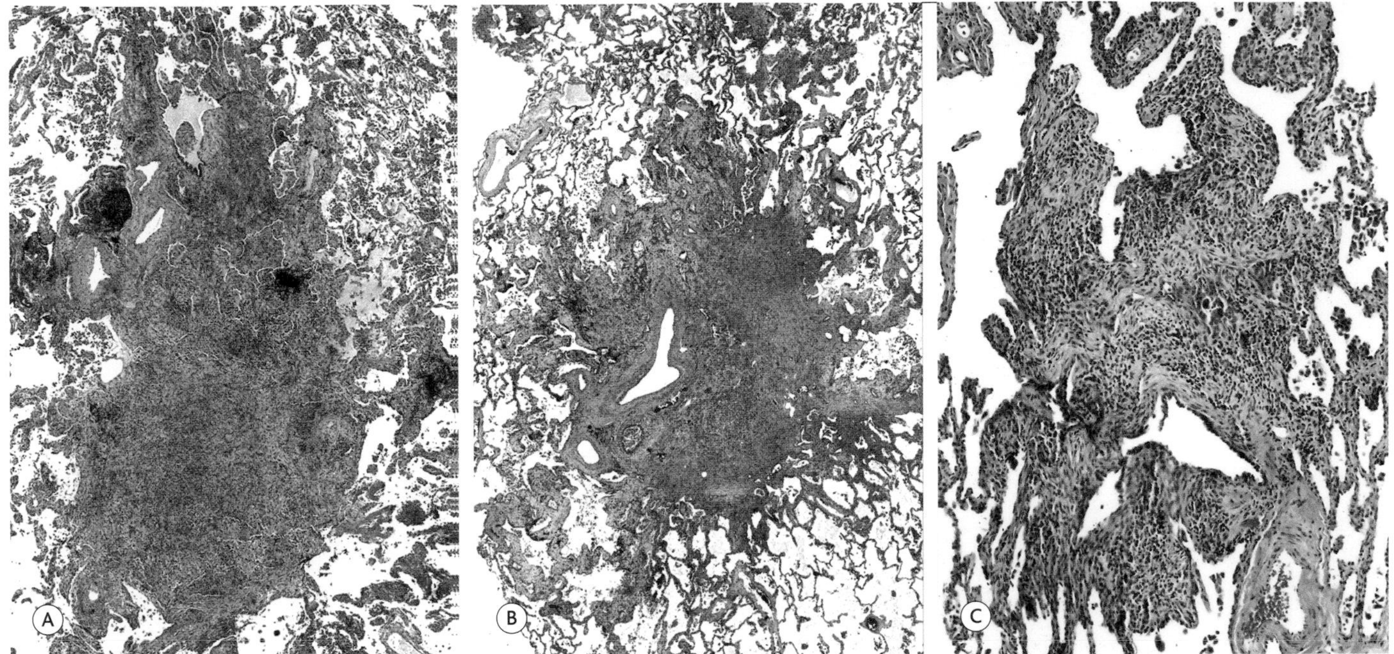

Fig. 8.39 **Pulmonary Langerhans cell histiocytosis (PLCH).** This image shows three different phases of the disease, with nodular cellular lesions (A,B) transitioning to (C) characteristically stellate morphology. The diagnosis of PLCH can frequently be made at scanning magnification, where one can easily appreciate the typical discrete, roughly symmetrical nodules, which have a stellate shape, a dense fibrotic core, and, frequently, a more cellular peripheral zone. The nodules involve the bronchiole and contain variable numbers of eosinophils and Langerhans cells.

will examine two frequent diseases, asthma and COPD, and two more rare, but well-defined diseases, panbronchiolitis and neuroendocrine cell hyperplasia with occlusive bronchiolar fibrosis (Aguayo–Miller disease). Emphysema will also be covered in this section, as it is a structural remodeling of the lung parenchyma that involves the small airways.

Asthma-associated airway diseases

In asthma inflammatory lesions are most prominent in the large airways but may also involve the small airways. The former lesions are those mainly seen in lobectomy and autopsy specimens from patients who die with status asthmaticus. Conversely, the small airway changes are more often observed in surgical specimens of peripheral lung.

In the bronchi, the classic changes consist of epithelial sloughing, mucus stasis, mural infiltration by eosinophils, smooth muscle hyperplasia, goblet cell metaplasia/hyperplasia, and basal membrane thickening[95–97] (Fig. 8.40, Table 8.14).

Some patients with asthma have prominent inflammatory small airways disease.[34,95,98] In addition to classic types of lesions, the small airways may also show several distinctive morphologic findings. These include chronic bronchiolitis, eosinophilic bronchiolitis, varicosity of bronchiolar lumens, bronchiolar metaplasia, constrictive bronchiolitis, and even features of bronchocentric granulomatosis (Figs 8.41–8.44).

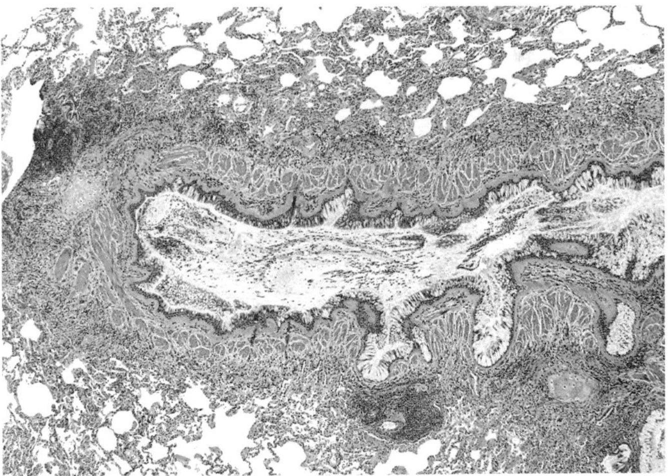

Fig. 8.40 **Asthmatic changes in a bronchus.** The lumen is occupied by mucus, the epithelium shows prominent goblet cell hyperplasia, the basal membrane is thick, smooth muscle is prominent, and there is a chronic inflammatory infiltrate extending through the bronchial wall.

Table 8.14 Pathologic findings in asthma

Mucus plugs
Mucosal eosinophils
Mucosal basement membrane thickening due to submembraneous collagen deposition
Distinctive inclusions in airway mucus: Charcot–Leyden crystals Creola bodies Curschmann's spirals
Epithelial shedding (desquamation)
Goblet cell metaplasia/hyperplasia
Squamous metaplasia
Airway wall edema
Bronchial mucus gland hyperplasia
Airway wall smooth muscle hyperplasia

Source: based on Dunnill et al.,[127] Aikawa et al.,[128] and Messer et al.[129]

In addition to these bronchial and bronchiolar alterations, there are four distinctive, albeit partially overlapping, asthma-associated lung diseases, that include eosinophilic pneumonia, allergic bronchial pulmonary fungal disease, mucoid impaction of bronchi, and bronchocentric granulomatosis.[99–101] Eosinophilic pneumonia is discussed in Chapters 5 and 7, whereas the remaining three diseases are described below.

Allergic bronchopulmonary fungal disease

In certain predisposed individuals, *Aspergillus* and other fungi may colonize the mucus of the respiratory tract and result in chronic inflammatory disease.[102] Other fungi implicated in the pathogenesis of this disorder include *Pseudallescheria boydii*, *Bipolaris* spp., *Torulopsis glabrata*, *Curvularia*, and *Lunata*. The hallmark of allergic bronchopulmonary fungal disease (ABFD) is the presence of

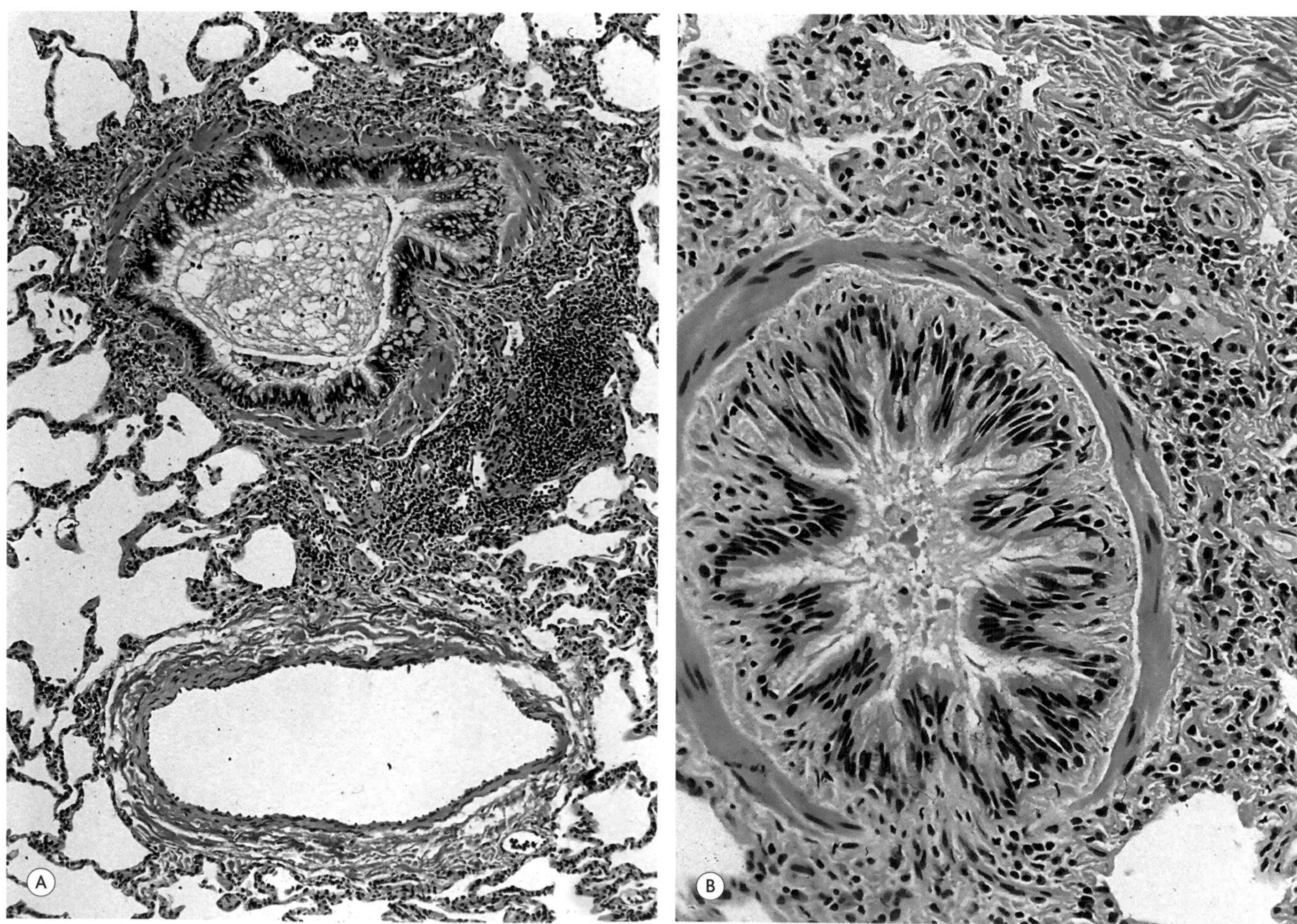

Fig. 8.41 **Constrictive bronchiolitis in asthma.** This asthmatic patient suffered from severe obstructive disease with a concurrent restrictive component. (A) The lung biopsy shows some of the usual features of asthma, as well as some scarring of the small airways. The bronchiole on the left is somewhat dilated, and has mucostasis. (B) The bronchiole on the right is smaller, shows subepithelial and adventitial fibrosis, and has inflammation with a prominent eosinophilic component.

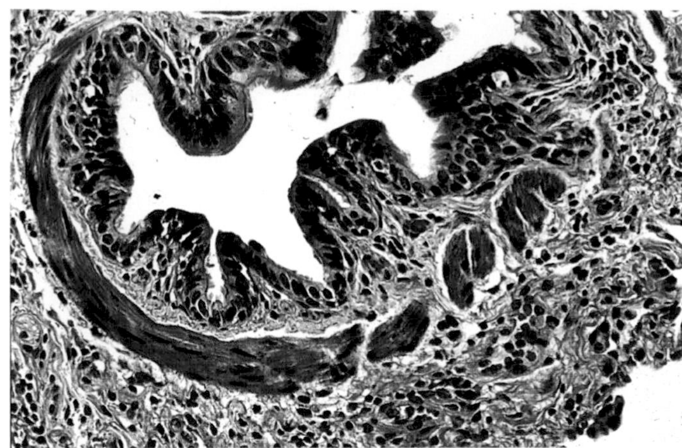

Fig. 8.42 **Constrictive bronchiolitis in asthma.** This bronchiole shows a very corrugated mucosa, with collagen fibers in the subepithelial connective tissue and also between the muscle fibers (trichrome stain).

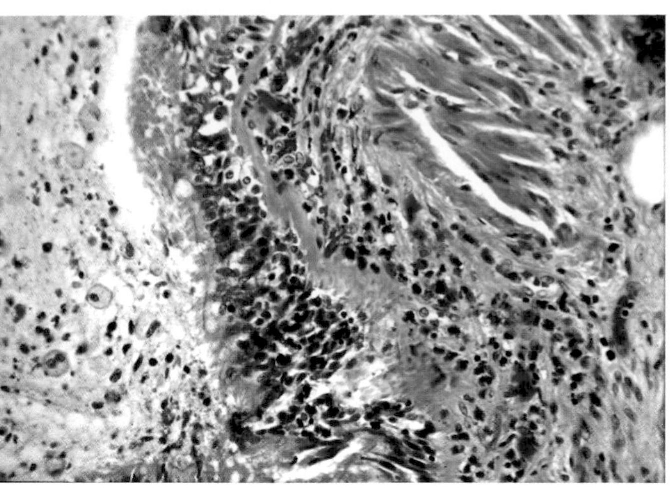

Fig. 8.44 **Fatal asthma.** This case illustrates several features of the asthmatic changes that may occur in the small airways. In a small bronchiole, there is a very prominent goblet cell metaplasia with mucostasis, and the basement membrane is thick and intensely eosinophilic. The smooth muscle layer is prominent.

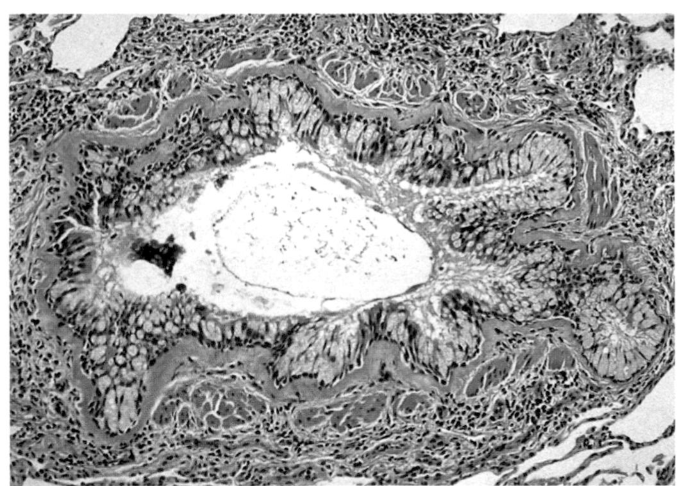

Fig. 8.43 **Bronchiolitis in asthma.** This bronchiole shows prominent goblet cell metaplasia and basement membrane thickening: the mucus in the lumen shows eosinophils and there is also an increased number of eosinophils in the epithelium and in the subepithelial connective tissue.

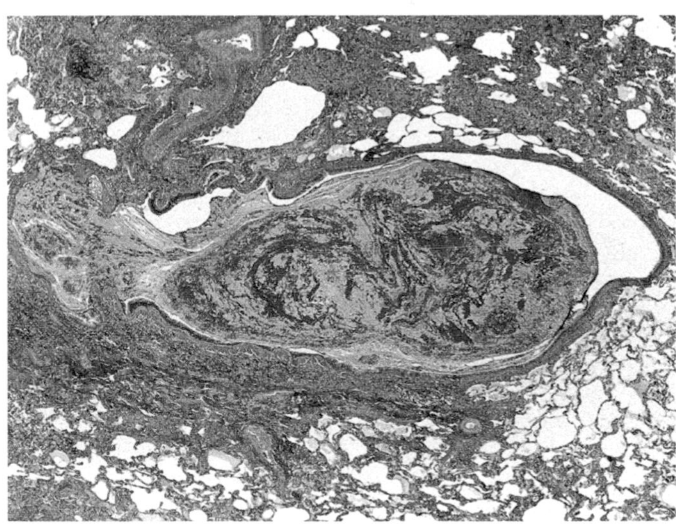

Fig. 8.45 **Allergic bronchopulmonary fungal disease.** Allergic mucin (mucus, eosinophils, and eosinophilic necrosis) is filling a distended bronchiole.

"allergic mucin."[103] Allergic mucin is characterized by the presence of eosinophils and eosinophil cytoplasmic granular debris (Fig. 8.45). Typically, one or more additional manifestations occur, such as mucoid impaction, bronchocentric granulomatosis, and eosinophilic pneumonia.[99,104,105] Calcium oxalate crystals may be present in the granular debris of allergic mucin, similar to that seen in sinus hypersensitivity to *Aspergillus* and other fungi in asthmatics. When allergic mucin is present, silver stains for fungal organisms are often helpful in confirming the diagnostic impression of ABFD. Because ABFD is considered an allergic manifestation, rather than a true infection, oral corticosteroids are often the treatment of choice.

Mucoid impaction of bronchi (MIB)

A distinctive clinicopathologic syndrome is characterized by the presence of extensive mucus plugging of the airways accompanied by airway dilatation.[100,106] The

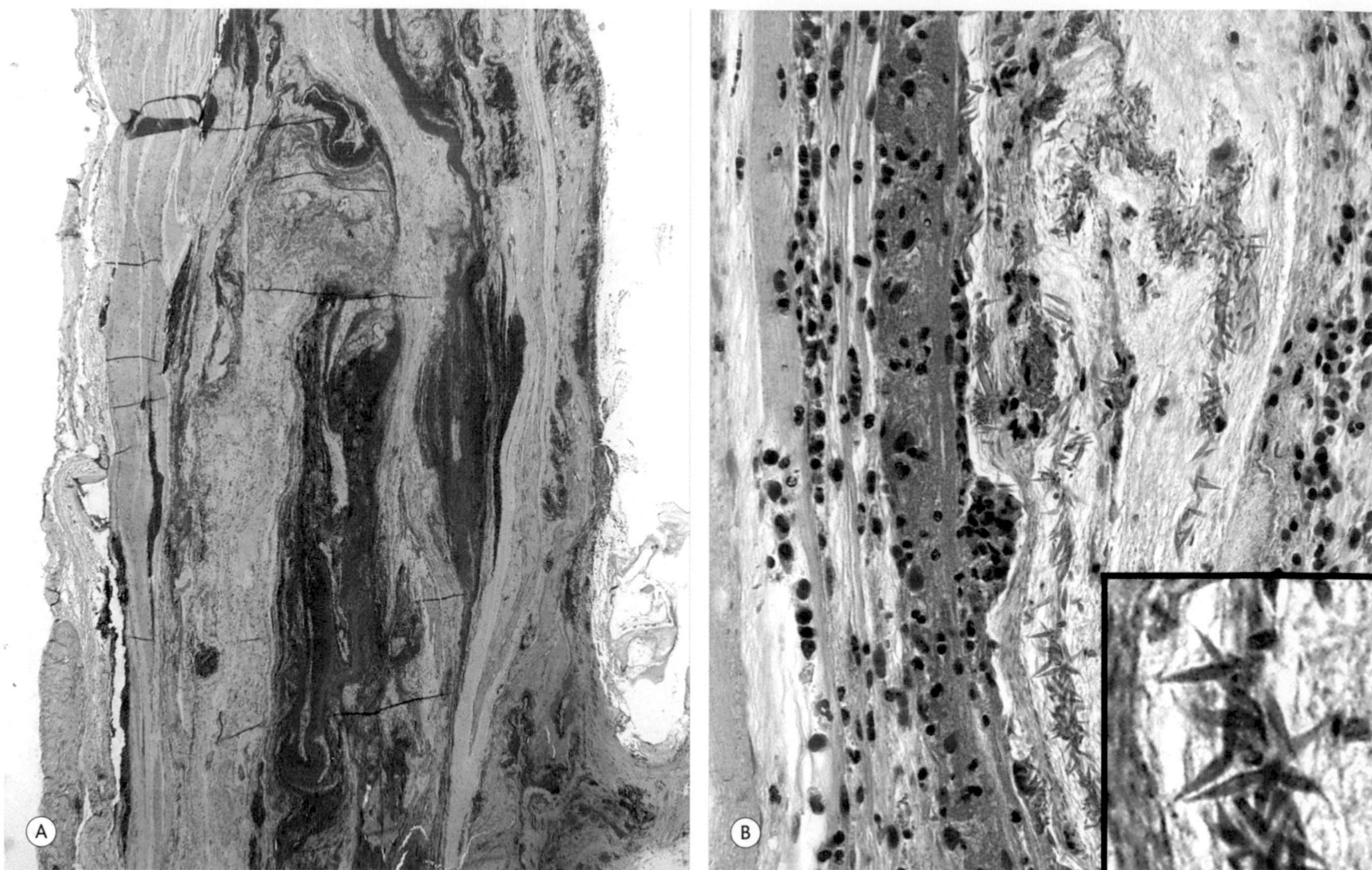

Fig. 8.46 **Mucoid impaction of bronchi.** (A) The characteristic laminated mucin. (B, and insert) At higher magnification, eosinophils and Charcot–Leyden crystals can be seen.

mucus of MIB has the appearance of allergic mucin. Mucoid impaction of bronchi is considered one of the major manifestations of allergic bronchopulmonary fungal disease.[99,104,105] Patients may be asymptomatic or may have obstructive pneumonia beyond the impaction.

Radiographic findings

Band-like or branching densities involving the upper lobes are characteristic findings ("gloved finger sign").[103] On occasion a solitary nodule may be produced. Branching strands of inspissated mucus may be coughed up by the patient and bronchoscopy may identify clues to the disease with the presence of impacted airways containing mucus.[107]

Pathologic findings

The affected bronchi are dilated and contain brownish to green mucus of tenacious consistency. Microscopically, the mucus has a laminated appearance (Fig. 8.46), with eosinophilic debris and Charcot–Leyden crystals (hexagonal brightly eosinophilic crystals). Asthmatic changes may be present in bronchoscopic biopsies from more central airways. Fungal stains may demonstrate hyphae, so it is useful to perform such stains whenever allergic mucin is found. Polarizable calcium oxalate crystals may also be present. Because mucus plugging can occur in a number of airway diseases, a distinctive laminated appearance should be present before the diagnosis is invoked.

Bronchocentric granulomatosis

Granulomatous inflammation associated with the airways can be generically considered a form of bronchocentric granulomatosis (BCG); however, this term is restricted to a distinctive form of granulomatous inflammation that surrounds and replaces bronchial walls and mucosa.[99,104,105] In bronchocentric granulomatosis, the lumen of the airway contains necrotic debris and palisaded histiocytes surround the lumen. Bronchocentric granulomatosis is not only confined to the larger bronchi but may also involve more distal bronchioles. Both infectious and non-infectious causes are described, and these are presented in Table 8.15.

Clinical manifestations

A useful distinguishing feature for separating infectious and non-infectious BCG is the presence or absence of asthma in the affected individual. Patients with asthma may present with exacerbation of their underlying airway disease accompanied by wheezing, cough, and fever. Bronchoscopy may identify mucoid impaction, with or without allergic mucin. In the non-asthmatic individual, infection should lead the differential diagnosis, even when special stains are negative in tissue sections.

Radiologic findings

In the non-asthmatic patient, given the propensity for infection as the etiology, the manifestations may be quite variable, ranging from localized consolidation to nodular parenchymal lesions on chest radiographs. Also, in the non-asthmatic patient, cavitation may be present in the nodules, attesting to the likelihood of an infectious etiology.[108] In the asthmatic patient the radiographic findings are often accompanied by the changes of mucoid impaction (branching opacities in a bronchial distribution).

Table 8.15 Common causes of bronchocentric granulomatosis

Allergic bronchopulmonary fungal disease
Bacterial infection, fungal infection, parasitic infestation
Rheumatoid arthritis
Wegener's granulomatosis
Necrotizing sarcoidosis

Pathologic findings

Destruction of the airway lumen is an important histologic manifestation of bronchocentric granulomatosis (Fig. 8.47). This feature is helpful in distinguishing peribronchial granulomas that occur in a number of infectious and non-infectious conditions (e.g. sarcoidosis). As in all cases of necrotizing granulomatosis inflammation, special stains for organisms should always be performed, even in the asthmatic patient where a hypersensitivity disease process is suspected. Rarely, Wegener's granulomatosis may be present in an exclusively airway-centered distribution, so clinical correlation and serologic studies may be useful. If the biopsy is from the middle lobe or lingula, consider middle lobe syndrome as an alternative diagnosis. Aspiration pneumonia is in the differential diagnosis and a careful search for foreign material is always advisable. The presence of conchoidal calcifications, or calcium oxalate crystals in isolation, is not a sign of aspiration, but can occur in any granulomatous inflammatory reaction. Vegetable material with thick cellular walls or meat (skeletal muscle fragments) implicates aspiration when it is present. Another feature helpful in excluding Wegener's granulomatosis is the presence of granulomas without necrosis (see Ch. 10). When granulomas are present without necrosis, Wegener's granulomatosis is an unlikely etiology.

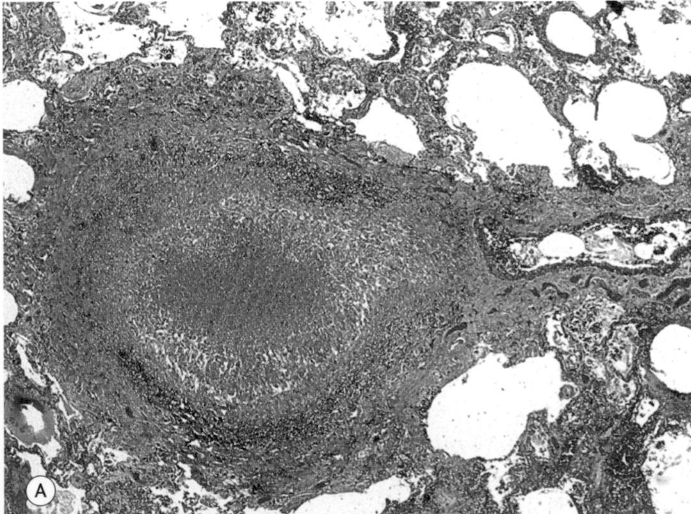

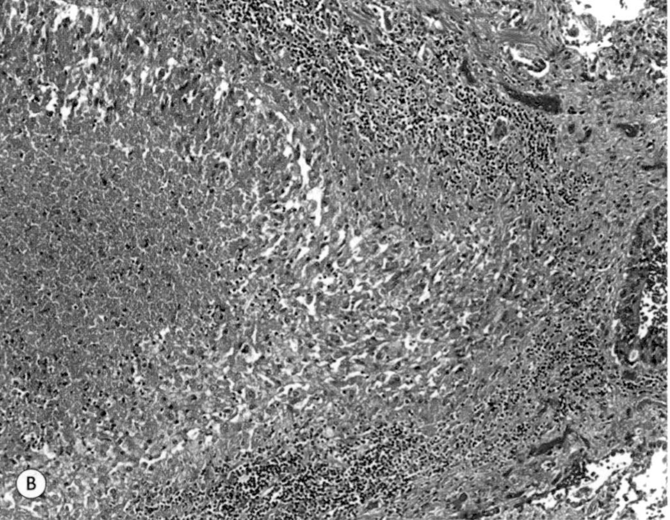

Fig. 8.47 **Bronchocentric granulomatosis.** (A) The disease is characterized by complete obliteration of the airway lumen and epithelium. (B) Note the prominent hystiocytic reaction at higher magnification.

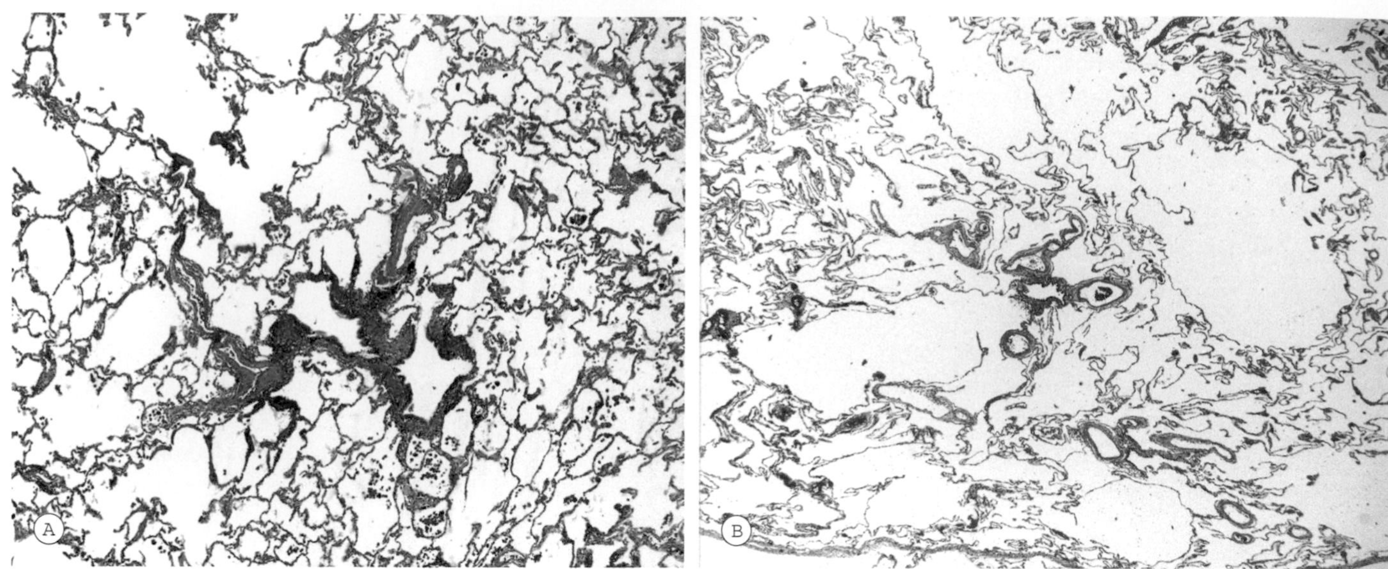

Fig. 8.48 **Emphysema.** The type and severity of emphysema may be difficult or impossible to determine on histologic grounds. (A) Here centriacinar emphysema is seen on the left and shows dilatation of the airspaces surrounding the bronchiole, whereas, (B) on the right, panacinar emphysema shows a more diffuse airspace dilatation.

Chronic obstructive pulmonary disease

Chronic obstructive pulmonary disease is a relatively common disease characterized by chronic airflow obstruction and small airways abnormalities.[109–111] The disease is usually related to cigarette smoking. The small airways in COPD are often subtly abnormal and this is the most common situation where one sees minor abnormalities of the bronchioles given the high prevalence of smoking.[112,113] Histologically, there is a minor degree of inflammation in the walls of bronchioles, including respiratory bronchioles, and there may be variable fibrosis, mucus stasis, loss of radial attachments, and bronchiolectasia (with dilatation and distortion). Emphysema and chronic bronchiolitis occur to variable degree in COPD.

Emphysema

Emphysema may be classified according to the part of the lung acinus that is primarily affected.[114] *Proximal (centrilobular, centriacinar) emphysema* involves the proximal part of the lung acinus; it is strongly associated with smoking; the respiratory bronchioles are enlarged and destroyed, and the enlarged airspaces are seen at the center of the secondary acinus; varying degrees of respiratory bronchiolitis may be present. *Panacinar emphysema* affects the whole acinus, and is characteristic of alpha-1-antitrypsin deficiency; the airspaces of the whole acinus are diffusely enlarged. *Distal (septal, pleural, localized) emphysema* affects the periphery of the acinus, most often beneath the pleura; it may be a cause of spontaneous pneumothorax in the young adult. *Irregular emphysema* may be seen in association with a lung scar, as those due to healed Langerhans cell histiocytosis, granulomatous inflammation, dust deposits, or pulmonary infarcts. Although gross examination of the lungs allows distinction between centriacinar and panacinar emphysema,[115,116] surgical lung pathology is not the primary method for diagnosing pulmonary emphysema. Noting the presence of emphysema on surgical wedge biopsies is reasonable, but it is not advisable to grade its severity (Fig. 8.48). The associated small airway and vascular changes may be prominent and include tortuosity.

Neuroendocrine cell hyperplasia with occlusive bronchiolar fibrosis (Aguayo–Miller disease)

Diffuse neuroendocrine cell hyperplasia of the bronchioles can be associated with partial or total occlusion of airway lumens by fibrous tissue and with chronic airflow obstruction (Figs 8.49 and 8.50).[93, 117] The disease is more frequent in women. Pathologically, the mildest lesions consist of linear zones of neuroendocrine cell hyperplasia with very focal subepithelial fibrosis. More obvious lesions consist of a plaque of eccentric fibrous tissue partially occluding the airway lumen. Sometimes the occlusion can be caused by a proliferation of neuroendocrine cells

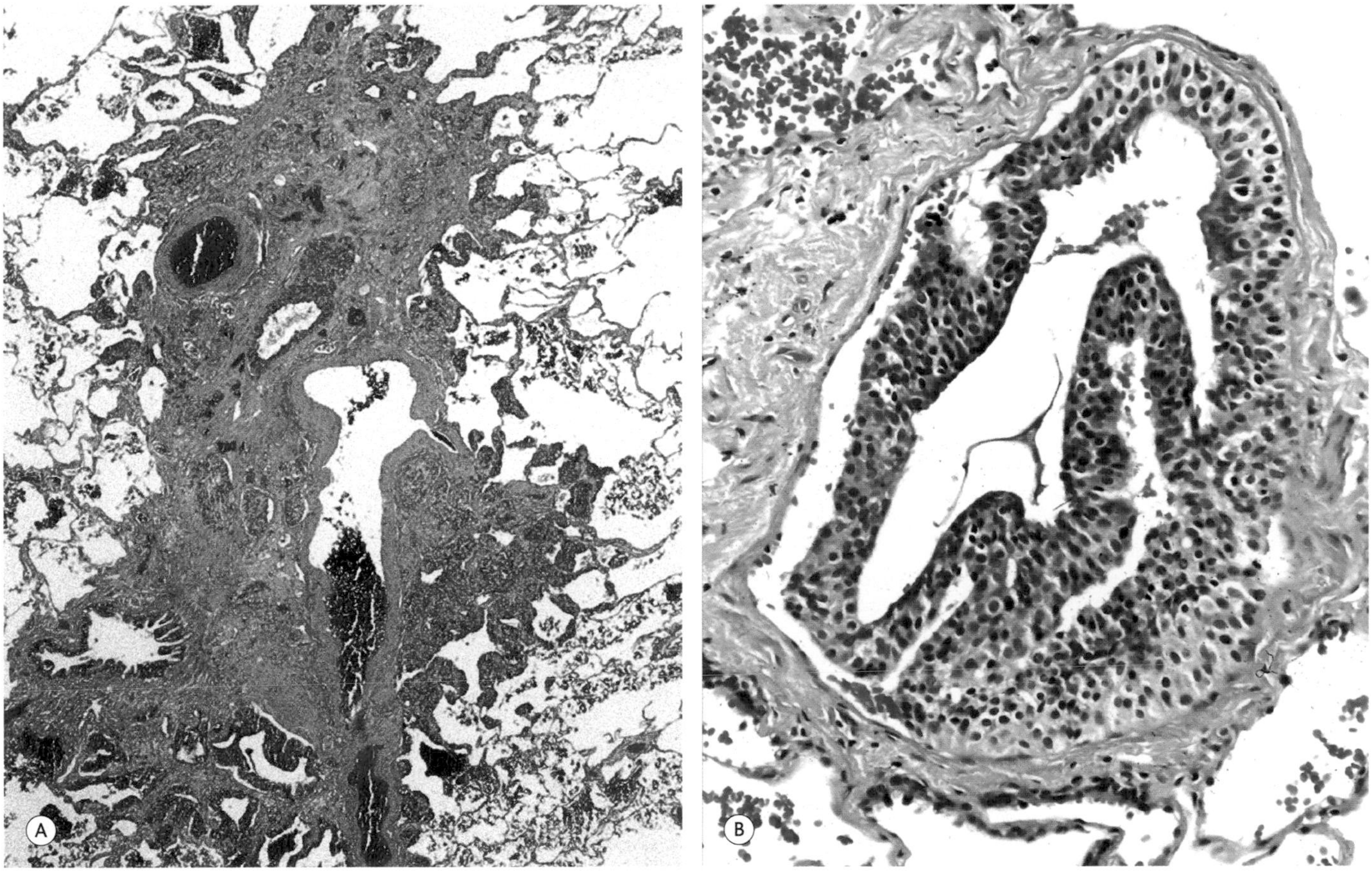

Fig. 8.49 **Aguayo–Miller disease.** These images are from a 74-year-old woman, who presented with dyspnea of recent onset and multiple pulmonary nodules, easily identified in the low-magnification view of the lung biopsy. (A) One of the nodules is composed of fibrous tissue encasing a small artery, some cellular nodules, and some small airways. The nodules are composed of neuroendocrine cells, demonstrable by their immunoreactivity for chromogranin-A and synaptophysin. The entrapped airways in the nodule show a narrowed lumen, with neuroendocrine cell hyperplasia that may protrude into the bronchiolar lumen. (B) Neuroendocrine cell hyperplasia in Aguayo–Miller disease is not only limited to airways associated with the nodules, but can also be found in isolated airways.

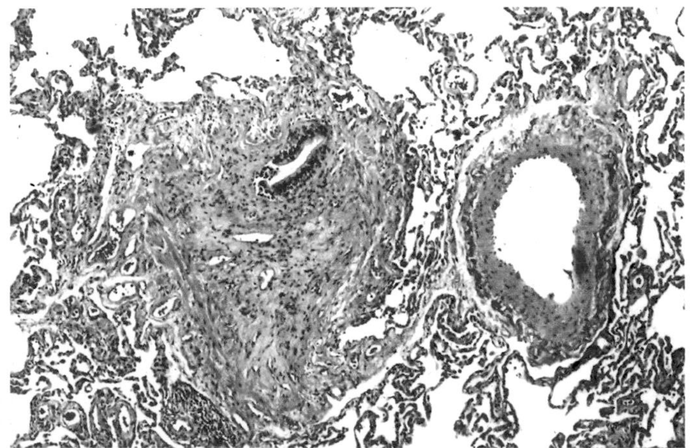

Fig. 8.50 **Aguayo–Miller disease.** Constrictive bronchiolitis. In Aguayo–Miller disease the clinical picture is dominated by obstructive physiology. In the present case, besides the neuroendocrine hyperplasia, in other bronchioles, there was prominent bronchiolar fibrosis with luminal narrowing.

within the airway epithelium. The most severely involved bronchioles show total occlusion of their lumens by fibrous tissue, with few visible neuroendocrine cells.

Diffuse panbronchiolitis

Diffuse panbronchiolitis (DPB), first described by Yamanaka et al.,[90] is a distinctive inflammatory condition characterized by chronic bronchiolitis associated with prominent interstitial vacuolated or "foamy" histiocytes in a peribronchiolar distribution (Fig. 8.51). Diffuse panbronchiolitis is seen more commonly in natives of Japan, Korea, and China and only rare cases have been described in non-Asian individuals.[88,118–122] Diffuse panbronchiolitis occurs with an age range of 20–60 years. Men are twice as commonly affected as women. Chronic productive cough and dyspnea are the typical presenting

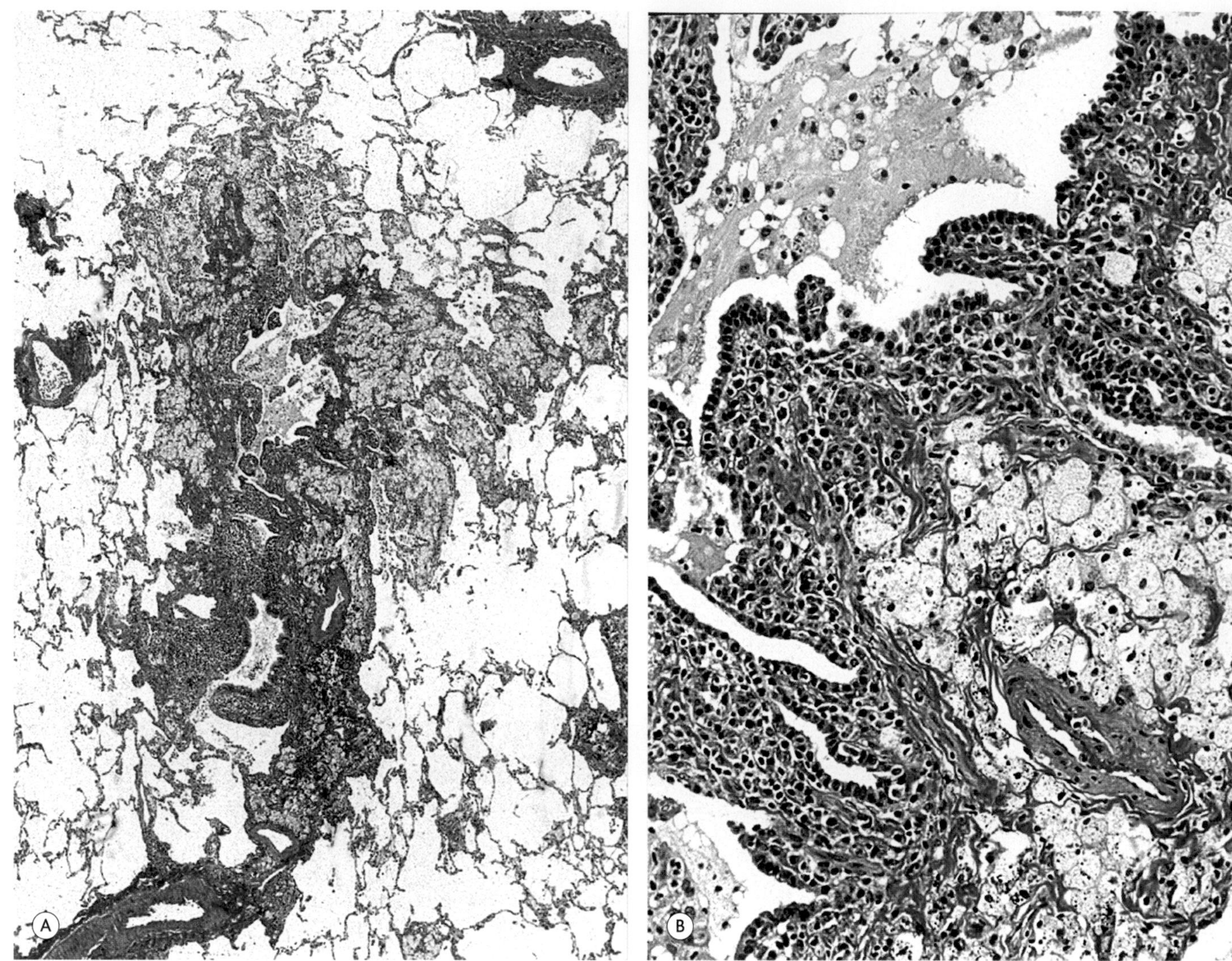

Fig. 8.51 **Diffuse panbronchiolitis.** (A) A low-magnification view shows a centrilobular nodule, composed of distinctive foamy macrophages distending the peribronchiolar septa, alveolar duct walls, and some alveolar septa. (B) This infiltration by pale foamy macrophages is more evident at higher magnification, and an associated chronic inflammatory infiltrate can be appreciated. This biopsy was taken from a Japanese man with a long history of chronic cough, sputum production, and dyspnea. A chest X-ray showed diffuse disseminated nodular shadows with hyperinflation. Pulmonary function testing showed an obstructive pattern with hypoxemia.

complaints, and most patients have sinusitis. A genetic susceptibility has been well documented over the years, and recently has been identified as a human leukocyte antigen (HLA)-associated major susceptibility gene, probably residing within the HLA-B locus on the short arm of chromosome 6 (6p21.3). HLA-B54 is the haplotype reported in Japanese patients and HLA-A11 is identified in those of Korean ancestry, suggesting that the DPB susceptibility locus is located between the HLA-B and HLA-A genes.[123,124]

REFERENCES

1. O'Regan A, Fenlon HM, Beamis JF Jr, et al.: Tracheobronchial amyloidosis. The Boston University experience from 1984 to 1999. Medicine (Baltimore) 2000; 79(2): 69–79.
2. Cordier JF, Loire R, Brune J: Amyloidosis of the lower respiratory tract. Clinical and pathologic features in a series of 21 patients. Chest 1986; 90(6): 827–831.
3. Papla B, Dubiel-Bigaj M: Tracheobronchial amyloidosis. Pol J Pathol 1998; 49(1): 27–34.
4. Weber AL: Radiologic evaluation of the trachea. Chest Surg Clin N Am 1996; 6(4): 637–673.
5. Herman DP, Colchen A, Milleron B, et al.: [The treatment of tracheobronchial amyloidosis using a bronchial laser. Apropos of a series of 13 cases]. Rev Mal Respir 1985; 2(1): 19–23.

6. Yang S, Chia SY, Chuah KL, et al.: Tracheobronchial amyloidosis treated with rigid bronchoscopy and stenting. Surg Endosc 2003; 17(4): 658–659.
7. Kalra S, Utz JP, Edell ES, et al.: External-beam radiation therapy in the treatment of diffuse tracheobronchial amyloidosis. Mayo Clin Proc 2001; 76(8): 853–856.
8. Fukumura M, Mieno T, Suzuki T, et al.: Primary diffuse tracheobronchial amyloidosis treated by bronchoscopic Nd–YAG laser irradiation. Jpn J Med 1990; 29(6): 620–692.
9. Masaoka A, Yamakawa Y, Niwa H, et al.: Pediatric and adult tracheobronchomalacia. Eur J Cardiothorac Surg 1996; 10(2): 87–92.
10. Jacobs IN, Wetmore RF, Tom LW, et al.: Tracheobronchomalacia in children. Arch Otolaryngol Head Neck Surg 1994; 120(2): 154–158.
11. Mair EA, Parsons DS: Pediatric tracheobronchomalacia and major airway collapse. Ann Otol Rhinol Laryngol 1992; 101(4): 300–309.
12. Nuutinen J: Acquired tracheobronchomalacia. Eur J Respir Dis 1982; 63(5): 380–387.
13. Tsunezuka Y, Sato H, Shimizu H: Tracheobronchial involvement in relapsing polychondritis. Respiration 2000; 67(3): 320–322.
14. Letko E, Zafirakis P, Baltatzis S, et al.: Relapsing polychondritis: a clinical review. Semin Arthritis Rheum 2002; 31(6): 384–395.
15. Karlikaya C, Yuksel M, Kilicli S, et al.: Tracheobronchopathia osteochondroplastica. Respirology 2000; 5(4): 377–380.
16. Meyer CN, Dossing M, Broholm H: Tracheobronchopathia osteochondroplastica. Respir Med 1997; 91(8): 499–502.
17. Vilkman S, Keistinen T: Tracheobronchopathia osteochondroplastica. Report of a young man with severe disease and retrospective review of 18 cases. Respiration 1995; 62(3): 151–154.
18. Travis WD, Colby TV, Koss MN, et al.: Non-neoplastic disorders of the lower respiratory tract. In: Atlas of nontumor pathology, Kind DW, Ed. 2002, Armed Forces Institute of Pathology, Washington, DC.
19. Dail DH: Bronchial and transbronchial diseases. In: Pulmonary pathology, Dail DHH, Hammar SP, Eds. 1988, Springer Verlag, New York, pp 79–119.
20. Thurlbeck W, Churg A, Eds: Pathology of the lung, 2nd edn. 1995, Thieme Medical Publishers, New York.
21. Barker AF, Bardana EJ Jr: Bronchiectasis: update of an orphan disease. Am Rev Respir Dis 1988; 137(4): 969–978.
22. Nicotra MB, Rivera M, Dale AM, et al.: Clinical, pathophysiologic, and microbiologic characterization of bronchiectasis in an aging cohort. Chest 1995; 108(4): 955–961.
23. Barker AF: Bronchiectasis. N Engl J Med 2002; 346(18): 1383–1393.
24. Tsang KW, Lam WK, Kwok E, et al.: *Helicobacter pylori* and upper gastrointestinal symptoms in bronchiectasis. Eur Respir J 1999; 14(6): 1345–1350.
25. Tsang KW, Lam SK, Lam WK, et al.: High seroprevalence of *Helicobacter pylori* in active bronchiectasis. Am J Respir Crit Care Med 1998; 158(4): 1047–1051.
26. Kang EY, Miller RR, Muller NL: Bronchiectasis: comparison of preoperative thin-section CT and pathologic findings in resected specimens. Radiology 1995; 195(3): 649–654.
27. Grenier P, Maurice F, Musset D, et al.: Bronchiectasis: assessment by thin-section CT. Radiology 1986; 161(1): 95–99.
28. Young K, Aspestrand F, Kolbenstvedt A: High resolution CT and bronchography in the assessment of bronchiectasis. Acta Radiol 1991; 32(6): 439–441.
29. Whitwell F: A study of the pathology and pathogenesis of bronchiectasis. Thorax 1952; 7: 213–239.
30. Kwon KY, Myers JL, Swensen SJ, et al.: Middle lobe syndrome: a clinicopathological study of 21 patients. Hum Pathol 1995; 26(3): 302–307.
31. Reich JM, Johnson RE: *Mycobacterium avium* complex pulmonary disease presenting as an isolated lingular or middle lobe pattern. The Lady Windermere syndrome. Chest 1992; 101(6): 1605–1609.
32. Wagner RB, Johnston MR: Middle lobe syndrome. Ann Thorac Surg 1983; 35(6): 679–686.
33. Fujita J, Ohtsuki Y, Suemitsu I, et al.: Pathological and radiological changes in resected lung specimens in *Mycobacterium avium intracellulare* complex disease. Eur Respir J 1999; 13(3): 535–540.
34. Colby TV: Bronchiolitis. Pathologic considerations. Am J Clin Pathol 1998; 109(1): 101–109.
35. Yousem SA: Small airways disease. Pathol Annu 1991; 26(Pt 2): 109–143.
36. Becroft D: Bronchiolitis obliterans, bronchiectasis and other sequelae of adenovirus type 21 infection in young children. J Clin Pathol 1971; 24: 72–79.
37. Becroft D: Histopathology of fatal adenovirus infection of the respiratory tract in young children. J Clin Pathol 1967; 20: 561–569.
38. Travis WD, Hoffman GS, Leavitt RY, et al.: Surgical pathology of the lung in Wegener's granulomatosis. Review of 87 open lung biopsies from 67 patients. Am J Surg Pathol 1991; 15(4): 315–333.
39. Colby TV, Leslie KO: Small airway lesions. In: Diagnostic pulmonary pathology, Cagle PT, Ed. 2000, Marcel Dekker, New York.
40. Wells AU, du Bois RM: Bronchiolitis in association with connective tissue disorders. Clin Chest Med 1993; 14(4): 655–666.
41. Howling SJ, Hansell DM, Wells AU, et al.: Follicular bronchiolitis: thin-section CT and histologic findings. Radiology 1999; 212(3): 637–642.
42. Nicholson AG, Colby TV, Wells AU: Histopathological approach to patterns of interstitial pneumonia in patient with connective tissue disorders. Sarcoidosis Vasc Diffuse Lung Dis 2002; 19(1): 10–17.
43. Yousem S, Colby T, Carrington C: Follicular bronchitis/ bronchiolitis. Hum Pathol 1985; 16: 700–706.
44. Nicholson AG, Wotherspoon AC, Diss TC, et al.: Reactive pulmonary lymphoid disorders. Histopathology 1995; 26(5): 405–412.
45. Fiche M, Caprons F, Berger F, et al.: Primary pulmonary non-Hodgkin's lymphomas. Histopathology 1995; 26(6): 529–537.
46. Roggeri A, Agostini L, Vezzani G, et al.: Primary malignant non-Hodgkin's lymphoma of the lung arising in mucosa-associated lymphoid tissue (MALT). Eur Respir J 1993; 6(1): 138–140.
47. Eschenbacher WL, Kreiss K, Lougheed MD, et al.: Nylon flock-associated interstitial lung disease. Am J Respir Crit Care Med 1999; 159(6): 2003–2008.
48. Boag AH, Colby TV, Fraire AE, et al.: The pathology of interstitial lung disease in nylon flock workers. Am J Surg Pathol 1999; 23(12): 1539–1545.
49. Kern DG, Kuhn C 3rd, Ely EW, et al.: Flock worker's lung: broadening the spectrum of clinicopathology, narrowing the spectrum of suspected etiologies. Chest 2000; 117(1): 251–259.
50. Kern DG, Crausman RS, Durand KT, et al.: Flock worker's lung: chronic interstitial lung disease in the nylon flocking industry. Ann Intern Med 1998; 129(4): 261–272.
51. Khoor A, Leslie KO, Tazelaar HD, et al.: Diffuse pulmonary disease caused by nontuberculous mycobacteria in immunocompetent people (hot tub lung). Am J Clin Pathol 2001; 115(5): 755–762.
52. Yousem SA: The histological spectrum of chronic necrotizing forms of pulmonary aspergillosis. Hum Pathol 1997; 28(6): 650–656.
53. Casey MB, Tazelaar HD, Myers JL, et al.: Noninfectious lung pathology in patients with Crohn's disease. Am J Surg Pathol 2003; 27(2): 213–219.
54. Camus P, Piard F, Ashcroft T, et al.: The lung in inflammatory bowel disease. Medicine (Baltimore) 1993; 72(3): 151–183.
55. Camus P, Colby TV: The lung in inflammatory bowel disease. Eur Respir J 2000; 15(1): 5–10.
56. Wang JL, Wang JB, Zhu YJ: Pyoderma gangrenosum with lung injury. Thorax 1999; 54(10): 953–955.
57. Vignon-Pennamen MD, Zelinsky-Gurung A, Janssen F, et al.: Pyoderma gangrenosum with pulmonary involvement. Arch Dermatol 1989; 125(9): 1239–1242.
58. Kruger S, Piroth W, Amo Takyi B, et al.: Multiple aseptic pulmonary nodules with central necrosis in association with pyoderma gangrenosum. Chest 2001; 119(3): 977–978.
59. Kasuga I, Yanagisawa N, Takeo C, et al.: Multiple pulmonary nodules in association with pyoderma gangrenosum. Respir Med 1997; 91(8): 493–495.
60. Fukuhara K, Urano Y, Kimura S, et al.: Pyoderma gangrenosum with rheumatoid arthritis and pulmonary aseptic abscess responding to treatment with dapsone. Br J Dermatol 1998; 139(3): 556–558.
61. Myers JL, Veal CF Jr, Shin MS, et al.: Respiratory bronchiolitis causing interstitial lung disease. A clinicopathologic study of six cases. Am Rev Respir Dis 1987; 135(4): 880–884.
62. Yousem S, Colby T, Gaensler E: Respiratory bronchiolitis-associated interstitial lung disease and its relationship to desquamative interstitial pneumonia. Mayo Clin Proc 1989; 64: 1373–1380.
63. Moon J, du Bois RM, Colby TV, et al.: Clinical significance of respiratory bronchiolitis on open lung biopsy and its relationship to smoking related interstitial lung disease. Thorax 1999; 54(11): 1009–1014.
64. Aubry MC, Wright JL, Myers JL: The pathology of smoking-related lung diseases. Clin Chest Med 2000; 21(1): 11–35, vii.

65. Fraig M, Shreesha U, Savici D, et al.: Respiratory bronchiolitis: a clinicopathologic study in current smokers, ex-smokers, and never-smokers. Am J Surg Pathol 2002; 26(5): 647–653.
66. Hartman TE, Tazelaar HD, Swensen SJ, et al.: Cigarette smoking: CT and pathologic findings of associated pulmonary diseases. Radiographics 1997; 17(2): 377–390.
67. Colby TV, Wistuba, II, Gazdar A: Precursors to pulmonary neoplasia. Adv Anat Pathol 1998; 5(4): 205–215.
68. Leslie KO, Colby TV: Pathology of lung cancer. Curr Opin Pulm Med 1997; 3(4): 252–256.
69. Nakahara R, Yokose T, Nagai K, et al.: Atypical adenomatous hyperplasia of the lung: a clinicopathological study of 118 cases including cases with multiple atypical adenomatous hyperplasia. Thorax 2001; 56(4): 302–305.
70. Weng S, Tsuchiya E, Satoh Y, et al.: Multiple atypical adenomatous hyperplasia of type II pneumonocytes and bronchiolo-alveolar carcinoma. Histopathology 1990; 16(1): 101–103.
71. Muir TE, Leslie KO, Popper H, et al.: Micronodular pneumocyte hyperplasia. Am J Surg Pathol 1998; 22(4): 465–472.
72. Leslie KO, Colby TV, Swensen SJ: Anatomic distribution and histopathologic patterns of interstitial lung disease. In: Interstitial lung disease, Schwartz MI, King TE, Eds. 2003, BC Decker, Hamilton, pp 31–53.
73. Davison A, Heard B, McAllister W, et al.: Cryptogenic organizing pneumonitis. Q J Med 1983; 52: 382–394.
74. Epler GR, Colby TV: The spectrum of bronchiolitis obliterans. Chest 1983; 83(2): 161–162.
75. Epler GR, Colby TV, McLoud TC, et al.: Bronchiolitis obliterans organizing pneumonia. N Engl J Med 1985; 312(3): 152–158.
76. Colby TV: Pathologic aspects of bronchiolitis obliterans organizing pneumonia. Chest 1992; 102(1 Suppl): 38S–43S.
77. Wright JL, Cagle P, Churg A, et al.: Diseases of the small airways. Am Rev Respir Dis 1992; 146(1): 240–262.
78. Paradis I, Yousem S, Griffith B: Airway obstruction and bronchiolitis obliterans after lung transplantation. Clin Chest Med 1993; 14(4): 751–763.
79. Estenne M, Maurer JR, Boehler A, et al.: Bronchiolitis obliterans syndrome 2001: an update of the diagnostic criteria. J Heart Lung Transplant 2002; 21(3): 297–310.
80. Yousem SA, Berry GJ, Cagle PT, et al.: Revision of the 1990 working formulation for the classification of pulmonary allograft rejection: Lung Rejection Study Group. J Heart Lung Transplant 1996; 15(1 Pt 1): 1–15.
81. Bando K, Paradis IL, Similo S, et al.: Obliterative bronchiolitis after lung and heart–lung transplantation. An analysis of risk factors and management. J Thorac Cardiovasc Surg 1995; 110(1): 4–13; discussion 13–14.
82. Cagle PT, Brown RW, Frost A, et al.: Diagnosis of chronic lung transplant rejection by transbronchial biopsy. Mod Pathol 1995; 8(2): 137–142.
83. Estenne M, Hertz MI: Bronchiolitis obliterans after human lung transplantation. Am J Respir Crit Care Med 2002; 166(4): 440–444.
84. Schlesinger C, Veeraraghavan S, Koss MN: Constructive (obliterative) bronchiolitis. Curr Opin Pulm Med 1998; 4(5): 288–293.
85. Schlesinger C, Meyer CA, Veeraraghavan S, et al.: Constrictive (obliterative) bronchiolitis: diagnosis, etiology, and a critical review of the literature. Ann Diagn Pathol 1998; 2(5): 321–334.
86. Kraft M, Mortenson RL, Colby TV, et al.: Cryptogenic constrictive bronchiolitis. A clinicopathologic study. Am Rev Respir Dis 1993; 148(4 Pt 1): 1093–1101.
87. Kraft M, Mortensen R, Colby T, et al.: Cryptogenic constrictive bronchiolitis. A clinicopathologic study. Am Rev Respir Dis 1992; 148: 1093–1101.
88. Myers JL, Colby TV: Pathologic manifestations of bronchiolitis, constrictive bronchiolitis, cryptogenic organizing pneumonia, and diffuse panbronchiolitis. Clin Chest Med 1993; 14(4): 611–622.
89. Douglas WW, Colby TV: Fume-related bronchiolitis obliterans. In: Diseases of the bronchioles, Epler GR, Ed. 1994, Raven Press, New York.
90. Yamanaka A, Saiki S, Tamura S, et al.: Problems in chronic obstructive bronchial diseases, with special reference to diffuse panbronchiolitis. Naika 1969; 23(3): 442–451.
91. Travis WD, Borok Z, Roum JH, et al.: Pulmonary Langerhans cell granulomatosis (histiocytosis X). A clinicopathologic study of 48 cases. Am J Surg Pathol 1993; 17(10): 971–986.
92. Webber D, Tron V, Askin F, et al.: S-100 staining in the diagnosis of eosinophilic granuloma of lung. Am J Clin Pathol 1985; 84(4): 447–453.
93. Aguayo S, Miller Y, Waldron JJ, et al.: Brief report: idiopathic diffuse hyperplasia of pulmonary neuroendocrine cells and airways disease. N Engl J Med 1992; 327: 1285–1288.
94. Miller R, Müller N: Neuroendocrine cell hyperplasia and obliterative bronchiolitis in patients with peripheral carcinoid tumors. Am J Surg Pathol 1995; 19: 653–658.
95. Hogg JC: Bronchiolitis in asthma and chronic obstructive pulmonary disease. Clin Chest Med 1993; 14(4): 733–740.
96. Kuwano K, Bosken CH, Pare PD, et al.: Small airways dimensions in asthma and in chronic obstructive pulmonary disease. Am Rev Respir Dis 1993; 148(5): 1220–1225.
97. Hogg JC: The pathology of asthma. Clin Chest Med 1984; 5(4): 567–571.
98. Hamid Q, Song Y, Kotsimbos TC, et al.: Inflammation of small airways in asthma. J Allergy Clin Immunol 1997; 100(1): 44–51.
99. Katzenstein A, Liebow A, Friedman P: Bronchocentric granulomatosis, mucoid impaction, and hypersensitivity reactions to fungi. Am Rev Respir Dis 1975; 111: 497–537.
100. Sanerkin NG, Seal RM, Leopold JG: Plastic bronchitis, mucoid impaction of the bronchi and allergic broncho-pulmonary aspergillosis, and their relationship to bronchial asthma. Ann Allergy 1966; 24(11): 586–594.
101. Sulavik SB: Bronchocentric granulomatosis and allergic bronchopulmonary aspergillosis. Clin Chest Med 1988; 9(4): 609–621.
102. Shah A, Panjabi C: Allergic bronchopulmonary aspergillosis: a review of a disease with a worldwide distribution. J Asthma 2002; 39(4): 273–289.
103. Aubry MC, Fraser R: The role of bronchial biopsy and washing in the diagnosis of allergic bronchopulmonary aspergillosis. Mod Pathol 1998; 11(7): 607–611.
104. Bosken CH, Myers JL, Greenberger PA, et al.: Pathologic features of allergic bronchopulmonary aspergillosis. Am J Surg Pathol 1988; 12(3): 216–222.
105. Jelihovsky T: The structure of bronchial plugs in mucoid impaction, bronchocentric granulomatosis and asthma. Histopathology 1983; 7(2): 153–167.
106. Urschel HC Jr, Paulson DL, Shaw RR: Mucoid impaction of the bronchi. Ann Thorac Surg 1966; 2(1): 1–16.
107. Angus RM, Davies ML, Cowan MD, et al.: Computed tomographic scanning of the lung in patients with allergic bronchopulmonary aspergillosis and in asthmatic patients with a positive skin test to *Aspergillus fumigatus*. Thorax 1994; 49(6): 586–589.
108. Ward S, Heyneman LE, Flint JD, et al.: Bronchocentric granulomatosis: computed tomographic findings in five patients. Clin Radiol 2000; 55(4): 296–300.
109. Niewoehner DE: The role of chronic bronchitis in the pathogenesis of chronic obstructive pulmonary disease. Semin Respir Infect 1988; 3(1): 14–26.
110. Niewoehner DE, Cosio MG: Chronic obstructive lung disease: the role of airway disease, with special emphasis on the pathology of small airways. Monogr Pathol 1978; 19: 160–179.
111. Thurlbeck W: Chronic airflow obstruction. In: Pathology of the lung, 2nd edn, Thurlbeck W, Churg A, Eds. 1995, Thieme Medical Publishers, New York, pp 739–825.
112. Jeffery PK: Comparison of the structural and inflammatory features of COPD and asthma. Giles F. Filley Lecture. Chest 2000; 117(5 suppl 1): 251S–260S.
113. Jeffery PK: Morphology of the airway wall in asthma and in chronic obstructive pulmonary disease. Am Rev Respir Dis 1991; 143(5 Pt 1): 1152–1158; discussion 61.
114. Cosio MG, Majo J: Overview of the pathology of emphysema in humans. Chest Surg Clin N Am 1995; 5(4): 603–621.
115. Bergin C, Muller N, Nichols DM, et al.: The diagnosis of emphysema. A computed tomographic–pathologic correlation. Am Rev Respir Dis 1986; 133(4): 541–546.
116. Wright JL: Emphysema: concepts under change – a pathologist's perspective. Mod Pathol 1995; 8(8): 873–880.
117. Miller RR, Muller NL: Neuroendocrine cell hyperplasia and obliterative bronchiolitis in patients with peripheral carcinoid tumors. Am J Surg Pathol 1995; 19(6): 653–658.
118. Homma H, Yamanaka A, Tanimoto S, et al.: Diffuse panbronchiolitis. Chest 1983; 83: 63–69.

119. Iwata M, Colby T, Kitaichi M: Diffuse panbronchiolitis: diagnosis and distinction from various pulmonary diseases with centrilobular interstitial foam cell accumulations. Hum Pathol 1994; 25: 357–363.
120. Poletti V, Pateli M, Poletti G, et al.: Diffuse panbronchiolitis observed in an Italian. Chest 1990; 98: 515–516.
121. Fisher MS Jr, Rush WL, Rosado-de-Christenson ML, et al.: Diffuse panbronchiolitis: histologic diagnosis in unsuspected cases involving North American residents of Asian descent. Arch Pathol Lab Med 1998; 122(2): 156–160.
122. Randhawa P, Hoagland MH, Yousem SA: Diffuse panbronchiolitis in North America. Report of three cases and review of the literature. Am J Surg Pathol 1991; 15(1): 43–47.
123. Matsuzaka Y, Tounai K, Denda A, et al.: Identification of novel candidate genes in the diffuse panbronchiolitis critical region of the class I human MHC. Immunogenetics 2002; 54(5): 301–309.
124. Keicho N, Ohashi J, Tamiya G, et al.: Fine localization of a major disease-susceptibility locus for diffuse panbronchiolitis. Am J Hum Genet 2000; 66(2): 501–507.
125. Lynch D: Imaging of diffuse parenchymal lung disease. In: Interstitial lung disease, Schwartz MI, King TE, Eds. 2003, BC Decker, Hamilton.
126. King TE: Bronchiolitis. In: Interstitial lung disease, Schwartz MI, King TE, Eds. 2003, BC Decker, Hamiton, pp 787–824.
127. Dunnill MS, Massarella GR, Anderson JA: A comparison of the quantitative anatomy of the bronchi in normal subjects, in status asthmaticus, in chronic bronchitis, and in emphysema. Thorax 1969; 24(2): 176–179.
128. Aikawa T, Shimura S, Sasaki H, et al.: Marked goblet cell hyperplasia with mucus accumulation in the airways of patients who died of severe acute asthma attack. Chest 1992; 101(4): 916–921.
129. Messer JW, Peters GA, Bennett WA: Causes of death and pathologic findings in 304 cases of bronchial asthma. Dis Chest 1960; 38: 616–624.

Pneumoconioses

Victor L Roggli   Kelly J Butnor

9

General introduction

Pneumoconiosis literally means dust in the lung, and has come to refer to diseases of the lung related to the inhalation of dusts. Pneumoconioses are for the most part due to the inhalation of inorganic dusts in the workplace, and the reaction of the lung to these dusts is generally fibrosis. These diseases typically evolve over several decades, although there are some exceptions to this rule. The pathologic findings in these conditions can resemble those of other fibrotic and granulomatous disorders of the lung, so the pathologist must be familiar with their diagnostic features. Although most of these disorders have no specific treatment, proper diagnosis is crucial for accurate determination of prognosis and, when indicated, compensation. The disorders covered in this chapter are listed in Table 9.1.

The toxicity, and hence fibrogenicity, of inorganic particulates is related to both the nature of the dust and the nature of the host response.[1] One important feature of particle toxicity is the aerodynamic diameter, with particles in the size range of 1–5 μm having the highest probability of deposition and retention within the respiratory tract. In addition, the total inhaled dose and intrinsic properties of the dust are important determinants of fibrosis. For example, crystalline silica is highly fibrogenic, whereas carbon is an innocuous, nuisance dust. Host factors include efficiency of clearance mechanisms and individual susceptibility. Many of the dusts have a characteristic reaction pattern or appearance in histologic sections, which permits an accurate diagnosis. The silicotic nodule and the asbestos body are familiar examples. Others are associated with a reaction pattern that may suggest the diagnosis, but a careful occupational history and/or supplemental analytical techniques may be required to confirm the diagnosis. Thus the histologic findings in berylliosis may closely resemble those of sarcoidosis.

Table 9.1 Pneumoconioses caused by inhalation of inorganic dusts

Silicosis:
Coal workers' pneumoconiosis
Asbestosis:
Silicatosis (silicate pneumoconiosis)
Talcosis (talc pneumoconiosis)
Siderosis
Aluminosis
Hard metal lung disease
Berylliosis
Rare earth (cerium oxide) pneumoconiosis

Analytical electron microscopy provides a powerful tool for identification of dusts in lung tissue samples, and these methods will be emphasized where appropriate.[2] An analytical electron microscope consists of a scanning or transmission electron microscope equipped with an energy dispersive spectrometer. Electron microscopic techniques may permit the detection of particles too small to be observed by light microscopy. Furthermore, energy dispersive X-ray analysis (EDXA) identifies the elemental composition of individual particulates, which can be critical to the identification and, in some cases, the source of the inhaled dust. However, it must be emphasized that the identification of a particular xenobiotic in lung tissue is in and of itself not proof of disease, and must be correlated with the pathologic response (if any) to the dust in routine histologic sections.

Silicosis

Introduction

Silicosis results from the inhalation of particles of crystalline silica. It is characterized by circumscribed areas of nodular fibrosis that tend to have the greatest profusion in the upper lung zones. Occupations with exposure to crystalline silica are summarized in Table 9.2.[3] In the past, very heavy exposures occurred from sandblasting. This type of exposure has been banned in most places. Soil in the extreme eastern and western portions of the United States is rich in alpha quartz (the most common form of crystalline silica). Silicotic nodules may be found in the thoracic lymph nodes and even within the lung parenchyma in farmers from these regions.

Table 9.2 Occupations with exposure to crystalline silica

Abrasive powder manufacture
Boiler scaling
Farming[a]
Firebrick manufacture
Foundry work
Mining[b]
Molding and grinding
Pottery and ceramic manufacture
Quarry work
Sandblasting
Stone masonry

[a] Soil in extreme eastern and western portions of United States.
[b] Coal, copper, gold, graphite, lead, mica, and tin.

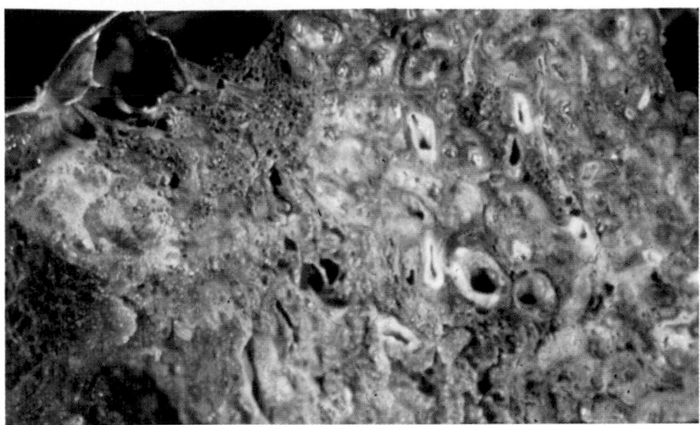

Fig. 9.1 **Silicosis.** Grossly, circumscribed areas of nodular fibrosis are firm and slate gray in appearance.

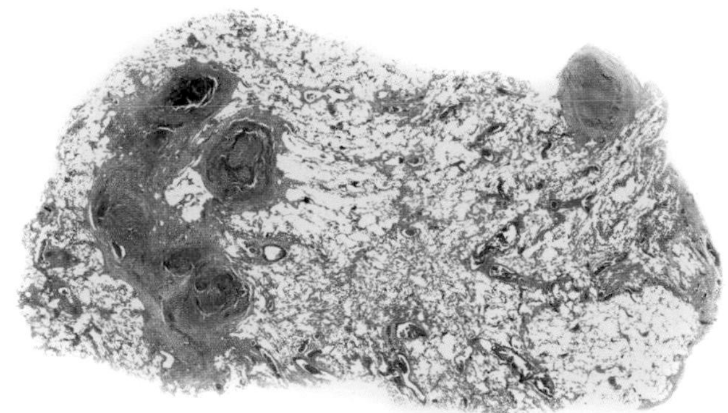

Fig. 9.2 **Silicosis.** At low magnification, silicotic nodules are sharply circumscribed and densely collagenous (Masson trichrome stain).

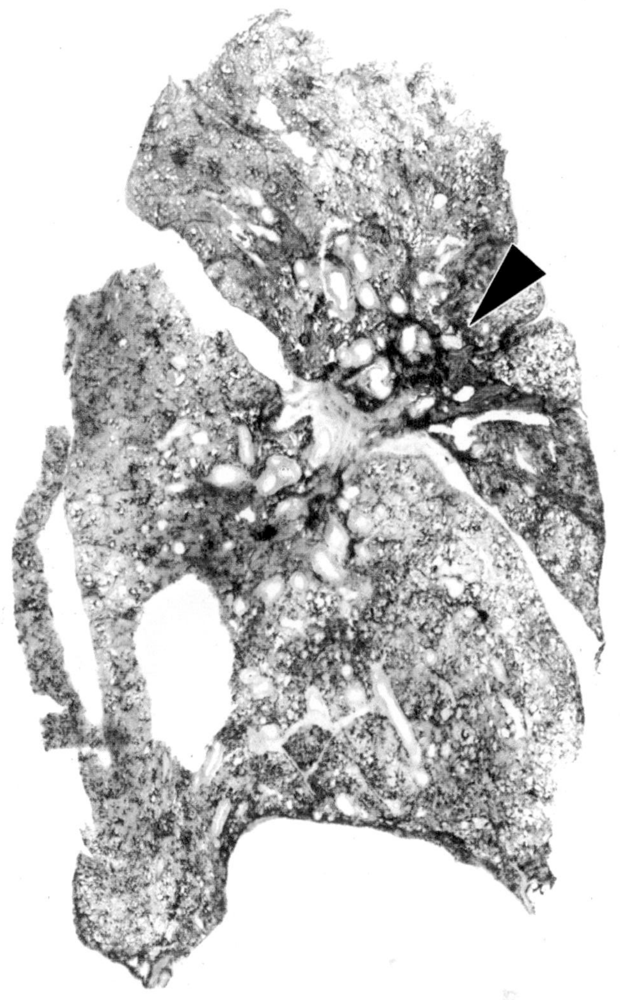

Fig. 9.3 **Conglomerate silicosis.** A Gough Wentworth section of lung from a tobacco field worker demonstrates confluent fibrosis in the upper lobe (arrow).

Clinical presentation

Patients range from asymptomatic with simple silicosis to markedly dyspneic with conglomerate silicosis. In conglomerate silicosis, hypoxemia and cor pulmonale may be fatal.

Pathologic findings

Silicotic nodules are firm and typically slate gray in appearance, measuring from a few millimeters to about 1 cm in diameter (Figs 9.1 and 9.2). As the disease progresses in severity, the nodules may become confluent (Figs 9.3 and 9.4). Areas of confluent fibrosis greater than 2 cm in maximum dimension are referred to as conglomerate silicosis. Cavitation may occur within areas of confluent fibrosis, and, when present, suggests the possibility of superimposed tuberculosis.

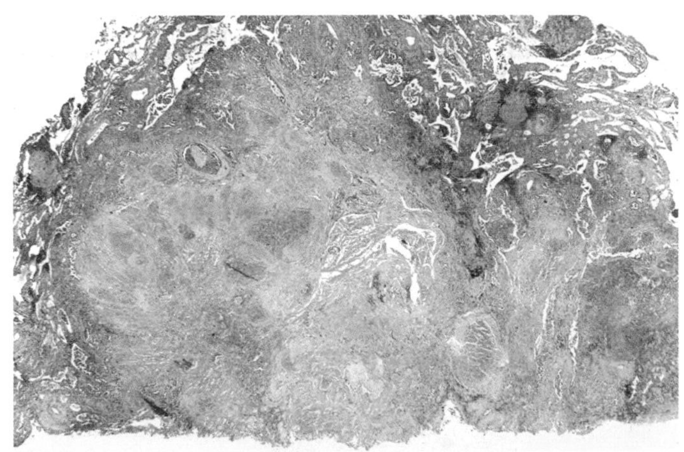

Fig. 9.4 **Conglomerate silicosis.** Multiple silicotic nodules have coalesced, forming an area of confluent fibrosis.

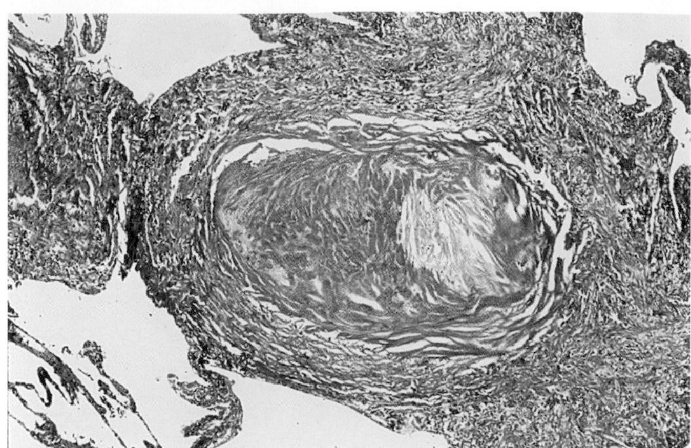

Fig. 9.5 **Silicosis.** A higher magnification view of a silicotic nodule shows the typical whorled appearance. Macrophages are present at the periphery of the nodule.

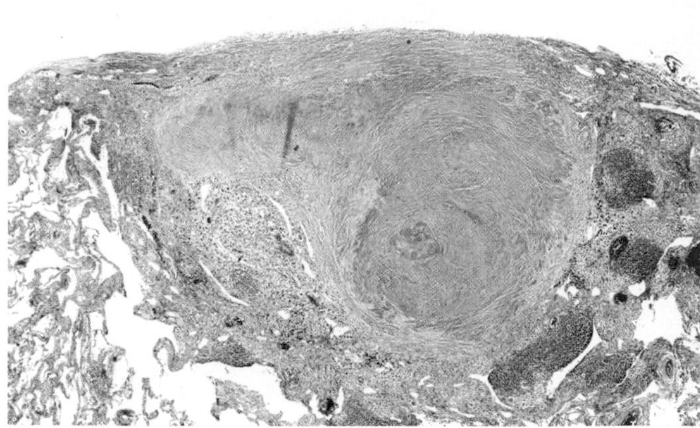

Fig. 9.7 **Silicosis.** The lung parenchyma underlying the pleura is a common location for silicotic nodules.

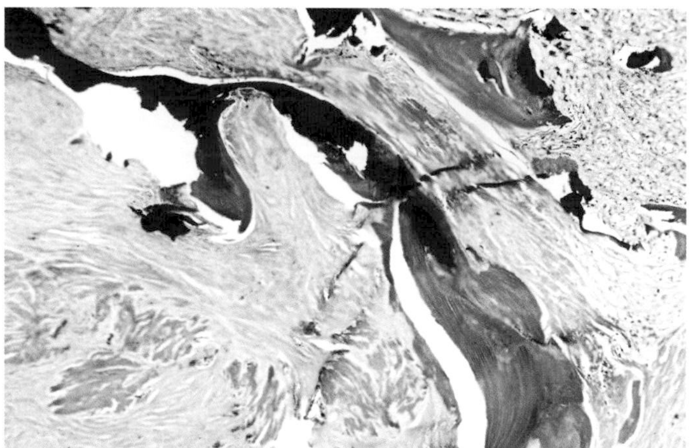

Fig. 9.6 **Silicosis.** A mature silicotic nodule exhibits partial ossification.

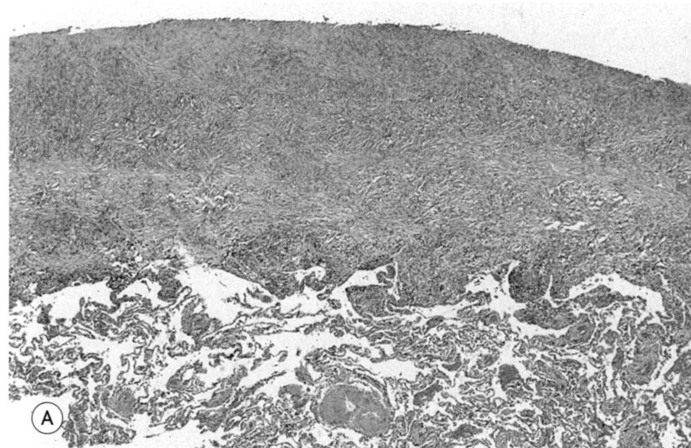

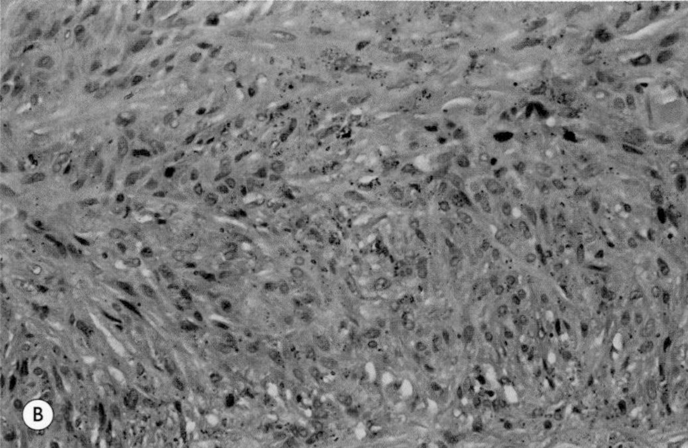

Fig. 9.8 **Pleural silicosis.** (A) In this example, pleural involvement manifests as dense fibrosis. (B) Higher magnification shows a cellular area consisting of fibroblasts and histiocytes. Polarizing microscopy showed numerous birefringent particulates.

The histologic hallmark of silicosis is the silicotic nodule.[4,5] This consists of a sharply circumscribed nodule of dense, whorled hyalinized collagen (Fig. 9.5). More loosely arranged collagen bundles are typically found at the periphery of the nodules. In earlier lesions, macrophages form a mantle around the fibrotic center. Older lesions may be calcified or even ossified (Fig. 9.6). The nodules may be present anywhere within the lung parenchyma, but are typically most numerous in the upper lung zones. Not uncommonly, they are concentrated beneath the pleura (Fig. 9.7). There may also be extensive pleural fibrosis (Fig. 9.8).[6] Nodules are frequently present

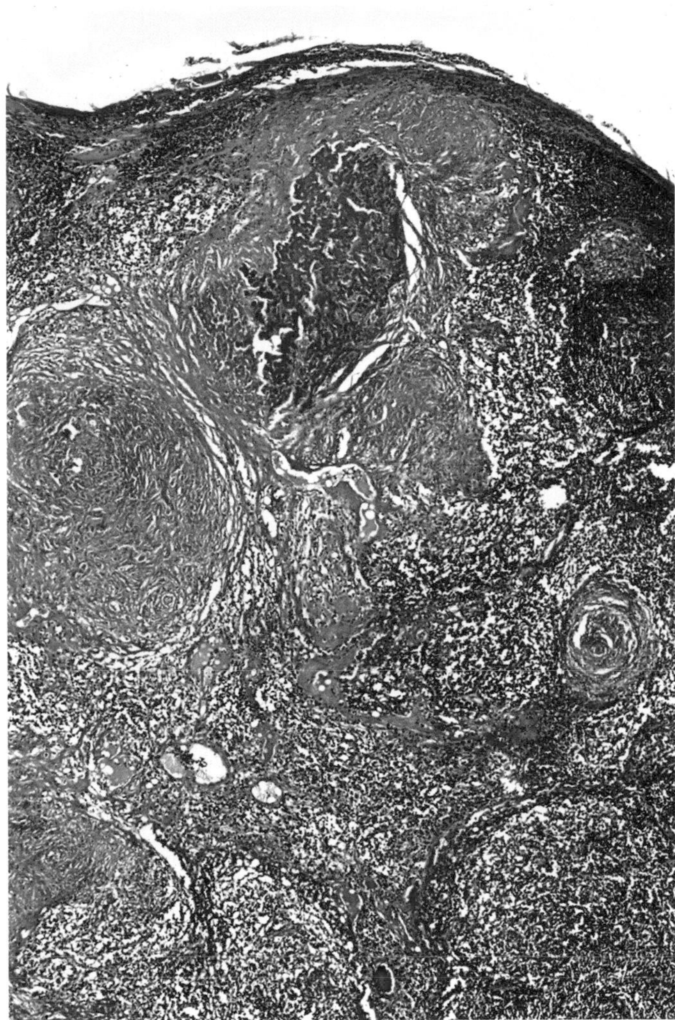

Fig. 9.9 **Silicosis.** Silicotic nodules within a lymph node characteristically contain centrally dense, hyalinized collagen surrounded by concentric whorls of more loosely arranged collagen bundles.

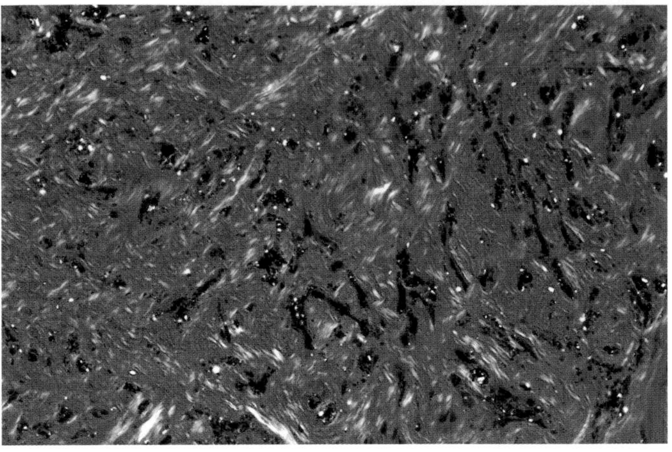

Fig. 9.11 **Silicosis.** Partial polarization of a silicotic nodule demonstrates faintly birefringent silica particles.

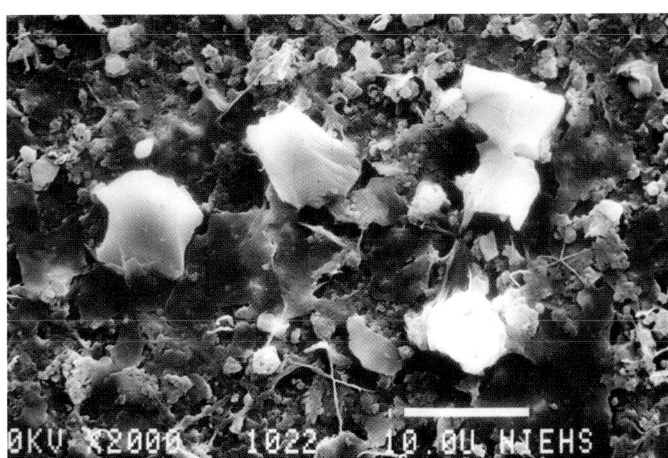

Fig. 9.12 **Silicosis.** Scanning electron microscopy demonstrates angulated silica particles.

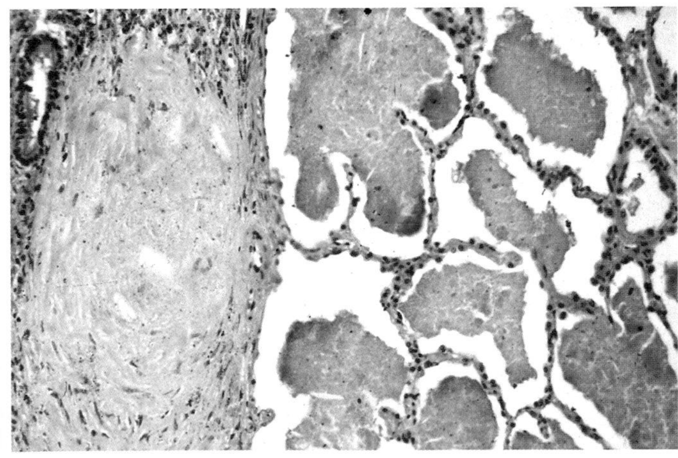

Fig. 9.10 **Acute silicosis.** Granular eosinophilic material fills alveoli, imparting an appearance similar to pulmonary alveolar proteinosis. Note the presence of a silicotic nodule at left. (Reprinted from Roggli and Shelburne,[1] with permission.)

within hilar lymph nodes (Fig 9.9). Patients with extremely high exposures to very fine silica particles may develop a pattern of lung injury closely resembling pulmonary alveolar proteinosis (Fig 9.10). This consists of granular eosinophilic material filling the alveoli, alveolar ducts, and bronchioles. Cholesterol clefts may be prominent within the intra-alveolar material. The granular proteinaceous exudate typically stains strongly positive with periodic acid Schiff (PAS).

Examination with polarizing microscopy shows faintly birefringent particulates within the fibrotic nodules (Fig. 9.11). Larger, brightly birefringent particles may also be seen, which represent silicates.[7] By scanning electron microscopy the particles appear angulated (Fig. 9.12).

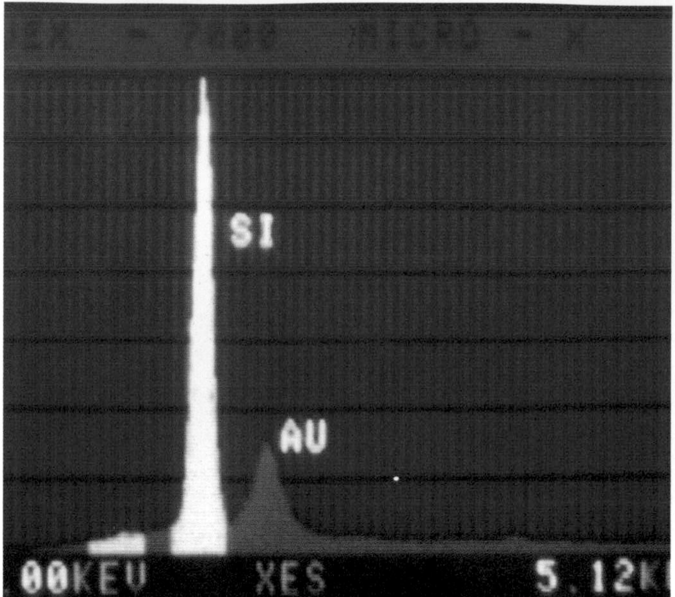

Fig. 9.13 **Silicosis.** Energy dispersive X-ray analysis (EDXA) spectrum shows a peak for silicon (Si). The peak for gold (Au) represents the coating applied to the specimen prior to electron microscopic examination.

Analytical electron microscopy with EDXA reveals peaks for silicon only (Fig. 9.13).

Differential diagnosis

Silicotic nodules must be distinguished from fibrotic nodules of healed or "burnt out" sarcoidosis and healed mycobacterial or fungal infections. The presence of multinucleate giant cells and the absence of significant dust deposits favor sarcoidosis. Sarcoid granulomas may contain fine needle-like or large platy birefringent particles representing endogenous calcium carbonates and oxalates, respectively (Fig. 9.14). These should not be confused with the foreign material of pneumoconiosis. Giant cells and necrosis favor an infectious etiology. Patients with silicosis are at increased risk for tuberculosis.[8] Both processes may be present simultaneously. This is most likely to occur in cases with conglomerate silicosis.

Extrathoracic location does not rule out a silicotic origin of a fibrous nodule, as silicotic nodules have been found in the liver, spleen, bone marrow, and abdominal lymph nodes.[9] This usually occurs in cases with advanced silicosis. The diagnostic yield of transbronchial biopsies in silicosis is low, probably because the firm circumscribed nodules are pushed aside by the biopsy forceps.

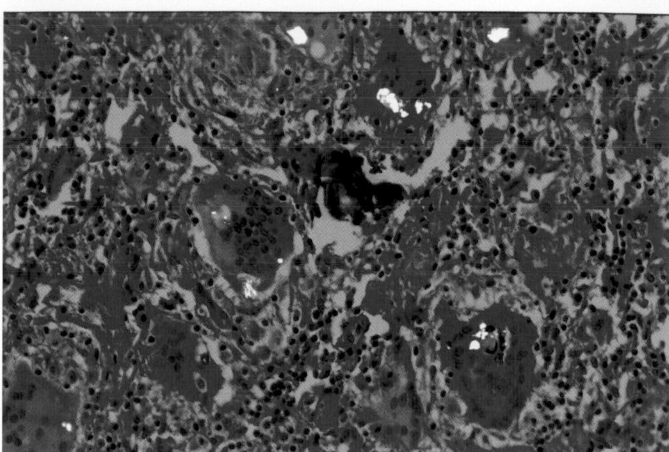

Fig. 9.14 **Birefringent particles in sarcoidosis.** In contrast to silicosis, this example of sarcoidosis contains large platy birefrigent particles, typical for endogenous calcium oxalate.

Coal workers' pneumoconiosis

Introduction

Coal workers' pneumoconiosis (CWP), also known as "black lung disease", occurs in individuals involved with the mining of coal. The nature of the disease is related to the intensity and duration of exposure, host factors, and the specific duties of the miner. Workers involved with drilling in the ceiling of the shaft or constructing communicating shafts are exposed to greater amounts of silica than those working at the coal face. Dust suppression measures have greatly reduced the incidence of progressive massive fibrosis (PMF), the advanced form of CWP.

Clinical presentation

Patients range from asymptomatic with simple coal workers' pneumoconiosis to markedly dyspneic with PMF. The latter is associated with hypoxemia and cor pulmonale and may be fatal.[10,11]

Pathologic findings

Coal workers' pneumoconiosis is characterized by increased pigmentation of the lung resulting from the deposition of coal dust (Figs 9.15–9.17). Accentuated pigmentation is present on the pleura and on cut surfaces of the lung, superimposed on a background of diffusely increased pigment. In some cases, palpable nodules are present within the lung parenchyma, usually most numerous in the upper lung zones. These nodules are grossly similar to silicotic nodules, except that they are

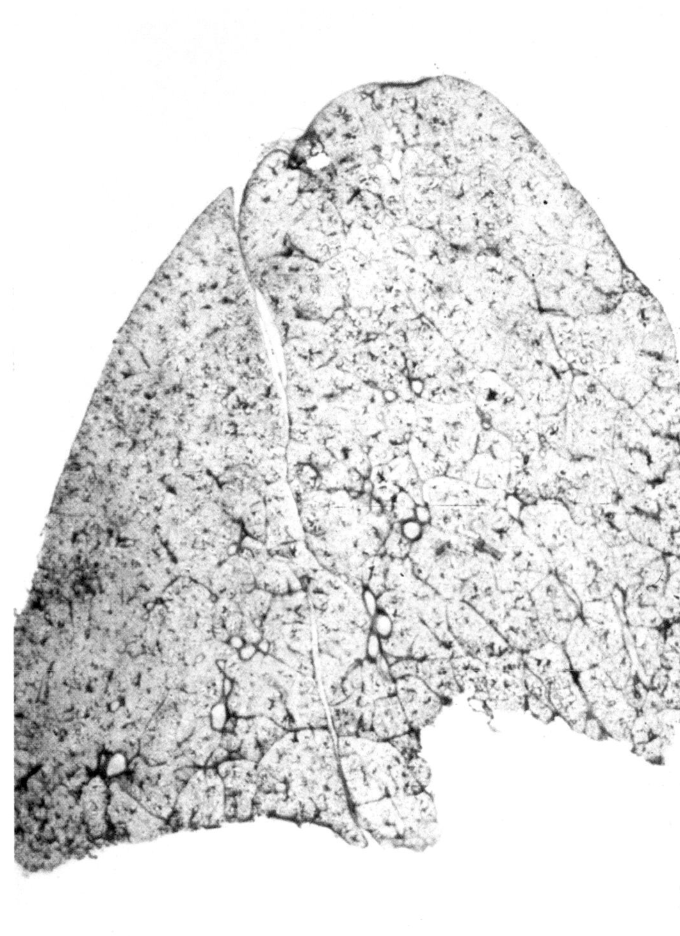

Fig. 9.15 **Normal lung.** A Gough–Wentworth section of a normal lung shows scattered minimal accumulations of anthracotic pigment and intact parenchyma. (Reprinted from Kleinerman et al.,[12] with permission.)

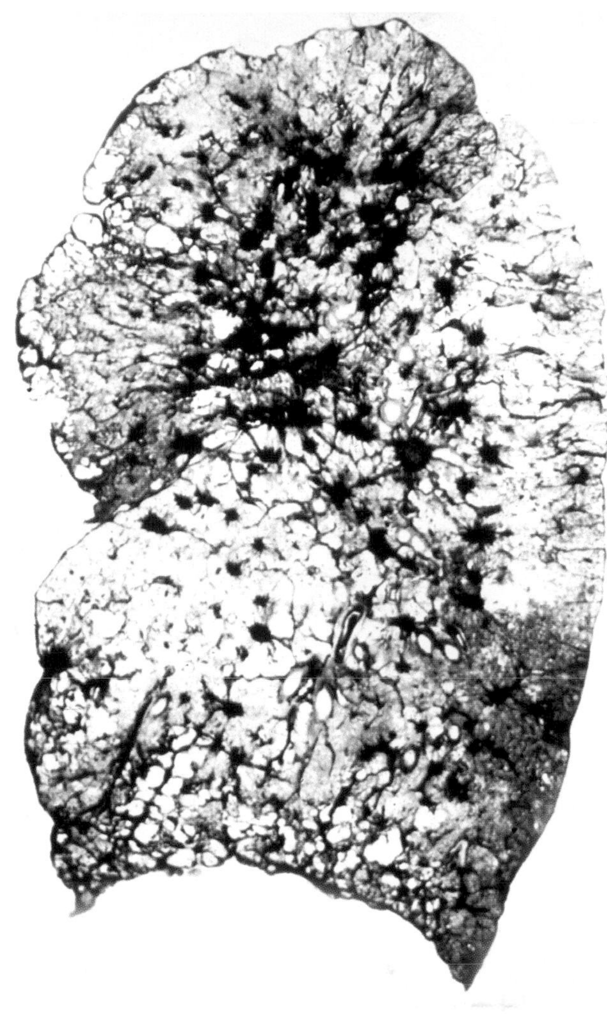

Fig. 9.16 **Simple coal workers' pneumoconiosis.** This thin section of lung demonstrates multiple small, circumscribed black nodules, predominantly in the upper lobe. (Reprinted from Kleinerman et al.,[12] with permission.)

black rather than slate gray (Fig. 9.18). In the most advanced cases of coal workers' pneumoconiosis, there are confluent areas of irregular fibrosis that are usually bilateral and in the upper to mid lung zones (see below). These areas are greater than 2 cm in maximum dimension and have the consistency of vulcanized rubber (Fig. 9.19). These are the lesions of PMF. Cavitation may occur within areas of PMF, and, when present, suggests superimposed tuberculosis.[12]

The histologic hallmark of coal workers' pneumoconiosis is the coal dust macule (Fig. 9.20). These macules consist of focal interstitial pigment deposition in the vicinity of respiratory bronchioles. Areas of emphysematous destruction, referred to as focal emphysema, are typically present at the periphery of the macule. Pigment-laden macrophages may be present within alveolar spaces. Pigment deposition may be identified anywhere along the lymphatic routes within the lung, including the secondary lobular septa and the pleura. Lymph nodes contain numerous pigmented macrophages and may also contain silicotic nodules. Silicotic nodules may also be present within the lung parenchyma, and have a collarette of pigmented macrophages, giving them a 'medusa-head' appearance (Fig 9.21). Areas of massive fibrosis (Fig. 9.22) consist of collagen bundles arranged in a haphazard distribution and intermixed with abundant pigment

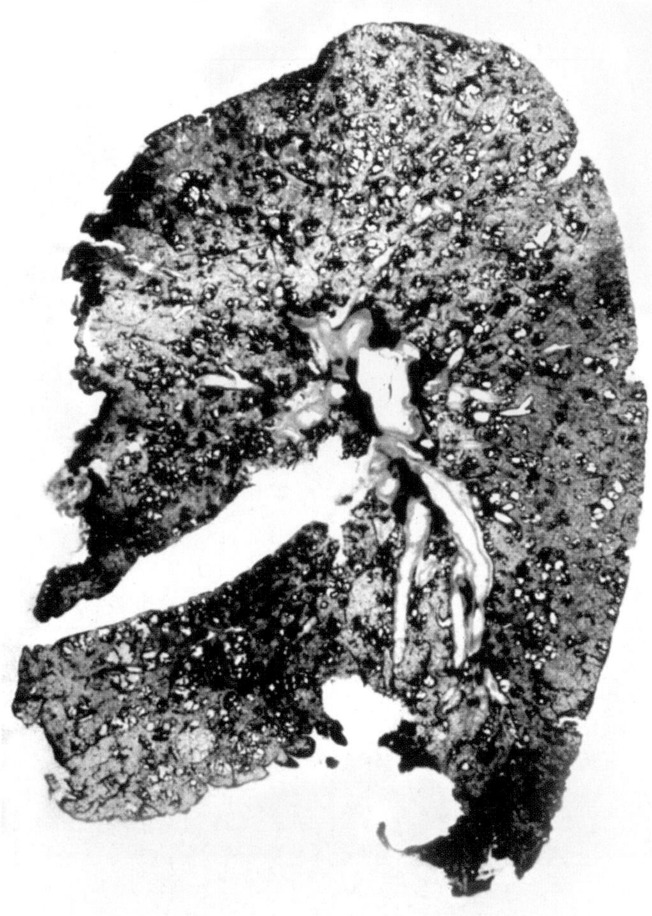

Fig. 9.17 **Simple coal workers' pneumoconiosis.** In contrast to the normal lung, this thin section shows diffusely increased pigment resulting from the deposition of coal dust. (Reprinted from Kleinerman et al.,[12] with permission.)

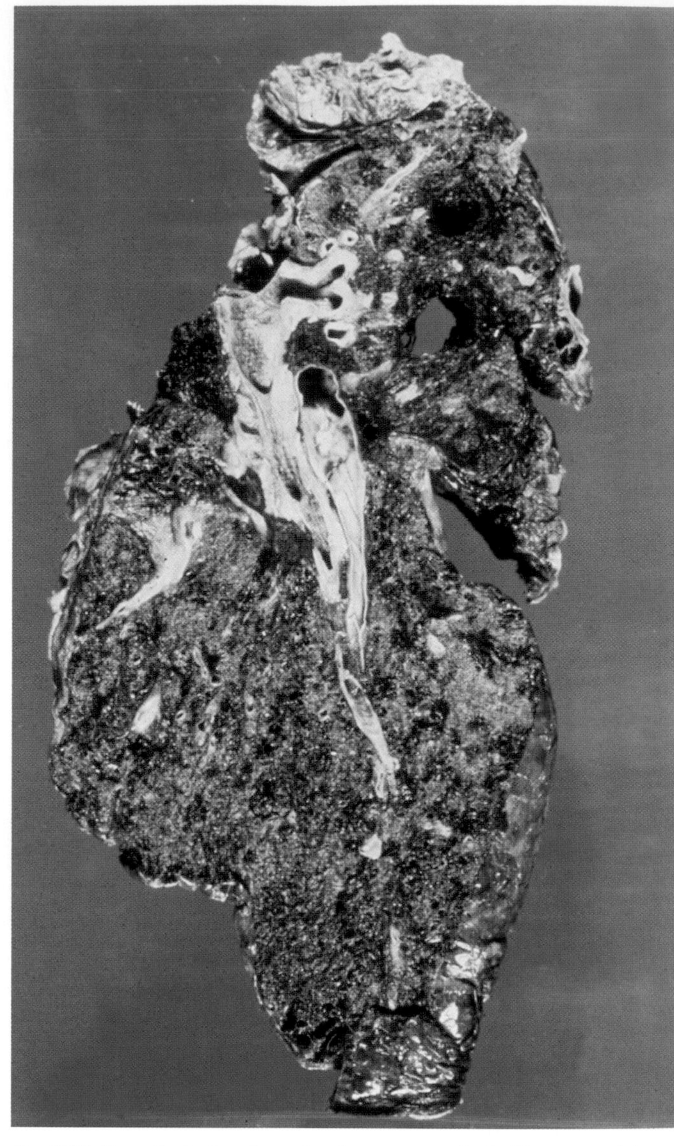

Fig. 9.19 **Complicated coal workers' pneumoconiosis.** The upper lobe contains a confluent irregular area of fibrosis with the consistency of vulcanized rubber. Central cavitation is present.

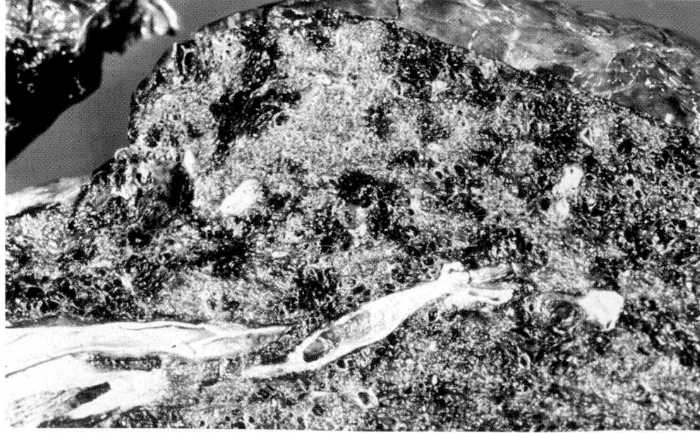

Fig. 9.18 **Simple coal workers' pneumoconiosis.** In addition to diffusely increased pigmentation, the lung parenchyma shows well-demarcated black nodules. Centrilobular emphysematous bullae are also present.

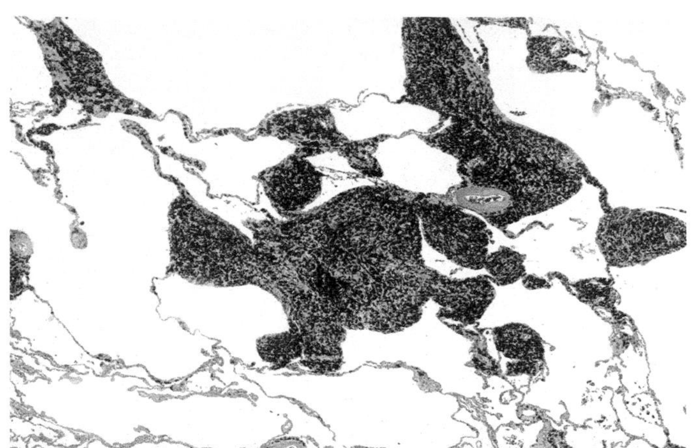

Fig. 9.20 **Simple coal workers' pneumoconiosis.** The coal dust macule is characterized by focal interstitial pigment deposition. In this example, destruction of the adjacent alveolar septa, termed focal emphysema, is also seen.

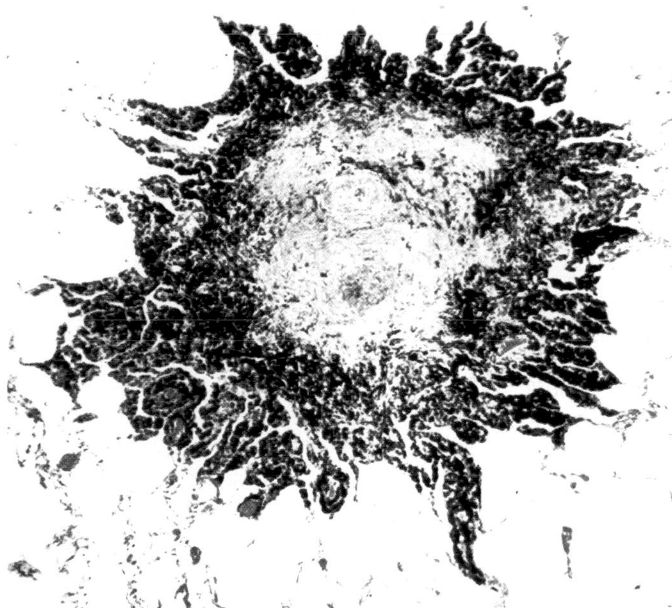

Fig. 9.21 **Simple coal workers' pneumoconiosis.** In this case of simple coal workers' pneumoconiosis, a collarette of pigmented macrophages gives this intraparenchymal silicotic nodule a "medusa-head" appearance.

(Figs 9.23 and 9.24). Vascular obliteration is common within areas of PMF, and ischemia may be the cause of cavitation in some cases.

Examination with polarizing microscopy typically shows numerous faintly to brightly birefringent particulates in a background of black pigment (Fig. 9.25). This appearance reflects the mixed nature of coal dust, which includes amorphous carbon, silicates, and silica. The latter is responsible for the formation of silicotic nodules and is

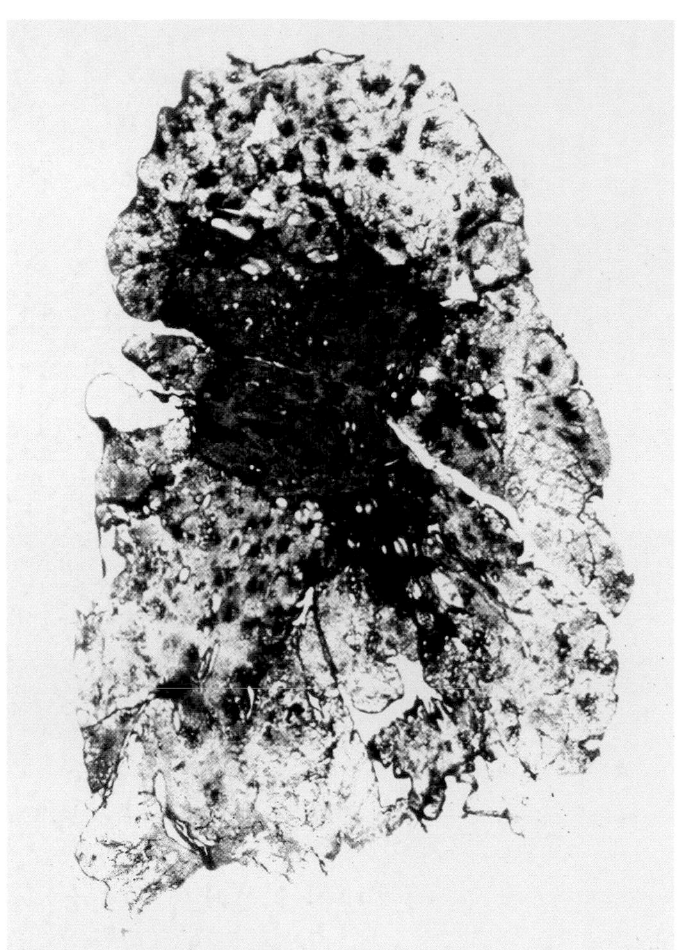

Fig. 9.22 **Complicated coal workers' pneumoconiosis.** A large black irregular fibrotic lesion has destroyed the perihilar lung parenchyma. (Reprinted from Kleinerman et al.,[12] with permission.)

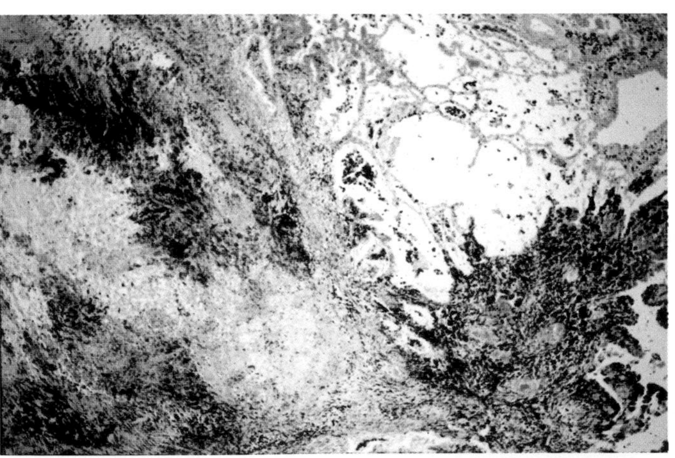

Fig. 9.23 **Complicated coal workers' pneumoconiosis.** In this example of progressive massive fibrosis, haphazardly arranged collagen bundles are interspersed with abundant pigment.

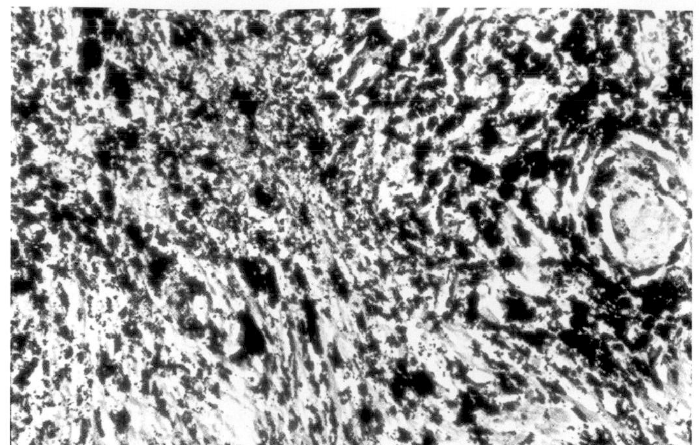

Fig. 9.24 **Complicated coal workers' pneumoconiosis.** A Masson trichrome stain highlights the collagenous composition of a heavily pigmented region of progressive massive fibrosis.

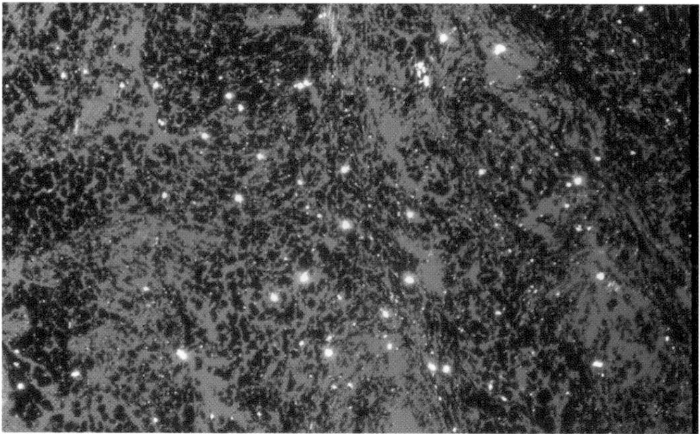

Fig. 9.25 **Coal workers' pneumoconiosis.** Partial polarization shows a mixture of faintly and brightly birefringent particles superimposed on black pigment.

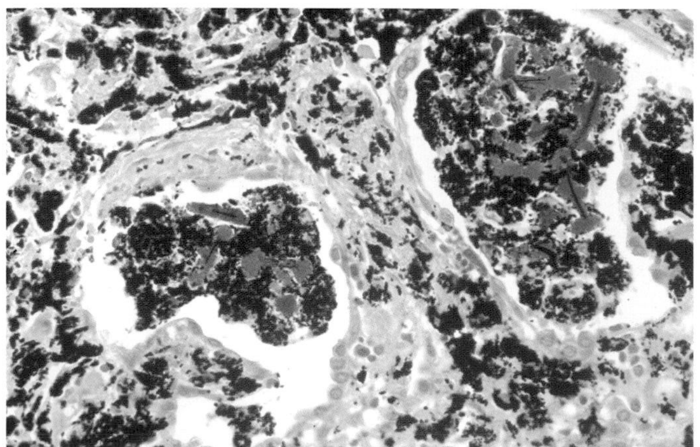

Fig. 9.26 **Coal workers' pneumoconiosis.** Along with pigmented macrophages, this case demonstrates numerous intra-alveolar ferruginous bodies.

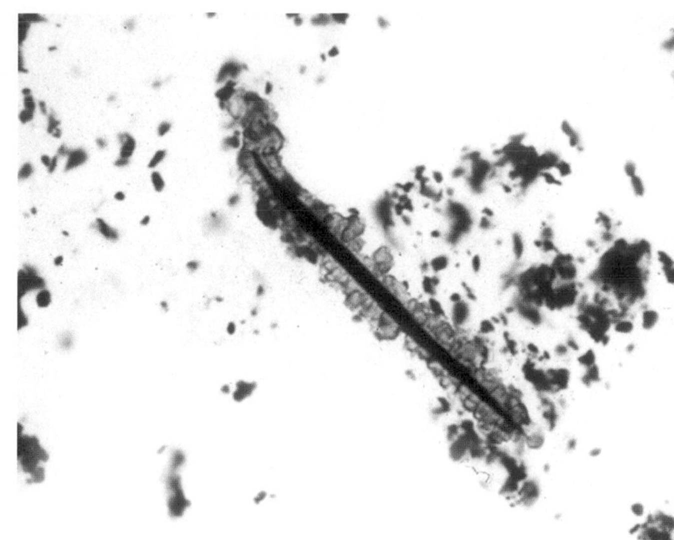

Fig. 9.27 **Coal workers' pneumoconiosis.** At higher magnification, the black carbonaceous core of this ferruginous, or pseudoasbestos, body is evident.

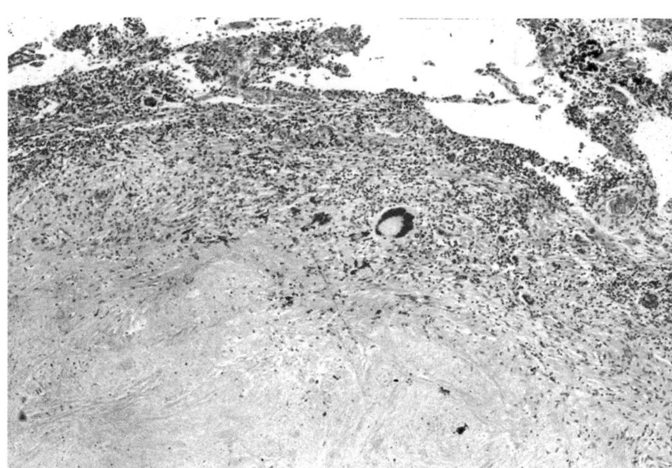

Fig. 9.28 **Coal workers' pneumoconiosis.** A caseous granuloma in this case of coal workers' pneumoconiosis was found to contain acid-fast bacilli.

an important factor in the genesis of PMF.[13] Coal workers may also have ferruginous bodies within their lungs, typically within the alveolar spaces (Fig 9.26). These may be distinguished from true asbestos bodies by virtue of their black carbonaceous core fiber (Fig 9.27).[14] Tuberculosis may also complicate CWP (Fig. 9.28).

Differential diagnosis

Coal workers' pneumoconiosis must be distinguished from anthracotic pigment deposition that occurs in urban dwellers and cigarette smokers, and from graphite workers' pneumoconiosis. The extent of pigmentation in normal subjects is a function of environmental exposure to carbon-containing dust and the lung's natural ability to cleanse itself. Distinction from coal workers' pneumoconiosis is somewhat a matter of degree, but the presence of true coal dust macules, as described above, is indicative of coal workers' pneumoconiosis. The finding of intra-alveolar anthracotic pigment-laden macrophages is also a useful feature, but may be absent in miners who have been retired for many years. Graphite workers' pneumoconiosis appears similar to coal workers' pneumoconiosis, but graphite is crystalline, whereas the carbon in coal is amorphous (Fig. 9.29). A giant cell reaction to the crystalline carbon of graphite assists in this distinction.[3] Transbronchial biopsies may be useful in the diagnosis of coal workers' pneumoconiosis, showing the typical changes described above. However, areas of nodular fibrosis or PMF may be missed by such biopsies. Therefore, transbronchial biopsy is not useful for assessing the severity of the disease.

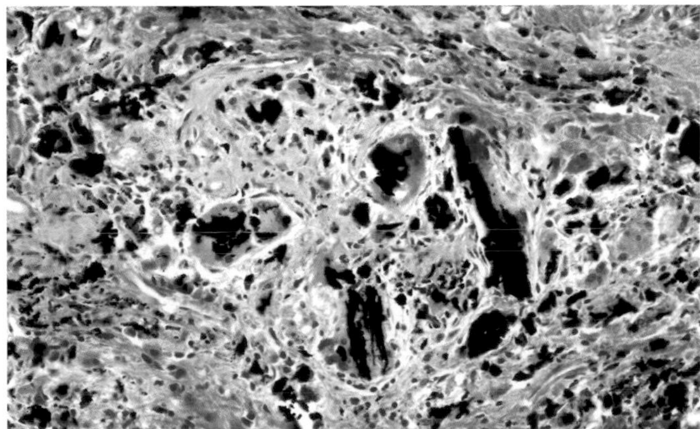

Fig. 9.29 **Graphite workers' pneumoconiosis.** While somewhat similar in appearance to coal workers' pneumoconiosis, graphite particles appear crystalline and elicit a giant cell reaction.

Asbestosis

Introduction

Asbestosis is defined as pulmonary interstitial fibrosis caused by the inhalation of asbestos fibers.[15,16] Substantial and significant exposures to asbestos can occur in a variety of occupational settings, including mining and milling of asbestos, the manufacture of asbestos-containing products, and the use of products containing asbestos. The latter includes such occupations as insulators, shipyard workers, railroad workers, power plant workers, US Navy or merchant marine seamen, oil or chemical refinery workers, construction workers, steel and other molten metal workers, and paper mill workers (Table 9.3). A few cases of asbestosis have also occurred among household contacts of asbestos workers, apparently as a consequence of asbestos brought home on the workers' clothing.

Table 9.3 Industries with exposure to asbestos

Industries with exposure to asbestos
Asbestos mining and milling
Asbestos products manufacture
Construction
Glass and ceramic manufacture
Insulation
Oil or chemical refineries
Paper mills
Power plants
Railroad
Ship building and repair
Steel and other molten metal manufacture
US Navy/merchant marines

Clinical presentation

Patients with asbestosis range from asymptomatic to severely dyspneic at rest. Hypoxemia and cor pulmonale may prove fatal in such patients. Pulmonary function tests typically show restrictive changes, and the diffusion capacity is reduced. Patients with asbestosis who smoke cigarettes have a markedly increased risk for developing lung cancer. Pleural plaques alone are rarely symptomatic, and should not be referred to as "asbestosis". Although the pleural and parenchymal changes caused by asbestos may be recognized on plain films, high-resolution computed tomography (CT) is considered to be more sensitive and specific.

Pathologic findings

The fibrosis in asbestosis is of a fine, reticular pattern and the lungs macroscopically range from normal to severely scarred and shrunken (Fig. 9.30) with evidence of honeycombing.[17,18] Diffuse visceral pleural fibrosis is frequently present, and is usually most severe in the lower lung zones. Parietal pleural plaques (Fig. 9.31) are present in the vast majority of cases and may be calcified. They are frequently bilateral. Although the pleural changes serve as a suggestive indicator of an asbestos etiology of pulmonary fibrosis, the term asbestosis should not be

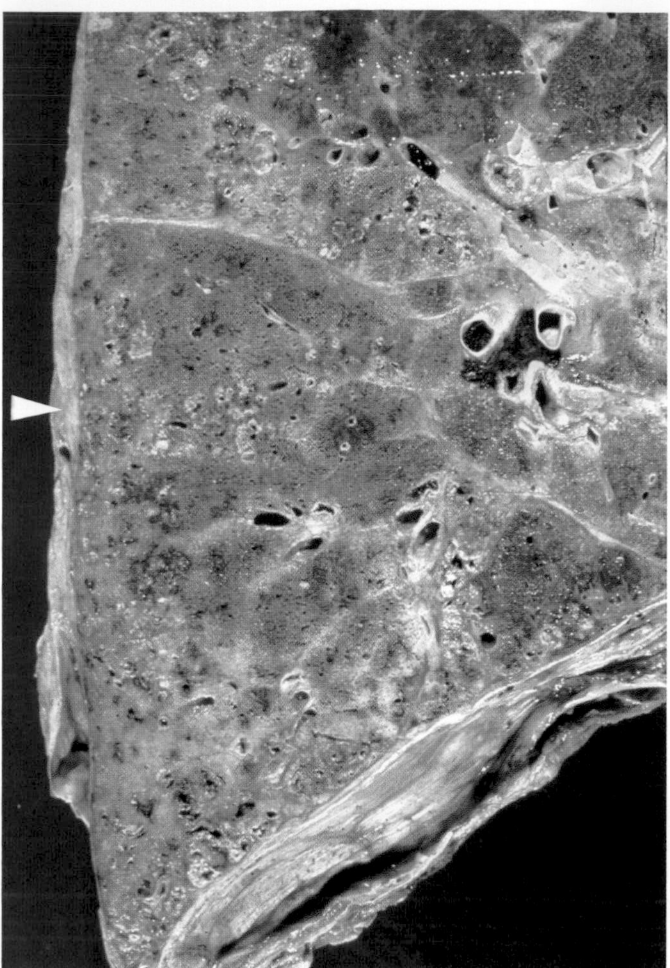

Fig. 9.30 **Asbestosis.** The lower lobe parenchyma shows patchy fibrosis. Visceral pleural thickening is also evident (arrow). (Reprinted from Roggli et al.,[16] with permission.)

applied to these pleural abnormalities when they occur in the absence of parenchymal disease.

Histologically, asbestosis consists of discrete foci of fibrosis in the walls of respiratory bronchioles accompanied by the presence of asbestos bodies (Figs 9.32A and 9.32B). As the fibrotic process progresses, it extends distally to the alveolar ducts and proximally to the membranous (terminal) bronchioles. In addition, the fibrosis extends radially to involve alveolar septa distant from the respiratory bronchiole (Fig. 9.33). In the most advanced cases, honeycomb fibrosis is present (Fig. 9.34), characterized by cysts 0.5–1.0 cm in diameter with fibrotic walls. The cysts are lined by bronchiolar epithelium and may contain pools of mucus. Alveolar macrophages may be so

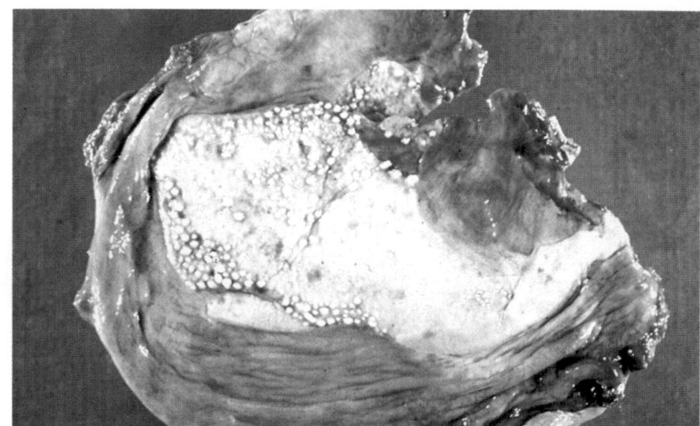

Fig. 9.31 **Pleural plaque.** The gross appearance has been likened to candle wax drippings.

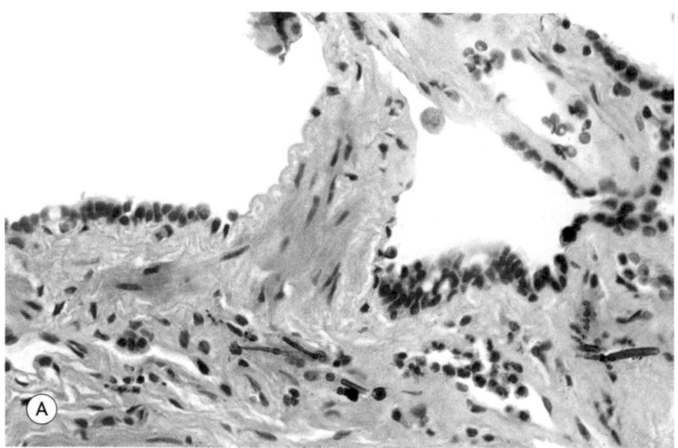

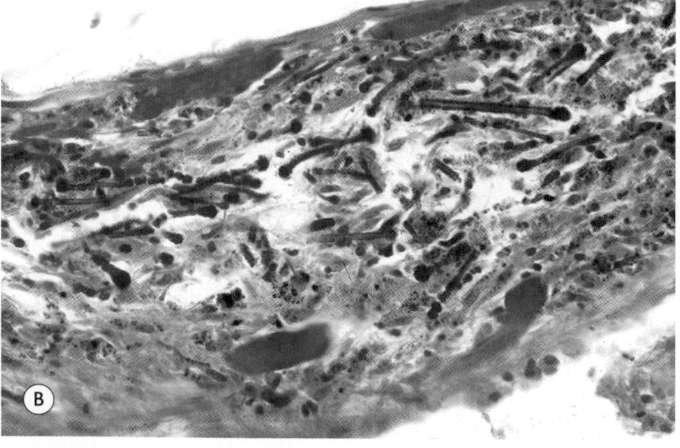

Fig. 9.32 **Asbestosis.** (A) The histologic hallmarks of asbestosis are peribronchiolar fibrosis accompanied by asbestos bodies. (B) Numerous asbestos bodies are present within a fibrotic alveolar septum in this case with heavy asbestos exposure. Note the variable beaded, rod-like, and dumbbell shapes.

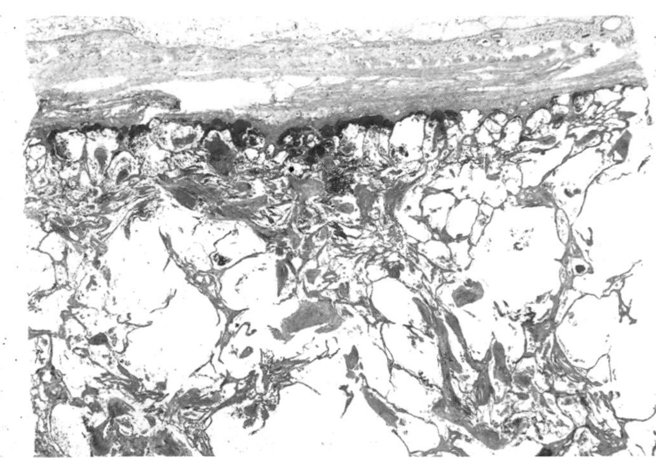

Fig. 9.33 **Asbestosis.** Peribronchiolar fibrosis extends into adjacent alveolar septa in this low-magnification view of moderate asbestosis. Centrilobular emphysema and visceral pleural fibrosis (top) are also seen.

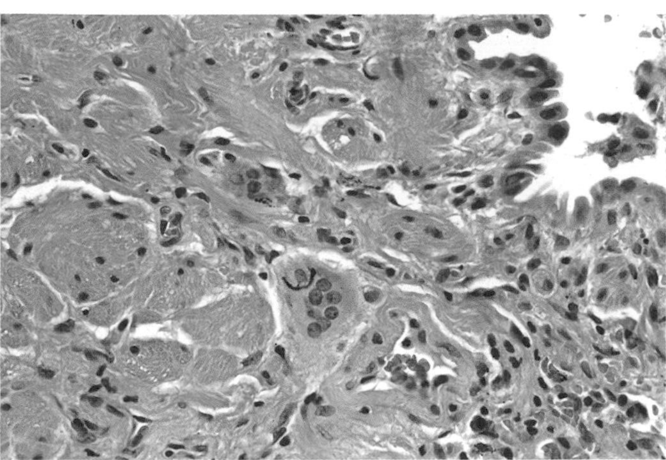

Fig. 9.35 **Asbestosis.** Within an interstitial giant cell lies a curvilinear asbestos body. Transbronchial biopsy.

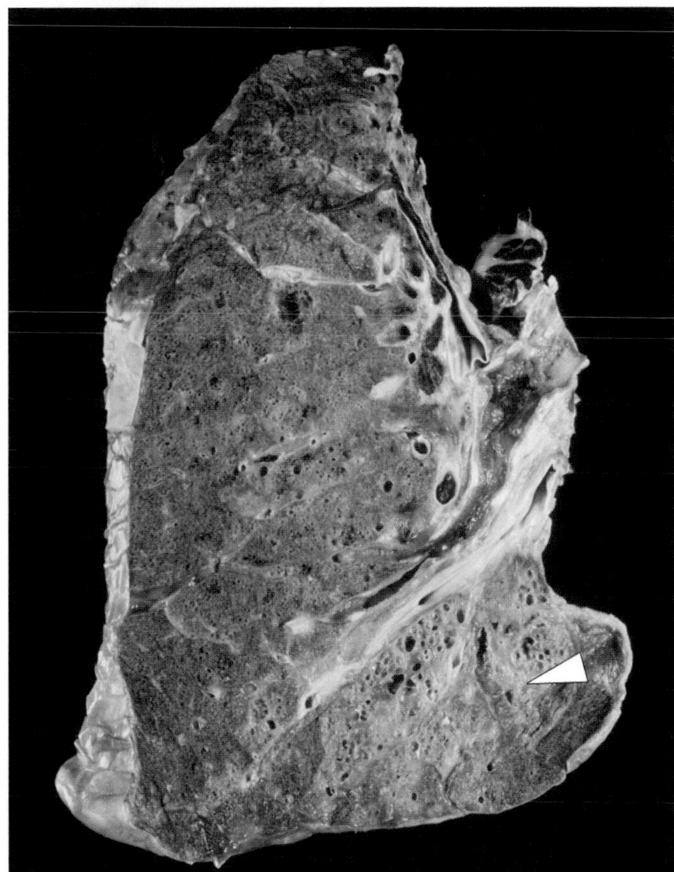

Fig. 9.34 **Asbestosis.** In a more advanced case, honeycombing is seen (arrow) in addition to lower lobe fibrosis.

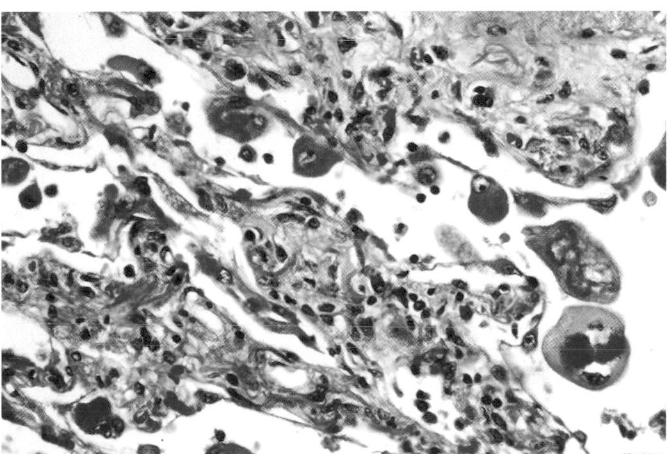

Fig. 9.36 **Asbestosis.** Type 2 pneumocytes demonstrating cytoplasmic hyaline.

prominent as to suggest a diagnosis of desquamative interstitial pneumonia. In some cases, multinucleate giant cells may be identified, either within the interstitium or alveolar spaces (Fig. 9.35). Rarely, hyperplastic alveolar type 2 pneumocytes may contain cytoplasmic hyaline (Fig. 9.36) reminiscent of that found in the cytoplasm of hepatocytes in alcoholic liver disease.

The hallmark of asbestos exposure is the asbestos body, a rod-like, beaded, or dumbbell-shaped structure with golden brown coating and a thin, translucent core.[19] Asbestos bodies are typically found in the peribronchiolar interstitium (Fig. 9.37), but, with heavy exposure, may be seen in the alveolar spaces (Fig. 9.38). Detection of asbestos bodies may be facilitated by the use of iron stains, which impart a deep blue color (Fig. 9.39). Asbestos bodies may also be seen in sputum (Fig. 9.40) and in thoracic lymph nodes (Fig. 9.41) of patients with heavy exposure to asbestos. Pleural plaques consist of layers of acellular hyalinized collagen, arranged in a "basket-weave" pattern (Fig. 9.42). Visceral pleural fibrosis may show this basket-weave pattern or appear as compact layers of

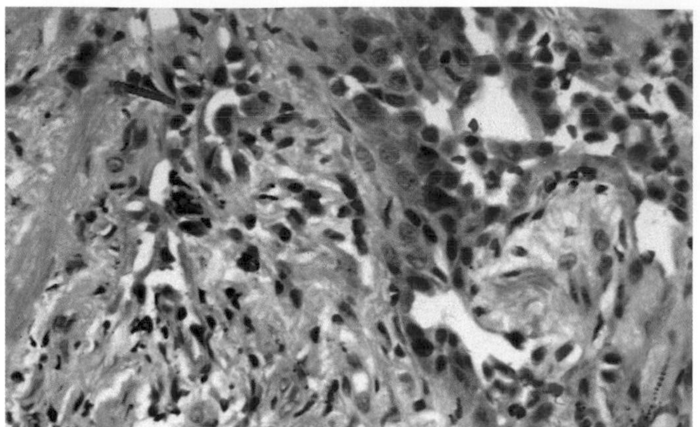

Fig. 9.37 **Asbestosis.** Asbestosis on a transbronchial biopsy, showing interstitial fibrosis and an asbestos body (upper left).

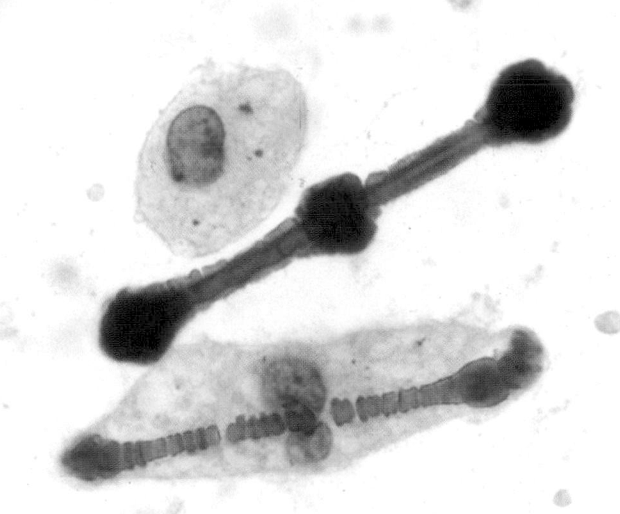

Fig. 9.40 **Asbestosis.** Asbestos bodies in a sputum cytology specimen.

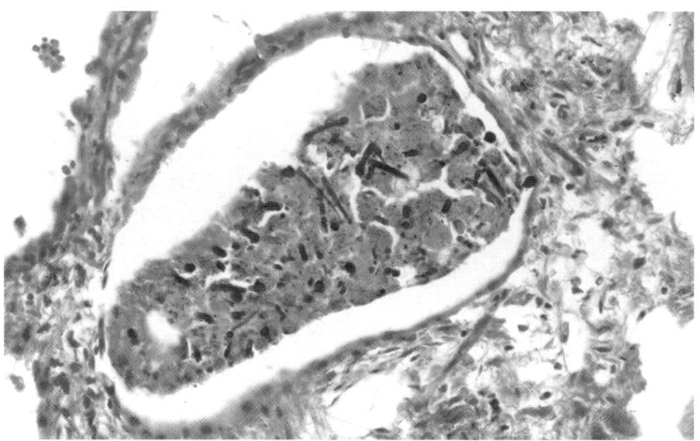

Fig. 9.38 **Asbestosis.** Asbestos bodies are present within an alveolar space in this case of severe asbestosis.

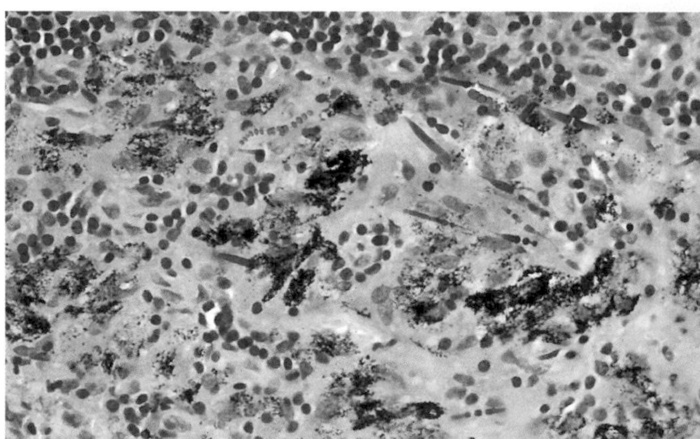

Fig. 9.41 **Asbestosis.** A section from thoracic lymph node from a heavily exposed individual contains numerous asbestos bodies.

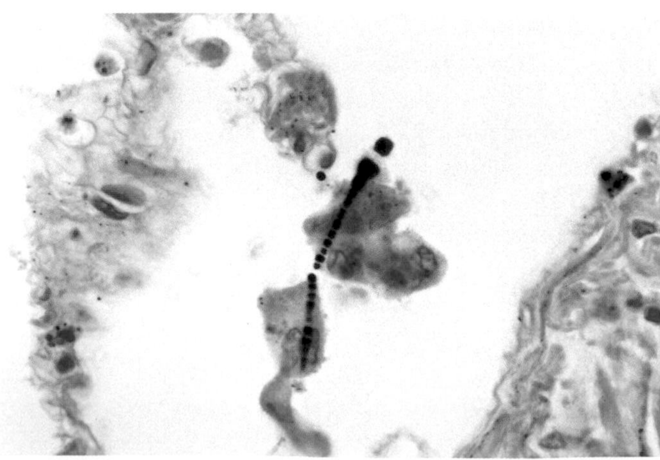

Fig. 9.39 **Asbestosis.** In this iron-stained section of lung, an asbestos body has a characteristic beaded morphology and deep blue color.

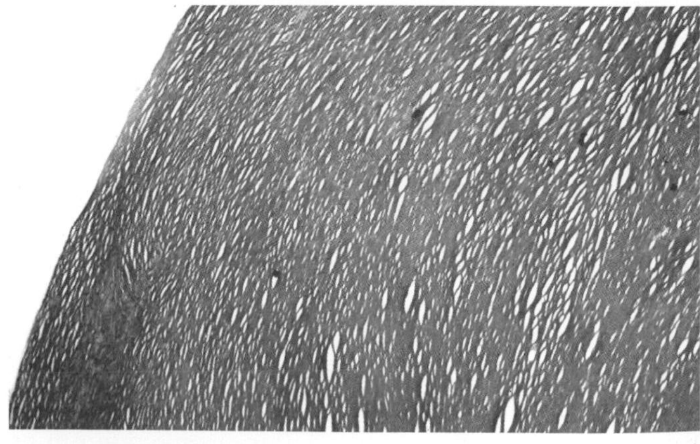

Fig. 9.42 **Pleural plaque.** Pleural plaque showing the typical composition of layers of acellular hyalinized collagen arranged in a "basket-weave" pattern.

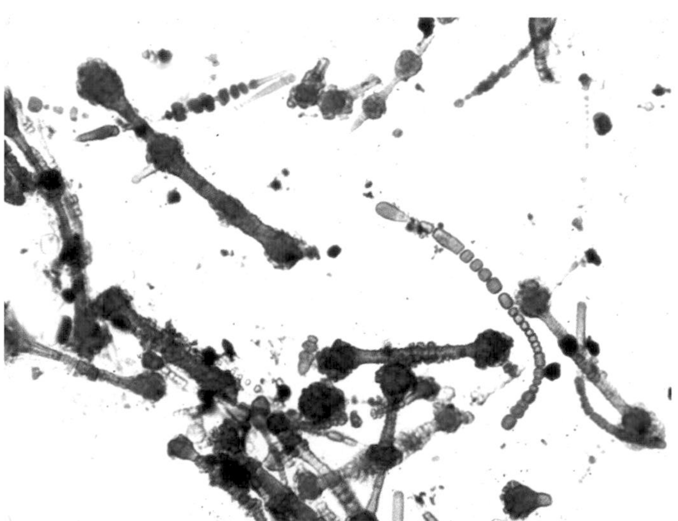

Fig. 9.43 **Asbestosis.** Asbestos bodies from a lung tissue digest on a Nuclepore® filter. (Reprinted from Roggli et al.,[16] with permission.)

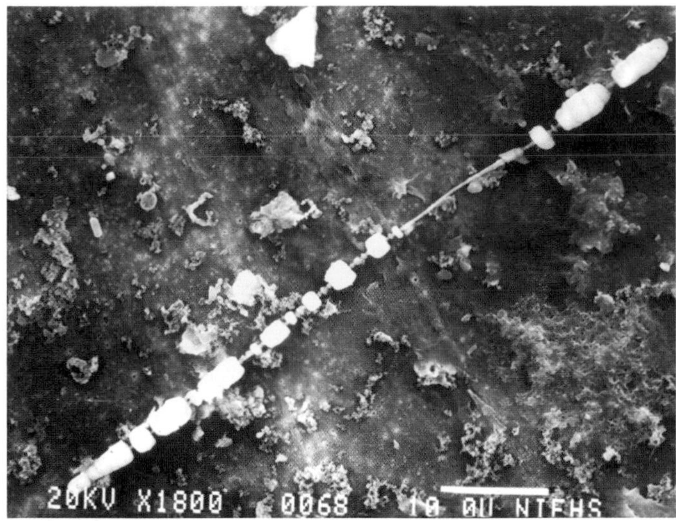

Fig. 9.44 **Asbestosis.** Scanning electron image of an asbestos body. Note the thin, beaded appearance.

collagen. A mild lymphocytic infiltrate sometimes accompanies the fibrosis.

Digestion procedures have been developed for quantifying the content of asbestos in lung tissue (Fig. 9.43). Any of the commercial forms of asbestos (chrysotile and/or amphiboles) may be identified in lung tissue from patients with asbestosis by means of analytical electron microscopy (Figs 9.44 and 9.45).[20] In cases where asbestos bodies are not identified in histologic sections, the fiber burden is virtually always more than two standard deviations below the mean value of cases with bona fide (histologically confirmed) asbestosis.[21] Polarizing

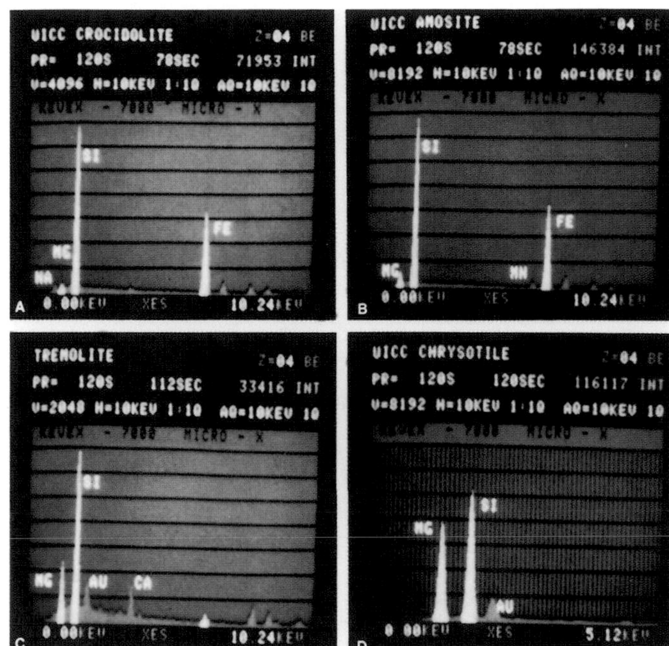

Fig. 9.45 **Asbestosis.** Energy dispersive X-ray analysis (EDXA) spectra for amosite (upper right), crocidolite (upper left), tremolite (lower left), and chrysotile (lower right). (Reprinted from Roggli,[19] with permission.)

microscopy is not useful for the detection of asbestos in histologic sections.

Differential diagnosis

Asbestosis must be distinguished from usual interstitial pneumonia (UIP) and other forms of diffuse pulmonary fibrosis on the one hand, and from the peribronchiolar fibrosis associated with cigarette smoking on the other. UIP is characterized by honeycomb changes, "fibroblastic foci", and the absence of asbestos bodies in histologic sections (see Ch. 7). Honeycomb changes are rare in asbestosis, and, in the authors' experience, true fibroblastic foci are also uncommon. Pleural changes are much more common in asbestosis. Peribronchiolar fibrosis associated with small airways' disease of cigarette smokers (respiratory bronchiolitis) tends to involve membranous (terminal) bronchioles and is often accompanied by mucus plugging and goblet cell metaplasia. Asbestos bodies are absent in respiratory bronchiolitis. Asbestos bodies must be distinguished from nonasbestos ferruginous bodies with broad yellow or black central cores (see Fig. 9.27) (also see Silicatosis section below). The use of transbronchial biopsies in the diagnosis of asbestosis is controversial.[16,20] In the authors' opinion, patients with diffuse pulmonary fibrosis on plain chest films or high-resolution CT who have pulmonary fibrosis and asbestos bodies on transbronchial biopsies can be reliably diagnosed with asbestosis.

Silicatosis (silicate pneumoconiosis)

Introduction

Silicatosis is caused by the inhalation of silicates. A variety of silicate minerals may be encountered in the workplace, usually in the setting of mining and quarry work. Silicates include talc (see Talcosis section below), vermiculite, mica, feldspar, kaolinite, bentonite, and fuller's earth.[3,22–25] Mixed dust pneumoconiosis occurs among patients exposed to a mixture of silica and non-fibrous silicates. Silicate pneumoconiosis has also been described in farm workers in areas with silica-rich soil.[26]

Clinical presentation

Patients with uncomplicated silicate pneumoconiosis are typically asymptomatic. With extensive fibrosis, patients may be short of breath and have restrictive changes on pulmonary function tests. In the rare case with massive fibrosis, hypoxemia and cor pulmonale may supervene.

Pathologic findings

Silicatosis is characterized by irregular deposits of collagen, predominantly in a peribronchiolar and perivascular distribution associated with numerous birefringent particulates.[5,27] The lungs may be macroscopically normal in mild disease, or firm and fibrotic (Fig. 9.46). In patients with significant exposure to silica, in addition to silicates, silicotic nodules and even massive fibrosis may also be present (Fig. 9.47). Paracicatricial emphysema may sometimes be seen adjacent to areas of fibrosis (Fig. 9.48).

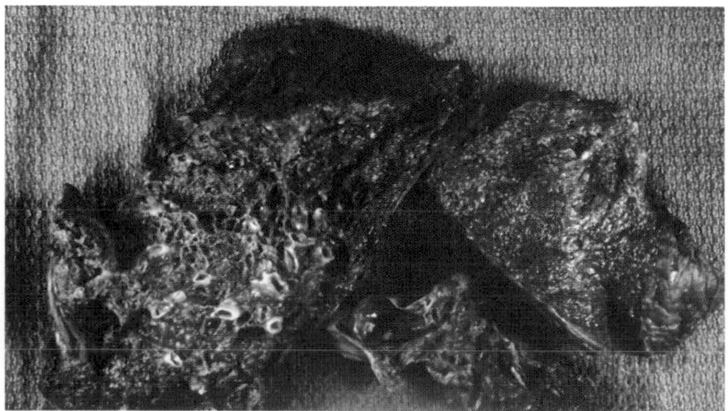

Fig. 9.46 **Silicatosis.** Grossly, this lung from a kaolinite worker shows scattered gray areas of fibrosis in addition to centrilobular emphysema.

The histologic findings in silicatosis include perivascular and peribronchiolar deposits of dust-laden macrophages (dust macules) (Fig. 9.49). Interstitial fibrosis may also be

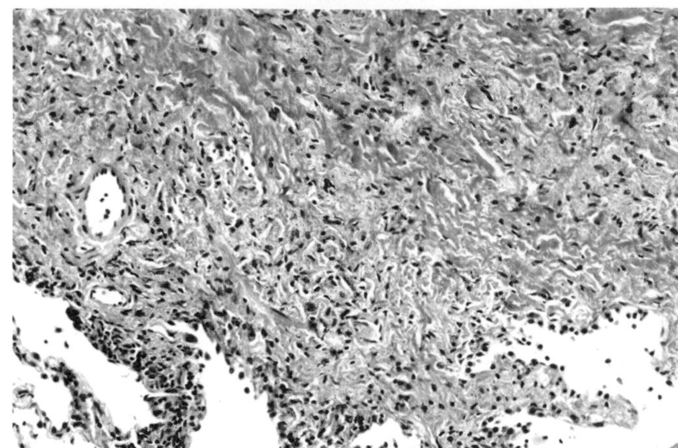

Fig. 9.47 **Silicatosis.** Area of massive fibrosis with deposits of dust-laden macrophages.

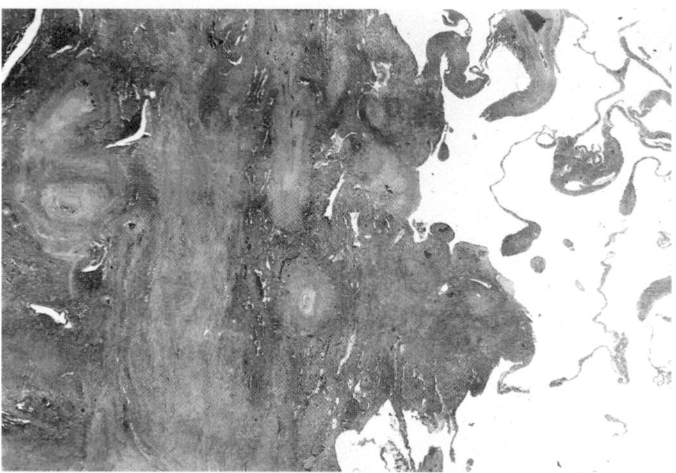

Fig. 9.48 **Silicatosis.** A section of lung from a patient with heavy exposure to kaolin dust demonstrates an area of massive fibrosis with paracicatricial emphysema.

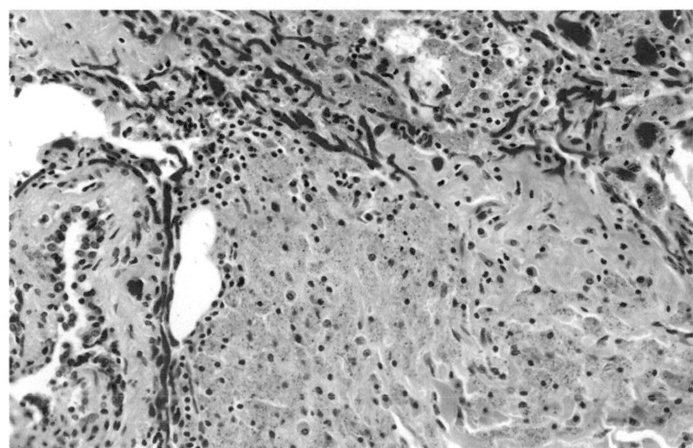

Fig. 9.49 **Silicatosis.** At higher magnification, the dust-laden macrophages appear gray-brown.

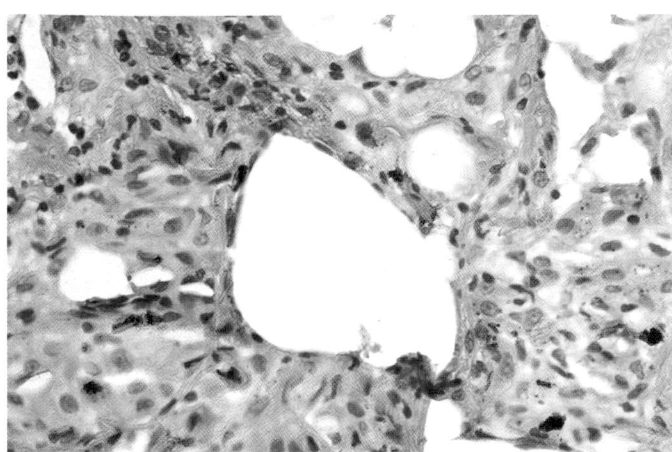

Fig. 9.50 **Silicatosis.** Pseudoasbestos ferruginous bodies accompany interstitial fibrosis in this case of silicatosis with exposure to feldspar. Transbronchial biopsy.

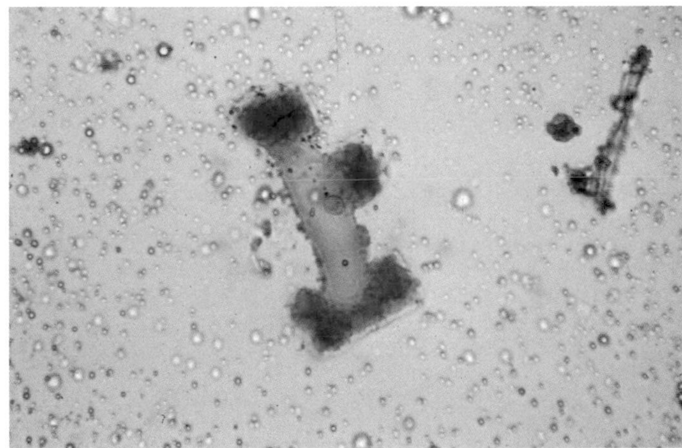

Fig. 9.51 **Silicatosis.** Higher magnification of pseudoasbestos bodies with broad yellow sheet-silicate cores.

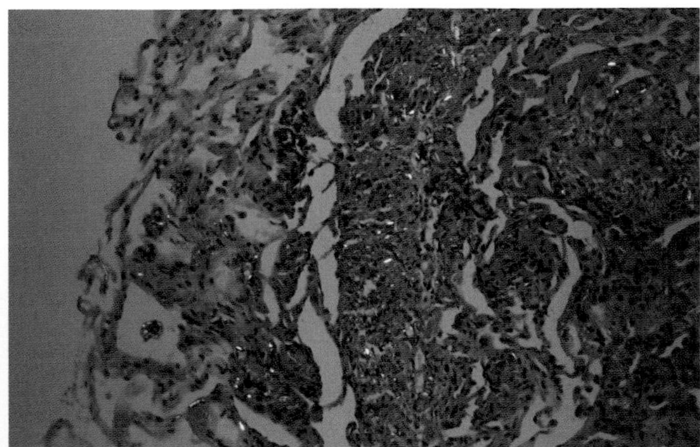

Fig. 9.52 **Silicatosis.** Partial polarization of a fibrotic area demonstrates brightly birefringent silicate particles.

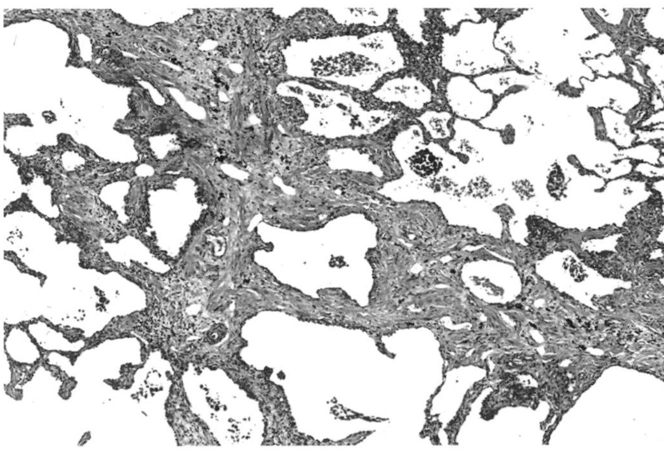

Fig. 9.53 **Mixed dust pneumoconiosis.** The peribronchiolar distribution of fibrosis seen in this case is typical of mixed dust pneumoconiosis.

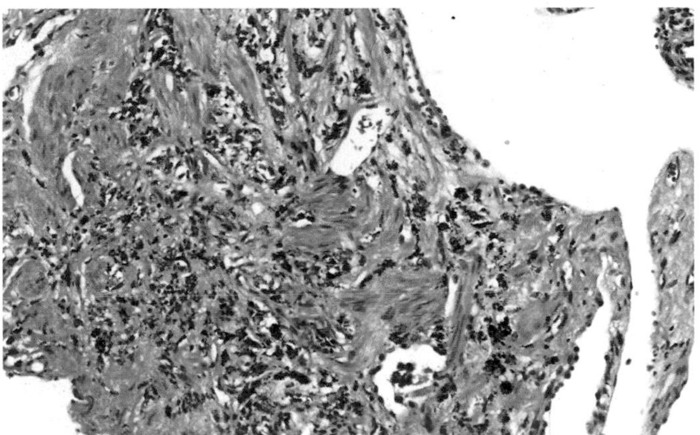

Fig. 9.54 **Mixed dust pneumoconiosis.** At higher magnification, dust deposits are evident in the peribronchiolar areas of fibrosis.

present, characterized by irregularly contoured, stellate lesions with variable collagenization. Non-asbestos ferruginous bodies with broad yellow sheet-silicate cores (Figs 9.50 and 9.51) may be observed in some cases.[14,27] Examination with polarizing microscopy typically demonstrates numerous brightly birefringent particulates (Fig. 9.52) associated with macrophages or within stellate lesions. Analytical electron microscopy shows numerous particulates, most of which consist of silicon combined with other elements, such as magnesium, aluminum, potassium, calcium, or iron.[28]

A special variant of silicatosis is mixed dust pneumoconiosis (MDP), defined as the occurrence of dust macules and stellate lesions producing so-called "mixed dust fibrotic nodules" (Figs 9.53 and 9.54), with or without silicotic nodules.[29] For a diagnosis of MDP, the macules and mixed dust fibrotic nodules should outnumber the silicotic nodules. If silicotic nodules predominate, the preferred diagnosis is silicosis. Analytical electron microscopy in MDP shows aluminum silicates with varying numbers of silica (SiO_2) particles.

Differential diagnosis

Silicatosis (silicate pneumoconiosis) must be distinguished from silicosis, usual interstitial pneumonia (UIP), and nonspecific interstitial pneumonia (NSIP). In cases with dust macules, mixed dust fibrotic lesions, and silicotic nodules, a diagnosis of silicosis should be made when silicotic nodules predominate. UIP has well-defined features that are not seen in silicate pneumoconiosis (see Ch. 7). However, a few scattered birefringent particulates may be found in lungs from the general population, including those with UIP and NSIP. Such findings should not be confused with silicate pneumoconiosis, in which numerous brightly birefringent silicate particles are present within the dust macules or mixed dust fibrotic lesions (Fig. 9.55).

Talcosis (talc pneumoconiosis)

Introduction

Talcosis, or talc pneumoconiosis, is a type of silicate pneumoconiosis with unique morphologic and clinical features. Talc is used in many industries. Typical exposures include mining and milling, as well as the rubber and steel industries. Exposures may also occur among individuals who use excessive amounts of talcum powder. Talc is a filler in many medications intended for oral consumption. It may reach the lungs by the vascular route in individuals who intravenously inject crushed tablets. Talc is also frequently used for pleurodesis and may be observed in radical extrapleural pneumonectomy or autopsy specimens from patients with malignant mesothelioma.

Clinical presentation

Patients are often asymptomatic, but fatal pulmonary fibrosis has been reported among talc miners and millers.[30] Intravenous drug abusers may develop pulmonary hypertension, massive fibrosis, or paracicatricial emphysema with spontaneous pneumothorax as a complication of massive intravascular deposits of talc within the lungs.[31,32]

Pathologic findings

Macroscopically, the lungs in talcosis may be normal or firm.[33,34] Histologically, patchy peribronchiolar and perivascular fibrosis is associated with abundant dust deposits. The particles within these deposits are needle-like and have a bluish-gray color (Fig. 9.56). Examination by polarizing microscopy shows numerous brightly birefringent, needle-like particles within giant cells (Fig. 9.57),

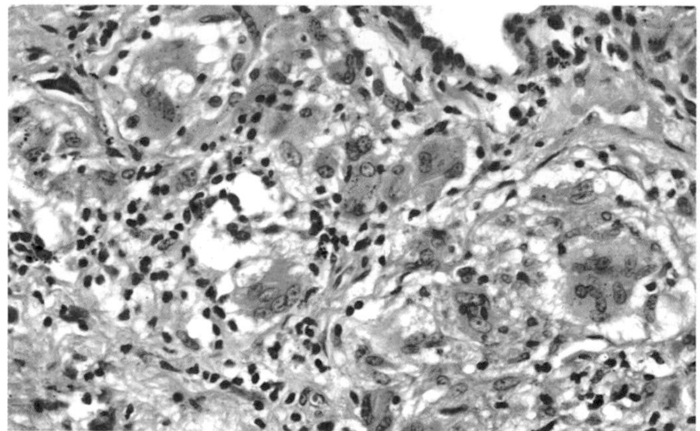

Fig. 9.56 **Talcosis.** In this example, needle-like talc particles are associated with an exuberant giant cell response.

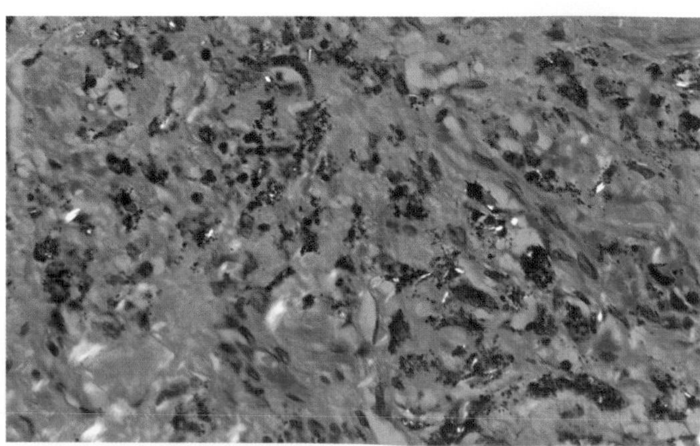

Fig. 9.55 **Mixed dust pneumoconiosis.** Partially polarized photomicrograph of a mixed dust fibrotic nodule showing particles with variable birefringence.

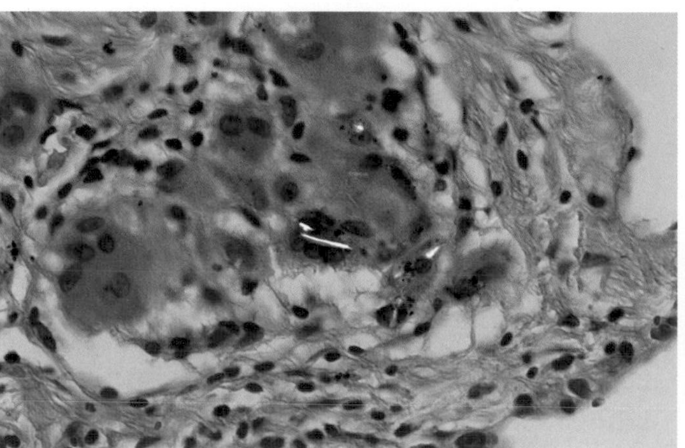

Fig. 9.57 **Talcosis.** Partially polarized view of talc, exhibiting a characteristic needle-like morphology.

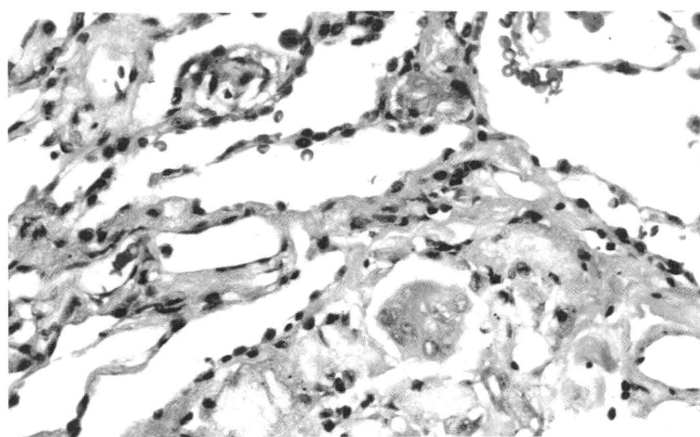

Fig. 9.58 **Intravenous talcosis.** Faintly blue-gray talc particles occupy cleft-like spaces. Note the presence of an asteroid body within a giant cell.

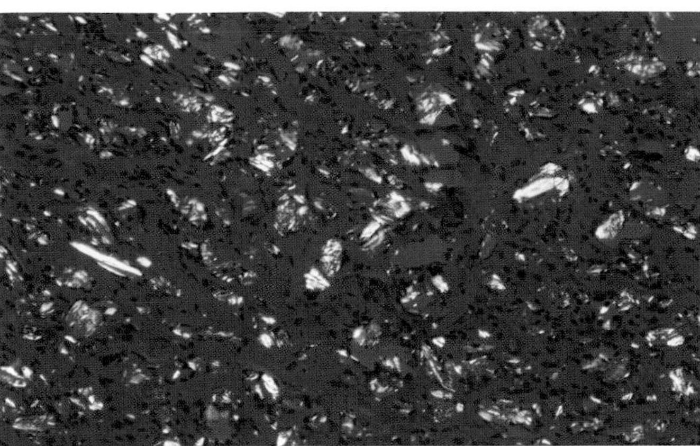

Fig. 9.61 **Talc pleurodesis.** Partial polarization of the above case shows numerous platy and needle-shaped birefringent talc particles.

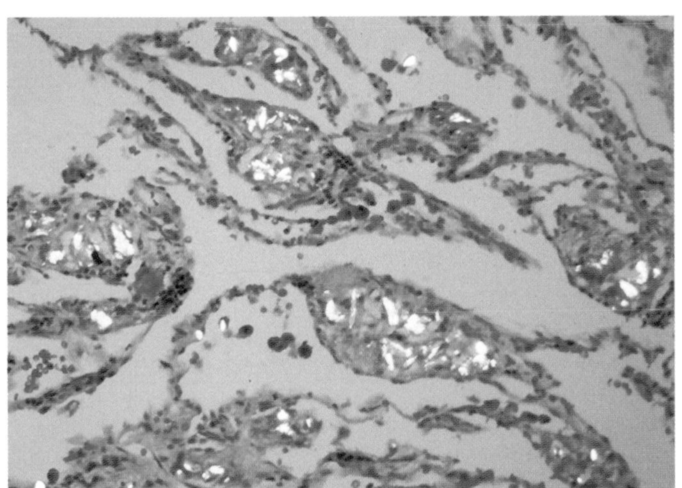

Fig. 9.59 **Intravenous talcosis.** Talc particles appear brightly birefringent under polarized light.

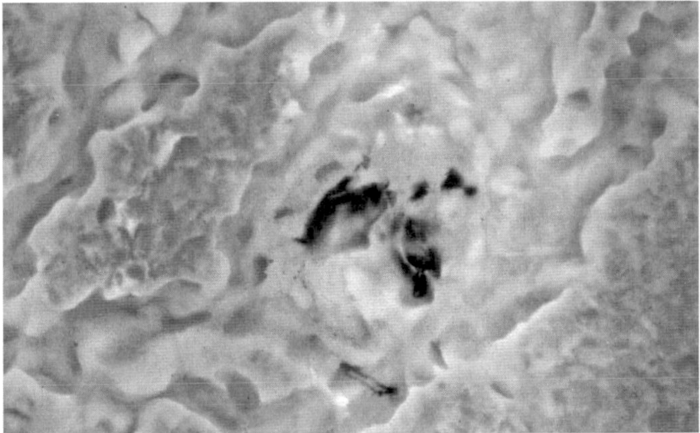

Fig. 9.62 **Talcosis.** In this backscatter electron image, talc has a platy appearance.

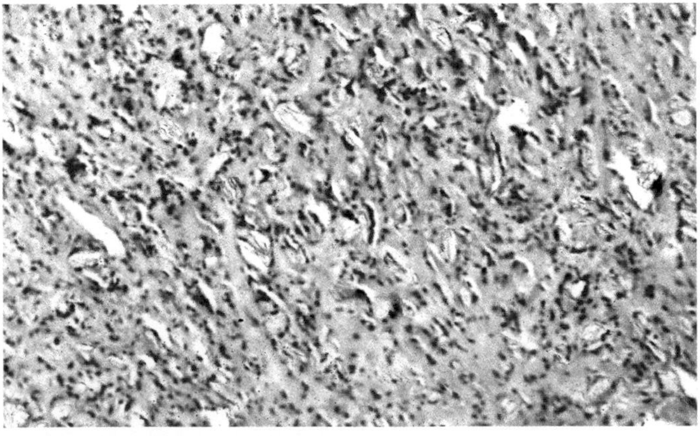

Fig. 9.60 **Talc pleurodesis.** Talc instilled into the pleural space for therapeutic purposes elicited a florid fibrohistiocytic response in this case from a patient with recurrent empyema.

granulomas, or foci of interstitial fibrosis. Multinucleate giant cells are variably present. In some cases, a granulomatous reaction may be present, resembling sarcoidosis. Ferruginous bodies with broad yellow sheet silicate-type cores may also be seen.[14] True asbestos bodies may also be observed in cases where talc is contaminated with substantial amounts of asbestos (anthophyllite or tremolite). Similarly, silicotic nodules may be seen when there is substantial contamination with quartz.

Intravenous drug abuse talcosis is characterized by the accumulation of numerous talc granulomas within the pulmonary vasculature and alveolar septal walls (Figs 9.58 and 9.59). Progressive massive fibrosis has been reported in some cases.[31] Concomitant paracicatricial emphysema may be pronounced.[32] Talc pleurodesis is characterized by deposits of talc (Figs 9.60 and 9.61) with pleural macrophages, accompanied by a giant cell reaction.[35]

Analytical electron microscopy in talcosis demonstrates platy particles composed of magnesium and silicon (Figs 9.62 and 9.63).[36]

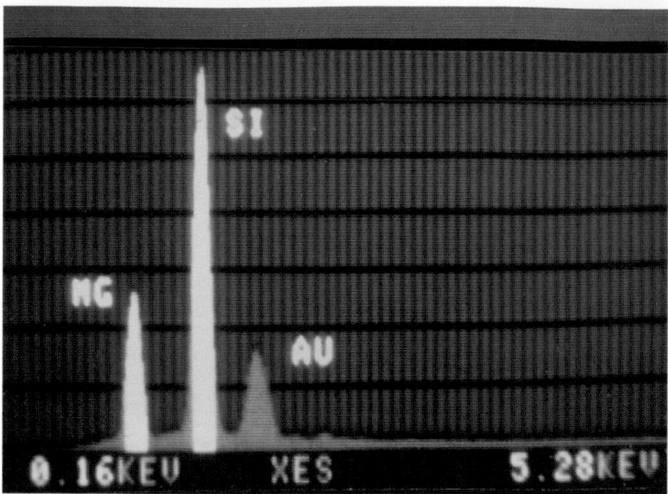

Fig. 9.63 **Talcosis.** Energy dispersive X-ray analysis (EDXA) spectrum of a talc particle demonstrating peaks for silica (Si) and magnesium (Mg). The peak for gold (Au) represents the coating applied to the specimen prior to electron microscopic examination.

Differential diagnosis

Inhalational talcosis must be distinguished from intravenous talcosis and from sarcoidosis. In inhalational talcosis, the deposits are primarily perivascular and peribronchiolar, and intra-alveolar pseudoasbestos bodies may be observed. In intravenous talcosis, talc deposits are intravascular and within alveolar capillary walls. The talc particles in intravenous talcosis are on average larger than those observed with inhalational talcosis. Often they are too large to be deposited by inhalation. Inhalational talcosis producing a prominent granulomatous reaction differs from sarcoidosis by the presence of numerous, long, needle-like birefringent crystals, as compared to the smaller and sparser needle-like particles in sarcoidosis. In difficult cases, analytical electron microscopy may be required to make the distinction. The fibrohistiocytic reaction to talc pleurodesis may superficially resemble areas of sarcomatoid mesothelioma. The distinction can be made by the presence of foreign body giant cells and numerous platy birefringent particles in talc pleurodesis.

Siderosis

Introduction

Siderosis refers to the accumulation of exogenous iron particulates within the lung parenchyma. Siderosis occurs primarily among hematite miners, iron foundry workers, and welders. Miners and foundry workers may be exposed to significant amounts of silica in the workplace, resulting in siderosilicosis, in which there are histologic features of both siderosis and silicosis.

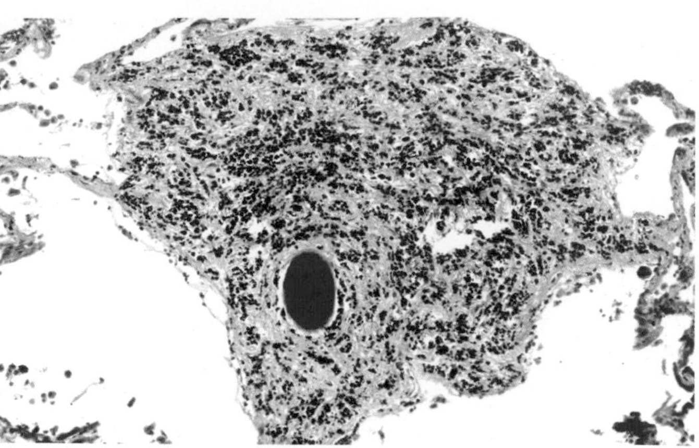

Fig. 9.64 **Siderosilicosis.** This case demonstrates welder's pigment, as well as nodular fibrosis typical of siderosilicosis.

Clinical presentation

Iron is minimally fibrogenic, so even patients with heavy exposures are typically asymptomatic. Chest X-rays may suggest interstitial fibrosis due to shadows cast by the deposits of iron pigment.[37] Patients with significant exposures to silica or asbestos in addition to iron may manifest clinical features related to the inhalation of such dusts.[38]

Pathologic findings

Iron pigment imparts a reddish-brown color to the lung parenchyma.[3,39] Because iron is a minimally fibrogenic dust, there is no increase in firmness in siderosis. However, in cases where there is concomitant exposure to significant amounts of silica or asbestos, excess collagen may be deposited (Fig. 9.64).

The histologic hallmark of siderosis is perivascular and peribronchiolar deposition of iron pigment (Fig. 9.65).[40] The pigment, which consists predominantly of iron oxide, typically is dark brown to black, often with a distinctive golden brown halo (Figs 9.66A and 9.66B). The pigment may be found in macrophages and/or the interstitium with very little fibrous response. As mentioned earlier, the finding of significant amounts of fibrosis should prompt a search for evidence of exposure to asbestos or silica (Fig. 9.67). Ferruginous bodies may be observed in some cases (Figs 9.68 and 9.70).[14] These may have black iron oxide cores, particularly in iron foundry workers (Fig. 9.71), or broad yellow sheet-silicate cores in welders

(Fig. 9.69). True asbestos bodies may also be observed if there has been significant exposure to asbestos, as with shipyard welders.

Iron oxide pigment is typically non-refringent when viewed with polarizing microscopy. Analytical electron microscopy demonstrates spherical particles with prominent peaks for iron (Figs 9.72 and 9.73).

Differential diagnosis

Siderosis must be distinguished from chronic passive congestion of the lungs, and from anthracosis (perivascular and peribronchiolar deposits of anthracotic pigment). Chronic passive congestion manifests as intra-alveolar accumulation of numerous hemosiderin-laden macrophages. Although both hemosiderin and exogenous iron pigment stain with Prussian blue, hemosiderin lacks the dark brown to black centers characteristic of iron oxide. At low magnification, iron oxide deposits may resemble anthracotic pigment. However, anthracotic pigment is black throughout and lacks the golden brown rim characteristic of iron oxide.

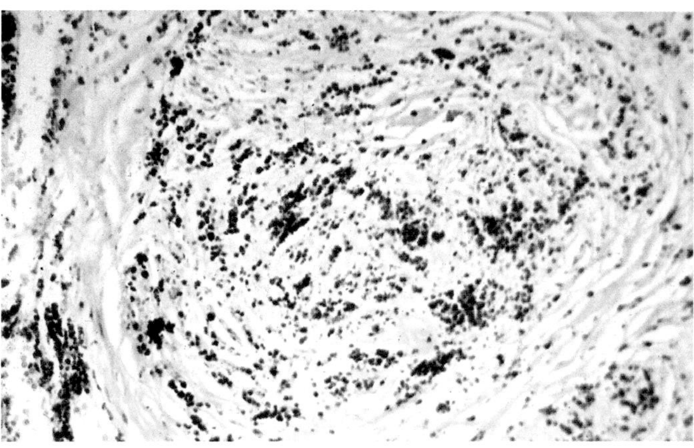

Fig. 9.67 **Siderosilicosis.** A Masson trichrome stain demonstrates the whorled appearance of this heavily pigmented silicotic nodule.

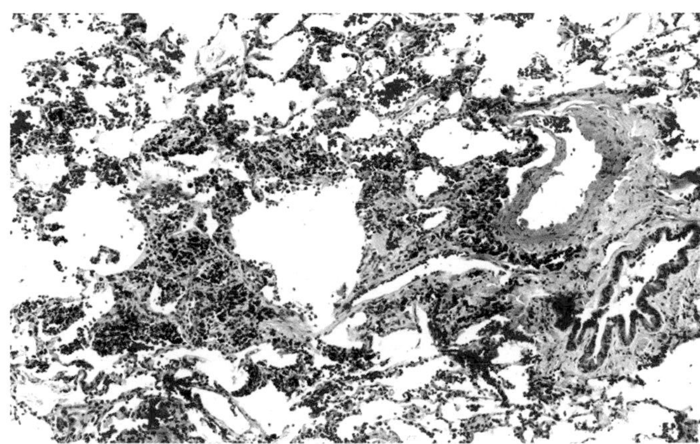

Fig. 9.65 **Siderosis.** Perivascular pigment deposition is seen in this histologic section taken from the lung of a welder.

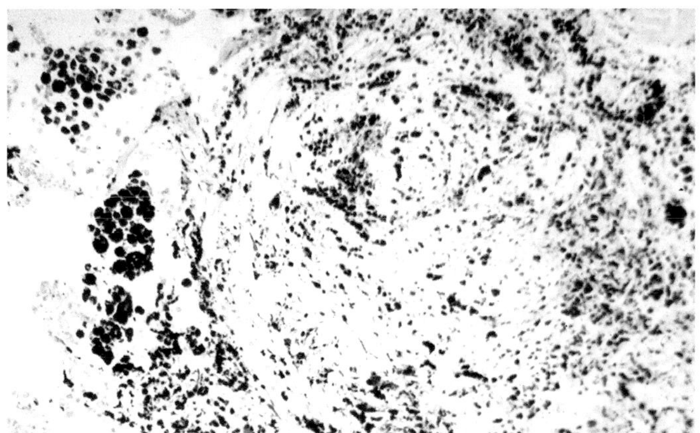

Fig. 9.68 **Siderosilicosis.** The iron pigment in the above case appears deep blue in this iron-stained section.

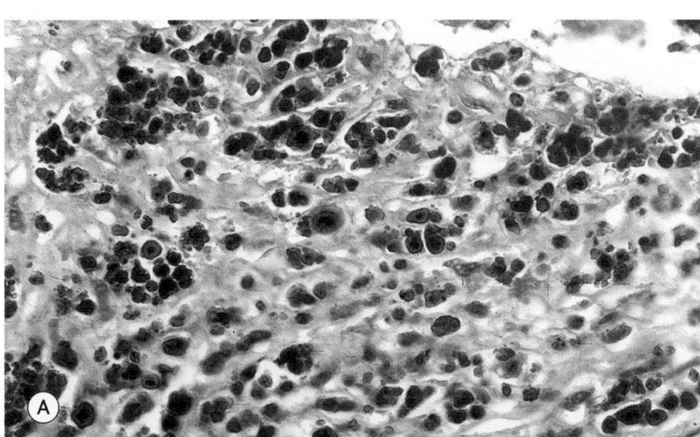

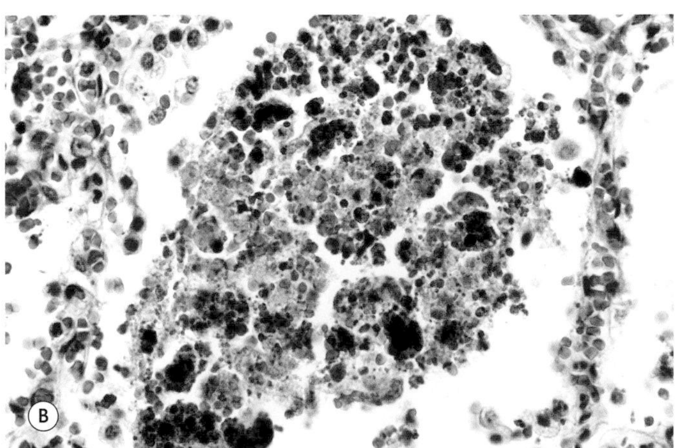

Fig. 9.66 **Siderosis.** (A) Detail of iron oxide, or welders' pigment, which appears brown-black with a golden brown halo. (B) In contrast to welders' pigment, hemosiderin is typically intra-alveolar and lacks black central cores.

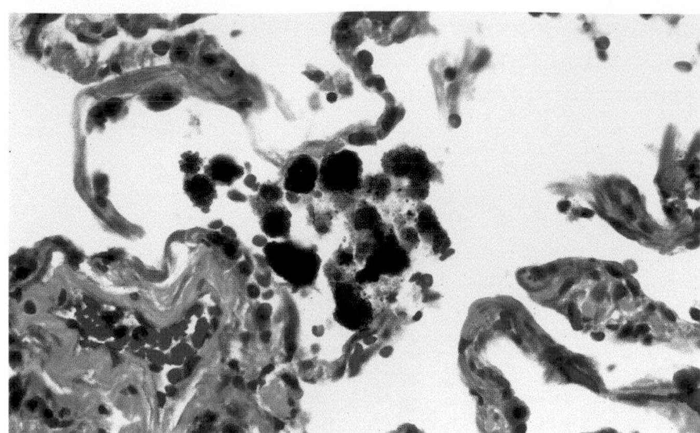

Fig. 9.69 **Siderosis.** Pseudoasbestos bodies with broad yellow sheet-silicate cores are seen in this case from a welder.

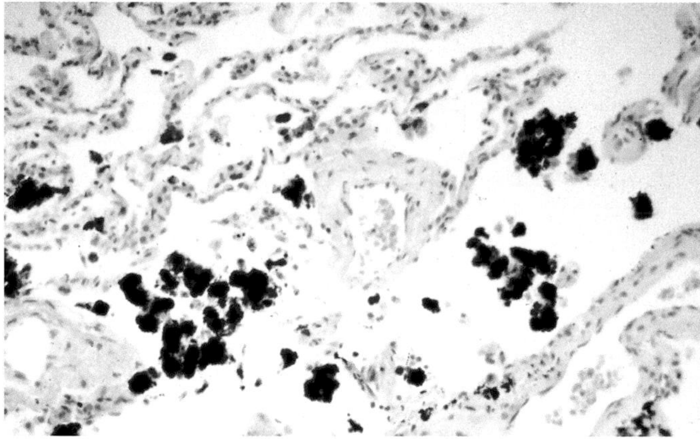

Fig. 9.70 **Siderosis.** Iron-stained section of the above case demonstrates numerous pseudoasbestos bodies.

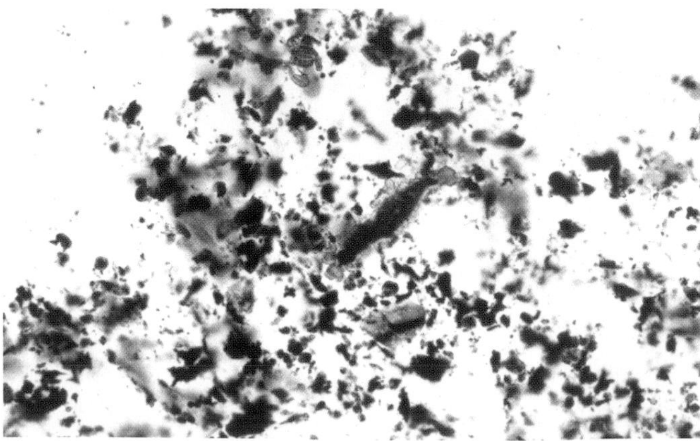

Fig. 9.71 **Siderosis.** Pseudoasbestos body on a tissue digestion filter from the lung of an iron foundry worker. Note the stout, irregular black iron oxide core.

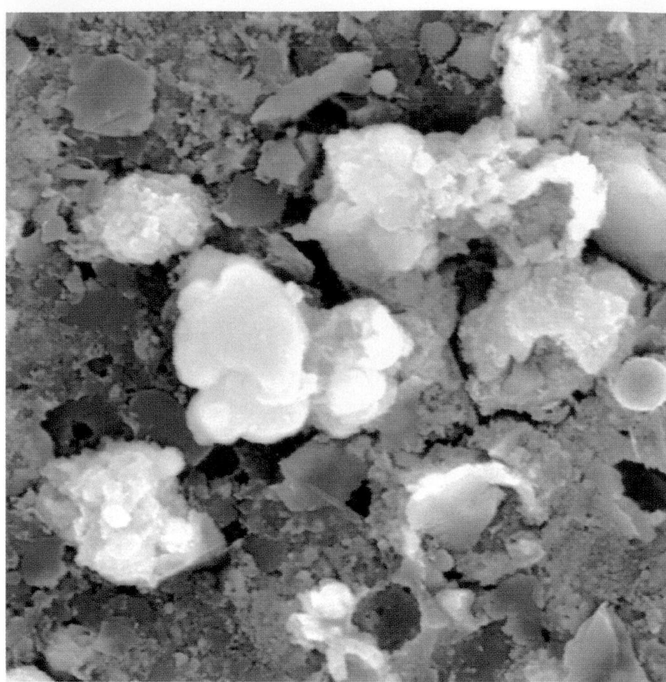

Fig. 9.72 **Siderosis.** Scanning electron micrograph of iron oxide particles from a welder's lung.

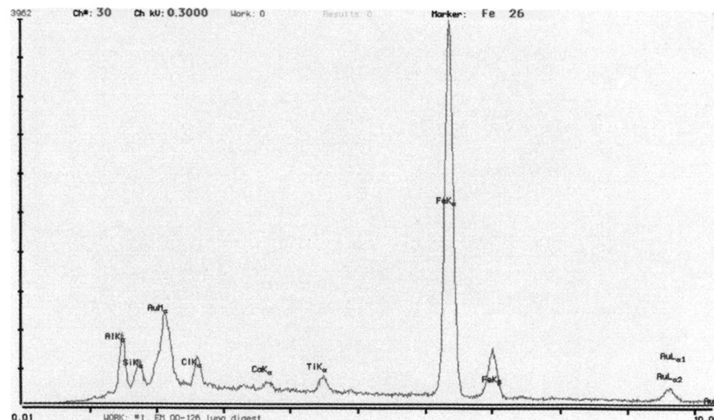

Fig. 9.73 **Siderosis.** Energy dispersive X-ray analysis (EDXA) spectrum of iron oxide particles, showing predominant peak for iron (Fe).

Aluminosis

Introduction

Aluminosis is lung disease caused by the inhalation of aluminum-containing dusts. While aluminum is a common component of our environment, aluminosis is a rare disease. Hypersensitivity to aluminum is believed to play a role in the pathogenesis of aluminosis. Substantial exposure to aluminum-containing dust may occur in the setting of aluminum smelting, manufacture of aluminum oxide abrasives, aluminum polishing, and aluminum arc-welding.[41–43]

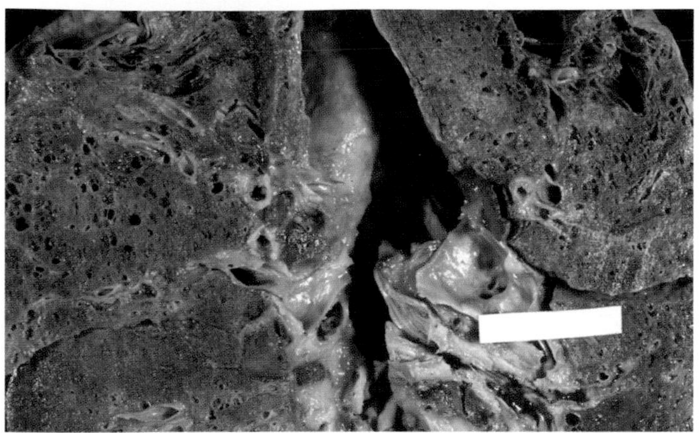

Fig. 9.74 **Aluminosis.** Scattered areas of fibrosis are present in the lungs of this aluminum arc welder.

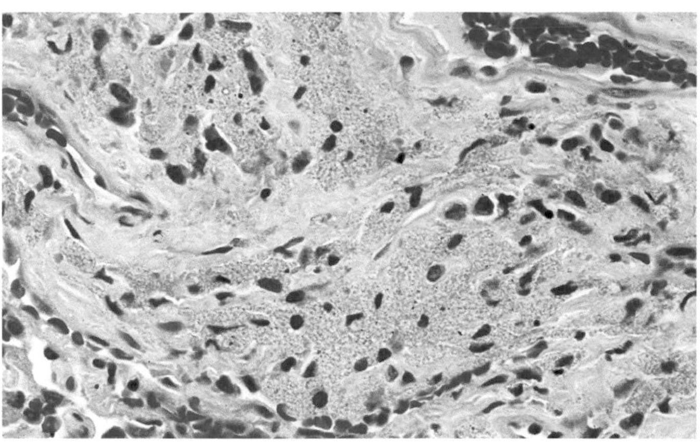

Fig. 9.76 **Aluminosis.** Detail of dust-laden macrophages, showing the gray-brown granular appearance typical of aluminum oxide.

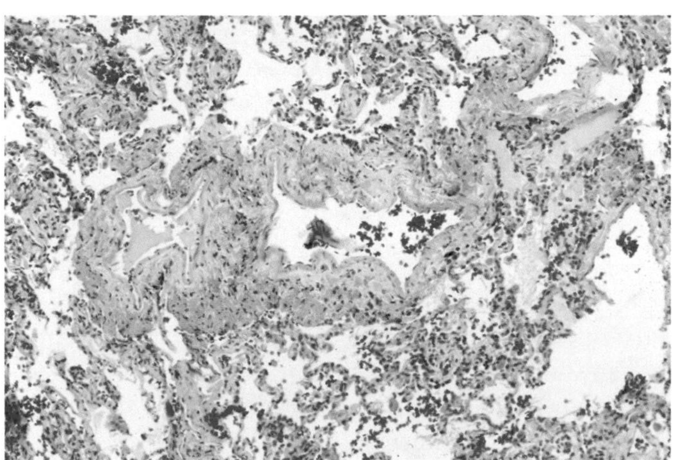

Fig. 9.75 **Aluminosis.** An accumulation of dust-laden macrophages surrounds a pulmonary vessel.

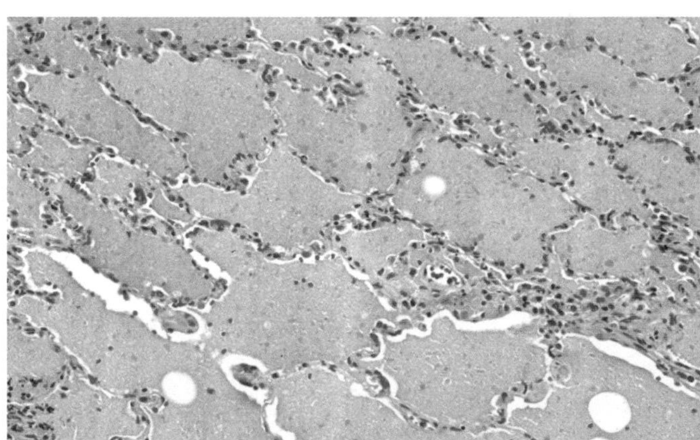

Fig. 9.77 **Aluminosis.** Amorphous eosinophilic material fills the alveoli in a pattern typical for pulmonary alveolar proteinosis. Interstitial accumulations of dust-laden macrophages are also present.

Clinical presentation

Cases in which interstitial fibrosis is the dominant tissue reaction may manifest as dyspnea on exertion and restrictive changes on pulmonary function tests. Fatal cases with severe interstitial fibrosis have been reported.[43]

Pathologic findings

Macroscopically, the lung parenchyma in aluminosis ranges from essentially normal to heavy and grayish black with dense fibrotic areas scattered throughout (Fig. 9.74).[3] A metallic sheen, resembling tarnished aluminum, has been described in some cases.

Histologic examination discloses perivascular and peribronchiolar accumulations of dust-laden macrophages (Fig. 9.75). The dust is refractile and gray to brown (Fig. 9.76). Tissue reaction to aluminum ranges from nil to interstitial fibrosis to granulomatous inflammation.[43–46] Cases with a prominent granulomatous response may resemble sarcoidosis. Areas resembling desquamative interstitial pneumonia may also be observed.[47] Rare cases have been described with an alveolar proteinosis-like pattern (Figs 9.77 and 9.78) similar to that seen in acute silicoproteinosis.[40]

The dust is non-refringent upon examination by polarizing microscopy. Analytical electron microscopy shows electron dense spherical particles (Figs 9.79 and 9.80) composed of aluminum (Fig. 9.81).

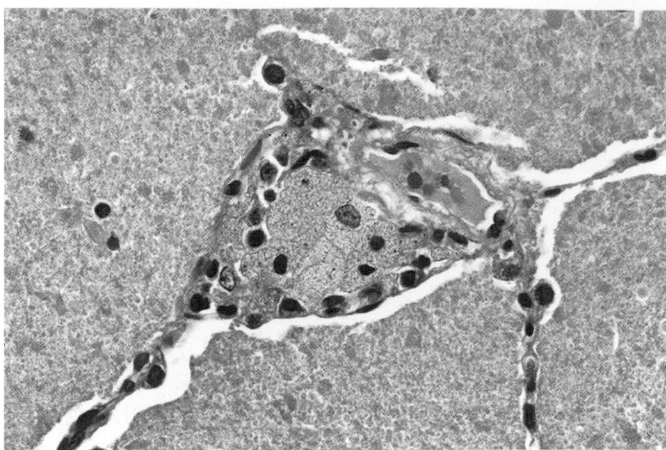

Fig. 9.78 **Aluminosis.** Higher magnification view, showing the characteristic gray-brown granular appearance of aluminum-laden macrophages.

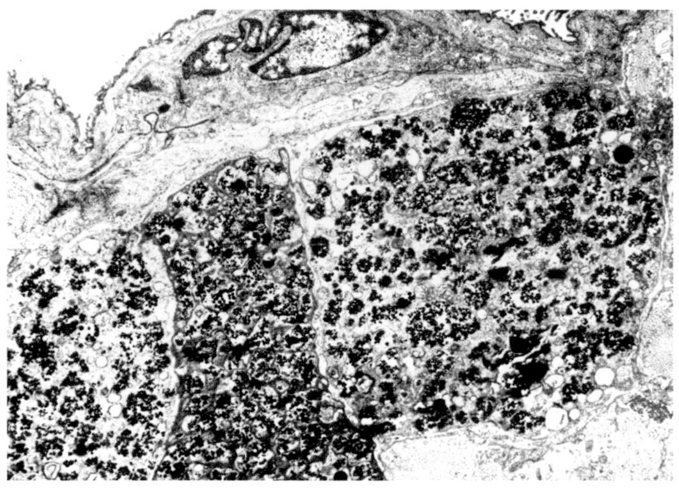

Fig. 9.79 **Aluminosis.** Transmission electron micrograph showing an alveolar type 2 cell overlying a dust-filled interstitial macrophage.

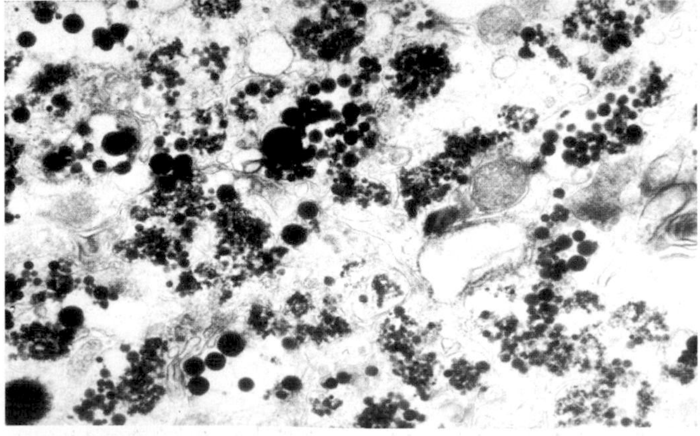

Fig. 9.80 **Aluminosis.** In this transmission electron micrograph of an aluminum-containing macrophage, the aluminum particles appear spherical and electron dense. (Reprinted from Roggli,[40] with permission.)

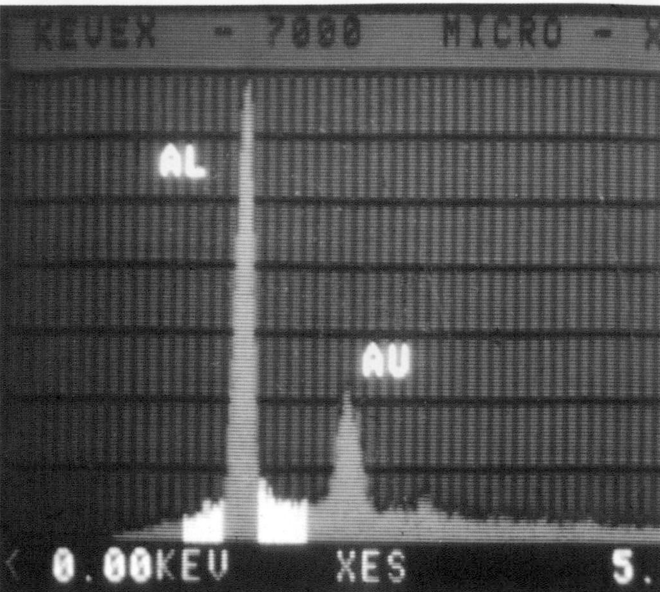

Fig. 9.81 **Aluminosis.** Energy dispersive X-ray analysis (EDXA) spectrum in a case of aluminosis demonstrates a peak for aluminum only (Al). The peak for gold (Au) represents the coating applied to the specimen prior to electron microscopic examination. (Reprinted from Roggli,[40] with permission.)

Differential diagnosis

Dust deposits of aluminum must be distinguished from kaolinite (a form of aluminum silicate; see Silicatosis section) and smokers' macrophages. The dust deposits in kaolin workers' pneumoconiosis are fine and tan, whereas aluminum is more refractile and gray to brown in color. In difficult cases, analytical electron microscopy may be required to make the distinction. Smokers' macrophages are located primarily within the alveolar spaces and are typically associated with scattered black dot-like carbon particles. Aluminum-induced granulomatosis must be considered in the differential diagnosis of sarcoidosis. In addition, aluminum exposure must be considered in cases with a pulmonary alveolar proteinosis pattern. In such cases, the presence of aluminum dust deposits is a useful differentiating feature.

Hard metal lung disease

Introduction

Tungsten carbide is used in the manufacture of cutting tools, drilling equipment, armaments, alloys, and ceramics (Table 9.4). Cobalt is used as a binder and may comprise up to 25% of the final product by weight. Hard metal lung disease occurs as a consequence of the inhalation of

Table 9.4 Uses for tungsten carbide

Alloys
Armaments
Ceramics
Circular saw blades
Cutting tools
Drilling equipment

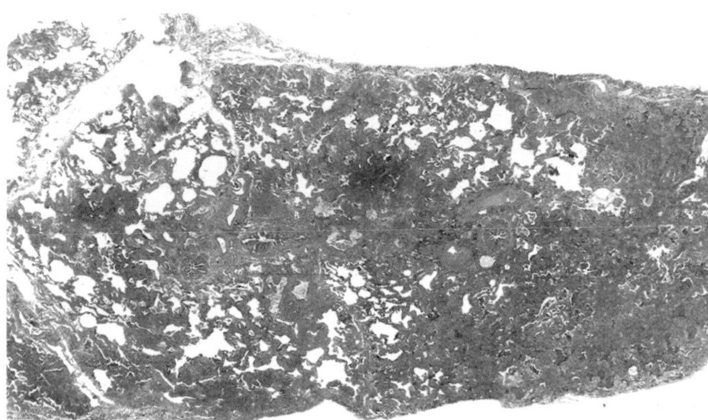

Fig. 9.82 **Hard metal pneumoconiosis.** At low magnification, the interstitium appears widened accompanied by alveolar filling.

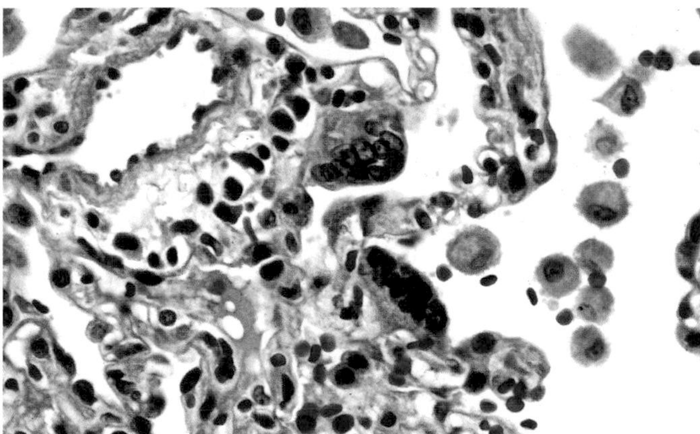

Fig. 9.83 **Hard metal pneumoconiosis.** This example demonstrates interstitial pneumonia with giant cells lining alveolar septa.

hard metal dust. Exposure may occur during the manufacturing process of hard metal-containing products or during their use.[48] Cobalt exposure has also been reported in diamond polishers who had no exposure to hard metal dust.[49,50]

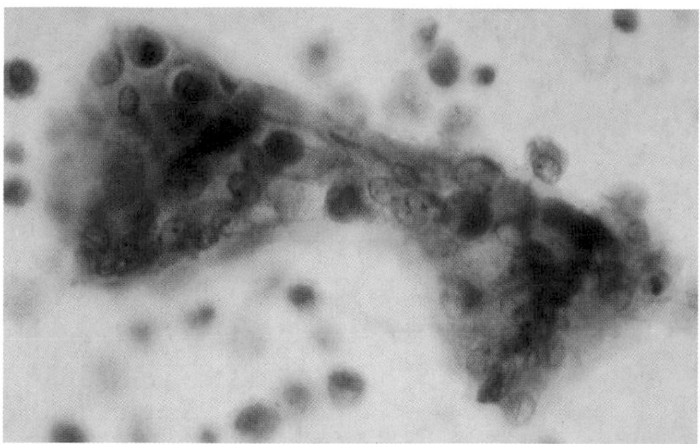

Fig. 9.84 **Hard metal pneumoconiosis.** A bronchoalveolar lavage fluid from a patient with hard metal pneumoconiosis demonstrates multinucleate giant cells. (Reprinted from Tabatowski et al.,[54] with permission.)

Clinical presentation

Workers with hard metal lung disease present with insidious onset of dyspnea and restrictive changes on pulmonary function tests with small lung volumes. Diffusely increased interstitial markings are observed on plain chest films and CT. Less than 1% of those exposed develop disease, which suggests that hypersensitivity to cobalt is the underlying pathogenetic mechanism. Workers may also present with asthma that predates interstitial lung disease by months to years. Hard metal lung disease has been reported to recur following lung transplantation,[51] without additional exposure.

Pathologic findings

Macroscopically, the lungs in hard metal lung disease are small and fibrotic. Microscopically, hard metal lung disease is synonymous with giant cell interstitial pneumonia (GIP),[52] once considered to be one of the "idiopathic" interstitial pneumonias. In this disorder, the alveolar septa are thickened and fibrotic, and lined by hyperplastic alveolar type 2 pneumocytes (Figs 9.82 and 9.83). A moderate chronic inflammatory infiltrate is present. Multinucleate giant cells are a conspicuous feature (Fig. 9.84), and are found both within the alveolar spaces and lining the alveolar septa. Alveolar macrophages are present in increased numbers, and in some cases a pattern reminiscent of desquamative interstitial pneumonia is observed (Fig. 9.85). Occasionally, the overall pattern mimics that of UIP, with areas of microscopic honeycombing (Figs 9.86 and 9.87). The fibrotic and inflammatory reaction may be accentuated around bronchioles.

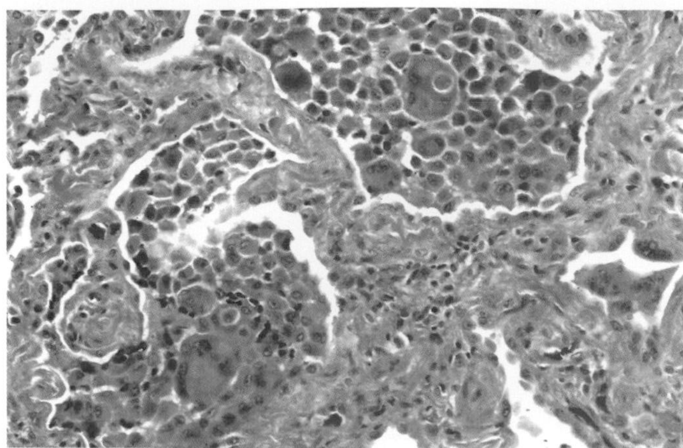

Fig. 9.85 **Hard metal pneumoconiosis.** Along with multinucleate giant cells, macrophages fill alveolar spaces in a pattern resembling desquamative interstitial pneumonia. (Reprinted from Roggli,[40] with permission.)

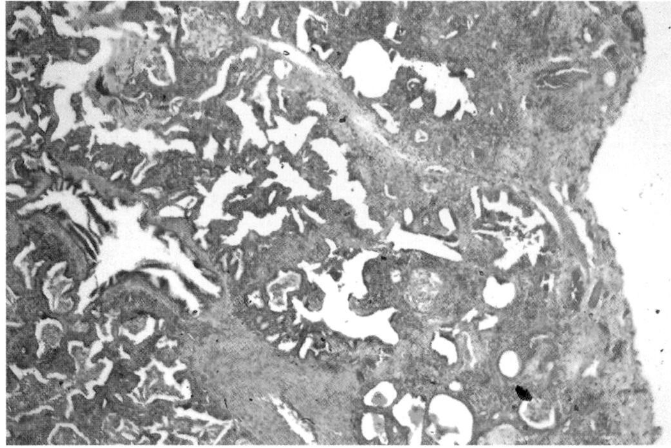

Fig. 9.86 **Hard metal pneumoconiosis.** The severe interstitial fibrosis with bronchiolar metaplasia and honeycombing in case of tungsten carbide pneumoconiosis are reminiscent of usual interstitial pneumonia.

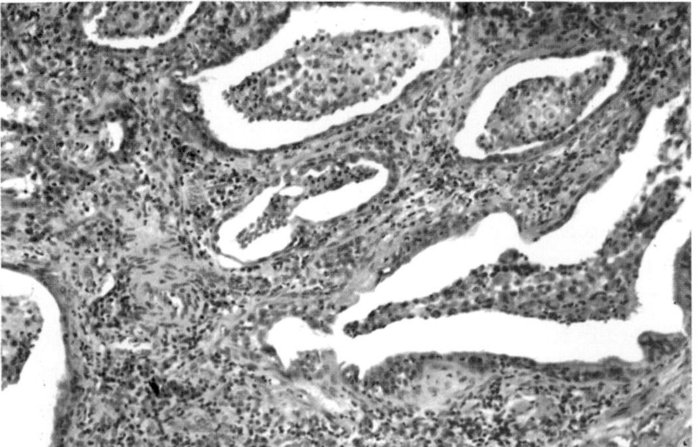

Fig. 9.87 **Hard metal pneumoconiosis.** Detail of the above case, showing honeycomb cysts filled with macrophages.

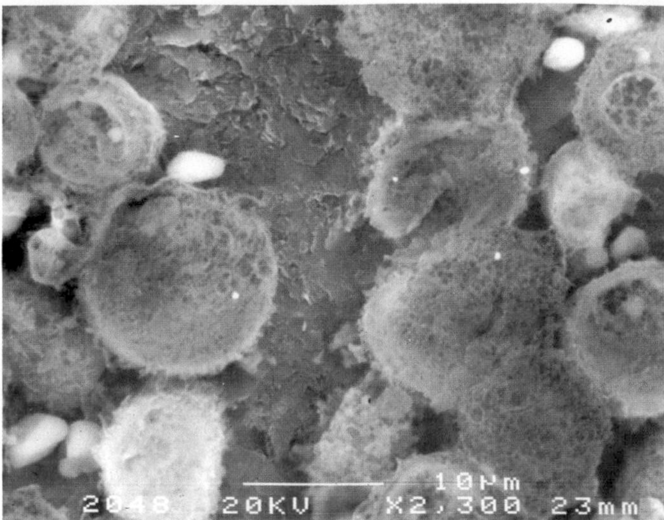

Fig. 9.88 **Hard metal pneumoconiosis.** Scanning electron image of alveolar macrophages shows small electron dense metal particles. (Case courtesy Dr. Frank Johnson and Dr. Jose Centano, AFIP, Washington, DC.)

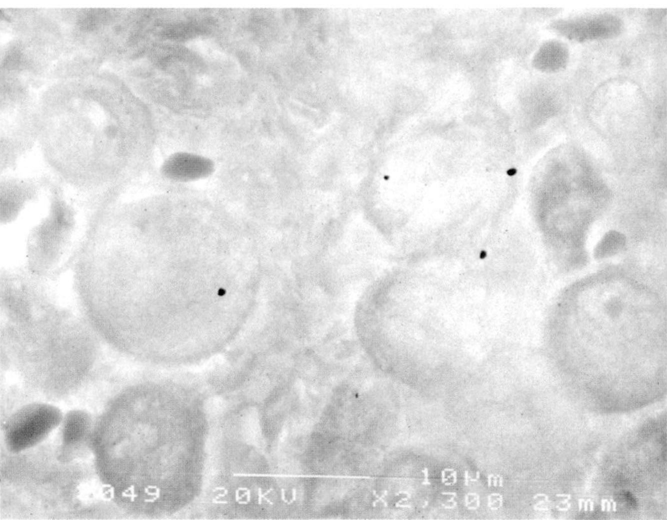

Fig. 9.89 **Hard metal pneumoconiosis.** The metal particles in the above case appear as dark dots in this backscatter electron micrograph. (Case courtesy Dr. Frank Johnson and Dr. Jose Centano, AFIP, Washington, DC.)

Dust deposits are not readily identified by either routine or polarizing light microscopy. The individual metal particles can be observed by analytical electron microscopy (Figs 9.88 and 9.89).[53] Tungsten particles are most common, followed by titanium and tantalum (Fig. 9.90). Cobalt, the suspected causative agent of the disease, may or may not be identified, since its water solubility makes it susceptible to removal from tissue.

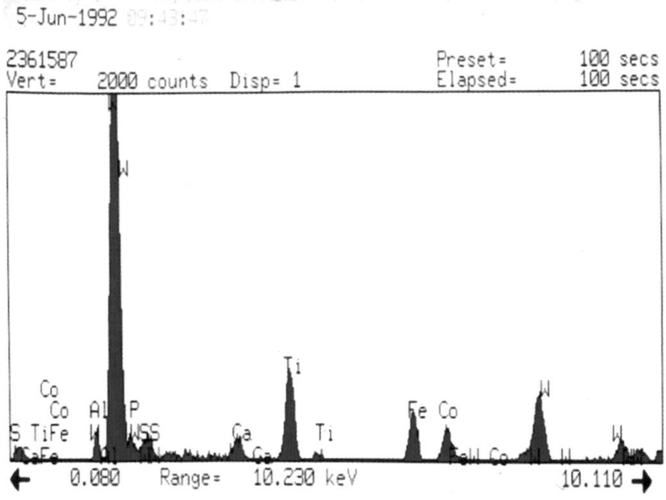

Fig. 9.90 **Hard metal pneumoconiosis.** Energy dispersive X-ray analysis (EDXA) spectrum demonstrates a large peak for tungsten, which is also known as wolfram (W). A small peak for cobalt (Co) is also present. (Case courtesy Dr. Frank Johnson and Dr. Jose Centano, AFIP, Washington, DC.)

Differential diagnosis

Hard-metal lung disease must be distinguished from UIP, desquamative interstitial pneumonia (DIP), and hypersensitivity pneumonitis. The presence of intra-alveolar and alveolar septal giant cells and the absence of honeycomb changes favor hard metal disease. In the absence of giant cells and an exposure history, analytical electron microscopy may be required to confirm the diagnosis. Desquamative interstitial pneumonia has a monotonous pattern with minimal interstitial fibrosis, and giant cells lining the alveolar septa are not a feature of DIP. Hypersensitivity pneumonitis is characterized by an interstitial chronic inflammatory infiltrate associated with small clusters of interstitial giant cells, as opposed to the intra-alveolar or alveolar septal giant cells of hard metal disease.

Transbronchial biopsy and bronchoalveolar lavage may be useful in the diagnosis of hard metal lung disease.[54] Analytical electron microscopy can be performed on either of these specimens and may demonstrate the characteristic profile of metallic elements.

Berylliosis

Introduction

Berylliosis is a granulomatous lung disease caused by the inhalation of beryllium-containing dust.[55,56] Beryllium is used in the aerospace industry in the manufacture of structural materials, guidance systems, optical devices,

Table 9.5 Uses of beryllium

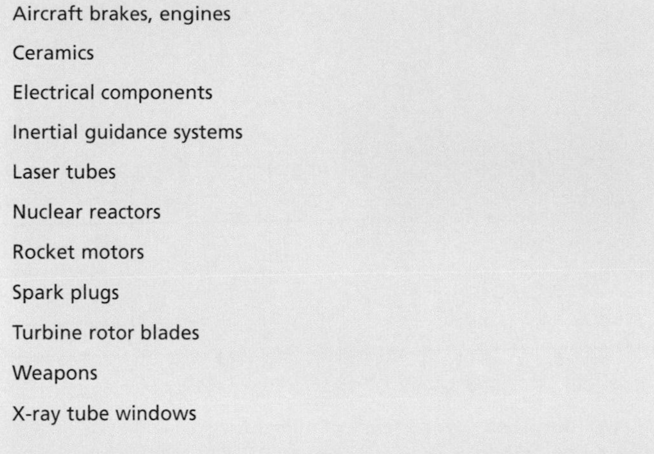

Uses of beryllium
Aircraft brakes, engines
Ceramics
Electrical components
Inertial guidance systems
Laser tubes
Nuclear reactors
Rocket motors
Spark plugs
Turbine rotor blades
Weapons
X-ray tube windows

rocket motor parts, and heat shields. It is also used in the manufacture of ceramic parts, thermal couplings, and crucibles, and as a controller in nuclear reactors (Table 9.5). Exposure may occur in any of these industries, as well as in the mining or extraction of beryllium ores.[57–59] Historically, beryllium was used in the manufacture of fluorescent light bulbs, which accounted for most of the initially reported cases of berylliosis.

Clinical presentation

Patients with berylliosis present with insidiously progressive dyspnea. Pulmonary function tests show restriction with diminished diffusing capacity. Plain films of the chest show a fibronodular process. Only about 1% of patients at risk develop the disease. Beryllium hypersensitivity has therefore been postulated as the likely pathogenetic mechanism, similar to the diseases caused by exposure to aluminum and hard metal. In-vitro reactivity of peripheral blood or bronchoalveolar lavage lymphocytes to beryllium salts has been used as part of the diagnostic work-up.[60]

Pathologic findings

Macroscopically, the lungs in chronic berylliosis are small and fibrotic, and may show honeycomb changes.[3] Bilateral hilar lymphadenopathy may be present. Microscopically, there are well-formed non-necrotizing granulomas (Figs 9.91–9.93). A chronic interstitial inflammatory infiltrate is typically present (Fig. 9.92). Granulomas may also be found in hilar lymph nodes. Schaumann bodies (Fig. 9.94) and asteroid bodies (Fig. 9.95) within multinucleate giant cells are observed in some cases.[39,40]

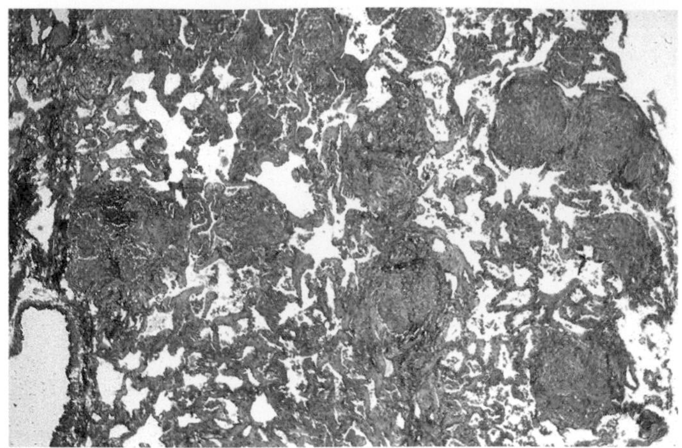

Fig. 9.91 **Berylliosis.** The presence of numerous granulomas is characteristic of berylliosis. (Case courtesy Dr. Fred Askin, Johns Hopkins, Baltimore, MD.)

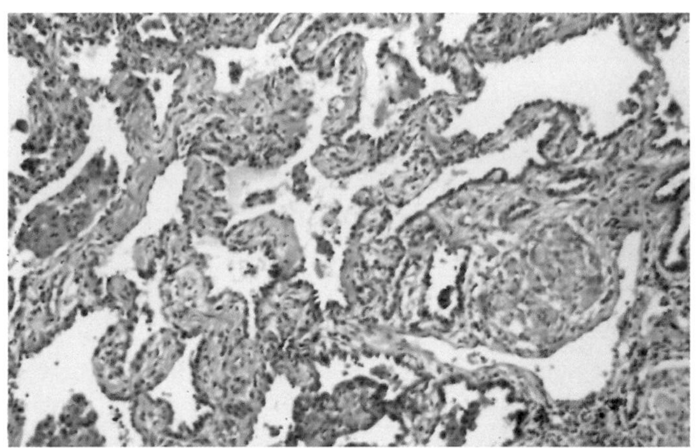

Fig. 9.92 **Berylliosis.** In addition to granulomatous inflammation, a chronic intersititial inflammatory infiltrate is seen. (Reprinted from Roggli,[40] with permission.)

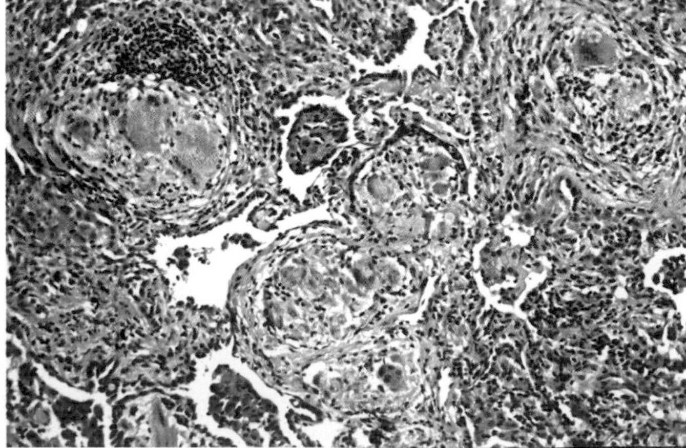

Fig. 9.93 **Berylliosis.** The granulomas in berylliosis are compact and lack necrosis. (Reprinted from Roggli et al.,[1] with permission.)

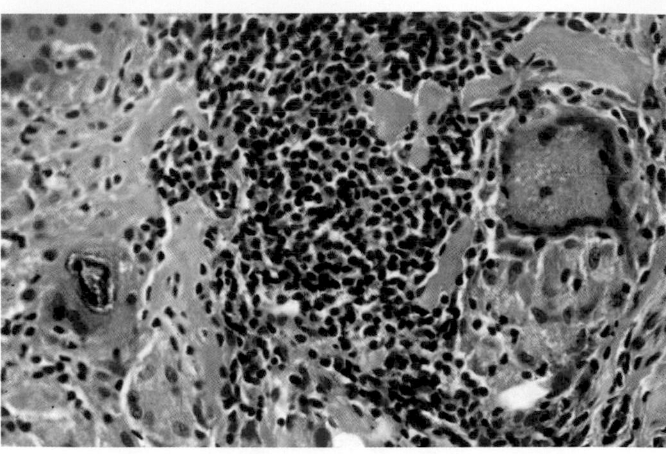

Fig. 9.94 **Berylliosis.** A Schaumann body, with its characteristic basophilic laminations, is observed within a giant cell (lower left). (Reprinted from Roggli,[40] with permission.)

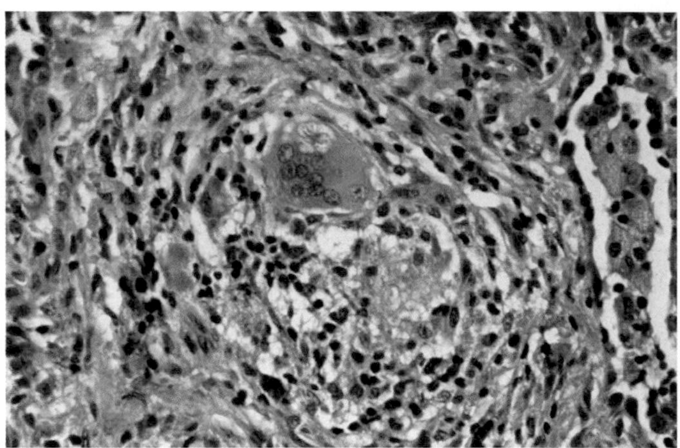

Fig. 9.95 **Berylliosis.** This granuloma features a giant cell containing an asteroid body (upper center). (Reprinted from Roggli,[40] with permission.)

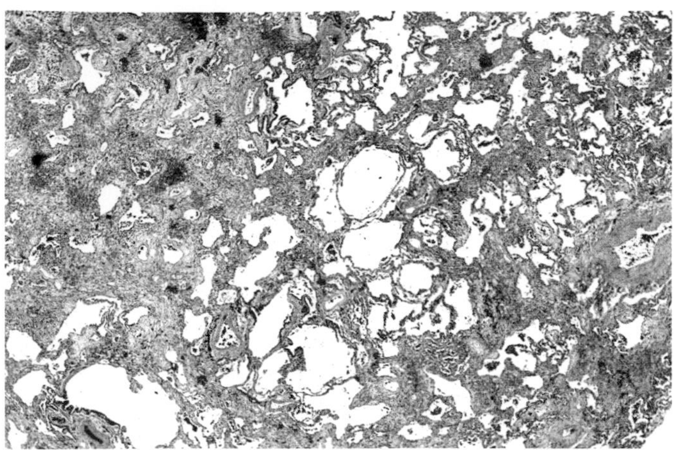

Fig. 9.96 **Rare earth pneumoconiosis.** There is diffuse interstitial fibrosis with honeycomb cyst formation in a pattern reminiscent of usual interstitial pneumonia.

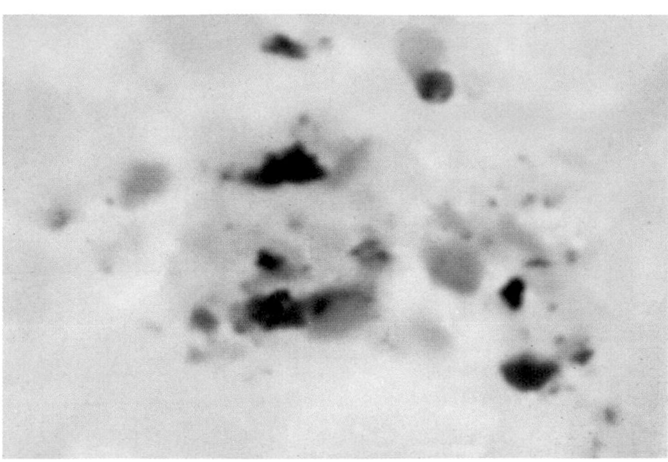

Fig. 9.97 **Rare earth pneumoconiosis.** Backscatter electron image of electron dense cerium oxide particles.

Beryllium is a lightweight metal that has recently been detected by analytical electron microscopy.[60a] Other techniques, such as wet chemical analysis, electron energy loss spectrometry, or ion or laser microprobe mass spectrometry may also be useful.[2] Polarizing microscopy is not useful in the diagnosis of berylliosis.

Differential diagnosis

Berylliosis must be distinguished from sarcoidosis and hypersensitivity pneumonitis. Sarcoidosis closely resembles berylliosis histologically, so a high index of suspicion for exposure to beryllium and a thorough occupational history are necessary in order to arrive at the correct diagnosis. Hypersensitivity pneumonitis is associated with a more intense lymphocytic interstitial and peribronchiolar infiltrate and lacks the well-formed granulomas observed in berylliosis.

Rare earth pneumoconiosis

Introduction

Rare earth (or cerium oxide) pneumoconiosis is an uncommon disease caused by the inhalation of rare earth metals, primarily cerium oxide. Only about 20 cases have been reported, and the pathological descriptions are sparse. Most patients with rare earth pneumoconiosis have been employed in settings with exposure to dust from carbon arc lamps. Two patients were exposed to cerium oxide in an extraction plant, two patients used cerium oxide rouge to polish lenses, and one patient was a producer of glass rubbing polish.[61–64]

Clinical presentation

Patients range from asymptomatic to having insidiously progressive dyspnea. Chest X-rays show a diffuse interstitial pattern. Pulmonary function tests show a restrictive or a mixed restrictive/obstructive pattern and reduced diffusion capacity. The rarity of this disease suggests hypersensitivity to cerium as the pathogenetic mechanism.

Pathologic findings

The histopathologic features range from granulomatous disease to interstitial fibrosis.[61] The fibrosis is similar to that observed with UIP (Fig. 9.96). Pigmented dust deposits may be observed with light microscopy, although these may be sparse. Cerium oxide is birefringent with polarizing microscopy. Analytical electron microscopy demonstrates rare earth metals, primarily cerium and to a lesser degree lanthanum, samarium, and neodymium (Figs 9.97 and 9.98).

Differential diagnosis

Rare earth pneumoconiosis is most readily confused with UIP or NSIP. Sarcoidosis may be considered if there is a

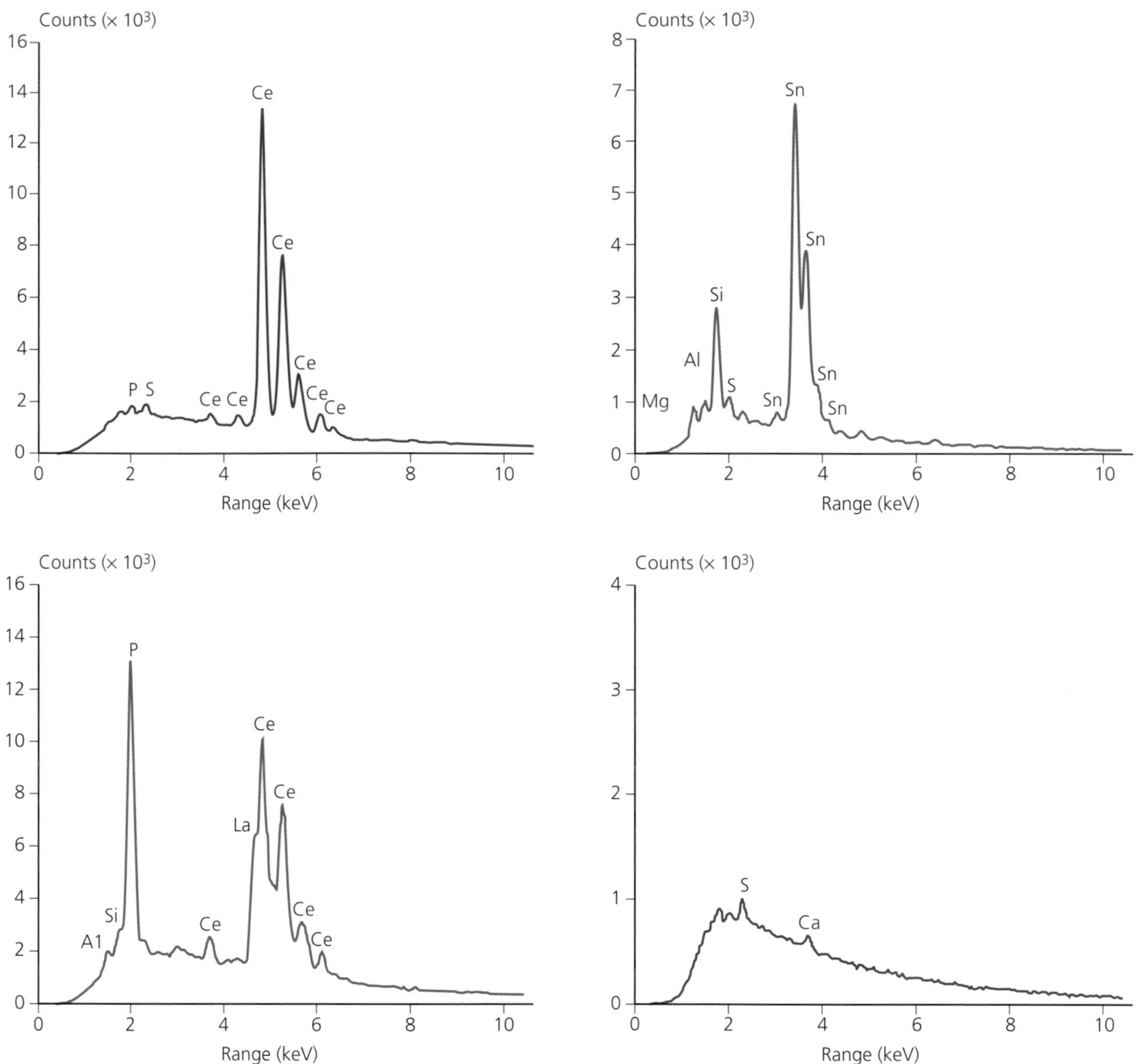

Fig. 9.98 **Rare earth pneumoconiosis.** Energy dispersive X-ray analysis (EDXA) spectra demonstrate peaks for rare earth metals, including cerium (Ce), upper left, and cerium plus lanthanum (La), lower left. Background is shown at lower right, and a tin particle (Sn) at upper right. (Reprinted from McDonald et al.,[61] with permission.)

prominent granulomatous reaction. The diagnosis can be made with a thorough occupational history and detection of rare earth compounds in lung tissue by analytical electron microscopy.

REFERENCES

1. Roggli VL, Shelburne JD: Pneumoconioses, Mineral and vegetable. In: Pulmonary pathology, 2nd edn, Dail DH, Hammar SP, Eds. 1994, Springer-Verlag, New York, pp 867–900.
2. Ingram P, Shelburne JD, Roggli VL, LeFurgey EA: Biomedical applications of microprobe analysis. 1999, Academic Press, San Diego.
3. Spencer H (Ed.): The pneumoconioses and other occupational lung diseases. In: Pathology of the lung, 4th edn, Vol. 1. 1985, Pergamon Press, Oxford, pp 413–510.
4. Churg A, Green FHY: Pathology of occupational lung disease, 2nd edn. 1998, Williams & Wilkins: Baltimore.
5. Craighead JE, Kleinerman J, Abraham JL, et al.: Diseases associated with exposure to silica and nonfibrous silicate minerals. Arch Pathol Lab Med 1988; 112: 673–720.
6. Zeren EH, Colby TV, Roggli VL: Silica-induced pleural disease: an unusual case mimicking mesothelioma. Chest 1997; 112: 1436–1438.
7. McDonald JW, Roggli VL: Detection of silica particles in lung tissue by polarizing light microscopy. Arch Pathol Lab Med 1995; 119: 242–246.
8. Cowie RL: The epidemiology of tuberculosis in gold miners with silicosis. Am J Respir Crit Care Med 1994; 150: 1460–1462.
9. Slavin RE, Swedo JL, Brandes D, Gonzalez-Vitale JC, Osornio-Vargas A: Extrapulmonary silicosis: a clinical, morphologic, and ultrastructural study. Hum Pathol 1985; 16: 393–412.
10. Vallyathan V, Brower PS, Green FHY, Attfield MD: Radiographic and pathologic correlation of coal workers' pneumoconiosis. Am J Respir Crit Care Med 1996; 154: 741–748.

11. Marine WM, Gurr D, Jacobsen M: Clinically important respiratory effects of dust exposure and smoking in British coal miners. Am Rev Respir Dis 1988; 137: 106–112.
12. Kleinerman J, Green FHY, Laquer W, et al.: Pathology standards for coal workers pneumoconiosis. Arch Pathol Lab Med 1979; 103: 375–432.
13. Pratt PC: Role of silica in progressive massive fibrosis in coal workers' pneumoconiosis. Arch Environ Health 1968; 16: 734–737.
14. Roggli VL: Asbestos bodies and non-asbestos ferruginous bodies. In: Pathology of asbestos-associated diseases, Roggli VL, Greenberg SD, Pratt PC, Eds. 1992, Little, Brown & Co., Boston, pp 39–75.
15. Hammar SP, Dodson RF: Asbestos. In: Pulmonary pathology, 2nd edn, Dail DH, Hammar SP, Eds. 1994, Springer-Verlag, New York, pp 901–983.
16. Roggli VL, Greenberg SD, Pratt PC, Eds: Pathology of asbestos-associated diseases. 1992, Little, Brown & Co., Boston.
17. Craighead JE, Abraham JL, Churg A, et al.: The pathology of asbestos-associated diseases of the lungs and pleural cavities: diagnostic criteria and proposed grading schema. Arch Pathol Lab Med 1982; 106: 544–596.
18. Roggli VL: Pathology of human asbestosis: a critical review. In: Advances in pathology, Vol. 2, Fenoglio-Preiser C, Ed. 1989, Year Book, Chicago, pp 31–60.
19. Roggli VL: The pneumoconioses: asbestosis. In: Pathology of pulmonary disease, Saldana MJ, Ed. 1994, Lippincott, Philadelphia, pp 395–410.
20. Churg A: Nonneoplastic disease caused by asbestos. In: Pathology of occupational lung disease, 2nd edn, Churg A, Green FHY, Eds. 1998, Williams & Wilkins, Baltimore, pp 277–338.
21. Roggli VL: Scanning electron microscopic analysis of mineral fiber content of lung tissue in the evaluation of diffuse pulmonary fibrosis. Scanning Microsc 1991; 5: 71–83.
22. Morgan WKC, Donner A, Higgins ITT, et al.: The effects of kaolin on the lung. Am Rev Respir Dis 1988; 138: 813–820.
23. Lapenas D, Gale P, Kennedy T, Rawlings W, Dietrich P: Kaolin pneumoconiosis: radiologic, pathologic, and mineralogic findings. Am Rev Respir Dis 1984; 130: 282–288.
24. Wagner JC, Pooley FD, Gibbs A, et al.: Inhalation of china stone and china clay dusts: relationship between the mineralogy of dust retained in the lungs and pathologic changes. Thorax 1986; 41: 190–196.
25. Landas SK, Schwartz DA: Mica-associated pulmonary interstitial fibrosis. Am Rev Respir Dis 1991; 144: 718–721.
26. Sherwin RP, Barman ML, Abraham JL: Silicate pneumoconiosis of farm workers. Lab Invest 1979; 40: 576–582.
27. Green FHY, Churg A: Diseases due to nonasbestos silicates. In: Pathology of occupational lung disease, 2nd edn, Churg A, Green FHY, Eds. 1998, Williams & Wilkins, Baltimore, pp 235–276.
28. Roub LW, Dekker A, Wagenblast HW, Reece GJ: Pulmonary silicatosis: A case diagnosed by needle-aspiration biopsy and energy-dispersive X-ray analysis. Am J Clin Pathol 72: 871–875, 1979.
29. Honma K, Abraham JL, Chiyotani K, et al.: Nikko criteria for mixed dust pneumoconiosis: definition, description and guidelines for pathological diagnosis and clinical correlation. J Pulmon Pathol (in press, 2004).
30. Vallyathan NV, Craighead JE: Pulmonary pathology in workers exposed to nonasbestiform talc. Hum Pathol 1981; 12: 28–35.
31. Crouch E, Churg A: Progressive massive fibrosis of the lung secondary to intravenous injection of talc: a pathologic and mineralogic analysis. Am J Clin Pathol 1983; 80: 520–526.
32. Pare JP, Cote G, Fraser RS: Long-term follow-up of drug abusers with intravenous talcosis. Am Rev Respir Dis 139: 233–241, 1989.
33. Bemer A, Gylseth B, Levy F: Talc dust pneumoconiosis. Acta Path Microbiol Scand A 1981; 89: 17–21.
34. Vallyathan NV: Talc pneumoconiosis. Respir Ther 1980; 10: 34–39.
35. Kennedy L, Sahn SA: Talc pleurodesis for the treatment of pneumothorax and pleural effusion. Chest 1994; 106: 1215–1222.
36. Miller A, Teirstein AS, Bader ME, Bader RA, Selikoff IJ: Talc pneumoconiosis: significance of sublight microscopic mineral particles. Am J Med 1971; 50: 395–402.
37. Sferlazza SJ, Beckett WS: The respiratory health of welders. Am Rev Respir Dis 1991; 143: 1134–1148.
38. Stern RM: The assessment of risk: application to the welding industry lung cancer. The International Institute of Welding Commission, VIII. Safety and Health Doc. IIW, VIII: 2034–2083. 1983, Danish Welding Institute: Copenhagen, pp 1–26.
39. Churg A, Colby TV: Diseases caused by metals and related compounds, In: Pathology of occupational lung disease, 2nd edn, Churg A, Green FHY, Eds. 1998, Williams & Wilkins, Baltimore, pp 77–128.
40. Roggli VL: Rare pneumoconioses: metalloconioses. In: Pathology of pulmonary disease, Saldana MJ, Ed. 1994, Lippincott, Philadelphia, pp 411–422.
41. Abramson MJ, Wlodarczyk JH, Saunders NA, Hensley MJ: Does aluminum smelting cause lung disease? Am Rev Respir Dis 1989; 139: 1042–1057.
42. Vallyathan V, Bergeron WN, Robichaux PA, Craighead JE: Pulmonary fibrosis in an aluminum arc welder. Chest 1982; 81: 372–374.
43. Jederlinic PJ, Abraham JL, Churg A, et al.: Pulmonary fibrosis in aluminum oxide workers: investigation of nine workers, with pathologic examination and microanalysis in three of them. Am Rev Respir Dis 1990; 142: 1179–1184.
44. Gilks B, Churg A: Aluminum-induced pulmonary fibrosis: Do fibers play a role? Am Rev Respir Dis 1987; 136: 176–179.
45. Chen W-J, Monnat RJ, Chen M, Moffet NK: Aluminum induced pulmonary granulomatosis. Hum Pathol 1978; 9: 705–711.
46. De Vuyst P, Dumortier P, Schandene L, et al.: Sarcoidlike lung granulomatosis induced by aluminum dusts. Am Rev Respir Dis 1987; 135: 493–497.
47. Herbert A, Sterling G, Abraham J, Corrin B: Desquamative interstitial pneumonia in an aluminum welder. Hum Pathol 1982; 13: 694–699.
48. Sprince NL, Oliver LC, Eisen EA, Greene RE, Chamberlin RI: Cobalt exposure and lung disease in tungsten carbide production: a cross-sectional study of current workers. Am Rev Respir Dis 1988; 138: 1220–1226.
49. Nemery B, Nagels J, Verbeken E, Dinsdale D, Demedts M: Rapidly fatal progression of cobalt lung in a diamond polisher. Am Rev Respir Dis 1990; 141: 1373–1378.
50. Nemery B, Casier P, Roosels D, Lahaye D, Demedts M: Survey of cobalt exposure and respiratory health in diamond polishers. Am Rev Respir Dis 1992; 145: 610–616.
51. Frost AE, Keller CA, Brown RW, et al.: Giant cell interstitial pneumonitis: disease recurrence in the transplanted lung. Am Rev Respir Dis 1993; 148: 1401–1404.
52. Ohori NP, Sciurba FC, Owens GR, Hodgson MJ, Yousem SA: Giant-cell interstitial pneumonia and hard-metal pneumoconiosis: a clinicopathologic study of four cases and review of the literature. Am J Surg Pathol 1989; 13: 581–587.
53. Stettler LE, Groth DH, Platek SF: Automated characterization of particles extracted from human lungs: three cases of tungsten carbide exposure. Scanning Electron Microscopy 1983; I: 439–448.
54. Tabatowski K, Roggli VL, Fulkerson WJ, et al.: Giant cell interstitial pneumonia in a hard-metal worker: cytologic, histologic and analytical electron microscopic investigation. Acta Cytolog 1988; 32: 240–246.
55. Meyer KC: Beryllium and lung disease. Chest 1994; 106: 942–946.
56. Kriebel D, Brain JD, Sprince NL, Kazemi H: The pulmonary toxicity of beryllium. Am Rev Respir Dis 1988; 137: 464–473.
57. Cullen MR, Kominsky JR, Rossman MD, et al.: Chronic beryllium disease in a precious metal refinery. Am Rev Respir Dis 1987; 135: 201–208.
58. Newman LS, Kreiss K, King TE, Seay S, Campbell PA: Pathologic and immunologic alterations in early stages of beryllium disease: re-examination of disease definition and natural history. Am Rev Respir Dis 1989; 139: 1479–1486.
59. Kotloff RM, Richman PS, Greenacre JK, Rossman MD: Chronic beryllium disease in a dental laboratory technician. Am Rev Respir Dis 1993; 147: 205–207.
60. Newman LS, Kreiss K: Nonoccupational beryllium disease masquerading as sarcoidosis: identification by blood lymphocyte proliferative response to beryllium. Am Rev Respir Dis 1992; 145: 1212–1214.
60a. Butnor KJ, Sporn TA, Ingram P, Gunasegarem S, Pinto JF, Roggli VL: Beryllium detection in human lung tissue using electron probe X-ray microanalysis. Mod Pathol 2003; 16: 1171–1177
61. McDonald JW, Ghio AJ, Sheehan CE, Bernhardt PF, Roggli VL: Rare earth (cerium oxide) pneumoconiosis: analytical scanning electron microscopy and literature review. Mod Pathol 1995; 8: 859–865.
62. Waring PM, Wating RJ: Rare earth deposits in a deceased movie projectionist: a new case of rare earth pneumoconiosis? Med J Aust 1990; 153: 726–730.
63. Sulotto F, Romano C, Berra A, et al.: Rare earth pneumoconiosis: a new case. Am J Ind Med 1986; 9: 567–575.
64. Husain MH, Dick JA, Kaplan YS: Rare earth pneumoconiosis. J Soc Occup Med 1980; 30: 15–19.

10

Pulmonary vasculitis and pulmonary hemorrhage

William D Travis   Kevin O Leslie

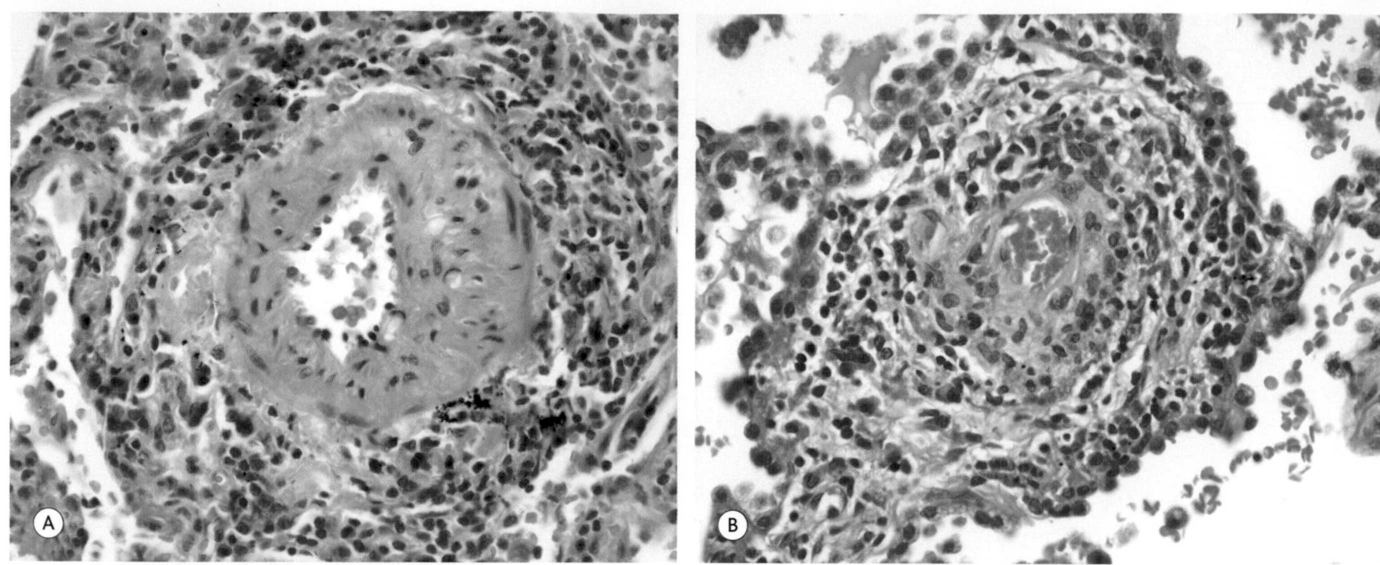

Fig. 10.1 **Vascular inflammation versus vasculitis.** A comparison of (A) vessel-associated inflammation and (B) true vasculitis. Note the disruption of the media by inflammatory cells in true vasculitis.

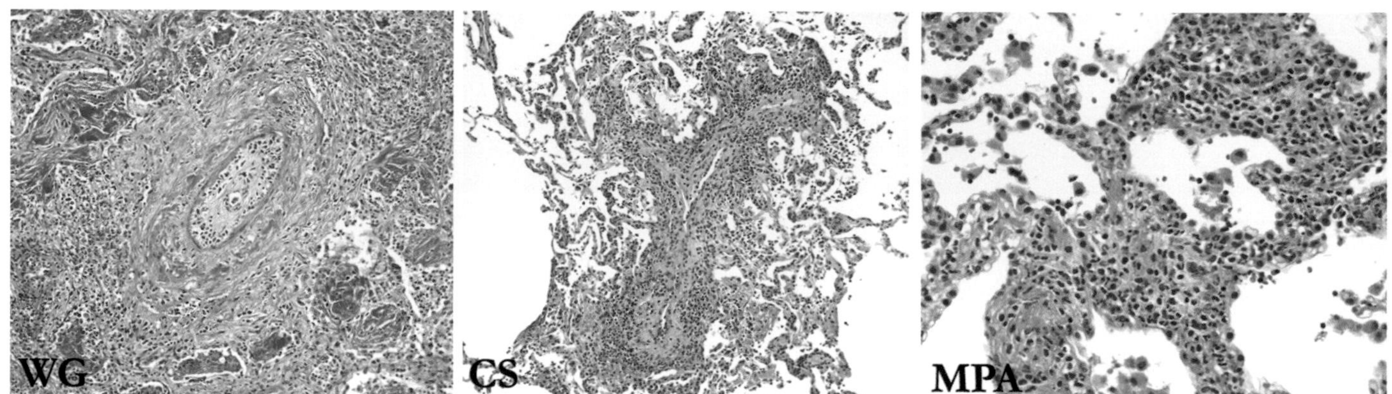

Fig. 10.2 **Common histopathologic manifestations of pulmonary vasculitis.** Three of the most common manifestations of pulmonary vasculitis: Wegener's granulomatosis (WG), Churg–Strauss syndrome (CS), and microscopic polyangiitis (MPA).

I. Pulmonary vasculitis

Inflammation of arteries and veins can occur in many inflammatory lung diseases, including infections. By convention, the diagnostic term "pulmonary vasculitis" is restricted to a relatively limited number of diseases in which vascular inflammation is felt to be the primary pathology. Most pulmonary vasculitides are felt to be immune-mediated diseases, although their etiology and pathogenesis remain unknown. By best estimates, the overall annual incidence of the major forms of vasculitis is 39 per million.[1]

When pulmonary vasculitis occurs, there is damage to the vessel wall, often accompanied by fibrin and sometimes, necrosis. Cuffing of blood vessels by inflammatory cells, a nonspecific finding, must be distinguished from infiltration of inflammatory cells into the media and intima of arteries and veins (Fig. 10.1).

A diagnosis of pulmonary vasculitis carries a strong implication for immediate therapeutic intervention (typically immunosuppression) and, as such, should never be made lightly. Furthermore, serologic data and clinical correlation with the pathologic findings is essential for a correct diagnosis. Typical examples of pulmonary vasculitis/capillaritis are shown in Fig. 10.2.

The general category of pulmonary vasculitis includes a number of different diseases that can be more easily understood by dividing them into three main groups (Table 10.1):

1. idiopathic vasculitic syndromes that commonly involve the lung (e.g. Wegener's granulomatosis),

Table 10.1 Pulmonary vasculitis syndromes

I. IDIOPATHIC VASCULITIS SYNDROMES WHICH COMMONLY AFFECT THE LUNG
Wegener's granulomatosis
Churg–Strauss angiitis and granulomatosis
Microscopic polyangiitis
II. IDIOPATHIC VASCULITIS SYNDROMES WHICH UNCOMMONLY AFFECT THE LUNG
Necrotizing sarcoid granulomatosis
Polyarteritis nodosa
Small vessel vasculitis
Takayasu's arteritis
Henoch–Shönlein purpura
Behçet's syndrome
Cryoglobulinemic vasculitis
Hypocomplementemic vasculitis
Idiopathic granulomatous arteritis
– Giant cell arteritis
– Disseminated visceral giant-cell angiitis
III. MISCELLANEOUS SYSTEMIC DISORDERS
Classical sarcoid
Collagen vascular disease
Inflammatory bowel disease
Malignancy
IV. DIFFUSE PULMONARY HEMORRHAGE SYNDROMES
V. SECONDARY OR LOCALIZED VASCULITIS
Pulmonary infection
Bronchocentric granulomatosis
Pulmonary hypertension
Interstitial lung diseases
– Chronic eosinophilic pneumonia
– Histiocytosis X
Inflammatory pseudotumors and pseudolymphomas
Sequestration
Embolic material (intravenous drug abuse)
Drug or toxic substances
Transplantation
Radiation
VI. VASCULAR INVOLVEMENT IN LYMPHOPROLIFERATIVE DISORDERS
Angiocentric immunoproliferative lesion (lymphomatoid granulomatosis)
Non-Hodgkin's lymphoma
Intravascular malignant lymphoma

Source: modified from Travis et al.[2]

2. vasculitic disorders that rarely involve the lung (a much larger number), and
3. miscellaneous conditions that produce pulmonary vascular inflammation.[2]

Wegener's granulomatosis (WG), Churg–Strauss syndrome (CSS), and microscopic polyangiitis (MPA) are the idiopathic vasculitis syndromes that commonly affect the lung, and these will be the primary focus here. The conditions of bronchocentric granulomatosis (BCG) and lymphomatoid granulomatosis traditionally have been grouped in the category of pulmonary "angiitis and granulomatosis"; however, neither of these entities is currently thought to be a vasculitic condition. BCG is a morphologic pattern of airway inflammation that occurs in a variety of conditions, especially infection, and lymphomatoid granulomatosis (also known as angiocentric immunoproliferative disorder), is now known to represent a lymphoproliferative disease in which prominent vascular involvement occurs.[3,4]

Idiopathic vasculitis syndromes that rarely affect the lung include such diseases as necrotizing sarcoid granulomatosis, Takayasu's arteritis, giant cell arteritis, and Behcet's syndrome. Necrotizing sarcoid granulomatosis (NSG) was formerly regarded as one of the major vasculitic syndromes but it is very rare and does not typically cause a systemic vasculitis, so it is now grouped under the syndromes that uncommonly affect the lung. Pulmonary vascular inflammation also occurs in a number of miscellaneous systemic disorders, in diffuse pulmonary hemorrhage syndromes (discussed later), and in a variety of secondary or localized forms.

It should come as no surprise that vasculitic syndromes pose major challenges to the surgical pathologist. First, like many non-neoplastic lung diseases, the diagnosis does not rest on pathology alone. Correlation between clinical, radiologic, and pathologic features is required for most of these entities. Secondly, because these are rare disorders, few pathologists have much experience with their diagnostic subtleties. Thirdly, the pathologic features of these infrequently encountered conditions overlap with common inflammatory lesions such as necrotizing infectious granulomas produced by mycobacteria or fungi. Since most vasculitis syndromes are treated with immunosuppressive agents, separation from infectious conditions is essential. Finally, in many cases, the histopathologic findings may not be "classical", thereby requiring the recognition of subtle clues in order to suspect the diagnosis.

Wegener's granulomatosis

Wegener's granulomatosis (WG) is a rare systemic inflammatory disease of unknown etiology that has vasculitis as a major manifestation. WG predominantly affects the upper and lower respiratory tract, and the kidneys.[5] Despite the term "granulomatosis", well-defined granulomas without necrosis (sarcoid-like) are not a feature of this disease. The necrotizing lesions of WG have a peripheral zone of palisaded histiocytes, contrasting with the more epithelioid histiocytes seen at the periphery

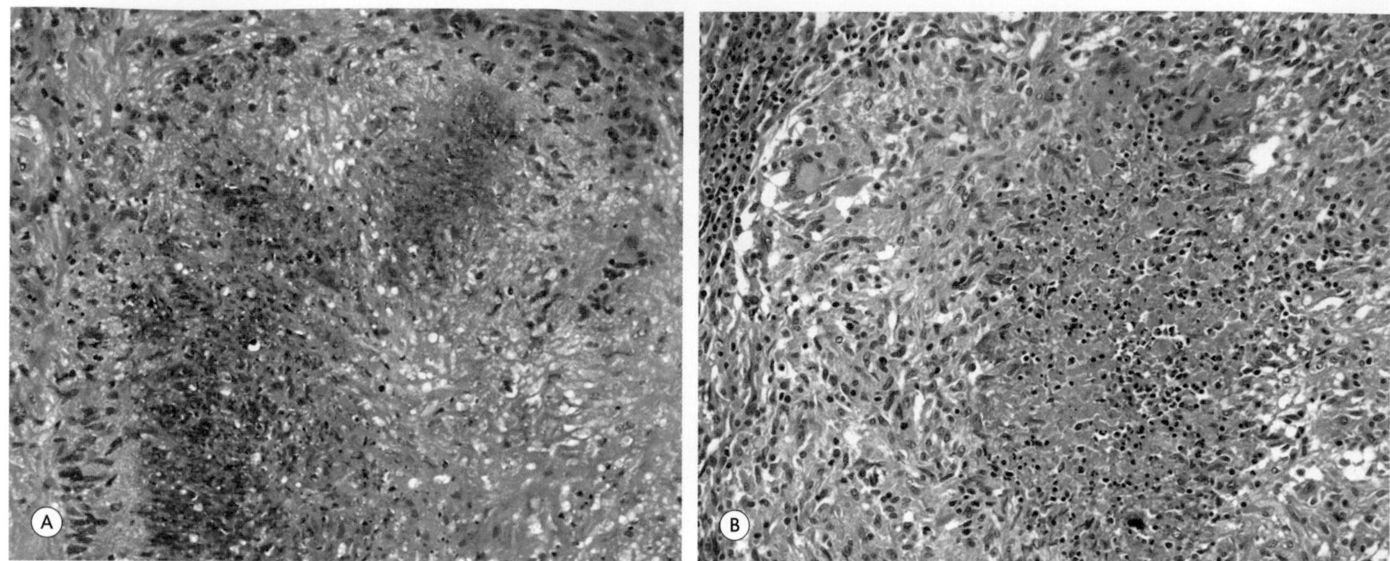

Fig. 10.3 **The granulomas of Wegener's granulomatosis (WG).** WG granulomas (A) tend to be more "pallisaded" than those seen in (B) granulomatous infection. Also note the blue (basophilic) appearance of the necrosis of WG, compared to the pink (eosinophilic) necrosis of infection.

of necrosis produced by mycobacteria or fungi (Fig. 10.3). In fact, when well-formed (sarcoid-like) granulomas without necrosis are present in a potential case of WG, another diagnosis should be considered (usually infection).

Clinical features

WG affects about 1 in every 3 million people in the United States[6] and 1 in 8.5 million people in the United Kingdom.[7] There is debate as to whether WG occurs more frequently during cold seasons, with some studies suggesting an increased occurrence in winter months.[7] Other studies have disputed these results.[6] In addition, an association between WG and infections remains unsubstantiated.[8]

WG occurs at any age, but typically it is a disease of adults, with a mean age of 50 years.[9–11] A list of the clinical manifestations of WG is presented in Table 10.2. Body sites most commonly affected are the head and neck region, followed by the lung, kidney, and eye.[9,12] Patients may experience a number of other complaints such as hoarseness, stridor, earache, hearing loss, otorrhea, cough, dyspnea, hemoptysis, or pleuritic pain. Pulmonary symptoms in the absence of upper respiratory tract manifestations are unusual. Destructive inflammation of the nose may result in a saddle nose deformity. In addition, patients may have more generalized systemic signs and symptoms, including arthralgias, fever, cutaneous lesions, weight loss, and peripheral neuropathy.[13] Rarely, WG may involve the salivary glands, pancreas, breast, mediastinum, gastrointestinal tract, prostate and urethra, vagina and cervix, heart, spleen, and peripheral or central nervous system.[14,15]

The most frequent abnormality on pulmonary function testing is airflow obstruction, often associated with a reduced diffusing capacity for carbon monoxide (DLCo), but restrictive or mixed patterns can occur. When significant airflow obstruction is identified, patients may be at risk for tracheal obstruction or lobar collapse by bronchial wall damage resulting from the disease.

Laboratory studies

Nonspecific abnormalities of general laboratory tests are often present in patients with WG. The most common of these include leukocytosis, thrombocytosis (>400,000/mm^3), marked elevation of the erythrocyte sedimentation rate (ESR), and normochromic, normocytic anemia. In the past decade, the diagnosis of WG has been dramatically aided by the discovery and use of the serum antineutrophil cytoplasmic antibodies (ANCA).[16–20]

Two major immunofluorescence patterns occur as expressions of ANCA (Fig. 10.4): the cytoplasmic or classical type (C-ANCA) and the perinuclear type (P-ANCA).[21] The C-ANCA pattern is associated with WG and is present in the vast majority of patients with active generalized disease. Partial or complete remission of disease is reflected in a lower frequency of a positive test, but 30–40% of patients in complete remission still have identifiable antibodies.[22] The P-ANCA pattern can be seen in a small percentage of patients with WG, but it is more characteristic of idiopathic necrotizing and crescentic

Table 10.2 Clinical manifestations of Wegener's granulomatosis

Manifestation	At presentation (%)	During course of disease (%)
Head & neck manifestations:	73	92
Sinusitis	51	85
Nasal Disease	36	68
Otitis Media	25	44
Hearing loss	14	42
Subglottic stenosis	8	16
Ear pain	1	14
Oral lesions	3	10
Pulmonary manifestations:	45	85
Infiltrates	23	66
Nodule	22	59
Cough	19	46
Hemoptysis	12	30
Infiltrates	10	28
Renal manifestations	18	77
Eye manifestations:	15	52
Conjunctivitis	5	18
Dacryocystitis	1	18
Scleritis	6	16
Proptosis	2	15
Eye pain	3	11
Visual loss	0	8
Retinal lesions	0	4
Corneal ulcers	0	1
Iritis	0	2
Systemic manifestations:		
Joints	32	67
Fever	23	50
Skin	13	46
Weight loss	15	35
Peripheral nervous system	1	15
Central nervous system	1	8
Pericarditis	2	6

Source: Hoffman et al.[9]

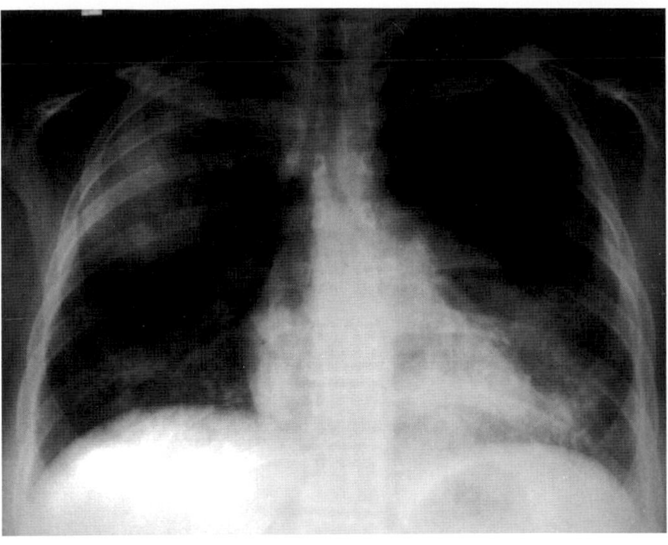

Fig. 10.5 **Wegener's granulomatosis chest radiographs.** PA chest radiograph in a patient with WG. Note the multifocal nodules, some of which appeared to cavitated. (Reprinted from Travis,[2] with permission.)

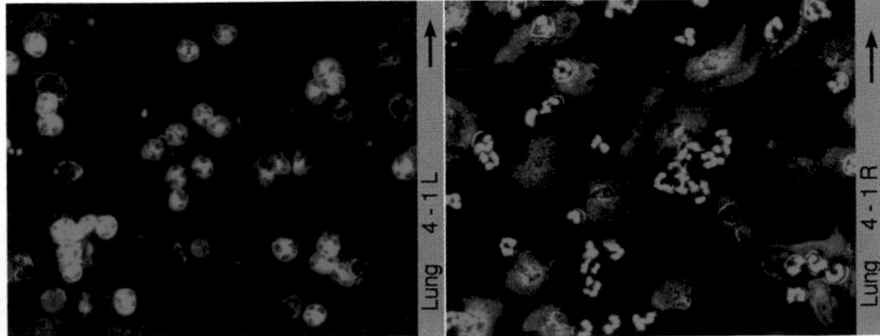

Fig. 10.4 **Antineutrophilic cytoplasmic antibody (ANCA) immunofluorescence.** Left panel: cytoplasmic staining of neutrophils characterizes the C-ANCA pattern. Right panel: perinuclear accentuation of staining is seen with the P-ANCA pattern. (Reprinted from Travis,[2] with permission.)

glomerulonephritis, MPA, polyarteritis nodosa (PAN), and CSS.[23]

The ANCA immunofluorescence patterns have been shown to correspond to specific antigen immunoreactivities: C-ANCA typically has specificity for proteinase 3, whereas most P-ANCAs have a specificity for myeloperoxidase. Recent studies have shown no significant difference in the lung biopsy findings from WG patients with C-ANCAs versus those with P-ANCAs.[24,25] Levels of C-ANCA in the bronchoalveolar lavage have not been shown to be a more specific predictor of WG or of the level of disease.[26] Importantly, the presence or absence of a positive serum test for C-ANCA alone is not sufficiently specific to make or exclude the diagnosis of WG.[27]

Radiologic features

Most patients with pulmonary disease have multiple opacities (Figs 10.5 and 10.6) in the form of well-marginated nodules or masses of varying size (0.5–10 cm). Lesions may wax and wane over time. Most occur in the lower lobes.[28–30] Poorly defined or even spiculated nodules may also be seen.[31] Cavitation of nodules occurs in 25 to 50% of cases, with cavity walls typically being thick and irregular. Such lesions may evolve into thin-walled cysts or disappear completely with therapy.[30,32] WG is often included in the differential diagnosis of interstitial lung disease because multifocal, ill-defined parenchymal consolidations can occur (with or without cavitation) and diffuse reticular and nodular interstitial opacities have also been reported.[30,33]

Patients with WG may present initially with pulmonary hemorrhage. In this setting, diffuse infiltrates on chest radiographs, and diffuse airspace opacities on computed tomograms are observed (Fig. 10.6). Pulmonary hemorrhage is a common presentation of WG in children, whereas pulmonary nodules occur less frequently in pediatric patients.[11]

Pleural effusion accompanies WG in 20–50% of cases, sometimes with focal pleural thickening. Hilar and/or mediastinal lymphadenopathy are unusual findings in WG, and, when significant, should raise concern for an alternate diagnosis. On rare occasions, WG occurs as a solitary pulmonary nodule (with or without cavitation), or as an isolated area of consolidation.[34]

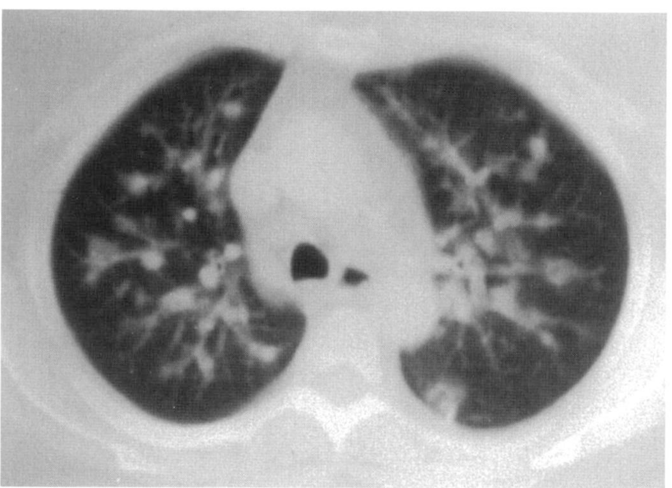

Fig. 10.6 **Wegener's granulomatosis: chest CT.** Chest CT (lung window) demonstrates multifocal, ill-defined small nodular opacities in close relationship to pulmonary arteries. Note the thick walls of these well-marginated lesions. (Reprinted from Travis,[2] with permission.)

Computed tomography (CT) provides optimal visualization of the number, location, and morphologic characteristics of the pulmonary abnormalities in WG. Well-marginated nodules and masses are typical findings, sometimes with spiculated borders. A "feeding" vessel is seen in 88% of nodules (Fig. 10.6), consistent with the angiocentric nature of this disorder.[35] Cavitation is identified in 50% of cases. Another very common finding in WG are wedge-shaped peripheral opacities mimicking the CT appearance of infarct. Other less common radiologic presentations include air bronchograms and the CT halo sign (ground glass opacity surrounding a pulmonary nodule or mass).[35,36] Stenosis of the trachea or large airways may occur in short or long segments and may be complicated by partial or complete lobar collapse.[33,37,38]

Pathologic features

WG is characterized by the presence of multiple bilateral pulmonary nodules, often with cavitation (Figs 10.6 and 10.7).[39] Solid nodular zones of consolidation with areas of punctate or geographic necrosis are typical findings (Fig. 10-7). WG can rarely present with a solitary lung lesion, but solitary granulomatous disease is always more likely to be of infectious origin.[40] When dealing with a solitary granulomatous lung nodule, a combination of both the classical histology and typical clinical/serologic findings of WG should be present before making a diagnosis.[34] Even when special stains for organisms and cultures are negative, most of these solitary lesions represent old fungal or mycobacterial infection. Rarely the lesions of WG may be centered on bronchi. When acute lung hemorrhage is prominent, the cut surface of the lung is bloody and dark red.

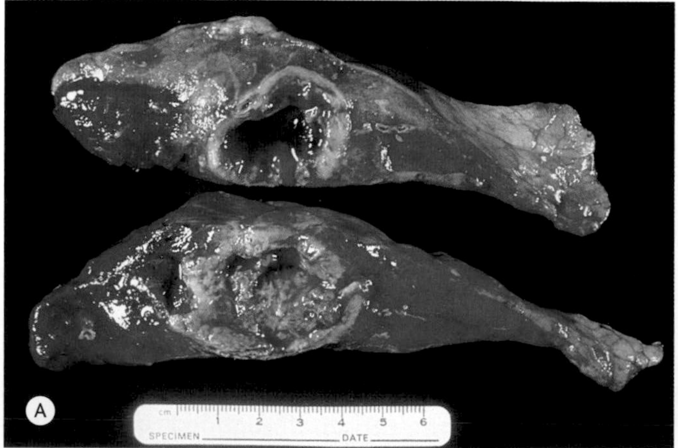

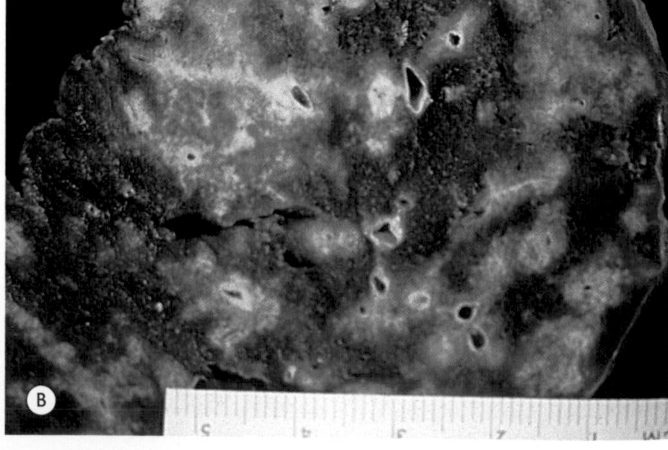

Fig. 10.7 **Wegener's granulomatosis: gross specimen.** Left, this necrotizing granuloma is cavitated with a necrotic center and an inflammatory border. Right: multiple scattered nodular foci of consolidation are present. Yellow-white areas represent necrosis. (Reprinted from Travis,[2] with permission.)

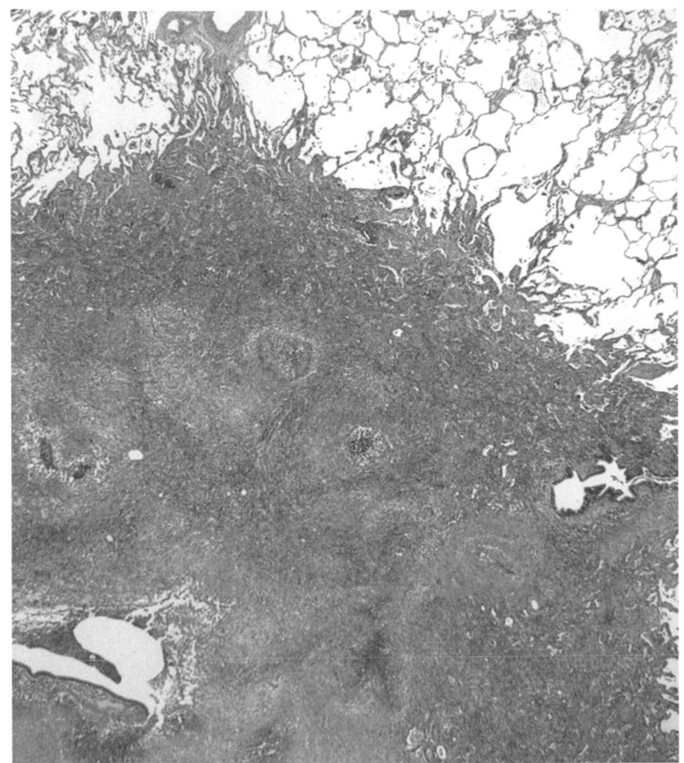

Fig. 10.8 **Wegener's granulomatosis: nodular lesions.** A nodular lesion of WG seen at scanning magnification shows the thick inflammatory wall surrounding irregular zones of basophilic necrosis. Note the airways and arteries visible within the lesion.

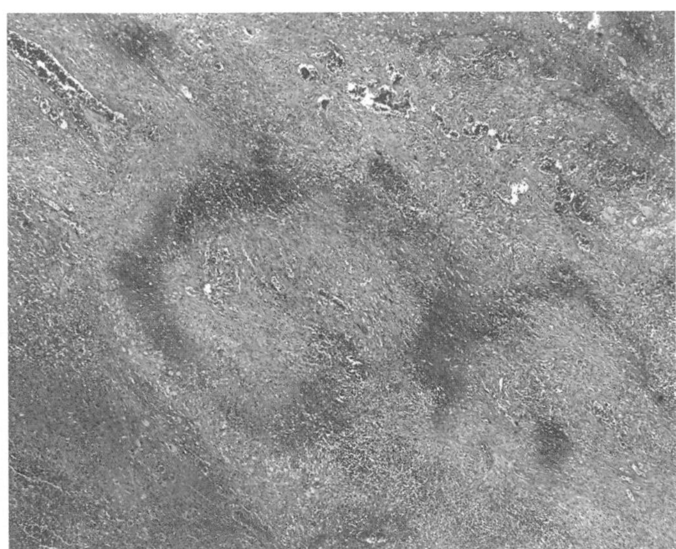

Fig. 10.9 **Wegener's granulomatosis: geographic necrosis.** The "geographic" basophilic necrosis of Wegener's granulomatosis can be appreciated at scanning magnification.

At scanning magnification, the pulmonary lesions of WG simulate their radiologic appearance (Fig. 10.8). The classical findings consist of nodular areas of consolidation with variable zones of necrosis. Major diagnostic criteria,

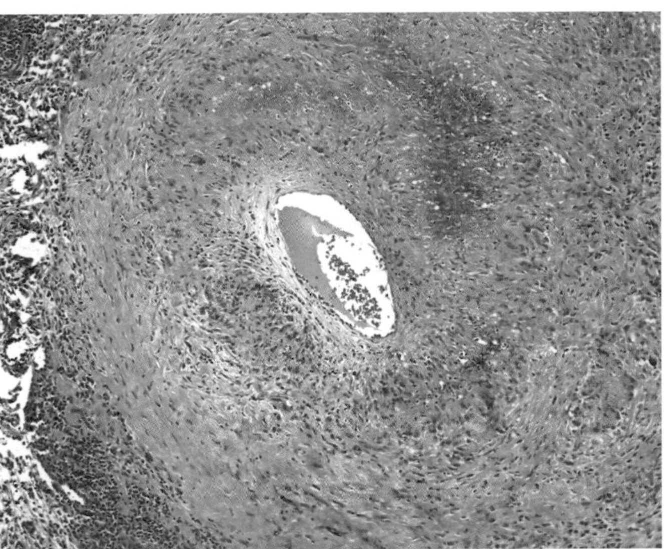

Fig. 10.10 **Wegener's granulomatosis vasculitis.** The vasculitis of Wegener's granulomatosis is characterized by necrotizing granulomas involving adventitia and media. This narrowed vessel shows palisaded granulomas with basophilic necrosis accompanied by inflammation and fibrosis of the adventitia.

presented in Table 10.3, include parenchymal necrosis (Fig. 10.9), vasculitis (Fig. 10.10), and granulomatous inflammation (Fig. 10.11). The accompanying inflammatory infiltrate is composed of neutrophils, lymphocytes, plasma cells, macrophages, giant cells, and eosinophils (Fig. 10.12). Parenchymal necrosis can take the form of neutrophilic microabscesses (Fig. 10.13) and/or large zones of geographic necrosis (see Fig. 10.9). The neutrophilic microabsceses seen in collagen are nearly pathognomonic of the disease and are best searched for in the adventitial collagen of larger arteries and veins, and also in the pleura overlying parenchymal disease. The smallest of these may be nothing more than a small collection of neutrophils surrounding a focus of degenerated, often hypereosinophilic, collagen.[39]

As illustrated in Fig. 10.9, the classical geographic necrosis of WG is typically basophilic, owing to the presence of numerous necrotic neutrophils. The necrotic centers of WG lesions often lack the "ghosted" image of lung structure, a diagnostic clue useful in the case with atypical features (Fig. 10.14). This probably occurs because the necrotic zones of WG are generally not the result of "infarct-like" zonal parenchymal necrosis, but rather occur by progressive expansion of collagen necrosis.

The "granulomatous" inflammation of WG typically includes giant cells scattered randomly or in loose aggregates (Fig.10.15). Also commonly observed are palisaded histiocytes (Fig. 10-16), giant cells lining the border of geographic necrosis or microabscesses, and

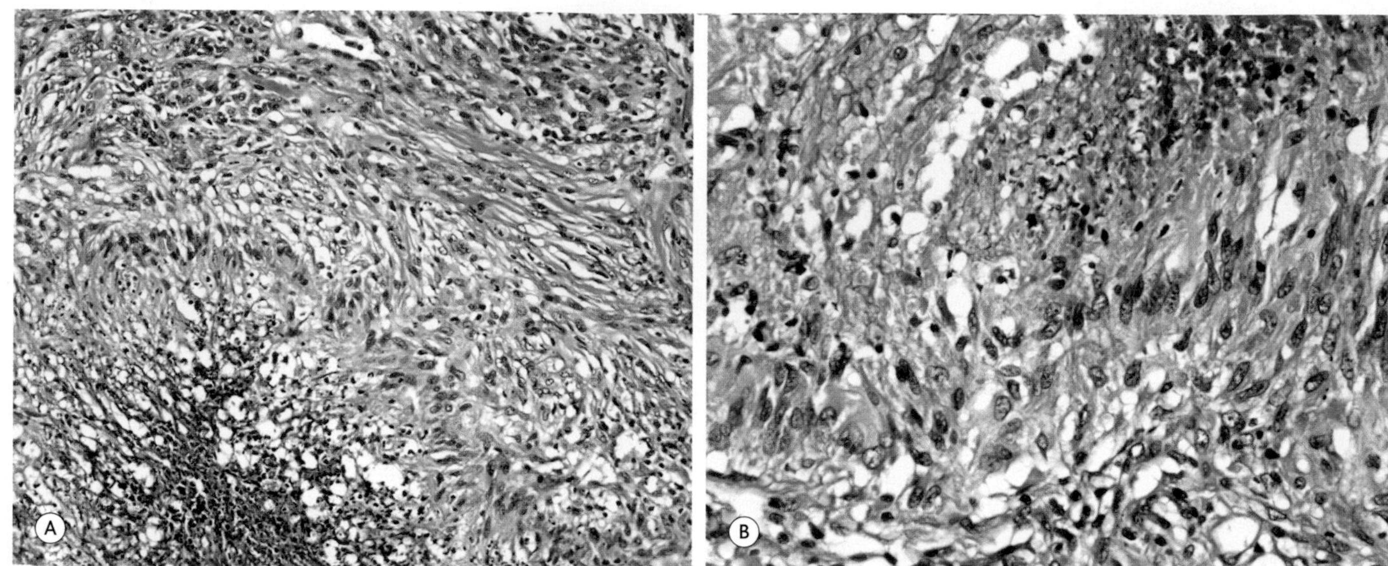

Fig. 10.11 **Wegener's granulomatosis: granulomatous inflammation.** (A) The granulomatous inflammation of WG generally has a palisaded configuration. (B) A closer view of palisaded histiocytes can be seen, bordering basophilic necrosis with nuclear debris.

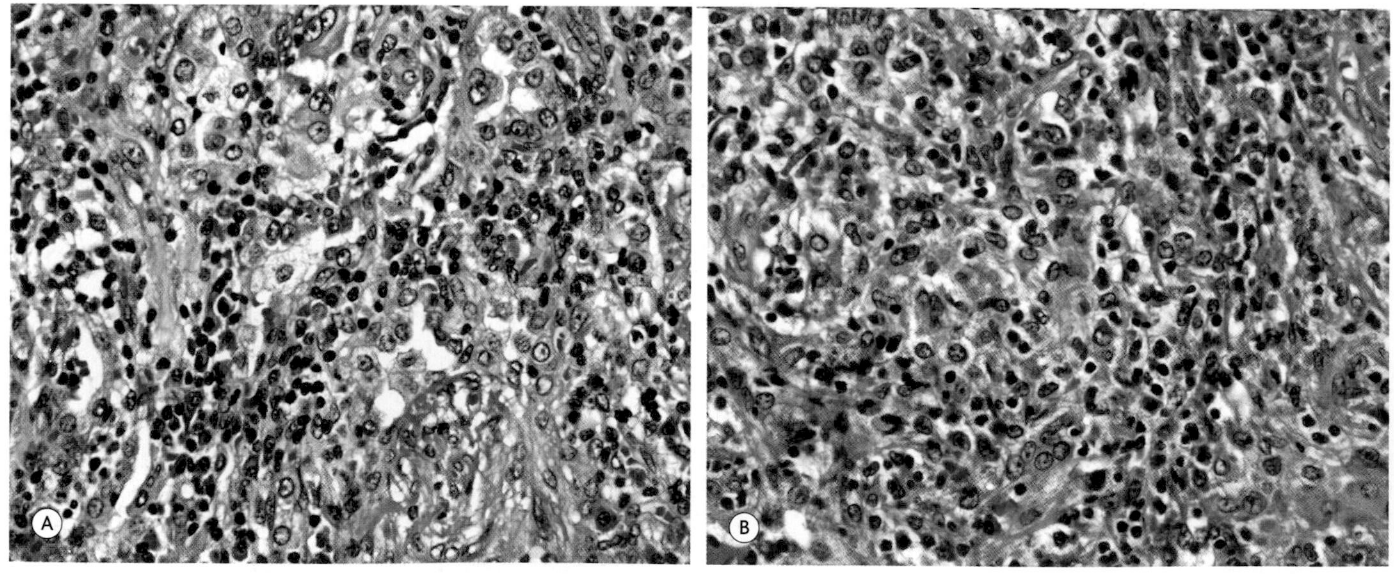

Fig. 10.12 **Wegener's granulomatosis-associated inflammation.** Inflammatory infiltrate of WG is generally mixed with (A) plasma cells, lymphocytes and (B) varying numbers of eosinophils.

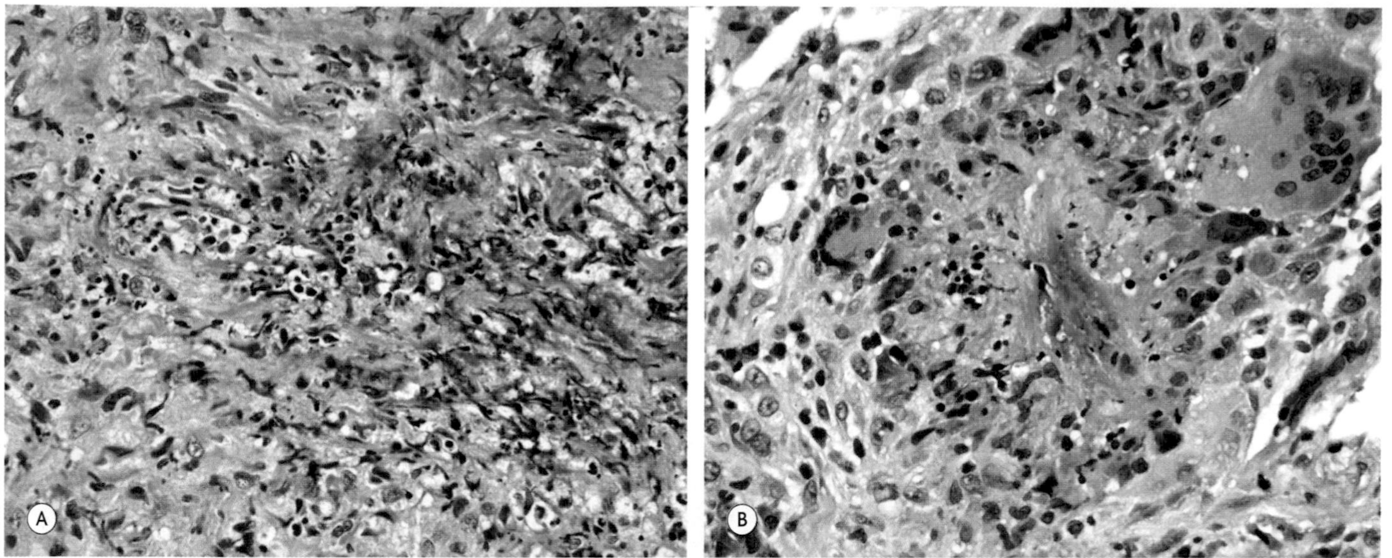

Fig. 10.13 **Wegener's granulomatosis: collagen necrosis.** Collagen necrosis is felt to be the primary pathologic event in WG. Zones of collagen necrosis can be (A) vague or discreet and (B) associated with giant cells and granulomatosis inflammation.

Table 10.3 Wegener's granulomatosis: major pathologic manifestations (diagnostic criteria)

I. VASCULITIS
   A. Arteritis, venulitis, capillaritis[a]
   B. Six types: acute, chronic, necrotizing granulomatous, non-necrotizing granulomatous, fibrinoid necrosis, cicatricial changes[b]

II. PARENCHYMAL NECROSIS
   A. Microabscess
   B. Geographic necrosis

III. GRANULOMATOUS INFLAMMATION (& MIXED INFLAMMATORY INFILTRATE)
   A. Microabscess surrounded by granulomatous inflammation
   B. Palisading histiocytes
   C. Scattered giant cells
   D. Poorly formed granulomas
   E. Sarcoid-like granulomas (rare)

Source: Travis et al.[2,39]
[a]Capillaritis was characterized primarily by acute inflammation. Veins and arteries demonstrated all the types of inflammation listed in IB.
[b]Cicatricial vascular changes are nonspecific and should not be used as a diagnostic criterion.

micrograngulomas consisting of small foci of palisaded histiocytes arranged in a cartwheel pattern, around a central nidus of necrosis[39](see Fig. 10.13). The presence of tightly cohesive, sarcoid-like granulomas is very rare in WG, and should suggest infection or necrotizing sarcoid. Also, the presence of granulomas without associated necrosis is a finding more in favor of an infectious etiology than WG.

The vasculitis of WG typically affects small arteries and veins with diameters up to 5 mm. When vasculitis is seen in the surgical biopsy, it most often occurs within the dense inflammatory infiltrate surrounding nodular or geographic areas of necrosis (Fig. 10.17). Vasculitis in WG may comprise a variety of inflammatory cells, including acute or chronic mural inflammation, necrotizing stellate granulomas, non-necrotizing stellate granulomas, and giant cells.[39] Cicatricial changes, consisting of mural fibrosis or luminal obliteration, may be seen in specimens following therapy. Destruction of the vascular elastic laminae is commonly observed (Fig. 10.18). Sometimes the inflammation is limited to the endothelium (endotheliolitis) and subendothelial aspect of the vessel wall. Despite these potential vascular changes, if necrotizing vasculitis is held as a requirement for the diagnosis, many cases of WG will be missed.

As mentioned, all types of inflammatory cells may occur in WG, including neutrophils, lymphocytes, plasma cells, eosinophils, histiocytes, and giant cells. Occasionally

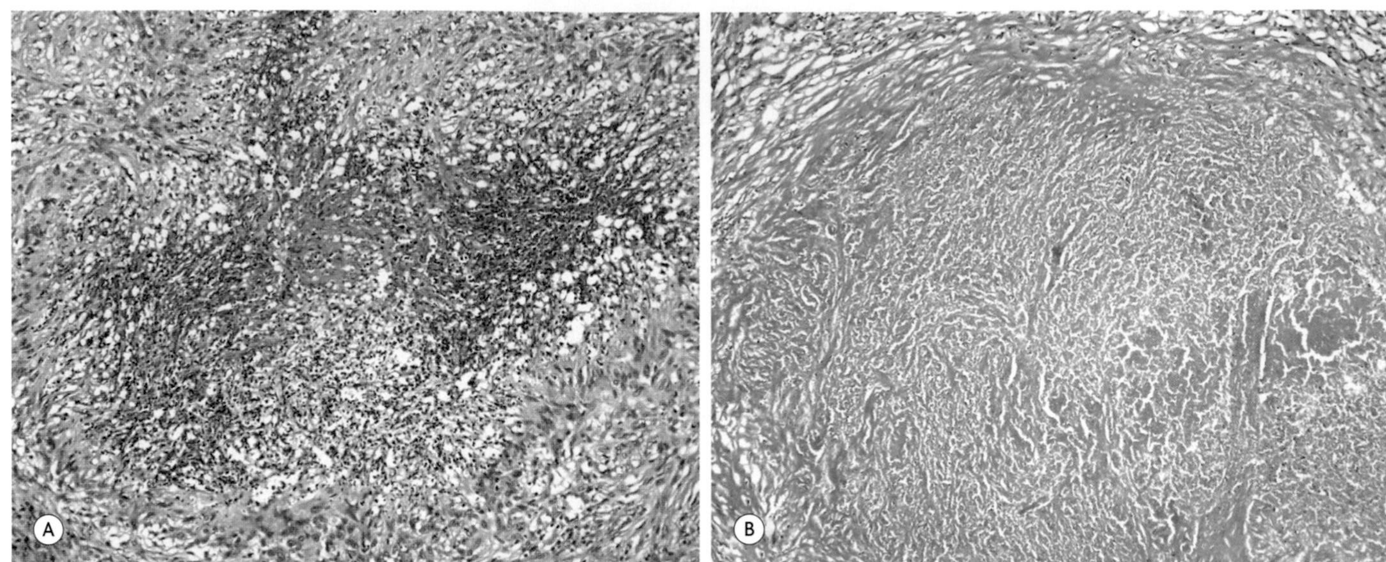

Fig. 10.14 **Wegener's granulomatosis: basophilic necrosis.** (A) The necrosis of WG is basophilic, owing to an abundance of nuclear debris. In necrotizing granulomatous infection (B) the necrosis typically has an eosinophilic appearance with some preservation of structure in areas of necrosis (this background structure visible within necrosis is often absent in WG).

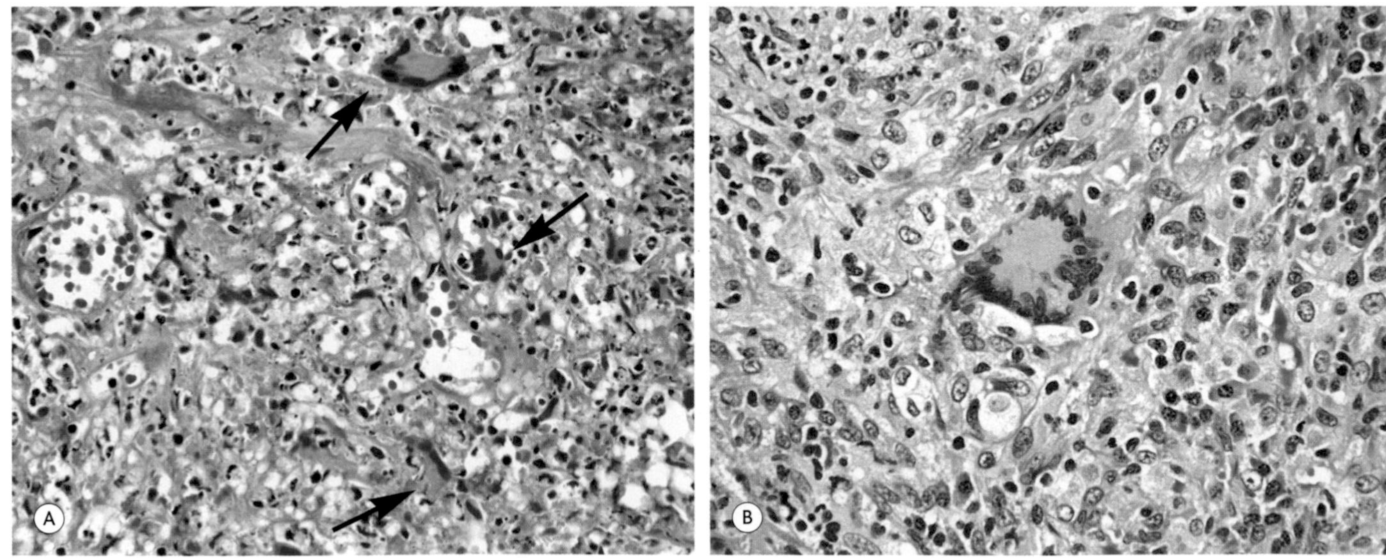

Fig. 10.15 **Wegener's granulomatosis: giant cells.** The giant cells of WG have smudged basophilic nuclei, often marginated at the periphery of the cell (A, arrows). A typical multinucleated giant cell of WG is seen in (B) at the periphery of necrosis (upper left).

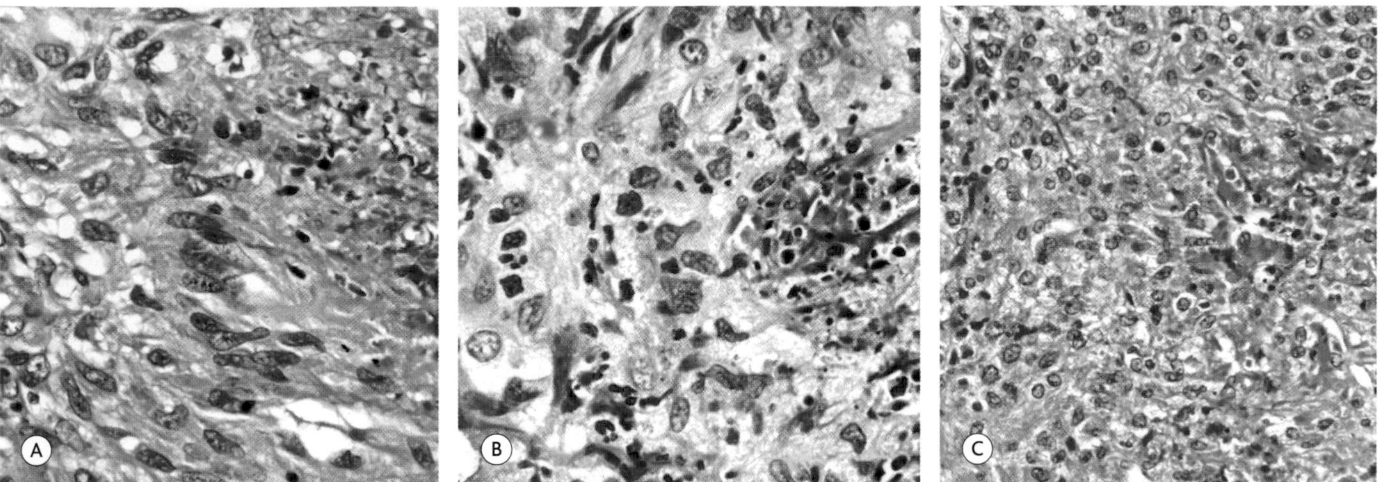

Fig. 10.16 **Wegener's granulomatosis: types of granulomatous inflammation.** Three examples of the "granulomatous" inflammation at the periphery of necrosis in Wegener's granulomatosis. (A) Palisaded histiocytes, (B) epithelioid histiocytes with little organization, (C) plump eosinophilic histiocytes.

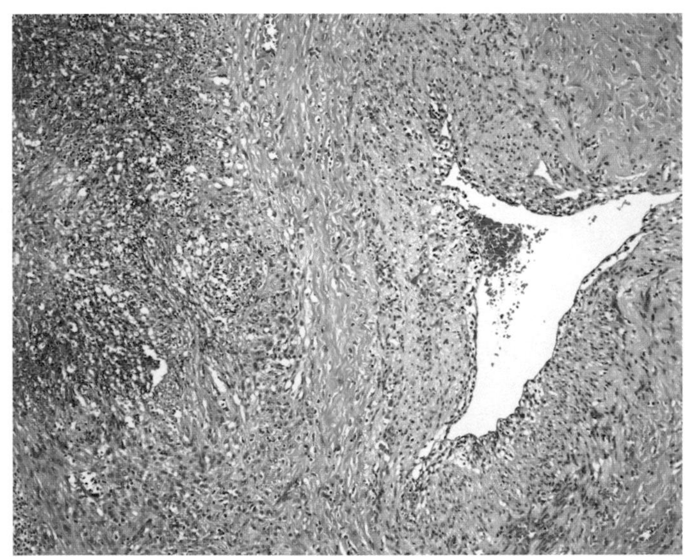

Fig. 10.17 **Wegener's granulomatosis: vasculitis.** Vasculitis at the edge of basophilic necrosis. Note, the adventitial fibrosis and expansion of the vascular media by inflammatory cells. Multinucleated giant cells can be seen at the interface of muscularis and adventitia, focally (lower right).

the inflammatory infiltrate consists mostly of lymphoid cells, but this is unusual. In such cases, distinction of WG from lymphomatoid granulomatosis may be difficult.

Another distinctive vascular manifestation of WG is capillaritis (Fig. 10.19). In many cases, capillaritis is only focally evident in the biopsy.[39] When capillaritis is prominent, it is distinctive and easily recognized. In the rare case of WG dominated by capillaritis, a careful search throughout the rest of the biopsy should be made for more typical findings of WG such as granulomas, foci of necrosis (such as neutrophilic microabscesses), multinucleated giant cells, and vasculitis affecting arterioles or veins.

In addition to these major histologic features, a variety of minor histologic features may be encountered (Table 10.4), including alveolar hemorrhage, interstitial fibrosis, lipoid pneumonia, organizing pneumonia, lymphoid hyperplasia, extravascular tissue eosinophils, and xanthomatous lesions. WG can also involve the airways, causing chronic bronchiolitis, acute bronchiolitis/bronchopneumonia, the histologic pattern of organizing pneumonia (see below), bronchocentric granulomatosis, follicular bronchiolitis, and bronchial stenosis.[39,41] Occasionally one of these minor lesions may be the dominant lung biopsy finding.[39] Diffuse pulmonary hemorrhage is a severe life-threatening manifestation of WG. The pattern of bronchocentric granulomatosis is another rare manifestation of WG encountered in 1% of cases.[39,41] Organizing pneumonia (Fig. 10.20) can be seen in 70% of lung biopsies from patients with WG[39] and rarely it may be sufficiently dominant that some have referred to this manifestation as the "bronchiolitis obliterans organizing pneumonia" or "BOOP" variant of WG.[39,42] This should not be confused with the idiopathic entity of BOOP (cryptogenic organizing pneumonia), but recognized as nonspecific secondary organization following alveolar injury related to the underlying lesions of WG.

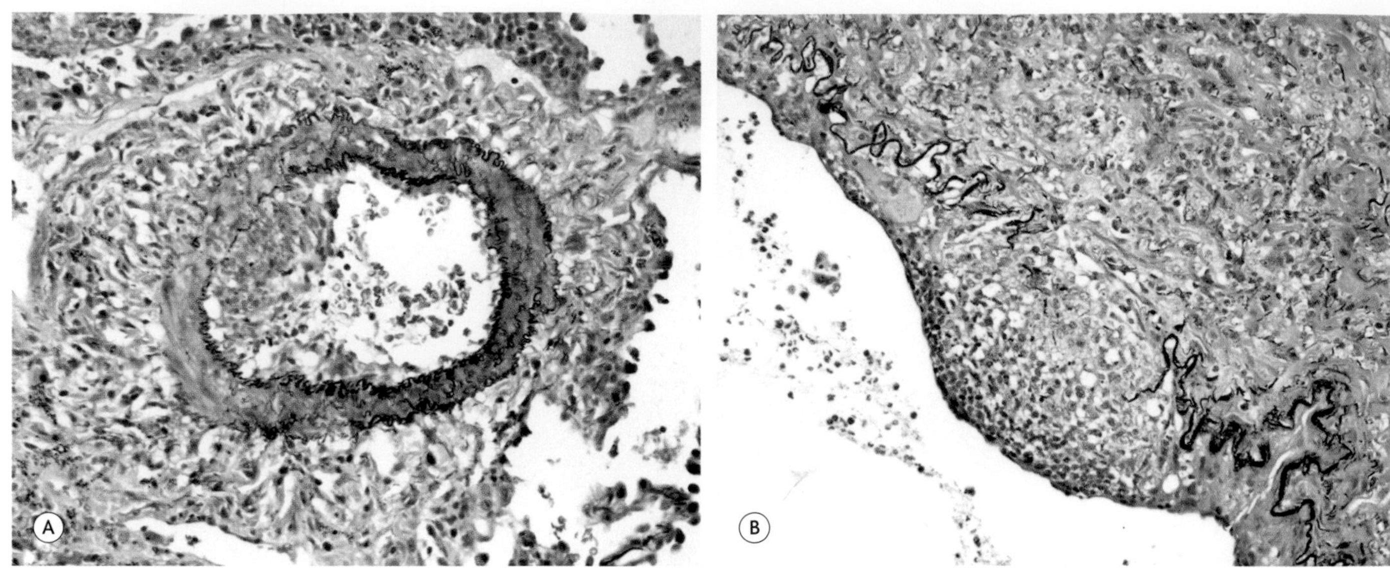

Fig. 10.18 **Wegener's granulomatosis: elastic tissue stains.** (A) Elastic tissue stains demonstrate disruption of the elastic lamina in involved arteries. (B) Granuloma displacing elastic lamina and protruding into the vessel lumen.

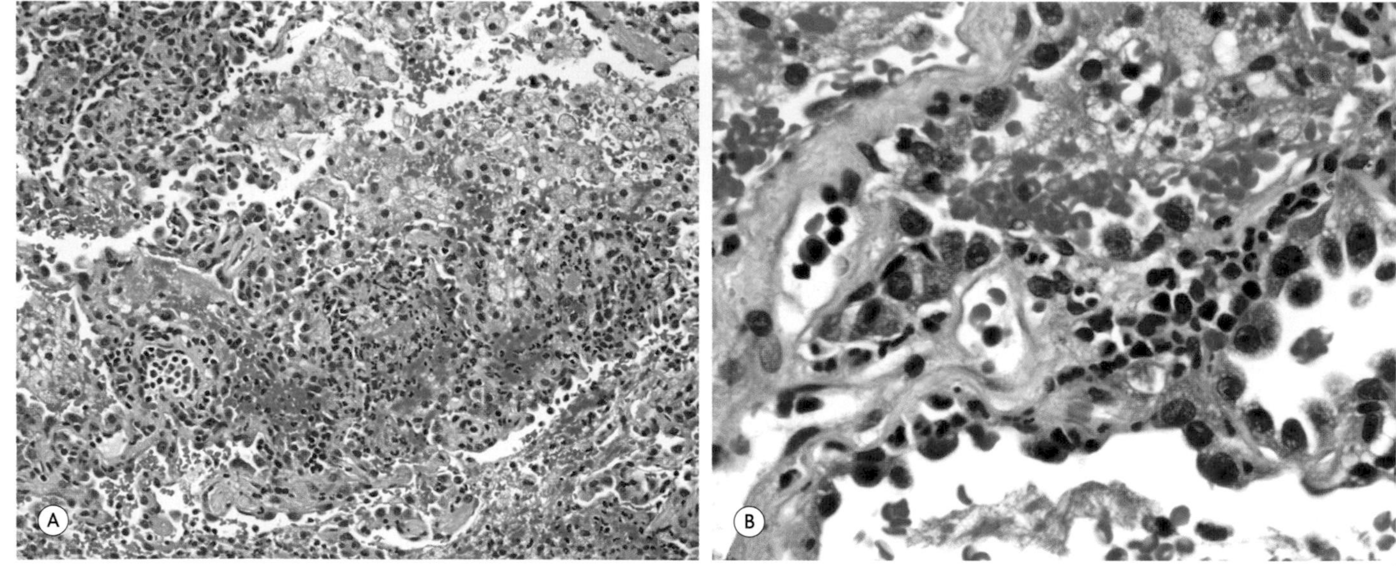

Fig. 10.19 **Wegener's granulomatosis: capillaritis.** (A) Capillaritis can be seen in Wegener's granulomatosis; at times this may be the dominant feature. (B) Higher magnification of an alveolar wall with increased neutrophils and disruption of capillaries. Note the hemosiderin aggregates in upper right.

The lung biopsy findings from patients with WG may not show classical histologic findings, especially if patients are either biopsied very early in the course of disease or following therapy.[39,43] Interstitial fibrosis (sometimes with scattered giant cells, but without necrosis) (Fig. 10.21), bronchial and/or bronchiolar scarring, and cicatricial vascular changes (Fig. 10.22), are common in lung biopsies from patients who have received therapy.[39,43]

Differential diagnosis

The differential diagnosis of WG in lung biopsies depends somewhat on the constellation of changes present and includes granulomatous infection,[40] lymphomatoid granulomatosis (LYG),[44,45] Churg–Strauss syndrome,[46–49] sarcoidosis, necrotizing sarcoid granulomatosis,[44,50,51] rheumatoid nodules,[51] bronchocentric granulomatosis,[41,51,52] and diffuse pulmonary hemorrhage syndromes.[53,54]

Table 10.4 Minor pathologic manifestations of Wegener's granulomatosis[a]

I. PARENCHYMAL
  A. Nodular interstitial fibrosis
  B. Endogenous lipoid pneumonia
  C. Alveolar hemorrhage
  D. Organizing intraluminal fibrosis
  E. Lymphoid aggregates
  F. Tissue eosinophils
  G. Xanthogranulomatous lesions
  H. Alveolar macrophage accumulation

II. BRONCHIAL/BRONCHIOLAR LESIONS
  A. Chronic bronchiolitis
  B. Acute bronchiolitis/bronchopneumonia
  C. Bronchiolitis obliterans or a BOOP histologic pattern[b]
  D. Bronchocentric granulomatosis
  E. Follicular bronchiolitis
  F. Bronchial stenosis

Source: Travis et al.[159] and Fernandes et al.[161]
[a]May uncommonly represent a dominant pathologic feature.
[b]BOOP = bronchiolitis obliterans with organizing pneumonia.

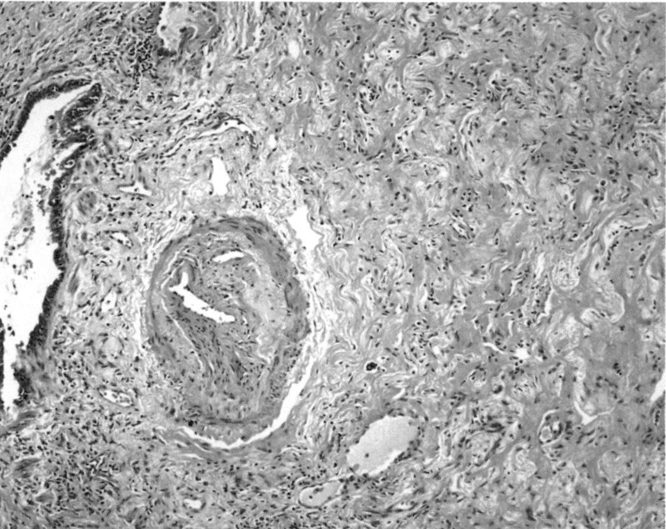

Fig. 10.21 **Wegener's granulomatosis: treatment effect.** Areas of lung fibrosis may occur in treated WG, frequently associated with parenchymal collapse (right). Here, a bronchiole and accompanying pulmonary artery show inflammatory sequela of WG.

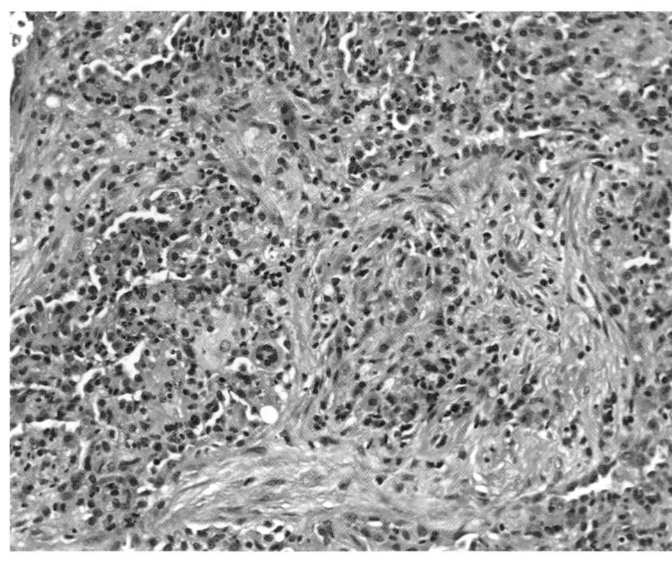

Fig. 10.20 **Wegener's granulomatosis: organizing pneumonia.** Organization may be prominent in WG and at times may be the dominant feature. Often capillaritis is evident, as are the "footprints" of prior hemorrhage (hemosiderin at center). Scattered multinucleated giant cells may be seen.

Occasionally, a form of diffuse large B-cell malignant lymphoma, commonly referred to as "lymphomatoid granulomatosis (LYG)" (see Ch. 15), can bear a striking resemblance to WG (Fig. 10.23). Like classical WG, LYG is characterized pathologically by the presence of multiple necrotic pulmonary nodules. Notwithstanding major clinical differences between these diseases, important histopathologic differences become evident at closer inspection. First, the necrosis in LYG typically has some areas of necrosis with pale shadows of large necrotic cells (dead lymphoma cells). Secondly, within the necrotic zones, and at the periphery of necrosis, medium-sized blood vessels can be seen whose outline is expanded by an angiocentric infiltration of lymphoid cells. LYG is a diffuse large B-cell lymphoma in which the B lymphoid cells are infected with Epstein–Barr virus (EBV) and associated with a T-lymphocyte-rich inflammatory reaction and vasculitis. In cases of high-grade LYG, the vasocentric infiltrate is mainly comprised of large atypical B cells. In lower-grade forms, the infiltrate may be polymorphous with more prominent T cells and a mixture of plasma cells and eosinophils. Immunohistochemistry for CD20 and CD3 highlights the large malignant B cells and background of inflammatory T cells. Immunohistochemistry for EBV latent membrane protein 1 (LMP-1) or in-situ hybridization for EBV are valuable diagnostic tools in this setting. Thirdly, LYG is a vasodestructive lymphoid neoplasm, so necrosis and obliteration of vessels is common; WG may show necrosis in vascular adventitia but wholesale medial necrosis in arteries and veins is unusual. Fourthly, the atypical cells of LYG often contain the Epstein–Barr virus,[3,55] a finding not expected in WG. Finally, granulomatous inflammation is comparatively rare in LYG, so the presence of granulomas in nodular lung lesions should suggest a diagnosis other than LYG (e.g. infection or WG).

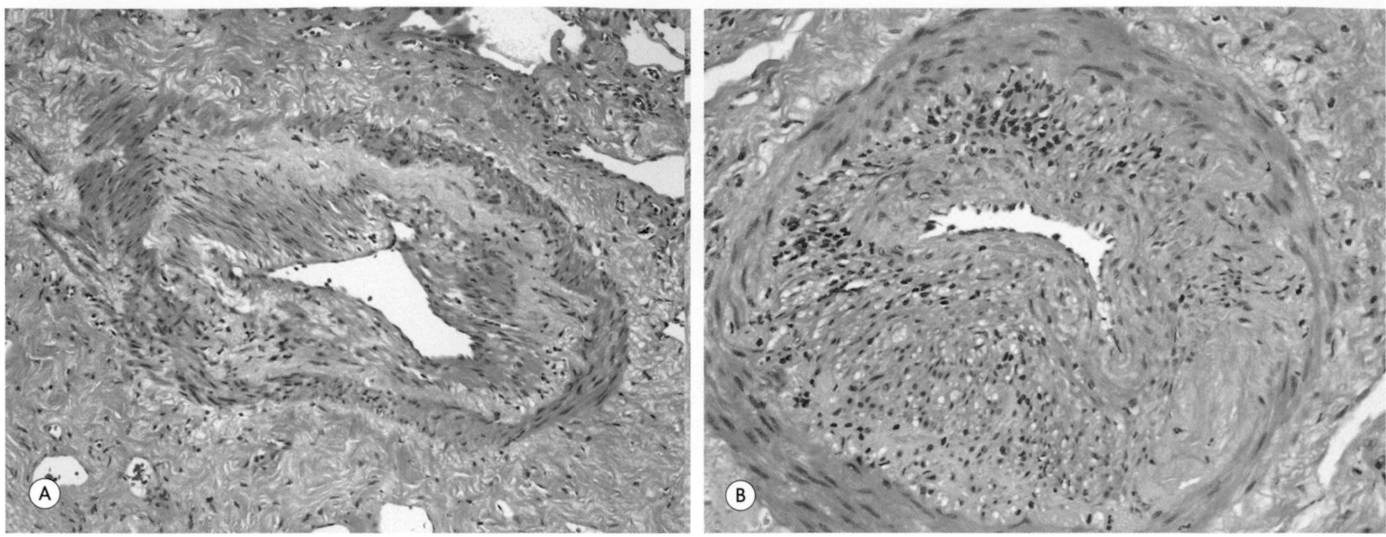

Fig. 10.22 **Wegener's granulomatosis: treatment effect.** (A) Treated WG may leave significant vascular scarring. (B) Remnants of the inflammatory infiltrate may persist within the vascular media. Note the giant cell within the media upper center.

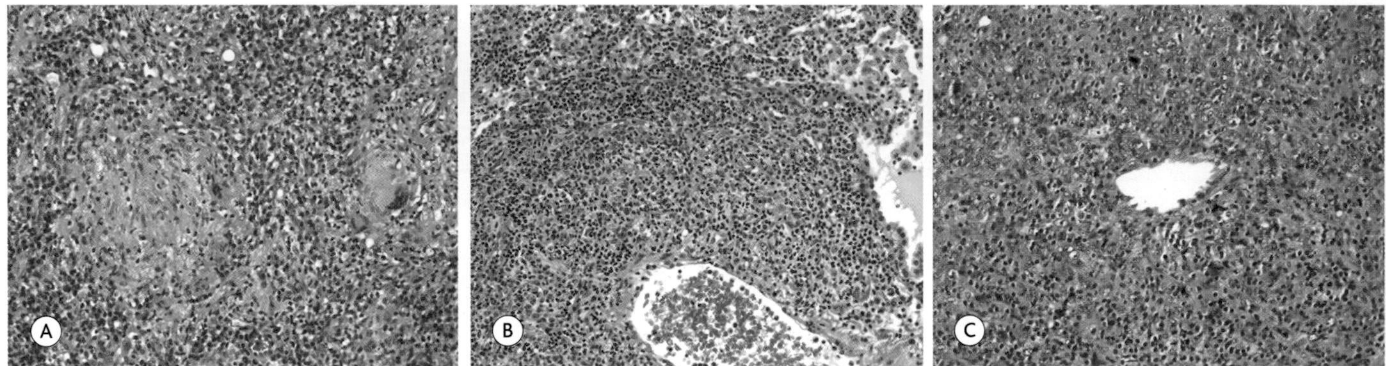

Fig. 10.23 **Wegener's granulomatosis differential diagnosis: prominent lymphoid infiltrates.** (A) Wegener's granulomatosis may be dominated by lymphocytes. When this occurs, differentiation from lymphoma (specifically, angiocentric lymphoma – B,C) may be difficult. Note the expansile appearance of the inflammatory infiltrate in B and C, with vessel wall destruction. Closer inspection will often reveal a degree of atypia in the lymphoid cells not seen in WG.

Prominent tissue eosinophilia occurs in about 5% of cases of WG (Fig. 10.24). When this occurs, the differential diagnosis should include Churg–Strauss syndrome (CSS – see below), along with fungal or parasitic infection.[46–49,56,57] Peripheral blood eosinophilia is characteristic of CSS and is uncommon in WG.[58] Also, asthma is not a characteristic feature of WG, although, rarely, asthmatic individuals may develop WG, presumably at a rate similar to that seen in the general population. The distinction between WG and CSS is usually straightforward, but some cases may require careful assessment of all of the clinical, pathologic, and laboratory data (Table 10.5).

Perhaps the most important, and often problematic, consideration in the diagnosis of WG is the exclusion of infection. Mycobacteria and fungi can cause necrotizing granulomatous inflammation and vasculitis resembling that seen in WG. Solitary necrotizing granulomas can be associated with vasculitis in 87% of mycobacterial lung infections and 57% of fungal lung infections.[40] Also, neutrophilic microabscesses are a feature of certain infections, such as blastomycosis and nocardiosis.

A number of important clues can be helpful in the approach to this differential diagnosis, even before special stains for organisms or culture data (which should be routinely ordered in such cases) are available. First, if the lesion is solitary, a high index of suspicion for infection is appropriate.[34] Secondly, WG does not tend to make granulomas without central necrosis,[39] except in the rare occurrence of infection superimposed on the necrotic center of a WG lesion. Thirdly, the necrosis of infection may show the "ghosted" outlines of underlying lung parenchyma, a finding uncharacteristic of WG. Fourthly, the patient with infection who simulates the multiple, bilateral nodular appearance of WG on radiologic studies is typically quite ill, with generalized systemic symptoms. In contrast, the WG patient may be relatively asymptomatic, despite numerous necrotic nodules in the lung. Finally, when strictly morphologic assessment fails to clarify the diagnosis, inquiry regarding the presence of sinonasal disease and/or renal disease, and serologic data (C-ANCA and P-ANCA) will usually resolve this quandry.

When WG presents with a predominantly bronchocentric pattern of lung involvement, bronchocentric granulomatosis (BCG) must be considered in the differential diagnosis.[39,41] Patients with bronchocentric WG should have other distinguishing features of WG, including renal or sinus involvement and a positive ANCA serology.

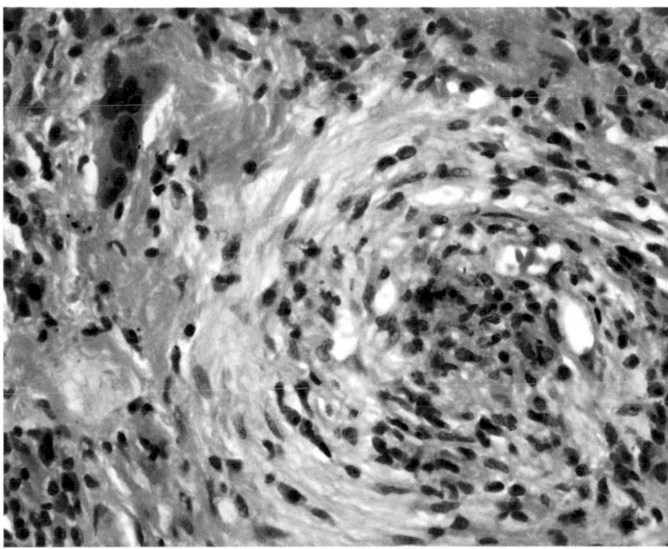

Fig. 10.24 **Wegener's granulomatosis: prominent eosinophils.** Eosinophils may be prominent in WG. When this occurs, the differential diagnosis includes Churg–Strauss syndrome. Here, a vessel is obliterated by inflammation and fibroblastic proliferation. Eosinophils are abundant. Note multinucleated giant cell in upper left.

Diagnosis of Wegener's granulomatosis

The histologic features of WG can be very suggestive of the diagnosis, but, as a general rule, it is extremely important to correlate the histopathology with clinical and serologic findings before making a definitive diagnosis on a lung biopsy specimen. The diagnosis can be impossible in cases where only partial clinical and/or pathologic criteria are present. In these situations a purely descriptive diagnosis with a differential diagnosis may be necessary. As mentioned earlier, ANCA serology can be helpful, as long as one keeps in mind that ANCAs are not specific for WG.[59] Moreover, when all other clinical and histopathologic findings are compelling for WG, the diagnosis is still possible despite negative ANCA studies.[27]

Treatment and prognosis

WG is commonly a fatal disease if left untreated, with up to 90% of patients dying within 2 years of diagnosis, most often from respiratory or renal failure. Fortunately, therapy with cyclophosphamide and prednisone is very effective in achieving remissions, with 85–90% of patients responding to therapy and approximately 75% experiencing complete remission.[60] The median time to remission is 12 months, although occasional patients require treatment for more than 2 years before all symptoms resolve. Even

Table 10.5 Distinguishing features: Wegener's granulomatosis vs Churg–Strauss syndrome

Clinical/pathologic feature	Wegener's granulomatosis	Churg–Strauss syndrome
Asthma	Rare	Characteristic (diagnostic criterion)
Eosinophilia:		
Peripheral	Up to 12%	Characteristic[a]
Tissue	Up to 6%	Characteristic[a]
Sinus disease	Destructive, often causing saddle nose deformity	Less severe, usually allergic rhinitis
Renal disease	More severe	Usually mild
Cardiac disease	Rare	Common
ANCA	Usually C-ANCA	Usually P-ANCA

[a] Eosinophilia may be fleeting and may be difficult to demonstrate during steroid therapy

in those patients who initially respond to therapy, relapses are common, with up to 50 of initial responders experiencing at least one relapse requiring another course of therapy. Trimethoprim–sulfamethoxazole, pulse cyclophosphamide, and methotrexate are also used to treat WG.[9,61–63] Trimethoprim–sulfamethoxazole may reduce relapses for those patients who are in remission.[64] The mechanism of this protective action is unknown. The outcome for WG seems to be significantly worse for patients over the age of 60, compared to younger patients, despite similar clinical manifestations and treatment regimen. Lung function frequently improves following treatment, but in some patients the diffusing capacity may never return to normal.

Churg–Strauss syndrome

Churg–Strauss syndrome (CSS) is a multisystem disorder characterized by the triad of asthma, peripheral blood eosinophilia, and vasculitis.[2,46,47,49,56–58,65,66] Although CSS was initially described by Churg and Strauss based on a series of autopsy cases,[46] it is now recognized primarily as a clinical entity. As such, most cases today are diagnosed on the basis of clinical findings rather than lung biopsy.[49]

In 1990, the American College of Rheumatology proposed two approaches to the diagnosis of CSS (ACR 1990 Criteria – Table 10.6), comprised of a traditional format classification and a classification tree.[67,68] According to the *traditional format classification*, six criteria are identified:

1. asthma
2. eosinophils greater than 10% of the white blood cell differential count
3. mononeuropathy (including multiplex) or polyneuropathy
4. non-fixed radiographic pulmonary infiltrates
5. paranasal sinus abnormalities
6. a biopsy containing a blood vessel with extravascular eosinophils.[67]

If four of six of these criteria are met, the diagnosis can be established with a sensitivity of 85% and a specificity of 99.7%.[67]

The major criteria used in the *classification tree* include: asthma, eosinophilia greater than 10%, and a history of allergy.[67] According to this method, patients with well-documented systemic vasculitis, but lacking a history of asthma, can be diagnosed with CSS if they have peripheral blood eosinophilia greater than 10%, and a history of allergy other than drug sensitivity.[67] This seems appropriate, since patients without asthma, but with a history of allergic disease, can develop CSS.[69–71] Both classification methods appear to be useful in the diagnosis, with greater sensitivity provided by the classification tree and greater specificity by the traditional approach.[67]

Table 10.6 Clinical manifestations of Churg–Strauss syndrome

Manifestation	Percent of patients
Pulmonary infiltrates	72
Mononeuritis multiplex	66
Abdominal pain	59
Arthritis/arthralgias	51
Mild/moderate renal disease	49
Purpura	48
Cardiac failure	47
Myalgia	41
Löffler's syndrome	40
Erythema/urticaria	35
Diarrhea	33
Pericarditis	32
Skin nodules	30
Pleural effusion	29
Hypertension	29
Central nervous system abnormalities	27
Gastrointestinal bleeding	18
Renal failure	9

Source: modified from Lanham and Churg.[57]

Clinical features

Despite over 40 years of study, the incidence and epidemiology of CSS remain unclear. Based on available (although limited) population-based studies, CSS is second only to WG as a major cause of systemic vasculitis, and CSS is the diagnosis in about 10% of patients who develop a major vasculitic syndrome.[1] The exact etiology of CSS is unknown; however, an autoimmune etiology is most likely.

CSS affects both sexes equally. The mean age at diagnosis is 50 years, but the systemic vasculitic phase is frequently evident in CSS patients in their late thirties. CSS mainly involves the upper respiratory tract, lungs, skin, and peripheral nerves.[47,49,57] Involvement of the heart and kidney also occurs and may be associated with a worse outcome.

CSS often progresses through three distinct phases. In the early, or *prodrome phase*, the disease manifests as allergic rhinitis, asthma, peripheral eosinophilia, and/or eosinophilic infiltrative disease.[47,49,57,58] Recurrent episodes of asthma may develop over a period of years prior to the onset of vasculitis and some data suggest that the interval between the onset of asthma and the subsequent vasculitis phase of the disease has a direct association with prognosis.[46,47,49] In the prodrome phase, tissue infiltration by eosinophils can affect the lungs or the gastrointestinal tract. Pulmonary manifestations may take the form of Löffler's syndrome, with fleeting pulmonary infiltrates or even chronic eosinophilic pneumonia.

The prodrome is followed by the *vasculitis phase.* During this phase, patients develop systemic signs and symptoms of vasculitis, such as mononeuritis multiplex and cutaneous leukocytoclastic vasculitis. P-ANCA is usually positive. The ACR criteria necessary for diagnosis only occur during this phase.[57] Unfortunately, most of the permanent damage is done by the disease during this phase. For this reason, when eosinophilic pneumonia occurs in an asthmatic patient, CSS should always be raised in the differential diagnosis, especially when prominent eosinophilic vasculitis is present in the lung biopsy. The vasculitis phase is followed by a *post-vasculitis phase.* Here, patients may experience neuropathy and hypertension, typically with persistent asthma and allergic rhinitis.[57,72] Proteinuria and gastrointestinal involvement are poor prognostic indicators.[73]

A major difference between CSS and WG is the frequency of cardiac and renal involvement. While the heart may be involved in both, up to 47% of CSS patients develop cardiac disease.[49,57] CSS can cause cardiac failure, pericarditis, hypertension, and acute myocardial infarction.[46,47,49] Also, while renal disease is characteristic in WG, it is less frequent and less severe in patients with CSS.[47,49,57,74]

Peripheral neuropathy, often in the form of mononeuritis multiplex, is seen in about two-thirds of patients with CSS. The most common cutaneous manifestation is leukocytoclastic vasculitis.[75] Sinonasal manifestations include nasal obstruction, nasal polyps, rhinnorhea, and thick intranasal crusts.[76] Central nervous system involvement can occur in 25% of cases.[49,57,66] Gastrointestinal hemorrhage and perforation are potential complications.[77] Serologically, CSS patients usually show the P-ANCA pattern, although C-ANCA can also be seen (the inverse of that seen in WG).[78] Elevated serum IgE is also a characteristic finding in CSS.[47–49,57]

A CSS-like syndrome develops as a rare complication in steroid-dependent asthmatics successfully treated with leukotriene receptor antagonists (e.g. pranlukast).[79–83] This complication probably is related to steroid withdrawal facilitated by the drugs, which unmasks underlying CSS, rather than a manifestation of the drugs. To this point, a similar unmasking of CSS has occurred in asthmatic patients whose withdrawal from oral steroids was facilitated by inhaled steroids.[83] Also, an unusual association between a CSS-like vasculitis and the illicit use of "free base" cocaine has been reported.[84]

There are no laboratory tests specific for CSS. Peripheral blood eosinophilia (usually 5000–9000/µl) is the most characteristic finding. Other nonspecific laboratory abnormalities include: normochromic, normocytic anemia, markedly elevated ESR, leukocytosis, elevated IgE level, and hypergammaglobulinemia. Bronchoalveolar lavage shows a high percentage of eosinophils (usually >33%). Pulmonary function abnormalities most often reflect the patient's underlying asthma.

Radiologic features

CSS most commonly manifests radiologically as multifocal lung parenchymal infiltrates that change in location and size over time (Fig. 10.25).[30,46,85] The infiltrates may also exhibit a peripheral distribution and thereby mimic those of chronic eosinophilic pneumonia. Lung involvement by pulmonary consolidation may be widespread. Diffuse miliary nodules have also been reported.[28,85] Cavitation of nodules is rare, and, when present, should suggest superimposed infection.[86] Eosinophilic pleural effusions may be seen in 29% of cases.[30,85] Hilar lymphadenopathy is infrequent. The chest radiograph can be normal in as many as 25% of patients.[30]

High-resolution computed tomography (HRCT) features of CSS most commonly consist of parenchymal opacifications (consolidation or ground glass attenuation),

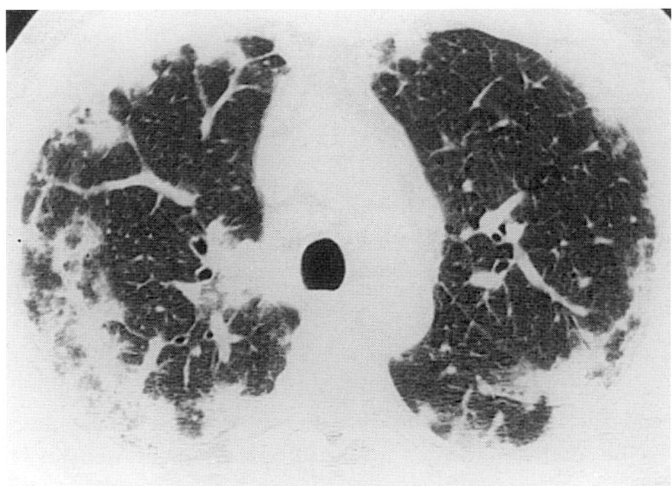

Fig. 10.25 **Churg–Strauss syndrome: chest CT.** Chest CT (lung window) in a patient with a 10-year history of asthma and peripheral eosinophilia demonstrates multifocal peripheral subpleural consolidations. The diagnosis of Churg–Strauss syndrome was confirmed at open lung biopsy. (Reprinted from Travis,[2] with permission.)

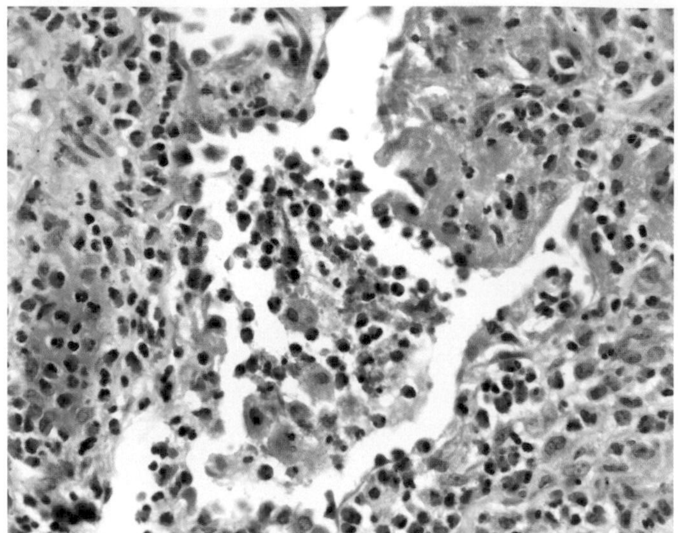

Fig. 10.26 **Churg–Strauss syndrome: eosinophilic pneumonia.** Eosinophilic pneumonia is the most consistent manifestation of CSS. Here, the triad of airspace eosinophils, eosinophilic macrophages with fibrin, and atypical alveolar lining cells can be easily appreciated.

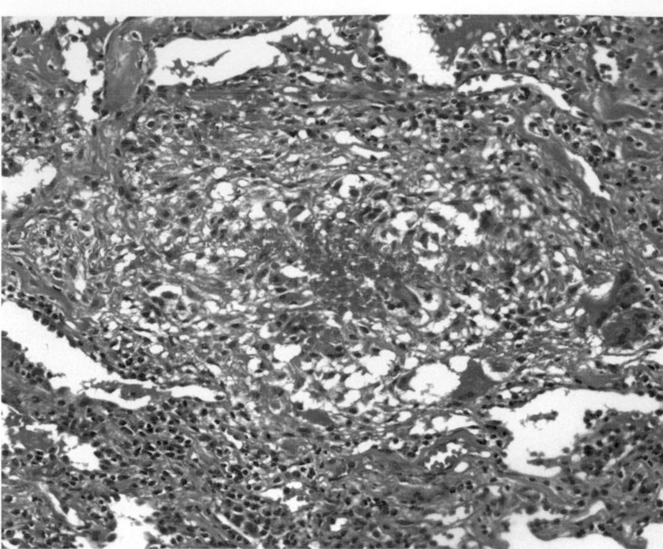

Fig. 10.27 **Churg–Strauss syndrome: allergic granulomas.** The characteristic "allergic granuloma" of CSS is illustrated. Note the vaguely palisaded histiocytes at the periphery of eosinophilic necrosis (center). Multinucleated giant cells may occur and typically have a brightly eosinophilic cytoplasm.

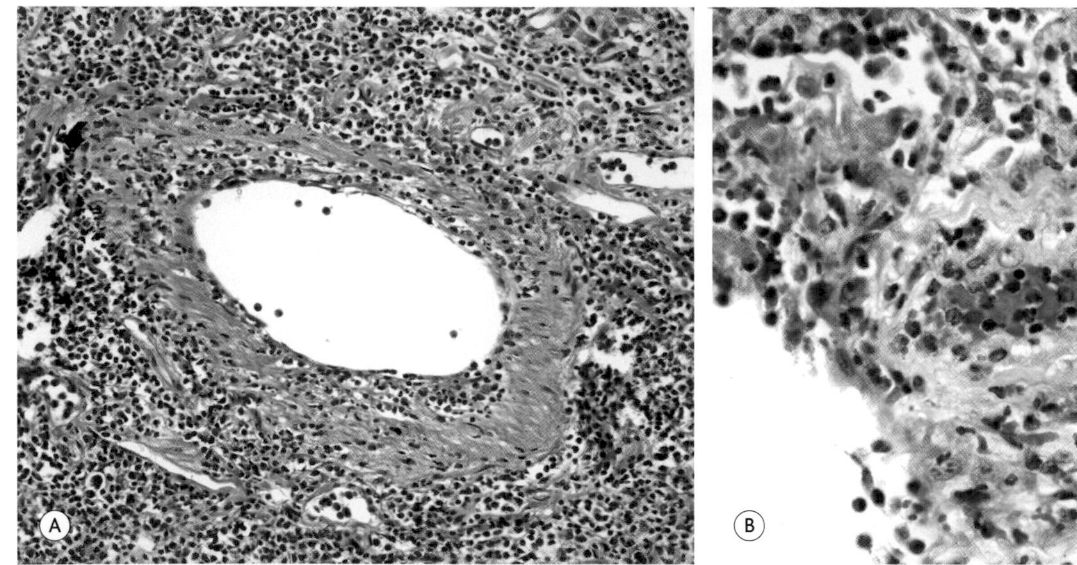

Fig. 10.28 **Churg–Strauss syndrome: vasculitis.** Vasculitis is characteristic in CSS. (A) A medium-sized artery infiltrated by eosinophils and scattered lymphocytes. (B) A venule infiltrated by eosinophils. Note fibrin and eosinophils in surrounding airspaces.

followed in frequency by pulmonary nodules, bronchial wall thickening or dilatation, interlobular septal thickening, or normal anatomy.[87] One reported case exhibited "stellate-shaped" peripheral pulmonary arteries and peribronchial and septal interstitial thickening. Small patchy opacities were also noted. These HRCT abnormalities correlated with eosinophilic infiltration and foci of eosinophilic pneumonia, respectively.[88]

Pathologic features

The findings on lung biopsy depend on the stage of the disease during which the biopsy is obtained and whether or not the patient has received therapy, particularly steroids. Lung biopsies from CSS patients in the full-blown vasculitic phase may show asthmatic bronchitis, eosinophilic pneumonia (Fig. 10.26), extravascular stellate granulomas (Fig. 10.27), and vasculitis (Fig. 10.28).[46,57] In

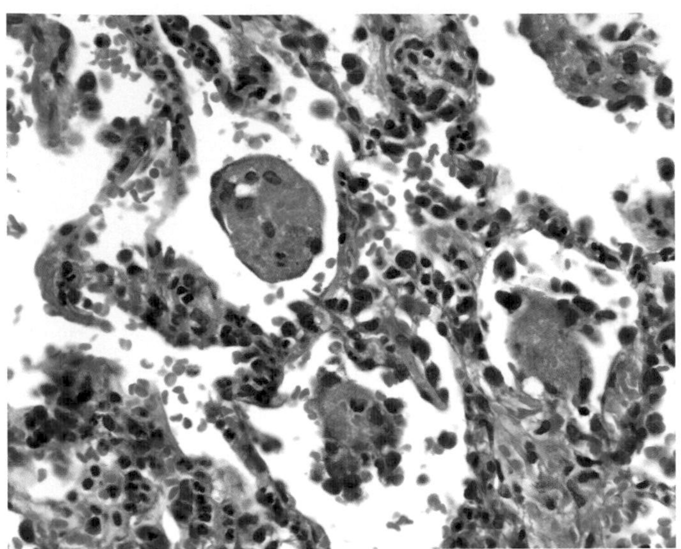

Fig. 10.29 **Churg–Strauss syndrome: pulmonary hemorrhage.** Diffuse pulmonary hemorrhage with capillaritis can occur in Churg–Strauss syndrome. Capillaritis is demonstrated here associated with aggregated airspace fibrin and eosinophils.

some cases, the inflammatory lesions extend along the pleura and interlobular septa. The extravascular granulomas have a border of palisaded histiocytes and multinucleated giant cells, surrounding a central necrotic zone replete with eosinophils and eosinophil cellular debris. Such lesions have been called "allergic granulomas". Vasculitis can affect arteries, veins, or capillaries. The vascular inflammatory infiltrates can be composed of chronic inflammatory cells, eosinophils, epithelioid cells, multinucleated giant cells, and/or neutrophils. Diffuse pulmonary hemorrhage and capillaritis (Fig. 10.29) can be seen.[74,89] In patients who are partially treated, the pathologic (and clinical) features may be incomplete.[85] Lung biopsy is not required for diagnosis if pulmonary infiltrates are present in association with other systemic findings that fulfill the required diagnostic criteria.

Differential diagnosis

The differential diagnosis of CSS includes eosinophilic pneumonia from any cause, Wegener's granulomatosis,[39] allergic bronchopulmonary fungal disease (ABPFD),[90] infection (especially parasitic and fungal),[91] Hodgkin's disease, and drug-induced vasculitis.[92]

Eosinophilic pneumonia and ABPFD lack systemic vasculitis, although some cases of eosinophilic pneumonia can show a mild non-necrotizing vasculitis, and "allergic granulomas" may be present. Features helpful in distinguishing CSS from WG are summarized in Table 10.5. Pathologic features similar to CSS can also be mimicked by certain parasitic infections, such as *Strongyloides stercoralis*[93] and *Toxocara canis*.[91] Therefore, parasitic infection should be carefully excluded when CSS is in the differential diagnosis on histopathologic grounds. Some fungal infections, especially *Aspergillus* spp. and *Coccidioides immitis* may be associated with granulomatous inflammation, prominent eosinophilia, and vasculitis. Rarely, Hodgkin's disease with prominent eosinophils and vascular inflammation, may be confused with CSS. Drugs such as carbamazepine can also cause a CSS-like syndrome, so attention should be paid to the patient's drug history.[92]

Treatment and prognosis

Most patients with CSS respond to systemic corticosteroids. In order to avoid irreversible organ injury, some authorities have favored treatment with cytotoxic immunosuppressive agents, such as cyclophosphamide, from the outset.[57] Azathioprine, interferon-alpha, and high-dose intravenous immune globulin have been used with apparent benefit in patients with severe, fulminant disease or in patients unresponsive to systemic corticosteroids. Plasma exchange occasionally has been used, but appears to have no added benefit to treatment with systemic corticosteroids, with or without the addition of cyclophosphamide.[94]

Patients who die from CSS typically have cardiac complications such as congestive heart failure or myocardial infarction. Other less common causes of death include renal failure, cerebral hemorrhage, gastrointestinal perforation or hemorrhage, status asthmaticus, and respiratory failure.[57,95]

Microscopic polyangiitis

Microscopic polyangiitis encompasses the spectrum of vasculitic disorders that previously had been called systemic necrotizing vasculitis, leukocytoclastic vasculitis, and hypersensitivity vasculitis.[96–99] A recent International Consensus Conference on the Nomenclature of Systemic Vasculitides[100,101] defined microscopic polyangiitis (MPA) as a vasculitis restricted to arterioles, venules, and capillaries.[100,101] The term "microscopic polyangiitis" was favored over "microscopic polyarteritis" since venules are affected as well as arterioles. MPA differs from polyarteritis nodosa (PAN) in that it involves arterioles, venules, and capillaries.

Clinical features

Systemic manifestations of MPA are more common than pulmonary manifestations, and include glomerulonephritis (97%), fever (62%), myalgia and arthralgia (52%), weight loss (45%), ear, nose, and throat symptoms (31%), and

Table 10.7 Microscopic polyangiitis: clinical features at presentation

Manifestation	Number (*n* = 29)	Percentage
Pulmonary	29	100
Dyspnea	26	90
Cough	26	90
Hemoptysis	23	79
Chest pain	5	17
Crackles	13	45
Renal	28	97
Fever (>37.5°C)	18	62
Weight loss	13	45
Musculoskeletal	15	52
Arthralgias	13	45
Arthritis	4	14
Myalgia	6	21
Ear, nose, and throat	9	31
Epistaxis	5	17
Sore throat	1	3
Mouth ulcers	2	7
Hearing loss	1	3
Skin	5	17
Purpura	4	14
Nodules	1	3
Erythema elevatum diutinum	1	3
Bullae	1	3
Hypertension	7	25
Ocular	7	25
Episcleritis	5	17
Xerophthlamia	2	7
Peripheral neuropathy	2	7
Gastrointestinal bleeding	1	3

Source: from Lauque et al.[102]

skin involvement (17%) (Table 10.7).[101,102] Approximately 50% of patients with MPA develop pulmonary involvement,[101] and such individuals are typically middle-aged or older (average = 56 ± 17 years) when this occurs. Women are affected slightly more often than men (female:male ratio 1.5:1).[102] Onset of symptoms is rapid in most patients, but up to 28% may have symptoms for more than 1 year prior to diagnosis.

Bronchoalveolar lavage typically shows acute hemorrhage and/or hemosiderin-laden macrophages when the lungs are involved. Kidney biopsies may show a necrotizing glomerulonephritis.[102] Over 80% of patients have a positive ANCA, most often P-ANCA.[101] Microscopic polyangiitis is the most common cause of so-called "pulmonary hemorrhage-renal syndrome".[101]

Radiographic features

The typical findings in MPA are manifestations of pulmonary hemorrhage. Bilateral alveolar infiltrates are seen on plain chest films and ground glass attenuation is seen on CT scans. The lower lung zones may be most frequently affected.[102]

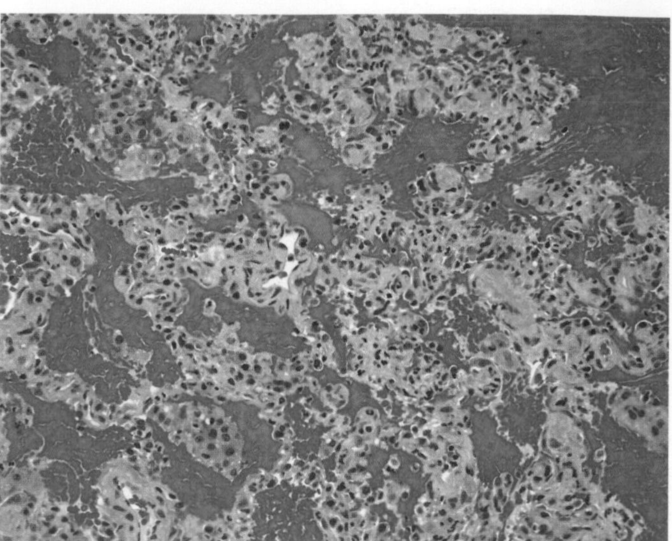

Fig. 10.30 **Microscopic polyangiitis: pulmonary hemorrhage.** Alveolar hemorrhage with capillaritis is a common manifestation of MPA.

Pathologic features

Surgical lung biopsies in MPA typically show pulmonary hemorrhage, hemosiderin-laden macrophages in alveolar spaces, and neutrophilic capillaritis (Fig. 10.30).[25,101] At scanning magnification, neutrophilic capillaritis often appears as scattered foci of increased alveolar wall cellularity, in a background of alveolar hemorrhage (Fig. 10.31). Closer inspection reveals the presence of neutrophils within the alveolar walls, sometimes spilling over into the surrounding alveolar spaces. In severe cases, the neutrophils may fill the alveoli and focally resemble an acute infectious pneumonia (Fig. 10.32). Identification of distinctive fibrinoid necrosis of capillary walls is often not possible. Alveolar fibrin may accompany the lesions of capillaritis, sometimes in a polypoid fashion (Fig. 10.33). As the lesions of capillaritis heal, polypoid plugs of organizing fibrosis may be seen, sometimes resulting in an organizing pneumonia pattern (Fig. 10.34), previously referred to as a BOOP-pattern. The presence of hemosiderin (typically within alveolar macrophages) is essential for an accurate diagnosis, since blood alone may be present in lung biopsies as an artifactual finding.

Hyaline membranes (Fig. 10.35) identical to those of diffuse alveolar damage (DAD) may also be seen.[25,103] In some cases it may be difficult to distinguish a hemorrhagic DAD from a diffuse pulmonary hemorrhage syndrome with capillaritis. Pulmonary fibrosis[24,25] and

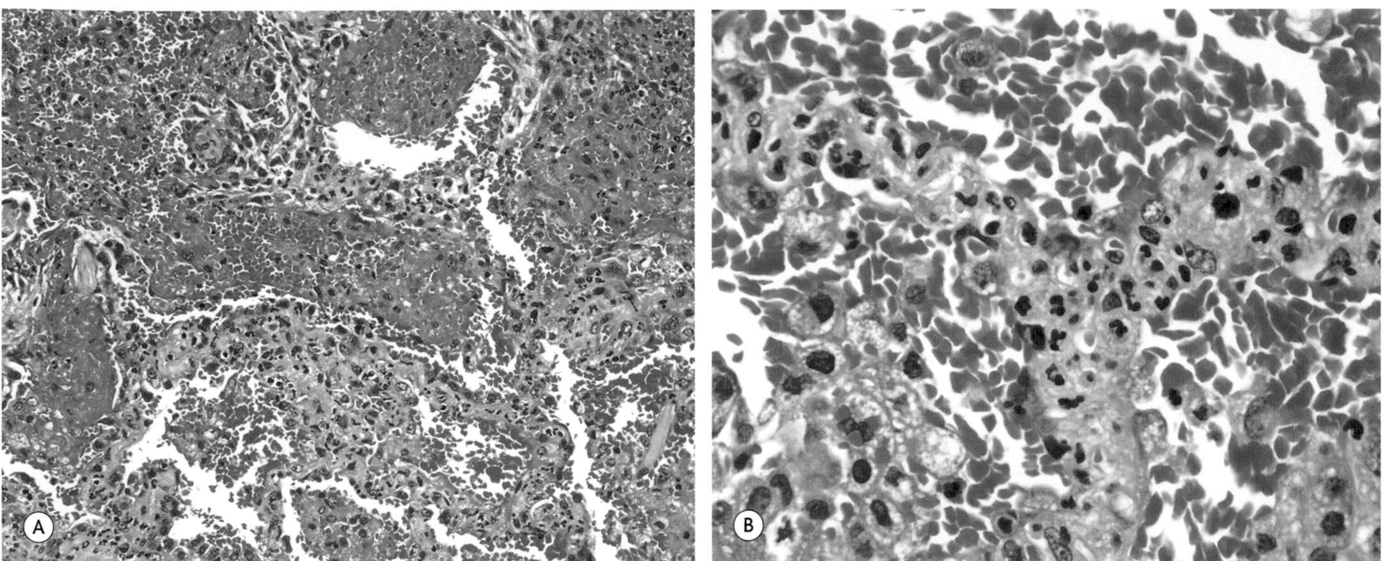

Fig. 10.31 **Microscopic polyangiitis: capillaritis.** The capillaritis of MPA can be quite diffuse (A). A higher magnification (B) shows fibrin and capillary disruption associated with neutrophils. Note hemosiderin-laden macrophages in adjacent airspaces (bottom left).

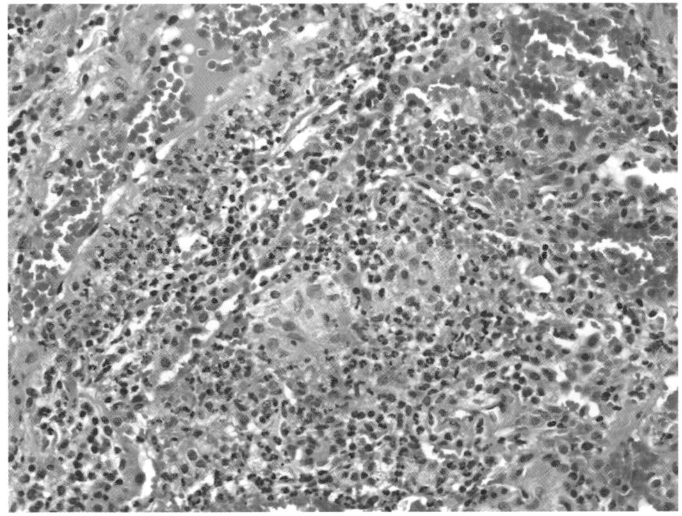

Fig. 10.32 **Microscopic polyangiitis: pseudobronchopneumonia.** Capillaritis may result in shedding of neutrophils into airspaces. When this occurs, neutrophilic acute bronchopneumonia may be simulated.

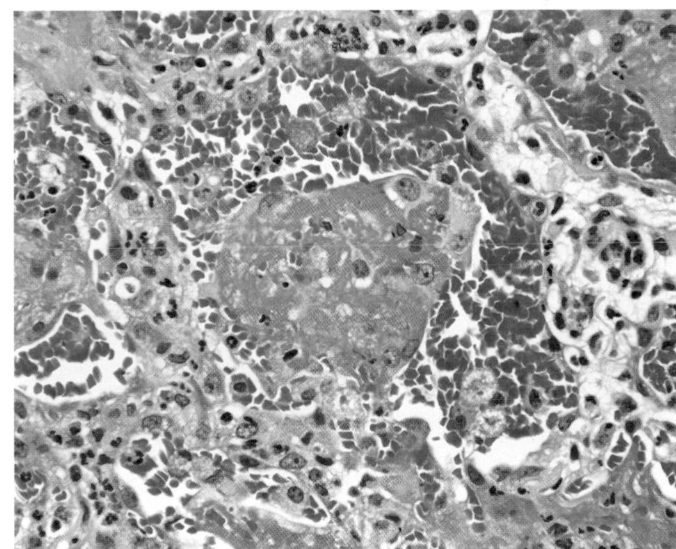

Fig. 10.33 **Microscopic polyangiitis: classical features.** The classical features of MPA include capillaritis with aggregated airspace fibrin and hemosiderin-laden macrophages.

progressive obstructive airway disease with emphysematous features[104,105] have also been reported in patients with MPA.

Differential diagnosis

The differential diagnosis of MPA includes hemorrhagic lung infections, Wegener's granulomatosis (WG) with prominent capillaritis, Goodpasture's disease, certain systemic collagen vascular diseases (e.g. SLE) and other small vessel vasculitides, such as Henoch–Schönlein purpura and cryoglobulinemia, and even certain rare drug reactions (e.g. diphenylhydantoin).[106]

WG typically has granulomatous inflammation, often consisting of palisaded histiocytes surrounding necrosis. *Pure capillaritis forms of WG cannot be reliably distinguished from MPA on histologic grounds.* In most of these instances, some areas of collagen necrosis will be present in WG. Unfortunately, granulomatous inflammation may not be included in the tissue sampled if a conservative approach

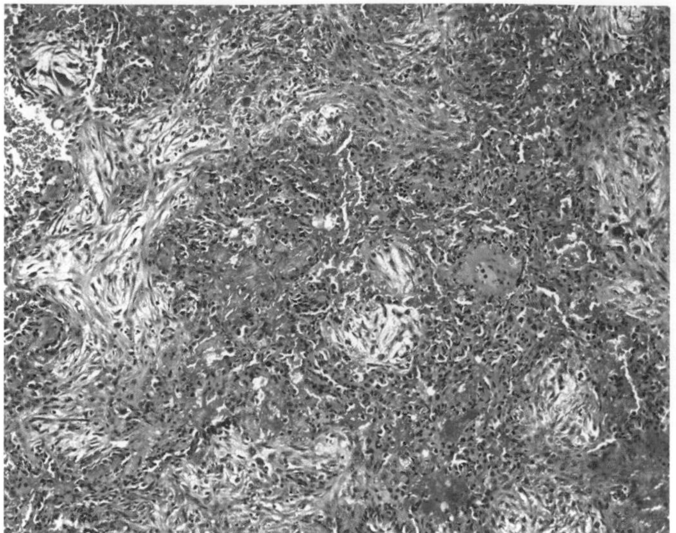

Fig. 10.34 **Microscopic polyangiitis: fibrin polyps.** Polypoid fibrin plugs may resolve with airspace organization. Airspace fibroblasts fill alveoli in this section from a biopsy in MPA. Note the cellular interstitium replete with neutrophils.

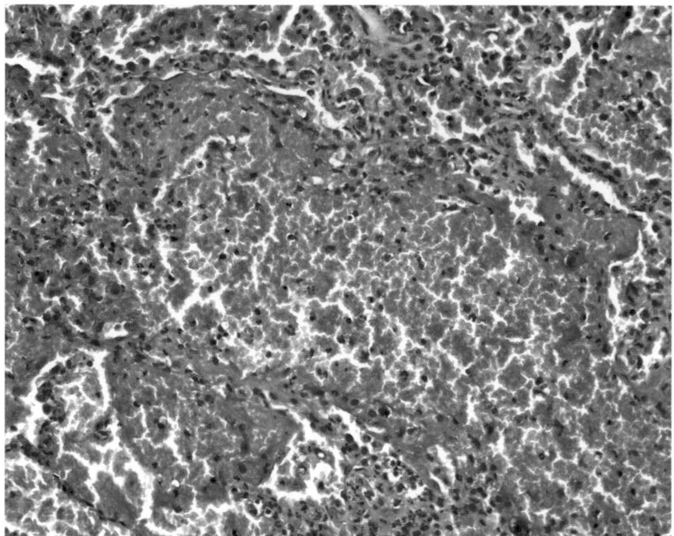

Fig. 10.35 **Microscopic polyangiitis: hyaline membranes.** Hyaline membranes may occur in MPA and other diffuse alveolar hemorrhage syndromes. Note the diffuse capillaritis evident here.

Table 10.8 Differential diagnosis of microscopic polyangiitis

Feature	Microscopic polyangiitis	Wegener's granulomatosis	Polyarteritis nodosa
Size of vessels			
Medium-sized arteries	Yes or No	Yes or No	Yes (bronchial arteries)
Arterioles, venules, capillaries	Yes	Yes	No
Granulomatous inflammation	No	Yes	No
Lung involvement	Common	Common	Uncommon
ANCA	Mostly P-ANCA	Mostly C-ANCA	Mostly P-ANCA

Table 10.9 Microscopic polyangiitis and other conditions associated with small vessel vasculitis [96,97,99,101,107]

IDIOPATHIC MICROSCOPIC POLYANGIITIS (SMALL VESSEL VASCULITIS)[a]
Systemic[101]
Localized pulmonary small vessel vasculitis[169]

SMALL VESSEL VASCULITIS ASSOCIATED WITH KNOWN CONDITIONS
Hypersensitivity vasculitis (drug-induced):[170]
- Penicillin
- Sulfonamides
- Diuretics
- Nonsteroidal anti-inflammatory agents
- Anticonvulsants

Infection:[98,99]
- Hepatitis B
- Upper respiratory tract streptococcal infections

Other diseases:
- Collagen vascular diseases[97,107]
- Malignancy[171,172]
- Henoch–Schönlein purpura[173–175]
- Mixed cryoglobulinemia[176–178]
- Pulmonary interstitial fibrosis in elderly patients[179]
- Cystic fibrosis[170]

Bone marrow transplantation[180]

Source: from Calabrese et al.,[96] Churg,[98] Swerlick and Lawley,[99] Jenette and Falk,[101] and Churg and Churg.[107]
[a]The terms microscopic polyangiitis, microscopic polyarteritis, and hypersensitivity vasculitis have all been used for idiopathic small vessel vasculitis syndromes.[96,101]

is taken to obtaining tissue biopsies in patients with WG. Moreover, on occasion, granulomas can be absent altogether in WG, or the biopsy may be obtained during a phase of disease where granulomas are not prominent. In these scenarios, clinical and serologic data are often helpful in separating these two diseases, even when biopsies cannot.

As mentioned earlier, MPA is distinguished from PAN by the involvement of vessels smaller than medium-sized arteries in microscopic polyangiitis, such as arterioles, venules, and capillaries (Table 10.8).[101]

Finally, MPA must be distinguished from a heterogeneous group of vasculitic disorders affecting venules, capillaries, and arterioles, some of which are associated with drugs or other agents (Table 10.9).[97–99,106,107] MPA is not associated with immune deposits in lung, as are some other types of small vessel vasculitis such as Henoch–Schönlein purpura, cryoglobulinemic vasculitis, serum sickness, and lupus

Table 10.10 Clinical and roentgenographic features of patients with necrotizing sarcoid granulomatosis[a]

	Liebow[116]	Saldana[181]	Churg[50]	Koss et al.[44]	Case reports[b]
No. of cases	11	30	32	13	8
Men:women	Approx. 1:1	12:18	1:4	3:10	3:5
Bilateral (%)	82	12	72	62	50
Solitary (%)	18*	88	22	15	25
Hilar adenopathy (%)	9	7	65	8	25
Cavitation (%)	NA	3	0	23	13
Patients with recurrence (%)	25	11	12	15	13
Died (%)	0	0	4[c]	0	13[d]

[a]Described as "localized, unilateral disease".
[b]Case reports.[109–111,117,118,182,183]
[c]One patient died of pneumonia several months post-resection of a solitary nodule.
[d]Patient died of oat cell carcinoma.
NA = data not available.

vasculitis.[100,101] Other conditions known to produce small vessel vasculitis (listed in Table 10.9) can typically be excluded on clinical and serologic grounds.

Treatment and prognosis

MPA is treated with immunosuppressive agents.[101] Lauque et al. treated a group of 29 patients using corticosteroids (100%), cyclophosphamide (79%), plasmapheresis (24%), dialysis (28%), and mechanical ventilation (10%).[102] Their 5-year survival rate was 68%, with causes of death equally divided between vasculitis and/or side-effects of treatment. Complete recovery occurred in most patients (69%), pulmonary function abnormalities persisted in 24%, and 11 patients relapsed, 2 of whom died of alveolar hemorrhage.[102]

Necrotizing sarcoid granulomatosis

Necrotizing sarcoid granulomatosis (NSG) is a rare granulomatous disease that primarily affects the lungs. Nodular masses of confluent sarcoid-like or epithelioid granulomas are seen in the lung parenchyma, often with extensive areas of necrosis and vasculitis. Debate continues over whether NSG is a vasculitic syndrome, a variant of sarcoidosis, or simply a manifestation of unusual infection. The principal argument against NSG being a vasculitic syndrome is that it is not a systemic vasculitic disorder and the lung pathology is primarily one of necrotizing granulomatous inflammation rather than vasculitis.

Clinical features

NSG is typically a disease of adults. A summary of case study clinical and radiologic features is presented in Table 10.10. The average age for patients who develop the disease is 50, but it can occur from adolescence to late adulthood.[2,14,108] Women develop NSG twice as often as men.[109,110] The usual presentation includes cough, fever, chest pain, dyspnea, malaise, and weight loss.[50,109,111] Up to one-quarter of patients may be asymptomatic at the time of diagnosis. Extrapulmonary manifestations are uncommon, with rare reports of uveitis and hypothalamic insufficiency.[51,112–114] Upper airway disease, glomerulonephritis, and systemic vasculitis are not expected findings. To date, positive ANCAs have not been reported in this disease.

Radiologic features

NSG usually manifests as bilateral, multifocal parenchymal nodular opacities. Nodules may be either well-marginated or have ill-defined borders (Fig. 10.36). Like the granulomas of sarcoidosis, lesions are typically located in a bronchovascular and subpleural distribution, but, unlike sarcoidosis, NSG lesions may be more numerous in the lower lung zones.[2,30,50,65,115] Solitary lesions and parenchymal consolidations may occur but are unusual manifestations.

On CT scans, cavitation and/or heterogeneous contrast enhancement of the lesions may be seen (Fig. 10.37), correlating with intra-lesional necrosis.[112] Pleural involvement with thickening or effusion may also be

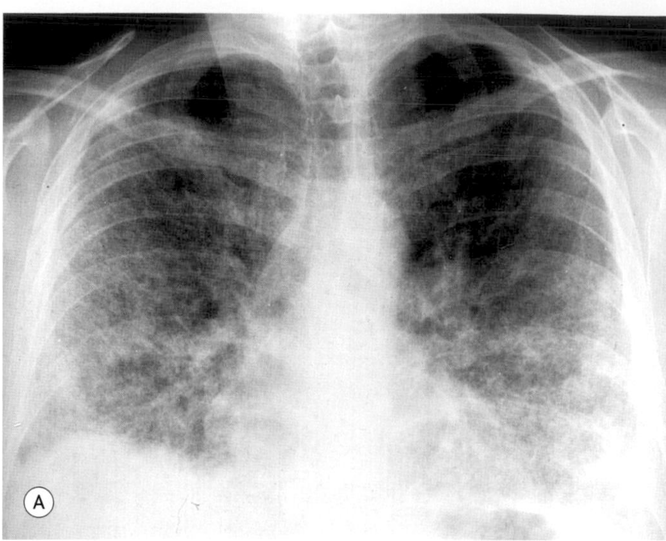

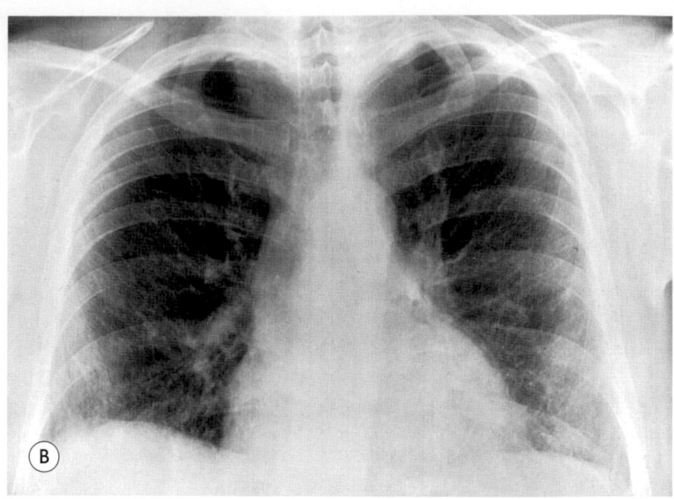

Fig. 10.36 **Necrotizing sarcoid granulomatosis: chest radiographs.** Radiographs from a 40-year-old male with fatigue, fever, and dyspnea. (A) PA chest radiograph demonstrates diffuse bilateral airspace consolidation with a predilection for the bases and the mid lung zones. (B) PA chest radiograph obtained following biopsy and steroid therapy demonstrates marked improvement with residual parenchymal consolidation in the lung periphery and lower lobes. (Reprinted from Travis,[2] with permission.)

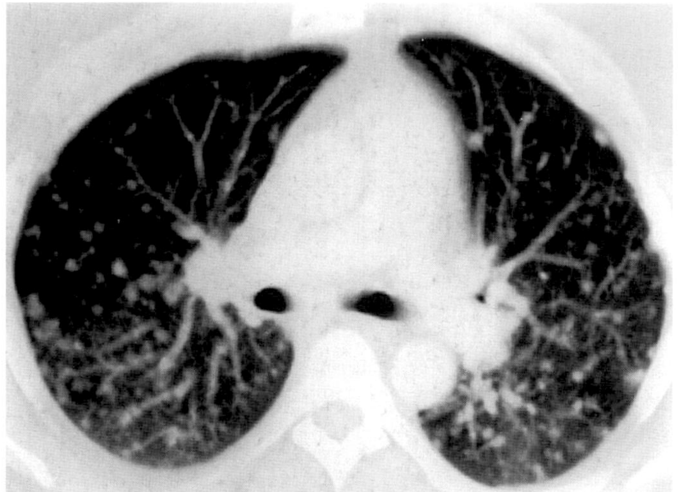

Fig. 10.37 **Necrotizing sarcoid granulomatosis: chest CT.** Chest CT (lung window) in a 41-year-old male with cough demonstrates multifocal small nodules. (Reprinted from Travis,[2] with permission.)

observed.[115] Hilar lymphadenopathy is variable and not seen as frequently as in sarcoidosis.[44]

Pathologic features

Confluent non-necrotizing granulomas form large nodules in the lung parenchyma (Fig. 10.38). Large zones of necrosis are present in the nodules (Fig. 10.39), and vasculitis (Fig. 10.40) is typically present. The granulomas in NSG resemble those of sarcoidosis, but for the presence of necrosis, with tight clusters of giant cells and epithelioid cells (Fig. 10.41). One can also see a sarcoidal pattern of lung involvement, with a lymphangitic distribution to the granulomas.[44,50,110] In addition to the large zones of necrosis, smaller foci of necrosis are often present.[44]

The vasculitis of NSG can affect both arteries and veins. Three patterns of vasculitis can be seen: necrotizing granulomas (Fig. 10.42), giant cell vasculitis (Fig. 10.43), and infiltration by chronic inflammatory cells.[116] Necrotizing granulomas may be present circumferentially along the vascular walls (Fig. 10.44).

Differential diagnosis

The differential diagnosis of NSG includes granulomatous infection, nodular sarcoidosis, and Wegener's granulomatosis. The most important of these, and the most difficult to exclude, is granulomatous infection,[44,51] especially since granulomatous infections caused by mycobacteria and fungi can produce both vasculitis and sarcoid-like granulomas.[39,40] Some regard NSG as representing the subset of sarcoidosis referred to as "nodular sarcoidosis", but true necrosis, as seen in NSG, is not typically present in the nodular form of sarcoidosis. The key features distinguishing NSG from WG are summarized in Table 10.11.

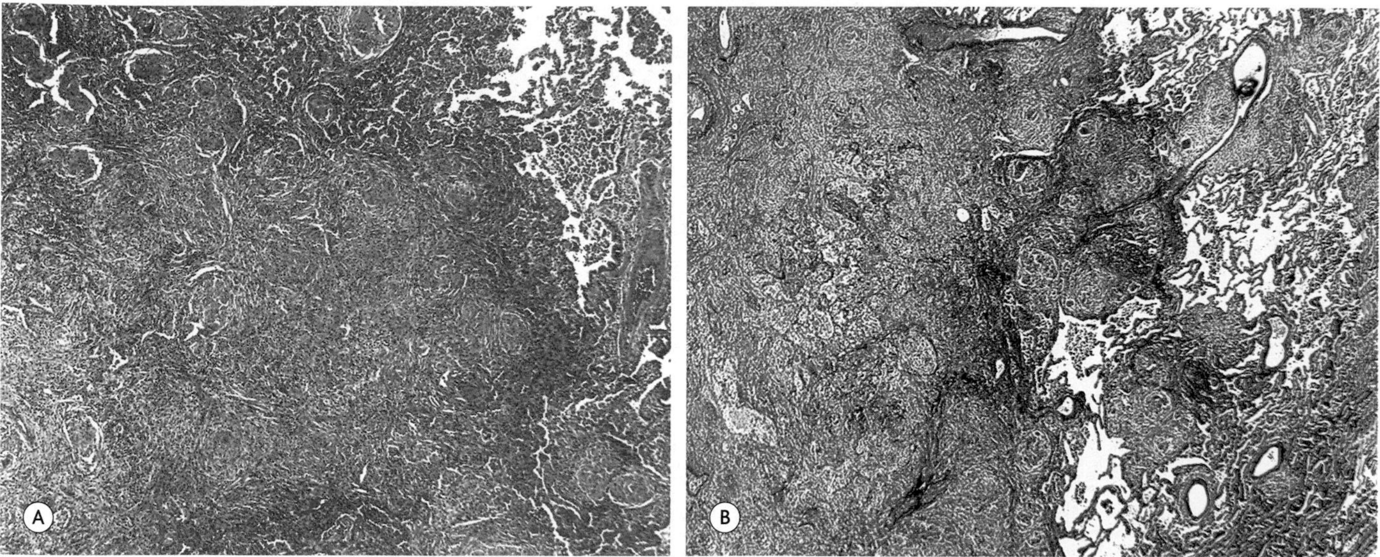

Fig. 10.38 **Necrotizing sarcoid granulomatosis: large nodules with variable necrosis.** Large parenchymal inflammatory nodules with necrosis are typically seen. (A) Confluent non-necrotizing granulomas are a dominant feature. (B) Elastic tissue stains help demonstrate vascular involvement within and around nodules (upper right, off center).

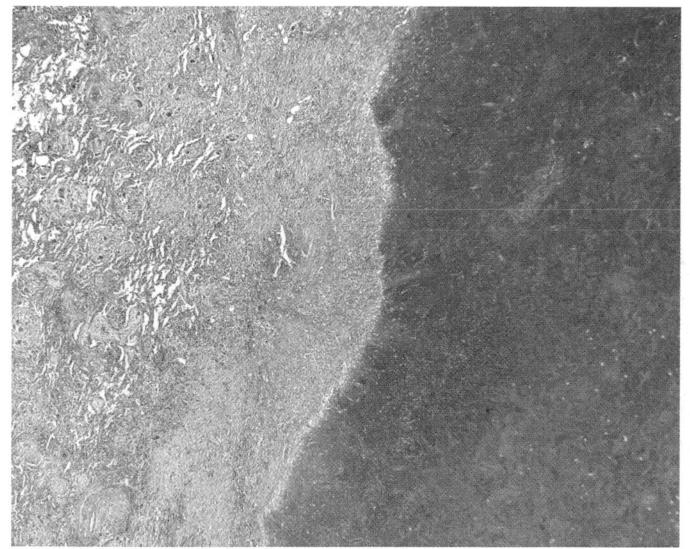

Fig. 10.39 **Necrotizing sarcoid granulomatosis: large zones of necrosis.** Large zones of necrosis may be seen in NSG (right).

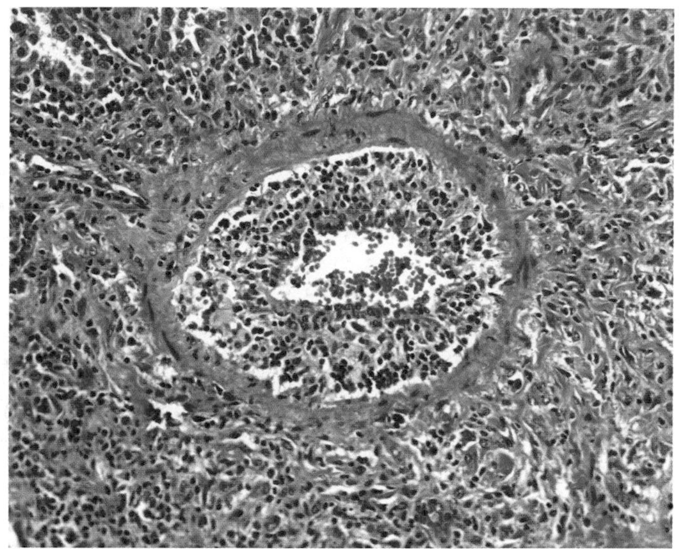

Fig. 10.40 **Necrotizing sarcoid granulomatosis: vasculitis.** Vasculitis is typically present. Here, lymphocytes and plasma cells infiltrate the media and subintimal region of a pulmonary artery. Note adventitial fibrosis.

Treatment and prognosis

The prognosis for patients with NSG is excellent.[110,117] Localized NSG can be cured by surgical resection alone. Patients with bilateral opacities or nodules may respond to systemic corticosteroids. A small percentage of patients will have persistent opacities[50,51] or will develop a relapse.[44,118] The only deaths reported in NSG have been due to opportunistic infections, so cytotoxic immunosuppression is generally not recommended.[50]

Vasculitis syndromes that uncommonly affect the lung

Giant cell (temporal) arteritis

Giant cell (temporal) arteritis (GCA) is a vasculitis that most commonly involves the temporal arteries in older individuals. Vascular lesions include giant cells, typically

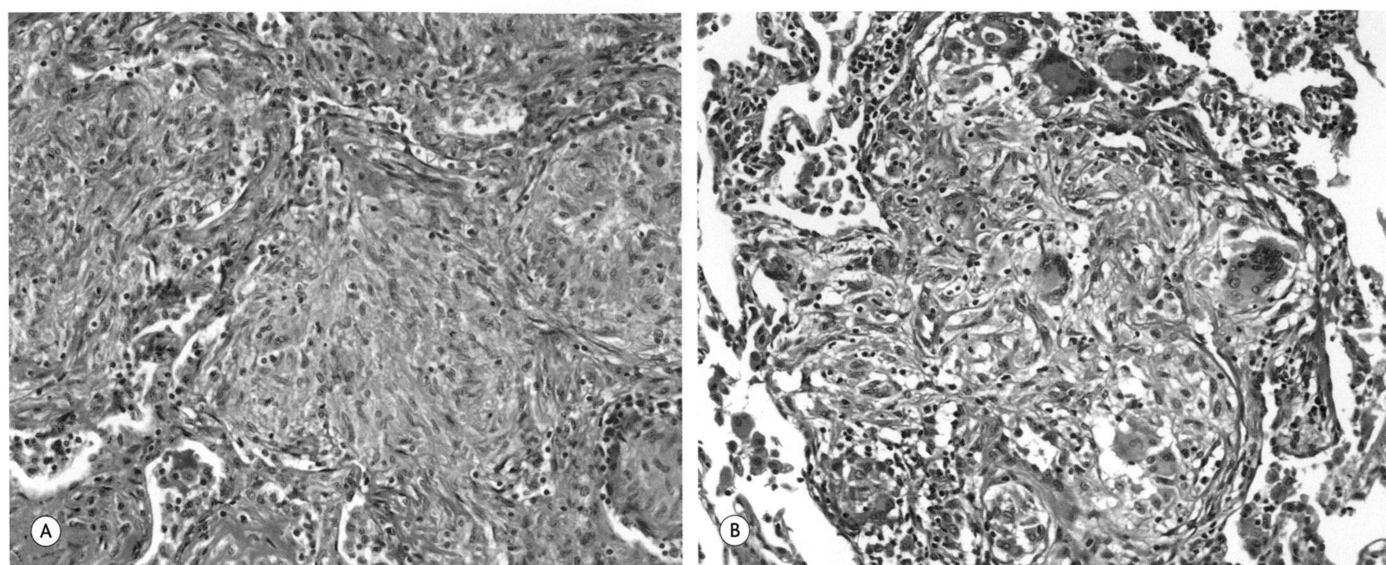

Fig. 10.41 **Necrotizing sarcoid granulomatosis: sarcoid-like granulomas.** (A) The granulomas of NSG resemble those of sarcoidosis. (B) Admixed multinucleated giant cells are typically seen.

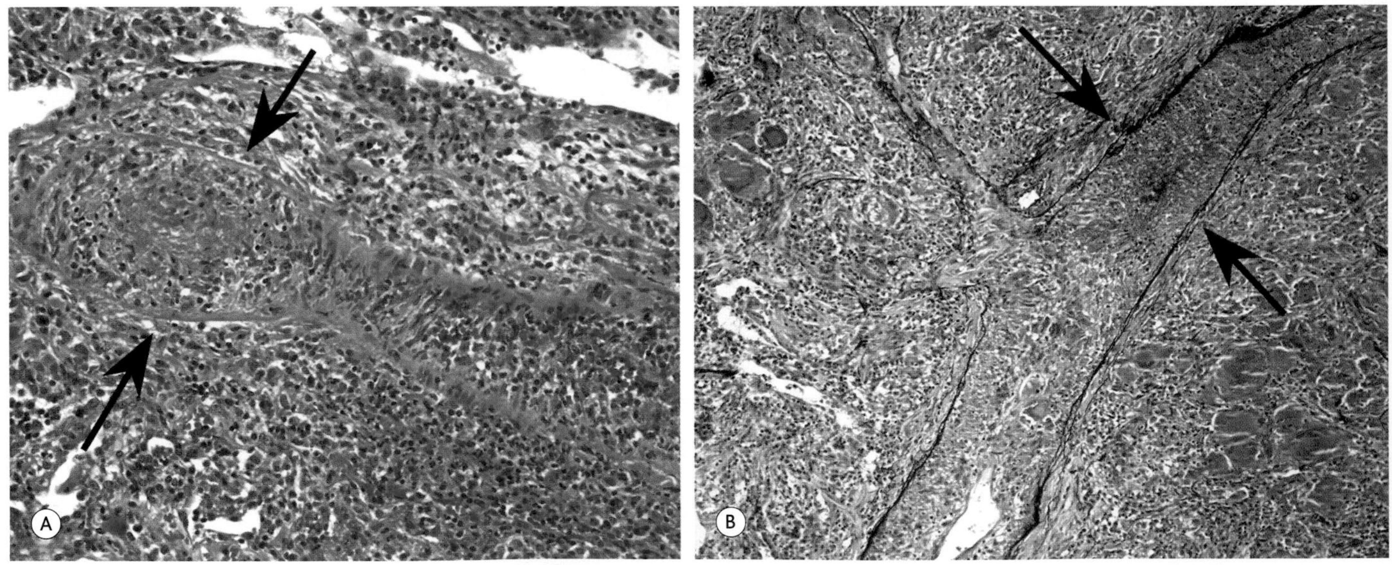

Fig. 10.42 **Necrotizing sarcoid granulomatosis: granulomatous vasculitis.** (A) Granulomatous vasculitis is a common pattern in NSG. (B) An elastic tissue stain is often helpful in defining distorted arteries within the inflammatory reaction.

centered on the vascular elastic lamina (Fig. 10.45). Lower respiratory tract involvement is extremely rare, although the disease can be associated with upper respiratory tract symptoms in about 10% of patients.[72] When the lungs are involved, patients may have nodules,[119,120] interstitial opacities,[121] and unilateral pleural effusions on chest radiographs.[72] Pulmonary arterial involvement is rarer still[122] but giant cell arteritis can affect the pulmonary trunk and main pulmonary arteries, as well as large and medium-sized intrapulmonary elastic arteries.[122] Histologically, the vasculitis shows medial and adventitial chronic inflammation with included giant cells. This causes destruction of the elastic laminae, sometimes with focal fibrinoid medial necrosis.[122] Bronchoscopic biopsies may show granulomatous inflammation of pulmonary arteries and fragmented elastic fibers.[119,122] GCA can be distinguished from WG, NSG, CSS, and granulomatous infections by the absence of parenchymal inflammation.[122] The temporal artery involvement and older age of the GCA patients distinguishes them from those with Takayasu's arteritis.[122]

A very rare disorder known as "idiopathic isolated pulmonary giant cell arteritis" has also been described.[123–125] The disease is limited to the lungs. Dyspnea on exertion may be a presenting finding, but patients usually lack hemoptysis, fever, or an elevated ESR. The vasculitis is

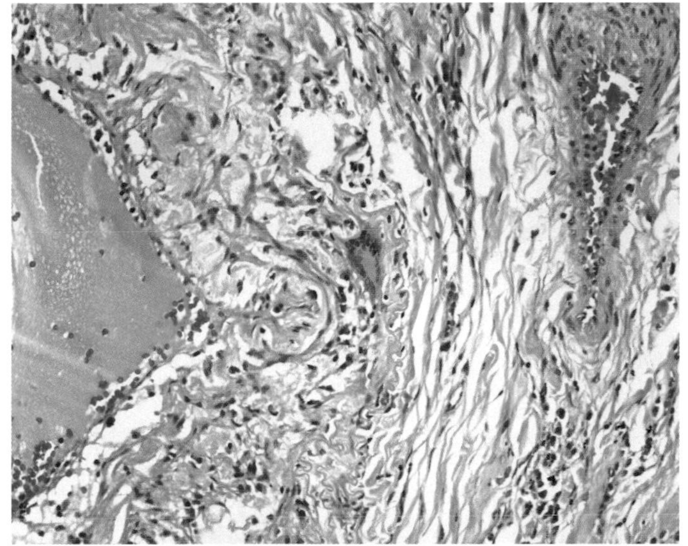

Fig. 10.43 **Necrotizing sarcoid granulomatosis: giant cells in arteries.** Giant cells may be a prominent component of the vasculitis.

Table 10.11 Distinguishing features: Wegener's granulomatosis vs necrotizing sarcoidosis

Clinical/pathologic feature	Wegener's granulomatosis	Necrotizing sarcoidosis
Lung involvement	66–85%	100%
Extrapulmonary involvement	90–100% ENT,[a] kidney, skin, neurologic	10% or less Ocular, neurologic
ANCA	Yes	No
Histology:		
– Sarcoidal granulomas	Rare	Characteristic
– Vasculitis	Characteristic	Characteristic

[a]ENT = ear, nose, and throat.

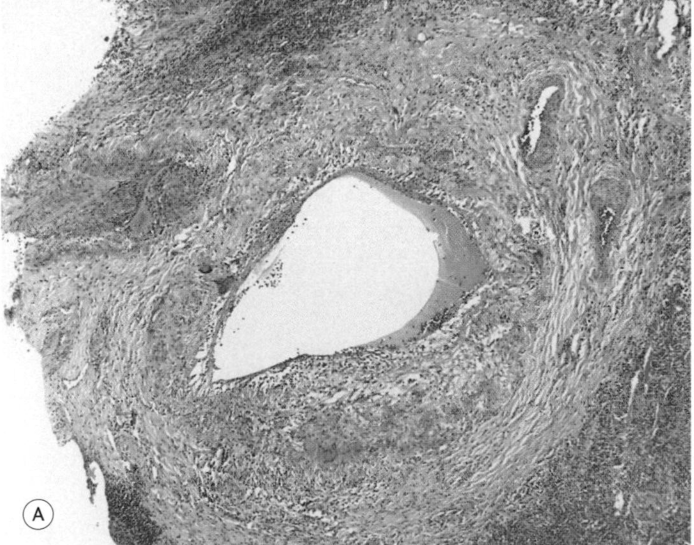

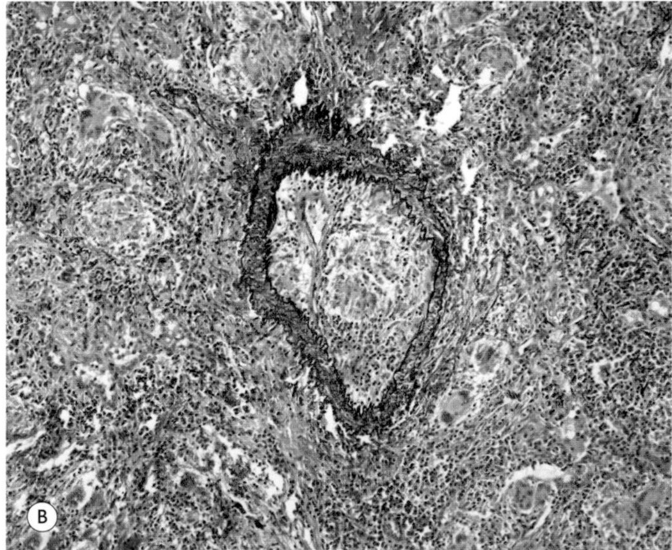

Fig. 10.44 **Necrotizing sarcoid granulomatosis: circumferential vascular envelopment.** (A) Granulomas may envelop arteries in a circumferential fashion in NSG. (B) An elastic tissue stain shows both subintimal granulomas, as well as granulomas involving the adventitia in a circumferential fashion.

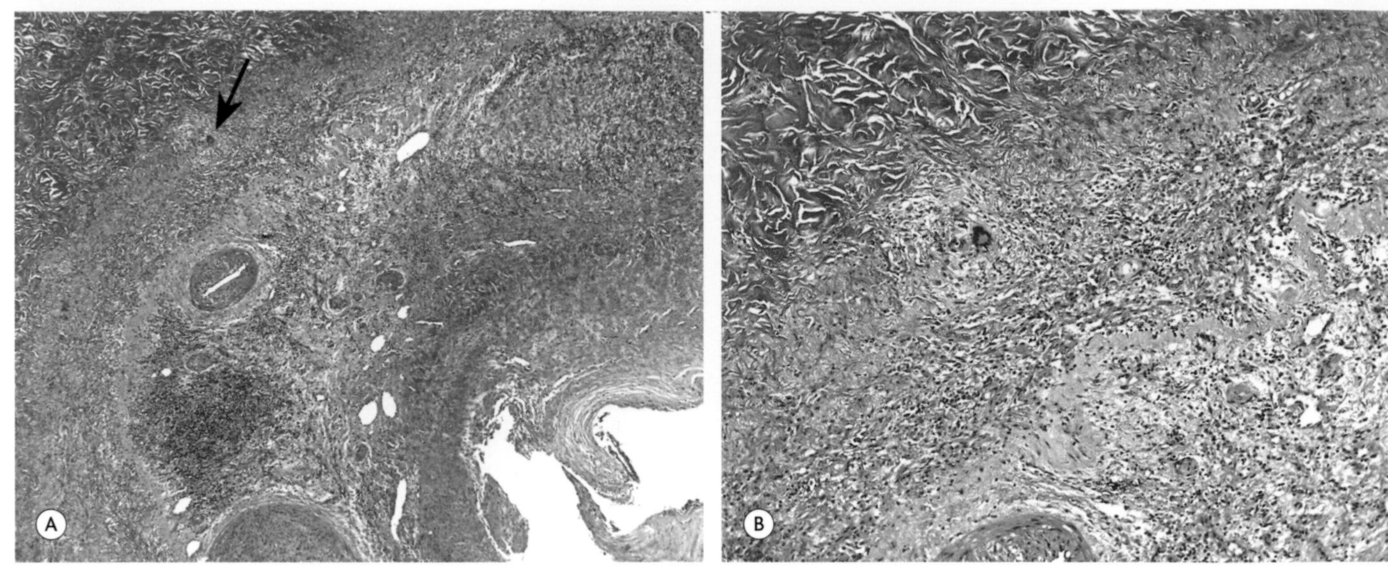

Fig. 10.45 **Giant cell arteritis: large pulmonary artery.** (A) A central pulmonary artery shows extensive medial damage. (B) The area designated by an arrow in (A) at higher magnification. Note the multinucleated giant cell and inflammation along the elastic lamina of the vessel.

usually an unsuspected finding that is seen first in a surgical or autopsy specimen.[123,124] Histologically, organized arterial thrombi with recanalization are identified and narrowing of large pulmonary arteries occurs. The vasculitis is characterized by a destructive inflammatory infiltrate of giant cells, histiocytes, and lymphocytes, causing fragmentation of elastic laminae.[123–125] Peripheral lung infarcts can occur.

Disseminated visceral giant cell angiitis is another rare form of giant cell arteritis that affects extracranial small arteries and arterioles, including those in the lung. This is a very rare condition, with only five reported cases in males, three of whom had lung involvement.[126,127] All of these cases were recognized as incidental autopsy findings.[126] Extracranial small arteries and arterioles were affected, and each patient had involvement of at least three of the following organs: heart, lung, kidneys, liver, pancreas, and stomach. The vasculitis showed prominent multinucleated giant cells of both the foreign body type and Langhans' types, but most of the inflammatory cells consisted of histiocytes, lymphocytes, and plasma cells. A relationship has been proposed between sarcoidosis and disseminated visceral giant cell arteritis, but the occurrence of these two manifestations together is so rare that it is difficult to be certain.[128–130]

Polyarteritis nodosa

Classical polyarteritis nodosa (PAN) is a vasculitis that involves arteries of medium and small size (Fig. 10.46). It can involve virtually any organ, but rarely affects the lungs. Most cases previously reported as PAN with lung involvement were probably examples of Churg–Strauss syndrome,[98,131–133] or possibly small vessel vasculitis (i.e. MPA). PAN differs from Churg–Strauss syndrome and MPA in that only arteries are affected. The tissue eosinophilia and extravascular granulomas characteristic of CSS are not seen. PAN differs from MPA in that medium-sized arteries are affected (primarily bronchial arteries),[7,133] whereas in MPA smaller arteries, venules, and capillaries typically manifest the disease.[100,101]

Takayasu's arteritis

Takayasu's arteritis (TA) is a vasculitis that primarily affects the aorta and its branches. The arteritis is comprised of lymphocytes, macrophages, and giant cells that infiltrate the adventitia, media and intima of these vessels.

Clinical features

TA most commonly affects women less than 40 years of age.[134] Pulmonary arteries are involved in 12–86% of patients with the disease,[134–137] and, rarely, pulmonary artery involvement may be the presenting manifestation.[138] TA may affect the kidneys, heart, skin, and gastrointestinal tract.[139] Because it is difficult to obtain tissue biopsy specimens from large vessels such as the aorta or pulmonary artery, the diagnosis is usually established by

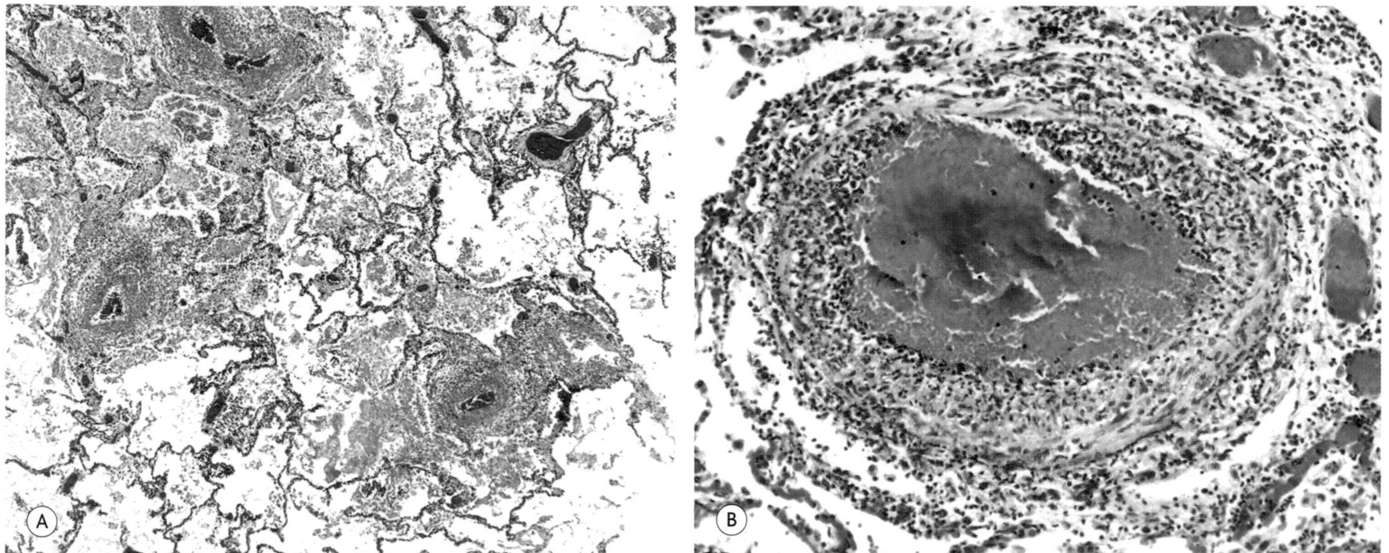

Fig. 10.46 **Polyarteritis nodosa arteritis.** (A) Arteries of medium and small size are typically involved in PAN. (B) A higher magnification of the vasculitis.

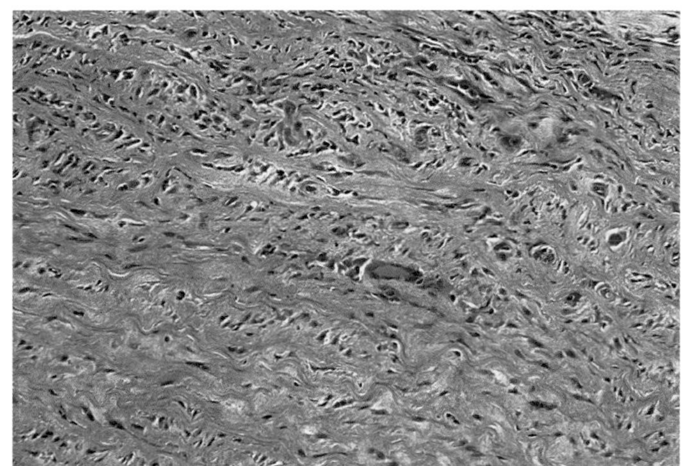

Fig. 10.47 **Takayasu's arteritis.** The wall of this pulmonary artery is infiltrated by lymphocytes and giant cells. (Reprinted from Travis,[2] with permission.)

angiography. Pulmonary artery stenosis, irregular narrowing, and occlusion may be seen.[135,136,140] Fistulas between pulmonary arteries and systemic arteries may occur.[141]

Radiographic features

CT scan findings in TA frequently include areas of low attenuation in the lung, presumably on the basis of regional hypoperfusion related to upstream arteritis.[142] Subpleural linear reticular changes and pleural thickening also occur.[142]

Pathologic features

TA affects the adventitia, media, and intima of large elastic pulmonary arteries (Fig. 10.47). Infiltration by lymphocytes, macrophages, and giant cells is characteristic. Thrombi may also be seen. There is progression to diffuse or nodular fibrosis of the artery wall with disintegration or loss of elastic fibers.[143,144] The fibrosis can result in stenosis or obliteration of the vascular lumen and cause aneurysm formation or dilatation of the artery. Matsubara et al. described a stenosis–recanalization phenomenon they called "blood vessels-in-blood vessels", occurring within the pulmonary elastic and muscular arteries.[144]

Treatment

Corticosteroid therapy is often effective, but some patients require the addition of a cytotoxic agent (e.g. cyclophosphamide) for management. Stenotic arterial lesions have been successfully corrected by surgical techniques.[145]

Behçet's syndrome

Behçet's syndrome is a multisystem inflammatory disorder characterized by skin lesions, oral and genital ulcers, and iridocyclitis. Debate continues over the nature of the disease. The etiology is unknown, but environmental, genetic, viral, bacterial, and immunologic factors have been implicated in its pathogenesis. The lung manifestations

Table 10.12 Behçet's syndrome – clinical criteria

Recurrent oral aphthosis
and
at least two of the following five clinical manifestations:
- Recurrent genital aphthosis
- Uveitis
- Synovitis
- Cutaneous vasculitis
- Meningoencephalitis
Absence of inflammatory bowel disease or other collagen vascular diseases

are clearly vasculitic, but an immune complex-mediated hypersensitivity reaction has been proposed for the mucocutaneous lesions, and an association with HLA-B51 has been identified.[146]

Clinical features

Behçet's syndrome has a worldwide distribution, but is most commonly a disease of the Mediterranean basin, the Middle East, and Japan.[147,148] The disease typically affects individuals between adolescence and middle age. The diagnosis is based primarily on clinical criteria (Table 10.12). The clinical feature that is common to all patients with Behçet's syndrome is recurrent painful aphthous oral or genital ulcers. Oral ulceration, occurring more than three times in 1 year, is required to meet the diagnostic criteria for the disease. These lesions must be distinguished from ulcers related to viral infection such as herpes simplex, and other diseases such as inflammatory bowel disease or systemic lupus erythematosus (SLE).

Symptoms of pulmonary involvement include dyspnea, cough, chest pain, and hemoptysis.[148] Males are more likely to develop lung manifestations, particularily hemoptysis.[148,149] The presence of circulating immune complexes in patients with active pulmonary disease suggests that immune complexes may be important in the pathogenesis of the lung involvement.[149,150]

Radiographic features

Airspace consolidation consistent with pulmonary hemorrhage, lung infarction, and pulmonary artery aneurysms may be seen when the lungs are involved.[151,152] Thoracic involvement in the patient with Behçet's syndrome can sometimes be suggested on CT images by the presence of thrombosis in the pulmonary arteries or in the superior vena cava. Characteristic aneurysms of the pulmonary arteries can also occur.[151,152] Pulmonary aneurysms and thromboses can be detected with angiography as well.[148]

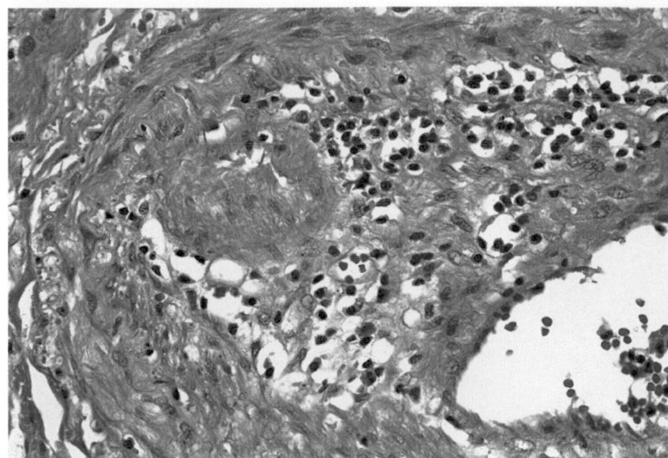

Fig. 10.48 **Behçet's syndrome: vasculitis.** The wall of this small artery is infiltrated by lymphocytes. (Reprinted from Travis,[2] with permission.)

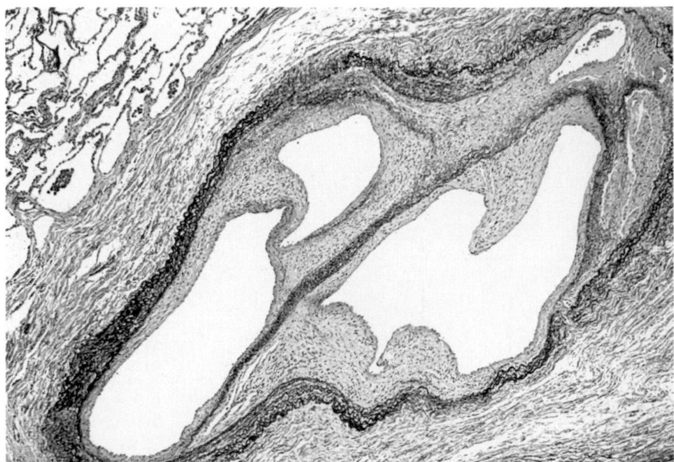

Fig. 10.49 **Behçet's syndrome: organizing thrombus.** The web of fibrosis traversing the lumen of this elastic artery is a recanalized thrombus. (Reprinted from Travis,[2] with permission.)

Pathologic features

Pulmonary involvement is characterized by a lymphocytic and necrotizing vasculitis that involves pulmonary arteries of all sizes, veins, and alveolar septal capillaries. (Fig. 10.48). Additional findings include aneurysms of elastic pulmonary arteries, arterial and venous thromboses (Fig. 10.49), pulmonary infarcts (Fig. 10.50), bronchial erosion by pulmonary artery aneurysms, and arterio-bronchial fistulas.[148,153,154] Perivascular adventitial fibrosis may be prominent. Collateral vessels lacking elastic lamellae may develop in the periadventitial fibrous

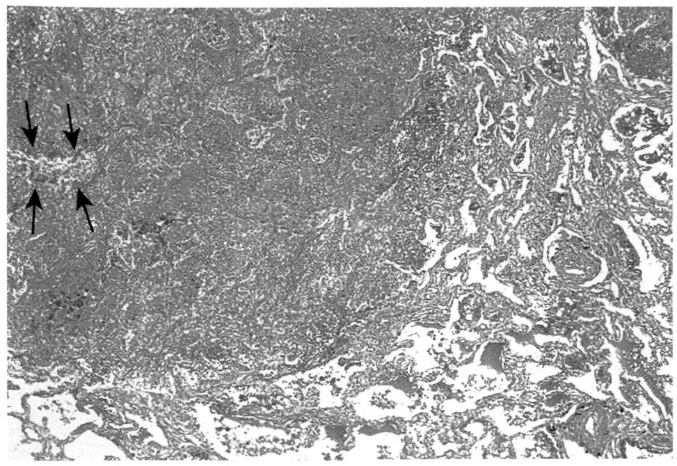

Fig. 10.50 **Behçet's syndrome: pulmonary infarct.** A pulmonary infarct can be seen here on elastic tissue stain. The arrows designate disrupted elastica of a pulmonary artery at the edge of a lung infarct (red).

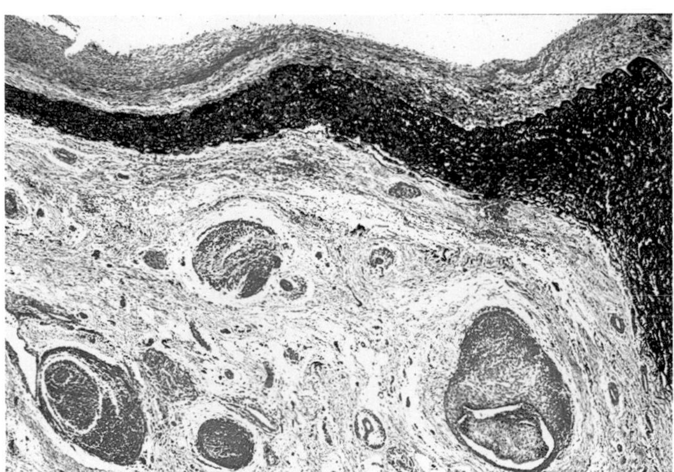

Fig. 10.51 **Beçhet's syndrome: collateral vessels.** The collateral vessels in the periadventitial tissues surrounding this large elastic artery lack elastic lamellae. (Reprinted from Travis,[2] with permission.)

tissues around thrombosed arteries and aneurysms (Fig. 10.51). Hemorrhage[155] and acute interstitial pneumonia[156] may occur as life-threatening pulmonary complications.

Treatment

A variety of treatments have been used to address the mucocutaneous manifestations of the disease, including oral colchicine, topical anesthetics, and corticosteroids (topical, intralesional, and/or systemic). Thalidomide and dapsone have also been shown to be effective. Aggressive immunosuppression with combined systemic corticosteroids and another agent (azathioprine, cyclophosphamide, cyclosporin, chlorambucil) may be necessary when significant ocular, neurologic, gastrointestinal, and vascular manifestations occur. Patients who develop thromboses require anticoagulation.[149] Severe hemoptysis may require surgical intervention.[155] The clinical course of Behçet's syndrome is characterized by exacerbations and remissions. Over time, the disease may decrease in severity.

Secondary vasculitis

Pulmonary infection and septic emboli

When pulmonary vessels are involved by inflammation and necrosis in the setting of infection, secondary vasculitis should always be a strong consideration. Certain bacterial pneumonias, especially those caused by *Pseudomonas aeruginosa*[157] and *Legionella pneumophila*,[158] are well known for their tendency to invade and produce necrosis of blood vessel walls. The necrotizing granulomas produced in response to fungal and mycobacterial infections commonly involve blood vessel walls, causing potential confusion with vascular involvement by Wegener's granulomatosis.[40] Necrotizing vasculitis can also be seen as a consequence of angioinvasive fungal infections in the immunocompromised patient, especially infections due to *Aspergillus* and *Mucor* spp. Such vasculitis may be granulomatous, and frequently causes pulmonary infarction. Pulmonary vasculitis can also accompany certain parasitic pulmonary infections such as *Dirofilaria immitis*, and *Schistosoma* and *Wuchereria* species. In HIV-infected patients, vasculitis can even be a rare complication of pneumocystis pneumonia.[159]

Classical sarcoidosis

Classical sarcoidosis can produce "granulomatous vasculitis" (typical sarcoid granulomas involving blood vessel walls) as an incidental histologic finding in surgical lung biopsies (see Ch. 7).[160]

On rare occasions, a systemic vasculitis can occur in patients with sarcoidosis. Fernandes et al. recently reported 6 patients with features of both sarcoidosis and systemic vasculitis, and reviewed 22 similar cases that had been previously reported.[161] The group included 13 children and 15 adults who developed fever, peripheral adenopathy, hilar adenopathy, rash, pulmonary parenchymal disease, musculoskeletal symptoms, and scleritis or iridocyclitis.[161]

Radiologic features

Arteriography demonstrated involvement of medium or large arteries in about half of the described patients, while the other half had findings of small vessel disease.[161]

Pathologic features

Pathologic findings consisted of sarcoid-like granulomas, sometimes with foci of necrosis, involving vessels in the skin, lymph node, lung, synovium, bone, bone marrow, liver, trachea, or sclera.

Therapy and prognosis

Patients may respond to prednisone alone; however, relapses tended to occur when the medication was tapered or withdrawn.[161]

II. Pulmonary hemorrhage

Hemorrhage in the lung may occur as a localized phenomenon or as a diffuse disease. Clinically significant hemorrhage is nearly always accompanied by hemoptysis. When blood is identified in the lung biopsy specimen, the question frequently arises as to whether it is a real finding or simply an artifact related to the procedure. Real pulmonary hemorrhage can be caused by a number of unrelated mechanisms. Pulmonary vasculitis and vasculitic syndromes, such as Goodpasture's syndrome, are important clinical causes of lung hemorrhage and typically require urgent therapy. Because the differential is broad, and the consequences of accurate diagnosis are significant, a diagnostic approach to pulmonary hemorrhage is presented here. A useful algorithm for this exercise is presented in Fig. 10.52.

Clinical view of pulmonary hemorrhage

The occurrence of hemoptysis is alarming to the patient and clinician alike. The potential causes of hemoptysis are presented in Table 10.13.[162] The distinction of localized from diffuse hemorrhage is important for management purposes, but is not always feasible. When classical symptoms of sudden unilateral chest pain followed by expectoration of bright red blood occurs, pulmonary embolus is usually high in the differential diagnosis. However, in most instances, the clinician must rely heavily on the radiologic findings in the approach to the patient with hemoptysis, since the physical examination is typically limited in defining the origin or extent of any hemorrhagic event. Bronchoscopy plays an important role as well in defining a potential localized source of bleeding and documenting the presence of hemosiderin-laden macrophages (siderophages) in lavage specimens examined under the microscope. Localized causes of pulmonary hemorrhage are often straightforward and include thromboembolism, tumor, abscess, bronchiectasis, and broncholithiasis. At times, localized hemorrhage may be life threatening, requiring lobectomy for control. In this situation, blood may be abundant in the lung parenchyma, but no exact origin for bleeding can be identified (analogous to colectomy for massive hemorrhage associated with diverticulosis). Diffuse pulmonary hemorrhage is more complicated in terms of etiology and will be the main focus here.

Morphologic approach to pulmonary hemorrhage

Not all patients with hemoptysis have histologic evidence of hemorrhage and, conversely, not all hemorrhage or hemosiderin seen in lung tissue is associated with hemoptysis or other evidence of lung hemorrhage. For the pathologist, the first step in the evaluation of extravascular blood seen in a biopsy specimen is to examine the context in which it occurs. Clinically significant hemorrhage rarely presents in biopsy specimens as blood alone. When intact red cells abound, the most common cause is trauma related to the biopsy procedure, especially in the case of thoracoscopic biopsies because of intraoperative manipulation.[163] Artifactual hemorrhage (Fig. 10.53) typically lacks fibrin, hemosiderin-laden macrophages, and cellular reactive changes in adjacent alveolar walls. Also, focal areas of organization may be seen within the airspaces in true hemorrhage and may be a useful marker for associated lung injury.

Unfortunately, the presence of siderophages alone is not sufficently specific for active hemorrhage in the absence of other more acute findings. Siderophages can occur as early as 2 days following an episode of alveolar hemorrhage, but can persist for weeks or even months after the event. Furthermore, the distinction of siderophages caused by hemorrhage from the pigmented macrophages seen in the lungs of cigarette smokers can be difficult on occasion.

The Prussian blue histochemical stain for iron is sometimes cited as a means of distinguishing siderophages from hemorrhage from macrophages seen in smokers (Fig. 10.54), but caution must be exerted, since so-called "smokers' macrophages" can have considerable amounts of stainable iron (Fig. 10.55). The pigment in smokers' macrophages tends to be finely granular, light brown in

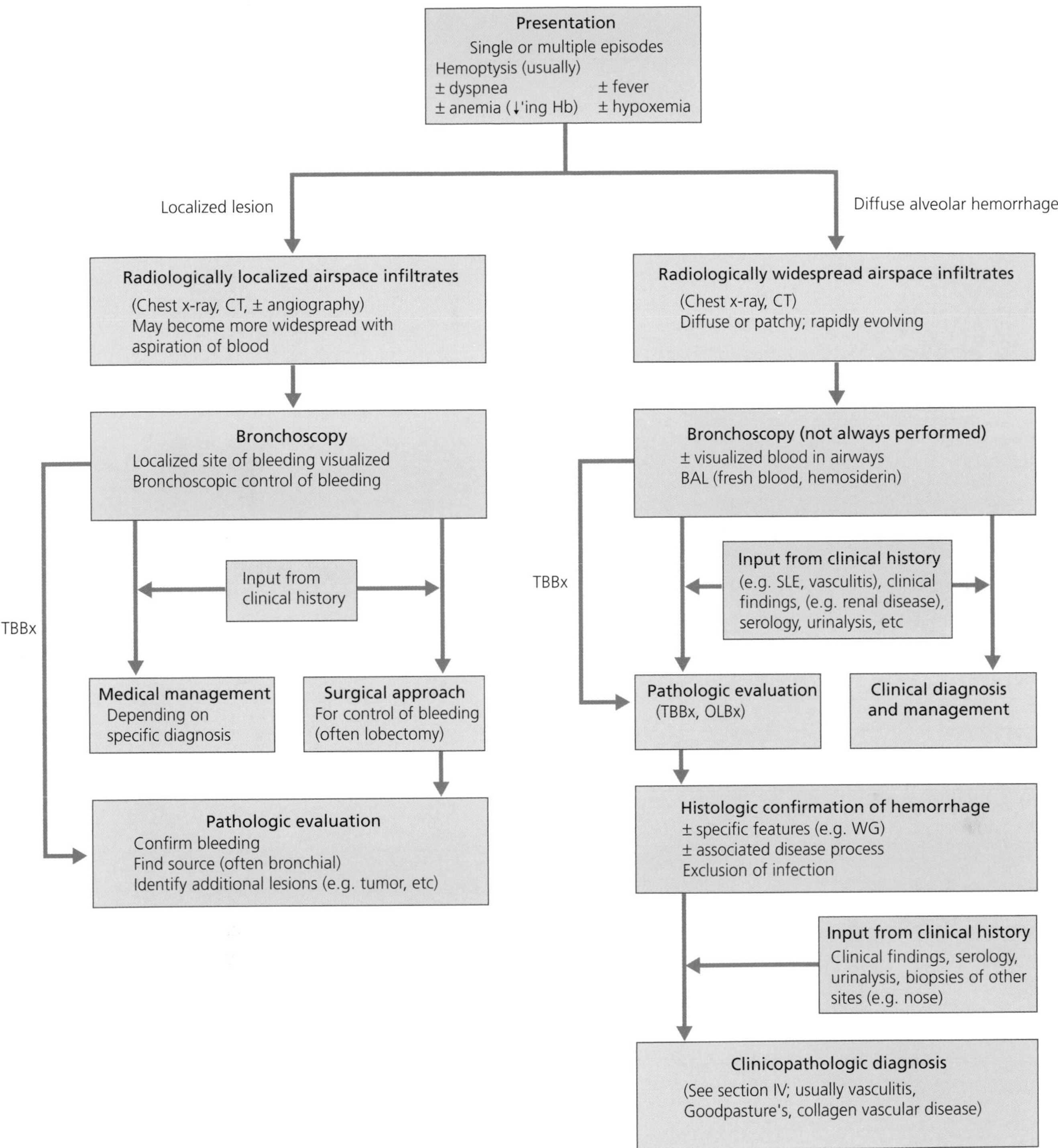

Fig. 10.52 **Diffuse alveolar hemorrhage: algorithm.** (Reprinted from Colby et al.,[162] with permission.)

color and typically has admixed punctate black pigment. True siderophages, on the other hand, are characterized by the presence of coarse, golden brown pigment that is minimally refractile (Fig. 10.56). Also, it is important to keep in mind that the Prussian blue stain reacts with other iron-associated substances in the lung, in addition to hemosiderin. Occupational dusts may contain iron and simulate siderophages in the patient with pneumoconiosis.

When all of the elements in the biopsy add up to real hemorrhage, and the patient has radiologic evidence of *diffuse* alveolar infiltrates, the differential diagnosis becomes one of diffuse alveolar hemorrhage (DAH). The potential causes of DAH are presented in Table 10.14[162]. It is useful to subdivide DAH by the presence or absence of

Table 10.13 Causes of hemoptysis

- **Infectious diseases**
  - Bacterial
    - Lung abscess[a]
    - Bronchitis[a]
    - Tuberculosis[a]
    - Bronchiectasis (including cystic fibrosis)
    - "Chronic pneumonia"
  - Viral
  - Fungal
    - Mycetoma
  - Parasitic
    - Paragonimiasis (in endemic areas)[a]
- **Cardiovascular diseases**
  - Left ventricular failure[a]
  - Pulmonary thromboembolism with infarction[a]
  - Mitral stenosis
  - Tricuspid endocarditis
  - Pulmonary hypertension
  - Aneurysms
    - Aortic aneurysm
    - Subclavian artery aneurysm
    - Left ventricular pseudoaneurysm
  - Vascular prostheses
  - Arteriovenous malformation
  - Portal hypertension
  - Absence of the inferior vena cava
  - Pulmonary artery agenesis with lung systemic vascularization
- **Neoplasms**
  - Pulmonary carcinoma
    - Squamous cell carcinoma
    - Small cell carcinoma
  - Carcinoid tumor
  - Tracheobronchial glad tumors
  - Metastatic carcinoma/sarcoma
- **Immunologic conditions**
  - Vasculitides
    - Wegener's granulomatosis
    - Systemic lupus erythematosus
    - Microscopic polyangiitis
  - Goodpasture's syndrome
  - Idiopathic pulmonary hemosiderosis
  - Other lung-renal syndromes
- **Trauma**
  - Aortic tear
  - Lung contusion
  - Lithotripsy
  - Ruptured bronchus
  - Tracheocarotid fistula
  - Bronchoscopy
  - Swan–Ganz catheterization
  - Lung biopsy
  - Transtracheal aspirate
  - Lymphangiography
  - Hickman catheter-induced cavabronchial fistula
- **Drugs and toxins**
  - Anticoagulants
  - Cocaine
  - Penicillamine
  - Trimellitic anhydride
  - Solvents
  - Amiodarone
- **Miscellaneous entities**
  - Increased bleeding tendency
    - Coagulopathy
    - Thrombocytopenia
  - Amyloidosis
  - Broncholithiasis
  - Endometriosis
  - Thoracic splenosis
  - Aspirated foreign body
  - Intralobar sequestration
  - Radiation
  - Lymphangiomyomatosis
  - Factitious
  - Bronchiolitis obliterans organizing pneumonia (BOOP)
  - Lipoid pneumonia

Source: from Colby et al[162] with permission (data adapted from Fraser et al.[184])
[a]Most common causes.

capillaritis. Rapidly evolving acute DAH is often accompanied by capillaritis and evokes a narrow differential diagnosis.

Diffuse alveolar hemorrhage

The histopathology of DAH is stereotypic, regardless of etiology. This fact is important for the surgical pathologist, since a specific diagnosis requires clinical and serologic data.[54] A generic designation such as "[Acute] and/or [organizing] pulmonary hemorrhage [with] or [without] capillaritis", followed by a differential diagnosis is often all that is required.

Most causes of DAH are immunologically mediated. Some of these diseases have specific patterns of immunoglobulin deposition that can be visualized in tissue sections using immunofluorescent staining of a specially prepared portion of the surgical lung biopsy. Performed correctly, the results of such staining can be diagnostically useful and visually striking. Fortunately, in practice today, immunofluorescent staining is rarely necessary for diagnosis because serologic studies are widely available and reasonably specific for the subtypes of DAH. For those forms of DAH mediated by immune complexes, deposits in the lung tissue can also be visualized ultrastructurally. Again, while historically interesting, electron microscopy really plays no role in the diagnosis of DAH today. A comparison of the major defined pulmonary vasculitis syndromes is presented in Table 10.15.[162]

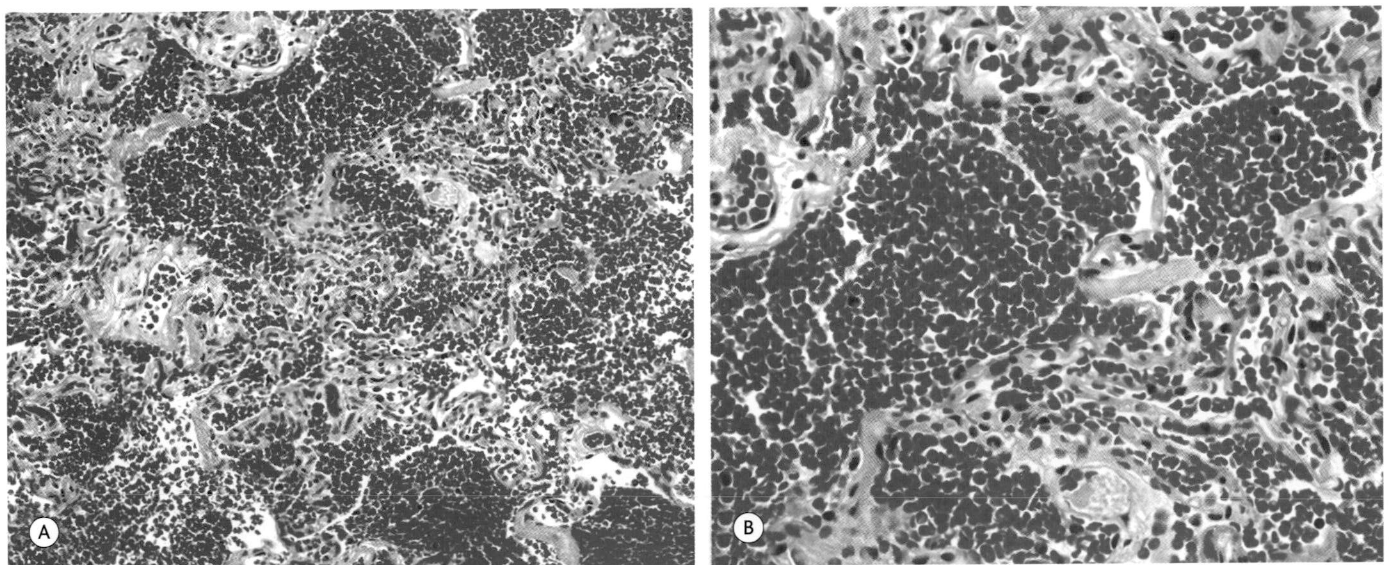

Fig. 10.53 **Diffuse alveolar hemorrhage: artifactual hemorrhage.** The distinction of artifactual hemorrhage into alveolar spaces from true hemorrhage can be difficult at times. (A) Artifactual hemorrhage in alveolar spaces. (B) Note the absence of fibrin and hemosiderin-laden macrophages. Also, the interstitium has no evidence of cellular reaction.

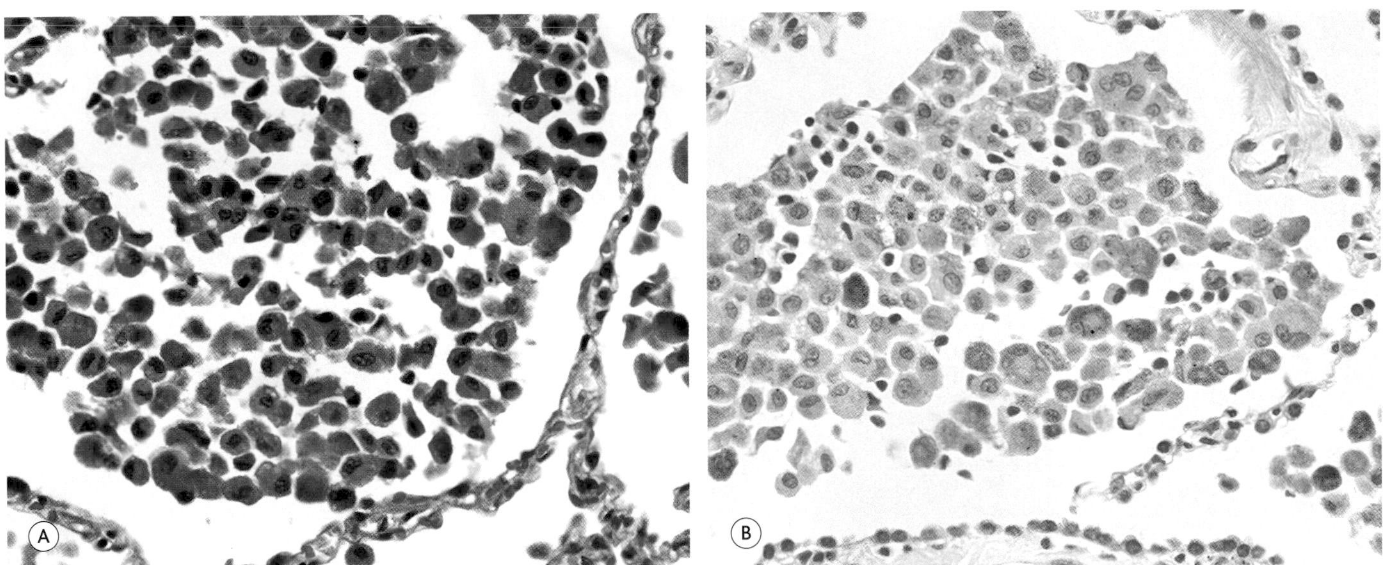

Fig. 10.54 **Diffuse alveolar hemorrhage: iron in smokers' macrophages.** (A) The pigmented macrophages of smokers can contain iron in their cytoplasm evident as granular brown material. (B) An iron stain will show this phenomenon.

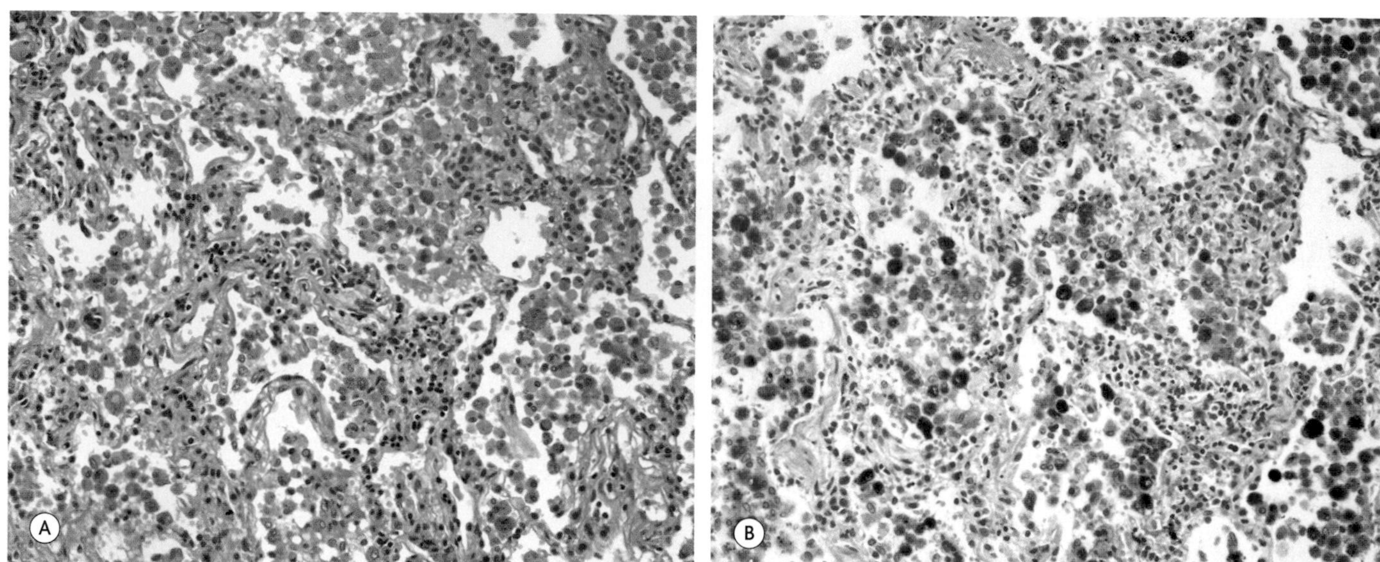

Fig. 10.55 **Diffuse alveolar hemorrhage: iron in smokers' macrophages.** (A) Caution is advised in interpreting pigment in macrophages. (B) Here, a smoker's macrophages contain abundant hemosiderin. Other findings of immunologically mediated hemorrhage are not seen.

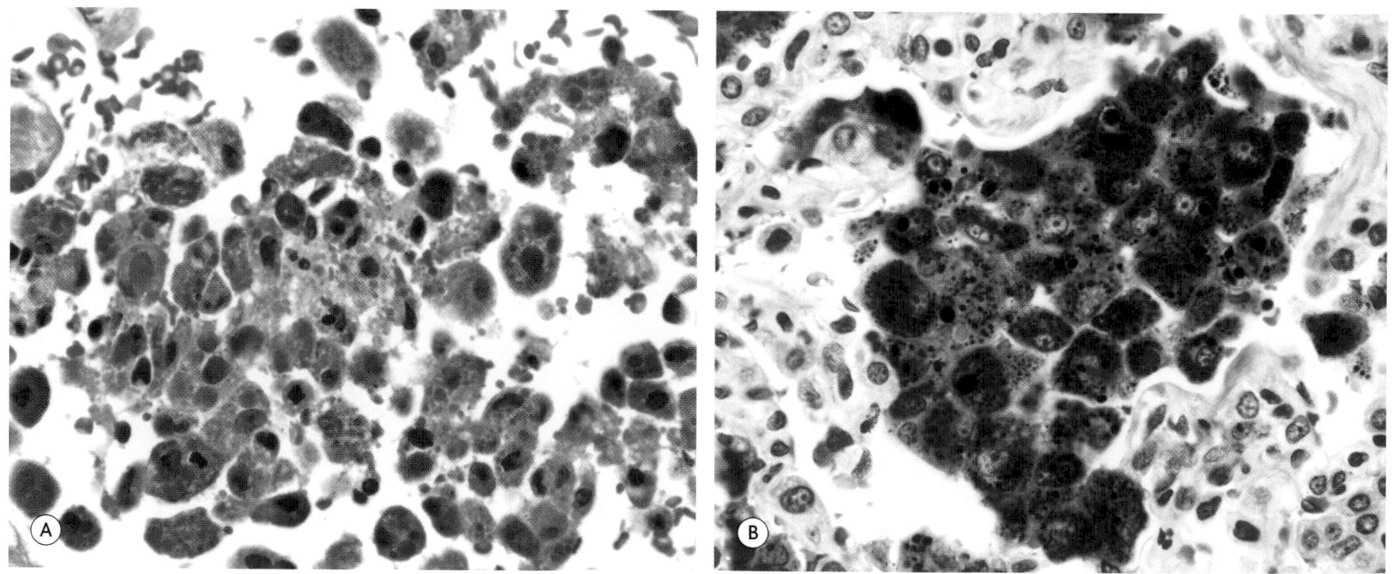

Fig. 10.56 **Diffuse alveolar hemorrhage: true hemosiderin-laden macrophages of hemorrhage.** (A) In contrast to smokers' macrophages with iron, true siderophages have granular refractile hemosiderin, which aggregates into large and small globular particles. (B) An iron stain accentuates this phenomenon.

Table 10.14 Causes of diffuse alveolar hemorrhage

With pulmonary capillaritis
- Wegener's granulomatosis
- Microscopic polyangiitis
- Isolated pulmonary capillaritis
- Connective tissue diseases
- Primary antiphospholipid syndrome
- Mixed cryoglobulinemia
- Behçet's syndrome
- Henoch–Schönlein purpura
- Goodpasture's syndrome
- Pauci-immune glomerulonephritis
- Immune complex-associated glomerulonephritis
- Drug-induced
- Acute lung allograft rejection

Without pulmonary capillaritis
- Idiopathic pulmonary hemosiderosis
- Systemic lupus erythematosus
- Goodpasture's syndrome
- Diffuse alveolar damage
- Penicillamine
- Trimellitic anhydride
- Mitral stenosis
- Coagulation disorders
- Pulmonary veno-occlusive disease
- Pulmonary capillary hemangiomatosis
- Lymphangioleiomyomatosis/tuberous sclerosis
- Human immunodeficiency virus infection
- Neoplasms (e.g. metastatic angiosarcoma, choriocarcinoma)

Source: from Colby et al.,[162] with permission.

Specific forms of diffuse alveolar hemorrhage

Goodpasture's syndrome (antiglomerular basement membrane antibody disease)

Goodpasture's syndrome (GS) affects individuals of all ages and both sexes, but the typical patient is a young male smoker.[164] Circulating antibodies directed against the non-collagenous domain of the alpha 3 chain of collagen type IV are identified in patient's with Goodpasture's syndrome. Using immunolocalization techniques, these antibodies can also be detected in the lung and kidney, where they are deposited in association with basement membranes. The histopathology of GS in the lung is not specific and resembles other diffuse alveolar hemorrhage syndromes (Fig. 10.57). Capillaritis may be present, but generally is not prominent.[165] Hyaline membranes may accompany the pulmonary hemorrhage of GS (Fig. 10.58).

Wegener's granulomatosis

A minority of patients with Wegener's granulomatosis (WG) present with pulmonary hemorrhage, although hemorrhage may occur in the course of the disease.[165] The typical systemic and serologic features of WG, as outlined

Table 10.15 Diffuse alveolar hemorrhage

	Goodpasture's syndrome	WG	MPA	SLE	IPH	Isolated pulmonary capillaritis	Henoch–Schönlein
Laboratory findings							
AGBA	Yes	No	No	No	No	No	No
C-ANCA	No	Usually	Occasional	No	No	No	NA
P-ANCA	No	Occasional	Usually	No	No	No	NA
ANA	No	No	No	Yes	No	No	NA
Extrapulmonary involvement							
Kidney	Yes	Often	Often	Often	No	No	Yes
Other organs	No	Often	Often	Sometimes	No	No	Yes
Pathologic findings							
Necrotizing capillaritis	Occasional, mild	Yes	Yes	Yes	Yes	Yes	Yes
Immunofluorescence	Linear	No	No	Granular	No	No	Yes
Electron-dense deposits	No	No	No	Yes	No	No	Yes

Abbreviations: AGBA, antiglomerular basement membrane antibody; WG, Wegener's granulomatosis; MPA, microscopic polyangiitis; SLE, systemic lupus erythematosus; IPH, idiopathic pulmonary hemosiderosis; NA, insufficient data.
Source: data from Lynch and Leatherman,[164] Schwarz et al,[168] Katzenstein,[185] and Jennette et al.[186]

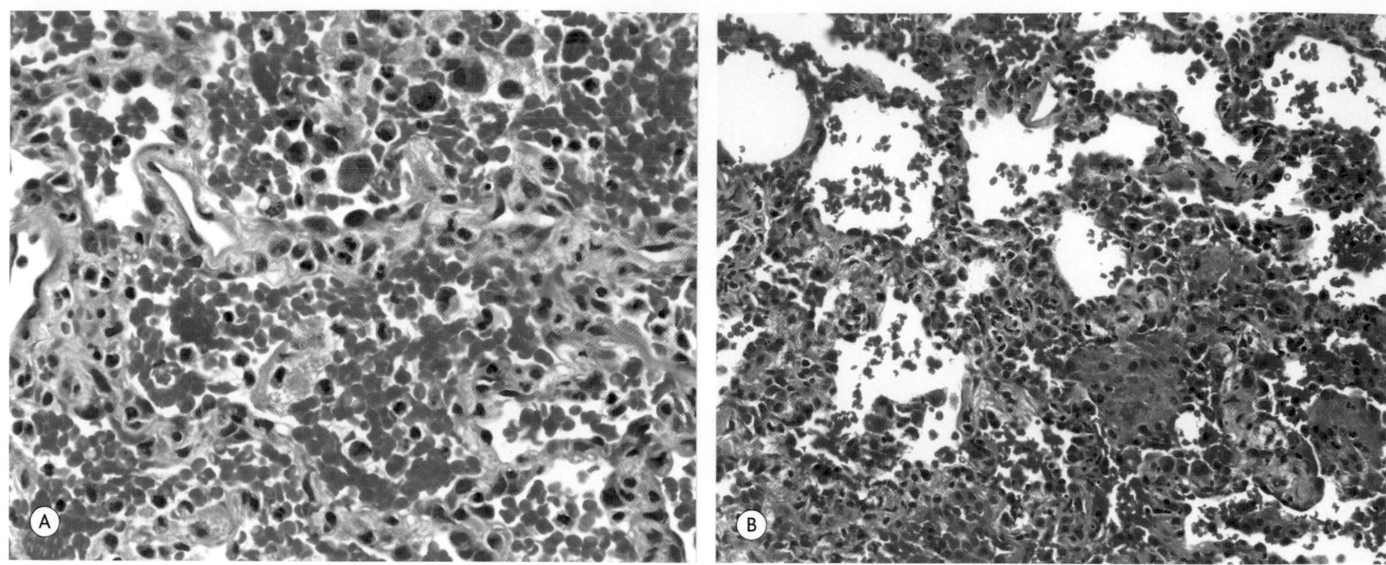

Fig. 10.57 **Goodpasture's syndrome: DAH with capillaritis.** (A) Alveolar hemorrhage with capillaritis is a typical finding of GS. (B) In some cases, the capillaritis may be quite cellular and prominent.

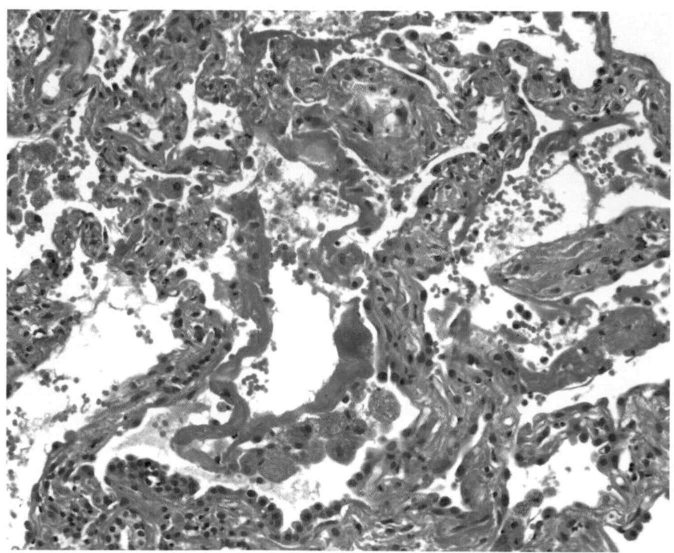

Fig. 10.58 **Goodpasture's syndrome: hyaline membranes.** As in other immune-mediated forms of alveolar hemorrhage, hyaline membranes may occur.

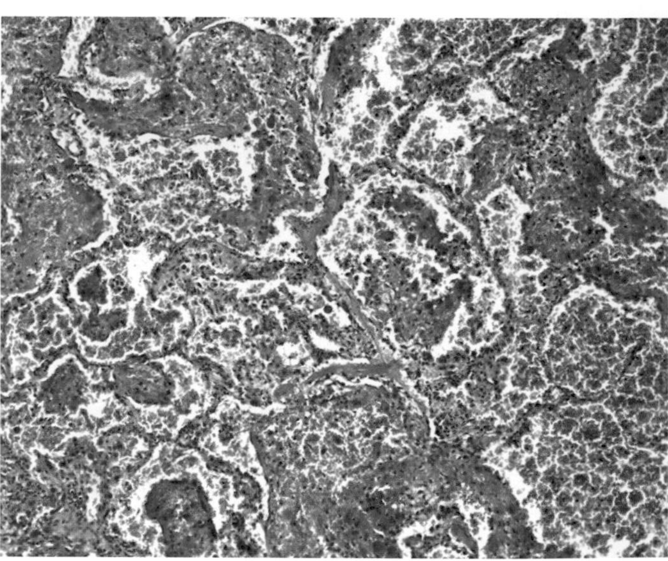

Fig. 10.59 **Wegener's granulomatosis: capillaritis.** Diffuse alveolar hemorrhage with capillaritis indistinguishable from other hemorrhage syndromes can be seen in WG. Here, airspace hemorrhage, fibrin, hemosiderin-laden macrophages, and capillaritis are all evident.

earlier, often accompany diffuse alveolar hemorrhage, making a clinical diagnosis possible even when the lung biopsy lacks diagnostic features. Diffuse alveolar hemorrhage in WG is often attended by dramatic capillaritis (Fig. 10.59). A careful search may reveal small foci of collagen necrosis, typically involving the adventitia of pulmonary arteries and the collagen surrounding bronchi and bronchioles. The presence of scattered giant cells may also be helpful in suggesting WG as a possible etiology for diffuse alveolar hemorrhage.

Microscopic polyangiitis

Microscopic polyangiitis has been discussed in detail earlier in this chapter. When alveolar hemorrhage dominates the presentation, distinction from alveolar hemorrhage in

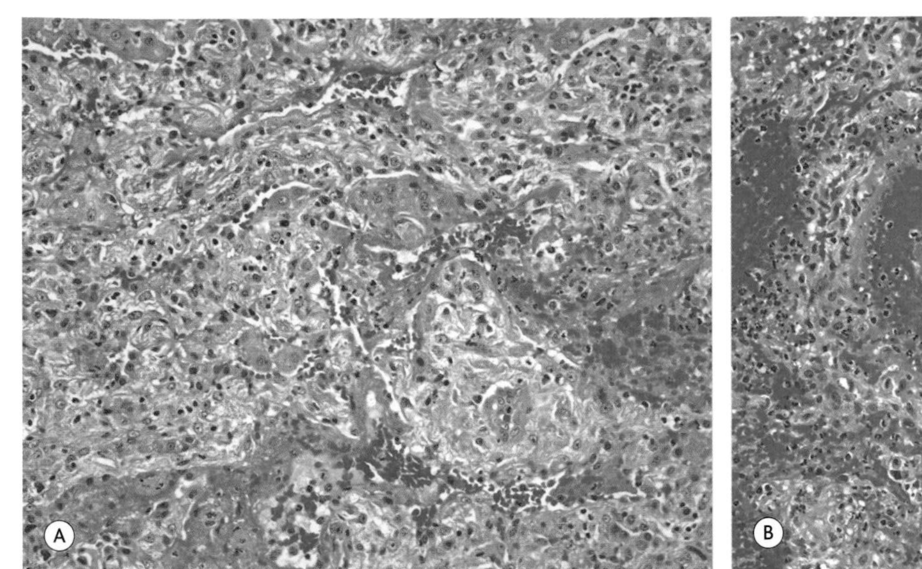

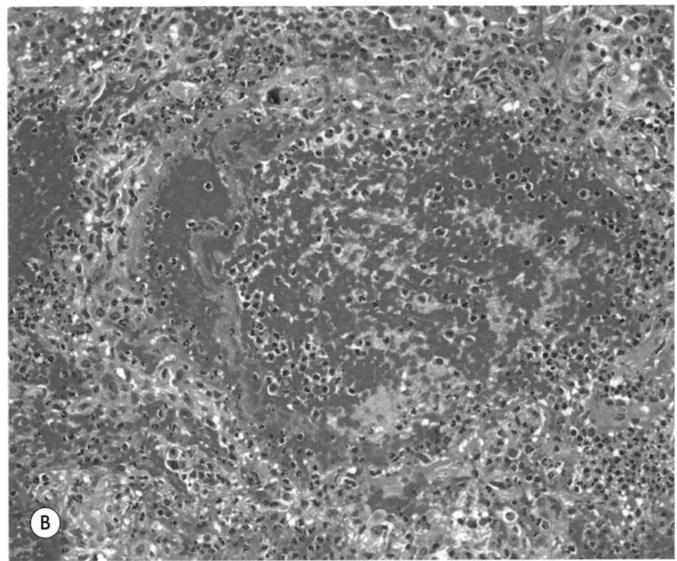

Fig. 10.60 **Microscopic polyangiitis: capillaritis.** (A) A case of microscopic polyangiitis, showing airspace fibrin and a cellular interstitium. (B) Another example, showing neutrophils filling alveolar spaces, resembling acute bronchopneumonia.

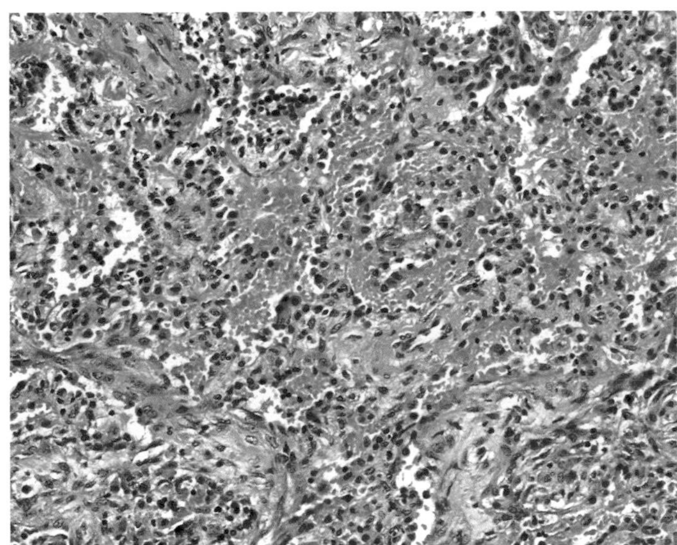

Fig. 10.61 **Systemic lupus erythematosus (SLE): capillaritis.** Alveolar hemorrhage with capillaritis can occur in SLE. Here, the picture is indistinguishable from that seen previously with GS, WG, and MPA.

Wegener's granulomatosis may be impossible on biopsy findings alone (Fig. 10.60). The frequency of extrathoracic site involvement in the two diseases and the common presence of P-ANCA in MPA usually suffice to differentiate them.

Systemic lupus erythematosus

Diffuse alveolar hemorrhage occurs more commonly in SLE than in any other connective tissue disease. Nevertheless, DHA is the presenting manifestation of the disease in only 11% of patients.[166] Patients with lupus nephritis are at increased risk for DHA. The histopathology of DAH in SLE is similar to that of other pulmonary hemorrhage syndromes, including the presence of capillaritis (Fig. 10.61).

Idiopathic pulmonary hemosiderosis

Idiopathic pulmonary hemosiderosis (IPH) affects children more commonly than adults and is characterized by recurrent episodes of DAH with hemoptysis. Patients are frequently anemic. An immunologic mechanism for the disease has not yet emerged and capillaritis is not seen. The histopathology of IPH is dominated by the presence of hemosiderin (Fig. 10.62). Interstitial widening with collagen deposition occurs over time.[167]

Henoch–Schönlein purpura

Like IPH, Henoch–Schönlein purpura affects children more often than adults.[106,164,166,168] Alveolar hemorrhage is rare and typically overshadowed by other systemic manifestations of the disease – such as involvement of the skin, joints, and kidneys. The histopathologic changes of pulmonary hemorrhage in Henoch–Schönlein pupura are nonspecific and resemble those of other pulmonary hemorrhage syndromes.

Isolated pulmonary capillaritis

Isolated pulmonary capillaritis is a rare form of diffuse alveolar hemorrhage in which no associated immunologic

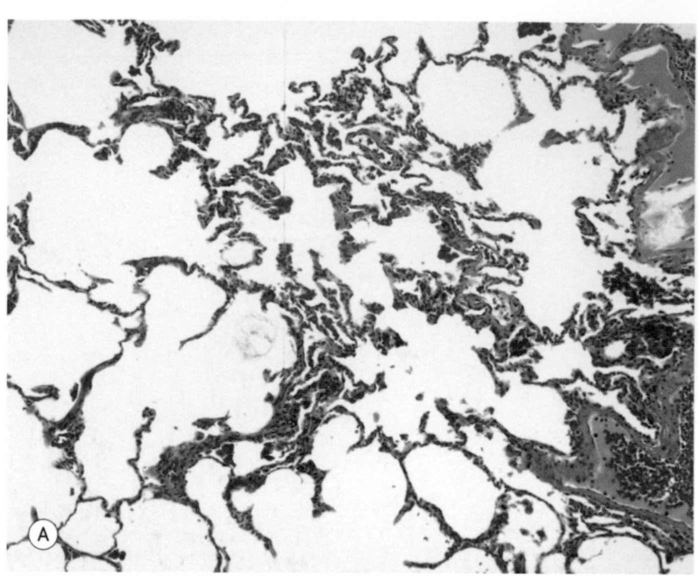

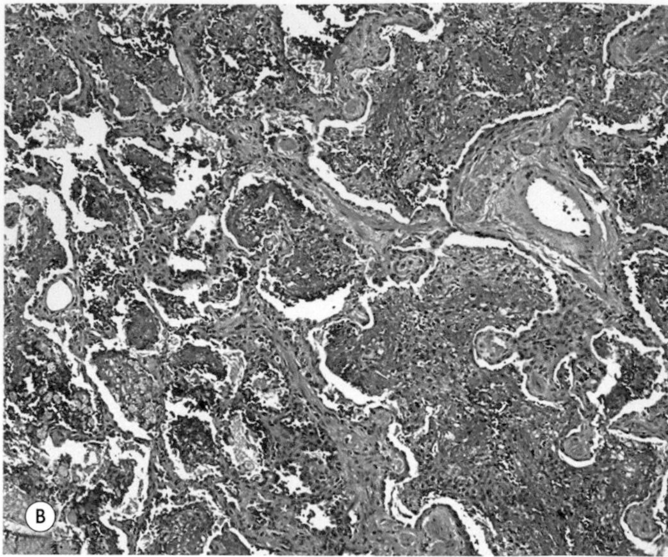

Fig. 10.62 **Idiopathic pulmonary hemosiderosis (IPH): mild hemosiderosis to fibrosis.** The hemosiderin deposition in IPH can be (A) mild or (B) prominently associated with interstitial thickening and airspace fibrin. Capillaritis and vasculitis are not expected findings in IPH.

or systemic manifestations are found. There may be overlap between this disorder, idiopathic pulmonary hemosiderosis in adults, and the group of diseases encompassed by Travis and coworkers as "idiopathic pulmonary hemorrhage".[54] The histopathology of isolated pulmonary capillaritis is similar to that of other alveolar hemorrhage syndromes that manifest capillaritis.

REFERENCES

1. Watts RA, Scott DG: Epidemiology of the vasculitides. Curr Opin Rheumatol 2003; 15(1): 11–16.
2. Travis W, Koss M: Vasculitis. In: Pulmonary pathology, Dail D, Hammar S, Eds. 1994, Springer-Verlag, New York, pp 1027–1095.
3. Guinee DJ, Jaffe E, Kingma D, et al.: Pulmonary lymphomatoid granulomatosis. Evidence for a proliferation of Epstein–Barr virus infected B-lymphocytes with a prominent T-cell component and vasculitis. Am J Surg Pathol 1994; 18: 753–764.
4. Nicholson A, Wotherspoon A, Diss T, et al.: Lymphomatoid granulomatosis: evidence that some cases represent Epstein–Barr virus-associated B-cell lymphoma. Histopathology 1996; 29: 317–324.
5. Wegener F: Generalized septic vascular diseases [translation]. Verh Dtsch Path Ges 1936; 29: 202–210.
6. Cotch M, Hoffman G, Yerg D, et al.: The epidemiology of Wegener's granulomatosis. Estimates of the five-year period prevalence, annual mortality, and geographic disease distribution from population-based data sources. Arthritis Rheum 1996; 39: 87–92.
7. Carruthers D, Watts R, Symmons D, et al.: Wegener's granulomatosis – increased incidence or increased recognition. Br J Rheumatol 1996; 35: 142–145.
8. George J, Levy Y, Kallenberg C, et al.: Infections and Wegener's granulomatosis – a cause and effect relationship. QJM 1997; 90: 367–373.
9. Hoffman G, Kerr G, Leavitt R, et al.: Wegener's granulomatosis: an analysis of 158 patients. Ann Intern Med 1992; 116: 488–498.
10. Roberti I, Reisman L, Churg J: Vasculitis in childhood. Pediatr Nephrol 1993; 7: 479–489.
11. Wadsworth D, Siegel M, Day D: Wegener's granulomatosis in children: chest radiographic manifestations. AJR Am J Roentgenol 1994; 163: 901–904.
12. Langford C, Hoffman G: Wegener's granulomatosis. Thorax 1999; 54: 629–637.
13. Colby T, Specks U: Wegener's granulomatosis in the 1990s – a pulmonary pathologists perspective. In: The lung. Current concepts, Churg A, Katzenstein A-L, Eds. 1993, Williams & Wilkins, Baltimore, pp 195–218.
14. Travis W: Common and uncommon manifestations of Wegener's granulomatosis. Cardiovasc Pathol 1994; 3: 217–225.
15. Goulart R, Mark E, Rosen S: Tumefactions as an extravascular manifestation of Wegener's granulomatosis. Am J Surg Pathol 1995; 19: 145–153.
16. Gross W, Csernok E: Immunodiagnostic and pathophysiologic aspects of antineutrophil cytoplasmic antibodies in vasculitis. Curr Opin Rheumatol 1995; 7: 11–19.
17. Jennette J, Falk R, Wilkman A: Anti-neutrophilic antibodies – a serologic marker for vasculitides. Ann Acad Med Singapore 1995; 24: 248–253.
18. Specks U: Pulmonary vasculitis. In: Interstitial lung disease, Schwarz M, King T, Eds. 1998, B.C. Decker, Inc., Hamilton, pp 507–534.
19. Gross W, Schnabel A, Trabandt A: New perspectives in pulmonary angiitis. From pulmonary angiitis and granulomatosis to ANCA associated vasculitis. Sarcoidosis Vasc Diffuse Lung Dis 2000; 17: 33–52.
20. Schultz D, Diego J: Antineutrophil cytoplasmic antibodies (ANCA) and systemic vasculitis: update of assays, immunopathogenesis, controversies, and report of a novel de novo ANCA-associated vasculitis after kidney transplantation. Semin Arthritis Rheum 2000; 29: 267–285.
21. Davenport A, Lock R, Wallington T: Clinical relevance of testing for antineutrophil cytoplasm antibodies (ANCA) with a standard indirect immunofluorescence ANCA test in patients with upper or lower respiratory tract symptoms. Thorax 1994; 49: 213–217.
22. Nölle B, Specks U, Lüdemann J, et al.: Anticytoplasmic autoantibodies: their immunodiagnostic value in Wegener's granulomatosis. Ann Intern Med 1989; 111: 28–40.
23. Jennette J, Charles L, Falk R: Anti-neutrophil cytoplasmic autoantibodies: disease associations, molecular biology, and pathophysiology. Int Rev Exp Pathol 1991; 32: 193–221.
24. Gal A, Salinas F, Staton GJ: The clinical and pathological spectrum of antineutrophil cytoplasmic autoantibody-related pulmonary disease.

A comparison between perinuclear and cytoplasmic antineutrophil cytoplasmic autoantibodies. Arch Pathol Lab Med 1994; 118: 1209–1214.
25. Gaudin P, Askin F, Falk R, et al.: The pathologic spectrum of pulmonary lesions in patients with anti-neutrophil cytoplasmic autoantibodies specific for anti-proteinase 3 and anti-myeloperoxidase [see comments]. Am J Clin Pathol 1995; 104: 7–16.
26. Schnabel A, Reuter M, Csernok E, et al.: Subclinical alveolar bleeding in pulmonary vasculitides: correlation with indices of disease activity. Eur Respir J 1999; 14(1): 118–124.
27. Jennings C, Jones N, Dugar J, et al.: Wegener's granulomatosis – a review of diagnosis and treatment in 53 patients. Rhinology 1998; 36(4): 188–191.
28. Feigin D: Vasculitis in the lung. J Thorac Imaging 1988; 3: 33–48.
29. Cordier J-F, Valeyre D, Guillevin L, et al.: Pulmonary Wegener's granulomatosis. A clinical and imaging study of 77 cases. Chest 1990; 97: 906–912.
30. Fraser, RS, Pare J, Fraser R, et al.: Diseases of altered immunologic activity. In: Synopsis of diseases of the chest, Fraser R, Pare J, Eds. 1994, WB Saunders, Philadelphia, pp 392–443.
31. Staples C: Pulmonary angiitis and granulomatosis. Radiol Clin North Am 1991; 29: 973–982.
32. Farrelly C: Wegener's granulomatosis: a radiological review of the pulmonary manifestations at initial presentation and during relapse. Clin Radiol 1982; 33: 545–551.
33. Aberle D, Gamsu G, Lynch D: Thoracic manifestations of Wegener granulomatosis: diagnosis and course. Radiology 1990; 174: 703–709.
34. Katzenstein A, Locke W: Solitary lung lesions in Wegener's granulomatosis. Pathologic findings and clinical significance in 25 cases. Am J Surg Pathol 1995; 19: 545–552.
35. Kuhlman J, Hruban R, Fishman E: Wegener granulomatosis: CT features of parenchymal lung disease. J Comput Assist Tomogr 1991; 15: 948–952.
36. Primack S, Hartman T, Lee K, et al.: Pulmonary nodules and the CT halo sign. Radiology 1994; 190: 513–515.
37. Daum T, Specks U, Colby T, et al.: Tracheobronchial involvement in Wegener's granulomatosis. Am J Respir Crit Care Med 1995; 151: 522–526.
38. Maguire R, Fauci A, Doppman J, et al.: Unusual radiographic features of Wegener's granulomatosis. AJR Am J Roentgenol 1978; 130: 233–238.
39. Travis W, Hoffman G, RY L, et al.: Surgical pathology of the lung in Wegener's granulomatosis. Review of 87 open lung biopsies from 67 patients. Am J Surg Pathol 1991; 15: 315–333.
40. Ulbright T, Katzenstein A: Solitary necrotizing granulomas of the lung: differentiating features and etiology. Am J Surg Pathol 1980; 4: 13–28.
41. Yousem SA: Bronchocentric injury in Wegener's granulomatosis: a report of five cases. Hum Pathol 1991; 22: 535–540.
42. Uner A, Rozum-Slota B, Katzenstein A: Bronchiolitis obliterans-organizing pneumonia (BOOP)-like variant of Wegener's granulomatosis. A clinicopathologic study of 16 cases. Am J Surg Pathol 1996; 20: 794–801.
43. Mark E, Flieder D, Matsubara O: Treated Wegener's granulomatosis: distinctive pathological findings in the lungs of 20 patients and what they tell us about the natural history of the disease. Hum Pathol 1997; 28: 450–458.
44. Koss M, Hochholzer L, Feigin D, et al.: Necrotizing sarcoid-like granulomatosis: clinical, pathologic, and immunopathologic findings. Human Pathol 1980; 11(5) (suppl): 510–519.
45. Lipford E Jr , Margolick J, Longo D, et al.: Angiocentric immunoproliferative lesions: a clinicopathologic spectrum of post-thymic T-cell proliferations. Blood 1988; 72: 1674–1681.
46. Churg J, Strauss L: Allergic granulomatosis, allergic angiitis and periarteritis nodosa. Am J Pathol 1951; 27: 277–294.
47. Chumbley L, Harrison E Jr , DeRemee R: Allergic granulomatosis and angiitis (Churg–Strauss syndrome). Report and analysis of 30 cases. Mayo Clin Proc 1977; 52: 477–484.
48. Koss M, Antonovych T, Hochholzer L: Allergic granulomatosis (Churg–Strauss syndrome). Am J Surg Pathol 1981; 5: 21–28.
49. Lanham J, Elkon K, Pusey C, et al.: Systemic vasculitis with asthma and eosinophilia: a clinical approach to the Churg–Strauss syndrome. Medicine (Baltimore) 1984; 63: 65–81.
50. Churg A, Carrington C, Gupta R: Necrotizing sarcoid granulomatosis. Chest 1979; 76: 406–413.
51. Churg A: Pulmonary angiitis and granulomatosis revisited. Hum Pathol 1983; 14: 868–883.
52. Koss M, Robinson R, Hochholzer L: Bronchocentric granulomatosis. Hum Pathol 1981; 12: 632–638.
53. Mark E, Ramirez J: Pulmonary capillaritis and hemorrhage in patients with systemic vasculitis. Arch Pathol Lab Med 1985; 109: 413–418.
54. Travis W, Colby T, Lombard C, et al.: A clinicopathologic study of 34 cases of diffuse pulmonary hemorrhage with lung biopsy confirmation. Am J Surg Pathol 1990; 14: 1112–1125.
55. Myers J, Kurtin P, Katzenstein A, et al.: Lymphomatoid granulomatosis. Evidence of immunophenotypic diversity and relationship to Epstein–Barr virus infection. Am J Surg Pathol 1995; 19: 1300–1312.
56. Churg J: Allergic granulomatosis and granulomatous-vascular syndromes. Ann Allergy 1963; 21: 619–628.
57. Lanham J, Churg J: Churg–Strauss syndrome. In: Systemic vasculitides, Churg A, Churg J, Eds. 1991, Igaku-Shoin, New York, pp 101–120.
58. Specks U, DeRemee R: Granulomatous vasculitis. Wegener's granulomatosis and Churg– Strauss syndrome. Rheum Dis Clin North Am 1990; 16: 377–397.
59. Fienberg R, Mark E, Goodman M, et al.: Correlation of antineutrophil cytoplasmic antibodies with the extrarenal histopathology of Wegener's (pathergic) granulomatosis and related forms of vasculitis. Hum Pathol 1993; 24: 160–168.
60. Fauci A, Haynes B, Katz P, et al.: Wegener's granulomatosis: prospective clinical and therapeutic experience with 85 patients over 21 years. Ann Intern Med 1983; 98: 76–85.
61. DeRemee R, McDonald T, Weiland L: Wegener's granulomatosis: observations on treatment with antimicrobial agents. Mayo Clin Proc 1985; 60: 27–32.
62. Langford C, Sneller M: New developments in the treatment of Wegener's granulomatosis, polyarteritis nodosa, microscopic polyangiitis, and Churg–Strauss syndrome. Curr Opin Rheumatol 1997; 9: 26–30.
63. Langford C, Sneller M: Update on the diagnosis and treatment of Wegener's granulomatosis. Adv Intern Med 2001; 46: 177–206.
64. Stegeman C, Tervaert J, de Jong P, et al.: Trimethoprim–sulfamethoxazole (co-trimoxazole) for the prevention of relapses of Wegener's granulomatosis. Dutch Co- Trimoxazole Wegener Study Group [see comments]. N Engl J Med 1996; 335: 16–20.
65. Travis W, Koss M: Pulmonary angiitis and granulomatosis: necrotizing sarcoid granulomatosis and Churg–Strauss syndrome. In: Pathology of pulmonary disease, Saldana M, Ed. 1994, JB Lippincott, Philadelphia, pp 803–809.
66. Sehgal M, Swanson J, DeRemee R, et al.: Neurologic manifestations of Churg–Strauss syndrome. Mayo Clin Proc 1995; 70: 337–341.
67. Masi A, Hunder G, Lie J, et al.: The American College of Rheumatology 1990 criteria for the classification of Churg–Strauss syndrome (allergic granulomatosis and angiitis). Arthritis Rheum 1990; 33: 1094–1100.
68. Lie J: Illustrated histopathologic classification criteria for selected vasculitis syndromes. American College of Rheumatology Subcommittee on Classification of Vasculitis. Arthritis Rheum 1990; 33: 1074–1087.
69. Sasaki A, Hasegawa M, Nakazato Y, et al.: Allergic granulomatosis and angiitis (Churg–Strauss syndrome). Report of an autopsy case in a nonasthmatic patient. Acta Pathol Jpn 1988; 38: 761–768.
70. Gambari P, Ostuni P, Lazzarin P, et al.: Eosinophilic granuloma and necrotizing vasculitis (Churg–Strauss syndrome) involving a parotid gland, lymph nodes, liver and spleen. Scand J Rheumatol 1989; 18: 171–175.
71. Lipworth B, Slater D, Corrin B, et al.: Allergic granulomatosis without asthma: a rare 'forme fruste' of the Churg–Strauss syndrome. Respir Med 1989; 83: 249–250.
72. Larson T, Hall S, Hepper N, et al.: Respiratory tract symptoms as a clue to giant cell arteritis. Ann Intern Med 1984; 101: 594–597.
73. Guillevin L, Lhote F, Gayraud M, et al.: Prognostic factors in polyarteritis nodosa and Churg–Strauss syndrome. A prospective study in 342 patients. Medicine (Baltimore) 1996; 75: 17–28.
74. Cluttterbuck E, Pusey C: Severe alveolar hemorrhage in Churg–Strauss syndrome. Eur J Respir Dis 1987; 71: 158–163.
75. Gibson L: Granulomatous vasculitides and the skin. Dermatol Clin 1990; 8: 335–345.

76. Olsen KD, Neel HB 3rd, Deremee RA, et al.: Nasal manifestations of allergic granulomatosis and angiitis (Churg–Strauss syndrome). Otolaryngol Head Neck Surg 1980; 88(1): 85–89.
77. Fraioli P, Barberis M, Rizzato G: Gastrointestinal presentation of Churg Strauss syndrome. Sarcoidosis 1994; 11: 42–45.
78. Harrison D, Simpson R, Kharbanda R, et al.: Antibodies to neutrophil cytoplasmic antigens in Wegener's granulomatosis and other conditions. Thorax 1989; 44: 373–377.
79. Churg J, Churg A: Zafirlukast and Churg–Strauss syndrome [letter; comment]. JAMA 1998; 279: 1949–1950.
80. Green R, Vayonis A: Churg–Strauss syndrome after zafirlukast in two patients not receiving systemic steroid treatment [letter]. Lancet 1999; 353: 725–726.
81. Holloway J, Ferriss J, Groff J, et al.: Churg–Strauss syndrome associated with zafirlukast [published erratum appears in J Am Osteopath Assoc 1998; 98(12): 676]. J Am Osteopath Assoc 1998; 98: 275–278.
82. Frosi A, Foresi A, Fozzoni M, et al.: Churg–Strauss syndrome and antiasthma therapy [letter; comment]. Lancet 1999; 353: 1102.
83. Wechsler M, Finn D, Gunawardena D, et al.: Churg–Strauss syndrome in patients receiving montelukast as treatment for asthma. Chest 2000; 117: 708–713.
84. Orriols R, Munoz X, Ferrer J, et al.: Cocaine-induced Churg–Strauss vasculitis. Eur Respir J 1996; 9: 175–177.
85. Churg A, Brallas M, Cronin S, et al.: Formes frustes of Churg–Strauss syndrome. Chest 1995; 108: 320–323.
86. Amundson D: Cavitary pulmonary cryptococcosis complicating Churg–Strauss vasculitis. South Med J 1992; 85: 700–702.
87. Worthy S, Muller N, Hansell D, et al.: Churg–Strauss syndrome: the spectrum of pulmonary CT findings in 17 patients. AJR Am J Roentgenol 1998; 170: 297–300.
88. Buschman D, Waldron J Jr , King TJ: Churg–Strauss pulmonary vasculitis. High-resolution computed tomography scanning and pathologic findings. Am Rev Respir Dis 1990; 142: 458–461.
89. Lai R, Lin S, NS L, et al.: Churg–Strauss syndrome presenting with pulmonary capillaritis and diffuse alveolar hemorrhage. Scand J Rheumatol 1998; 27: 230–232.
90. Travis W, Kwon-Chung K, Kleiner D, et al.: Unusual aspects of allergic bronchopulmonary fungal disease: report of two cases due to *Curvularia* organisms associated with allergic fungal sinusitis. Hum Pathol 1991; 22: 1240–1248.
91. Brill R, Churg J, Beaver P: Allergic granulomatosis associated with visceral larva migrans. Am J Clin Pathol 1953; 23: 1208–1215.
92. Imai H, Nakamoto Y, Hirokawa M, et al.: Carbamazepine-induced granulomatous necrotizing angiitis with acute renal failure. Nephron 1989; 51: 405–408.
93. Strazzella W, Safirstein B: Asthma due to parasitic infestation. N J Med 1989; 89: 947–949.
94. Guillevin L, Cohen P, Gayraud M, et al.: Churg–Strauss syndrome. Clinical study and long-term follow-up of 96 patients. Medicine (Baltimore) 1999; 78: 26–37.
95. Abu-Shakra M, Smythe H, Lewtas J, et al.: Outcome of polyarteritis nodosa and Churg–Strauss syndrome. An analysis of twenty-five patients. Arthritis Rheum 1994; 37: 1798–1803.
96. Calabrese L, Michel B, Bloch D, et al.: The American College of Rheumatology 1990 criteria for the classification of hypersensitivity vasculitis. Arthritis Rheum 1990; 33: 1108–1113.
97. Churg J: Nomenclature of vasculitic syndromes: a historical perspective. Am J Kidney Dis 1991; 18: 148–153.
98. Leavitt R, Travis W, Fauci A: Vasculitis. In: Respiratory disease in the immunosuppressed host, Shelhamer J, Pizzo P, Parrillo J, et al., Eds. 1991, JB Lippincott, Philadelphia, pp 703–727.
99. Swerlick R, Lawley T: Small-vessel vasculitis and cutaneous vasculitis. In: Systemic vasculitides, Churg A, Churg J, Eds. 1991, Igaku-Shoin, New York, pp 193–201.
100. Jennette J, Falk R, Andrassy K, et al.: Nomenclature of systemic vasculitis. Arthritis Rheum 1994; 37: 187–192.
101. Jennette J, Falk R: Small-vessel vasculitis. N Engl J Med 1997; 337: 1512–1523.
102. Lauque D, Cadranel J, Lazor R, et al.: Microscopic polyangiitis with alveolar hemorrhage. A study of 29 cases and review of the literature. Groupe d'Etudes et de Recherche sur les Maladies Orphelines; Pulmonaires. Medicine (Baltimore) 2000; 79: 222–233.
103. Akikusa B, Kondo Y, Irabu N, et al.: Six cases of microscopic polyarteritis exhibiting acute interstitial pneumonia [published erratum appears in Pathol Int 1995; 45(11): 901]. Pathol Int 1995; 45: 580–588.
104. Brugiere O, Raffy O, Sleiman C, et al.: Progressive obstructive lung disease associated with microscopic polyangiitis. Am J Respir Crit Care Med 1997; 155: 739–742.
105. Schwarz M, Mortenson R, Colby T, et al.: Pulmonary capillaritis. The association with progressive irreversible airflow limitation and hyperinflation. Am Rev Respir Dis 1993; 148: 507–511.
106. Green R, Ruoss S, Kraft S, et al.: Pulmonary capillaritis and alveolar hemorrhage. Update on diagnosis and management. Chest 1996; 110(5): 1305–1316.
107. Churg J, Churg A: Idiopathic and secondary vasculitis: A review. Mod Pathol 1989; 2: 144–160.
108. Tauber E, Wojnarowski C, Horcher E, et al.: Necrotizing sarcoid granulomatosis in a 14-yr-old female. Eur Respir J 1999; 13: 703–705.
109. Beach R, Corrin B, Scopes J, et al.: Necrotizing sarcoid granulomatosis with neurologic lesions in a child. J Pediatr 1980; 97: 950–953.
110. Singh N, Cole S, Krause P, et al.: Necrotizing sarcoid granulomatosis with extrapulmonary involvement. Clinical, pathologic, ultrastructural, and immunologic features. Am Rev Respir Dis 1981; 124: 189–192.
111. Stephen J, Braimbridge M, Corrin B, et al.: Necrotizing 'sarcoidal' angiitis and granulomatosis of the lung. Thorax 1976; 31: 356–360.
112. Niimi H, Hartman T, Muller N: Necrotizing sarcoid granulomatosis: computed tomography and pathologic findings. J Comput Assist Tomogr 1995; 19: 920–923.
113. Le Gall F, Loeuillet L, Delaval P, et al.: Necrotizing sarcoid granulomatosis with and without extrapulmonary involvement. Pathol Res Pract 1996; 192: 306–313.
114. Dykhuizen R, Smith C, Kennedy M, et al.: Necrotizing sarcoid granulomatosis with extrapulmonary involvement. Eur Respir J 1997; 10: 245–247.
115. Chittock D, Joseph M, Paterson N, et al.: Necrotizing sarcoid granulomatosis with pleural involvement. Clinical and radiographic features. Chest 1994; 106: 672–676.
116. Liebow A: The J. Burns Amberson lecture – pulmonary angiitis and granulomatosis. Am Rev Respir Dis 1973; 108: 1–18.
117. Rolfes D, Weiss M, Sanders M: Necrotizing sarcoid granulomatosis with suppurative features. Am J Clin Pathol 1984; 82: 602–607.
118. Spiteri M, Gledhill A, Campbell D, et al.: Necrotizing sarcoid granulomatosis. Br J Dis Chest 1987; 81: 70–75.
119. Rodat O, Buzelin F, Weber M, et al.: Manifestations broncho-pulmonaires de la maladie de Horton: A propos d'une observation. Rev Med Interne 1983; 4: 225–230.
120. Bradley J, Pinals R, Blumenfeld H, et al.: Giant cell arteritis with pulmonary nodules. Am J Med 1984; 77: 135–140.
121. Karam G, Fulmer J: Giant cell arteritis presenting as interstitial lung disease. Chest 1982; 82: 781–789.
122. Ladanyi M, Fraser R: Pulmonary involvement in giant cell arteritis. Arch Pathol Lab Med 1987; 111: 1178–1180.
123. Wagenaar S, Westermann C, Corrin B: Giant cell arteritis limited to large elastic pulmonary arteries. Thorax 1981; 36: 876–877.
124. Wagenaar S, van den Bosch J, Westermann C, et al.: Isolated granulomatous giant cell vasculitis of the pulmonary elastic arteries. Arch Pathol Lab Med 1986; 110: 962–964.
125. Okubo S, Kuneida T, Ando M, et al.: Idiopathic isolated pulmonary arteritis with chronic cor pulmonale. Chest 1988; 94: 665–666.
126. Lie J: Disseminated visceral giant cell arteritis. Histopathologic description and differentiation from other granulomatous vasculitides. Am J Clin Pathol 1978; 69: 299–305.
127. Morita T, Kamimura A, Koizumi F: Disseminated visceral giant cell arteritis. Acta Pathol Jpn 1987; 37: 863–870.
128. Marcussen N, Lund C: Combined sarcoidosis and disseminated visceral giant cell vasculitis. Path Res Pract 1989; 184: 325–330.
129. Shintaku M, Mase K, Ohtsuki H, et al.: Generalized sarcoidlike granulomas with systemic angiitis, crescentic glomerulonephritis, and pulmonary hemorrhage. Report of an autopsy case. Arch Pathol Lab Med 1989; 113: 1295–1298.
130. Lie J: Combined sarcoidosis and disseminated visceral giant cell angiitis: a third opinion (letter). Arch Pathol Lab Med 1991; 115: 210–211.
131. DeRemee R, Weiland L, McDonald T: Respiratory vasculitis. Mayo Clin Proc 1980; 55: 492–498.
132. Leavitt R, Fauci A: Pulmonary vasculitis. Am Rev Respir Dis 1986; 134: 149–166.

133. Rosen S, Falk R, Jennette J: Polyarteritis nodosa, including microscopic form and renal vasculitis. In: Systemic vasculitides, Churg A, Churg J, Eds. 1991, Igaku-Shoin, New York, pp 57–77.
134. Arend W, Michel B, Bloch D, et al.: The American College of Rheumatology 1990 criteria for the classification of Takayasu arteritis. Arthritis Rheum 1990; 33: 1129–1134.
135. He N, Liu F, Wu E, et al.: Pulmonary artery involvement in aorto-arteritis. An analysis of DSA. Chin Med J (Engl) 1990; 103: 666–672.
136. Sharma S, Kamalaka T, Rajani M, et al.: The incidence and patterns of pulmonary artery involvement in Takayasu's arteritis. Clin Radiol 1990; 42: 177–181.
137. Sharma S, Rajani M, Shrivastava S, et al.: Non-specific aorto-arteritis (Takayasu's disease) in children. Br J Radiol 1991; 64: 690–698.
138. Nakabayashi K, Kurata N, Nangi N, et al.: Pulmonary artery involvement as first manifestation in three cases of Takayasu arteritis. Int J Cardiol 1997; 54: S177–S83.
139. Sharma B, Jain S, Sagar S: Systemic manifestations of Takayasu arteritis: the expanding spectrum. Int J Cardiol 1997; 54(suppl): S149–S154.
140. Lie J: Takayasu's arteritis. In: Systemic vasculitides, Churg A, Churg J, Eds. 1991, Igaku-Shoin, New York, pp 159–179.
141. Horimoto M, Igarashi K, Aoi K, et al.: Unilateral diffuse pulmonary artery involvement in Takayasu's arteritis associated with coronary–pulmonary artery fistula and bronchial–pulmonary artery fistula: a case report. Angiology 1991; 42: 73–80.
142. Takahashi K, Honda M, Furuse M, et al.: CT findings of pulmonary parenchyma in Takayasu arteritis. J Comput Assist Tomogr 1996; 20: 742–748.
143. Rose A, Sinclair-Smith C: Takayasu's arteritis. A study of 16 autopsy cases. Arch Pathol Lab Med 1980; 104: 231–237.
144. Matsubara O, Yoshimura N, Tamura A, et al.: Pathological features of the pulmonary artery in Takayasu arteritis. Heart Vessels 1992; 7: 18–25.
145. Jakob H, R V, Stangl G, et al.: Surgical correction of a severely obstructed pulmonary artery bifurcation in Takayasu's arteritis. Eur J Cardiothorac Surg 1990; 4: 456–458.
146. Direskeneli H: Behçet's disease: infectious aetiology, new autoantigens and HLA-B51. Ann Rheum Dis 2001; 60(11): 996–1002.
147. Fairley C, Wilson J, Barraclough D: Pulmonary involvement in Behçet's syndrome. Chest 1989; 96: 1428–1429.
148. Raz I, Okon E, Chajek-Shaul T: Pulmonary manifestations in Behçet's syndrome. Chest 1989; 95: 585–589.
149. Efthimiou J, Johnston C, Spiro S, et al.: Pulmonary disease in Behçet's syndrome. Q J Med 1986; 58: 259–280.
150. Gamble C, Wiesner K, Shapiro R, et al.: The immune complex pathogenesis of glomerulonephritis and pulmonary vasculitis in Behçet's disease. Am J Med 1979; 66: 1031–1039.
151. Ahn J, Im J, Ryoo J, et al.: Thoracic manifestations of Behçet syndrome: radiographic and CT findings in nine patients. Radiology 1995; 194: 199–203.
152. Tunaci A, Berkmen Y, Gokmen E: Thoracic involvement in Behçet's disease: pathologic, clinical, and imaging features. AJR Am J Roentgenol 1995; 164: 51–56.
153. Slavin R, de Groot W: Pathology of the lung in Behçet's disease. Case report and review of the literature. Am J Surg Pathol 1981; 5: 779–788.
154. Lakhanpal S, Tani K, Lie J, et al.: Pathologic features of Behçet's syndrome: a review of Japanese autopsy registry data. Hum Pathol 1985; 16: 790–795.
155. Salamon F, Weinberger A, Nili M, et al.: Massive hemoptysis complicating Behçet's syndrome: the importance of early pulmonary angiography and operation. Ann Thorac Surg 1988; 45: 566–567.
156. Corren J: Acute interstitial pneumonia in a patient with Behcet's syndrome and common variable immunodeficiency [clinical conference]. Ann Allergy 1990; 64: 15–20.
157. Soave R, Murray H, Litrenta M: Bacterial invasion of pulmonary vessels. *Pseudomonas* bacteremia mimicking pulmonary thromboembolism with infarction. Am J Med 1978; 65: 864–867.
158. Winn W, Myerowitz R: The pathology of the *Legionella* pneumonias. A review of 74 cases and the literature. Hum Pathol 1981; 12: 401–422.
159. Travis W, Pittaluga S, Lipschik G, et al.: Atypical pathologic manifestations of *Pneumocystis carinii* pneumonia in the acquired immune deficiency syndrome. Review of 123 lung biopsies from 76 patients with emphasis on cysts, vascular invasion, vasculitis, and granulomas. Am J Surg Pathol 1990; 14: 615–625.
160. Takemura T, Matsui Y, Saiki S, et al.: Pulmonary vascular involvement in sarcoidosis: a report of 40 autopsy cases. Hum Pathol 1992; 23: 1216–1223.
161. Fernandes S, Singsen B, Hoffman G: Sarcoidosis and systemic vasculitis. Semin Arthritis Rheum 2000; 30: 33–46.
162. Colby T, Fukuoka J, Ewaskow S, et al.: Pathologic approach to pulmonary hemorrhage. Ann Diagn Pathol 2001; 5: 309–319.
163. Kadokura M, Colby T, Myers J: Pathologic comparison of video-assisted thoracic surgical biopsy with traditional open lung biopsy. J Thorac Cardiovasc Surg 1995; 109: 494–498.
164. Lynch J, Leatherman J: Alveolar hemorrhage syndromes. In: Fishman's pulmonary diseases and disorders, Fishman A, Ed. 1998, McGraw-Hill, New York, pp 1193–1210.
165. Lombard C, Colby T, Elliott C: Surgical pathology of the lung in antibasement membrane antibody-associated Goodpasture's syndrome. Human Pathol 1989; 20: 445–451.
166. Specks U: Diffuse alveolar hemorrhage syndromes. Opin Rheumatol 2001; 13: 12–17.
167. Cutz E: Idiopathic pulmonary hemosiderosis and related disorders in infancy and childhood. Perspect Pediatr Pathol 1987; 11: 47–81.
168. Schwarz M, Cherniak R, King T: Diffuse alveolar hemorrhage and other rare infiltrative disorders. In: Textbook of respiratory medicine, Murray J, Nadel J, Eds. 2000, WB Saunders, Philadelphia, pp 1733–1755.
169. Jennings C, King T, Tuder R, et al.: Diffuse alveolar hemorrhage with underlying isolated, pauciimmune pulmonary capillaritis. Am J Respir Crit Care Med 1997; 155: 1101–1109.
170. Finnegan M, Hinchcliffe J, Russell-Jones D, et al.: Vasculitis complicating cystic fibrosis. Q J Med 1989; 72: 609–621.
171. Fortin P, Esdaile J: Vasculitis and malignancy. In: Systemic vasculitides, Churg A, Churg J, Eds. 1991, Igaku-Shoin, New York, pp 327–341.
172. Komadina K, Houck R: Polyarteritis nodosa presenting as recurrent pneumonia following splenectomy for hairy-cell leukemia. Semin Arthritis Rheum 1989; 18: 252–257.
173. Fiegler W, Siemoneit K: Pulmonary manifestations in anaphylactoid purpura (Henoch- Schönlein syndrome). ROFO Fortschr Geb Rontgenstr Nuklearmed 1981; 134: 269–272.
174. Marandian M, Ezzati M, Behvad A, et al.: Pulmonary involvement in Schönlein–Henoch's purpura. Arch Fr Pediatr 1982; 39: 255–257.
175. White R: Henoch–Schönlein purpura. In: Systemic vasculitides, Churg A, Churg J, Eds. 1991, Igaku-Shoin, New York, pp 203–217.
176. Bombardieri S, Paoletti P, Ferri C, et al.: Lung involvement in essential mixed cryoglobulinemia. Am J Med 1979; 66: 748–756.
177. Churg J: Cryoglobulinemic vasculitis. In: Systemic vasculitides, Churg A, Churg J, Eds. 1991, Igaku-Shoin, New York, pp 293–298.
178. Monti G, Galli M, Cereda U, et al.: Mycosis fungoides with mixed cryoglobulinemia and pulmonary vasculitis. A case report. Boll Ist Sieroter Milan 1987; 66: 324–328.
179. Nada A, Torres V, Ryu J, et al.: Pulmonary fibrosis as an unusual clinical manifestation of a pulmonary–renal vasculitis in elderly patients. Mayo Clin Proc 1990; 65: 847–856.
180. Seiden M, O'Donnell W, Weinblatt M, et al.: Vasculitis with recurrent pulmonary hemorrhage in a long-term survivor after autologous bone marrow transplantation. Bone Marrow Transplant 1990; 6: 345–347.
181. Saldana M: Necrotizing sarcoid granulomatosis: clinicopathologic observations in 24 patients [Abstract]. Lab Invest 1978; 38: 364.
182. Chabalko J: Solitary lung lesion with cavitation due to necrotizing sarcoid granulomatosis. Del Med J 1986; 58: 15–16.
183. Fisher M, Christ M, Bernstein J: Necrotizing sarcoid-like granulomatosis: radiologic–pathologic correlation. J Can Assoc Radiol 1984; 35: 313–315.
184. Fraser R, Muller N, Colman N, et al.: Fraser and Parè's diagnosis of diseases of the chest. In. (ed), Vol 4. 1999, WB Saunders, Philadelphia.
185. Katzenstein A: Alveolar hemorrhage syndromes. In: Surgical pathology of non-neoplastic lung disease, Katzenstein A, Askin F, Eds. 1997, WB Saunders, Philadelphia, pp 153–159.
186. Jennette J, Thomas D, Falk R: Microscopic polyangiitis (microscopic polyarteritis). Semin Diagn Pathol 2001; 18: 3–13.

Pulmonary hypertension

11

Andrew Churg   Joanne L Wright

Introduction

Biopsies for evaluation of pulmonary hypertension are relatively uncommon, and in the past have sometimes been viewed as offering little therapeutic benefit. However, as argued by Wagenvoort,[1] biopsies in patients with pulmonary hypertension serve three purposes:

- They can establish the nature of the underlying lesion. This is potentially important information, since patients with purely thrombotic lesions appear to have a much better prognosis than patients with plexogenic arteriopathy or veno-occlusive disease.[2]
- Occasionally, the lung lesions shed light on the type of underlying congenital cardiac abnormality.
- The lesions seen in the lung biopsy provide an indication of potential reversibility.

This information is important in deciding whether to perform corrective surgery in congenital heart disease[1] and appears to be of value in predicting response to vasodilator therapy.[3]

Morphologic features of the pulmonary vasculature

Pulmonary arteries

Any diagnosis of pulmonary hypertension requires recognition of the different types of vessels seen in the lung. This is aided by the use of elastic tissue stains, which should be a routine approach when a biopsy or larger specimen shows potential vascular disease. Knowledge of the structure of the normal pulmonary vascular bed is important when assessing biopsy material.[4,5] Branches of the *pulmonary artery* run with the bronchi and then the bronchioles. Arteries associated with the bronchi are typically larger than 1 mm diameter and have a fairly extensive elastic fiber meshwork in their walls. *Muscular pulmonary arteries* (Fig. 11.1) are usually associated with bronchioles and measure between 100 and 1000 µm. They are frequently abnormal in pulmonary hypertension. Elastic stain (Fig. 11.2) shows that they have both an internal and an external elastic lamina. In the normal lung the diameter of a muscular pulmonary artery and its accompanying airway should be about the same. Below a diameter of about 100 µm, the pulmonary artery branches lose the internal elastica and are termed *arterioles*. Arterioles run adjacent to the alveolar ducts and can be found as a corner vessel by the alveolar saccules, but should not be found in alveolar walls. A well-defined mesh of capillaries arranged in a single layer of rings and spokes forms the gas exchange system in the alveoli (Fig. 11.3).[6]

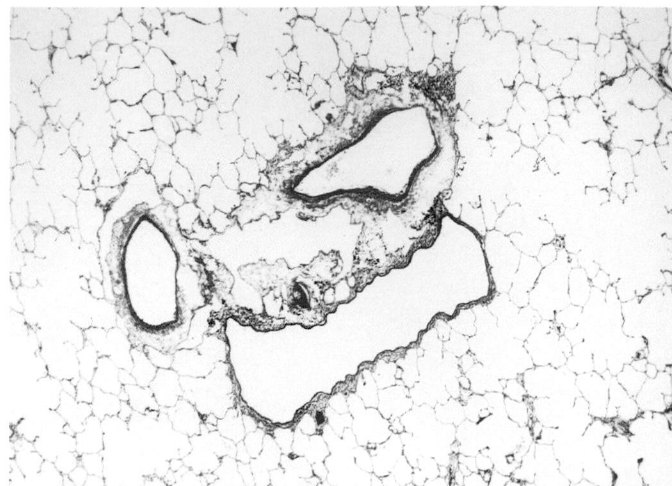

Fig. 11.1 Normal muscular pulmonary artery branches accompanying a bronchiole.

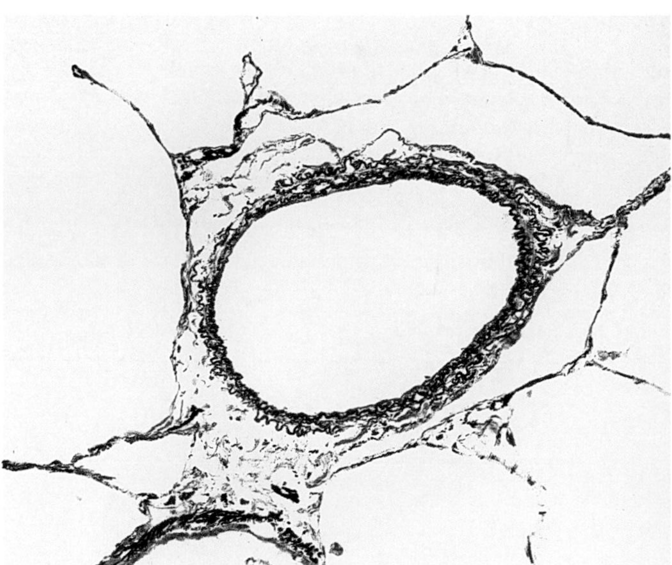

Fig. 11.2 Elastic stain of a normal small muscular pulmonary artery showing double elastic laminae surrounding a fairly thin muscular layer. The intima is unobtrusive.

Pulmonary veins

Normal *pulmonary veins* have only a single elastica and a thin layer of muscle. Veins are best identified by anatomic location. Larger pulmonary veins run in the interlobular septa (Fig. 11.4). Smaller veins are found associated with the alveolar saccules and are indistinguishable by morphology from pulmonary arterioles; thus, the identification of a small vessel as a vein often requires tracing it back through several sections until it joins a

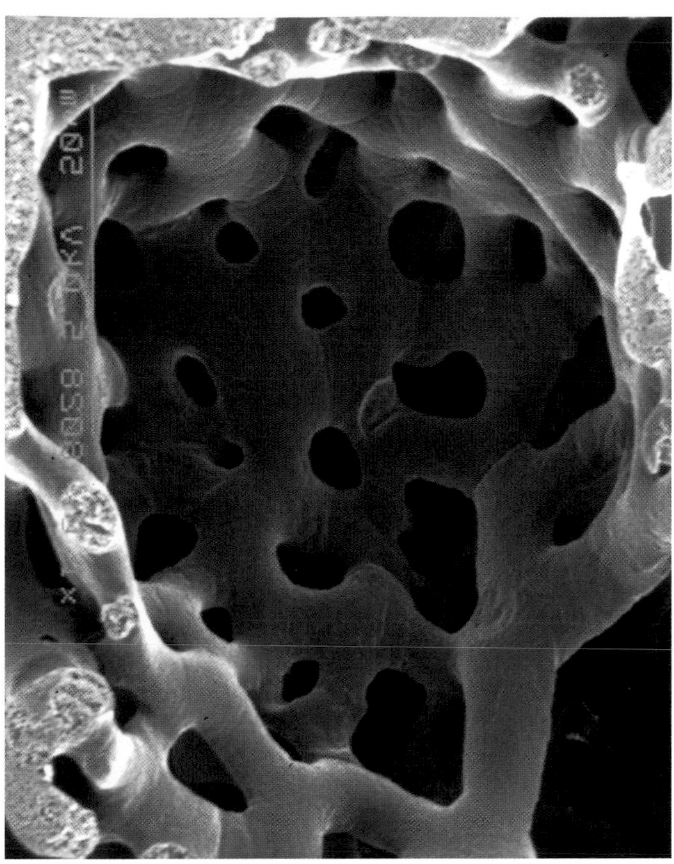

Fig. 11.3 Methacrylate vascular cast of an alveolus showing the mesh of capillaries (scanning electron micrograph).

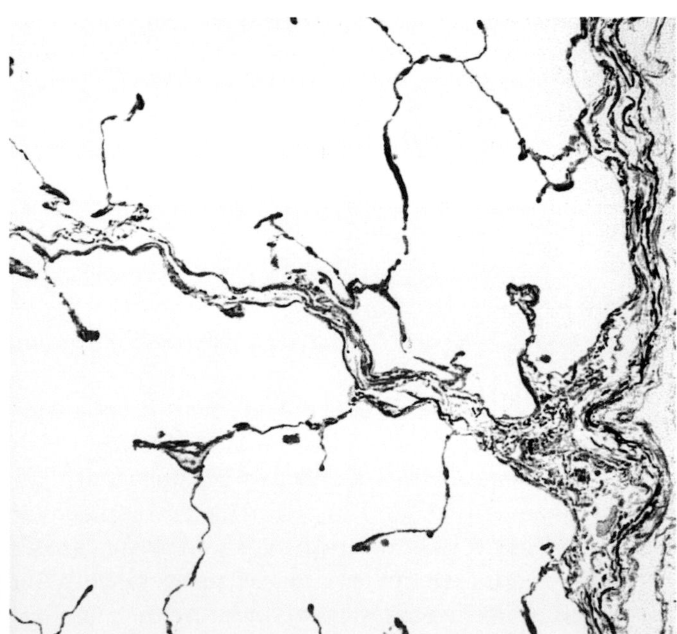

Fig. 11.4 Elastic stain of a normal pulmonary vein running in the interlobular septum. Note the single elastica, a characteristic finding of pulmonary veins.

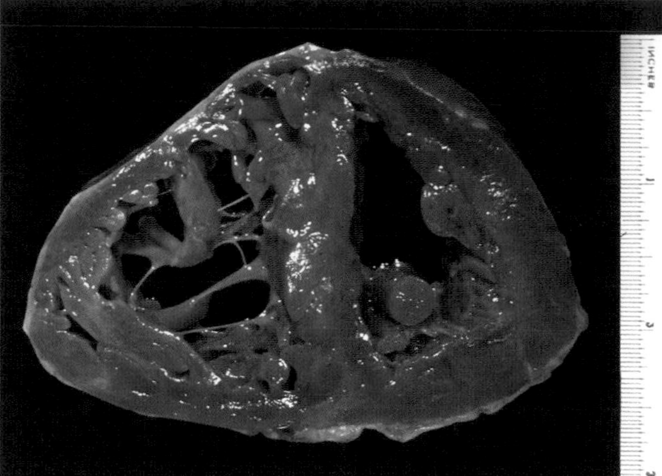

Fig. 11.5 Cross section of heart at autopsy from a patient with pulmonary hypertension secondary to fenfluramine/phentermine use. Note the markedly thickened right ventricle.

definite vein in an interlobular septum. Of note, in pulmonary venous hypertension, the larger veins may acquire both a double elastica and additional muscle and resemble muscular arteries, but the location in the septa indicates their true nature.

Bronchial arteries

Bronchial arteries are found in the walls of the larger bronchi. They are usually heavily muscularized and have a prominent internal elastica and a less well-defined external elastica. Bronchial arteries may develop longitudinal muscle bands, a feature helpful in identification. Bronchial arteries are systemic vessels at systemic pressure, and areas where they anastomose with the pulmonary circulation (around bronchiectatic foci, in plexogenic arteriopathy) there may be foci of hemorrhage.

Recognition of right ventricular hypertrophy

A quick, but relatively inaccurate, determination of ventricular hypertrophy can be made by simple measurement of the right ventricular wall muscle thickness (Fig. 11.5). Measurements obtained from a normal adult population should be approximately 2–3 mm, with measurements greater than 5 mm thought to represent hypertrophy.[7] Partitioning of the heart into right ventricle and left ventricle plus septum[8] provides a sensitive estimation of ventricular hypertrophy, with a weight of 65 g or greater considered abnormal.[7] Although a portion of the septum will enlarge with the right ventricle, a ratio of left ventricular weight/right ventricular weight of less than 1.9 is considered to represent right ventricular hypertrophy. Obviously, such ratios are only useful if there is no enlargement of the left ventricle.

Microscopic examination of the right ventricle does not show the generalized increase of fibrosis that can be found in left ventricular hypertrophy. Detailed measurement of the myocytes will demonstrate enlarged fiber diameters,[9] but this finding may be too subtle to recognize visually.

Classification of pulmonary hypertension

The normal pressure (in mmHg) in the pulmonary artery is 20/12 (mean = 15) at sea level, and 38/14 (mean = 25) at approximately 15,000 ft altitude. In general, a mean arterial pressure of 20 at sea level is considered abnormal, whereas at 15,000 ft, a pressure of >25 is considered abnormal. Pulmonary hypertension is defined clinically as a mean pulmonary artery pressure at rest of greater than 25 mmHg, or a mean pressure greater than 30 mmHg during exercise.[10] Pulmonary hypertension may be a manifestation of a primary pulmonary vascular disease, or may be secondary to other (nonvascular) diseases in the lung, but the morphologic patterns seen in the vessels in pulmonary hypertension are fairly limited, and thus clinical correlation is required for a specific diagnosis.

A variety of schemes for classification of pulmonary hypertension have been proposed.[2,11–16] We show a simplified scheme in Table 11.1. Some authors have argued that there is no real difference between thrombotic and plexogenic arteriopathy, largely because thrombotic lesions may be found in both.[14] However, we believe, as Wagenvoort and Mulder[17] have argued, that there are very clear clinical and morphologic differences among the entities shown in Table 11.1, and that thrombosis is a secondary phenomenon in most types of pulmonary hypertension (see below).

Table 11.1 Classification of pulmonary hypertension

A. Plexogenic arteriopathy:
   - Idiopathic ("primary")
     - Associated with congenital heart disease with left-to-right shunts
     - Associated with collagen vascular disease
     - Associated with cirrhosis
   - Secondary to drug use
     - Dexfenfluramine, fenfluramine/phentermine ("FenPhen")
     - Aminorex
   - Associated with HIV infection

B. Thrombotic and embolic pulmonary hypertension:
   - Associated with recurrent thromboemboli or in-situ thromboses
   - Associated with sickle cell disease
   - Associated with IV drug abuse (injection of insoluble foreign particles)
   - Associated with tumor emboli

C. Associated with interstitial lung disease, emphysema, or other intrinsic lung disease

D. Associated with chronic hypoxia

E. Pulmonary veno-occlusive disease

F. Pulmonary venous hypertension:
   - Left-sided cardiac disease, especially mitral stenosis
   - Atrial myxomas
   - Sclerosing mediastinitis
   - Congenital cardiac malformations affecting venous outflow

G. Pulmonary capillary hemangiomatosis

In pulmonary hypertension associated with anorectic agents, the pulmonary vascular lesions are associated with cardiac valvular lesions, predominately on the left side of the heart.[18,19] In those patients who develop their pulmonary hypertension in association with HIV disease, the majority can be directly related to HIV infection; other cofactors include liver disease and coagulation abnormalities. There is a wide age range of the affected population. The interval between HIV infection and clinical presentation of pulmonary hypertension may be up to 3 years, but after presentation the prognosis is poor.[20,21]

Clinical features

The features of pulmonary hypertension in general are very nonspecific. Patients typically describe progressive shortness of breath, which is particularly marked during exercise. Syncopal episodes, presumably related to cardiac arrhythmias, may occur. Chest pain is usually a sign of right-sided cardiac ischemia and is seen late in the course in those who develop cor pulmonale. Similarly, abdominal discomfort is a sign of right heart failure with progressive liver congestion.

Radiographic features

Plain chest film early in the disease may be totally normal; with more advanced disease, enlarged pulmonary arteries become apparent (Fig. 11.6), and with the development of cor pulmonale, the right ventricle may be visibly enlarged. With long-standing pulmonary hypertension, calcification of the large arteries, presumably representing atherosclerosis, can be seen. Computed tomography (CT) scanning allows measurements of the diameters of the main pulmonary artery; in general, if the diameter of the

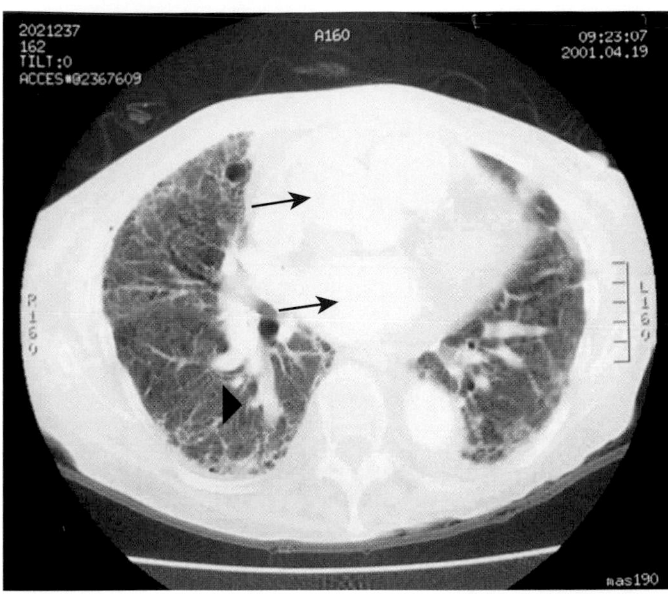

Fig. 11.6 CT scan from a patient with severe pulmonary hypertension. The long arrows mark the enlarged pulmonary arteries. Note the pruned appearance of the vessels as they extend peripherally (arrowhead).

pulmonary artery is larger than that of the ascending aorta, there is a high probability of pulmonary hypertension.[22] Angiography classically demonstrates vascular "pruning" in which the vessels have a simplified branching pattern.

Morphologic features

Plexiform lesions were first clearly characterized by Heath and Edwards.[16] The term "plexogenic pulmonary arteriopathy" was coined by Wagenvoort[11] to describe a morphologic response pattern that sometimes, but not always, is characterized by the formation of peculiar thrombi with multiple small channels, i.e. "plexiform lesions". However, plexiform lesions are the end result of a series of vascular changes, and a given case of plexogenic arteriopathy may show only the lower-grade changes without formation of plexiform lesions.

Plexogenic arteriopathy primarily affects muscular arteries and arterioles, but larger arteries may demonstrate increased atherosclerosis, a finding that may be seen in pulmonary hypertension of any cause or in the absence of hypertension. Statistically, however, the most common cause of atherosclerosis in the pulmonary artery is severe systemic atherosclerosis.[23]

The vascular changes in the muscular arteries and arterioles in plexogenic arteriopathy appear to reflect, in general, the level of pulmonary artery pressure, and to a lesser extent the length of time hypertension has been present; thus, in a broad sense, higher-grade lesions (see below) are found in individuals with higher pulmonary artery pressures. However, the correlations are not exact and only lower-grade lesions may be found in some cases with quite marked pulmonary hypertension. There is also some controversy about the order in which different lesions develop.[2,13,14,16] It is our belief that the original Heath and Edwards classification[16] is incorrect and that the actual sequence of changes is that proposed by Wagenvoort and Wagenvoort,[11] as follows.

Grade I: muscular hypertrophy

Muscular hypertrophy appears as thickening of the walls of muscular arteries, often with obvious narrowing of the lumens (Fig. 11.7). Elastic stain shows that the space between the internal and external elastica has become widened by the new muscle. Normal pre-acinar muscular pulmonary arteries should have, in the fully distended state, a ratio of medial thickness to vessel diameter of 1–2%, although in the smaller muscular arteries 30–100 μm in external diameter, the percent medial thickness may be up to 5%.[24] Muscular hypertrophy in small arteries is often accompanied by *muscularization of arterioles*, such that the arteriole acquires both a double elastica and muscle between the elasticas (Fig. 11.8). Muscularized arterioles thus come to resemble ordinary muscular arteries, but are found in the lung parenchyma, a clue to the correct diagnosis, since arteries are normally present only next to accompanying airways.

Grade II: intimal proliferation

In this stage, proliferation of intimal cells leads to a thickened intima superimposed on a thickened muscular media (Fig. 11.9). The intimal cells do not show any special organization.

Grade III: concentric laminar intimal fibrosis

In this stage the intima is markedly thickened and organized in a series of concentric bands of collagen and spindle-shaped cells which lend a whorled appearance (Fig. 11.10). The lumen is often dramatically narrowed.

Grade IV: necrotizing vasculitis

As a result of markedly increased pressure, the arterial wall may become necrotic. The typical pattern is that of *fibrinoid necrosis* with eosinophilic granular necrotic material replacing the normal arterial wall (Fig. 11.11). Inflammatory cells, usually polymorphonuclear leukocytes but sometimes eosinophils, may be present. Elastic stains show that, typically, the internal elastic is destroyed.

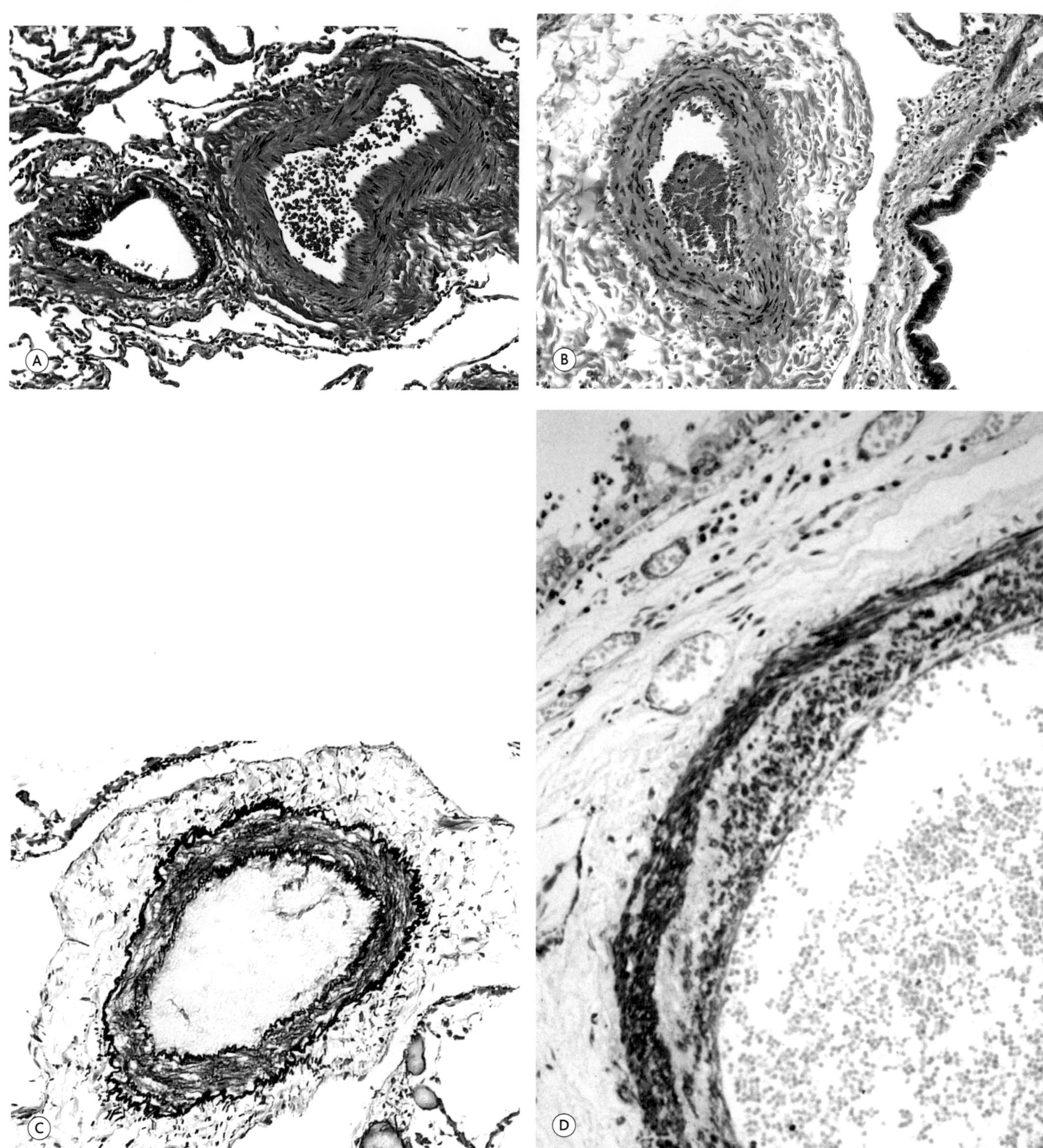

Fig. 11.7 **Muscular hypertrophy in pulmonary hypertension.** (A) Muscular pulmonary artery branches showing muscular hypertrophy. In normal bronchovascular bundles, airways and vessels are about the same size; here, the vessel is larger and very thick walled. Note the obviously increased muscle area on the elastic stain (C). Muscular hypertrophy of this type may be seen in pulmonary hypertension of any cause and by itself does not indicate a diagnosis of plexogenic arteriopathy. (B) Thickened muscular media is very obvious at higher magnification. (C) Increase in muscle well demonstrated on elastic stain. (D) Occasionally smooth muscle proliferation occurs in the intima in pulmonary hypertension; when this occurs the muscle bundles run longitudinally, as here (smooth muscle actin stain).

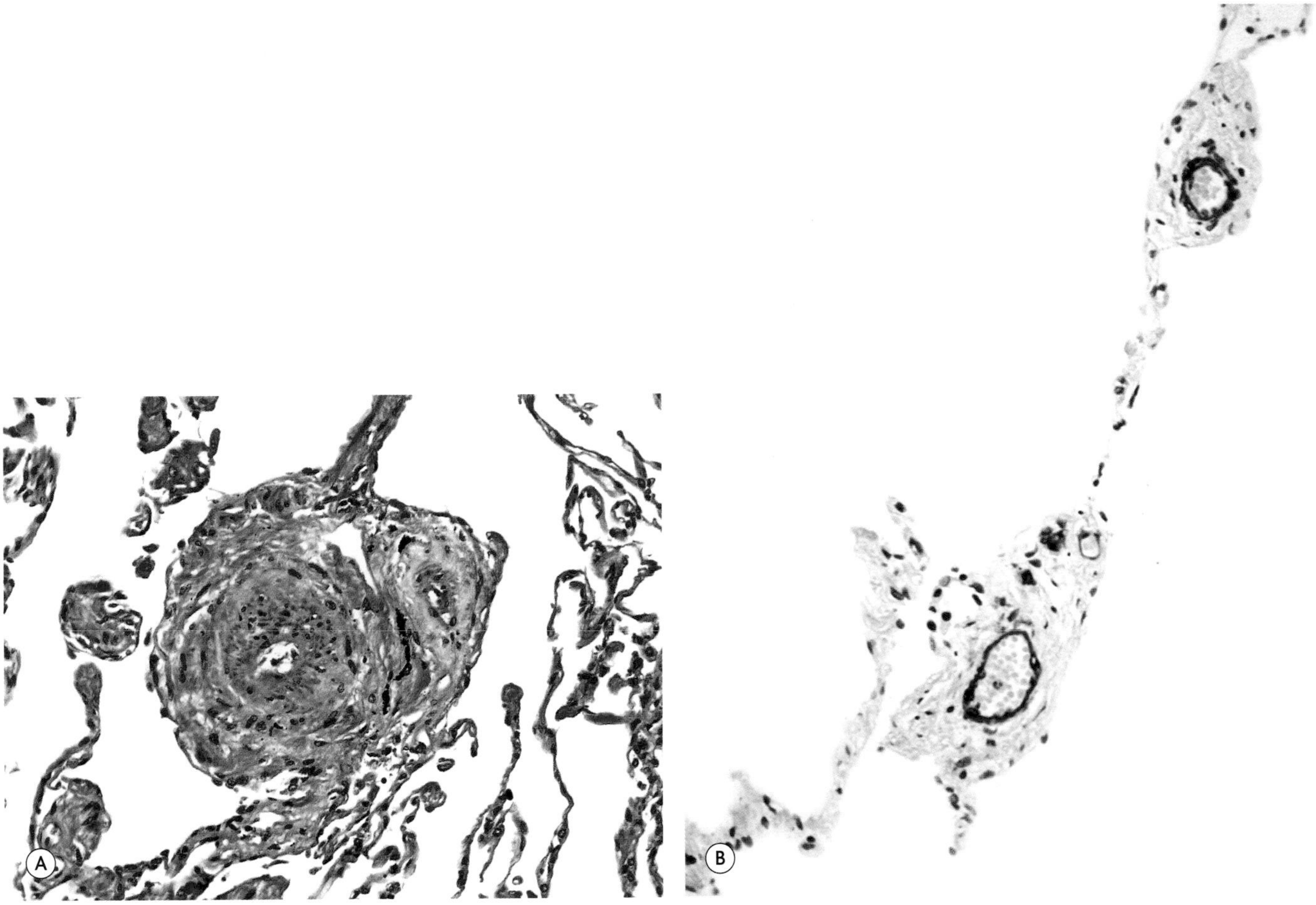

Fig. 11.8 (A) Severe muscular hypertrophy in a very small arterial branch. (B) Smooth muscle actin stain of alveolar corner arterioles, showing complete muscular media in a case of pulmonary hypertension. Ordinarily these vessels do not have a complete muscular media.

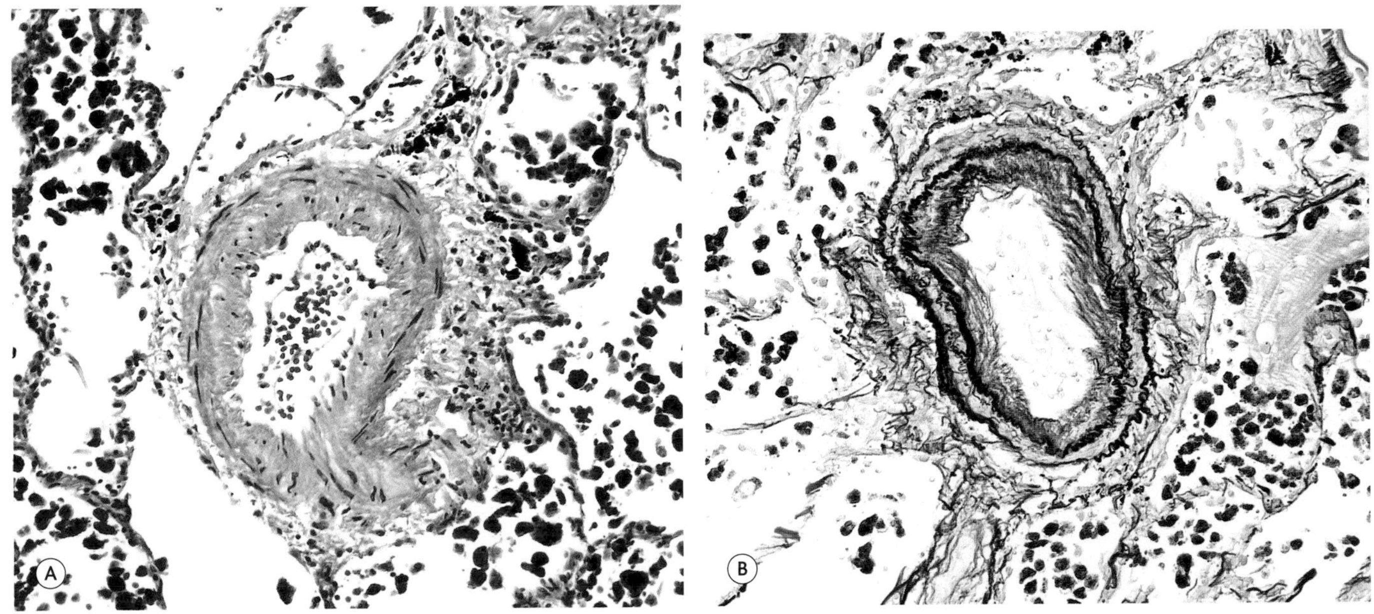

Fig. 11.9 **Mild intimal proliferation.** (A,B) The elastic stain (B) is required to separate this process from muscular hypertrophy.

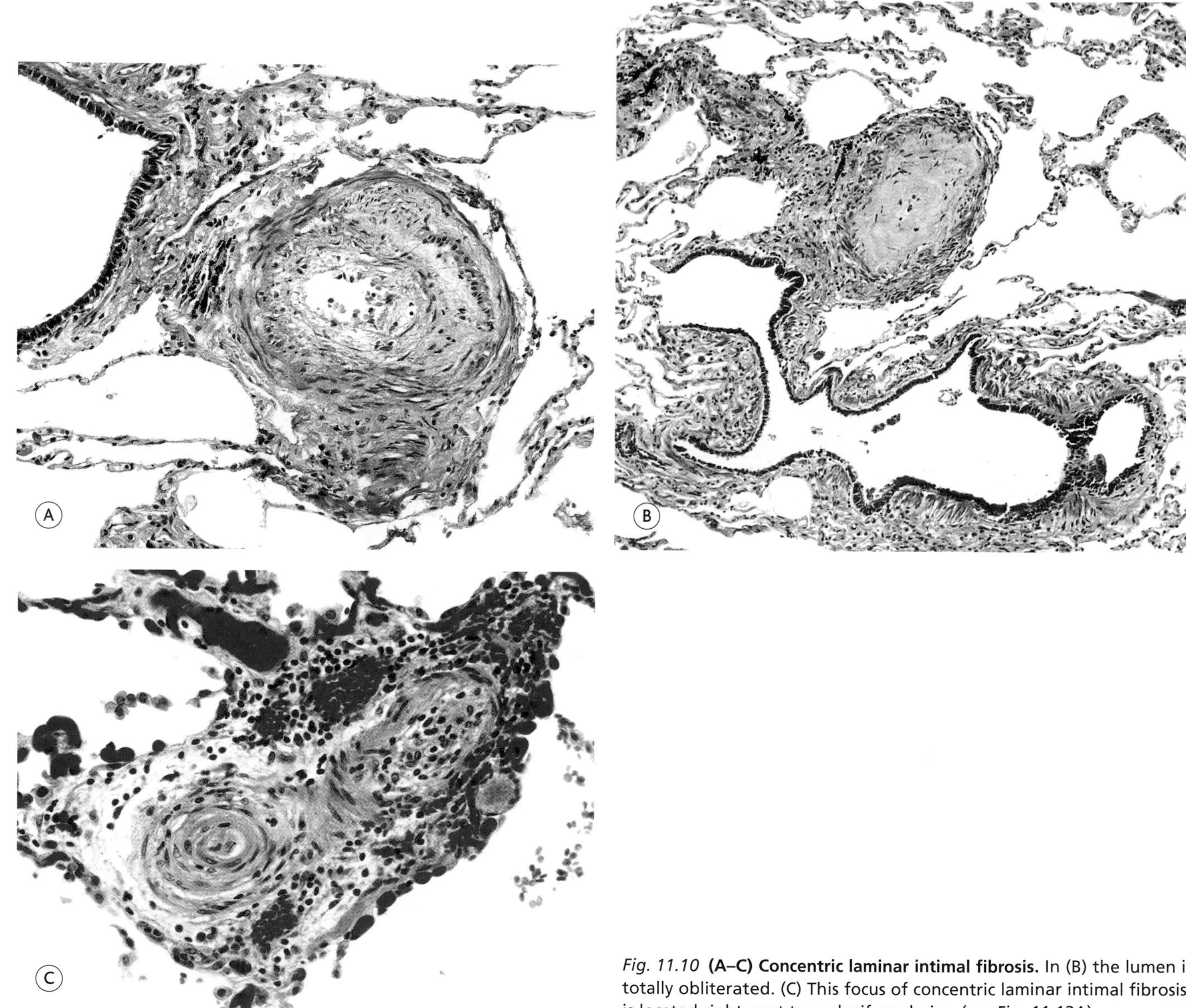

Fig. 11.10 **(A–C) Concentric laminar intimal fibrosis.** In (B) the lumen is totally obliterated. (C) This focus of concentric laminar intimal fibrosis is located right next to a plexiform lesion (see Fig. 11.12A).

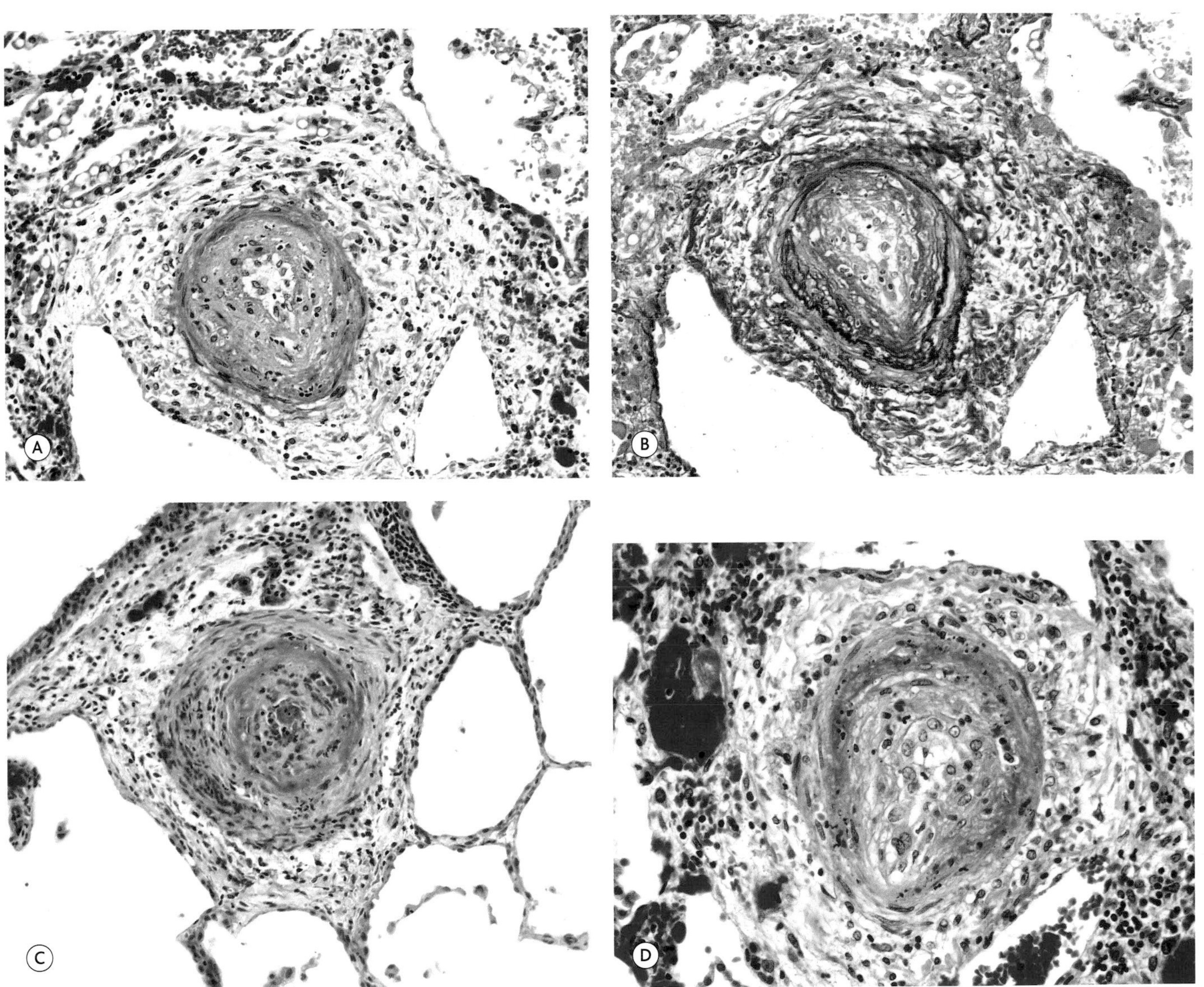

Fig. 11.11 **(A–D) Necrotizing vasculitis.** Note the combination of inflammatory cells and pink material (fibrinoid necrosis) in the vessel wall in (A) and (B) the partial loss of the internal elastica in the matching section. In (C) a small thrombus is present in the lumen. In (D) the process at higher power is shown.

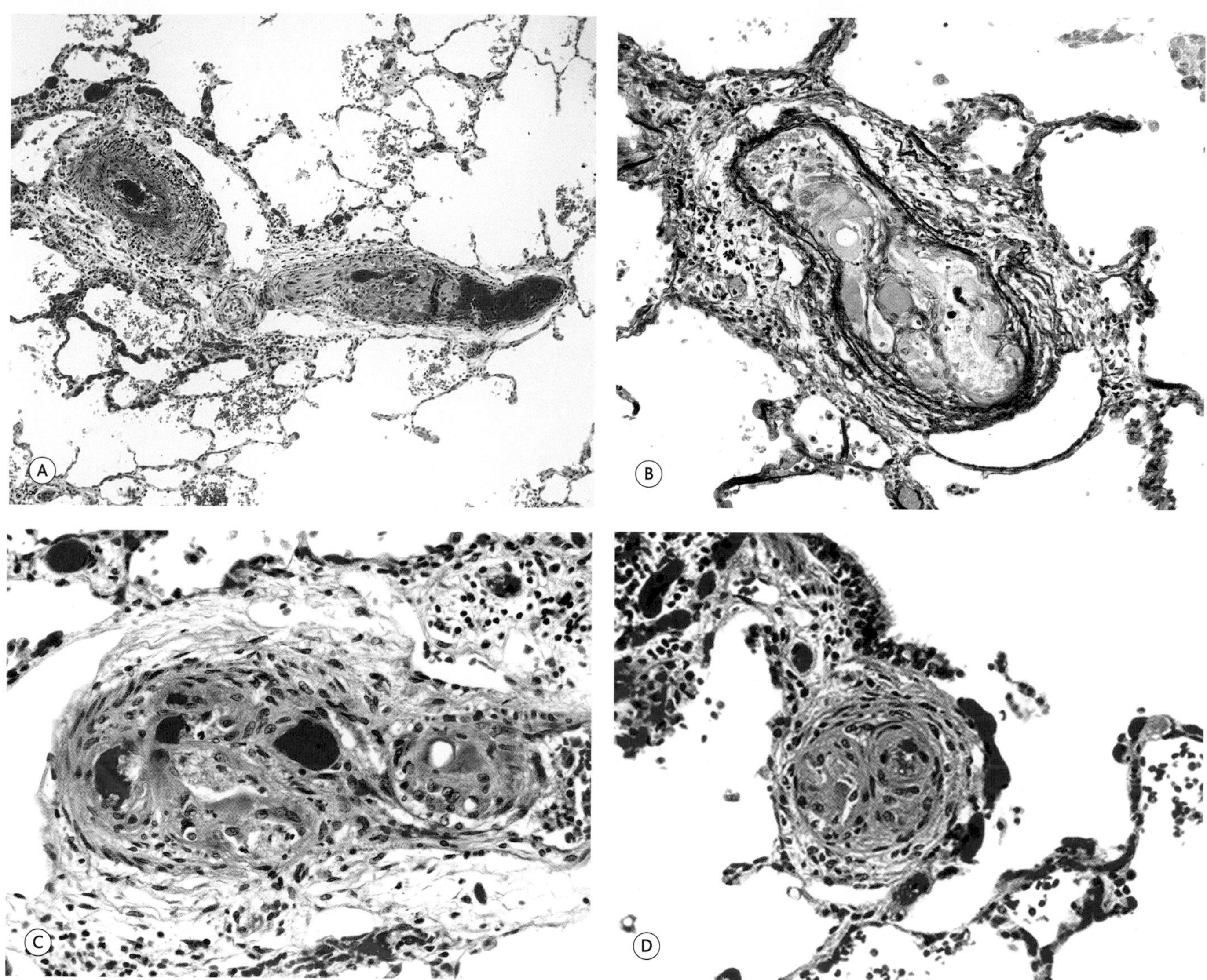

Fig. 11.12 **Plexiform lesions.** (A) Low-power view showing fibrinoid necrosis in one branch of the artery, concentric laminar intimal fibrosis best seen in the middle of the field, and a plexiform lesion cut in longitudinal section. (B) Elastic stain of plexiform lesion showing the typical combination of multiple small capillary channels and loss of the internal elastica. (C) Similar image on hematoxylin and eosin (H&E) stain. (D) Plexiform lesion seen in cross section. The plexiform lesion appears to represent organization and thrombosis in arteries that have developed necrotizing vasculitis.

Grade V: plexiform lesions

Plexiform lesions are typically found in small muscular arteries at branch points. The artery immediately proximal to the plexiform lesion often shows marked muscular hypertrophy and intimal hyperplasia. In the plexiform lesion itself the vessel is often dilated and the lumen is characteristically filled with capillary channels that very much resemble a fairly cellular organizing thrombus (Fig. 11.12). However, in contradistinction to most thrombi, where the elastic laminae are intact,[2] elastic stains show that the inner elastica is typically destroyed in the region of the plexiform lesion, and this is a useful feature in a case where a question of thrombotic vs plexogenic arteriopathy arises. This set of findings reflect the fact that plexiform lesions are actually the result of fibrinoid necrosis of the vessels, with subsequent thrombosis and organization. The acute plexiform lesions may show small fibrin thrombi and small numbers of inflammatory cells in the capillary channels; as the lesions age, they scar and become paucicellular. Plexiform lesions are usually not very numerous and can be widely scattered within the lung parenchyma; thus, a certain amount of hunting may be required to demonstrate them.

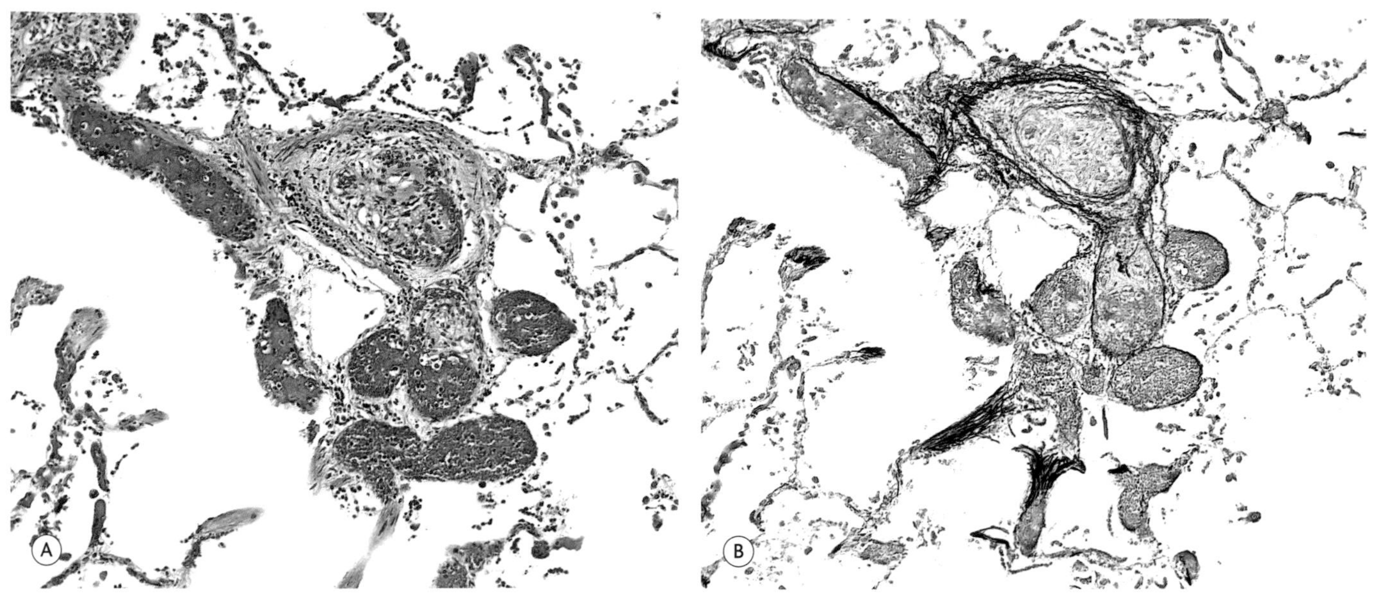

Fig. 11.13 **Dilatation lesions.** (A–B) The dilatation lesions appear as thin-walled blood-filled channels. Dilatation lesions develop distal to plexiform lesions, shown here at the top of the field.

Table 11.2 Reversible and irreversible lesions

Potentially reversible	Not reversible
Muscular hypertrophy	Marked concentric lamellar fibrosis
Intimal proliferation	Fibrinoid necrosis
Mild concentric lamellar fibrosis	Plexiform lesions
	Dilatation and angiomatoid lesions

Grade VI: dilatation and angiomatoid lesions

These arterial lesions are located distal to plexiform lesions and probably are related to changes in flow produced by the plexiform lesions. They consist of thin-walled, often dilated and tortuous, channels with a single elastic; these channels are not of obvious arterial structure, but their origin can be proved by tracing back through serial sections (Fig. 11.13). Dilatation and angiomatoid lesions may rupture, with resulting pulmonary hemorrhage, and in some instances these lesions appear to anastomose with the bronchial circulation, thus exposing these relatively weak structures to systemic arterial pressures.

Clinical correlations

As noted in the Introduction, assessment of reversibility or potential for response to treatment is an important reason for performing lung biopsies in patients with pulmonary hypertension. However, the question of what features actually predict reversibility is controversial. As a first approximation, lesions can be separated as shown in Table 11.2.

Wagenvoort[12,13] and Palevsky et al.[3] have more recently suggested that simple qualitative assessment of the types of lesions present is inadequate by itself for predicting response, and that quantitative measurements are required, particularly measurements of intimal proliferation. For example, Palevsky et al.[3] found that an average intimal area of more than 18% of the vascular cross section predicted a poor response to therapy. The interested readers should consult the appropriate references.[2,3,13,25]

The long-term outlook for patients with pulmonary hypertension caused by plexogenic arteriopathy tends to be poor, with deaths from cor pulmonale or sudden arrhythmias. In some forms of congenital heart disease hypertension may be reversed by repair of the cardiac defect. In adults, transplantation is, at present, the only known cure.

Differential diagnosis

Higher-grade lesions in the plexogenic arteriopathy group are distinctive and not easily confused with other diseases. Systemic necrotizing vasculitis (microscopic polyangiitis, Wegener's granulomatosis) may produce fibrinoid necrosis of vessels, but is not associated with lower-grade vascular changes or with plexiform lesions.

It should be remembered that some degree of muscular arterial hypertrophy is seen in virtually all forms of pulmonary hypertension, including some cases of veno-occlusive disease and venous hypertension secondary to mitral stenosis or other cardiac lesions.[2] Thus, the finding of muscular hypertrophy as the only vascular abnormality does not necessarily mean that the patient has plexogenic arteriopathy.

Conversely, low-grade morphologic changes, especially muscular hypertrophy, are not necessarily good predictors of either the degree or even the presence of pulmonary hypertension. In our experience, biopsies from patients with interstitial lung disease frequently appear to show muscular arterial hypertrophy, even when cardiac catheterization shows normal pressures. There is also an aging effect on the vessels with increasing intimal fibrosis.[26] Thus, caution should be exercised in the individual case when interpreting apparently low-grade lesions, particularly when the morphologic changes occur in a setting not suggestive of pulmonary hypertension.

A further problem in interpretation is that thrombotic lesions, presumably reflecting in-situ thromboses caused by abnormal flow, are now recognized as a finding in many different morphologic types of pulmonary hypertension[2,3,17] (see morphologic description in the next section), and certainly may be found in plexogenic arteriopathy. This does not invalidate the notion that plexogenic arteriopathy is morphologically separate from thrombotic hypertension.[17]

Thrombotic and emboli hypertension

Clinical features

Typically, this form of hypertension is characterized by the insidious onset of shortness of breath without clinical evidence of pulmonary emboli (hence, thrombotic hypertension is sometimes included in the differential of 'primary' pulmonary hypertension). However, there may be a history of prior events that suggest the diagnosis; for example, recurrent sickle crises, a history of IV drug abuse, or known episodes of thromboembolism.

Radiographic features

The radiographic features are not specific, but angiogram or CT with contrast may reveal large emboli or sometimes evidence of multiple small thrombi, with apparent abrupt ending of the vessels.

Pathologic findings

Pathologic findings vary with the type of underlying lesion. In classic thrombotic or thromboembolic hypertension, thrombi in various stages of organization, mostly old, are seen in branches of the small muscular pulmonary arteries. Of note, both elastic laminae are usually intact in thrombotic disease, as opposed to the destruction of the internal elastic in plexiform lesions.[2] Larger arteries may show "webs" (Fig. 11.14), which are simply organized thrombi with channels large enough to be seen grossly. Some cases of thrombotic/emboli hypertension demonstrate thrombi in the main branches of the pulmonary artery, sometimes with webs as well; these patients often have underlying (non-hypertensive) lung disease or left-sided cardiac disease, as well as peripheral vascular thromboses.[27]

A helpful feature that should alert the pathologist to the presence of thrombi and emboli is the finding of *eccentric* intimal proliferation and/or intimal fibrosis in arterial vessels (Fig. 11.15); these lesions represent old small organizing thrombi. Both eccentric lesions and recanalized thrombi may be seen in pulmonary hypertension of other causes.[17] However, the concentric intimal proliferation seen in plexogenic arteriopathy is not a feature of thrombotic hypertension.

Patients with sickle cell disease may develop thrombi in their pulmonary arterial branches during sickle crises, and recurrent episodes can lead to a form of thrombotic pulmonary hypertension. The lesions look like organizing thrombi, but close examination reveals the presence of sickled cells (Fig. 11.16).

Intravenous injection of licit drugs intended for oral use, or sometimes of illicit drugs such as heroin or cocaine,[28] tends to produce deposits of insoluble filler material from the drug in the small muscular arteries. In mild disease, small numbers of birefringent particles are seen in the lumens or in the arterial walls (Fig. 11.17), presumably having been incorporated into organizing thrombi. With injection of large amounts of drug, the inflammatory and thrombotic reaction to the particles leads to formation of peculiar thrombus-like formations with capillary channels called angiothrombotic lesions.[29] These are probably just peculiar in situ thrombi caused by large numbers of particles. They more or less completely obstruct the arterial branch, and accumulation of such lesions leads to pulmonary hypertension. Polarized light examination reveals the particulate matter, with differences depending on the exact nature of the filler used to make the drug tablet. Starch appears as Maltese cross-like images; talc as brightly birefringent plates; and microcrystalline cellulose as PAS-positive rectangular crystals

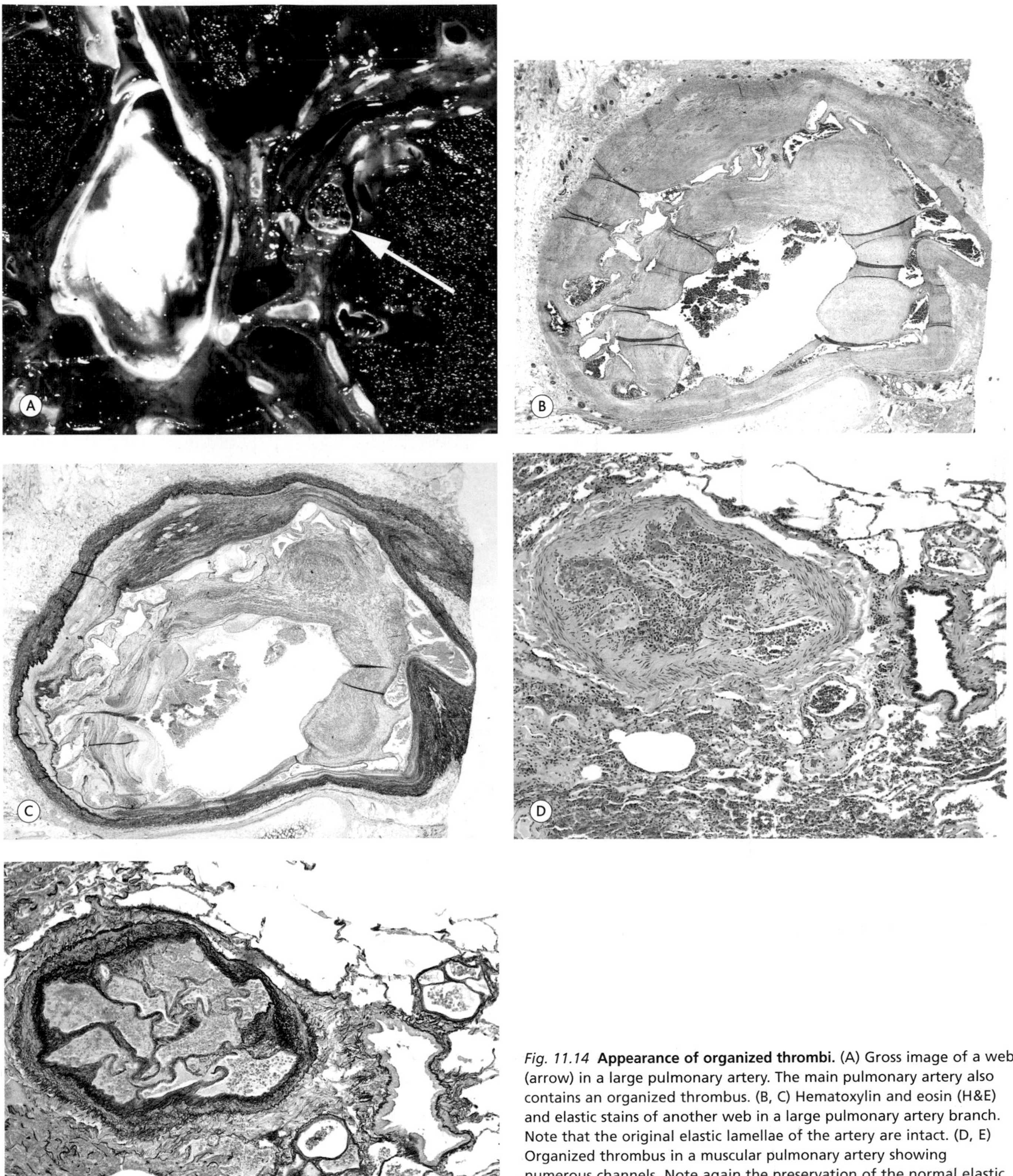

Fig. 11.14 **Appearance of organized thrombi.** (A) Gross image of a web (arrow) in a large pulmonary artery. The main pulmonary artery also contains an organized thrombus. (B, C) Hematoxylin and eosin (H&E) and elastic stains of another web in a large pulmonary artery branch. Note that the original elastic lamellae of the artery are intact. (D, E) Organized thrombus in a muscular pulmonary artery showing numerous channels. Note again the preservation of the normal elastic structure in the arterial wall. Most thrombi do not disturb the arterial wall structure, as opposed to the destructive process that leads to plexiform lesions.

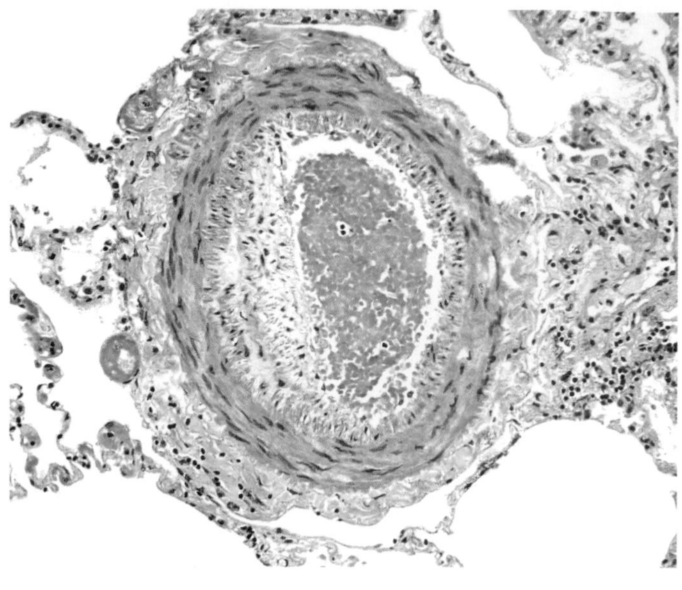

Fig. 11.15 Eccentric intimal proliferation representing an old thrombus. Compare with the concentric intimal proliferation of plexogenic arteriopathy in Figs 11.9 and 11.10.

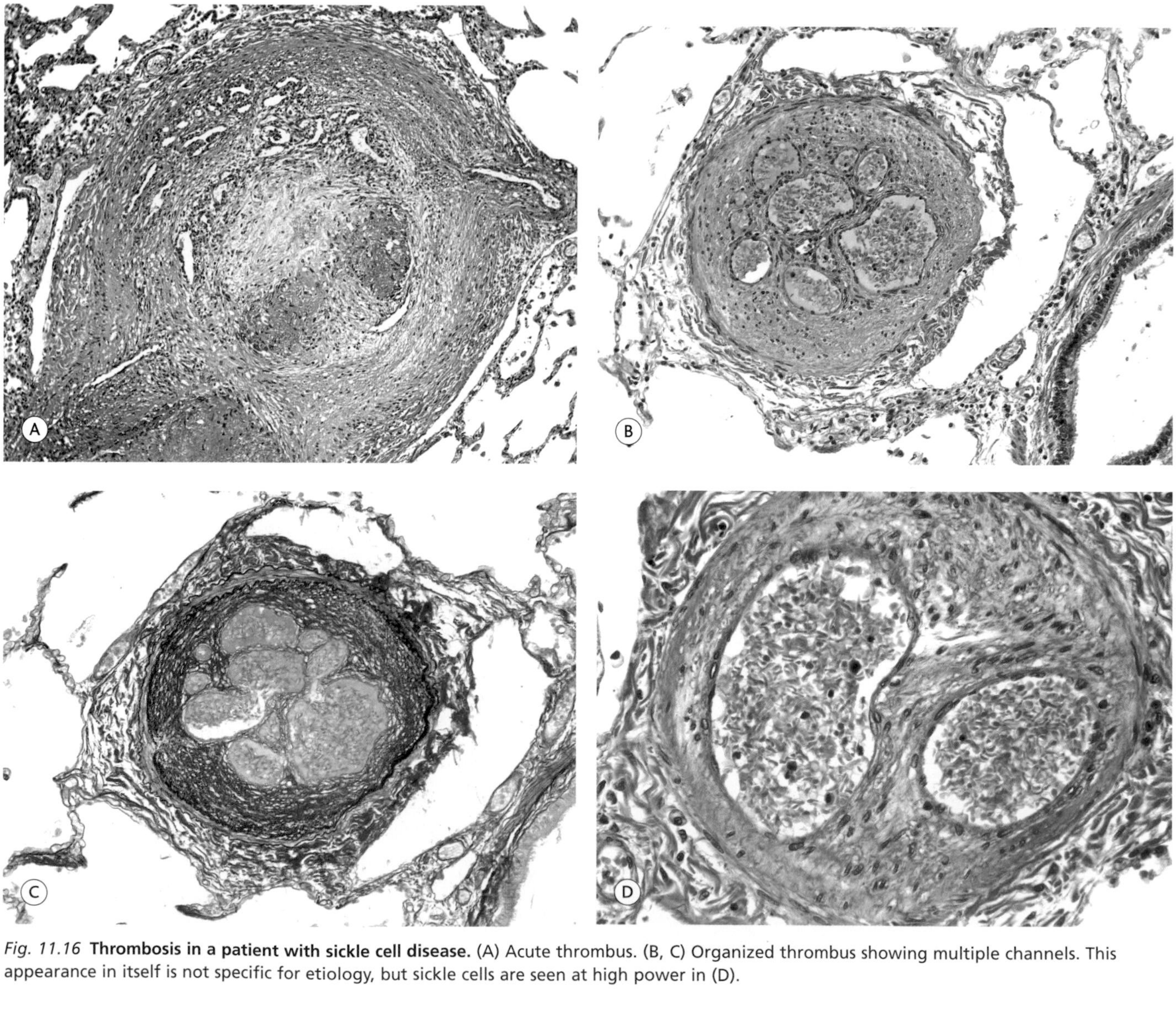

Fig. 11.16 **Thrombosis in a patient with sickle cell disease.** (A) Acute thrombus. (B, C) Organized thrombus showing multiple channels. This appearance in itself is not specific for etiology, but sickle cells are seen at high power in (D).

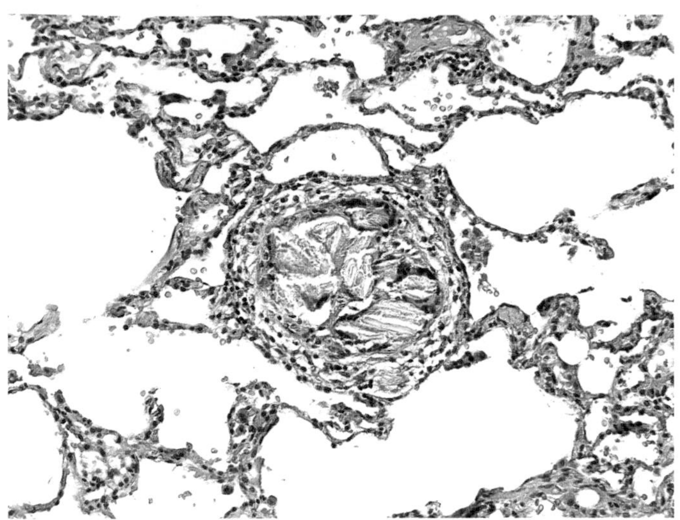

Fig. 11.17 Organized thrombus and birefringent particles in a muscular pulmonary artery from an IV drug abuser.

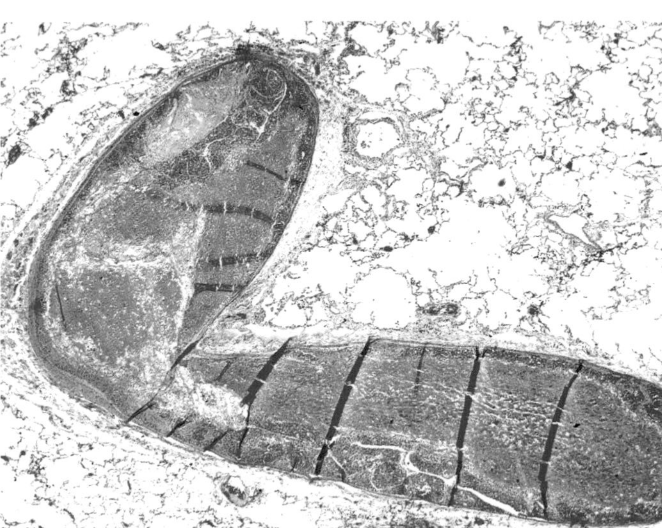

Fig. 11.18 Filling of pulmonary artery branches by tumor emboli from a hepatocellular carcinoma.

that are also birefringent. For illicit drugs, exact identification of the filler may not be possible.

Pulmonary hypertension may develop as a result of filling of the small arterial branches with tumor emboli (Fig. 11.18). Radiographically or pathologically visible metastases may or may not be present. Pulmonary hypertension in this setting has been most commonly reported with lung, breast, stomach, ovarian, and hepatocellular carcinomas.[27]

Clinical correlation

In most of these conditions there is no specific therapy. However, when pulmonary hypertension is caused by large vessel, especially main pulmonary artery, thrombi, surgical removal of the thrombi may reverse the hypertension.

Differential diagnosis

As noted, scattered thrombi are fairly common in other types of pulmonary hypertension such as plexogenic arteriopathy, and the presence of thrombi or eccentric intimal lesions does not automatically indicate a diagnosis of thrombotic and embolic hypertension. Although it has been claimed that plexiform lesions can, rarely, be seen in thrombotic and embolic hypertension,[30] we believe that such cases in fact represent plexogenic arteriopathy with more than the usual number of thrombi. Thus, it is important to be sure that typical plexogenic lesions are not present and to demonstrate the presence of *multiple* thrombi or emboli when making a diagnosis of thrombi or embolic hypertension.

Pulmonary veno-occlusive disease and other types of pulmonary venous hypertension

Clinical features

Like other forms of pulmonary hypertension, pulmonary veno-occlusive disease (PVOD) is characterized by the insidious onset of shortness of breath, often associated with a nonproductive cough. Clubbing has been identified in some patients. There is a wide age range of affected subjects, with the mean age less than 50, and including a significant proportion of children. Patients with PVOD do not have clinical evidence of thrombotic or embolic disease, but may have small hemoptyses.

Radiographic features

On plain films, patients with advanced disease show pulmonary artery enlargement and, with cor pulmonale, right ventricular hypertrophy. A helpful finding in PVOD is the presence of prominent Kerley B lines and mild-to-moderate interstitial infiltrates. The CT scan shows distinctly thickened interlobular septa.[31]

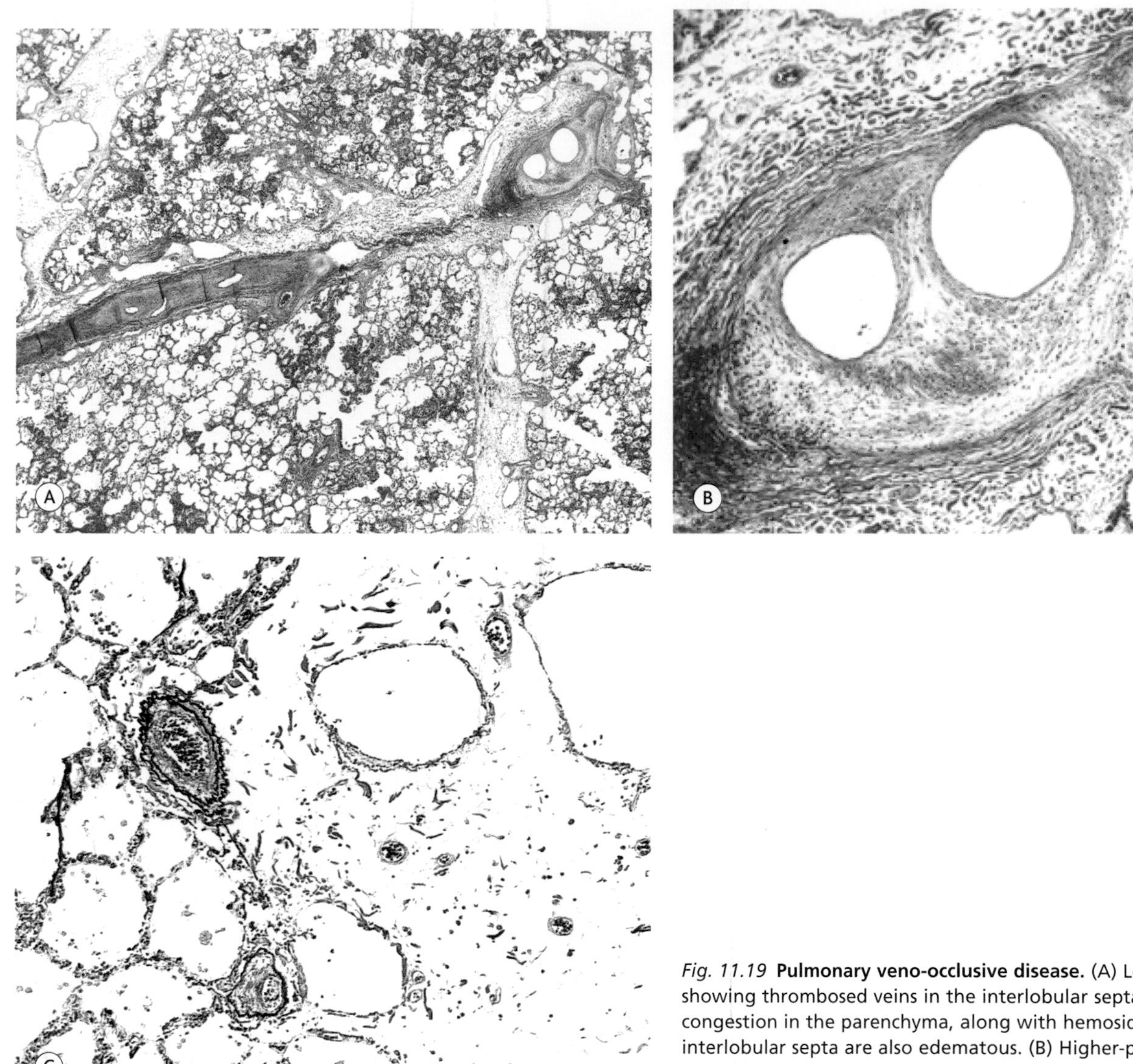

Fig. 11.19 **Pulmonary veno-occlusive disease.** (A) Low-power view showing thrombosed veins in the interlobular septa and intense congestion in the parenchyma, along with hemosiderin pigment. The interlobular septa are also edematous. (B) Higher-power view of an organized thrombus in a large vein. (C) Elastic stain demonstrating arterialized veins and marked edema in the interlobular septa.

Pathologic findings

The fundamental lesion in PVOD is thrombosis, typically old thrombosis, of small pulmonary veins and venules. This is best seen in veins in the interlobular septa (Fig. 11.19) where the location ensures that the structure is indeed a vein. With increasing pressure, such veins may become arterialized, i.e. they develop a double elastic lamina and a distinct layer of muscle (Fig. 11.19C), and are thus distinguishable from arteries only by their location.

The venules in PVOD are often thrombosed as well, but this may be difficult to document. Venous hypertension of any cause is associated with intimal fibrosis and lumenal narrowing of the veins and venules, but in PVOD the lumen of small venules may simply be obliterated by fibrous tissue (Fig. 11.20). Use of elastic stains is mandatory to find such vessels, and once small vessels with apparent lumenal obliteration are found, these may need to be traced back through several sections until they connect with a vein in an interlobular septum, thus proving their nature. The diagnosis of PVOD can be exceedingly difficult in cases where only small venules are affected.

The vascular changes in PVOD do not occur in isolation. The interlobular septa are generally edematous and the lymphatics prominently dilated (Fig. 11.19). A peculiar, usually mild, form of interstitial fibrosis which

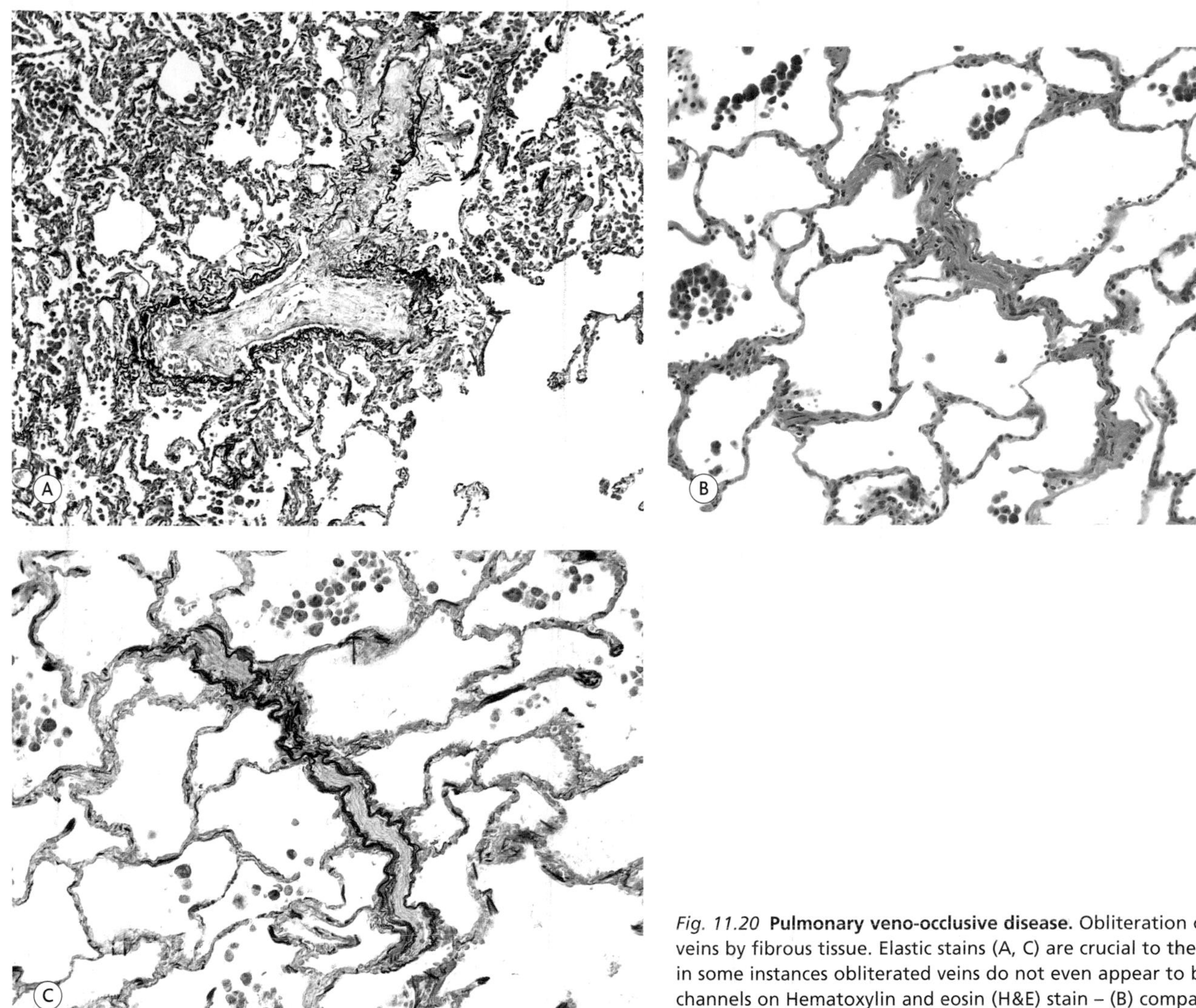

Fig. 11.20 **Pulmonary veno-occlusive disease.** Obliteration of small veins by fibrous tissue. Elastic stains (A, C) are crucial to the diagnosis; in some instances obliterated veins do not even appear to be vascular channels on Hematoxylin and eosin (H&E) stain – (B) compare the same image by elastic stain in (C).

tends to be more marked in the very periphery of the lung under the pleura (Fig. 11.21) is common in PVOD. The fibrosis is fairly homogeneous, paucicellular, and raises the morphologic question of a chronic interstitial pneumonia. Accompanying the fibrosis are usually very small foci of acute or old hemorrhage with hemosiderin-laden macrophages (Fig. 11.21B). The combination of mild, homogeneous fibrosis and small hemorrhages should bring the diagnosis of PVOD to mind and prompt examination of the veins in the interlobular septa.

Arterial changes may be present in PVOD. These consist of muscular hypertrophy and sometimes mild intimal fibrosis. Another change that may be seen in PVOD, but also in any disease characterized by repeated pulmonary hemorrhage, is so-called *endogenous pneumoconiosis*. This consists of coating of elastic fibers by iron and calcium, with a resulting appearance that resembles a ferruginous body (Fig. 11.21C) of the type seen in asbestosis. Foci of dystrophic ossification may also be present, but are a fairly nonspecific marker of venous hypertension (see below).

Clinical correlation

Most cases of PVOD have no known cause, but small numbers of cases have been reported in patients given chemotherapeutic agents.[32] In general, the prognosis is poor and, at present, transplantation offers the only hope

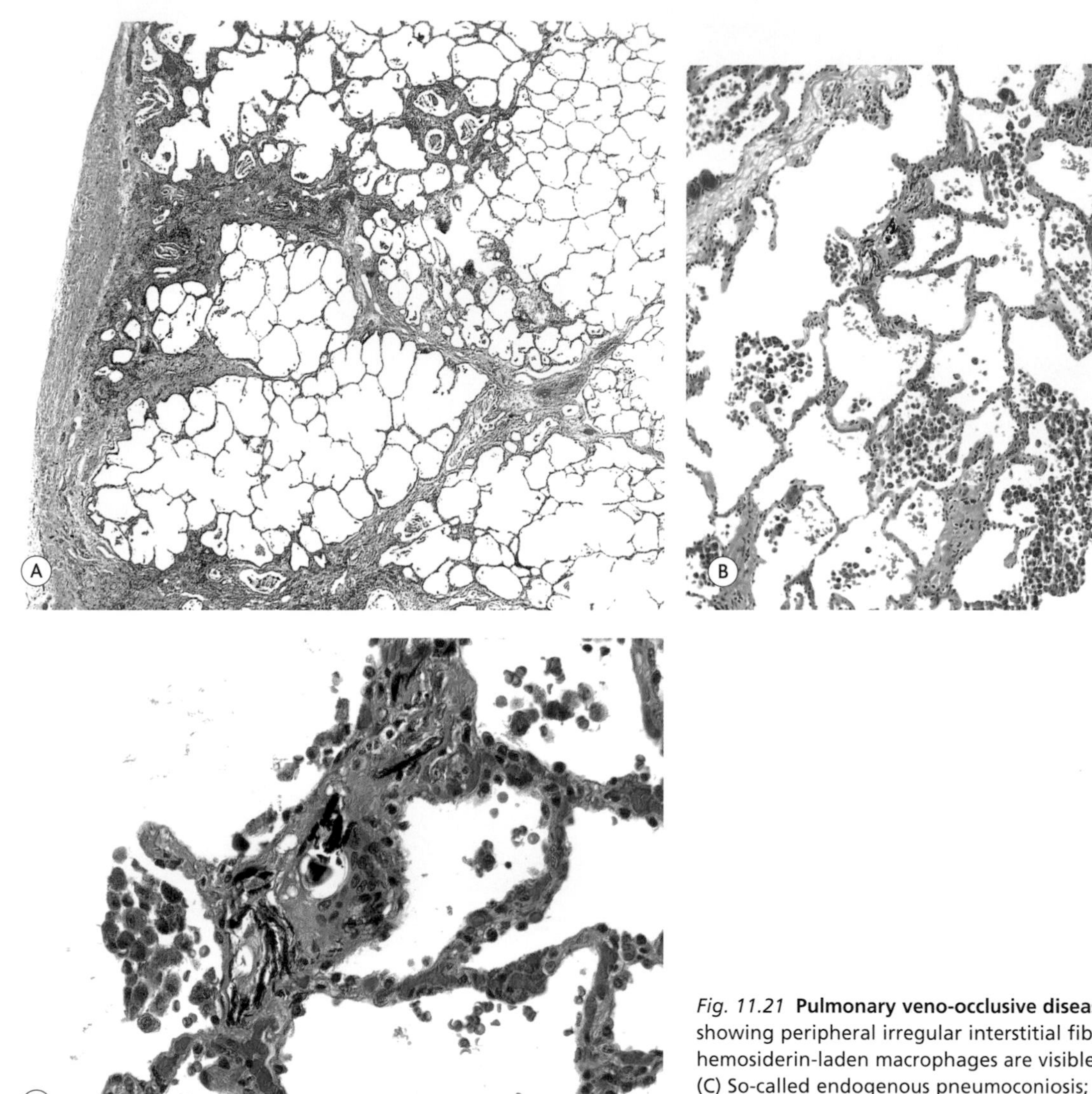

Fig. 11.21 **Pulmonary veno-occlusive disease.** (A) Low-power view showing peripheral irregular interstitial fibrosis. (B) Fine fibrosis and hemosiderin-laden macrophages are visible in the higher-power view. (C) So-called endogenous pneumoconiosis; i.e. encrustation of elastic fibers by iron and calcium and reactive multinucleated giant cells. This lesion may be seen in any cause of chronic pulmonary hemorrhage.

of cure. Vasodilator therapy must be approached with caution since it may induce severe pulmonary edema.

Differential diagnosis

PVOD is the most dramatic and severe form of *pulmonary venous hypertension*. Venous hypertension may also be seen in patients with left-sided heart disease, especially mitral stenosis, and, rarely, atrial myxomas; in conditions such as sclerosing mediastinitis in which the pulmonary veins are obliterated or narrowed in the mediastinum; and in some types of congenital cardiac malformations where the major pulmonary veins are abnormal or absent. Intimal fibrosis in the small pulmonary veins and venules, mild interstitial inflammation and edema, small hemorrhages, 'endogenous pneumoconiosis', and dystrophic ossification are common in all these conditions, and muscular hypertrophy in the small pulmonary arterial branches may be present as well (Fig. 11.22). However, true venous obliteration, the hallmark of PVOD, is absent. Idiopathic interstitial pneumonias and even real pneumoconioses come into the differential diagnosis, as indicated above.

Pulmonary capillary hemangiomatosis

Clinical and radiographic features

Pulmonary capillary hemangiomatosis (PCH) is a very rare disease, mostly seen in adults. The usual nonspecific signs of pulmonary hypertension are present and small

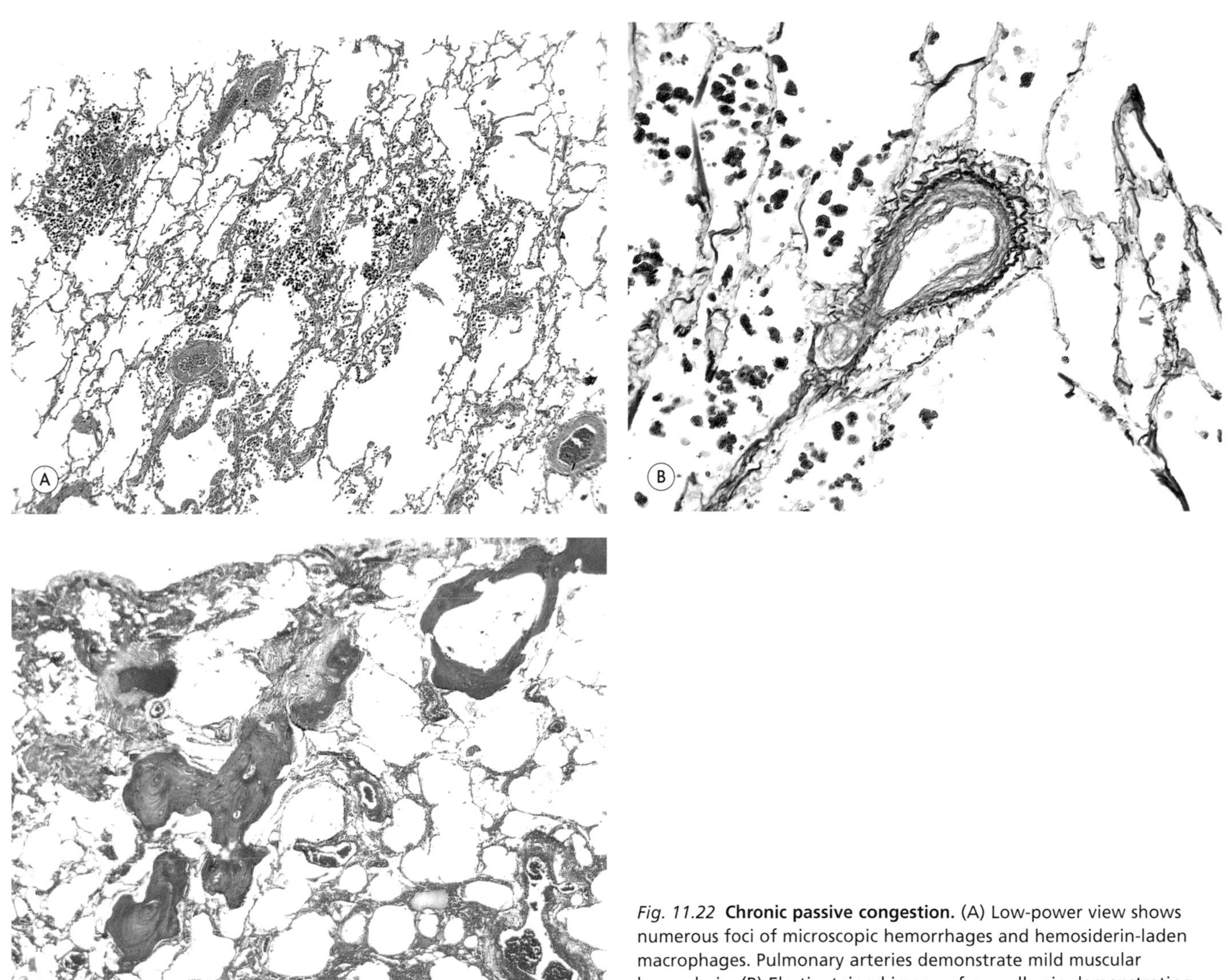

Fig. 11.22 **Chronic passive congestion.** (A) Low-power view shows numerous foci of microscopic hemorrhages and hemosiderin-laden macrophages. Pulmonary arteries demonstrate mild muscular hyperplasia. (B) Elastic stained image of a small vein demonstrating intimal proliferation. This is a nonspecific finding that can be seen in venous hypertension but is also commonly observed as an aging effect. (C) Ossification in the parenchyma, a common finding with venous stasis.

hemoptyses may occur. Chest radiography demonstrates interstitial infiltrates, with thickened interlobular septa.[33]

Pathologic findings

PCH is characterized by proliferation of dilated capillary-sized channels along and in the alveolar walls (Fig. 11.23). In this it resembles a very severe form of passive congestion, but careful examination shows that there appears to be duplicate or multiple capillary channels in an alveolar wall, something not present in passive congestion.[34] The proliferating capillary channels extend into arterioles and venules, producing a peculiar pattern of capillary proliferation within the walls of the larger vessel with resulting lumenal narrowing or obliteration; it is this involvement of larger vessels that is thought to produce pulmonary hypertension. Often there is an admixture of very abnormal areas of lung with extensive capillary proliferation combined with perfectly normal appearing lung, again a helpful finding in separating capillary hemangiomatosis from passive congestion (the latter should be more homogeneous). Small acute and old hemorrhages may be present, as may muscular hypertrophy in small pulmonary arteries.

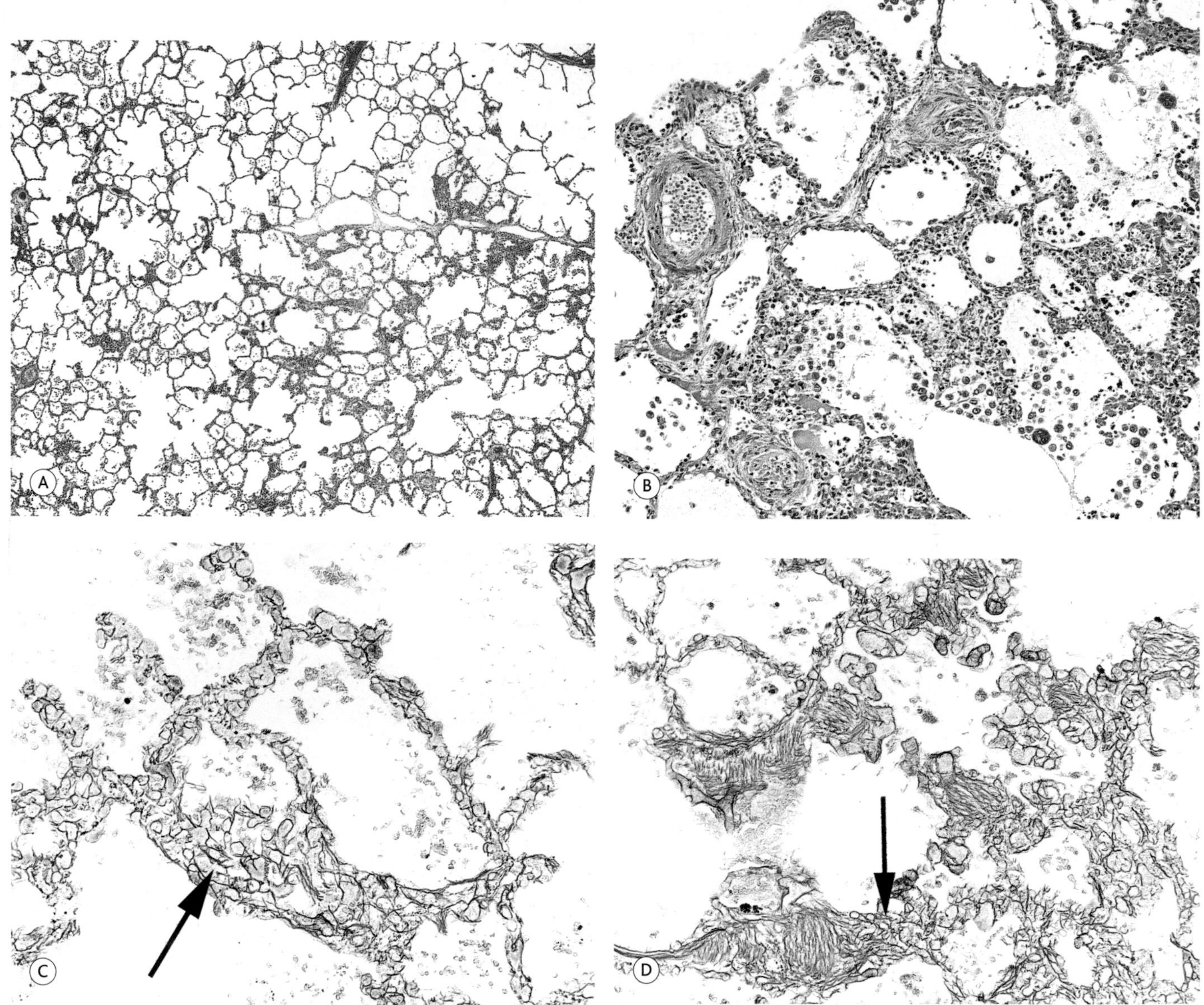

Fig. 11.23 **Pulmonary capillary hemangiomatosis.** (A) Low-power view showing what at first glance appears to be marked congestion. (B) Higher-power image demonstrates thickened alveolar walls caused by proliferating capillaries. (C) Proliferating capillary channels are better demonstrated in this reticulum stain, and are shown to invade into the walls of a small vein (arrow). (D) Reticulum stain shows capillaries invading wall of airway (arrow).

Clinical correlation

The etiology of PCH is not known, but the lesion behaves much like a very-low-grade vascular sarcoma. Some patients have been treated with transplantation.

Pulmonary hypertension secondary to other forms of intrinsic lung disease

Pulmonary hypertension is commonly found associated with different forms of non-vascular intrinsic lung disease, including emphysema, bronchiectasis, usual interstitial pneumonia, and any other conditions that produce extensive scarring of the parenchyma or that produce chronic hypoxia. In emphysema, claims have been made that hypertension is secondary to loss of capillary bed, although this may not be correct, and vascular changes may be caused by direct effects of cigarette smoke on the vasculature or by local hypoxic vasoconstriction. The reasons for the development of pulmonary hypertension in the other conditions listed is unclear, although in some instances hypertension is probably caused by destruction of the vascular bed. The development of cor pulmonale is common in all of these diseases and may be the cause of death.

In all of these settings, the vascular changes consist of muscular hypertrophy of the small pulmonary arteries, often with extension of muscle into the arterioles. Sometimes, mild intimal proliferation is present.

REFERENCES

1. Wagenvoort CA: Lung biopsy specimens in the evaluation of pulmonary vascular disease. Chest 1980; 77: 614–625.
2. Pietra GG, Edwards WD, Kay JM, et al. Histopathology of primary pulmonary hypertension. Circulation 1989; 80: 1198–1206.
3. Palevsky HI, Schloo BL, Pietra GG, et al. Primary pulmonary hypertension. Vascular structure, morphometry, and responsiveness to vasodilator agents. Circulation 1989; 80: 1207–1220.
4. Wagenvoort CA, Wagenvoort N: Pulmonary vascular bed: normal anatomy and responses to disease. In: Pulmonary vascular diseases: lung biology in health and disease, Moser KM, Ed. 1979, Marcel Dekker, New York, pp 1–110.
5. Rabinovitch M: Morphology of the developing pulmonary bed: pharmacologic implications. Pediatr Pharm 1985; 5: 31–48.
6. Schraufnagel DE: Corrosion casting of the lung for scanning electron microscopy. In: Electron microscopy of the lung, C. Lenfant C, Ed. 1990, Marcel Dekker, New York, pp 257–297.
7. Murphy ML, Bone RC: Cor pulmonale in chronic bronchitis and emphysema. 1984, Future Publishing, New York.
8. Fulton RM, Hutchinson EC, Jones AM: Ventricular weight in cardiac hypertrophy. Br Heart J 1952; 14: 413–420.
9. Ishikawa S, Fattal GA: Functional morphometry of myocardial fibres in cor pulmonale. Am Rev Respir Dis 1972; 105: 358–367.
10. Fishman AP: Pulmonary hypertension and cor pulmonale. In: Pulmonary diseases and disorders, 2nd edn, Fishman AP, Ed. 1988, McGraw-Hill, New York.
11. Wagenvoort CA, Wagenvoort N: Pathology of pulmonary hypertension. 1977, John Wiley and Sons, New York.
12. Wagenvoort CA: Lung biopsies in the differential diagnosis of thromboembolic versus primary pulmonary hypertension. Prog Resp Res 1980; 13: 16–21.
13. Wagenvoort CA: Grading of pulmonary vascular lesions – a reappraisal. Histopathology 1981; 5: 595–598.
14. Pietra GG, Ruttner JR: Specificity of pulmonary vascular lesions in primary pulmonary hypertension. A reappraisal. Respiration 1982; 52: 81–85.
15. Burke AP, Farb A, Virmani R: The pathology of primary pulmonary hypertension. Mod Pathol 1991; 4: 269–277.
16. Heath D, Edwards JE: The pathology of hypertensive pulmonary vascular disease. Circulation 1958; 18: 533–543.
17. Wagenvoort CA, Mulder RGH: Thrombotic lesion in primary plexogenic arteriopathy: similar pathogenesis or complication? Chest 1993; 103: 844–849.
18. Abenhaim L, Moride UY, Brenot F, et al.: Appetite-suppressant drugs and the risk of primary pulmonary hypertension. N Engl J Med 1996; 335: 609–616.
19. Fishman AP: Aminorex to Fen/Phen: an epidemic foretold. Circulation. 1999; 99:156–161.
20. Mehta NJ, Khan LA, Mehta RN, Sepkowitz DA: HIV-related pulmonary hypertension: analytic review of 131 cases. Chest 2000; 118: 1133–1141.
21. Pellicelli AM, Barbaro G, Palmieri F, et al.: Primary pulmonary hypertension in HIV patients: a systematic review. Angiology 2001; 51: 31–41.
22. Ng CS, Wells AU, Padley SP: A CT sign of chronic pulmonary arterial hypertension: the ratio of main pulmonary artery to aortic diameter. J Thorac Imaging 1999; 14: 270–278.
23. Moore GW, Smith RR, Hutchins GM: Pulmonary artery atherosclerosis: correlation with systemic atherosclerosis and hypertensive pulmonary vascular disease. Arch Pathol Lab Med 1982; 106: 378–380.
24. Meyrick B: The structure and ultrastructure of the pulmonary microvasculature. In: The pulmonary circulation in health and disease, Will JA, Dawson CA, Weir EK, Buckner CK, Eds. 1987, Academic Press, New York.
25. Yamaki S, Wagenvoort CA: Plexogenic pulmonary arteriopathy: significance of medial thickness with respect to advanced pulmonary vascular lesions. Am J Pathol 1981; 105: 70–75.
26. Fernie JM, Lamb D: Effects of age and smoking on intima of muscular pulmonary arteries. J Clin Pathol 1986; 39: 1204–1208.
27. Katzenstein A-L: Pulmonary hypertension and other vascular disorders. In: Katzenstein and Askin's surgical pathology of non-neoplastic lung disease, 3rd edn. 1997, WB Saunders, Philadelphia, pp 322–360.
28. Yakel DL, Eisenberg MJ: Pulmonary artery hypertension in chronic intravenous cocaine users. Am Heart J 1995; 130: 398–390.
29. Tomashefski JF, Hirsch CS: The pulmonary vascular lesions of intravenous drug abuse. Hum Pathol 1980; 11: 133–145.
30. Moser KM, Bloor CM: Pulmonary vascular lesions occurring in patients with chronic major vessel thromboembolic pulmonary hypertension. Circulation 1981; 210: 507–511.
31. Holcomb BS, Loyd JE, Ely W, et al.: Pulmonary veno-occlusive disease. Chest 2000; 118: 1671–1679.
32. Lombard C, Churg A, Winokur A: Pulmonary veno-occlusive disease following therapy for malignant neoplasms. Chest 1987; 92: 871–876.
33. Al-Fawaz IM, Al Mobiareek KF, Al-Suhaibani M, Ashour M: Pulmonary capillary hemangiomatosis. Pediatr Pulmonol 1995; 19: 243–248.
34. Tron V, Magee F, Wright J, et al.: Pulmonary capillary hemangiomatosis. Human Pathol 1986; 17: 1144–1150.

12

Pathology of lung transplantation

Andras Khoor Samuel A Yousem

Introduction

Lung transplantation may offer longer survival and improved quality of life to patients with end-stage lung disease. The most common procedure performed is single-lung transplantation, followed by heart–lung and bilateral/double-lung transplantation.[1] Indications for lung transplantation are listed in Table 12.1. Living donor single lobe transplantation may be a viable alternative to cadaveric lung transplantation for selected patients.[2] Currently, the 1-year survival for patients with pulmonary allografts is approximately 70%; the 5-year survival is somewhat below 50%.[1]

Complications of lung transplantation may be related to:

- the operation itself (reimplantation response, harvest injury, anastomotic complications)
- the host's immunologic response to the allograft (rejection)
- the immunosuppressive therapy used to prevent rejection (infection, post-transplant lymphoproliferative disorders).

Table 12.1 Most common indications for lung transplant procedures

Transplant procedure	Most common indications
Heart–lung	Congenital heart disease Primary pulmonary hypertension Cystic fibrosis
Adult single lung	Chronic obstructive pulmonary disease Idiopathic pulmonary fibrosis
Adult bilateral/double lung	Cystic fibrosis Chronic obstructive pulmonary disease Primary pulmonary hypertension Idiopathic pulmonary fibrosis
Pediatric lung	Cystic fibrosis Primary pulmonary hypertension

Source: modified from Hosenpud et al.[1]

Other complications, such as organizing pneumonia and recurrence of the original disease, may also occur. For diagnostic purposes, time interval after transplantation can be divided arbitrarily into immediate (within 4 days), early (4 days to 1 month), and late (beyond 1 month) post-transplant period.[3] The differential diagnostic possibilities for each period are listed in Table 12.2.

Post-transplant lung (transbronchial) biopsies can be performed as surveillance of rejection and for a specific clinical indication. The role of surveillance biopsies remains controversial.[4] The histopathologic findings most commonly encountered in a post-transplant transbronchial biopsy include acute rejection, cytomegalovirus (CMV) infection, airway-centered inflammation, pneumonia, bronchiolitis obliterans, harvest injury, invasive aspergillosis, and post-transplant lymphoproliferative disorders.[4]

Operation-related complications

Reimplantation response

Unavoidable transplantation-related injuries, including surgical trauma, denervation, lymphatic interruption, and ischemia, result in what has been called reimplantation response.[5]

Table 12.2 Complications of lung transplantation

Post-transplantation period	Operation-related complications	Rejection	Immunosuppression-related complications	Other complications
Immediate (within 4 days)	Reimplantation response Harvest injury Arterial anastomotic obstruction Venous anastomotic obstruction Airway dehiscence	Hyperacute rejection	Bacterial pneumonia	
Early (4 days to 1 month)	Arterial anastomotic obstruction Venous anastomotic obstruction Airway dehiscence Large airway stenosis	Acute rejection	Infection (bacterial, viral, fungal, *Pneumocystis jerovici*)	
Late (beyond 1 month)	Large airway stenosis	Acute rejection Chronic airway rejection	Infection (bacterial, viral, fungal, *Pneumocystis jerovici*) Post-transplant lymphoproliferative disorders	Organizing pneumonia Recurrence of the primary disease

Time period

Reimplantation response begins within 48 hours and usually peaks on the 4th post-transplant day.

Clinical presentation

Clinical signs include worsening oxygenation, and decreased lung compliance.

Radiologic findings

Radiographs show diffuse alveolar and interstitial infiltrates, which are most prominent in the perihilar region.

Diagnosis

The diagnosis is made by exclusion. Appropriate investigations may include bronchoalveolar lavage (BAL) and transbronchial biopsy to exclude early acute rejection.

Pathologic findings

Histologically, alveolar and interstitial edema and scattered neutrophils are seen, with hyaline membranes developing over time.[6]

Treatment and prognosis

The treatment is supportive and may require mechanical ventilation. Reimplantation response may resolve within a few days, but may last as long as several weeks.

Harvest injury

Harvest injury, also known as preservation or reperfusion injury, is a consequence of prolonged periods of donor organ preservation under anoxic conditions. It presents as primary graft failure with acute deterioration of lung function shortly after revascularization of the pulmonary allograft.

Time period

Respiratory decline becomes apparent within 24 hours after transplantation.

Clinical presentation

Clinical signs of harvest injury include rapidly progressive pulmonary edema, and markedly diminished pulmonary compliance.

Radiologic findings

Radiographically, diffuse bilateral pulmonary infiltrates are seen.

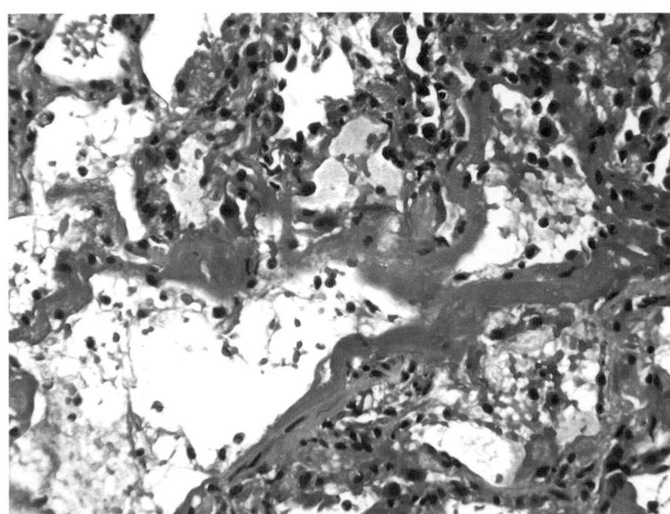

Fig. 12.1 Acute diffuse alveolar damage due to harvest injury. The key to the diagnosis is the presence of hyaline membranes.

Diagnosis

The diagnosis is made by exclusion of other causes of primary graft failure, including hyperacute rejection, pulmonary venous obstruction, fluid overload, and infection. In particular, donor sepsis or shock can manifest in the recipient within hours or days after transplant, despite little abnormality in the donor prior to harvest. Harvest injury differs from reimplantation response by the severity of symptoms, and may simply represent a more severe form of acute lung injury; i.e. diffuse alveolar damage (DAD).

Pathologic findings

The histologic correlate of clinical harvest injury is DAD. The acute phase is characterized by densely eosinophilic hyaline membranes, interstitial edema, occasional fibrin thrombi, and scattered neutrophils in the alveolar septa (Fig. 12.1). In the organizing phase, the hyaline membranes are incorporated into the alveolar septa, which become thickened by fibroblast rich connective tissue (Fig. 12.2).

Histologic differential diagnosis

Factors that may cause DAD in a lung transplant patient are listed in Table 12.3. Immunofluorescent studies are helpful in separating harvest injury from hyperacute rejection. Harvest injury lacks the presence of immunoglobulin (Ig) and complement deposits, whereas IgG and complement can be detected in the alveolar septa in hyperacute rejection. Hyperacute rejection can present as a leukocytoclastic vasculitis affecting small vessels, accompanied by alveolar hemorrhage.

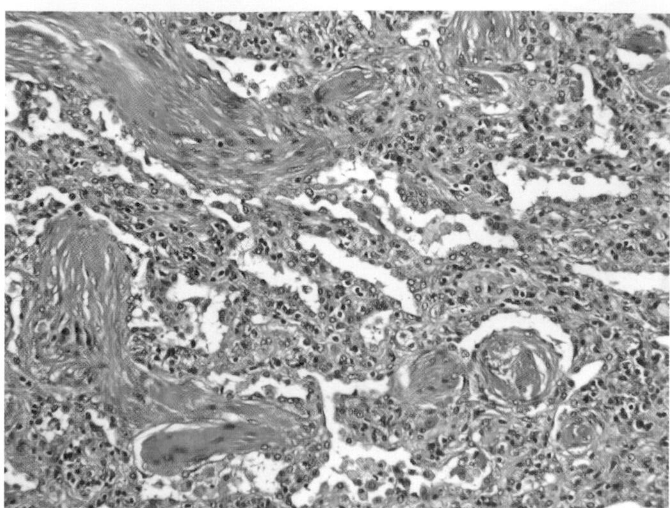

Fig. 12.2 Organizing diffuse alveolar damage as a result of harvest injury. In the absence of residual hyaline membranes, the history can aid the diagnosis.

Table 12.3 Common causes of diffuse alveolar damage in the pulmonary allograft

Harvest injury
Hyperacute rejection
Severe acute rejection
Infection

Fortunately, today, acute rejection is not a major concern during the immediate post-transplant period. Because any infection can present as DAD in an immunocompromised patient, special stains should always be performed to rule out this possibility.

Treatment and prognosis

Harvest injury leading to primary graft failure is a very serious complication of lung transplantation and has a high mortality rate.[7]

Arterial anastomotic obstruction

The incidence of pulmonary arterial anastomotic obstruction after lung transplantation is relatively low.[8] Causes include narrowed anastomosis, with or without thrombus formation, resulting from suboptimal surgical anastomoses[9] and excessive length of donor or recipient pulmonary artery with kinking/torsing of the anastomosis.

Time period

Arterial anastomotic obstruction usually occurs during the first week after transplantation.

Clinical presentation

Signs and symptoms include dyspnea, hypoxemia, and elevated pulmonary arterial pressure.

Diagnosis

The diagnosis is suggested by reduced perfusion in the allograft by ventilation/perfusion (V/Q) scan and can be confirmed by echocardiogram or pulmonary angiography. Large areas of infarction may be present. Pathologic confirmation is usually not required.

Venous anastomotic obstruction

Minor abnormalities of the pulmonary venous anastomosis are relatively common complications of lung transplantation.[10,11] Occlusive thrombus formation is relatively rare, but may have catastrophic consequences, including allograft failure and stroke.

Time period

Venous anastomotic obstruction usually presents in the immediate post-transplant period, but has been reported to occur as late as the eighth postoperative day.[8]

Clinical presentation

Typical features include unilateral frothy pulmonary edema and other signs and symptoms of outflow obstruction.

Radiologic findings

Chest X-ray reveals diffuse unilateral interstitial edema.

Diagnosis

Diagnosis is made by transesophageal echocardiogram.[10–12]

Pathologic findings

The specimen from the surgical revision may include a thrombus. Biopsy of the lung obtained at the same time may show congestion, and venous engorgement.

Treatment

Venous anastomotic obstruction is considered a surgical emergency and revision of the anastomosis with removal of any associated thrombus is required to prevent irreversible injury to the lung allograft.[3]

Airway dehiscence

In the early years of lung transplantation, airway dehiscence due to ischemia of the donor bronchus was a major cause of morbidity and mortality.[13] Improvement in surgical techniques, including telescoped anastomoses, reduced immunosuppression and better allograft preservation, has reduced the incidence of lethal airway dehiscence to approximately 0.6%.[14]

Time period

Airway dehiscence may develop in the first few weeks after transplantation.

Diagnosis

Ischemia and necrosis of the bronchus can be diagnosed by direct visualization with a bronchoscope.

Pathologic findings

Biopsies show coagulation necrosis of the bronchial mucosa, submucosa, and cartilage. Superimposed bacterial or fungal infection may produce neutrophilic infiltrates, and thereby enhance necrosis and dehiscence of the anastomosis.

Treatment

Surgical options are limited, but may include anastomotic revision, retransplantation, or stent placement.

Large airway stenosis

Large airway stenosis at the anastomosis site results from excessive growth of granulation tissue, often in response to the combined effects of bronchial ischemia, rejection, and infection. Improved surgical techniques and better allograft preservation have reduced the incidence of large airway stenosis. Currently, it occurs in approximately 3.3% of bronchial anastomoses.[14]

Nonanastomotic large airway stenosis has also been described.[15,16] The pathogenesis of this lesion is unclear, but it may represent a response to ischemic damage, alloreactive injury, or infection.

Time period

Bronchial stenosis usually occurs a few months after the transplant, but has been described as early as 8 days.[9]

Clinical presentation

Clinical findings include dyspnea, retained secretions, recurrent pneumonia, and decline in spirometry, all of which can mimic chronic airway rejection.

Diagnosis

Bronchoscopic examination provides the diagnosis, with biopsies providing confirmatory histology.

Pathologic findings

Common findings include prominent granulation tissue, fibrosis, and squamous metaplasia.

Treatment

Large airway stenosis is treated with stent placement or repetitive dilatations.

Rejection

Except in the case of monozygotic twins, donors and recipients are genetically different and express different histocompatibility antigens. This results in rejection of the allograft by the recipient's immune system. Multiple immunologic processes are involved, creating a spectrum of rejection responses. In 1990, a "working formulation for the classification of pulmonary allograft rejection" was introduced.[17] In 1995, a group of international experts revised the original working formulation.[18] This revision has become a generally accepted scheme for the grading of pulmonary allograft rejection (Table 12.4). Although hyperacute rejection is not included in the working formulation, it will be discussed here for completeness sake.

Table 12.4 Working formulation for classification and grading of pulmonary allograft rejection

A. Acute rejection Grade 0 – None Grade 1 – Minimal Grade 2 – Mild Grade 3 – Moderate Grade 4 – Severe	with/without	B. Airway inflammation –lymphocytic bronchitis/bronchiolitis
C. Chronic airway rejection – bronchiolitis obliterans a. Active b. Inactive		
D. Chronic vascular rejection – accelerated graft vascular sclerosis		

Source: from Yousem et al.[18]

Hyperacute rejection

Hyperacute rejection is a rare, but potentially fatal, complication of lung transplantation. It involves anti-donor antibodies that have developed in the recipient before transplantation. When transplantation occurs, the preformed antibodies bind to endothelial surfaces of the allograft and activate inflammatory and coagulation cascades. Recipients with a high titer of "panel-reactive" and anti-endothelial antibodies are at the highest risk for developing hyperacute rejection.[19]

Time period

Clinical signs are noticeable within minutes to hours after transplantation.

Clinical presentation

The clinical features include pulmonary edema, progressive respiratory failure, and pleural effusion.

Radiologic findings

Complete opacification of the pulmonary allograft is seen.

Diagnosis

The diagnosis is based on the clinical findings and a positive donor-specific IgG crossmatch. Although histologic confirmation is usually not necessary, an intraoperative lung biopsy may be performed.

Pathologic findings

At the time of the Lung Rejection Study Group meeting in 1995, there were not enough data available to define hyperacute rejection.[18] Recent studies have indicated that histologic features of hyperacute rejection include DAD, interstitial neutrophilia, extensive fibrin thrombi, and vasculitis.[19,20] Immunofluorescent studies reveal deposition of IgG and complement in the alveolar septa.[19,20]

Histologic differential diagnosis

From the pathologist's perspective, vasculitis and positive immunofluorescent studies separate hyperacute rejection from harvest injury.

Acute rejection

Most lung transplant patients experience episodes of acute rejection. This is a cell-mediated process, in contrast to the humoral-mediated process of hyperacute rejection.

Time period

Acute rejection may occur as early as 3 days and as late as several years after transplantation. The majority of acute rejection episodes begin within the first 3 months after transplantation.

Clinical presentation

Clinical features may include low-grade fever, cough, dyspnea, crackles, and adventitious sounds on auscultation. Features suspicious for rejection include a more than 10% decrease in the forced expiratory volume in 1 minute (FEV_1), and hypoxemia.

Radiologic findings

Radiologic abnormalities include perihilar or lower lung zone alveolar and interstitial infiltrates, septal lines, subpleural edema, peribronchial cuffing, and pleural effusion. In cases of a single-lung transplant, the ventilation perfusion (V/Q) lung scan will show decreased perfusion to the allograft.

Diagnosis

Clinical features may suggest acute rejection, but a transbronchial biopsy is usually required to confirm the diagnosis and rule out infection. If biopsy from multiple sites is technically impossible, biopsies of the lower lobes should be performed, since they appear to be more informative.[21]

Pathologic findings

The hallmark of acute rejection is the presence of perivascular mononuclear cell infiltrates. Although the process may involve the conducting airways, the histologic diagnosis is based solely on changes in the alveolated parenchyma.[18] If airway inflammation is present, it should be noted[18] (see below).

Acute rejection is graded according to the density and extent of the perivascular infiltrates, and the presence or absence of secondary pneumocyte damage (Table 12.5). Rejection-type infiltrates usually involve more than one vessel, but a single perivascular infiltrate should be evaluated by the same criteria as multiple infiltrates as follows:

1. Minimal acute rejection (Grade A1) is characterized by infrequent, 2–3 cell thick perivascular mononuclear cell infiltrates (Fig. 12.3).
2. In mild acute rejection (Grade A2), the perivascular mononuclear cell infiltrates become thicker, denser, and usually more frequent (Fig. 12.4).

Table 12.5 Grading acute rejection

Grade of acute rejection	Histologic criteria	Cellular composition	Comments
A0 – None	Normal pulmonary parenchyma		
A1 – Minimal	Perivascular mononuclear cell infiltrates, 2–3 cells thick (not obvious at low magnification)	Small round, plasmacytoid, and transformed lymphocytes	The perivascular infiltrates are usually infrequent
A2 – Mild	Perivascular mononuclear cell infiltrates, more than 3 cells thick (easily seen at low magnification)	Same as A1, with macrophages, and eosinophils	The perivascular infiltrates are usually frequent. Endothelialitis and airway inflammation are often present
A3 – Moderate	Perivascular mononuclear cell infiltrates, similar to A2, with extension into alveolar septa and air spaces	Same as A2, with occasional neutrophils	Endothelialitis and airway inflammation are usually present
A4 – Severe	Diffuse mononuclear cell infiltrates, similar to A3, with prominent pneumocyte damage	Same as A3	The pneumocyte damage is commonly associated with hyaline membranes

Source: modified from Yousem et al.[18]

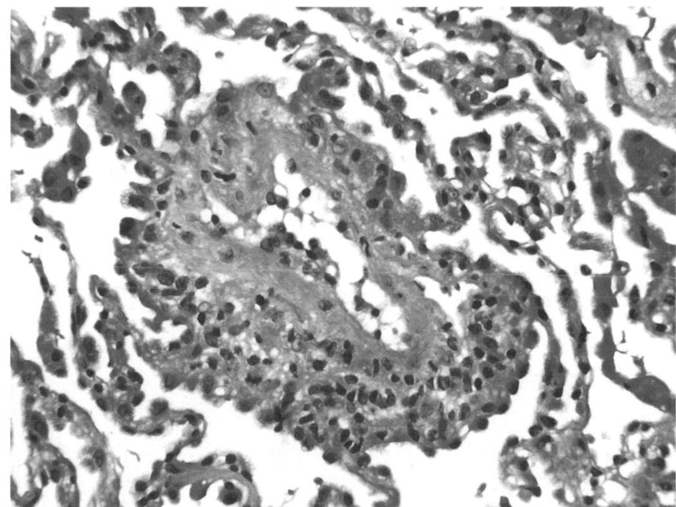

Fig. 12.3 Minimal acute rejection (A1) with sparse perivascular mononuclear cell infiltrate.

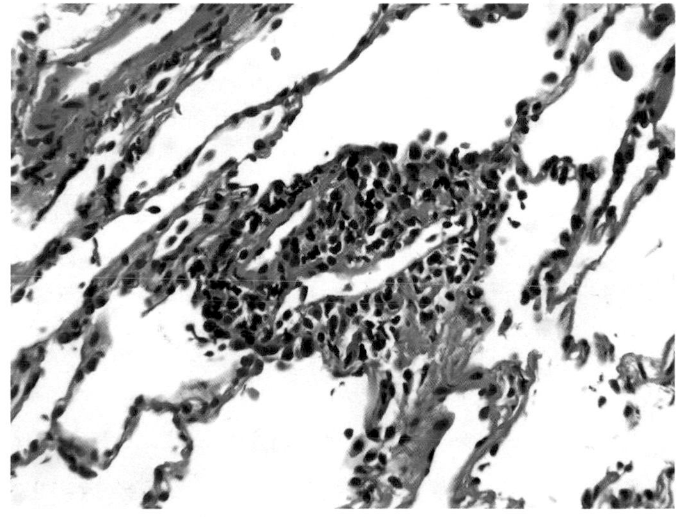

Fig. 12.4 **Mild acute rejection (A2).** The mononuclear cell infiltrate is denser and is more than 3 cell layers thick. However, it is limited to the perivascular area.

3. In moderate acute rejection (Grade A3), the infiltrates extend into the alveolar septa and air spaces (Fig. 12.5).
4. In severe acute rejection (Grade A4), the mononuclear cell infiltrates are associated with pneumocyte damage. The latter often manifests as diffuse alveolar damage with hyaline membranes (Fig. 12.6).

The composition of the cellular infiltrates also changes with increasing severity of rejection. In minimal acute rejection, the perivascular infiltrates are composed predominantly of small, round, plasmacytoid, and transformed lymphocytes. As the rejection advances in intensity, the infiltrates contain more activated lymphocytes, macrophages, eosinophils, and neutrophils. Also subendothelial and peribronchiolar infiltrates become more pronounced.

In higher-grade rejection, the inflammatory cells permeate through the vessels with extension to the endothelium, giving rise to endothelialitis. In 30% of mild and 60% of moderate acute rejection, there is also associated airway inflammation.

A rare form of acute rejection also exists. This is characterized by abundant eosinophils, which may obscure the mononuclear cells in the perivascular infiltrates.

Histologic differential diagnosis

Perivascular and interstitial mononuclear cell infiltrates are not specific for acute rejection.[18] Differential diagnostic considerations include infections, especially CMV pneumonia and *Pneumocystis carinii (jiroveci)* pneumonia (PCP),[22–25] and post-transplant lymphoproliferative disorders[26] (Table 12.6). Some histologic features may favor infection over acute rejection[27] (Table 12.7). Cultures and special stains may be helpful in the diagnosis of mycobacterial, fungal, and *Pneumocystis jiroveci* infections. Viral pneumonias can be confirmed by cultures, as well as serologic, immunohistochemical or molecular hybridization techniques.

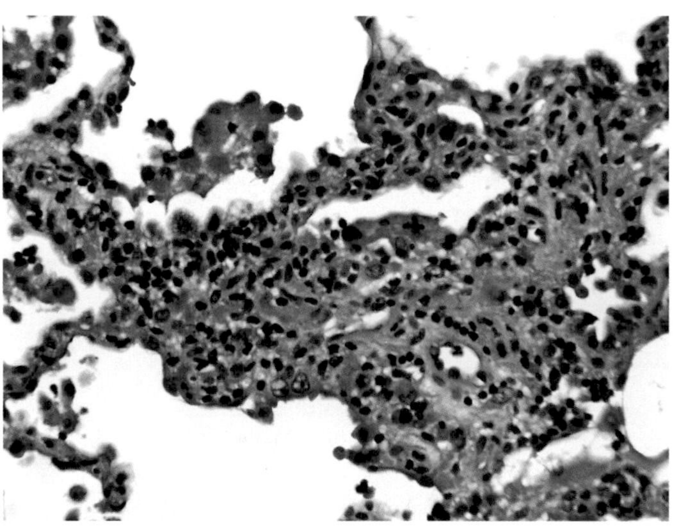

Fig. 12.5 In moderate acute rejection (A3), the perivascular infiltrate extends into the alveolar septa.

In some cases, histologic features of acute rejection and infection coexist. In these cases, the pathologist should attempt to decide which is dominant, and guide the clinician by favoring one over the other. Follow-up biopsy after appropriate antimicrobial therapy is also recommended, so that any acute rejection component can be reassessed.[18] The differential diagnosis between acute rejection and post-transplant lymphoproliferative disorders will be discussed later.

Treatment and prognosis

The discrimination of minimal and mild acute rejection has important therapeutic implications. Currently, most transplant centers do not treat asymptomatic minimal acute rejection, whereas higher-grade rejections are treated. The treatment typically consists of bolus therapy with intravenous steroids, which may be supplemented by temporary increases in the maintenance immunosuppression regimen. In at least 80% of the cases, acute rejection is successfully treated. However, 15–20% of acute rejection episodes persist or recur, presenting a particularly difficult management problem for the clinician.[28,29] When this occurs, intensified immuno-

Table 12.6 Differential diagnoses of perivascular and interstitial mononuclear cell infiltrates

Acute rejection
Infection
Post-transplant lymphoproliferative disorders

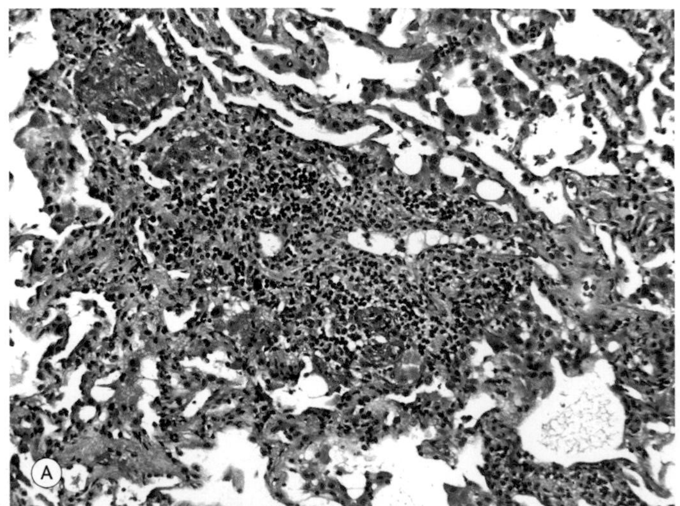

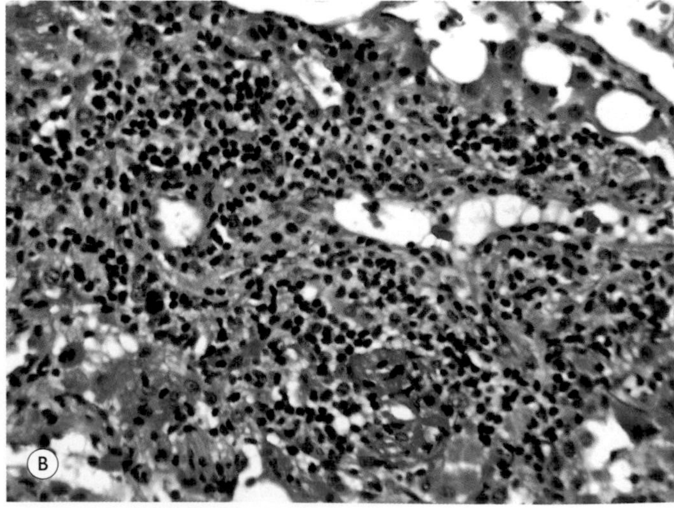

Fig. 12.6 In severe acute rejection (A4), the perivascular infiltrates lead to lung injury. The latter manifests as fibrinous exudates and hyaline membranes in this case. (A) Lower magnification. (B) Higher magnification.

Table 12.7 Histologic features favoring infection over acute rejection

Histologic features	Infection favored
Predominant alveolar septal infiltrates as compared to perivascular infiltrates	Any infection
Abundant neutrophils	Bacterial pneumonia, cytomegalovirus (CMV) pneumonia, or candidiasis
Abundant eosinophils	Fungal infection
Nuclear or cytoplasmic inclusions	Viral pneumonia
Multinucleation	Respiratory syncytial virus, or parainfluenza virus pneumonia
Punctate zones of necrosis	Herpes simplex virus, varicella-zoster virus, or CMV pneumonia
Granulomatous inflammation	Mycobacterial, fungal, or *Pneumocystis jiroveci* infection
Frothy intra-alveolar exudates	*Pneumocystis jiroveci* pneumonia

Source: modified from Zander,[27] with permission granted by Marcel Dekker.

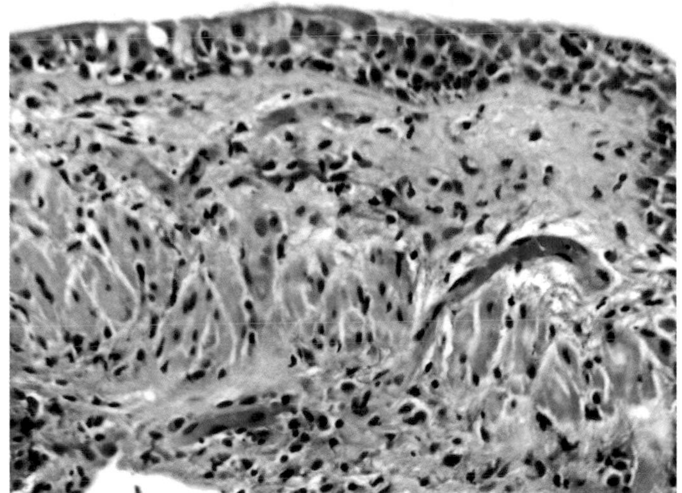

Fig. 12.7 Minimal lymphocytic bronchitis (B1) with sparse mononuclear cells in the submucosa.

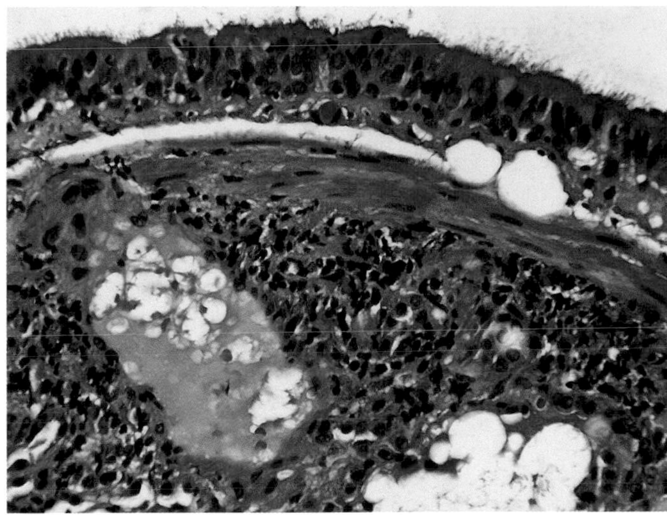

Fig. 12.8 Mild lymphocytic bronchitis (B2) with band-like mononuclear cell infiltrates in the submucosa.

suppression with one or more agents is usually attempted. However, it has been shown that patients with persistent, recurrent, or late (occurring at least 3 months post-transplant) acute rejection are at an increased risk for developing chronic airway rejection.[30]

Airway inflammation – lymphocytic bronchitis/bronchiolitis

As discussed earlier, the diagnosis of acute rejection is based on the presence of intraparenchymal perivascular mononuclear cell infiltrates. However, airway inflammation may also represent an alloreactive injury and may be a harbinger of chronic airway rejection.[31,32] Therefore, the presence of combined large and small airway inflammation (lymphocytic bronchitis and bronchiolitis) should be noted in the pathology report.[18]

Pathologic findings

Some transplant centers may elect to grade airway inflammation, whereas others prefer to acknowledge only its presence or absence[18] (Figs 12.7 and 12.8). Criteria for grading airway inflammation are listed in Table 12.8.

Histologic differential diagnosis

There are many causes of lymphocytic bronchitis and bronchiolitis (Table 12.9). Infections, particularly those caused by viral, bacterial, mycoplasmal, fungal, and chlamydial organisms, may mimic the airway inflammation related to acute rejection.[6,33–36]

Because of the loss of cough reflex and tracheal sensitivity, lung transplant patients are predisposed to recurrent aspiration. The diagnosis of aspiration is

Table 12.8 Grading airway inflammation

Grade	Airway inflammation
B0 – No airway inflammation	None
B1 – Minimal airway inflammation	Rare mononuclear cells in the submucosa
B2 – Mild airway inflammation	Band-like infiltrates of mononuclear cells and eosinophils in the submucosa
B3 – Moderate airway inflammation	Similar to B2, with extension into the epithelium, and epithelial cell necrosis
B4 – Severe airway inflammation	Similar to B3, with dissociation of epithelium from the basement membrane, ulceration, and fibrinopurulent exudates
BX – Ungradable	Sampling problems, infection, tangential cutting, etc.

Source: modified from Yousem et al.[18]

Table 12.9 Differential diagnoses of airway inflammation (lymphocytic bronchitis and bronchiolitis)

Airway inflammation related to acute rejection
Infection
Aspiration
Bronchus-associated lymphoid tissue
Previous biopsy site
Ischemia

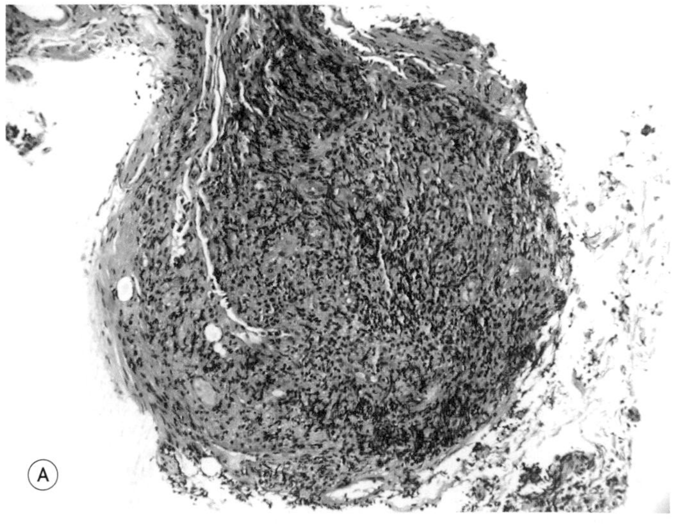

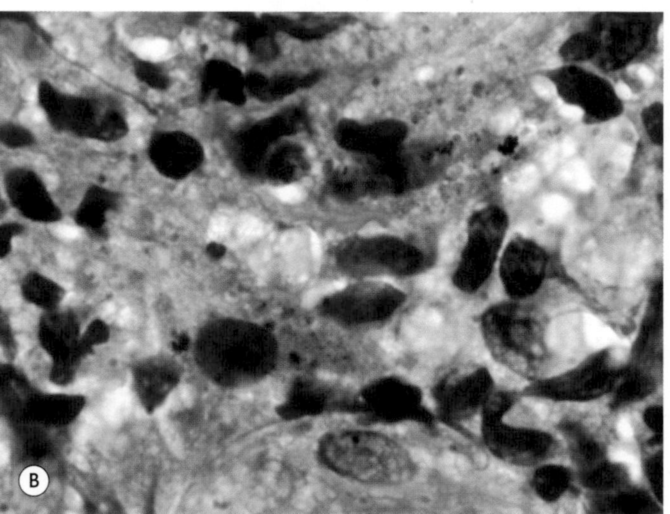

Fig. 12.9 **Bronchus-associated lymphoid tissue (BALT).** (A) It is well circumscribed and (B) contains tingible body macrophages.

supported by identification of exogenous material (typically food particles), and associated foreign body-type giant cell reactions.

Bronchus-associated lymphoid tissue (BALT) is well circumscribed, contains tingible body macrophages, and is unassociated with epithelial injury or eosinophils, as would be expected in airway rejection[18] (Fig. 12.9). BALT is located beneath the epithelium of large airways.

Chronic airway rejection – bronchiolitis obliterans

Bronchiolitis obliterans is the most significant long-term complication of lung transplantation, with a prevalence of 30–50% and an associated mortality rate of 25%.[37] The terminology is somewhat confusing. In the transplantation literature, the term bronchiolitis obliterans is applied to the histologic changes of chronic airway rejection. How-

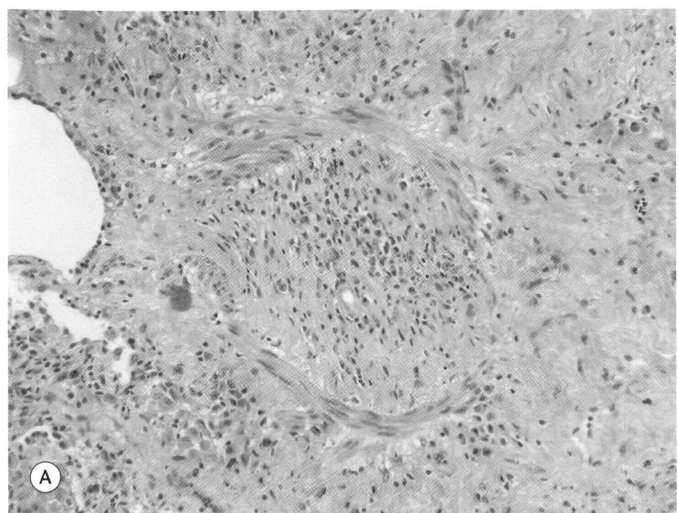

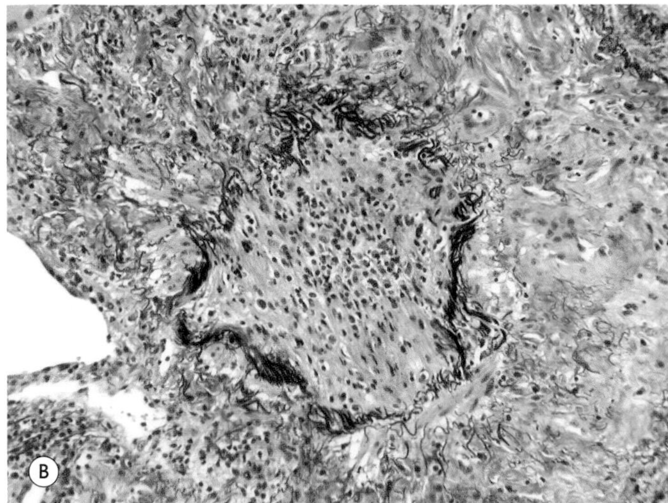

Fig. 12.10 **Bronchiolitis obliterans.** Scar tissue obliterates the lumen of a bronchiole, which can be recognized by the presence of smooth muscle and elastic fibers in the wall. (A) Hematoxylin & eosin stain. (B) Elastic van Gieson stain.

ever, in nontransplant settings, histologically similar lesions are termed "constrictive bronchiolitis obliterans" or "obliterative bronchiolitis."[38,39] The name is less important than the understanding that bronchiolitis obliterans of chronic airway rejection is both clinically and histologically different from the acute lung injury pattern previously known as bronchiolitis obliterans organizing pneumonia (BOOP).[38,39] The terminology for BOOP has recently changed; the current preferred term is "cryptogenic organizing pneumonia."[40] Transplant bronchiolitis obliterans shares many pathogenetic features with the graft-versus-host reaction seen in the lungs of bone marrow recipients.[41]

Time period

Bronchiolitis obliterans is most frequently diagnosed between the 9th and 15th post-transplant months.[41] It rarely develops during the first 3 months, but has been reported as early as 2 months after transplantation.[41]

Clinical presentation

Bronchiolitis obliterans often develops insidiously with vague general symptoms, and nonproductive cough. Later, progressive dyspnea on exertion becomes the dominant complaint. At this later stage, pulmonary function tests show a decline in the FEV_1 as compared to a previously established post-transplant baseline.

Radiologic findings

Chest radiographs are typically unremarkable until later in the disease, when a variable pattern of bronchiectasis, is accompanied by airway tapering/obliteration and zones of hyperinflation. These changes reflect the peculiar nature of chronic airway rejection – proximal bronchiectasis (dilatation) with distal bronchiolitis obliterans (constriction).

Table 12.10 Grading chronic airway rejection

Grade	Histologic features
Ca – Bronchiolitis obliterans, active	Dense fibrous scarring with intrabronchiolar and peribronchiolar mononuclear cell infiltrates
Cb – Bronchiolitis obliterans, inactive	Dense fibrous scarring without cellular infiltrates

Source: modified from Yousem et al.[18]

Diagnosis

In symptomatic patients, a transbronchial biopsy is usually performed to confirm the diagnosis. The reported yield of these biopsies varies from 5 to 100%. Some centers also perform surveillance transbronchial biopsies on asymptomatic patients to detect early bronchiolitis obliterans.

Pathologic findings

In the context of lung transplantation, the term bronchiolitis obliterans refers to hyalinized fibrous plaques present in the submucosa of small airways.[6,18,33] They lead to partial or complete luminal compromise (Fig. 12.10). The scar tissue may be concentric or eccentric and may be associated with destruction of the smooth muscle wall. If there is an accompanying infiltrate of mononuclear inflammatory cells, the process is termed "active" (Table 12.10). If no inflammatory cells are present,

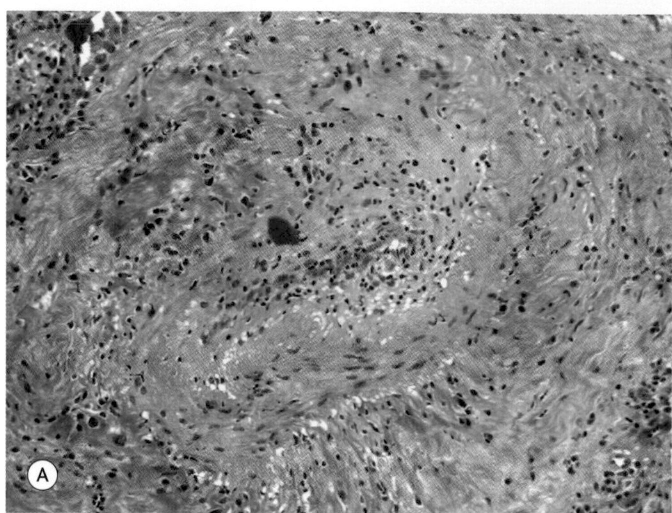

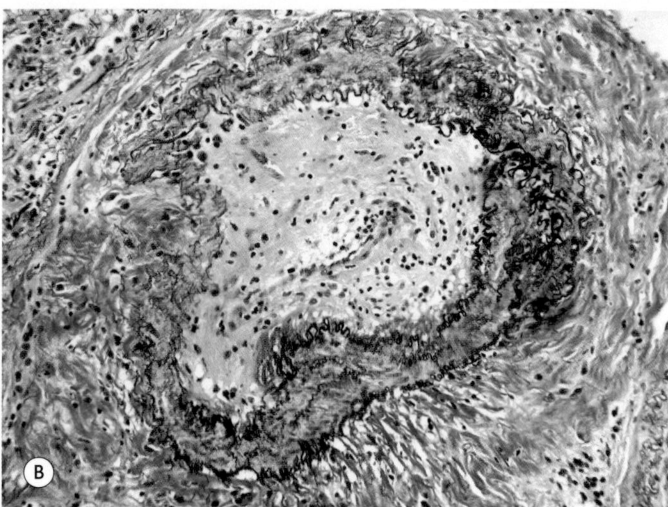

Fig. 12.11 **Chronic vascular rejection (accelerated vascular sclerosis).** Intimal proliferation occludes the lumen of a muscular pulmonary artery, which can be recognized by the presence of two elastic laminae. (A) Hematoxylin & eosin stain (H&E) stain. (B) Elastic van Gieson stain.

the term inactive is applied. Bronchiolitis obliterans often produces mucostasis or postobstructive (endogenous lipid) pneumonia.[6,18,33]

Histologic differential diagnosis

Transplant bronchiolitis obliterans involves the small airways. Large airway fibrosis is a nonspecific finding and should not be considered as evidence of chronic airway rejection.[18] Organizing pneumonia pattern is manifested as fibromyxoid connective tissue plugs within the lumina of bronchioles and alveoli.[42] These loose edematous polyps should be distinguished from the dense eosinophilic scars of transplant bronchiolitis obliterans.

Treatment and prognosis

Because this disorder is most probably of immunologic origin, advances in transplant immunology that create better tolerance between the donor and recipient, as well as efforts to prevent CMV infection and airway ischemic injury, will probably be effective preventive measures. Augmented immunosuppression appears to be of some benefit in treating bronchiolitis obliterans, but it is far from optimal. Avoiding this complication of lung transplantation may require better use of current immunosuppressive medications, or the development of novel immunosuppressive strategies.[41]

Chronic vascular rejection – accelerated graft vascular sclerosis

The significance of chronic vascular rejection is unclear. It is known that certain vascular changes correlate with the presence of bronchiolitis obliterans in pulmonary allografts.[18] Furthermore, pulmonary vascular changes correlate with the presence of accelerated coronary artery disease in combined heart–lung transplant patients.[43]

Pathologic findings

In chronic vascular rejection, there is fibrointimal thickening in arteries and veins[18] (Fig. 12.11). There may also be an "active" inflammatory component consisting of subendothelial, intimal, or medial, predominantly lymphoid, mononuclear cell infiltrates.

Infection

Bacterial infections

Bacterial infections of the lower respiratory tract in the setting of lung transplantation may manifest as acute bronchitis or bronchopneumonia. Gram-negative infections, especially those caused by Pseudomonas spp., account for about 75% of bacterial pneumonias. Other reported bacteria include a wide range of nosocomial organisms. Legionellosis is rarely reported.[44]

Time period

Bacterial infections can occur shortly after transplantation, presumably due to transmission of bacteria from the donor. Nevertheless, the risk of bacterial infection persists throughout the lifetime of the allograft.

Clinical presentation

The clinical findings include fever, cough, purulent sputum, shortness of breath, rales on auscultation, hypoxemia, leukocytosis, and decline in spirometry.

Radiologic findings

New or increasing infiltrates on chest X-ray, often localized, are common manifestations of bacterial pneumonias.

Diagnosis

Most of the clinical features of transplant-associated pneumonia are nonspecific and largely modified by the patient's immunocompromised status. Bronchoalveolar lavage and transbronchial biopsy are often performed in the evaluation of new infiltrates. Culture results are often an important part of the diagnostic work-up.

Pathologic findings

In acute bronchitis, neutrophils infiltrate the bronchial mucosa. This may be associated with mucosal ulceration and intraluminal neutrophils. As in the normal host, acute pneumonia is recognized by the presence of neutrophils within the alveolar spaces (Fig. 12.12).

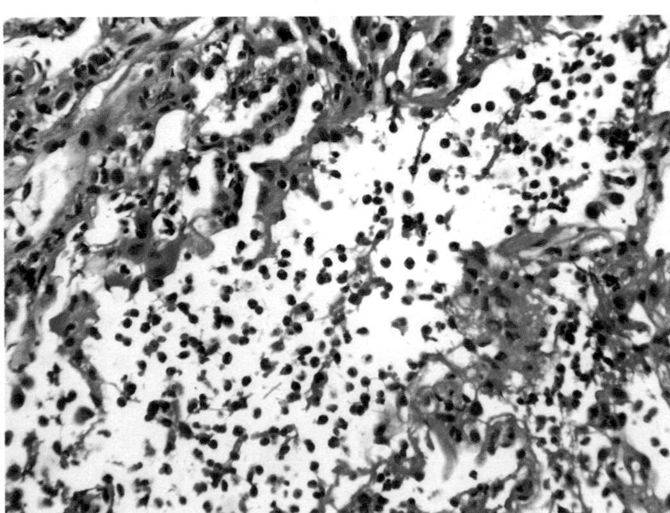

Fig. 12.12 **Acute pneumonia.** Neutrophil granulocytes are present in the alveolar spaces.

Histologic differential diagnosis

The composition of inflammatory infiltrates distinguishes bacterial infection from acute rejection. Bacterial infection is characterized by the presence of neutrophils, whereas mononuclear cells (mainly lymphoid cells) are seen predominantly in acute rejection.

Treatment and prognosis

Organism-specific management is essential. The use of broad-spectrum antibiotics, prior to identification of an organism, should include agents effective against *Pseudomonas* spp.

Viral infections

Lung transplant recipients are prone to viral infections, in particular CMV pneumonia, because of their immunocompromised status. Donor-recipient mismatch, with the donor being seropositive and the recipient seronegative for CMV, poses the highest risk for the development of CMV pneumonia. Without CMV prophylaxis, the incidence of CMV pneumonia in this group is 83%. With prophylaxis, the incidence falls to 55.6%.[45,46] Seropositive recipients of a seropositive or negative donor are at intermediate risk of acquiring active CMV pneumonia, whereas seronegative recipients of a seronegative donor are at lowest risk.

Herpes simplex virus (HSV) infections are also a potential problem in lung transplantation. Such infections have been reduced remarkably with the routine use of acyclovir or ganciclovir prophylaxis.

Other viruses responsible for respiratory infections include adenovirus, respiratory syncytial virus, influenza virus, parainfluenza virus, and varicella-zoster virus.[47–49]

Time period

Cytomegalovirus infection occurs most frequently between 2 weeks and 4 months after transplantation. Herpes simplex virus infection usually begins as oral ulcers or tracheitis during the first post-transplant month.

Clinical presentation

Fever, malaise, myalgias, chills, abdominal discomfort, cough, and shortness of breath are frequent symptoms of CMV pneumonia. Physical examination may reveal crackles or may be normal. Other features include hypoxemia, and decline in spirometry. Fortunately, pneumonia caused by HSV is now rare, thanks to routine prophylaxis. The clinical features are similar to those of CMV pneumonia.

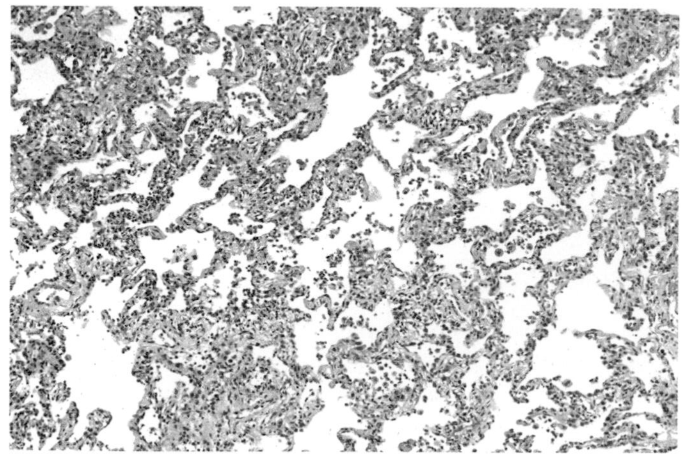

Fig. 12.13 **Cytomegalovirus (CMV) pneumonia.** Mononuclear cells infiltrate the alveolar septa diffusely with no perivascular accentuation.

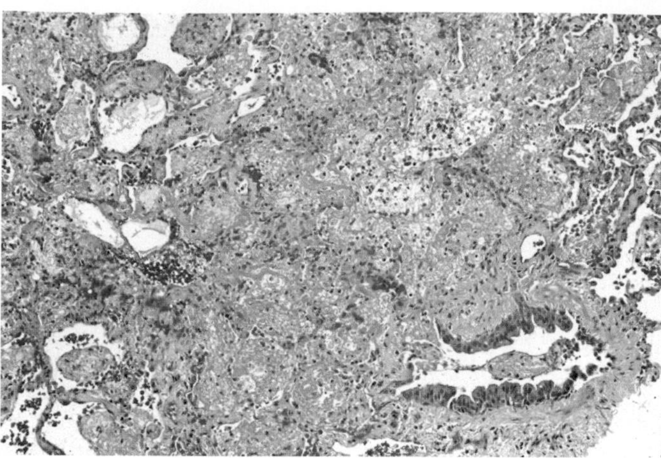

Fig. 12.15 Herpes simplex virus (HSV) pneumonia with an area of necrosis.

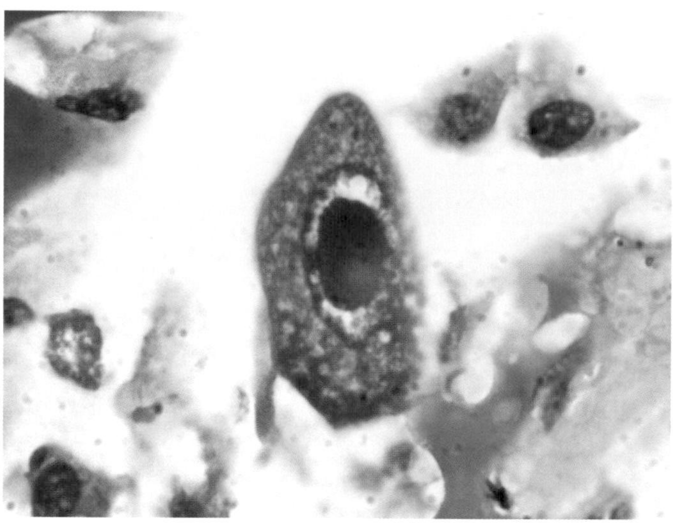

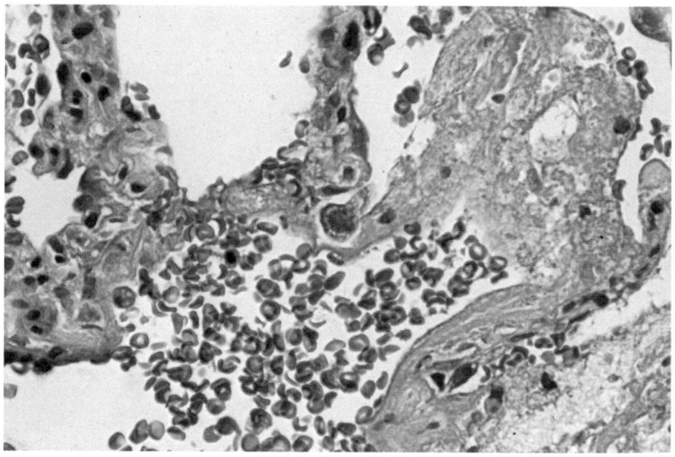

Fig. 12.14 **Cytopathic effects characteristic of cytomegalovirus (CMV) infection.** Both nuclear and cytoplasmic inclusions are present, but the latter are less apparent.

Fig. 12.16 Higher-power view of herpes simplex virus (HSV) pneumonia, showing a nuclear inclusion.

Radiologic findings

Chest radiographs may show reticular or reticulonodular infiltrates, but may be clear in up to two-thirds of patients.

Diagnosis

The diagnosis of viral pneumonia is often impossible on clinical grounds alone: BAL and transbronchial biopsy play important roles in establishing the diagnosis.

Pathologic findings

Recognizing tissue responses and cytopathic effects may help in identifying viral infections (see Ch. 6). Tissue responses to viral pathogens range from minimal non-specific inflammation to overwhelming DAD. Most cases of CMV infection show interstitial pneumonia with a mixed lymphocytic and polymorphonuclear cell infiltrate[22] (Figs 12.13 and 12.14). Zonal necrosis may be seen with herpes simplex, varicella-zoster, and CMV pneumonia (Figs 12.15 and 12.16). Cytomegalovirus may also be associated with neutrophilic microabscesses. Necrotizing bronchiolitis may be features of adenovirus, influenza, and respiratory syncytial virus infection. Some characteristic viral cytopathic effects are listed in Table 12.11. These cytopathic effects, however, can be sparse or absent.

Immunohistochemistry, in-situ hybridization and polymerase chain reaction (PCR) techniques can be used to identify many viruses and have largely replaced electron microscopy in this role[50] (Fig. 12.17). Immunohistochemistry is performed routinely in some centers to rule out insidious CMV infection, where only rare positive cells may occur.

Table 12.11 Viruses and their cytopathic effects

Virus	Cytopathic effect
Cytomegalovirus	Cytomegaly, nuclear and cytoplasmic inclusions
Herpes simplex virus	Nuclear inclusions
Varicella-zoster virus	Nuclear inclusions
Adenovirus	Smudge cells, nuclear inclusions
Respiratory syncytial virus	Occasional multinucleation, cytoplasmic inclusions
Influenza virus	None
Parainfluenza virus	Occasional multinucleation, cytoplasmic inclusions

Source: modified from Katzenstein,[50] with permission granted by WB Saunders.

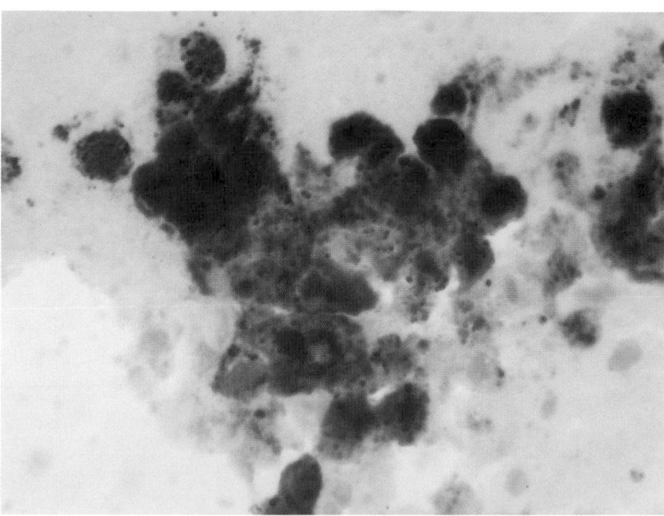

Fig. 12.17 **Herpes simplex virus (HSV) infection.** Paraffin immunoperoxidase studies reveal HSV-positive cells.

Histologic differential diagnosis

The histologic differential diagnosis of viral pneumonia includes acute rejection.[22] Both processes can exhibit perivascular and interstitial mononuclear cell infiltrates. However, perivascular infiltrates predominate in acute rejection and alveolar septal infiltrates are more prominent in viral infection (see Table 12.7). The presence of CMV inclusions is indicative of CMV pneumonia, but attention to other histologic details is necessary to exclude comorbid acute rejection and bronchiolitis obliterans, which are frequently associated with CMV infection.

Fungal infections

Fungal infections are less frequent than other infections in the transplant patient, but have a high mortality rate when they do occur. The fungal species most commonly encountered in lung transplant biopsies include *Aspergillus* and *Candida*.[45] Cryptococcosis, histoplasmosis, coccidioidomycosis, and mucormycosis have also been reported.[45,51,52] Fungal organisms may colonize the respiratory tract or cause overt infection.[53,54] Prolonged antibiotic therapy predisposes patients to disseminated candidiasis.

Time period

Fungal infections are most commonly seen between 2 weeks and 2 months after transplantation.

Clinical presentation

The clinical picture is not specific. Fungal pneumonias may present with fever, leukocytosis, and hypoxemia.

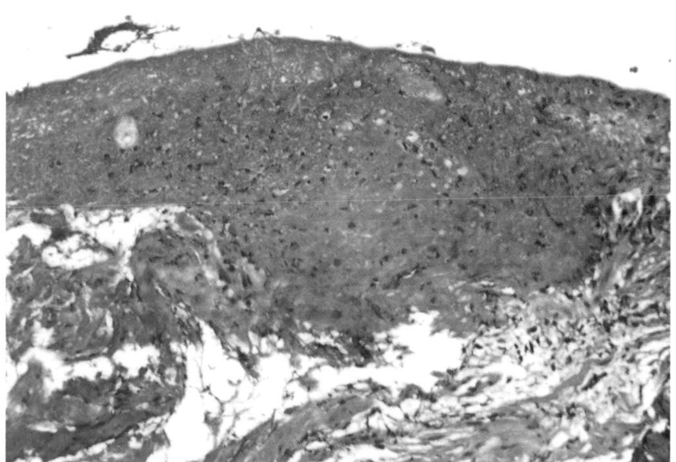

Fig. 12.18 Bronchial mucosal necrosis and associated *Aspergillus* infection. There is no significant inflammation.

Radiologic findings

Radiographically, pulmonary infiltrates with consolidation or cavitary nodules may be seen.

Diagnosis

The diagnosis is most often made by a combination of clinical features and the recovery of fungal organisms from BAL, transbronchial biopsy, blood, or other body fluids.

Pathologic findings

Fungal species may be a source of bronchial anastomotic infections (Figs 12.18 and 12.19). *Aspergillus* pneumonia is

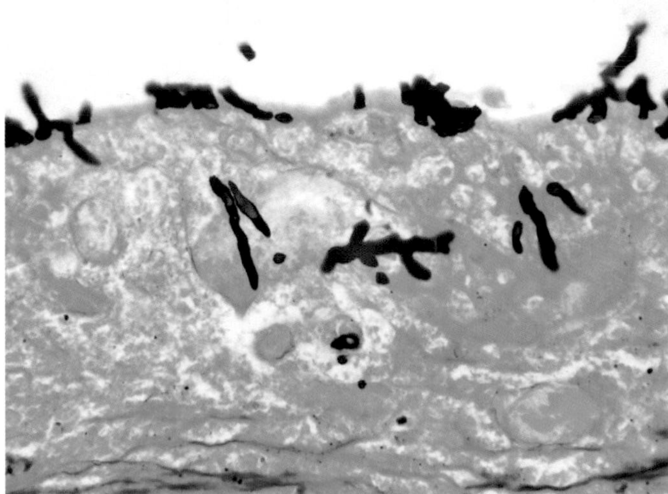

Fig. 12.19 Gomori's methenamine silver stain performed on the case shown in Fig. 12.18 reveals fungal organisms compatible with *Aspergillus* spp.

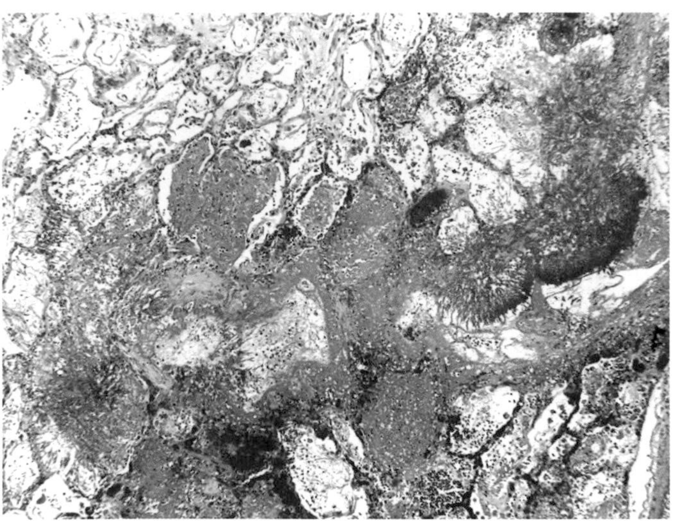

Fig. 12.20 Aspergillus pneumonia with an area of infarction.

characterized by hemorrhagic infarction, and sparse inflammatory cell infiltrates (Figs 12.20 and 12.21). Long, septate hyphae, with 45° branching points, invade blood vessels and permeate alveolar septa. *Candida* infection produces neutrophilic infiltrates and is associated with abscess formation. Clusters of pseudohyphae and yeast forms are often found in the center of abscesses.

Pneumocystis pneumonia (PCP)

Although recent studies have strongly suggested that *Pneumocystis jiroveci* is a fungus, we discuss pneumocystis pneumonia separately from other fungal infections for didactic purposes. Without prophylaxis, pneumocystis

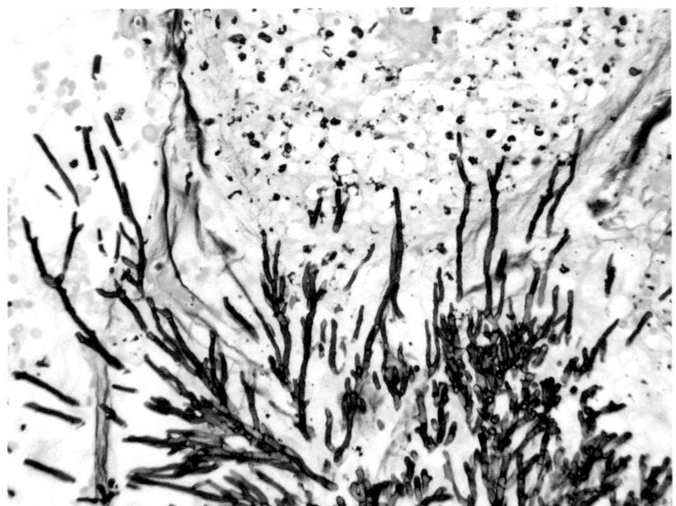

Fig. 12.21 Gomori's methenamine silver stain performed on the case shown in Fig. 12.20 shows vasoinvasive fungal elements compatible with *Aspergillus* spp.

pneumonia occurs in nearly all lung transplant recipients.[55] Fortunately, thanks to the routine use of prophylaxis, it is rarely seen today in this patient population.

Time period

Historically, infections were most common around the seventh post-transplant week.

Clinical presentation

The clinical presentation is nonspecific and includes cough, fever, dyspnea, and hypoxemia.

Radiologic findings

Radiographically, diffuse pulmonary infiltrates are seen.

Diagnosis

Since *Pneumocystis* cannot be grown in culture, the diagnosis is usually made by indentification of the organisms in lavage fluid. Rarely, a transbronchial lung biopsy is required.

Pathologic findings

The classic histologic picture of interstitial pneumonia with frothy intra-alveolar exudates, seen in patients with acquired immunodeficiency syndrome, is rarely encountered in lung transplant patients (Figs 12.22 and 12.23). In these patients, pneumocystis pneumonia more often manifests as DAD and the organisms are typically

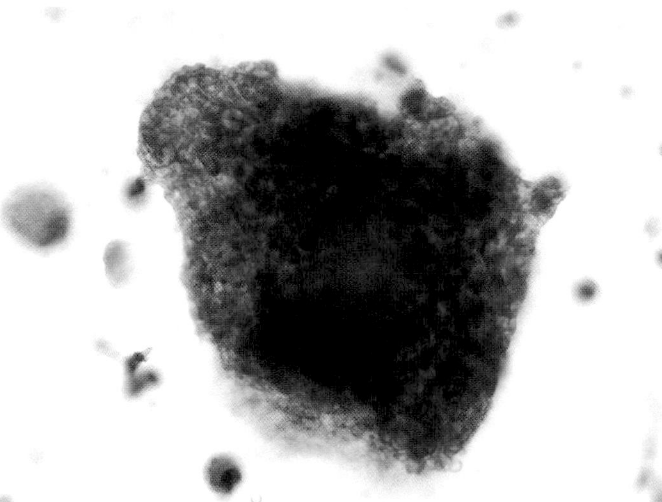

Fig. 12.22 Pneumocystis jiroveci pneumonia, bronchoalveolar lavage. Frothy exudate can be seen.

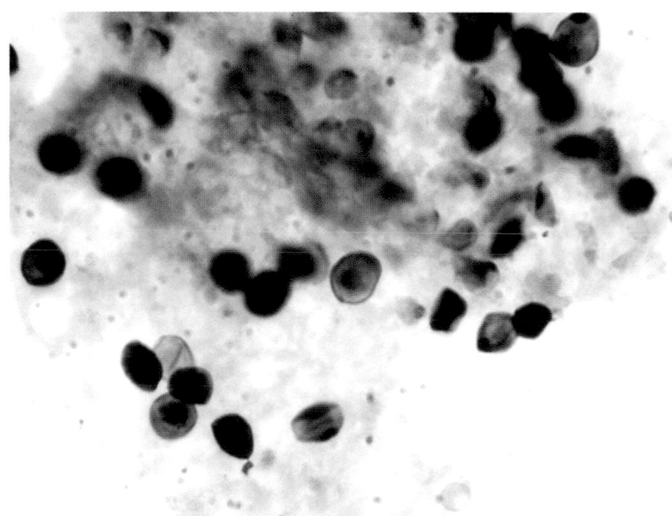

Fig. 12.23 Gomori's methenamine silver stain performed on the case shown in Fig. 12.22 reveals *Pneumocystis jiroveci* organisms.

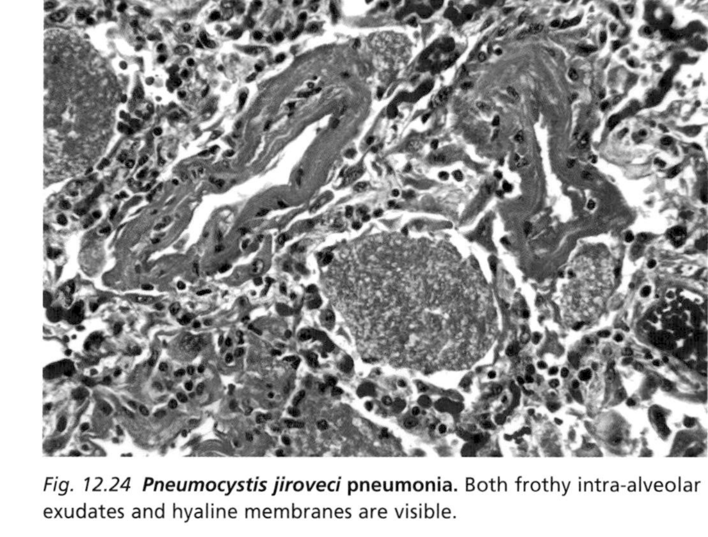

Fig. 12.24 ***Pneumocystis jiroveci*** **pneumonia.** Both frothy intra-alveolar exudates and hyaline membranes are visible.

embedded in the prominent hyaline membranes (Fig. 12.24). Granulomatous inflammation is a less common manifestation of infection with *Pneumocystis*.

Post-transplant lymphoproliferative disorders

Post-transplant lymphoproliferative disorders (PTLDs) is a lymphoid proliferation that develops in an allograft recipient as a consequence of immunosuppression.[56] Characteristics of PTLDs somewhat vary with allograft types, and immunosuppressive regimens. PTLDs are relatively more common among pulmonary allograft recipients, as a result of higher levels of immunosuppression.[26] In this population, the occurrence of PTLD may be as high as 5%.

The majority of PTLDs are associated with primary or reactivated Epstein–Barr virus (EBV) infection and appear to represent EBV-induced B-cell or rarely T-cell proliferations. EBV-seronegative recipients who develop primary EBV infection have a higher incidence of PTLD. Approximately 20% of PTLDs are EBV-negative. The etiology of EBV-negative cases is unknown, but the fact that some of them respond to decreased immunosuppression suggests that they are also related to decreased immune competence.

Time period

The mean interval to PTLD following lung transplantation is 3 months, but disease has been reported as early as 1 month after transplantation.

Clinical presentation

Primary EBV infection often presents as a mononucleosis-like illness with fever, and sore throat. Pulmonary involvement by PTLD may cause shortness of breath or may be discovered incidentally on a routine chest X-ray. Simultaneous involvement of extrapulmonary sites may result in diarrhea, due to involvement of the gastrointestinal tract, and dysphagia, due to involvement of the tonsils. Physical examination may reveal lymphadenopathy, enlarged tonsils, splenomegaly, and crackles on chest auscultation. In some cases, the physical examination may be entirely normal.

Radiologic findings

Thoracic manifestations are present in most lung transplant recipients with PTLD.[57] The most common radiologic finding is multiple pulmonary nodules. Other findings include a solitary nodule, multifocal alveolar infiltrates, and hilar or mediastinal adenopathy.

Diagnosis

The diagnosis is usually suspected on the basis of the clinical and radiologic findings, but clinical differentiation from granulomatous infections and acute rejection requires transbronchial or surgical lung biopsy.

Pathologic findings

PTLDs comprise a spectrum ranging from lymphoid hyperplasias to lymphomas. Several classification schemes have been proposed.[58–62] The Classification by the World Health Organization (WHO) is now widely accepted and is presented in Table 12.12.[56]

Specimen evaluation for the diagnosis of PTLD should include routine morphology, immunophenotyping, preservation of tissue for potential molecular genetic studies, and detection of EBV infection.[56,63] Flow cytometry or frozen section immunohistochemistry is more useful in determining cell lineage and clonality than paraffin section immunohistochemistry. If immunophenotyping studies show polytypic immunoglobulin, clonality can be further assessed by molecular genetic studies, which are capable of identifying polyclonal or monoclonal gene rearrangement. Epstein–Barr virus infection can be detected using immunohistochemistry for latent membrane protein (LMP-1), but in-situ hybridization for EBV-encoded nuclear RNA (EBER) is considered the gold standard.

Table 12.12 The World Health Organization Classification of Post-transplant Lymphoproliferative Disorders (PTLDs)

1. Early lesions
   - Reactive plasmacytic hyperplasia
   - Infectious mononucleosis-like
2. Polymorphic PTLD
3. Monomorphic PTLD (classify according to lymphoma classification)
   - B-cell neoplasms
     - Diffuse large B-cell lymphoma (immunoblastic, centroblastic, anaplastic)
     - Burkitt/Burkitt-like lymphoma
     - Plasma cell myeloma
     - Plasmacytoma-like lesions
   - T-cell neoplasms
     - Peripheral T-cell lymphoma, not otherwise specified
     - Other types
4. Hodgkin lymphoma (HL) and Hodgkin lymphoma-like PTLD

Source: modified from Harris et al.,[56] with permission granted by IARC Press.

Early lesions

Early lesions of PTLD include plasmacytic hyperplasia and infectious mononucleosis-like PTLD. These lesions usually arise in lymph nodes or Waldeyer's ring and only rarely involve true extranodal sites such as the lung. They are characterized by some degree of architectural preservation of the involved tissue,[56] but they differ from typical reactive follicular hyperplasia in having a diffuse proliferation of plasma cells. Plasmacytic hyperplasia PTLD is distinguished by numerous plasma cells and rare immunoblasts, whereas infectious mononucleosis-like lesion has the typical morphologic features of infectious mononucleosis in the lymph node: namely, paracortical expansion and numerous immunoblasts in a background of T cells and plasma cells.

Immunophenotypic studies show an admixture of polyclonal B cells, plasma cells, and T cells. EBV-positive immunoblasts are typically present.

Polymorphic post-transplant lymphoproliferative disorders

Polymorphic PTLDs are destructive lesions that efface the architecture of lymph nodes or form destructive extranodal masses.[56] In contrast to most lymphomas, polymorphic PTLDs show the full extent of B-cell maturation and are composed of immunoblasts, plasma cells, small and intermediate-sized lymphocytes, and centrocyte-like cells. Scattered large, bizarre cells (atypical immunoblasts) and areas of necrosis may also be present. Polymorphic PTLDs were at one time subdivided into "polymorphic B-cell hyperplasia" and "polymorphic B-cell lymphoma." Today this separation is not deemed necessary, since both have similar clinical features. Immunophenotyping studies typically show a mixture of B and T cells. Most of the cases are monoclonal, at least by molecular genetic studies. EBV-positive immunoblasts are present in the majority of cases.

Monomorphic B-cell post-transplant lymphoproliferative disorders

Monomorphic B-cell PTLDs are characterized by nodal architectural effacement or tumoral growth in extranodal sites, with confluent sheets of large, transformed cells.[56] These tumors should be diagnosed as B-cell lymphomas and should be classified according to lymphoma classification guidelines. However, the term PTLD should also

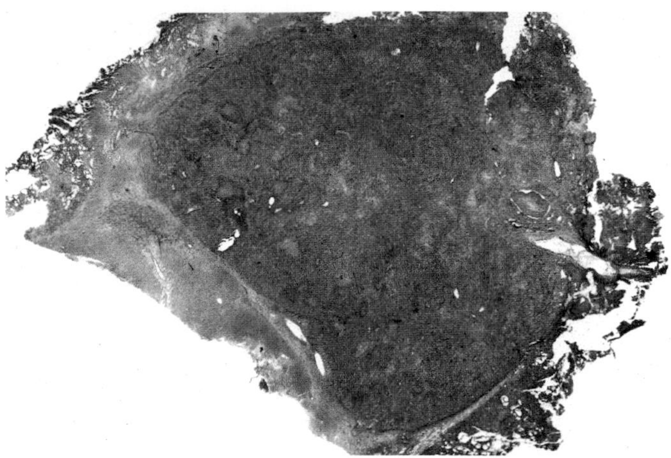

Fig. 12.25 Panoramic view of monomorphic B-cell post-transplant lymphoproliferative disorder (PTLD), showing a mass-like lesion in the pulmonary parenchyma.

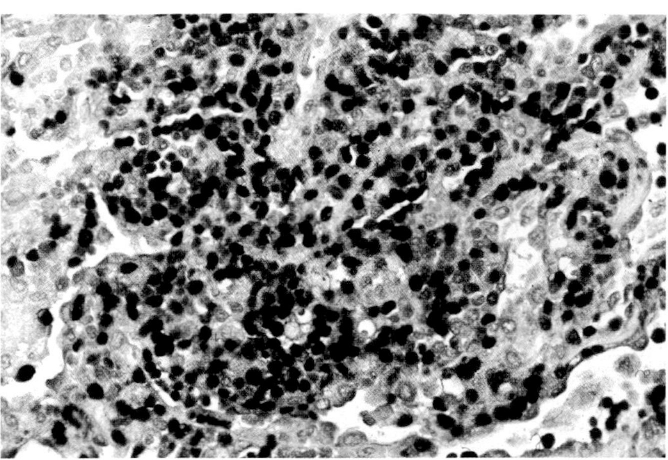

Fig. 12.27 In-situ hybridization studies performed on a case of B-cell post-transplant lymphoproliferative disorder (PTLD) reveal numerous cells that are positive for EBV-encoded nuclear RNA.

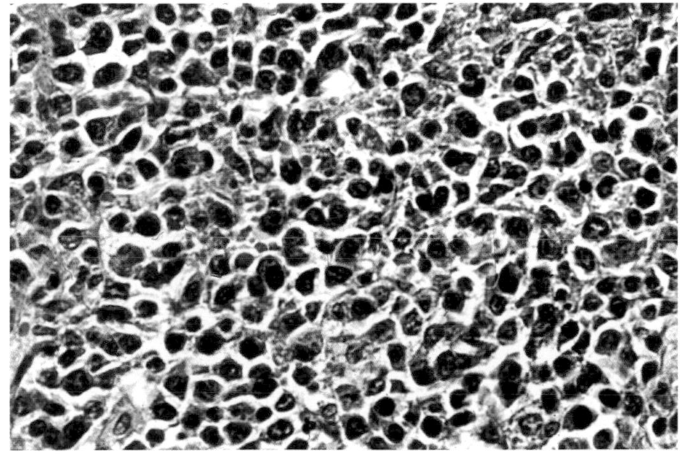

Fig. 12.26 Higher magnification of B-cell post-transplant lymphoproliferative disorder (PTLD), showing morphologic features of a diffuse large B-cell lymphoma.

appear in the diagnosis. The majority of B-cell PTLDs have morphologic features of diffuse large B-cell lymphoma (Figs 12.25-12.27). A minority may be classified as Burkitt lymphoma, plasma cell myeloma, or plasmacytoma-like lesions. Immunophenotyping studies of monomorphic B-cell PTLD show B-cell-associated antigen expression (CD19, CD20, CD79a).[56] Many cases co-express antigens usually associated with T cells (CD43, CD45RO). The majority of cases are monoclonal and EBV-positive. Monomorphic B-cell PTLDs often contain oncogene or tumor suppressor gene alterations (N-ras gene codon 61 point mutation, p53 gene mutation, or c-myc gene rearrangement).[60]

Monomorphic T-cell post-transplant lymphoproliferative disorders

T-cell lymphomas have been reported in allograft recipients. Similar to monomorphic B-cell PTLDs, monomorphic T-cell PTLDs have sufficient atypia to be recognized as neoplastic, and should be classified according to the standard lymphoma classification. Monomorphic T-cell PTLDs express pan-T-cell antigens. Most of the reported cases are EBV-negative.

Hodgkin lymphoma and Hodgkin lymphoma-like post-transplant lymphoproliferative disorders

Both classical Hodgkin lymphoma and cases of Hodgkin lymphoma-like PTLD have been reported in allograft recipients. Cases of classical Hodgkin lymphoma express CD15 and CD30. Hodgkin lymphoma-like PTLDs often have an atypical immunophenotype with B-cell antigen expression. Virtually all cases are EBV-positive. A small proportion of PTLDs are of T-cell lineage. Unlike B-cell PTLDs, T-cell PTLDs are not considered EBV-driven and are histologically similar to T-cell lymphomas that occur in the general population.

Histologic differential diagnosis

Acute rejection may be considered in the differential diagnosis of PTLDs, especially in small biopsy samples. Detection of EBV infection is most helpful in this respect. A sheet-like monomorphous infiltrate with a mononuclear composition of more than 25% B cells and more than 30% large lymphoid cells also favors PTLD over acute rejection.[64]

Treatment and prognosis

Early lesions often regress, either spontaneously or with reduction of immunosuppression. The prognosis is excellent in general, but rare cases progress to polymorphic or monomorphic PTLD. Polymorphic, and less often, monomorphic PTLDs may also regress with reduction of immunosuppression. However, a proportion of cases of both types fail to regress and require cytotoxic chemotherapy. Overall, the mortality of PTLDs in solid organ allograft recipients is approximately 60%.

Other complications

Cryptogenic organizing pneumonia

Cryptogenic organizing pneumonia, previously known as bronchiolitis obliterans organizing pneumonia (BOOP), occurs as a response to acute lung injury. In lung transplant recipients, it is commonly associated with aspiration, infection, and acute rejection.[42,65–67] However, organizing pneumonia is not a component of, and does not necessarily predispose to, chronic airway rejection (bronchiolitis obliterans).

Time period

The time from transplant to onset of cryptogenic organizing pneumonia ranges from 2 to 43 months.

Clinical presentation

The clinical findings are nonspecific and may include cough, dyspnea, fever, hypoxemia, and a decline in pulmonary function.

Radiologic findings

The chest X-ray may be normal, or show localized or diffuse infiltrates.

Diagnosis

Cryptogenic organizing pneumonia is a histologic diagnosis and requires transbronchial or surgical lung biopsy.

Pathologic findings

Fibromyxoid plugs of granulation tissue are seen within small airways, and airspaces, typically in a patchy distribution (Fig. 12.28).

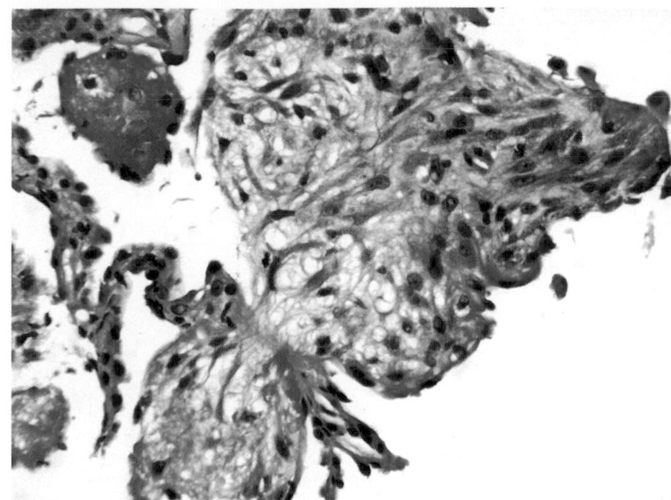

Fig. 12.28 Organizing pneumonia with intra-alveolar fibroblastic plugs.

Histologic differential diagnosis

In organizing DAD, the fibroblastic proliferation involves the interstitium rather than the airspaces and remnants of hyaline membranes may be seen.[42] However, organizing pneumonia and DAD are both acute lung injury patterns and features of both may be present in a given case. Airspace fibromyxoid tissue can also be seen in organizing infectious pneumonia and healing rejection, especially higher-grade rejection following steroid therapy. Separation of organizing pneumonia from transplant bronchiolitis obliterans has been discussed earlier.

Recurrence of the primary disease

A relatively small percentage of transplant patients are at risk for recurrence of their primary disease following lung transplantation. Sarcoidosis is the most common disease to recur.[68] Other reported cases include recurrence of lymphangioleiomyomatosis,[69,70] diffuse panbronchiolitis,[71] giant cell interstitial pneumonia,[72] desquamative interstitial pneumonia,[73] intravenous talc granulomatosis,[74] and bronchioloalveolar carcinoma.[75]

Clinical features

Recurrence of the primary disease is usually an incidental finding on transbronchial biopsy or autopsy. However, symptomatic cases have also been described.

Diagnosis

The diagnosis depends on transbronchial or other biopsy samples.

REFERENCES

1. Hosenpud JD, Bennett LE, Keck BM, Boucek MM, Novick RJ: The Registry of the International Society for Heart and Lung Transplantation: eighteenth official report – 2001. J Heart Lung Transplant 2001; 20: 805–815.
2. Woo MS, MacLaughlin EF, Horn MV, et al.: Living donor lobar lung transplantation: the pediatric experience. Pediatr Transplant 1998; 2: 185–90.
3. Nizami I, Frost AE: Clinical diagnosis of transplant-related problems. In: Diagnostic pulmonary pathology, Cagle PT, Ed. 2000, Marcel Dekker, New York, pp 485–499.
4. Hopkins PM, Aboyoun CL, Chhajed PN, et al.: Prospective analysis of 1,235 transbronchial lung biopsies in lung transplant recipients. J Heart Lung Transplant 2002; 21: 1062–1067.
5. Prop J, Ehrie MG, Crapo JD, Nieuwenhuis P, Wildevuur CR: Reimplantation response in isografted rat lungs. Analysis of causal factors. J Thorac Cardiovasc Surg 1984; 87: 702–711.
6. Tazelaar HD, Yousem SA: The pathology of combined heart-lung transplantation: an autopsy study. Hum Pathol 1988; 19: 1403–1416.
7. Bando K, Paradis IL, Komatsu K, et al.: Analysis of time-dependent risks for infection, rejection, and death after pulmonary transplantation. J Thorac Cardiovasc Surg 1995; 109: 49–59.
8. Clark SC, Levine AJ, Hasan A, et al.: Vascular complications of lung transplantation. Ann Thorac Surg 1996; 61: 1079–1082.
9. Griffith BP, Magee MJ, Gonzalez IF, et al.: Anastomotic pitfalls in lung transplantation. J Thorac Cardiovasc Surg 1994; 107: 743–754.
10. Leibowitz DW, Smith CR, Michler RE, et al.: Incidence of pulmonary vein complications after lung transplantation: a prospective transesophageal echocardiographic study. J Am Coll Cardiol 1994; 24: 671–675.
11. Schulman LL, Anandarangam T, Leibowitz DW, et al.: Four-year prospective study of pulmonary venous thrombosis after lung transplantation. J Am Soc Echocardiogr 2001; 14: 806–812.
12. Huang YC, Cheng YJ, Lin YH, Wang MJ, Tsai SK: Graft failure caused by pulmonary venous obstruction diagnosed by intraoperative transesophageal echocardiography during lung transplantation. Anesth Analg 2000; 91: 558–560.
13. Shennib H, Massard G: Airway complications in lung transplantation. Ann Thorac Surg 1994; 57: 506–511.
14. Alvarez A, Algar J, Santos F, et al.: Airway complications after lung transplantation: a review of 151 anastomoses. Eur J Cardiothorac Surg 2001; 19: 381–387.
15. Yousem SA, Paradis IL, Dauber JA, et al.: Large airway inflammation in heart-lung transplant recipients – its significance and prognostic implications. Transplantation 1990; 49: 654–656.
16. Hasegawa T, Iacono AT, Orons PD, Yousem SA: Segmental nonanastomotic bronchial stenosis after lung transplantation. Ann Thorac Surg 2000; 69: 1020–1024.
17. Yousem SA, Berry GJ, Brunt EM, et al.: A working formulation for the standardization of nomenclature in the diagnosis of heart and lung rejection: Lung Rejection Study Group. The International Society for Heart Transplantation. J Heart Transplant 1990; 9: 593–601.
18. Yousem SA, Berry GJ, Cagle PT, et al.: Revision of the 1990 working formulation for the classification of pulmonary allograft rejection: Lung Rejection Study Group. J Heart Lung Transplant 1996; 15:1–15.
19. Choi JK, Kearns J, Palevsky HI, et al.: Hyperacute rejection of a pulmonary allograft. Immediate clinical and pathologic findings. Am J Respir Crit Care Med 1999; 160: 1015–1018.
20. Frost AE, Jammal CT, Cagle PT: Hyperacute rejection following lung transplantation. Chest 1996; 110: 559–562.
21. Hasegawa T, Iacono AT, Yousem SA: The anatomic distribution of acute cellular rejection in the allograft lung. Ann Thorac Surg 2000; 69: 1529–1531.
22. Nakhleh RE, Bolman RM 3rd, Henke CA, Hertz MI: Lung transplant pathology. A comparative study of pulmonary acute rejection and cytomegaloviral infection. Am J Surg Pathol 1991; 15: 1197–1201.
23. Marshall SE, Lewiston NJ, Kramer MR, et al.: Prospective analysis of serial pulmonary function studies and transbronchial biopsies in single-lung transplant recipients. Transplant Proc 1991; 23: 1217–1219.
24. Stewart S: Pathology of lung transplantation. Semin Diagn Pathol 1992; 9: 210–219.
25. Tazelaar HD: Perivascular inflammation in pulmonary infections: implications for the diagnosis of lung rejection. J Heart Lung Transplant 1991; 10: 437–441.
26. Randhawa PS, Yousem SA, Paradis IL, et al.: The clinical spectrum, pathology, and clonal analysis of Epstein–Barr virus-associated lymphoproliferative disorders in heart-lung transplant recipients. Am J Clin Pathol 1989; 92: 177–185.
27. Zander DS: Transplant-related pathology. In: Diagnostic pulmonary pathology, Cagle PT, Ed. 2000, Marcel Dekker, New York, pp 461–484.
28. Keenan RJ, Iacono A, Dauber JH, et al.: Treatment of refractory acute allograft rejection with aerosolized cyclosporine in lung transplant recipients. J Thorac Cardiovasc Surg 1997; 113: 335–341.
29. Shennib H, Mercado M, Nguyen D, et al.: Successful treatment of steroid-resistant double-lung allograft rejection with Orthoclone OKT3. Am Rev Respir Dis 1991; 144: 224–226.
30. Valentine VG, Robbins RC, Wehner JH, et al.: Total lymphoid irradiation for refractory acute rejection in heart-lung and lung allografts. Chest 1996; 109: 1184–1189.
31. Hirt SW, You XM, Moller F, et al.: Development of obliterative bronchiolitis after allogeneic rat lung transplantation: implication of acute rejection and the time point of treatment. J Heart Lung Transplant 1999; 18: 542–548.
32. Yousem SA: Lymphocytic bronchitis/bronchiolitis in lung allograft recipients. Am J Surg Pathol. 1993; 17: 491–496.
33. Yousem SA, Burke CM, Billingham ME: Pathologic pulmonary alterations in long-term human heart-lung transplantation. Hum Pathol 1985; 16: 911–923.
34. Scott JP, Higenbottam TW, Clelland CA, et al.: The natural history of chronic rejection in heart-lung transplant recipients: a clinical, pathological, and physiological review of 29 long-term survivors. Transplant Proc 1990; 22: 1474–1476.
35. Scott JP, Sharples L, Mullins P, et al.: Further studies on the natural history of obliterative bronchiolitis following heart-lung transplantation. Transplant Proc 1991; 23: 1201–1202.
36. Yousem SA, Dauber JH, Griffith BP: Bronchial cartilage alterations in lung transplantation. Chest 1990; 98: 1121–1124.
37. Bando K, Paradis IL, Similo S, et al.: Obliterative bronchiolitis after lung and heart-lung transplantation. An analysis of risk factors and management. J Thorac Cardiovasc Surg 1995; 110: 4–14.
38. Myers JL, Colby TV: Pathologic manifestations of bronchiolitis, constrictive bronchiolitis, cryptogenic organizing pneumonia, and diffuse panbronchiolitis. Clin Chest Med 1993; 14: 611–622.
39. Colby TV: Bronchiolitis. Pathologic considerations. Am J Clin Pathol 1998; 109: 101–109.
40. American Thoracic Society/European Respiratory Society International Multidisciplinary Consensus Classification of the Idiopathic Interstitial Pneumonias. This joint statement of the American Thoracic Society (ATS), and the European Respiratory Society (ERS) was adopted by the ATS board of directors, June 2001 and by the ERS Executive Committee, June 2001. Am J Respir Crit Care Med 2002; 165: 277–304.
41. Paradis I, Yousem S, Griffith B: Airway obstruction and bronchiolitis obliterans after lung transplantation. Clin Chest Med 1993; 14: 751–763.
42. Yousem SA, Duncan SR, Griffith BP: Interstitial and airspace granulation tissue reactions in lung transplant recipients. Am J Surg Pathol 1992; 16: 877–884.
43. Yousem SA, Paradis IL, Dauber JH, et al.: Pulmonary arteriosclerosis in long-term human heart-lung transplant recipients. Transplantation 1989; 47: 564–569.
44. Marchevsky A, Hartman G, Walts A, et al.: Lung transplantation: the pathologic diagnosis of pulmonary complications. Mod Pathol 1991; 4: 133–138.
45. Kramer MR, Marshall SE, Starnes VA, et al.: Infectious complications in heart-lung transplantation. Analysis of 200 episodes. Arch Intern Med 1993; 153: 2010–2016.
46. Gould FK, Freeman R, Taylor CE, et al.: Prophylaxis and management of cytomegalovirus pneumonitis after lung transplantation: a review of experience in one center. J Heart Lung Transplant 1993; 12: 695–699.
47. Paradis IL, Williams P: Infection after lung transplantation. Semin Respir Infect 1993; 8: 207–215.

48. Holt ND, Gould FK, Taylor CE, et al.: Incidence and significance of noncytomegalovirus viral respiratory infection after adult lung transplantation. J Heart Lung Transplant 1997; 16: 416–419.
49. Ohori NP, Michaels MG, Jaffe R, Williams P, Yousem SA: Adenovirus pneumonia in lung transplant recipients. Hum Pathol 1995; 26: 1073–1079.
50. Katzenstein A-LA: Katzenstein and Askin's surgical pathology of non-neoplastic lung disease, Vol. 13, 3rd edn. 1997, WB Saunders, Philadelphia, 1997.
51. Kanj SS, Welty-Wolf K, Madden J, et al.: Fungal infections in lung and heart-lung transplant recipients. Report of 9 cases and review of the literature. Medicine (Baltimore) 1996; 75: 142–156.
52. Hunstad DA, Cohen AH, St Geme JW 3rd: Successful eradication of mucormycosis occurring in a pulmonary allograft. J Heart Lung Transplant 1999; 18: 801–804.
53. Cahill BC, Hibbs JR, Savik K, et al.: Aspergillus airway colonization and invasive disease after lung transplantation. Chest 1997; 112: 1160–1164.
54. Nunley DR, Gal AA, Vega JD, et al.: Saprophytic fungal infections and complications involving the bronchial anastomosis following human lung transplantation. Chest 2002; 122: 1185–1191.
55. Gryzan S, Paradis IL, Zeevi A, et al.: Unexpectedly high incidence of *Pneumocystis carinii* infection after lung-heart transplantation. Implications for lung defense and allograft survival. Am Rev Respir Dis 1988; 137: 1268–1274.
56. Harris NL, Swerdlow SH, Frizzera G, Knowles DM: Post-transplant lymphoproliferative disorders. In: Pathology and genetics of tumours of haematopoietic and lymphoid tissues, Jaffe ES, Harris NL, Stein H, Vardiman JW, Eds. 2001, IARC Press, Lyon.
57. Pickhardt PJ, Siegel MJ, Anderson DC, Hayashi R, DeBaun MR: Chest radiography as a predictor of outcome in posttransplantation lymphoproliferative disorder in lung allograft recipients. AJR Am J Roentgenol 1998; 171: 375–382.
58. Frizzera G, Hanto DW, Gajl-Peczalska KJ, et al.: Polymorphic diffuse B-cell hyperplasias and lymphomas in renal transplant recipients. Cancer Res 1981; 41: 4262–4279.
59. Nalesnik MA, Jaffe R, Starzl TE, et al.: The pathology of posttransplant lymphoproliferative disorders occurring in the setting of cyclosporine A-prednisone immunosuppression. Am J Pathol 1988; 133: 173–192.
60. Knowles DM, Cesarman E, Chadburn A, et al.: Correlative morphologic and molecular genetic analysis demonstrates three distinct categories of posttransplantation lymphoproliferative disorders. Blood 1995; 85: 552–565.
61. Chadburn A, Cesarman E, Knowles DM: Molecular pathology of posttransplantation lymphoproliferative disorders. Semin Diagn Pathol 1997; 14: 15-26.
62. Chadburn A, Chen JM, Hsu DT, et al.: The morphologic and molecular genetic categories of posttransplantation lymphoproliferative disorders are clinically relevant. Cancer 1998; 82: 1978–1987.
63. Harris NL, Ferry JA, Swerdlow SH: Posttransplant lymphoproliferative disorders: summary of Society for Hematopathology Workshop. Semin Diagn Pathol 1997; 14: 8–14.
64. Rosendale B, Yousem SA. Discrimination of Epstein–Barr virus-related posttransplant lymphoproliferations from acute rejection in lung allograft recipients. Arch Pathol Lab Med 1995; 119: 418–423.
65. Abernathy EC, Hruban RH, Baumgartner WA, Reitz BA, Hutchins GM: The two forms of bronchiolitis obliterans in heart-lung transplant recipients. Hum Pathol 1991; 22: 1102–1110.
66. Chaparro C, Chamberlain D, Maurer J, et al.: Bronchiolitis obliterans organizing pneumonia (BOOP) in lung transplant recipients. Chest 1996; 110: 1150–1154.
67. Siddiqui MT, Garrity ER, Husain AN: Bronchiolitis obliterans organizing pneumonia-like reactions: a nonspecific response or an atypical form of rejection or infection in lung allograft recipients? Hum Pathol 1996; 27: 714–719.
68. Collins J, Hartman MJ, Warner TF, et al.: Frequency and CT findings of recurrent disease after lung transplantation. Radiology 2001; 219: 503–509.
69. O'Brien JD, Lium JH, Parosa JF, et al.: Lymphangiomyomatosis recurrence in the allograft after single-lung transplantation. Am J Respir Crit Care Med 1995; 151: 2033–2036.
70. Collins J, Muller NL, Kazerooni EA, et al.: Lung transplantation for lymphangioleiomyomatosis: role of imaging in the assessment of complications related to the underlying disease. Radiology 1999; 210: 325–332.
71. Baz MA, Kussin PS, Van Trigt P, et al.: Recurrence of diffuse panbronchiolitis after lung transplantation. Am J Respir Crit Care Med 1995; 151: 895–898.
72. Frost AE, Keller CA, Brown RW, et al.: Giant cell interstitial pneumonitis. Disease recurrence in the transplanted lung. Am Rev Respir Dis 1993; 148: 1401–1404.
73. Verleden GM, Sels F, Van Raemdonck D, et al.: Possible recurrence of desquamative interstitial pneumonitis in a single lung transplant recipient. Eur Respir J 1998; 11: 971–974.
74. Cook RC, Fradet G, English JC, et al.: Recurrence of intravenous talc granulomatosis following single lung transplantation. Can Respir J 1998; 5: 511–514.
75. Garver RI Jr, Zorn GL, Wu X, et al.: Recurrence of bronchioloalveolar carcinoma in transplanted lungs. N Engl J Med 1999; 340: 1071–1074.

13

Neuroendocrine neoplasms of the lung

Mark R Wick   Kevin O Leslie   Jon H Ritter   Stacey E Mills

Introduction

The concept of a "diffuse neuroendocrine system" (DNS) is not a new one. Feyrter developed this paradigm in 1938,[1] in a philosophical attempt to unify tumors in several anatomic locations which had potential secretory functions and similar morphologic characteristics. Pearse refined and renamed the cellular network in question 35 years later,[2] coining the designation of "APUD" system (for Amine Precursor Uptake and Decarboxylation) to describe its shared biochemical attributes. Inherent in the latter scheme was the presumption that all "APUD" cells – and tumors deriving from them (i.e. "APUDomas") – emanated from the remnants of the neural crest. In light of these and other observations, continuing nosologic revisionism over the past 10 years has pushed many pathologists away from such traditional diagnostic terms as "carcinoid" and "islet cell tumor" in describing certain potentially malignant but low-grade neoplasms of the neuroendocrine system,[3,4] although "traditionalists" do remain.[5] Similarly, the classification of poorly differentiated lesions has changed as well. This chapter will attempt to outline the current foundations of existing classification schemes for neuroendocrine tumors, and will (hopefully) allow the reader to come away with a simplified – and therefore practical – understanding of this confusing area of oncology.

Terminology pertaining to neuroendocrine neoplasms

There is, perhaps, no other single aspect of neuroendocrine neoplasia that is as perplexing as the pathologic terminology that has been used to describe it. Such terms as "bronchial adenoma," "carcinoid," "atypical carcinoid," "Kulchitsky cell carcinoma," "argentaffinoma," "APUDoma," "atypical endocrine carcinoma," "oat cell carcinoma," "medullary thyroid carcinoma," "islet cell tumor,"and "cutaneous Merkel cell carcinoma" (group 1) have all been employed historically in this context, in addition to "neuroblastoma," "esthesioneuroblastoma," "olfactory neuroblastoma," "medulloblastoma," "pineoblastoma," "retinoblastoma," "paraganglioma," "pheochromocytoma," "chemodectoma," and "glomus jugulare tumor" (group 2).[6–10]

This diverse lexicon reflects a basic division of neuroendocrine tumors into two broad categories– epithelial (group 1) and neural (group 2).[6] With that piece of information in hand, one can then go on to structure a much more user-friendly and straightforward classification scheme, which , in fact, has made significant inroads in the pathology literature.

Another crucial concept in understanding the categorization and clinical behavior of neuroendocrine neoplasms is that all of them are at least potentially malignant tumors, regardless of whether they belong to group 1 or group 2.[9] Moreover, in selected subgroups (e.g. classical "carcinoid" tumor, extra-adrenal paraganglioma, and pheochromocytoma [intra-adrenal paraganglioma)], one cannot reliably use macroscopic or microscopic characteristics of the tumors to predict whether they will behave innocuously or aggressively. Therefore, it follows logically that the modifier "benign" should not ever be applied in conjunction with any of the above-cited diagnostic terms. For example, even with regard to appendiceal or classical bronchial "carcinoids" – generally regarded as defining the "low" end of the spectrum of biologic behavior in this context[11–13] – there are many well-documented examples of metastasizing lesions that can be found in the literature on these tumors.

Current terminological recommendations are, therefore, different from those that might have pertained even 10 years ago, or from those with which some practitioners may feel "comfortable." The designation of *neuroendocrine carcinoma* has been proposed as a replacement for all of the various above-cited group 1 terms, with modifiers of well-differentiated (grade I/III); moderately differentiated (grade II/III); and poorly differentiated (grade III/III) being appended as appropriate.[9,12,14] In contrast, most of the traditional rubric has been retained in reference to group 2 tumors, such that *extra-adrenal paraganglioma; intra-adrenal paraganglioma (pheochromocytoma); sympatheticoadrenal neuroblastoma* (and congeners [e.g. ganglioneuroblastoma]); *olfactory neuroblastoma; retinoblastoma*; and *primitive neuroectodermal tumor* (PNET) are now the recommended terms for the categorization of this constellation of lesions.[9] In reporting on a biopsy or resection specimen, the pathologist can then work within this framework – using further descriptive comments and summaries of the aggregate literature on each tumor – to provide the clinician with an outline of expected behavior for each neoplasm based on its individual nuances.

There are two notable exceptions to the paradigm that has just been outlined. Pituitary adenomas and parathyroid adenomas are, of course, completely benign in the vast majority of cases, and it would be a mistake to label them as "grade 1 neuroendocrine carcinomas." With that said, however, it must be acknowledged that aggressive pituitary adenomas exist, and rare carcinomas also may be encountered in each location.

Distribution and pathogenesis of neuroendocrine neoplasia

If one refers to basic textbooks on human embryogenesis, a common theme that is seen in all anatomic sites is that of a neuroendocrine or neuroectodermal stage of differentiation during early organ development.[6,15,16] Because it is currently thought that oncogenesis partially (and aberrantly) recapitulates normal embryologic development, this information is central to our understanding of why neuroendocrine and neuroectodermal neoplasms have been reported in virtually every topographic location. It is true that some of the latter are, by far, more commonly hosts to such tumors, for unknown reasons. For example, the lung is the most common site of neuroendocrine carcinogenesis, where the process is clearly related etiologically to cigarette smoking and is associated with partial deletion of the short arm of chromosome 3.[17] However, identical sporadic primary neoplasms in other organs have, as yet, not been linked with any definitive pathogenetic factors.[18] Group 2 neoplasms in the "peripheral primitive neuroectodermal" category similarly demonstrate a uniform balanced translocation between chromosomes 11 and 22,[19,20] with synthesis of a unique gene product (p30/32 glycoprotein) that is recognized by a particular set of monoclonal antibodies (e.g. 12E7 and O13).[20]

Still other neuroendocrine carcinomas and group 2 tumors (especially neuroblastoma and retinoblastoma) occur in definite Mendelian-heritable – typically autosomal-dominant – patterns, as seen in multiple endocrine neoplasia (MEN) type 1 (pancreatic and thymic group 1 tumors) and MEN2 (medullary thyroid carcinoma and also group 2 tumors [pheochromocytomas]).[9,11,21,22] Ongoing work has elucidated the locations of at least some operative aberrant gene complexes in such disorders (e.g. the MEN2A locus on chromosome 10 and deletion of the Rb-1 "anti-oncogene" on chromosome 13 in heritable bilateral retinoblastoma),[17,19,23] but *sporadic* examples of the tumors cited above do not necessarily exhibit the same karyotypic or gene-sequence abnormalities.[24] Clearly, more work is needed to provide a complete picture of the molecular disturbances at play,[14,25] but this is an exciting area for current and future development because it may yield clinical tests that could be used in early diagnosis and treatment.

Other pathologic aspects of neuroendocrine neoplasia

Up to this point, this discussion has focused on "pure" neuroendocrine and neuroectodermal neoplasms. Increasingly in recent years, however, it has been recognized that human malignancies much more often show mixed or "divergent" differentiation than was ever appreciated in the past. Accordingly, oncologists are now faced with such diagnoses as "adenocarcinoma/squamous carcinoma/transitional cell carcinoma with neuroendocrine features" or, more simply, "mixed adenocarcinoma–small cell neuroendocrine carcinoma".[26–33] In the former of these scenarios, the pathologist is attempting to convey the concept that the tumor at hand looks like conventional squamous carcinoma, adenocarcinoma, or transitional cell carcinoma with a routine hematoxylin and eosin (H&E) stain, but that additional studies (e.g. ultrastructural or immunohistochemical) have demonstrated the presence of submicroscopic neuroendocrine differentiation in the neoplastic cells. In some organ systems such as the lung, it is presently thought that such a constellation of findings portends a more aggressive course of certain tumor types (e.g. "large cell anaplastic pulmonary carcinoma with neuroendocrine features"),[34] but generic extrapolation of this model to other tissues would not be scientifically justified at this time and, in fact, appears to be definitely invalid in some specific settings.[31,33] In the situation where one sees a truly mixed carcinoma at a light microscopic level, pathologists are describing the juxtaposition and admixture of two distinct histologic patterns such as adenocarcinoma and small cell neuroendocrine carcinoma.[29,30] Again, using tumors of the lung as examples, it would be expected that the responses to therapy and behavior of such mixed lesions would also be a hybrid of those attending each component (i.e. adenocarcinoma or small cell carcinoma) in pure form.[37,35–38] Nonetheless, uniform validation of that premise and delineation of optimal therapeutic approaches for each of these "amalgam" tumors have yet to occur.

Pathologic recognition of neuroendocrine differentiation

Several techniques are available that allow the pathologist to diagnose neuroendocrine differentiation in poorly differentiated malignant neoplasms of the lung and other sites. These methods are considered in the following sections.

Standard morphologic examination

By virtue of the histologic appearance of some tumors, a neuroendocrine phenotype is obvious. Ready examples include classic pulmonary small cell carcinoma and central bronchial "carcinoid" tumor. The standard cytomorphologic features of small cell carcinoma are well-known, and

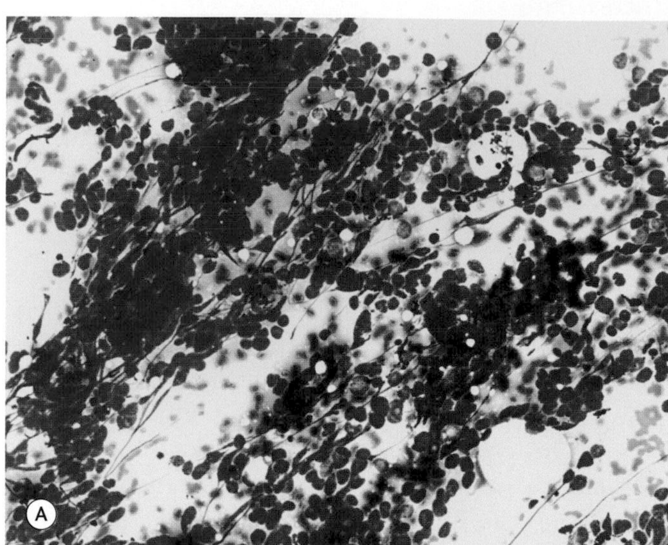

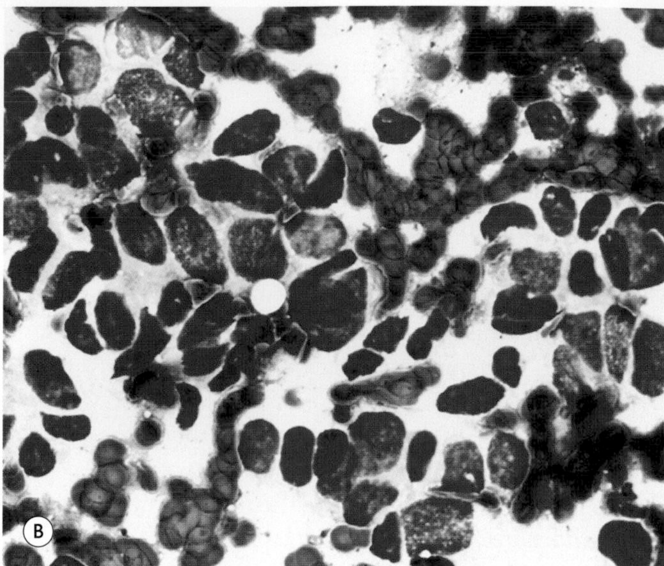

Fig. 13.1 (A) Fine-needle aspiration biopsy of small-cell neuroendocrine carcinoma of the lung, showing characteristic crush artifact, nuclear "molding," high nucleocytoplasmic ratios, and a relative lack of nuclei. (B) Nuclear "molding" and dispersed nuclear chromatin are better seen in this image of the same tumor.

include hyperchromatic nuclei with dispersed chromatin, inconspicuous nucleoli, and a tendency for the nuclei to mold to one another (Fig. 13.1). The cells are oval or carrot-shaped with scant cytoplasm, and often there is marked crush artifact. Extensive necrosis is often observed, with either a geographic pattern or with the dropout of individual cells (i.e. apoptosis). Likewise, bronchial "carcinoid" features stippled nuclear chromatin, and a distinctly organoid growth pattern, with formation of rosettes, trabeculae, or ribbons ("festoons")[39] (Fig. 13.2).

In such cases, special stains, electron microscopy, and other adjunctive diagnostic techniques are merely confirmatory. In fact, because small cell neuroendocrine carcinomas (SCNCs) often fail to exhibit ultrastructural or immunohistologic markers of endocrine differentiation due to sampling artifacts and other factors, one may actually engender confusion on the part of clinicians by obtaining negative results in those studies. Our practice in dealing with endobronchial biopsies showing groups of small round cells with crush artifact is simply to obtain immunostains for cytokeratin and leukocyte common antigen (CD45) (see below). The aim of this approach is simply to address generic cellular lineage, with the conclusion that small cell epithelial lesions with the specified characteristics represent SCNCs.

Adjunctive procedures become more valuable when one encounters large cell pulmonary malignancies that do not have prototypical neuroendocrine characteristics.

Histochemical methods

Histochemical techniques are still valuable in selected settings, although in current practice they have been supplanted by newer technologies. In specific reference to neuroendocrine lesions, such techniques rely on the ability of endocrine cells to reduce silver solutions and form insoluble precipitates in tissue sections. The available methods are broadly subdivided into two groups: namely, argentaffin and argyrophil stains.[40–42]

Argentaffin techniques depend on the presence of endogenous cellular reducing agents. The most widely used among them is the Fontana–Masson stain, which is only variably reactive with pulmonary neuroendocrine neoplasms. Argyrophilic methods are those in which an exogenous reducing agent is added, such as in the Grimelius or Churukian–Schenk procedures. They are typically positive in the majority of well-differentiated neuroendocrine tumors of the lung (Fig. 13.3), with much lesser reactivity in high-grade carcinomas such as SCNC.[42]

Electron microscopy

The ultrastructural hallmark of neuroendocrine neoplasms in the lung and elsewhere is the presence of cytoplasmic neurosecretory granules (NSGs). These are rounded structures that consist of a central dense core, a peripheral lucent halo, and a single delimiting outer membrane. They vary from 30 to 300 nm in diameter, and may occur singly or in clusters[42,43–54,54a] (Fig. 13.4). Budding of NSGs

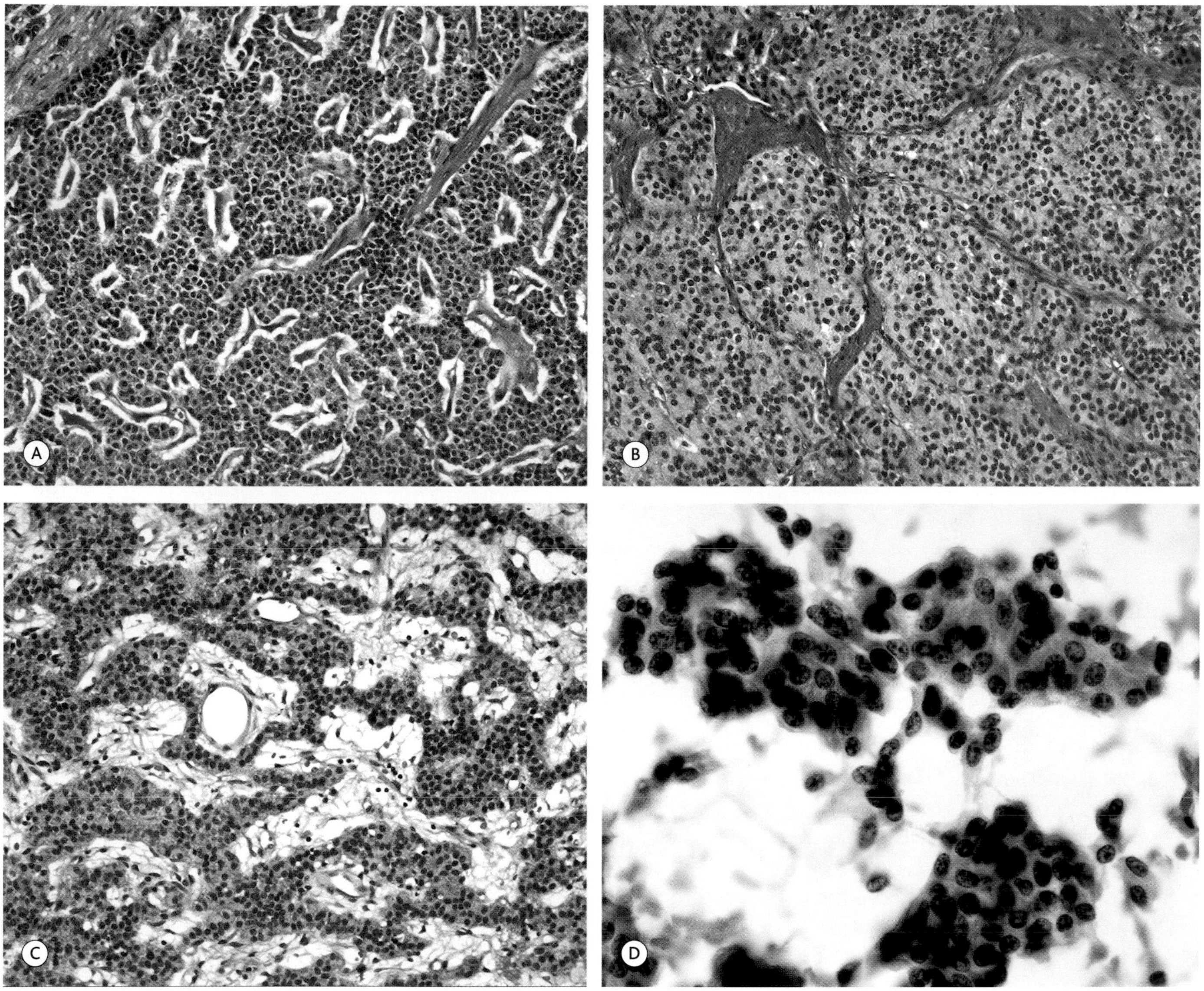

Fig. 13.2 Characteristic growth patterns in neuroendocrine carcinoma, including (A,B) insular cellular arrangement and (C) insular and ribboning growth. (D) Insulae are seen in fine-needle aspiration biopsy specimens as well.

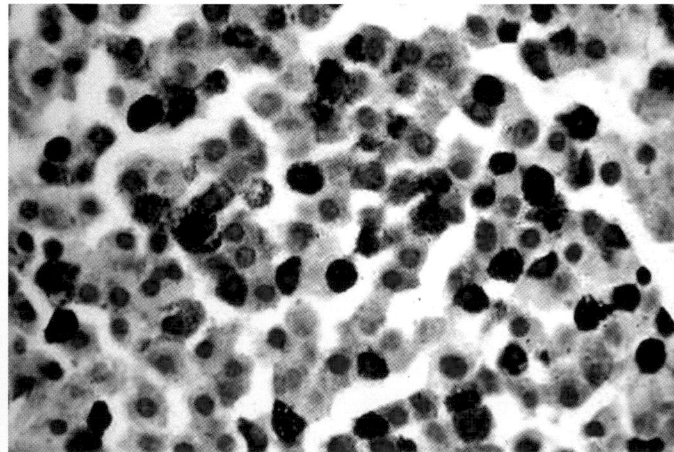

Fig. 13.3 Argyrophil-reactivity of neuroendocrine carcinoma with the Churukian–Schenck method.

from prominent Golgi apparatus is occasionally observed. One drawback of electron microscopy is that the number of granules, and the number of cells *containing* granules, tends to be greatest in well-differentiated tumors and lowest in poorly differentiated lesions (where they are most needed for diagnosis!). Also, electron microscopy is capable of examining only relatively few cells in any given tumor. However, it is still a highly useful technique if sufficient time and care are invested in a thorough search for dense core granules. In a study by Nagle et al.,[40] ultrastructural analysis documented neuroendocrine differentiation in all of 41 putative neuroendocrine lesions, whereas a significant percentage was negative for endocrine markers using immunohistochemical techniques.

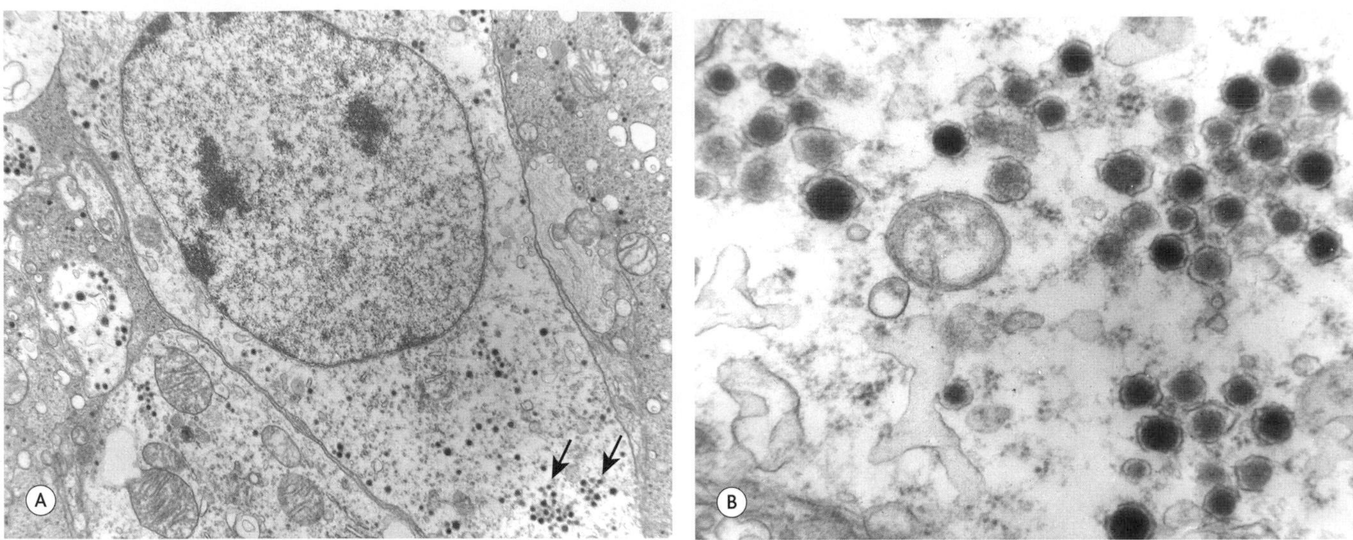

Fig. 13.4 (A) Electron micrograph of neuroendocrine carcinoma of the lung, demonstrating numerous cytoplasmic dense-core (neurosecretory) granules (arrows). (B) These inclusions are demonstrable even in specimens retrieved from paraffin blocks.

Immunohistology

Advances in immunohistochemistry over the last 15 years have yielded powerful tools for the pathologist in recognizing neuroendocrine differentiation.[44,50,54–59] Advantages of this approach include a relatively low cost, rapid turnaround time, the ability to perform studies on routinely processed tissue, and the capacity to rapidly screen a large number of cells as opposed to the limited number that can be seen by electron microscopy. The following markers represent those with greatest utility in this context.

Intermediate filament proteins

Group I neuroendocrine neoplasms manifest uniform immunoreactivity for keratin, especially keratin classes 8 and 18.[60] To a lesser extent, keratin 19 is also observed in neuroendocrine carcinomas (NECs) in general. Pulmonary NECs may label for keratin 20 as well, but only in <10% of cases.[61] Keratin proteins are generally well-recognized by several commercial monoclonal antibodies, especially CAM5.2 and MFN116. Monospecific reagents directly against only one keratin class polypeptide are also available, but are not necessary in this specific context. In the authors' opinion, the optimal approach to the detection of keratin in *any* poorly differentiated neoplasm, neuroendocrine or otherwise, is to prepare a *mixture* of monoclonal antikeratin antibodies with partially overlapping and partially distinctive keratin class specificities. When reagents of this type are used on paraffin sections, together with properly-performed proteolytic digestion or microwave (heat)-mediated epitope "retrieval" methods, the detectability of keratin in neuroendocrine carcinomas should approximate 100%, even in essentially "undifferentiated" tumors (e.g. small cell neuroendocrine carcinoma).[62] Another feature of keratin reactivity in many NECs is that a distinctive punctate or globoid perinuclear zone of positivity is observed.[63] This result (Fig. 13.5) is simultaneously diagnostic of both epithelial *and* neuroendocrine differentiation in a small cell malignancy, and obviates the need for other "neuroendocrine markers." Keratin is not typically expected in group II neuroendocrine neoplasms, although some

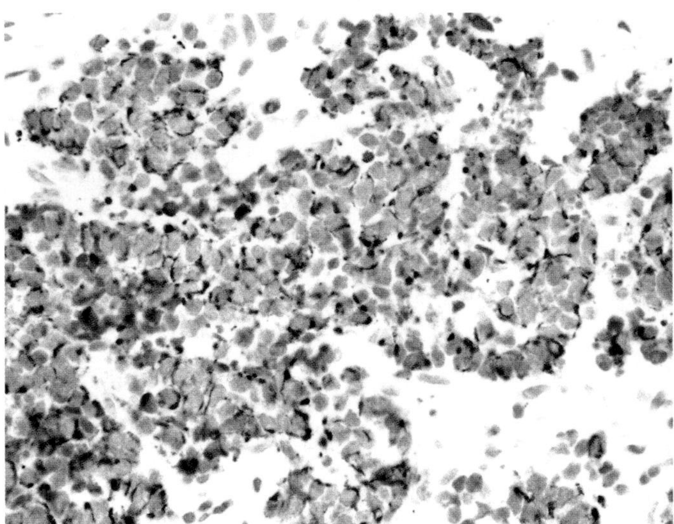

Fig. 13.5 Paranuclear "dot"-like immunoreactivity for keratin in small cell pulmonary neuroendocrine carcinoma. This pattern concurrently establishes the epithelial and the neuroendocrine nature of the tumor in question.

lesions in that group have indeed shown its presence in an "aberrant" manner.[64–67] The foremost example of that phenomenon is represented by PNET with "divergent" differentiation (also known as "polyphenotypic small cell tumor"), an example of which is the "desmoplastic small round cell tumor".[68–70] In most cases of keratin expression in more nondescript PNETs, reactivity for that protein is focal, unlike its pattern in NECs; in addition, vimentin expression tends to be mutually exclusive in PNETs and NECs. Nonetheless, problems in differential diagnosis may arise between those classes of neuroendocrine tumors, sometimes necessitating cytogenetic evaluation to distinguish between them.[71]

Neurofilament protein (NFP) is variably coexpressed by NECs,[72–75] but that determinant is seen as the sole intermediate filament in the majority of differentiated group II neuroendocrine tumors such as paragangliomas and pheochromocytomas, as well as some neuroblastomas.[76–78] Unfortunately, NFP is not well-visualized in paraffin sections, even with epitope retrieval technology, and it is most reliably evaluated in frozen material. Vimentin also may be evident in the cells of paragangliomas in approximately 50% of cases,[78] and it is the *only* intermediate filament that can be detected in primitive group II tumors such as neuroblastoma and PNET.[67] That is also true in Ewing's sarcoma, a tumor that is in the same family as PNET. Vimentin is only exceptionally present in NECs, as stated above. Eusebi et al.[79] have recently described three NECs that coexpressed keratin and desmin, as a reflection of divergent (sarcomatoid) rhabdomyoblastic differentiation. This same proclivity is regularly seen in desmoplastic small round cell tumors, in which keratin, desmin, and vimentin are commonly present concomitantly in the same neoplastic cells.[68–70]

Glial fibrillary acidic protein (GFAP) is not an expected reactant in either NEC or PNET. In the central nervous system, therefore, this marker is helpful in differential diagnosis with small cell malignant gliomas,[80] most of which are reactive for GFAP. That fact is all the more important because a proportion of glial tumors manifest aberrant keratin reactivity,[81] and also express vimentin.

Chromogranins

Chromogranins are matrical proteins that are associated with neurosecretory granules, and, as such, they are absolutely specific for neuroendocrine differentiation.[82–84] These polypeptides have been subdivided biochemically into two groups, A and B,[85,86] with the latter being synonymous with secretogranin-I. Conceptually, every cell that packages peptides into neurosecretory granules must synthesize either chromogranin-A (CGA) or chromogranin-B (CGB); hence, a screening reagent incorporating antibodies to both of those proteins would be extremely useful diagnostically. Unfortunately, reliable commercial anti-CGB products have not been introduced thus far. The most widely used anti-CGA antibody is clone LK2H10.[87] This reagent was raised against pheochromocytoma cells, and shows excellent reactivity with paraffin sections (Fig. 13.6). The major shortcoming of anti-CGA is twofold. First, because neuroendocrine cells or tumors may preferentially synthesize CGB, CGA obviously cannot be regarded as a "universal" marker of such elements. Secondly, the detectability of *both* CGA and CGB is directly related to the number of neurosecretory granules in any given neuroendocrine cell population. If one is dealing with poorly differentiated malignancies having only scant numbers of such organelles, immunostains for CGA and CGB will be predictably negative in the majority of cases. Therefore, one may legitimately conclude that a tumor has neuroendocrine properties if it can be labeled for a chromogranin, but negative results do not *exclude* that possibility, particularly in high-grade neoplasms.

Synaptophysin

Synaptophysin is a 38 kDa molecule that is associated with the synaptic vesicles of neurons and cells with neuroendocrine or neuroectodermal characteristics.[77,88–91] Monoclonal antibodies to this marker have been used widely in diagnostic surgical pathology and cytopathology with good success, particularly in conjunction with epitope

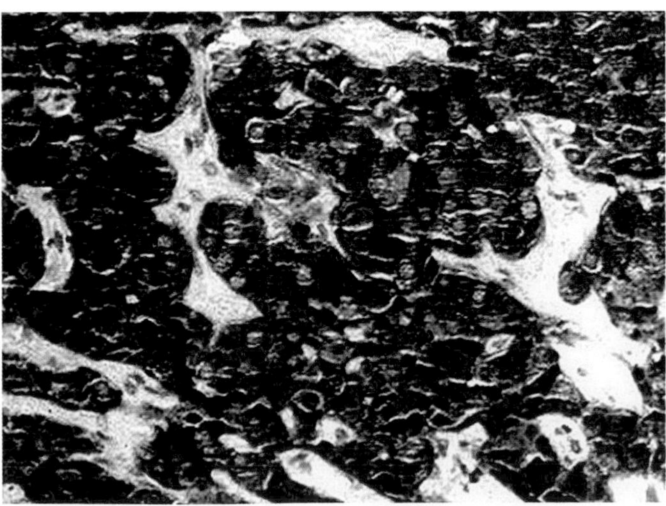

Fig. 13.6 Immunoreactivity for chromogranin-A in neuroendocrine carcinoma of the lung.

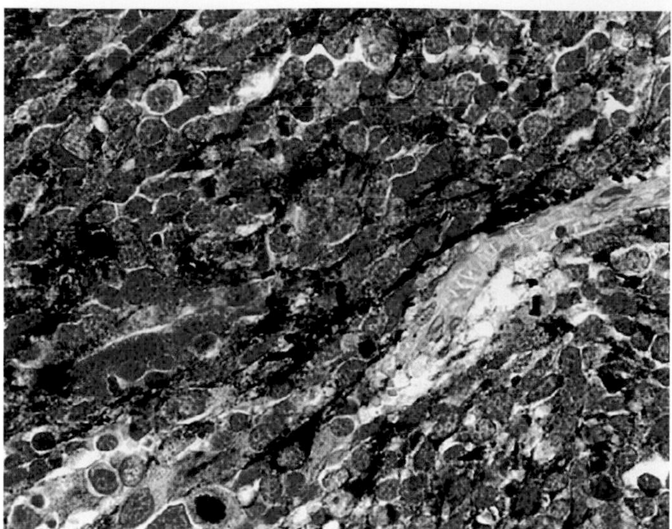

Fig. 13.7 Immunolabeling for synaptophysin in pulmonary neuroendocrine carcinoma.

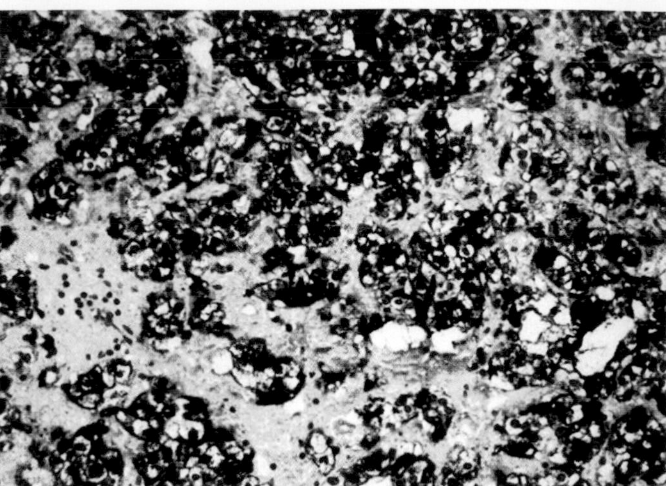

Fig. 13.8 Immunoreactivity for CD56 (neural cell adhesion molecule) in neuroendocrine carcinoma of the lung.

retrieval techniques (Fig. 13.7). In light of its subcellular associations, one might assume that synaptophysin would have a synonymous tissue distribution to that of the chromogranins; however, in practicality, that is not true. Thus, a sizable proportion of neuroendocrine neoplasms will label for CGA or CGB, but not synaptophysin, and the converse of that relationship also applies.[92] Thus, anti-synaptophysins and anti-chromogranins should be conceptualized as complementary reagents.

Loy et al. have challenged the specificity of chromogranins and synaptophysin as markers of neuroendocrine lineage, in a study using ultrastructure as the standard for definition of that lineage.[58] However, in the authors' opinion, the concept behind that analysis was flawed. Sampling bias (a significant problem in fine structural evaluations) probably accounted for those cases in which immunoreactivity was observed for the specified endocrine markers, but no neurosecretory granules were identified by electron microscopy.

CD57 (Leu-7)

CD57 was originally characterized as a marker for natural killer lymphocytes, and is recognized by monoclonal antibody HNK-1,[93] among others. Subsequently, shared epitopes of this molecule have been detected immunohistochemically in normal constituents and tumors of the brain, peripheral nervous system, soft tissues, prostate gland, thymus, and the DNS.[94–100] In specific reference to neuroendocrine neoplasms, CD57 appears to bind to a matrical component of neurosecretory granules that is distinct from both CGA and CGB.[101] As such, it both corroborates and extends the sensitivity of chromogranin immunostains in many clinical settings. Nonetheless, because of the imperfect specificity of Leu-7, it cannot be used as confidently as a "stand-alone" neuroendocrine marker. Moreover, it suffers from the same failings in sensitivity as those of CGA and CGB that relate to the density of neurosecretory granules in poorly differentiated tumors.

Neural cell adhesion molecule (NCAM; CD56)

The monoclonal antibodies 123C3 and JLP5B9 recognize formalin-preserved epitopes of CD56, or neural cell adhesion molecule, a cell membrane protein that has a role in the cohesiveness of cells in the peripheral and central nervous systems.[102–108] In likeness to synaptophysin, NCAM is also distributed among neuroendocrine and neuroectodermal cells and tumors (Fig. 13.8). Indeed, several studies have shown that NCAM is a sensitive marker of endocrine lineage in small cell carcinoma of the lung, as well as extrapulmonary sites.[105–107] Nonetheless, it is not absolutely specific for neuroendocrine differentiation, inasmuch as a minority (up to 25%) of ovarian surface carcinomas, renal cell carcinomas, non-endocrine lung cancers, and endometrial carcinomas will demonstrate CD56-immunoreactivity.[107] Despite this caveat, antibodies to NCAM are useful additions to diagnostic panels for endocrine tumors. Reagents raised against the *polysialylated* form of CD56 are said to be the most sensitive among this group.[104]

Neuron-specific (gamma-dimer) enolase

"Neuron-specific" enolase (NSE) is a gamma-dimeric form of 14-3-2 protein, a glycolytic enzyme that is present in neurons and cells of the DNS.[109] It is thought to be associated with the formation of intercellular synapses in the nervous system. NSE was one of the first markers to be used in diagnostic immunohistochemistry as a general indicator of putative neuroendocrine differentiation.[109–111] Indeed, heteroantisera to NSE are very sensitive in that regard, labeling virtually all neuronal and neuroendocrine proliferations regardless of the level of cellular differentiation.[111] Nevertheless, the specificity of those reagents is poor, owing to cross-reactivity between gamma-dimers and heterodimers (e.g. alpha-gamma; alpha-beta) of NSE that are expressed by non-neuroendocrine neoplasms of many different types.[112] In reaction to that problem, monoclonal antibodies to NSE have been developed and tested,[113] but these have generally manifested a low degree of sensitivity and have not enjoyed widespread usage. An alternative approach to lessening the cross-reactivity of anti-NSE heteroantisera is to absorb them with acetone-fixed, pulverized human tissues known to contain high levels of the alpha or beta forms of the molecule. However, that approach is time-consuming and somewhat demanding technically, and likewise has not been embraced in clinical practice. Currently, antibodies to NSE are primarily utilized as "screens" for endocrine differentiation,[114–116] and reactivity with them is usually pursued further by applying other neuroendocrine immunostains, as described above and below.

Protein gene product 9.5 (PGP9.5)

PGP9.5 is a protein that removes ubiquitin (an intracellular regulatory protein) from other proteins and protects them from degradation by proteases. It is expressed widely within cells and tumors of the DNS, and therefore has been applied as an immunohistochemical marker of neuroendocrine differentiation.[117–119] Nevertheless, the general distribution of PGP9.5 in human neoplasms has shown that it is not particularly specific for an endocrine lineage; in particular, non-small cell carcinomas of the lung that lack neuroendocrine morphologic patterns and contain no neurosecretory granules on ultrastructural analysis have been PGP9.5-positive in approximately 55% of cases in some series.[120] Thus, the practical utility of this marker is similar to that of NSE.

Specific neuropeptides

Specific neuropeptides, such as adrenocorticotropic hormone, gastrin, insulin, somatostatin, calcitonin, "whole" bombesin and its C-terminal flanking peptide, leu- and met- enkephalins, etc., were the initial molecular moieties that were evaluated immunohistochemically, in efforts to substantiate the neuroendocrine nature of selected epithelial human neoplasms.[92] Today, these markers have been largely relegated to a secondary role in the pathologic assessment of tumors in the DNS. Antibodies to such peptides are of academic interest in correlating clinical endocrinopathies with histopathologic findings, but are not nearly sensitive enough to serve as screening reagents. Another potential but limited application is in the delineation of "occult" (non-endocrinopathy-related) peptide production by neuroendocrine tumors, which may serve as the basis for serologic monitoring of tumor growth and activity.

CD99 (MIC2; p30/32 protein)

The membranocytoplasmic protein known as CD99 in the hematopoietic antigen cluster designation is the same molecule that has been called MIC2 or p30/32 protein.[121] The function of this moiety is uncertain at the present time, but it is empirically known to be expressed in virtually all PNETs and Ewing's sarcomas[121,122] (Fig. 13.9). The specificity of CD99 antibodies for a neuroectodermal lineage is not absolute, however, because they may also label a minority (<15%) of alveolar rhabdomyosarcomas as well as the overwhelming majority (90%) of lymphoblastic lymphomas.[123] CD99 is observed in up to 20% of neuroendocrine carcinomas in some body sites as well.[124,125] This is an important fact, because it may obscure the difference between NEC and PNET in selected instances; this is particularly true in light of the potential for keratin reactivity that both lesions have. On the other hand, *differentiated* group II neuroendocrine

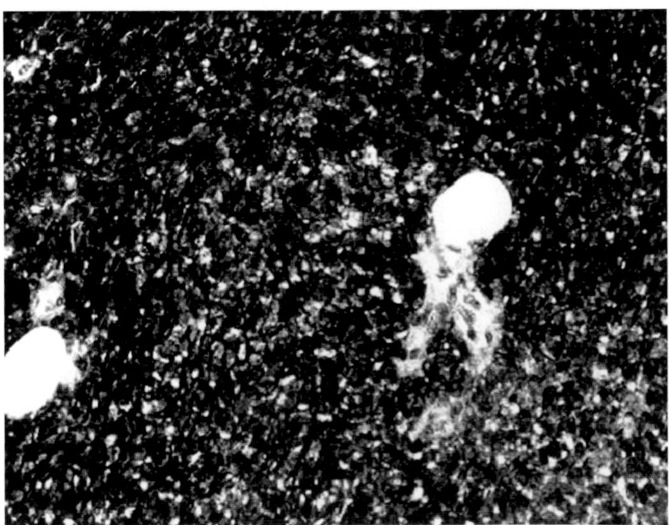

Fig. 13.9 Immunolabeling for CD99 (MIC2 protein) in primitive neuroectodermal tumor. This marker can also be observed in neuroendocrine carcinomas.

tumors, such as paragangliomas, are non-reactive for this determinant.

Other reagents

Several other antibodies have been developed that have immunohistochemical properties that overlap those of LK2H10 (anti-CGA). These include both polyclonal and hybridoma reagents. A monoclonal antibody designated HISL-19 by Krisch et al.[126] is thought to manifest neuroendocrine specificity. The determinant that it recognizes is proteinaceous but seems to be nonidentical to chromogranin. This statement is based on the relative strength of reactivity of HISL-19 with several neuroendocrine tissues, which is dissimilar to that of LK2H10. Moreover, some nonendocrine tissues and tumors, such as the gallbladder epithelium and adenocarcinomas of the lung, stomach, and endometrium, are labeled by the former reagent but not the latter. These differences notwithstanding, HISL-19 does appear to bind to a neurosecretory granule-related moiety, inasmuch as neoplasms with few of these granules (parathyroid adenoma, melanoma, neuroblastoma, and oat cell lung cancer) are only weakly stained but others with numerous granules (pituitary adenoma, pheochromocytoma, medullary thyroid carcinoma, carcinoid, and islet cell tumor) are labeled intensely. Western immunoblot analyses have shown that the target of HISL-19 is not neuron-specific enolase. [126]

Lloyd et al. have employed monoclonal antibodies to adrenaline (epinephrine) and noradrenaline (norepinephrine) in the study of similar neuroendocrine neoplasms.[127] In general, pheochromocytomas displayed adrenaline alone, but extra-adrenal paragangliomas exhibited reactivity for adrenaline and noradrenaline, or noradrenaline only. Neuroblastomas, carcinoids, pituitary adenomas, pancreatic endocrine tumors, and parathyroid adenomas also showed positivity for noradrenaline. These authors emphasized the point that catecholamine-positive neoplasms also expressed reactivity with LK2H10, implying that stains for adrenaline and noradrenaline did not add appreciably to diagnostic information obtained with antichromogranin.

Haspel and colleagues found that mice infected with reovirus type I often developed autoimmune syndromes featuring polyendocrinopathies.[128] Spleen cells from such animals were used as the substrates for hybridoma production, and two of the resulting monoclonal antibodies (5B5 and 5B8) showed reactivity with human anterior pituitary cells in frozen and Bouin's-fixed specimens.[128] Further immunostaining results in normal and neoplastic human tissues were not provided, but it was thought that 5B5 and 5B8 recognized discrete hormonal products, such as growth hormone, based on competitive inhibition studies.

The absence of preceding discussion on S100 protein may seem surprising, because of the still-common belief that this marker is associated with neuroendocrine tumors. In reality, that is not so. The only endocrine neoplasm that reproducibly contains S100 protein-positive cells is paraganglioma, and the immunoreactive elements therein are actually "sustentacular" cells rather than tumor cells.[78] It has been contended that sustentacular elements decrease in density when paragangliomas undergo malignant change,[129] but that is an uncertain tenet in reference to individual cases.

Yet another recently characterized reagent is that known as antithyroid transcription factor-1 (TTF1).[129a–g] This intranuclear protein is expressed not only by thyroid epithelium but also by glandular cells of the lung, pulmonary adenocarcinomas, and neuroendocrine carcinomas of the lung (Fig. 13.10). Among the last of these lesional groups, small cell carcinoma and large cell neuroendocrine carcinomas have the highest incidence of reactivity (in approximately 85–90% of cases). Interestingly, however, extrapulmonary high-grade neuroendocrine carcinomas likewise show a tendency to be TTF1-positive in many organ sites (bladder, uterine cervix, prostate, gastrointestinal tract), and therefore this marker can be considered to represent an "adjunct" neuroendocrine determinant, if additional studies for thyroid-related and lung-associated labels are negative. Obviously, then, TTF1 *cannot* be employed reliably to distinguish metastatic

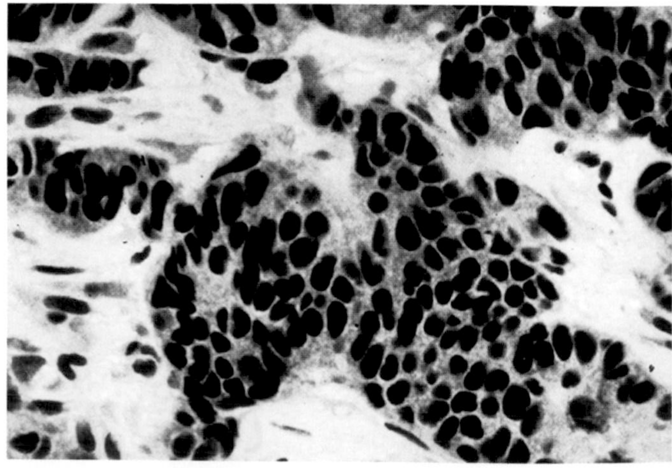

Fig. 13.10 Nuclear immunoreactivity for thyroid transcription factor-1 (TTF-1) in pulmonary neuroendocrine carcinoma.

Table 13.1 WHO classification of pulmonary neuroendocrine lesions

1) Submacroscopic pulmonary neuroendocrine lesions
   a) Tumorlet
   b) Neuroendocrine body
2) Common tumors with a light-microscopic neuroendocrine appearance
   a) Carcinoid tumor
   b) Atypical carcinoid/well-differentiated neuroendocrine carcinoma
   c) Large cell neuroendocrine carcinoma (intermediate cell neuroendocrine carcinoma)
   d) Small cell carcinoma
      i) Pure small cell carcinoma (oat cell and intermediate variants)
      ii) Small cell/large cell neuroendocrine carcinoma
      iii) Combined small cell/non-small cell carcinoma
3) Non-small cell carcinoma with neuroendocrine features (neuroendocrine differentiation detected only by immunostaining or electron microscopy)
4) Uncommon primary tumors with neuroendocrine differentiation
   a) Amphicrine neoplasms
   b) Blastoma with neuroendocrine differentiation
   c) Primitive neuroectodermal tumors

Source: from Travis et al.[130]

Table 13.2 Alternative classification of neuroendocrine proliferations of the lung

I. Neuroendocrine hyperplasias – microscopic tumorlet, neuropeithelial body

II. Type I neoplastic lesions (neuroendocrine carcinomas (NECs))
   - Grade I NEC (formerly called "classic carcinoid")
   - Grade II NEC (formerly called "atypical carcinoid" or "well-differentiated neuroendocrine carcinoma")
   - Grade III NEC (further characterized by cell size as small cell neuroendocrine carcinoma or large cell neuroendocrine carcinoma, or mixtures thereof)
   - Mixed neuroendocrine/non-neuroendocrine carcinomas
   - Non-small cell carcinoma with occult neuroendocrine differentiation

III. Type II neoplastic lesions (paraganglioma, primitive neuroectodermal tumor, and neuroblastoma)

neuroendocrine carcinoma of the lung from other neuroendocrine malignancies.

Specific features of pulmonary neuroendocrine proliferations

Before further discussion of specific neuroendocrine proliferations in the lung, a general consideration of their current nosology is in order. Travis et al. have recently provided a classification scheme for pulmonary neoplasms in general through the auspices of the World Health Organization (WHO) (Table 13.1).[130]

A central tenet in our thinking, as expressed in the Introduction, is that we believe that all neuroendocrine proliferations of the lung are at least potentially malignant. The only exceptions to this statement are represented by pulmonary tumorlets and the neuroepithelial bodies, which are considered to be hyperplastic rather than neoplastic in nature. As others have done before us,[131] we have espoused the scheme shown in Table 13.2 as more appropriate than the WHO paradigm in the general categorization of neuroendocrine lesions.

The following points constitute our rationale for this type of classification:

1. From 5 to 15% of classical bronchial "carcinoids" may metastasize to regional lymph nodes, and at least 1–2% may be fatal.[5] These tumors thus have low-grade biologic attributes, and can usually be cured by complete resection, but their malignant potential is not nil. However, these data clearly escape many observers, who equate the term "carcinoid" with a benign process.
2. The term "atypical carcinoid" is fraught with interpretative problems, because it is still regarded erroneously as a variant of *classical* carcinoid by many clinicians. In essence, this is a reflection of the fact that many pathologists tend to use the term "atypical," particularly in cytopathology, to describe benign but morphogically abnormal cells. By contrast, "atypical carcinoid" (grade II neuroendocrine carcinoma) is an undeniably aggressive malignancy, with a 5-year mortality of at least 35%.[5] Moreover, the term "atypical carcinoid" has taken on a nebulous quality, with a general lack of agreement on necessary criteria for that diagnosis. Some use the term for any neuroendocrine lesion of the lung that is not a central classic "carcinoid" or a small cell carcinoma.
4. Large-cell neuroendocrine carcinomas appear to be unquestionably high-grade tumors behaviorally and histologically. Referring to these neoplasms as "moderately differentiated" or "intermediate,"[12] underestimates their biologic potential. In addition, use of the term "intermediate" is confounding in this specific context, because it has been employed in the past in reference to variants of small cell carcinoma of the lung.[35]
5. The time has probably come to re-examine the venerated dichotomy of surgical or non-surgical treatment pertaining to non-small cell- and small cell carcinomas of the lung, respectively. Although they are rare, pathologic stage I SCNCs are surgically

treatable lesions;[131] conversely, high-grade large cell neuroendocrine carcinomas could benefit from chemotherapeutic approaches that are usually applied to SCNC.[4] However, these issues are unsettled, and are likely to remain so as long as the traditional small cell/non-small cell carcinoma paradigm is rigidly followed.

6. The argument is often made that clinicians understand only the "traditional" terms for neuroendocrine neoplasms, and therefore they should remain in the lexicon of pathologists. In contrast, our sense is rather that clinical physicians do *not* understand well the biologic potential of pulmonary neuroendocrine proliferations, and that several terms which have been used for years serve only to perpetuate myths.

At this time, we make the diagnosis of "neuroendocrine carcinoma," followed by its grade, for *all* type I (epithelial) neuroendocrine tumors of the lung. In a parenthetical comment, the traditional terminology is usually given as well to facilitate transitions in nomenclature. At some point in the future, it should be possible to omit the older terminology altogether.

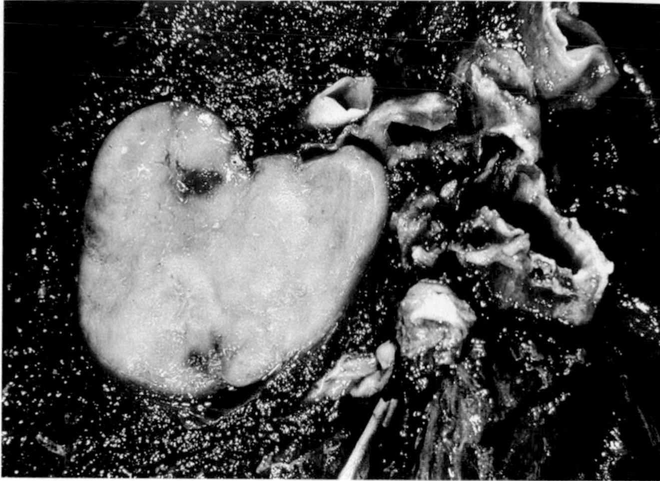

Fig. 13.11 This yellow-white mass in the peripheral pulmonary parenchyma had the histologic image of a grade I neuroendocrine carcinoma ("classical carcinoid").

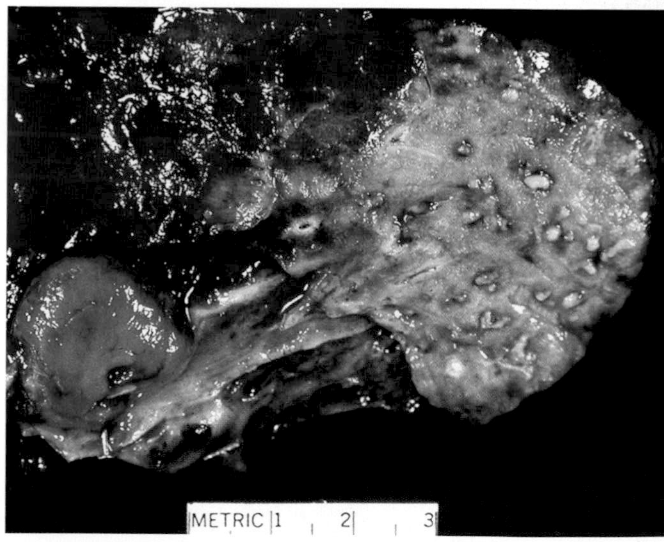

Fig. 13.12 This endobronchial mass (far left) with intact overlying mucosa represents a central grade I neuroendocrine carcinoma of the lung ("classical carcinoid"). The lesion caused bronchial luminal obstruction with attendant post obstructive pneumonia (right).

Grade I neuroendocrine carcinoma ("classical carcinoid")

Bronchopulmonary "carcinoid" (grade I neuroendocrine carcinoma (NEC)) was initially considered to be an "adenoma" of the bronchus,[132] a term that unfortunately persists in the lexicon of some individuals. The similarity of this lesion to gastrointestinal carcinoids, so named as "carcinoma-like tumors" and described 30 years earlier, was then noted. Although the majority of classic carcinoids are centrally located, approximately 10–20% are found in the periphery of the lung[11,12,15,45,133–138] (Fig. 13.11). An anatomic landmark that is commonly used to distinguish central and peripheral tumors is the cartilaginous airways; those neoplasms associated with such structures are considered to be central, and others without that relationship are considered to be peripheral.[134]

Clinical features

Grade I NECs with typical histologic features are rarely diagnostic problems. They usually grow as polypoid intraluminal masses with an intact overlying epithelium (Fig. 13.12), or one demonstrating squamous metaplasia.[45,133,134] This pattern explains a common clinical presentation, which is that of localized airway obstruction. Patients manifest with wheezing, cough, or pneumonia. They almost never develop the carcinoid syndrome, presumably because the tumors in question are incapable of synthesizing the biochemical substances responsible for its pathogenesis. Rare individuals with grade I NEC have associated Cushing's syndrome or other endocrinopathies, owing to ectopic neuropeptide production by the neoplasm.[139–145] A proposed association between pulmonary carcinoids and sarcoidosis has also been made.[146]

Localized obstruction also dominates the radiographic picture, with evidence of obstructive pneumonia or

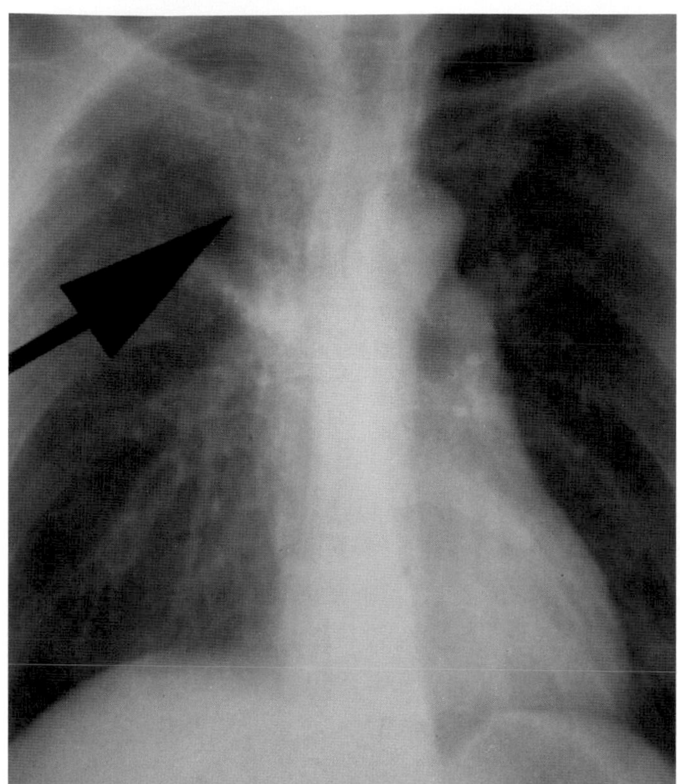

Fig. 13.13 Bronchial obstruction by central low-grade neuroendocrine carcinoma caused segmental atelectasis of the right upper lobe, as seen in this chest radiograph (arrow).

atelectasis (Fig. 13.13). Occasionally, a central mass with a dumbbell-like configuration will be seen on plain films, and computed tomographic (CT) scans usually demonstrate a lesion within and adjacent to a large airway.[147]

Men and women are approximately equally affected by pulmonary "carcinoids"; although all age groups may develop grade I pulmonary NECs, young to middle-aged adults account for the majority of cases. The lesions therefore appear at substantially lower ages than those associated with other pulmonary carcinomas.

Peripheral carcinoids are subpleural, small, and well circumscribed.[134,137,138] As such, they often present only as incidental findings, lacking the propensity to produce the obstructive changes of their central counterparts. Instead, the differential diagnosis of a "coin lesion" is encountered. Radiographically, such entities as granulomas, hamartomas, or peripheral adenocarcinomas enter consideration. Some studies have shown a predominance of peripheral grade I NECs in the right middle lobe, and a greater number of female patients have those tumors as compared to central neuroendocrine carcinomas of the lung.[137,138]

Gross and microscopic pathologic findings

"Classic carcinoids" are typically 2–4 cm in maximum dimension. The lesions vary in color from tan-yellow to dark red, and they lack obvious internal necrosis and hemorrhage. Central tumors display diverse growth patterns, including trabecular, ribboning, insular, and solid sheet-like configurations[11,133,134] (Fig. 13.14). A delicate fibrovascular stroma is present, sometimes with associated matrical amyloid deposition.[148] Rare lesions may contain metaplastic bone or cartilage.[11] The latter findings are postulated to reflect the production of factors related to TGF-beta or various bone morphogenetic proteins.[134] Tumor cell cytoplasm is relatively abundant, and may be strikingly granular and oncocytic or even clear.[149–152] Eccentricity of the nuclei can yield a plasmacytoid cellular image, particularly in fine-needle aspiration biopsy specimens (Fig. 13.15). A papillary configuration has also been reported.[11,153] Other variants of grade I NEC produce melanin,[154,155] and some are said to contain S100 protein-immunoreactive sustentacular cells, as more typically seen in paragangliomas.[156] An exceptional case presented by Skinner and Ewen featured diffuse replacement of the lung parenchyma by carcinoid tumor cells.[157]

Peripheral carcinoids may be morphologically identical to central tumors, in which case the diagnosis is usually made without difficulty. Nonetheless, peripheral grade I NECs are often singular in demonstrating a prominent spindle cell growth pattern.[137,138] (Fig. 13.16).

Differential diagnostic considerations

The intraluminal growth pattern of grade I pulmonary NEC can be simulated by salivary gland-like tumors such as mucoepidermoid carcinoma; mesenchymal lesions, including peripheral nerve sheath tumors and rare inflammatory pseudotumors; and some metastatic neoplasms. Most of these possibilities present little difficulty histologically. Nonetheless, problems may arise occasionally in separating carcinoids from well-differentiated adenocarcinomas, higher-grade neuroendocrine carcinomas, primary pulmonary paragangliomas, and "solid" adenoid cystic carcinomas, particularly in small transbronchial biopsies which may demonstrate significant artifactual distortion. Distinction from "atypical" carcinoids will be discussed in more detail subsequently. However, uniform nuclear features, the lack of significant mitotic activity, abundant cytoplasm, and the absence of necrosis are all indicative of grade I NEC rather than a grade II tumor.[3,5,135] Because of the well-differentiated nature of classical carcinoids, one can expect almost all of

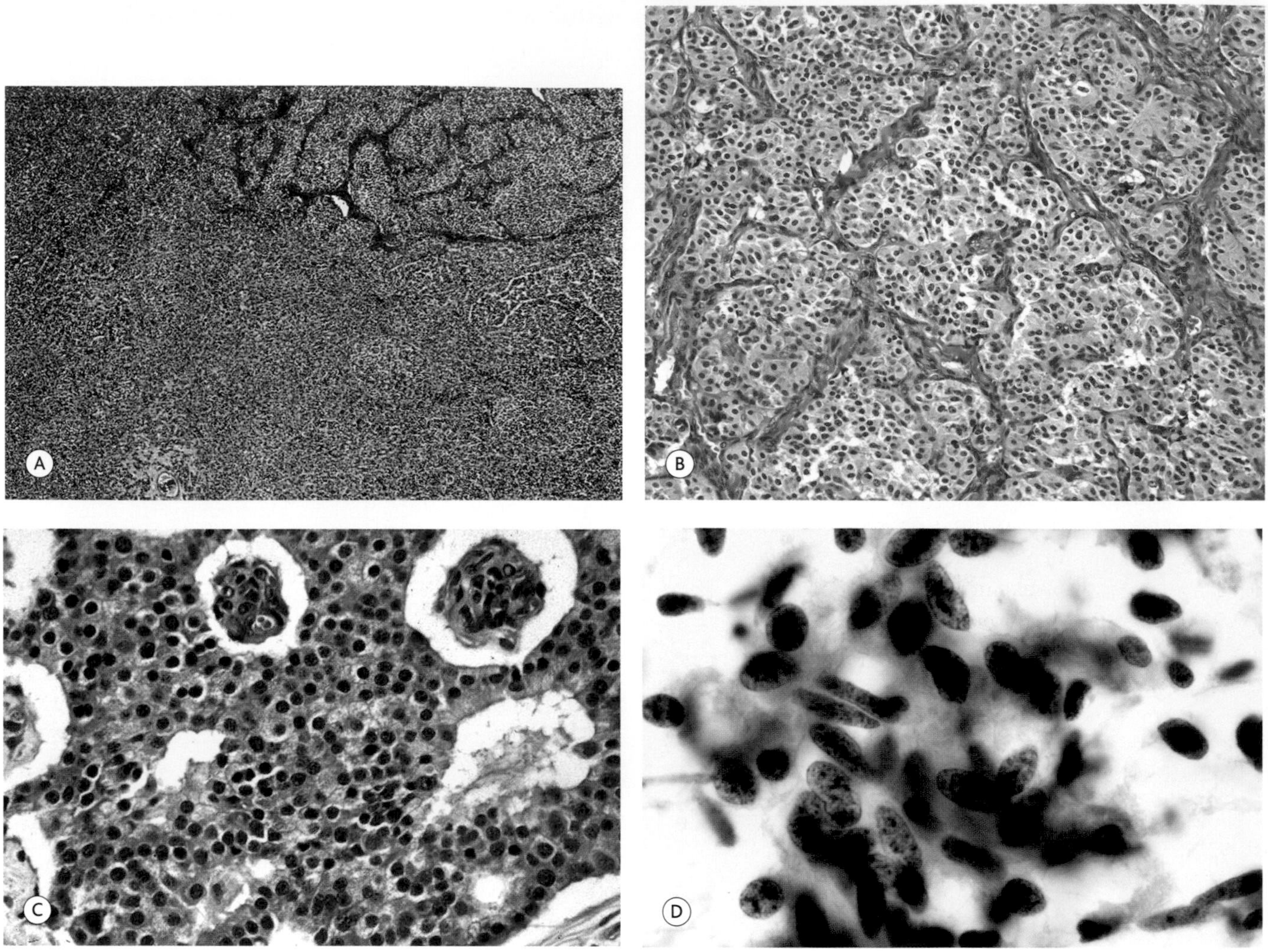

Fig. 13.14 Grade I neuroendocrine carcinoma (classical carcinoid) may assume several growth patterns, including (A) mixed medullary-insular, (B) insular, (C) pseudoglandular, and (D) spindle cell (in a fine-needle aspiration biopsy specimen).

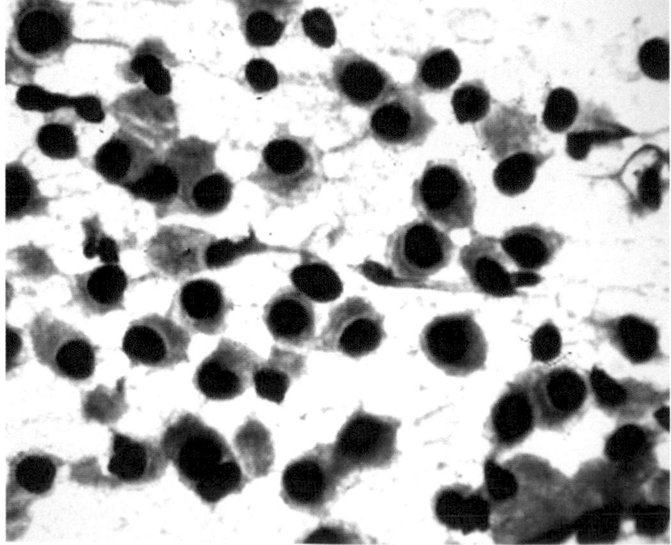

Fig. 13.15 Fine-needle aspirates of low-grade neuroendocrine carcinomas may show dyshesive cells with plasmacytoid configurations, causing potential confusion with hematopoietic proliferations.

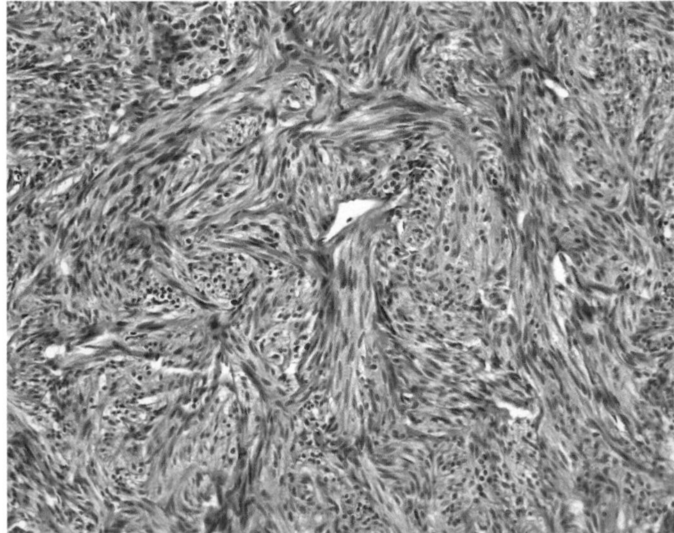

Fig. 13.16 Spindle cell growth in a peripheral low-grade neuroendocrine carcinoma of the lung.

them to be diffusely reactive for keratin, chromogranin-A, synaptophysin, and CD57,[4,156] whereas none of the other diagnostic alternatives show that immunophenotypic profile. The p53 gene, as studied by immunohistochemical or genetic analysis, is infrequently mutated in grade I NEC,[158] as opposed to higher-grade neuroendocrine tumors.[159]

Spindle cell growth in grade I NECs raises a dissimilar set of differential diagnostic considerations. These include fibrous and smooth muscle neoplasms, fibrous pseudotumors, primary or metastatic spindle cell melanomas, and metastatic medullary thyroid carcinomas. Careful attention to nuclear detail in spindle cell carcinoids shows a retention of the typical stippled chromatin pattern, and nucleoli are small and inconspicuous. The lesions also express the majority of immunohistologic markers seen in central carcinoids, as detailed above. A combination of morphologic and adjunctive studies should be capable of excluding most of the differential diagnostic considerations mentioned above, but metastatic medullary thyroid carcinoma is virtually indistinguishable from grade I pulmonary NEC on pathologic grounds.[148]

A similar issue is the separation of tumorlets (Fig. 13.17) from peripheral carcinoids. This is an arbitrary distinction, because immunohistochemical and ultrastructural studies indicate that the cells of these two lesions are essentially identical.[160–162] Also, there is debate over whether tumorlets represent true neoplasms, or are instead hyperplasias of respiratory neuroendocrine cells.[15,161,163] They generally occur within and around small bronchioles, and typically have a spindle cell composition. Although such tumorlets, which may number in the hundreds in some cases, are said to occur most often in diseased lungs with such associated lesions as bronchiectasis or pulmonary fibrosis,[160–164] they also may arise in otherwise normal lungs.[162] In any event, an arbitrary size of 4 mm or less has been suggested for tumorlets; larger lesions are considered to be peripheral carcinoids.[161] A continuum for such proliferations was suggested by Miller and Muller,[165] who found that peripheral carcinoid tumors were often associated with diffuse neuroendocrine cell hyperplasia and airway obstruction. A particular pitfall associated with tumorlets is that they may be misdiagnosed as much more aggressive lesions in small biopsy specimens, especially when clinical data are ignored or unavailable.[166,167]

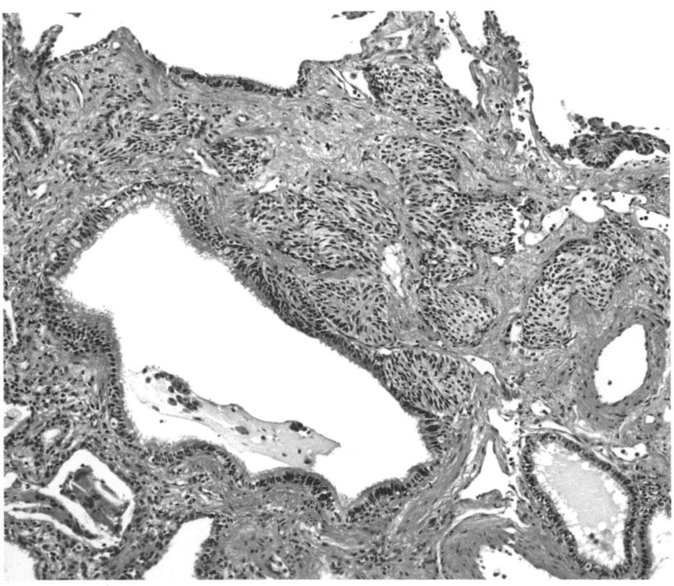

Fig. 13.17 This neuroendocrine tumorlet (NT) has the same architectural and cytologic features as those of low-grade neuroendocrine carcinoma of the lung; however, NTs are microscopic in scope and are associated with chronic lung disease, unlike their neoplastic counterpart.

Treatment and outcome

The clinical outcome in cases of central grade I NECs of the lung is generally excellent.[5,11,45] Complete excision is the treatment of choice, possibly necessitating lobectomy or sleeve resection.[168] Conservative endobronchial excision is generally associated with an unacceptable rate of local recurrence.[168–171]

It should be emphasized that a peripheral location or a spindle cell growth pattern do not, in and of themselves, equate with "atypical" morphology in grade I NECs of the lung. The prognosis for low-grade spindle cell peripheral lesions is equivalent to that of their central relatives, despite a slightly higher rate of lymph node metastasis in some series.[45,137,138]

Figures for the incidence of metastasis differ widely, and depend on two major variables. These include the definition of peribronchial lymph node metastasis (i.e. direct invasion of nodes versus embolic metastatic involvement) and histologic purity of the primary lesion. Some studies with high rates of metastasis for classic "carcinoid" have improperly included higher-grade neuroendocrine lesions. Quoted metastatic rates vary from 1 to 20%; a figure of ~5–10% is probably closest to the actual incidence, and most secondary implants involve adjacent peribronchial or hilar lymph nodes.[5,170–172] It is this behavioral attribute that leads us, as well as others, to consider central pulmonary carcinoids as irrefutable carcinomas.[131] Distant metastases may also occur rarely, and there is a tendency for spread to the bones, liver, skin, or brain.[45,171,172] Interestingly, osseous metastases are typically blastic.[173] Flow cytometric measurement of DNA content in grade I NECs is not helpful in predicting metastatic potential.[135,174]

The overall survival of patients with grade I NEC of the lung is in excess of 90–95% at 5 years.[5,45,134,170–172] Metastatic disease may be palliated using interleukin or somatostatin analogues,[38,175] and surgical excision of secondary implants can also be considered, given the slow growth of this tumor type.

Grade II neuroendocrine carcinoma ("atypical carcinoid")

The term "atypical carcinoid" was first used by Arrigoni et al. in 1972.[176] Those authors reviewed 216 bronchial carcinoids seen at the Mayo Clinic, and they found 23 with unusual features including pleomorphism, mitotic activity, nuclear hyperchromatism with increased nucleo-cytoplasmic ratios, and evidence of spontaneous necrosis or hemorrhage. In the original series, 70% of the lesions metastasized and 7 individuals (30%) died of their tumors. A diversity of terms has subsequently entered the literature on this lesion, including 'Kulschitzky cell carcinoma"[177] and "well-differentiated neuroendocrine carcinoma,"[12,15,172,177–184] and criteria for their definition are still being debated.[3,5,35,184a]

Clinical findings

"Atypical carcinoids" of the lung are usually >3 cm in maximum dimension. Other characteristics include an etiological link to cigarette smoking, differing from the epidemiological features of grade I NECs.[5,176–191] Grade II tumors are more likely to be peripherally located in the lung (Fig. 13.18) as compared with "classic" carcinoids; in fact, the former lesions have been so situated in the majority of cases in several studies.[176–191] Potential associations with Cushing's syndrome[191a] and the Eaton–Lambert syndrome[191b] also apply to these lesions.

Pathologic findings

With the exception of the possible gross identification of hemorrhage or necrosis, and a tendency to be slightly larger, the lesions were difficult, if not impossible, to distinguish from typical carcinoids by clinical, radiographic, or gross pathologic evaluation (Fig. 13.19). The pathologic requirements for a diagnosis of "atypical carcinoid" have varied from study to study, but most have included mitotic activity and necrosis. We currently utilize the criteria of El Naggar et al.[135] to define grade II neuroendocrine carcinoma of the lung (Fig. 13.20), preferring that term to "atypical carcinoid" but stipulating that the two are conceptually synonymous. Those requirements center on the following points:

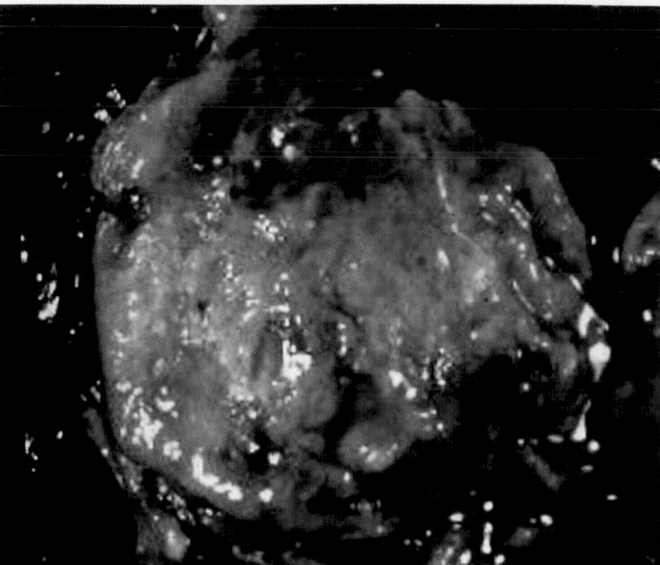

Fig. 13.18 Grade II neuroendocrine carcinoma (atypical carcinoid) is usually peripherally located in the lung parenchyma, and may contain areas of hemorrhage or necrosis, as seen in this gross photograph.

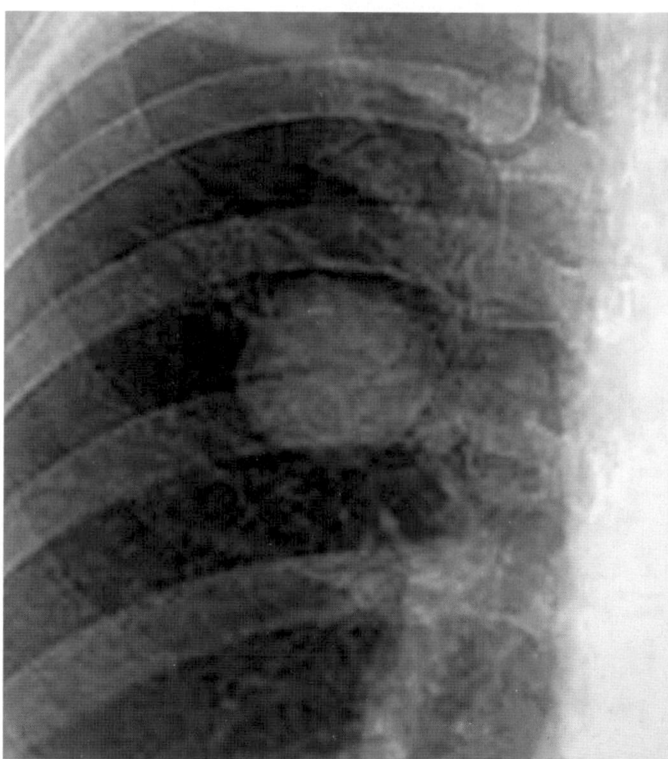

Fig. 13.19 Chest radiography of grade II neuroendocrine carcinomas of the lung (atypical carcinoids) shows features that are essentially identical to those associated with grade I tumors.

- mitotic rate of 5 or more division figures per 10 high power (×400) fields
- discernible nuclear pleomorphism
- at least focal necrosis; and
- at least focal loss of an organoid growth pattern.

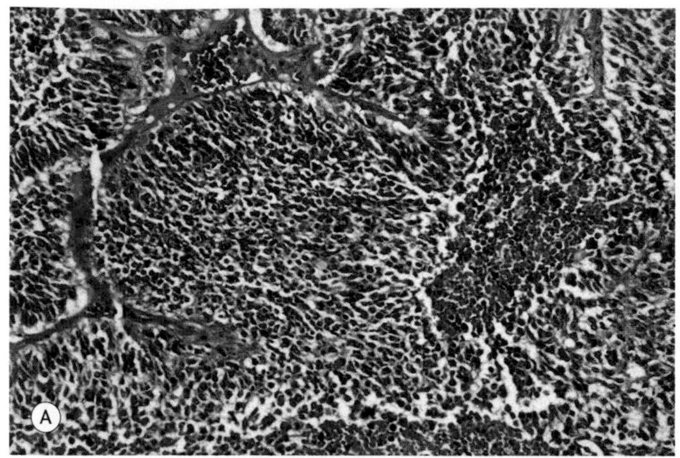

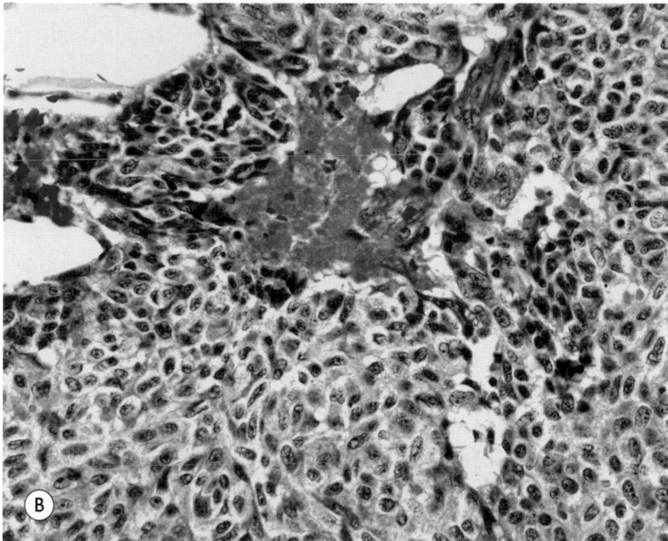

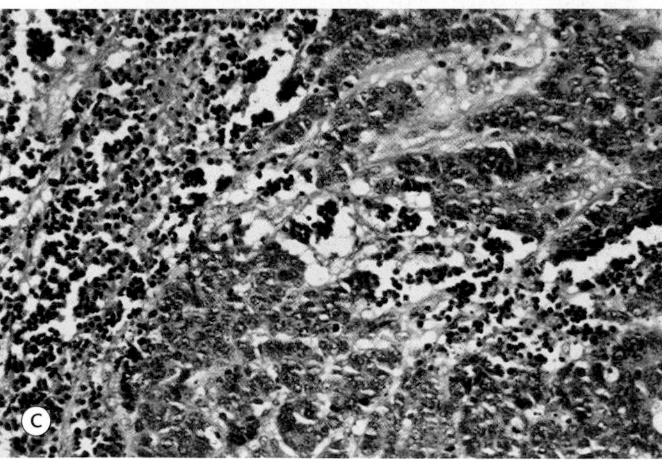

Fig. 13.20 (A–C) Grade II neuroendocrine carcinomas exhibit organoid growth patterns but show notable mitotic activity and areas of spontaneous necrosis, unlike grade I tumors.

Spindle cell change in grade II NECs of the lung is potentially seen but rather uncommon.[190] As observed by Yousem and colleagues,[3,192] a requirement for *at least two* of these criteria is more reasonable than basing the diagnosis of grade II NEC on only one feature, in a lesion that is otherwise a classic carcinoid of the lung.

Immunohistochemical studies reveal some differences between grade I NEC and grade II NEC of the lung. As expected of more poorly differentiated tumors, "atypical carcinoids" tend to express fewer markers of neuroendocrine differentiation or to demonstrate more focal labeling for them; such markers as synaptophysin, chromogranin-A, and CD57 are usually less impressive in grade II lesions.[91,116,119,193,194] Reactivity for specific neuropeptides – e.g. bombesin, calcitonin, adrenocorticotropic hormone (ACTH) – is relatively uncommon.[195] Mutant p53 protein is demonstrable by immunostaining in some atypical carcinoids, as opposed to its absence in the great majority of typical carcinoids but in likeness to its presence in most small cell carcinomas.[158,196,197]

Ultrastructural analysis of grade II NEC shows fewer neurosecretory granules as compared to grade I neuroendocrine neoplasms.[182] Cytogenetic analysis also has demonstrated multiple karyotypic abnormalities in grade II NEC but not in classic carcinoid,[198–201] paralleling the flow cytometric incidences of aneuploidy in the two tumor types.[135,192,202]

Differential diagnosis

Aside from its separation from other neuroendocrine lesions, the differential diagnosis of grade II NEC also includes poorly differentiated non-neuroendocrine carcinomas of the lung.[44,50,53,185] In particular, selected examples of high-grade adenocarcinoma may simulate the microscopic configuration of "atypical carcinoids," and "basaloid carcinoma" (basaloid squamous cell carcinoma)[202a] is *regularly* confused with grade II NEC. The nuclear characteristics of those lesions differ from one another, in that non-neuroendocrine tumors do not manifest the dispersed chromatin seen in "atypical carcinoids," instead showing more vesicular nuclei with often-prominent nucleoli (Fig. 13.21). Immunohistochemical studies *may* assist with differential diagnosis in this context, but, because some grade II NECs lack reactivity for endocrine markers, and, conversely, selected non-neuroendocrine carcinomas of the lung *do* demonstrate their presence, this technique is problematic. Electron microscopy is still probably the surest technique for separating grade II NEC from its non-neuroendocrine diagnostic simulators.

Treatment and clinical outcome

A vexing problem is which diagnostic label to assign a neuroendocrine pulmonary tumor with only one indicator of potentially aggressive behavior, such as angiolymphatic

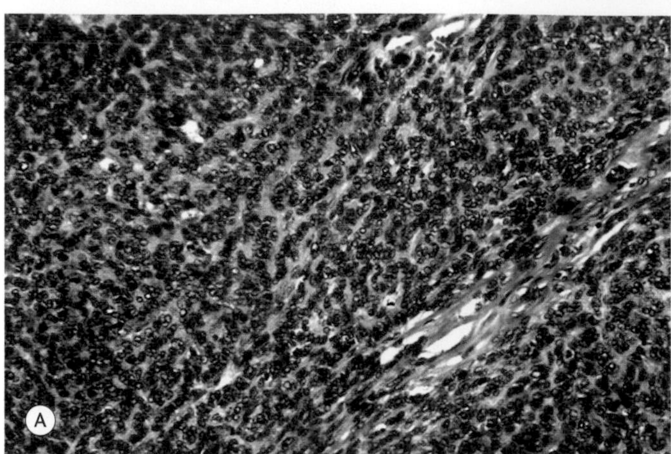

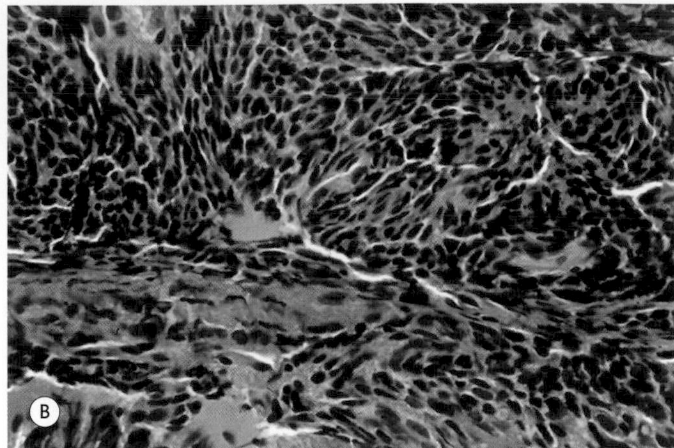

Fig. 13.21 Basaloid squamous carcinoma of the lung is also composed of polygonal (A) and spindle-shaped (B) tumor cells, potentially like those of neuroendocrine carcinomas, but the former tumors have more vesicular nuclear chromatin and prominent nucleoli. Their immunophenotypes also lack positivity for endocrine markers, and no neurosecretory granules are present on electron microscopy.

invasion, brisk mitotic activity, aneuploidy, or large size. None of these features independently appears to warrant adjuvant therapy, but it is probably prudent to suggest that they *may* be associated with an adverse outcome and that the patient be carefully monitored for recurrence. Special techniques may provide some additional information. In a flow cytometric analysis by El Naggar and colleagues, approximately 80% of 'atypical carcinoids' were aneuploid, whereas 80% of classical carcinoids were diploid.[135] Also, grade II lesions were more likely to have an S-phase fraction greater than 7%. Both of these factors were statistically linked to a worse outcome. However, in that analysis, the most significant predictor was accurate morphologic separation into grade I and grade II categories. Rush et al.,[181] Jackson-York & coworkers,[202] and Travis et al.[203] have concluded that accurate classification of these tumors is more important in prognosis than DNA content. Other factors said to significantly decrease survival in cases of "atypical carcinoid" include the presence of lymph node metastases, vascular invasion, and overall tumor size > 3 cm.[5,134,176–191,203]

Lymph node metastases are found at the time of diagnosis in 30–50% of cases, and roughly 25% of patients with grade II NEC of the lung will have remote metastatic disease at presentation.[5,190,191,204] As in cases of small cell neuroendocrine carcinoma, the brain is a common site for metastasis and recurrence. Importantly, the mortality from this neoplasm is in the range 30–50% at 2 years.[5,134,176–191] Rush et al.[181] have reported 5- and 10-year survival of 60 and 40%. Obviously, these figures reflect a different biologic potential than those of classic carcinoid on the one hand, and small cell carcinoma on the other. The use of adjunctive therapy in the management of grade II NEC of the lung is still an unsettled issue.[205,205a] Some researchers have suggested that chemotherapy or irradiation or both are beneficial in this setting, but there has been no consensus on that point. The difficulty in securing diagnostically "pure" study populations for treatment evaluations has likely contributed to this uncertainty concerning therapeutic recommendations.

Grade III neuroendocrine carcinoma, small cell type

Small cell carcinoma is probably the best-recognized neuroendocrine neoplasm in this discussion, accounting for about 25% of all lung carcinomas.[32] That diagnostic entity is generally traced to Barnard's description in 1926 of "oat cell carcinoma";[206] although the tumor had been felt to be a lymphoma or sarcoma prior to that time, he accurately recognized its epithelial nature. In 1959, Azzopardi refined the pathologic description of SCNC.[207]

Clinical features

Small cell neuroendocrine carcinoma of the lung has many potential modes of clinical presentation. These include symptoms and signs like those of other common carcinomas of the lung, such as cough, hemoptysis, weight loss, anorexia, fatigue, and the syndrome of hypertrophic osteoarthropathy.[208,209] In addition, however, unusual findings such as hyponatremia, hypercalcemia, or Cushing's syndrome may emanate from ectopic production by the tumor of antidiuretic hormone, parathyroid hormone-like peptides (PTHLPs), and ACTH, respectively.[141,145,208,210,211] Rarely, individuals with SCNC manifest the Eaton–Lambert (pseudomyasthenia)

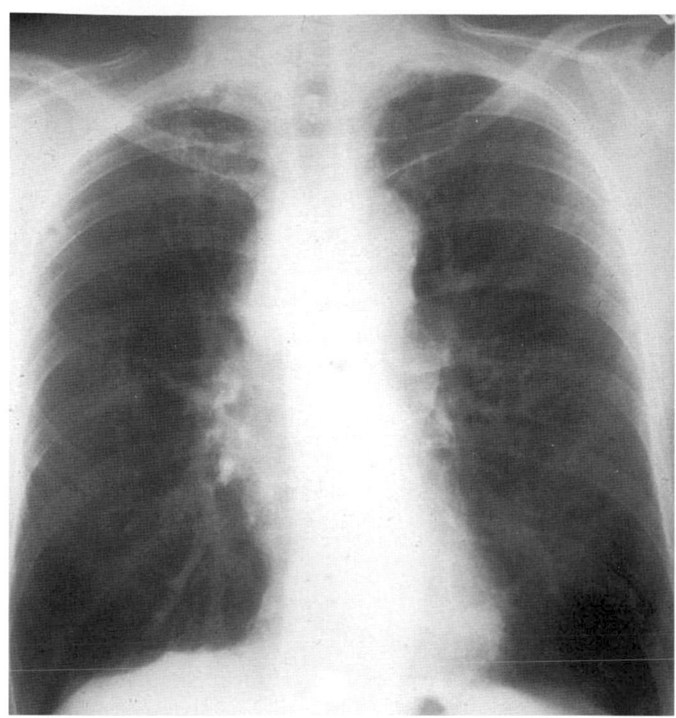

Fig. 13.22 Chest radiograph of small cell neuroendocrine carcinoma of the lung, showing a right hilar mass with mediastinal widening.

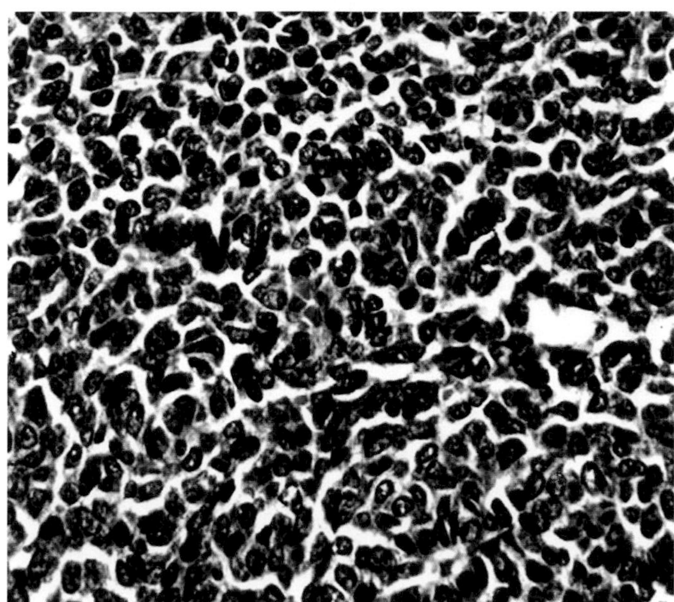

Fig. 13.23 "Oat cell" variant of small cell pulmonary neuroendocrine carcinoma, demonstrating angular, carrot-shaped nuclear profiles and hyperchromatic nuclei.

syndrome owing to paraneoplastic interference with neuromuscular function;[212,213] retinopathy, central and peripheral neuropathies, encephalitis, glomerulonephritis, cutaneous reactions, sarcoid-like granulomatous lesions, and systemic vasculitis also have been reported in this context.[213–220] Massive hepatomegaly with liver failure,[221] myelophthisic anemia,[222,223] or seizure activity and headaches[224] are additional clinical constellations that relate to the effects of distant visceral metastases at initial diagnosis.

Chest radiographic findings may be relatively unremarkable, or they may demonstrate the presence of a central hilar (or, more rarely, a peripheral intrapulmonary) mass (Fig. 13.22). Obstructive pneumonia is a potential complication; peribronchial or mediastinal lymphadenopathy is common and may be massive in scope.[147,208] Pleural effusions typically signify the presence of serosal metastases of SCNC, and rarely the tumor may so markedly involve the pleura that it produces a peripulmonary "rind" like that seen in association with mesotheliomas.[225]

Pathologic findinqs

The macroscopic features of SCNC are such that the tumor bears more resemblance to a lymphoma than to other carcinomas. The cut section of the lesion is typically uniformly gray-tan and fleshy, with possible small areas of necrosis or hemorrhage.

Microscopically, SCNC exhibits a spectrum of morphologic appearances.[207,226–235] Classical "oat cell" tumors are relatively rare, accounting for only 10–20% of cases.[226,227] Oat cell morphology (Fig. 13.23), with bluntly-fusiform, carrot-shaped cells, nuclear molding, and crush artifact, is more often seen in bronchial biopsies or fine-needle aspiration biopsies than in resected neoplasms or lymph node metastases. Tumor cell size is in the range of 1.5–3.0 times the diameter of non-neoplastic lymphocytes.[235] The so-called "intermediate cell" variant of SCNC (Fig. 13.24) accounts for approximately 75% of cases, and may be combined with oat cell areas.[228–231] Cell size in the former subtype is more variable, but may be as much as twice that seen in oat cell SCNC. Nuclear molding and crush artifact are less conspicuous; the tumor cells also may show small nucleoli, but they maintain the marked hyperchromatism and granular chromatin that are seen in other forms of SCNC. There may be blunt spindle cell change, and the cells may show pseudorosette formation, or grow in distinct ribbons. Other recognized types are those of combined small cell–large cell neuroendocrine carcinoma,[232,236,236a] and mixtures of SCNC with either adenocarcinoma or squamous carcinoma (Fig. 13.25).[27] All variations share the tendency to show prominent apoptosis, brisk mitotic activity, scant amphophilic cytoplasm, and the so-called "Azzopardi phenomenon," which is the accretion of basophilic nucleic acid around intratumoral blood vessels.[226,227] (Fig. 13.26).

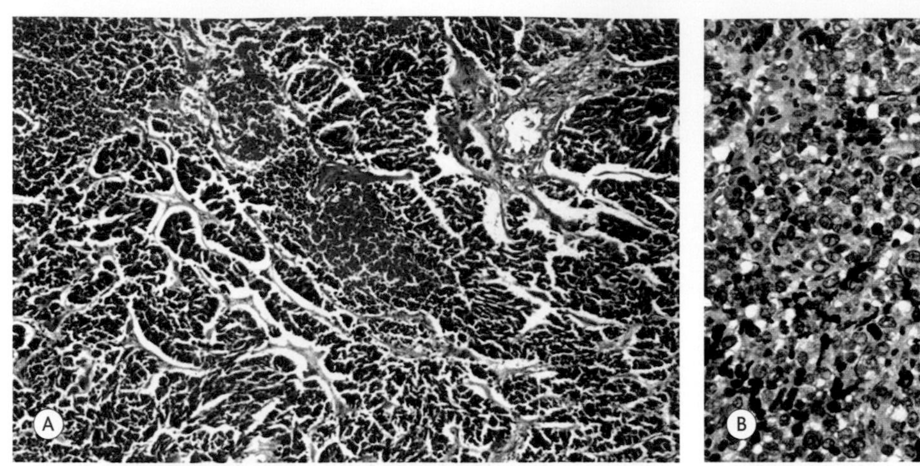

Fig. 13.24 "Intermediate" variant of grade III neuroendocrine carcinoma, small cell type. The tumor cells grow in a discernibly organoid fashion (A) and are more regular in shape and size (B) than those of the oat cell subtype. However, the distinction between histologic variants of small cell neuroendocrine carcinoma has no clinical importance.

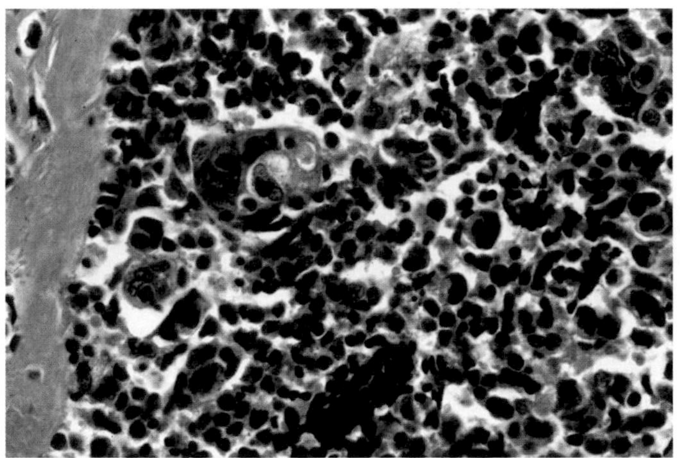

Fig. 13.25 Divergent glandular differentiation is apparent in this small cell neuroendocrine carcinoma (left upper central aspect of figure).

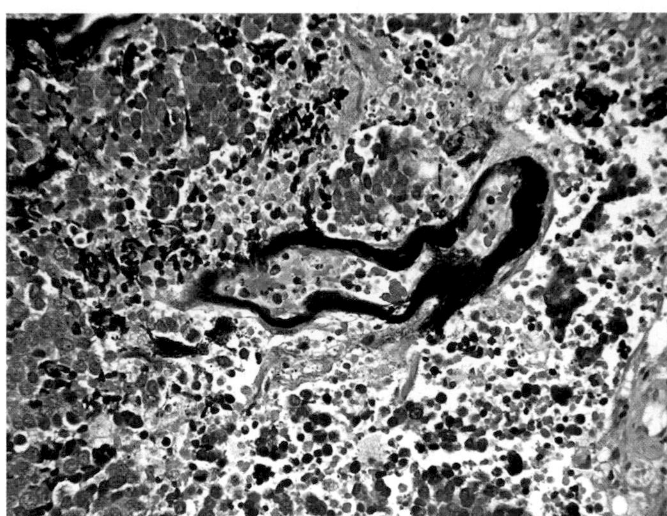

Fig. 13.26 The "Azzopardi phenomenon" is represented by accretion of densely basophilic, smudgy nucleic acid material adjacent to intratumoral blood vessels in small cell neuroendocrine carcinoma.

In our opinion, differences in cytomorphology in SCNC have little or no prognostic importance, based on a synthesis of the aggregated literature on this topic.[208,228-231,237,238] Instead, it is necessary to be familiar with the microscopic subtypes to avoid misdiagnosis. The presence of some variation in nuclear size, small nucleoli, and a modest amount of cytoplasm should not prevent one from making a diagnosis of small cell carcinoma, recognizing that these features are seen regularly in the intermediate variant of SCNC, especially in cytologic preparations.[236a] This is particularly true in fine-needle aspirate material.[234,238ab,239]

Another difficulty that one may face is the identification of SCNC in biopsies of peripheral lung nodules, as seen in approximately 10% of cases.[240] In that setting, the fear among many pathologists is that the lesion may in fact represent a lower-grade neuroendocrine lesion. This difficulty is best resolved by close attention to cytologic details. Marked nuclear hyperchromatism, brisk apoptosis, and scanty cytoplasm usually allow one to comfortably exclude a lower-grade lesion. Secondly, and more importantly, evidence has emerged which suggests that surgical therapy is indeed appropriate for peripheral high-grade but low-stage NECs of the lung.[240–246] As stated earlier in this discussion, rigid adherence to the dogma of "surgery for non-small cell carcinoma; no surgery for small cell carcinoma" is probably improperly restrictive. Smit et al. studied 20 patients with resected small cell carcinoma of stages I, II, and III.[243] The median survival in that series was 29 months for stage I and II tumors, and 20 months for stage III lesions. Another review of this topic has also been published by Mentzer and colleagues.[242] Whether surgery should precede or follow chemotherapy, or be accompanied by irradiation, are other contextual topics of debate.[208,247,248] Nonetheless, we believe that sufficient data are now available to suggest that all low-stage NECs of the lung should be resected, *regardless of grade.*

Yet another conundrum in fine-needle aspirates, limited biopsies, or frozen sections is the distinction between SCNC and high-grade large cell NEC of the lung;[248ab] indeed, the two forms of grade III may coexist in the same tumor mass, yielding the neoplastic variant known as "combined small cell carcinoma."[235,236,236a,248c] In light of comments in the preceding paragraph, it should be apparent that the separation of these two forms of high-grade NEC has dubious significance, in our opinion, with regard to the suitability of surgical management. Use of the designation "high-grade neuroendocrine carcinoma" is an equitable solution to the problem at hand; whether or not the lesion is then excised should be decided by the clinical stage rather than by cytologic details.

Differential diagnosis

The diagnosis of SCNC in biopsy material involves the exclusion of lymphoid infiltrates as well as other types of carcinoma that may be composed of small basaloid cells.[226,227,249,249a] As stated previously, broadly reactive keratin antibody mixtures label essentially all SCNCs, in many cases with a characteristic dot-like pattern of cytoplasmic staining. Hence, a simple two-antibody panel to cytokeratin and CD45 is effective in showing that a morphologically indeterminate small cell tumor is epithelial.[55] Extremely rare reports of apparent CD45 reactivity in SCNC[250] underscore the inadvisability of relying on only one immunostain diagnostically. In our experience, a more difficult question is the exclusion of basaloid squamous cell carcinoma, particularly in a small biopsy.[202a] The keratin labeling pattern described above may be helpful, and an extended panel of antibodies to chromogranin-A, NCAM, synaptophysin (Fig. 13.27), and CD57 can be applied as well. The latter will identify approximately 80% of all SCNCs.[55,193] Incidentally, we do not subscribe to the premise that there are "small cell neuroendocrine" and "small cell 'undifferentiated' carcinomas," but rather believe that some poorly differentiated tumors simply fail to express overt neuroendocrine differentiation to a degree detectable by our current methods.[55,251] Again, one should keep in mind the fact that clinical stage is the best determinant of whether surgery is advisable, and, in that framework, it becomes less crucial to separate SCNC from basaloid squamous carcinoma in biopsy specimens.

Treatment and clinical outcome

Over the years, SCNC has emerged as a clinically distinctive entity. As virtually all physicians are aware, long-term survival of patients with this neoplasm is rare; it is seen in less than 5% of cases in most centers,[205a,208,247,248,251ab] with rare exceptions.[251c] A staging system centered on the terms "limited" and "extensive" small cell carcinoma has now been supplanted by American Joint Committee on Cancer (AJCC) staging, in which stage I, II, and III correspond to the old "limited" stages, and "extensive" disease is stage IV.[208] Staging is a powerful parameter, and virtually the only reliable indicator of clinical outcome for pulmonary SCNC. Indeed, as we have stated repeatedly above, low-stage tumors are potentially resectable;[240–246] chemotherapy with or without irradiation can be given postoperatively as "consolidation" treatment.[208]

Naturally, many factors have been investigated as possible prognostic indicators in small cell carcinoma. As stated above, we do not believe that cytologic subdivision into "oat cell" and "intermediate cell" SCNC is prognostically contributory, despite the claims of some other authors.[238] *Mixed* SCNC (SCNC admixed with squamous carcinoma, adenocarcinoma, etc.) and *combined* SCNC (SCNC admixed with large cell neuroendocrine carcinoma) do, however, appear to be more refractory to therapy.[208] Vollmer et al. have suggested that an ultrastructural loss of desmosomes was associated with more aggressive behavior in SCNC, but that observation has not been the focus of practical application. DNA-ploidy

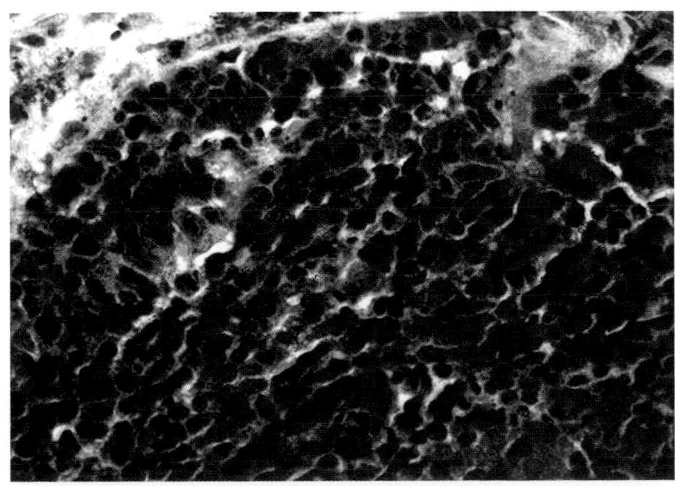

Fig. 13.27 Diffuse immunoreactivity for synaptophysin in grade III neuroendocrine carcinoma of the lung, small cell type.

analysis similarly does not seem to contribute significant information.[202] Numerous cytogenetic abnormalities are now reported in SCNC of the lung; one of the most common is a deletion of 3p,[253–256] suggesting that area may harbor potential tumor suppressor loci. Other abnormalities that have commonly been seen include deletions of 5q, 9p, 11p, 13q, and 17p.[256,257] Proto-oncogenes implicated include *c-myc, n-myc, myb, c-kit, c-src,* and *c-jun.*[254,256] At least two tumor suppressor genes – namely, p53 and the retinoblastoma gene – may play a role in SCNC carcinogenesis.[25,254,256] As mentioned in the discussion on grade I and grade II NECs of the lung, the p53 gene is more often mutated in small cell carcinoma than it is in lower-grade lesions. Other molecules, including p-glycoprotein (the multidrug resistance protein), CD99, and *bcl-2* protein have likewise been investigated as possible prognosticators.[254,256] Unfortunately, there is little practical information to be garnered from those studies at this time.

Grade III neuroendocrine carcinoma, large cell type (large cell neuroendocrine carcinoma)

The diagnosis of "large cell neuroendocrine carcinoma" (LCNC) is a relatively new addition to the nomenclature pertaining to pulmonary carcinomas. Travis et al.[203] proposed that this term be used for tumors that show morphologic features of neuroendocrine differentiation by light microscopy, but which do not fit into the categories of grade I NEC, grade II NEC, or SCNC. Thus, LCNCs are, by definition, different lesions than non-small cell lung cancers that demonstrate evidence of neuroendocrine differentiation *only* by immunohistochemical or ultrastructural studies;[26,34] those will be discussed subsequently in this chapter, under the rubric of "large cell carcinomas with 'occult' neuroendocrine differentiation." LCNC is also synonymous with neoplasms that have been called "intermediately differentiated neuroendocrine carcinoma" by Warren and co-workers.[12,54a] As we have already stated, we believe that use of the modifier "intermediate" for these cases is ill-chosen, because it introduces confusion with the "intermediate" cellular variant of SCNC. We prefer the term grade III NEC, large cell type, to refer to LCNC cases, for reasons that are specified below. Other authors have endorsed that usage.[256a]

Clinical features

The clinical attributes of LCNCs are hybrids of those attending adenocarcinoma of the lung and SCNC. In series by Travis et al.[5,203] and others,[205a,251ab,257,258,258a–c] LCNCs almost always occur in heavy smokers, as does small cell carcinoma. Symptoms and signs are generally most like those of non-neuroendocrine carcinoma; however, again in likeness to SCNC, examples of the Eaton–Lambert syndrome[259] and paraneoplastic retinopathy[260] also have been reported in connection with grade III large cell NEC. Although a minority of LCNC cases present as central masses, they tend to be situated in the mid-to-peripheral lung fields. Oddly, despite a high histologic grade, most LCNCs present as T1 or T2 tumors without lymph node metastases or evidence of systemic spread.[5,258]

Pathologic findings

Grossly, pulmonary grade III NEC of the large cell type varies in maximum dimension from 1 to >10 cm, and often demonstrates central necrosis, with or without dystrophic calcification.[5,257,258] Microscopically, it typically shows extensive coagulative necrosis that is obvious on low-power examination (Fig. 13.28). At slightly higher magnification, one often sees an insular or ribboning growth pattern in the tumor between the necrotic zones. The individual neoplastic cells are larger than those of grade II lesions, with moderate-to-abundant amphophilic cytoplasm. In some instances, tumor cells are granular and eosinophilic; Chetty et al. have reported rare examples with "rhabdoid" cytologic features, in which globular hyaline cytoplasmic inclusions were apparent in the tumor cells,[261] and Khalifa and colleagues documented an example of LCNC with divergent sarcomatoid (spindle cell) differentiation.[261a] Nuclei in LCNC are more pleomorphic than those of SCNC or grade II NEC;

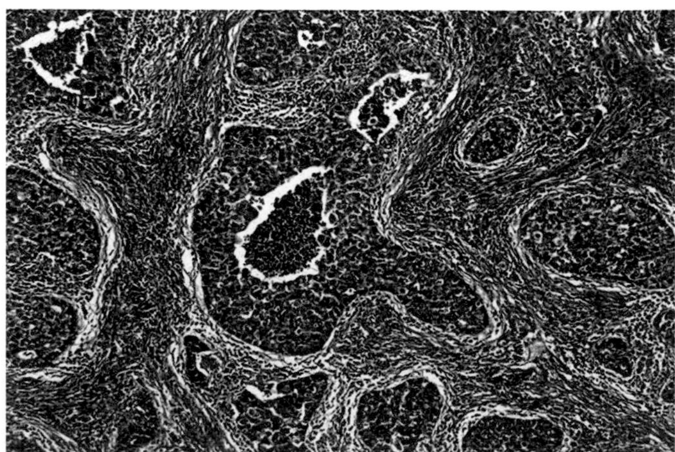

Fig. 13.28 Organoid growth with multiple foci of geographic necrosis, in high-grade pulmonary neuroendocrine carcinoma, large cell type (large cell neuroendocrine carcinoma).

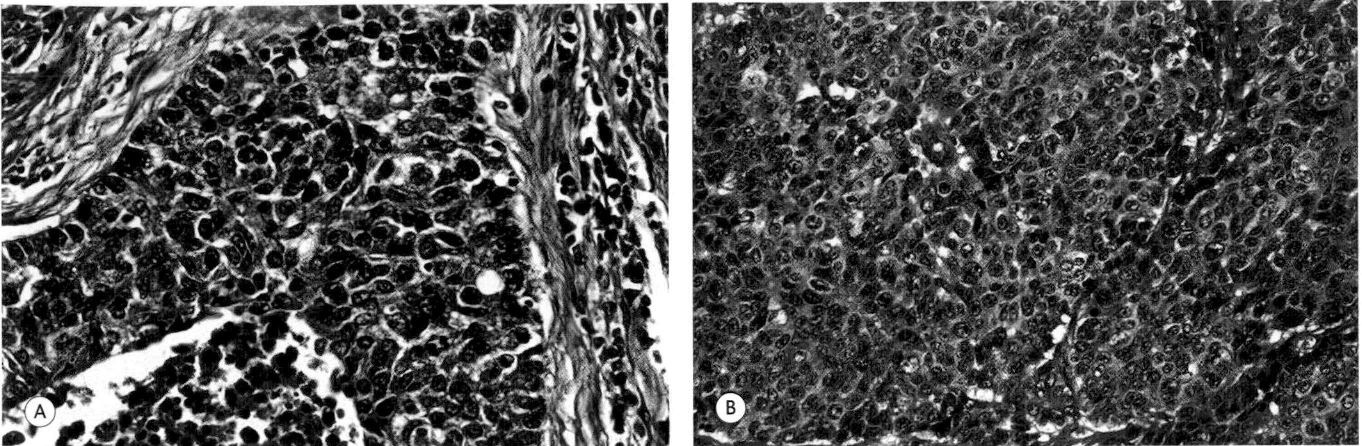

Fig. 13.29 Foci of geographic necrosis (A) and relatively prominent nucleoli (B) in large cell neuroendocrine carcinoma.

nucleoli are variable in prominence and nuclear chromatin is more heterogeneous as well, varying from granular to vesicular in nature (Fig. 13.29). The mitotic rate in LCNC is brisk, usually measuring in excess of 10 division figures per 10 high-power microscopic fields, and sometimes being in the range of 50–100.[5] All cases show reactivity for cytokeratin, and immunoreactivity is observed in *almost* all cases for at least one neuroendocrine marker.[5,257] Similarly, electron microscopy shows the presence of dense core granules in large cell grade III NEC.[5,203,258b]

Differential diagnosis

These lesions may be challenging to recognize correctly. In the past, examples of LCNC were probably assigned to one of three other diagnostic categories: namely, "atypical carcinoid"; "non-small cell carcinoma, not further specified"; or "large cell undifferentiated carcinoma." A distinction from grade II NEC can usually be made by attention to several features. First, the cells of LCNC tend to be larger, and there is more nuclear pleomorphism. Chromatin in "atypical carcinoid" tends to be granular and nucleoli are small;[261b] in contrast, the chromatin of LCNC is not uncommonly vesicular, and nucleoli are often prominent. Nucleocytoplasmic ratios in grade II tumors are actually higher than those of LCNCs. Necrosis in the latter tumor type is generally extensive and infarct-like, versus more punctate or limited confluent necrosis in grade II NEC. Mitotic activity is another key feature in this diagnostic comparison. As outlined by Travis and colleagues, LCNC has a high mitotic rate (>50/10 high-power fields); accordingly, those authors suggested that cases with >10 mitoses/10 high-power fields probably represent LCNC, whereas "atypical carcinoid" is more likely to show a figure of ≤10.[5,203,261b] However, we prefer to assess the *overall* microscopic configuration of the lesion in question in making that distinction, rather than relying on only one pathologic parameter. Despite that caveat, some examples of pulmonary neuroendocrine tumors are still encountered where it is virtually impossible to assign a label of grade II NEC versus LCNC with certainty.

Separation of LCNC from non-neuroendocrine non-small cell carcinomas depends primarily on the presence or absence of endocrine morphologic features, as enumerated above. As referenced earlier, we believe that the low-power appearance of grade III large cell NEC is one of the most helpful indicators of the proper diagnosis. Extensive zonal necrosis, producing a "jig-saw puzzle" pattern, is often visible. Prompted by this feature, which, of course, can be mimicked by the appearance of necrotic squamous cell carcinomas or poorly differentiated adenocarcinomas, one then examines the lesion for organoid growth and neuroendocrine nuclear features. In contrast to our discussion of SCNC, special techniques do play an often-important part in the diagnosis of LCNC of the lung. Ultrastructural studies are useful in demonstrating neurosecretory granules.[5,262] By immunohistochemical analysis, all cases of grade III large cell NEC should demonstrate keratin reactivity and many are carcino-embryonic antigen-positive as well.[5,203,257] Virtually all LCNCs react with antibodies to NSE; of more specific markers, chromogranin-A is the most consistently detected antigen. Antibodies to CD57 and synaptophysin stain fewer cases.

This discussion raises several points. First, given the vagaries of immunohistochemistry and neoplasia, one could predict that cases will be encountered with classic morphologic features of LCNC, but which will fail to demonstrate any "neuroendocrine" markers. Electron

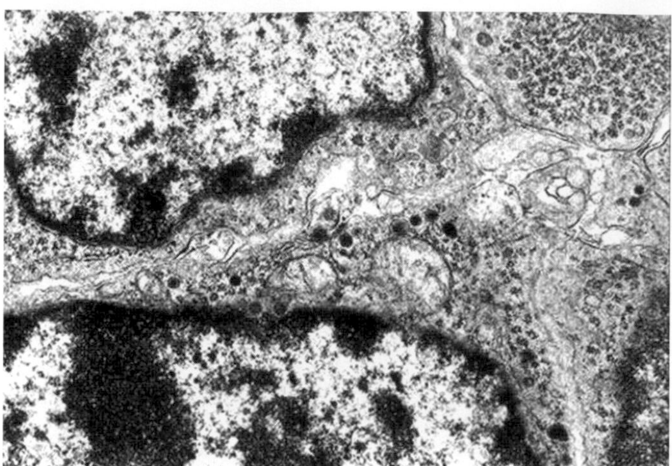

Fig. 13.30 Large cell grade III neuroendocrine carcinomas of the lung may require ultrastructural study to document their endocrine nature. This example shows the presence of scattered neurosecretory granules (center of figure).

microscopic examination is advisable in such cases (Fig. 13.30). It *is* probably necessary to provide some corroborating evidence of neuroendocrine differentiation before making an interpretation of LCNC, because some basaloid squamous cell carcinomas[202a] and other non-neuroendocrine large cell carcinomas may mimic LCNC in selected instances.[26,34] Conversely, however, if no light microscopic features exist to support the diagnosis of LCNC, immunostaining results and ultrastructural analysis should *not* be used to make the diagnosis. It has been well-documented that generic non-small cell lung neoplasms may contain cells with endocrine characteristics,[26,34] as will be considered subsequently.

Even though they are both forms of grade III NEC, LCNC and SCNC can usually be distinguished from one another readily in surgical material. The fact that they are, indeed, different tumor entities is supported by the observations of Ullmann et al., showing that dissimilar genotypes are present in LCNC and SCNC.[262a] The larger cell size, polygonal shape, lower nucleocytoplasmic ratios, nucleolation, and more irregular chromatin in LCNCs should make this separation a relatively straightforward one in most cases. Nevertheless, it must again be remembered that the two cytologic forms of high-grade NEC will occasionally coexist, in "combined small cell carcinomas."[35,235,236] Moreover, in cytologic material, the cited distinction between SCNC and LCNC is sometimes very challenging. Yang et al.[238a] have described three potential images of LCNC in fine-needle aspiration specimens, one of which closely simulates that of SCNC. The presence of prominent nucleoli is a helpful clue to the recognition of LCNC in that particular setting.[238ab]

Treatment and clinical outcome

The aggressive behavior of grade III large cell NECs of the lung cannot be overstated. Only 1 of 10 patients studied by Warren et al.[12] was alive at 2 years' follow-up, despite the fact that all of the cases were stage I (T1 or 2/N0/M0). All of the patients in series by Travis and colleagues[5,203] had either died of their tumors or were likely to do so at the same time point. Another report by Rush et al.[181] quoted respective 5- and 10-year survival rates of 33% and 11% for LCNC. Dresler and colleagues studied a series of 40 non-small cell neuroendocrine carcinomas, including 23 LCNC as defined here. The survival for stage I cases in that series was 18% at 40 months, representing a figure that was significantly worse than those attending similarly staged adenocarcinomas or squamous carcinomas.[258] Surprisingly, if one examines the survival of patients with resected low-stage SCNCs,[240–246] which are usually peripheral, the survival is better than that of individuals with LCNC. Likewise, the latter tumor type is more aggressive than "atypical carcinoid."[5,181,203,258]

Travis et al. and Rush and coworkers both performed flow cytometric DNA analysis on cases of grade III large cell NEC of the lung.[5,181] Both groups found no prognostic value in those studies.

The optimal therapy for these lesions is unsettled, in large part because there has been a frustrating tendency for both pathologists and clinicians to inappropriately push LCNC into generic non-small cell carcinoma treatment protocols rather than evaluating them as a separate tumor entity. Inasmuch as LCNCs tend to present as low-stage lesions,[258,258a–d] most can (and probably should) be surgically resected. However, there have been no randomized trials to address the value of postoperative chemotherapy or irradiation. Most patients with grade III large cell NEC appear to fail with either distant metastases or intrathoracic recurrence;[5,203,257,258] thus, both of those adjunctive treatment modalities would appear to have some intuitive merit. Anecdotal experience suggests that LCNCs respond unimpressively to standard chemotherapy regimens used for SCNC, and, with selected exceptions, tumors representing "combined small cell carcinomas" (SCNC/LCNC in the same tumor mass) have also had a poor response to such treatment.[35,208,235,236] In that regard, it is intriguing that expression of the multidrug resistance protein seems to be relatively common in grade III large cell NECs.[263] In summary, definitive recommendations for therapy in LCNC cases must await prospective studies of that topic.

Composite (mixed) neuroendocrine/ non-neuroendocrine carcinomas

The concept of overtly "mixed" or "divergent" differentiation has been recognized increasingly in the past few years, using conventional light microscopy.[27,264] Although this pattern is, perhaps, most frequently encountered in the gut and the lung,[230,264,265] composite epithelial tumors with a partial neuroendocrine phenotype have been observed in a wide variety of organ sites. The biologic significance of mixed neuroendocrine differentiation is still being studied, but it appears to depend on the location of the particular neoplasm being considered as well as the level of cytological anaplasia inherent in that tumor.[248c,264]

In specific reference to these neoplasms, a bewildering array of terms have been used to describe them, many of which are still in use. These include "stem cell carcinoma," "amphicrine carcinoma," "composite carcinoma (small cell carcinoma/adenocarcinoma or squamous cell carcinoma)," and "carcinoid with glandular differentiation."[264,266–277] Needless to say, many people are confused by this diverse lexicon, and they are accordingly uncertain as to how to treat the neoplasms in question. In our view, because mixtures of neuroendocrine carcinoma (with variable levels of differentiation, including high-grade tumors) and squamous cell carcinoma, adenocarcinoma, transitional carcinoma, or spindle cell carcinoma have been documented in malignant epithelial neoplasms of the lung, pancreas, stomach, duodenum, small bowel, colon, rectum, pancreas, liver, biliary tree, urinary bladder, prostate, uterine cervix and endometrium, ovaries, breast, skin, thyroid, salivary glands, and larynx,[51,266–277] it would seem most straightforward to use descriptive terminology diagnostically, such as "combined neuroendocrine carcinoma–adenocarcinoma" (Fig. 13.31) or "combined neuroendocrine carcinoma–squamous cell carcinoma," along with comments in surgical pathology reports that summarize the morphologic details and expected behavioral attributes of the lesion being studied.

Clinical findings

Virtually any carcinoma in the lung can potentially be found to have a neuroendocrine component, which can have the image of grade I, II, or III NEC. Hence, there are no specific clinical features that can be ascribed to "combined" neuroendocrine/non-neuroendocrine tumors. Nonetheless, it is of some interest that mixtures of squamous carcinoma or adenocarcinoma with NEC are most commonly seen in biopsies that are taken *after therapy*,[278] suggesting that effective treatment of the neuroendocrine cell population may allow for "overgrowth" of a theretofore minor non-endocrine component.

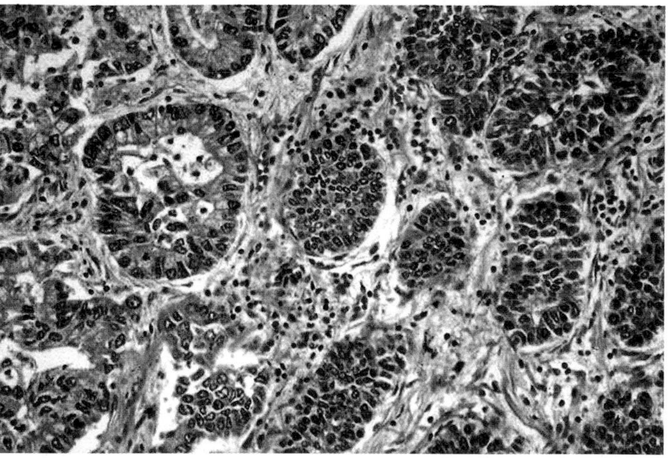

Fig. 13.31 Combined adenocarcinoma (left of figure) and grade II neuroendocrine carcinoma (right side of figure) of the lung.

Pathologic features

As opposed to poorly differentiated carcinomas in which neuroendocrine differentiation is "occult," and therefore discernible only by application of immunohistology or electron microscopy,[279] it is important to remember that those tumors considered in this section are recognizable as mixed by conventional microscopy. *All* of the neuroendocrine tumor types (i.e. grade I NEC; grade II NEC; small cell or large cell grade III NEC) that have been discussed up to this point may be components of combined carcinomas in the lung.

If one wishes to perform special studies out of interest, it should be expected that a spectrum of findings will be encountered. Some tumors will demonstrate truly bifid differentiation – exhibiting, for example, true glandular and neuroendocrine features in the same neoplastic cells[264,266] – whereas others will display admixtures of cellular elements with mutually exclusive ultrastructural or immunophenotypic properties. For practical purposes, these differences do not appear to have any meaning from mechanistic or clinical points of view. The latter comment also brings to mind discussions in the pertinent literature over whether divergent neuroendocrine lesions are "collision" tumors or not.[264] Given the fact that virtually *all* neoplasms derive from transformed stem cells, regardless of anatomic site, it would appear much more logical to conclude that divergent growth simply emanates from dissimilar (and largely unknown) post-transformational modulators of differentiation.[280,280a]

Differential diagnosis

Because of the unique histologic appearances of combined carcinomas with neuroendocrine elements, differential diagnostic considerations are limited. These generally concern making a distinction between poorly differentiated NEC components and high-grade portions of "pure" adenocarcinomas or squamous cell carcinomas with variable microscopic patterns that *simulate* neuroendocrine differentiation.[249] Ultrastructural and immunohistochemical markers of neuroendocrine differentiation should be pursued if that particular question exists.

Treatment and clinical outcome

Mixed neuroendocrine/non-neuroendocrine carcinomas generally have more adverse prognoses than those attending histologically "pure" tumors,[27,208,276] including lesions with grade I NEC components, which are very rare.[277] Thus, therapy must be chosen to address *all* of the cellular elements in these composite neoplasms, but with the expectation that response to treatment will likely be blunted and survival will be worse than that of patients with pathologically homogeneous lesions.

Non-small cell lung carcinomas with occult neuroendocrine differentiation

Beginning in the 1980s, several investigators have noted the presence of neuroendocrine features (e.g. neurosecretory granules; immunoreactivity for endocrine peptides) in lung tumors that otherwise had the microscopic appearances of poorly differentiated squamous cell carcinoma and adenocarcinoma, or large cell "undifferentiated" carcinoma.[26,279,281–288,288a–d] With those observations, controversies began over diagnostic terms that should be appended to such neoplasms, as well as their behavioral attributes.

The notion that there may be a variety of cell types in any given neoplasm has steadily gained recognition over the past decade. Tumors of the skin, genitourinary tract, gastrointestinal tract, lung, and many other sites all share this potential, which is best-termed "multidirectional differentiation."[264] "Occult" neuroendocrine lesions are no different than others with glandular or squamous differentiation in this context, in the sense that very poorly differentiated neoplasms may not show light microscopic patterns that indicate the presence of any of these cellular lineages.[289] Their "hidden" characteristics can only be detected by adjunctive pathologic techniques; as we have stated previously, that practical point of difference nosologically separates LCNC (which has microscopically overt neuroendocrine features) and "large cell carcinoma with occult neuroendocrine differentiation" (which does not).

Clinical findings

Pulmonary carcinomas with occult neuroendocrine differentiation (OND) are not substantially any different clinically than "pure" non-neuroendocrine malignancies of the lung, in reference to the symptoms and signs they produce. The only exceptional aspect of lung cancer with OND is the occasional example which demonstrates a paraneoplastic phenomenon that can be ascribed to production of an endocrine substance. For example, the authors have observed several examples of poorly differentiated adenocarcinoma of the lung associated with the watery diarrhea–hypokalemia syndrome, in which immunoreactivity for vasoactive intestinal polypeptide (VIP) was found in the tumor cells. Similarly, hypercalcemia or hypercortisolism may relate to ectopic production of PTHRPs or ACTH by such neoplasms.

Pathologic features

As stated above, pulmonary squamous cell carcinomas and adenocarcinomas with OND are no different macroscopically or histologically than their counterparts that lack any endocrine features.[279,282–284,290] In specific reference to large cell "anaplastic" carcinomas of the lung with OND,[26,34,281,287,288] the tumor cells are at least twice as large as those of SCNC. By definition, those lesions lack overt glandular or squamous differentiation, and have rather monomorphic nuclei with dispersed or vesicular chromatin and prominent nucleoli. Small foci of necrosis may be seen, but it lacks the infarct-like configuration of that seen in LCNC. Similarly, manifestations of organoid growth (e.g. insulae; ribbons; cords; rosettes) are absent in large cell carcinomas with OND. Still other tumors with occult neuroendocrine elements may show more unusual histologic patterns, such as sarcomatoid differentiation[241] or a blastomatous configuration (e.g. as in "well-differentiated adenocarcinoma simulating fetal lung").[291,292]

There is some debate over the "best" method to document OND in lung carcinomas.[58,293] Some observers argue that ultrastructure should be the standard technique,[58] but, as discussed earlier, sampling problems interfere with the reliability of that procedure. Putative nonspecificity of neuroendocrine determinants such as chromogranin and synaptophysin is not a problem in our view, because we believe that publications which raised such concerns[58] contained conceptual flaws. They were

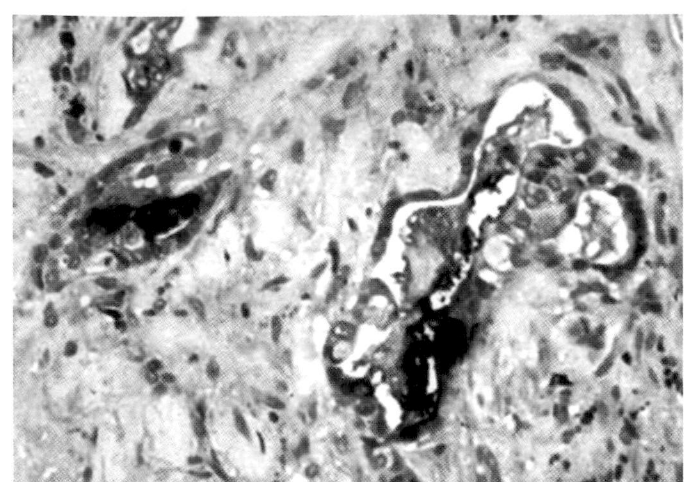

Fig. 13.32 "Occult" neuroendocrine differentiation in adenocarcinoma of the lung, manifested by immunoreactivity for chromogranin-A.

based on electron microscopy as the "validating" technology, ignoring the effects of sampling just cited. In our view, positivity for either of the two immunomarkers just cited (Fig. 13.32) does reliably predict the presence of neuroendocrine differentiation.

Differential diagnosis

The differential diagnosis of squamous cell carcinomas or adenocarcinomas with OND is principally with that of similar tumors which *lack* endocrine features. On the other hand, large cell carcinoma with OND must be distinguished both from large cell "undifferentiated" lung carcinoma and LCNC, primarily by electron microscopy and immunohistology.[34] In addition, large cell carcinomas may be sufficiently nebulous morphologically that metastatic melanoma, poorly differentiated sarcoma with epithelioid features, and large cell lymphoma also enter into diagnostic consideration. Again, adjunctive pathologic studies will usually be required to address those possibilities.[294]

Treatment and clinical outcome

The optimal therapy for pulmonary carcinomas with OND is still open to question. Some investigators have concluded that neuroendocrine differentiation justifies the use of therapeutic approaches like those employed in SCNC cases, whereas other authors have demurred on that point.[295–299] Similarly, there is no consensus on whether any prognostic value may be derived from the identification of "occult" neuroendocrine differentiation in lung cancers of various pathologic types, with contradictions in published studies on that point.[297–299] At the present time, all that can be said with confidence is that surgical excision is still the foundation of treatment in low-stage cases.[34,299]

Primary intrapulmonary paraganglioma

Paraganglioma (PG) is a distinctly uncommon lesion in the population at large,[300] and it is vanishingly rare as a primary pulmonary tumor, with less than 25 reported cases in the world literature.[301–310,310a] The demographic profiles of patients with this neoplasm are somewhat variable, depending on the topographic location of the lesion and its possible occurrence in genetic syndrome complexes.

Clinical features

In sporadic cases of PG in the lung and elsewhere, males predominate and usually come to diagnostic attention in middle life (between the ages of 40 and 50).[300–310] In contrast, females outnumber males in the context of the "type 2" multiple endocrine neoplasia (MEN) syndromes, and they are recognized as having a paraganglioma approximately 15 years earlier.[300] The latter of these observations may simply reflect the fact that family members in kindreds with MEN are usually regularly screened for constituent tumors from childhood onward.[311] Paragangliomas have been described in virtually all organ sites, including the orbits, nasal cavity, thyroid, heart, urinary bladder, gallbladder, liver, biliary system, kidneys, prostate, urethra, spermatic cord, uterus, ovaries, vagina, vulva, cauda equina, and lungs; primary pulmonary tumors are among the rarest.[300]

Functionality of PGs in these diverse locations is only sporadic. Biosynthetic tumors may present themselves with episodic or sustained hypertension; hypertensive crisis or "malignant hyperthermia" upon induction of general anesthesia; episodic nausea, weakness, cardiac arrhythmias, pallor, flushing, headache, diaphoresis, anxiety, or localized pain; or cardiovascular decompensation with heart failure. Reflections of neuropeptide production may include Cushing's syndrome with PGs that synthesize ACTH, or the watery diarrhea–hypokalemia complex (Verner–Morrison syndrome) with neoplasms that manufacture VIP. Occasional examples also have apparently produced a PTHRP, with associated hypercalcemia, or an erythropoietin-like moiety in linkage with paraneoplastic polycythemia. Finally, rare patients with PG and associated systemic abnormalities may have von Recklinghausen's disease (neurofibromatosis) or the Beckwith–Wiedemann syndrome (hemihypertrophy and macroglossia).[300]

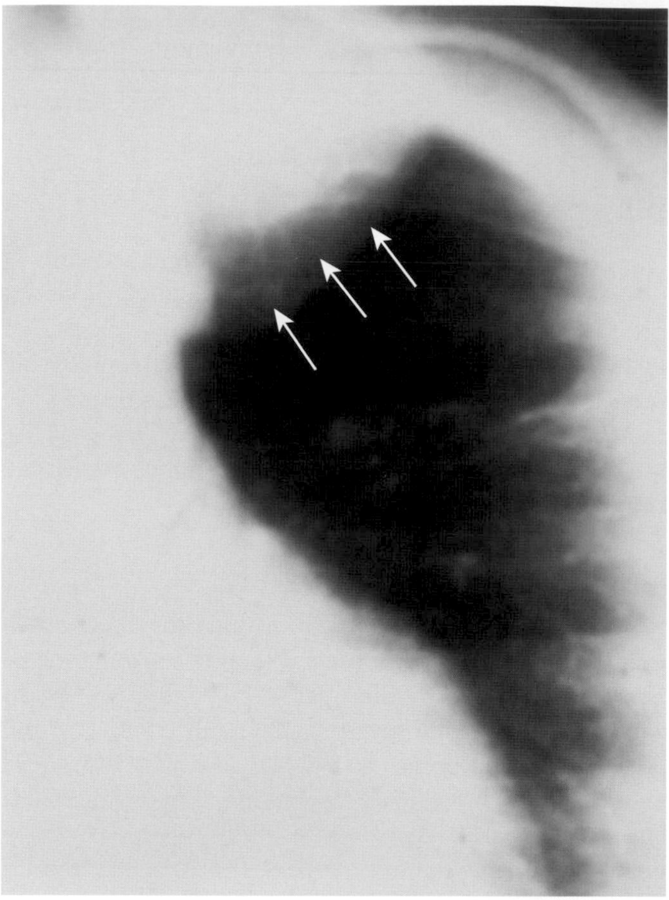

Fig. 13.33 Chest radiograph of intrapulmonary paraganglioma, represented by a left apical mass (arrows).

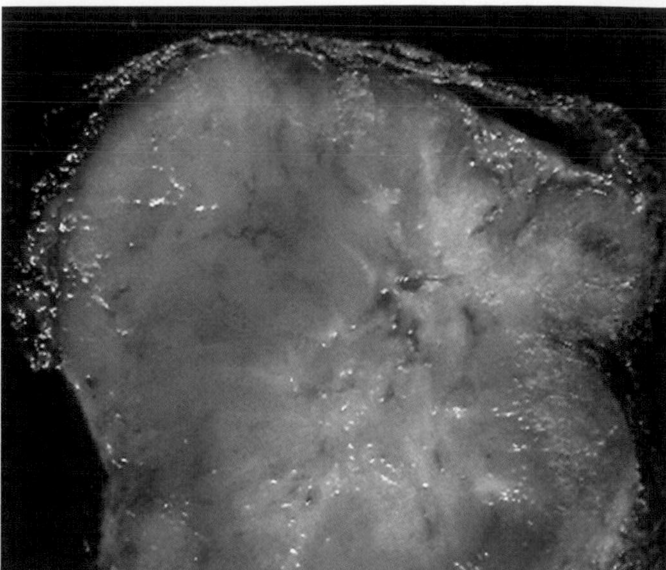

Fig. 13.34 Gross photograph of resected intrathoracic paraganglioma, showing a relatively nondescript reddish-yellow lobulated tumor.

Non-functional tumors become manifest only through the appearance of a steadily enlarging mass, with other symptoms and signs thereof being dependent upon the anatomic location of the lesion. In the lung, PGs that impinge on large airways produce complaints relating to obstruction (such as cough or stridor), but peripheral non-functional lesions are typically found incidentally on screening chest radiographs[301–310] (Fig. 13.33).

Pathologic features

Grossly, PGs are typically spherical or slightly lobulated masses that range from a few millimeters to several centimeters in greatest dimension. They may be either centrally or peripherally located in the lung. Their cut surfaces are bloody in most cases because of dense intralesional vascularity, and the tumor tissue itself may be gray, pink, lavender, brown, or mottled (Fig. 13.34). Characteristically, immersion of fresh tissue in Bouin's fixative or another picric acid-containing solution will cause the specimen to assume a brownish appearance. In general, PG is a circumscribed lesion with a partial or complete fibrous capsule; hence, the surgeon will report that the lesion was relatively easy to dissect from contiguous structures. However, approximately 10–20% of tumors demonstrate local infiltration of adjacent tissues,[300] and these may therefore be submitted to the surgical pathology laboratory in a fragmented state or with adherent structures attached to their peripheral aspects. An important step in the initial pathologic evaluation of PG is not only to do standard three-dimensional measurement of the lesion but also to *weigh* it after dissecting extraneous soft tissue that may be attached. Secondly, one should pay special attention to whether a PG appears to be multinodular or multifocal. This is because multicentricity of such neoplasms correlates well with a syndromic association.

The histopathologic characteristics of pulmonary PGs are also variable. The peculiar nesting configuration of the tumor cells, separated by prominent fibrovascular stromal septa (so-called zellballen) (Fig. 13.35) is actually poorly developed in many of these lesions. In the lung in particular, this feature leads to considerable difficulty in the separation of PG from carcinoid tumors (which, of course, are far more common). Aside from the organoid growth pattern of PGs, they are also marked by a tendency toward nuclear pleomorphism, the common presence of intranuclear "pseudoinclusions" (invaginations of cytoplasm), intercellular hyaline globules, accumulations of intercellular proteinaceous material resembling thyroid colloid, potential spindle cell or oncocytic change, and elements resembling ganglion cells[310a,312]

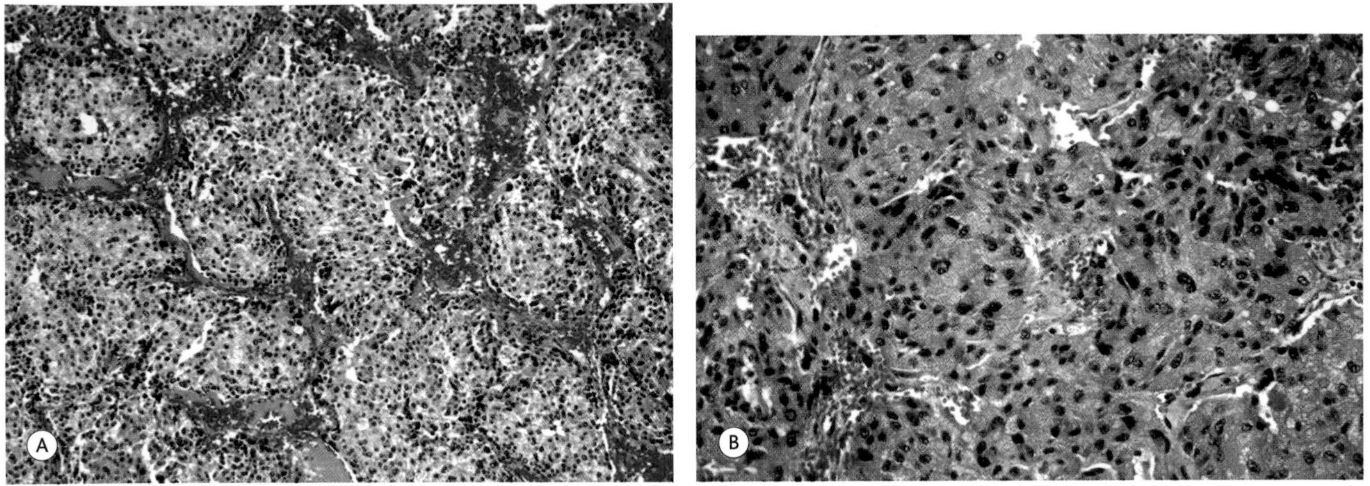

Fig. 13.35 The formation of distinct cell groups (zellballen) may be conspicuous (A) or relatively vague (B) in paraganglioma.

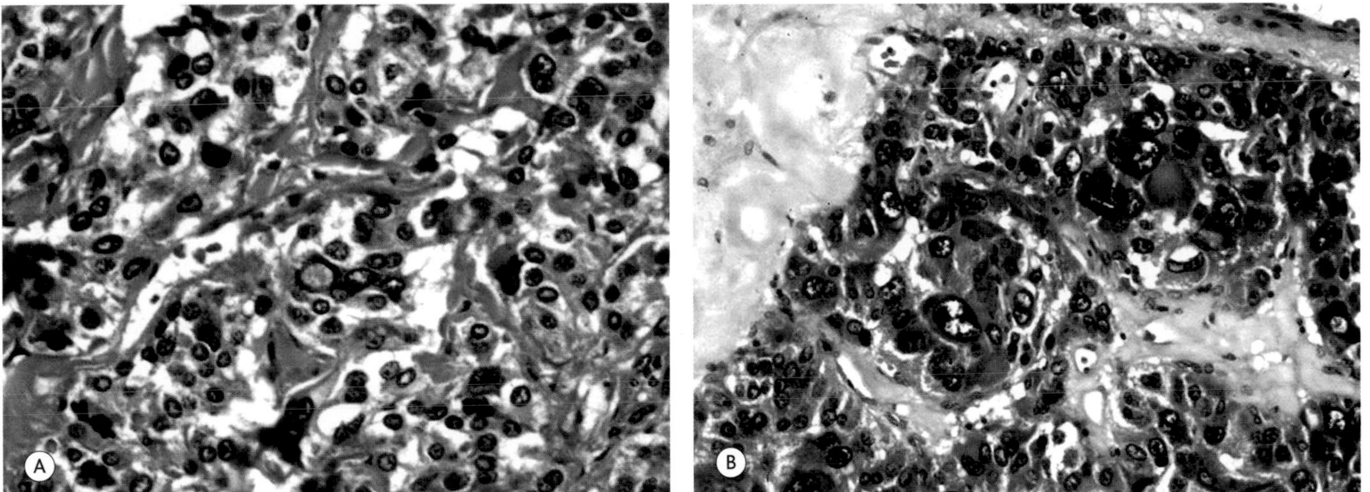

Fig. 13.36 Intranuclear pseudoinclusions (A) and nuclear pleomorphism with eosinophilic cytoplasmic inclusions (B) in paraganglioma.

(Fig. 13.36). Mitotic figures are seen in approximately 45% of benign PGs and 65% of malignant lesions, regardless of location; hence, they are not useful in and of themselves in predicting tumor behavior. Similarly, although vascular invasion is apparent in one-fifth of malignant PGs, it is also evident in 5–6% of benign tumors.[312] Thus, it should be apparent that requests for a definitive diagnosis of PG in the frozen section laboratory are impossible to satisfy, particularly in reference to pulmonary tumors.

Relatively few PGs have been subjected to fine-needle aspiration and cytologic assessment.[313–315] However, a report on this topic by Gonzalez-Campora et al.[314] showed that such tumors commonly exhibited marked anisokaryosis, a tendency to form acini or follicles, and intranuclear invaginations of cytoplasm like those seen in papillary thyroid carcinoma. Nuclear pleomorphism has not been correlated with adverse behavior; in fact, malignant PGs have tended to display *less* nuclear variability than did their benign counterparts.[312]

Differential diagnosis

Special studies are typically needed to bolster the histologic diagnosis of PG in visceral locations, especially in the lung. Other considerations in pulmonary cases center on neuroendocrine *carcinoma*, as well as metastatic malignant PG originating at another site. Electron microscopy is still a useful modality in this context, in that the neurosecretory granules of paraganglion cell tumors generally differ from those of other neuroendocrine cells and neoplasms.[300] They feature an unusual, "blister"-like configuration, where the internal submembranous "halos" of the granules are obviously eccentric and appear

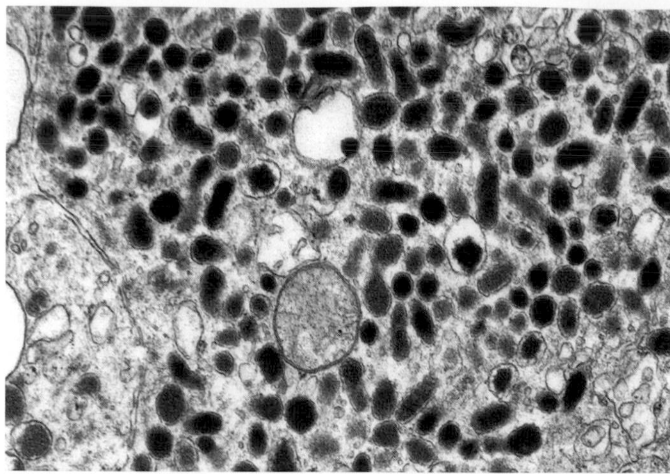

Fig. 13.37 Electron photomicrograph of paraganglioma showing irregularly placed dense cores in neurosecretory granules, giving some of them a "blister-like" image.

to emanate from the dense core in a bubble-like fashion (Fig. 13.37). Otherwise, the cells of PGs are similar to those of the dispersed neuroendocrine system, showing prominent Golgi complexes and rough endoplasmic reticulum, macular intercellular junctions, and only incomplete pericellular basal lamina.[316]

Immunohistologically, most examples of PG have a distinctive intermediate filament protein (IFP) profile that is not shared by other neoplasms except for neuroblastomas.[75,317] This features the presence of neurofilament protein, with or without vimentin, to the exclusion of other IFPs. It should be noted that neurofilament protein may be difficult to demonstrate in formalin-fixed, paraffin-embedded tissues, so that in practical terms, the majority of routinely processed PGs do not manifest *any* detectable IFP.[317] This observation is useful in making the distinction between PG (and other "type 2" [neural] neuroendocrine tumors) and "type 1" (epithelial) neoplasms that often are considered in differential diagnosis and which uniformly exhibit keratin positivity.[55] We have not found keratin proteins in PGs, in the lung or elsewhere. This is in stark contrast to the figure of 30% that has been cited by some authors for keratin positivity in PG,[65] and which we believe to be a reflection of procedural shortcomings. Occasional examples of PG may also show focal immunoreactivity for glial fibrillary acidic protein, but they uniformly lack desmin.[75] Virtually *all* PGs are diffusely and intensely positive for chromogranin-A and synaptophysin, whereas beta-tubulin and microtubule-associated protein are only focally seen in such lesions and are instead characteristic of neuroblastic and ganglioneuromatous neoplasms.[55,82,88,89] Other immunodeterminants that can be detected in PGs include ACTH (approximately 30%); VIP (40%); Leu- or Met-enkephalins (50–60%); calcitonin (<5%); CD57 (50%); and beta-endorphin (10%).[74,78,92]

A word is in order regarding "minute pulmonary chemodectoma" (MPC) as a differential diagnostic consideration in this context. That is necessary because "chemodectoma" is a term that was formerly used in reference to PG.[300] In fact, MPCs have no relationship to the paraganglion system whatsoever. They are small peripheral pulmonary parenchymal aggregations of polygonal or bluntly fusiform cells, often with a concentric configuration. Immunohistochemical studies of MPCs have demonstrated a similarity to meningothelial rather than neuroendocrine tissues, with reactivity for vimentin and epithelial membrane antigen.[320] Moreover, analyses of cellular clonality in such lesions have demonstrated that they are polyclonal and probably reactive in nature,[321] rather than neoplastic, as true of PGs.

One other recent development should be mentioned in reference to paragangliomas. It has now been shown conclusively that both familial (MEN2-related) and selected sporadic examples of this tumor demonstrate mutations in the *ret* gene.[311] These take the form of (Cys634–>Arg) in MEN2A and (Met918–>Thr) in MEN2B. Whether or not this information enters the diagnostic sphere in the near future must await further technical developments and clinical correlation.

Treatment and clinical outcome

The most contentious aspect of PGs is the prediction of their often-capricious behavior. In the lung, the great majority of primary paraganglionic tumors have been benign biologically, but occasional examples have metastasized to regional lymph nodes or other viscera.[301–310]

At one extreme, some authors such as Neville have stated that a diagnosis of malignant PG can only be made after metastasis has occurred; others have claimed that pathologic mitotic figures or vascular invasion;[312] lessened immunoreactivity for selected neuropeptides (particularly neuropeptide Y);[322] or loss of intratumoral S100 protein-positive sustentacular cells[129,323] could be correlated with aggressive behavior. These concepts are, admittedly, still in evolution. Some reports concerning the biology of PG have, however, provided additional useful information. Based on the results of logistical regression analyses, it would now appear certain that mitotic activity, nuclear atypia, and vascular or capsular invasion are of little or no use as individual parameters in the prognostication of PGs.[312] Similarly, Lack,[300] Linnoila and colleagues,[312] and Gonzalez-Campora et al.[324] all found no statistically significant association between static or flow cytometric DNA aneuploidy and behavior in paraganglion cell tumors, with only Pang and Tsao demurring on the latter point.[325] Multiparametric assessment of 16 non-microscopic and histologic features by Linnoila and associates showed that 4 of them were the most predictively useful.[312] These included an extra-adrenal location, coarse macroscopic nodularity of the tumor, confluent tumor necrosis on microscopic examination, and an absence of intercellular hyaline globules. Among 120 PGs in that series, 71% of the biologically malignant lesions showed 2 or 3 of the 4 specified features, whereas 89% of the benign tumors manifested 0 or 1 of them. Accordingly, there was a >95% probability that more than 70% of PGs could be correctly classified using this paradigm.[312] In our opinion, such an approach is, in fact, the recommended one. It can be used by any pathologist and does not require the availability of special equipment.

Primary primitive neuroectodermal tumors of the lung

Primitive neuroectodermal tumors (PNETs) are most commonly seen as primary soft tissue tumors. In the thorax, they typically affect the pleura and chest wall, and are known as "Askin's tumors." In the lung, only three examples of PNET have been well-documented as primary tumors by Imamura et al.[326] and Mikami et al.,[326a] and information on primary intrapulmonary lesions is accordingly only anecdotal. The neoplasms were seen in persons who were 17, 30, and 41 years of age, who presented with nodular intrapulmonary masses. Characteristic t(11;22) chromosomal translocations and expression of CD99 were observed in each neoplasm, and they lacked immunoreactivity for keratin, myogenic markers, and S100 protein. After surgical excision and appropriate chemotherapy, two of the patients were alive and free of disease after 16 and 22 months; the other was lost to follow-up.

Differential diagnosis is principally with SCNC – which should be uniformly keratin-positive[55] and lack t(11;22) – and *metastatic* PNET arising in other locations and involving the lung secondarily. Another possibility is that of small cell primary or metastatic pulmonary synovial sarcoma, which represents a particular interpretative trap because it shares potential immunoreactivity for CD99 with PNET.[326b] However, the cytogenetic profiles of those lesions are mutually exclusive; synovial sarcoma lacks t(11;22) and instead consistently exhibits a t(X;18) chromosomal translocation.

Primary neuroblastoma of the lung

Neuroblastoma (NB) continues to represent an important neoplasm in the sphere of pediatric oncology. It is the fourth most frequently encountered malignancy in children, behind leukemia, lymphoma, and aggressive central nervous system tumors.[300,327,328] The great majority of NBs (and congeners thereof) are encountered in the first decade of life, with no particular predilection for either sex and only rare cases in adults.[329,330] Paradoxically, however, the only examples of *primary intrapulmonary* NB that have thus far been reported have been in three patients over the age of 20 years.[331,332]

Clinical features

Generally speaking, symptoms and signs of these neoplasms typically relate to the presence of an enlarging mass, and, in the lung, they are therefore most closely allied to interference with the function of structures on which the lesions impinge, such as major bronchi. In unusual instances, paraneoplastic phenomena like those seen with more differentiated autonomic neural tumors – i.e. paragangliomas – may be seen at presentation in association with NBs.[333–335] In one case of pulmonary ganglioneuroblastoma reported by Hochholzer et al., signs of a multiple endocrine neoplasia syndrome were also observed.[332]

Pathologic findings

The gross pathologic attributes of neuroblastic tumors are variable. Undifferentiated NB has a prototypical gray-white, encephaloid appearance. In lesions with partial ganglionic differentiation, nodules of more "fleshy" tissue are noted as discrete foci in the cut surfaces of the lesion. Other potential gross features of neuroblastic neoplasms include a hemangioma-like image because of extreme intratumoral hemorrhage; extensive cystic change; and diffuse or localized calcification that is often readily apparent upon sectioning the mass.[336]

The microscopic characteristics of these tumors likewise form a continuum.[336–340] At one pole, one encounters classical undifferentiated small round cell tumors with little or no discernible stroma and no attempts at neural rosette formation (Fig. 13.38). Moving further along the spectrum of differentiation, the next group of neuroblastomas begins to exhibit background "neuropil," a fibrillary eosinophilic matrix that represents the elaboration of numerous cytoplasmic extensions by the tumor cells (Fig. 13.39). Often, Homer Wright rosettes – having a fibrillary non-luminal center – are also encountered. The separation between NB and *ganglio-*

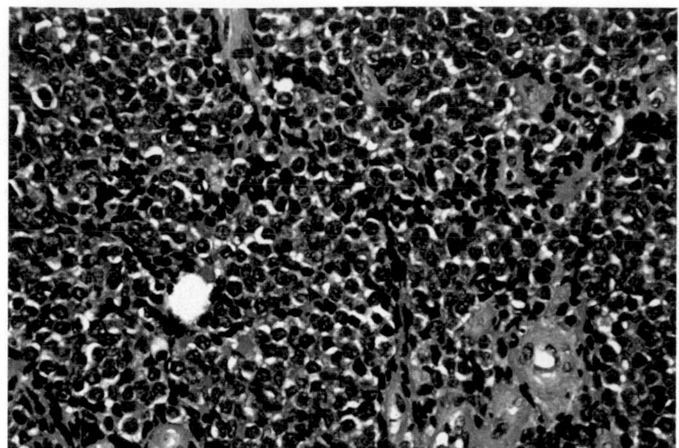

Fig. 13.38 Solid, undifferentiated growth of small round anaplastic tumor cells in neuroblastoma. This appearance is similar to that of high-grade neuroendocrine carcinoma.

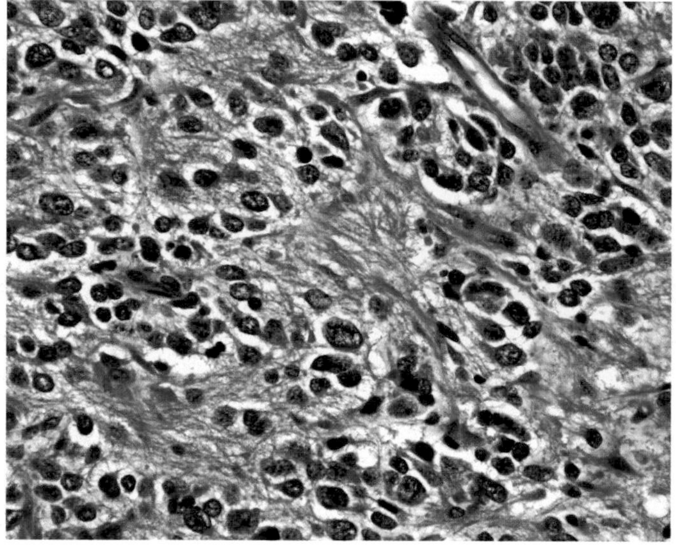

Fig. 13.39 Differentiating neuroblastoma, exhibiting the formation of fibrillar eosinophilic cytoplasmic extensions (neuropil).

neuroblastoma requires the presence of definable ganglion cell differentiation in the latter neoplasms, but where they begin and "differentiating neuroblastoma" ends is more art than science. This statement is limited to so-called "diffuse ganglioneuroblastomas" ("differentiating stromal-poor neuroblastomas" of Shimada et al.),[340] because, as enunciated above, stromal-*rich* tumors look most like ganglioneuromas (composed of mature ganglion cells and spindled Schwann cell-like elements) rather than predominantly small cell proliferations. Stromal-rich neoplasms that are not nodular (i.e. CGNB) are further subdivided into "well-differentiated" lesions, with only a few randomly dispersed neuroblastic cells

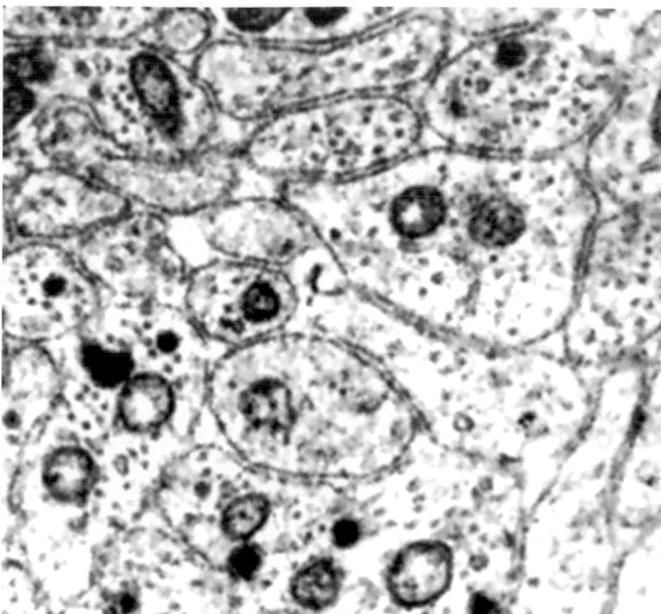

Fig. 13.40 Electron photomicrograph of neuroblastoma, demonstrating interdigitating cytoplasmic extensions, each of which contains microtubules, or synaptic-neurosecretory granules, or both. This constellation of findings would not be expected in epithelial neuroendocrine neoplasms.

punctuating the image of a ganglioneuroma, and "intermixed" tumors that contain small nests of neuroblasts having sharp interfaces with the surrounding ganglionic/ Schwannian tissue.

Differential diagnosis

Differential diagnosis with other small round cell tumors is principally a problem in examples of "undifferentiated" NB.[336] In that setting, electron microscopy demonstrates characteristically elongated cell processes containing microtubular complexes in neuroblastic tumors, with or without presynaptic vesicles or dense-core granules as well[341] (Fig. 13.40).

Immunohistologically, most neuroblastic neoplasms express only neurofilament protein among all of the intermediate filament (IF) types, and, because that marker is usually not well-preserved in formalin-fixed tissues, no IFs are demonstrable in the majority of cases.[342] In contrast, SCNC, an important consideration in adults, is uniformly keratin-positive.[62,63] Synaptophysin is usually present in NB, ganglioneuroblastomas, and ganglioneuromas,[88,89] but chromogranin-A is much less commonly observed.[82] Neuron-specific enolase is a sensitive marker for NB (and as such may have limited utility in identifying bone marrow micrometastases[343]), but it suffers from a lack of specificity and may also be seen in PNETs as well as some cases of rhabdomyosarcoma.[111] The once-difficult distinction between NB and PNET has now been facilitated by the availability of antibodies to the MIC-2 protein and beta-2-microglobulin, both of which are seen in PNET but not NB.[294] Likewise, immunoreactivity for muscle-specific actin and/or desmin characterizes rhabdomyoblastic neoplasms and is not expected in NB.[294] This observation principally comes into play in examples of "anaplastic" NB that may resemble embryonal rhabdomyosarcoma on conventional microscopy.[344]

Treatment and clinical outcome

In specific reference to the three reported cases of primary intrapulmonary neuroblastoma, two patients were alive and well, 1 and 2.5 years after surgical resection and chemotherapy.[331,332] The other individual died shortly after admission to hospital.

In much more general terms, two histologic parameters with prognostic significance should be additionally recorded in evaluating neuroblastic neoplasms. These include the level of ganglionic differentiation (<5% or ≥5%)[336–340] and the "mitotic-karyorrhectic index" (MKI).[340,345,346] The last-cited analyte refers to the number of mitotic or karyorrhectic nuclei that are counted in an evaluation of 5000 tumor cells in "neuropil-free" areas of any given tumor. Needless to say, the daunting prospect of assessing that many cells has dissuaded many pathologists from embracing the Shimada system with enthusiasm. However, common practice has shown that a reasonable estimation of the MKI can be obtained with simple pattern matching approaches. With data on differentiation and MKI in hand, prognostic substratification of stromal-poor neoplasms can then be accomplished, within appropriately age-, location-, and stage-matched tumor groups.[347]

Accurate classification and prognostication of neuroblastic tumors mandates the availability of detailed data on clinical, macroscopic, and histologic levels. Moreover, biochemical observations – as derived from the clinical chemistry laboratory – may provide additional nuances in this context in any given case.[348] The presence of vanillacetic acid in the urine (as opposed to homovanillic acid or vanillyolmandelic acid) worsens the clinical outlook, as do elevated serum levels of ferritin, lactate dehydrogenase, NSE, chromogranin-A, and creatine kinase isozyme BB.[348] On the other hand, elevated somatostatin levels in serum or tumor tissue have been linked to a *better* prognosis.[349]

In regard to other adjunctive modalities of pathologic evaluation as they are applied to neuroblastic tumors, three of them have been used increasingly in the past decade. Cytogenetic assessment (requiring submission of fresh tissue, although current fluorescence–in-situ-hybridization methods may change that) has shown aberrations (deletions; rearrangements) in chromosome 1p in most cases of NB and ganglioneuroblastoma,[350] possibly aiding differential diagnosis with other small cell tumors that lack such abnormalities. In a prognostic vein, it has been found that aneuploidy, hyperdiploidy, and near-tetraploidy in neuroblastic neoplasms correlate with *improved* prognosis, in contrast to the norm for most other malignant tumors.[336,345] Conversely, DNA-diploid lesions tend to behave aggressively. Likewise, increased copy numbers of the oncogene N-*myc* are also biologically detrimental in neuroblastomas.[351–354] This marker can be assessed directly by Southern blot methodology or indirectly by Northern/Western blots or in-situ hybridization. Immunohistology for the protein product of N-*myc* can also be done on fresh tissue with generally acceptable results. The *RET* gene, which is important in prognosis in other neuroendocrine tumors, also appears to correlate with neuronal differentiation in neuroblastoma and, therefore, roughly with prognosis.[355] Lastly, preliminary work has shown that the immunolabeling index for Ki-67 (an indicator of cell replication) is inversely correlated with the length of survival in neuroblastoma cases;[356] furthermore, loss of expression of the *Trk-A* gene and/or CD44 by the tumor cells is also associated with high stage at diagnosis and a poor outcome.[354]

REFERENCES

1. Feyrter F: Uber diffuse endokrine epitheliale organe. 1938, JA Barth, Leipzig, pp 1–334.
2. Pearse AGE: The APUD cell concept and its implications in pathology. Pathol Annu 1974; 9: 27–41.
3. Yousem SA: Pulmonary carcinoid tumors and well-differentiated neuroendocrine carcinomas: is there room for an atypical carcinoid? Am J Clin Pathol 1991; 95: 763–764.
4. Hasleton PS, Bostanci G: Pulmonary carcinoid and related tumors. Rocz Akad Med Bialymst 1997; 42(suppl 1): 28–42.
5. Travis WD, Rush W, Flieder DB, et al.: Survival analysis of 200 pulmonary neuroendocrine tumors with clarification of criteria for atypical carcinoid and its separation from typical carcinoid. Am J Surg Pathol 1998; 22: 934–944.
6. Lloyd RV: Endocrine pathology. 1990, Springer-Verlag, New York, pp 1–151.
7. Lee JE, Evans DB: Advances in the diagnosis and treatment of gastrointestinal neuroendocrine tumors. Cancer Treat Res 1997; 90: 227–238.
8. Warner RR: Gut neuroendocrine tumors. Curr Ther Endocrinol Metab 1997; 6: 606–614.
9. Mendelsohn G: Diagnosis and pathology of endocrine diseases. 1988, JB Lippincott, Philadelphia, pp 1–205.
10. Argani P, Erlandson RA, Rosai J: Thymic neuroblastoma in adults: report of three cases with special emphasis on its association with the syndrome of inappropriate secretion of antidiuretic hormone. Am J Clin Pathol 1997; 108: 537–543.

11. Hasleton PS, Al-Saffar N: The histological spectrum of bronchial carcinoid tumors. Appl Pathol 1989; 7: 205–218.
12. Warren WH, Faber LP, Gould VE: Neuroendocrine neoplasms of the lung: a clinicopathologic update. J Thorac Cardiovasc Surg 1989; 98: 321–332.
13. Glasser CM, Bhagavan BS: Carcinoid tumors of the appendix. Arch Pathol Lab Med 1980; 104: 272–275.
14. Rusch VW, Klimstra DS, Venkatraman ES: Molecular markers help characterize neuroendocrine lung tumors. Ann Thorac Surg 1996; 62: 798–809.
15. Gould VE, Linnoila RI, Memoli VA, Warren WH: Neuroendocrine components of the bronchopulmonary tract. Lab Invest 1983; 49: 519–537.
16. Shackney SE, Shankey TV: Common patterns of genetic evolution in human solid tumors. Cytometry 1997; 29: 1–27.
17. Yunis JJ: Genes and chromosomes in the pathogenesis and prognosis of human cancers. Adv Pathol Lab Med 1989; 2: 147–188.
18. Galanis E, Frytak S, Lloyd RV: Extrapulmonary small cell carcinoma. Cancer 1997; 79: 1729–1736.
19. Fletcher JA: Cytogenetic aberrations in malignant soft tissue tumors. Adv Pathol Lab Med 1991; 4: 235–246.
20. Dehner LP: Primitive neuroectodermal tumor and Ewing's sarcoma. Am J Surg Pathol 1993; 17: 1–13.
21. Simpson NE, Kidd KK, Goodfellow PJ, et al.: Assignment of multiple endocrine neoplasia type 2A to chromosome 10 by linkage. Nature 1987; 328: 528–530.
22. Komminoth P: Multiple endocrine neoplasia type 1 and 2: 1997 diagnostic guidelines & molecular pathology. Pathologe 1997; 18: 286–300.
23. Komminoth P: Multiple endocrine neoplasia type 1 & 2: from morphology to molecular pathology 1997. Verh Dtsch Ges Pathol 1997; 81: 125–138.
24. Eng C, Mulligan LM: Mutations of the RET protooncogene in the multiple endocrine neoplasia type 2 syndromes, related sporadic tumors, & Hirschsprung's disease. Hum Mutations 1997; 9: 97–109.
25. Cagle PT, El-Naggar AK, Xu HJ, et al.: Differential retinoblastoma protein expression in neuroendocrine tumors of the lung: potential diagnostic implications. Am J Pathol 1997; 150: 393–400.
26. McDowell EM, Wilson TS, Trump BF: Atypical endocrine tumors of the lung. Arch Pathol Lab Med 1981; 105: 20–28.
27. Adelstein DJ, Tomashefski JF: Mixed small-cell and non-small-cell lung cancer. Chest 1986; 89: 699–704.
28. Hishima T, Fukayama M, Hayashi Y, et al.: Neuroendocrine differentiation in thymic epithelial tumors, with special reference to thymic carcinoma & atypical thymoma. Hum Pathol 1998; 29: 330–338.
29. Usuda H, Emura I, Naito M, Hirono T: Peripheral lung carcinomas associated with central fibrosis and mixed small cell and other histologic components. Pathol Int 1995; 45: 940–946.
30. Robertson NJ, Rahamim J, Smith ME: Carcinosarcoma of the esophagus showing neuroendocrine, squamous, and glandular differentiation. Histopathology 1997; 31: 263–266.
31. McWilliam LJ, Manson C, George NJ: Neuroendocrine differentiation and prognosis in prostatic adenocarcinoma. Br J Urol 1997; 80: 287–290.
32. Leslie KO, Colby TV: Pathology of lung cancer. Curr Opin Pulm Med 1997; 3: 252–256.
33. Bosman FT: Neuroendocrine cells in non-endocrine tumors: what does it mean? Verh Dtsch Ges Pathol 1997; 81: 62–72.
34. Wick MR, Berg LC, Hertz MI: Large cell carcinoma of the lung with neuroendocrine differentiation. Am J Clin Pathol 1992; 97: 796–805.
35. Radice PA, Matthews MJ, Ihde DC, et al.: The clinical behavior of mixed small cell/large cell bronchogenic carcinoma compared to pure small cell subtypes. *Cancer* 1982; 50: 2894–2902.
36. Fushimi H, Kikui M, Morino H, et al.: Histologic changes in small cell lung carcinoma after treatment. Cancer 1996; 77: 278–283.
37. Wiseman GA, Kvols LK: Therapy of neuroendocrine tumors with radiolabeled MIBG and somatostatin analogues. Semin Nucl Med 1995; 25: 272–278.
38. DiBartolomeo M, Bajetta E, Buzzoni R, et al., & the ITMO Association: Clinical efficacy of octreotide in the treatment of metastatic neuroendocrine tumors. Cancer 1996; 77: 402–408.
39. Saldiva PHN, Capelozzi VL, Battlehner CN: Neuroendocrine tumors of the lung. In: Pathology of lung tumors, Corrin B, Ed. 1997, Churchill-Livingstone, New York, pp 55–70.
40. Nagle RB, Payne CM, Clark VA: Comparison of the usefulness of histochemistry and ultrastructural cytochemistry in the identification of neuroendocrine neoplasms. Am J Clin Pathol 1986; 85: 289–296.
41. Samsonov VA: Carcinoid lung tumors: clinicomorphologic characteristics and diagnosis. Arkh Patol 1995; 57: 20–24.
42. Kogan EA, Sekamova SM, Mazurenko NN, Bogatyrev VN: Peripheral small cell carcinoma, atypical and typical lung carcinoids. Arkh Patol 1991; 53: 42–48.
43. Erlandson RA: Diagnostic transmission electron microscopy of tumors. 1994, Raven Press, New York, pp 123–125.
44. Carey FA, Save VE: Neuroendocrine differentiation in lung cancer. J Pathol 1997; 182: 9–10.
45. Soga J, Yakuwa Y: Bronchopulmonary carcinoids: an analysis of 1875 reported cases with special reference to a comparison between typical carcinoids and typical varieties. Ann Thorac Cardiovasc Surg 1999; 5: 211–219.
46. Dardick I, Christensen H, Stratis M: Immunoelectron microscopy for chromogranin A in small cell neuroendocrine carcinoma of lung. Ultrastruct Pathol 1996; 20: 361–368.
47. Yang GC: Mixed small cell/large cell carcinoma of the lung: report of a case with cytologic features and ultrastructural correlation. Acta Cytol 1995; 39: 1175–1181.
48. Taccagni GL, Rovere E, Terreni MR, Gambini S, Cantaboni A: Divergent differentiative histogenetic lines in lung tumors: identification of histotypes with pure and mixed ultrastructural phenotype and their prognostic significance. Ultrastruct Pathol 1995; 19: 61–73.
49. Mount SL, Taatjes DJ, von Turkovich M, Tindle BH, Trainer TD: Diagnostic immunoelectron microscopy in surgical pathology: assessment of various tissue fixation and processing protocols. Ultrastruct Pathol 1993; 17: 547–556.
50. Przybylowski P, Mlynarczyk W, Blotna-Filipiak M, Biczysko W: Application of electron microscopy and immunocytochemistry in lung cancer diagnosis. Folia Morphol 1993; 52: 191–200.
51. Tsubota YT, Kawaguchi T, Hoso T, Nishino E, Travis WD: A combined small cell and spindle cell carcinoma of the lung: report of a unique case with immunohistochemical and ultrastructural studies. Am J Surg Pathol 1992; 16: 1108–1115.
52. Pilotti S, Patriarca C, Lombardi L, Scopsi L, Rilke F: Well-differentiated neuroendocrine carcinoma of the lung: a clinicopathologic and ultrastructural study of 10 cases. Tumori 1992; 78: 121–129.
53. Dardick I, Yazdi HM, Brosko C, Rippstein P, Hickey NM: A quantitative comparison of light and electron microscopic diagnoses in specimens obtained by fine needle aspiration biopsy. Ultrastruct Pathol 1991; 15: 105–129.
54. Muller KM, Fisseler-Eckhoff A: Small cell bronchial cancer – pathologic anatomy. Langenbecks Arch Chir Suppl Kongressbd 1991; 534–543.
554a. Warren WH, Gould VE: Neuroendocrine tumors of the bronchopulmonary tract: a reappraisal of their classification after 20 years. Surg Clin North Am 2002; 82: 525–540.
55. Wick MR: Immunohistology of neuroendocrine and neuroectodermal tumors. Semin Diagn Pathol 19(4): 207–218.
56. Brambilla E, Veale D, Moro D, et al: Neuroendocrine phenotype in lung cancers: comparison of immunohistochemistry with biochemical determination of enolase isoenzymes. Am J Clin Pathol 1992; 98: 88–97.
57. Broers JL, Mijnheere EP, Rot MK, et al.: Novel antigens characteristic of neuroendocrine malignancies. Cancer 1991; 67: 619–633.
58. Loy TS, Darkow GVD, Quesenbery JT: Immunostaining in the diagnosis of pulmonary neuroendocrine carcinomas. An immunohistochemical study with ultrastructural correlations. Am J Surg Pathol 1995; 19: 173–182.
59. Tome Y, Hirohashi S, Noguchi M, et al.: Immunocytologic diagnosis of small-cell lung cancer in imprint smears. Acta Cytologica 1991; 35: 485–490.
60. Miettinen M: Keratin immunohistochemistry: update of applications and pitfalls. Pathol Annu 1993; 28(2): 113–143.
61. Chan JKC, Suser S, Wenig BM, et al.: Cytokeratin 20 immunoreactivity distinguishes Merkel cell (primary cutaneous neuroendocrine) carcinomas and salivary gland small cell carcinomas from small cell carcinomas of various sites. Am J Surg Pathol 1997; 21: 226–234.

62. Battifora H: Diagnostic uses of antibodies to keratins: a review and immunohistochemical comparison of seven monoclonal and three polyclonal antibodies. Prog Surg Pathol 1988; 8: 1–16.
63. Battifora H, Silva EG: The use of antikeratin antibodies in the immunohistochemical distinction between neuroendocrine (Merkel cell) carcinoma of the skin, lymphoma, and oat cell carcinoma. Cancer 1986; 58: 1040–1046.
64. Labrousse F, Leboutet MJ, Petit B, et al.: Cytokeratin expression in paragangliomas of the cauda equina. Clin Neuropathol 1999; 18: 208–213.
65. Chetty R, Pillay P, Jaichand V: Cytokeratin expression in adrenal pheochromocytomas and extraadrenal paragangliomas. J Clin Pathol 1998; 51: 477–478.
66. Marley EF, Liapis H, Humphrey PA, et al.: Primitive neuroectodermal tumor of the kidney – another enigma: a pathologic, immunohistochemical, and molecular diagnostic study. Am J Surg Pathol 1997; 21: 354–359.
67. Moll R, Lee I, Gould VE, et al.: Immunocytochemical analysis of Ewing's tumors: patterns of expression of intermediate filaments and desmosomal proteins indicate cell type heterogeneity and pluripotential differentiation. Am J Pathol 1987; 127: 288–304.
68. Thorner P: Intraabdominal polyphenotypic tumor. Pediatr Pathol Lab Med 1996; 16: 161–169.
69. Gerald WL, Ladanyi M, de Alava E, et al.: Clinical, pathologic, and molecular spectrum of tumors associated with t(11;22)(p13;q12): desmoplastic small round cell tumor and its variants. J Clin Oncol 1998; 16: 3028–3036.
70. Ordonez NG: Desmoplastic small round cell tumor. II. An ultrastructural and immunohistochemical study with emphasis on new immunohistochemical markers. Am J Surg Pathol 1998; 22: 1314–1327.
71. Winters JL, Geil JD, O'Connor WN: Immunohistology, cytogenetics, and molecular studies of small round cell tumors of childhood: a review. Ann Clin Lab Sci 1995; 25: 66–78.
72. Broers JL, Carney DN, de Ley L, Vooijs GP, Ramaekers FCS: Differential expression of intermediate filament proteins distinguishes classic from variant small-cell lung cancer cell lines. Proc Natl Acad Sci USA 1985; 82: 4409–4413.
73. Merot Y, Margolis RJ, Dahl D, Saurat JH, Mihm MC Jr: Coexpression of neurofilament and keratin proteins in cutaneous neuroendocrine carcinoma cells. J Invest Dermatol 1986; 86: 74–77.
74. Moran CA, Suster S, Fishback N, Koss MN: Mediastinal paragangliomas: a clinicopathologic and immunohistochemical study of 16 cases. Cancer 1993; 72: 2358–2364.
75. Kimura N, Nakazato Y, Nagura H, Sasano N: Expression of intermediate filaments in neuroendocrine tumors. Arch Pathol Lab Med 1990; 114: 506–510.
76. Hirose T, Scheithauer BW, Lopes MB, et al.: Olfactory neuroblastoma: an immunohistochemical, ultrastructural, and flow cytometric study. Cancer 1995; 76: 4–19.
77. Miettinen M: Synaptophysin and neurofilament proteins as markers for neuroendocrine tumors. Arch Pathol Lab Med 1987; 111: 813–818.
78. Johnson TL, Zarbo RJ, Lloyd RV, Crissman JD: Paragangliomas of the head and neck: immunohistochemical neuroendocrine and intermediate filament typing. Mod Pathol 1988; 1: 216–223.
79. Eusebi V, Damiani S, Pasquinelli G, et al.: Small cell neuroendocrine carcinoma with skeletal muscle differentiation. Am J Surg Pathol 2000; 24: 223–230.
80. Friede RL, Janzer RC, Roessmann U: Infantile small cell gliomas. Acta Neuropathol 1982; 57: 103–110.
81. Oh D, Prayson RA: Evaluation of epithelial and keratin markers in glioblastoma multiforme: an immunohistochemical study. Arch Pathol Lab Med 1999; 123: 917–920.
82. Wilson RS, Lloyd RV: Detection of chromogranin in neuroendocrine cells with a monoclonal antibody. Am J Pathol 1984; 115: 458–468.
83. Settleman J, Fonseca R, Nolan J, Angeletti RH: Relationship of multiple forms of chromogranin. J Biol Chem 1985; 260: 1645–1651.
84. O'Connor DT: Chromogranin: widespread immunoreactivity in polypeptide hormone-producing tissues and in serum. Regul Pept 1983; 6: 263–280.
85. Eriksson B, Arnberg H, Oberg K, et al.: A polyclonal antiserum against chromogranin A and B – a new sensitive marker for neuroendocrine tumors. Acta Endocrinol 1990; 122: 145–155.
86. Woussen-Colle MC, Gourlet P, Vandermeers A, et al.: Identification of a new chromogranin B fragment (314-365) in endocrine tumors. Peptides 1995; 16: 231–236.
87. Lloyd RV, Wilson RS: Specific endocrine marker defined by a monoclonal antibody. Science 1983; 222: 628–630.
88. Gould VE, Lee I, Wiedenmann B, et al.: Synaptophysin: a novel marker for neurons, certain neuroendocrine cells, and their neoplasms. Hum Pathol 1986; 17: 979–983.
89. Buffa R, Rindi G, Sessa F, et al.: Synaptophysin immunoreactivity and small clear vesicles in neuroendocrine cells and related tumors. Mol Cell Probes 1987; 1: 367–381.
90. Stridsberg M: The use of chromogranin, synaptophysin, and islet amyloid polypeptide as markers for neuroendocrine tumors. Ups J Med Sci 1995; 100: 169–199.
91. Poola I, Graziano SL: Expression of neuron-specific enolase, chromogranin A, synaptophysin, and Leu-7 in lung cancer cell lines. J Exp Clin Cancer Res 1998; 17: 165–173.
92. Erlandson RA, Nesland JM: Tumors of the endocrine/neuroendocrine system: an overview. Ultrastruct Pathol 1994; 18: 149–170.
93. Lipinski M, Braham K, Caillaud JM, Carlu C, Tursz T: HNK-1 antibody detects an antigen expressed on neuroectodermal cells. J Exp Med 1983; 158: 1775–1780.
94. Tsutsumi Y: Leu-7 immunoreactivity as a histochemical marker for paraffin-embedded neuroendocrine tumors. Acta Histochem Cytochem 1984; 17: 15–21.
95. Bunn PA Jr, Linnoila I, Minna JD, Carney D, Gazdar AF: Small cell lung cancer, endocrine cells of the fetal bronchus, and other neuroendocrine cells express the Leu-7 antigenic determinant present on natural killer cells. Blood 1985; 65: 764–768.
96. Perentes E, Rubinstein LJ: Immunohistochemical recognition of human nerve sheath tumors by anti-Leu 7 (HNK-1) monoclonal antibody. Acta Neuropathol 1985; 68: 319–324.
97. Abenoza P, Manivel JC, Swanson PE, Wick MR: Synovial sarcoma: ultrastructural study and immunohistochemical analysis by a combined PAP/ABC procedure. Hum Pathol 1986; 17: 1107–1115.
98. Rusthoven JJ, Robinson JB, Kolin A, Pinkerton PH: The natural killer cell associated HNK-1 (Leu-7) antibody reacts with hypertrophic and malignant prostatic epithelium. Cancer 1985; 56: 289–293.
99. May EE, Perentes E: Anti-Leu 7 immunoreactivity with human tumors: its value in the diagnosis of prostatic adenocarcinoma. Histopathology 1987; 11: 295–304.
100. Kodama T, Watanable S, Sato Y, Shimosato Y, Miyazawa N: An immunohistochemical study of thymic epithelial tumors. I. Epithelial component. Am J Surg Pathol 1986; 10: 26–33.
101. Tischler AS, Mobtaker H, Mann K, et al.: Anti-lymphocyte antibody Leu-7 (HNK-1) recognizes a constituent of neuroendocrine granule matrix. J Histochem Cytochem 1986; 34: 1213–1216.
102. Lantuejoul S, Moro D, Michalides RJ, Brambilla C, Brambilla E: Neural cell adhesion molecules (NCAM) and NCAM-PSA expression in neuroendocrine lung tumors. Am J Surg Pathol 1998; 22: 1267–1276.
103. Kaufmann O, Georgi T, Dietel M: Utility of 123C3 monoclonal antibody against CD56 (NCAM) for the diagnosis of small cell carcinomas on paraffin sections. Hum Pathol 1997; 28: 1373–1378.
104. Del Rio M, Demoly P, Koros AM, et al.: JLP5B9: new monoclonal antibody against polysialylated neural cell adhesion molecule is of value in phenotyping lung cancer. J Immunol Meth 2000; 233: 21–31.
105. Hage R, Elbers HR, Brutel de la Riviere A, van den Bosch JM: Neural cell adhesion molecule expression: prognosis in 889 patients with resected non-small cell lung cancer. Chest 1998; 114: 1316–1320.
106. Jaques G, Auerbach B, Pritsch M, et al.: Evaluation of serum neural cell adhesion molecule as a new tumor marker in small cell lung cancer. Cancer 1993; 72: 418–425.
107. Seldeslagh KA, Lauweryns JM: NCAM expression in the pulmonary neural and diffuse neuroendocrine cell system. Microsc Res Tech 1997; 37: 69–76.
108. Kwa HB, Verheijen MG, Litvinov SV, et al.: Prognostic factors in resected non-small cell lung cancer: an immunohistochemical study of 39 cases. Lung Cancer 1996; 16: 35–45.
109. Tapia FJ, Barbosa AJA, Marangos PJ, et al.: Neuron-specific enolase is produced by neuroendocrine tumors. Lancet 1981; 2: 808–811.
110. Wick MR, Scheithauer BW, Kovacs K: Neuron-specific enolase in neuroendocrine tumors of the thymus, bronchus, and skin. Am J Clin Pathol 1983; 79: 703–707.

111. Carlei F, Polak JM: Antibodies to neuron-specific enolase for the delineation of the entire diffuse neuroendocrine system in health and disease. Semin Diagn Pathol 1984; 1: 59–70.
112. Haimoto H, Takahashi Y, Koshikawa T, Nagura H, Kato K: Immunohistochemical localization of gamma-enolase in normal human tissues other than nervous and neuroendocrine tissues. Lab Invest 1985; 52: 257–263.
113. Thomas P, Battifora H, Manderino GL, Patrick J: A monoclonal antibody against neuron-specific enolase: immunohistochemical comparison with a polyclonal antiserum. Am J Clin Pathol 1987; 88: 146–152.
114. Vinores SA, Bonnin JM, Rubinstein LJ, Marangos PJ: Immunohistochemical demonstration of neuron-specific enolase in neoplasms of the CNS and other tissues. Arch Pathol Lab Med 1984; 108: 536–540.
115. DeLellis RA: Endocrine tumors. In: Diagnostic immunopathology, 1st edn, Colvin RB, Bhan AK, McCluskey RT, Eds. 1988, Raven Press, New York, pp 301–338.
116. Said JW, Vimadalal S, Nash G, et al.: Immunoreactive neuron-specific enolase, bombesin, and chromogranin-A as markers for neuroendocrine lung tumors. Hum Pathol 1985; 16: 236–240.
117. Rode J: PGP 9.5 – a new marker for vertebrate neurons and neuroendocrine cells. Brain Res 1983; 278: 224–228.
118. Gosney JR, Gosney MA, Lye M, Butt SA: Reliability of commercially available immunocytochemical markers for identification of neuroendocrine differentiation in bronchoscopic biopsies of bronchial carcinoma. Thorax 1995; 50: 116–120.
119. Addis BJ, Hamid Q, Ibrahim NB, et al.: Immunohistochemical markers of small cell carcinoma and related neuroendocrine tumors of the lung. J Pathol 1987; 153: 137–150.
120. Hibi K, Westra WH, Borges M, et al.: PGP9.5 as a candidate tumor marker for non-small cell lung cancer. Am J Pathol 1999; 155: 711–715.
121. Amann G, Zoubek A, Salzer-Kuntschik M, Windhager R, Kovar H: Relation of neurological marker expression and EWS gene fusion types in MIC2/CD99-positive tumors of the Ewing family. Hum Pathol 1999; 30: 1058–1064.
122. Dehner LP: Primitive neuroectodermal tumors and Ewing's sarcoma. Am J Surg Pathol 1993; 17: 1–13.
123. Soslow RA, Bhargava V, Warnke RA: MIC2, TdT, *bcl*-2, and CD34 expression in paraffin-embedded high-grade lymphoma/acute lymphoblastic leukemia distinguishes between distinct clinicopathologic entities. Hum Pathol 1997; 28: 1158–1165.
124. Lumadue JA, Askin FB, Perlman EJ: MIC2 analysis of small cell carcinoma. Am J Clin Pathol 1994; 102: 692–694.
125. Nicholson SA, McDermott MB, Swanson PE, Wick MR: CD99 and cytokeratin-20 in small-cell and basaloid tumors of the skin. Appl Immunohistochem Mol Morphol in press.
126. Krisch K, Buxbaum P, Horvat G, et al.: Monoclonal antibody HISL-19 as an immunocytochemical probe for neuroendocrine differentiation. Its application in diagnostic pathology. Am J Pathol 1986; 123: 100–108.
127. Lloyd RV, Sisson JC, Shapiro B, Verhofstad AA: Immunohistochemical localization of epinephrine, norepinephrine, catecholamine-synthesizing enzymes, and chromogranin in neuroendocrine cells and tumors. Am J Pathol 1986; 125: 45–64.
128. Haspel MV, Onodera T, Prabhakar BS, et al.: Multiple organ-reactive monoclonal autoantibodies. Nature 1983; 304: 73–76.
129. Unger P, Hoffman K, Pertsemlidis D, et al.: S100 protein-positive sustentacular cells in malignant and locally aggressive adrenal pheochromocytomas. Arch Pathol Lab Med 1991; 115: 484–487.
129a. Sturm N, Rossi G, Lantuejoul S, et al.: Expression of thyroid transcription factor-1 in the spectrum of neuroendocrine cell lung proliferations with special interest in carcinoids. Hum Pathol 2002; 33: 175–182.
129b. Oliveira AM, Tazelaar HD, Myers JL, Erickson LA, Lloyd RV: Thyroid transcription factor-1 distinguishes metastatic pulmonary from well-differentiated neuroendocrine tumors of other sites. Am J Surg Pathol 2001; 25: 815–819.
129c. Ordonez NG: Value of thyroid transcription factor-1 immunostaining in distinguishing small cell lung carcinomas from other small cell carcinomas. Am J Surg Pathol 2000; 24: 1217–1223.
129d. Kaufmann O, Dietel M: Expression of thyroid transcription factor-1 in pulmonary and extrapulmonary small cell carcinomas and other neuroendocrine carcinomas of various primary sites. Histopathology 2000; 36: 415–420.
129e. Agoff SN, Lamps LW, Philip AT, et al.: Thyroid transcription factor-1 is expressed in extrapulmonary small cell carcinomas but not in other extrapulmonary neuroendocrine tumors. Mod Pathol 2000; 13: 238–242.
129f. Folpe AL, Gown AM, Lamps LW, et al.: Thyroid transcription factor-1: immunohistochemical evaluation in pulmonary neuroendocrine tumors. Mod Pathol 1999; 12: 5–8.
129g. Zamecnik J, Kodet R: Value of thyroid transcription factor-1 and surfactant apoprotein A in the differential diagnosis of pulmonary carcinomas: a study of 109 cases. Virchows Arch A 2002; 440: 353–361.
130. Travis WD, Colby TV, Corrin B, Shimosato Y, Brambilla E: Histological typing of lung & pleural tumours (International Histological Classification of Tumours). 1999, World Health Organization, Geneva, Switzerland. pp 1–55.
131. Hofler H: Neuroendocrine tumors of the lung. Verh Dtsch Ges Pathol 1997; 81: 118–124.
132. Kramer R: Adenoma of the bronchus. Ann Otol Rhinol Laryngol 1930; 39: 689–695.
133. Carter D, Eggleston JC: Tumors of the lower respiratory tract. In: Atlas of tumor pathology, second series, Fascicle 17. Armed Forces Institute of Pathology, Washington, DC, pp 162–188.
134. Colby TV, Koss MN, Travis WD: Tumors of the lower respiratory tract. In: Atlas of tumor pathology, second series, Fascicle 13. 1995, Armed Forces Institute of Pathology, Washington, DC, pp 287–318.
135. El-Naggar AK, Ballance W, Abdul Karim FW, et al.: Typical and atypical bronchopulmonary carcinoids: Am J Clin Pathol 1991; 95: 828–834.
136. McCaughan BC, Martini N, Bains MS: Bronchial carcinoids: review of 124 cases. J Thorac Cardiovasc Surg 1985; 89: 8–17.
137. Abdi EA, Goel R, Bishop S, Bain GO: Peripheral carcinoid tumours of the lung: a clinicopathologic study. J Surg Oncol 1988; 39: 190–196.
138. Ranchod M, Levine GD: Spindle cell carcinoid tumors of the lung: a clinicopathologic study of 35 cases. Am J Surg Pathol 1980: 4: 315–331.
139. Zarate A, Kovacs K, Flores M, et al.: ACTH and CRF-producing bronchial carcinoid associated with Cushing's syndrome. Clin Endocrinol 1986; 24: 523–529.
140. Findling JW, Tyrrell JB: Occult ectopic secretion of corticotropin. Arch Intern Med 1986; 146: 929–933.
141. Ankotche A, Raffin-Sanson ML, Mosnier-Pudard H, Bertagna X, Luton JP: Ectopic ACTH secretion: a heterogeneous entity. Presse Med 1997; 26: 1330–1333.
142. Shrager JB, Wright CD, Wain JC, et al.: Bronchopulmonary carcinoid tumors associated with Cushing's syndrome: a more aggressive variant of typical carcinoid. J Thorac Cardiovasc Surg 1997; 114 : 367–375.
143. Oliaro A, Filosso PL, Casadio C, et al.: Bronchial carcinoid associated with Cushing's syndrome. J Cardiovasc Surg 1995; 36: 511–514.
144. White A, Clark AJ: The cellular and molecular basis of the ectopic ACTH syndrome. Clin Endocrinol 1993; 39: 131–141.
145. Liu TH, Liu HR, Lu ZL, et al.: Thoracic ectopic ACTH-producing tumors with Cushing's syndrome. Zentrabl Pathol 1993; 139: 131–139.
146. Levy NT, Rubin J, DeRemee RA, et al.: Carcinoid tumors and sarcoidosis – does a link exist? Mayo Clin Proc 1997; 72: 112–116.
147. Flieder DB, Vazquez VF: Lung tumors with neuroendocrine morphology: a perspective for the new millenium. Radiol Clin North Am 2000; 38: 563–577.
148. Al-Kaisa N, Abdul-Karim FW, Mendelsohn G, Jacobs G: Bronchial carcinoid tumor with amyloid stroma. Arch Pathol Lab Med 1988; 112: 211–214.
149. Scharifker D, Marchevsky A: Oncocytic carcinoid tumor of lung: an ultrastructural analysis. Cancer 1981: 47: 530–532.
150. Sklar JL, Churg A, Bensch KG: Oncocytic carcinoid tumor of the lung. Am J Surg Pathol 1980; 4: 287–292.
151. Ritter JH, Nappi O: Oxyphilic proliferations of the respiratory tract and paranasal sinuses. Semin Diagn Pathol 1999; 16: 105–116.
152. Gaffey MJ, Mills SE, Frierson HF Jr, Askin FB, Maygarden SJ: Pulmonary clear cell carcinoid tumor: another entity in the differential diagnosis of pulmonary clear cell neoplasia. *Am J Surg Pathol* 1998; 22: 1020–1025.
153. Mark EJ, Quay SC, Dickerson GR: Papillary carcinoid tumor of the lung. Cancer 1981; 48: 316–324.
154. Grazer R, Cohen SM, Jacobs JB, Lucas P: Melanin-containing peripheral carcinoid tumor of the lung. Am J Surg Pathol 1982; 6: 73–78.

155. Carlson JA, Dickersin GR: Melanotic paraganglioid carcinoid tumor: a case report and review of the literature. Ultrastruct Pathol 1993; 17: 353–372.
156. Al-Khafaji B, Noffsinger AE, Miller MA, et al.: Immunohistologic analysis of gastrointestinal and pulmonary carcinoid tumors. Hum Pathol 1998; 29: 992–999.
157. Skinner C, Ewen SWB: Carcinoid lung: diffuse pulmonary infiltration by a multifocal bronchial carcinoid. Thorax 1976; 31: 212–219.
158. Lohmann DR, Fesseler B, Putz B, et al.: Infrequent mutations of the p53 gene in pulmonary carcinoid tumors. Cancer Res 1993; 53: 5797–5801.
159. Jiang SX, Kameya T, Shinada J, Yoshimura H: The significance of frequent and independent p53 and *bcl-2* expression in large cell neuroendocrine carcinoma of the lung. Mod Pathol 1999; 12: 362–369.
160. Pelosi G, Zancanaro C, Sbabo L, et al.: Development of innumerable neuroendocrine tumorlets in pulmonary lobe scarred by intralobar sequestration: immunohistochemical and ultrastructural study of an unusual case. Arch Pathol Lab Med 1992; 116: 1167–1174.
161. Canessa PA, Santini D, Zanelli M, Capecchi V: Pulmonary tumorlets and microcarcinoids in bronchiectasis. Monaldi Arch Chest Dis 1997; 52: 138–139.
162. Ramon-Capilla M, Arnau-Obrer A, Navarro-Ibanez R, et al.: Pulmonary tumorlet: report of 5 cases. Arch Bronchopneumonol 1996; 32: 489–491.
163. Zanetta G, Zanoni M, Colombo F: Argentaffin pulmonary tumorlets. Tumori 1979; 65: 761–766.
164. Watanabe H, Kobayashi H, Honma K, Ohnishi Y, Iwafuchi M: Diffuse panbronchiolitis with multiple tumorlets: a quantitative study of the Kultschitzky cells and the clusters. Acta Pathol Jpn 1985; 35: 1221–1231.
165. Miller RR, Muller NL: Neuroendocrine cell hyperplasia and obliterative bronchiolitis in patients with peripheral carcinoid tumors. Am J Surg Pathol 1995; 19: 653–658.
166. Satoh Y, Fujiyama J, Ueno M, Ishikawa Y: High cellular atypia in a pulmonary tumorlet: report of a case with cytologic findings. Acta Cytol 2000; 44: 242–246.
167. Higashiyama M, Doi O, Kodama K, et al.: A case of pulmonary tumorlet with tuberculoma misdiagnosed as small cell lung carcinoma by transbronchial lung biopsy. Kyobu Geka 1995; 48: 165–168.
168. Shah R, Sabanathan S, Mearns J, Richardson J, Goulden C: Carcinoid tumor of the lung. J Cardiovasc Surg 1997; 38: 187–189.
169. DiGiorgio A, Tocchi A, Puntillo G, et al.: Tracheobronchial carcinoids: current therapeutic trends. Ann Ital Chir 1990; 61: 405–409.
170. Huwer H, Kalweit G, Kruger B, Straub U, Schafers HJ: Bronchopulmonary carcinoids: surgical therapy and prognosis. Pneumonologie 1996; 50: 786–789.
171. Ferguson MK, Landreneau RJ, Hazelrigg SR, et al.: Long-term outcome after resection for bronchial carcinoid tumors. Eur J Cardiothorac Surg 2000; 18: 156–161.
172. Warren WH, Gould VE, Faber LP, Kittle CF, Memoli VA: Neuroendocrine neoplasms of the bronchopulmonary tract: a classification of the spectrum of carcinoid to small cell carcinoma and intervening variants. J Thorac Cardiovasc Surg 1985; 89: 819–825.
173. Ashraf MH: Bronchial carcinoid with osteoblastic metastases. Thorax 1977; 32: 509–511.
174. Padberg BC, Woenckhaus J, Hilger G, et al.: DNA cytophotometry and prognosis in typical and atypical bronchopulmonary carcinoids: a clinicomorphologic study of 100 neuroendocrine lung tumors. Am J Surg Pathol 1996; 20: 815–822.
175. Lissoni P, Barni S, Tacini G, et al.: Immunoendocrine therapy with low-dose subcutaneous interleukin-2 plus melatonin of locally advanced or metastatic endocrine tumors. Oncology 1995; 52: 163–166.
176. Arrigoni MG, Woolner LB, Bernatz PE: Atypical carcinoid tumors of the lung. J Thorac Cardiovasc Surg. 1972; 64: 413–421.
177. Paladugu RR, Benefield JR, Pak HY, et al.: Bronchopulmonary Kulchitzky cell carcinomas: a new classification scheme for typical and atypical carcinoids. Cancer 1985; 55: 1303–1311.
178. Lequaglie C, Patriarca C, Cataldo I, et al.: Prognosis of resected well-differentiated neuroendocrine carcinoma of the lung. Chest 1991; 100: 1053–1056.
179. Memoli V: Well-differentiated neuroendocrine carcinoma: a designation comes of age. Chest 1991; 100: 892.
180. Garcia-Yuste M, Matilla JM, Alvarez-Gago F, et al.: Prognostic factors in neuroendocrine lung tumors. Ann Thorac Surg 2000; 70; 258–263.
181. Rush W, Zeren H, Griffin JL, et al.: Histologic subtypes of neuroendocrine carcinoma: prognostic correlations [abstract]. Lab Invest 1995; 72: 153A.
182. Warren WH, Memoli Va, Gould VE: Immunohistochemical and ultrastructural analysis of bronchopulmonary neuroendocrine neoplasms. II. Well-differentiated neuroendocrine carcinomas. Ultrastruct Pathol 1984; 7: 185–199.
183. Warren WH, Memoli VA, Gould VE: Well differentiated and small cell neuroendocrine carcinomas of the lung: two related but distinct clinicopathologic entities. Virch Arch B Cell Pathol 1988; 55: 299–310.
184. Warren WH, Memoli VA, Jordan AG, et al.: Re-evaluation of pulmonary neoplasms resected as small cell carcinomas: significance of distinguishing between well-differentiated and small cell neuroendocrine carcinomas. Cancer 1990; 65: 1003–1010.
185. Carter D, Yesner R: Carcinomas of the lung with neuroendocrine differentiation. Semin Diagn Pathol 1985; 2: 235–254.
186. Oliaro A, Donati G, Filosso PL, Ruffini E: Neuroendocrine tumors of the lung. Minerva Chir 2000; 66: 7–16.
187. Slodkowska J, Langfort R, Rudzinski P, Kupis W: Typical and atypical pulmonary carcinoids: pathologic and clinical analysis of 77 cases. Pneumonol Alergol Pol 1998; 66: 297–303.
188. Pareja E, Arnau A, Aartigues E, et al.: Bronchial carcinoid tumors: a prospective study. Arch Bronchopneumonol 1998; 34: 71–75.
189. Balli M, Fabris GA, Dewar A, Hornall D, Sheppard MN: Atypical carcinoid tumor: a study of 33 cases with prognostic features. Histopathology 1994; 24: 363–369.
190. Mills SE, Walker AN, Cooper PH, et al.: Atypical carcinoid tumor of the lung: a clinicopathologic study of 17 cases. Am J Surg. Pathol 1982; 6: 643–654.
191. Grote TH, Macon WR, Davis B, et al.: Atypical carcinoid of the lung: a distinct clinicopathologic entity. Chest 1988; 93: 370–375.
191a. Burns TM, Juel VC, Sanders DB, Phillips LH II: Neuroendocrine lung tumors and disorders of the neuromuscular junction. Neurology 1999; 52: 1490–1491.
192. Yousem SA, Taylor SR: Typical and atypical carcinoid tumors of lung. A clinicopathologic and DNA analysis of 20 tumors. Modern Pathol 1990; 3: 502–507.
193. Guinee DG Jr, Fishback NF, Koss MN, Abbondanzo SL, Travis WD: The spectrum of immunohistochemical staining of small cell lung carcinoma in specimens from transbronchial and open-lung biopsies. Am J Clin Pathol 1994; 102: 406–414.
194. Slodkowska J: The value of immunohistochemical identification of neuroendocrine differentiation in non-small cell lung carcinoma. Rocz Akad Med Bialymst 1997; 42(suppl 1): 23–27.
195. Al-Saffar N, White A, Moore M, Hasleton PS: Immunoreactivity of various peptides in typical and atypical bronchopulmonary carcinoid tumors. Br J Cancer 1988; 58: 762–766.
196. Couce ME, Bautista D, Costa J, Carter D: Analysis of K-*ras*, N-*ras*, H-*ras*, and p53 in lung neuroendocrine neoplasms. Diagn Mol Pathol 1999; 8: 71–79.
197. Roncalli M, Doglioni C, Springall DR, et al.: Abnormal p53 expression in lung neuroendocrine tumors. Diagnostic and prognostic implications. Diag Molec Pathol 1992; 1: 129–135.
198. Anbazhagan R, Tihan T, Bornman DM, et al.: Classification of small cell lung cancer and pulmonary carcinoid by gene expression profiles. Cancer Res 1999; 59: 5119–5122.
199. Onuki N, Wistuba II, Travis WD, et al.: Genetic changes in the spectrum of neuroendocrine lung tumors. Cancer 1999; 85: 600–607.
200. Ullmann R, Schwendel A, Klemen H, et al.: Unbalanced chromosomal aberrations in neuroendocrine lung tumors as detected by comparative genomic hybridization. Hum Pathol 1998; 29: 1145–1149.
201. Johansson M, Heim S, Mandahl N, et al.: Cytogentic analysis of six bronchial carcinoids. Cancer Gen Cytogen 1993; 66: 33–38.
202. Jackson-York GL, David BH, Warren WH, et al.: Flow cytometric DNA content analysis in neuroendocrine carcinoma of the lung. Cancer 1991; 68: 374–379.
202a. Brambilla E, Moro D, Veale D, et al.: Basal cell (basaloid) carcinoma of the lung: a new morphologic and phenotypic entity with separate prognostic significance. Hum Pathol 1992; 23: 993–1003.
203. Travis WD, Linnoila RI, Tsokos MG, et al.: Neuroendocrine tumors of the lung with proposed criteria for large-cell neuroendocrine

carcinoma: an ultrastructural, immunohistochemical, and flow cytometric study of 35 cases. Am J Surg Pathol 1991; 15: 529–553.
204. McBurney RP, Kirklin JW, Woolner LB: Metastasizing bronchial adenomas. Surg Gynecol Obstet 1953; 96: 482–492.
205. Marty-Ane CH, Costes V, Pujol JL, et al.: Carcinoid tumors of the lung: do atypical features require aggressive management? Annu Thorac Surg 1995; 59: 78–83.
205a. Carretta A, Ceresoli GL, Arrigoni G, et al.: Diagnostic and therapeutic management of neuroendocrine lung tumors: a clinical study of 44 cases. Lung Cancer 2000; 29: 217–225.
206. Barnard WG. The nature of the "oat cell sarcoma" of the mediastinum. J Pathol Bacteriol 1926; 29: 241–244.
207. Azzopardi JG: Oat cell carcinoma of the bronchus. J Pathol Bacteriol 1959; 78: 513–519.
208. Cook RM, Miller YE, Bunn PA Jr: Small cell lung cancer: etiology, biology, clinical features, staging, and treatment. Curr Probl Cancer 1993; 17: 69–141.
209. Perkins PJ: Delayed onset of secondary hypertrophic osteoarthropathy. Am J Roentgenol 1978; 130: 561–562.
210. Johnson BE, Chute JP, Rushin J, et al.: A prospective study of patients with lung cancer and hyponatremia of malignancy. Am J Respir Crit Care Med 1997; 156: 1669–1678.
211. Takai E, Yano T, Iguchi H, et al.: Tumor-induced hypercalcemia and parathyroid hormone-related protein in lung carcinoma. Cancer 1996; 78: 1384–1387.
212. Ferroir JP, Milleron B, Ropert A, et al.: Atypical paraneoplastic myasthenic syndrome: Lambert–Eaton syndrome or myasthenia? Rev Pneumonol Clin 1999; 55: 168–170.
213. Posner JB: Paraneoplastic syndromes: a brief review. Ann NY Acad Sci 1997; 835: 83–90.
214. Thirkill CE: Lung cancer-induced blindness. Lung Cancer 1996; 14: 253–264.
215. Usalan C, Emri S: Membranoproliferative glomerulonephritis associated with small cell lung carcinoma. Int Urol Nephrol 1998; 30: 209–213.
216. Brenner S, Golan H, Gat A, Bialy-Golan A: Paraneoplastic subacute cutaneous lupus erythematosus: report of a case associated with cancer of the lung. Dermatology 1997; 194: 172–174.
217. Hsu CW, Wang HC, Lu JY: Small cell lung carcinoma associated with paraneoplastic limbic encephalitis. J Formos Med Assoc 1999; 18: 368–371.
218. Kamiyoshihara M, Hirai T, Kawashima O, Ishikawa S, Morishita Y: Sarcoid reactions in primary pulmonary carcinoma: report of seven cases. Oncol Rep 1998; 5: 177–180.
219. Conejo-Mir JS, Casals M, Carciandia C, et al.: Cutaneous sarcoid granulomas with oat cell carcinoma of the lung. Dermatology 1995; 191: 59–61.
220. Ponge T, Boutoille D, Moreau A, et al.: Systemic vasculitis in a patient with small-cell neuroendocrine bronchial cancer. Eur Respir J 1998; 12: 1228–1229.
221. Krauss EA, Ludwig PW, Sumner HW: Metastatic carcinoma presenting as fulminant hepatic failure. Am J Gastroenterol 1979; 72: 651–654.
222. Horlyck A, Henriques U, Jakobsen A: The value of bone marrow examination in small cell carcinoma. Acta Oncol 1994; 33: 909–911.
223. Tritz DB, Doll DC, Ringenberg QS, et al.: Bone marrow involvement in small cell lung cancer: clinical significance and correlation with routine laboratory values. Cancer 1989; 63: 763–766.
224. Nguyen LN, Maor MH, Oswald MJ: Brain metastases as the only manifestation of an undetected primary tumor. Cancer 1998; 83: 2181–2184.
225. Falconieri G, Zanconati F, Bussani R, DiBonito L: Small cell carcinoma of lung simulating pleural mesothelioma: report of 4 cases with autopsy confirmation. Pathol Res Pract 1995; 191: 1147–1152.
226. Yesner R: Small cell tumors of the lung. Am J Surg Pathol 1983; 7: 775–785.
227. Carter D: Small cell carcinoma of the lung. Am J Surg Pathol 1983; 7: 787–795.
228. Aisner SC, Finkelstein DM, Ettinger DS, et al.: The clinical significance of variant morphology small cell carcinoma of the lung. J Clin Oncol 1990; 8: 402–408.
229. Bepler G, Neumann K, Holle R, et al.: Clinical relevance of histologic subtyping in small cell lung cancer. Cancer 1980; 45: 74–79.
230. Hirsch FR, Matthews MJ, Aisner SC, et al.: Histopathologic classification of small cell lung cancer: changing concepts and terminology. Cancer 1988; 62: 973–977.
231. Hirsch FR, Matthews MJ, Yesner R: Histopathologic classification of small cell carcinoma of the lung: comments based on an interobserver examination. Cancer 1982; 50: 1360–1366.
232. Magum MD, Greco FA, Hainsworth JD, et al.: Combined small cell and non-small cell lung cancer. J Clin Oncol 1989; 7: 607–612.
233. Sehested M, Hirsch FR, Osterlind K, et al.: Morphologic variations of small cell lung cancer: a histopathologic study of pretreatment and posttreatment specimens in 104 patients. Cancer 1986; 57: 805–807.
234. Thomas JS, Lamb D, Ashcroft T, et al.: How reliable is the diagnosis of lung cancer using small biopsy specimens? Report of a UKCCCR Lung Cancer Working Party. Thorax 1993; 48: 1135–1139.
235. Vollmer RT: The effect of cell size on the pathologic diagnosis of small and large cell carcinomas of the lung. Cancer 1982; 50: 1380–1383.
236. Fushimi H, Kukui M, Morino H, et al.: Detection of large cell component in small cell lung carcinoma by combined cytologic and histologic examinations and its clinical implication. Cancer 1992; 70: 599–605.
236a. Nicholson SA, Beasley MB, Brambilla E, et al.: Small cell lung carcinoma (SCLC): a clinicopathologic study of 100 cases with surgical specimens. Am J Surg Pathol 2002; 26: 1184–1197.
237. Facilone F, Cimmino A, Assennato G, et al.: What is the prognostic significance of histomorphology in small cell lung carcinoma? Pathologica 1993; 85: 387–393.
238. Fraire AE, Johnson EH, Yesner R, et al.: Prognostic significance of histopathologic subtype and stage in small cell lung cancer. Hum Pathol 1992; 23: 520–528.
238a. Yang YJ, Steele CT, Ou XL, Snyder KP, Kohman LJ: Diagnosis of high-grade pulmonary neuroendocrine carcinoma by fine-needle aspiration biopsy: nonsmall-cell or small-cell type? Diagn Cytopathol 2001; 25: 292–300.
238b. Nicholson SA, Ryan MR: A review of cytologic findings in neuroendocrine carcinomas including carcinoid tumors with histologic correlation. Cancer 2000; 90: 148–161.
239. Tome Y, Hirohashi S, Noguchi M, et al.: Immunocytologic diagnosis of small cell lung cancer in imprint smears. Acta Cytol 1991; 35: 485–490.
240. Gephardt GN, Grady KJ, Ahmad M, et al.: Peripheral small cell undifferentiated carcinoma of the lung: clinicopathologic features of 17 cases. Cancer 1988; 61: 1002–1008.
241. Hamzik J, Vrastyak J, Janik M, et al.: Surgical treatment of small cell pulmonary carcinoma. Rozhledy V Chir 1994; 73: 106–109.
242. Mentzer SJ, Reilly JJ, Sugarbaker DJ: Surgical resection in the management of small cell carcinoma of the lung. Chest 1993; 103(suppl): 349S–351S.
243. Smit EF, Croen HJ, Timens W, deBoer WJ, Postmus PE: Surgical resection for small cell carcinoma of the lung: a retrospective study. Thorax 1994; 49: 20–22.
244. Ishida T, Nishino T, Oka T, et al.: Surgical treatment of patients with small cell carcinoma of the lung: a histochemical and immunohistochemical study. J Surg Oncol 1989; 40: 188–193.
245. Shepherd FA, Ginsberg RJ, Feld R, Evans WK, Johansen E: Surgical treatment for limited small-cell lung cancer: the University of Toronto Lung Oncology Group experience. J Thorac Cardiovasc Surg 1991; 101: 385–393.
246. Shepherd FA, Ginsberg RJ, Patterson GA, et al.: Is there ever a role for salvage operations in limited small cell lung cancer? J Thorac Cardiovasc Surg 1991; 101: 196–200.
247. Bunn PA Jr, Carney DN: Overview of chemotherapy for small cell lung cancer. Semin Oncol 1997; 24(2 suppl 7): S69–S74.
248. Comis RL: Developments in therapy for extensive disease small cell lung cancer. Semin Oncol 1992; 19(6 suppl 13): 45–50.
248a. Marchevsky AM, Gal AA, Shah S, Koss MN: Morphometry confirms the presence of considerable nuclear size overlap between "small cells" and "large cells" in high-grade pulmonary neuroendocrine neoplasms. Am J Clin Pathol 2001; 116: 466–472.
248b. Wiatrowska BA, Krol J, Zakowski MF: Large-cell neuroendocrine carcinoma of the lung: proposed criteria for cytologic diagnosis. Diagn Cytopathol 2001; 24: 58–64.
248c. Brambilla E, Lanteujoul S, Sturm N: Divergent differentiation in neuroendocrine lung tumors. Semin Diagn Pathol 2000; 17: 138–148.

249. Warren WH, Gould VE: Differential diagnosis of small cell neuroendocrine carcinoma of the lung. Chest Surg Clin N Am 1997; 7: 49–63.

249a. Brambilla E, Travis WD, Colby TV, Corrin B, Shimosato Y: The new World Health Organization classification of lung tumors. Eur Respir J 2001; 18: 1059–1068.

250. Nandedkar MA, Palazzo J, Abbondanzo SL, Lasota J, Miettinen M: CD45 (leukocyte common antigen) immunoreactivity in metastatic undifferentiated and neuroendocrine carcinoma: a potential diagnostic pitfall. Mod Pathol 1998; 11: 1204–1210.

251. Copple B, Wright SE, Moatamed F: Electron microscopy in small cell lung carcinomas: clinical correlations. J Clin Oncol 1984; 2: 910–916.

251a. Garcia-Yuste M, Matilla JM, Alvarez-Gago T, et al.: Prognostic factors in neuroendocrine lung tumors: a Spanish multicenter study: Spanish multicenter study of neuroendocrine tumors of the lung of the Spanish Society of Pneumonology and Thoracic Surgery (EMETNE-SEPAR). Ann Thorac Surg 2000; 70: 258–263.

251b. Cooper WA, Thourani VH, Gal AA, et al.: The surgical spectrum of pulmonary neuroendocrine neoplasms. Chest 2001; 119: 14–18.

251c. Huang Q, Muzitansky A, Mark EJ: Pulmonary neuroendocrine carcinomas: a review of 234 cases and a statistical analysis of 50 cases treated at one institution using a simple clinicopathologic classification. Arch Pathol Lab Med 2002; 126: 545–553.

252. Vollmer RT, Shelburne JD, Igelhart JD: Intercellular junctions and tumor stage in small cell carcinoma of the lung. Hum Pathol 1986; 18: 22–27.

253. Hosoe S, Shigedo Y, Ueno K, et al.: Detailed deletion mapping of the short arm of chromosome 3 in small cell and non-small cell carcinoma of the lung. Lung Cancer 1994; 20: 297–305.

254. Vuitch F, Sekido Y, Fong K, et al.: Neuroendocrine tumors of the lung: pathology and molecular biology. Chest Surg Clin N Am 1997; 7: 21–47.

255. Kovatich A, Friedland DM, Druck T, et al.: Molecular alterations to human chromosome 3q loci in neuroendocrine lung tumors. Cancer 1998; 83: 1109–1117.

255a. Flieder DB: Neuroendocrine tumors of the lung: recent developments in histopathology. Curr Opin Pulm Med 2002; 8: 275–280.

256. Williams CL: Basic science of small cell lung cancer. Chest Surg Clin N Am 1997; 7: 1–19.

257. Jiang SX, Kameya T, Shoji M, et al.: Large cell neuroendocrine carcinoma of the lung: a histologic and immunohistochemical study of 22 cases. Am J Surg Pathol 1998; 22: 526–537.

258. Dresler CM, Ritter JH, Patterson GA, et al.: Clinical-pathologic analysis of 40 patients with large cell neuroendocrine carcinoma of the lung. Ann Thorac Surg 1997; 63; 180–185.

258a. Takei H, Asamura H, Maeshima, et al.: Large cell neuroendocrine carcinoma of the lung: a clinicopathologic study of eighty-seven cases. J Thorac Cardiovasc Surg 2002; 124: 285–292.

258b. Jung KJ, Lee KS, Han J, et al.: Large cell neuroendocrine carcinoma of the lung: clinical, CT, and pathologic findings in 11 patients. J Thorac Imaging 2001; 16: 156–162.

258c. Iyoda A, Hiroshima K, Toyozaki T, et al.: Clinical characterization of pulmonary large-cell neuroendocrine carcinoma and large-cell carcinoma with neuroendocrine morphology. Cancer 2001; 91: 1992–2000.

258d. Shin AR, Shin BK, Choi JA, et al.: Large-cell neuroendocrine carcinoma of the lung: radiologic and pathologic findings. J Comput Assist Tomogr 2000; 24: 567–573.

259. Demirer T, Ravits J, Aboulafia D: Myasthenic (Eaton–Lambert) syndrome associated with pulmonary large cell neuroendocrine carcinoma. South Med J 1994; 87: 1186–1189.

260. Stanford MR, Edelstein CE, Hughes JD, et al.: Paraneoplastic retinopathy in association with large cell neuroendocrine bronchial carcinoma. Br J Ophthalmol 1995; 79: 617–618.

261. Chetty R, Bhana B, Batitang S, Govender D: Lung carcinoma composed of rhabdoid cells. Eur J Surg Oncol 1997; 23: 432–434.

261a. Khalifa M, Hruby G, Ehrlich L, Danjoux C, Perez-Ordonez B: Combined large cell neuroendocrine carcinoma and spindle cell carcinoma of the lung. Ann Diagn Pathol 2001; 5: 240–245.

261b. Oliaro A, Filosso PL, Donati G, Ruffini E: Atypical bronchial carcinoids: review of 46 patients. J Cardiovasc Surg 2000; 41: 131–135.

262. Franklin WA: Diagnosis of lung cancer: pathology of invasive and preinvasive neoplasia. Chest 2000; 117(4 suppl 1): 80S–89S.

262a. Ullmann R, Petzmann S, Sharma A, Cagle PT, Popper HH: Chromosomal aberrations in a series of large-cell neuroendocrine carcinomas: unexpected divergence from small-cell carcinoma of the lung. Hum Pathol 2001; 32: 1059–1063.

263. Lai SL, Goldstein LJ, Gottesman MM, et al.: MDR1 gene expression in lung cancer. J Natl Cancer Inst USA 1989; 81: 1144–1150.

264. DeLellis RA, Tischler AS. Wolfe HJ: Multidirectional differentiation in neuroendocrine neoplasms. J Histochem Cytochem 1984; 32: 899–904.

265. Gaffey MJ, Mills SE, Lack EE: Neuroendocrine carcinoma of the colon and rectum. Am J Surg Pathol 1990; 14: 1010–1023.

266. Chejfec G, Capella C, Solcia E, et al.: Amphicrine cells, dysplasias, and neoplasias. Cancer 1985; 56: 2683–2690.

267. Eusebi V, Capella C, Bondi A, et al.: Endocrine-paracrine cells in pancreatic exocrine carcinomas. Histopathology 1981; 9: 599–613.

268. Groben P, Reddick R, Askin FB: The pathologic spectrum of small cell carcinoma of the cervix. Int J Gynecol Pathol 1985; 4: 42–47.

269. Hales M, Rosenau W, Okerlund MD, Galante M: Carcinoma of the thyroid with a mixed medullary and follicular pattern. Cancer 1982; 50: 1352–1359.

270. Lewin K: Carcinoid tumors and the mixed (composite) glandular-endocrine cell carcinomas. Am J Surg Pathol 1987; 11(suppl 1): 71–76.

271. Manivel JC, Wick MR, Sibley RK: Neuroendocrine differentiation in Mullerian neoplasms. Am J Clin Pathol 1986; 86: 438–443.

272. McCluggage WG, Napier SS, Primrose WJ, Adair A, Toner PG: Sinonasal neuroendocrine carcinoma exhibiting amphicrine differentiation. Histopathology 1995; 27: 79–82.

273. Mills SE, Wolfe JT, Weiss MA, et al.: Small cell undifferentiated carcinoma of the urinary bladder. Am J Surg Pathol 1987; 11: 606–617.

274. Reid JD, Yuh SL, Petrelli M, Jaffe R: Ductoinsular tumors of the pancreas. Cancer 1982; 49: 908–915.

275. Silva EG, Mackay B, Goepfert H, et al.: Endocrine carcinoma of the skin (Merkel cell carcinoma). Pathol Annu 1984; 19(1): 1–30.

276. Brambilla E, Lanteujoul S, Sturm N: Divergent differentiation in neuroendocrine lung tumors. Semin Diagn Pathol 2000; 17: 138–148.

277. Sen F, Borczuk AC: Combined carcinoid tumor of the lung: a combination of carcinoid and adenocarcinoma. Lung Cancer 1998; 21: 53–58.

278. Frank GA, Trakhtenberg AK, Boguslavskii VM: The prognosis of small cell carcinoma and malignant carcinoid of the lung. Vopr Onkol 1989; 35: 192–198.

279. Mooi WJ, Dewar A, Springall D, et al.: Non-small cell lung carcinomas with neuroendocrine features: a light microscopic, immunohisto-chemical, and ultrastructural study of 11 cases. Histopathology 1988; 13: 329–337.

280. Otto WR: Lung stem cells. Int J Exp Pathol 1997; 78: 291–310.

280a. Huang J, Behrens C, Wistuba II, Gazdar AF, Jagirdar J: Clonality of combined tumors. Arch Pathol Lab Med 2002; 126: 437–441.

281. Piehl MR, Gould VE, Warren WH, et al.: Immunohistochemical identification of exocrine and neuroendocrine subsets of large cell lung carcinomas. Pathol Res Pract 1988; 183: 675–682.

282. Neal MH, Kosinski R, Cohen P, et al.: Atypical endocrine tumors of the lung: a histologic, ultrastructural, and clinical study of 19 cases. Hum Pathol 1986; 17: 1264–1277.

283. Visscher DW, Zarbo RJ, Trojanowski JQ, et al.: Neuroendocrine differentiation in poorly differentiated lung carcinomas: a light microscopic and immunohistologic study. Mod Pathol 1990; 3: 508–512.

284. Skov BG, Sorenson JB, Hirsch FR , et al.: Prognostic impact of histologic demonstration chromogranin A and neuron specific enolase in pulmonary adenocarcinoma. Ann Oncol 1991; 2: 355–360.

285. Linnoila RI, Gazdar AF. Non-small cell lung carcinoma with neuroendocrine features. Anat Pathol 1990; 18: 1–5.

286. Linnoila RI, Mulshine JL, Steinberg SM, et al.: Neuroendocrine differentiation in endocrine and nonendocrine lung carcinomas. Am J Clin Pathol 1988; 90: 641–652.

287. Hammond ME, Sause WT: Large cell neuroendocrine tumors of the lung: clinical significance and histopathologic definition. Cancer 1985; 56: 1624–1629.

288. Berendsen HH, Deleij L, Poppema S: Clinical characterization of non-small cell lung cancer tumors showing neuroendocrine differentiation features. J Clin Oncol 1989; 7: 1614–1629.

288a. Hiroshima K, Iyoda A, Shibuya K, et al.: Prognostic significance of neuroendocrine differentiation in adenocarcinoma of the lung. Ann Thorac Surg 2002; 73: 1732–1735.

288b. Carnaghi C, Rimassa L, Garassino I, Santoro A: Clinical significance of neuroendocrine phenotype in non-small-cell lung cancer. Ann Oncol 2001; 12(suppl 2): S119–S123.
288c. Baldi A, Groger AM, Esposito V, et al.: Neuroendocrine differentiation in non-small-cell lung carcinomas. In Vivo 2000; 14: 109–114.
288d. Fresvig A, Qvigstad G, Halvorsen TB, Falkmer S, Waldum HL: Neuroendocrine differentiation in bronchial carcinomas of classic squamous cell type: an immunohistochemical study of 29 cases applying the tyramide signal amplification technique. Appl Immunohistochem Mol Morphol 2001; 9: 9–13.
289. Churg A: The fine structure of large cell undifferentiated carcinoma of the lung: evidence for its relation to squamous cell carcinomas and adenocarcinomas. Hum Pathol 1978; 9: 143–156.
290. Baldi A, Groger AM, Esposito V, et al.: Neuroendocrine differentiation in non-small cell lung carcinomas. In Vivo 2000; 14: 109–114.
291. Nakatani Y, Kitamura H, Inayama Y, et al.: Pulmonary adenocarcinoma of the fetal lung type: a clinicopathologic study indicating differences in histology, epidemiology, and natural history of low-grade and high-grade forms. Am J Surg Pathol 1998; 22: 399–411.
292. Chetritt J, Fiche M, Cassagnau E, et al.: Pulmonary endodermal tumor resembling fetal lung: low grade adenocarcinoma of the fetal lung type. Ann Pathol 1999; 19: 116–118.
293. Abbona G, Papotti M, Viberti L, et al.: Chromogranin A gene expression in non-small cell lung carcinomas. J Pathol 1998; 186: 151–156.
294. Leong ASY, Wick MR, Swanson PE: Immunohistology & electron microscopy of anaplastic & pleomorphic tumors. 1997, Cambridge University Press, Cambridge, UK, pp 161–208.
295. Graziano SL, Mazid R, Newman N, et al.: The use of neuroendocrine immunoperoxidase markers to predict chemotherapy response in patients with non-small-cell lung cancer. J Clin Oncol 1989; 7: 1398–1406.
296. Hainsworth JD, Johnson DH, Greco FA: Poorly-differentiated neuroendocrine carcinoma of unknown primary site: a newly recognized clinicopathologic entity. Ann Intern Med 1988; 109: 364–371.
297. Hainsworth JD, Wright EP, Johnson DH, et al.: Poorly differentiated carcinoma of unknown primary site: clinical usefulness of immunoperoxidase staining. J Clin Oncol 1991; 9: 1931-1938.
298. Schleusener J, Tazelaar H, Jung S: Neuroendocrine differentiation correlates with survival in chemotherapy treated non-small cell lung cancer [abstract]. Lab Invest 1995; 72: 153A.
299. Wertzel H, Grahmann PR, Bansbach S, et al.: Results after surgery in undifferentiated large cell carcinoma of the lung: the role of neuroendocrine expression. Eur J Cardiothorac Surg 1997; 12: 698–702.
300. Lack EE: Pathology of adrenal & extraadrenal paraganglia. 1994, WB Saunders, Philadelphia, pp 1–350.
301. Goodman ML, Laforet EG: Solitary primary chemodectomas of the lung. Chest 1972; 61: 48–60.
302. Siingh G, Lee RE, Brooks DH: Primary pulmonary paraganglioma: report of a case and review of the literature. Cancer 1977; 40; 2286–2289.
303. DeLuise VP, Holman CW, Gray GF: Primary pulmonary paraganglioma. NY State J Med 1977; 77: 2270–2271.
304. Hangartner JR, Loosemore TM, Burke M, Pepper JR: Malignant primary pulmonary paraganglioma. Thorax 1989; 44: 154–156.
305. Dusseldorf M, Straaten HG: Primary pulmonary paraganglioma. Zentralbl Chir 1990; 115: 1575–1578.
306. Lemonick DM, Pai PB, Hines GL: Malignant primary pulmonary paraganglioma with hilar metastasis. J Thorac Cardiovasc Surg 1990; 99: 563–564.
307. Vuorela AL, Anttinen J: Primary chemodectoma of the lung. Am J Roentgenol 1993; 161: 1111–1112.
308. Hagemeyer O, Gabius HJ, Kayser K: Paraganglioma of the lung –developed after exposure to nuclear radiation by the Tschernobyl atomic reactor accident? Respiration 1994; 61: 236–239.
309. Skodt V, Jacobsen GK, Helsted M: Primary paraganglioma of the lung: report of two cases and review of the literature. APMIS 1995; 103: 597–603.
310. Saeki T, Akiba T, Joh K, et al.: An extremely large solitary primary paraganglioma of the lung: report of a case. Surg Today 1999; 29: 1195–1200.
310a. Hironaka M, Fukayama M, Takayashiki N, et al.: Pulmonary gangliocytic paraganglioma: case report and comparative immunohistochemical study of related neuroendocrine neoplasms. Am J Surg Pathol 2001; 25: 688–693.
311. Rossel M, Pasini A, Chappuis S, et al.: Distinct biological properties of two RET isoforms activated by MEN2A and MEN2B mutations. Oncogene 1997; 14: 265–275.
312. Linnoila RI, Keiser HR, Steinberg SM, Lack EE: Histopathology of benign versus malignant sympathoadrenal paragangliomas: clinicopathologic study of 120 cases including unusual histologic features. Hum Pathol 1990; 21: 1168–1180.
313. Engzell V, Franzen S, Zajicek J: Aspiration biopsy of tumors of the neck. II. Cytologic findings in 13 cases of carotid body tumors. Acta Cytol 1971; 15: 25–30.
314. Gonzalez-Campora R, Otal-Salaverri C, Panea-Flores P, et al.: Fine needle aspiration cytology of paraganglionic tumors. Acta Cytol 1988; 32: 386–390.
315. Hood IC, Qizilbash AH, Young JEH, Archibald SD: Fine needle aspiration biopsy cytology of paragangliomas. Acta Cytol 1983; 27: 651–657.
316. Fournel P, Boucheron S, Baril A, Gounot J, Emonot A: Intrapulmonary chemodectoma: a new case with ultrastructural study. Rev Pneumonol Clin 1986; 42: 250–253.
317. Trojanowski JQ: Neurofilament and glial filament proteins. In: Monoclonal antibodies in diagnostic immunohistochemistry, Wick MR, Siegal GP, Eds. 1988, Marcel Dekker, New York, pp 115–146.
318. Ichinose H, Hewitt RL, Drapanas T: Minute pulmonary chemodectoma. Cancer 1971; 28: 692–700.
319. Churg AM, Warnock ML: So-called "minute pulmonary chemodectoma": a tumor not related to paragangliomas. Cancer 1976; 37: 1759–1769.
320. Gaffey MJ, Mills SE, Askin FB: Minute pulmonary meningothelial-like nodules: a clinicopathologic study of so-called minute pulmonary chemodectoma. Am J Surg Pathol 1988; 12: 167–175.
321. Niho S, Yokose T, Nishiwaki Y, Mukai K: Immunohistochemical and clonal analysis of minute pulmonary meningothelial-like nodules. Hum Pathol 1999; 30: 425–429.
322. Helman LJ, Cohen PS, Averbuch SD, et al.: Neuropeptide Y distinguishes benign from malignant pheochromocytoma. J Clin Oncol 1989; 7: 720–725.
323. Schroder HD, Johannsen L: Demonstration of S100 protein in sustentacular cells of pheochromocytomas and paragangliomas. Histopathology 1986; 10: 1023–1033.
324. Gonzalez-Campora R, Diaz-Cano S, Lerma-Puertas E, et al.: Paragangliomas: static cytometric studies of nuclear DNA patterns. Cancer 1993; 71: 820–824.
325. Pang LC, Tsao KC: Flow cytometric DNA analysis for the determination of malignant potential in adrenal and extra-adrenal pheochromocytomas or paragangliomas. Arch Pathol Lab Med 1993; 117: 1142–1147.
326. Imamura F, Funakoshi T, Nakamura S, et al.: Primary primitive neuroectodermal tumor of the lung: report of two cases. Lung Cancer 2000; 27: 55–60.
326a. Mikami Y, Nakajima M, Hashimoto H, et al.: Primary pulmonary primitive neuroectodermal tumor (PNET): a case report. Pathol Res Pract 2001; 197: 113–119.
326b. Hummel P, Yang GC, Kumar A, et al.: PNET-like features of synovial sarcoma of the lung: a pitfall in the cytologic diagnosis of soft tissue tumors. Diagn Cytopathol 2001; 24: 283–288.
327. Jaffe N: Neuroblastoma: review of the literature and an examination of factors contributing to its enigmatic character. Cancer Treat Rev 1976; 3: 61–82.
328. Young JL Jr, Miller RW: Incidence of malignant tumors in children. J Pediatr 1975; 86: 254–258.
329. Kilton LJ, Aschenbrener C, Burns CP: Ganglioneuroblastoma in adults. Cancer 1976; 37: 974–983.
330. Nagashima Y, Miyagi Y, Tanaka Y, et al.: Adult ganglioneuroblastoma of the anterior mediastinum. Pathol Res Pract 1997; 193: 727–732.
331. Cooney TP: Primary pulmonary ganglioneuroblastoma in an adult: maturation, involution, and the immune response. Histopathology 1981; 5: 451–463.
332. Hochholzer L, Moran CA, Koss MN: Primary pulmonary ganglioneuroblastoma: a clinicopathologic and

immunohistochemical study of two cases. Ann Diagn Pathol 1998; 2: 154–158.

333. Kaplan SJ, HolbrookCT, McDaniel HG, et al.: Vasoactive intestinal peptide secreting tumors of childhood. Am J Dis Childhood 1980; 134: 21–24.

334. Kenny FM, Stavrides A, Voorhess ML, Klein R: Cushing's syndrome associated with adrenal neuroblastoma. Am J Dis Childhood 1967; 113: 611–615.

335. Ikuno N, Shimokawa I, Nakamura T, Ishizaka Y, Ikeda T: *RET* oncogene expression correlates with neuronal differentiation of neuroblastic tumors. Pathol Res Pract 1995; 191: 92–99.

336. Dehner LP: Pathologic anatomy of classic neuroblastoma, including prognostic factors and differential diagnosis. In: Neuroblastoma: tumor biology & therapy, Pochedly C, Ed. 1990, CRC Press, Boca Raton, pp 111–143.

337. Hughes M, Marsden HB, Palmer MK: Histologic patterns of neuroblastoma related to prognosis and clinical stage. Cancer 1974; 34: 1706–1711.

338. Makinen J: Microscopic patterns as a guide to prognosis of neuroblastomas in childhood. Cancer 1972; 29: 1637–1646.

339. McLaughlin JE, Urich H: Maturing neuroblastoma and ganglioneuroblastoma: a study of four cases with long survival. J Pathol 1977; 121: 19–26.

340. Shimada H, Chatten J, Newton WA Jr, et al.: Histopathologic prognostic factors in neuroblastic tumors. J Natl Cancer Inst 1984; 73: 405–416.

341. Hicks MJ, Mackay B: Comparison of ultrastructural features among neuroblastic tumors: maturation from neuroblastoma to ganglioneuroma. Ultrastruct Pathol 1995; 19: 311–322.

342. Molenaar WM, Baker DL, Pleasure D, Lee VMU, Tronajowski JQ: The neuroendocrine and neural profiles of neuroblastomas, ganglioneuroblastomas, and ganglioneuromas. Am J Pathol 1990; 136: 375–382.

343. Crary GS, Singleton TP, Neglia JP, et al.: Detection of metastatic neuroblastoma in bone marrow biopsy specimens with an antibody to neuron-specific enolase. Mod Pathol 1992; 5: 308-314.

344. Cozzutto C, Carbone A: Pleomorphic (anaplastic) neuroblastoma. Arch Pathol Lab Med 1988; 112: 621–625.

345. Berthold F, Trechow R, Utsch S, Zieschang J: Prognostic factors in metastatic neuroblastoma: a multivariate analysis of 182 cases. Am J Pediatr Hematol Oncol 1992; 14: 207–215.

346. Joshi VV, Chatten J, Sather HN, Shimada H: Evaluation of the Shimada classification in advanced neuroblastoma with a special reference to the mitosis-karyorrhexis index. Mod Pathol 1991; 4: 139–147.

347. Coldman AJ, Fryer CJH, Elwood JM, Sonley MJ: Neuroblastoma: influence of age at diagnosis, stage, tumor site, and sex on prognosis. Cancer 1980; 46: 1896–1901.

348. Gitlow SE, Dziedzic LB, Strauss L, et al.: Biochemical and histologic determinants in the prognosis of neuroblastoma. Cancer 1973; 32: 898–905.

349. Kogner P, Borgstrom P, Bjellerup P, et al.: Somatostatin in neuroblastoma and ganglioneuroma. Eur J Cancer 1997; 33: 2084–2089.

350. Hayashi Y, Kanda N, Inaba T, et al.: Cytogenetic findings and prognosis in neuroblastoma with emphasis on marker chromosome 1. Cancer 1989; 63: 126–132.

351. Berthold F, Sahin K, Hero B, et al.: The current contribution of molecular factors to risk estimation in neuroblastoma patients. Eur J Cancer 1997; 33: 2092–2097.

352. Brodeur GM, Seeger RC, Sather H, et al.: Clinical implications of oncogene activation in human neuroblastomas. Cancer 1986; 58: 541–545.

353. Hashimoto H, Daimaru Y, Enjoji M, Nakagawara A: N-*myc* gene product expression in neuroblastoma. J Clin Pathol 1989; 42: 52–55.

354. Kramer K, Cheung NK, Gerald WL, et al.: Correlation of *myc*-N amplification, *Trk-A* and CD44 expression with clinical stage in 250 patients with neuroblastoma. Eur J Cancer 1997; 33: 2098–2100.

355. Ikuno N, Shimokawa I, Nakamura T, Ishizaka Y, Ikeda T: *RET* oncogene expression correlates with neuronal differentiation of neuroblastic tumors. Pathol Res Pract 1995; 191: 92–99.

356. Graham D, Magee H, Kierce B, et al.: Evaluation of Ki-67 reactivity in neuroblastoma using paraffin-embedded tissue. Pathol Res Pract 1995; 191: 87–91.

14

Sarcomas and sarcomatoid neoplasms of the lungs and pleural surfaces

Mark R Wick   Kevin O Leslie   Lisa A Cerilli   Stacey E Mills

Introduction

Primary malignant pleuropulmonary tumors showing sarcomatoid features are exceedingly uncommon. Overwhelmingly, such lesions are typically epithelial in nature; neoplasms with a mesenchymal lineage in the lung and pleura are most often proven to be *secondary*, emanating from deep soft tissue sites or the female genital tract.

In fact, *because* of the rarity of this category of pleuropulmonary malignancies, relatively few data exist in the literature regarding the morphologic or clinical details of such lesions. Hence, one can correctly anticipate that most pulmonologists, oncologists, radiologists, and pathologists are unfamiliar with intrathoracic tumors composed of spindled and pleomorphic cells.

This chapter summarizes the clinicopathologic information pertaining to such lesions. It devotes exclusive attention to *malignant* lesions, because virtually all benign mesenchymal neoplasms of the lung and pleura are straightforward diagnostic entities. "Pseudotumors" are considered in another portion of this book. Nevertheless, those pathologic categories and other lesions will indeed be mentioned in the context of differential diagnosis. The entities that are discussed are arranged in order of frequency, to give the reader a sense of their relative incidences.

Part I. Sarcomatoid carcinoma of the lung

Although they are rare in an absolute sense, sarcomatoid carcinomas represent the most common spindle cell malignancies of the airways.[1,2] True sarcomas are very infrequently seen in the tracheobronchial tree.[1–9,9a] Therefore, one usually considers a cytologically atypical spindle cell tumor of the lung to be a sarcomatoid carcinoma (SC) unless thorough immunohistological and ultrastructural studies indicate otherwise. This review will discuss neoplasms in this general category, using information taken from the pertinent literature as well as the personal experience of the authors.

Historical and terminological considerations

Controversy has existed for some time concerning the mechanisms through which obvious foci of carcinoma of the lung are admixed with malignant but nondescript spindle cell elements or tissues with a "committed" sarcomatous differentiation pattern. Also, purely spindle cell and pleomorphic pulmonary carcinomas are recognized nosologically but are incompletely characterized at a molecular level.

Morphologically similar tumors have been given a variety of designations in the upper and lower respiratory tracts. These diagnostic terms have included "blastoma," "sarcomatoid carcinoma," "spindle cell carcinoma," "squamous cell carcinoma with pseudosarcomatous stroma," "pseudosarcoma," and "carcinosarcoma," based largely on the specific microscopic attributes of the lesions in question and the conceptual leanings of the authors describing them.[10–35]

Over 60 years ago, Saphir and Vass[36] assessed the literature then extant on "carcinosarcomas," and concluded that they represented primary epithelial malignancies which had undergone divergent differentiation ("tumor metaplasia"). Their paper cited several reported lesions of the lung. Thereafter, opposing publications on "histogenesis" espoused the opinion that biphasic neoplasms of the airways were "collision" tumors, or that they reflected the proliferation of non-neoplastic mesenchymal tissue components that were induced by the carcinomatous elements.[37–39] At the turn of the last century, Krompecher[40] and others[41] had held to the same theories as those of Saphir and Vass.

In the last two decades, results of studies using electron microscopy, immunohistology, and "molecular" assays of clonality have tended to support the foresighted views of those pioneers convincingly. Hence, it is believed currently that blastomas, carcinosarcomas, carcinomas with pseudosarcomatous stroma, and sarcomatoid carcinomas comprise a single morphological spectrum of basically epithelial tumors, regardless of their anatomic locations.[29,29a,29b] "Biphasic sarcomatoid carcinoma" and "monophasic sarcomatoid carcinoma" have been proposed as replacements for the former designations of carcinosarcoma and spindle cell carcinoma, respectively.[28,29,29c] In the latest iteration of the World Health Organization nosological scheme, such lesions are included in the category designated "carcinoma with pleomorphic, sarcomatoid, or sarcomatous elements".[29b]

Clinicopathologic features of pulmonary sarcomatoid carcinomas

Clinical attributes

Sarcomatoid carcinomas (SCs) much more often arise in the large bronchi and peripheral lung fields than in the trachea, although the authors have indeed seen some lesions that took origin above the carina. The majority of individuals with pulmonary SC are men, and most have

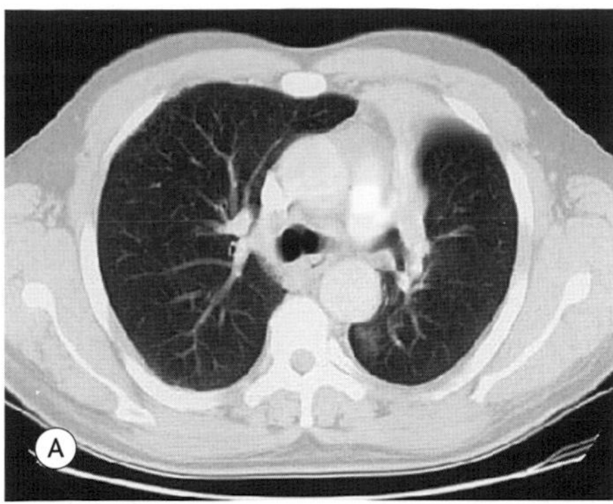

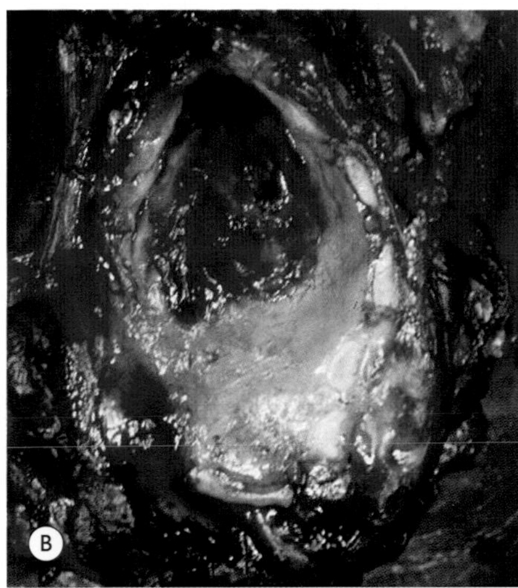

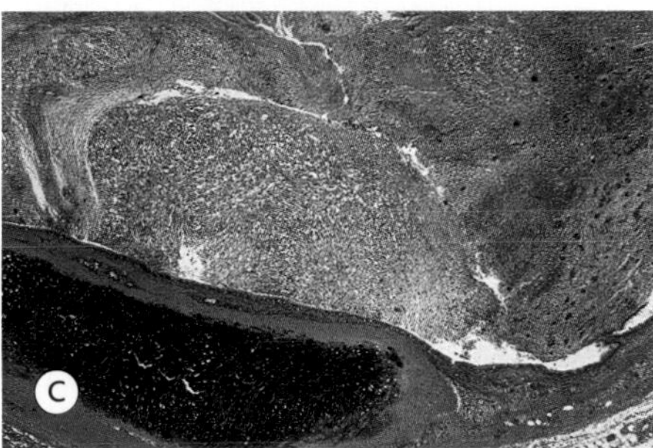

Fig. 14.1 (A) Computed tomogram showing an endobronchial mass in the left mainstem bronchus. (B,C) Resection of the lung demonstrated an endoluminal neoplasm that proved to be a sarcomatoid carcinoma.

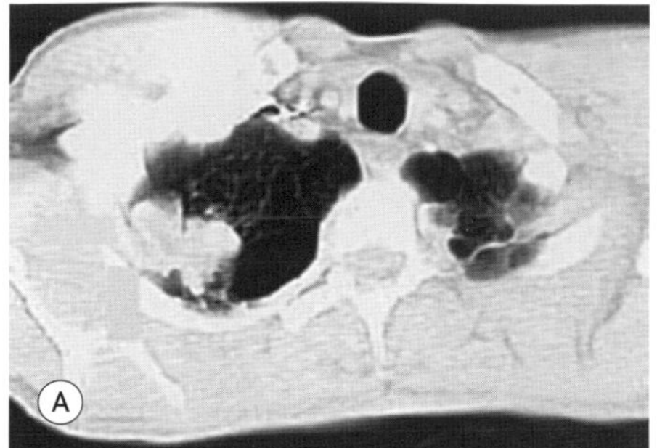

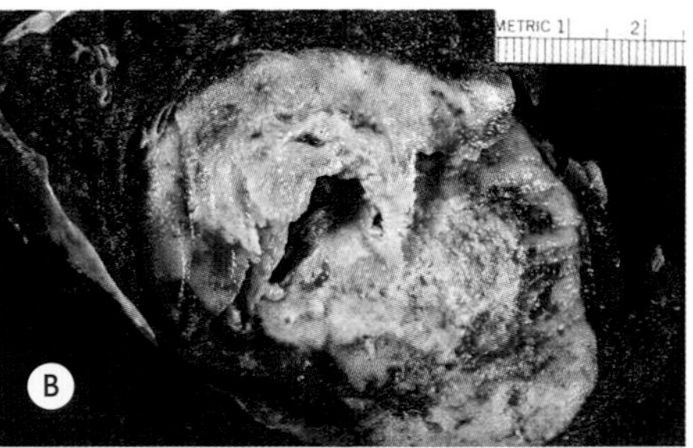

Fig. 14.2 (A) Peripheral sarcomatoid carcinoma of the right lung, as seen on a computed tomogram, and (B) in a lobectomy specimen. The tumor demonstrates prominent central necrosis.

a history of heavy smoking.[10,19,19a] The average patient age is 60 years.[28] Clinical signs and symptoms produced by these tumors are directly associated with their specific locations. Endoluminal lesions in large tubular airways characteristically cause refractory or recurrent pneumonia in the corresponding distal parenchyma, or they are associated with progressive dyspnea, cough, hemoptysis, and audible expiratory rhonchi over the affected lung field.[10–13,19,37–39,42,43] In contrast, SC in the peripheral lung often manifests no symptoms or, alternatively, presents with chest pain caused by invasion of the pleura and extrapulmonary soft tissue.[19] As might be expected, central endobronchial tumors are smaller than peripheral SCs; their average sizes are 6 cm and >10 cm, respectively[38,44] (Fig. 14.1).

In spite of their anaplastic nature, sarcomatoid carcinomas of the lung are surgically resectable in roughly 90% of cases,[19,28] and approximately one-half of patients with such neoplasms present with stage I disease. Paradoxically, however, the prognosis of pulmonary SC is still dismal. Overall 5-year survival is 20%, with a slightly better figure being associated with small, central endobronchial lesions.[19,28,44] Metastatic SC of the lung involves the same organ sites that are affected by more usual forms of lung cancer: namely, the opposite lung, liver, bones, adrenal glands, and brain.[38,43] The metastases may exhibit either carcinomatous or sarcoma-like histologic configurations.[38] Adjuvant radiation treatment and chemotherapy have been used in many cases of pulmonary SC, but these measures have provided little benefit in general.[10,28,30]

Macroscopic features

Grossly, the lesions of pulmonary SC that are >5 cm in size tend to exhibit central necrosis and hemorrhage, and they also demonstrate irregular permeation of the surrounding lung parenchyma[28,29] (Fig. 14.2). Tumors

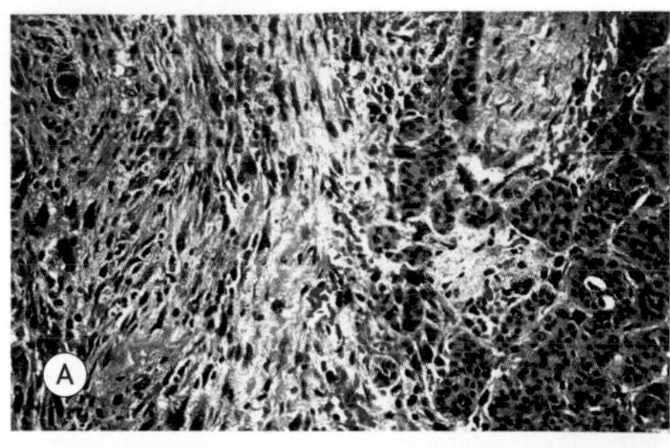

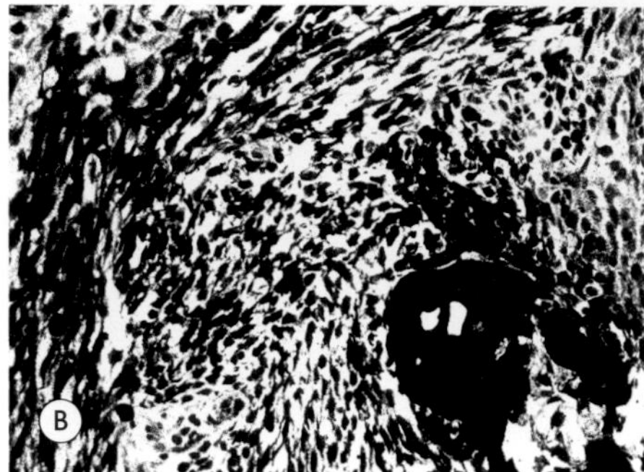

Fig. 14.3 (A) Homologous biphasic sarcomatoid carcinoma of the lung, showing overtly epithelial growth apposed to sarcoma-like pleomorphic elements. (B) An immunostain for keratin demonstrates reactivity in both neoplastic components.

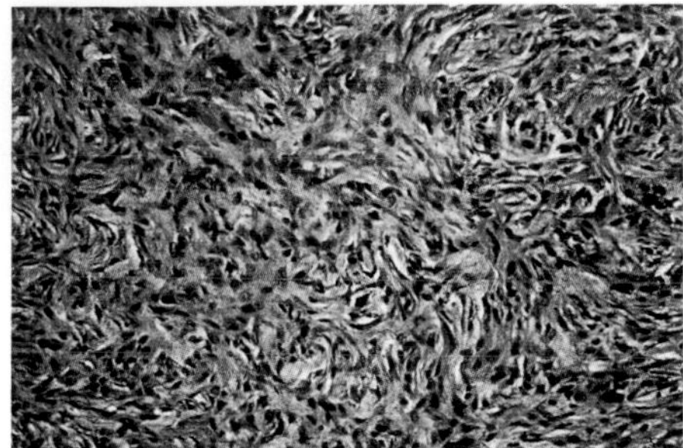

Fig. 14.4 Storiform growth of neoplastic fusiform and pleomorphic cells in sarcomatoid carcinoma of the lung, simulating malignant fibrous histiocytoma.

that are smaller and located within bronchial confines often exhibit a polypoid appearance and are attached to the subjacent mucosa by a relatively narrow stalk of tissue;[44] SCs in the peripheral lung parenchyma may have the gross appearance of conventional adenocarcinomas.[29]

Histologic characteristics

Biphasic sarcomatoid carcinomas of the lung can be divided into two subgroups, based on the nature of the stromal elements in each lesion. These variants may be called homologous and heterologous SCs.

Homologous biphasic sarcomatoid carcinomas

Variants of SC that were formerly called "spindle cell carcinomas" are constituted microscopically by a predominance of nondescript spindled and pleomophic cells, admixed with a minor, obviously carcinomatous, component. The latter portion of such lesions is generally inconspicuous and variably distributed; in roughly 40% of cases such foci are very rare, and require extensive sampling to document their presence. The general appearance of the carcinomatous elements is that of a well- to moderately-differentiated squamous malignancy in most instances, whereas adenosquamous, adenocarcinomatous, large cell undifferentiated, or neuroendocrine carcinoma is seen in a minority of cases[10,45–47,47a] (Fig. 14.3). Rare examples of this tumor type show mixtures of several carcinoma morphotypes.[46] Zones of transition between epithelial and sarcoma-like components are usually evident, at least focally.

The sarcomatoid elements of this subtype of SC lack specialized differentiation into identifiable myogenic, chondroosseous, or vasoformative tissues by standard light microscopy, and, as such, are homologous to the lung ("organ-appropriate"). They are composed of markedly heterogeneous cells with nuclear atypia and variably growth patterns. The corresponding microscopic images range from those of fibromatosis-like or low-grade fibrosarcoma-like areas – with relatively bland nuclear features, sparse mitoses, moderate-to-rich matrical collagen deposition, and a "herringbone" pattern – to others in which pleomorphic giant cells are mixed with fusiform elements showing dense cellularity, coarse chromatin, prominent nucleoli, and numerous mitoses[10–12,19,28,37] (Fig. 14.4). The last of these descriptions is closely similar to that attending spindle cell-pleomorphic malignant fibrous histiocytoma (MFH) of the soft tissues.[46] Neoplastic spindle cells often infiltrate the submucosa of small and medium-sized bronchi, which nonetheless tend to retain their mural cartilage plates and mucosal integrity.[28,29]

Sarcoma-like elements in some biphasic "spindle cell carcinomas" may include cytologically bland, osteoclast-like giant cells[44,48,49] (Fig. 14.5). The latter are admixed with atypical fusiform cells or more uniform polygonal tumor cells. Another variant histologic pattern is that in which bluntly fusiform tumor cells surround discrete zones of necrosis, producing a necrotizing granuloma-like image. Rare examples of SC may demonstrate extravasated erythrocytes between relatively bland spindled tumor cells, simulating the characteristics of Kaposi's sarcoma.[28]

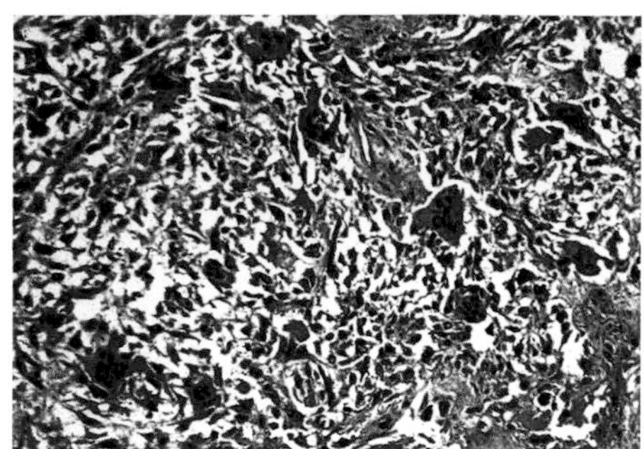

Fig. 14.5 Osteoclast-like giant cells are interspersed with the neoplastic spindle cells of this sarcomatoid pulmonary carcinoma.

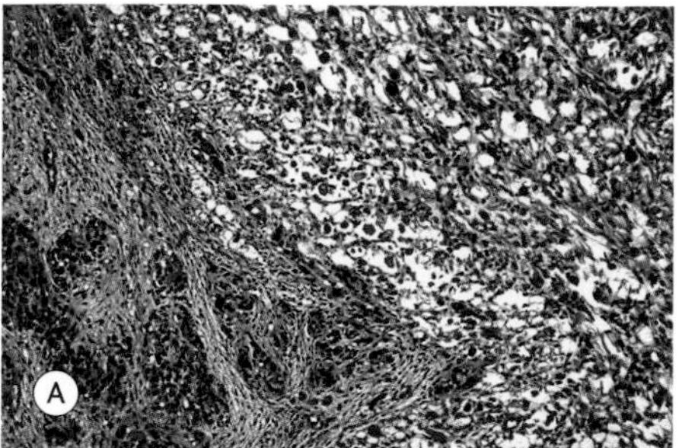

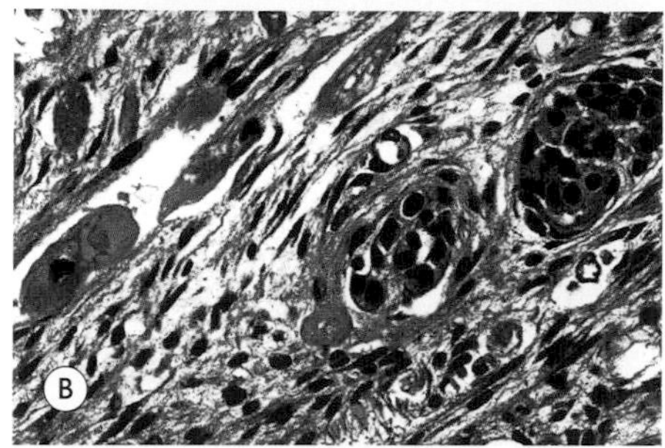

Fig. 14.6 (A) Heterologous biphasic sarcomatoid carcinoma of the lung, showing obviously epithelial elements juxtaposed to (B) rhabdomyoblast-like elements with cytoplasmic cross-striations.

Heterologous biphasic sarcomatoid carcinomas

Other biphasic sarcomatoid neoplasms differ from the descriptions just given, in regard to their content of focal myogenous or chondroosseous differentiation. Thus, they are analogous to the heterologous form of malignant mixed müllerian tumors of the uterus, ovaries, and other female genital sites.[50,51] Those neoplasms may exhibit microscopic foci that simulate embryonal or adult-type pleomorphic rhabdomyosarcoma, containing proliferations of closely apposed compact round with a slightly myxoid background, or large "strap" cells with cytoplasmic eosinophilia and cross-striations, respectively[10–12,28,29,38,44] (Fig. 14.6). Other heterologous SCs contain components that closely imitate the histologic features of osteosarcoma or chondrosarcoma.[19,29] In light of this information, it is easy to understand why lesions with such microscopic features were felt to be carcinosarcomas in the past, and are still so designated by some observers even today. The obviously carcinomatous elements in these lesions usually take the form of squamous carcinoma, but lesions with glandular or neuroendocrine differentiation have also been reported.[10,46,47] Transitional zones between obvious epithelial foci, nondescript sarcomatoid areas, and myosarcoma-like components are often evident.

With regard to the relationship between biologic behavior and histologic appearance, there is no difference in the clinical evolution of homologous and heterologous biphasic pulmonary SCs. A distinction is made between those lesions only to reflect their synonymity with sarcomatoid epithelial tumors in other body sites.[50,51]

Monophasic sarcomatoid carcinomas

Some sarcomatoid carcinomas display no conventional light microscopic evidence of epithelial differentiation whatsoever. A carcinomatous nature for these neoplasms is discerned only after immunohistochemical or ultrastructural evaluations have been done, but it is usually suspected beforehand because of the clinical and gross characteristics of the lesions.[28]

Most tumors in this category are constituted exclusively of cell populations like those in the sarcoma-like components of biphasic SCs. These potentially include foci that have an unremarkable spindle cell or pleomorphic image (Fig. 14.7), as well as areas imitating rhabdomyosarcoma, osteosarcoma, or other morphologic appearances that do not correspond to native tissues in the non-neoplastic lung. Because of the monomorphic nature of the tumor variants under discussion here – which lack any attributes of conventional lung carcinomas histologically – the corresponding diagnosis suggested by the World Health Organization criteria for pulmonary neoplasms[52] (based only on hematoxylin and eosin (H&E) stains and conventional histologic examination) would be that of a primary pulmonary *sarcoma*. The latter point has made the existence of monophasic sarcomatoid carcinoma of the lung somewhat contentious. Nevertheless, we have no doubt of its validity as a reproducible pathologic entity, and other authors appear to concur.[29a]

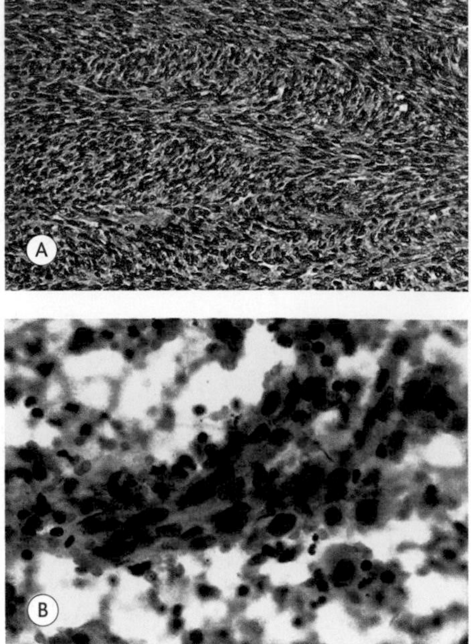

Fig. 14.7 (A) Monophasic spindle cell sarcomatoid carcinoma of the lung, simulating fibrosarcoma or monophasic synovial sarcoma. (B) A fine-needle aspiration specimen from this case demonstrates loosely cohesive aggregates of the spindle cells, and may be viewed as a generic image of all lesions discussed in this chapter.

Special variants of sarcomatoid carcinoma of the lung

There are three subtypes of SC of the lung that are deserving of additional discussion. These include the tumor known as "pulmonary blastoma," pseudoangiosarcomatous carcinoma, and inflammatory sarcomatoid carcinoma.

Pulmonary blastoma

Since its initial description by Barnett and Barnard[53] and a later discussion by Spencer,[54] pulmonary blastoma (PB) has been regarded by some observers as the pulmonary counterpart of primitive childhood tumors of other organs.[55–61] This view has been fostered in part by confusion of PB with *pleuro*pulmonary blastoma (PPB), the latter of which is primarily seen in adolescent patients.[62–68] PB is a biphasic neoplasm, containing a mixture of tubular epithelial cell profiles and compact groupings of nondescript bluntly fusiform cells with a blastema-like configuration[31,62,65] (Fig. 14.8). These resemble the elements of renal Wilms' tumors.[69] On the other hand, PPB altogether lacks epithelial differentiation and may

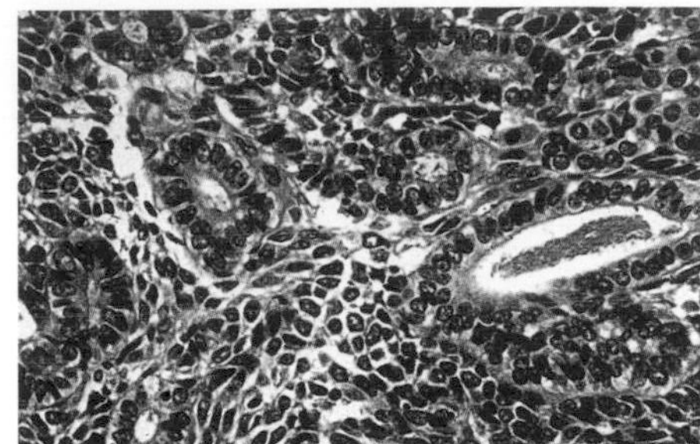

Fig. 14.8 Pulmonary "blastoma," showing an admixture of fetal glands and undifferentiated spindle cell elements. This tumor is a special morphological form of sarcomatoid carcinoma.

instead show divergent mesenchymal differentiation into myogenous or chondroosseous tissues.[65] Morever, PB shows no particular disease associations, whereas PPB is linked in a familial fashion to a number of other malignant neoplasms.[67]

If one carefully excludes examples of PPB from consideration, it becomes clear that PB is seen *overwhelmingly* in adults, and its clinical characteristics are superimposable on those of ordinary lung cancers and other pulmonary SCs. This realization allows one to more easily embrace an alternative view of the nature of PB that was advanced in the past by Souza et al.,[70] Stackhouse and colleagues,[10] and Millard,[71] among others. Those authors had the opinion that PB is merely a special, usually peripheral parenchymal form of pulmonary sarcomatoid carcinoma ("carcinosarcoma"), rather than a blastemal neoplasm which contains truly embryonal tissues. We also espouse the latter premise.

Returning to the particular microscopic attributes of PB, it should be noted that this tumor may demonstrate the same range of epithelial and mesenchymoid differentiation that is seen in other biphasic pulmonary SCs.[31,57,72] The epithelial elements in PB resemble fetal pulmonary pseudoglands (a misnomer), composed of stratified columnar cells with glycogen-rich clear cytoplasm and high nucleocytoplasmic ratios.[57,72–74] Luminal mucin may be present in those cellular arrays, and squamous morules are sometimes also evident.[57] Interestingly, "occult" neuroendocrine differentiation is a rather common finding in the epithelial components of PB, with potential histochemical argyrophilia and immunoreactivity for neuroendocrine markers.[75,76] There is a significant sharing of microscopic features between classical PB and the tumor described as "pulmonary endodermal tumor resembling fetal lung" or alternatively as "well-differentiated adenocarcinoma simulating fetal lung" (Fig. 14.9). It differs only in its relative lack of a malignant stromal component and more frequent synthesis of a particular oncofetal polypeptide – alpha-fetoprotein.[31,73,75–78] We believe that the latter lesion merely represents a polar extreme of the same continuum of neoplasms in which PB resides: namely, that of sarcomatoid carcinomas in general.

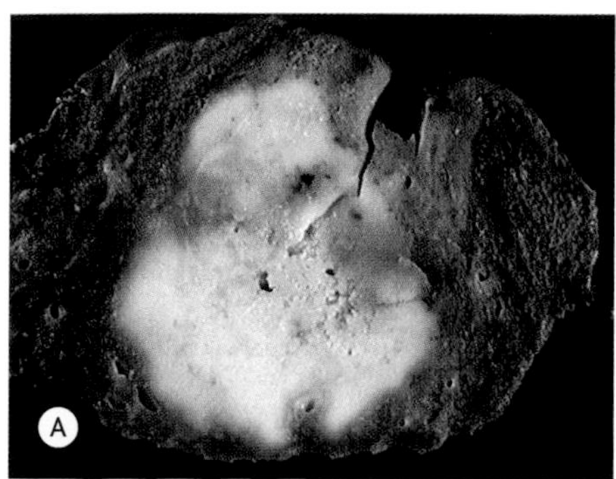

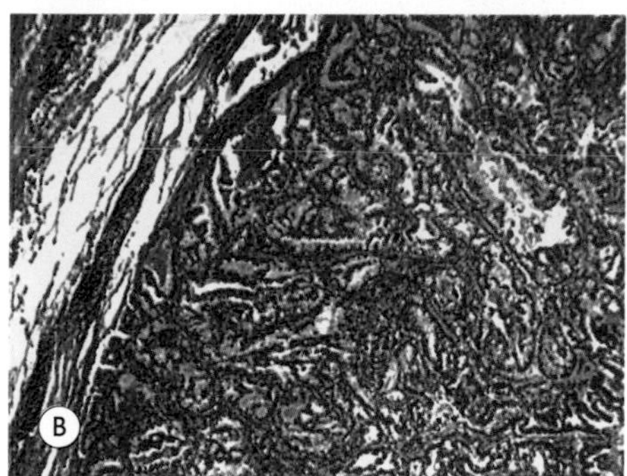

Fig. 14.9 Gross (A) and microscopic (B) images of fetal-type adenocarcinoma of the lung, representing a monophasic epithelial variant of "pulmonary blastoma." (Courtesy of Dr Samuel A Yousem, University of Pittsburgh Medical Center, Pittsburgh, PA.)

The elements of PB showing mesenchymoid differentiation are, as stated earlier, usually nondescript morphologically and blastema- or fibroblast-like. However, examples of this tumor have been documented in which heterologous rhabdomyoblastoid, leiomyosarcomatoid, or apparent chondroosseous tissues were present.[57,72] This observation serves to further solidify the relatedness of PB and other sarcomatoid pulmonary carcinomas, as do reports of some tumors in which "typical" PB was admixed with homologous or heterologous biphasic SC, as described above.[70,79,81]

The clinical behavior of PB is difficult to determine with certainty, because of the aforementioned contamination of some series with cases of PPB. However, mortality figures of 30–70% have been reported, with death usually being due to distant metastases.[55,57,72] Secondary deposits of PB may have a purely epithelial, purely mesenchymal-like, or biphasic appearance, as true of other sarcomatoid carcinomas.

Pseudoangiosarcomatous carcinoma

The authors have studied several lung tumors in which obvious squamous cell carcinoma was admixed with areas demonstrating interanastomosing channels mantled by anaplastic, plump, epithelioid cells, focally grouped into pseudopapillae. Because the open spaces in these areas contained erythrocytes and focally formed blood lakes, the histologic appearance was that of biphasic SC in which an angiosarcomatoid component was admixed with overt squamous carcinoma.[82] (Fig. 14.10). These neoplasms are felt to represent the pulmonary counter-

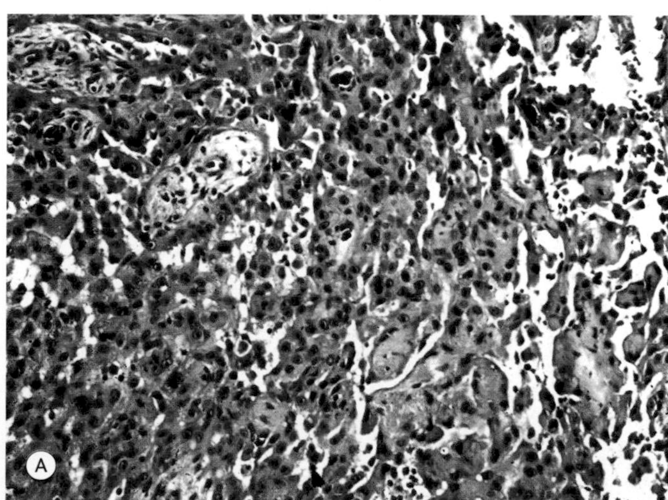

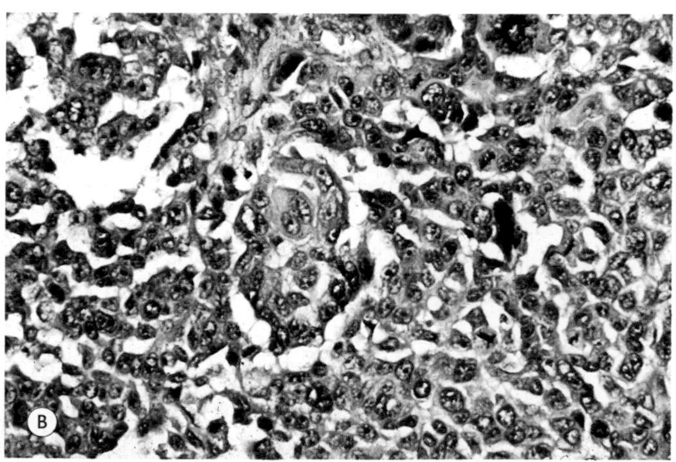

Fig. 14.10 (A) Pseudoangiosarcomatous sarcomatoid carcinoma of the lung, demonstrating dyscohesion of the neoplastic cells in a fashion simulating the image of angiosarcoma. (B) A focus of more obviously carcinomatous growth is apparent in the center of this figure.

parts of pseudovascular adenoid squamous cell carcinoma, as seen in the skin, breast, thyroid gland, and other organs.[29,82–87] This is a tumor type that is known to *simulate* true angiosarcoma but lacks actual endothelial differentiation. Thus, "pseudoangiosarcomatous carcinoma" (PASC) would be an apt synonym.[84]

Primary pulmonary angiosarcoma is, comparatively, a very rare lesion, comprising only 10% of true sarcomas of the lung in one report from the Mayo Clinic.[4] Mainly anecdotal reports of this tumor exist in the remaining literature, and not all of them satisfy rigorous diagnostic criteria.[88–96] Metastases *to* the lung from angiosarcomas arising in extrapulmonary sites are much more common, including examples that have originated in the heart, great vessels, or extrathoracic viscera.[88]

Similar to reports on previously cited pseudovascular carcinomas in other body sites, two publications have specifically considered squamous cell carcinomas of the lung that imitated angiosarcomas. The first, by Banerjee et al.,[84] showed that such tumors produced clinical symptoms and signs resembling those of ordinary types of lung cancer. They presented in the fifth to seventh decades of life; were associated with cigarette smoking, complaints of cough, weight loss, and dyspnea; and were visible on chest radiographs as well-defined central or peripheral parenchymal masses. In another series by Nappi and coworkers,[82] the tumors were essentially identical microscopically to pseudovascular squamous carcinomas of the breast and skin. Important differences between PASC and true pleuropulmonary angiosarcoma include an absence of atypical endothelial cells in stromal blood vessels surrounding the tumor mass in PASCs; less infiltrative growth through the interstitium of the lung; and, perhaps most importantly, the presence of small foci of morphologically obvious squamous cell carcinoma in most PASCs.[82]

The behavioral features of PASC are similar to those of other sarcomatoid pulmonary carcinomas. The patients studied by Nappi et al. developed distant metastases to the bones, liver, adrenal glands, and contralateral lung, and died after follow-up periods of 5 to 34 months.

Inflammatory sarcomatoid carcinoma

Much attention has been given to a group of space-occupying lesions in the lung that carry the popular but inaccurate designation of "inflammatory pseudotumors" (IPs).[89–102] These proliferations may occur in children or adults, and have been divided into "fibrohistiocytic," "plasma cell granulomatous," and "focal organizing pneumonia" types, based on their individual clinicopathological features. The nomenclature used for this group of lesions has been well-summarized by Koss[102] and Matsubara et al.[94] There is still some controversy over whether such lesions are neoplastic or reactive in nature.[103] However, the bulk of available information indicates that IPs are relatively innocuous clinical imitators of malignant neoplasms.[102] Occasional cases have been linked causally to specific infectious organisms,[104,105] but the etiologic factors associated with most pulmonary IPs are uncertain.

In contrast, primary sarcomatoid carcinoma is generally regarded as a neoplasm which may simulate pleuropulmonary mesenchymal *malignancies*, and it is typically not mentioned in discussions on the pathologic differential diagnosis of IPs. This is so because SC usually demonstrates obvious cytologic anaplasia, and lacks a significant component of inflammatory cells. Indeed, the morphologic distinction between IPs and *all* bronchogenic carcinomas (including SC) has been portrayed by some authors as an uncomplicated process.[93,96] However, we have observed several examples of pulmonary SC which exhibited surprisingly bland morphologic appearances, and which, as a result, were separable from IP *only* by thorough study and adjunctive pathologic techniques. These have been designated as examples of "inflammatory sarcomatoid carcinoma" (ISC).[106]

Examples of ISC are composed of variably densely apposed spindle cells with only modest pleomorphism, arranged haphazardly or in fascicular and storiform patterns. The stroma is at least partially myxoid in some cases, and may be prominently so. The tumors demonstrate an irregular, spiculated interface with the surrounding lung; the adjacent parenchyma exhibits interstitial fibrosis, and small nodular infiltrates of mature lymphocytes are admixed with dense collagenous tissue at the periphery of ISCs (Fig. 14.11). Focally hyalinized, keloidal-type collagen is admixed with the tumor cells in the central portions of some of these tumors, with or without small foci of central necrosis. Vascular invasion and luminal obliteration by neoplastic cells may be apparent; similarly, bronchial submucosal infiltration is another potential observation. ISCs do not contain appreciable stromal neutrophils, eosinophils, or xanthoma cells, but a moderate number of lymphocytes and plasma cells can be seen.

Cytologically, the nuclei of the tumor cells in ISCs are relatively uniform in size and spindle-shaped, with coarse chromatin and occasional small nucleoli (Fig. 14.12). Cytoplasm is moderate in amount and amphophilic. Mitoses generally average ≤ 2 per 10 high-power (×400) fields, and pathologic division figures are absent. Thorough sampling of the tumor tissue in cases of ISC

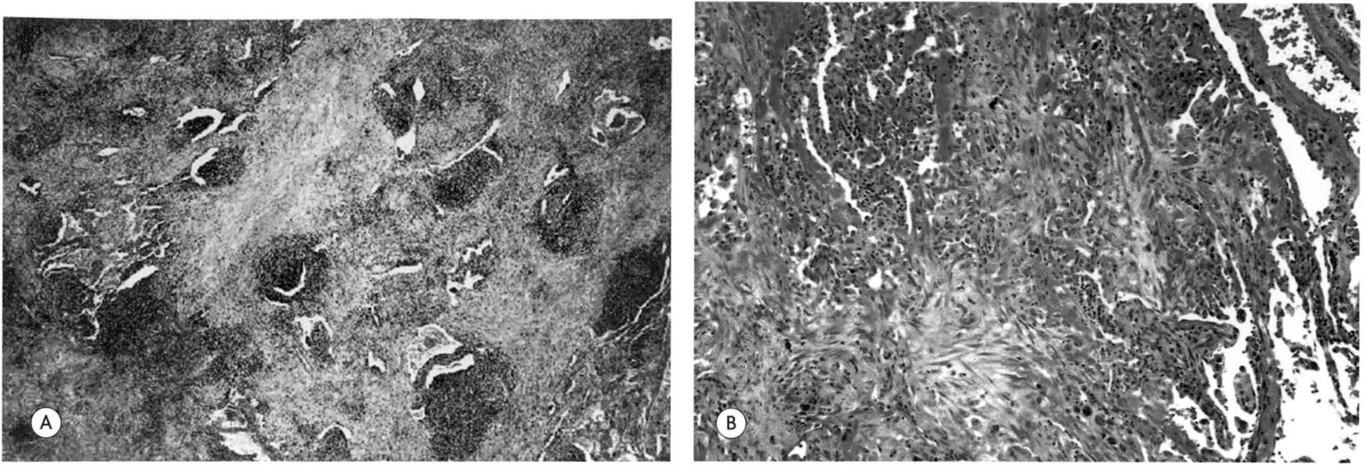

Fig. 14.11 (A) Inflammatory sarcomatoid carcinoma of the lung, showing brisk intratumoral and peritumoral chronic inflammation and (B) a bland proliferation of fibroblast-like cells at the periphery.

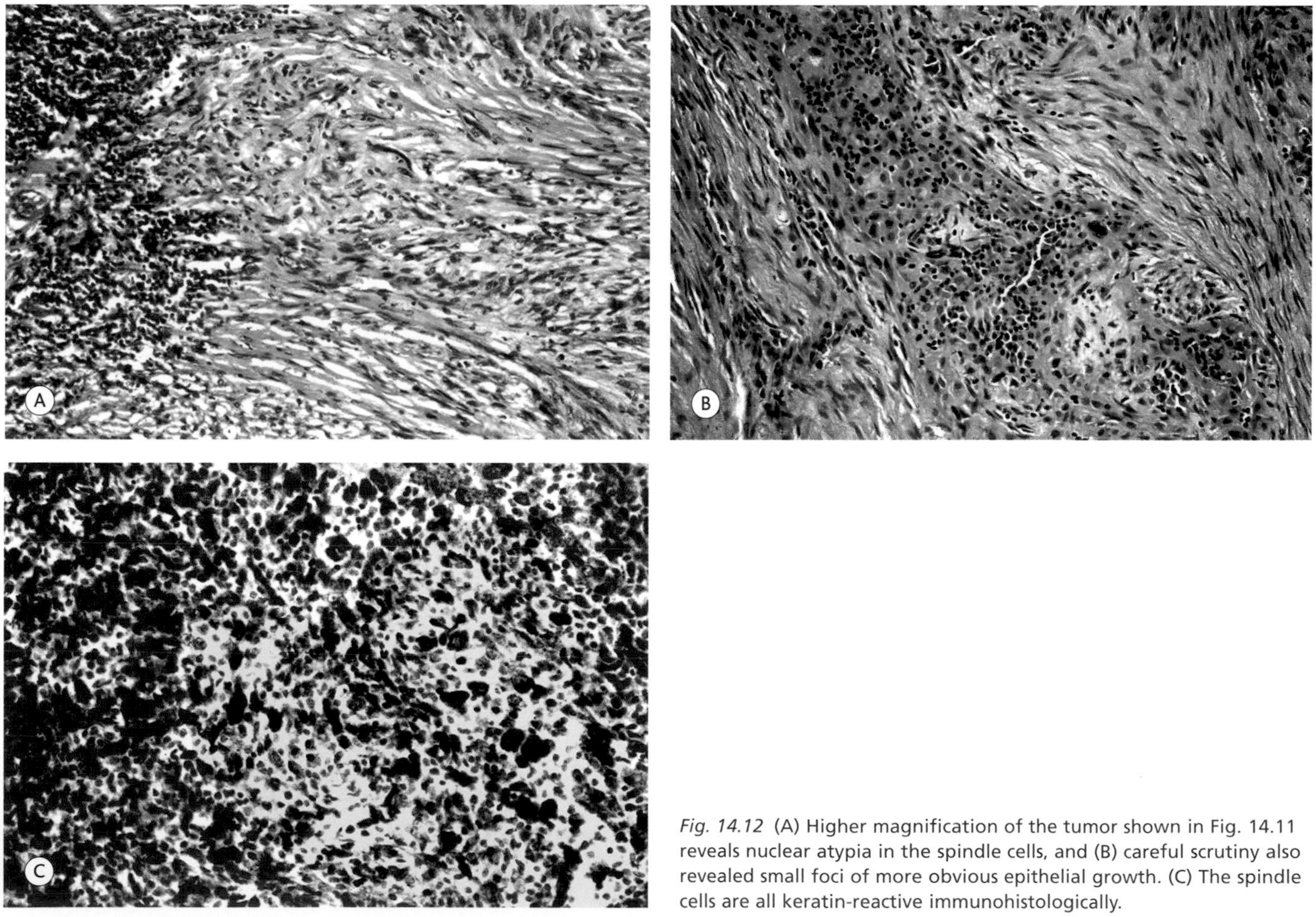

Fig. 14.12 (A) Higher magnification of the tumor shown in Fig. 14.11 reveals nuclear atypia in the spindle cells, and (B) careful scrutiny also revealed small foci of more obvious epithelial growth. (C) The spindle cells are all keratin-reactive immunohistologically.

typically demonstrates minute foci of cohesive epithelioid cells, suggesting the diagnosis of squamous carcinoma on conventional histologic grounds. However, some ISCs lack such foci and are recognizable as carcinomas only with special pathologic evaluations (Fig. 14.12C).[106]

Pleurotropic ("pseudomesotheliomatous") sarcomatoid carcinoma

Occasional examples of SC are distinctive not because of their histologic attributes, but because of their macroscopic appearances. In particular, a small subset of these neoplasms arises in the very periphery of the pulmonary parenchyma and grows preferentially into the pleura that encases the lungs.[106ab] This produces clinical symptoms and signs that are indistinguishable from those of malignant mesothelioma; hence, the names "pleurotropic" or "pseudomesotheliomatous" carcinoma.[106b] Moreover, the microscopic features of pleurotropic SC (PSC) are basically superimposable with those of biphasic or sarcomatoid mesotheliomas.

Even though there is no real clinical value in making the distinction between PSC and mesothelioma, with regard to efficacy of treatment or prognosis, legal ramifications of these diagnoses are worthy of comment. Because of the potential causal linkage of mesothelioma with occupational-level amphibole asbestos exposure, some patients with that tumor are eligible for monetary compensation. However, there is no convincing evidence whatsoever to link PSC with asbestos, and its etiology appears to be identical to that of "routine" forms of lung cancer.

Results of adjunctive pathologic studies

Accounts of the electron microscopic and immunohistologic characteristics of pulmonary SC have not been altogether uniform. Some authors have preferred the view that such data in fact confirm the existence of true "carcinosarcomas,"[107–109] whereas others have felt that this information instead supports the concept of a pathologic continuum that is predicated on carcinoma in pure form.[11,13,30,110–114] We strongly prefer the second of these opinions.

It is true that the sarcoma-like elements in SC of the airways do not uniformly exhibit the ultrastructural presence of intercellular junctions and tonofibrils, or immunoreactivity for keratin or epithelial membrane antigen (EMA) in fusiform and pleomorphic tumor cells. In fact, these generic markers of epithelial differentiation may be seen only extremely focally in such neoplastic components, and we have even seen isolated examples in which cell membrane-based EMA reactivity was obvious but keratin positivity was altogether absent. Humphrey et al. observed cytoplasmic tonofibrils or keratin positivity in the sarcomatoid elements of only 3 of 8 pulmonary SCs.[11] However, it should be noted that the latter study was performed with a single heteroantiserum to high molecular weight keratin, representing a relatively insensitive means of immunodetection. In our previously published experience with sarcomatoid carcinomas of the respiratory tract,[28] 81% were ultrastructurally or immunohistochemically proven (with a mixture of monoclonal antikeratin antibodies [AE1/AE3/CAM5.2/MAK-6]) to be wholly epithelial in nature, and other authors have recorded similar findings.[110–114]

The fact that features of epithelial differentiation are present *at all* in the sarcomatoid elements of these neoplasms strongly supports the premise that respiratory tract SC is a basically carcinomatous lesion "in transition."[115] This concept has been well-accepted in reference to "dedifferentiated" sarcomas of the soft tissue, in which clonal evolution is thought to account for a change in the morphology as well as the immunophenotype of the progenitor lesion.[116] Lessons learned in the latter sphere – as well as recent molecular biologic assessments of clonality in SCs[117] – have direct corollaries in the context under discussion here. We have observed the coexpression of vimentin (a "primordial" intermediate filament) in *all* examples of keratin-positive SC of the airways, and a minority of these lesions are additionally labeled for desmin (the intermediate filament of myogenous cells) and muscle-specific actin in the same cells that contain the other two filament proteins.[28] Collagen type IV is also seen surrounding individual tumor cells in most instances. Markers of neuroendocrine differentiation – such as chromogranin-A, CD57, and synaptophysin – likewise may be seen in selected lesions in their overtly epithelial components,[45,47] and S100 protein is apparent in foci resembling chondroid tissue by conventional microscopy.[2] In contrast, von Willebrand factor and CD31 are typically absent in PASC, whereas one or both of those endothelial determinants would be expected in true pleuropulmonary angiosarcomas.[83]

These accrued observations coincide with ultrastructural findings reported by Battifora in two cases of SC – which demonstrated the coincidence of desmosomes, tonofibrils, and collagen production in the same neoplastic cells – implying the presence of multilinear differentiation.[118] Thus, SC can be viewed basically as an epithelial neoplasm with divergent mesenchymal differentiation, in which carcinoma cells acquire the potential to express a mesenchymal phenotype at light microscopic, ultrastructural, and immunohistologic levels. The pathogenetic bases for this peculiarity are currently unknown, but the practical deduction to be gleaned from this construct is that *all* SCs of the respiratory tract should be treated clinically as poorly differentiated carcinomas.

Wakely has reviewed the characteristics of pulmonary spindle cell tumors as seen in fine-needle aspiration biopsy specimens (see Fig. 14.7).[118a] He concluded that adjunctive pathologic studies, such as those discussed above, were virtually mandatory before definitive diagnoses could be reached in that context.

Differential diagnosis of sarcomatoid carcinoma

The differential diagnosis of sarcomatoid carcinomas of the airways principally centers on the exclusion of true sarcomas, as discussed in the remainder of this chapter. As a particular word of caution, it should be noted that synovial sarcoma (SS) and sarcomatoid mesothelioma may be virtually identical to SC as seen with the electron microscope or in immunophenotypic evaluations. The marked propensity for SS to affect children, adolescents, and young adults, and its typical t(X;18) cytogenetic aberration[119,120] (not seen in carcinomas) are crucial points in its distinction from SC of the upper airways, and nuances of histologic appearance and radiographic characteristics are also valuable in this specific differential diagnostic setting. Similarly, roentgenologic findings are more helpful than morphologic observations in making the distinction between SC and spindle cell or biphasic mesothelioma. The ultrastructural profiles of the latter two lesions are, for all intents and purposes, superimposable on one another,[1,2,121] and, aside from selective reactivity for calretinin in mesotheliomas, the same comment applies to their immunophenotypes.

Part II: True primary sarcomas of the lung

Kaposi's sarcoma

The recent natural history of Kaposi's sarcoma (KS) is a sad testimony to the global impact of the acquired immunodeficiency syndrome (AIDS). Before the 1980s, KS was a relatively rare neoplasm outside of Africa and the Mediterranean basin. Moreover, with relatively uncommon exceptions, this lesion was a cutaneous proliferation that uncommonly involved the viscera.[122] However, today with particular regard to the intrathoracic organs, KS is – in most large metropolitan areas of the world – the commonest of all pulmonary sarcomas.[123] Whereas initial presentation of this tumor in the bronchopulmonary tract was an almost-unknown phenomenon prior to the advent of AIDS, it is currently a well-recognized variation of the latter disease.[124]

Clinical summary

In the context just mentioned, most patients with KS of the lung (KSL) are homosexual men,[124–131] and more uncommonly include those in other high-risk groups for AIDS such as intravenous drug abusers. Most individuals with KS generally have other symptoms and signs of AIDS, such as weight loss, fever, night sweats, fatigue, lymphadenopathy, and opportunistic infections. However, fever may be directly caused by KS in the lungs. There has been a case report of an AIDS patient with persistent pyrexia for which no source of infection was found, but which finally resolved after radiation therapy.[132] *Cutaneous* KS is usually detected early in its clinical evolution, but identical tumors of the bronchial mucosa and lung parenchyma typically have grown to a volume sufficient to produce symptoms, and, therefore, are relatively advanced at the time of diagnosis.[133] Presenting complaints which are specific to the neoplasm include dyspnea, stridor (when endobronchial lesions are present), cough, and hemoptysis, which may be massive.[124]

On bronchoscopic examination, nodular or flat bluish-red discolorations in the mucosa are seen, some of which may be actively bleeding. This bronchoscopic appearance is usually considered diagnostic, and endobronchial lesions are not generally biopsied. The diagnostic yield of transbronchial biopsies is usually quite low, and unless they are deep enough, KSL will be missed because the mucosa itself is usually uninvolved.[134] In addition, bronchoscopy is necessary to exclude other causes of pulmonary infiltrates, especially infections. Open lung biopsies are diagnostically more productive, but they are not absolutely sensitive.

Radiographic findings on chest X-rays may be nonspecific, showing only ill-defined interstitial infiltrates (Fig. 14.13). An alveolar filling pattern is usually evident only if the patient has suffered hemoptysis and aspirated blood, but pleural effusions or pneumothorax may be seen in cases where the lesion involves the serosal surfaces as well as the lung parenchyma.[135,136] Mediastinal adenopathy is not common, but, if it is present, this can be very helpful in separating KS from *Pneumocystis jiroveci* infection, because the latter does not cause adenopathy. Computed tomographic (CT) scans and magnetic resonance images (MRIs) generally provide no more information than the chest radiographs. In summary, the

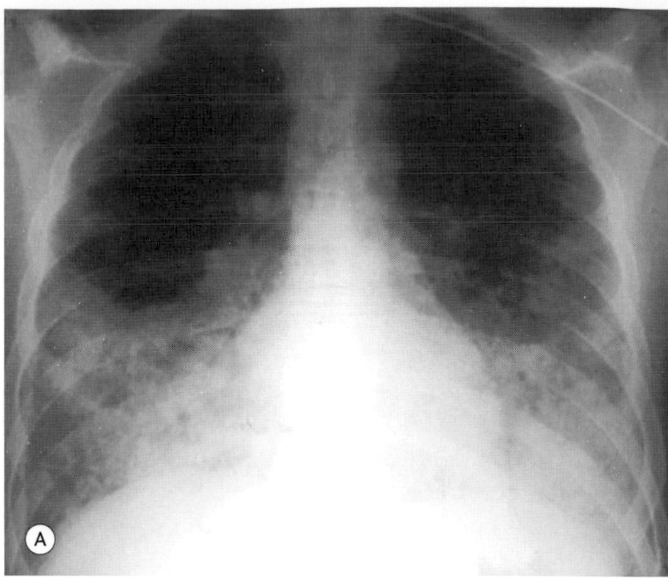

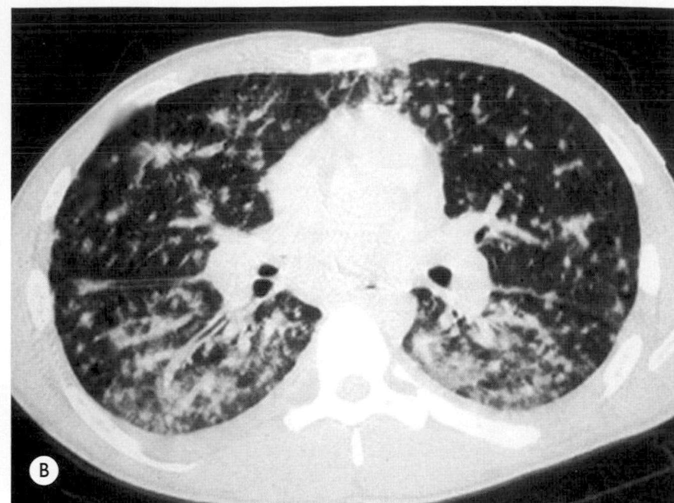

Fig. 14.13 A relatively nondescript reticulonodular interstitial infiltrate is seen on conventional (A) chest radiographs and (B) computed tomography, in a patient with acquired immunodeficiency syndrome. The clinical differential diagnosis of such a pattern would include infection as well as neoplasia, but pulmonary Kaposi's sarcoma was the ultimate interpretation in this case.

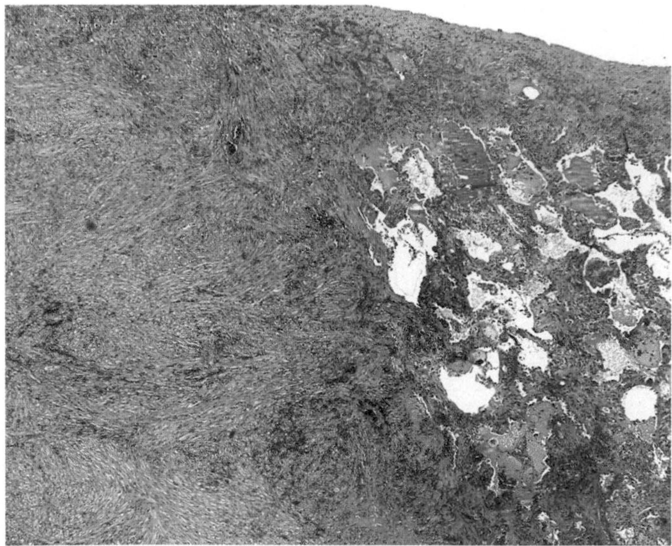

Fig. 14.14 Low-magnification image of pulmonary Kaposi's sarcoma, showing a nodular proliferation of spindle cells and neovascular spaces (left) that permeates the pulmonary interstitium (right).

presence of bilateral pleural effusions and bilateral interstitial infiltrates with ill-defined nodularity is suggestive of pulmonary KS, especially in a patient with known tumor elsewhere.[125,126]

Pathologic findings

As alluded to above, it is distinctly uncommon for the pathologist to be able to make a definitive diagnosis of KSL on a transbronchial biopsy specimen. Usually, a wedge biopsy is necessary, as obtained via video-guided thoracoscopy or a limited thoracotomy.[134] On gross examination, this type of specimen exhibits numerous hemangiomatoid or ecchymosis-like zones of bluish-red discoloration in the parenchyma, with ill-defined borders.

In the lung, KS shows a tendency to grow along pre-existing fibrous intrapulmonary septa, and it also concentrates around small tubular airways and blood vessels (Fig. 14.14). The tumor comprises a mixture of ectatic, thin-walled blood vessels that "dissect" or push through the pulmonary interstitial collagen, together with haphazardly arranged fascicles of spindle cells that show only modest nuclear atypia and may contain cytoplasmic vacuoles.[124,134] Extravasated erythrocytes and hemosiderin pigment are common in and around the tumor masses (Fig. 14.15). Pleural KS "layers" itself over the submesothelial mantle of connective tissue, effacing the mesothelium itself in doing so.

Mitotic activity is variable in PKSL, but it is usually detectable. If it is present at all, necrosis is limited in scope and visible only on microscopy.

Therapy and prognosis

Regardless of its occurrence in AIDS or in non-HIV-related cases, the presence of KS in the lung is prognostically ominous. Virtually all patients with visceral disease will die within 2 years, from infection if not from

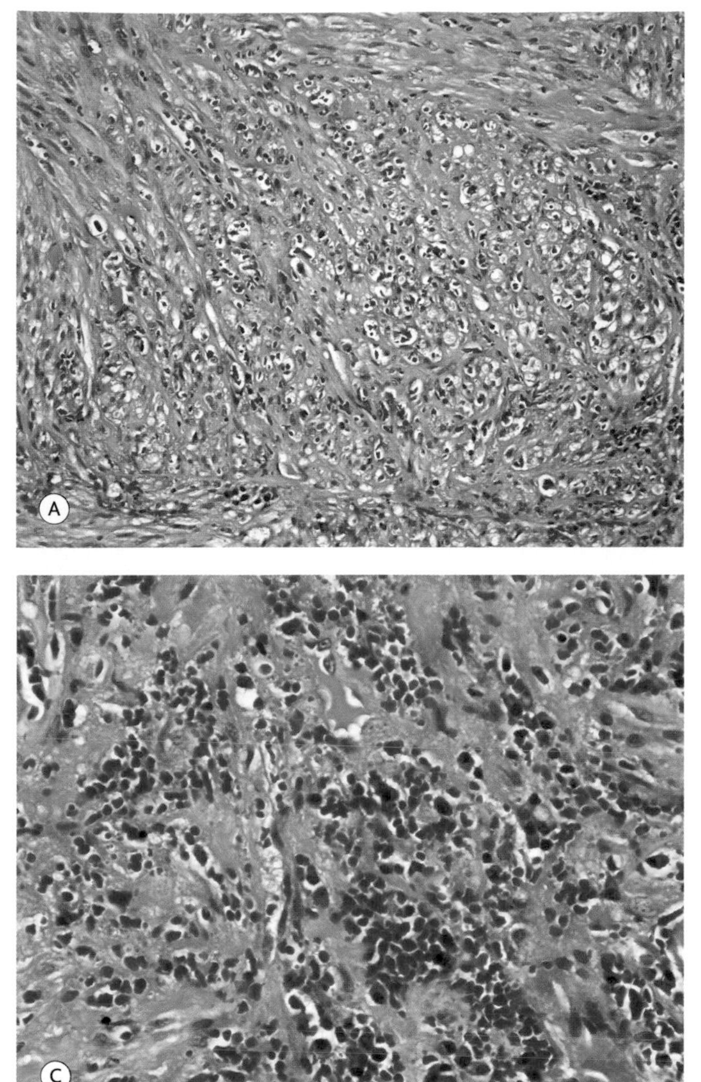
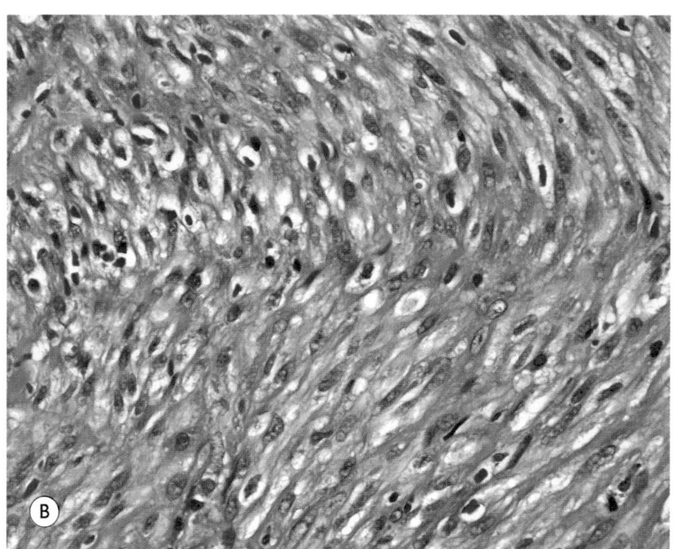

Fig. 14.15 (A) Kaposi's sarcoma of the lung, demonstrating formation of interanastomosing vascular channels, (B) foci of solid spindle cell growth, and (C) areas with extravasation of erythrocytes into the stroma and deposition of hemosiderin pigment.

KS itself.[123,129,131] Because of the multiplicity of KS, surgical resection is not a realistic option in the management of patients with this neoplasm. Chemotherapy is considered the treatment of choice, with a relatively good response rate and relatively rapid improvement within 2–4 weeks.[20] Chemotherapy regimens in the few published therapeutic trials designed specifically for pulmonary KS have primarily included Adriamycin, bleomycin, and vincristine.[124,137–139] Gill et al. found an 85% response with combination chemotherapy in a group of 13 patients.[138] Patients who benefited from this treatment included those who achieved at least partial responses. Complete response is defined by the following three criteria:

- direct bronchoscopy revealing complete disappearance of KS lesions in the tracheobronchial tree
- a normal chest X-ray
- resolution of all other sites of disease.

A partial response is characterized by the same three points, except that the degree of resolution is not total.[137,138]

Despite fairly good results with combination chemotherapy, patients with pulmonary KS do not have long survival. In the trial reported by Gill et al., the median survival for responders was slightly but significantly longer than that of nonresponders (10 versus 6 months, respectively). However, considerable overlap between the 2 groups was present.[138]

Other more experimental (and inconclusive) approaches have included the administration of zidovudine, interferon, and other antiviral compounds.[122,128,129] Radiotherapy may provide palliation of symptoms, but is non-curative. The most important piece of data in prognosticating cases of KSL is the serologic HIV status of the patient, inasmuch as AIDS is currently a uniformly lethal illness.

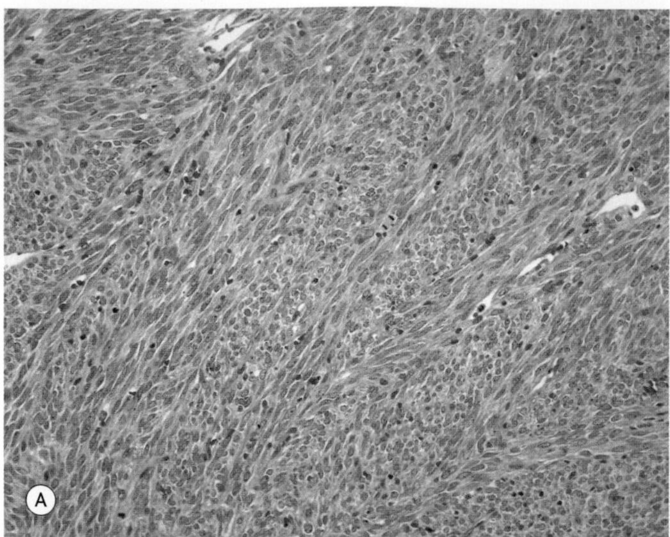

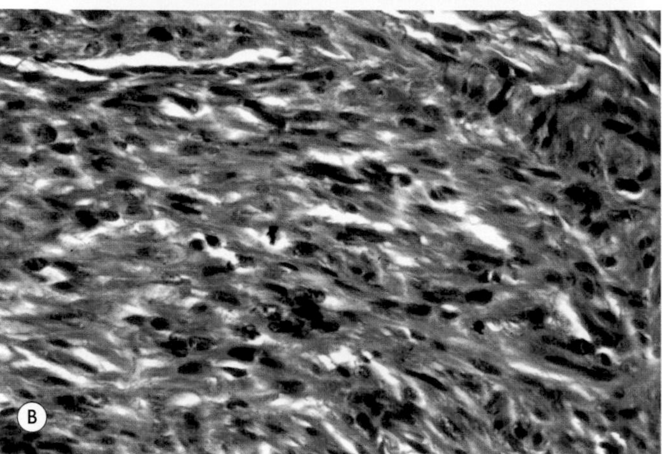

Fig. 14.16 (A) Pulmonary fibrosarcoma, represented by a cellular proliferation of atypical spindle cells. (B) Mitotic activity is apparent on high magnification.

Fibrosarcoma

Primary fibrosarcoma of the lung (FSL), like its soft tissue counterpart, is defined as a fibroblastic spindle cell neoplasm without any evidence of specialized cellular differentiation. Although it has been cited – along with leiomyosarcoma – as the most common primary pulmonary sarcoma,[140] FSL was, and probably still is, over-diagnosed.[141] Two separate studies from the Mayo Clinic cited two different time-dependent incidence figures for fibrosarcoma of the lung. From 1950 to 1978, it constituted 50% of all primary pulmonary sarcomas,[142] but only 20% in the decade 1980 to 1990.[143] As considered above, it is our belief that the great majority of pulmonary "fibrosarcomas" are actually sarcomatoid *carcinomas*. Only those tumors which have been subjected to rigorous and specialized pathologic examination should be accepted as bona fide examples of this rare sarcoma variant.

Clinical summary

Guccion and Rosen studied 13 cases of fibrosarcoma of the lung, which were divided into "endobronchial" and "intrapulmonary" types.[140] This classification scheme was said to have clinical and prognostic importance. In conjunction with a review of 48 reported cases in the literature, the authors just cited found that the majority of "endobronchial" FSLs occurred in children and young adults, whereas "parenchymal" tumors predominated in middle-aged and elderly patients. In contrast, Pettinato and associates reported three parenchymal tumors in two newborns and a 6-month old infant.[144] There was roughly an equal distribution by gender among endobronchial lesions; however, most intraparenchymal neoplasms occurred in men. All endobronchial FSLs in a series reported by the Armed Forces Institute of Pathology (AFIP) produced symptoms of cough, hemoptysis, or chest pain; some of the parenchymal cases did so as well, but others were asymptomatic.[140] Thoracic imaging studies of FSL usually show discrete, homogenous masses. However, one reported pulmonary fibrosarcoma simulated a bronchogenic cyst clinically and radiographically.[145] Gladish et al.[9a] have observed that fibrosarcoma is much more likely to arise in the soft tissue of the chest wall and *secondarily* involve the lung, than it is to show the converse of that relationship.

Pathologic findings

Endobronchial fibrosarcomas are smaller than microscopically similar tumors in the parenchyma; the former variants usually measure <3 cm and the latter range from 3.5 to 23 cm in greatest dimension. Parenchymal masses are typically well-delimited and lobulated with frequent areas of necrosis and hemorrhage.

FSL is histologically identical to its soft tissue counterparts, and characteristically shows sheets and intertwining fascicles of spindle-shaped cells with a typical "herringbone" growth pattern and discernible stromal collagenogenesis (Fig. 14.16). The tumor cells contain oval to elongated, hyperchromatic nuclei, and scant amphophilic cytoplasm with ill-defined cellular borders. In addition, some areas may have a slightly epithelioid appearance – in which the tumor cells are more ovoid than spindled – and others may show significant pleomorphism that merges with the image of malignant fibrous histiocytoma (Fig. 14.17). Mitotic activity is variable.

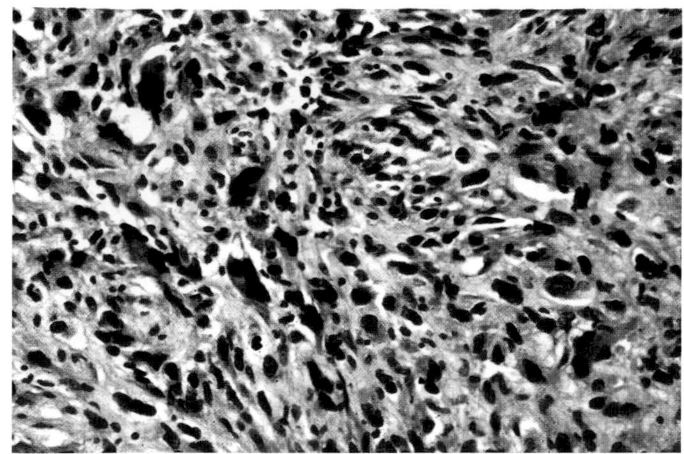

Fig. 14.17 This image from another case of high-grade intrapulmonary fibrosarcoma shows more nuclear pleomorphism in the tumor cells, overlapping the appearance of malignant fibrous histiocytoma.

Electron microscopic and immunohistochemical studies are required to confirm the fibroblastic nature of these neoplasms. The tumor cells in FSL are characterized by abundant rough endoplasmic reticulum and free ribosomes, as well as the production of extracellular collagen fibers that may be aligned at right angles to the tumor cell membranes. There should be no detectable myofilaments, pericellular basal lamina, or intercellular junctions in lesions thought to represent FSL. Because there are no specific immunological markers for fibroblasts, the diagnosis of fibrosarcoma is one of immunohistologic exclusion. Tumor cells in FSL generally stain only for vimentin, a primitive intermediate filament protein, and they lack all myogenous, neural, and endothelial markers.[144,146,147]

Therapy and prognosis

Although resection is the treatment of choice, many surgically treated fibrosarcomas of the lungs do recur, and survival after this event is short, with patient fatality usually eventuating within 2 years.[140] Three cases seen at the Mayo Clinic between 1980 and 1990 occurred in young women whose lesions all recurred within 15 months following surgical excision.[143] In contrast, primary bronchopulmonary fibrosarcomas in children appear to have a relatively favorable prognosis and behave only as low-grade malignancies.[144,145] The 5 patients with pediatric FSL reported by Pettinato et al. all had complete surgical removal of their tumors, and 4 were disease-free after 4–9 years. The fifth case in that series had insignificant follow-up.[144] The efficacy of adjunctive chemotherapy and irradiation has not yet been proven.

Primary pulmonary leiomyosarcoma

The most common anatomic locations for leiomyosarcomas in general are the uterus, gastrointestinal tract, and soft tissue, in order of relative frequency. Primary *pulmonary* leiomyosarcomas (PPLMS) are extremely uncommon and presumably take their origins from bronchial or pulmonary vascular smooth muscle. Only three cases of leiomyosarcoma were found among roughly 10,000 primary malignancies of the lung at one large American medical center between 1980 and 1990.[143] Because *secondary* pulmonary involvement by malignant smooth muscle tumors is a relatively frequent event, the diagnosis of PPLMS absolutely requires exclusion of an occult extrathoracic neoplasm presenting with a single "herald" metastasis to the lung.

Clinical summary

A series of 19 PPLMSs seen at the AFIP was divided into those neoplasms which were predominantly endobronchial and others that were intraparenchymal, in analogy to pulmonary fibrosarcomas.[140] The majority of these tumors in children are endobronchial in nature,[148,149] whereas those in adults are not. In contrast to leiomyosarcomas of the soft tissue – which occur most commonly in women – patients in the aforementioned report from the AFIP were almost exclusively males. However, another survey that reviewed 92 cases of PPLMS in the literature found a male-to-female ratio of 2.5, suggesting that the paramilitary study just cited was biased demographically by its affiliation with the armed services.[150] In contrast to carcinoma of the lung, leiomyosarcoma is not associated with cigarette smoking or other potential inhalant carcinogens. Most patients with PPLMS (particularly its endobronchial form) are symptomatic, often complaining of cough, hemoptysis, or chest pain. However, intraparenchymal lesions may be discovered incidentally on chest radiographs. Roentgenographically, PPLMS usually takes the form of a discrete mass, sometimes with cavitation or cyst formation that is best seen by CT of the thorax.[140,151,152]

Pathologic findings

Parenchymal tumors range from 3 to 15 cm in maximum dimension; they are well-circumscribed, white to yellowish tan, and variably firm. Cut surfaces of these neoplasms commonly show hemorrhagic and necrotic areas. Endobronchial tumors are often smaller than the intraparenchymal lesions, presumably because of confinement by the bronchial walls.[153]

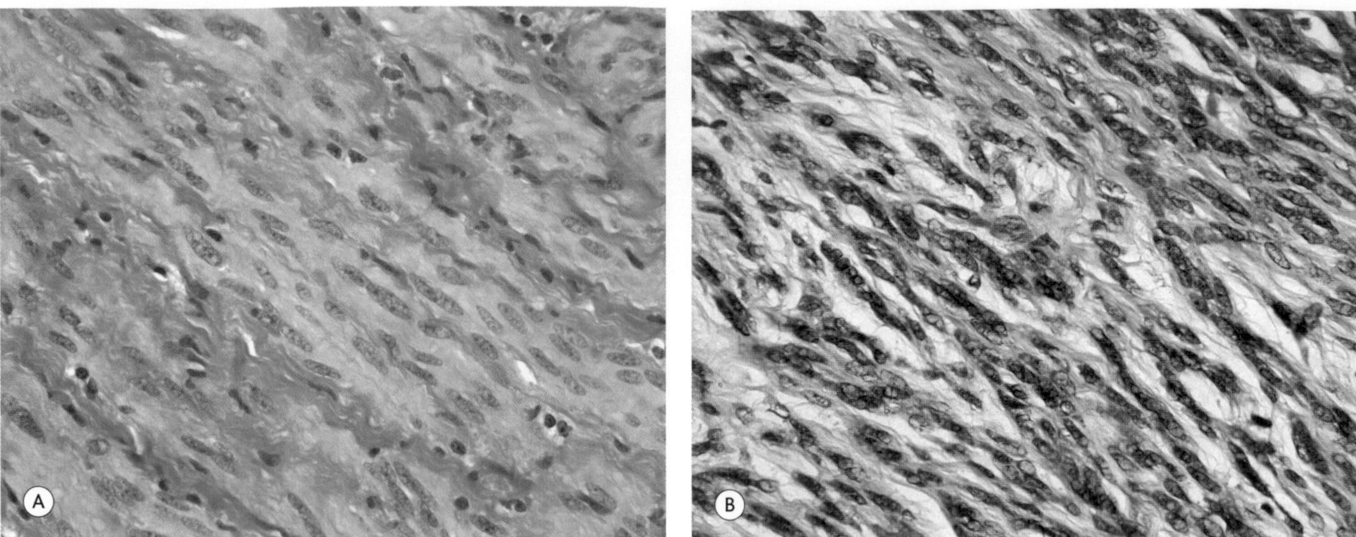

Fig. 14.18 (A) Primary leiomyosarcoma of the lung, showing fascicular growth of atypical spindle cells with blunt-ended nuclei and fibrillary cytoplasm. (B) The densely cellular nature of the tumor is better seen here.

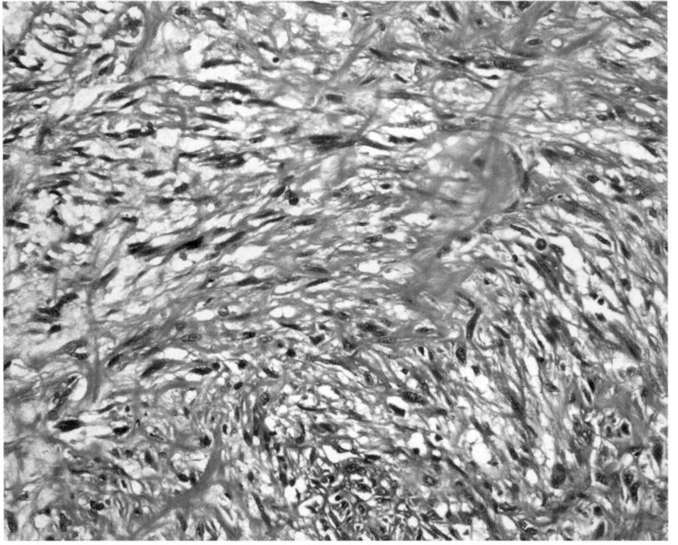

Fig. 14.19 Myxoid change in primary pulmonary leiomyosarcoma (top right and bottom left of photograph).

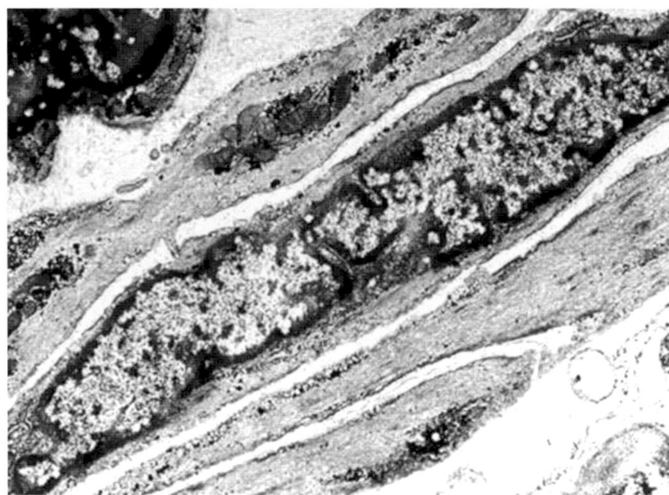

Fig. 14.20 Electron photomicrograph of pulmonary leiomyosarcoma, demonstrating cytoplasmic thin filaments, pericellular basal lamina, and cytoplasmic dense bodies.

Microscopy discloses histologic features that mirror those of leiomyosarcomas elsewhere in the body. On low-power magnification, there are interlacing fascicles of spindled cells which are arranged haphazardly, yielding a "whorled" appearance (Fig. 14.18). The neoplastic cells have cigar-shaped nuclei with blunt ends, a moderate amount of cytoplasm, and indistinct cell borders. Fascicles cut in cross section demonstrate characteristic intracellular perinuclear lucencies.[153–156] Prominent myxoid stromal change may be observed[157] (Fig. 14.19).

The differential diagnosis of PPLMS includes fibrosarcoma and malignant schwannoma, as well as sarcomatoid carcinoma. Electron microscopy and immunohistochemistry are again helpful in confirming the smooth muscle nature of a spindle cell neoplasm.[155] Ultrastructural features of leiomyogenous differentiation include cytoplasmic dense bodies punctuating skeins of thin filaments, subplasmalemmal dense plaques, plasmalemmal pinocytotic vesicles, and pericellular basal lamina (Fig. 14.20). Immunoreactivity for desmin, muscle specific actin, or smooth muscle actin is also characteristic of the tumor cells in PPLMS.[158]

Therapy and prognosis

The natural history of PPLMS and its responses to various therapeutic regimens are difficult to predict because of the rarity of this neoplasm. However, there is generally a consensus that surgical resection is the treatment of choice,[150,153–155] and that it produces a survival rate of 45–50% at 5 years. Survival for as long as 15–30 years has been documented in PPLMS cases.[140,142] However, pulmonary leiomyosarcomas appear to be relatively resistant to irradiation and chemotherapy.[150,156] Various prognostic variables have been discussed in connection with these lesions.[140,142] Endobronchial tumors are thought to be less aggressive than parenychmal neoplasms, largely because the former tend to be smaller and are diagnosed earlier. It follows, therefore, that tumor size is an important indicator of biological behavior for *all* pulmonary leiomyosarcomas. The scope of mitotic activity may affect prognosis as well. In an AFIP series on PPLMS, a mitotic rate of 8 or less per 10 high-power fields was associated with infrequent metastasis and a generally favorable clinical outcome.[140]

Epithelioid hemangioendothelioma

In 1975, Dail and Liebow reported the first cases of an unusual pulmonary neoplasm that they called "intravascular bronchioloalveolar tumor" (IVBAT). This name reflected their original hypothesis that the lesion in question was an epithelial tumor: specifically, a bronchioloalveolar carcinoma variant showing prominent vascular invasion.[159,160] Four years thereafter, Corrin et al. alternatively proposed an endothelial origin for this tumor based on the results of ultrastructural studies.[161] Subsequent evaluations by other authors have confirmed the vascular histogenesis of the "IVBAT." Indeed, in 1982, Weiss and Enzinger described a series of soft tissue tumors that were histologically identical to IVBAT, and these authors were the first to use the term "epithelioid hemangioendothelioma" (EH) for these lesions to emphasize their distinctively epithelioid (or "histiocytoid") cytological features.[162] In addition to the lungs and soft tissues, EH also primarily occurs in the bone and liver.

Clinical summary

EH of the lung is a neoplasm that arises predominantly in female patients; women account for roughly 80% of all cases.[160,163,164] It primarily occurs in young adults, with approximately 50% being less than 40 years of age; only 10% are older than 50 years at diagnosis.[165] Many affected persons are asymptomatic, and their tumors are detected incidentally on chest radiographs. Patients who have tumor-related complaints usually present with pleuritic pain, dyspnea, and cough. Case reports have also documented alveolar hemorrhage as a presenting sign of pulmonary EH,[166,167] and it may simulate thromboembolic disease symptomatically as well.[168] Chest radiographs commonly show numerous, small nodular lesions throughout both lung fields (Fig. 14.21). Therefore, EH enters the roentgenographic differential diagnosis of multiple pulmonary nodules in asymptomatic young women, together with metastatic germ cell tumors,

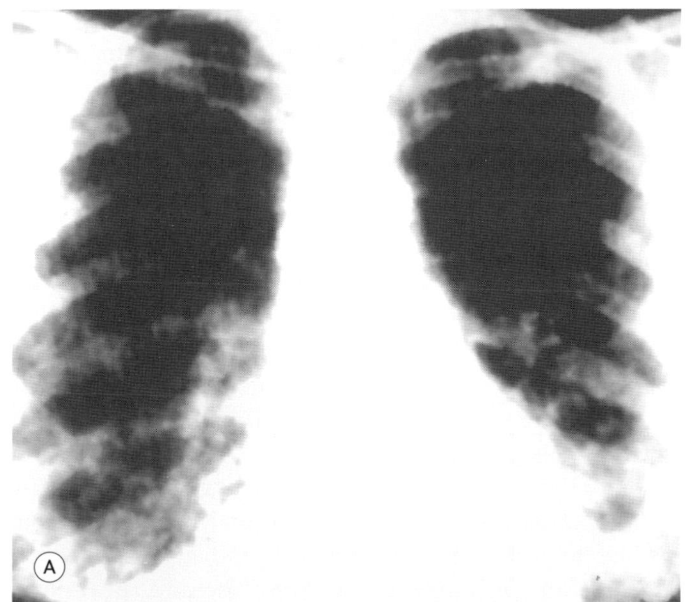

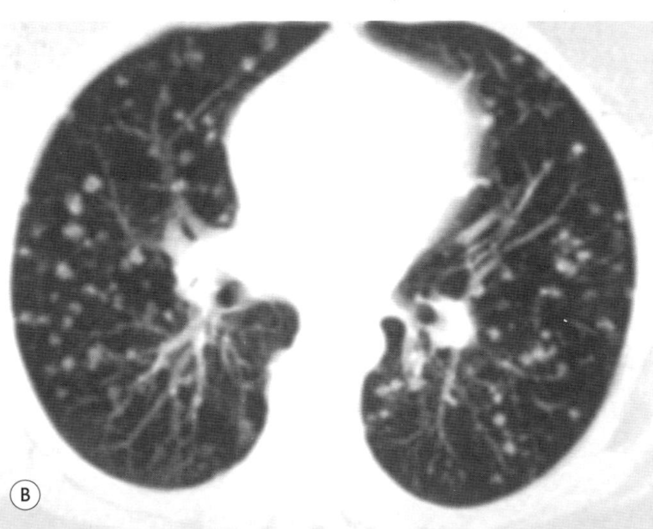

Fig. 14.21 Multiple nodular densities are seen throughout both lung fields (A) on plain film radiography and (B) computed tomography in this case of primary pulmonary epithelioid hemangioendothelioma.

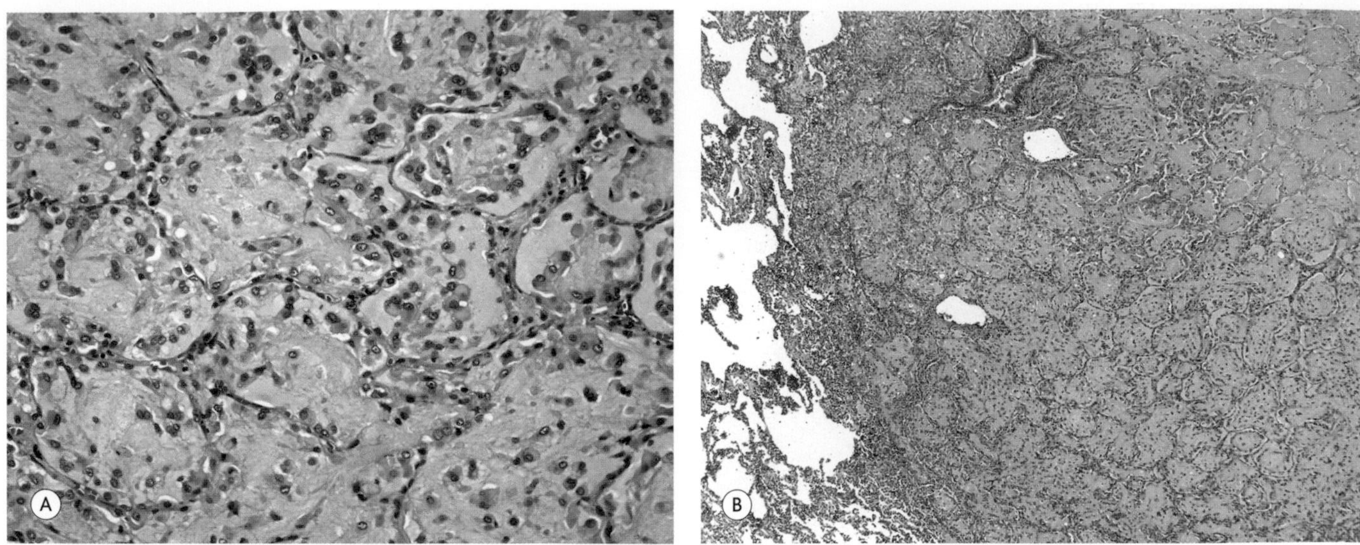

Fig. 14.22 (A) Epithelioid cells are set in a homogeneous myxofibrous stroma in this case of epithelioid hemangioendothelioma of the lung. (A and B) The tumor grows in a lepidic fashion through the alveolar pores of Kohn, yielding a micronodular image. Secondary alveolar pneumocytic proliferation is also evident.

chondroid pulmonary hamartomas, multiple arteriovenous malformations of the lung, deposits of "benign metastasizing leiomyoma," and malignant lymphoma.[169]

Pathologic findings

The pathologic diagnosis of EH is almost always made by open lung biopsy, inasmuch as transbronchial biopsy is usually ineffectual because of sampling constraints. Most nodules of EH are discrete and usually measure less than 2 cm. They are grayish-white to tan and have a chondroid macroscopic consistency. More nodules are typically seen on histologic examination than are apparent grossly. Microscopically, EH is typified by multiple oval or round nodules with hypocellular, sclerotic, or necrotic centers[160,163] (Fig. 14.22B). These are surrounded by rims of viable, more cellular tissue that is associated with a myxohyaline fibrous stroma. The neoplastic cell population is composed of plump, epithelioid cells which are the histologic hallmark of EH (Fig. 14.23). They have centrally located, round-to-oval nuclei and ample amounts of eosinophilic cytoplasm. Often, intracytoplasmic vacuoles are evident, which should raise the possibility of endothelial differentiation on light microscopy. Tumoral involvement of arterioles, venules, and lymphatics is variable within the tumor nodules as well as other distant sites. EH commonly shows an intra-alveolar pattern of growth secondary to tumor extension through the pores of Kohn, and surgical margins may be, therefore, difficult to ascertain on gross examination if a limited resection of the lesion is attempted.

Ultrastructural and immunohistochemical evaluation can be of great assistance in confirming the endothelial origin of EH.[161,163,170–173] Briefly, ultrastructural features of this tumor include cytoplasmic vacuoles, Weibel–Palade bodies (Fig. 14.24), cell membranous pinocytotic vesicles, and pericellular basal lamina.[172] Histochemical and immunological markers of endothelial differentiation – such as anti-von Willebrand factor, *Ulex europaeus* I lectin, anti-CD31, and anti-CD34 – are helpful in labeling the neoplastic cells in virtually all examples of EH.[174]

Therapy and prognosis

Surgery is usually not feasible as effective treatment for EH because of its tendency to show intrapulmonary multicentricity. Unfortunately, irradiation and chemotherapy likewise have been of little benefit.[160,163] Nevertheless, EH is generally an indolent neoplasm that is classified as a "borderline" malignancy. It is associated with a protracted clinical course and potential survival of several years after diagnosis.[170] Most patients do eventually succumb to the tumor and die of respiratory failure secondary to progressive parenchymal replacement. Adverse prognostic factors that predict a more rapid decline in pulmonary function include prominent symptoms at the time of presentation, radiographic demonstration of extensive intravascular, endobronchial,

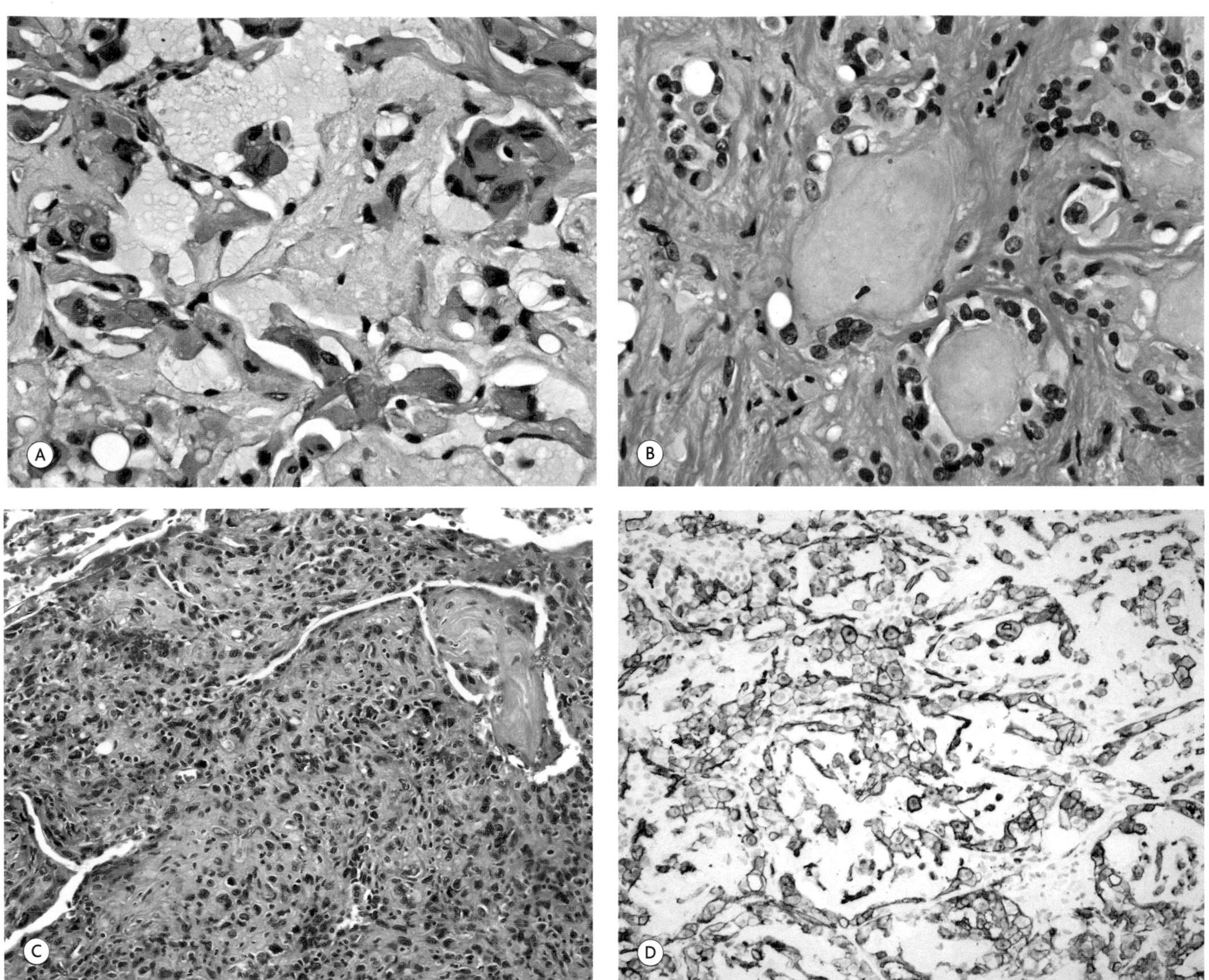

Fig. 14.23 (A, B) The epithelioid nature of the tumor cells in pulmonary epithelioid hemangioendothelioma (PEH) is well-seen in these photograph, as well as the tumor's myxofibrous stroma. (B) The neoplastic cells in grade I PEH are bland cytologically, and some have intracytoplasmic lumina. (C) Grade II PEH demonstrates a greater degree of nuclear atypia and may show mitotic activity as well. (D) Immunoreactivity for CD31, indicating the endothelial nature of PEH.

or pleural spread of the tumor,[160] and the presence of fusiform tumor cells.[164]

The general predilection of EH for women, a reported association of primary hepatic EH with oral contraceptives, and the lack of effective therapy for this tumor have prompted some investigators to explore the possibility of treatment involving hormonal modulation. These tumors have been examined for possible expression of estrogen and progesterone receptor proteins, as well as other estradiol-binding moieties. Ohori et al. analyzed 5 cases of pulmonary EH for steroid hormone receptors by immunohistochemical methods, using paraffin-embedded material.[175] Only one case showed apparent binding of estradiol. Our own unpublished experience with the immunohistologic characteristics of pulmonary EH has disclosed no reactivity with monoclonal antibodies against estrogen and progesterone receptor proteins. Thus, we believe that hormonal therapies are unlikely to produce significant results in this setting.

Hemangiopericytoma

As first described in 1942 by Stout and Murray,[176] hemangiopericytoma (HPC) is an uncommon, potentially malignant neoplasm that shows apparent differentiation towards the phenotype of pericytes. These are cells with

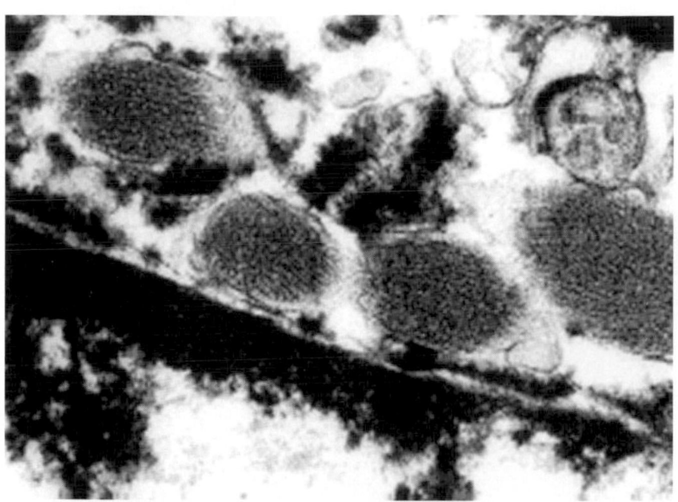

Fig. 14.24 Numerous Weibel–Palade bodies – which have the appearance of lysosomal-like inclusions with internal striations – are present in epithelioid hemangioendothelioma in this electron photomicrograph. These organelles are the intracellular packaging sites for von Willebrand factor.

long cytoplasmic processes which surround capillaries and serve a vasoregulatory function. HPC occurs most commonly in the deep muscles of the thigh, the pelvic fossa, and the retroperitoneum. However, 5–10% of all hemangiopericytomas are said to present as primary pulmonary tumors.[153,177] It must be remembered that the lungs and the bones are the anatomic sites that most frequently harbor metastases of HPC,[178] and therefore a primary extrapulmonary tumor must be excluded before a diagnosis of a primary HPC can be rendered safely.

Clinical summary

Pulmonary HPC affects men and women equally, and most commonly arises in middle adulthood. The peak incidence of this lesion is in the fifth decade of life, although individuals as young as 4 years and as old as 73 years have been reported.[179,180] Some tumors are detected incidentally on radiographic studies without causing pulmonary symptoms; six of 18 cases in one series fit this scenario.[181] Alternatively, presenting symptoms may include hemoptysis, chest pain, cough, and dyspnea, and, more rarely, pulmonary osteoarthropathy.[181]

Various radiographic imaging studies have been utilized in studying this neoplasm. Although angiography has usually not been performed, vascular contrast studies of HPC generally show a characteristic intralesional "blush".[182] No other pathognomonic features are evident in chest roentgenograms, CT scans, and MRIs of hemangiopericytomas of the lung.[180,183] Plain film X-rays typically show a discrete, homogeneously dense mass with lobulated contours. On CT images, however, HPC is *heterogeneous*. Central low-density areas are evident that correspond to necrotic foci, and an apparent capsule may be seen at the interface with surrounding lung parenchyma. MRIs also show intratumoral heterogeneity with respect to tissue density, and are apparently more sensitive in depicting intralesional hemorrhage. These images were found to be the most useful in delineating the potential plane of surgical separation between an HPC and surrounding soft tissue in one report.[184] In summary, a radiologic diagnosis of pulmonary HPC may be suspected in a middle-aged person lacking pulmonary symptoms, but whose radiographic imaging studies reveal a large, lobulated, sharply marginated, variably dense mass that does not cause compression atelectasis.[183]

Pathologic findings

Hemangiopericytomas of the lung can attain large sizes, and lesions measuring up to 18 cm have been documented. The typical gross appearance of this tumor is that of a well-circumscribed, yellow to tan-brown mass with a pseudocapsule, and areas of internal necrosis and hemorrhage. Histologic sections typically show a relatively monomorphous cellular proliferation that surrounds thin-walled, anastomosing vascular channels that are lined by a single endothelial layer (Fig. 14.25). These blood vessels often (but not always) assume gaping, "staghorn," or "antler-like" configurations (Fig. 14.26). The population of neoplastic cells is uniform, with oval compact nuclei and ill-defined cytoplasm.[153] Mitotic

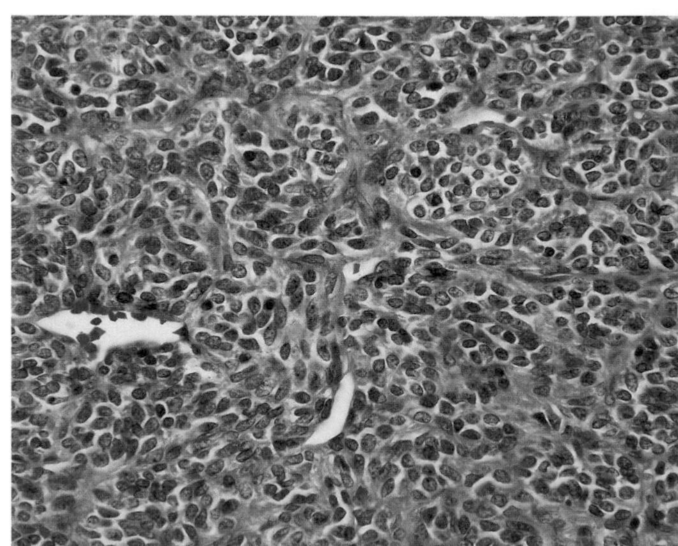

Fig. 14.25 Pulmonary hemangiopericytoma, showing ill-defined clusters of bluntly fusiform tumor cells and prominent stromal blood vessels.

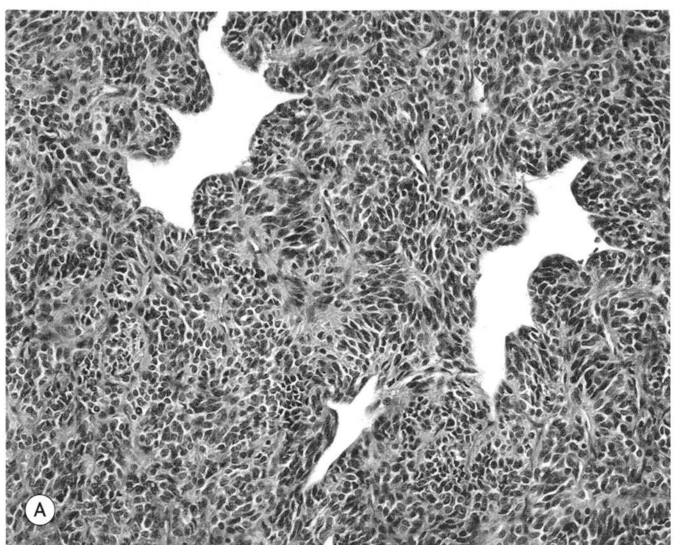
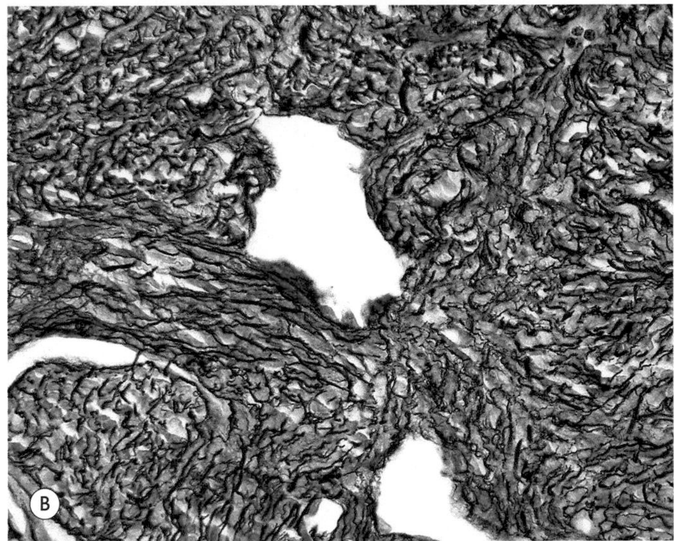

Fig. 14.26 (A) "Staghorn"-shaped blood vessels in primary pulmonary hemangiopericytoma. (B) Individual tumor cells are invested by reticulin fibers in HPC (reticulin stain method).

activity and areas of necrosis and hemorrhage are noted frequently. Vascular invasion of large pulmonary vessels, however, is uncommon. With regard to the latter features, some pathologists have, in the past, rendered a diagnosis of "benign hemangiopericytoma" if necrosis, hemorrhage, and mitoses were absent. In our view, this approach is dangerous. We have seen cases of pulmonary HPC with exceedingly bland histologic profiles in which metastasis nonetheless supervened. Accordingly, it is advised that *each* report on this tumor should carry the statement that HPC is at least *potentially* malignant behaviorally.[178,181]

Pulmonary HPC has sometimes been overdiagnosed because other neoplasms may show foci that resemble the former lesion. In this regard, pathologists will do well to remember that in their seminal report, Stout and Murray admonished others to make the diagnosis of HPC *by ultimate exclusion*.[176] The histologic differential diagnosis includes sarcomatoid carcinoma, synovial sarcoma, pleuropulmonary solitary fibrous tumors, fibrous histiocytomas, and mesenchymal chondrosarcoma,[178] and distinctions between these neoplasms are best made by ancillary studies. Electron microscopy can confirm the pericytic nature of HPC through the demonstration of polygonal cells with cytoplasmic processes, pinocytotic vesicles, basal lamina, and a paucity of other organelles.[146,178] Hemangiopericytoma is a neoplasm that is devoid of most immunohistochemical markers except for vimentin, collagen type IV, and CD57.[46] Endothelial stains such as *Ulex europaeus* I, CD31, and factor VIII-related antigen highlight the lining of intralesional vascular spaces, but do not label the surrounding tumor cells. Silver impregnation techniques highlight a complex reticulin matrix with individual cell investment.

Therapy and prognosis

As in the management of soft tissue HPC, complete surgical excision is the mainstay of therapy for primary pulmonary tumors of this type. However, it is known that intraoperative rupture of pulmonary HPC is prone to occur (especially those which are adherent to the chest wall); as expected, this complication results in early local recurrence, as reported by Van Damme et al., and should therefore be avoided at all costs.[180] Chemotherapy and irradiation have not been shown to be *consistently* effective adjuvant modalities, but they may have some role to play in management.[185,186] A study by Jha et al. on the general role of radiation therapy in treating HPC showed that postoperative irradiation was useful for local tumor control, for salvage therapy after local recurrence, and for palliation.[187] Tumors <5 cm in maximum dimension exhibit a better response than those that are larger than 10 cm.[188]

As mentioned above, hemangiopericytomas in general are well known for their unpredictable biologic behavior. Postoperative survival has ranged from 10 weeks to 18 years.[180,188] Even with apparently complete surgical resection, HPC recurs locally in approximately 50% of cases within 2 years,[181,184,189] and later recurrences are not uncommon. Clinical and histologic features that have been cited as prognostically useful[178,179,184] include the presence of symptoms at presentation; mitotic activity of ≥4 mitoses per 10 high-power microscopic fields; spontaneous tumor necrosis; vascular invasion; and tumor size >5 cm. In one series, metastases were seen in one-third of tumors that measured >5 cm, and in two-thirds of those >10 cm.[179] However, Yousem and Hochholzer did not find any single histologic or clinical feature that was statistically significant in reliably predicting the clinical course of *primary pulmonary* HPC.[181]

Malignant fibrous histiocytoma

Malignant fibrous histiocytoma is a common, extensively studied soft tissue sarcoma of older adults that develops most frequently in the extremities and the retroperitoneum. In a series of 200 cases by Weiss and Enzinger,[190] the lungs were the most common site of *metastases*. Thus, exclusion of an occult soft tissue tumor is once again necessary before a diagnosis of primary pulmonary malignant fibrous histiocytoma (PPMFH) can be made. A review of Mayo Clinic cases found only 4 examples among 10,134 tumors arising in the lung.[143] Currently, there are less than 50 reported cases of PPMFH in the English literature.[190–200]

Clinical summary

In general, malignant fibrous histiocytoma is a neoplasm of patients who are in late middle age, with a median of 54 years. However, its occasional occurrence in children and young adults has also been reported.[191,200] No consistent predilection for either gender is seen. Previous irradiation is a pathogenetic risk factor for tumors arising in soft tissue, and the literature similarly contains sporadic reports of PPMFH presenting in patients who have received radiation therapy previously. Clinical and radiographic features of this tumor are nonspecific, and a distinction from the much more common epithelial tumors of the lungs absolutely requires tissue examination. The majority of patients present with symptoms of cough, chest pain, hemoptysis, or dyspnea. Chest X-rays generally show a solitary mass with a nondescript appearance and a relatively homogeneous density on CT or MRI studies.[199]

Pathologic findings

Most examples of PPMFH are intraparenchymal, but occasional endobronchial lesions have also been observed.[191] There is apparently no predilection for any particular lobe of either lung. These tumors are usually large, ranging up to 25 cm in maximum dimension,[201] with an average size of 6–7 cm. They are well-circumscribed, lobular, and white-tan, and not uncommonly contain central necrosis or cavitation on macroscopic examination.

Histologically, PPMFH is characterized by fusiform and pleomorphic elements that are arranged in storiform, fascicular, or medullary patterns (Fig. 14.27). As the name "malignant fibrous histiocytoma" implies, this tumor was originally thought to be composed of malignant fibroblast-like and the histiocytoid cells; however, it now appears that there is little if any relationship between the neoplastic elements and true histiocytes. Fusiform tumor cells contain elongated nuclei and relatively scant cytoplasm, and the histiocytoid cells have round-to-oval nuclei with a moderate quantity of amphophilic cytoplasm (Fig. 14.28). A hallmark of most lesions in this category is the presence of large, bizarre, often-multinucleated cells with irregular contours. Mitoses, including atypical forms, are easily found and number from 5 to 30 per 10 high-power microscopic fields.[146]

The differential diagnosis of PPMFH by light microscopy includes primary or secondary pleomorphic sarcomas (e.g. "dedifferentiated" leiomyosarcoma and pleomorphic rhabdomyosarcoma), metastatic malignant melanoma, and sarcomatoid carcinoma.[9a] Immunohistochemical and electron microscopic studies can be employed to separate these pathologic entities.[192–196,201] Ultrastructurally, PPMFH shows fibroblastic and histiocyte-like differentiation, with abundant rough endoplasmic reticulum, numerous lysosomes, and a variable number of small cytoplasmic lipid droplets. Desmosomes, tonofibrils, elongated cell processes, myogenous filament skeins, and cytoplasmic dense bodies are absent. PPMFH expresses vimentin, but is devoid of other specialized markers of myogenous, neural, or epithelial differentiation, on immunohistologic analyses.[146]

Therapy and prognosis

The rarity of PPMFH again serves as an impediment to assessments of optimal treatment for this tumor. Surgical resection is currently the recommended treatment of choice, even if the lesion in question shows limited extrapulmonary spread to the intrathoracic great vessels or soft tissue.[202] Adjunctive chemotherapy and irradiation have not proven to be effective in the few published cases of PPMFH in which these treatments have been employed.[191,201] In one series of 22 examples,[191] 7 of 15 patients who underwent radical surgical resection suffered relapses and died from metastatic disease. There was recurrence in the lungs and pleura, as well as

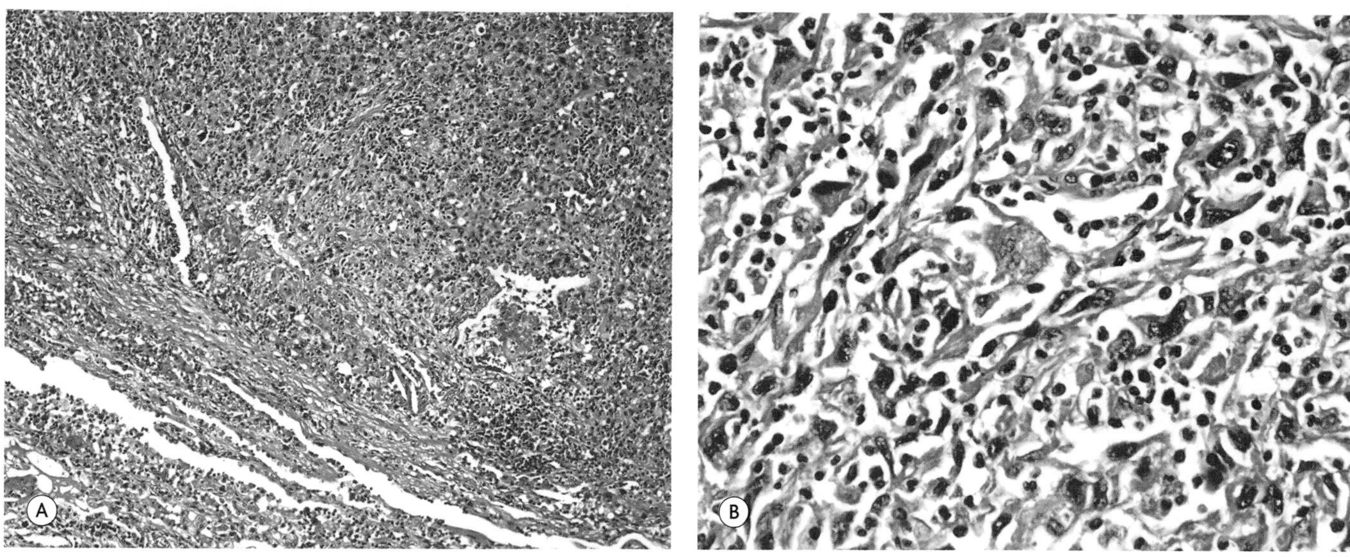

Fig. 14.27 (A) Primary pulmonary malignant fibrous histiocytoma, showing a disorganized proliferation of atypical spindle cells and pleomorphic elements that entraps alveolar airspaces. (B) Marked nuclear pleomorphism and multinucleation are focally present in the lesion.

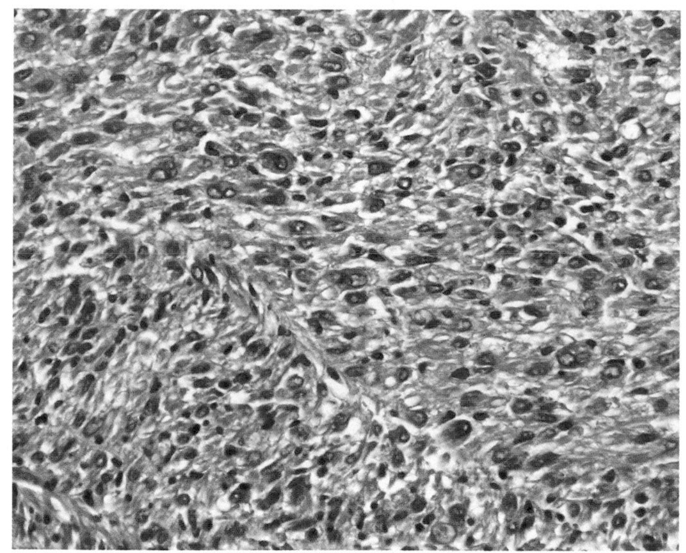

Fig. 14.28 This example of primary pulmonary malignant fibrous histiocytoma shows a more epithelioid cell population that could cause diagnostic confusion with poorly differentiated carcinoma.

metastasis to the liver and brain; almost all of these events occurred within 12 months of diagnosis. However, survivals as long as 5–10 years have been documented in a few patients with PPMFH.[191,193]

Potential adverse prognostic factors include an advanced clinical or pathologic stage at presentation (with mediastinal, chest wall, or carinal involvement), prominent symptoms at diagnosis, incompleteness of excision, and tumor recurrence. Histologic findings have not been found to affect behavior.

Rhabdomyosarcoma

For practical purposes, primary rhabdomyosarcoma of the lung (RMSL) is a tumor that is confined to the pediatric population. In adults, tumors resembling rhabdomyosarcoma are almost invariably examples of sarcomatoid carcinoma,[1,2] and this fact should be borne in mind in interpreting all but the most recent literature on this topic. Moreover, this is another sarcoma type which much more commonly arises outside of the lungs, and the probability that one is dealing with metastasis *to* the pulmonary parenchyma is therefore important to remember.

Clinical summary

To date, there are less than 20 well-documented examples of bona fide intrapulmonary rhabdomyosarcoma in the pertinent literature. They all occurred in patients who were in the first two decades of life, and most were in children under 10 years of age.[203–206] Symptoms and signs of RMSL may be nonspecific, including cough, wheezing, and dyspnea, or the patient may present with spontaneous pneumothorax.[207] The latter relates to a peculiar tendency of RMSL to associate itself with cystic lesions of the lungs.[204,205,208] When these cysts rupture, pneumothorax results. The underlying lesions in such cases of RMSL have included congenital cystic adenomatoid malformations and peripheral bronchogenic cysts.[208]

Roentgenographic studies may demonstrate a single, nondescript, intraparenchymal mass that is homogeneous on CT or MRI analyses, or they may reveal the presence

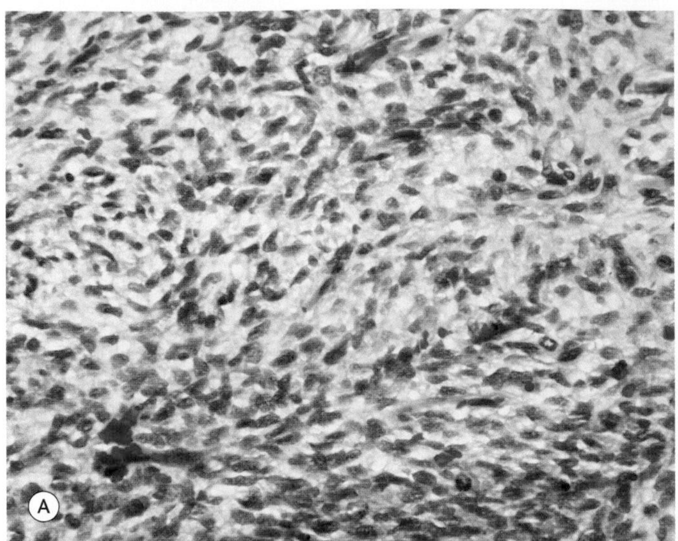

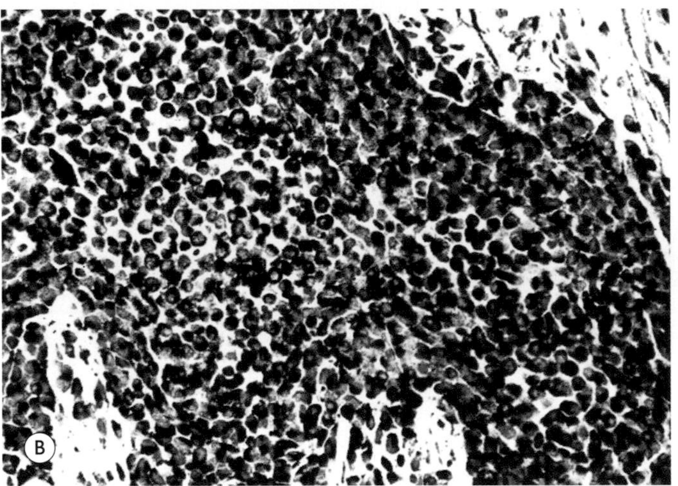

Fig. 14.29 (A) Embryonal rhabdomyosarcoma (ERMS) of the lung, which presented as an endobronchial lesion in a child. The tumor comprises hyperchromatic small cells with modestly irregular nuclear outlines, set in a myxoid stroma. (B) Immunoreactivity for desmin is intense in another example of ERMS.

of a mass in the wall of a cyst. The second of these scenarios is much more likely to result in a correct diagnosis by the radiologist.

Pathologic findings

As mentioned above, RMSL may be associated with preexisting cysts of the lung such as congenital cystic adenomatoid malformations or intrapulmonary bronchogenic cysts. Hence, the latter lesions should always be examined – at least cursorily – for a malignant component, despite the extreme rarity of the latter complication.

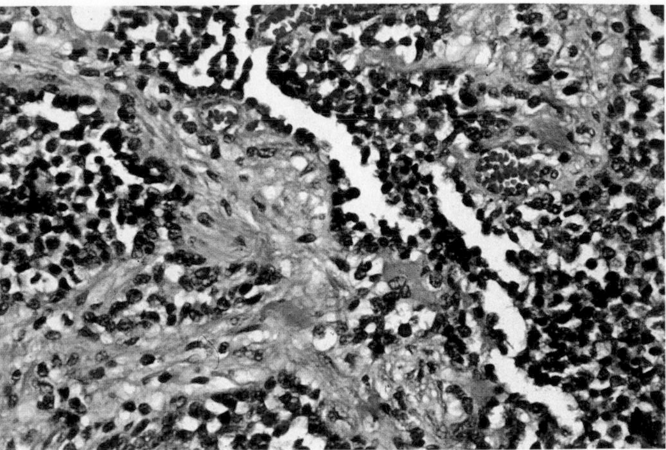

Fig. 14.30 Alveolar rhabdomyosarcoma of the lung, composed of undifferentiated small round cells that lack cohesion and form cleft-like or alveolar spaces.

Pulmonary rhabdomyosarcomas have most often assumed an embryonal or an alveolar growth pattern,[204,205] (Figs 14.29 and 14.30) although pleomorphic tumors, which are usually encountered in the soft tissues of adults, have been reported in the lung.[209] These neoplasms are typically composed of small round cells that are configured in one of three ways. These include "solid" sheet-like clusters with no further distinguishing morphologic attributes; dyscohesive groups with internal pseudolumina or alveoli; and "botryoid" proliferations in which a polypoid lesion (usually within a bronchial lumen) shows a zonation into hypocellular and hypercellular cellular strata (so-called "cambium" layers).[210] In contradistinction to other small round cell tumors of children, RMSL demonstrates a moderate degree of cellular pleomorphism and anisonucleosis. Nuclear chromatin is usually coarse and clumped; cytoplasm is scanty and amphophilic or eosinophilic; and mitoses and apoptotic cells are easily found. Small foci of spontaneous necrosis are also present.

Particularly in those lesions that have an embryonal "solid" appearance histologically, special pathologic studies are nearly always necessary to procure a definitive diagnosis. Moreover, these analyses should also be done in *all* putative cases in adults, for reasons mentioned above. Histochemical stains show that striated muscle tumors contain abundant glycogen, as determined with the periodic acid–Schiff method with and without diastase digestion. Electron microscopically, rhabdomyosarcoma is characterized by the focal presence of intermediate filament whorls in the cytoplasm, sometimes with the addition of "thick" filaments in aggregates that resemble primitive muscular Z-bands

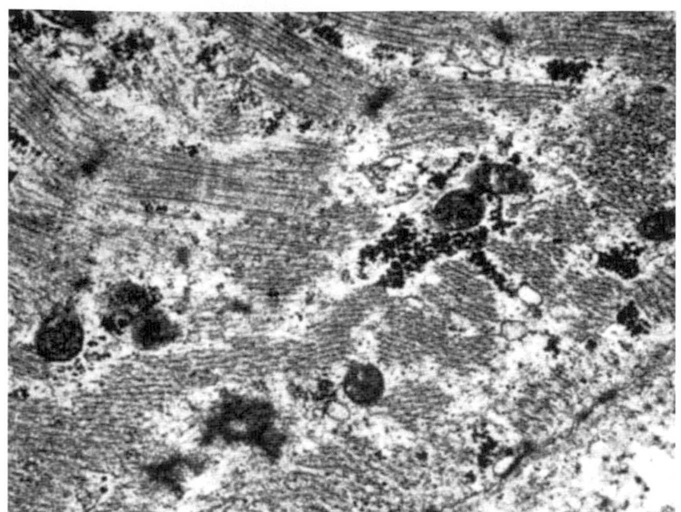

Fig. 14.31 Electron photomicrograph of pulmonary rhabdomyosarcoma, showing cytoplasmic sarcomeric differentiation with formation of Z-bands.

(Fig. 14.31). Furthermore, cytoplasmic glycogen is present and pericellular basal lamina can be visualized. This constellation of fine structural attributes excludes other small cell tumors from diagnostic consideration.[211] By immunohistology, RMSL is found to express one or more myogenous determinants, such as desmin, tropomyosin, titin, muscle-specific actin, "fast" myosin, or Z-band protein.[212] Vimentin is also uniformly found, but markers of epithelial differentiation – such as keratin and EMA – must be *absent* in order to make the diagnosis.

Therapy and prognosis

The great majority of reported cases of RMSL have been treated surgically, with the usual addition of post-operative irradiation and standard chemotherapy such as that used by the InterGroup Rhabdomyosarcoma Study.[203–209] However, there are no controlled studies to determine whether or not this protocol is the optimal approach to management. Once again, the extreme rarity of the lesion in question interferes with the design of the most efficacious therapeutic regimen.

Prognostically, the fact that RMSL is a *visceral* manifestation of rhabdomyosarcoma is an adverse clinical variable, along with the probability that such tumors may attain a size of several centimeters before coming to clinical attention. Pathologic features that have been associated with unfavorable tumoral behavior include the focal or global presence of an alveolar growth pattern, and the existence of areas that resemble adult-type pleomorphic rhabdomyosarcoma.[213]

Chondrosarcoma of the respiratory tract

Chondrosarcomas are uncommon, but well-documented in the supporting tissues of both the upper and lower airways. Indeed, although cartilaginous malignancies are usually observed in the proximal long bones of adults, visceral lesions of this type have been reported in a variety of locations. As one would expect, there are few if any examples of primary pulmonary chondrosarcoma (PPCS) that involve the most distal portion of the respiratory tract, because cartilaginous support for the bronchi ends at the level of subsegmental bronchi.[214–216] Accordingly, most PPCSs affect the trachea and major bronchial divisions,[217–219] and chondrosarcomas that are seen in the peripheral lung fields should be carefully examined radiologically to make certain that they are not extensions of contiguous bony lesions in the sternum, vertebral bodies, or ribs.

In contrast to statements pertaining to most other sarcomas of the lung, it is virtually unknown for chondroid malignancies to metastasize while they are still occult in peripheral osseous or soft tissue sites. Thus, once a pathologic diagnosis of chondrosarcoma has been established for a lesion that clearly involves the airway, it may safely be considered to have arisen at that location.

Clinical summary

Patients with PPCS are adults, with no predilection of the tumor for either gender. They may present with slowly evolving stridor, wheezing, cough, vague chest pain, or episodes of hemoptysis.[216,217] Systemic complaints are not encountered. Tracheobronchoscopy usually demonstrates a smooth, nodular, glistening mass that stretches and attenuates the overlying mucosa but does not ulcerate it. Attempted biopsy of the mass through the bronchoscope is usually unsuccessful, because of the firm consistency of the tumor and difficulty of sampling submucosal lesions in general.[214]

Radiographically, there may be no visible abnormalities on plain films if the neoplasm is predominantly or exclusively intraluminal in a large airway. Other examples of PPCS are manifest simply as sharply circumscribed, lobulated masses that may contain flecks of central calcification or cystic change.[219] The latter findings are more graphically displayed in CT or MRI studies.[217]

Pathologic findings

Chondrosarcomas of the lung differ significantly from pulmonary chondroid hamartomas on microscopic

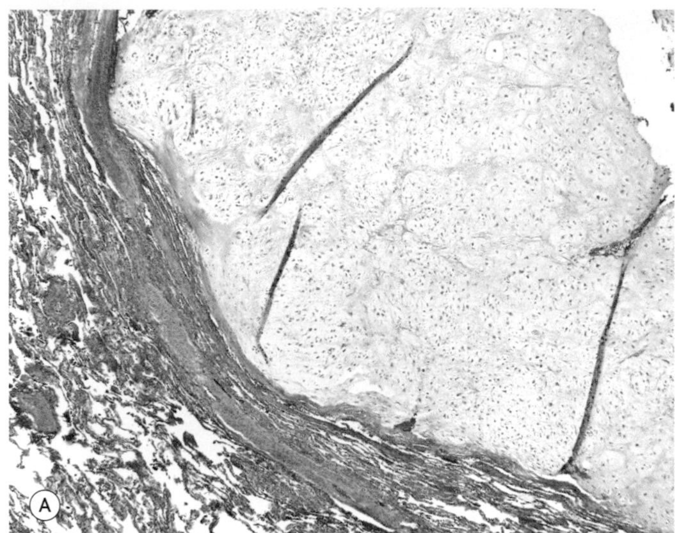

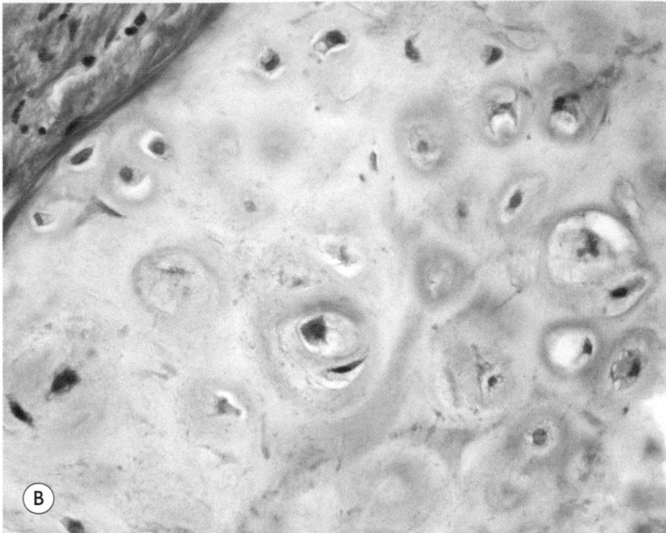

Fig. 14.32 **Low-grade chondrosarcoma of the carina.** (A,B) The constituent neoplastic chondrocytes are minimally atypical, but this particular lesion grossly demonstrated obvious destruction of the wall of the airway and justified a malignant diagnosis.

grounds. The latter lesions typically entrap small tubular airways and are composed of extremely well-differentiated chondrocytes. In contrast, PPCS exhibits at least modest nuclear pleomorphism, nuclear crowding, and cellular binucleation, and does *not* contain respiratory epithelial profiles.[214,216] (Fig. 14.32). Despite the statements just made, most chondrosarcomas of the lung *are* well-differentiated tumors. Hence, a striking degree of nondescript spindle cell growth or cellular anaplasia in a cartilage-forming tumor should instead invoke concerns over a probable diagnosis of sarcomatoid carcinoma with "divergent" chondroid areas.[1,2] Mesenchymal chondrosarcomas,[215] represented by small cell neoplasms of childhood with resemblances to Ewing's sarcoma (see below) (Fig. 14.33) are rare and special variants that differ from the descriptions just given above. They comprise sheets of small lymphocyte-like cells, often punctuated by hemangiopericytoid blood vessels, with interposed islands of embryonal-type cartilage.

With these features in mind, there are few other differential diagnostic considerations in cases of PPCS. Thus, special histochemical, ultrastructural, and immunohistochemical assessments are not usually needed to establish a confident diagnosis.

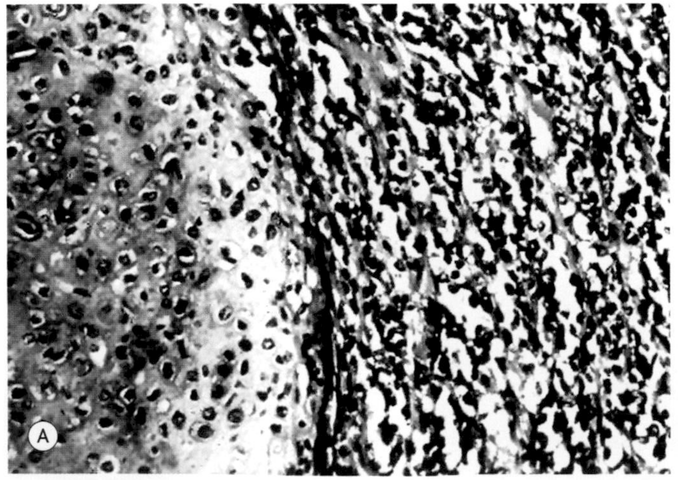

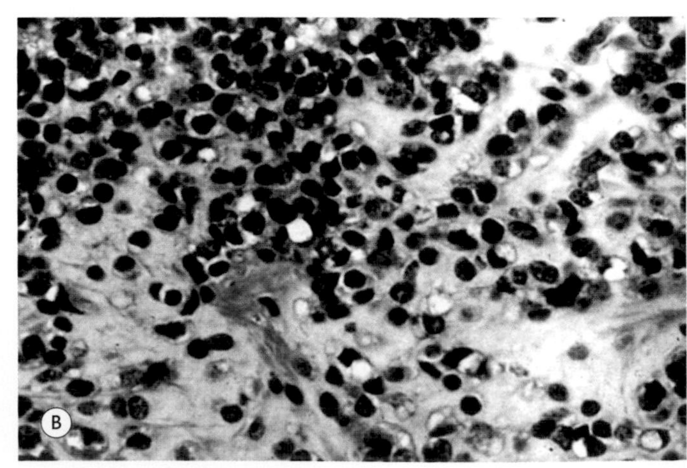

Fig. 14.33 (A) Mesenchymal chondrosarcoma of the lung, showing a juxtaposition of chondroid islands and undifferentiated small round tumor cells. (B) Elsewhere in the mass, a more gradual transition between the two components was present.

Therapy and prognosis

Primary chondrosarcomas of the airway are best treated by surgical ablation. Because these are slowly growing and generally low-grade malignancies, such intervention carries with it a good chance of long-term survival if the tumor can be completely extirpated.[217] Chemotherapy and irradiation are ineffectual in treating PPCS, and probably incur more morbidity than is acceptable in the treatment of an indolent sarcoma.

In extrapolation from bone tumor pathology, there are only two features that correlate with a risk of recurrence or metastasis of chondrosarcoma: a tumor size of >5 cm and vascular invasion by the neoplastic cells. There is no evidence that adjuvant treatment of patients with these risk factors in any way improves the clinical outlook. Indeed, it is our opinion that reoperation to remove any recurrent masses is the most sensible approach to patient management in this context.

Primary pulmonary synovial sarcoma

Although synovial sarcoma (SS) is primarily a peripheral soft tissue tumor, it is also potentially seen as a primary pleuropulmonary lesion. Published reports of approximately 40 cases have now attested to that fact.[158,220–227] Because of the range of histologic and radiographic appearances associated with SS, it enters into differential diagnosis with several other neoplasms in the lung and pleura.

Clinical findings

The basic symptoms and signs that are associated with primary pulmonary SS are no different than those attending bronchogenic carcinomas, except they are seen in a younger age group (mean – 38.5 years). Chest pain, cough, shortness of breath, and hemoptysis may be encountered, but, in one series, one-quarter of all patients were asymptomatic.[220] Men and women are relatively equally likely to develop SS of the lung. Roentgenographically, there is usually little to point the radiologist toward a specific diagnosis of SS in the lung, which may arise in any segment of any pulmonary lobe. However, some cases will show flocculent or particulate calcification on plain film radiographs or computed tomograms. Cystic change may also be noted, and a minority of lesions are clearly associated with a major bronchus.[220–227]

Pathologic findings

The microscopic spectrum of synovial sarcomas of the lung parallels that seen in similar tumors of peripheral soft tissue.[228] Classically, "biphasic" SS is composed of fascicles of compact spindle cells arranged in interweaving or "herringbone" fascicles, punctuated by clefts or overtly gland-like spaces that are lined by cuboidal to low columnar tumor cells (Fig. 14.34). The latter inclusions may contain mucoid matrical material and may also demonstrate squamous or goblet-cell metaplasia. Nuclei of the neoplastic cells in both components are generally monomorphic, with dispersed chromatin and

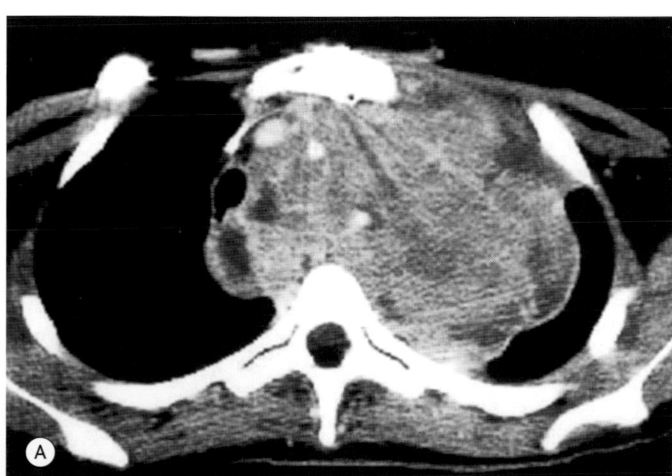

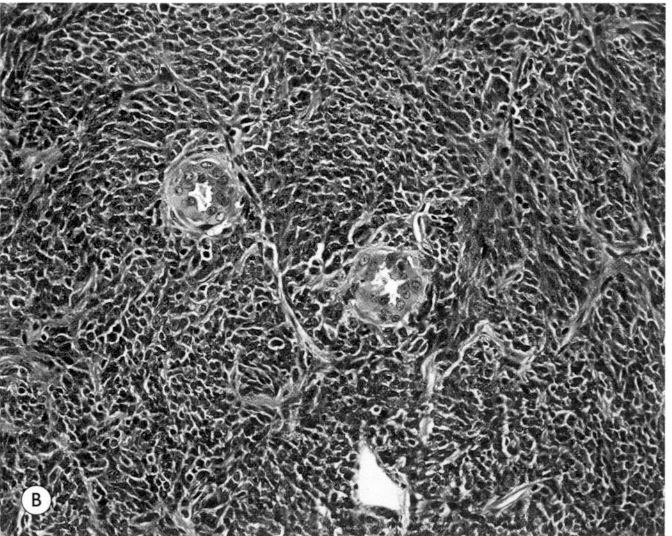

Fig. 14.34 (A) CT scan of primary pulmonary synovial sarcoma showing a large mass nearly filling the left hemithorax. (B) photomicrograph of biphasic synovial sarcoma of the lung. The tumor contains gland-like epithelial structures punctuating a neoplastic spindle cell proliferation. Diagnostic confusion with biphasic sarcomatoid carcinoma is possible.

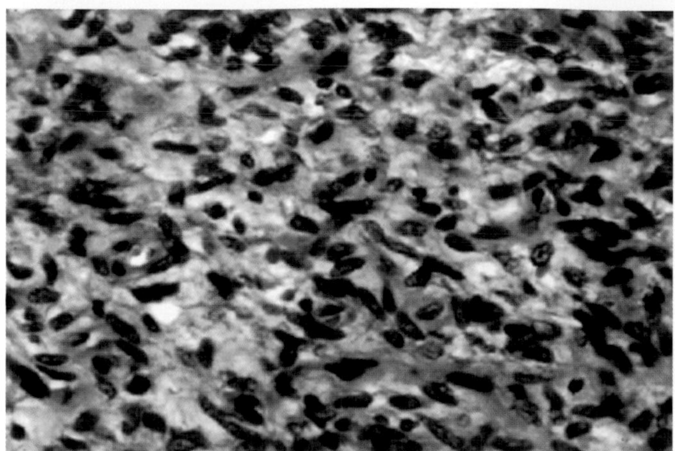

Fig. 14.35 **Myxoid stroma in synovial sarcoma.** This feature is again potentially shared with sarcomatoid carcinomas.

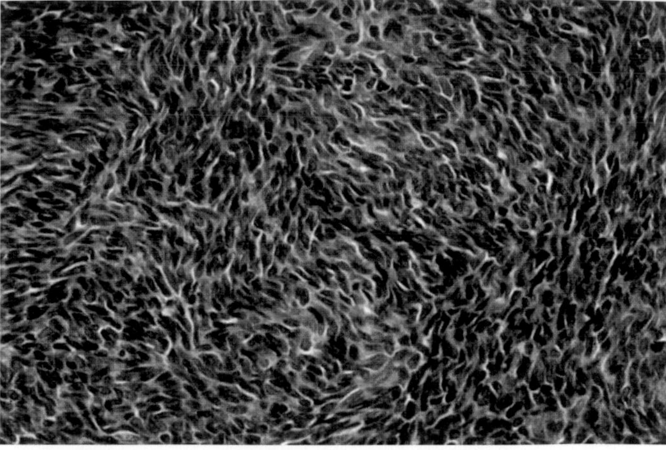

Fig. 14.36 **Monophasic spindle cell synovial sarcoma.** The image shown here overlaps with that of sarcomatoid carcinomas as well as other sarcoma morphotypes.

inconspicuous nucleoli. Cytoplasm is sparse in the fusiform cellular elements. In contrast, a moderate quantity of amphophilic, eosinophilic, or vacuolated cytoplasm is apparent in gland-like foci. Mitotic activity is greatly variable, may be surprisingly scant, and only rarely features the presence of "atypical" division figures. Intercellular calcifications (sometimes with a psammomatous configuration) may be scattered randomly throughout the tumor, or be clustered in discrete foci, or be lacking altogether. The finding of necrosis is likewise highly variable. Tumoral stroma can be overtly collagenous, delicate and fibrovascular, or myxoid (Fig. 14.35). Besides the prototypic form of biphasic SS, another with an admixture of solid polygonal cell clusters and spindle cell zones is recognized.[228]

The existence of "monophasic" SS is now accepted. This variant may be composed entirely of fusiform elements, epithelioid polygonal cells that may or may not demonstrate obvious gland-like differentiation, or sheets of small round cells.[220] Monophasic *spindle* cell SS is more common by far (Fig. 14.36), and recognition of it as a distinct entity has resulted in reclassification of many "fibrosarcomas" of the soft tissues and other sites. It is now realized that the great majority of sarcomas with a "herringbone" spindle cell constituency are actually synovial rather than fibroblastic, as traditionally taught.[212] Another key feature to the recognition of monophasic spindle cell SS is the presence of a "staghorn" pattern of intratumoral vascularity.[228] Divergent differentiation, simulating osteogenic, neural, or squamous lesions, is another pathologic facet of monophasic SS that may cause diagnostic consternation.[220]

Electron microscopy and immunohistology have shown that SS is actually an epithelial proliferation, with ultrastructurally well-formed junctional complexes between the tumor cells.[212,228] Reticulin stains are often useful in outlining epithelioid cell clusters when they are present but indistinct. Immunostains for keratin and epithelial membrane antigen (EMA) can be used to similar advantage, but these determinants are also commonly seen together with vimentin in the *spindle* cells of biphasic or monophasic SS. CD99, calretinin, and *bcl*-2 protein are often observed in SS as well.[228] An exciting development is the knowledge that SS shows a characteristic t(X;18) chromosomal translocation (Fig. 14.37), which can be assessed using traditional cytogenetic tech-

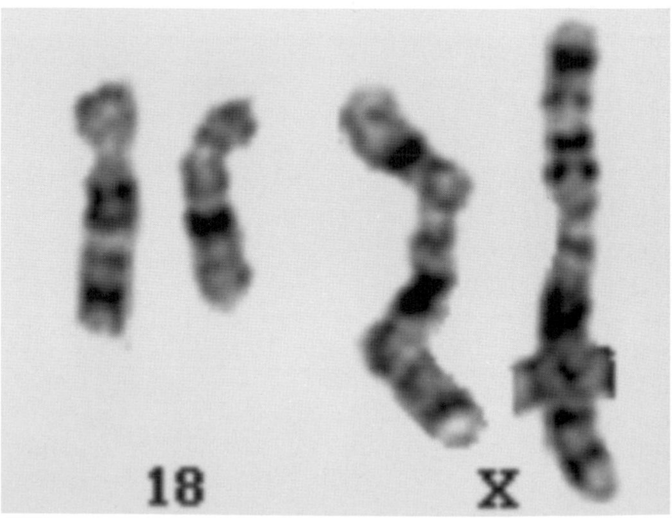

Fig. 14.37 Karyotypic preparation of tumor tissue from primary pulmonary synovial sarcoma, showing the t(X;18) chromosomal translocation that typifies this neoplasm.

niques or fluorescence in-situ hybridization (FISH).[222,223] This karyotypic aberration produces a selective fusion transcript known as *SYT-SSX*, and the polymerase chain reaction can be employed to detect it diagnostically, using suitable primer pairs of nucleotides.[227]

The major differential diagnostic alternatives to primary SS in the lung are *metastatic* synovial sarcoma from soft tissue sites, hemangiopericytoma, fibrosarcoma, mesothelioma, and sarcomatoid carcinoma. Among these possibilities, only SS shows the aforementioned t(X;18) chromosomal abnormality, making cytogenetic evaluation, with or without other adjunctive studies, highly desirable in this context.

Therapy and prognosis

The long-term outlook for patients with SS of the lung is guarded at best. In a series reported by Zeren et al., 14 of 18 patients had died of their tumors or were likely to do so at a mean follow-up period of 12.5 years.[220] In general, this neoplasm has the ability to recur locally or demonstrate distant metastasis many years after its initial diagnosis; indeed, follow-up shows that tumor-related mortality continues to accrue up to 20 years after presentation.[228]

Recommended therapy for primary pulmonary SS is predicated on radical surgical extirpation. The efficacy of adjuvant radiation treatment and chemotherapy is somewhat controversial.

Other primary pulmonary sarcomas

In addition to those tumors that have been previously considered, there are other sarcoma morphotypes that may be encountered in the lungs. These include *liposarcoma*,[229] *angiosarcoma*,[230] *malignant peripheral nerve sheath tumor*,[153,158,232] and *osteosarcoma*.[233] Less than 10 cases each of these neoplasms have been documented in the literature, making it impossible to present their clinicopathologic attributes as if they were thoroughly studied and well-characterized.

However, a few generalizations do appear to be appropriate. First, liposarcomas and malignant schwannomas of the lung have been primarily documented as tumors that have an endobronchial component, potentially producing airway obstruction. In contrast, this feature is not part of the profile of either angiosarcoma or osteosarcoma. Secondly, both angiosarcoma-*like* and osteosarcoma-*like epithelial* neoplasms are vastly more common in the respiratory tract than true sarcomas with those respective microscopic patterns.[2] Thus, the pathologist must be certain to address the likelihood of sarcomatoid carcinoma under such circumstances. Finally, therapy for those rare lesions in this category that *have* proven to be primary in the lungs is completely anecdotal, and has been based on extrapolation from treatment used for histologically similar neoplasms in osseous and soft tissue sites.

Part III: Primary malignant melanomas of the lung

Melanomas arising primarily in the lung are extraordinarily rare; the literature contains sparse reports on this topic.[234–242,242ab] The largest series is from the AFIP, consisting of 8 cases seen over a period of many years.[234] Although rigorous criteria have been proposed for primary malignant melanoma of the lung (PMML), this interpretation cannot be established with absolute certainty because of the well-known capacity for spontaneous regression of primary melanomas in mucosal or cutaneous sites. In order to consider a diagnosis of PMML seriously, there obviously must be no prior history of a potentially malignant pigmented tumor of the skin or ocular uveal tract. Moreover, clinical examination for possibly occult melanomas in the integument, nailbeds, eyes, nasal cavity, paranasal sinuses, oral cavity, esophagus, anus, rectum, vulva, and leptomeninges should not show any extrapulmonary lesions. In fact, some authors have suggested that a case of PMML can be regarded as bona fide only retrospectively, after a postmortem examination has excluded another source of a primary melanoma.[235–237] Hence, it is self-evident that this diagnosis can never be considered irrefutable during life.

As to the fundamental question of the origin of primary melanoma in the respiratory tract, some have stressed that the tracheobronchial tree is, in fact, of endodermal derivation – in similarity to the oral cavity and the esophagus – where well-documented primary melanomas have originated.[237] Nonetheless, these tumors are generally thought to be neuroectodermal, and their presence in endodermal or mesodermal sites is therefore problematic with reference to "classical" histogenetic theory. We instead subscribe to the "stem cell" theory of neoplasia – wherein embryologic constructs are essentially irrelevant – to explain the phenomenon under discussion here. In that vein, it is interesting that some *benign* proliferations of the lung also demonstrate partial or global melanocytic differentiation: namely, clear-cell "sugar" tumor, angiomyolipoma, and lymphangioleiomyomatosis.[242c–g]

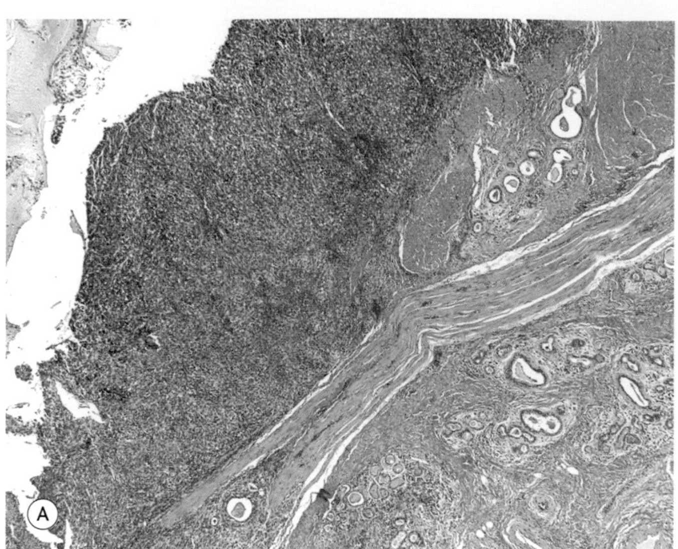
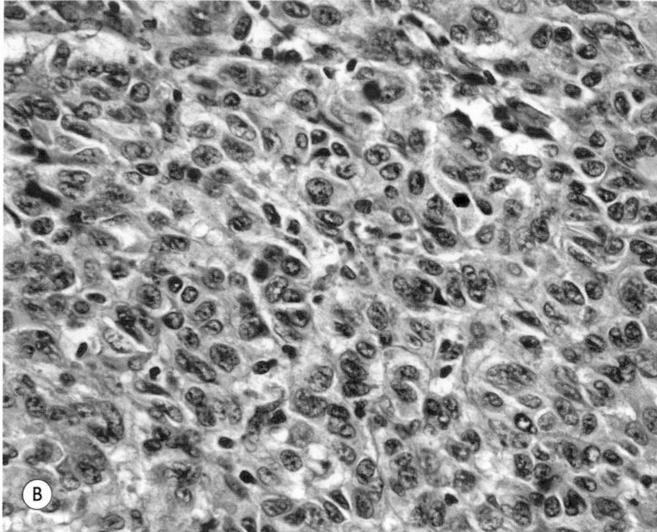

Fig. 14.38 (A,B) Apparently primary malignant melanoma of the lung, represented by an amelanotic proliferation of pleomorphic tumor cells within a bronchus. Immunohistologic studies were necessary to support the presence of melanocytic differentiation in this case.

Clinical summary

The ages of reported patients with PMML have ranged from 29 to 80 years. Because of the rarity of this lesion, no meaningful statements can be made regarding gender-related incidence figures. Some patients with broncho-pulmonary melanoma have been asymptomatic, whereas others have presented with hemoptysis, dyspnea, or cough.[234–242] Plain-film radiographic examinations generally have shown abnormalities only if the tumors were in the pulmonary parenchyma; in other words, endobronchial tumors are visible only on CT or MRI studies.

Pathologic findings

In several reported cases of PMML, the lesions have been centered in large airways, including the trachea and major bronchi.[234,248,249,240,242] Grossly, these tumors are generally polypoid, endoluminal masses that are partially or completely obstructing, or they present as nodules within the lung parenchyma, which range from 1 to 4.5 cm in greatest dimension. In addition, they are characteristically colored, in shades of brown or black.

Histologically, PMMLs are composed of heterogeneously pigmented and variably pleomorphic cells that range from epitheloid to fusiform in configuration with occasional gigantiform figures; overtly sarcoma-like lesions are certainly part of the repertoire of these neoplasms (Fig. 14.38). An important microscopic feature that further supports a primary origin in the respiratory tract is the presence of a cytologically atypical in-situ melanocytic proliferation in adjacent bronchial mucosa, which may be metaplastic[234,237] (Fig. 14.39). Electron microscopic studies showing the presence of cytoplasmic premelanosomes (Fig. 14.40), or immunohistochemical negativity for keratin and labeling for S100 protein, HMB-45 antigen, Melan-A/MART-1, or tyrosinase are useful in confirming the presence of melanocytic differentiation [234] and excluding the differential diagnoses of anaplastic carcinoma or sarcoma.

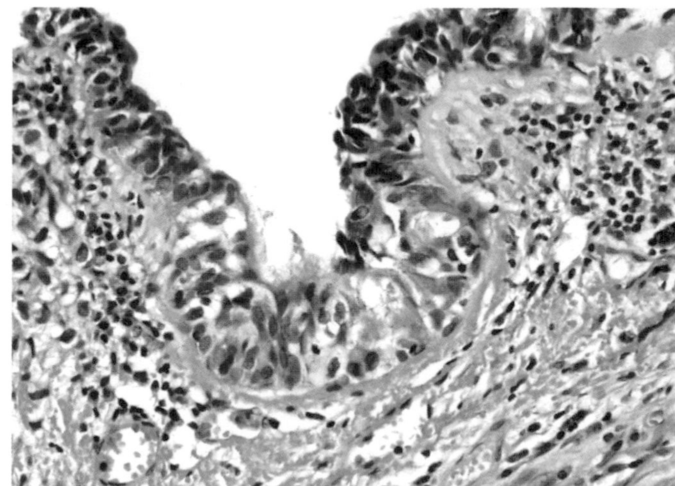

Fig. 14.39 In-situ malignant melanoma of the bronchial mucosa. The tumor cells are scattered throughout the epithelium randomly.

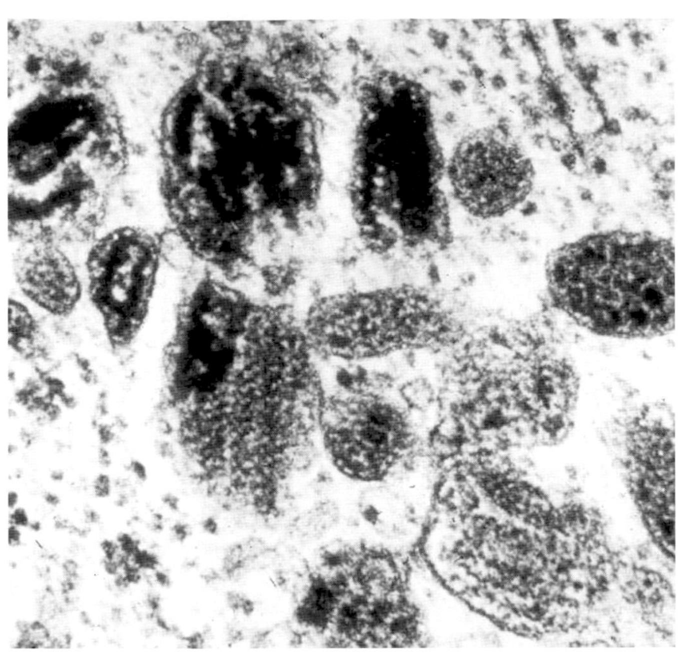

Fig. 14.40 Electron photomicrograph of malignant melanoma, demonstrating the presence of cytoplasmic premelanosomes. These inclusions are diagnostic.

Therapy and prognosis

Most documented cases of PMML have fared extremely poorly, with the majority of patients dying within 1 year of diagnosis.[234,237–239,241] Reid and Mehta reported one individual who survived 11 years after surgery;[240] however, there was no mention in the latter study of clinical evaluations which were designed to exclude other primary sites of origin, and no in-situ melanocytic proliferation was found in the pulmonary resection specimen. Thus, the latter case is doubtful as a verifiable PMML. Most patients have undergone surgical resections of their tumors, although a few have received irradiation or chemotherapy.[235] In extension of therapeutic results obtained in cases of other primary melanomas of the viscera, it must be concluded that long-term survival of patients with PMML is an idiosyncratic and unlikely event.

Part IV: Sarcomas of the pulmonary arterial trunk

Although it is technically not part of the respiratory tract, the pulmonary arterial trunk is an appropriate topic for this discussion that centers on intrathoracic mesenchymal malignancies. For over 70 years, it has been known that this vascular segment may serve as the point of origin for sarcomas with diverse histologic features, and clinical manifestations which are just as variable.[243] To date, approximately 150 cases of pulmonary trunk sarcoma (PTS) have been documented.[9a,243–245]

Clinical summary

Patients with PTS are adults in middle life or beyond, with no predilection for either gender. They present with a panoply of potential symptoms and signs, the most common of which simulate the findings of right-sided cardiac failure or pulmonary thromboembolic disease. Patients often complain of intractable cough, progressive dyspnea, and dull chest pain that may increase with exertion; cardiac tamponade has rarely been observed.[245] Neck veins may be distended, a loud precordial systolic heart murmur may be audible at the upper left sternal border, and the patient may manifest the complete clinical scenario of anasarca.[246,247] However, cardiac imaging studies demonstrate no evidence of ventricular hypokinesis or perfusion abnormalities.[248]

In the era before modern angiography, echocardiography, CT, and specialized radionuclide scans, the diagnosis of PTS was usually made for the first time at autopsy.[243] However, current imaging modalities are now capable of revealing the tumor in question rather easily[248] (Fig. 14.41). It takes the form of a partially obstructing, endoluminal mass at the level of the right ventricular outlet or above it, and may extend over a span of several centimeters. Attachment of the lesion to the arterial wall is variable in character, and may be either sessile or

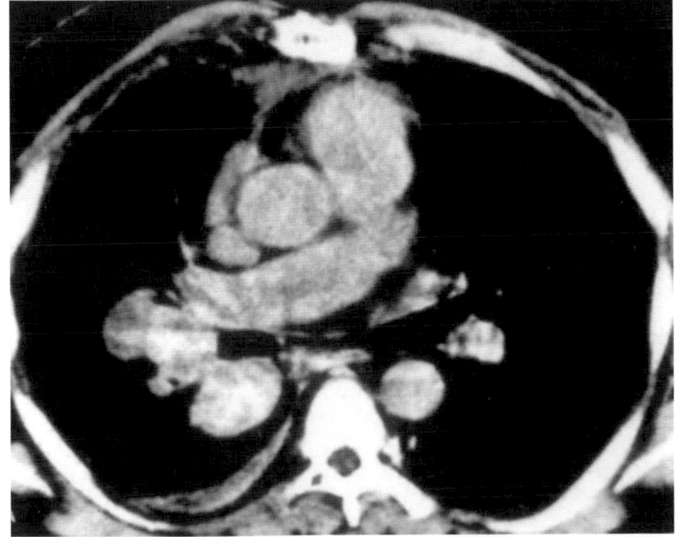

Fig. 14.41 Computed tomogram showing a mass within the pulmonary trunk, representing pulmonary trunk sarcoma.

pedunculated. The neoplasm is typically somewhat heterogeneous in density and greatly heterogeneous in size, from case to case.

Pathologic findings

The preoperative diagnosis of PTS is typically one that may not involve the pathologist, inasmuch as biopsy of an intravascular mass in the right ventricular outlet is a challenging procedure. Thus, his first encounter with such lesions may be in the frozen section laboratory during a definitive surgical procedure. In this context, it is important to realize that a firm diagnosis of a particular sarcoma type (or even of a malignancy) may not be an easy proposition. Some PTSs take the form of rather paucicellular myxoid proliferations with surprisingly bland cytologic characteristics, whereas others are anaplastic tumors that defy easy classification under the microscope[243] (Fig. 14.42). The proffered pathologic interpretations in the literature on PTS include such diagnoses as "undifferentiated sarcoma," "angiosarcoma," "leiomyosarcoma," "rhabdomyosarcoma," "fibromyxosarcoma," "fibrosarcoma," "chondrosarcoma," "osteosarcoma," "hemangioendothelioma," "malignant fibrous histiocytoma," and "malignant mesenchymoma."[247,247a–h] What one is able to glean from this apparently confusing list is that the histologic spectrum and pathologic grades of PTS are broadly distributed, such that no two individual lesions look quite the same under the microscope. Beyond that, pathologists take a great deal of interest in speculating on the mechanistic *"reasons"* for this diversity, but this issue has admittedly little clinical import at the present time.

With respect to differential diagnosis, the majority of PTSs have the characteristics of high-grade spindle cell or pleomorphic sarcomas, which, in current parlance, would usually be grouped together under the rubric of "malignant fibrous histiocytoma." However, some low-grade fibromyxoid variants can closely simulate an intracardiac myxoma or organizing mural thrombus.[243] Close attention to cytologic detail is the only certain method for distinguishing between such possibilities.

Therapy and prognosis

Because of the dominance of autopsy reports in the earliest literature on PTS, the recommended therapy for this tumor must still be considered evolutionary. At the present time, providing that a firm radiologic diagnosis can be made or a frozen section interpretation of sarcoma can be rendered, the surgeon may perform an en bloc resection of the pulmonary trunk and its luminal tumor contents, followed by interposition of a synthetic graft.[249] This is probably the most definitive approach to operative therapy, inasmuch as it is difficult to determine the boundaries of intramural tumor growth by visual inspection. The latter point makes more limited vascular resections and reconstructions a tenuous enterprise.

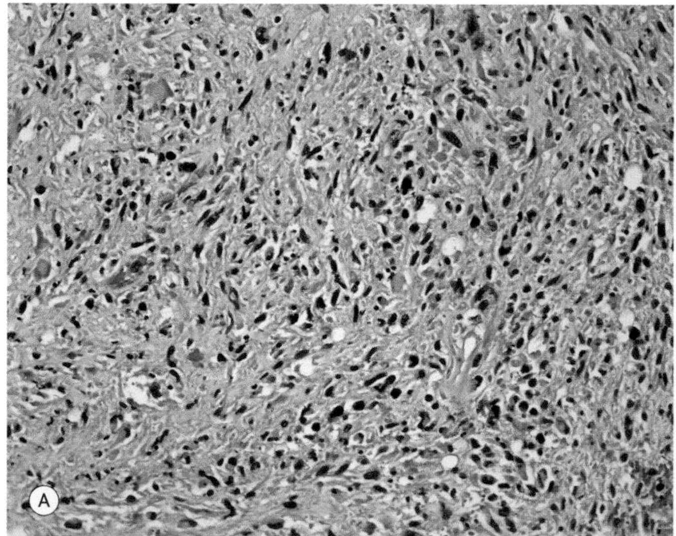

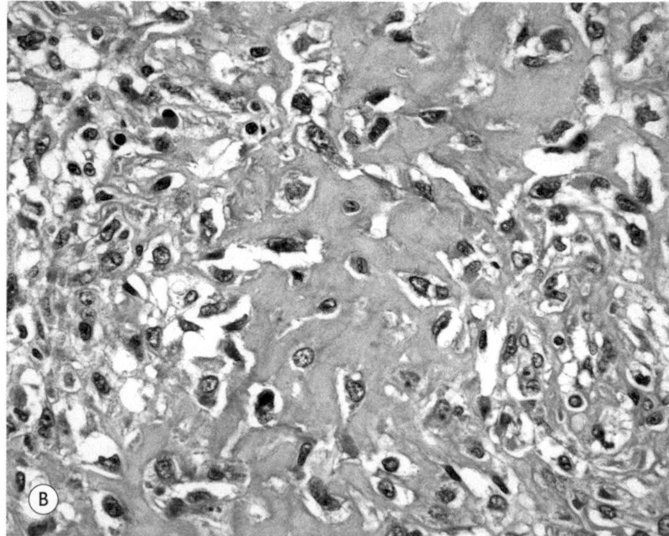

Fig. 14.42 These microscopic images of a case of pulmonary trunk sarcoma demonstrate (A) one area that resembles malignant fibrous histiocytoma histologically, (B) whereas another focus in the lesion shows obvious formation of osteoid. The exact nosologic classification of such tumors is often difficult.

Extension of the tumor through the wall of the pulmonary artery is the single most important piece of pathologic information in cases of PTS, inasmuch as histologic grading does not appear to correlate with tumor behavior in a consistent fashion.[243,247] In addition, the surgeon's or radiologist's estimation of whether the lesion is pendunculated or sessile has considerable importance. Tumors with a narrow stalk tend to "flutter" in the stream of ejected blood in the ventricular outflow tract, and pieces of the neoplasm may be embolized into the lungs.[250] This phenomenon is not as common with lesions that assume a broadly based sessile macroscopic growth pattern.

Cases demonstrating metastasis or obvious extravascular spread of PTS may be managed with irradiation or chemotherapy. However, there are no unified recommendations for the use of these treatments, and their implementation has produced discouraging results thus far.

Part V: Tumors of the pleura

Sarcomatoid malignant mesothelioma

Clinical summary

Regardless of histologic subtype – sarcomatoid or otherwise – the clinical features of intrathoracic mesothelioma are the same.[251–253] Malignant mesothelioma of the pleura typically affects adult men, although women and children are certainly represented in the patient population with this neoplasm.[253,254] The most common presenting symptoms and signs are pleuritic-type chest pain and shortness of breath, with a pleural effusion on chest radiographs. The lesion most commonly takes the form of multiple nodules and plaques in the serosal surfaces, but may occasionally be represented by a solitary mass. Later in the clinical course, encasement of the lung by confluent neoplastic tissue is seen (Figs 14.43 and 14.44). An influenza-like syndrome is occasionally reported in association with pleural mesothelioma. In likeness to examples of *peritoneal* mesothelioma that have been linked causally to chronic recurrent peritonitis in the context of familial Mediterranean fever,[255] the authors have observed several pleural tumors that arose in the background of chronic pleuritis in patients with a connective tissue disease (e.g. lupus erythematosus). Roughly 50–60% of pleural mesotheliomas can be objectively related to prior occupational-level asbestos exposure.[256] In those instances, 85-90% of patients will show the presence of pleural plaques or pleural calcifications, or quantitative pulmonary asbestos fiber burdens clearly in excess of the background, serving as tangible markers of such exposure.[257–263] Those findings are regarded as vastly more reliable than patients' historical accounts of occupational conditions, and should be sought in all instances before concluding objectively that a given mesothelioma is indeed asbestos-related etiologically.

Other accepted pathogenetic factors in mesothelioma cases include inhalation exposure to erionite (a mineral restricted to the Mideastern part of the world), chronic infection of the pleural spaces (e.g. in tuberculous pleuritis), and prior therapeutic irradiation of the thorax.[264,265] Substantial recent interest has centered on the potential role of simian virus-40 in this setting,[266] but conclusions on whether that agent is indeed causative in any way are premature. At least 40% of pleural mesotheliomas are idiopathic.[256]

Pathologic findings

In considering the pathologic appearances of overtly malignant mesothelial tumors, a surprising variety of patterns has emerged over time, and these have expanded the traditional categorical outline which theretofore included "epithelioid," "biphasic," and "sarcomatoid" mesotheliomas.[253,267,268] The epithelioid subgroup has now been enlarged to include mesothelial malignancies that have a wholly clear cell, oncocytoid or granular cell, tubulopapillary, large polygonal cell, polyhedral stromal mucin-producing, "medullary" epithelioid, or even small cell appearance.[267] The differential diagnostic potentialities raised by such images are numerous, including metastatic non-small cell carcinomas of various primary origins, metastatic melanoma, pleural sarcomas with an epithelioid or small round cell appearance, and even metastatic small cell neuroendocrine carcinoma. In reference to biphasic MM – with epithelioid and sarcoma-like elements – primary synovial sarcoma of the pleura has now been well-characterized as an important diagnostic alternative.[269] Indeed, in the absence of data showing the characteristic t(X;18) chromosomal translocation of synovial sarcoma, which is associated with production of *SYT-SSX* fusion transcripts,[270] its separation from MM can be extremely challenging. This is so because the immunophenotypes of the two tumors are largely overlapping.[271] Monophasic sarcomatoid mesothelioma potentially simulates a range of spindle cell sarcoma morphotypes that may affect the pleura, again including monophasic synovial sarcoma, but also fibrosarcoma, malignant fibrous histiocytoma, rhabdomyosarcoma, chondrosarcoma, osteosarcoma, leiomyosarcoma, and

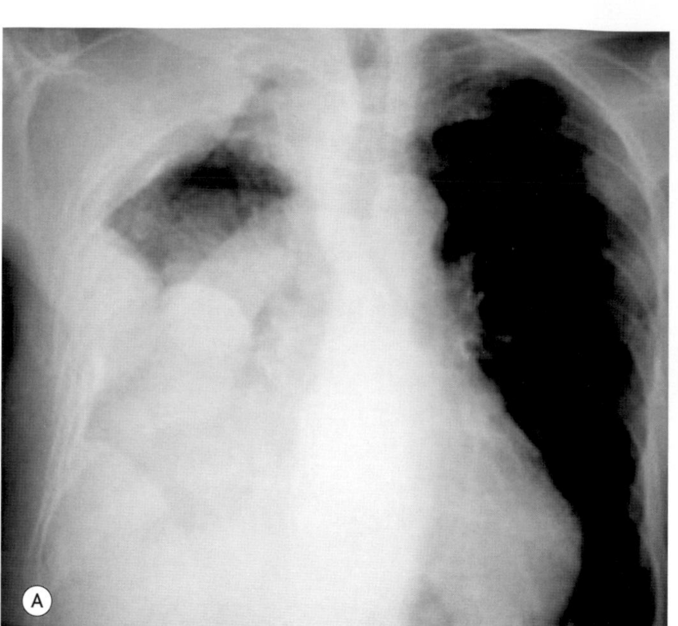

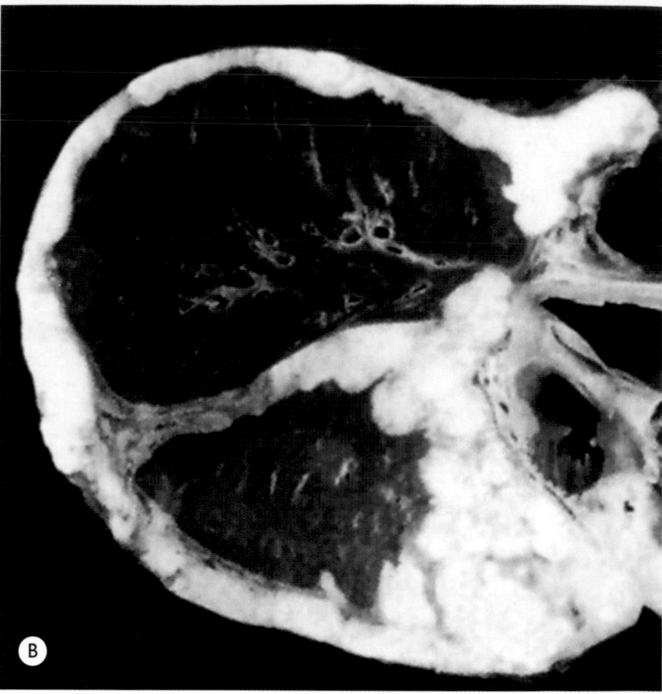

Fig. 14.43 (A) Chest radiograph of a right pleural malignant mesothelioma of the sarcomatoid type, showing loculated pleural effusion and multinodular pleural thickening. (B) An extrapleural pneumonectomy specimen in this case demonstrates circumferential encasement of the lung by tumor tissue, as well as extension into the interlobar septa.

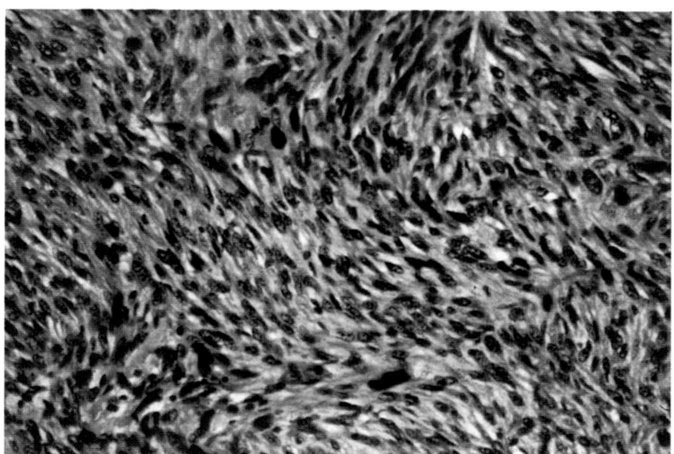

Fig. 14.44 Microscopic image of sarcomatoid malignant mesothelioma, showing a disorganized proliferation of highly atypical spindle cells. Metastatic or pleurotropic sarcomatoid carcinoma and true sarcomas of the pleura are differential diagnostic alternatives.

malignant peripheral nerve sheath tumor.[1,272–276] "Pseudomesotheliomatous" secondary pleural carcinomas with a sarcomatoid phenotype also enter the differential diagnosis in a meaningful fashion, as referenced earlier in this discussion. The histomorphologic findings in that particular differential diagnostic group of tumors have been summarized previously.

In specific reference to sarcomatoid mesotheliomas, the basic image of those lesions is virtually identical to that associated with sarcomatoid carcinoma of the lung.[277–282] Indeed, cases in which a tumor mass involves both the peripheral lung and the pleura will require immunohistologic evaluation in order for a distinction to be made with definition between those tumor types. As such, sarcomatoid mesotheliomas are comprised exclusively by overtly malignant spindle cells and pleomorphic elements, with or without such heterotopic tissue as osteoid, cartilage, muscle, or osteoclast-like giant cells. Two special variants of sarcomatoid mesothelioma merit further consideration: namely, the "lymphohistiocytoid" subtype[283,284] and desmoplastic mesothelioma.[285–291] These are respectively characterized by sheets of large cells with vesicular nuclear chromatin, prominent nucleoli, and abundant admixed lymphocytes (Fig. 14.45); and by relatively bland neoplastic spindle cells that are set in a densely collagenized fibrohyaline matrix with a so-called "patternless pattern" of growth (Fig. 14.46). Differential diagnosis in the latter instance is with fibrous (or fibrohyaline) pleuritis, in which case the presence of focally dense and atypical cellular growth, necrosis, obvious invasion of lung or soft tissue, or metastasis points to a diagnosis of mesothelioma.[290] On

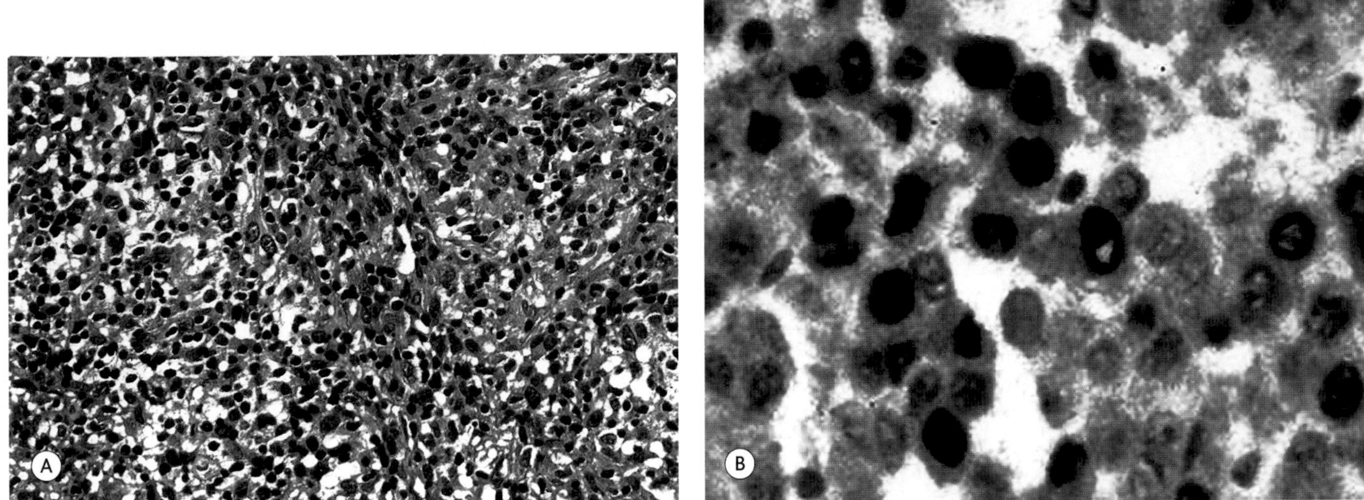

Fig. 14.45 (A, B) Lymphohistiocytoid sarcomatoid mesothelioma, showing anaplastic tumor cells admixed with numerous mature lymphocytes.

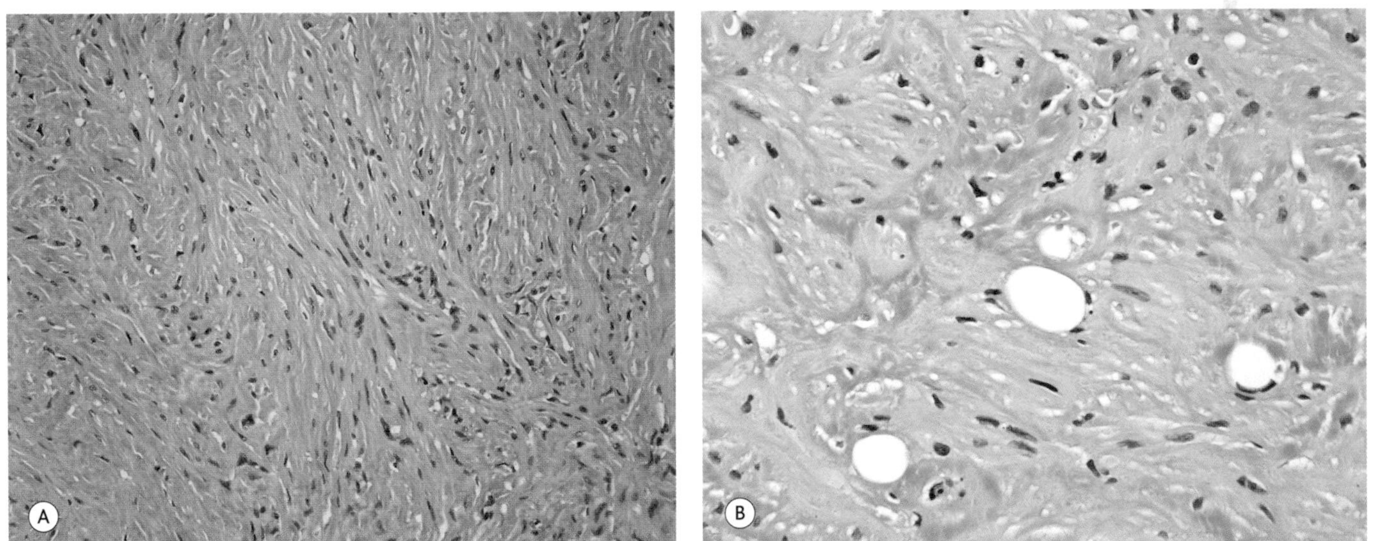

Fig. 14.46 (A, B) Desmoplastic sarcomatoid malignant mesothelioma, composed of minimally atypical spindle cells set in a densely hyalinized collagenous stroma. A distinction from fibrous pleurisy is often difficult.

the other hand, "lymphohistiocytoid" mesotheliomas may be confused with malignant lymphoma, inflammatory myofibroblastic (pseudo-)tumor of the pleura, or metastatic lymphoepithelioma-like carcinoma.[283,284]

This information brings one to a consideration of adjunctive pathologic studies in the objectification of a diagnosis of MM. In regard to this important topic, it should be remembered that there are definite roles for a *number* of laboratory analyses, including but not limited to histochemistry, immunohistology, electron microscopy, fluorescent in-situ hybridization (FISH), the polymerase chain reaction (PCR) using appropriately chosen primers, and traditional cytogenetic evaluations.[251–263,292,293] Although most attention has been paid in recent years to the immunohistochemical separation of epithelioid MM from metastatic adenocarcinoma,[294,295] the panel of markers used for that purpose is generally *not* helpful in the differential diagnosis of *non*-epithelioid (i.e. sarcomatoid) MM variants, with selected exceptions. Standard approaches to separating MM from adenocarcinoma include immunostains for keratin (either "pan-keratin" or keratin 5/6); epithelial membrane antigen; thrombomodulin; HBME-1; calretinin; WT-1; tumor-associated glycoprotein-72 (recognized by B72.3); carcinoembryonic antigen; CD15; Ber-EP4; BG8; and MOC-31, with expected reactivity in MM primarily including any of the first six of those determinants.[296] Electron microscopy is still extremely useful in this particular context, inasmuch as the long, branching, bushy microvilli that one associates with mesothelial cells are best represented in epithelioid MM.[297] Neither immunohistology nor electron microscopy is nearly as helpful in the realm of biphasic or sarcomatoid tumors, and an entirely different set of morphologic and immunophenotypic variables must be assessed in those lesions. For example, keratin, WT-1, and calretinin assume much greater value in the differential diagnosis of sarcomatoid MM,[296,298] because the principal interpretative alternatives are those of true sarcoma or solitary fibrous tumor, and sarcoma-like mesotheliomas may divergently express some mesenchymal markers such as desmin and muscle actin isoforms.[299,300] Moreover, FISH or PCR for *SYT-SSX* transcripts may be necessary to separate such entities as synovial sarcoma (which are also reactive for keratin and potentially for calretinin) from MM with certainty.[270,271] Ultrastructural analyses are likewise not very helpful in that setting, because sarcomatoid MM tends to lose the specialized features of epithelial cells when it assumes a spindle cell appearance.[282,301] Rarely, sarcomatoid mesotheliomas also may resemble solitary fibrous tumors of the pleura; in those cases, CD34 immunoreactivity tends to exclude a diagnosis of MM.[302]

Therapy and prognosis

The natural history of malignant pleural mesothelioma is an adverse one. The usual survival of patients with that tumor is less than 15 months, with death occurring because of cardiorespiratory embarrassment or pulmonary superinfection.[251,252,303] A peculiarity of this neoplasm is its tendency to grow through surgical defects in the chest wall, either represented by thoracotomy incisions or thoracostomy sites. Metastases outside the thorax are rare, although they have been reported in a small minority of cases in such sites as liver, bones, and skin.[304] Treatment is generally supportive, inasmuch as irradiation and chemotherapy produce little survival benefit.[305] Extrapleural pneumonectomy is a controversial surgical approach to mesothelioma; its proponents claim a definite decrease in mortality in the operative group, as compared with stage- and age- matched controls managed by other means.[306] However, those observations have not been supported by other studies.[307]

Primary pleural sarcomas

Sarcomas are as rare in the pleura as they are in the lungs. Most neoplasms that take the generic appearance of malignant mesenchymal tumors in the serosae of the thorax are, in actuality, epithelial lesions. They may either represent metastatic sarcomatoid carcinomas or variants of malignant mesothelioma, as considered above. In addition, there are only a limited number of definable clinicopathologic entities to consider in this specific anatomic location. These include fibrosarcoma, malignant solitary (localized) fibrous tumor of the pleura, leiomyosarcoma, synovial sarcoma, Askin's malignant thoracopulmonary small round cell tumor, pleuropulmonary blastoma, Kaposi's sarcoma, epithelioid hemangioendothelioma, and angiosarcoma. Extraordinarily rare examples of granulocytic sarcoma (extramedullary tumefactive acute myeloid leukemia),[308] malignant peripheral nerve sheath tumor,[275] mesenchymal chondrosarcoma,[309] myxoid chondrosarcoma,[310] liposarcoma,[311,312] and extraosseous osteosarcoma[313] have been documented as apparently primary pleural tumors, but information on such lesions is anecdotal.

Pleural fibrosarcoma and malignant solitary (localized) fibrous tumor

A review of the literature on serosal neoplasms reveals few examples of well-documented primary pleural fibrosarcoma (PPFS).[314] The latter is only arbitrarily distinguished from malignant solitary (localized) fibrous tumor (MSFT) of the pleura by its clinical growth pattern, which is diffuse rather than localized. However, in other respects, these two tumor entities are virtually identical to one another; in fact, some examples of PPFS have apparently evolved *from* solitary fibrous tumors of the pleura.[315–320] Although some authors prefer to separate malignant fibrous tumors of the pleura into "true" fibrosarcoma and MFH-like tumors,[321] all of these lesions will herein be considered as a single group because of their closely similar clinicopathologic attributes.

Clinical summary

Pleural fibrosarcoma and MSFT arise in adult patients over a wide range of ages (15–75 years), with a male-to-female ratio of 3:1. They may be associated with dull or pleuritic chest pain, dyspnea, cough, systemic flu-like symptoms, and digital clubbing.[321,322] In addition, a small proportion of patients may manifest paraneoplastic hypoglycemia because of the production of an insulin-like peptide by the tumor cells.[322,323] It appears that

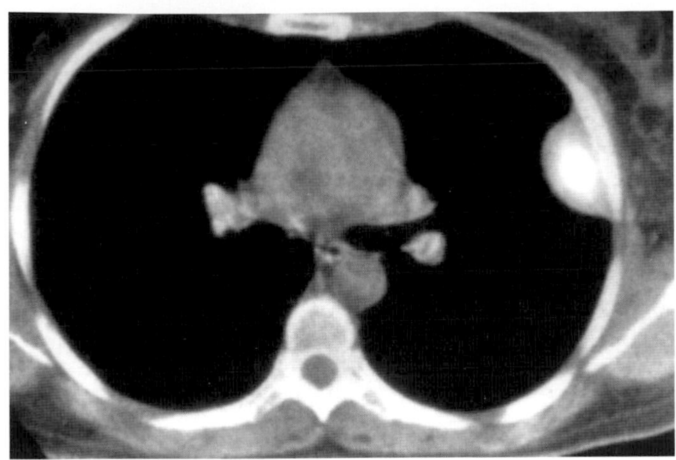

Fig. 14.47 Computed tomogram showing left pleural-based mass, which proved to be a malignant solitary fibrous tumor.

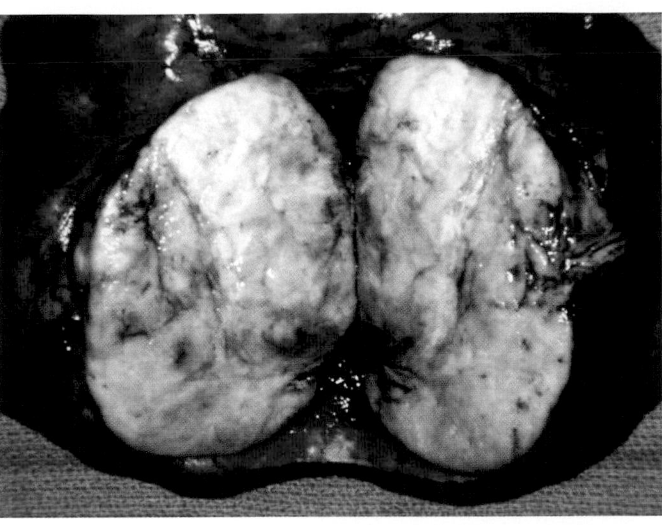

Fig. 14.48 Gross photograph of excised malignant solitary fibrous tumor of the pleura, demonstrating internal foci of necrosis.

pleural sarcomas have no association with prior asbestos exposure (in contradistinction to a proportion of malignant mesotheliomas).[280] Other potential etiologies of these lesions are unsettled at the present time, but some authors have reported a putative pathogenetic linkage to chronic tuberculous pleuritis and prior pyothorax.[324,325]

Radiographic studies in cases of PPFS commonly demonstrate the presence of a unilateral pleural effusion, which may be massive.[322,326] In addition, a dominant mass and diffuse but irregular thickening of the pleura are usually evident, and are especially well-seen with CT or MRI studies.[326] Based on clinical data, it is not possible to distinguish PPFS from diffuse malignant mesothelioma, and tissue procurement is mandatory for this purpose. On the other hand, MSFT are typically well-circumscribed, pleural-based masses on chest X-rays; they usually show rounded contours, but may occasionally be lobulated[322] (Fig. 14.47). Most measure between 1 and 10 cm in maximal dimension. In contrast to *benign* solitary fibrous pleural tumors, MSFTs are less often pedunculated, and usually attain a larger size. Moreover, the latter lesion has a higher likelihood of involving the parietal pleura or mediastinum, or of demonstrating "inverting" growth into the subjacent lung parenchyma.[315,322]

Pathologic findings

The macroscopic appearance of PPFS is virtually identical to that of diffuse malignant mesothelioma: i.e. as a "rind" of solid tissue that encases the lung and restricts its movement. These tumors commonly extend into interlobar fissures and intrapulmonary interstitial septa as well.[314–323] On the other hand, MSFTs are sessile or pedunculated localized masses that are most often seen in the upper portions of either hemithorax. They have bosselated, fleshy, tan-gray cut surfaces, usually with foci of spontaneous necrosis and hemorrhage[315,322] (Fig. 14.48).

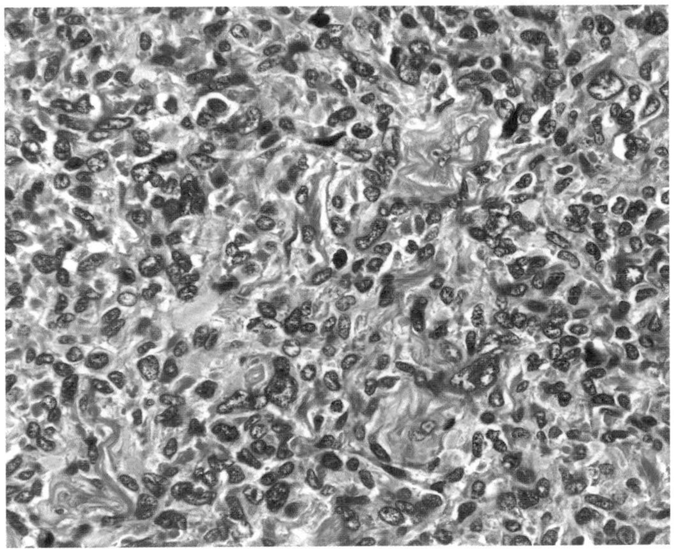

Fig. 14.49 Microscopic image of malignant solitary fibrous tumor of the pleura, showing an atypical spindle cell proliferation.

Microscopically, one sees a dense proliferation of spindle cells with high nuclear-to-cytoplasmic ratios, coarse chromatin, nuclear irregularity, and prominent nucleoli. Mitotic activity is typically brisk, and foci of spontaneous hemorrhage and necrosis may be evident as well (Fig. 14.49). The neoplastic cells may be arranged in a storiform fashion and show moderately-to-markedly

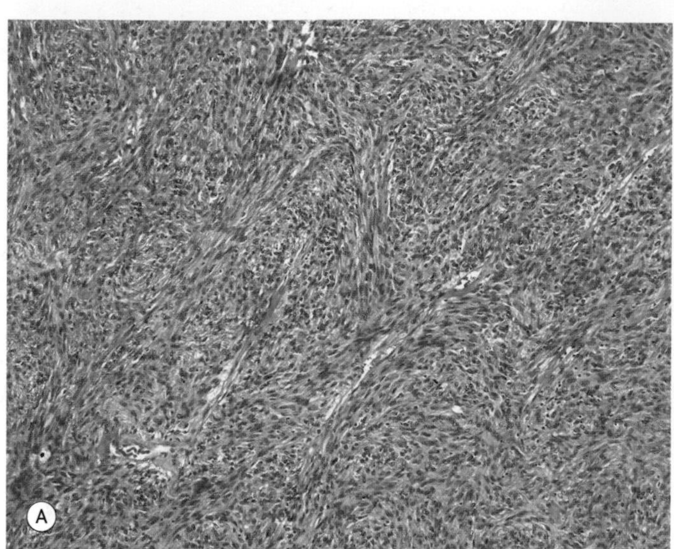

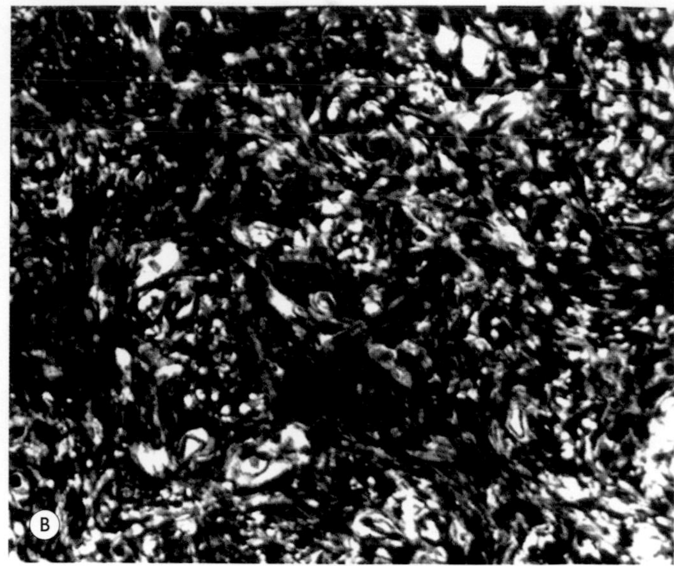

Fig. 14.50 (A) A "herringbone" pattern of densely cellular growth and mitotic activity are present in this malignant solitary (localized) fibrous tumor (MSFT) of the pleura. (B) The lesion is immunoreactive for CD34, although a proportion of MSFTs lose that marker.

pleomorphic cytologic features, calling to mind the histologic attributes of MFH (see above).[314,322] In other cases, they are aligned in a fascicular "herringbone" configuration, as in pulmonary fibrosarcomas (Fig. 14.50). The subjacent lung is involved by tumor only if it extends downward from the pleura via the intrasegmental fibrous septa, and there is no association with pleural fibrohyaline plaques, the presence of intraparenchymal asbestos fibers, or asbestosis. MSFT may contain areas that resemble *benign* solitary fibrous pleural tumors, in which more bland spindle cell aggregates are enmeshed in hyalinized, keloidal-type collagen.[322] A "staghorn" stromal vascular pattern is common in such areas as well.

Electron microscopy shows only primitive, fibroblast-like characteristics of the neoplastic cells. They are loosely apposed and surrounded in part by collagen fibers; cytoplasmic contents are rudimentary, and include the basic metabolic organelles as well as abundant free polyribosomes and rough endoplasmic reticulum. There is no ultrastructural evidence of epithelial or myogenous differentiation. Similarly, immunohistologic assessment of PPFS and MSFT demonstrates reactivity for vimentin alone, to the exclusion of actin, desmin, keratin, and EMA.[314–316] In contrast, true mesotheliomas (including sarcomatoid variants) uniformly express epithelial markers.[298] In contrast to *benign* SFTs, some MSFTs may lack immunoreactivity for CD34.[320]

Therapy and prognosis

PPFS is not often treatable by surgical means, owing to its diffuse nature. The only operative procedure that can be attempted in such circumstances is extrapleural pneumonectomy, which generally is associated with a very high level of morbidity and mortality. Radiotherapy and chemotherapy (including intrapleural instillation of pharmaceuticals) may play a role in palliation of symptoms, but unfortunately they are not curative treatments. Death is due to progressive respiratory compromise, and PPFS also may involve the pericardium and produce cardiac embarrassment.[327] Actuarial 1-year survival was only 39% in one series where multimodality therapy was employed.[321]

MSFT, on the other hand, is amenable to complete surgical resection in a high proportion of cases; in a series from the AFIP, 45% of such lesions were cured by excision alone.[322] Most of these were pedunculated, well-localized masses that involved only a small area of the pleural surface, and the authors of the latter report therefore suggested that resectability was the single most favorable prognostic feature in MSFT cases. Those lesions that do go on to recur may involve the contralateral pleura, the lung parenchyma, and other viscera. Interestingly, relapses often still take the form of *localized* masses rather than disseminating along the pleural surface, and even patients with persistent tumor may go on to survive for extended periods of time.[280] Irradiation and chemotherapy do not appear to offer any benefits in this setting, and may even *shorten* the survival of patients with MSFT.[322]

Primary pleural leiomyosarcoma

Leiomyosarcomas are extremely rare as primary pleural neoplasms, with less than 15 well-documented cases in the literature.[328,329] Only one series of such tumors has been reported, by Moran and colleagues.[328]

Clinical summary

Patients with primary pleural leiomyosarcoma present in a similar fashion to those with mesothelioma, except that a greater proportion have had asymptomatic lesions. Radiographically, pleural effusions have not been observed consistently in association with such tumors, the majority of which appeared as solitary, solid, unilateral masses measuring up to 18 cm in greatest dimension. Some examples have encased the lung completely, simulating malignant mesothelial tumors.[328]

Pathologic findings

As in other anatomic sites, pleural leiomyosarcomas are characterized by fascicles and whorls of atypical spindle cells, featuring fusiform nuclei, fibrillary eosinophilic cytoplasm, nuclear pleomorphism, and mitotic activity. Necrosis is also frequently encountered as well. The tumors invade the lung parenchyma, or the soft tissues of the chest wall, or both.

Ultrastructural analyses have shown typical findings of smooth muscle differentiation in such tumors, including plasmalemmal dense plaques, pinocytotic vesicles, cytoplasmic thin filaments punctuated by dense bodies, and pericellular basal lamina. Immunohistologically, pleural leiomyosarcomas are reactive for vimentin, desmin, muscle-specific actin, and alpha-isoform actin,[328] yielding potential immunophenotypic overlap with sarcomatoid carcinoma or mesothelioma. However, in our experience, keratin, epithelial membrane antigen, and calretinin are uniformly absent, providing points of difference from the latter two epithelial tumors.

Therapy and prognosis

Because of the rarity of these lesions, only anecdotal information is available on the biology of primary pleural leiomyosarcomas. Moran et al. advocated surgical ablation, but found that two of five such lesions they studied could not be resected completely.[328] The merits of adjuvant therapeutic modalities are as yet unstudied.

Askin's tumor (primitive neuroectodermal tumor) and desmoplastic small round cell tumor

In 1979, Askin and colleagues described a peculiar thoracic neoplasm that was seemingly limited to children, adolescents, and young adults.[330] This lesion arises from the pleura or the extrapleural intercostal soft tissue, and was originally named the "malignant small cell tumor of the thoracopulmonary region." Since then, it has become known more simply as "Askin's tumor," or, alternatively – because the neoplasm has been shown to exhibit neuroepithelial differentiation – thoracopulmonary "primitive neuroectodermal tumor" (TPNET).[331–342] Prior to its seminal description, it is likely that this lesion was included among cases of Ewing's sarcoma of the thorax or "peripheral neuroblastoma."[343] Primary PNET of the lung is considered elsewhere in this monograph, but Askin's tumor is considered to be separate from that entity and will therefore be discussed at this point. A related neoplasm is known as "desmoplastic small round cell tumor"(DSRCT) of the serosal surfaces. It was originally described in the peritoneum, and is more common there by far, but several examples have been described in the pleura as well.[344–346]

Clinical summary

Askin's tumor and DSRCT demonstrate a peak incidence during the second decade of life (mean age 15 years), and shows a slight male predilection. Isolated cases of TPNETs in infants and in older adults have also been documented.[344–349] These neoplasms may present as asymptomatic masses in the chest wall, or produce symptoms of cough, unilateral chest pain, and dyspnea or tachypnea. Pleural effusion is a common complication, and may be detected on physical examination or by radiography of the thorax.[331] Although they have been confused with classical neuroblastoma in some reports, Askin's tumors and DSRCTs are *not* associated with elevations of catecholamine metabolite levels in the urine or blood, nor do they produce the opsoclonus-myoclonus syndrome.[339,347]

Chest X-rays and other imaging studies typically show a large mass that may be pleural-based or centered in the thoracic soft tissue, with secondary extension into the pleural space (Fig. 14.51). TPNETs and DSRCTs often reach a size of >10 cm at the time of initial diagnosis, and they demonstrate ill-defined interfaces with the subjacent lung or surrounding tissues.[350]

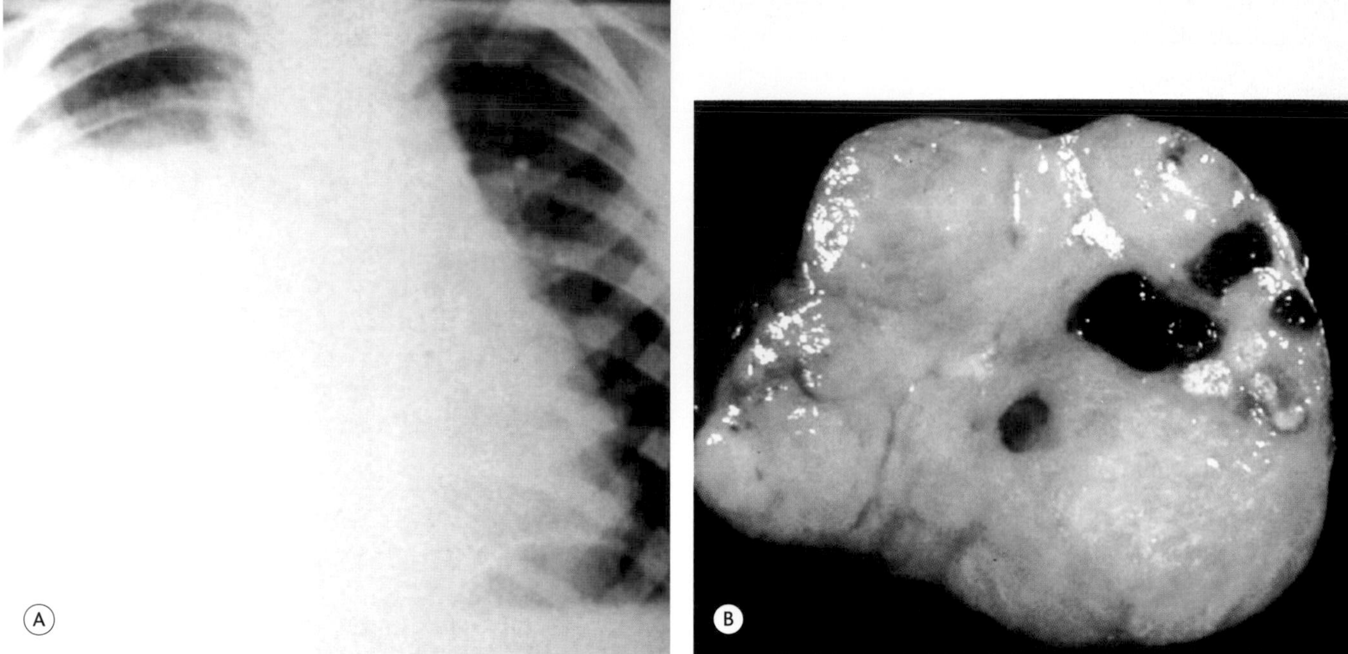

Fig. 14.51 **Askin's tumor (primitive neuroectodermal tumor) of the right hemithorax in a young child, as seen in a plain film chest radiograph.** (A) The lesion is massive and replaces much of the right lung field. (B) Partial excision of the lesion yielded a fleshy mass demonstrating internal foci of necrosis.

Pathologic findings

Askin's tumor is one of the prototypical small round cell neoplasms of children, and may be confused with several other tumor entities by the pathologist.[339] At a macroscopic level, TPNET is lobulated with fleshy, relatively soft, tan-gray cut surfaces that may show foci of hemorrhage and necrosis.[330] Microscopically, it exhibits cellular monomorphism, with round-to-oval nuclei, even distribution of chromatin, indistinct nucleoli, and variable mitotic activity (Fig. 14.52). Stromal blood vessels are numerous and form a discernible network within the tumor mass; matrical hemorrhage also may be manifest[330–347] (Fig. 14.53). One of the most characteristic findings of TPNET on conventional microscopy is the presence of neural-type cellular "rosettes," wherein tumor cells are disposed radially around small virtual tissue spaces[330,331] (Fig. 14.54). Histochemically, Askin's tumor may or may not contain abundant glycogen with the periodic acid–Schiff (PAS) method, although in the original series on this lesion, only PAS-negative neoplasms were accepted to facilitate separation from classical Ewing's sarcoma.

DSRCT differs from the description just given in that it features aggregates of small monomorphic tumor cells that are set in a much more fibrogenic stroma than that seen in Askin's tumor. The growth pattern is also more organoid than in conventional TPNET.[344–346] Although no obvious evidence of myogenous differentiation is apparent at a conventional morphologic level, immunostains typically show coreactivity for vimentin, desmin, and keratin in DSRCT (Fig. 14.55),[345] and ultrastructural studies also support the presence of bifid epithelial-myogenic differentiation.

Special studies of biopsy or resection specimens are mandatory to recognize TPNET and DSRCT properly and exclude other diagnostic possibilities. Those include mesenchymal chondrosarcoma, small cell synovial sarcoma, hemangiopericytoma, and metastatic small cell neuroendocrine carcinoma; the last of these possiblities is unlikely in the usual patient group with TPNET. Along with other peripheral neuroepithelial neoplasms, TPNET and DSRCT demonstrate characteristic t(11:22) chromosomal translocations[331,351] (Fig. 14.56). By electron microscopy, they demonstrate blunt cytoplasmic processes that contain dense-core granules or microtubules; these

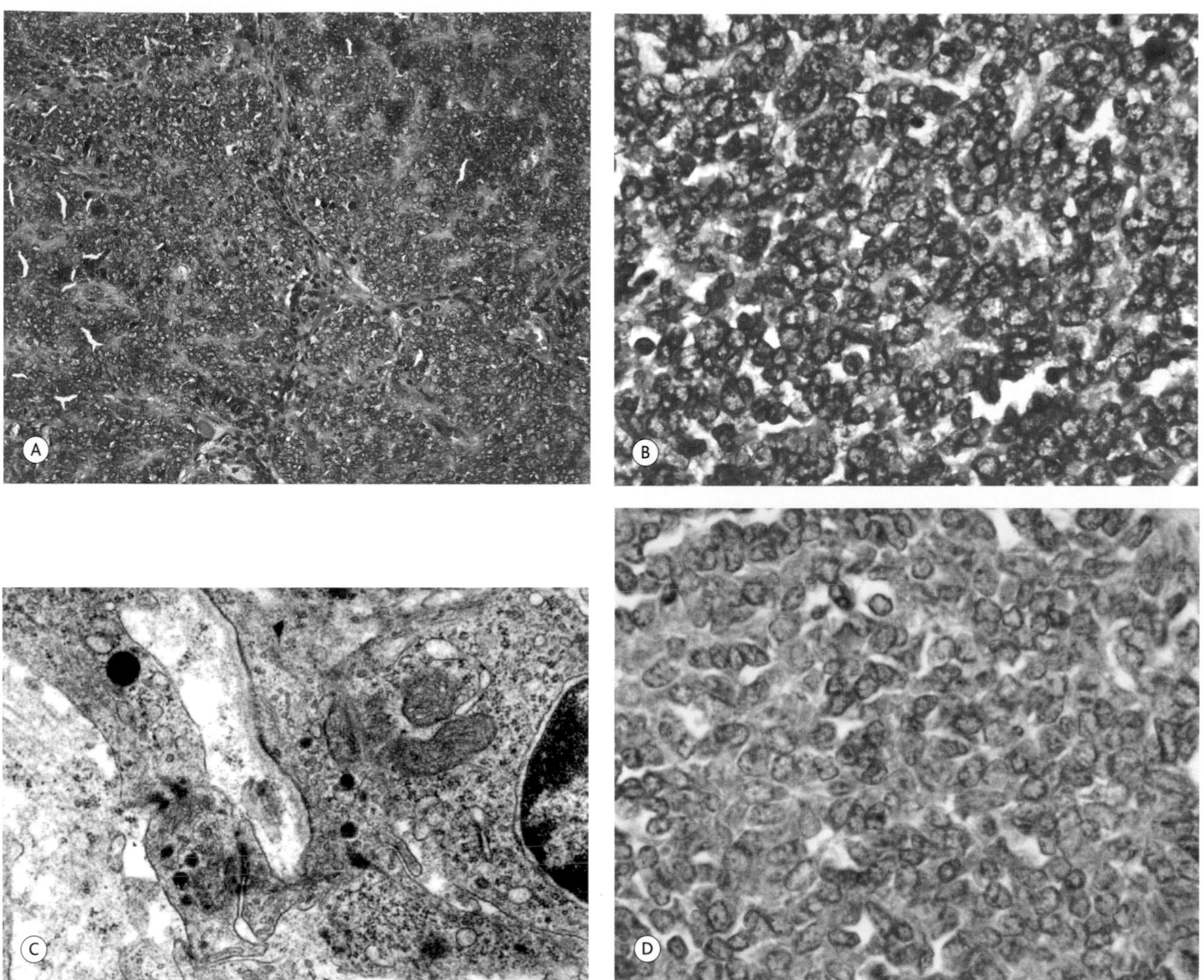

Fig. 14.52 (A) Microscopic image of primitive neuroectodermal tumor (PNET), showing a densely cellular poliferation of monomorphic small round cells. (B) The neoplastic cells have scant cytoplasm and dispersed nuclear chromatin. (C) An electron micrograph of the lesion shows primitive cytoplasmic extensions that contain neurosecretory-type or synaptic vesicles. (D) Immunoreactivity for CD99 (MIC2 protein) is also present.

characteristics are seen in classical neuroblastoma as well, but not in other small round cell tumors.[339] Immunohistochemically, TPNET and DSRCT are related to Ewing's tumor in that they show reactivity for synaptophysin as well as CD99.[352] Askin's tumor and DSRCT may be distinguished from classical neuroblastoma immunophenotypically; the former lesion is reactive for both beta$_2$-microglobulin and CD99,[345] whereas the latter tumor is not.

Therapy and prognosis

The most important prognostic procedure in cases of TPNET or DSRCT is that of accurate staging. Using a scheme devised by the National Cancer Institute, stage I tumors are defined as those measuring <5 cm in maximum diameter that can be completely excised; stage II lesions are <5 cm and are grossly resectable but show positive microscopic margins; stage III neoplasms are

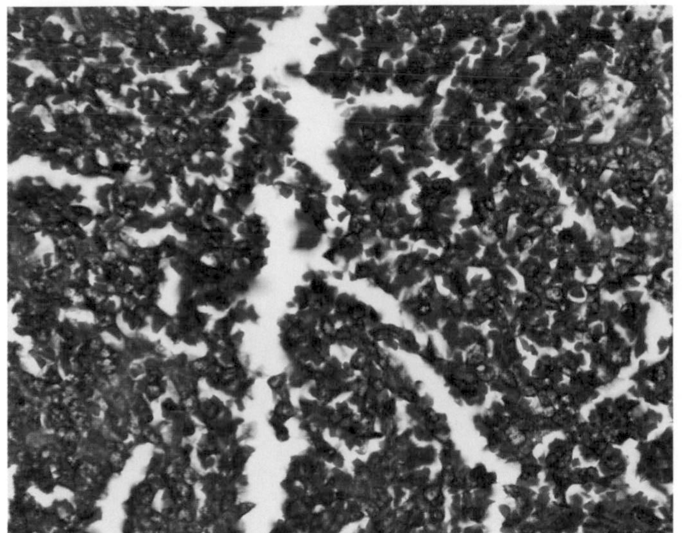

Fig. 14.53 A markedly vascular stroma is apparent in this Askin's tumor (primitive neuroectodermal tumor), with extravasation of erythrocytes.

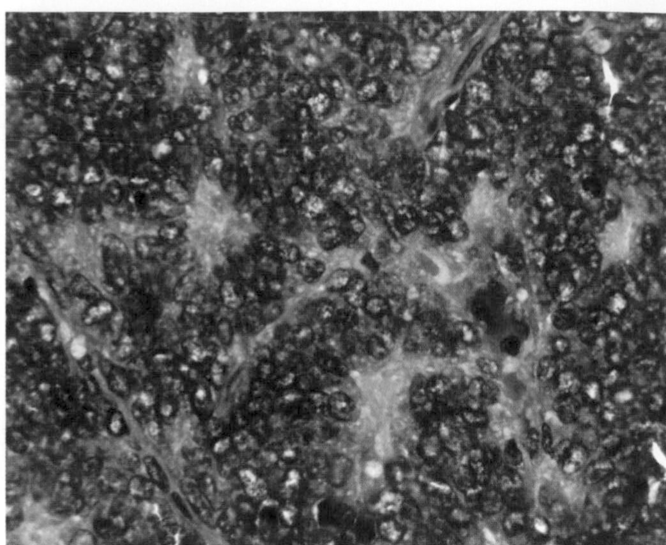

Fig. 14.54 Primitive intercellular rosettes are present in this Askin's tumor (primitive neuroectodermal tumor).

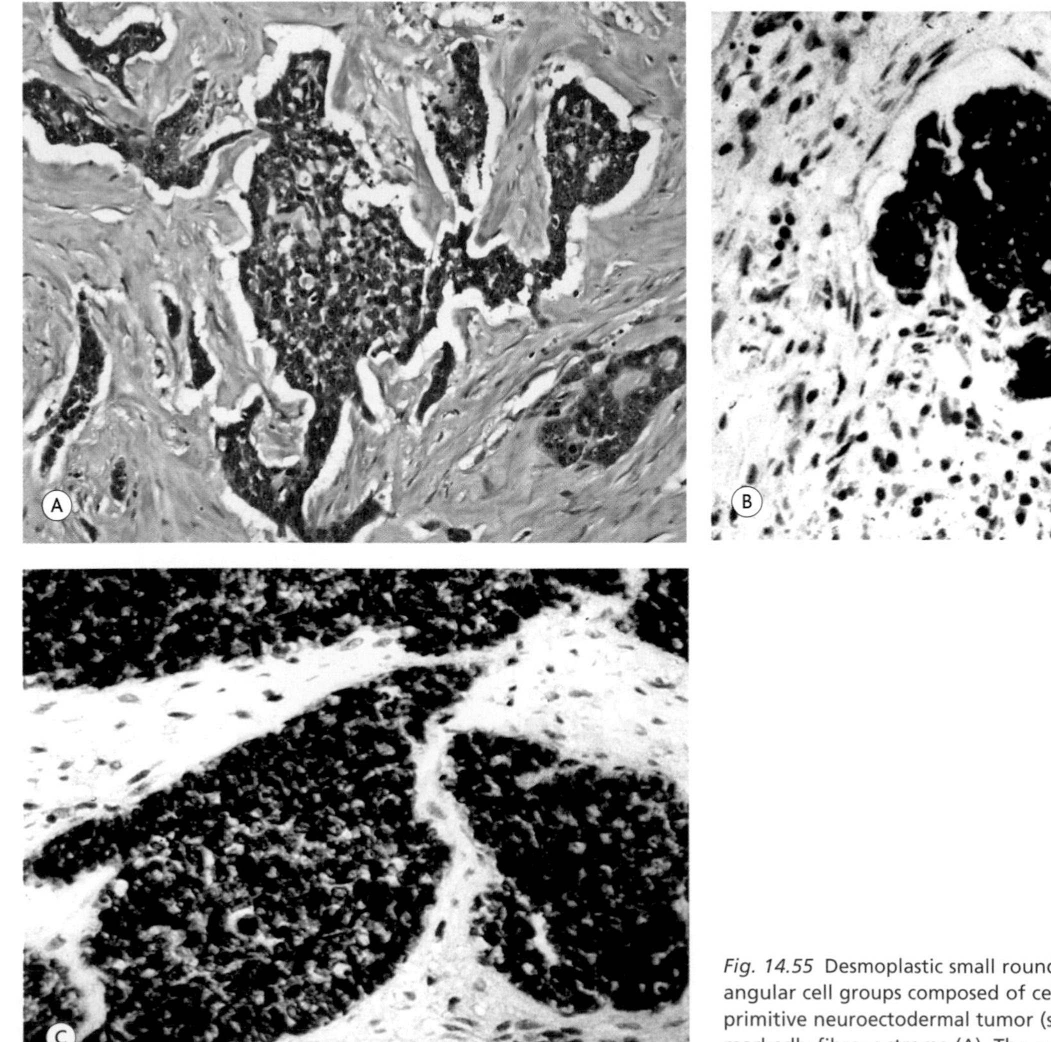

Fig. 14.55 Desmoplastic small round cell tumor of the pleura, in which angular cell groups composed of cells like those of "ordinary" primitive neuroectodermal tumor (see Figs 14.52–14.54) are set in a markedly fibrous stroma (A). The neoplastic cells are concurrently immunoreactive for keratin (B) and desmin (C).

Fig. 14.56 The characteristic t(11;22) chromosomal translocation of primitive neuroectodermal tumor is seen in this karyotypic preparation.

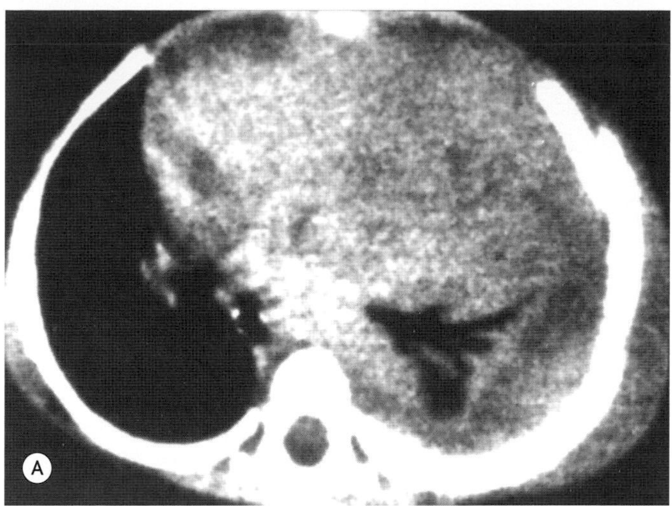

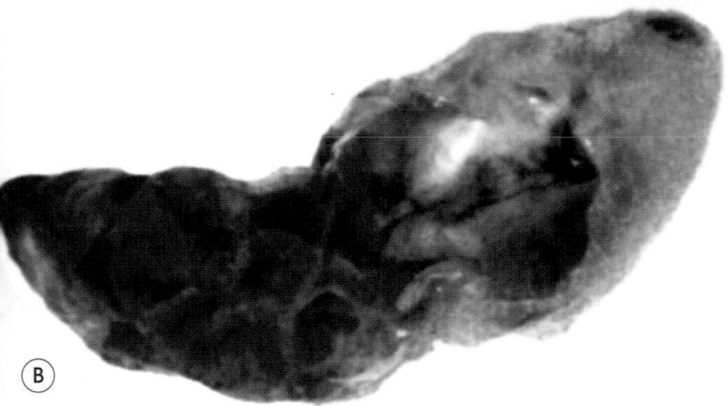

Fig. 14.57 (A) Computed tomogram of pleuropulmonary blastoma (PPB) in a young adult, showing effacement of much of the left hemithorax. (B) Internal cystic change is apparent in this PPB.

>5 cm, and are non-resectable; and stage IV primitive neuroectodermal tumors have metastasized to extrapleural sites.[331] Low stage has shown a direct correlation with long-term survival after surgical removal and intensive cyclical postoperative treatment with irradiation and chemotherapy, using protocols that are similar to those employed for Ewing's sarcoma.[332,353] Stage III and IV Askin's tumors and DSRCTs are probably best managed non-surgically, as there are no data to support a role for debulking surgery in such circumstances.[331]

A sobering aspect of the therapy for TPNET and DSRCT is that it undeniably subjects patients who become survivors to the risk of a second malignancy. Intensive radiation to the chest wall may be followed years later by a post-radiation sarcoma in approximately 1% of cases, and Farhi et al. have described several examples of post-chemotherapy myelodysplastic syndrome and acute leukemia in this context.[354]

Pleuropulmonary blastoma

Until 1988, a group of anaplastic mesenchymal tumors of the peripheral lung and pleura in children had been grouped together under the rubric of "pediatric pulmonary blastoma." Nonetheless, Manivel et al.[62] showed that such lesions differed from typical pulmonary blastomas in adults, which comprise a subset of sarcomatoid *carcinomas*. The childhood tumors were found to be more often primary in the pleura; they also showed a histologic resemblance to soft tissue sarcomas. Because of these important points of difference from adult pulmonary "blastomas," the pediatric lesions were reclassified as *pleuro*pulmonary blastomas (PPB).

Clinical summary

Pleuropulmonary blastomas arise most often in the first decade of life, without a distinct preference for males or females. However, examples have been reported of this tumor in patients as old as 36 years of age.[62–68,355–365] Cough, chest pain, weight loss, and dyspnea or tachypnea are the most common presenting complaints of PPB.[62,361] Evidence of a pleural effusion may also be found on physical examination. It appears that this neoplasm may be part of certain "cancer families," in which other soft tissue sarcomas, variants of Wilms' tumor, and cystic nephromas may be seen in other members of the kindred.[66,67,361,362]

Radiological studies typically demonstrate the presence of a large, irregularly outlined mass in the thorax, which may have its epicenter in the pleura, the mediastinal soft tissue, or the peripheral lung parenchyma. These lesions can be massive – sometimes effacing an entire hemithorax – and they demonstrate internal variation in density on CT (Fig. 14.57) or MRI studies. Some examples may show focal internal calcification or obvious cyst formation.[62,361,363,364]

Pathologic findings

"Classical" PPB is grossly fleshy and tan-pink or gray upon prosection, with frequent foci of internal hemorrhage and punctate necrosis; overt cystification is also seen in many cases. Chondroid areas may be apparent on macroscopic examination of the mass, and areas of calcification may be manifest as "grittiness" that is encountered when sectioning the lesion.

Dehner and coworkers[65,361] have subclassified PPBs into three groups, based on the extent of cystic change that they demonstrate. Type I tumors are predominantly cystic; type II lesions are mixed solid and cystic; and type III PPBs are predominantly solid. Cystic foci are lined by modified respiratory epithelium that is typically bland cytologically, and the surrounding stroma is variably myxoid and relatively hypocellular. Microscopically, one sees a heterogeneous mixture of growth patterns that are admixed with one another in various solid regions of these tumors. Some foci resemble MFH (Fig. 14.58); others take on a rhabdomyosarcomatous appearance; and still other areas have the features of fibrosarcoma, liposarcoma, chondrosarcoma, or osteosarcoma.[62,361] Some observers may wish to apply the term "malignant mesenchymoma" to PPB, but such a designation has generally fallen from favor in current nosology. Importantly, *epithelial* foci are absent in PPB, in contrast to their dominance in so-called adult pulmonary blastoma.[62,65,361] Immunohistochemical and ultrastructural studies demonstrate findings that are in accord with the aforementioned microscopic features, and they again fail to reveal epithelial characteristics in these lesions.[62]

The pathologic differential diagnosis of PPB concerns sarcomatoid carcinoma of the lung and pleura, sarcomatoid mesothelioma with divergent differentiation, and rhabdomyosarcoma arising in congenital pulmonary cysts or teratoid tumors involving the pleura. The absence of keratin in PPB excludes pulmonary "blastoma," other forms of carcinoma, mesothelioma, and germ cell tumors from further consideration. Secondary malignancy in congenital cysts is somewhat more arbitrarily distinguished from pleuropulmonary blastomatous tumors, but, if thorough sampling fails to identify non-myogenic sarcomatous elements, that interpretation would be favored.

Therapy and prognosis

PPB is a relatively rare tumor; therefore, organized protocol studies of therapy are still in evolution. In general, however, it is obvious that this neoplasm is a highly aggressive lesion that requires every effort at surgical extirpation, followed by intensive irradiation and chemotherapy.[361] Because of the histologic characteristics of the tumor, which are like those of de-novo soft tissue sarcomas, it would seem appropriate to employ drug combinations that are directed towards the various histologic components of PPB (e.g. rhabdomyosarcoma, MFH, osteosarcoma, etc.). Surgical debulking of the tumor mass should also be considered in individual cases where complete resection is not thought to be feasible. Dehner and colleagues have related morphologic findings in PPBs to prognosis; predominantly cystic lesions have the best outlook, whereas type II and type III neoplasms are aggressive and often prove fatal within 2 years of diagnosis.[361] Interestingly, Wright has also reported a case wherein successive recurrences of a PPB showed progressive transformation from type I to type III morphology.[365]

Vascular sarcomas of the pleura

As mentioned previously, angiosarcoma, Kaposi's sarcoma, and epithelioid hemangioendothelioma may take origin in the pleura as well as in the pulmonary parenchyma. The general clinical attributes of these lesions have been described above. It is notable that the most common initial sign of angiosarcoma and KS of the pleura is the presence of a bloody pleural effusion.[230] Gross examination of the tumor at thoracotomy shows multiple soft, hemorrhagic, red-violet, nodular pleural implants in examples of angiosarcoma and KS. However, epithelioid hemangioendothelioma is virtually identical to malignant mesothelioma at a macroscopic level, and pathologic study is necessary to distinguish between them.[366] As is true of their intrapulmonary counterparts, KS and angiosarcoma of the pleura are associated with a dismal prognosis, whereas patients with epithelioid hemangioendothelioma may survive for prolonged periods of time.[366]

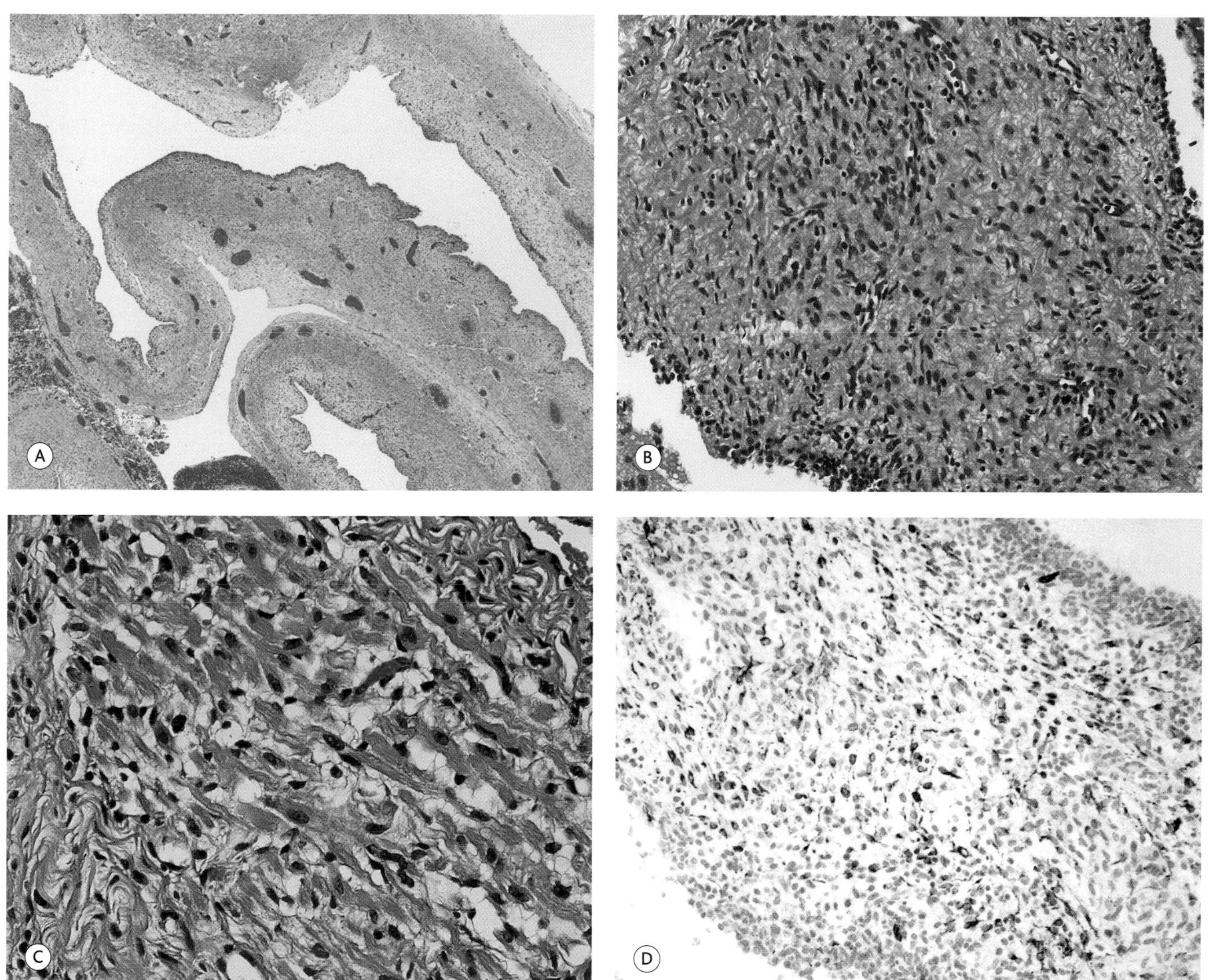

Fig. 14.58 Examples of pleuropulmonary blastoma, demonstrating cyst formation in a low grade example (A, B), Rhabdomyoblasts (C), immunohistologic reaction using anti-desmin antibodies (D). No epithelial elements are present.

REFERENCES

1. Huang JC, Ritter JH, Wick MR: Malignant nonepithelial neoplasms of the lungs and pleural surfaces. In: Comprehensive textbook of thoracic oncology, Aisner J, et al., Eds. 1996, Williams & Wilkins, Baltimore, pp 815–849.
2. Wick MR, Ritter JH, Humphrey PA: Sarcomatoid carcinomas of the lung: a clinicopathologic review. Am J Clin Pathol 1997; 108: 40–53.
3. Steele RH: Lung tumors: a personal review. Diagn Histopathol 1983; 6: 119–123.
4. Nascimento AG, Unni KK: Sarcomas of the lung. Mayo Clin Proc 1982; 57: 355–359.
5. Guccion JG, Rosen SH: Bronchopulmonary leiomyosarcomas and fibrosarcomas: a study of 32 cases and review of the literature. Cancer 1972; 30: 835–847.
6. Przygodzki RM, Moran CA, Suster S, Koss MN: Primary pulmonary rhabdomyosarcomas: a clinicopathologic and immunohistochemical study of three cases. Mod Pathol 1995; 8: 658–661.
7. Suster S: Primary sarcomas of the lung. Semin Diagn Pathol 1995; 12: 140–157.
8. Zeren H, Moran CA, Suster S, Fishback NF, Koss MN: Primary pulmonary sarcomas with features of monophasic synovial sarcoma: a clinicopathological, immunohistochemical, and ultrastructural study of 25 cases. Hum Pathol 1995; 26: 474–480.
9. Gaertner E, Zeren EH, Fleming MV, Colby TV, Travis WD: Biphasic synovial sarcomas arising in the pleural cavity: a clinicopathologic study of five cases. Am J Surg Pathol 1996; 20: 36–45.
9a. Gladish GW, Sabloff BM, Munden RF, et al.: Primary thoracic sarcomas. Radiographics 2002; 22: 621–637.
10. Stackhouse EM, Harrison EG Jr, Ellis FH Jr: Primary mixed malignancies of lung: carcinosarcoma and blastoma. J Thorac Cardiovasc Surg 1969; 57: 385–399.
11. Humphrey PA, Scroggs MW, Roggli VL, Shelbourne JD: Pulmonary carcinoma with a sarcomatoid element. Hum Pathol 1988; 19: 155–165.
12. Ishida T, Tatsishi M, Kaneko S, et al.: Carcinosarcoma and spindle-cell carcinoma of the lung. J Thorac Cardiovasc Surg 1990; 100: 844–852.
13. Matsui K, Kitagawa M: Spindle cell carcinoma of the lung: a clinicopathologic study of three cases. Cancer 1991; 67: 2361–2367.
14. Leventon GS, Evans HL: Sarcomatoid squamous cell carcinoma of the mucous membranes of the head and neck. Cancer 1981; 48: 994–1003.
15. Piscioli F, Aldovini D, Bondi A, Eusebi V: Squamous cell carcinoma with sarcoma-like stroma of the nose and paranasal sinuses: report of two cases. Histopathology 1984; 8: 633–639.
16. Lane N: Pseudosarcoma (polypoid sarcoma-like masses) associated with squamous cell carcinoma of the mouth, fauces, and larynx: report of ten cases. Cancer 1957; 10: 19–41.
17. Lasser KH, Naeim F, Higgins J, et al.: "Pseudosarcoma" of the larynx. Am J Surg Pathol 1979; 3: 397–404.
18. Lambert PR, Ward PH, Berci G: Pseudosarcoma of the larynx: a comprehensive analysis. Arch Otolaryngol 1980; 106: 700–708.
19. Davis MP, Eagan RT, Weiland LH, Pairolero PC: Carcinosarcoma of the lung: Mayo Clinic experience and response to chemotherapy. Mayo Clin Proc 1984; 59: 598–603.
19a. Chang YL, Lee YC, Shih JY, Wu CT: Pulmonary pleomorphic (spindle) cell carcinoma: peculiar clinicopathologic manifestations different from ordinary non-small-cell carcinoma. Lung Cancer 2001; 34: 91–97.
20. Fung CH, Lo JW, Yonan TN, et al.: Pulmonary blastoma: an ultrastructural study with brief review of literature and discussion of pathogenesis. Cancer 1977; 39: 153–163.
21. Heffner DK, Hyams VJ: Teratocarcinosarcoma (malignant teratoma?) of the nasal cavity and paranasal sinuses: a clinicopathologic study of 20 cases. Cancer 1984; 53: 2140–2154.
22. Patterson SD, Ballard RW: Nasal blastoma: a light and electron microscopic study. Ultrastruct Pathol 1980; 1: 487–494.
23. Minckler DS, Meligro CH, Norris HT: Carcinosarcoma of the larynx. Cancer 1970; 26: 195–200.
24. Goellner JR, Devine KD, Weiland LH: Pseudosarcoma of the larynx. Am J Clin Pathol 1973; 59: 312–326.
25. Farrell DJ, Cooper PN, Malcolm AJ: Carcinosarcoma of the lung associated with asbestosis. Histopathology 1995; 27: 484–486.
26. Berho M, Moran CA, Suster S: Malignant mixed epithelial/mesenchymal neoplasms of the lung. Semin Diagn Pathol 1995; 12: 123–139.
27. Reynolds S, Jenkins G, Akosa A, Roberts CM: Carcinosarcoma of the lung: an unusual cause of empyema. Respir Med 1995; 89: 73–75.
28. Nappi O, Glasner SD, Swanson PE, Wick MR: Biphasic and monophasic sarcomatoid carcinomas of the lung: a reappraisal of "carcinosarcomas" and "spindle cell carcinomas." Am J Clin Pathol 1994; 102: 331–340.
29. Nappi O, Wick MR: Sarcomatoid neoplasms of the respiratory tract. Semin Diagn Pathol 1993; 10: 137–147.
29a. Nakajima M, Kasai T, Hashimoto H, Iwata Y, Manabe H: Sarcomatoid carcinoma of the lung: a clinicopathologic study of 37 cases. Cancer 1999; 86: 608–616.
29b. Brambilla E, Travis WD, Colby TV, Corrin B, Shimosato Y: The new World Health Organization classification of lung tumors. Eur Respir J 2001; 18: 1059–1068.
29c. Terzi A, Gorla A, Piubello Q, Tomezzoli A, Furlan G: Biphasic sarcomatoid carcinoma of the lung: report of 5 cases and review of the literature. Eur J Surg Oncol 1997; 23: 457.
30. Ro JY, Chen JL, Lee JS, et al.: Sarcomatoid carcinoma of the lung: immunohistochemical and ultrastructural studies of 14 cases. Cancer 1992; 69: 376–386.
31. Koss MN: Pulmonary blastomas. Cancer Treat Res 1995; 72: 349–362.
32. Miller RR, Champagne K, Murray RC: Primary pulmonary germ cell tumor with blastomatous differentiation. Chest 1994; 106: 1595–1596.
33. Huwer H, Kalweit G, Straub U, et al.: Pulmonary carcinosarcoma: diagnostic problems and determinants of prognosis. Eur J Cardiothorac Surg 1996; 10: 403–407.
34. Melissari M, Giordano G, Gabrielli M: Immunohistochemical and ultrastructural study of a case of carcinosarcoma (biphasic sarcomatoid carcinoma) of the lung with rhabdomyoblastic differentiation. Pathologica 1997; 89: 412–419.
35. Pankowski J, Grodzki T, Janowski H, Parafiniuk W, Wojcik J: Carcinosarcoma of the lung: report of three cases. J Cardiovasc Surg 1998; 39: 121–125.
36. Saphir O, Vass A: Carcinosarcoma. Am J Cancer 1938; 33: 331–359.
37. Sarma DP, Deshotels SJ Jr: Carcinosarcoma of the lung. J Surg Oncol 1982; 19: 216–218.
38. Bergmann M, Ackerman LV, Kemler RL: Carcinosarcoma of the lung: review of the literature and report of two cases treated by pneumonectomy. Cancer 1951; 4: 919–929.
39. Kakos GS, Williams TE Jr, Assor D, Vasko JS: Pulmonary carcinosarcoma: etiologic, therapeutic, and prognostic considerations. J Thorac Cardiovasc Surg 1971; 61: 777–783.
40. Krompecher E: Der drusernartige Oberflachen-Epitheliakrebscarcinom epitheliale Adenoides. Beitr Pathol 1900; 28: 1–41.
41. Herxheimer G, Reinke F: Carcinoma sarcomatodes: pathologie des Krebses. Ergebn Allg Pathol Pathol Anat 1912; 16: 280–282.
42. Moore TC: Carcinosarcoma of the lung. Surgery 1961; 50: 886–893.
43. Cabarcos A, Gomez-Dorronsoro M, Lobo-Beristain JL: Pulmonary carcinosarcoma: a case study and review of the literature. Br J Dis Chest 1985; 79: 83–90.
44. Ludwigsen E: Endobronchial carcinosarcoma. Virchows Arch A Pathol Anat 1977; 373: 293–302.
45. Rainosek DE, Ro JY, Ordonez NG, Kulaga AD, Ayala AG: Sarcomatoid carcinoma of the lung: a case with atypical carcinoid and rhabdomyosarcomatous components. Am J Clin Pathol 1994; 102: 360–364.
46. Fishback NF, Travis WD, Moran CA, et al.: Pleomorphic (spindle/giant cell) carcinoma of the lung: a clinicopathologic correlation of 78 cases. Cancer 1994; 73: 2936–2945.
47. Tsubota YT, Kawaguchi T, Hoso T, Nishino E, Travis WD: A combined small cell and spindle cell carcinoma of the lung: report of a unique case with immunohistochemical and ultrastructural studies. Am J Surg Pathol 1992; 16: 1108–1115.
47a. Khalifa M, Hruby G, Ehrlich L, Danjoux C, Perez-Ordonez B: Combined large cell neuroendocrine carcinoma and spindle cell carcinoma of the lung. Ann Diagn Pathol 2001; 5: 240–245.
48. Oyasu R, Battifora HA, Buckingham WB, Hidvegi D: Metaplastic

squamous cell carcinoma of bronchus simulating giant cell tumor of bone. Cancer 1977; 39: 1119–1128.
49. Love GL, Droca PJ: Bronchogenic sarcomatoid squamous cell carcinoma with osteoclast-like giant cells. Hum Pathol 1983; 14: 1004–1006.
50. Colombi RP: Sarcomatoid carcinomas of the female genital tract (malignant mixed müllerian tumors). Semin Diagn Pathol 1993; 10: 169–175.
51. George E, Manivel JC, Dehner LP, Wick MR: Malignant mixed Müllerian tumors: an immunohistochemical study of 47 cases with histogenetic considerations and clinical correlation. Hum Pathol 1991; 22: 215–223.
52. Travis WD, Colby TV, Corrin B, Shimosato Y, Brambilla E: Histological typing of lung & pleural tumours (International Histological Classification of Tumours). 1999, World Health Organization, Geneva, Switzerland, pp 1–55.
53. Barnett NR, Barnard WG: Some unusual thoracic tumors. Br J Surg 1945; 32: 447–457.
54. Spencer H: Pulmonary blastoma. J Pathol Bacteriol 1961; 82: 161–165.
55. Francis D, Jacobsen M: Pulmonary blastoma. Curr Top Pathol 1983; 73: 265–294.
56. Ohtomo K, Araki T, Yashiro N, Iio M: Pulmonary blastoma in children. Radiology 1983; 147: 101–104.
57. Gal AA, Marchevsky AM, Koss MN: Unusual tumors of the lung. In: Surgical pathology of lung neoplasms, Marchevsky AM, Ed. 1990, Marcel Dekker, New York, pp 325–388.
58. Jetley NK, Bhatnagar V, Krishna A, et al.: Pulmonary blastoma in a neonate. J Pediatr Surg 1988; 23: 1009–1010.
59. Jimenez JF: Pulmonary blastoma in childhood. J Surg Oncol 1987; 334: 87–93.
60. Senac MO Jr, Wood BP, Isaacs H, et al.: Pulmonary blastoma: a rare childhood malignancy. Radiology 1991; 179: 743–746.
61. Cohen M, Emms M, Kaschula ROC: Childhood pulmonary blastoma: a pleuropulmonary variant of the adult pulmonary blastoma. Pediatr Pathol 1991; 11: 737–739.
62. Manivel JC, Priest JR, Watterson J, et al.: Pleuropulmonary blastoma: the so-called pulmonary blastoma of childhood. Cancer 1988; 62: 1516–1526.
63. Hachitanda Y, Aoyama C, Sato JK, et al.: Pleuropulmonary blastoma in childhood: a tumor of divergent differentiation. Am J Surg Pathol 1993; 17: 382–391.
64. Seballos RM, Klein RL: Pulmonary blastoma in children: report of two cases and review of the literature. J Pediatr Surg 1994; 29: 1553–1556.
65. Dehner LP: Pleuropulmonary blastoma is *the* pulmonary blastoma of childhood. Semin Diagn Pathol 1994; 11: 144–151.
66. Delahunt B, Thomson KJ, Ferguson AF, et al.: Familial cystic nephroma and pleuropulmonary blastoma. Cancer 1993; 71: 1338–1342.
67. Sciot R, Dal-Cin P, Brock P, et al.: Pleuropulmonary blastoma (pulmonary blastoma of childhood): genetic link with other embryonal malignancies? Histopathology 1994; 24: 559–563.
68. Schmaltz C, Sauter S, Opitz O, et al.: Pleuropulmonary blastoma: a case report and review of the literature. Med Pediatr Oncol 1995; 25: 479–484.
69. Re GG, Hazen-Martin DJ, Sens DA, Garvin J: Nephroblastoma (Wilms' tumor): a model system of aberrant renal development. Semin Diagn Pathol 1994; 11: 125–135.
70. Souza RC, Peasley ED, Takaro T: Pulmonary blastomas: a distinctive group of carcinosarcomas of the lung. Ann Thorac Surg 1965; 1: 259–268.
71. Millard M: Lung, pleura, & mediastinum. In: Pathology, Anderson WAD, Ed., Vol. 2, 6th edn. 1971; CV Mosby, St. Louis, pp 875–997.
72. Koss MN, Hochholzer L, O'Leary T: Pulmonary blastomas. Cancer 1991; 67: 2368–2381.
73. Takahasi H, Tanaka K, Uchida Y, et al.: A case of pulmonary blastoma composed of histological features of both pulmonary blastoma and pulmonary endodermal tumor resembling fetal lung. J Jpn Assn Thorac Surg 1995; 43: 1217–1222.
74. Babycos PB, Daroca PJ Jr: Polypoid pulmonary endodermal tumor resembling fetal lung: report of a case. Mod Pathol 1995; 8: 303–306.
75. Kodama T, Shimosato Y, Watanabe S, et al.: Six cases of well-differentiated adenocarcinoma simulating fetal lung tissues in pseudoglandular stage: comparison with pulmonary blastoma. Am J Surg Pathol 1984; 8: 735–744.
76. Kradin RL, Young RH, Dickersin RG, Kirkham SE, Mark EJ: Pulmonary blastoma with argyrophil cells lacking sarcomatous features (pulmonary endodermal tumor resembling fetal lung). Am J Surg Pathol 1982; 6: 165–172.
77. Manning JT, Ordonez NG, Rosenberg HS, Walker WE: Pulmonary endodermal tumor resembling fetal lung. Arch Pathol Lab Med 1985; 109: 48–50.
78. Muller-Hermelink HK, Kaiserling E: Pulmonary adenocarcinoma of fetal type: alternating differentiation argues in favor of a common endodermal stem cell. Virchows Arch A 1986; 409: 195–210.
79. Olenick SJ, Fan CC, Ryoo JW: Mixed pulmonary blastoma and carcinosarcoma. Histopathology 1994; 25: 171–174.
80. Roth JA, Elquezabel A: Pulmonary blastoma evolving into carcinosarcoma: a case study. Am J Surg Pathol 1978; 2: 407–413.
81. Jacobsen M, Francis D: Pulmonary blastoma: a clinicopathologic study of eleven cases. Acta Pathol Microbiol Immunol Scand [A] 1980; 88: 151–160.
82. Nappi O, Swanson PE, Wick MR: Pseudovascular adenoid squamous cell carcinoma of the lung: clinicopathologic of three cases and comparison with true pleuropulmonary angiosarcoma. Hum Pathol 1994; 25: 373–378.
83. Ritter JH, Mills SE, Nappi O, Wick MR: Angiosarcoma-like neoplasms of epithelial organs: true endothelial tumors or variants of carcinoma? Semin Diagn Pathol 1995; 12: 270–282.
84. Banerjee SS, Eyden BP, Wells S, et al.: Pseudoangiosarcomatous carcinoma: a clinicopathological study of seven cases. Histopathology 1992; 21: 13–23.
85. Nappi O, Wick MR, Pettinato G, Ghiselli R, Swanson PE: Pseudovascular adenoid squamous cell carcinoma of the skin: a neoplasm that may be mistaken for angiosarcoma. Am J Surg Pathol 1992; 16: 429–438.
86. Eusebi V, Lamovec J, Cattani MG, et al.: Acantholytic variant of squamous cell carcinoma of the breast. Am J Surg Pathol 1986; 10: 855–861.
87. Mills SE, Gaffey MJ, Watts JC, et al.: Angiomatoid carcinoma and "angiosarcoma" of the thyroid gland: a spectrum of endothelial differentiation. Am J Clin Pathol 1994; 102: 322–330.
88. Umiker W, Iverson L: Postinflammatory "tumors" of the lung. J Thorac Surg 1954; 28: 55–63.
89. Titus J, Harrison EG Jr, Clagett O, Anderson MV, Kuaff LY: Xanthomatous and inflammatory pseudotumors of the lung. Cancer 1962; 15: 522–538.
90. Mandelbaum I, Brashear RE, Hull MT: Surgical treatment and course of pulmonary pseudotumor (plasma cell granuloma). J Thorac Cardiovasc Surg 1981; 82: 77–82.
91. Berardi RS, Lee SS, Chen HP, Stines GJ: Inflammatory pseudotumors of the lung. Surg Gynecol Obstet 1983; 156: 89–96.
92. Chen HP, Lee SS, Berardi RS: Inflammatory pseudotumor of the lung: ultrastructural and light microscopic study of a myxomatous variant. Cancer 1984; 54: 861–865.
93. Maples MD, Adkins RB Jr, Graham BS, Dao H, Scott HW Jr: Pseudotumor of the lung. Am Surg 1985; 51: 84–88.
94. Matsubara O, Tan-Liu NS, Kenney RM, Mark EJ: Inflammatory pseudotumors of the lung: progression from organizing pneumonia to fibrous histiocytoma or to plasma cell granuloma in 32 cases. Hum Pathol 1988; 19: 807–814.
95. Machicao CN, Sorensen K, Abdul KF, et al.: Transthoracic needle aspiration biopsy in inflammatory pseudotumors of the lung. Diagn Cytopathol 1989; 5: 400–403.
96. Ishida T, Oka T, Nishino T, et al.: Inflammatory pseudotumor of the lung in adults: radiographic and clinicopathological analysis. Ann Thorac Surg 1989; 48: 90–95.
97. Barbareschi M, Ferrero S, Aldovini D, et al.: Inflammatory pseudotumor of the lung: immunohistochemical analysis on four new cases. Histol Histopathol 1990; 5: 205–211.
98. Kobzik L: Benign pulmonary lesions that may be misdiagnosed as malignant. Semin Diagn Pathol 1990; 7: 129–138.
99. Vujanic GM, Dojcinov D: Inflammatory pseudotumor of the lung in children. Pediatr Hematol Oncol 1991; 8: 121–129.
100. Daudi FA, Lees GM, Higa TE: Inflammatory pseudotumors of the lung: two cases and a review. Can J Surg 1991; 34: 461–464.
101. Nonomura A, Mizukami Y, Matsubara F, et al.: Seven patients with plasma cell granuloma (inflammatory pseudotumor) of the lung,

including two with intrabronchial growth: an immunohistochemical and electron microscopic study. Intern Med 1992; 31: 756–765.
102. Koss MN: Tumor-like conditions of lung. Adv Pathol Lab Med 1994; 7: 123–150.
103. Pettinato G, Manivel JC, DeRosa N, Dehner LP: Inflammatory myofibroblastic tumor (plasma cell granuloma): clinicopathologic study of 20 cases with immunohistochemical and ultrastructural observations. Am J Clin Pathol 1990; 94: 538–546.
104. Lipton JH, Fong TC, Gill MJ, Burgess K, Elliott PD: Q fever inflammatory pseudotumor of the lung. Chest 1987; 92: 756–757.
105. Bishopric GA, D'Agay MF, Schlemmer B, Sarfati E, Brocheriou C: Pulmonary pseudotumor due to *Corynebacterium equi* in a patient with the acquired immunodeficiency syndrome. Thorax 1988; 43: 486–487.
106. Wick MR, Ritter JH, Nappi O: Inflammatory sarcomatoid carcinoma of the lung: report of three cases and clinicopathologic comparison with inflammatory pseudotumors in adult patients. Hum Pathol 1995; 26: 1014–1021.
106a. Hartmann CA, Schutze H: Mesothelioma-like tumors of the pleura: a review of 72 autopsy cases. Cancer Res Clin Oncol 1994; 120: 331–347.
106b. Shah IA, Salvatore JR, Kummet T, Gani OS, Wheeler LA: Pseudomesotheliomatous carcinoma involving pleura and peritoneum: a clinicopathologic and immunohistochemical study of three cases. Ann Diagn Pathol 1999; 3: 148–159.
107. Huszar M, Herczeg E, Lieberman Y, et al.: Distinctive immunofluorescent labeling of epithelial and mesenchymal elements of carcinosarcoma with antibodies specific for different intermediate filaments. Hum Pathol 1984; 15: 532–538.
108. Zimmerman KG, Sobonya RE, Payne CM: Histochemical and ultrastructural features of an unusual pulmonary carcinosarcoma. Hum Pathol 1981; 12: 1046–1051.
109. Koss MN, Hochholzer L, Frommelt RA: Carcinosarcomas of the lung: a clinicopathologic study of 66 patients. Am J Surg Pathol 1999; 23: 1514–1526.
110. Yousem SA, Wick MR, Randhawa P, Manivel JC: Pulmonary blastoma: an immunohistochemical comparison to fetal lung in its pseudoglandular stage. Am J Clin Pathol 1990; 93: 167–175.
111. Matsui K, Kitagawa M, Miwa A: Lung carcinoma with spindle cell components: sixteen cases examined by immunohistochemistry. Hum Pathol 1992; 23: 1289–1297.
112. Addis BJ, Corrin B: Pulmonary blastoma, carcinosarcoma, and spindle-cell carcinoma: an immunohistochemical study of keratin intermediate filaments. J Pathol 1985; 147: 291–301.
113. Suster S, Huszar M, Herczeg E: Spindle-cell carcinoma of the lung: immunocytochemical and ultrastructural study of a case. Histopathology 1987; 11: 871–878.
114. Berean K, Truong LD, Dudley AW Jr, Cagle PT: Immunohistochemical characterization of pulmonary blastoma. Am J Clin Pathol 1988; 89: 773–777.
115. Wick MR, Swanson PE: Acarcinosarcomas – current perspectives and a historical review of nosological concepts. Semin Diagn Pathol 1993; 10: 118–127.
116. Brooks JJ: The significance of double phenotypic patterns and markers in human sarcomas. Am J Pathol 1986; 125: 113–123.
117. Thompson L, Chang B, Barsky SH: Monoclonal origins of malignant mixed tumors (carcinosarcomas). Am J Surg Pathol 1996; 20: 277–287.
118. Battifora H: Spindle-cell carcinoma: ultrastructural evidence of squamous origin and collagen production by the tumor cells. Cancer 1976; 37: 2275–2282.
118a. Wakely PE Jr: Pulmonary spindle cell lesions: correlation of aspiration cytopathology and histopathology. Ann Diagn Pathol 2001; 5: 216–228.
119. Roberts CA, Seemayer TA, Neff JR, et al.: Translocation (X;18) in primary synovial sarcoma of the lung. Cancer Genet Cytogenet 1996; 88: 49–52.
120. Kaplan MA, Goodman MD, Satish J, Bhagavan BS, Travis WD: Primary pulmonary sarcoma with morphologic features of monophasic synovial sarcoma and chromosome translocation t(X;18). Am J Clin Pathol 1996; 105: 195–199.
121. Kung IT, Thallas V, Spencer EJ, Wilson SM: Expression of muscle actins in diffuse mesotheliomas. Hum Pathol 1995; 26: 565–570.
122. Wick MR: Kaposi's sarcoma unrelated to the acquired immunodeficiency syndrome: a review. Curr Opin Oncol 1991; 3: 377–383.
123. Ognibene FP, Shelhamer JH: Kaposi's sarcoma. Clin Chest Med 1988; 9: 459–465.
124. Garay SM, Belenko M, Fazzini E, Schinella R: Pulmonary manifestations of Kaposi's sarcoma. Chest 1987; 91: 39–43.
125. White DA, Matthay RA: Noninfectious pulmonary complications of infection with the human immunodeficiency virus. Am Rev Respir Dis 1989; 140: 1763–1787.
126. Meduri GU, Stover DE, Lee M, et al.: Pulmonary Kaposi's sarcoma in the acquired immune deficiency syndrome: clinical, radiographic, and pathologic manifestations. Am J Med 1986; 81: 11–18.
127. Purdy LJ, Colby TV, Yousem SA, Battifora H: Pulmonary Kaposi's sarcoma: premortem histologic diagnosis. Am J Surg Pathol 1986; 10: 301–311.
128. Cadranel J, Naccache J, Wislez M, Mayaud C: Pulmonary malignancies in the immunocompromised patient. Respiration 1999; 66: 289–309.
129. Katariya K, Thurer RJ: Malignancies associated with the immunocompromised state. Chest Surg Clin N Am 1999; 9: 63–77.
130. Smith C, Lilly S, Mann KP, et al.: AIDS-related malignancies. Ann Med 1998; 30: 323–344.
131. Hannon FB, Easterbrook PJ, Padley S, et al.: Bronchopulmonary Kaposi's sarcoma in 106 HIV-1-infected patients. Int J STD AIDS 1998; 9: 518–525.
132. Bach MC, Bagwell SP, Fanning JP: Primary pulmonary Kaposi's sarcoma in the acquired immunodeficiency syndrome: a cause of persistent pyrexia. Am J Med 1988; 85: 274–275.
133. Hanno R, Owen LG, Callen JP: Kaposi's sarcoma with extensive silent internal involvement. Int J Dermatol 1979; 18: 718–721.
134. Gal AA, Koss MN, Hartmann B, Strigle S: A review of pulmonary pathology in the acquired immune deficiency syndrome. Surg Pathol 1988; 1: 325–346.
135. O'Brien RF, Cohn DL: Serosanguineous pleural effusions in AIDS-associated Kaposi's sarcoma. Chest 1989; 96: 460–466.
136. Floris C, Sulis ML, Bernascani M, et al.: Pneumothorax in pleuropulmonary Kaposi's sarcoma related to acquired immune deficiency syndrome. Am J Med 1989; 87: 123–124.
137. Ireland-Gill A, Espina BM, Akil B, Gill PS: Treatment of acquired immunodeficiency syndrome-related Kaposi's sarcoma using bleomycin-containing combination chemotherapy regimens. Semin Oncol 1992; 19(2 suppl 5):32–37.
138. Gill PS, Akil B, Colletti P, et al.: Pulmonary Kaposi's sarcoma: clinical findings and results of therapy. Am J Med 1989; 87: 57–61.
139. Ognibene FP, Steis RG, Macher AM, et al.: Kaposi's sarcoma causing pulmonary infiltrates and respiratory failure in the acquired immunodeficiency syndrome. Ann Intern Med 1985; 102: 471–475.
140. Guccion JG, Rosen SH: Bronchopulmonary leiomyosarcoma and fibrosarcoma: a study of 32 cases and review of the literature. Cancer 1972; 30: 836–847.
141. Enzinger FM, Weiss SW: Fibrosarcoma. In: Soft tissue tumors, 2nd edn. 1988, CV Mosby, St. Louis, pp 201–222.
142. Nascimento AG, Unni KK, Bernatz PE: Sarcomas of the lung. Mayo Clin Proc 1982; 57: 355–359.
143. Miller DL, Allen MS: Rare pulmonary neoplasms. Mayo Clin Proc 1993; 68: 492–498.
144. Pettinato G, Manivel JC, Saldana MJ, Peyser J, Dehner LP: Primary bronchopulmonary fibrosarcoma of childhood and adolescence: reassessment of a low-grade malignancy. Hum Pathol 1989; 20: 463–471.
145. Goldthorn JF, Duncan MH, Kosloske AM, Ball WS: Cavitating primary pulmonary fibrosarcoma in a child. J Thorac Cardiovasc Surg 1986; 91: 932–934.
146. Wick MR, Manivel JC: Primary sarcomas of the lung. In: Textbook of uncommon cancer, Williams CJ, Krikorian JG, Green MR, Raghavan D, Eds. 1988, John Wiley & Sons, New York, pp 335–381.
147. Logrono R, Filipowicz EA, Eyzaguirre EJ, Sawh RN: Diagnosis of primary fibrosarcoma of the lung by fine needle aspiration and core biopsy. Arch Pathol Lab Med 1999; 123: 731–735.
148. Beluffi G, Bertolotti P, Mietta A, Manara G, Luisetti M: Primary leiomyosarcoma of the lung in a girl. Pediatr Radiol 1986; 16: 240–244.
149. Jimenez JF, Uthman EO, Townsend JW, Gloster ES, Seibert JJ: Primary bronchopulmonary leiomyosarcoma in childhood. Arch Pathol Lab Med 1986; 110: 348–351.

150. Yellin A, Rosenman Y, Lieberman Y: Review of smooth muscle tumours of the lower respiratory tract. Br J Dis Chest 1984; 78; 337–351.
151. Lillo-Gil R, Albrechtsson U, Jakobsson B: Pulmonary leiomyosarcoma appearing as a cyst: report of one case and review of the literature. Thorac Cardiovasc Surgeon 1985; 33: 250–252.
152. Yu H, Ren H, Miao Q, et al.: Pulmonary leiomyosarcoma: report of three cases. Chin Med J 1996; 11: 191–194.
153. Attanoos RL, Appleton MA, Gibbs AR: Primary sarcomas of the lung: a clinicopathological and immunohistochemical study of 14 cases. Histopathology 1996; 29: 29–36.
154. Morgan PGM, Ball J: Pulmonary leiomyosarcomas. Br J Dis Chest 1980; 74: 245–252.
155. Wick MR, Scheithauer BW, Piehler JM, Pairolero PC: Primary pulmonary leiomyosarcomas: a light and electron microscopic study. Arch Pathol Lab Med 1982; 106: 510–514.
156. Chaudhuri MR: Primary leiomyosarcoma of the lung. Br J Dis Chest 1973; 67: 75–80.
157. Koizumi N, Fukuda T, Ohnishi Y, et al.: Pulmonary myxoid leiomyosarcoma. Pathol Int 1995; 45: 879–884.
158. Keel SB, Bacha E, Mark EJ, Nielsen GP, Rosenberg AE: Primary pulmonary sarcoma: a clinicopathologic study of 26 cases. Mod Pathol 1999; 12: 1124–1131.
159. Dail DH, Liebow AA: Intravascular bronchioloalveolar tumor [abstract]. Am J Pathol 1975; 78 :6a.
160. Dail DH, Liebow AA, Gmelich JT, et al.: Intravascular, bronchiolar, and alveolar tumor of the lung (IVBAT). Cancer 1983; 51: 452–464.
161. Corrin B, Manners B, Millard M, Weaver L. Histogenesis of so-called "intravascular bronchioloalveolar tumour." J Pathol 1979; 128: 163–167.
162. Weiss SW, Enzinger FM: Epithelioid hemangioendothelioma: a vascular tumor often mistaken for a carcinoma. Cancer 1982; 50: 970–981.
163. Weiss SW, Ishak KG, Dail DH, Sweet DE, Enzinger FM: Epithelioid hemangioendothelioma and related lesions. Semin Diagn Pathol 1986; 3: 259–287.
164. Kitaichi M, Nagai S, Nishimura K, et al.: Pulmonary epithelioid hemangioendothelioma in 21 patients, including three with partial spontaneous regression. Eur Respir J 1998; 12: 89–96.
165. Rock MJ, Kaufman RA, Lobe TE, Hensley SD, Moss ML: Epithelioid hemangioendothelioma of the lung (intravascular bronchioloalveolar tumor) in a young girl. Pediatr Pulmonol 1991; 11: 181–186.
166. Carter EJ, Bradburne RM, Jhung JW, Ettensohn DB: Alveolar hemorrhage with epithelioid hemangioendothelioma: a previously unreported manifestation of a rare tumor. Am Rev Respir Dis 1990; 142: 700–701.
167. Briens E, Caulet-Maugendre S, Desrues B, et al.: Alveolar hemorrhage revealing epithelioid hemangioendothelioma. Respir Med 1997; 91: 111–114.
168. Yi ES, Auger WR, Friedman PJ, Morris TA, Shin SS: Intravascular bronchioloalveolar tumor of the lung presenting as pulmonary thromboembolic disease and pulmonary hypertension. Arch Pathol Lab Med 1995; 119: 255–260.
169. Ross GJ, Violi L, Friedman AC, Edmonds PR, Unger E: Intravascular bronchioloalveolar tumor: CT and pathologic correlation. J Comput Assist Tomogr 1989; 13: 240–243.
170. Bhagavan BS, Murthy MSN, Dorfman HD, Eggleston JC: Intravascular bronchiolo-alveolar tumor (IVBAT): a low-grade sclerosing epithelioid angiosarcoma of lung. Am J Surg Pathol 1982; 6: 41–52.
171. Corrin B, Harrison WJ, Wright DH: The so-called intravascular bronchioloalveolar tumour of lung (low grade sclerosing angiosarcoma). Diagn Histopathol 1983; 6: 229–237.
172. Corrin B, Dewar A, Simpson CG: Epithelioid hemangioendothelioima of the lung. Ultrastruct Pathol 1996; 20: 345–347.
173. Buggage RR, Soudi N, Olson JL, Busseniers AE: Epithelioid hemangioendothelioma of the lung: pleural effusion cytology, ultrastructure, and brief literature review. Diagn Cytopathol 1995; 13: 54–60.
174. Bollinger BK, Laskin WB, Knight CB: Epithelioid hemangioendothelioma with multiple site involvement: literature review and observations. Cancer 1994; 73: 610–615.
175. Ohori NP, Yousem SA, Sonmez-Alpan E, Colby TV: Estrogen and progesterone receptors in lymphangioleiomyomatosis, epithelioid hemangioendothelioma, and sclerosing hemangioma of the lungs. Am J Clin Pathol 1991; 96: 529–535.
176. Stout AP, Murray MR: Hemangiopericytoma: a vascular tumor featuring Zimmerman's pericytes. Ann Surg 1942; 116: 26–33.
177. Meade JB, Whitwell F, Bickford BJ, Waddington JKB: Primary haemangiopericytoma of lung. Thorax 1974; 29: 1–15.
178. Enzinger FM, Weiss SW: Hemangiopericytoma. In: Soft tissue tumors, 2nd edn. 1988, CV Mosby, St. Louis, pp 596–613.
179. Shin MS, Ho KJ: Primary hemangiopericytoma of lung: radiography and pathology. AJR 1979; 133: 1077–1083.
180. Van Damme H, Dekoster G, Creemers E, Hermans G, Limet R: Primary pulmonary hemangiopericytoma: early local recurrence after perioperative rupture of the giant tumor mass (two cases). Surgery 1990; 108: 105–109.
181. Yousem SA, Hochholzer L: Primary pulmonary hemangiopericytoma. Cancer 1987; 59: 549–555.
182. Yaghmai I: Angiographic manifestations of soft-tissue and osseous hemangiopericytomas. Radiology 1978; 126: 653–659.
183. Halle M, Blum U, Dinkel E, Brugger W: CT and MR features of primary pulmonary hemangiopericytomas. J Comput Assist Tomogr 1993; 17: 51–55.
184. Rusch VW, Shuman WP, Schmidt R, Laramore GE: Massive pulmonary hemangiopericytoma: an innovative approach to evaluation and treatment. Cancer 1989; 64: 1928–1936.
185. Kiefer T, Wertzel H, Freudenberg N, Hasse J: Long-term survival after repetitive surgery for malignant hemangiopericytoma of the lung with subsequent systemic metastases: case report and review of the literature. Thorac Cardiovasc Surg 1997; 45: 307–309.
186. Wong PP, Yagoda A: Chemotherapy of malignant hemangiopericytoma. Cancer 1978; 41: 1256–1260.
187. Jha N, McNeese M, Barkley HT, Kong J: Does radiotherapy have a role in hemangiopericytoma management? Report of 14 new cases and a review of the literature. Int J Radiat Oncol Biol Phys 1987; 13: 1399–1402.
188. Mira JG, Chu FCH, Fortner JG: The role of radiotherapy in the management of malignant hemangiopericytoma: report of eleven new cases and review of the literature. Cancer 1977; 39: 1254–1259.
189. Hansen CP, Francis D, Bertelsen S: Primary hemangiopericytoma of the lung: case report. Scand J Thor Cardiovasc Surg 1990; 24: 89–92.
190. Weiss SW, Enzinger FM. Malignant fibrous histiocytoma: an analysis of 200 cases. Cancer 1978; 41: 2250–2266.
191. Yousem SA, Hochholzer L: Malignant fibrous histiocytoma of the lung. Cancer 1987; 60: 2532–2541.
192. McDonnell T, Kyriakos M, Roper C, Mazoujian G: Malignant fibrous histiocytoma of the lung. Cancer 1988; 61: 137–145.
193. Lee JT, Shelburne JD, Linder J: Primary malignant fibrous histiocytoma of the lung: a clinicopathologic and ultrastructural study of five cases. Cancer 1984; 53: 1124–1130.
194. Bedrossian CW, Verani R, Unger KM, Salman J: Pulmonary malignant fibrous histiocytoma: light and electron microscopic studies of one case. Chest 1979; 75: 186–189.
195. Kern WH, Hughes RK, Meyer BW, Harley DP: Malignant fibrous histiocytoma of the lung. Cancer 1979; 44: 1793–1801.
196. Chowdhury LN, Swerdlow MA, Jao W, Kathpalia S, Desser RK: Postirradiation malignant fibrous histiocytoma of the lung: demonstration of alpha-1-antitrypsin-like material in neoplastic cells. Am J Clin Pathol 1980; 74: 820–826.
197. Kimizuka G, Okuzawa K, Yarita T: Primary giant cell malignant fibrous histiocytoma of the lung: a case report. Pathol Int 1999; 49: 342–346.
198. Barbas CS, Capelozzi VL, Takagaki TY, deCarvalho CR, Barbas-Fiho JV: Primary malignant fibrous histiocytoma of the lung: report of a case with bronchial brushing cytologic features. Acta Cytol 1997; 41: 919–923.
199. Halyard MY, Camoriano JK, Culligan JA, et al.: Malignant fibrous histiocytoma of the lung: report of four cases and review of the literature. Cancer 1996; 78: 2492–2497.
200. Shah SJ, Craver RD, Yu LC: Primary malignant fibrous histiocytoma of the lung in a child: a case report and review of literature. Pediatr Hematol Oncol 1996; 13: 531–538.

201. Juettner FM, Popper H, Sommersgutter K, Smolle J, Friehs GB: Malignant fibrous histiocytoma of the lung: prognosis and therapy of a rare disease: report of two cases and review of the literature. Thorac Cardiovasc Surg 1987; 35: 226–231.
202. Higashiyama M, Doi O, Kodama K, et al.: Successful surgery of malignant fibrous histiocytoma in the lung with gross extension into the right main pulmonary artery. Thorac Cardiovasc Surg 1993; 41: 73–76.
203. McDermott VG, MacKenzie S, Hendry GM: Case report: primary intrathoracic rhabdomyosarcoma: a rare childhood malignancy. Br J Radiol 1993; 66: 937–941.
204. Schiavetti A, Dominici C, Matrunola M, et al.: Primary pulmonary rhabdomyosarcoma in childhood: clinicobiologic features in two cases with review of the literature. Med Pediatr Oncol 1996; 26: 201–207.
205. Noda T, Todani T, Watanabe Y, et al.: Alveolar rhabdomyosarcoma of the lung in a child. J Pediatr Surg 1995; 30: 1607–1608.
206. Hancock BJ, DiLorenzo M, Youssef S, et al.: Childhood primary pulmonary neoplasms. J Pediatr Surg 1993; 28: 1133–1136.
207. Allan BT, Day DL, Dehner LP: Primary pulmonary rhabdomyosarcoma of the lung in children: report of two cases presenting with spontaneous pneumothorax. Cancer 1987; 59: 1005–1011.
208. Murphy JJ, Blair GK, Fraser GC, et al.: Rhabdomyosarcoma arising within congenital pulmonary cysts: report of three cases. J Pediatr Surg 1992; 27: 1364–1367.
209. Lee SH, Rengaciary SS, Paramesh J: Primary pulmonary rhabdomyosarcoma: a case report and review of the literature. Hum Pathol 1981; 12: 92–96.
210. Eriksson A, Thunell M, Lundquist G: Pedunculated endobronchial rhabdomyosarcoma with fatal asphyxia. Thorax 1982; 37: 390–391.
211. Triche TJ, Askin FB, Kissane JM: Neuroblastoma, Ewing's sarcoma, and the differential diagnosis of small round blue cell tumors. In: Pathology of neoplasia in children and adolescents, Finegold M, Ed. 1986, WB Saunders, Philadelphia, pp 145–195.
212. Wick MR, Swanson PE, Manivel JC: Immunohistochemical analysis of soft tissue sarcomas: comparisons with electron microscopy. Appl Pathol 1988; 6: 169–196.
213. Dehner LP: Soft tissue, peritoneum, and retroperitoneum. In: Pediatric surgical pathology, 2nd edn. 1987, Williams & Wilkins, Baltimore, pp 869–938.
214. Sun CCJ, Kroll M, Miller JE: Primary chondrosarcoma of the lung. Cancer 1982; 50: 1864–1866.
215. Kurotaki H, Tateoka H, Takeuchi M, et al.: Primary mesenchymal chondrosarcoma of the lung: a case report with immunohistochemical and ultrastructural studies. Acta Pathol Jpn 1992; 42: 364–371.
216. Hayashi T, Tsuda N, Iseki M, et al.: Primary chondrosarcoma of the lung: a clinicopathologic study. Cancer 1993; 72: 69–74.
217. Morgan AD, Salama FD: Primary chondrosarcoma of the lung: case report and review of the literature. J Thorac Cardiovasc Surg 1972; 64: 460–466.
218. Fallahnejad M, Harrell D, Tucker J, et al.: Chondrosarcoma of the trachea: report of a case and five-year followup. J Thorac Cardiovasc Surg 1973; 65: 210–213.
219. Parker LA, Molina PL, Bignault AG, Fidler ME: Primary pulmonary chondrosarcoma mimicking bronchogenic cyst on CT and MRI. Clin Imaging 1996; 20: 181–183.
220. Zeren H, Moran CA, Suster S, Fishback NF, Koss MN: Primary pulmonary sarcomas with features of monophasic synovial sarcoma: a clinicopathological, immunohistochemical, and ultrastructural study of 25 cases. Hum Pathol 1995; 26: 474–480.
221. Yoon GS, Park SY, Kang GH, Kim OJ: Primary pulmonary sarcoma with morphologic features of biphasic synovial sarcoma: a case report. J Korean Med Sci 1998; 13: 71–76.
222. Kaplan MA, Goodman MD, Satish J, Bhagavan BS, Travis WD: Primary pulmonary sarcoma with morphologic features of monophasic synovial sarcoma and chromosome translocation t(X;18). Am J Clin Pathol 1996; 105: 195–199.
223. Roberts CA, Seemayer TA, Neff JR, et al.: Translocation t(X;18) in primary synovial sarcoma of the lung. Cancer Genet Cytogenet 1996; 88: 49–52.
224. Sekeres M, Vasconcelles MJ, McMenamin M, Rosenfeld-Darling M, Bueno R: Two patients with sarcoma. Case 1: Synovial cell sarcoma of the lung. J Clin Oncol 2000; 18: 2341–2342.
225. Zaring RA, Roepke JE: Pathologic quiz case: pulmonary mass in a patient presenting with a hemothorax. Diagnosis: primary pulmonary biphasic synovial sarcoma. Arch Pathol Lab Med 1999; 123: 1287–1289.
226. Bacha EA, Wright CD, Grillo HC, et al.: Surgical treatment of primary pulmonary sarcomas. Eur J Cardiothorac Surg 1999; 15: 456–460.
227. Hisaoka M, Hashimoto H, Iwamasa T, Ishikawa K, Aoki T: Primary synovial sarcoma of the lung: report of two cases confirmed by molecular detection of SYT-SSX fusion gene transcripts. Histopathology 1999; 34: 205–210.
228. Fisher C: Synovial sarcoma. Ann Diagn Pathol 1998; 2: 401–421.
229. Sawamura K, Hashimoto T, Nanjo S, et al.: Primary liposarcoma of the lung. J Surg Oncol 1982; 19: 243–246.
230. Yousem SA: Angiosarcoma presenting in the lung. Arch Pathol Lab Med 1986; 110: 112–115.
231. Segal SL, Lenchner GS, Cicchelli AV, et al.: Angiosarcoma presenting as diffuse alveolar hemorrhage. Chest 1988; 94: 214–216.
232. Bartley TD, Arean VM: Intrapulmonary neurogenic tumors. J Thorac Cardiovasc Surg 1965; 50: 114–123.
233. Reingold IM, Amromin GD: Extraosseous osteosarcoma of the lung. Cancer 1971; 28: 491–498.
234. Wilson RW, Moran CA: Primary melanoma of the lung: a clinicopathologic and immunohistochemical study of eight cases. Am J Surg Pathol 1997; 21: 1196–1202.
235. Ost D, Joseph C, Sogoloff H, Menezes G: Primary pulmonary melanoma: case report and literature review. Mayo Clin Proc 1999; 74: 62–66.
236. Jensen OA, Egedorf J: Primary malignant melanoma of the lung. Scand J Resp Dis 1967; 48: 127–135.
237. Salm R: A primary malignant melanoma of the bronchus. J Path Bact 1963; 85: 121–126.
238. Bagwell SP, Flynn SD, Cox PM, Davison JA: Primary malignant melanoma of the lung. Am Rev Respir Dis 1989; 139: 1543–1547.
239. Carstens PHB, Kuhns JG, Ghazi C: Primary malignant melanomas of the lung and adrenal. Hum Pathol 1984; 15: 910–914.
240. Reid JD, Mehta VT: Melanoma of the lower respiratory tract. Cancer 1966; 19: 627–631.
241. Robertson AJ, Sinclair DJM, Sutton PP, Guthrie W: Primary melanocarcinoma of the lower respiratory tract. Thorax 1980; 35: 158–159.
242. Reed RJ, Kent EM: Solitary pulmonary melanomas: two case reports. J Thorac Cardiovasc Surg 1964: 48: 226–231.
242a. Gephardt GN: Malignant melanoma of the bronchus. Hum Pathol 1981; 12: 671–673.
242b. Ozdemir N, Cangir AK, Kutlay H, Yavuzer ST: Primary malignant melanoma of the lung in an oculocutaneous albino patient. Eur J Cardiothorac Surg 2001; 20: 864–867.
242c. Hashimoto T, Oka K, Hakozaki H, et al.: Benign clear cell tumor of the lung. Ultrastruct Pathol 2001; 25: 479–483.
242d. Gaffey MJ, Mills SE, Askin FB, et al.: Clear cell tumor of the lung: a clinicopathologic, immunohistochemical, and ultrastructural study of eight cases. Am J Surg Pathol 1990; 14: 248–259.
242e. Kuhnen C, Preisler K, Muller KM: Pulmonary lymphangioleiomyomatosis: morphologic and immunohistochemical findings. Pathologe 2001; 22: 197–204.
242f. Ferrans VJ, Yu ZX, Nelson WK, et al.: Lymphangioleiomyomatosis (LAM): a review of clinical and morphological features. J Nippon Med Sch 2000; 67: 311–329.
242g. Ito M, Sugamura Y, Ikari H, Sekine L: Angiomyolipoma of the lung. Arch Pathol Lab Med 1998; 122: 1023–1025.
243. McGlennen RC, Manivel JC, Stanley SJ, et al.: Pulmonary artery trunk sarcoma: a clinicopathologic, ultrastructural, and immunohistochemical study of four cases. Mod Pathol 1989; 2: 486–494.
244. Tanaka I, Masuda R, Inoue M, et al.: Primary pulmonary artery sarcoma: report of a case with complete resection and graft replacement, and review of 47 surgically-treated cases reported in the literature. Thorac Cardiovasc Surg 1994; 42: 64–68.
245. Al-Robaish A, Lien DC, Slatnik J, Nguyen GK: Sarcoma of the pulmonary artery trunk: report of a case complicated with hemopericardium and cardiac tamponade. Can J Cardiol 1995; 11: 707–709.

246. Sethi GK, Slaven JE, Kepes JJ: Primary sarcoma of the pulmonary artery. J Thorac Cardiovasc Surg 1972; 63: 587–596.
247. Baker PB, Goodwin RA: Pulmonary artery sarcoma. Arch Pathol Lab Med 1985; 109: 35–40.
247a. Weijmer MC, Kummer JA, Thijs LG: Case report of a patient with an intimal sarcoma of the pulmonary trunk presenting as a pulmonary embolism. Neth J Med 1999; 55: 80–83.
247b. Pagni S, Passik CS, Riordan C, D'Agostino RS: Sarcoma of the main pulmonary artery: an unusual etiology for recurrent pulmonary emboli. J Cardiovasc Surg 1999; 40: 457–461.
247c. Babatasi G, Massetti M, Agostini D, et al.: Leiomyosarcoma of the heart and great vessels. Ann Cardiol Angiol 1998; 47: 451–458.
247d. Fujii H, Osako M, Otani H, et al.: Primary pulmonary artery sarcoma. Jpn Circ J 1998; 62: 379–381.
247e. Babatasi G, Massetti M, Galateau F, Khayat A: Pulmonary artery trunk leiomyosarcoma. Thorac Cardiovasc Surg 1998; 46: 45–47.
247f. Mazzucco A, Luciani GB, Bertolini P, et al.: Primary leiomyosarcoma of the pulmonary artery: diagnostic and surgical implications. Ann Thorac Surg 1994; 57: 222–225.
247g. Johansson L, Carien B: Sarcoma of the pulmonary artery: report of four cases with electron microscopic and immunohistochemical examinations, and review of the literature. Virchows Arch A 1994; 424: 217–224.
247h. Ramp U, Gerharz CD, Iversen S, et al.: Sarcoma of the pulmonary artery: report of two cases and a review of the literature. J Cancer Res Clin Oncol 1992; 118: 551–556.
248. Hynes JK, Smith HC, Holmes DR: Pulmonary artery sarcoma: preoperative diagnosis noninvasively by two-dimensional echocardiography. Circulation 1983; 67: 459–477.
249. Lyerly HK, Reves JG, Sabiston DC: Management of primary sarcomas of the pulmonary artery and reperfusion intrabronchial hemorrhage. Surg Gynecol Obstet 1986; 163: 291–298.
250. Bleisch VR, Kraus FT: Polypoid sarcoma of the pulmonary trunk. Cancer 1980; 46: 314–321.
251. Law MR, Gregor A, Hodson ME, Bloom HJ, Turner-Warwick M: Malignant mesothelioma of the pleura: a study of 52 treated and 54 untreated patients. Thorax 1984; 39: 25–259.
252. Adams VI, Unni KK, Muhm JR, et al.: Diffuse malignant mesothelioma of pleura: diagnosis and survival in 92 cases. Cancer 1986; 58: 1540–1551.
253. Grondin SC, Sugarbaker DJ: Malignant mesothelioma of the pleural space. Oncology 1999; 13: 919–932.
254. Coffin CM, Dehner LP: Mesothelial and related neoplasms in children and adolescents: a clinicopathologic and immunohistochemical analysis of eight cases. Pediatr Pathol 1992; 12: 333–347.
255. Gentiloni N, Febbraro S, Barone C, et al.: Peritoneal mesothelioma in recurrent familial peritonitis. J Clin Gastroenterol 1997; 24: 276–279.
256. Walz R, Koch HK: Malignant pleural mesothelioma: some aspects of epidemiology, differential diagnosis, and prognosis. Histological and immunohistochemical evaluation and followup of mesotheliomas diagnosed from 1964 to January 1985. Pathol Res Pract 1990; 186: 124–134.
257. Bianchi C, Brollo Ramani L, Zuch C: Pleural plaques as risk indicators for malignant pleural mesothelioma: a necropsy-based study. Am J Ind Med 1997; 32: 445–449.
258. Sanden A, Jarvholm B: A study of possible predictors of mesothelioma in shipyard workers exposed to asbestos. J Occup Med 1991; 33: 770–773.
259. Hasan FM, Nash G, Kazemi H: The significance of asbestos exposure in the diagnosis of mesothelioma: a 28-year experience from a major urban hospital. Am Rev Respir Dis 1977; 115: 761–768.
260. Hasan FM, Nash G, Kazemi H: Asbestos exposure and related neoplasia: the 28-year experience of a major urban hospital. Am J Med 1978; 65: 649–654.
261. Grant DC, Seltzer SE, Antman KH, Finberg HJ, Koster K: Computed tomography of malignant pleural mesothelioma. J Comput Assist Tomogr 1983; 7: 626–632.
262. Kishimoto T, Ono T, Okada K, Ito H: Relationship between number of asbestos bodies in autopsy lung and pleural plaques on chest x-ray film. Chest 1989; 95: 549–552.
263. Navratil M, Trippe F: Prevalence of pleural calcification in persons exposed to asbestos dust, and in the general population in the same district. Environ Res 1972; 5: 210–216.
264. Peterson JT, Greenberg SD, Buffler P: Non-asbestos-related malignant mesothelioma: a review. Cancer 1984; 54: 951–960.
265. Cavazza A, Travis LB, Travis WD, et al.: Post-irradiation malignant mesothelioma. Cancer 1996; 77: 1379–1385.
266. Strickler HD, Goedert JJ, Fleming M, et al.: Simian virus 40 and pleural mesothelioma in humans. Cancer Epidemiol Biomarkers Prev 1996; 5: 473–475.
267. Wick MR, Mills SE: Mesothelial proliferations: an increasing morphological spectrum. Am J Clin Pathol 2000; 113: 619–622.
268. Law MR, Hodson ME, Heard BE: Malignant mesothelioma of the pleura: relation between histological type and clinical behavior. Thorax 1982; 37: 810–815.
269. Gaertner E, Zeren EH, Fleming MV, Colby TV, Travis WD: Biphasic synovial sarcomas arising in the pleural cavity: a clinicopathologic study of five cases. Am J Surg Pathol 1996; 20: 36–45.
270. Argani P, Zakowski MF, Klimstra DS, Rosai J, Ladanyi M: Detection of the *SYT-SSX* chimeric RNA of synovial sarcoma in paraffin-embedded tissue and its application in problematic cases. Mod Pathol 1998; 11: 65–71.
271. Miettinen M, Limon J, Niezabitowski A, Lasota J: Calretinin and other mesothelioma markers in synovial sarcoma: analysis of antigenic similarities and differences with malignant mesothelioma. Am J Surg Pathol 2001; 25: 610–617.
272. Attanoos RL, Biggs AR: Pathology of malignant mesothelioma. Histopathology 1997; 30: 403–418.
273. Andrion A, Mazzuco G, Bernardi P, Mollo F: Sarcomatous tumor of the chest wall with osteochondroid differentiation: evidence of mesothelial origin. Am J Surg Pathol 1989; 13: 707–712.
274. Yousem SA, Hochholzer L: Malignant mesothelioma with osseous and cartilaginous differentiation. Arch Pathol Lab Med 1987; 111: 62–66.
275. Okamoto T, Yokota S, Shinkawa K, et al.: Pleural malignant mesothelioma with osseous, cartilaginous, and rhabdomyogenic differentiation. Nihon Kokyuki Gakkai Zasshi 1998; 36: 696–701.
276. Ordonez NG, Tornos C: Malignant peripheral nerve sheath tumor of the pleura with epithelial and rhabdomyoblastic differentiation: report of a case clinically simulating mesothelioma. Am J Surg Pathol 1997; 21: 1515–1521.
277. Corson JM: Pathology of diffuse malignant pleural mesothelioma. Semin Thorac Cardiovasc Surg 1997; 9: 347–355.
278. Avellini C, Alampi G, Cocchi V, et al.: Malignant sarcomatoid mesothelioma of the pleura: a histological and immunohistochemical study of a case. Pathologica 1991; 83: 335–340.
279. Cagle PT, Truong LD, Roggli VL, Greenberg SD: Immunohistochemical differentiation of sarcomatoid mesotheliomas from other spindle cell neoplasms. Am J Clin Pathol 1989; 92: 566–571.
280. Carter D, Otis CN: Three types of spindle cell tumors of the pleura: fibroma, sarcoma, and sarcomatoid mesothelioma. Am J Surg Pathol 1988; 12: 747–753.
281. Montag AG, Pinkus GS, Corson JM: Keratin protein immunoreactivity of sarcomatoid and mixed types of diffuse malignant mesothelioma: an immunoperoxidase study of 30 cases. Hum Pathol 1988; 19: 336–342.
282. Hammar SP, Bolen JW: Sarcomatoid pleural mesothelioma. Ultrastruct Pathol 1985; 9: 337–343.
283. Khalidi HS, Medeiros LJ, Battifora H: Lymphohistiocytoid mesothelioma: an often misdiagnosed variant of sarcomatoid malignant mesothelioma. Am J Clin Pathol, in press.
284. Henderson DW, Attwood HD, Constance TJ, Shilkin KB, Steele RH: Lymphohistiocytoid mesothelioma: a rare lymphomatoid variant of predominantly sarcomatoid mesothelioma. Ultrastruct Pathol 1988; 12: 367–384.
285. Mangano WE, Cagle PT, Churg A, Vollmer RT, Roggli VL: The diagnosis of desmoplastic malignant mesothelioma and its distinction from fibrous pleurisy: a histologic and immunohistochemical analysis of 31 cases including p53 immunostaining. Am J Clin Pathol 1998; 110: 191–199.
286. Wilson GE, Hasleton PS, Chatterjee AK: Desmoplastic malignant mesothelioma: a review of 17 cases. J Clin Pathol 1992; 45: 295–298.
287. Crotty TB, Colby TV, Gay PC, Pisani RJ: Desmoplastic malignant mesothelioma masquerading as sclerosing mediastinitis: a diagnostic dilemma. Hum Pathol 1992; 23: 79–82.
288. Epstein JI, Budin RE: Keratin and epithelial membrane antigen immunoreactivity in nonneoplastic fibrous pleural lesions:

implications for the diagnosis of desmoplastic mesothelioma. Hum Pathol 1986; 17: 514–519.
289. Cantin R, Al-Jabi M, McCaughey WT: Desmoplastic diffuse mesothelioma. Am J Surg Pathol 1982; 6: 215–222.
290. Colby TV: The diagnosis of desmoplastic malignant mesothelioma. Am J Clin Pathol 1998; 110: 135–136.
291. Colby TV: Malignancies in the lung and pleura mimicking benign processes. Semin Diagn Pathol 1995; 12: 30–44.
292. Center R, Lukeis R, Dietzsch E, Gillespie M, Garson OM: Molecular deletion of 9p sequences in non-small cell lung cancer and malignant mesothelioma. Genes Chromosomes & Cancer 1993; 7: 47–53.
293. Cheng JQ, Jhanwar SC, Lu YY, Testa JR: Homozygous deletions within 9p21-p22 identify a small critical region of chromosomal loss in human malignant mesotheliomas. Cancer Res 1993; 53: 4761–4763.
294. Brown RW, Clark GM, Tandon AK, Allred DC: Multiple-marker immunohistochemical phenotypes distinguishing malignant pleural mesothelioma from pulmonary adenocarcinoma. Hum Pathol 1993; 24: 347–354.
295. Riera JR, Astengo-Osuna C, Longmate JA, Battifora H: The immunohistochemical diagnostic panel for epithelial mesothelioma: a reevaluation following heat-induced epitope retrieval. Am J Surg Pathol 1997; 21: 1409–1419.
296. Ordonez NG: Role of immunohistochemistry in differentiating epithelial mesothelioma from adenocarcinoma: review and update. Am J Clin Pathol 1999; 112: 75–89.
297. Burns TR, Greenberg D, Mace ML, Johnson EH: Ultrastructural diagnosis of epithelial malignant mesothelioma. Cancer 1985; 56: 2036–2040.
298. Cury PM, Butcher DN, Corrin B, Nicholson AG: The use of histological and immunohistochemical markers to distinguish pleural malignant mesothelioma and in situ mesothelioma from reactive mesothelial hyperplasia and reactive pleural fibrosis. J Pathol. 1999; 189: 251–257.
299. Kung IT, Thallas V, Spencer EJ, Wilson SM: Expression of muscle actins in diffuse mesotheliomas. Hum Pathol 1995; 26: 565–570.
300. Hurliman J: Desmin and neural marker expression in mesothelial cells and mesotheliomas. Hum Pathol 1994; 25: 753–757.
301. Klima M, Bossart MI: Sarcomatous type of malignant mesothelioma. Ultrastruct Pathol 1983; 4: 349–358.
302. Flint A, Weiss SW: CD34 and keratin expression distinguishes solitary fibrous tumor (fibrous mesothelioma) of pleura from desmoplastic mesothelioma. Hum Pathol 1995; 26: 428–431.
303. Huncharek M, Kelsey K, Mark EJ, et al.: Treatment and survival in diffuse malignant pleural mesothelioma: a study of 83 cases from the Massachusetts General Hospital. Anticancer Res 1996; 16(3A): 1265–1268.
304. Machin T, Mashiyama ET, Henderson JA, McCaughey WT: Bony metastases in desmoplastic pleural mesothelioma. Thorax 1988; 43: 155–156.
305. Chahinian AP, Antman K, Goutsou M, et al.: Randomized phase II trial of cisplatin with mitomycin or doxorubicin for malignant mesothelioma by the Cancer & Leukemia Group B. J Clin Oncol 1993; 11: 1559–1565.
306. Sugarbaker DJ, Garcia JP, Richards WG, et al.: Extrapleural pneumonectomy in the multimodality therapy of malignant pleural mesothelioma results in 120 consecutive patients. Ann Surg 1996; 224: 288–296.
307. DaValle MJ, Faber LP, Kittle CF, Jensik RJ: Extrapleural pneumonectomy for diffuse malignant mesothelioma. Ann Thorac Surg 1986; 42: 612–618.
308. Lee MJ, Grogan L, Meehan S, Breatnach E: Pleural granulocytic sarcoma: CT characteristics. Clin Radiol 1991; 43: 57–59.
309. Luppi G, Cesinaro AM, Zoboli A, Morandi U, Piccinini L: Mesenchymal chondrosarcoma of the pleura. Eur Respir J 1996; 9: 840–843.
310. Goetz SP, Robinson RA, Landas SK: Extraskeletal myxoid chondrosarcoma of the pleura: report of a case clinically simulating mesothelioma. Am J Clin Pathol 1992; 97: 498–502.
311. Okby NT, Travis WD: Liposarcoma of the pleural cavity: clinical and pathologic features of 4 cases with a review of the literature. Arch Pathol Lab Med 2000; 124: 699–703.
312. Wong WW, Pluth JR, Grado GL, Schild SE, Sanderson DR: Liposarcoma of the pleura. Mayo Clin Proc 1994; 69: 882–885.
313. Stark P, Smith DC, Watkins GE, Chun KE: Primary intrathoracic extraosseous osteogenic sarcoma: report of three cases. Radiology 1990; 174: 725–726.
314. Moran CA, Suster S, Koss MN: The spectrum of histologic growth patterns in benign and malignant fibrous tumors of the pleura. Semin Diagn Pathol 1992; 9: 169–180.
315. Ali SZ, Hoon V, Hoda S, Heelan R, Zakowski MF: Solitary fibrous tumor: a cytologic–histologic study with clinical, radiologic, and immunohistochemical correlations. Cancer 1997; 81: 116–121.
316. Hanau CA, Miettinen M: Solitary fibrous tumor: histological and immunohistochemical spectrum of benign and malignant variants presenting at different sites. Hum Pathol 1995; 26: 440–449.
317. Mezzetti M, Augusti A: Fibrosarcoma of the pleura: circumscribed primary pleural neoplasms. Arch Ital Chir 1969; 95: 544–555.
318. Meyer M, Krause U: Solitary fibrous tumors of the pleura. Chirurg 1999; 70: 979–952.
319. Vallat-Decouvelaere AV, Dry SM, Fletcher CDM: Atypical and malignant solitary fibrous tumors in extrathoracic locations: evidence of their comparability to intrathoracic tumors. Am J Surg Pathol 1998; 22: 1501–1511.
320. Yokoi T, Tsuzuki T, Yatabe Y, et al.: Solitary fibrous tumor: significance of p53 and CD34 immunoreactivity in its malignant transformation. Histopathology 1998; 32: 423–432.
321. Myoui A, Aozasa K, Iuchi K, et al.: Soft tissue sarcoma of the pleural cavity. Cancer 1991; 68: 1550–1554.
322. England DM, Hochholzer L, McCarthy MJ: Localized benign and malignant fibrous tumors of the pleura. Am J Surg Pathol 1989; 13: 640–658.
323. Fukasawa Y, Takada A, Tateno M, et al.: Solitary fibrous tumor of the pleura causing recurrent hypoglycemia by secretion of insulin-like growth factor II. Pathol Int 1998; 48: 47–52.
324. Theegarten D, Meisel M: Malignant fibrous histiocytoma of the thoracic wall in the area of a tuberculous pleural callosity. Pneumonologie 1993; 47: 458–460.
325. Watanabe S, Hitomi S, Nakamura T, et al.: A clinical study of six surgically-treated patients with malignant tumors arising from chronic pleuritis and pyothorax. Nippon Kyobu Geka Gakkai Zasshi 1989; 37: 281–286.
326. Saiffudin A, DaCosta P, Chalmers AG, et al.: Primary malignant localized fibrous tumors of the pleura: clinical, radiological, and pathological features. Clin Radiol 1992; 45: 13–17.
327. Toochika H, Kiminok K, Tagawa Y, et al.: Malignant fibrous histiocytoma of the chest cavity: report of four resected cases. Nippon Kyobu Geka Gakkai Zasshi 1990; 38: 647–653.
328. Moran CA, Suster S, Koss MN: Smooth muscle tumors presenting as pleural neoplasms. Histopathology 1995; 27: 227–234.
329. Gibbs AR: Smooth muscle tumors of the pleura. Histopathology 1995; 27: 295–296.
330. Askin FB, Rosai J, Sibley RK, et al.: Malignant small cell tumor of the thoracopulmonary region in childhood. Cancer 1979; 43: 2438–2451.
331. Israel MA: Peripheral neuroepithelioma. In: Textbook of uncommon cancer, Williams CJ, Krikorian JG, Green MR, Rhagavan D, Eds. 1988, John Wiley & Sons, New York, pp 683–690.
332. Jurgens H, Bier V, Harms D, et al.: Malignant peripheral neuroectodermal tumors. Cancer 1988; 61: 349–357.
333. Dang NC, Siegel SE, Phillips JD: Malignant chest wall tumors in children and young adults. J Pediatr Surg 1999; 34: 1773–1778.
334. Promnitz S, Petri F, Schulz HJ, Gellert K: Askin's tumor: a rare entity. Case report with references to the literature. Pneumonologie 1999; 53: 393–399.
335. Liptay MJ, Fry WA: Malignant bone tumors of the chest wall. Semin Thorac Cardiovasc Surg 1999; 11: 278–284.
336. Kabiri H, El-Fakir Y, Mahassini N, et al.: Malignant small cell thoracic pulmonary tumor. Rev Pneumonol Clin 1999; 55: 21–25.
337. Taneli C, Genc A, Erikci V, Yuce G, Balik E: Askin tumors in children: a report of four cases. Eur J Pediatr Surg 1998; 8: 312–314.
338. Sallustio G, Pirronti T, Lasorella A, et al.: Diagnostic imaging of primitive neuroectodermal tumor of the chest wall (Askin tumor). Pediatr Radiol 1998; 28: 697–702.
339. Askin FB, Perlman EJ: Neuroblastoma and peripheral neuroectodermal tumors. Am J Clin Pathol 1998; 109(4 suppl 1): S23–S30.
340. Sabate JM, Franquet T, Parellada JA, Monill JM, Oliva E: Malignant

neuroectodermal tumor of the chest wall (Askin tumor): CT and MR findings in eight patients. Clin Radiol 1994; 49: 634–638.
341. Shamberger RC, Tarbell NJ, Perez-Atayde AR, Grier HE: Malignant small round cell tumor (Ewing's-PNET) of the chest wall in children. J Pediatr Surg 1994; 29: 179–185.
342. Winer-Muram HT, Kauffman WM, Gronemeyer SA, Jennings SG: Primitive neuroectodermal tumors of the chest wall (Askin tumors): CT and MR findings. Am J Roentgenol 1993; 161: 265–268.
343. Dehner LP: Soft tissue sarcomas of childhood. Natl Cancer Inst Monogr 1981: 56: 43–59.
344. Sapi Z, Szentirmay Z, Orosz Z: Desmoplastic small round cell tumor of the pleura: a case report with further cytogenetic and ultrastructural evidence of "mesothelioblastemic" origin. Eur J Surg Oncol 1999; 25: 633–634.
345. Parkash V, Gerald WL, Parma A, Miettinen M, Rosai J: Desmoplastic small round cell tumor of the pleura. Am J Surg Pathol 1995; 19: 659–665.
346. Bian Y, Jordan AG, Rupp M, et al.: Effusion cytology of desmoplastic small round cell tumor of the pleura: a case report. Acta Cytol 1993; 37: 77–82.
347. Sarkar MR, Bahr R: The Askin tumor. Chirurg 1992; 63: 973–976.
348. Contesso G, Llombart-Bosch A, Terrier P, et al.: Does malignant small round cell tumor of the thoracopulmonary region (Askin tumor) constitute a clinicopathologic entity? Cancer 1992; 69: 1012–1020.
349. Takahashi K, Dambara T, Uekusa T, et al.: Massive chest wall tumor diagnosed as Askin tumor: successful treatment by intensive combined modality therapy in an adult. Chest 1993; 104: 287–288.
350. Fitzgibbons JF, Feldhaus SJ, McNamara LF, Langdon RM Jr: Diagnostic features and treatment of the Askin tumor – malignant small cell tumor of the thoracopulmonary region: a case report. Nebr Med J 1993; 78: 2–6.
351. Kushner BH, LaQuaglia MP, Cheung NK, et al.: Clinically critical impact of molecular genetic studies in pediatric solid tumors. Med Pediatr Oncol 1999; 33: 530–535.
352. Dehner LP: Peripheral neuroectodermal tumor and Ewing's sarcoma. Am J Surg Pathol 1993; 17: 1–13.
353. Miser JS, Kinsella TJ, Triche TJ, et al.: Treatment of peripheral neuroepithelioma in children and young adults. J Clin Oncol 1987; 5: 1752–1758.
354. Farhi DC, Odell CA, Shurin SB: Myelodysplastic syndrome and acute myeloid leukemia after treatment for solid tumor of childhood. Am J Clin Pathol 1993; 100: 270–275.
355. Cohen M, Kaschula RO: Primary pulmonary tumors in childhood: a review of 31 years' experience and the literature. Pediatr Pulmonol 1992; 14: 222–232.
356. Hill DA, Sadeghi S, Schultz MZ, Burr JS, Dehner LP: Pleuropulmonary blastoma in an adult: an initial case report. Cancer 1999; 85: 2368–2374.
357. Szczesny T, Hussein N, Szczesna A: Pulmonary blastoma and related primary malignant pulmonary neoplasms. Pneumonol Alergol Pol 1999; 67: 263–270.
358. Romeo C, Impellizzeri P, Grosso M, Vitarelli E, Gentile C: Pleuropulmonary blastoma: long-term survival and literature review. Med Pediatr Oncol 1999; 33: 372–376.
359. Benouachane T, El-Khorassani M, Nachef MN, et al.: Pleuropulmonary blastoma: report of 4 cases. Rev Mal Respir 1999; 16: 390–394.
360. Baraniya J, Desai S, Kane S, et al.: Pleuropulmonary blastoma. Med Pediatr Oncol 1999; 32: 52–56.
361. Priest JR, McDermott MB, Bhatia S, et al.: Pleuropulmonary blastoma: a clinicopathologic study of 50 cases. Cancer 1997; 80: 147–161.
362. Priest JR, Watterson J, Strong L, et al.: Pleuropulmonary blastoma: a marker for familial disease. J Pediatr 1996; 128: 220–224.
363. Lopez-Andreu JA, Ferris-Tortajada J, Gomez J: Pleuropulmonary blastoma and congenital cystic malformations. J Pediatr 1996; 129: 773–775.
364. Tagge EP, Mulvihill D, Chandler JC, et al.: Childhood pleuropulmonary blastoma: caution against nonoperative management of congenital lung cysts. J Pediatr Surg 1996; 31: 187–190.
365. Wright JR: Pleuropulmonary blastoma: a case report documenting transition from type I (cystic) to type III (solid). Cancer 2000; 88: 2853–2858.
366. Lin BT, Colby TV, Gown AM, et al.: Malignant vascular tumors of the serous membranes mimicking mesothelioma: a report of 14 cases. Am J Surg Pathol 1996; 20: 1431–1439.

Hematolymphoid proliferations involving the lung

15

Madeleine D Kraus   Mark R Wick

As a consequence of advances in cytogenetics and molecular biology, and greater understanding of the immune system, the diagnosis and classification of hematologic conditions has undergone substantial evolution in the past 10 years. The nosology of non-Hodgkin's lymphomas (NHLs), in particular, has been brought into alignment with modern concepts of normal B- and T-cell maturation, and much of the terminology relates tumors to their non-neoplastic lymphoid counterparts. In light of these factors, a mastery of the diagnosis of lymphoma and leukemia requires an understanding of the molecular and immunologic underpinnings of their pathogenesis.

Normal lymphoid tissue in the lung and the concept of mucosa-associated lymphoid tissue

The lung contains an extensive lymphatic network that channels antigen-rich lymphatic fluid centripetally towards parenchymal, septal, hilar, and mediastinal lymph nodes. Organized lymphoid tissue in the periphery of the normal lung is limited to sparse submucosal aggregates of lymphocytes and intrapulmonary lymph nodes, but it is more substantial centrally[1,2] along bronchioles and central airways.[3–5] Inhaled particulate matter is trapped in the mucus layer of proximal airways and some passes across patches of specialized epithelium where it initiates the primary and secondary immune response. The lymphoid hyperplasia that results has been termed "acquired mucosa-associated lymphoid tissue" (MALT);[6,7] it includes secondary follicles with prominent germinal centers and a broad marginal zone of activated and memory B cells that are primed to recognize and neutralize antigens (Fig. 15.1). Acquired MALT has a distinctive immuno-architecture with four compartments: B-cell-rich follicles, the follicular mantle and marginal zones, and T-cell-rich interfollicular regions.

As stated above, the accurate diagnosis of benign lymphoid proliferations and the classification of lymphomas are based on the morphologic, immunologic, and genetic features that the lesional cells share with normal B- and T-lymphocytes (Fig. 15.2). According to this paradigm, the characteristic features that are used to diagnose follicular lymphoma (i.e. a mixture of centrocytes and centroblasts; CD10 and *bcl*-6 expression) resemble those of the cells in benign germinal centers, whereas those of mantle cell lymphomas and marginal zone lymphomas recapitulate specific aspects of mantle and marginal zone lymphocytes, respectively.

Special studies that are useful in the evaluation of hematolymphoid proliferations

Immunohistochemistry

Immunophenotypic analysis of tissue sections has become an essential part of the evaluation of hematolymphoid proliferations, in both nodal and extranodal sites. Not

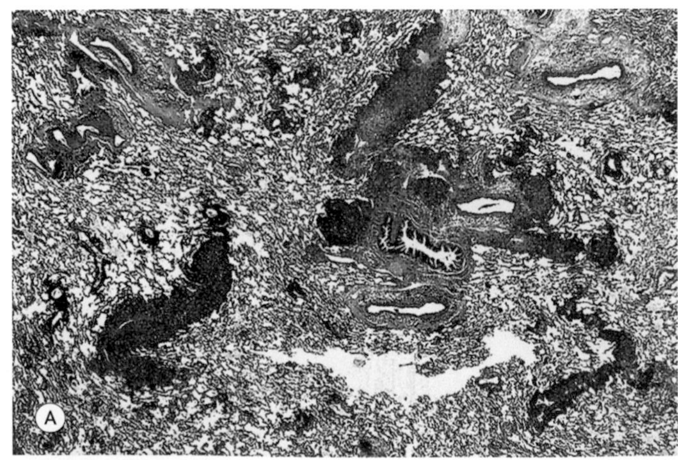

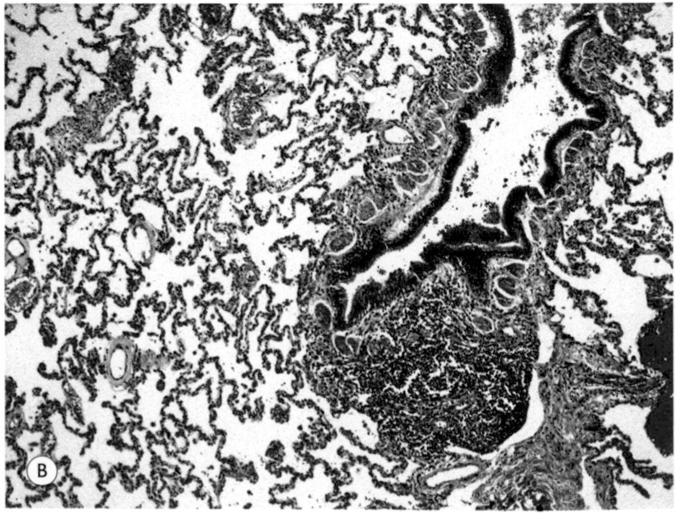

Fig. 15.1 (A) Benign mucosa-associated lymphoid tissue accumulates adjacent to airways after exposure to immunogenic material. The proliferation represents a mixture of B- and T-lineage lymphocytes, with a structure that loosely recapitulates the germinal centers (B) and paracortex as found in reactive lymph nodes.

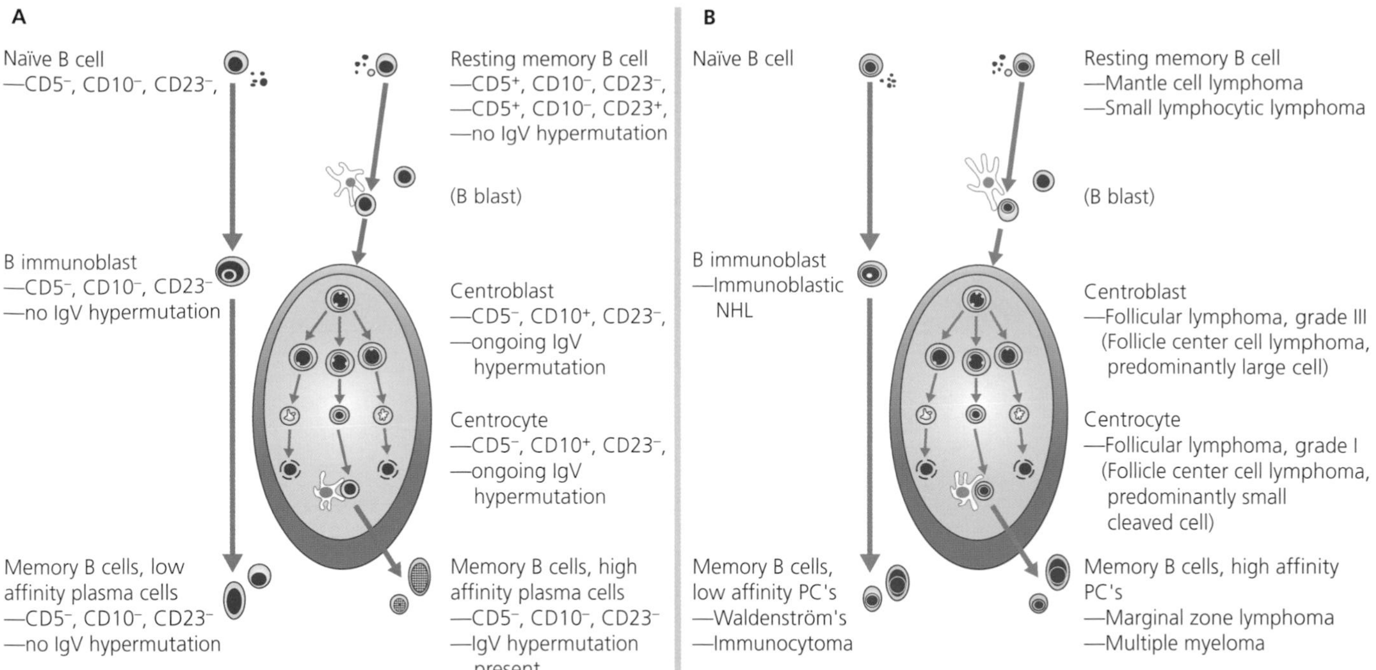

Fig. 15.2 (A) The stages of development found in the ontogeny of the primary and secondary immune response form the basis of the classification of B-cell neoplasms. The stages most relevant to pulmonary lymphomas range from the circulating naïve B cell (upper left) to the mature, high-affinity plasma cell (lower right), and are associated with specific phenotypic profiles. (B) The immunophenotype of B-cell lymphomas closely approximate specific stages of B-cell development, and it is the principal means by which these lymphomas are recognized.

only is this technique helpful in assessing the lineage of the infiltrate (Table 15.1) but it also provides the basis from which inferences about the reactive or neoplastic nature of the proliferation can be made. Some combinations of markers indicate that the lesional cells are neoplastic,[8] while other immunoprofiles provide the necessary information to classify a particular lymphoma as a specific tumor subtype (Table 15.2).[9,10] Accurate categorization of lymphomas cannot be achieved with the results of a single test or stain, but, rather, it reflects the integration of several data. In consequence, a panel approach is necessary (Table 15.3), regardless of whether fresh or formalin-fixed tissue is available as a substrate.

Analytic flow cytometry

The concepts underlying flow cytometry (FCM) are identical to those of tissue section-based immunohistochemistry, except that a fluorescing (rather than precipitating) chromogen is attached to cells that are dispersed in fluid. A broader array of surface antigens is available for diagnostic use in FCM, and by generation of a more detailed antigenic profile, the pathologic process can be classified more accurately.[11,12] An additional advantage that FCM has over immunohistologic phenotyping is that three or four markers can be evaluated simultaneously in specific cell populations, permitting thorough evaluation even when only a limited amount of tissue is available. One drawback to FCM is that the phenotype and morphologic features of the analyzed cells cannot be reviewed together. Therefore, judgments regarding immuno-architecture are not possible. Most flow cytometry laboratories have established panels that focus on specific, predefined clinical scenarios and the identification of immunophenotypic profiles that are classically associated with common disease entities (Table 15.3).[13]

Molecular genetics

Specialized techniques such as polymerase chain reaction (PCR) analysis may be applied to paraffin-embedded material or archival snap-frozen tissue to document clonality, define lineage, and assess for the presence of viral infection(s).[14] Clonality is evaluated by examination of areas of the immunoglobulin heavy- and light-chain loci or T-cell receptor α/β or γ loci that are rearranged during normal lymphoid development.[15,16] Southern blot analysis, which was previously the "gold standard" in molecular analysis of lymphomas, is less commonly done currently because of the labor-intensive nature of the testing and a long turnaround time of 1–2 weeks. For all

Table 15.1 Antibodies useful in the evaluation of hematolymphoid proliferations in the lung

Marker	Description
B-cell lineage markers	
CD10	Positive in follicle center cell NHL (not lineage specific; also present on some epithelial tumors)
CD19	Early B-cell marker (also present on B-LBL; not present on plasma cells)
CD20	Mature B-cell marker (not present on B-LBL; most plasma cells negative)
CD23	Activated B cells
CD74	Mature B cells
CD79a	Immature and mature B cells (present on B-LBL as well as plasma cells)
PAX5	Immature B cells, including lymphoblasts, mature B cells; negative in plasma cells
CD138	Plasma cells, some cases of classic Hodgkin's lymphoma
IgD	Cytoplasmic immunoglobulin heavy chain, present in benign mantle cells, some lymphomas
κ, λ	Cytoplasmic κ and λ immunoglobulin light chains
T-cell lineage markers	
CD1a	Some T cells (thymocytes), Langerhans cells
CD2	Pan T-cell marker
CD3	T cells
CD4	Helper/suppressor T cells
CD5	Preferential T-cell marker (also positive in some B-cell neoplasms)
CD7	T cells, some NK cells
CD8	Cytotoxic T cells
CD16[a]	Natural killer cells, granulocytes
CD43	Preferential T-cell marker (also positive in some B-cell neoplasms)
CD45RO	T cells, some macrophages
CD56	Natural killer cells and some T cells
CD57	Natural killer cells and some T cells
Monocyte/macrophage/accessory cell markers	
CD1a	Some T cells (thymocytes), Langerhans cells
CD15	Granulocytes, also positive in Hodgkin's lymphoma
CD21	Follicular dendritic cells, some B cells
CD68	Macrophages, monocytes
s100	Langerhans cells, melanoma, paracortical dendritic cells
Miscellaneous markers	
ALK	Positive on some peripheral T-cell lymphomas
EBV–LMP	Epstein–Barr virus latent membrane protein
EBNA-1[a]	Epstein–Barr virus nuclear antigen 1
EBNA-2[a]	Epstein–Barr virus nuclear antigen 2
bcl6	A transcriptional regulator positive only in germinal center B cells as well as some lymphoblasts
bcl2	An antiapoptosis protein positive in virtually all lymphoid proliferations ***except*** benign germinal center B cells
cyclin D1	A cell cycle regulator positive in mantle cell lymphoma
CD45	Leukocyte common antigen (LCA)
Oct2	A transcription factor in some B and T cells, also present in L&H type Reed–Sternberg cells
TdT	Terminal deoxynucleotidyl transferase (TdT), a marker of the blastic stage of differentiation
EMA	Epithelial membrane antigen (positive in some large cell lymphomas and in some plasmacytomas)

B-LBL = lymphoblastic lymphoma; NHL = non-Hodgkin's lymphoma; NK = natural killer.
[a]Not available for paraffin section immunohistochemistry.

molecular analyses, it is important to note that clonality is used to help define neoplasia, but a *lack* of clonality does not prove that a lesion is benign and reactive. For example, low tumor cell numbers in "lymphomatoid granulomatosis" and T-cell-rich B-cell lymphomas may yield apparently non-clonal results because of the dilutional effects of reactive cells in the sample being evaluated. Similarly, non-B-, non-T-cell malignancies such as natural killer cell lymphomas and myeloid leukemias will yield a polyclonal profile because the lesional cells do not contain rearrangements of either B- or T-cell receptor genes.

Cytogenetics

Many types of non-Hodgkin's lymphoma have recurring chromosomal translocations that can be identified with classical cytogenetic techniques. Recent technical advances and the development of commercially available probes now permit fluorescent in-situ hybridization (FISH)

Table 15.2 Immunophenotypic profiles associated with lymphoid neoplasia

Phenotypic findings indicative of lymphoid neoplasia
Aberrant gain of a preferential T-cell marker on a proliferation of B cells:
Aberrant expression of CD5 is the hallmark of small lymphocytic lymphoma and mantle cell lymphoma
Aberrant expression of CD43 is often seen in small lymphocytic lymphoma, less common in mantle cell lymphoma
A restricted pattern of a single immunoglobulin light chain:
A profoundly skewed ratio (e.g. 10:1 or 1:10) of kappa-positive or lambda-positive cells provides strong support for the presence of a monoclonal population of B cells (considered definitional of B cell neoplasia)
Aberrant loss of a maturation or stage-specific marker:
Absence of CD5 and CD7 on a population of T cells is abnormal and is commonly seen in peripheral T-cell lymphomas
Absence of both CD4 and CD8 is abnormal outside of the thymus, and is commonly seen in T γ/δ lymphomas
Phenotypic findings helpful in classifying morphologically malignant lymphoid proliferations
TdT expression:[a] supports classification as a lymphoblastic lymphoma
cyclin D1 expression: supports classification as mantle cell lymphoma
***bcl-6* expression:** supports classification as a lymphoma of follicle center cell origin
CD21 expression: when it highlights a disrupted follicular dendritic cell meshwork indicative of colonization, can assist in diagnosing marginal zone ("MALT/BALT") lymphomas of the lung

[a]Since benign cortical and medullary thymocytes are TdT+, great care should be taken in evaluating small biopsies of hilar or midline intrathoracic masses.

Table 15.3 A panel approach to the immunophenotypic analysis of pulmonary hematolymphoid proliferations

Small lymphoid proliferations with a diffuse architecture:
Paraffin sections: CD3 or CD45ro, CD20, CD43, CD45RO, cyclin D1, cytokeratin
Fresh tissue/flow cytometry: CD3, CD19, CD20, CD5, CD10, CD23, sIg κ/λ
Small lymphoid proliferations with nodular component:
Paraffin sections: CD3 or CD45ro, CD20, CD43, CD45RO, cyclin D1, *bcl6*, cytokeratin
Fresh tissue/flow cytometry: CD3, CD19, CD20, CD5, CD10, CD23, sIg κ/λ
Small lymphoid proliferations with plasmacytic differentiation:
Paraffin sections: CD3 or CD45ro, CD20, CD21, CD43, cIg κ/λ, EMA, cytokeratin
Fresh tissue/flow cytometry: CD3, CD19, CD20, CD5, CD10, CD23, sIg κ/λ, CD138, cIg κ/λ
Large lymphoid proliferations with plasmacytic differentiation:
paraffin sections: CD3 or CD45ro, CD20, CD74, CD75, CD45, kappa, lambda
fresh tissue/flow cytometry: CD3, CD19, CD20, CD5, CD10, CD23, CD138, sIg κ/λ, cIg κ/λ
Bimorphic small cell and very large cell populations:
paraffin sections: CD20, CD45ro, CD15, CD30, CD57
fresh tissue/flow cytometry: CD3, CD19, CD20, CD5, CD10, CD23, sIg κ/λ

cIg κ/λ = cytoplasmic kappa and lambda immunoglobulin (can be assessed in paraffin sections or on fresh tissue); sIg κ/λ = surface kappa and lambda immunoglobulin (evaluation of expression requires fresh tissue); EMA = epithelial membrane antigen.

studies for some karyotypic abnormalities. These can be applied to archival touch preparations which have been made from fresh lesional tissue, or even from interphase nuclei extracted from paraffin-embedded material (Fig. 15.3). The most common and clinically relevant karyotypic changes related to NHL are given in Table 15.4.

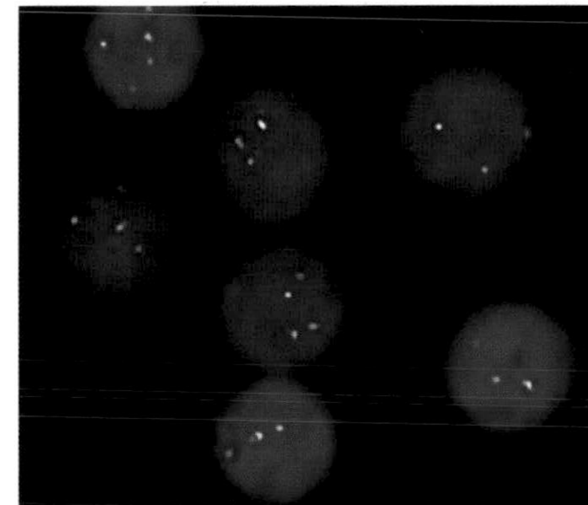

Fig. 15.3 Air-dried touch preparations of fresh tissue can provide sufficient nuclei for fluorescent in-situ hybridization studies to be performed. In this case of mantle cell lymphoma, a CCND1/IgH fusion probe was used to search for the t(11;14) (q13;q32) chromosomal translocation.

Reactive lymphoid hyperplasia

Because it is constantly exposed to exogenous antigens, the lung is commonly involved in reactive inflammatory conditions.[17] Hyperplasia of the MALT of the lung occurs in the setting of autoimmune conditions or otherwise-altered immunity such as acquired immunodeficiency syndrome (AIDS) and congenital immunodeficiency states. Disorders in this group may be sufficiently extensive anatomically to produce symptoms such as cough or dyspnea, or they may be detected incidentally

Table 15.4 Cytogenetic analyses associated with hematolymphoid proliferations in the lung

Disease	Abnormality	Implicated loci
B-cell chronic lymphocytic leukemia	trisomy 12[a]	
T-cell prolymphocytic leukemia	inv 14	
Follicle center cell lymphoma	t(14;18)[a]	IgH – *bcl-2*
Mantle cell lymphoma	t(11;14)[a]	*bcl-1* – IgH
MALT lymphoma	trisomy 3[a] t(11;18)	 *API2 – MLT*
B-cell large cell lymphoma	t(3q27;V)	*bcl-6* – variable partners
Burkitt's lymphoma	t(2;8)[a] t(8;14)[a] t(8;22)[a]	IgL – *c-myc* *c-myc* – IgH *c-myc* – IgL
T-cell anaplastic large cell lymphoma	t(2;5)[a]	NPM – *alk*

[a]Presence of this karyotypic abnormality can be evaluated via interphase FISH analysis on touch preparations from lesional fresh tissue.

during radiologic procedures done for other reasons. The three main patterns of hyperplasia – follicular bronchiolitis, nodular lymphoid hyperplasia, and diffuse lymphoid hyperplasia (lymphoid interstitial pneumonia) – may be seen in isolation or they may coexist in the same specimen.

Follicular bronchiolitis

Follicular bronchiolitis (FB) is slightly more common in males than in females.[18] It involves the lungs bilaterally and produces an interstitial pattern of involvement on chest radiographs.[19] This disorder is most commonly seen in patients with congenital or acquired immunodeficiency, collagen vascular disease, or chronic obstructive pulmonary disease,[20,21] and may be observed as a denovo condition or at the periphery of localized infectious processes in the lung. Microscopically, the key feature of FB is an eccentric peribronchiolar accumulation of lymphoid tissue that distorts and narrows the bronchiolar lumina. The structure of benign MALT is preserved, with germinal centers, crisply demarcated mantle zones, and mixed lymphocytic and histiocytic components at the interface with normal lung parenchyma.[22] There is negligible interstitial involvement away from the bronchioles and the airspaces are uninvolved (Fig. 15.4), features that distinguish FB from lymphoid interstitial pneumonia.[18,20] Immunophenotypic findings are identical to those seen in nodular lymphoid hyperplasia (see below) and the two differ only in the quantity of the lymphoid infiltrate.

Nodular lymphoid hyperplasia

In past literature on the topic, "nodular lymphoid hyperplasia" (NLH) has been used synonymously with "pseudolymphoma."[22–25] However, the latter is an outdated and confusing term that should be avoided diagnostically because it creates uncertainty over whether the lesion in question is actually neoplastic.[26] NLH is most commonly seen in adults, some of whom have altered immune states (collagen vascular diseases, other autoimmune disorders, or AIDS).[27–31] The reticular or reticulonodular appearance of NLH on chest films correlates with the histologic finding of lymphoid infiltrates that form expansive but circumscribed nodular aggregations along the course of bronchovascular bundles (Fig. 15.5).

Follicular (germinal center-based) lymphoid hyperplasia with interfollicular lymphoplasmacytosis is the histologic hallmark of NLH. Either a nodular or a diffuse architecture predominates, depending on the relative abundance of germinal centers.[18,22] In contrast to follicular *lymphoma*, the germinal centers in NLH are widely spaced; they also vary in size, exhibit tinctorial polarity, and are demarcated by a mantle zone that is composed of cytologically bland small lymphoid cells. Lymphocytes and plasma cells fill the interfollicular zones, which may also contain patchy accumulations of histiocytes. Lesional foci of NLH are sharply demarcated from the surrounding lung parenchyma (Fig. 15.6), without a tendency to extend along lobar septa or into alveolar walls. Destructive lymphoepithelial lesions, Dutcher bodies (eosinophilic intranuclear deposits of immunoglobulin), and follicular colonization by atypical lymphocytes are absent.

The *bcl*-6+, CD20+ B lymphocytes in the follicles of NLH are definitionally polytypic, as are lesional plasma cells and IgD+ mantle cells. The interfollicular areas are rich in CD3+, CD45RO+ T cells. CD21 staining in NLH highlights the compact nature of the follicular dendritic cell network (Fig. 15.7). A disrupted appearance, particularly if it is associated with a significant *bcl*-2+, *bcl*-6– population of B cells within the follicles, or an increase in the number of interfollicular B cells, should suggest a diagnosis of marginal zone lymphoma (Table 15.5).[32] Cyclin D1 staining will be negative in interfollicular and mantle cells, helping in difficult cases to exclude mantle cell lymphoma (Table 15.6). In contrast to follicular bronchiolitis, NLH forms masses in the lung.[20] A distinction between NLH and lymphoid interstitial pneumonia may be difficult, particularly in small

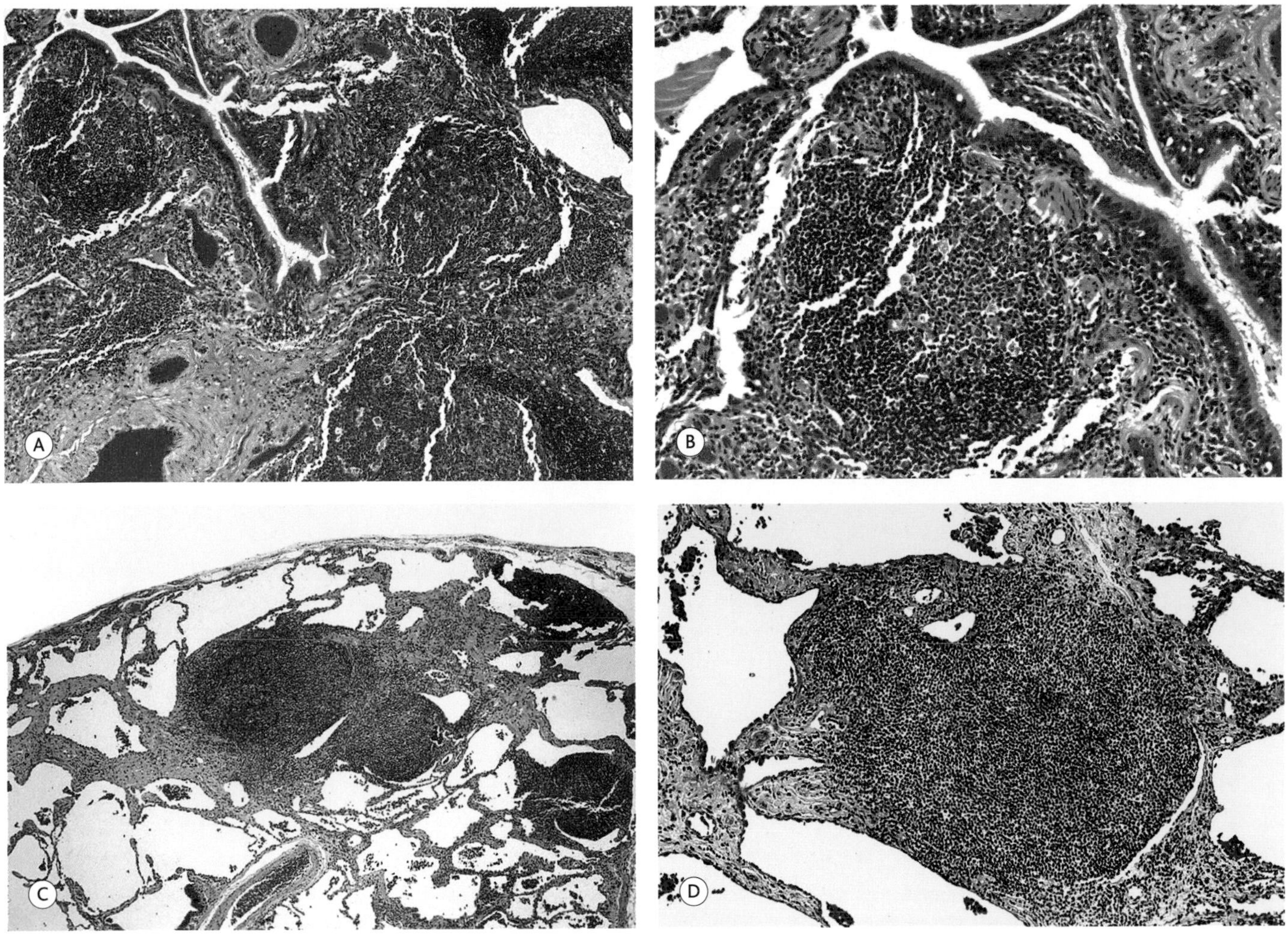

Fig. 15.4 (A–D) Eccentric accumulation of lymphocytes around airways is the principal morphologic finding in follicular bronchiolitis. Note the abrupt termination and discrete nature of the proliferation, which does not track along alveolar septa as lymphoid interstitial pneumonitis often does.

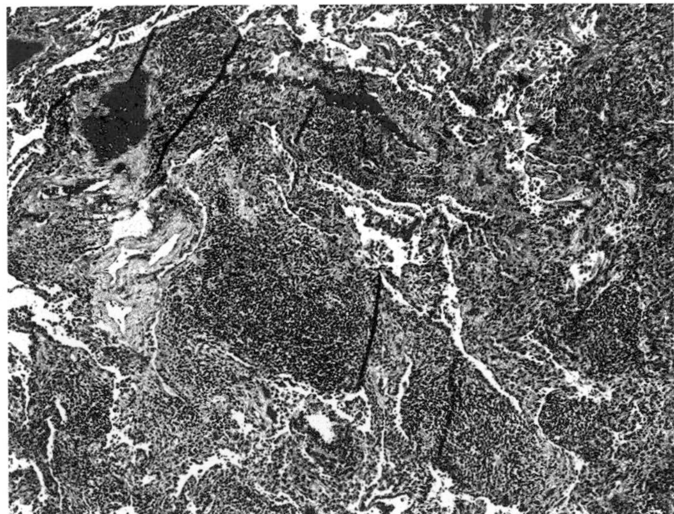

Fig. 15.5 Nodular lymphoid hyperplasia is a more discrete mass-forming lymphoid proliferation that is denser than the focal accumulations of benign mucosa-associated lymphoid tissue illustrated in Fig. 15.1. It retains a germinal center–mantle–paracortex structure.

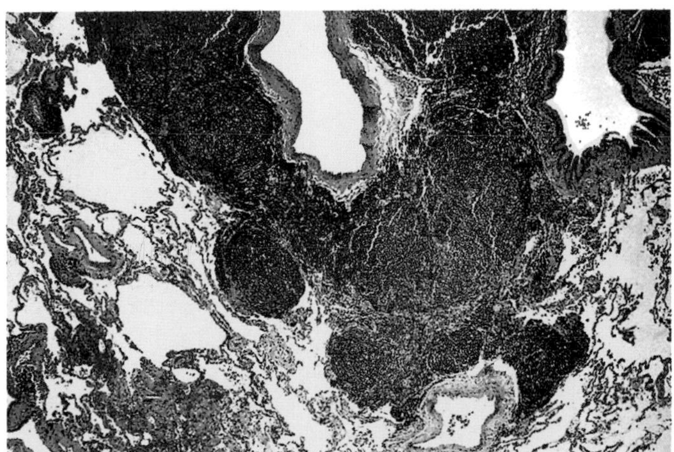

Fig. 15.6 Sharp circumscription is a common feature of nodular lymphoid hyperplasia (NLH), which is often present more proximally than follicular bronchiolitis. NLH also does not extend along alveolar septa.

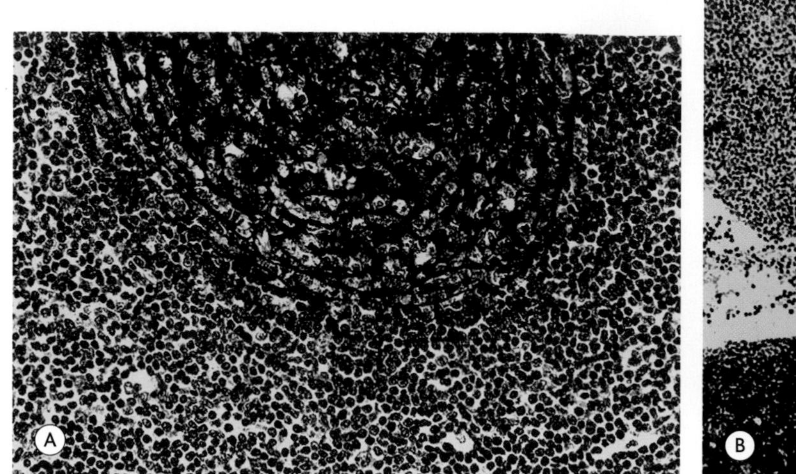

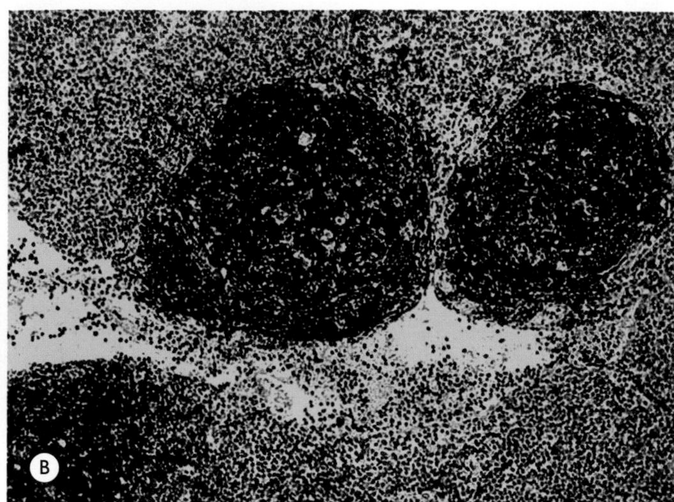

Fig. 15.7 (A) CD21 immunostaining accentuates the presence of well-circumscribed arrays of follicular dendritic cells in nodular lymphoid hyperplasia (NLH), and the processes of those cells terminate sharply at the interface between the mantle and the interfollicular regions. A moth-eaten or disrupted appearance would raise the possibility of follicular colonization, a process that is characteristic of marginal zone lymphoma. (B) The nodules of NLH are composed primarily of CD20+ B cells, with the rest of the lymphoid component, including interstitial elements, being constituted by CD3+ T cells.

Table 15.5 Differential diagnosis of marginal zone lymphoma from benign lymphoid proliferations in the lung

	Nodular lymphoid hyperplasia	Lymphoid interstitial pneumonia	Marginal zone lymphoma
Clinical features	Adults > children ± altered immune state	Common in children, association with immunodeficiency	Adults ≫ children, association with immunodeficiency
Location of infiltrates	Peribronchiolar, septal, patchy, may be multifocal	Interstitial, patchy, may be multifocal	Mass-like or patternless, typically unifocal
Architecture	Diffuse effacement of lung parenchymal structures Germinal centers often present but colonization is not	Expansion of tissue planes by lymphoid infiltrate Germinal centers may be present but colonization is not	Complete effacement of normal lung parenchyma. Germinal centers often present, and often disrupted by infiltrate of monocytoid or centrocytoid cells ("colonization")
Cellular composition	Polymorphous array of lymphocytes, plasma cells No Dutcher bodies	Polymorphous array of lymphocytes, plasma cells No Dutcher bodies	Germinal centers are surrounded by broad marginal zone with variable proportions of centrocytoid, Monocytoid, or plasmacytoid cells. ± Dutcher bodies within lymphoplasmacytoid cells
Immunophenotype	Polytpic pattern of light-chain expression. CD5, 10, 23 negative CD21 accentuates presence of well-defined germinal centers No lymphoepithelial lesions on cytokeratin stain	Polytypic pattern of light-chain expression. CD5, CD10, CD23 negative CD21 may accentuate well-defined germinal centers No lymphoepithelial lesions on cytokeratin stain	Monotypic light-chain pattern CD5, CD10, CD23 negative CD21 identifies disrupted FDC network due to influx of bcl2+, bcl6(-) cells (colonization) Lymphoepithelial lesions present and easy to identify even on routine stains

Table 15.6 Morphologic and phenotypic differences amongst B-cell lymphomas

Disease	Phenotype CD19	CD20	CD5	CD10	CD23	CD43	sIg	cIg	CD138	CD21	TdT	*bcl*-6	cyclin D1	CD15	CD30	PAX5	D138
B-LBL	+	–	–	±	–	–	–	±	–	–	+	–	–	–	–	+	–
B-SLL	+	+	+	–	+	±	dim	–	–	–	–	–	–	–	–	+	–
MCL	+	+	+	–	–	±	int	–	–	–	–	–	+	–	–	+	–
FCCL	+	+	–	+	–	–	brt	–	–	FDC	–	+	–	–	–	+	–
BL	+	+	–	+	–	–	brt	–	–	–	–	+	–	–	–	+	–
MaZL	+	+	–	–	–	–	int	±	–	FDC	–	–	–	–	–	+	–
B-LCL																	
typical	+	+	±	±	–	±	+	±	–	–	–	+	–	–	±	+	–
TCRBCL	+	+	NS	±	–	NS	+	±	–	–	–	±	–	–	±	+	–
IVL	+	+	±	–	–	NS	+	±	–	–	–	NS	–	–	±	+	–
PCY	–	–	–	–	–	–	–	+	+	–	–	–	–	–	±	–	+

B-LBL = lymphoblastic lymphoma
B-SLL = small lymphocytic lymphoma
MCL = mantle cell lymphoma
FCCL = follicle center cell lymphoma
BL = Burkitt's lymphoma
dim = dimly positive
MaZL = marginal zone lymphoma
B-LCL = large cell lymphoma
TCRBCL = T-cell-rich B-cell lymphoma
IVL = intravascular lymphoma
PCY = plasmacytoma
int = intermediate intensity positive
+ = lesional cells are almost always positive
– = lesional cells are almost always negative
± = lesional cells positive in some cases
FDC = only follicular dendritic cells positive
NS = not studied
brt = bright intensity positive

biopsies, although the latter of those conditions has a primary interstitial localization with extensive infiltration of alveolar walls, whereas the former does not.

Diffuse lymphoid hyperplasia – lymphoid interstitial pneumonia

As part of the spectrum of pulmonary lymphoid hyperplasia, lymphoid interstitial pneumonia (LIP) affects both children and adults, and it is diagnosed with increased frequency in patients with altered immune states. These include autoimmune diseases, AIDS,[33] collagen vascular disorders, chronic infections with Epstein–Barr virus (EBV) or mycoplasma,[34,35] congenital immunodeficiency states,[36] patients who have undergone bone marrow transplantation (BMT), and familial dysimmunity.[37–40] In some series, females are disproportionately affected.[18] Patients present with cough and shortness of breath, and radiologic studies usually disclose bilateral basilar patchy opacities or reticulonodular infiltrates.[22,41,42] A subset of individuals with LIP shows systemic symptoms such as fever and weight loss, and many will have polyclonal hypergammaglobulinemia.

In contrast to FB and NLH, the infiltrates of LIP have a dominant interstitial pattern of distribution (Fig. 15.8); however, the constituent cellular components are otherwise similar.[9,18,43,44] Small, cytologically bland lymphocytes and intermingled plasma cells distend the alveolar walls, with accentuation along bronchovascular bundles and lobular septae (Figs 15.9–15.11). Aggregates of histiocytes or poorly formed granulomas may be present as well,[45] but neutrophils and eosinophils are scarce. Germinal centers, although they may be present, are generally few in number.[18,45] An intraepithelial component that mimicks the lymphoepithelial lesions of MALT lymphomas has been described in LIP. Coalescence of cellular infiltrates in and around the microvasculature has also been noted in LIP, but true *angiodestruction* is not part of this condition.[18,45]

The cellular infiltrate that distends the alveolar walls in LIP is composed primarily of T cells, with relatively few intermingled B lymphocytes.[45] Both the plasma cells and the small lymphocytes exhibit a polytypic pattern of cytoplasmic and surface light-chain immunoglobulin expression. Residual germinal centers, when they are present, show a compact array of CD21+ follicular dendritic cells and are rich in CD20+, *bcl*-2–, *bcl*-6+ centrocytes. These findings contrast to the *bcl*-2+, *bcl*-6– B cells that are associated with follicular colonization by marginal zone lymphoma. AIDS-related lesions often demonstrate immunoreactivity for the p21 protein of human immunodeficiency virus (Fig. 15.12).

Lung infiltrates that are secondary to acute EBV-related infectious mononucleosis may resemble LIP, but the latter disorder seldom has a lymphangitic pattern, and never shows the population of activated immunoblasts that typifies mononucleosis.[35] The presence of occasional

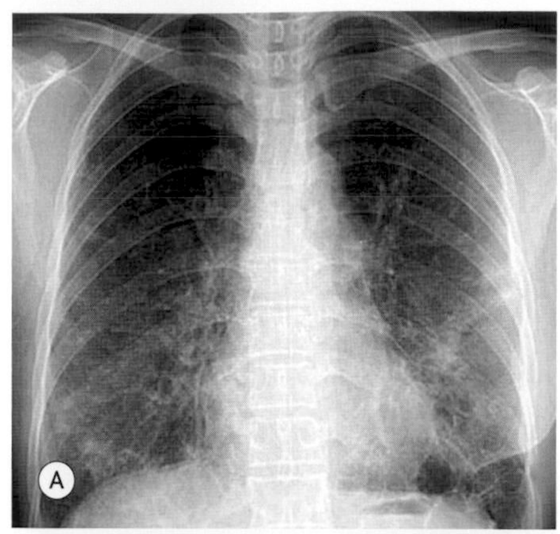

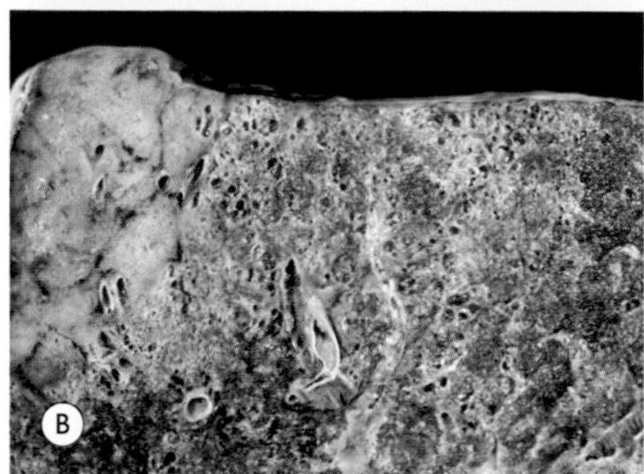

Fig. 15.8 Lymphoid interstitial pneumonia is a diffuse interstitial process, as manifested radiographically (A) and on gross examination of the disease at autopsy (B).

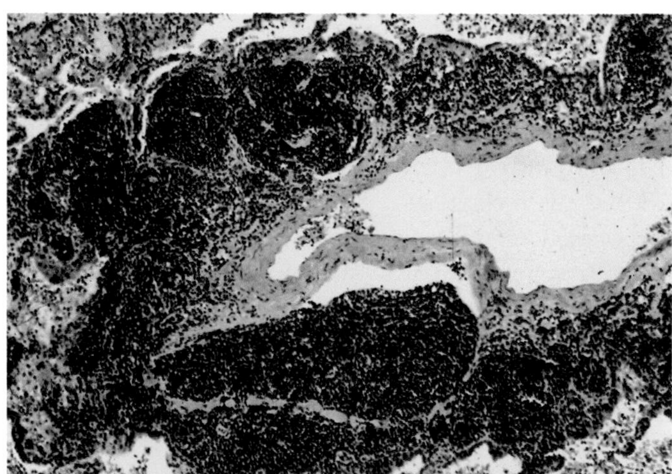

Fig. 15.9 Lymphoid interstitial pneumonia lacks the mass-forming qualities of nodular lymphoid hyperplasia as well as the nodularity of the latter condition.

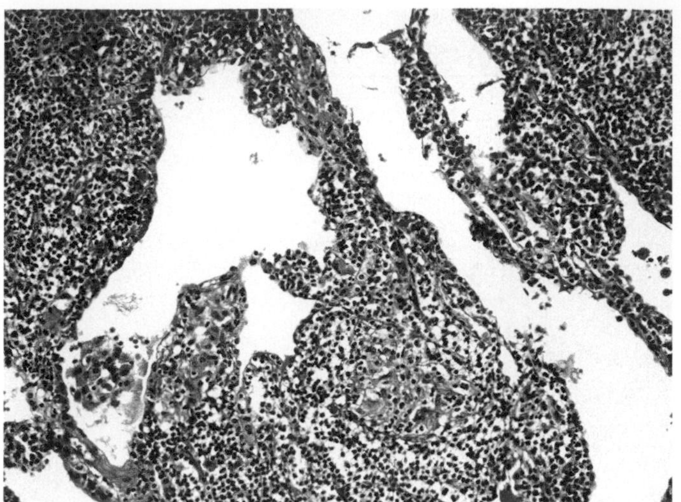

Fig. 15.10 Lymphoid interstitial pneumonia expands interalveolar septa and focally forms microaggregates of constituent lymphocytes.

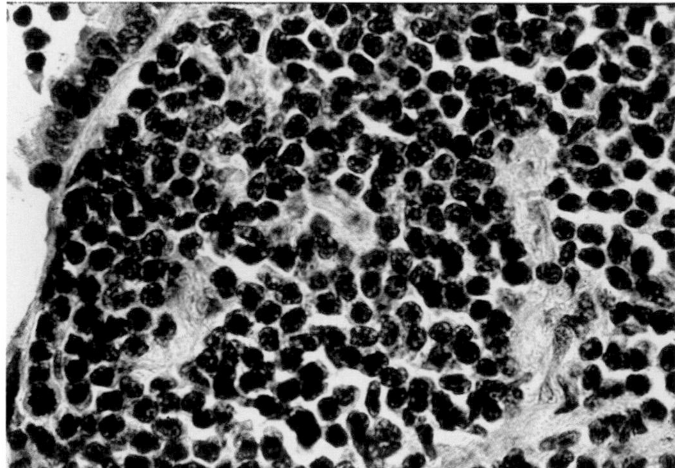

Fig. 15.11 Lymphoid interstitial pneumonia demonstrates a composition by morphologically mature lymphocytes. Most are CD3-positive T cells, a helpful feature in distinguishing it from marginal zone lymphoma.

germinal centers and focal intraepithelial accumulations of lymphocytes may prompt consideration of a marginal zone MALT lymphoma, but the bilateral and interstitial (rather than unifocal and mass-forming) nature of LIP, as well as the lack of a dominant and monotypic B-cell population in interfollicular areas, provides a strong objective means of excluding such neoplasms.[46] Fibrosis, intra-alveolar accumulations of foamy macrophages, foci of bronchiolitis obliterans, and a peribronchiolar and non-interstitial accentuation of the infiltrate suggest extrinsic allergic alveolitis ("hypersensitivity pneumonitis"). Because of the interstitial distribution, dominant T-cell constituency, and cytologic heterogeneity of LIP, distinction from a pulmonary presentation of systemic lymphomas is seldom an issue. In difficult cases, or when diagnostic material is limited, immunohistochemical evaluation will usually permit a definite diagnosis to be made (see Table 15.6).

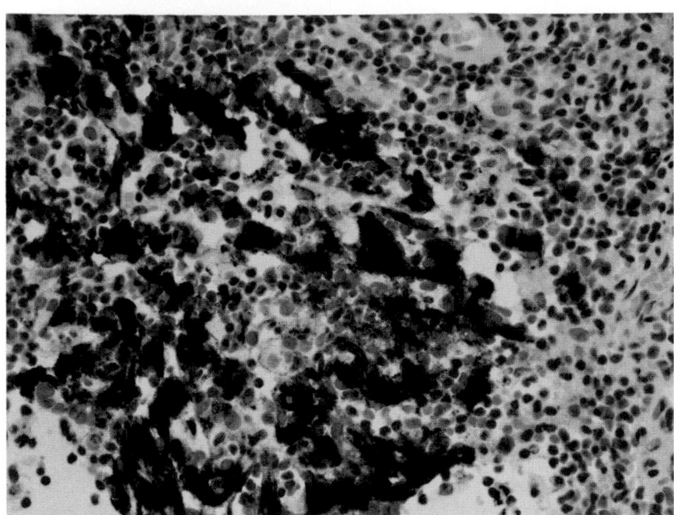

Fig. 15.12 Examples of lymphoid interstitial pneumonia that occur in the context of the acquired immunodeficiency syndrome usually demonstrate immunoreactivity for the p21 protein of human immunodeficiency virus.

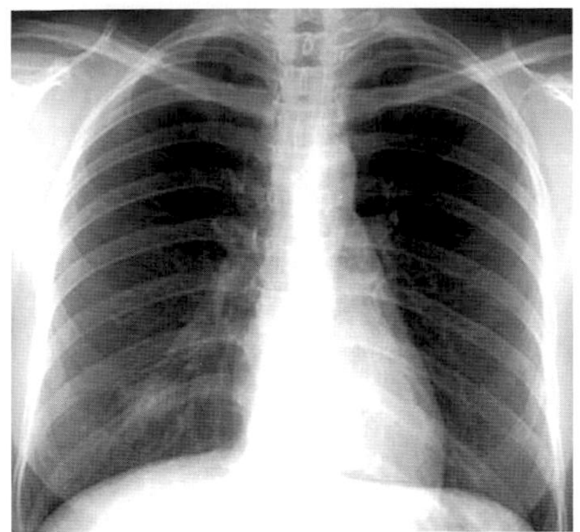

Fig. 15.13 This chest radiograph of a patient with marginal zone lymphoma shows a nodule in the mid-right lung field.

The prognosis for patients with LIP is variable, ranging from complete resolution to death caused by superimposed infection or renal failure. Comorbid conditions also contribute to the high mortality that has been associated with this disease.[47] A subset of LIP cases progresses to end-stage pulmonary fibrosis with "honey-comb" change. Hence, in those instances, the prognosis is actually worse than it is for a neoplastic simulator of LIP: namely, marginal zone lymphoma. The reportedly increased risk of developing lymphoma in LIP likely relates, at least in part, to the fact that many cases previously interpreted as LIP were in fact lymphomas ab initio.

Primary pulmonary lymphoma

The lung is a relatively common site in which extranodal lymphomas arise, following the gastrointestinal tract, skin, and nervous system in incidence.[48] Regardless of the histologic type of pulmonary lymphoma, adults are most commonly affected; indeed, children rarely develop this disease.[49–51] The designation of primary pulmonary lymphoma (PPL) is restricted to denovo lymphomas that present with limited disease in the lungs. Other than hilar node involvement, no evidence of extrapulmonary disease should be evident on staging procedures that are done at presentation or after a period of observation. Various intervals of clinical surveillance have been proposed before considering a diagnosis of pulmonary lymphoma.[27,52,53] Strictly defined, it is my opinion that patients with PPL should have little disease-related morbidity and essentially no disease-related mortality[54,55] at 6 months after initial detection.

Lymphomas of B-cell lineage

Primary pulmonary marginal zone lymphoma

Although it was not recognized as a distinct type of NHL until the early 1990s, marginal zone lymphoma (MaZL) of MALT type is now felt to be the commonest type of PPL. Indeed, it accounts for most examples of so-called "MALToma" of the lung, which represents a heterogeneous aggregation of lesions. Unlike MaZL of the stomach, thyroid, and salivary glands, however, it has an inconstant association with infectious agents or specific autoimmune conditions.[31,56,57] Recent studies have shown that 40% of cases contain a t(11;18) chromosomal translocation that involves API2 and MALT1, contrasting to other non-gastric MALT-type lymphomas which rarely harbor this aberration and arise much more often in the setting of autoimmunity. Although some patients with MaZL are entirely asymptomatic, many present with a cough, fever,[58] or unexplained weight loss.[48] Radiologic studies most commonly disclose the presence of solitary or multiple[59] discrete nodules[17,50,60,61] (Figs 15.13 and 15.14). Results of serum protein electrophoresis are abnormal in up to 30% of patients, and staging reveals extrathoracic disease in one-third of patients. The disease is almost entirely restricted to adults, although rare examples of pulmonary MaZL have indeed been described in children.[46]

Following the model of benign MALT, MaZL is composed of cells that morphologically and immuno-phenotypically resemble the mature B cells that form the outer rim of the malpighian corpuscles of the spleen, and

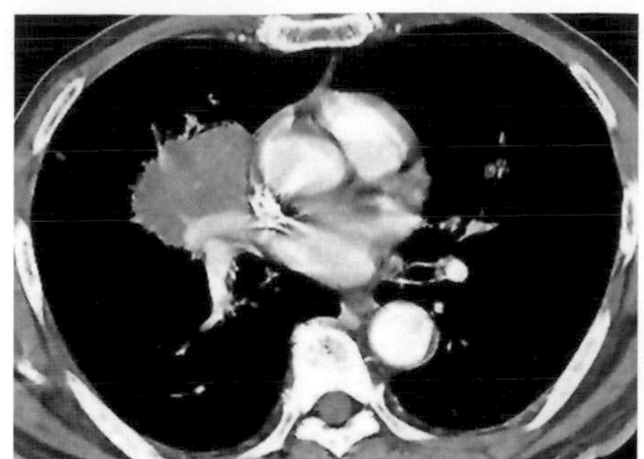

Fig. 15.14 A computed tomogram in a case of marginal zone pulmonary lymphoma shows a nodular mass in the right parahilar lung field.

their counterparts in Peyer's patches of the terminal ileum.[8,9,48,62,63] On scanning microscopy, MaZL may have a nodular or a diffuse pattern, and, at its periphery, the lesion may extend along intact alveolar walls in a discontinuous fashion (Fig. 15.15). Occasionally, a "beaded" image is noted. Nodularity is usually inconspicuous but, when present, it corresponds to the presence of residual benign germinal centers that have been infiltrated ("colonized") by tumor cells to various degrees.[49] The bulk of the neoplastic proliferation in MaZL is present between the nodules. It is composed of a mixture of small, resting lymphocytes; monocytoid cells with oval or reniform nuclei, condensed chromatin, and moderate quantities of cytoplasm; and plasmacytoid forms[66,67] (Fig. 15.16).

Because of their ontogenic relationship to lymphocytes that "home" to mucosal surfaces, tumor cells in MaZL

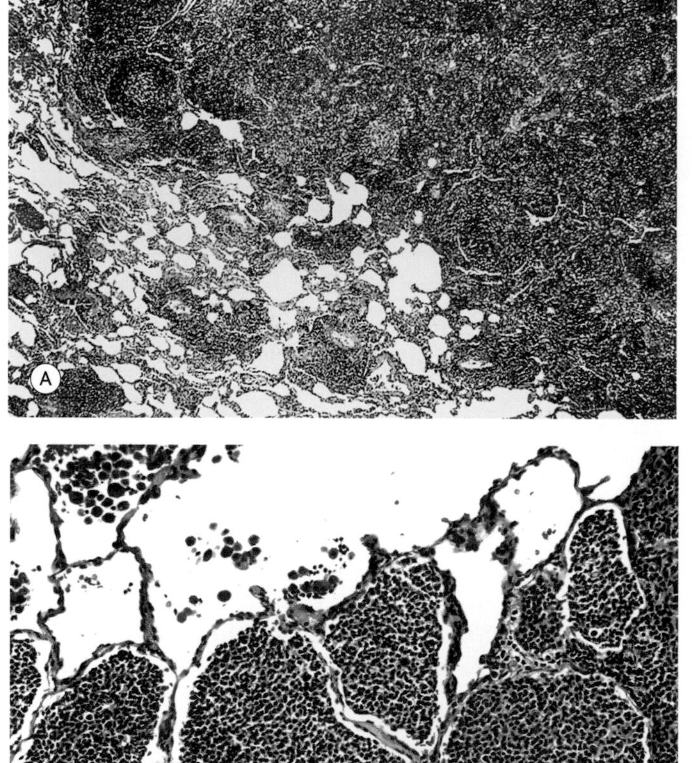

Fig. 15.15 (A) Marginal zone lymphoma distorts the lung parenchyma as a patchy or mass-forming process. (B) At its periphery it involves alveolar spaces; one may also see small nodular accumulations of lymphoid cells around bronchovascular bundles, potentially yielding a beaded motif if extensive enough.

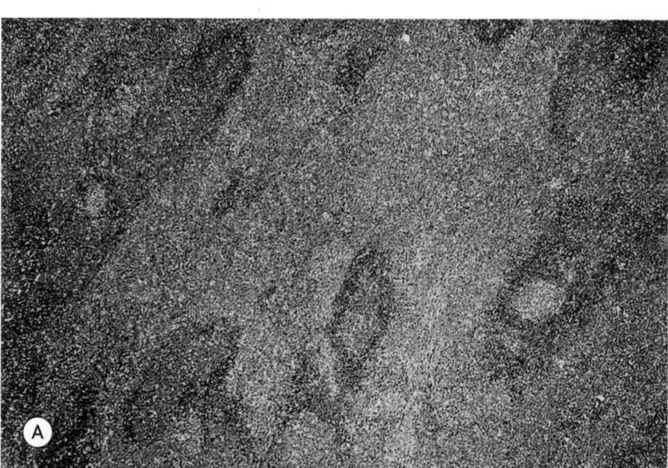

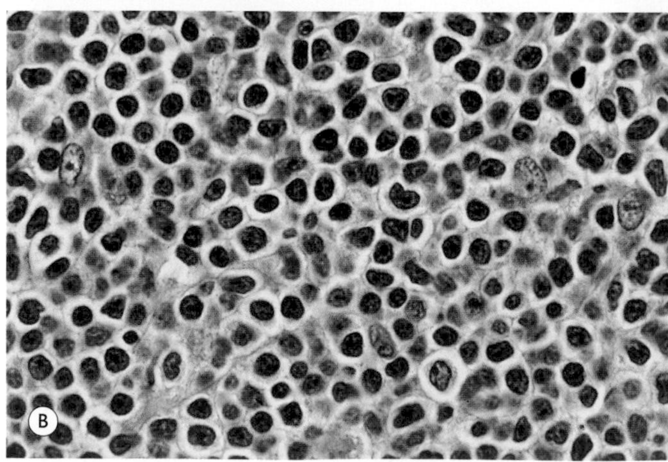

Fig. 15.16 Both within and between follicular aggregates, the lymphocytes in marginal zone lymphoma are B cells. The pale staining of the monocytoid and plasmacytoid interfollicular cells in this tumor type (A) is striking, and serves as a clue to the diagnosis. (B) Marginal zone lymphomas often have a monocytoid appearance, with the lesional cells having reniform or indented nuclei and moderate amounts of cytoplasm.

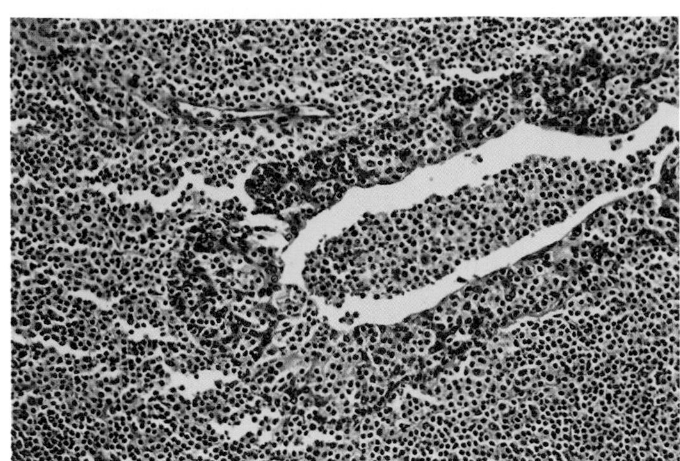

Fig. 15.17 The cells of marginal zone lymphoma commonly surround and permeate tubular airways, such that the bronchiolar epithelium is destroyed – the so-called "lymphoepithelial lesion."

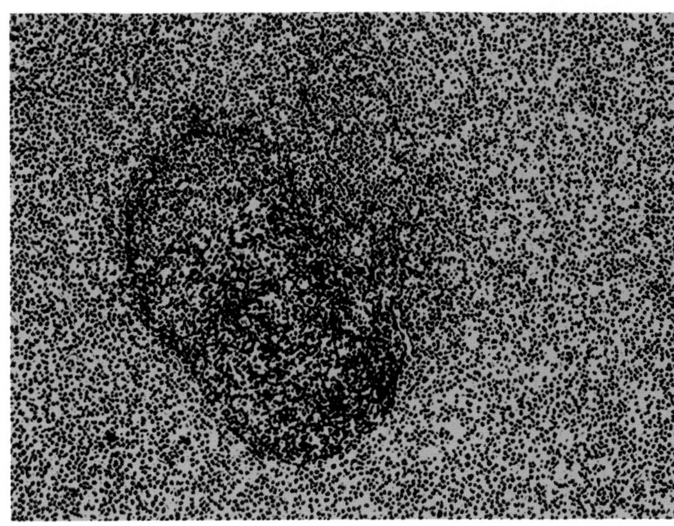

Fig. 15.18 Follicular colonization by bcl-2+, bcl-6– B cells occurs in extranodal marginal zone lymphomas. This distends and disrupts the normally circumscribed follicular dendritic cell meshwork (CD21 stain, avidin–biotin complex method).

have a tendency to form destructive "lymphoepithelial lesions" (Fig. 15.17); these feature the colonization of epithelial structures by neoplastic lymphoid cells, with degenerative changes in the epithelium. They are a characteristic feature of this disease, although not independently diagnostic of neoplasia.[8,9] In some cases, a monocytoid morphologic image is dominant, but in others the tumor cells most closely resemble centrocytes in germinal centers. Transbronchial biopsies should be approached with caution, because plasmacytoid differentiation in MaZL may be so striking superficially that a diagnosis of plasmacytoma is suggested. With fuller representation of the lesion, as in a wedge biopsy specimen, a concomitant lymphoid component is often identified that permits accurate classification. Occasional cases may contain amyloid deposits or intracytoplasmic crystalline immunoglobulin.[7,63,65,66]

The lesional cells of MaZL are CD19+ and CD20+, but they do not coexpress CD5, CD10, CD23, terminal deoxynucleotidyltransferase (TdT), cyclin-D1, or *bcl*-6. In small biopsies, a keratin immunostain may help to identify lymphoepithelial lesions, and the combination of CD21, *bcl*-2, and *bcl*-6 stains will highlight germinal centers that are colonized and overrun by tumor cells.[65] In MaZL, these structures are *bcl*-2+, *bcl*-6– and have a disrupted network of follicular dendritic cells[67,68] (Fig. 15.18). The protein expression of *bcl*-10 has been shown to correlate with the presence of molecular evidence of the t(11;18) (API2/MALT1) translocation, and a positive result for that marker in paraffin-section immunohistochemistry can be a helpful adjunct.[69]

MaZL resembles pulmonary NLH, but the latter condition has a polymorphous population of lymphoid cells in interfollicular areas; benign, "uncolonized" germinal centers with a *bcl*-2–, *bcl*-6+ phenotype; and T-cell predominance in interfollicular areas (see Table 15.5), unlike MaZL. Small biopsies of MaZL may show some degree of morphologic overlap with LIP, but MaZL tends to efface normal structures and does not manifest the predominant interstitial localization that is associated with LIP. A distinction of MaZL from other lymphomas rests on immunophenotyping (see Tables 15.3 and 15.6), although colonization of germinal centers and heterogeneity of the lesional infiltrate are two features that favor MaZL.

Primary pulmonary large cell lymphoma with B-cell differentiation

Large cell lymphoma of B-cell type (B-LCL) is the second most common type of PPL (17,49), and it most commonly affects adults in the sixth and seventh decades of life (Fig. 15.19). Patients present with cough or dyspnea, but hemoptysis is rare. Most intrapulmonary lesions of B-LCL are solitary, solid, and off-white in color on gross examination, and they have discrete borders with the adjacent normal lung parenchyma (Fig. 15.20). A subset of B-LCL cases arises by transformation of preexisting or concurrent low-grade NHLs such as MaZL, small lymphocytic lymphoma, and follicular lymphoma. Rapidly proliferating tumors may exhibit central cavitation on computed tomographic (CT) images, corresponding to the presence of necrosis.

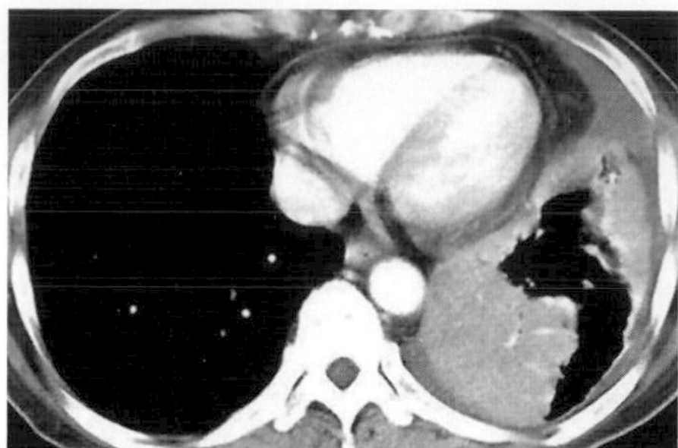

Fig. 15.19 This computed tomogram of the thorax demonstrates a large cavitating mass in the left lung field, representing a large cell lymphoma with B-cell differentiation.

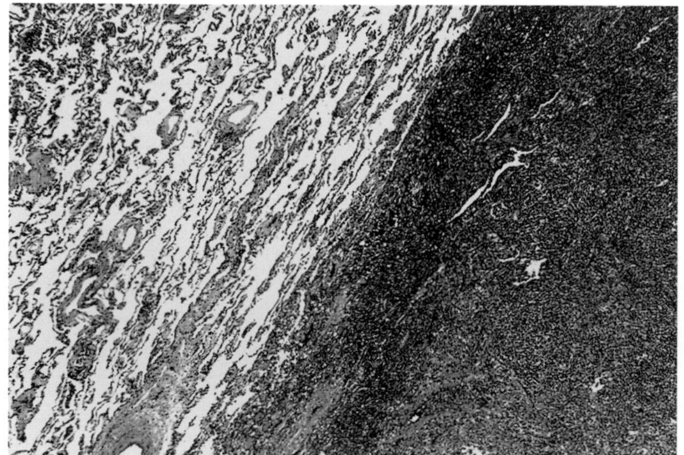

Fig. 15.20 A large B-cell lymphoma almost invariably has a sharp interface with the normal lung.

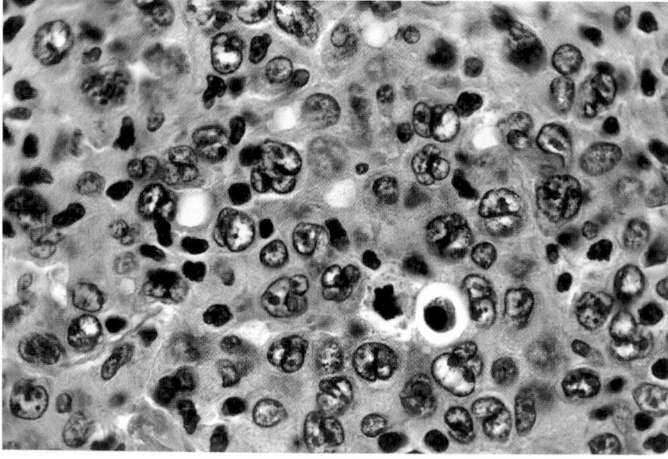

Fig. 15.21 Polylobated variants of large B-cell lymphoma (B-LCL) have coarse chromatin and highly irregular nuclear shapes. This morphology may also be seen in primary mediastinal B-LCL; hence, correlation with radiologic studies must be undertaken to determine whether the process is confined to the lung or not.

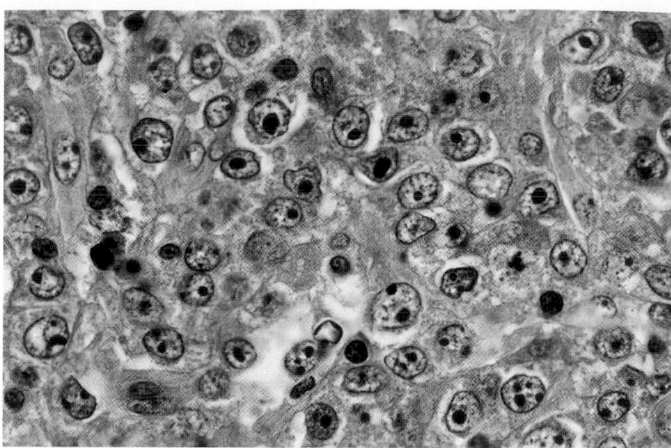

Fig. 15.22 The majority of the cells in the immunoblastic subtype of B-cell lymphoma have solitary centrally placed eosinophilic nucleoli, thick nuclear membranes, and moderate amounts of pale or amphophilic cytoplasm.

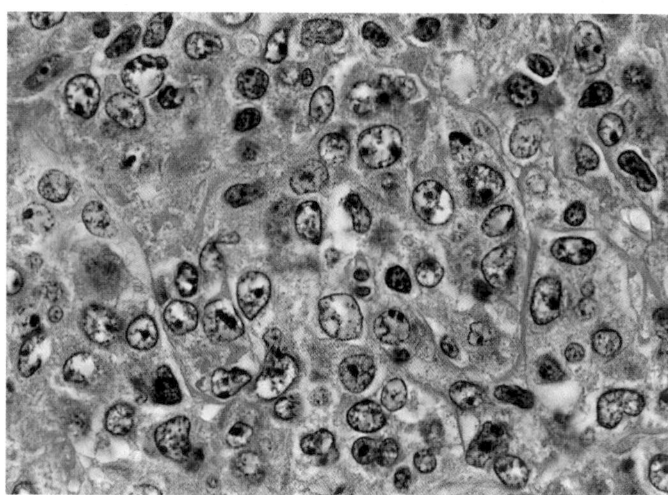

Fig. 15.23 The centroblastic variant of B-cell large cell lymphoma shows irregular nuclear configurations, coarse chromatin, and distinct but not prominent nucleoli. Intermingled centrocytes suggest a low-grade follicular origin.

The neoplastic nature of B-LCL is readily evident from the dominant population of obviously atypical large cells, as well as the destruction of lung parenchyma. The lesional cells are large (measuring 20–30 mm) and they form confluent but dyshesive sheets (Figs 15.21 and 15.22). Cytologic features vary from case to case, but in most instances the tumor cells have coarse chromatin, distinct nucleoli, and abundant amphophilic cytoplasm (Fig. 15.23). Essentially, all examples of B-LCL are CD19+,

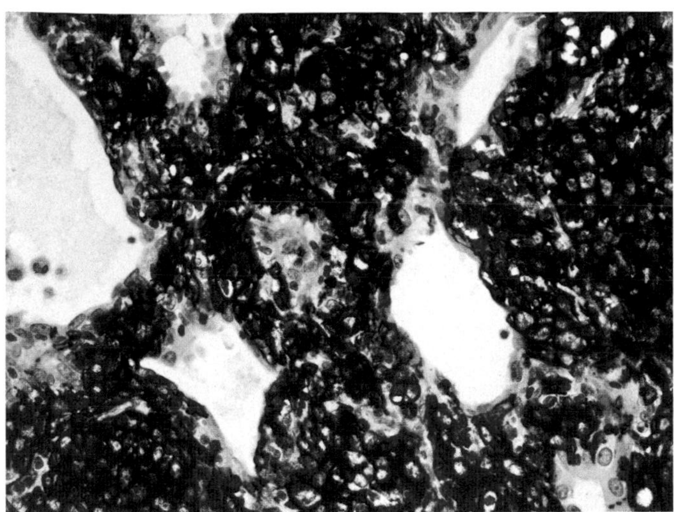

Fig. 15.24 Immunoreactivity for CD20 is strong in this B-cell large cell lymphoma of the lung.

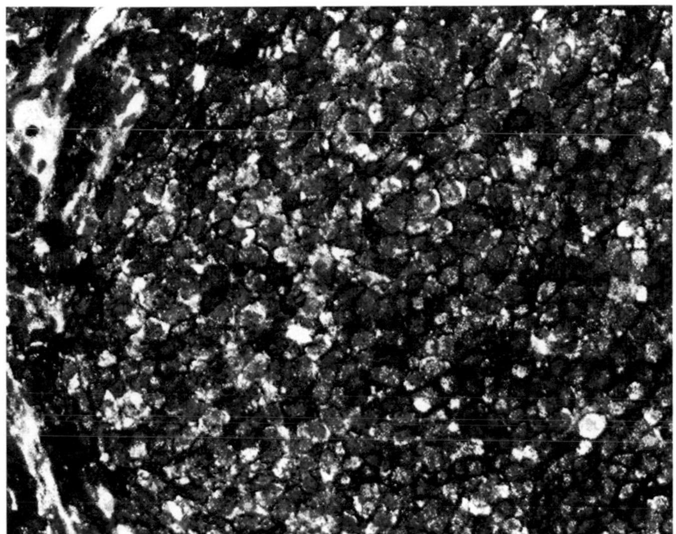

Fig. 15.25 Another example of large cell B-cell pulmonary lymphoma manifests strong immunostaining for CD10, reflecting a follicular nature.

CD20+ (Fig. 15.24), and CD79a+, and those with a follicle center cell origin also express CD10 and *bcl*-6 (Fig. 15.25).[67] Tumor cells in the immunoblastic variant of B-LCL contain vesicular chromatin, thick nuclear membranes, prominent and centrally placed eosinophilic nucleoli, and abundant amphophilic cytoplasm: that morphologic variant may be associated with a worsened prognosis.[67] An intravascular ("angiotropic") variant of B-LCL – also known as "intravascular lymphomatosis" (IL) or "malignant angioendotheliomatosis" – is also recognized in the World Health Organization (WHO) classification of lymphomas and other schema (Figs 15.26 and 15.27).

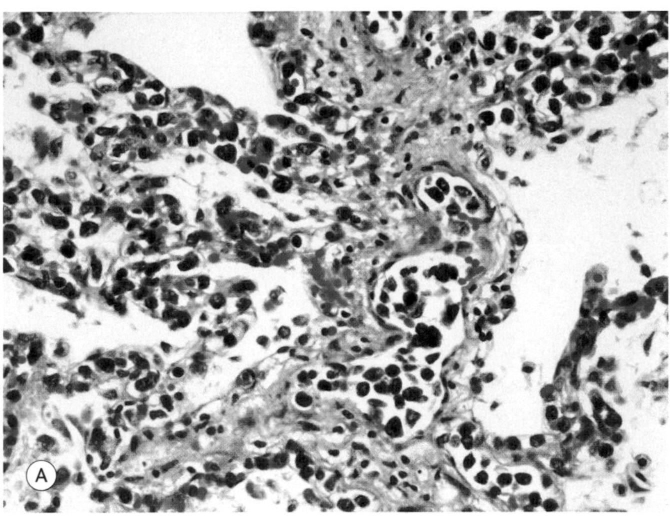

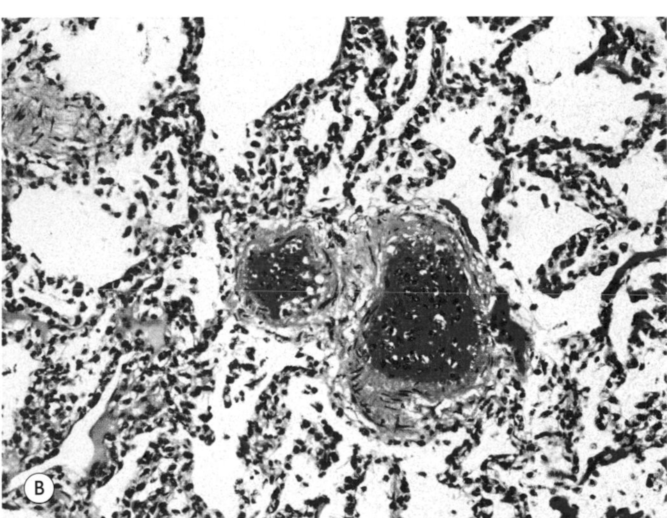

Fig. 15.26 (A,B) On routine stains, intravascular large B-cell lymphoma (IVL) involves the lung in a surreptitious manner within tubular vessels and alveolar septal capillaries.

Although IL may have prominent pulmonary manifestations, that disease is not restricted to the lung and should be regarded as an aggressive, systemic lymphoma from the outset.[70]

Differential diagnostic considerations based on morphologic analysis include primary or metastatic carcinomas, metastatic melanoma, and other epithelioid malignancies. These are generally separable from one another by immunophenotypic analysis, with or without FCM. Some cases of B-LCL may have a high content of reactive T cells or histiocytes (so-called "T-cell-rich large B-cell lymphoma" (TcRBCL) (Fig. 15.28),[71–75] and may be impossible to distinguish from lymphoepithelioma-like carcinomas or Hodgkin's lymphoma without immunostains.

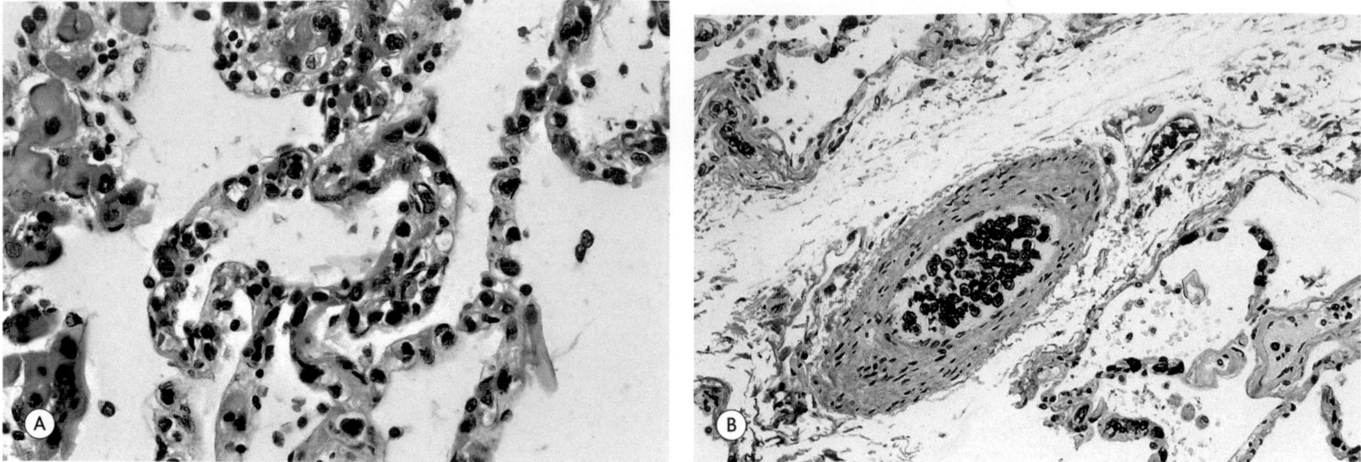

Fig. 15.27 (A) Septal capillary involvement by intravascular lymphomatosis is better seen here. (B) Immunostaining for CD20 demonstrates the presence of the tumor cells.

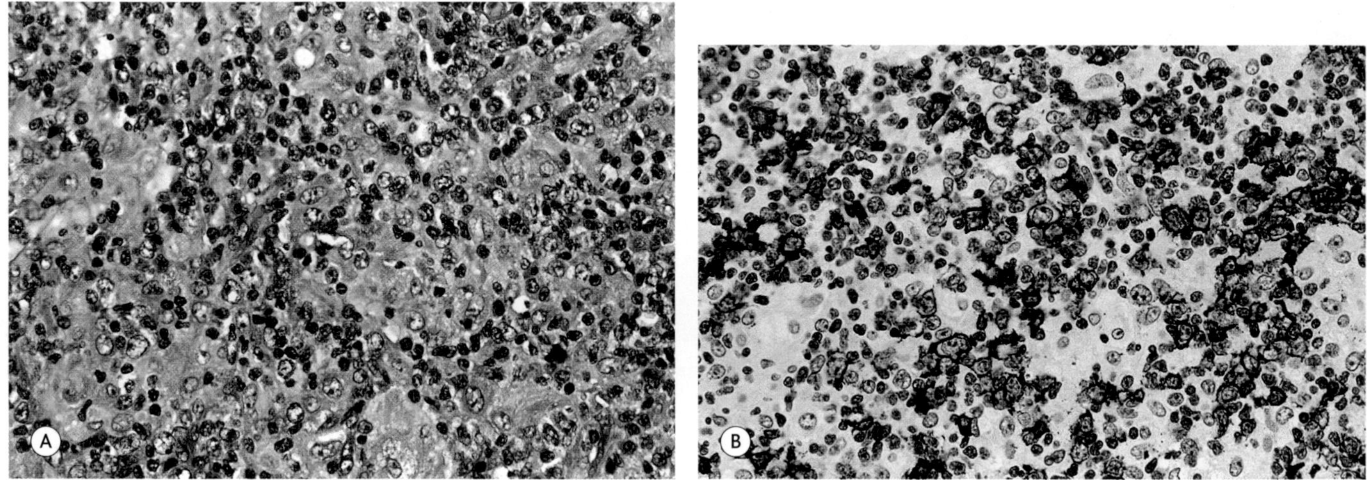

Fig. 15.28 (A) The lesional cells of T-cell and/or histiocyte-rich large B-cell lymphoma are masked by the reactive infiltrate, but (B) the neoplastic cells can be highlighted with immunostains for CD20.

Primary pulmonary plasmacytoma

Extraosseous plasmacytomas are uncommon, and they usually involve the upper aerodigestive tract.[63,64,76] Primary pulmonary plasmacytomas are far less common than secondary involvement of the lungs by a disseminated plasma cell dyscrasia (i.e. multiple myeloma). Intrapulmonary plasma cell tumors exhibit discrete demarcation from the surrounding parenchyma. They are typically brown or dark tan and fleshy on cut section.[77] Amyloid deposition may be evident macroscopically in the form of white nodules or streaks in large tumors.[78,79] Microscopically, plasmacytomas are composed of syncytia of plasma cells with no residual germinal centers and negligible numbers of intermingled small lymphocytes (Figs 15.29–15.31). Occasionally, the lesional cells in plasmacytomas show a pleomorphic or anaplastic appearance (Figs 15.32 and 15.33) and they may imitate the image of bronchogenic carcinoma or metastatic melanoma. Nonetheless, the amphophilic cytoplasm and paranuclear clear zone ("Hof") of plasma cells is usually represented in sufficient numbers of cells to suggest the correct diagnosis.

FCM analysis of plasmacytomas usually yields confusing results. Plasma cells are terminally differentiated B cells, and, as such, they are usually negative for CD45 (leukocyte common antigen), as well as the B-cell markers

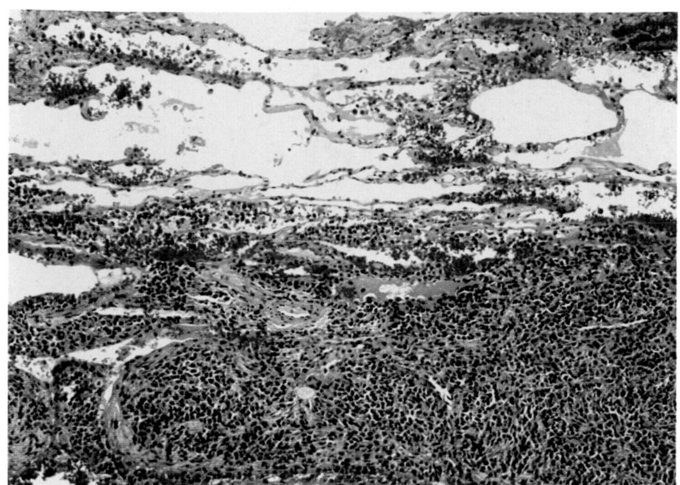

Fig. 15.29 Plasmacytoma of the lung, showing a relatively sharp interface with the surrounding parenchyma.

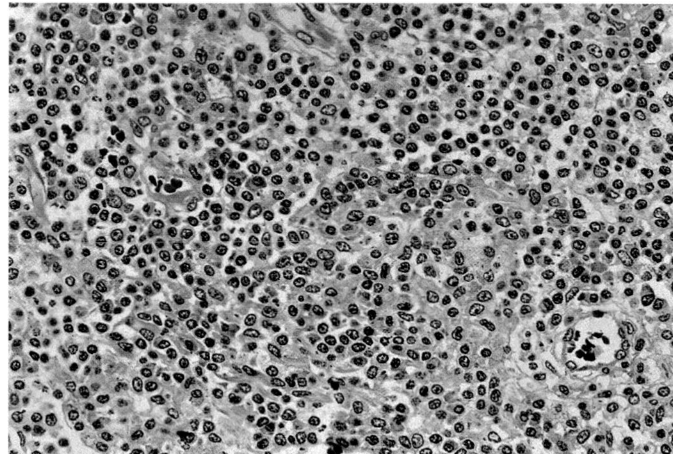

Fig. 15.30 Pulmonary plasmacytoma has the morphology of extra-osseous myeloma, being composed of plasma cells with coarse chromatin, eccentric nuclei, paranuclear "Hofs," and a moderate amount of amphophilic cytoplasm.

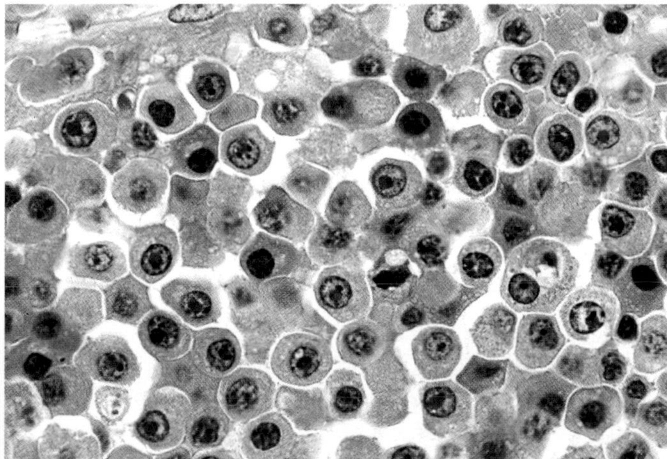

Fig. 15.31 Occasionally, extraosseous plasmacytoma shows prominent nucleoli. This form of the tumor closely resembles so-called "plasmablastic lymphoma," but the latter neoplasm is CD20+, CD45+, and surface immunoglobulin-positive, unlike the cells of plasmacytomas.

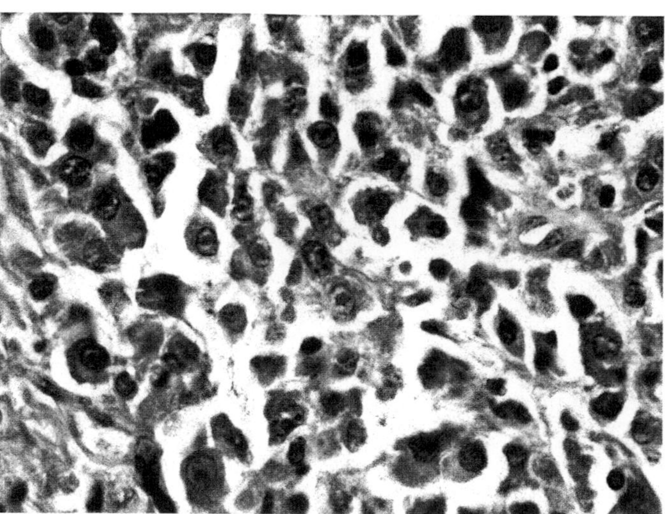

Fig. 15.32 So-called "anaplastic" plasmacytoma shows cellular pleomorphism and the presence of nucleoli.

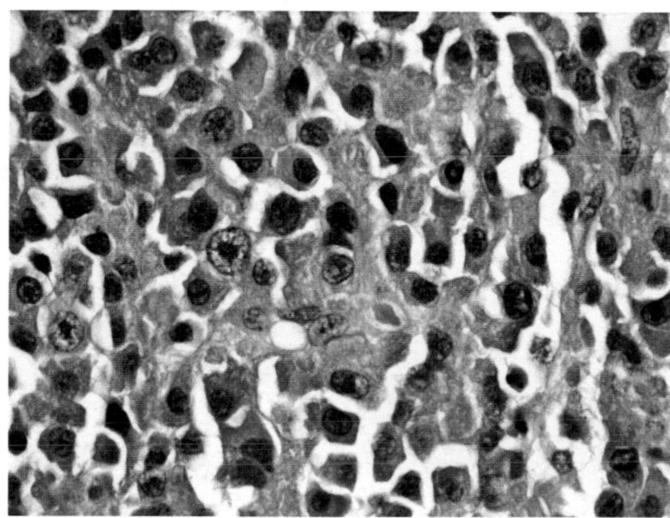

Fig. 15.33 Another example of "anaplastic" pulmonary plasmacytoma is shown in this photograph.

PAX-5, CD19, and CD20. Moreover, they do not have sufficient quantities of surface immunoglobulin to yield positive results by FCM[67] (see Table 15.6). Adjunctive diagnosis rests on the demonstration of CD138 positivity in plasmacytomas (Fig. 15.34) and a restricted pattern of cytoplasmic immunoglobulin expression that can be seen well by paraffin-section immunohistology (Fig. 15.35). Other markers that may be present in neoplastic plasma cells include CD30 and epithelial membrane antigen (EMA), but neither one of those determinants is lineage specific. Moreover, both of them should be interpreted in the context of panel studies that include immunostains for keratin, S100 protein, and other lineage-related markers.

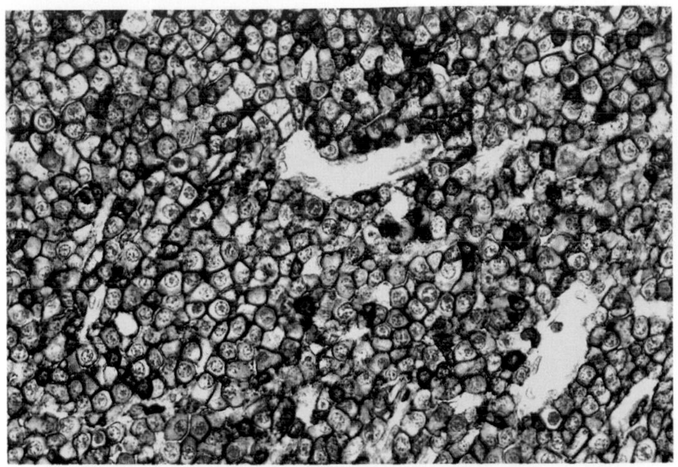

Fig. 15.34 Both benign and neoplastic plasma cells are positive for CD138 (syndecan-1), as depicted here, whereas most lymphomas are not.

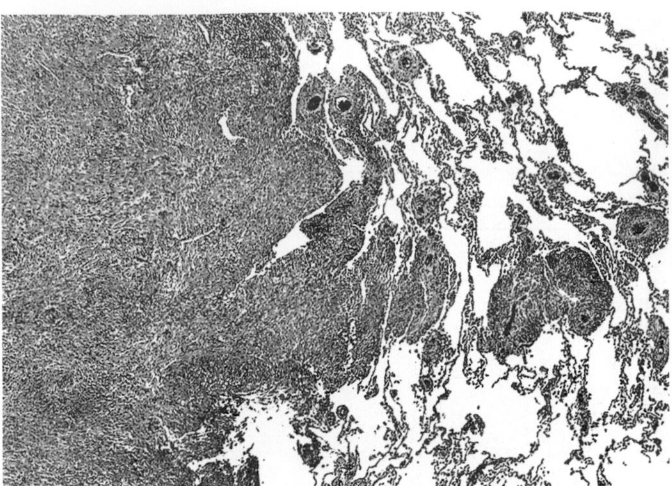

Fig. 15.36 Amyloid deposition, as shown here, is an uncommon intrapulmonary manifestion of myeloma/plasmacytoma.

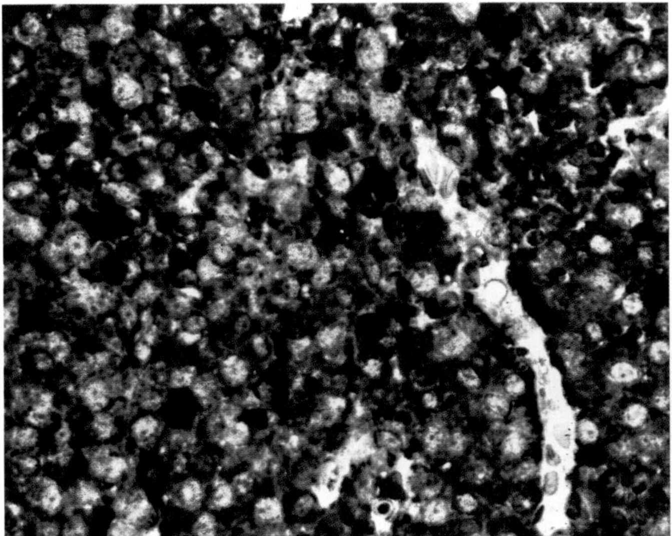

Fig. 15.35 Monotypic immunostaining for kappa (κ) light-chain immunoglobulin is seen in the cytoplasm of tumor cells in this pulmonary plasmacytoma. There was no reactivity for lambda (λ) light-chain protein.

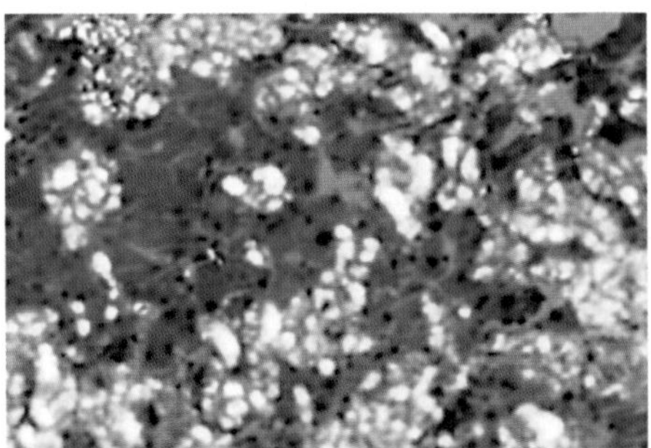

Fig. 15.37 The nature of amyloid can be confirmed by observation of bright green birefringence on polarization microscopy, after Congo red staining.

When more than 20–30% of a plasmacytic proliferation is composed of small lymphocytes, consideration should be given to alternative diagnoses of small lymphocytic lymphoma (SLL), lymphoplasmacytic lymphoma (LPL), or primary pulmonary MaZL.[66,69] All of those proliferations have a CD45+, CD20+, surface immunoglobulin+ immunoprofile, whereas plasmacytomas are negative for those markers (see Table 15.6). Additional findings that favor MaZL include colonized germinal centers and a polymorphous array of monocytoid, centrocytoid, and plasmacytoid cells.[65] If residual germinal centers are detected in the setting of extreme plasmacytosis, the possibility of MaZL is again raised and the plasma cell variant of Castleman's disease is another consideration.[80] Because it is impossible to distinguish between solitary primary intrapulmonary plasmacytoma and pulmonary involvement by a systemic plasma cell dyscrasia (multiple myeloma), all patients with biopsy-proven plasmacytomas in the lungs should be fully evaluated with serum and urine protein electrophoresis, skeletal radiographic surveys, and bone marrow biopsies.

Patients with known plasma cell dyscrasias may develop nodular deposits of amyloid in the lung parenchyma.[79] These may be solitary or multiple, but patients with pulmonary amyloidomas are usually asymptomatic. Microscopically, the stromal material in such lesions is homogenously eosinophilic and non-fibrillary, and it may contain intermingled lymphocytes, plasma cells, and transitional lymphoplasmacytoid forms (Fig. 15.36); polarization microscopy after staining with the Congo red method yields "apple-green" birefringence (Fig. 15.37). It is important to note that accumulations of

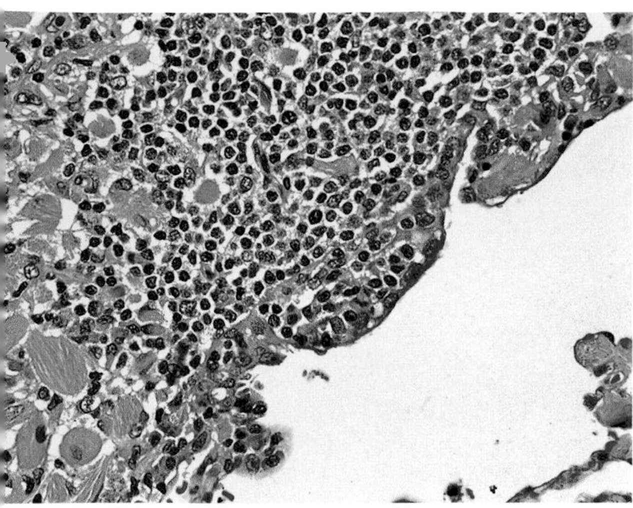

15.38 Crystal-storing histiocytosis is a very rare manifestion of unoglobulin deposition in the lung. The proliferation shows a ete interface with normal lung parenchyma.

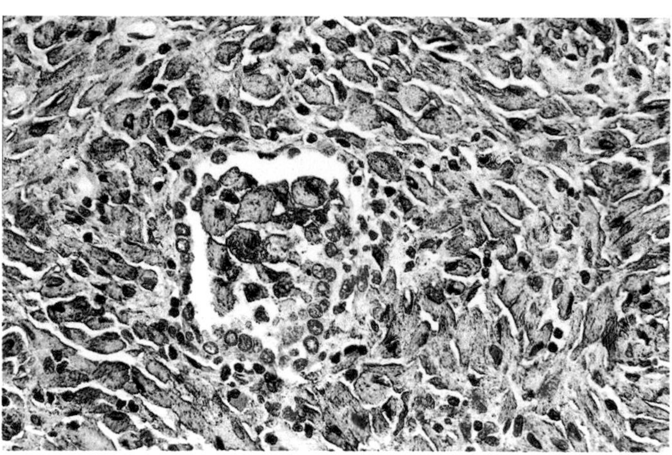

Fig. 15.40 The constituent histiocytes in crystal-storing histiocytosis demonstrate monotypic immunostaining for light-chain immunoglobulin. This case shows strong labeling for lambda light-chain protein immunoglobulin. Immunostains for myogenic markers were negative.

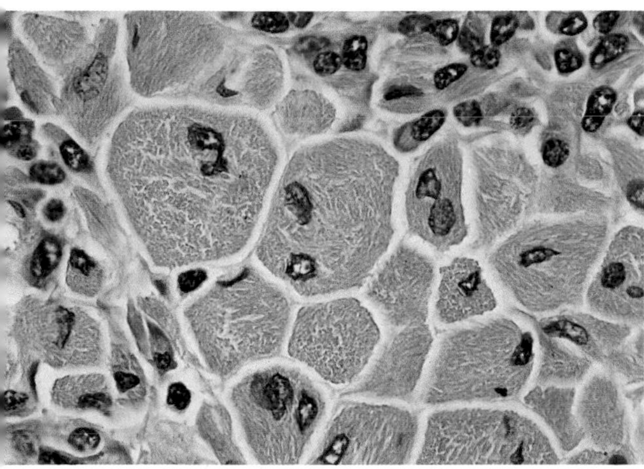

15.39 Crystal-storing histiocytosis, complicating a case of marginal lymphoma with extensive plasmacytic differentiation. The unoglobulin-bearing histiocytes are reminiscent of the cells found dult-type rhabdomyomas of soft tissue.

yloid in the lung may also be seen in association with ZL and lymphoplasmacytoid lymphoma, as well as in ents with no evidence of neoplasia whatsoever.[79]

Crystal-storing histiocytosis (CSH) is another rare distinctive form of monotypic immunoglobulin osition that histologically imitates the image of adult odomyoma. Bones, spleen, lymph nodes, stomach, mus, sinonasal mucosa, and the lungs have all been ed as sites of infiltration in CSH, by mass-forming liferations of large polygonal histiocytes. These contain e crystalloids that label with the periodic acid–Schiff phosphotungstic acid–hematoxylin techniques (Figs 15.38 and 15.39). CSH can be distinguished from rhabdomyoma and plasmacytoma phenotypically because it is CD68+, CD138–, and negative for muscle-specific actin. Furthermore, the cytoplasmic crystalloids are immunoreactive for immunoglobulin light chains, usually of the kappa type (Fig. 15.40).[66,81–83]

Lymphomatoid granulomatosis (angiocentric immunoproliferative lesions)

Although most cells in the lesions of "lymphomatoid granulomatosis" (LYG; also known as "angiocentric immunoproliferative lesions," "polymorphic reticulosis," and "midline lethal granuloma") are T lymphocytes, recent studies have shown that the *neoplastic* elements in this disorder are represented by a clonal population of EBV-infected B cells.[84,85] Consequently, LYG is best considered ontogenetically in the category of B-lineage lymphoproliferative disorders. It is a disease that primarily affects adults, and, because it has an etiologic relationship to EBV infection, many cases arise in the setting of immunodeficiency. In most cases, there is a prodromal phase of fever and nonspecific symptoms that may relate to pulmonary or sinonasal disease (e.g. cough and epistaxis); the skin and the central nervous system may also be involved.[86–88] Radiologic studies in patients with LYG usually disclose the presence of multiple nodular pulmonary opacities, with or without cavitation (Figs 15.41 and 15.42), but mediastinal lymphadenopathy is rare. In resected lung specimens, the tumoral masses are centrally located and have a homogenous white–gray color on cut section.

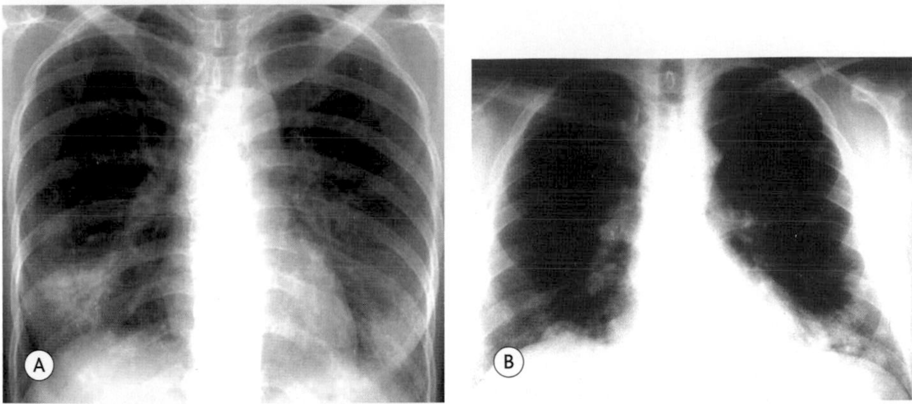

Fig. 15.41 (A,B) "Lymphomatoid granulomatosis" (angiocentric immunoproliferative lesions) shows multinodular infiltrates throughout either or both lung fields on plain-film radiographs.

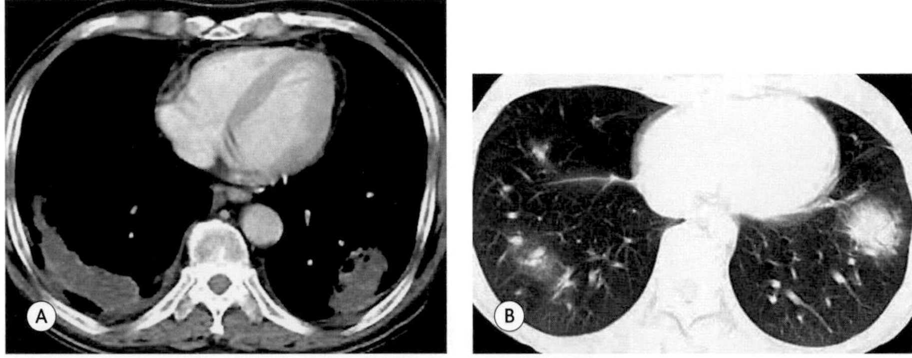

Fig. 15.42 (A,B) The multinodular quality of lymphomatoid granulomatosis is well-seen in these thoracic computed tomograms.

Extensive necrosis and preferential perivascular localization of the lesional lymphoid cells are the histologic hallmarks of LYG.[66,82] Three categories or "grades" of this disease have been codified, and they correspond roughly with clinical aggressivity. At the low end of the spectrum, in **grade I LYG,** the cellular proliferation is polymorphous and composed of cytologically bland small lymphocytes, plasma cells, histiocytes, and occasional eosinophils (Fig. 15.43). Large lesional B cells are also present, but they represent no more than 1% of the total cell population. Such elements have coarse chromatin, distinct nucleoli, and moderate amounts of amphophilic cytoplasm. LYG of all grades is angiocentric, with accumulations of viable cells around arterioles and venules, and angiodestructive, with mural vascular invasion, luminal occlusion, and vascular disruption. Endothelial cells in affected vessels are plump ("activated"). Necrosis may be present in grade I LYG, although it should be focal. Cytologic atypia – with irregular nuclear contours, nuclear hyperchromasia, nucleomegaly, and nucleoli – is seen in the lymph component in **grade II LYG**, together with more obvi necrosis (Fig. 15.44). However, large centroblas immunoblastic cells in grade II lesions are still relativ widely dispersed and difficult to find on rout microscopy. **Grade III LYG** has all of the hallmarks high-grade NHL – with a high content of mitotic active large atypical cells and necrosis (Fig. 15.45) – the small lymphoid component persists to some ext The angiocentric component takes on a monomorp quality and there is nuclear atypia in all of the constitu lymphocytes in grade III lesions.[67,89,90]

The bulk of the lymphoid component in LYC composed of CD2+, CD3+, CD4+ T-helper lymphocy with lesser numbers of CD8+ T-killer cells and CD CD56+ natural killer cells. CD79a and CD20 labelin present in the large cell component only, and those markers help to identify lesional cells that may not readily evident on hematoxylin and eosin (H&E) sta EBV-latent membrane protein expression and E

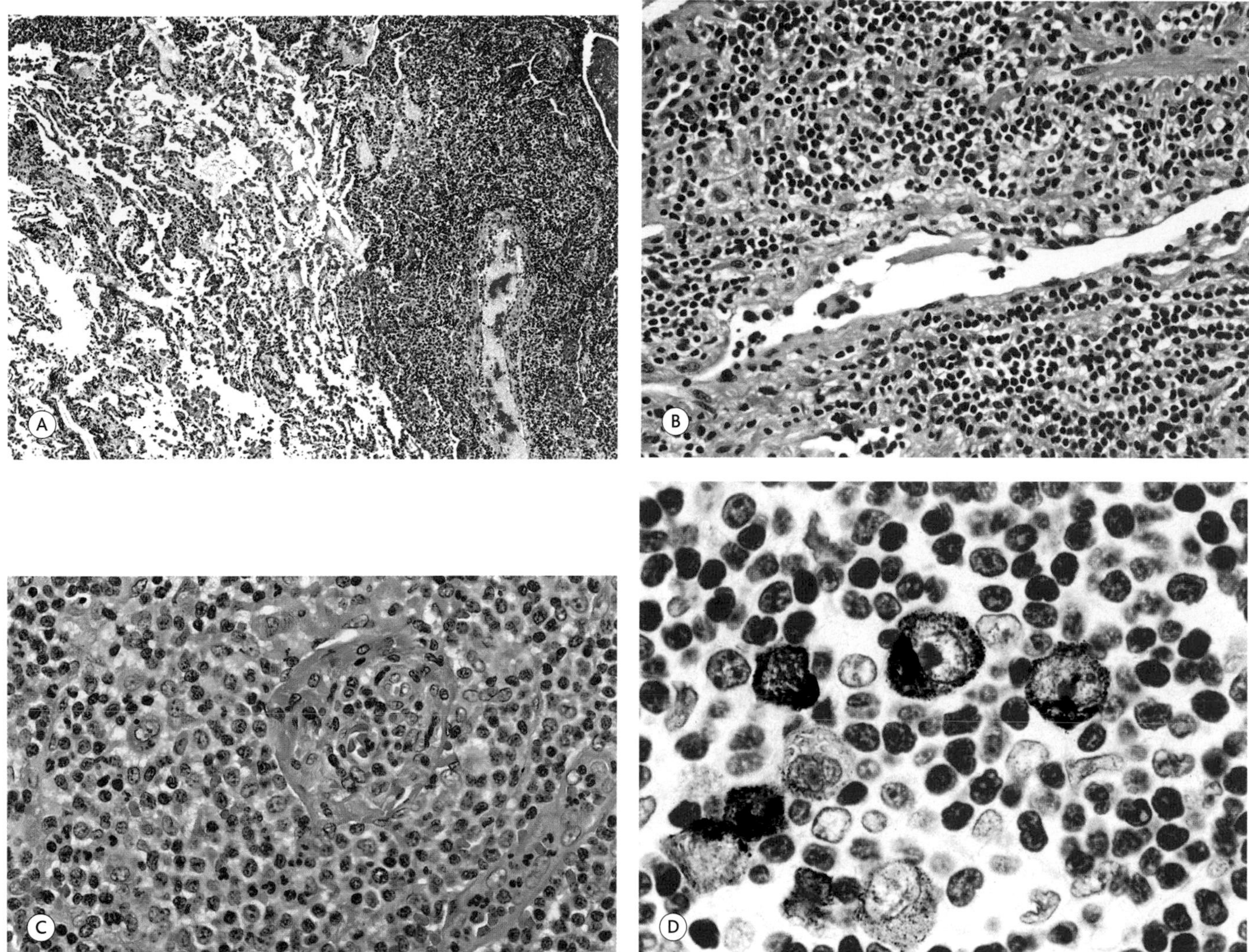

Fig. 15.43 (A–C) Grade I lymphomatoid granulomatosis features infiltrates of modestly atypical lymphocytes that surround intrapulmonary blood vessels, often adhering to their endothelial surfaces. (D) Immunostains for CD20 demonstrate reactivity in widely scattered larger cells in the infiltrates. The remaining elements have a T-lymphocytic phenotype.

encoded ribonucleotides (EBERs; detected by in-situ hybridization) are present in the large B cells of LYG but not in intralesional T cells.[67]

Wegener's granulomatosis shows some degree of histologic similarity to LYG, but it lacks large CD20+ B cells and contains neutrophil-rich zones of necrosis with true granulomas and multinucleated histiocytic giant cells. Other inflammatory conditions that may resemble LYG include Varicella-zoster-related viral pneumonia and bronchocentric granulomatosis, but both of those disorders lack the vasocentricity and lymphocyte-rich, neutrophil/eosinophil-poor cell population that typifies all grades of LYG.

Because LYG shows a bimorphic population of large cells in a polymorphous background of lymphocytes, Hodgkin's lymphoma and TcRBCL should also be considered in its differential diagnosis. However, TcRBCL rarely manifests necrosis and does not exhibit angiocentricity or angiodestruction, and is EBV(–). The lung is a very unusual site for the primary presentation of Hodgkin's disease (see below). Large lymphoid elements in that condition are reactive for CD15 and CD30, but they lack CD20, CD45, and CD79a, as seen in LYG.

In contrast to LYG, peripheral T-cell lymphomas (PTCLs) lack the presence of atypical large CD20+ cells, and they demonstrate significant cytologic atypia in both small and large lymphoid elements. Moreover, there is usually an aberrant loss of at least one stage-specific pan-T-cell marker (e.g. CD2, CD3, CD5, or CD7) (Table 15.7), and PTCL usually shows clonal T-cell receptor gene rearrangements by PCR analysis.

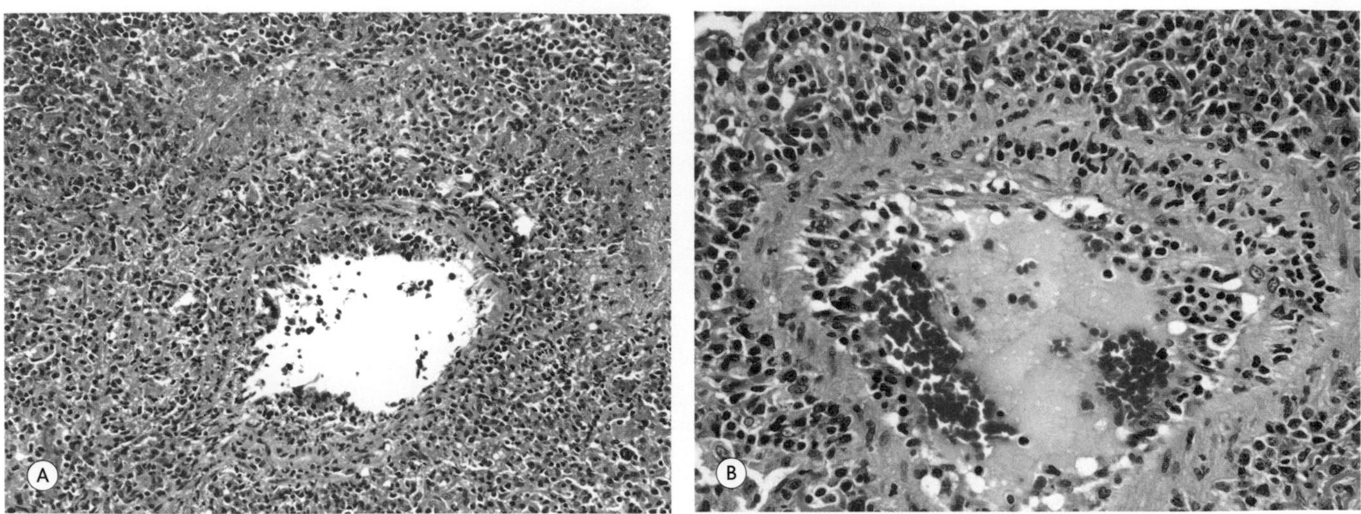

Fig. 15.44 (A,B) Grade II lymphomatoid granulomatosis demonstrates a moderate degree of nuclear atypia in many of the cells in the perivascular intrapulmonary infiltrate.

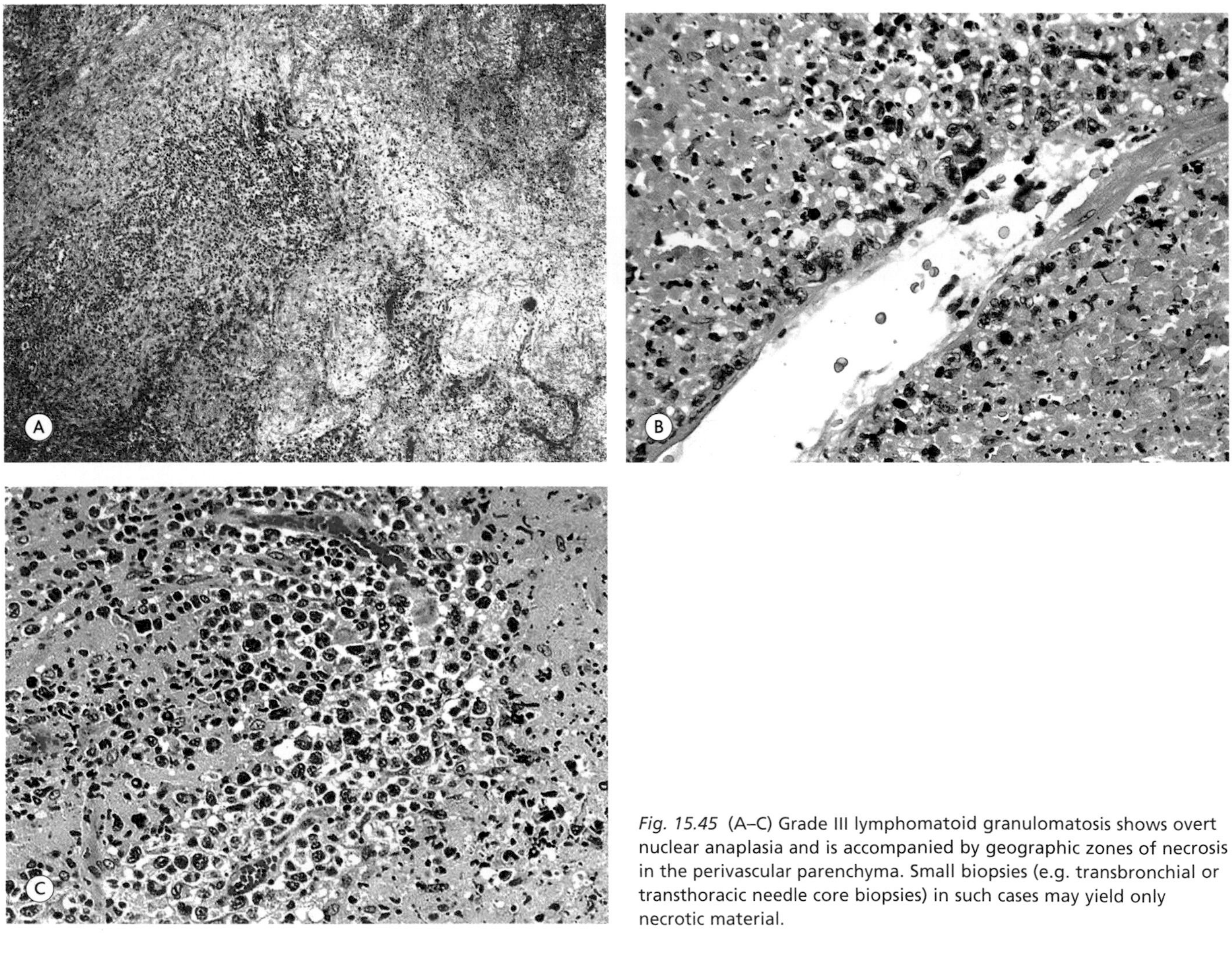

Fig. 15.45 (A–C) Grade III lymphomatoid granulomatosis shows overt nuclear anaplasia and is accompanied by geographic zones of necrosis in the perivascular parenchyma. Small biopsies (e.g. transbronchial or transthoracic needle core biopsies) in such cases may yield only necrotic material.

Table 15.7 Morphologic and phenotypic differences among T- and T/NK-cell lymphomas

Disease	Phenotype CD2	CD3	[CD4+8-]	[CD4-8+]	CD5	CD7	CD16/56	CD43	CD45ro	TdT	*bcl*-6	CD15	CD30	LCA
T-LBL	+	+	common	rare	D	D	– –	+	+	+	±	–	–	dim
T-SLL/LGL	+	+	common	rare	D	D	± +	+	+	–	–	–	–	+
PTCL, NOS	+	+	common	rare	D	D	– –	±	+	–	–	–	±	+
ALCL														
T-cell type	+	+	common	rare	D	D	± ±	+	+	–	–	–	+	+
Null-cell type	–	–	–	–	–	–	– –	–	–	–	–	–	+	+
NK cell tumor	–	C	–	–	–	–	+ +	–	–	–	–	–	–	+

LBL = lymphoblastic lymphoma
SLL = small lymphocytic lymphoma
PTCL = peripheral T cell lymphoma
NOS = not otherwise specified
NK = natural killer cell lymphoma
LGL = large granular lymphocytic leukemia
ALCL = anaplastic large cell lymphona

+ = lesional cells are almost always positive
– = lesional cells are almost always negative
± = lesional cells positive in some cases
D = lesional cells often lose this antigen in the course of malignant transformation
C = cytoplasmic staining only with polyclonal CD3 antibody (epsilon epitope)

Pulmonary lesions of true natural killer cell lymphoma (NKCL) may exhibit virtually complete morphologic overlap with LYG. Nevertheless, although the cells in that tumor may be positive for *cytoplasmic* CD3 (ε epitope) by paraffin-section immunohistochemistry, they lack all other pan-T-cell markers, including *surface* CD3, and have a CD16+, CD56+ immunophenotype. Those characteristics are sufficient to distinguish NKCL from LYG consistently.

Post-transplant lymphoproliferative disorders

The immunosuppressed state that is necessary after organ transplantation predisposes transplant recipients to the development of lymphoid proliferations. These are often EBV-related and they usually demonstrate a B-lymphocytic lineage[91] (Table 15.8). For most patients, the disease is systemic at the time it is detected clinically; however, in many lung transplant cases, lesions of post-transplantation lymphoproliferative disorder (PTLD) arise in, and remain confined to, the allograft itself.[91] Radiographic findings vary from bilateral reticulonodular infiltrates to single or multiple discrete nodules or masses (Figs 15.46 and 15.47), with the latter being most common in patients with high-grade histologic lesions.[92,93]

The classification of PTLDs requires integration of morphologic, phenotypic, and genetic data.[67] Polymorphous PTLD is composed of a mixture of lymphocytes, plasma cells, and transitional lymphoplasmacytoid forms[94,95] (Figs 15.48 and 15.49). In this context, a polytypic pattern of immunoglobulin light-chain expression and a lack of clonality on Southern blot analysis are compatible with categorization of the process as "polymorphous B-cell hyperplasia."[96] If there is, instead, a monotypic population of B cells by FCM, or if gene rearrangement studies identify a clonal population, morphologically heterogeneous infiltrates are best diagnosed as "polymorphous post-transplant B-cell lymphomas." Many examples of PTLD do have a monomorphic appearance, and a histologic image which is identical to that of de-novo large cell lymphoma or Burkitt's lymphoma occurring in immunocompetent patients[86] (Figs 15.50 and 15.51).[92,95–98] Regardless of their microscopic features, the lymphoid cells in most cases of PTLD contain Epstein–Barr virus, which can be detected either immunohistochemically or with in-situ hybridization methods (Fig. 15.52). T-lineage PTLDs also occur, and a number have been shown to be of a special (T-γ/δ hepatosplenic) type.[99]

Generally speaking, polymorphic PTLDs are more likely than their monomorphic counterparts to regress if immunosuppression is reduced or withheld. Consequently, classification plays an important role in initial treatment planning, and as an important indicator of prognosis.[97,98] It is important to recognize, however, that transplant patients can develop lymphomas of any type, and that lineage and clonality should be evaluated fully in every case.

Differential diagnostic considerations in suspected PTLD cases are few, because the lymphoid nature of the proliferation is readily apparent histologically and immunophenotypic studies usually yield straightforward results. Difficulty may arise if only a transbronchial biopsy has been obtained, because the volume of lesional

Table 15.8 Histologic, phenotypic and genetic characteristics of post-transplant lymphoproliferative disorders (PTLDs)

	P-BCH	P-BCL	M-BLCL	M-BL	M-BPCY
Cellular composition	Mixture of small lymphs, plasma cells, and occasional large centroblastic and immunoblastic cells	Mixture of small lymphs, plasma cells, and occasional large centroblastic and immunoblastic cells	Uniform population of centroblastic or immunoblastic type large cells	Uniform population of intermediate-sized cells with coarse chromatin, multiple distinct nucleoli and moderate quantities of eosinophilic or amphophilic cytoplasm	Uniform population of plasmacytic or plasmablastic cells with coarse chromatin; moderate or abundant quantities of amphophilic cytoplasm
Histologic grade	Low (occasional mitoses no necrosis)	Low (occasional mitoses, no necrosis)	High (increased mitoses ± necrosis)	High (numerous mitoses, necrosis often present)	May be low or high ± mitoses, necrosis
sIg expression	Polytypic	Monotypic	Monotypic (some cases sIg neg)	Monotypic	Most cases sIg neg
cIg expression	Polytypic	Monotypic	Usually cIg neg (some cases monotypic)	Usually cIg neg	Monotypic
Clonal IgH/IgL loci rearrangements	None	Present	Present	Present	Present
Mutational analysis of c-myc/n-myc	Normal	Normal	Often mutated	Often mutated	Often mutated
Outcome	May resolve spontaneously with reduced immunosuppression	May resolve spontaneously with reduced immunosuppression	Less likely to resolve without systemic chemotherapy	Unlikely to resolve without systemic chemotherapy	Unlikely to resolve without systemic chemotherapy; often fatal

P-BCH = polymorphous B-cell hyperplasia
P-BCL = polymorphous B-cell lymphoma
M-BLCL = monomorphous B-cell large cell lymphoma
M-BL = monomorphous Burkitt's lymphoma
M-BPCY = monomorpous B-cell plasmacytoma
neg = negative
cIg = cytoplasmic immunoglobulin
sIg = surface immunoglobulin

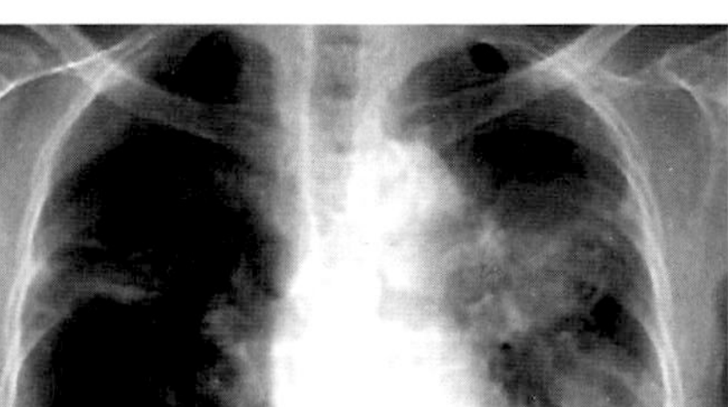

Fig. 15.46 This example of post-transplant lymphoproliferative disorder shows multiple nodular and infiltrative parenchymal lesions throughout both lung fields. The patient had had a renal transplant 5 months previously.

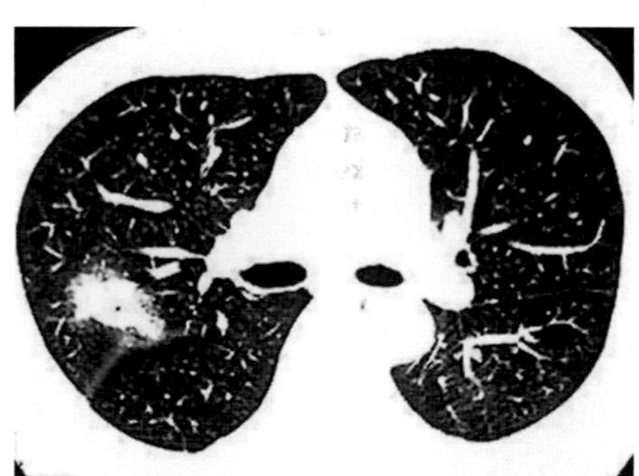

Fig. 15.47 Another case of post-transplant lymphoproliferative disorder, represented by a nodular lesion in the right lung in this computed tomogram.

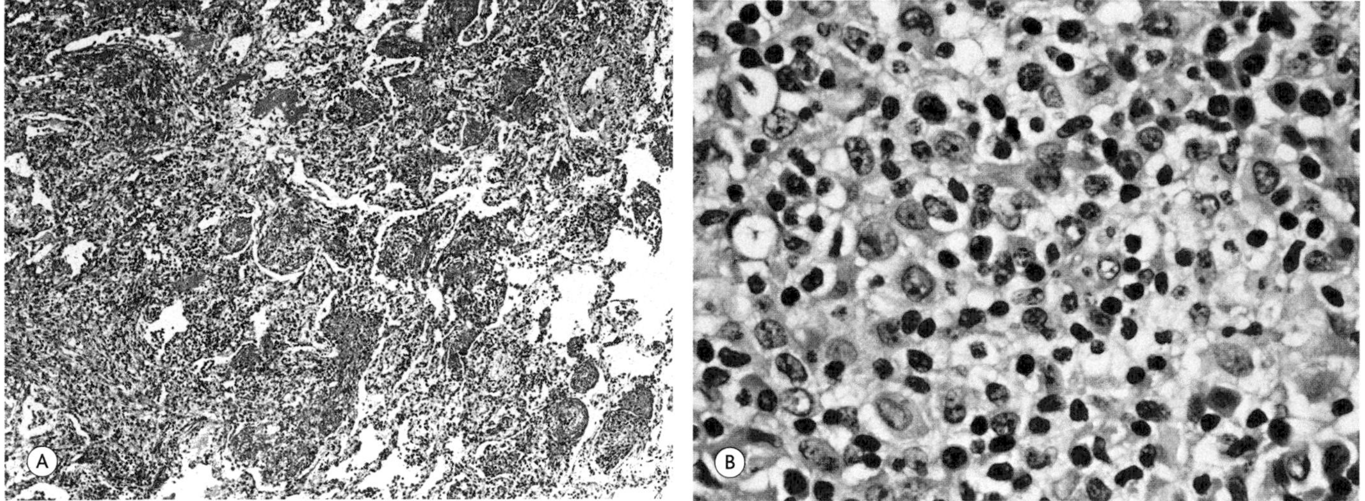

Fig. 15.48 Polymorphous post-transplant lymphoproliferative disorder in the lung, showing (A) an alveolar and interstitial infiltrate of (B) hematopoietic elements with lymphoplasmacytic features.

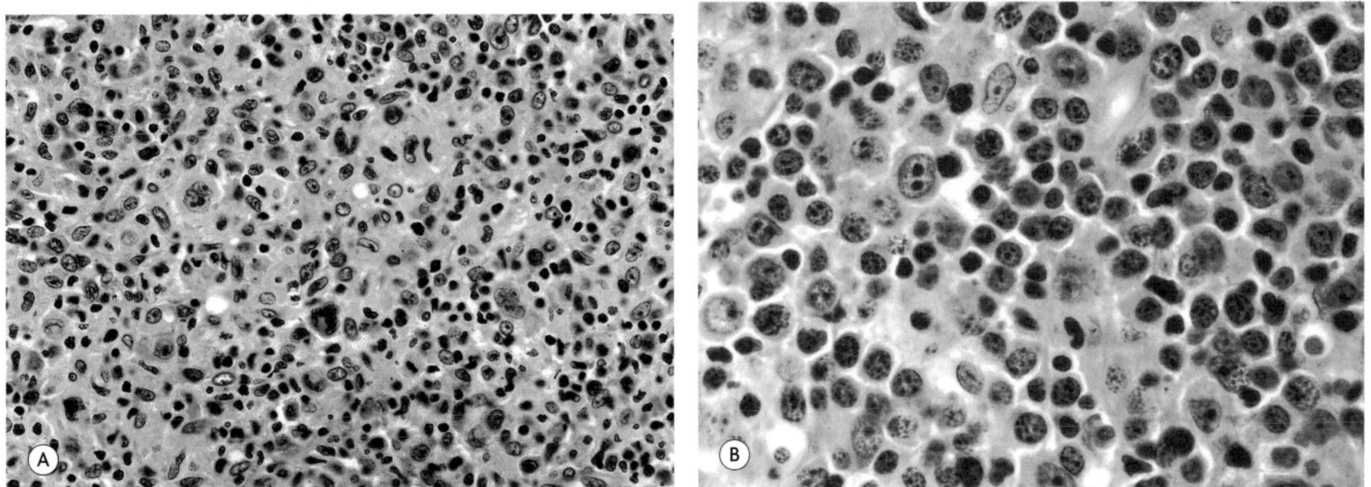

Fig. 15.49 (A) Polymorphous post-transplant lymphoproliferative disorder may demonstrate an admixture of atypical mononuclear cells, plasma cells, and Reed–Sternberg cell-like elements, or (B) a prominent histiocytic component together with lymphocytes and plasma cells. This process is driven by infection with the Epstein–Barr virus; it is polyclonal and not associated with mutations of proto-oncogenes such as c-myc.

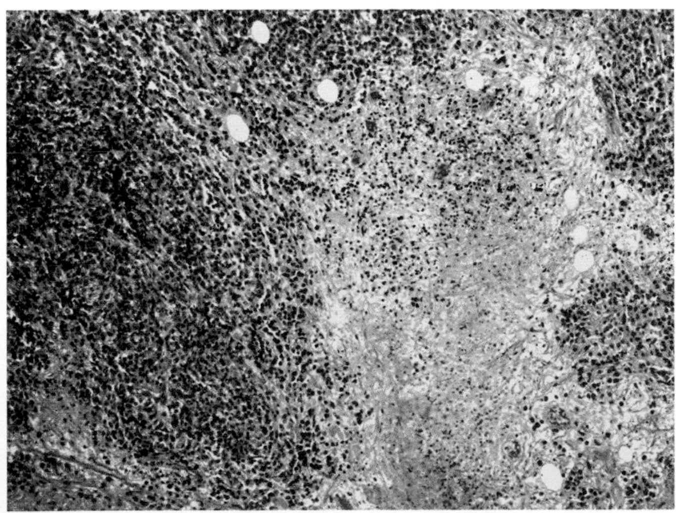

Fig. 15.50 High-grade monotypic post-transplant lymphoproliferative disorder in the lung, showing an infiltrate of atypical large cells in a field of geographic necrosis.

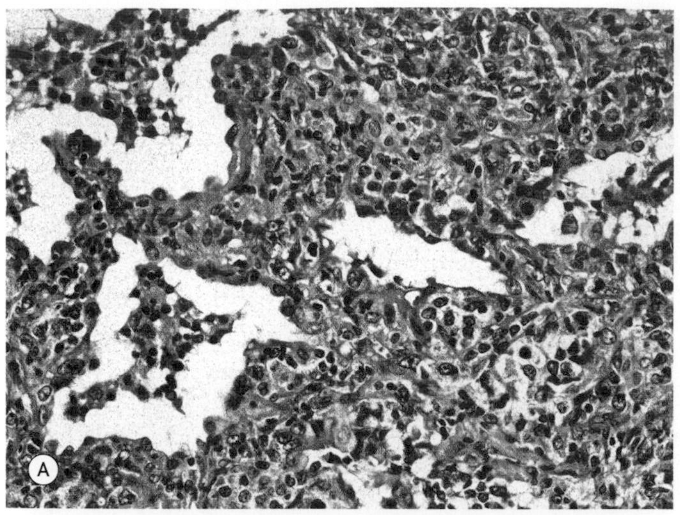

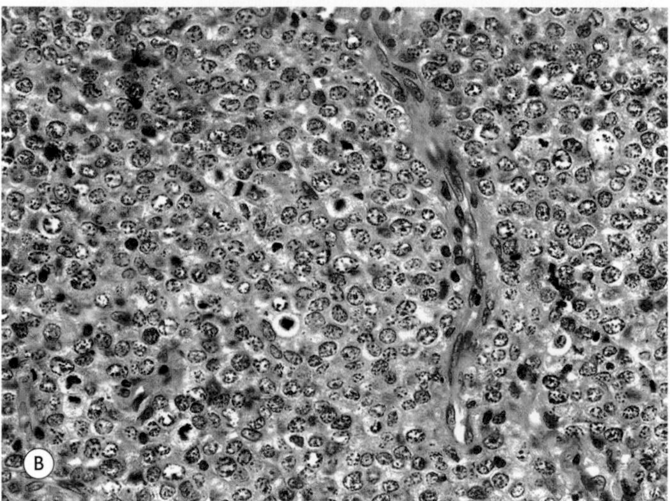

Fig. 15.51 (A) The lesional cells of high-grade monotypic post-transplant lymphoproliferative disorder (PTLD) expand and distort the interalveolar septa. They show obvious nuclear anaplasia (B) and were monoclonal genotypically and immunophenotypically.

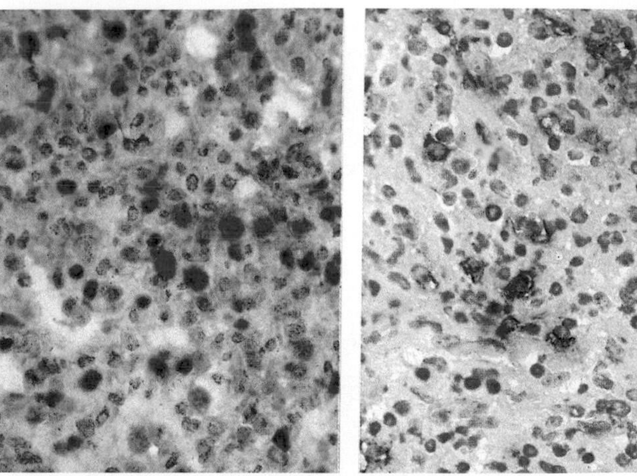

Fig. 15.52 In-situ hybridization for Epstein–Barr virus-related ribonucleic acid (left) or immunostaining for Epstein–Barr virus latent membrane protein (right) usually yields positive results in post-transplant lymphoproliferative disorder of the lung.

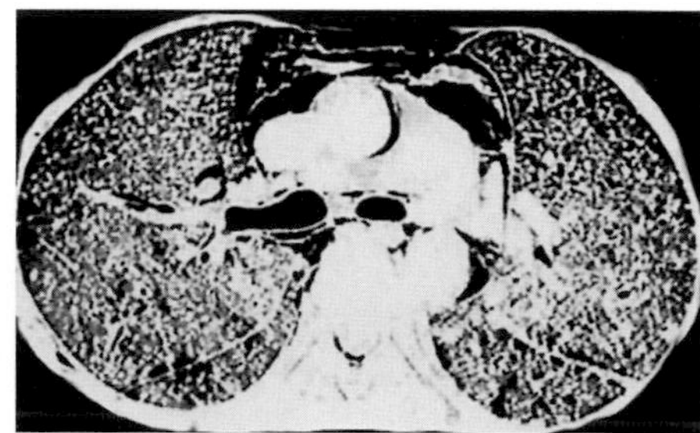

Fig. 15.53 Peripheral T-cell lymphoma of the lung, assuming a radiographic pattern which simulates that of miliary tuberculosis in this computed tomogram.

infiltrate may be too limited to make a meaningful histologic classification into polymorphic or monomorphic categories, or to fully exclude other diseases such as lymphomatoid granulomatosis, Hodgkin's lymphoma, or non-neoplastic disorders such as viral pneumonia (particularly due to cytomegalovirus).

Primary pulmonary lymphomas of T-cell lineage

Most patients with peripheral T-cell lymphoma (PTCL) are clinically ill at presentation, and may have features such as high fevers, rash, and pulmonary infiltrates that suggest the presence of infection. Bilateral miliary intrapulmonary nodules simulating mycobacterial infection (Fig. 15.53)[100] or reticulonodular infiltrates imitating interstitial disease have been reported, and mass lesions mimicking bronchogenic carcinoma are also relatively frequently observed. A common feature to both precursor- and mature T-cell lymphomas is that there is a systemic distribution of disease at presentation,[101] so the lung is seldom biopsied for initial diagnosis.

Anaplastic large cell lymphoma (ALCL) with T-cell differentiation

Several cases of primary pulmonary ALCL of T- or null-cell type have been reported,[102–104] all of which were associated with mass lesions; some presented as solitary endobronchial lesions that were associated with stridor.[102] Microscopically, ALCL is formed by diffuse sheets of

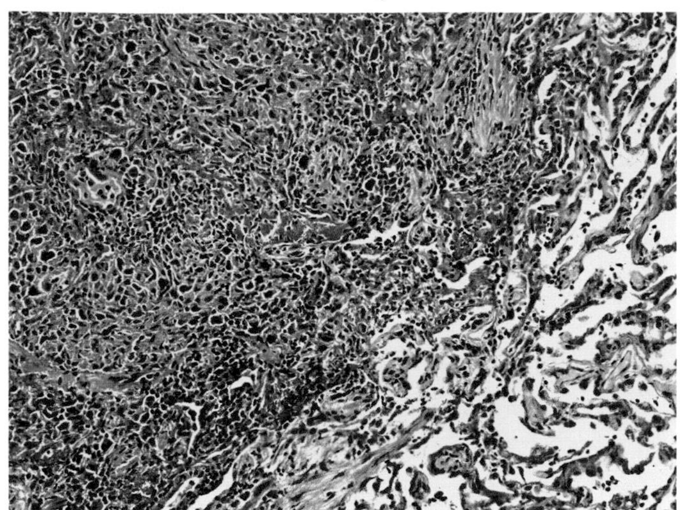

Fig. 15.54 Anaplastic large cell lymphoma presents as a primary pulmonary tumor only very rarely, and it may show a deceptively sharp interface with the surrounding lung parenchyma.

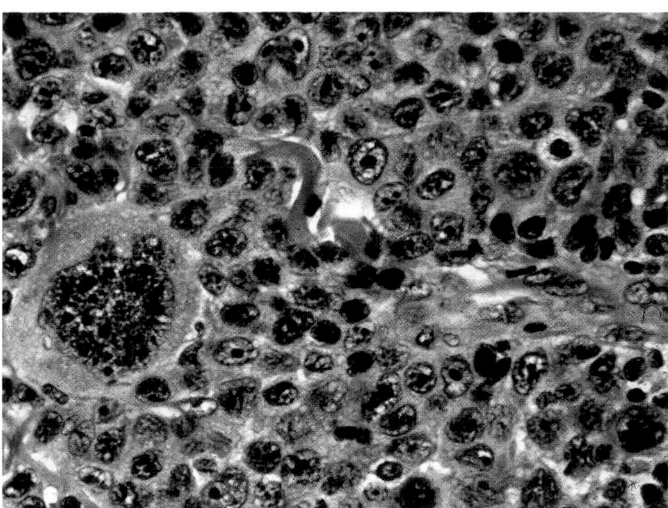

Fig. 15.56 Extreme nuclear pleomorphism and multinucleation are evident in the tumor cells of this intrapulmonary anaplastic large cell lymphoma.

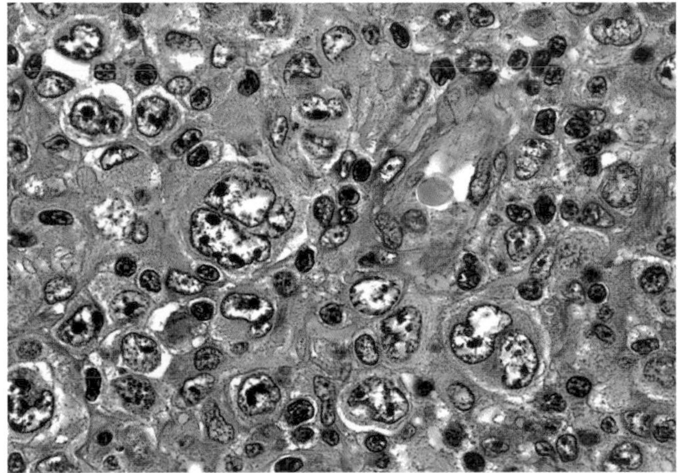

Fig. 15.55 Anaplastic large-cell lymphoma often has morphologic features which are reminiscent of carcinomas or melanomas.

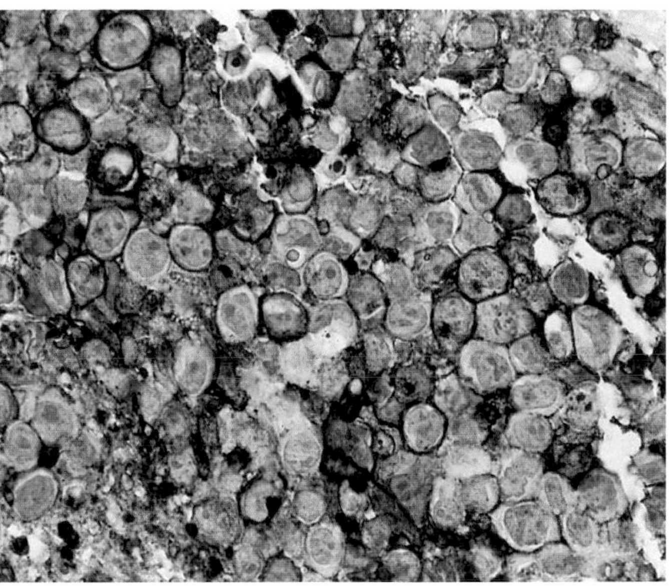

Fig. 15.57 The CD30+ phenotype, as shown in this immunostain, when taken in conjunction with either phenotypic or molecular evidence of T-cell lineage, establish the diagnosis of the T-cell type of anaplastic large cell lymphoma.

large and multifocally bizarre cells with pleomorphic nuclei and abundant cytoplasm, and a similarity to carcinoma or melanoma may be striking (Figs 15.54–15.56). Careful attention to the periphery of the lesion may disclose a dyshesive array of intra-alveolar tumor cells, representing a helpful cue that the disease may be of hematolymphoid origin. The majority of these cases are positive for a pan-T-cell marker such as CD2, CD3, or CD45RO, although some may be negative for all of those antigens ("null cell phenotype") or negative for CD45. CD30 reactivity (Fig. 15.57) is considered a virtual sine qua non for this entity. ALK-1 expression (Fig. 15.58) can be documented immunohistochemically in a proportion of ALCL cases, and it correlates with the presence of a t(2;5) chromosomal translocation involving the *nucleophosmin* and *ALK* genes. Because so few cases of pulmonary ALCL have been reported, predictions of outcome are difficult. Preliminary data suggest that the risk of progression to systemic disease and death is high, even when ALCL presents with strictly defined stage IE disease (primary extranodal disease limited to one non-nodal site) in the lung.[102,105]

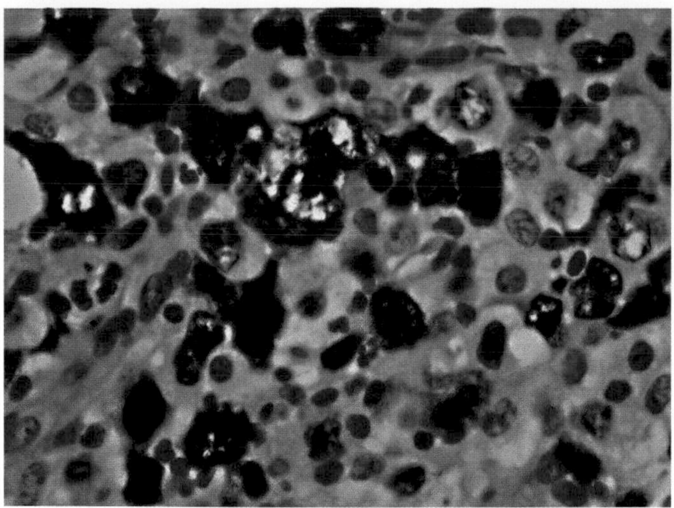

Fig. 15.58 A subset of anaplastic large cell lymphomas demonstrate immunoreactivity for the ALK-1 protein, associated with a t(2;5) chromosomal translocation.

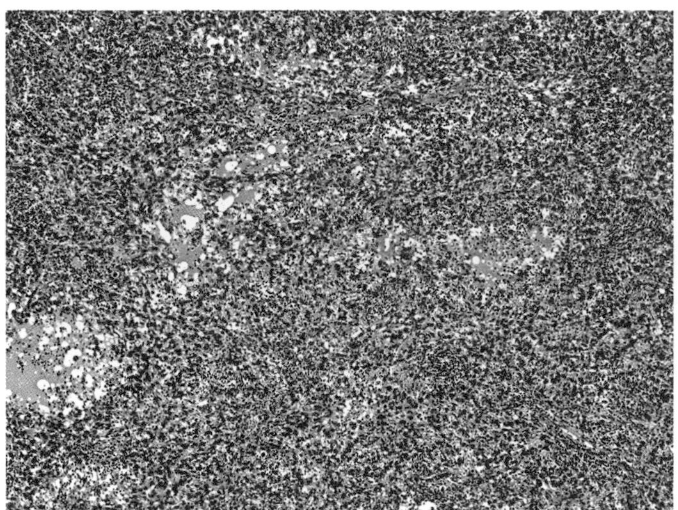

Fig. 15.59 Follicular dendritic cell sarcoma of the lung, showing an infiltrate of atypical mononuclear cells that are bluntly fusiform. The lesion effaces the pulmonary parenchyma.

Follicular dendritic cell tumors

Follicular dendritic cell sarcoma (FDCS) is a rare tumor that typically arises in lymph nodes in adults.[106–110] It is composed of bluntly fusiform cells that are arranged in short fascicles, whorls, storiform profiles, or pseudo-epithelial clusters, admixed with small lymphocytes and plasma cells (Figs 15.59 and 15.60). Nuclei in such lesions are vesicular, and nucleoli are distinct (Fig. 15.61). The overall microscopic image of FDCS superficially resembles that of inflammatory malignant fibrous histiocytoma or spindle cell thymoma.[111] Immunophenotypically, dendritic

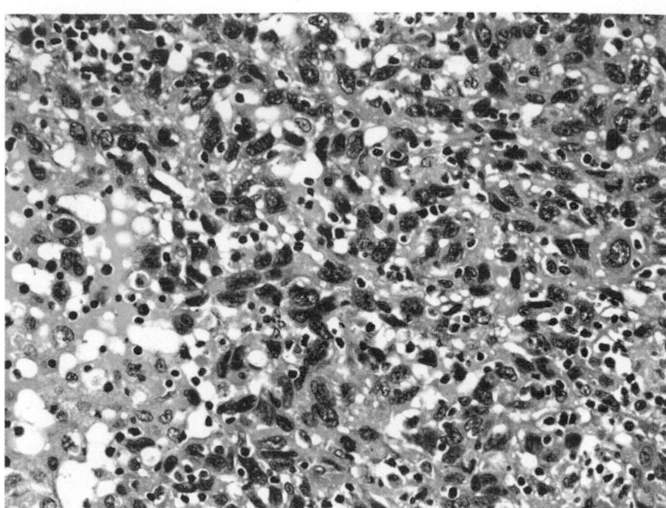

Fig. 15.60 Fusiform tumor cells in follicular dendritic cell sarcoma are intermixed with mature lymphocytes.

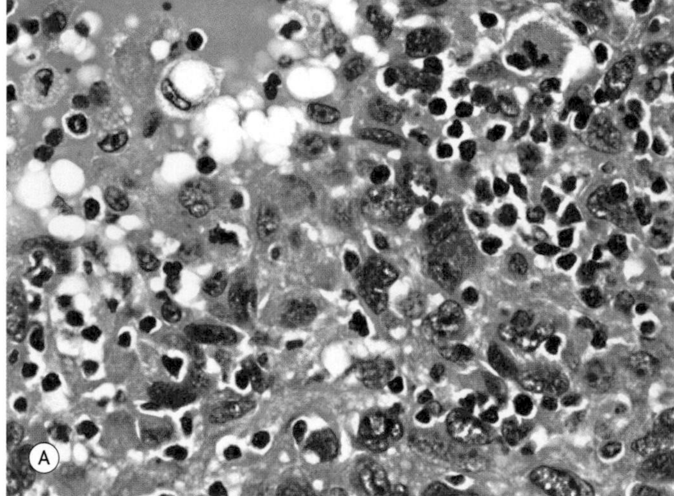

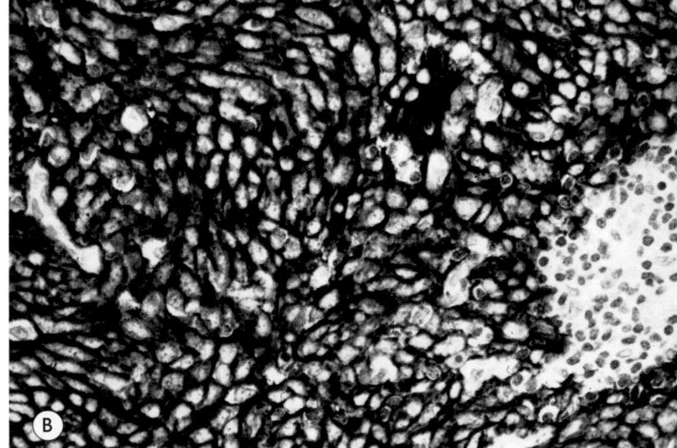

Fig. 15.61 (A) The neoplastic cells in follicular dendritic cell sarcoma show vesicular chromatin and discernible nucleoli. (B) They are diffusely immunoreactive for CD21, as shown here, as well as CD35.

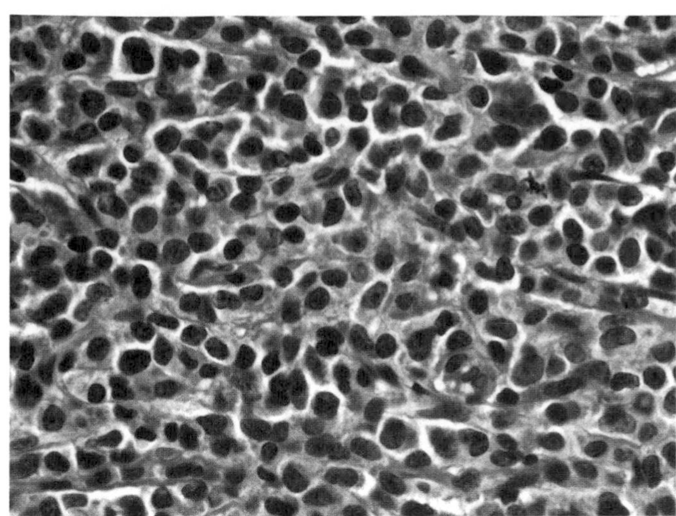

Fig. 15.62 The lung may be secondarily involved by any type of B-cell lymphoma. Follicular lymphoma is demonstrated in this image, in which the tumor cells have folded or twisted nuclear profiles.

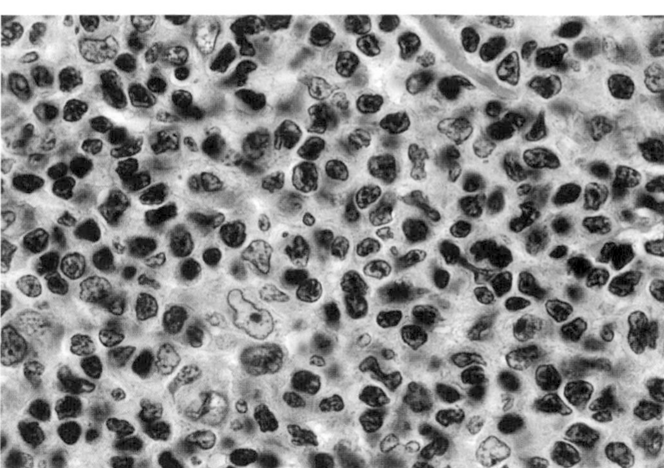

Fig. 15.63 Another example of intrapulmonary follicular lymphoma, showing irregular nuclear contours.

cell tumors are nonreactive for keratin and CD45, but they express vimentin, CD21, CD35, and desmoplakin. Epithelial membrane antigen CD68, and S100 protein may also be observed in some cases.[108,109]

One apparently primary example of FDCS in the lung has been reported by Shah et al.,[112] as a 9.5 cm tan-white dominant mass with smaller "satellite" nodules in the parenchyma, pleura, and regional lymph nodes. In addition, one may observe metastases *to* the lung from FDCSs originating in other anatomic sites.[111]

The long-term prognosis for patients with such lesions is guarded, inasmuch as FDCS may recur up to 20 years after presentation.[109,111] Because of the rarity of this tumor, its optimal therapy has yet to be defined.

Systemic lymphoproliferative disorders that involve the lung

The term **secondary pulmonary non-Hodgkin's lymphoma** refers to an NHL that is seen in the lung in a patient who has prior or concurrent nodal lesions of lymphoma, or develops evidence of systemic lymphoma up to 6 months after presentation. The diagnostic criteria for evaluating lymph node biopsies should be applied in the lung in these instances.[67,104] Patients with secondary pulmonary lymphoma are staged using the Ann Arbor criteria, and their prognosis is determined by both stage and histologic type. It is important to note that there are several specific types of lymphoma that seldom remain localized to the lung (see Table 15.6), and, even if initial staging discloses no extrapulmonary sites of disease, the patient should be followed very closely with the expectation that additional anatomic sites will demonstrate involvement.

Secondary pulmonary B-lineage lymphoma

In the United States, follicular lymphoma, small lymphocytic lymphoma, and mantle cell lymphoma are the most common systemic lymphomas to secondarily involve the lung. Careful attention to cytologic detail, a broad panel of immunohistochemical evaluations, and, above all, the clinical history, are necessary to provide an accurate diagnosis in most cases (see Table 15.6). Although B-cell lymphomas may remain localized for a variable period of time, all such tumors have a very high risk of dissemination. Clues to the diagnosis of follicular lymphoma include a mixture of small, intermediate, and large cells and cleaved nuclear contours, including irregularly cleaved, elongated "twisted towel"-shaped, and gourd-shaped nuclei (Figs 15.62 and 15.63).[113] Mantle cell lymphoma, by contrast, is composed of monotonous small lymphocytes with condensed chromatin and minimally irregular nuclear profiles (Fig. 15.64).[114] Small lymphocytic lymphoma, although it is similar to mantle cell lymphoma cytologically (Figs 15.65 and 15.66), has a second cell population of para-immunoblastic and immunoblastic elements, which often accumulate in pale-staining areas of the lesion (so-called "proliferation centers").[115] MaZL frequently involves the lung secondarily after presentation in other mucosal sites, and, like secondary B-cell large cell NHL, it cannot be distinguished from a primary pulmonary lymphoma on purely morphologic grounds. Immunohistochemical studies are central to an accurate diagnosis and classification for all these conditions (see Table 15.6).

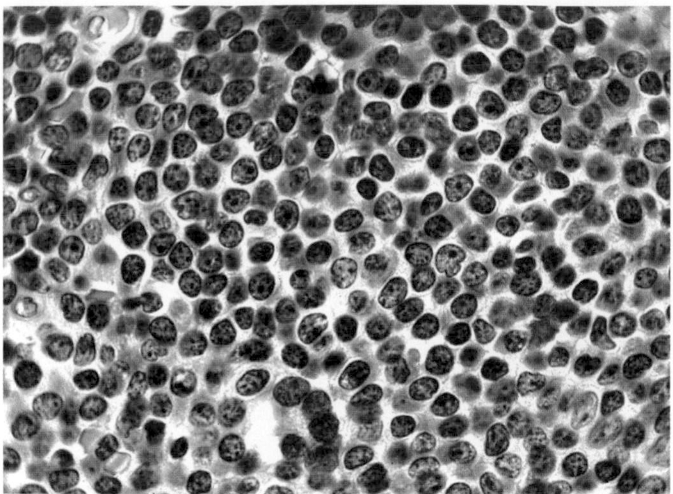

Fig. 15.64 Mantle cell lymphoma of the lung, showing a composition by relatively mature and monomorphic small lymphoid cells. This tumor has also been known in the past as "centrocytic lymphoma" or "lymphocytic lymphoma with intermediate differentiation." A chromosomal translocation t(11;14) in mantle cell lymphoma involves the bcl-1 locus on chromosome 11 and the immunoglobulin heavy-chain locus on chromosome 14. It leads to overexpression of the PRAD-1 gene, which encodes cyclin-D1. Hence, nuclear immunolabeling for the latter protein is a reproducible diagnostic marker for mantle cell lymphoma.

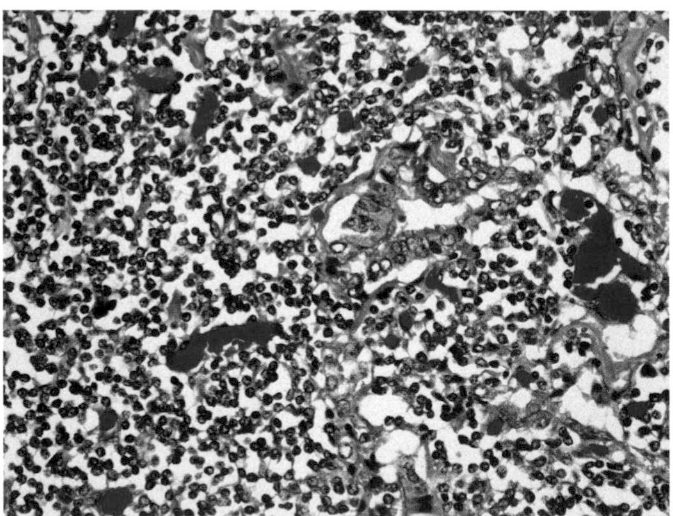

Fig. 15.65 Small lymphocytic lymphoma (SLL) is shown here involving the lung. It is morphologically similar to mantle cell lymphoma but is often accompanied by a leukemic component. Moreover, SLL lacks cyclin-D1 immunoreactivity, and instead shows labeling for CD5, CD20, and CD43. Flow cytometric studies of SLL also should demonstrate positivity for CD23.

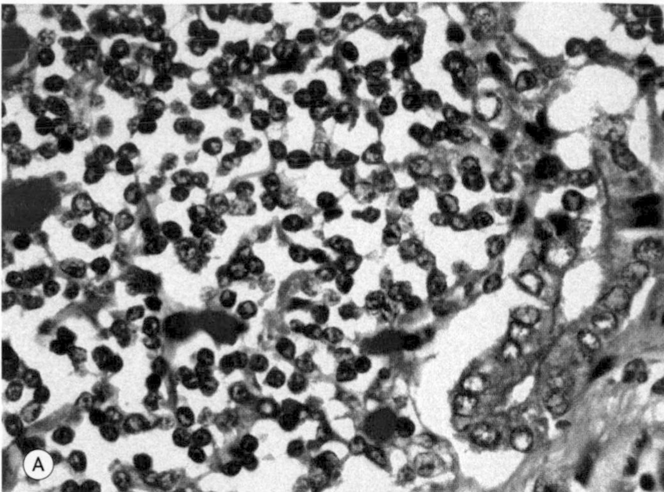

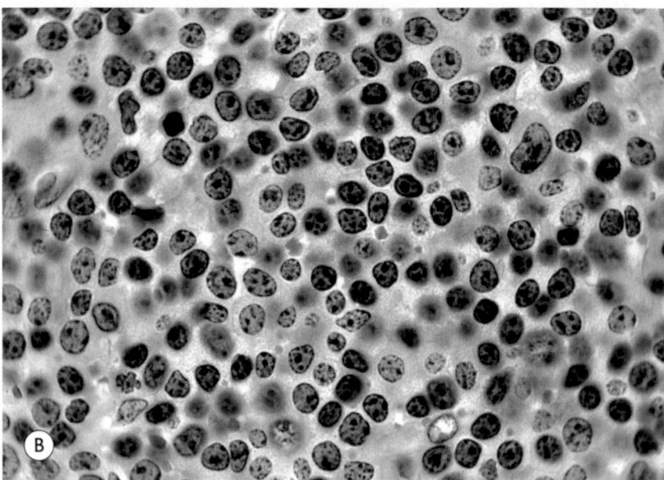

Fig. 15.66 (A,B) The similarity of tumor cells in small lymphocytic lymphoma to mature non-neoplastic B lymphocytes is well shown here.

Secondary pulmonary T-lineage lymphomas

As indicated previously, the vast majority of T-cell lymphomas are systemic disorders at presentation, and the criteria established for morphologic evaluation of lymph node biopsies[67,104] are appropriate for application to the lung as well. Clinical, histologic, immunophenotypic, viral, cytogenetic, site-specific, and other data contribute to defining several specific types of PTCL, including T-cell prolymphocytic leukemia (T-PLL),[116] angio-immunoblastic type PTCL (AILD-PTCL),[117] and T-cell ALCL. Those PTCLs that are not felt to be distinct entities on the basis of clinical, phenotypic, or genotypic data are further described by the predominant cell population that is observed.[118] The histologic hallmarks of most otherwise-unclassifiable PTCLs are a spectrum of atypical small, intermediate, and large cells with irregular nuclear shapes and clear cytoplasm; hypervascularity; and tissue eosinophilia[105,119] (Figs 15.67–15.70).

Regardless of the precise category of disease, PTCLs are non-reactive for the lymphoblast-stage marker TdT, and they are positive for at least one pan-T-cell marker such as CD3 and CD45RO. There is variable reactivity for CD2, CD5, and CD7 (Figs 15.71 and 15.72). Most PTCLs

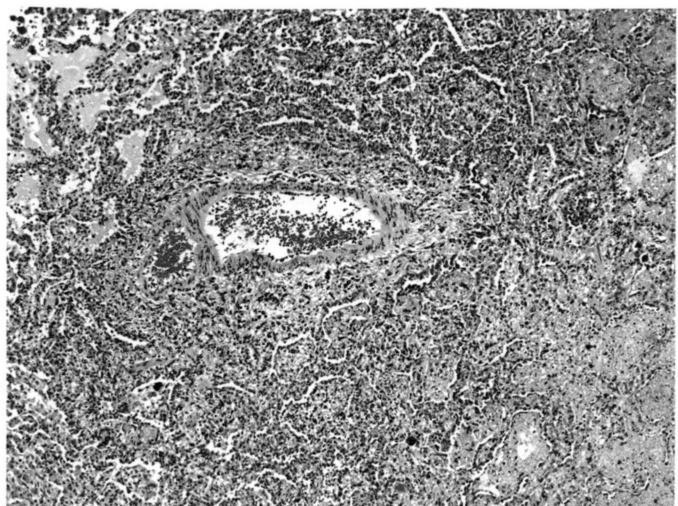

Fig. 15.67 Peripheral T-cell lymphoma of the lung, growing in an interstitial pattern with a tendency to confluence.

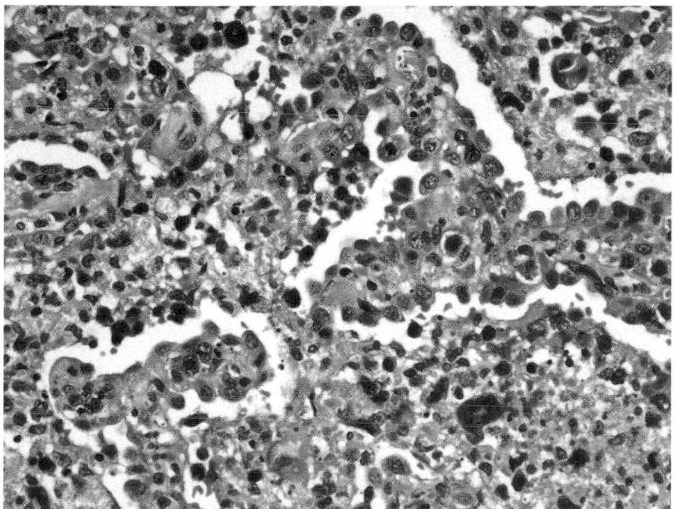

Fig. 15.68 Interalveolar septa are expanded and distorted by obviously atypical lymphoid cells in peripheral cell lymphoma of the lung.

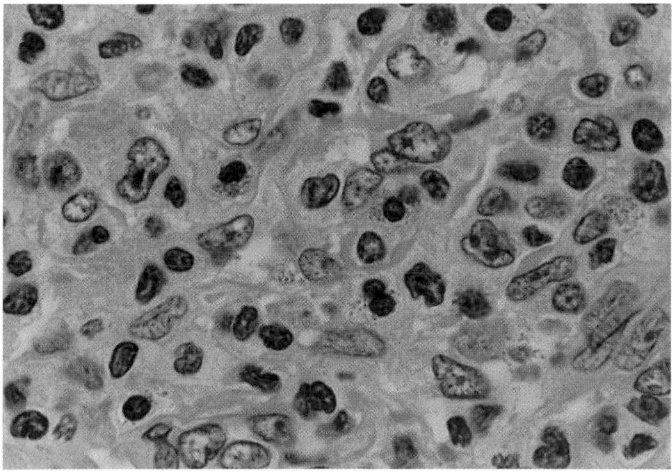

Fig. 15.69 The morphologic triad of a spectrum of small, intermediate, and large atypical cells with pale cytoplasm; hypervascularity; and eosinophilia is often present in peripheral T-cell lymphoma, as shown here.

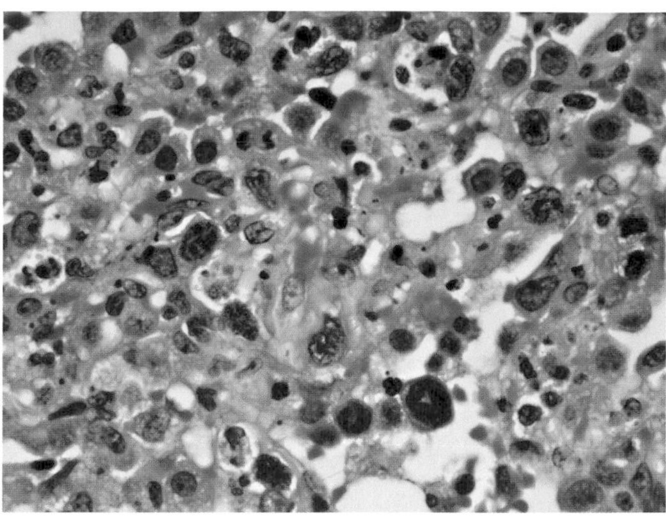

Fig. 15.70 Markedly irregular nuclear contours and nuclear hyperchromasia are present in the tumor cells of this intrapulmonary peripheral T-cell lymphoma.

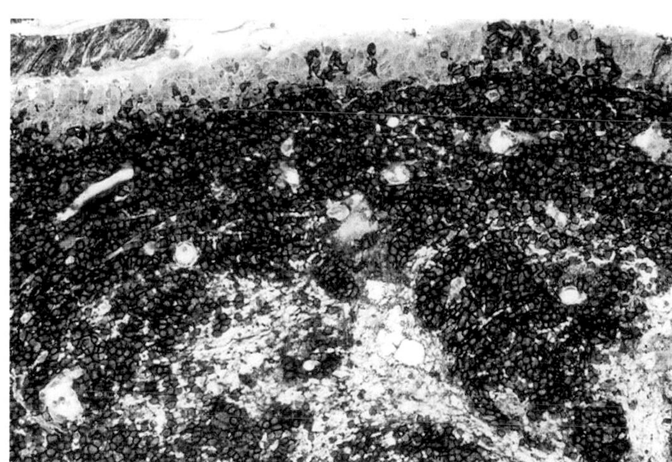

Fig. 15.71 Expression of the pan-T-cell marker CD3 is present in the vast majority of tumor cells in this intrapulmonary peripheral T-cell lymphoma.

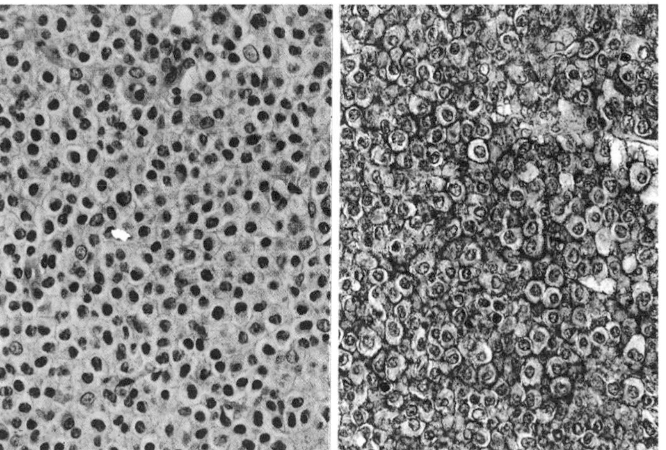

Fig. 15.72 Many cases of peripheral T-cell lymphoma show a selective loss of one or more pan-T-cell markers, as detected in paraffin-section immunostains. Here, CD7 is lacking in the tumor cells (left) but CD5 is present (right).

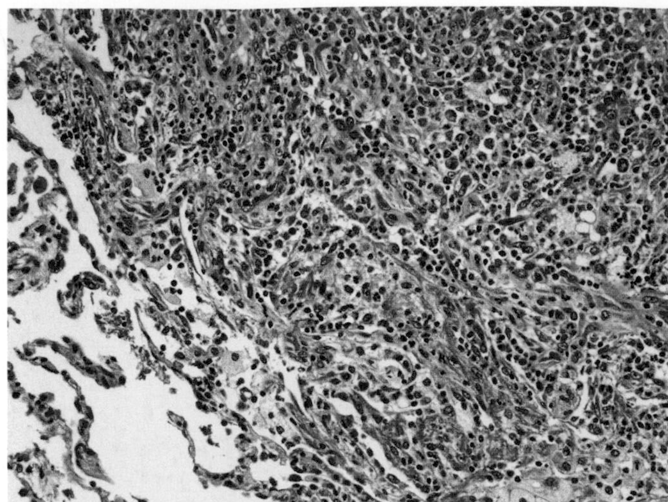

Fig. 15.73 Intrapulmonary Hodgkin's lymphoma, showing a polymorphous lymphoid infiltrate in this wedge biopsy. Reed–Sternberg cells with multilobated nuclear profiles are seen focally.

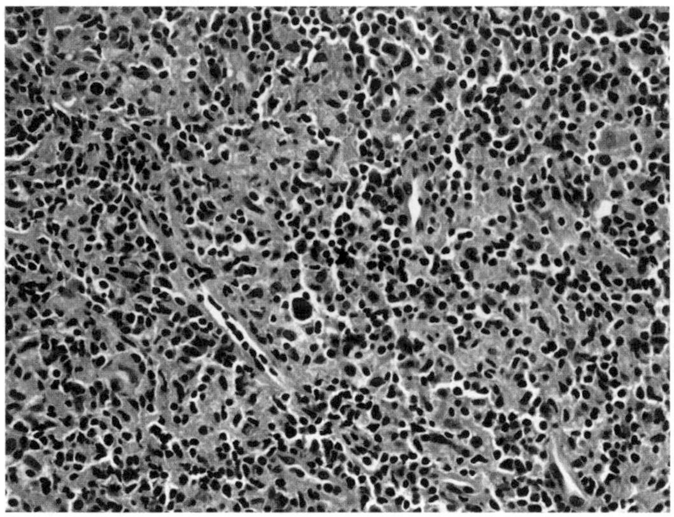

Fig. 15.74 A "mummified" Reed–Sternberg cell with smudged nuclear chromatin is seen in the center of this field, from a lesion of intrapulmonary Hodgkin's lymphoma.

have a [CD4+, CD8–] T-helper-cell phenotype, with no more than 10% having a [CD4–, CD8+] T-cytotoxic-cell or [CD4+, CD8+] ("double positive") or [CD4–, CD8–] ("double negative") profile[119] (see Table 15.7). "Aberrant antigen loss" is easiest to detect via multicolor FCM, where the tumor cells can be studied for three or four markers at the same time. Immunohistochemistry on serial sections from paraffin blocks can also disclose this phenotypic shift.[120] ALCL may be distinguished from other T-cell large cell lymphomas by its reactivity for ALK-1 on immunostaining, or by observation of the t(2;5) translocation involving the *npm* and *ALK* genes. There

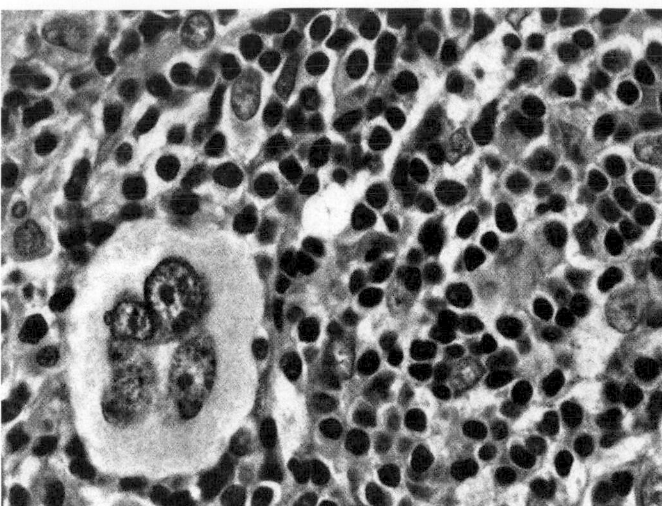

Fig. 15.75 A large Reed–Sternberg cell stands away from a background of small lymphoid elements in this example of Hodgkin's lymphoma.

are no immunostains that specifically characterize T-PLL, but that disease is associated with karyotypic abnormalities involving chromosome 14.[121]

Pulmonary involvement by Hodgkin's disease

Hodgkin's lymphoma (HL) is a tumor of lymphoid lineage,[122,123] the key characteristic of which is that the truly neoplastic cells in the lesion are numerically sparse. In the REAL and WHO classifications there are two main diagnostic and prognostic categories – classic HL and lymphocyte predominance HL (LPHL) – based on the phenotype of the lesional cells as well as the nature of the background inflammatory infiltrate. Most patients with pulmonary HL present with concomitant cervical, mediastinal, or supraclavicular lymphadenopathy, or combinations thereof, and the diagnosis is therefore established by lymph node biopsy. In very rare instances, however, clinical, pathologic, and radiologic assessment discloses the presence of only pulmonary disease.[124–127]

Although the identification of the large and pleomorphic "Reed–Sternberg" (RS) cells in HL is easy in generous biopsy specimens (Figs 15.73 and 15.74), those cells may be difficult or impossible to find in transbronchial or transthoracic needle core biopsies of the lung. RS cells may be seen in other clinical contexts, including small lymphocytic lymphoma–chronic lymphocytic leukemia and acute infectious mononucleosis, and they cannot be used as the *only* criterion for diagnosis. In classic HL the background infiltrate ranges from a monotonous population of cytologically bland small T lymphocytes to a polymorphous mixture of lymphocytes, histiocytes, plasma cells, eosinophils, and neutrophils (Figs 15.75 and

15.76). Immunohistologic analysis typically yields a CD15+, CD30+, CD20–, CD45RO–, CD45– Oct2–, BOB.1– phenotype in HL (Fig. 15.77), but weak or focal CD20 reactivity may be present in some cases[128] (Table 15.9). In the lung, differential diagnostic considerations for classic HL include inflamed solitary fibrous tumors of the pleura, and inflammatory myofibroblastic tumor – pseudotumor.

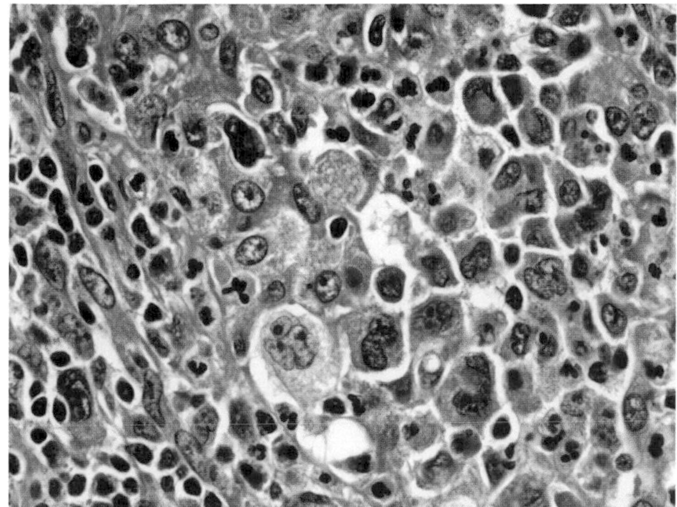

Fig. 15.76 Reed–Sternberg cells in this case of Hodgkin's lymphoma are admixed with eosinophils, lymphocytes, plasma cells, and rare neutrophils.

To date, the 'non-classic' subtype of Hodgkin's lymphoma – LPHL – has not been reported as a primary lung tumor. That disease is typically localized to a single lymph node at presentation, and it pursues an indolent clinical course. The vast majority of patients demonstrate a survival which is similar to that of age-matched individuals without LPHL.[129] Great care should be taken in evaluating lung biopsies with histologic features that may suggest LPHL. That is true because the immunophenotype of so-called "L&H" RS cell variants in LPHD (CD15–, CD30–, CD20+, CD45RO–, CD45+ Oct2+, BOB.1+) (Table 15.9) is identical to that seen in TcRBCL.[130,131] Procurement of a large tissue specimen is essential to resolve this diagnostic issue, because the tumor milieu helps to define the disease at least as much as the nature of the lesional cells.

Extramedullary myeloid tumors (tumefactive acute leukemia)

Extramedullary myeloid tumors (EMTs; also known as "granulocytic sarcomas") are constituted by proliferating

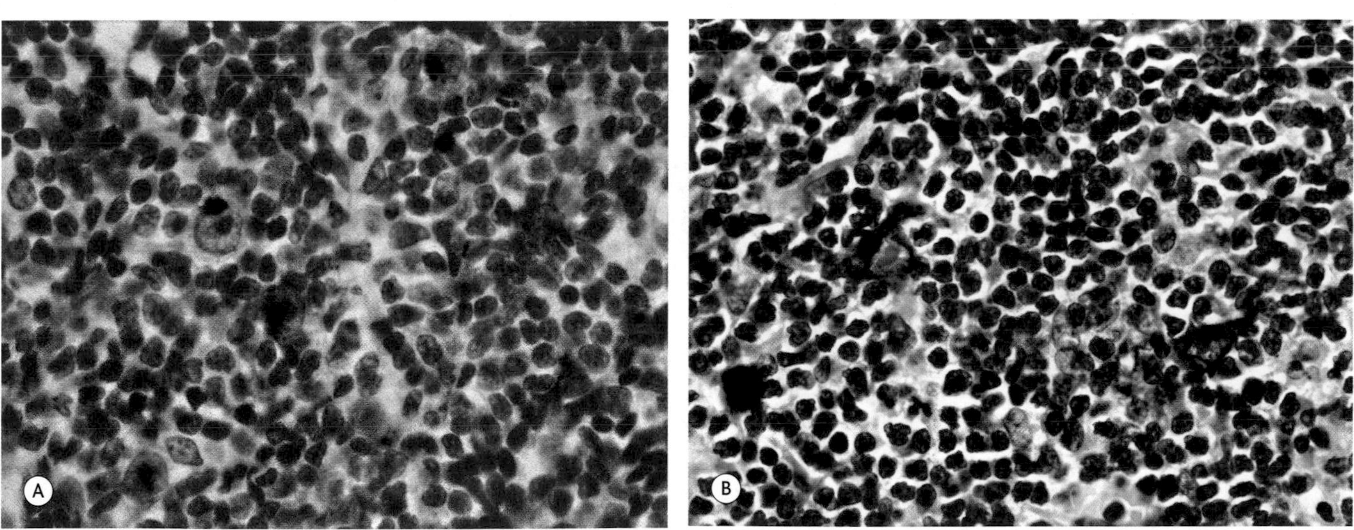

Fig. 15.77 Immunoreactivity for CD15 (A) and CD30 (B) is typical of Reed–Sternberg cells and their variants in Hodgkin's lymphoma; however, they lack CD45, as seen in non-Hodgkin's lymphomas.

Table 15.9 Phenotypic differences between classic Hodgkin's disease (HD) and lymphocyte predominant Hodgkin's disease (LP-HD)

	CD20	CD2	CD3	sIg	cIg	CD21	*bcl*-6	cyclin-D1	CD15	CD30	LCA	Oct2/BOB.1
Classic HD	–	–	–	–	–	–	±	–	+	+	–	–
LP-HD	+	–	–	–	±	FDC	+	–	–	–	+	+

+ Reed–Sternberg cells and variants are almost always positive
– Reed–Sternberg cells and variants are almost always negative
± Reed–Sternberg cells and variants positive in some cases
FDC positive in disrupted follicular dendritic cells

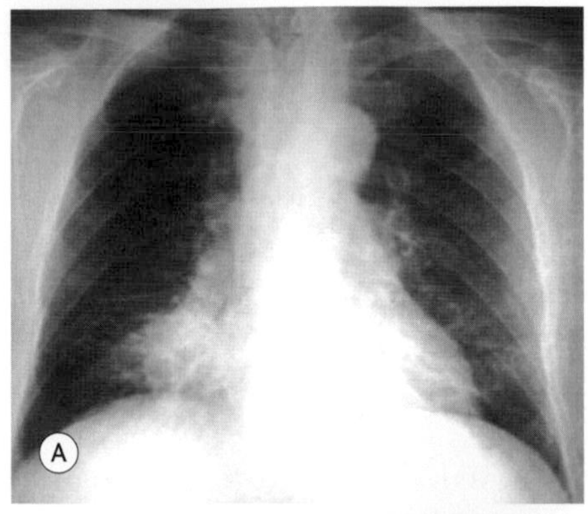

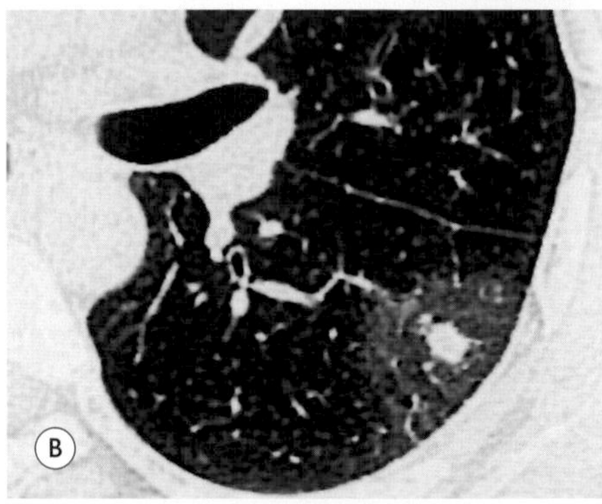

Fig. 15.78 (A) Intrapulmonary and mediastinal masses are present on this plain-film chest radiograph, in a case of extramedullary myeloid tumor (EMT; "granulocytic sarcoma") involving the lungs. (B) A vaguely defined peripheral nodule is seen in this computed tomogram of the lung, in another example of EMT.

and neoplastic (clonal) myeloid cells that exhibit only limited differentiation. By definition, they arise outside the bone marrow but usually develop during the course of systemic myeloproliferative diseases. The latter, in particular, are represented by the myelogenous leukemias, but they also include myelodysplasias and the "hypereosinophilic syndrome."[132–137] EMT may represent the initial manifestation of leukemia at a time when the marrow is still morphologically normal ("aleukemic leukemia");[138,139] in this circumstance, one observes a mass lesion in various locations, the symptoms of which typically relate to its mechanical presence in any given site. Peripheral myelogenous leukemia develops after variable time periods, but, in extraordinary cases, it may never appear. In other instances, EMTs represent a form of acute transformation of chronic myelogenous leukemia or relapses of treated acute leukemia.[132]

Demographic information associated with EMTs is superimposable on that attending myelogenous leukemia in general. The majority of patients with both of those conditions are adults, with a median age of 60 years at presentation, simply because non-lymphocytic leukemia is uncommon in pediatric practice. The overall incidence of EMT is estimated at 0.7 cases per million children in the general population per year, and 2.0 cases per million adults per year.[132]

Many examples of EMT arise in bones, but a significant proportion of cases occur elsewhere and virtually any visceral site – including the lungs[133,134] (Fig. 15.78) – may serve as host to tumefactive leukemic masses. Associated pulmonary symptoms and signs have included pleural effusions, chest pain, and cough.

EMT is most frequently misdiagnosed when this tumor develops in a patient who lacks pre-existing hematologic abnormalities. It may be confused microscopically with NHL, as well as undifferentiated carcinoma, rhabdomyosarcoma, Ewing's sarcoma, Langerhans cell disease, multiple myeloma, and benign inflammatory conditions, attesting to the variability of potential clinical and histologic presentations of this neoplasm.

Gross examination of excised EMTs reveals a distinctive macroscopic image that accounts for one of the earliest names for such lesions: namely, that of "chloroma." That designation relates to the greenish color that these tumors have when exposed to room air. This peculiar characteristic is explained by a pigmented greenish breakdown product of myeloperoxidase in the cells of EMTs. Otherwise, the gross appearance of EMT is indistinguishable from that of non-Hodgkin's lymphoma.

Histologically, three variants of EMT are recognized: blastic, "intermediate," and differentiated.[132] In the first of those, one observes sheets of anaplastic round or polyhedral cells that distort or efface the architecture of whichever tissue they colonize. The neoplastic elements generally have large vesicular nuclei (sometimes with cleaved or folded nuclear membranes), discernible nucleoli, and nondescript amphophilic or basophilic cytoplasm (Figs 15.79 and 15.80). Occasionally, one may observe scant scattered cells that demonstrate sparse cytoplasmic granulation. Background inflammatory cells in the blastic form of EMT are banal, usually comprising mature lymphocytes and histiocytes. This "hiatus" between the tumor cells and reactive elements may be a helpful clue to the non-lymphoid nature of the lesion in cases that are initially thought to represent lymphomas.

Compared with "blastic" variants of EMT, its intermediate subtype exhibits a more balanced mixture of myeloblastic and promyelocytic cells; some cases also show the rare presence of more differentiated granulocytes, particularly eosinophilic myelocytes. Differentiated tumors could be termed "promyelocytomas" because

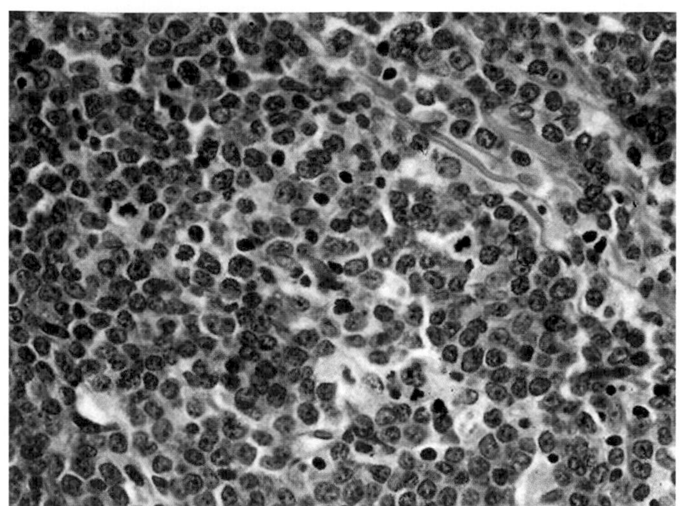

Fig. 15.79 Extramedullary myeloid tumor of the lung, represented by primitive lymphocyte-like cells with distinct nucleoli. The myeloid nature of the lesion is not obvious morphologically.

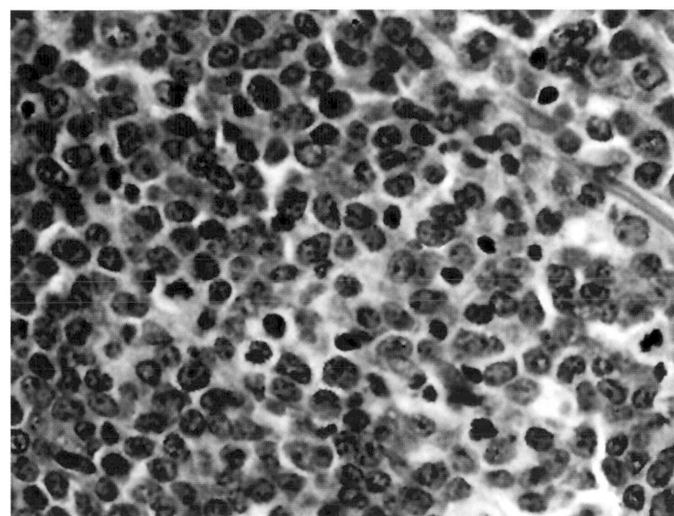

Fig. 15.80 Irregular nuclear contours, apoptotic figures, and numerous mitoses are apparent in this extramedullary myeloid tumor.

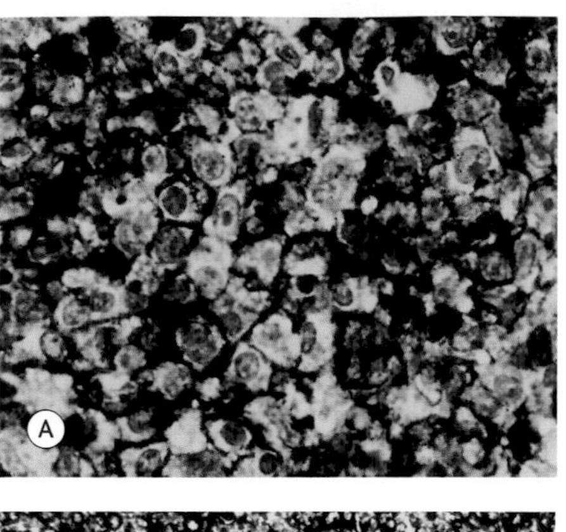

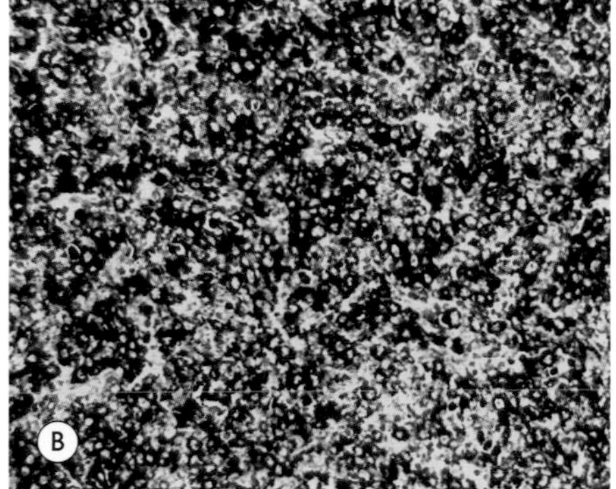

Fig. 15.81 (A) Immunoreactivity for CD43 and (B) myeloperoxidase is apparent in most cases of extramedullary myeloid tumor.

they show a preponderance of those cells, and granulated myelocytes are also easily found.

Ultimately, the definitive diagnosis of EMTs depends on the results of histochemical and immunohistologic studies. Histochemical methods that yield positivity in such lesions include the myeloperoxidase reaction, the naphthol–ASD–chloroacetate esterase (von Leder) technique, and the Sudan black B procedure. Air-dried cytologic smears are optimal for the application of these analyses, but the von Leder method (and, with lesser success, the benzidine technique) can also be applied to paraffin sections. It must be remembered that the enzymes being assessed are contained in primary myeloid granules; hence, the fewer of those structures the cells of any given EMT possess, the less likely they are to manifest histochemical positivity. Overall, we have seen reactivity with the von Leder stain in <30% of blastic EMTs; 30–50% of "intermediate" tumors; and >50% of differentiated lesions.

Markers that yield immunoreactivity in the majority of EMT cases include lysozyme (muramidase), CD43, CD45, and myeloperoxidase (Fig. 15.81). Antibodies to CD15, CD34, CD68, CD117, neutrophil elastase, and MAC387 may also label myeloid leukemias but do so more variably or less intensely. The main problem in this context is that "myeloid" antibodies typically are not included in panels that are intended for lineage typing of presumed cases of lymphoma. Put another way, it would appear that CD45 reactivity in an "undifferentiated" malignant tumor seldom evokes a prospective consideration of the lesion under discussion here, despite the voluminous literature on EMT. Therefore, as sensitive as some "myeloid" antibodies may be for the recognition of granulocytic precursors, they may be of little practical use in this context because they are rarely employed.

Goldstein et al.[140] posited that staining patterns existed with commonly used "lymphoid" reagents which would allow informed observers to suspect a diagnosis of EMT. They further proposed that if this postulate proved to be true, knowledge of such phenotypes could be used to obtain a second tier of immunostains intended to recognize myeloid cells with more definition. Their results indicated a consistent lack of reactivity for CD20 and specific pan-T-cell markers in EMT, suggesting that a CD45+ tumor lacking reactivity for those determinants should be suspected of possibly representing an EMT, which is especially true if the tumor in question does express CD43.

In the circumstances just cited, one can then go on to apply appropriate "myeloid" or "myelomonocytic" markers to the further characterization of putative examples of EMT. In this specific context, immunoreactivity for either lysozyme or myeloperoxidase is both sensitive and specific for myeloid differentiation.[125,133] Further substantiation of a hematopoietic lineage can be obtained by adding antibodies to CD15, CD68, CD34, CD117, MAC387, neutrophil elastase, von Willebrand's factor, FLI-1, and glycophorin A in additional evaluations. If, on the other hand, all of those reagents produce no labeling of the tumor, it can safely be considered as a non-myeloid lymphoreticular neoplasm. The most common example of the latter would be a T-cell lymphoma expressing only CD45 and CD43.

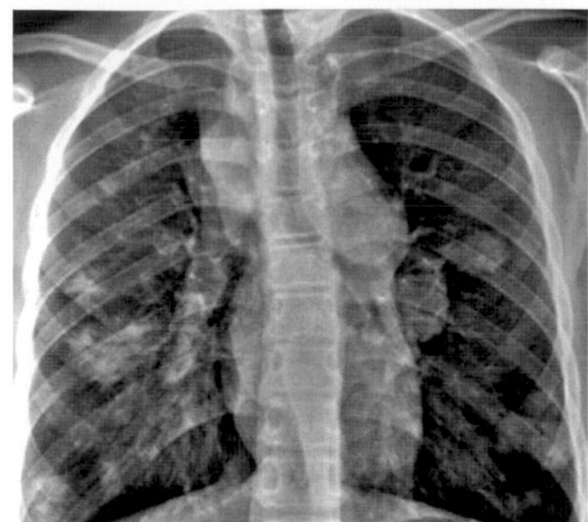

Fig. 15.82 Multiple intrapulmonary nodules and prominent intrathoracic lymphadenopathy are evident in this plain-film chest radiograph from a case of systemic Castleman's disease.

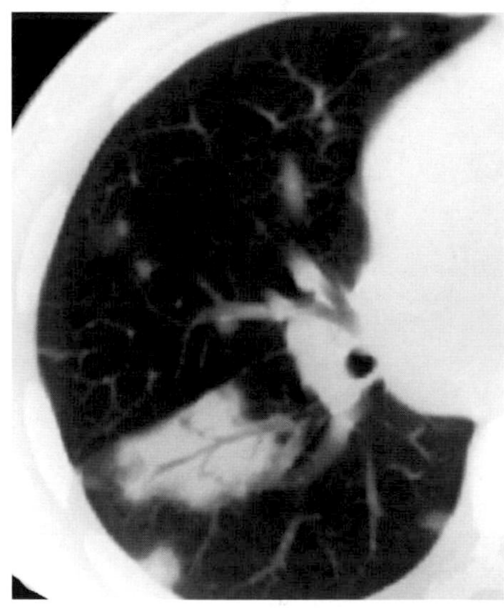

Fig. 15.83 This computed tomogram shows nodular intraparenchymal lesions in the right-lung field in another case of pulmonary Castleman's disease.

Castleman's disease

Castleman's disease – also known as angiofollicular lymphoid hyperplasia or giant lymph node hyperplasia – may rarely affect the lungs, either as part of a multiorgan-based proliferation[141–149] or as an isolated lesion.[150–152] Patients with pleuropulmonary involvement by disseminated disease of this type are typically young or middle-aged adults with mean age of 43 years; most have systemic symptoms and signs such as fever, anemia, weight loss, and malaise. Polyclonal hypergammaglobulinemia, elevations in the erythrocyte sedimentation rate, and hypoalbuminemia are also common, as is intrathoracic lymphadenopathy.[153]

On the other hand, reported individuals with unicentric (organ-limited) Castleman's disease of the lung have been asymptomatic.[150–152] Nodular intrapulmonary masses were discovered in those instances on radiographic studies as incidental findings, except for one case in which recurrent pleural effusion was also evident.[153]

Radiographs of the chest in patients with multicentric Castleman's disease (MCD) demonstrate intrathoracic lymph node enlargement with pleural or intrapulmonary nodules in most instances (Figs 15.82 and 15.83); cystic changes in the parenchyma and thickening of interlobular septa or bronchovascular bundles are also possible. Occasionally, subpleural nodules, ground glass attenuation of the parenchyma, airspace consolidation, or bronchiectasis may be observed.[142,143,148,154] Interstitial nephritis, secondary amyloidosis, and the POEMS syndrome – including *p*olyneuropathy, *o*rganomegaly, *e*ndocrinopathy, *m*onoclonal gammopathy, and *s*kin lesions (cutaneous glomeruloid hemangiomas) – has also been reported in association with MCD of the lung.[141,143]

The gross image of Castleman's disease is that of a tan-gray mass with variable degrees of internal vascularity

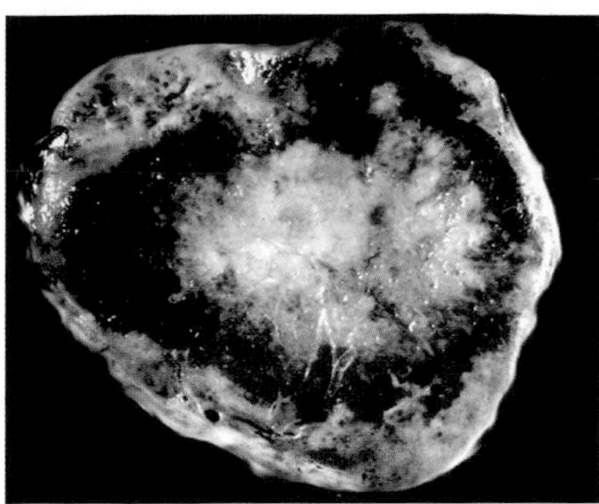

Fig. 15.84 Gross photograph of Castleman's disease, showing a tan-pink nodular lesion with obvious internal vascularity.

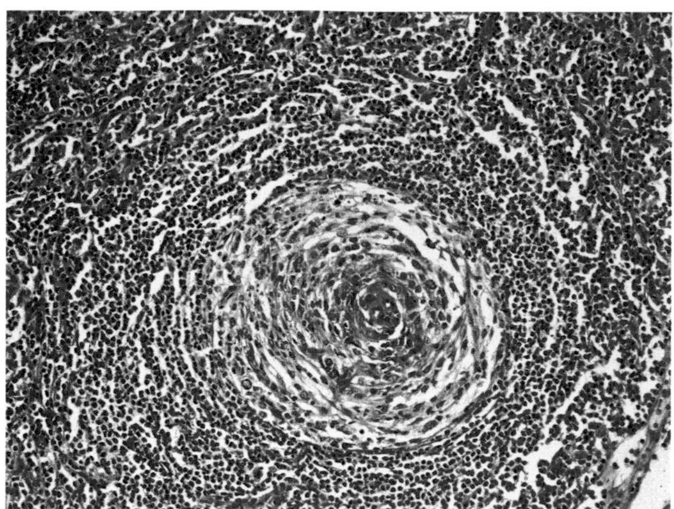

Fig. 15.86 Concentric arrays of small lymphoid cells surround distorted germinal center-like structures (GCLS) in Castleman's disease. The central aspects of the GCLS contain prominent blood vessels.

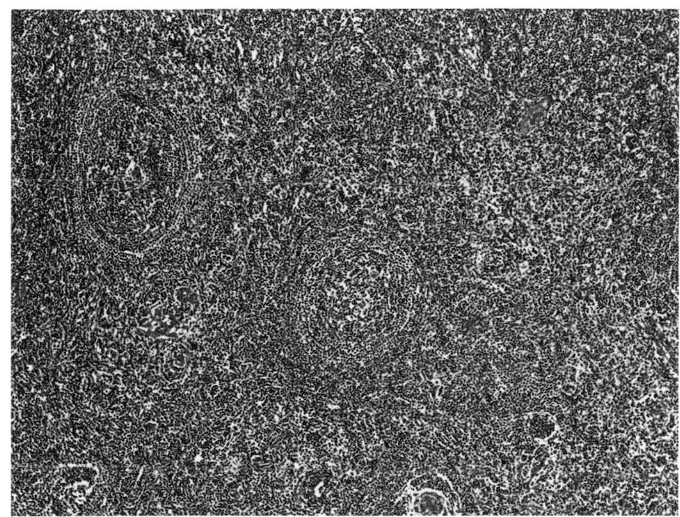

Fig. 15.85 The scanning microscopic image of Castleman's disease features the presence of closely set follicular structures having prominent lymphoid mantles. The appearance is similar to that of progressive germinal transformation of lymph nodes.

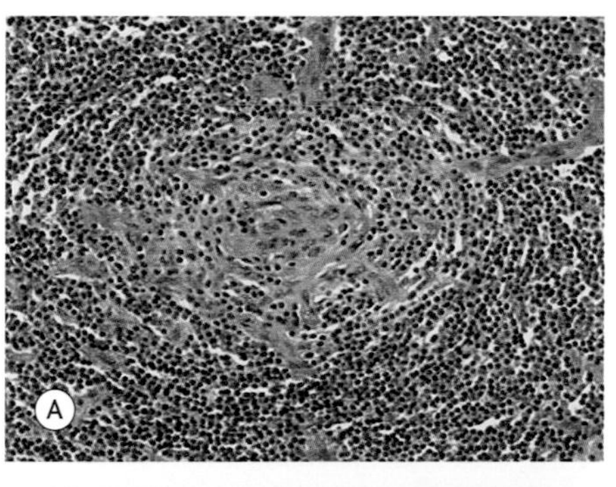

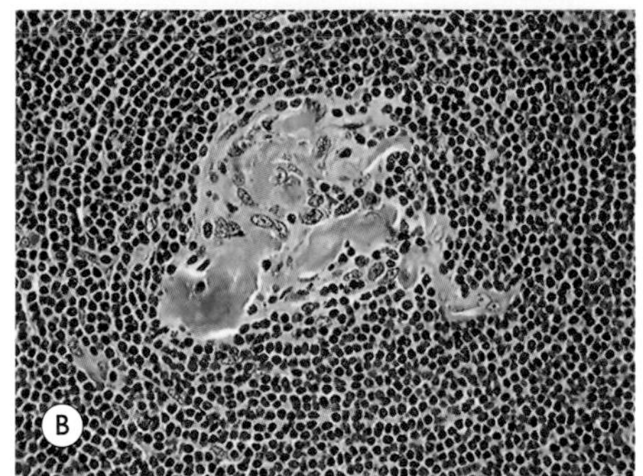

Fig. 15.87 (A) Vascular proliferation and (B) hyalinization are easily seen in the germinal center-like structures of hyaline-vascular type Castleman's disease.

(Fig. 15.84). Histologically, two subtypes of Castleman's disease have been delineated: the hyaline-vascular form and the plasmacellular variant. On scanning microscopy, both of these subtypes show an image that resembles progressive follicular transformation in lymph nodes (Fig. 15.85). Follicular aggregates of lymphoid cells are surrounded by concentric ("onion skin") arrays of small lymphocytes – representing altered mantle zones – which merge with one another (Fig. 15.86). In hyaline-vascular Castleman's disease, the interfollicular areas of the proliferation may also contain scattered plasma cells, immunoblasts, and eosinophils. Central aspects of lesional follicles in that condition demonstrate a proliferation of small blood vessels with prominently hyalinized walls (Fig. 15.87), yielding an appearance which sometimes has been likened to that of a miniature lollipop. Micro-aggregates of plump CD21+ follicular dendritic cells with vesicular nuclei (Fig. 15.88) may also be seen in the follicles.

Plasmacellular Castleman's disease is typically the form that one observes in MCD affecting the lungs. It differs from the hyaline-vascular variant in exhibiting

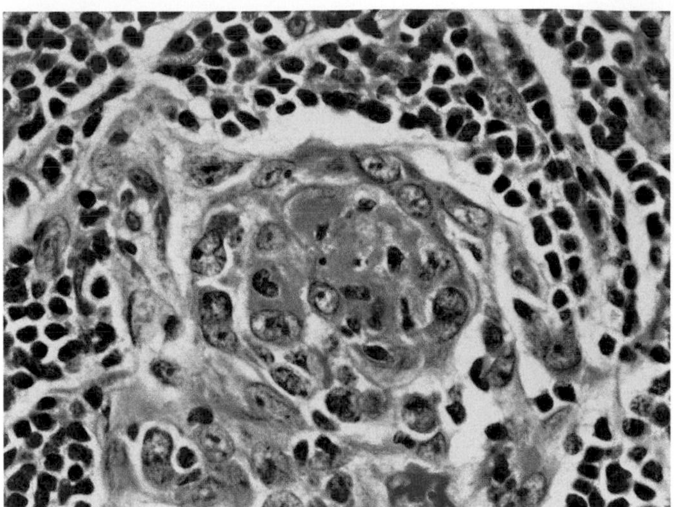

Fig. 15.88 Plump follicular dendritic cells are numerous in a germinal center-like structure in this example of Castleman's disease.

sheets of mature plasma cells between the transformed follicular structures (Fig. 15.89), together with numerous small blood vessels. No hyalinized vessels are apparent in the follicle centers. The plasma cells are usually polytypic for light-chain immunoglobulins immunohistochemically, but occasional cases may show monotypism for either lambda or kappa light-chain proteins. The lung parenchyma surrounding the lesions of plasmacellular Castleman's disease may also present the image of lymphoid interstitial pneumonia,[144] or it may demonstrate mature plasmacytic infiltrates.

Etiologically, Castleman's disease of the plasmacellular type may be linked to infection with human immunodeficiency virus,[155] human herpesvirus-8,[156] or Epstein–Barr virus.[157] Those agents can be detected best in the lesional tissue by using FISH or PCR. Some examples of the plasmacellular variant will also demonstrate clonal rearrangement of immunoglobulin heavy-chain genes or the T-cell-receptor genes.[151,158]

The prognosis of unicentric, lung-limited Castleman's disease is good, and simple excision of the mass is typically curative.[150–152] On the other hand, MCD has a much more guarded outlook.[149] It may persist for a long period of time, causing substantial morbidity. In addition, patients with that disorder have an increased risk of developing other neoplasms such as outright Hodgkin's or non-Hodgkin's lymphomas,[155,159,160] plasmacytomas,[155] and Kaposi's sarcoma.[155]

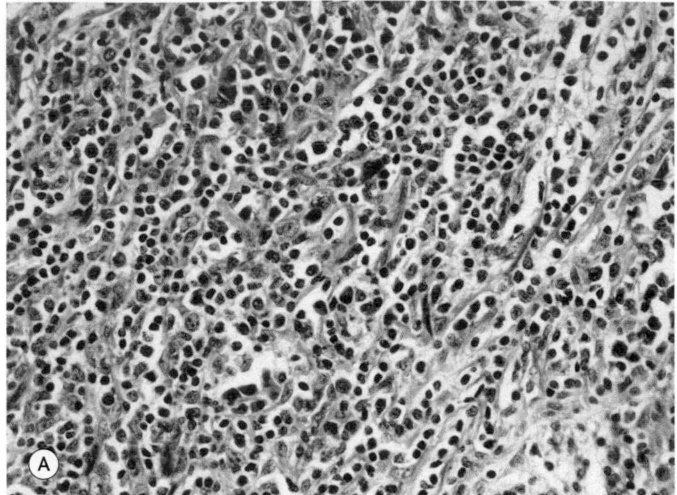

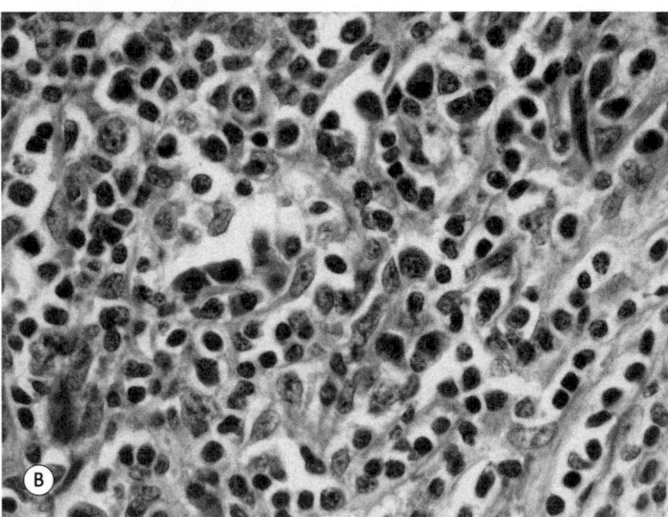

Fig. 15.89 (A,B) Sheets of mature plasma cells and lymphocytes separate the germinal center-like structures in cases of plasmacellular Castleman's disease. This variant is the most likely to be multicentric and to affect viscera such as the lungs.

REFERENCES

1. Colby TV, Yousem SA: Pulmonary histology for the surgical pathologist. Am J Surg Pathol 1988; 12: 223–239.
2. Kradin RL, Spririn PW, Mark EJ: Intrapulmonary lymph nodes. Chest 1985; 87: 662–667.
3. Gould SJ, Isaacson PG: Bronchus associated lymphoid tissue (BALT) in human fetal and infant lung. J Pathol 1993; 169: 229–234.
4. Bienstock J, Befus D: Gut and bronchus associated lymphoid tissue Am J Anat 1984; 170: 437–445.
5. Richmond I, Pritchard GE, Ashcroft T, et al.: Bronchus associated lymphoid tissue in human lung – its distribution in smokers and nonsmokers.Thorax 1993; 48: 1130–1134.
6. Harris NL: Extranodal lymphoid infiltrates and mucosa-associated lymphoid tissue: a unifying concept. Am J Surg Pathol 1991; 15: 879–884.
7. Isaacson PG, Norton AJ: Extranodal lymphomas. 1994, Churchill Livingstone, London.
8. Kurtin PJ: How do you distinguish benign from malignant extranodal small B cell proliferations? Am J Clin Pathol 1999; 111(Suppl 1): S119–S126.

9. Harris NL: Extranodal lymphoid infiltrates and mucosa associated lymphoid tissue (MALT). Am J Surg Pathol 1991; 15: 879–884.
10. Weiss LM, Yousem SA, Warnke RA: Non-Hodgkin's lymphomas of the lung. A study of 19 cases emphasizing the utility of frozen section immunologic studies in differential diagnosis. Am J Surg Pathol 1985; 9: 480–490.
11. Fuhr JE, Kattine AA, Sullivan TA. Nelson HS Jr: Flow cytometric analysis of pulmonary fluids and cells for the detection of malignancies. Am J Pathol 1992; 141: 211–215.
12. Jennings CD, Foon KA: Recent advances in flow cytometry: application to the diagnosis of hematologic malignancy. Blood 1997; 90: 2863–2892.
13. Zaer FS, Brayland RC, Aanxer DS, Iturraspe JA, Almasri NM: Multi-parametric flow cytometry in the diagnosis and characterization of low grade pulmonary mucosa-associated lymphoid tissue lymphomas. Mod Pathol 1998; 11: 525–532.
14. Nicholson AG, Wotherspoon AC, Diss C, et al.: Pulmonary B cell non-Hodgkin's lymphomas. The value of immunohistochemistry and gene analysis in diagnosis. Histopathology 1995; 26: 395–403.
15. Phillipe B, Delfau-Larue MH, Epardeau B, et al.: B cell pulmonary lymphoma: gene rearrangement analysis of bronchoalveolar lymphocytes by PCR. Chest 1999; 115: 1242–1247.
16. Schwaiger A, Prior C, Weyrer K, et al.: Non-Hodgkin's lymphoma of the lung diagnosed by gene rearrangement from bronchoalveolar lavage fluid: a fast and non-invasive method [Letter to the Editor]. Blood 1991; 77: 2538–2539.
17. Li G, Hansmann M-L, Zwingers , Lennert K: Primary lymphomas of the lung: morphological, immunohistochemical, and clinical features. Histopathology 1990; 16: 519–531.
18. Nicholson AG, Wotherspoon AC, Diss TC, et al.: Reactive pulmonary lymphoid disorders. Histopathology 1995; 26: 405–412.
19. Yousem SA: The pulmonary pathologic manifestations of the CREST syndrome. Hum Pathol 1990; 21: 467–474.
20. Yousem SA, Colby TV, Carrington CB: Follicular bronchitis – bronchiolitis. Hum Pathol 1985; 16: 700–706.
21. Kinnane BT, Mansell AL, Zwerdling RG, Lapey A, Shannon DC: Follicular bronchitis in the pediatric population. Chest 1993; 104: 1183–1186.
22. Kobzik L: Benign pulmonary lesions that may be misdiagnosed as malignant. Semin Diagn Pathol 1990; 7: 129–138.
23. Addis BJ, Hyjek E, Isaacson PG: Primary pulmonary lymphoma: a reappraisal of its histogenesis and its relationship to pseudolymphoma and lymphoid interstitial pneumonia. Histopathology 1988; 12: 1–17.
24. Kradin RL, Mark EJ: Benign lymphoid disorders of the lung with a theory regarding their development. Hum Pathol 1983; 14: 857–867.
25. Koss M, Hochholzer L, Nichols PW, Wehund WD, Lazarus AA: Primary non-Hodgkin's lymphoma and pseudolymphoma of the lung: a study of 161 patients. Hum Pathol 1983; 14: 1024–1038.
26. Abbondanzo SL, Rush W, Bijwaard KE, Koss MN: Nodular lymphoid hyperplasia of the lung: a clinicopathologic study of 14 cases. Am J Surg Pathol 2000; 24: 587–597.
27. Julsrud PR, Brown LR, Li CY, Rosenow EC III, Crowe JK: Pulmonary processes of mature-appearing lymphocytes: pseudolymphoma, well-differentiated lymphocytic lymphoma, and lymphocytic interstitial pneumonitis. Radiology 1978; 127: 289–296.
28. Thompson GP, Utz, JP, Rosenow EC, Meyers JL, Swensen SJ: Pulmonary lymphoproliferative disorders. Mayo Clin Proc 1993; 68: 804–817.
29. Blanco R, McLaren B, Davis B, Steele P, Smith R: Systemic lupus erythematosus-associated lymphoproliferative disorder: report of a case and discussion in light of the literature. Hum Pathol 1997; 28: 980–985.
30. Deheinzelin D, Capelozzi VL, Kairalla RA, et al.: Interstitial lung disease in primary Sjögren's syndrome. Clinical-pathological evaluation and response to treatment. Am J Respir Crit Care Med 1996; 154: 794–799.
31. Hansen LA, Prakash UBS, Colby TV: Pulmonary lymphoma in Sjögren's syndrome. Mayo Clin Proc 1989; 64: 920–931.
32. Begueret H, Vergier B, Parrens M, et al.: Primary lung small cell lymphoma versus lymphoid hyperplasia: evaluation of diagnostic criteria in 26 cases. Am J Surg Pathol 2002; 26: 76–81.
33. Marchevsky A, Rosen MJ, Chrystal G, Kleinerman J: Pulmonary complications of the acquired immunodeficiency syndrome: a clinicopathologic study of 70 cases. Hum Pathol 1985; 16: 659–670.
34. Reddy A, Lyall EG, Crawford DH: Epstein–Barr virus and lymphoid interstitial pneumonitis: an association revisited. Ped Infect Dis J 1998; 17: 82–83.
35. Meyers JL, Peiper SC, Katzenstein A-L: Pulmonary involvement in infectious mononucleosis: histopathologic features and detection of Epstein–Barr virus related DNA sequences. Mod Pathol 1989; 2: 444–448.
36. Sacco O, Fregonese B, Picco P, et al.: Common variable immunodeficiency presenting in a girl as lung infiltrates and mediastinal adenopathies leading to severe "superior vena cava" syndrome. Eur Resp J 1996; 9:1958–1961.
37. Fishback N, Koss M: Update on lymphoid interstitial pneumonitis. Curr Opin Pulm Med 1996; 2: 429–433.
38. Joshi VV, Oleske JM, Minnefor AB, et al.: Pathologic pulmonary findings in children with the acquired immunodeficiency syndrome: a study of ten cases. Hum Pathol 1985; 16: 241–246.
39. Joshi VV, Kauffman S, Oleske JM, et al.: Polyclonal polymorphic B-cell lymphoproliferative disorder with prominent pulmonary involvement in children with acquired immune deficiency syndrome. Cancer 1987; 59:1455–1462.
40. Joshi VV, Gagnon GA, Chadwick EG, et al.: The spectrum of mucosa-associated lymphoid tissue lesions in pediatric patients infected with HIV: a clinicopathologic study of six cases. Am J Clin Pathol 1997; 107: 592–600.
41. Koss MN: Pulmonary lymphoid disorders. Semin Diagn Pathol 1995; 12: 158–171.
42. Koss MN, Hochholzer L, Langloss JM, et al.: Lymphoid interstitial pneumonia: clinicopathologic and immunopathologic findings in 18 cases. Pathology 1987; 19: 178–185.
43. Herbert A, Walters MT, Cawley MID, Godfrey RC: Lymphocytic interstitial pneumonia identified as lymphoma of mucosa associated lymphoid tissue. J Pathol 1985; 146: 129–138.
44. Liebow AA, Carrington CB: Diffuse pulmonary lymphoreticular infiltrations associated with dysproteinemia. Med Clin North Am 1973; 57: 809–843.
45. Nicholson AG, Kim H, Corrin B, et al.: The value of classifying interstitial pneumonitis in childhood according to defined histological patterns. Histopathology 1998; 33: 203–211.
46. Teruya-Feldsein J, Temeck BK, Sloas MM, et al.: Pulmonary malignant lymphoma of mucosa associated lymphoid tissue in a pediatric HIV+ patient. Am J Surg Pathol 1995; 19: 357–363.
47. Zwerski S, Witebsky FG, Conville PS, Gill VJ, Freifeld AG: Fatal Nocardia pulmonary infection in a child with acquired immunodeficiency syndrome and lymphoid interstitial pneumonitis. Pediatr Infect Dis J 1997; 16: 1088–1089.
48. Burke JS: Are there site-specific differences among the MALT lymphomas – morphologic, clinical? Am J Clin Pathol 1999; 111 (Suppl 1): S133–S143.
49. Fiche M, Capron F, Berger F, et al.: Primary pulmonary non-Hodgkin's lymphomas. Histopathology 1995; 26: 529–537.
50. Habermann TM, Ryu JH, Inwards DJ, Kurtin PJ: Primary pulmonary lymphoma. Sem Oncol 1999; 26: 307–315.
51. Peterson H, Snider HL, Yam LT, et al.: Primary pulmonary lymphoma. Cancer 1985; 56: 805–813.
52. L'Hoste RJ, Fillipa DA, Leiberman PH, Bretsky S: Primary pulmonary lymphomas. Cancer 1984; 54: 1397–1406.
53. Rush WL, Andriko JA, Taubenberger JK, et al.: Primary anaplastic large cell lymphoma of the lung: a clinicopathologic study of five patients. Mod Pathol 2000; 13: 1285–1292.
54. Thieblemont C, Bastion Y, Berger F, et al.: Mucosa-associated lymphoid tissue gastrointestinal and nongastrointestinal lymphoma behavior: analysis of 108 patients. J Clin Oncol 1997; 15: 1624–1630.
55. Zinzani PL, Magagnoli M, Ascani S, et al.: Nongastrointestinal mucosa-associated lymphoid tissue (MALT) lymphomas: clinical and therapeutic features of 24 localized patients. Ann Oncol 1997; 8: 883–886.
56. Royer B, Cazals-Hatem D, Sibilia J, et al.: Lymphomas in patients with Sjögren's syndrome are marginal zone B-cell neoplasms, arise in diverse extranodal and nodal sites, and are not associated with viruses. Blood 1997; 90: 766–775.
57. Luppi M, Longo G, Ferrari MG, et al.: Additional neoplasms and HCV infection in low-grade lymphoma of MALT type. Br J Haem 1996; 94: 373–375.

58. Chow WH, Ducheine Y, Hilfer J, Brandstetter RD: Chronic pneumonia. Primary malignant non-Hodgkin's lymphoma of the lung arising in mucosa-associated lymphoid tissue. Chest 1996; 110: 838–840.
59. Elenitoba-Johnson K, Medeiros LJ, Khorsand J, King TC: Lymphoma of the mucosa-associated lymphoid tissue of the lung. A multifocal case of common clonal origin. Am J Clin Pathol 1995;103: 341–345.
60. O'Donnell PG, Jackson SA, Tung KT, et al.: Radiological appearances of lymphomas arising from mucosa-associated lymphoid tissue (MALT) in the lung. Clin Radiol 1998; 53: 258–263.
61. Cordier JF, Chailleux E, Lauque D, et al.: Primary pulmonary lymphomas – a clinical study of 70 cases in non-immunocompromised patients. Chest 1993; 103: 201–208.
62. Harris NL, Isaacson PG: What are the criteria for distinguishing MALT from non-MALT lymphomas at extranodal sites? Am J Clin Pathol 1999; 111 (Suppl 1) S126-S132.
63. Hussong JW. Perkins SL. Schnitzer B. Hargreaves H. Frizzera G. Extramedullary plasmacytoma. A form of marginal zone cell lymphoma? Am J Clin Pathol 1999; 111: 111–116.
64. Prasad ML, Charney DA, Sarlin J, Keller SM: Pulmonary immunocytoma with massive crystal storing histiocytosis: a case report with review of literature. Am J Surg Pathol 1998; 22: 1148–1153.
65. Isaacson PG, Wotherspoon AC, Diss T, Pan LX: Follicular colonization in B cell lymphoma of mucosa associated lymphoid tissue. Am J Surg Pathol 1991; 819–828.
66. Chetty R, Close PM, Timme AH, et al.: Primary biphasic lymphoplasmacytic lymphoma of the lung. A mucosa associated lymphoid tissue lymphoma with compartmentalization of plasma cells in the lung and lymph node. Cancer 1992; 69: 1124–1129
67. Jaffe ES, Harris NL, Stein H, Vardiman JW (Eds): Pathology and genetics: WHO classification of tumours of hematopoeitic and lymphoid tissue. 2001, IARC Press, Geneva.
68. Kurtin PJ, Myers JL, Adlakha H, et al.: Pathologic and clinical features of primary pulmonary extranodal marginal zone B-cell lymphoma of MALT type. Am J Surg Pathol 2001; 25: 997–1008.
69. Okabe M, Inagaki H, Ohshima K, et al.: API2-MALT1 fusion defines a distinctive clinico-pathologic subtype in pulmonary extranodal marginal zone B cell lymphoma of mucosa-associated lymphoid tissue. Am J Pathol 2003; 162: 1113–1122.
70. Kraus MD, Jones DM, Bartlett NL: Angiotrophic lymphoma and endocrinopathy: a report of four cases and a review of the literature. Am J Med 1999; 107: 169–176.
71. Chittal SM, Brousset P, Voigt J-J, DelSol G: Large B-cell lymphoma rich in T-cells and simulating Hodgkin's disease. Histopathology 1991; 19: 211–220.
72. De Wolf-Peetes, Pittaluga S: T cell rich B cell lymphoma a morphologic variant of a variety of non-Hodgkin's lymphomas or a clinicopathologic entity? Histopathology 1995; 26: 383–385.
73. Brousset P, Chittal SM, Schlaifer D, DelSol: T-cell-rich B-cell lymphoma in the lung. Histopathology 1995; 26: 371–373.
74. Rudiger T, Ott G, Ott MM, Muller-Deubert SM, Muller-Hermelink HK: Differential diagnosis between classic Hodgkin's lymphoma, T cell rich B cell lymphoma, and paragranuloma by paraffin immunohistochemistry. Am J Surg Pathol 1998; 22: 1184–1191.
75. Delabie J, Vandenberghe E, Kennes C, et al.: Histiocyte-rich B-cell lymphoma. Am J Surg Pathol 1992; 16: 37–48.
76. Amin R: Extramedullary plasmacytoma of the lung. Cancer 1985; 56: 152–156.
77. Kazzaz B, Dewar A, Corrin B: An unusual pulmonary plasmacytoma. Histopathology 1992; 21: 285–287.
78. Morinaga S, Watanabe H, Gemma A, et al.: Plasmacytoma of the lung associated with nodular deposits of immunoglobulin. Am J Surg Pathol 1987; 11: 989–995.
79. Dacic S, Colby TV, Yousem SA: Nodular amyloidoma and primary pulmonary lymphoma with amyloid production: a differential diagnostic problem. Mod Pathol 2000; 12: 934–940.
80. Danon AD, Krishnan J, Frizzera G: Morpho-immunophenotypic diversity of Castleman's disease, hyaline-vascular type: with emphasis on a stroma-rich variant and a new pathogenetic hypothesis. Virchows Arch 1993; 423; 369–382.
81. Lebeau A, Zeindl-Eberhart E, Muller EC, et al. Generalized crystal-storing histiocytosis associated with monoclonal gammopathy: molecular analysis of a disorder with rapid clinical course and review of the literature. Blood 2002; 100: 1817–1827
82. Jones D, Bhatia VK, Krausz T, Pinkus GS: Crystal-storing histiocytosis: a disorder occurring in plasmacytic tumors expressing immunoglobulin kappa light chain. Hum Pathol 1999; 30: 1441–1448.
83. Prasad ML, Charney DA, Sarlin J, Keller SM: Pulmonary immunocytoma with massive crystal storing histiocytosis: a case report with review of literature. Am J Surg Pathol 1998; 22: 1148–1153.
84. Guinee D, Jaffe E, Kingma D, et al.: Pulmonary lymphomatoid granulomatosis – evidence for a proliferation of Epstein–Barr virus infected B-lymphocytes with a prominent T-cell component and vasculitis. Am J Surg Pathol 1994; 18: 753–764.
85. Wilson WH, Kingma DW, Raffeld M, Wittes RE, Jaffe ES: Association of lymphomatoid granulomatosis with Epstein–Barr viral infection of B-lymphocytes and response to interferon alpha 2b. Blood 1996; 87: 4531–4537.
86. Nicholson AG, Wotherspoon AC, Diss TC, et al.: Lymphomatoid granulomatosis: evidence that some cases represent Epstein–Barr virus-associated B-cell lymphoma. Histopathology 1996; 29: 317–324.
87. Koss MN, Hochholzer L, Langloss JM, Wehunt WD, Lazarus AA: Lymphomatoid granulomatosis: a clinicopathologic and immunopathologic study of 42 patients. Pathology 1986; 18: 283–288.
88. Meyers JL, Kurtin PJ, Katzenstein ALA, et al.: Lymphomatoid granulomatosis: evidence of immunophenotypic diversity and relationship to Epstein–Barr virus infection. Am J Surg Pathol 1995; 19: 1300–1312.
89. Guinee DG, Perkins SL, Travis WD, et al.: Proliferation and cellular phenotype in lymphomatoid granulomatosis: implications of a higher proliferation index in B cells. Am J Surg Pathol 1998; 22: 1093–1100.
90. Katzenstein AL, Carrington G, Liebow AA: Lymphomatoid granulomatosis: a clinicopathologic study of 152 cases. Cancer 1979; 43: 360–373.
91. Randhawa PS, Yousem SA, Paradis IL, et al.: The clinical spectrum, pathology and clonal analysis of Epstein–Barr virus-associated lymphoproliferative disorders in heart–lung transplant recipients. Am J Clin Pathol 1989; 92: 177–185.
92. Harris NL, Ferry JA, Swerdlow SH: Post-transplant lymphoproliferative disorders: summary of Society for Hematopathology workshop. Semin Diagn Pathol 1997; 14: 8–14.
93. Chadburn A, Suciu-Foca N, Cesarman E, et al.: Post-transplantation lymphoproliferative disorders arising in solid organ transplant recipients are usually of recipient origin. Am J Pathol 1995; 147: 1862–1870.
94. Frizzera G, Hanto DW, Gajl-Peczalska KJ, et al.: Polymorphic diffuse B-cell hyperplasias and lymphomas in renal transplant recipients. Cancer Res 1981; 41: 4262–4279.
95. Swerdlow SH: Post-transplant lymphoproliferative disorders: a working classification. Curr Diagn Pathol 1997; 4: 28–36.
96. Knowles DM, Cesarman E, Chadburn A, et al.: Correlative morphologic and molecular genetic analysis demonstrates three distinct categories of posttransplantation lymphoproliferative disorders. Blood 1995; 85: 552–565.
97. Chadburn A, Chen JM, Hsu DT, et al.: The morphologic and molecular genetic categories of posttransplantation lymphoproliferative disorders are clinically relevant. Cancer 1998; 82: 1978–1987.
98. Chadburn A, Cesarman E, Knowles DM: Molecular pathology of posttransplantation lymphoproliferative disorders. Semin Diagn Pathol 1997; 14: 15–26.
99. Steurer M, Stauder R, Grunewald K, et al.: Hepatosplenic gamma delta-T-cell lymphoma with leukemic course after renal transplantation. Hum Pathol 2002; 33: 253–258.
100. Close PM, Macrae MB, Hammad JM, et al.: Anaplastic large cell Ki-1 lymphoma: pulmonary presentation mimicking tuberculosis. Am J Clin Pathol 1993; 99: 631–636.
101. Armitage JO: The non-Hodgkin's lymphoma classification project: a clinical evaluation of the International Lymphoma Study Group classification of non-Hodgkin's lymphoma. Blood 1997; 89: 3909–3918.
102. Chott A, Kaserer K, Augustin I, et al.: Ki-1-positive large cell lymphoma. A clinicopathologic study of 41 cases. Am J Surg Pathol 1998; 14: 439–448.
103. Chadburn A, Cesarman E, Jagirdar J, et al.: CD30 (Ki-1) positive anaplastic large cell lymphomas in individuals infected with the human immunodeficiency virus. Cancer 1993; 72: 3078–3090.
104. Harris NJ, Jaffe ES, Stein H, et al.: A revised European–American classification of lymphoid neoplasms: a proposal from the International Lymphoma Study Group. Blood 1994; 84: 1361–1392.

105. Armitage JO, Weisenburger DD, for the Non Hodgkin's Lymphoma Classification Project: New approach to classify non-Hodgkin's lymphomas: clinical features of the major histologic subtypes. J Clin Oncol 1998; 16: 2780–2795.
106. Hollowood K, Pease C, Mackay AM, Fletcher CDM: Sarcomatoid tumors of lymph nodes showing follicular dendritic cell differentiation. J Pathol 1991; 163: 205–216.
107. Fonseca R, Yamakawa M, Nakamura S, et al.: Follicular dendritic cell sarcoma and interdigitating reticulum cell sarcoma: a review. Am J Hematol 1998; 59: 161–167.
108. Perez-Ordonez B, Rosai J: Follicular dendritic cell tumor: review of the entity. Semin Diagn Pathol 1998; 15: 144–154.
109. Chan JKC, Fletcher CDM, Nayler SJ, Cooper K: Follicular dendritic cell sarcoma: clinicopathologic analysis of 17 cases suggesting a malignant potential higher than currently recognized. Cancer 1997; 79: 294–313.
110. Perez-Ordonez B, Erlandson RA, Rosai J: Follicular dendritic cell tumor: report of 13 additional cases of a distinctive entity. Am J Surg Pathol 1996; 20: 944–955.
111. Choi PC, To KF, Lai FM, et al.: Follicular dendritic cell sarcoma of the neck: report of two cases complicated by pulmonary metastases. Cancer 2000; 89: 664–672.
112. Shah RN, Ozden O, Yeldandi A, et al.: Follicular dendritic cell tumor presenting in the lung: a case report. Hum Pathol 2001; 32: 745–749.
113. Warnke RA, Weiss LM, Chan JKC, Cleary ML, Dorfman RF: Tumors of the lymph nodes and spleen. In: Atlas of tumor pathology, Fascicle 14, 3rd Series, Armed Forces Institute of Pathology. 1995, American Registry of Pathology Press, Washington, DC.
114. Banks PM, Chan J, Cleary M, et al.: Mantle cell lymphoma: a proposal for unification of morphologic, immunologic, and molecular data. Am J Surg Pathol 1992; 16: 637–642.
115. Cheson BD, Bennet JM, Grever M, et al.: National Cancer Institute-sponsored working group for chronic lymphocytic leukemia: revised guidelines for diagnosis and treatment. Blood 1996; 12: 4990–4997.
116. Matutes E, Brito-Babapulle V, Swansbury J, et al.: Clinical and laboratory features of 78 cases of T-prolymphocytic leukemia. Blood 1991; 78: 3269–3274.
117. Frizzera G, Kaneko Y, Sakurai M: Angioimmunoblastic lymphadenopathy and related disorders: a retrospective look in search of definitions. Leukemia 1989, 3: 1–5.
118. Suchi T, Lennert K, Tu LY, et al.: Histopathology and immunohistochemistry of peripheral T cell lymphomas: a proposal for their classification. J Clin Pathol 1987; 40: 995–1015.
119. Pinkus GS, O'Hara CJ, Said JW: Peripheral/post-thymic T cell lymphomas: a spectrum of disease. Clinical, pathologic and immunologic features of 78 cases. Cancer 1990; 65: 971–998.
120. Picker LJ, Weiss LM, Medeiros LJ, Wood GS, Warnke RA: Immunophenotypic criteria for the diagnosis of non-Hodgkin's lymphomas. Am J Pathol 1987; 128: 181–201.
121. Arcaroli JJ, Dave BJ, Pickering DL, et al.: Is a duplication of 14q32 a new recurrent chromosomal alteration in B-cell non-Hodgkin lymphoma? Cancer Genet Cytogenet 1999; 113: 19–24.
122. Marafioti T, Hummel M, Anagnostopoulos I, et al.: Origin of nodular lymphocyte-predominant Hodgkin's disease from a clonal expansion of highly mutated germinal-centre B cells. N Engl J Med 1997; 337: 453–458.
123. Ohno T, Stribley JA, Gang Wu MA, et al.: Clonality in nodular lymphocyte-predominant Hodgkin's disease. N Engl J Med 1997; 337: 459–466.
124. Kern WGH, Crepeau AG, Jones JC: Primary Hodgkin's disease of the lung. Cancer 1961; 1151–1165.
125. Radin AI: Primary pulmonary Hodgkin's disease. Cancer 1990; 65: 550–563.
126. Yousem SA, Weiss LM, Colby TV: Primary pulmonary Hodgkin's disease: a clinicopathologic study of 15 cases. Cancer 1986; 57: 1217–1224.
127. Harper PG, Fisher C, McLennan K, Souhami RL: Presentation of Hodgkin's disease as an endobronchial lesions. Cancer 1984; 53: 147–150.
128. Harris NL: Hodgkin's lymphomas: classification, diagnosis, and grading. Semin Hematol 1999; 36: 220–232.
129. Bodis S, Kraus MD, Pinkus GS, et al.: Clinical presentation and outcome in lymphocyte predominance Hodgkin's disease. J Clin Oncol 1997; 15: 3060–3066.
130. Brousset P, Chittal SM, Schlafer D, Delsol G: T cell rich B cell large cell lymphoma in the lung. Histopathology 1995; 26; 371–373.
131. Kraus MD, Haley JC: Lymphocyte predominance Hodgkin's disease: the utility of bcl6 and CD57 in diagnosis and differential diagnosis. Am J Surg Pathol 2000; 24: 1068–1078.
132. Nappi O, Boscaino A, Wick MR: Extramedullary hematopoietic proliferations, extraosseous plasmacytomas, and ectopic splenic implants (splenosis). Semin Diagn Pathol 2003; 20: 338–356.
133. Takasugi JE, Godwin JD, Marglin SI, Petersdorf SH: Intrathoracic granulocytic sarcomas. J Thorac Imaging 1996; 11: 223–230.
134. Nieman RS, Barcos M, Berard C: Granulocytic sarcoma: a clinicopathologic study of 61 biopsied cases. Cancer 1981; 48: 426–437.
135. Wong KF, Chan JKC, Chan JC, Lam SY: Acute myeloid leukemia presenting as granulocytic sarcoma of the lung. Am J Hematol 1993; 43: 77–78.
136. Byrd JC, Edenfield WJ, Dow NS, Aylesworth C, Dawson N: Extramedullary myeloid cell tumors in myelodysplastic syndromes: not a true indication of impending acute myeloid leukemia. Leuk Lymphoma 1996; 21: 153–159.
137. Hicsonmez G, Cetin M, Yenicesu J, et al.: Evaluation of children with myelodysplastic syndromes: importance of extramedullary disease as a presenting symptom. Leuk Lymphoma 2000; 42 : 665–674.
138. Sisack MJ, Dunsmore K, Sidhu-Malik N: Granulocytic sarcoma in the absence of myeloid leukemia. J Am Acad Dermatol 1997; 37: 308–311.
139. Meis JM, Butler JJ, Osborne BM: Granulocytic sarcoma in non-leukemic patients. Cancer 1986; 58: 2697–2709.
140. Goldstein NS, Ritter JH, Argenyi ZB, et al.: Granulocytic sarcoma: potential diagnostic clues from immunostaining patterns seen with anti-lymphoid antibodies. Int J Surg Pathol 1995; 2: 199–206.
141. Iyonaga K, Ichikado K, Muranaka H, et al.: Multicentric Castleman's disease manifesting in the lung: clinical, radiographic, and pathologic findings and successful treatment with corticosteroid and cyclophosphamide. Intern Med 2003; 42: 182–186.
142. Buckley J, Shaw PJ, Cartledge JD, Miller RF: Multicentric plasma cell variant Castleman's disease mimicking intrapulmonary malignancy. Sex Transm Infect 2002; 78: 304–305.
143. Johkoh T, Muller NL, Ichikado K, et al.: Intrathoracic multicentric Castleman disease: CT findings in 12 patients. Radiology 1998; 209: 477–481.
144. Sato T, Wakabayashi Y, Hirasawa A, et al.: Multicentric Castleman's disease accompanied with both lymphoid interstitial pneumonia and interstitial nephritis. Jpn J Clin Hematol 1994; 35: 1322–1328.
145. Bragg DG, Chor PJ, Murray KA, Kjeldsberg CR: Lymphoproliferative disorders of the lung: histopathology, clinical manifestations, and imaging features. Am J Roentgenol 1994; 163: 273–281.
146. Pejaver RK, Watson AH: Castleman's disease. Respir Med 1994; 88: 309–311.
147. Epstein DM, Glickstein MF: Pulmonary lymphoproliferative disorders. Radiol Clin North Am 1989; 27: 1077–1084.
148. Glickstein MF, Kornstein MJ, Pietra GG, et al.: Nonlymphomatous lymphoid disorders of the lung. Am J Roentgenol 1986; 147: 227–237.
149. Frizzera G, Banks PM, Massarelli G, Rosai J: A systemic lymphoproliferative disorder with morphologic features of Castleman's disease: pathological findings in 15 patients. Am J Surg Pathol 1983; 7: 211–231.
150. Ferrozzi F, Tognini G, Spaggiari E, Pavone P: Focal Castleman's disease of the lung: MRI findings. Clin Imaging 2001; 25: 400–402.
151. Spedini C, Lombardi C, Lanzani G, Di Fabio D, Chiodera PL: Castleman's disease presenting as an asymptomatic solitary pulmonary nodule. Monaldi Arch Chest Dis 1995; 50: 363–365.
152. Joynt GH, Pantalony D: Angiofollicular lymph node hyperplasia of the lung simulating carcinoma: pseudolymphoma with inflammatory changes. Can J Surg 1975; 18: 536–541.
153. Awotedu AA, Otulana BA, Ukoli CO: Giant lymph node hyperplasia of the lung (Castleman's disease) associated with recurrent pleural effusion. Thorax 1990; 45: 775–776.
154. Ko SF, Ng SH, Hsieh MJ, et al.: Castleman disease of the pleura: experience with eight surgically-proven cases. Ann Thorac Surg 2003; 76: 219–224.
155. Oksenhendler E, Boulanger E, Galicier L, et al.: High incidence of Kaposi sarcoma-associated herpesvirus-related non-Hodgkin lymphoma in patients with HIV infection and multicentric Castlelman disease. Blood 2002; 99: 2331–2336.

156. Cathomas G: Human herpesvirus 8: a new virus discloses its face. Virchows Arch 2000; 436: 195–206.
157. Hanson CA, Frizzera G, Patton DF, et al.: Clonal rearrangement for immunoglobulin and T-cell-receptor genes in systemic Castleman's disease: association with Epstein–Barr virus. Am J Pathol 1988; 131: 84–91.
158. Hall PA, Donaghy M, Cotter FE, Stansfeld AG, Levison DA: An immunohistochemical and genotypic study of the plasma cell form of Castleman's disease. Histopathology 1989; 14: 333–346.
159. Caussinus E, Meggetto F, Delsol G, Brousset P: Simultaneous occurrence of Epstein–Barr virus associated Hodgkin's disease and HHV8-related multicentric Castleman's disease: a fortuitous event? J Clin Pathol 2001; 54: 790–791.
160. Molinie V, Perie G, Melo I, et al.: Association of Castleman's disease and Hodgkin's disease: eight cases and review of the literature. Ann Pathol 1994; 14: 384–391.

16

Non-neuroendocrine carcinomas (excluding "sarcomatoid" carcinoma) and salivary gland analogue tumors of the lung

Cesar A Moran   Kevin O Leslie   Mark R Wick

Carcinoma of the lung is a growing public health problem of worrisome proportions, not only in the United States but also on the international scene.[1–5] The American Cancer Society has estimated that over 170,000 new cases of lung cancer will be encountered each year in the United States in the foreseeable future. This unfortunate reality owes to the continuing use of cigarettes, cigars, and pipes by a significant fraction of the world population, and the now-undeniable causal relationship between inhaled tobacco smoke and pulmonary carcinoma.[1–7] To make matters even worse, it has been shown that persons who are in constant and close proximity to heavy smokers, either at home or in the workplace, inhale sufficient "sidestream" smoke to place them at definite risk of developing lung cancer even if they have never smoked themselves.[6,8,9] The pathogenetic influence of other potential etiologic agents (e.g. human papillomavirus, radon, and pneumoconiosis-related minerals) on pulmonary carcinogenesis also continues to undergo analysis.[3,10] Women now develop cancer of the lung on a rough numerical parity with men, and the mortality of that disease in both sexes is so high that it represents the leading worldwide cause of death related to malignancy.[2,5,6]

The goal of this chapter is to provide a summary of the pathologic features of recognized lung carcinoma morphotypes. In addition, specific issues relating to differential diagnosis and evolving conceptual topics will be considered. Difficult subjects are given a relatively disproportionate volume of space in the ensuing discussion, with concise treatment of those that are familiar to surgical pathologists. In the interest of conserving space, the results of several adjunctive pathologic techniques including electron microscopy, flow cytometry, genetic analysis, and morphometry will also not be discussed here.

The nosology of lung cancer and diagnostic effects of sampling methods

Seventy-five years ago, the first attempt at morphologic classification of lung cancer was undertaken by Marchesani (cited in Ref. 10). This scheme, outlining the now-classical categories of squamous cell carcinoma, adenocarcinoma, and small cell "undifferentiated" and large cell "undifferentiated" carcinomas, is still widely recognized and has gone through several iterations over the ensuing decades. In recent times, a pragmatic, clinically attuned movement has been enjoined wherein a more simplified system was embraced, dividing malignant epithelial tumors of the lung into "small cell" and "non-small cell" carcinomas. At the same time, research by pathologists has resulted in ever-greater refinement of morphologic categorization, and the interface between the practical needs of the operating suite and data generated in the clinical laboratory has therefore become problematic. In light of this situation, a prognostically oriented nosologic scheme for lung cancer was devised by the Veterans Administration Lung Group in 1991[11] it has since been modified by other organizations.

Whether any given pathologist elects to use one or another of these systems is a decision that should be made after consultation with clinical colleagues. In any event, non-standard designations for pulmonary carcinomas (i.e. those that are not sanctioned by the World Health Organization[10]) should be well-defined in surgical pathology reports, with pertinent references being provided in cases that are particularly uncommon or conceptually contentious.

A particular problem that must be recognized forthrightly by everyone involved in treating lung cancer is the common heterogeneity that it may demonstrate at a light microscopic level. The literature is now well-supplied with reports of admixtures of virtually all of the lung carcinoma histotypes with one another in the same tumor mass.[3,12,13] An analysis by Roggli and colleagues[14] demonstrated such heterogeneity in fully 66% of a consecutive series of lung cancers, and others have reported similar findings. This biologic diversity may attain prognostic importance in the future, particularly in light of recent work that appears to affirm the impact of histologic features on tumor evolution.[15] In any event, neoplastic heterogeneity is a practical diagnostic problem for surgeons and medical oncologists, because small biopsies will often fail to represent "divergent" tumor elements as a consequence of sampling bias. At a time when ever more limited methods of tissue procurement are being advanced, it is clear that substantial discrepancies will be observed between biopsy results and examination of resection specimens in the surgical pathology laboratory. That is not to imply that such techniques as fine-needle aspiration biopsy should not be used, because they are extremely helpful in planning therapy in many cases. Nonetheless, the potential limitations of *all* sampling procedures must be weighed carefully against their benefits.

Clinicopathologic features of non-neuroendocrine pulmonary carcinomas, excluding "sarcomatoid" carcinoma

Squamous cell carcinoma

Probably because of changes in the smoking habits of the public, with a greater preference for filtered cigarettes in the last 35 years,[7] squamous cell carcinoma (SCC) is no longer the most common type of lung cancer and has been eclipsed by adenocarcinoma in recent years.[13,16] However, SCC has retained its classical clinicopathologic attributes in those cases in which it is seen. These include a tendency for multifocal but clonal in-situ disease in the bronchial mucosa, often preceding the appearance of a discrete mass by several years, and a propensity to arise in large central airways that are proximal to the subsegmental bronchi. Because of the common presence of an endobronchial tumor mass, obstructive pneumonia is a relatively common accompaniment of this neoplasm, albeit by no means pathognomonic of it. "Pure" SCC may certainly take origin in the peripheral pulmonary parenchyma as well, and rare examples are even subpleural.[3]

Squamous cancer of the lung has an irregular, often friable, gray-white cut surface, commonly showing a large area of central necrosis, with or without cavitation (Fig. 16.1). The surrounding pulmonary parenchyma is frequently tethered to the mass, giving it a "spiculated" appearance that may be well seen on radiographic images. Microscopically, SCC is defined by its resemblance to stratified squamous epithelium of the upper airway, but with disordered architectural and cytologic maturation.

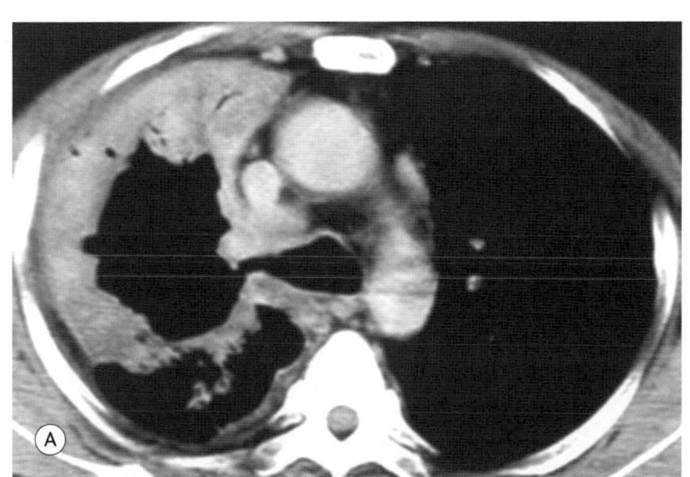

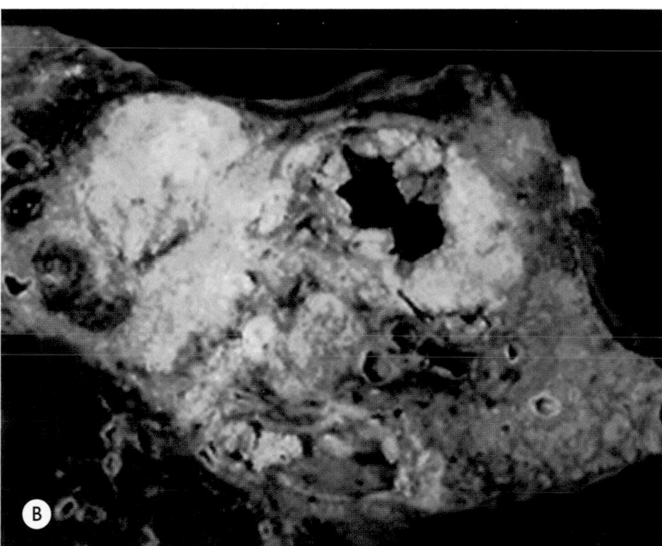

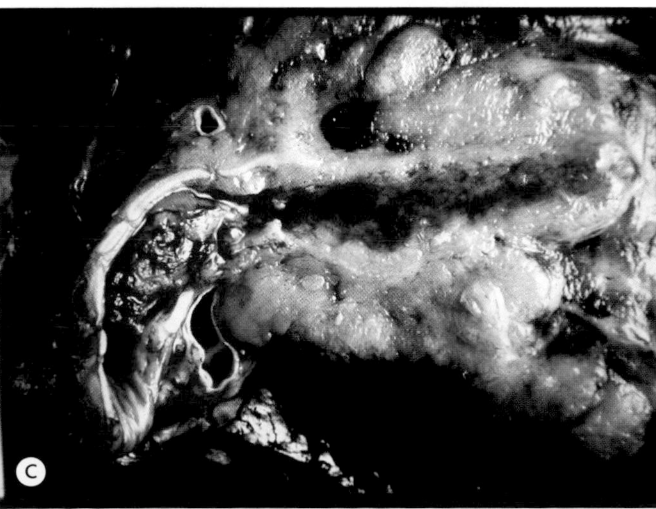

Fig. 16.1 (A) Thoracic computed tomogram showing a large centrally cavitary squamous cell carcinoma of the right lung. (B) Gross photograph of squamous cell carcinoma of the lung, demonstrating characteristic central necrotic cavitation. (C) Close-up view of another example of squamous cell carcinoma.

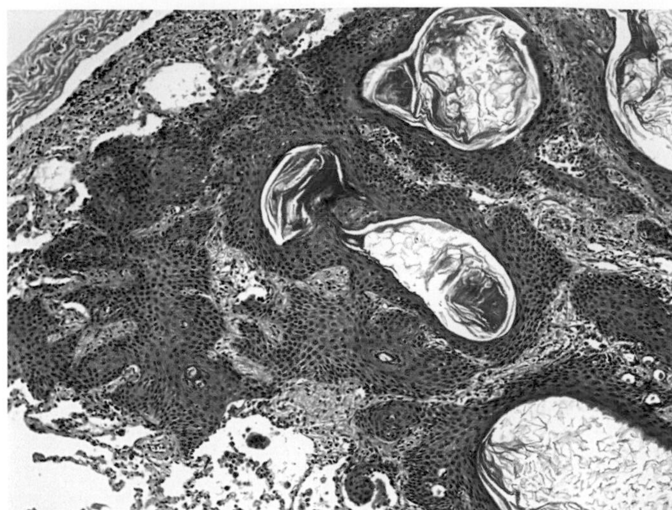

Fig. 16.2 Photomicrograph of well-differentiated squamous carcinoma, showing obvious keratinization.

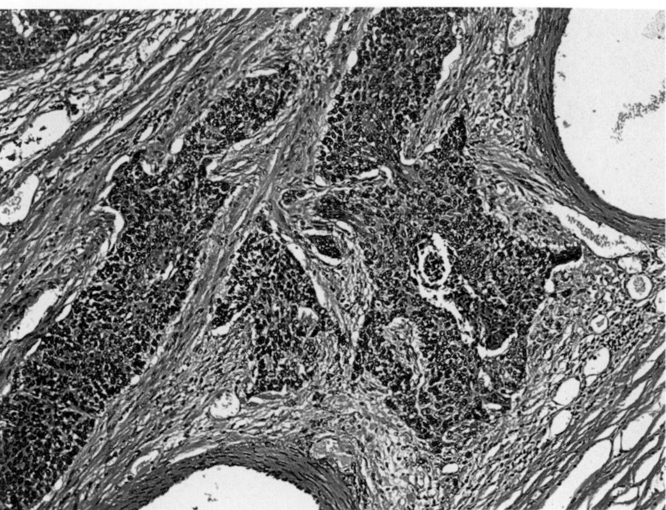

Fig. 16.4 Poorly differentiated squamous carcinoma showing only focal keratinization and a predominant composition by primitive epithelial cells.

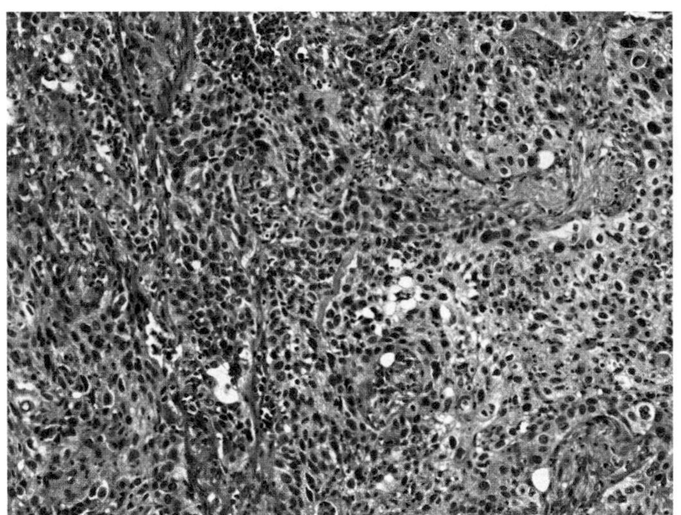

Fig. 16.3 Poorly differentiated squamous carcinoma comprising groups of relatively primitive polygonal cells, invading the soft tissue of the chest wall.

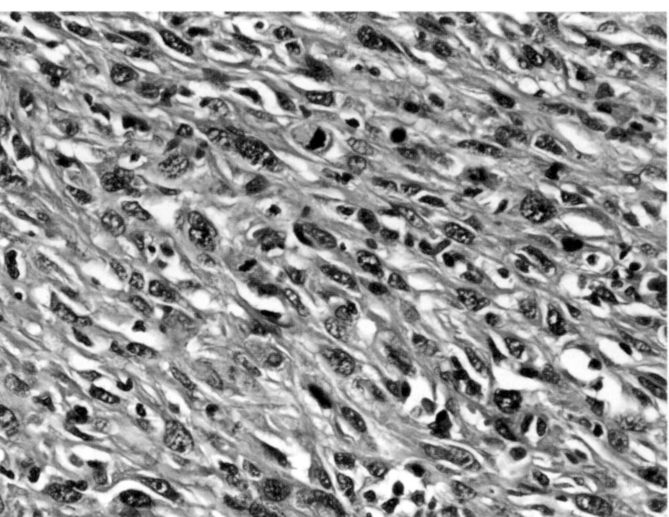

Fig. 16.5 Poorly differentiated pulmonary squamous carcinoma with sarcomatoid features, presenting difficulty in recognition of the lesion as epithelial in nature.

Anucleate keratin and squamous pearls are observed in only the better-differentiated of these lesions, which account for a minority of pulmonary carcinomas (Fig. 16.2). Poorly differentiated SCC (Figs 16.3–16.5) may be extremely difficult for the pathologist to distinguish from high-grade adenocarcinomas, small cell carcinomas, or large cell undifferentiated carcinomas, inasmuch as all of them commonly take the form of rather nondescript proliferations of primitive epithelioid cells of varying size, arranged in nests and sheets with no other distinguishing features. In the absence of special studies, one may have to use the default terminology of "poorly differentiated carcinoma, not further specified," in the frozen section laboratory and in reference to small biopsies of such lesions. Recognized and distinct subtypes of poorly differentiated SCC include spindle cell and pleo-

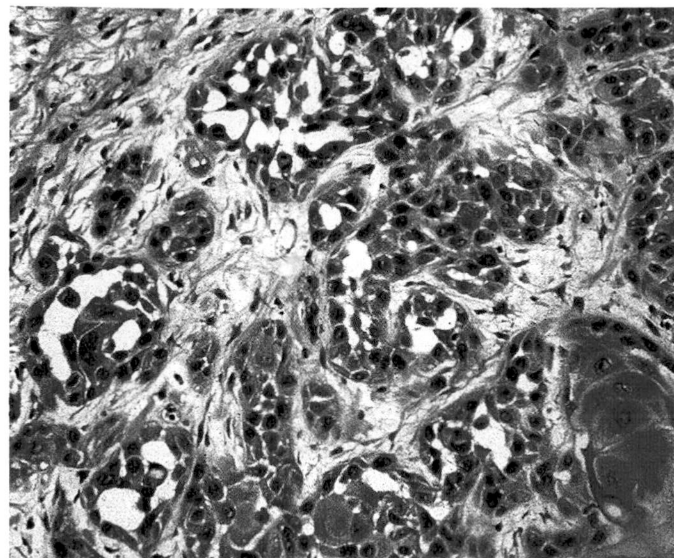

Fig. 16.6 Adenoid (pseudoglandular/acantholytic) squamous cell carcinoma of the lung, demonstrating dyshesion of the tumor cells in such a way that the lesion focally resembles a gland-forming neoplasm.

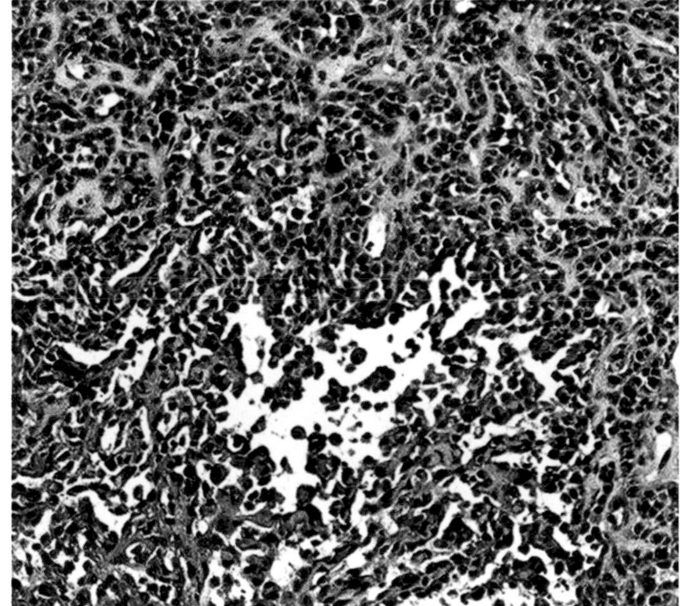

Fig. 16.7 This adenoid squamous cell carcinoma subtype is called "angiosarcoma-like" or "pseudovascular" because its particular version of intercellular dyshesion simulates the image of an endothelial malignancy.

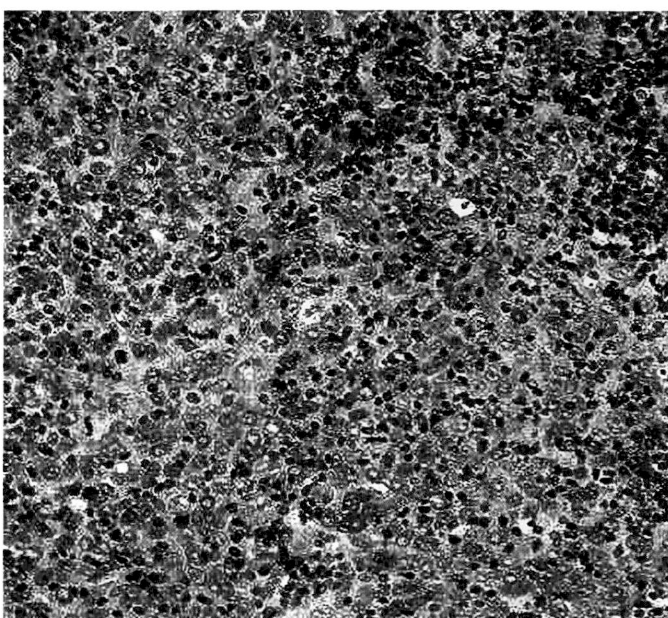

Fig. 16.8 Lymphoepithelioma-like squamous carcinoma of the lung, showing syncytia of polygonal neoplastic cells with vesicular nuclear chromatin and prominent nucleoli, which are interspersed with mature lymphocytes. This tumor variant is also considered a subtype of large cell undifferentiated carcinoma by some observers.

morphic forms[17] (see Ch. 14); adenoid (pseudoglandular) variants (Fig. 16.6);[18] a pseudovascular (angiosarcoma-like) subtype (Fig. 16.7);[18,19] "lymphoepithelioma-like" carcinoma (Fig. 16.8);[20] and a basaloid form (Fig. 16.9) ("small cell squamous carcinoma" or "basaloid squamous carcinoma")[21] that is analogous to primary poorly differentiated squamous carcinoma of the anorectum, hypopharynx, thymus, and other anatomic sites. Other than presenting special problems in microscopic differential diagnosis, these tumor variants have no singular clinical significance.

Adenocarcinoma

As stated earlier, adenocarcinoma (ACA) has now successfully eclipsed SCC as the most common form of monodifferentiated lung cancer. In North America and Europe, most ACAs are predominantly peripheral parenchymal masses; however, interestingly, histologically identical lesions in India and Asia are as likely to be central as peripheral in location. Grossly, ACA typically has an irregularly lobulated configuration, with a gray-white cut surface (Fig. 16.10). Anthracotic pigment is commonly entrapped in the tumor mass as well, but foci of necrosis and hemorrhage are seen only in large (>5 cm) lesions. A relationship to tubular airways is only rarely obvious. Close inspection may also demonstrate the presence of "satellitotic" nodules around the main tumor mass; in fact, however, this phenomenon may be a reflection of the tendency for pulmonary ACA to be synchronously or metachronously multifocal, either in

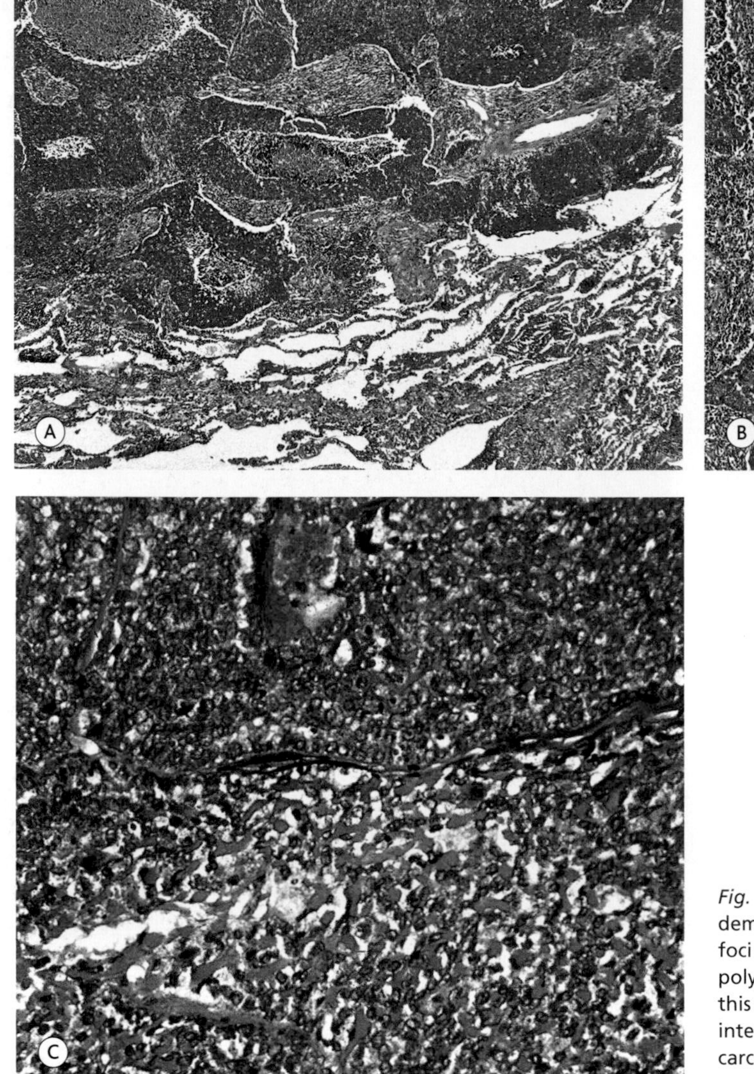

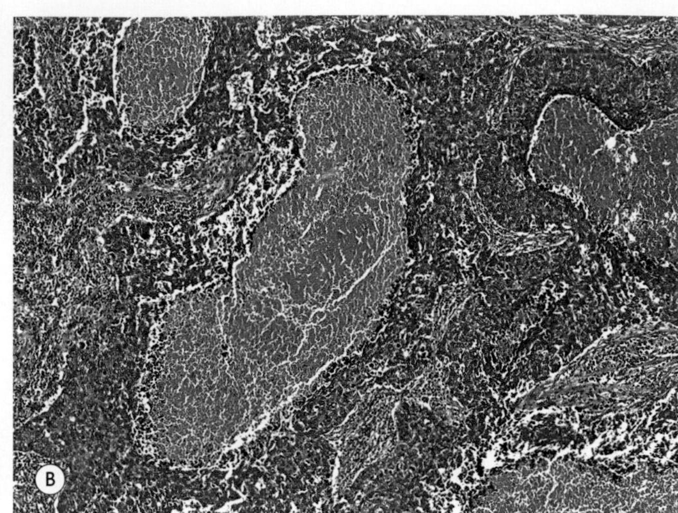

Fig. 16.9 (A) Basaloid squamous carcinoma of the lung, demonstrating a typically organoid growth pattern with prominent foci of geographic necrosis and a composition dominated by small polyhedral cells. (B) Zones of centrilobular necrosis are well seen in this image of basaloid squamous carcinoma. (C) Deposition of intercellular basal lamina is relatively common in basaloid squamous carcinoma, potentially causing confusion with such other tumor entities as adenoid cystic carcinoma.

one lobe of the lung or in both lungs. The latter statement applies particularly to a special subtype of ACA: namely, bronchioloalveolar carcinoma (BAC; see below). One peculiar and uncommon macroscopic presentation of pulmonary ACA that merits special mention is its "pseudomesotheliomatous" form, wherein the pleurotropic growth of extremely peripheral intrapulmonary tumors creates a "rind" of tumor tissue surrounding the lung (Fig. 16.11). This virtually perfectly simulates the appearance of mesothelioma, both intraoperatively and on radiographic imaging studies.[22–24]

Microscopically, there are four principal subtypes of pulmonary ACA:

- acinar (the most common, Fig. 16.12)
- papillary (Fig. 16.13)
- bronchioloalveolar (see below)
- solid (Fig. 16.14).[25]

However, additional variants exist, such as sarcomatoid (see Ch. 14); fetal (Fig. 16.15); well-differentiated mucinous ("colloid") (Fig. 16.16); signet-ring-cell (Fig. 16.17); clear cell (Fig. 16.18); and enteric (intestinal-like) (Fig. 16.19).[26–30] In some cases, because of the overlap between these histologic groups and the appearances of *metastatic* adenocarcinomas in the lung, it may be extremely difficult for the pathologist to separate primary from secondary lesions. This is particularly true of enteric and signet-ring-cell tumors, which can closely imitate the attributes of gastric or colorectal carcinomas (see Ch. 17).

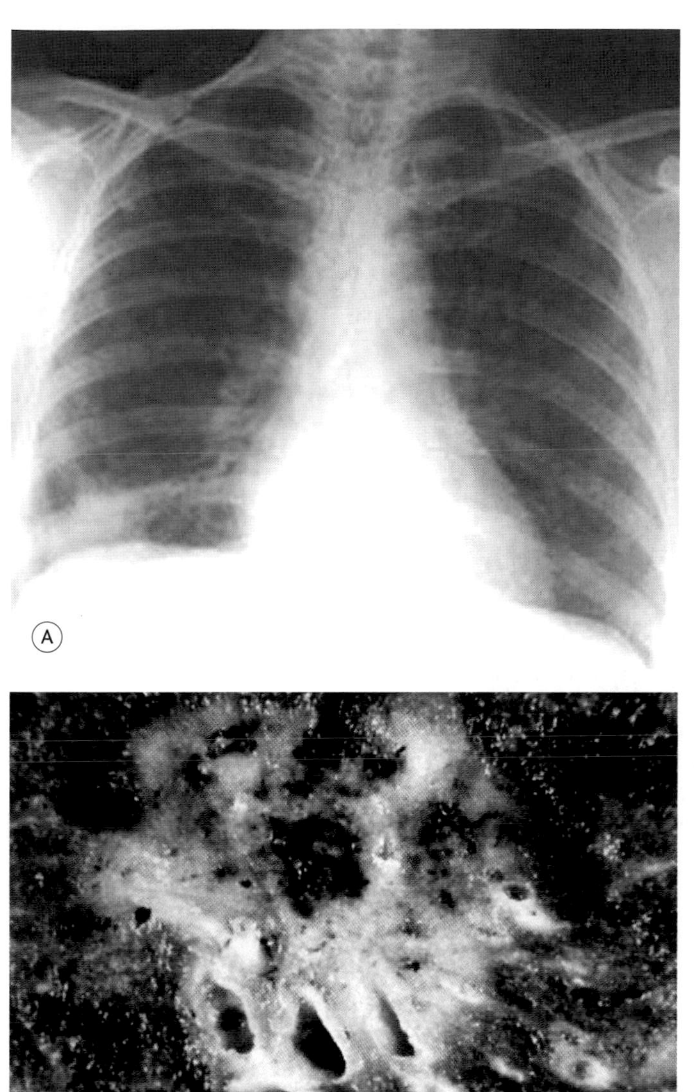

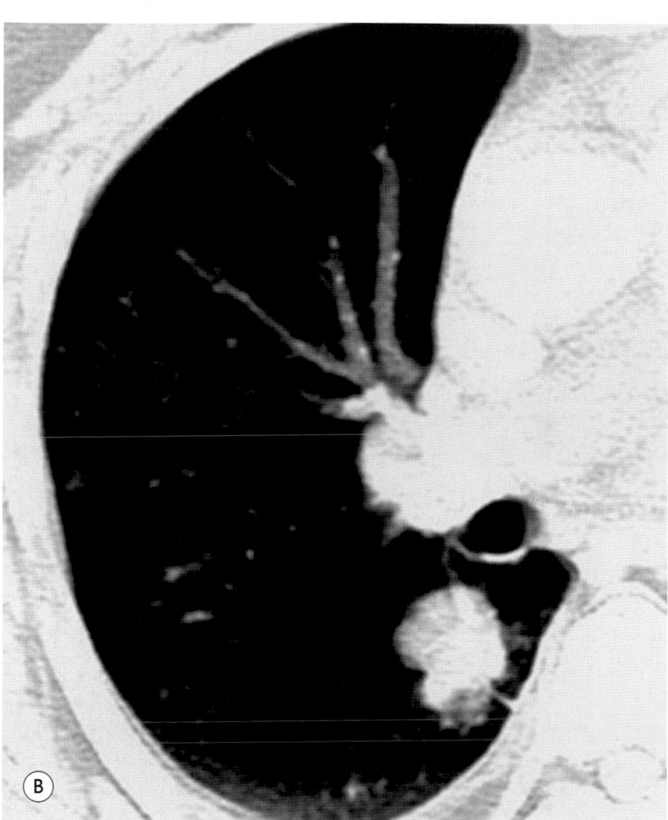

Fig. 16.10 (A) Plain-film chest radiograph showing a solitary peripheral nodular mass in the right lower lung field, representing primary adenocarcinoma. (B) This computed tomograph from another case of primary pulmonary adenocarcinoma shows a "spiculated" mass in the right lung field. (C) A gross photograph of resected pulmonary adenocarcinoma demonstrates the irregular ("spiculated") periphery of the lesion and foci of entrapped anthracotic pigment.

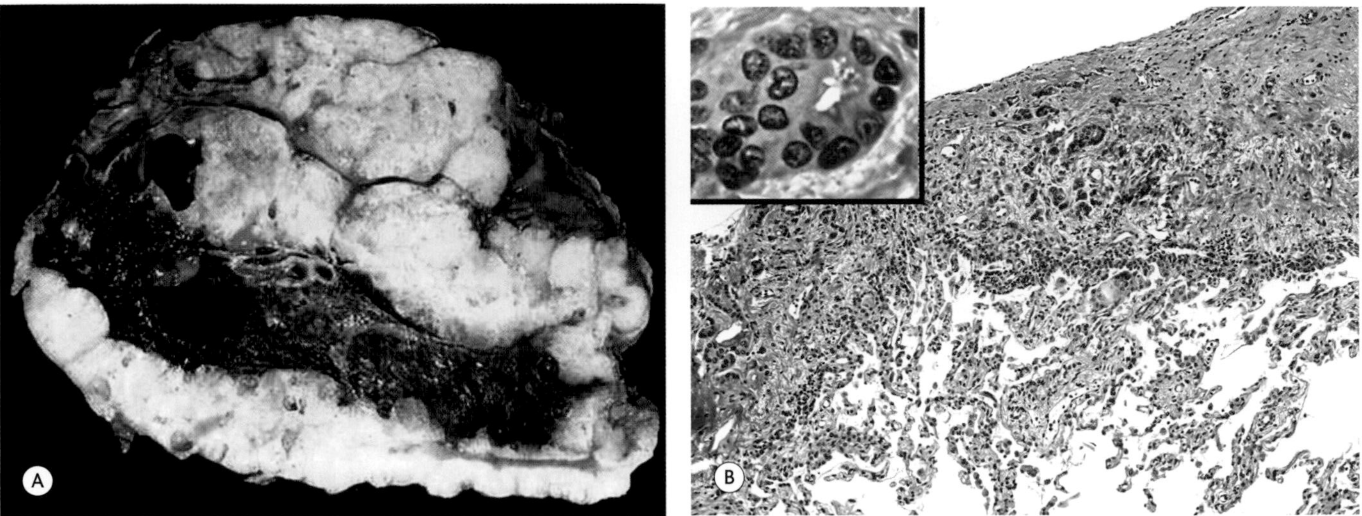

Fig. 16.11 (A) This gross photograph of a "pseudomesotheliomatous" (pleurotropic) adenocarcinoma of the lung shows a neoplasm that encompasses the lung parenchyma, yielding a macroscopic image which is identical to that of true mesothelioma. (B) Glandular arrays of tumor cells are present in the pleura in the absence of a definable intraparenchymal lesion, in "pseudomesotheliomatous" adenocarcinoma of the lung. (B [inset]) High magnification view of an infiltrating malignant gland in pleurotropic adenocarcinoma.

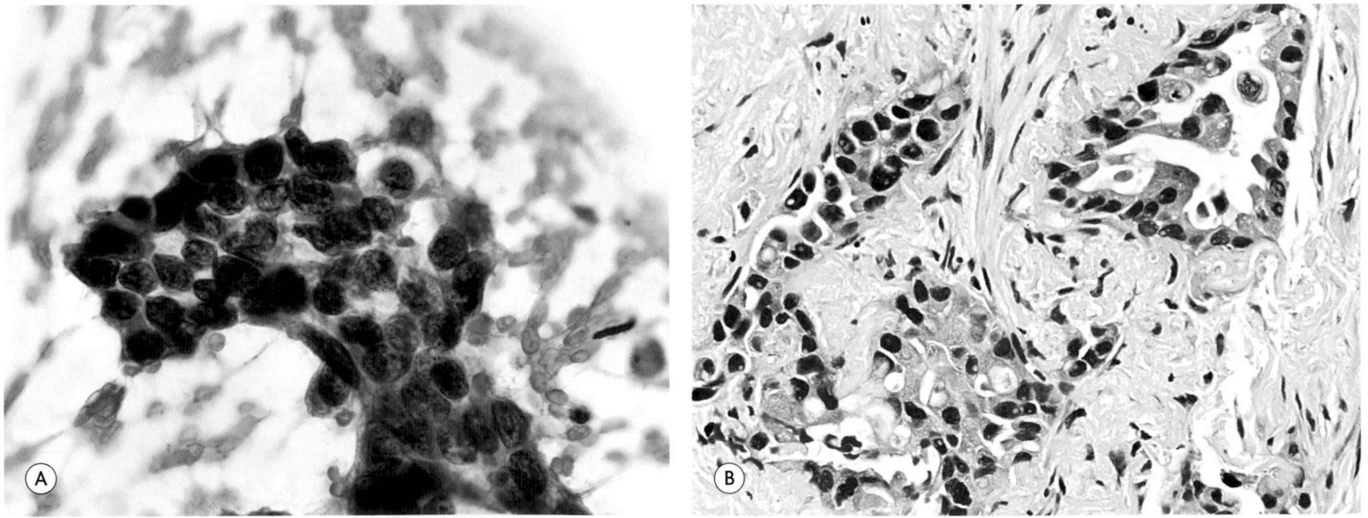

Fig. 16.12 (A) A fine-needle aspiration specimen from acinar-type primary adenocarcinoma of the lung shows a three-dimensional cell group comprising atypical polygonal cells with prominent nucleoli. (B) This well-differentiated acinar (usual-type) adenocarcinoma of the lung demonstrates easily seen formation of glandular lumina.

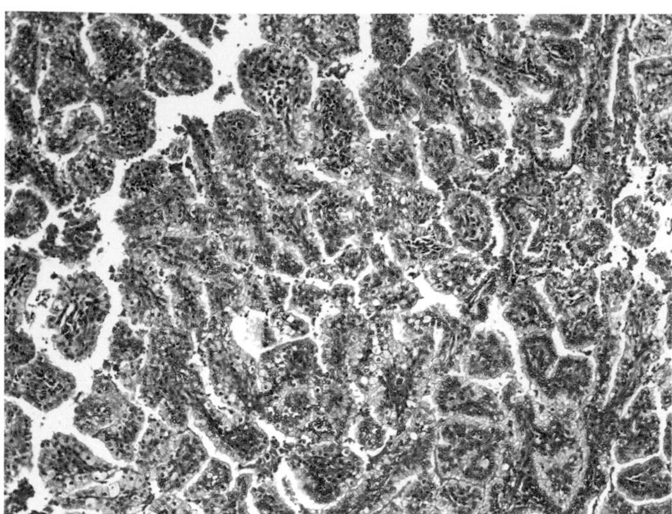

Fig. 16.13 A minority of primary adenocarcinomas of the lung show papillary differentiation, as shown in this photomicrograph.

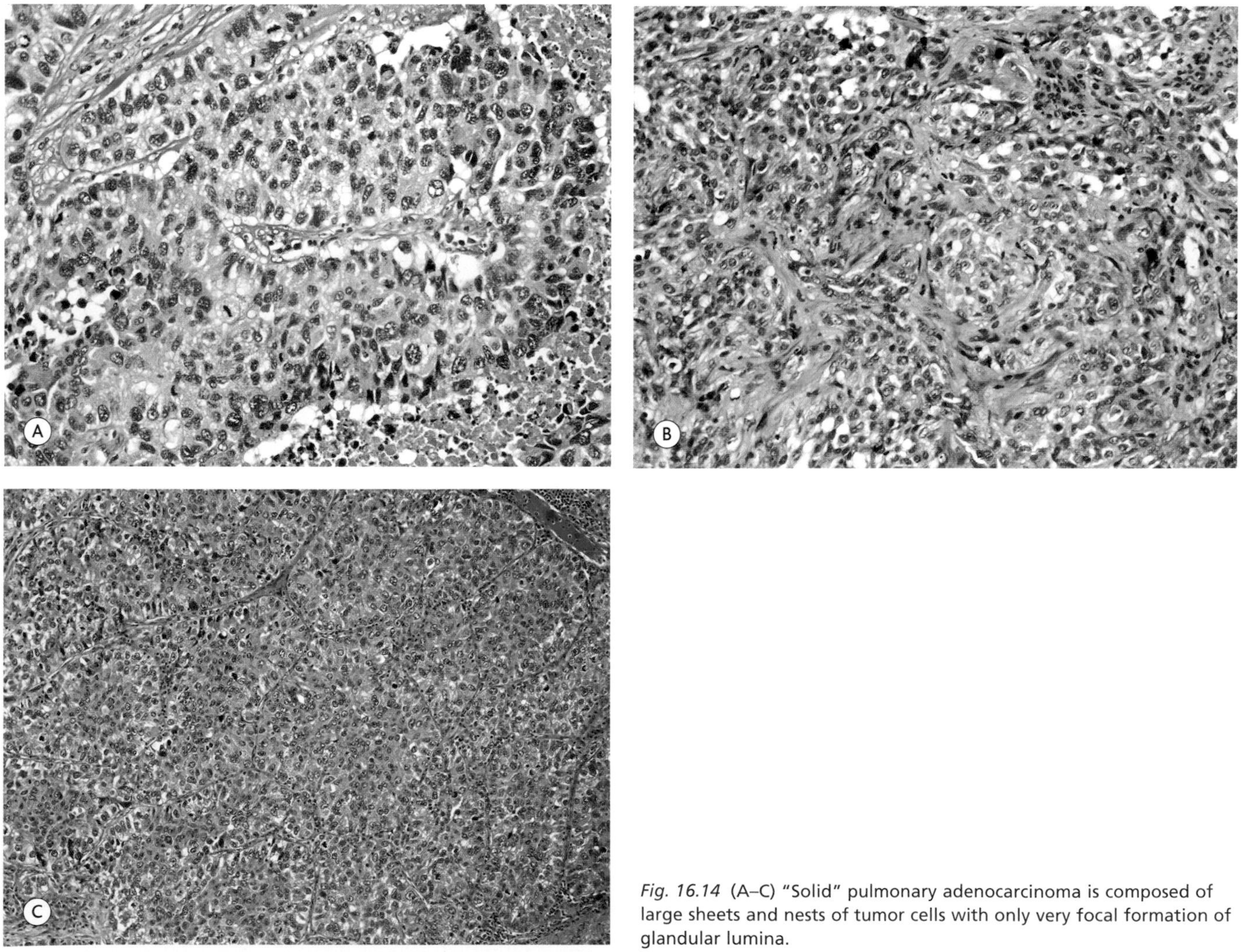

Fig. 16.14 (A–C) "Solid" pulmonary adenocarcinoma is composed of large sheets and nests of tumor cells with only very focal formation of glandular lumina.

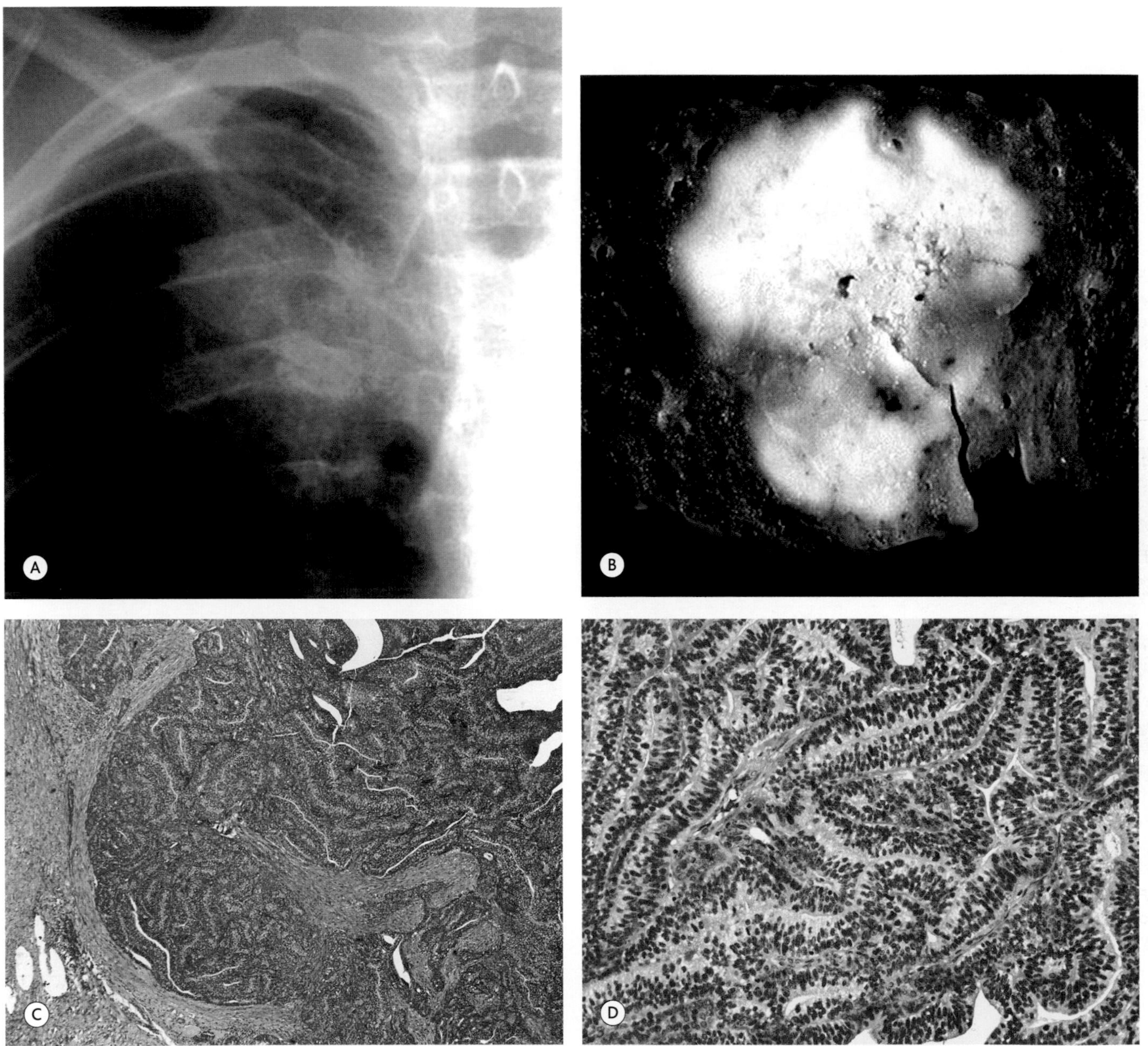

Fig. 16.15 (A) "Fetal" adenocarcinoma of the lung is considered to be in the same family of tumors as pulmonary "blastoma," and is shown here in an adult patient as a peripheral nodule in the right upper lung field on a plain-film radiograph. (B) The resected tumor is a solid, relatively well-demarcated and homogeneous mass. (C,D) Microscopically, fetal adenocarcinoma comprises closely apposed glandular arrays made up of compact columnar cells, resembling those seen in embryonic lungs (Figures A and B courtesy of Dr Samuel A. Yousem, University of Pittsburgh Medical Center, Pittsburgh, PA).

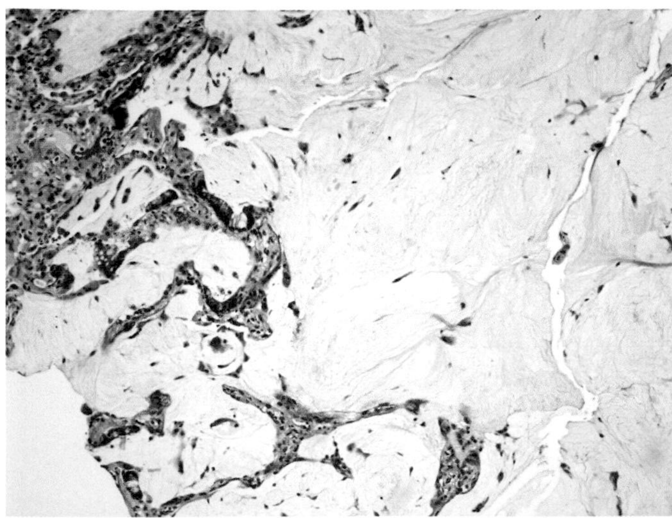

Fig. 16.16 Primary "colloid"-type adenocarcinoma of the lung shows nests of polyhedral tumor cells that are suspended in pools of copious extracellular mucin. This image is analogous to that seen in primary lesions of the breast, gastrointestinal tract, and skin.

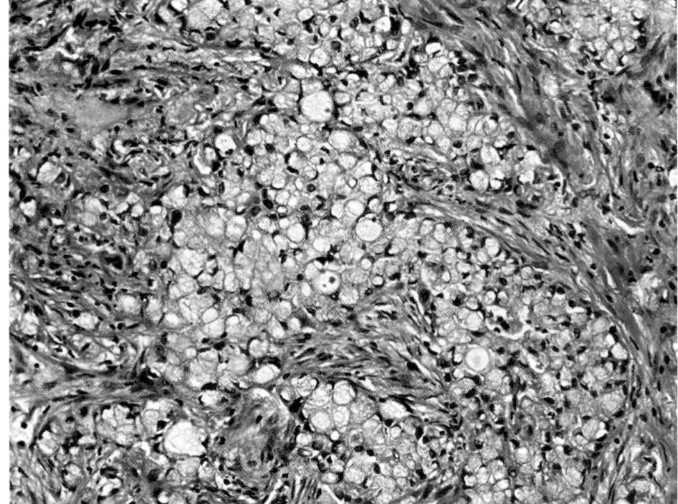

Fig. 16.17 This rare primary pulmonary adenocarcinoma is composed of tumor cells with prominent intracytoplasmic mucin vacuoles, yielding a "signet-ring-cell" appearance.

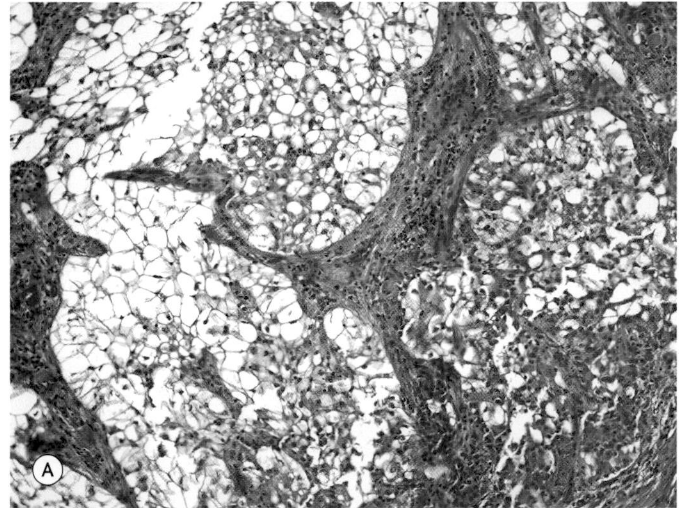

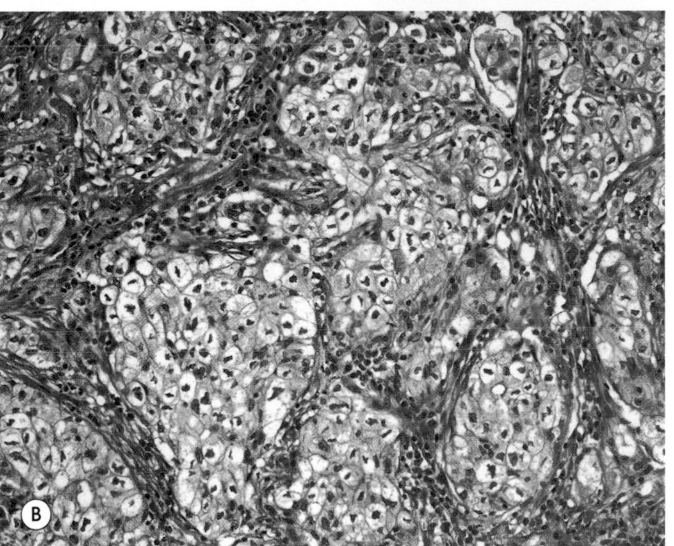

Fig. 16.18 (A) Clear cell change in primary pulmonary adenocarcinoma. This feature may lead to consideration of a metastatic lesion, particularly one arising in the kidney. (B) Higher magnification of another case of clear cell change in a primary pulmonary adenocarcinoma.

Psammoma bodies can also be seen in primary papillary adenocarcinomas of the lung,[31] and these structures therefore raise the question of whether one is instead viewing a solitary metastasis from an occult tumor of the thyroid, ovary, or other locations wherein psammomatous carcinomas are potentially found. Needless to say, in cases featuring multifocality of adenocarcinoma in more than one lobe, this problem is even more striking. Special studies, including electron microscopy and immunohistology, are helpful in resolving this differential diagnosis. Ultimately, however, diagnostic reliance is also placed on such banal characteristics as peritumoral fibrosis and inflammation, which are generally more common in primary pulmonary lesions than in metastases.

Pulmonary ACA may rarely involve the bronchial epithelium diffusely in a pagetoid fashion (Fig. 16.20).[32] Whether this represents intraepithelial spread of the tumor or multifocal synchronous growth is an open question, but pagetoid lesions are excrutiating management problems because of the difficulty in obtaining tumor-free bronchial margins.

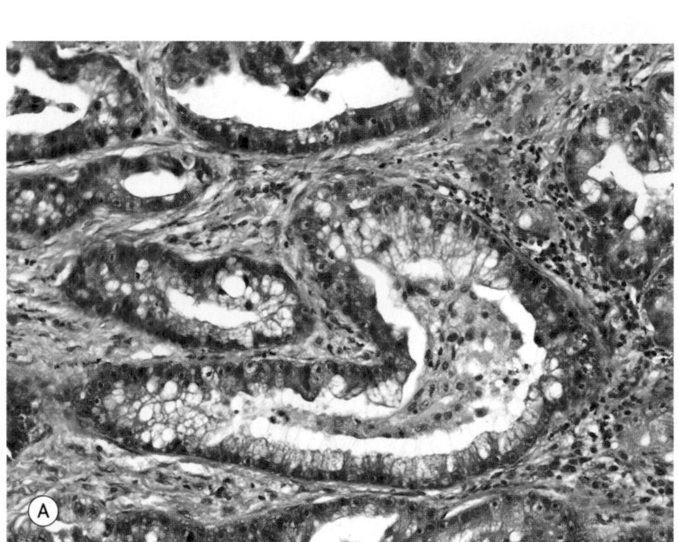

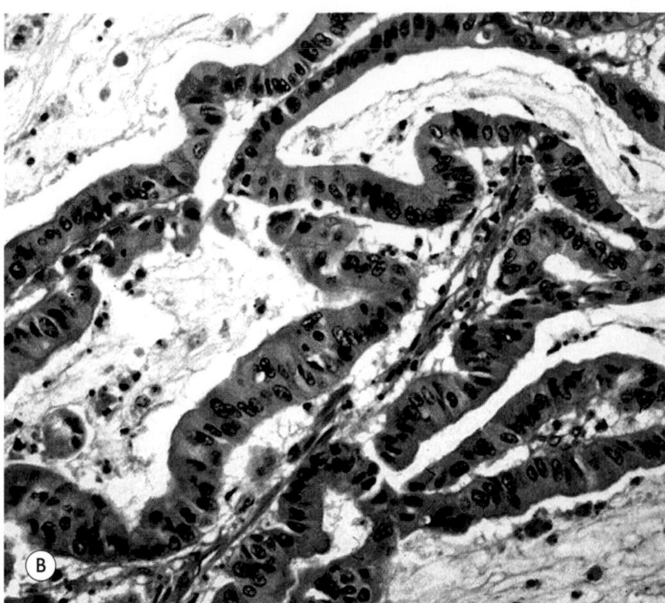

Fig. 16.19 (A,B) "Enteric" primary adenocarcinoma of the lung, featuring a composition by low-columnar tumor cells with basally oriented nuclei and mucin production. The overall image of the lesion is reminiscent of a neoplasm arising in the gastrointestinal tract.

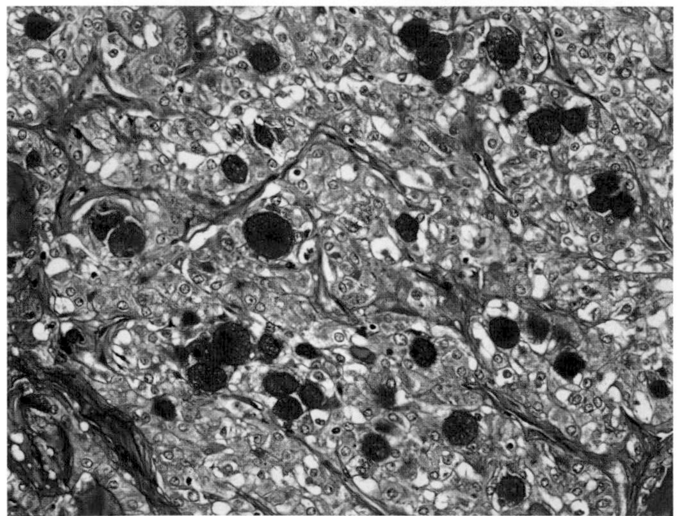

Fig. 16.20 This section, stained with the digested periodic acid-Schiff technique for mucin, shows "pagetoid" involvement of non-neoplastic but hyperplastic bronchial epithelium by adenocarcinoma cells. A typical adenocarcinomatous mass lesion was present in the nearby parenchyma.

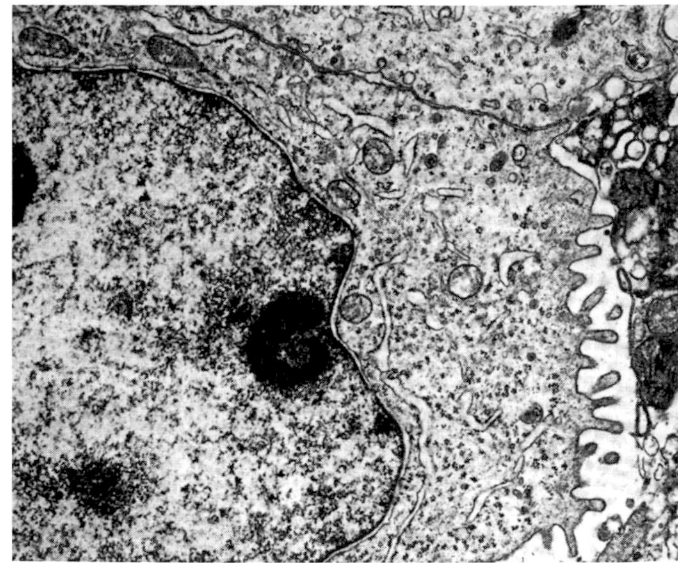

Fig. 16.21 Electron photomicrograph of "pseudomesotheliomatous" adenocarcinoma in the pleura, demonstrating short, non-branching cell surface microvilli, structures typical of adenocarcinoma but not mesothelioma.

"Pseudomesotheliomatous" (pleurotropic) adenocarcinomas are indeed separable from true mesotheliomas using adjuvant pathologic techniques, particularly immunophenotyping and electron microscopy (Figs 16.21 and 16.22; Table 16.1).[33] Nonetheless, whether this exercise has any more than academic significance is an open question. At present, available therapies for both of these tumor types are suboptimal to say the least, and the only real significance of the differential diagnosis in question may be a medicolegal one. The latter comment refers to the fact that, in the absence of asbestosis, pleurotropic adenocarcinoma has no proven causal relationship to asbestos exposure.

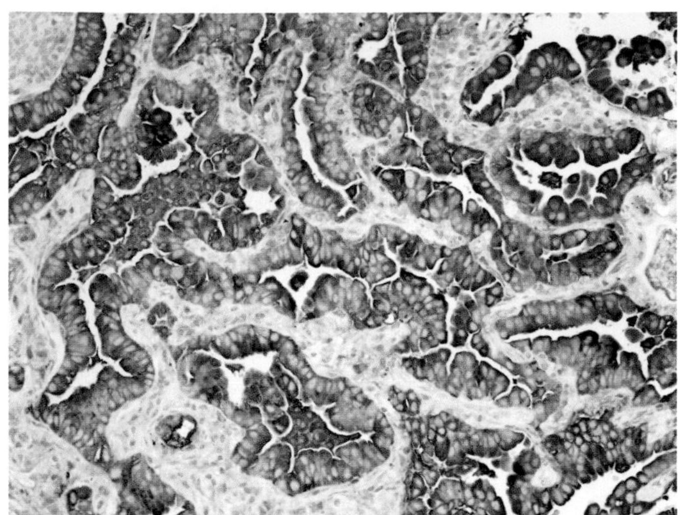

Fig. 16.22 The tumor depicted in Fig. 16.21 shows diffuse immunoreactivity for carcinoembryonic antigen, as expected in most adenocarcinomas of the lung.

Bronchioloalveolar carcinoma

Bronchioloalveolar carcinoma of the lung was initially described in the 1800s, but was most fully characterized as a distinct entity by Liebow in 1960.[34] Since that time, BAC has been the subject of intense interest and controversy. In particular, the pathologic criteria that apply to the diagnosis of this tumor entity, and how its histologic attributes relate to prognosis, represent perhaps the two most contentious issues.[35–43]

There are no particular distinguishing demographic features that are associated with BAC, vis-à-vis other adenocarcinomas of the lung. They tend to occur in elderly individuals, with an essentially equal distribution by gender.[36,43] Contrary to reports made in the 1970s[41] – before such phenomena as "passive" tobacco exposure were recognized – there *is* a definite relationship between cigarette smoking and the genesis of this tumor, as true of

Table 16.1 Role of immunohistochemical reagents used to distinguish between epithelial mesothelioma and adenocarcinoma

Antibody	Mesothelioma Result	%	Adenocarcinoma Result	%
BG8	+	4%	+	88%
MoAb 44-3A6	+	100%	+	8%
Factor VIII	±	Rare	–	N.S.
Surfactant apoprotein	–	–	+	62%
Anti Lewis antigen	+	11%	+	76%
Tn antigen	–	–	+	62%
E-cadherin	+	10%	+	77%
TTF-1	+	68%	+	100%
MoAb SM3	+	52%	+	100%
Secretory component (SC)	+	0–62%	+	60%
Pregnancy specific protein	+	0–6%	+	34–59%
CA 19-9	–	–	+	39%
OV632	+	85–91%	+	20–63%
NSE	+	96%	N.S.	N.S.
CD57	+	70%	N.S.	N.S.
Mab 45	+	N.S.	+	N.S.
HEA-125	–	–	+	75%
Anti BRG	–	–	+	83%
ICAM-1	+	100%	N.S.	N.S.
VCAM	+	87%	N.S.	N.S.
Parathyroid hormone	+	84%	+	11%
CD44H	+	91%	+	45%
IOB 3	–	–	+	100%

Source: modified from Moran et al.[150]
N.S. = not studied or not specified; MoAb = monoclonal antibody; NSE = neuron-specific enolase; ICAM = intercellular adhesion molecule; VCAM = vascular cell adhesion molecule; BRG = retinoblastoma-gene-related protein; other abbreviations are monoclonal antibody designations and have no expanded names.

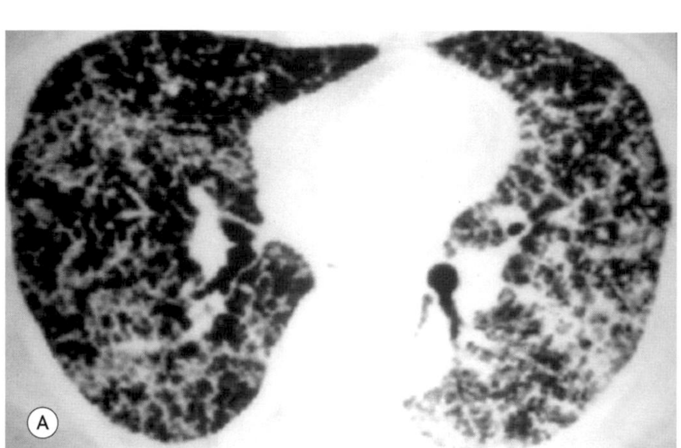

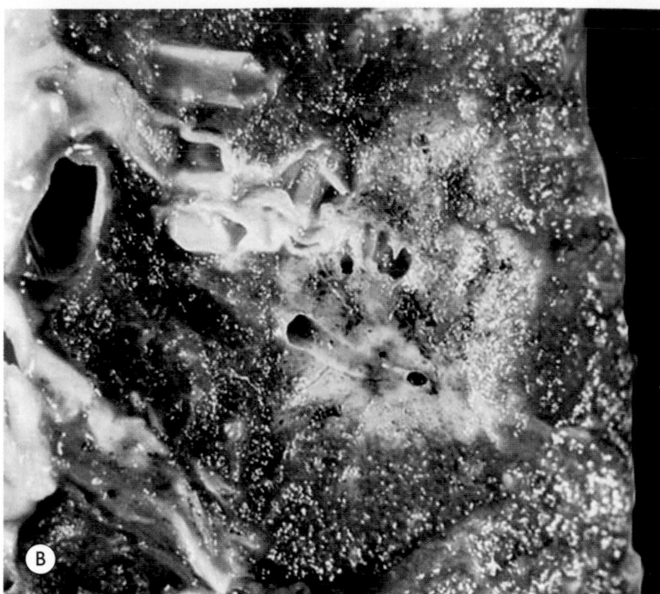

Fig. 16.23 (A) Bilateral reticulonodular and consolidative lesions are seen in this thoracic computed tomogram from a patient with bronchioloalveolar carcinoma, resembling the changes of an infiltrative non-neoplastic lung disease. (B) This gross photograph from a similar case shows the permeative nature of the tumor in the lung parenchyma.

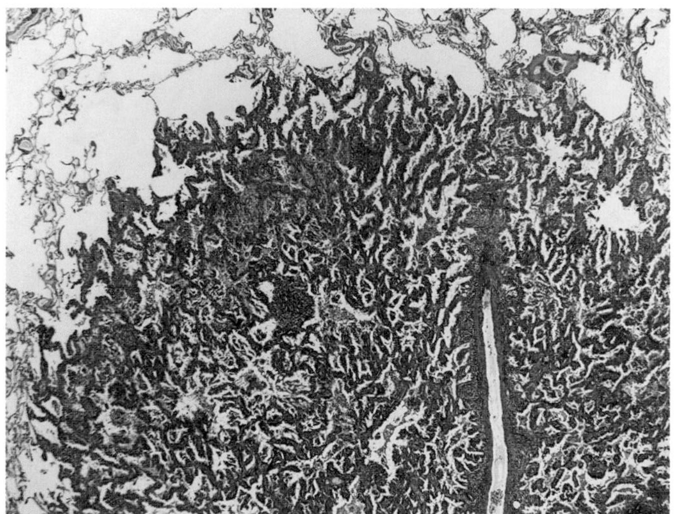

Fig. 16.24 A scanning photomicrograph of solitary bronchioloalveolar carcinoma shows an image which is similar to that of ordinary pulmonary adenocarcinoma.

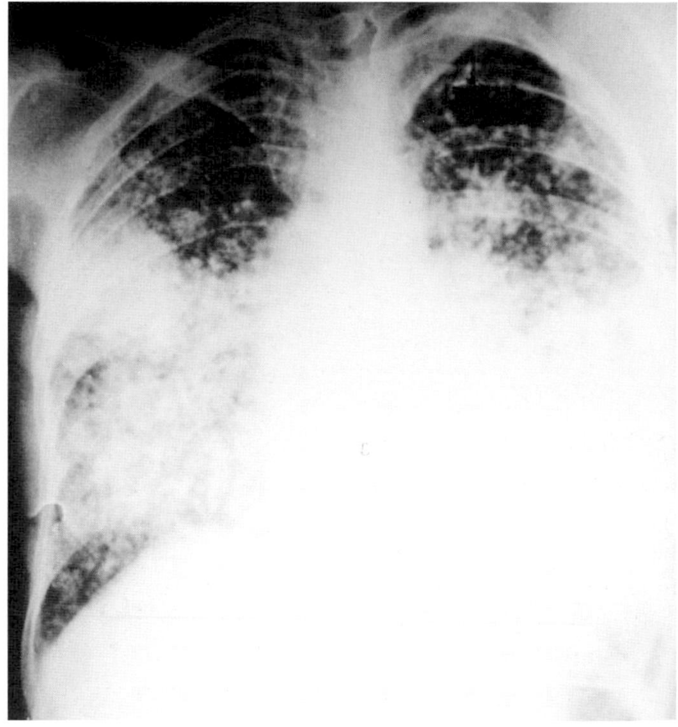

Fig. 16.25 Multifocal-synchronous bronchioloalveolar carcinoma, presenting as multiple rounded nodules throughout both lung fields and simulating the radiographic appearance of metastatic disease.

virtually all pulmonary carcinomas. Nonetheless, BAC is indeed over-represented (with regard to other histotypes of lung cancer) in patients who have never smoked and who have never lived with smokers. The latter point has raised the issue of whether other etiologic factors – in particular, infection with human papillomavirus – might account for the genesis of some BACs. However, data generated by Yousem et al.[11] make the latter possibility seem unlikely.

Radiologically and clinically, three discrete subsets of patients with BAC are recognized.[43,44] These include individuals who have chest X-ray findings and clinical complaints suggesting the presence of pneumonia (fever, productive cough, and lobar or segmental consolidation) (Fig. 16.23), as well as some patients with a solitary peripheral mass lesion (Fig. 16.24) and others with *multiple* rounded densities throughout one or both lung fields (Fig. 16.25).

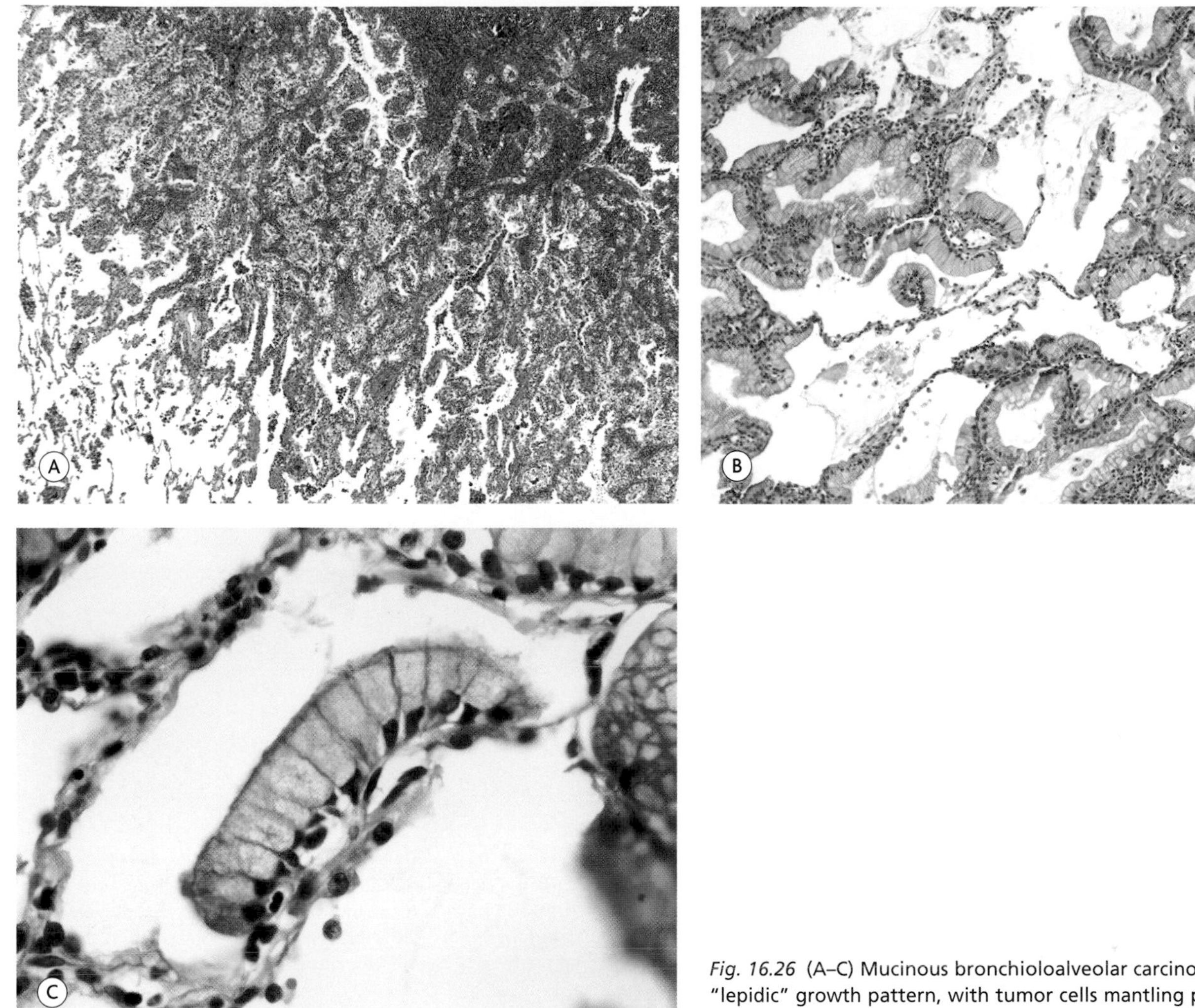

Fig. 16.26 (A–C) Mucinous bronchioloalveolar carcinoma shows a "lepidic" growth pattern, with tumor cells mantling pre-existing alveolar septa, and production of abundant extracellular mucin.

On computed tomograms, the latter lesions may assume a "cheerio" shape, in that they commonly demonstrate small central areas of cavitation. Hence, BAC may simulate an infectious disease, or represent a nondescript "coin" lesion of the lung, or imitate the pattern of metastases *to* the lung from an occult visceral neoplasm.

Histologically, two distinct cytologic subtypes of BAC are recognized: mucinous and non-mucinous.[35,36,40] These are of importance because of their clinical associations. Mucinous tumors (Fig. 16.26) are those that tend to assume a pseudopneumonic or multifocal/multinodular clinical appearance, whereas non-mucinous BAC (Fig. 16.27) is more commonly a solitary lesion. Furthermore, stage for stage, non-mucinous variants may show a more favorable clinical evolution.[40] The criteria for distinction of BAC from *type ordinaire* pulmonary adenocarcinoma have been debated. The authors restrict the use of this diagnosis to neoplasms which demonstrate a mantling of pre-existing airspaces ("lepidic growth") by single layers or limited strata and micropapillae of only modestly atypical cuboidal or columnar epithelial cells, with or without intracellular or extracellular mucin production. Intranuclear inclusions of cytoplasm containing surfactant proteins are also common.[45] Save for mucin production, such characteristics are shared by both of the forms of BAC: namely, mucinous and non-mucinous (serous). Moreover, there must be *no* sclerosis or inflammation within or around the lesion if it is to be considered a bona fide BAC. This demanding definition differs from that of some other observers, who have accepted the existence of a "sclerosing" BAC subtype.[46] Justification for more narrow requirements is gained from biologic data, which show a worse behavior of "sclerosing" BAC than that of non-fibrotic tumors.[35] Indeed, Clayton,[36] who has devoted much attention to BAC, has stated that:

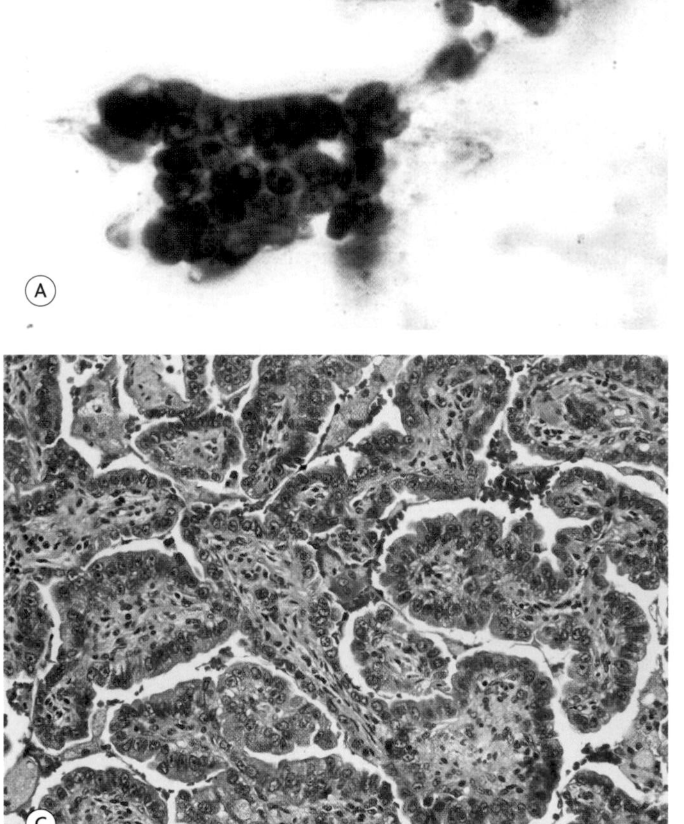

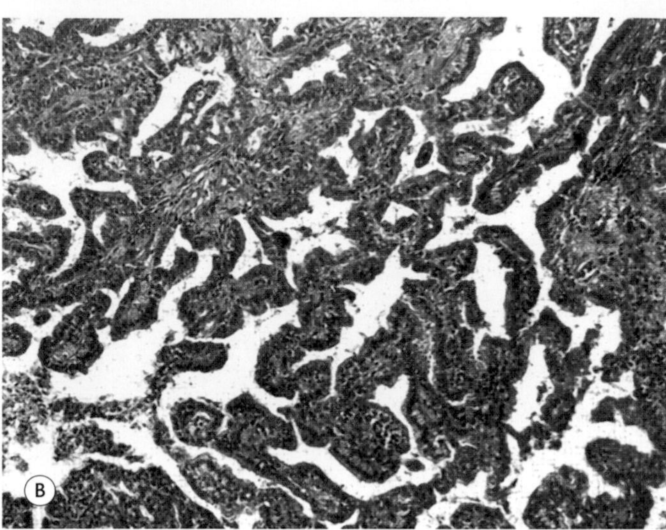

Fig. 16.27 (A) Fine-needle aspiration biopsy specimen from non-mucinous bronchioloalveolar carcinoma (BAC), showing relatively bland and homogeneous polygonal cells that are arranged in three-dimensional profiles. (B) Non-mucinous BAC shows mantling of alveolar septa by well-differentiated low-columnar tumor cells. (C) Small micropapillary structures may also be seen in non-mucinous BAC, and intranuclear invaginations of cytoplasm ("pseudoinclusions") are potentially visible.

bronchioloalveolar carcinomas with sclerosis should be classified with other peripheral adenocarcinomas.

Another traditional point of discussion pertaining to the microscopic features of BAC (particularly its mucinous form) is that this neoplasm is said to disseminate within the lung by "aerogenous" means. That is to say, it has been felt that tumor cells are detached from a "mother lesion" and spread to other foci in the pulmonary parenchyma by the process of inhalation and exhalation. Some molecular analyses, however, have cast doubt on that premise and instead suggest that the lesions are multiclonal.[47]

With respect to other lesions that may be confused pathologically with BAC, they include foci of florid type II pneumocytic hyperplasia surrounding areas of diffuse alveolar damage[48] and interstitial fibrosing pneumonitides or organizing pulmonary infarcts;[49] the proliferation known as "atypical adenomatous alveolar hyperplasia" (see below);[50] and the unicentric neoplasms known as "papillary alveolar adenoma" and "sclerosing hemangioma."[51] The latter two entities are bland cytologically and show a sharp interface with the surrounding pulmonary parenchyma, unlike BAC. Another point that was often raised in the older literature on BAC concerned the great difficulty with which metastases *to* the lung could be distinguished from the former neoplasm. It is still true that there are currently no immunohistologic or ultrastructural markers that can be used with absolute certainty to distinguish BAC from all extrapulmonary adenocarcinomas, and this separation must ultimately rest on careful analysis of conventional clinicopathologic data.

Prognostically, patients with multifocal BACs have an outlook that is much worse than that of patients with unicentric tumors of this type, quite simply because the former lesions are inoperable. Furthermore, mucinous tumors tend to behave more aggressively – with a higher incidence of extrapulmonary metastasis – than non-mucinous BAC when they are matched by size and stage.[35,36] Overall, non-mucinous tumors measuring under 3 cm in maximum dimension have a good prognosis, approximating 90% at 5 years. It should be remembered that the natural history of BAC is more protracted than that of more conventional pulmonary adenocarcinomas, and tumor-related fatalities will continue to accrue even at 10 years after diagnosis.[35,41] Nevertheless, in an often-cited study by Manning et al.,[40] the 5-year survival of non-mucinous BAC was 72%, whereas only 26% of patients with mucinous tumors survived at that point.

Atypical adenomatous alveolar hyperplasia and its relationship to bronchioloalveolar carcinoma

Kitamura et al.[52] have recently addressed the conceptual mechanistic relationship between topographically small atypical glandular proliferations of the lung – "atypical adenomatous alveolar hyperplasia" (AAAH) – and BAC. Their model appears to demonstrate a stepwise progression from atypical adenomatous hyperplasia to BAC, with further evolution to invasive growth. This concept has been advanced before, especially by Miller and colleagues, who postulated that such a stepwise process existed in the lung in analogy to the adenoma–carcinoma sequence in the colon.[53]

Atypical adenomatous hyperplasia must be differentiated from reactive or regenerative pneumocytic lesions, at one end of the spectrum, and from small bona fide adenocarcinomas, at the other. With regard to separation of AAAH from various reactive lesions, Kitamura and coworkers have emphasized the tendency of reactive lesions to include multiple cell types, including type II pneumocytes, ciliated cells, and mucinous cells, and they have described the relatively more conspicuous interstitial inflammation and edema in localized interstitial pneumonitis.[52] Additional criteria that are found to be helpful in this context involve assessment of the lesional borders and patterns of fibrosis. There is a tendency for lesions of AAAH to be more sharply circumscribed and for the mild interstitial fibrosis and inflammation to stop at the same boundary as the atypical alveolar cells. Conversely, reactive lesions tend to be less well defined, and the interstitial scarring extends beyond the areas of alveolar cell atypia. The individual cells in AAAH, although less homogeneous than those in BAC, tend to be more uniformly atypical than those of reactive hyperplasias (Fig. 16.28). It should be remembered that a variety of chemotherapeutic agents can induce striking degrees of cytologic atypia, and this phenomenon is a well-documented pitfall in exfoliative cytology.[49,54] The authors have also seen several examples of pneumocytes

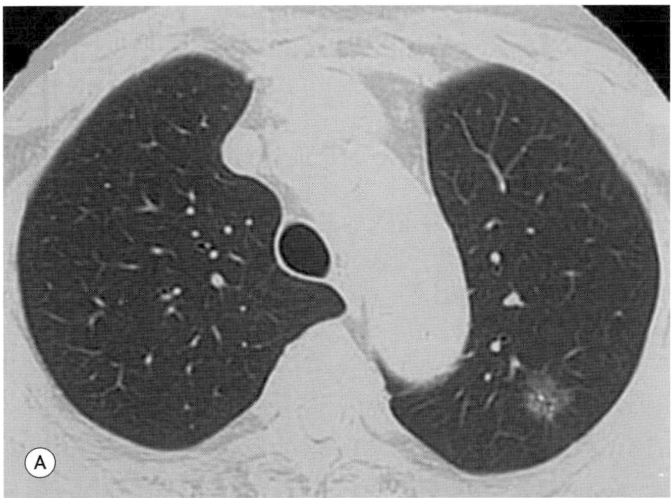

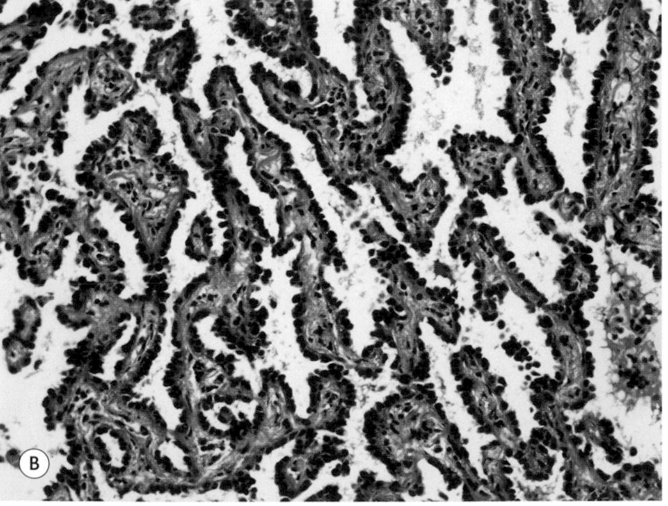

Fig. 16.28 (A) This computed tomograph of the chest shows a vague density in the left lung field, which was felt to represent "atypical adenomatous alveolar hyperplasia" (AAAH) after excision and pathologic examination. (B) The image of AAAH is shown here, and is virtually identical to that of non-mucinous bronchioloalveolar carcinoma (see Fig. 16.27). Indeed, the separation of those entities is probably more semantic than real.

with intranuclear cytoplasmic inclusions in clear-cut cases of organizing phase diffuse alveolar damage; hence their presence should not be viewed as pathognomonic of neoplasia.

It is the authors' view that the distinction between AAAH and small BAC is a conceptually arbitrary one. Standard criteria that have been cited as useful in this task include uniformly atypical nuclei, large lesional size, and complex growth with budding or tufting of tumor cells in the alveolar spaces in BAC but not AAAH.[50,55] Kitamura et al. suggested that a nuclear area of less than 40 μm^2 and a lesional diameter of less than 5 mm could effectively identify AAAH, as opposed to small BAC.[52] Miller[56] also proposed a cut-off of 5 mm to separate "bronchioloalveolar cell adenoma" from BAC.

Nevertheless, morphometric and immunohistologic analyses have shown a synonymity rather than a disparity between AAAH and BAC.[57,58] Similarly, molecular studies, while showing some differences in statistical groups, have demonstrated many more shared features than differences.[59,60]

The most important consideration of this discussion concerns the clinical significance of AAAH. In practice, this lesion is not appreciated until microscopic sections arrive on the pathologist's desk, and they are seen in four main contexts:

- in sections of a wedge biopsy specimen of a non-neoplastic disease
- in wedge resection margins of a peripheral carcinoma
- in "random" sections of a lobe with another, discrete carcinoma
- as suspected nodules of multifocal tumor along with at least one other documented peripheral adenocarcinoma.

To develop some understanding of the importance of atypical lesions, several points must be kept in mind. First, inasmuch as most AAAH lesions are found in patients undergoing resection of an obvious cancer, it is nearly an insurmountable challenge to arrive at any conclusions concerning their biology. This is so because the outcome of those cases will be determined by the characteristics of the macroscopically obvious tumors. Atypical adenomatous alveolar hyperplasia lesions tend to be multifocal throughout both lungs but may be inapparent on gross examination, and can be easily missed even with current radiologic imaging techniques. Therefore, short of bilateral lung transplantation, it is impossible to say what would constitute adequate surgical resection of such lesions. Given these realities, it is best for pathologists to be pragmatically conservative in the diagnosis of clinically inapparent AAAH as small BACs, despite the above-cited conceptual considerations. It is important to emphasize, however, that such lesions can be multifocal and have a relationship with subsequent multicentric BAC, underscoring the need for close follow-up to identify the possible appearance of metachronous tumors. On the other hand, proliferations that represent grossly observed lesions with compellingly atypical cytology should be designated as outright carcinomas.

Adenocarcinomas associated with scars

In the relatively recent past, it was taught that fibrous scarring in the lung – seen as a consequence of pneumonia, interstitial fibroproliferative diseases, or pneumoconioses – predisposed to adenocarcinoma and had a directly causative role in the genesis of that tumor type.[61] Nevertheless, several investigators have concluded that the central fibrosis seen in "scar adenocarcinomas" (Fig. 16.29) is formed *following* initiation of the carcinoma, and is the product of the tumor cells themselves.[62–64] At a practical level, there is no reason to suspect that fibrosing conditions in the lung are, in and of themselves, preneoplastic. With particular reference to asbestosis and silicosis, special forms of pulmonary interstitial fibrosis, the authors' redaction of the aggregated literature leads to the conclusion that carcinomas of the lung arise *only* in patients with those conditions who are also, or have been, cigarette smokers. In that scenario, it is further believed that smoking is the principal carcinogenic factor.

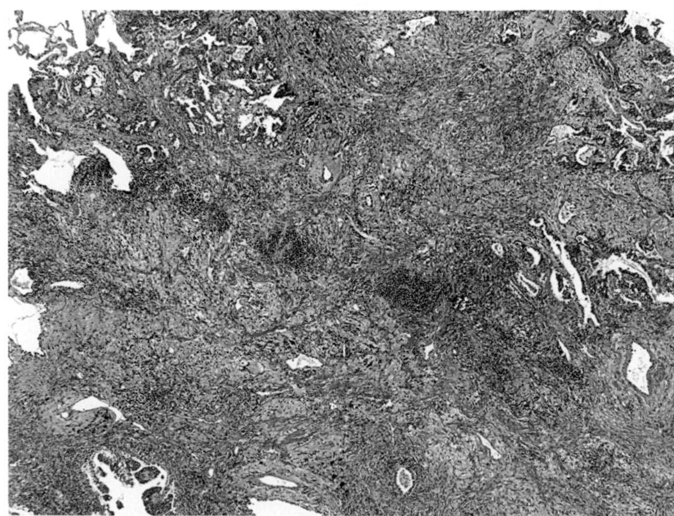

Fig. 16.29 A broad zone of fibroelastotic "scarring" is seen in the center of this pulmonary adenocarcinoma. It has been shown that matrical changes such as this are a product of the tumor rather than a pre-existing condition.

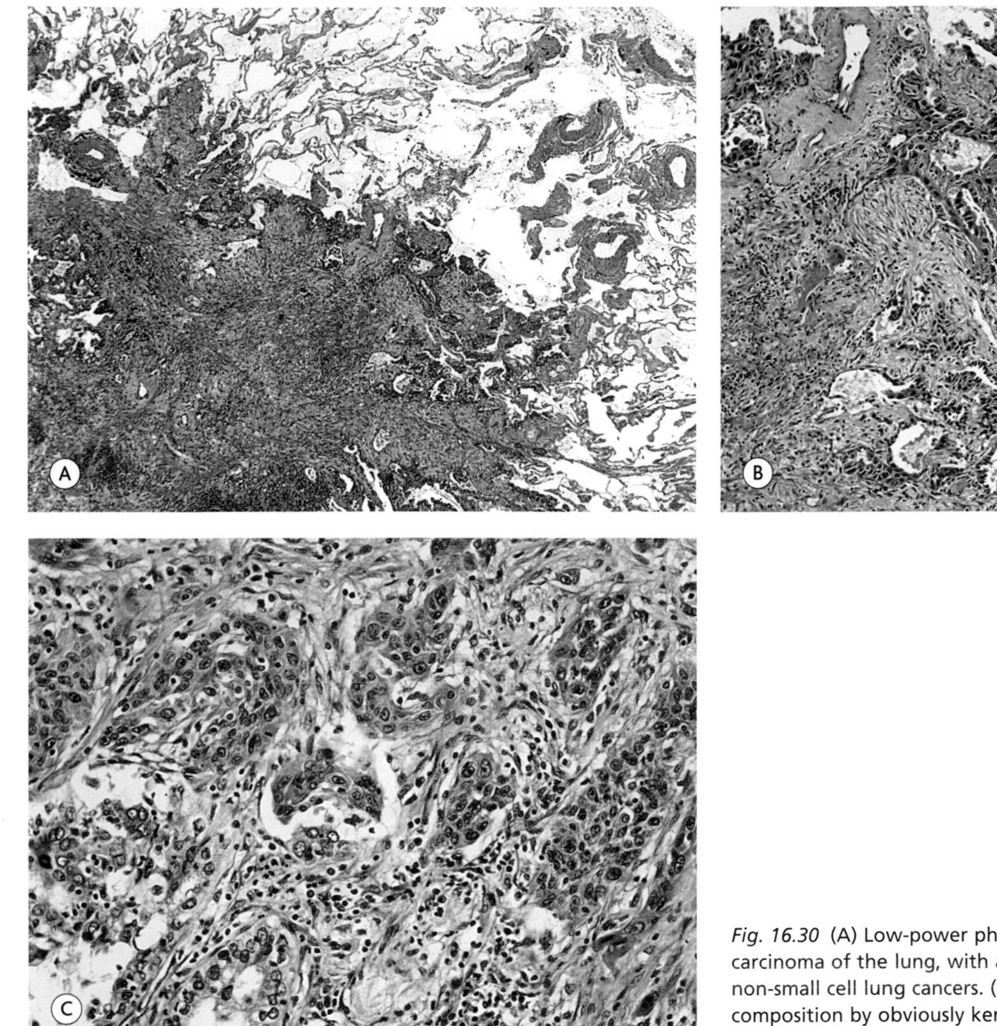
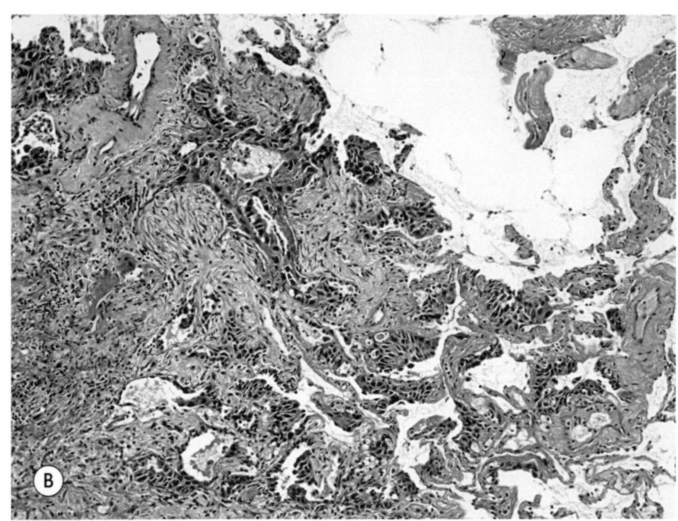

Fig. 16.30 (A) Low-power photomicrograph of adenosquamous carcinoma of the lung, with a configuration like that of other non-small cell lung cancers. (B,C) Closer inspection shows a bifid composition by obviously keratinizing squamous elements and gland-forming tumor cells, which are intimately admixed.

Adenosquamous carcinoma

Adenosquamous carcinoma (ASC) is a "composite" tumor, exhibiting simultaneous squamous and glandular differentiation in the same mass (Fig. 16.30). It accounts for no more than 5% of all lung cancers in most surgical series.[65–67] The clinical, radiographic, and gross pathologic attributes of ASC are most similar to those of "pure" adenocarcinomas of the lung. A point of contention in regard to this lesion is whether it is synonymous with high-grade mucoepidermoid carcinoma of the salivary glandular type. The authors' opinion is that those two neoplasms are typically separable from one another. Salivary gland analogue tumors in the lung, as considered subsequently, tend to arise in the large central airways, in contrast to the propensity for ASC to be peripheral. In addition, foci of lower-grade mucoepidermoid carcinoma are often present in the former, but not the latter, of these tumor types. The prognosis of pulmonary ASC is said to be rather adverse. In studies reported by Ishida & colleagues and Takamori et al., the survival of patients with adenosquamous tumors was statistically worse than that of individuals with "pure" adenocarcinomas or squamous cell carcinomas.[65,67]

Large cell undifferentiated carcinoma

Large cell undifferentiated carcinomas (LCUCs) account for approximately 15% of all lung cancers.[68] As mentioned earlier in this discussion, diagnostic use of the term "non-small cell carcinoma" has produced some confusion between poorly differentiated SCC, poorly differentiated ACA, poorly differentiated ASC, and true LCUC. Accordingly, it has been suggested that the designation of "large cell carcinoma" should be employed restrictively as a synonym for LCUC.

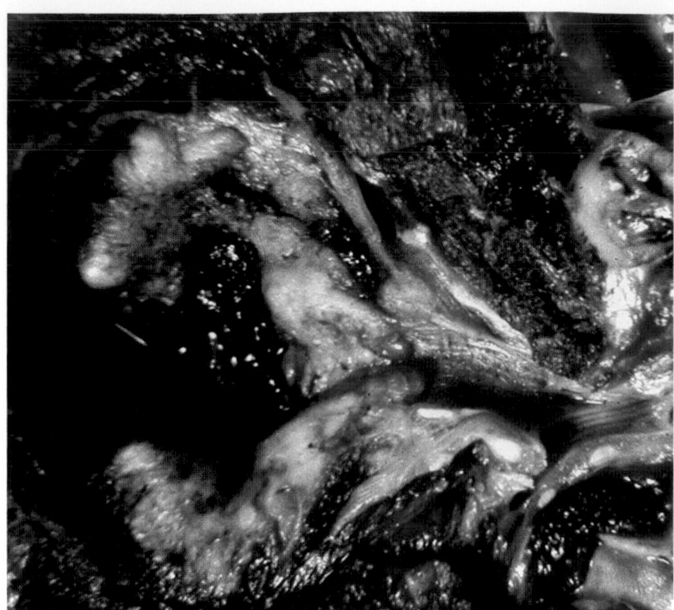

Fig. 16.31 Gross photograph of large cell undifferentiated carcinoma of the lung, showing a fleshy tan-pink mass with no other distinguishing features.

Large cell undifferentiated carcinomas are typically >5 cm in maximum dimension, have a white-gray cut surface (which may be lobulated and resemble "fish flesh," thus potentially simulating the appearance of a sarcoma or a hematolymphoid lesion) (Fig. 16.31), and are rarely multicentric. Internal necrosis is a relatively common feature. Approximately 50% demonstrate a connection to a large tubular airway.

Histologically, LCUCs show a composition of large polygonal cells with vesicular chromatin, prominent nucleoli, discernible cytoplasmic borders, and a lack of glandular differentiation or keratinization (Fig. 16.32). They are typically arranged in sheets or large clusters, potentially exhibiting foci of central necrosis. Two distinctive subtypes of large cell carcinoma also exist – giant cell carcinoma and clear cell carcinoma.

Giant cell carcinoma was initially thought to be a separate clinicopathologic entity unto itself,[69,70] but that philosophy is no longer thought to be valid.[71] Microscopically, this variant of LCUC is composed of extremely pleomorphic large tumor cells, which are often multinucleated (Fig. 16.33). There is a regular admixture of polymorphonuclear leukocytes with the neoplastic elements, even in the absence of necrosis, suggesting tumoral synthesis of leukocyte cytokines such as granulocyte colony stimulating factor.[72] Parenthetically, this phenomenon can also be associated with *systemic* neutrophilia in association with giant cell subtype of LCUC. Neoplastic "cannibalism" may also be observed, wherein the giant tumor cells appear to engulf one another.

Primary clear cell carcinoma of the lung (CCCL) is a diagnosis of exclusion, and it is likely that tumors with both squamous and glandular differentiation are included in that group. A number of other clear cell neoplasms of the lung, including some "carcinoids," the so-called benign "sugar tumor," metastatic renal cell carcinoma, and metastatic "balloon cell" melanoma, must also be considered before making an interpretation of CCCL.[29,73–77] This can be accomplished by a combination of radiographic, electron microscopic, and immunohistologic evaluations, which should be done invariably in each instance. The overall clinicopathologic attributes of CCCL are comparable to those of LCUC, not otherwise specified.

In recent years, it has been suggested that a subset of pulmonary large cell carcinomas which shows neuroendocrine differentiation (as detected by electron microscopy or immunohistology) should be nosologically separated from truly undifferentiated large cell tumors.[78–81] Hence, the terms "exocrine large cell carcinoma" (another synonym for LCUC) and "endocrine large cell carcinoma" have entered use.[80] In the authors' opinion, "endocrine large cell carcinomas" are best specified as either *high-grade neuroendocrine carcinomas, large cell type* or *large cell carcinomas with occult neuroendocrine differentiation*, and these two entities are considered in more detail in another chapter on neuroendocrine neoplasms of the lung. Finally, a recent report has documented the existence of large cell undifferentiated lung cancers that have a "rhabdoid" phenotype[82] with eosinophilic hyaline inclusions in the cytoplasm and large vesicular nuclei with prominent nucleoli (Fig. 16.34). It is likely that this image represents a final common pathway of clonal evolution ("dedifferentiation") in carcinomas of the lung, as in other neoplasms demonstrating a rhaboid configuration.[83]

Salivary gland-type tumors of the lung

Primary salivary gland-type tumors of the lung (SGTTLs) are unusual, comprising no more than 1% of all pulmonary neoplasms.[84] Moreover, their diagnosis may pose a problem not only because of their rarity but also because in small biopsies it is relatively easy to consign them to the broad category of "non-small cell carcinoma." That would be unfortunate, because the clinical behavior of SGTTLs can be quite different from that of conventional

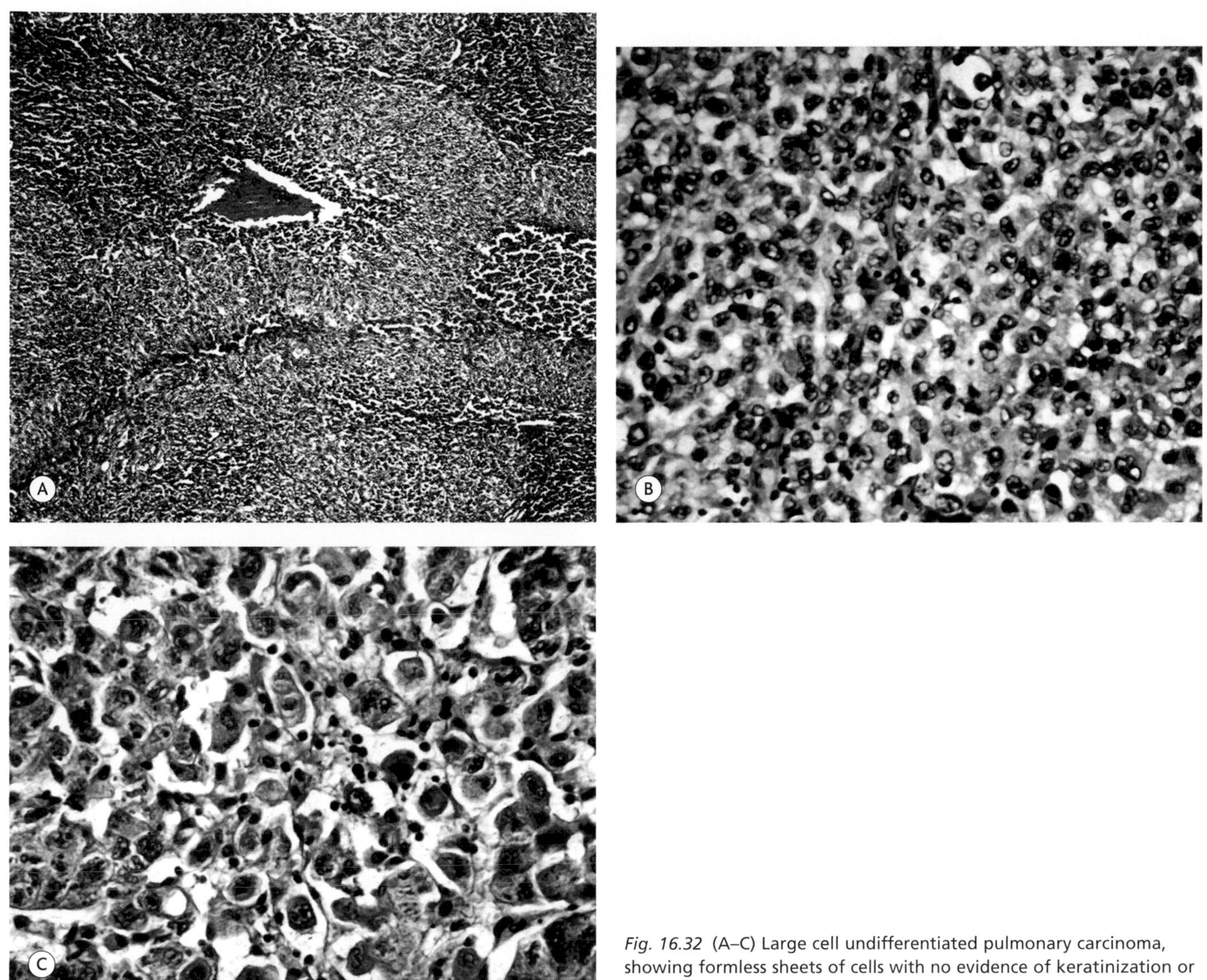

Fig. 16.32 (A–C) Large cell undifferentiated pulmonary carcinoma, showing formless sheets of cells with no evidence of keratinization or gland formation.

lung cancers. This family of tumors shares a similar immunohistochemical profile to that of ordinary pulmonary carcinomas, a fact which tends to negate that modality of study in differential diagnosis.

Interestingly, if one attempts to make correlations between the occurrence of SGTTLs and histologically identical tumors in the salivary glands, one finds differences rather than similarities. For instance, neoplasms that are seen very commonly in the salivary glands, such as pleomorphic adenoma (mixed tumor), are only rarely seen in the lung. In fact, most SGTTLs are malignant lesions, justifying their inclusion in this chapter. Furthermore, some histologic features that are commonly observed in pulmonary salivary gland analogue tumors do not necessarily parallel those of their counterparts in the salivary glands themselves.

Specific salivary gland-type tumors of the lung

Mucoepidermoid carcinoma

Mucoepidermoid carcinoma (MEC) is the most common of the SGTTLs and may be encountered in any age group; however, most cases have been seen in adults.[85–93] In a series of cases reported by Yousem and Hochholzer,[93] 58 patients ranged from 9 to 78 years of age, with a male-to-female distribution of almost 1.5:1. When the tumors

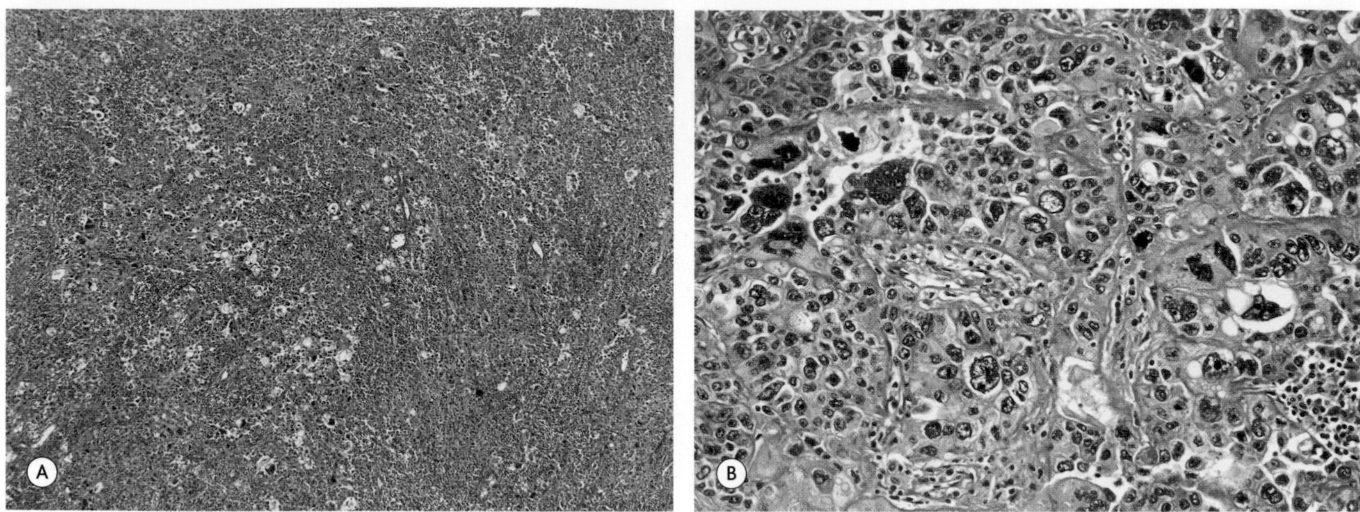

Fig. 16.33 Giant cell carcinoma of the lung: (A) showing sheets of undifferentiated tumor cells, like those shown in Fig. 16.32, with the exception that (B) large neoplastic multinucleated cells are also present.

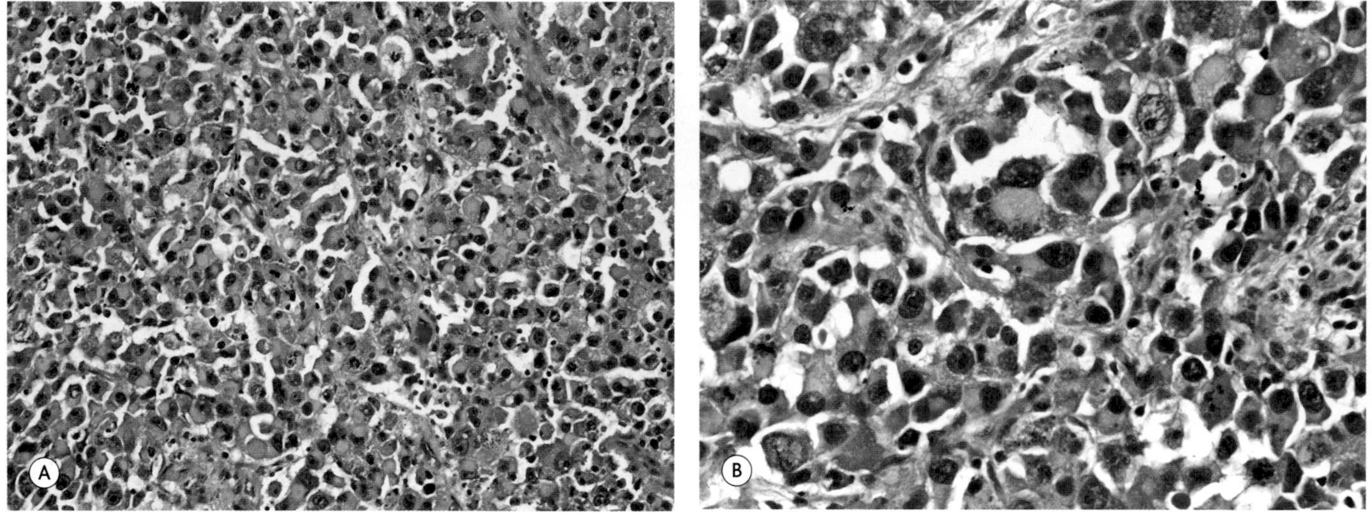

Fig. 16.34 (A,B) Large cell undifferentiated lung carcinoma with a "rhabdoid" phenotype, in which globular eosinophilic cytoplasmic inclusions displace the nuclei of the tumor cells.

were separated into low- and high-grade lesions, no preference for any particular age group was noted for either group. Nevertheless, the great majority of these tumors belong in the low-grade category. Clinical complaints in patients with MECs are dependent on the size and the location of the neoplasms. Large central tumors cause symptoms of obstruction, with pneumonia, dyspnea, or chest pain. More peripheral lesions may be asymptomatic and are discovered with routine chest radiography.

MECs classically present as exophytic endobronchial tumors and are potentially >5 cm in greatest diameter. They are usually well circumscribed with smooth overlying mucosal surfaces. On cut section, these tumors are tan-gray or yellow. They are solid or cystic, or both, and may show overtly mucoid features (Fig. 16.35). There is no topographic predilection for any particular pulmonary lobe or segment.

Mucoepidermoid carcinomas of the lung are classified into low-grade and high-grade tumors morphologically,

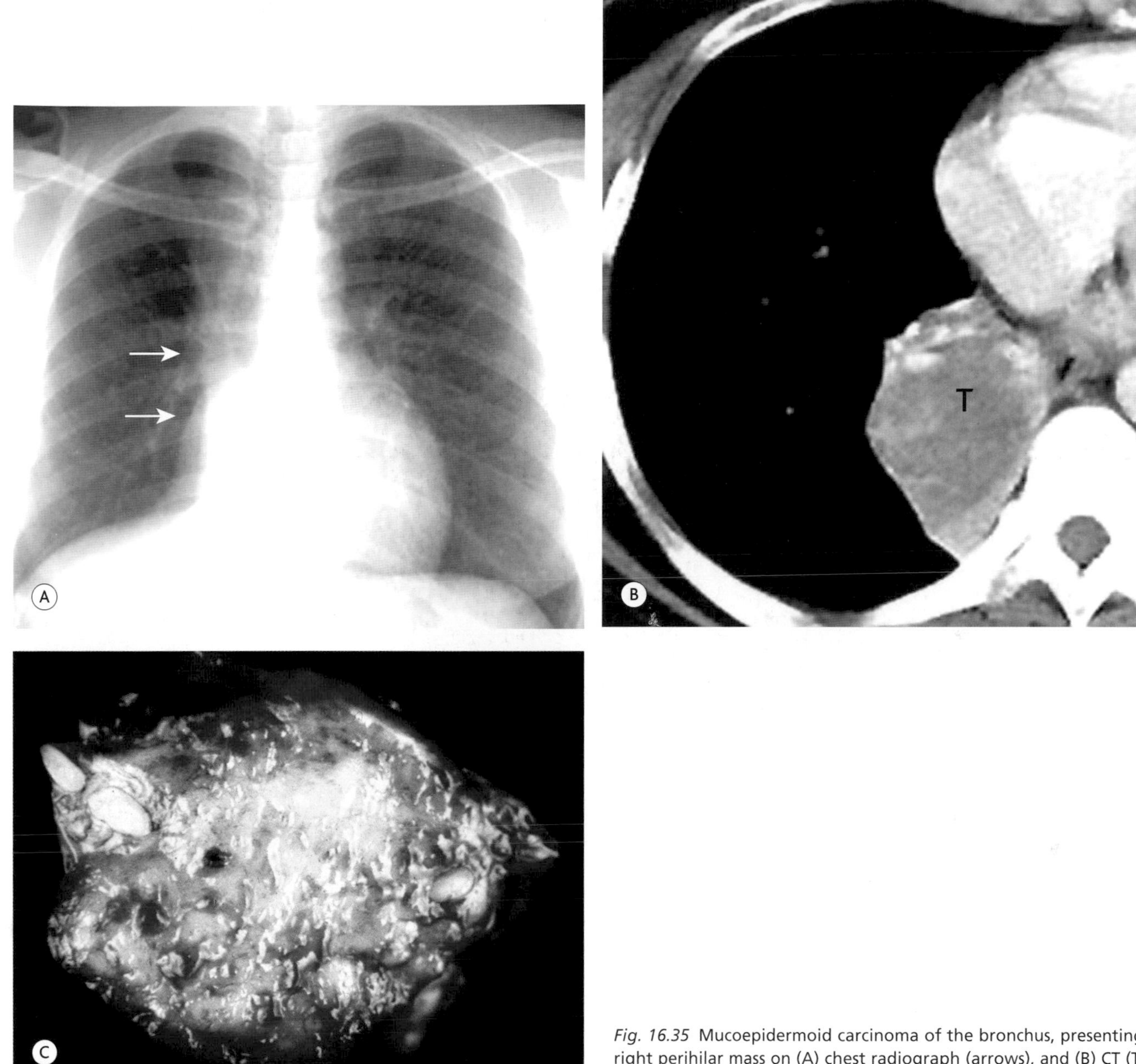

Fig. 16.35 Mucoepidermoid carcinoma of the bronchus, presenting as a right perihilar mass on (A) chest radiograph (arrows), and (B) CT (T), and (C) as seen in the resected lung.

principally based on their cytologic features. In low-grade lesions, the panoramic appearance is one of a neoplasm, with cystic and solid areas in close association with a tubular airway (Fig. 16.36). On closer inspection of the solid areas, it is possible to identify clear cells, squamoid cells, or transitional (intermediate) polygonal cells. These elements are interspersed with areas in which there are mucus-secreting glandular cells. Most examples of MEC do not contain large foci of keratinization. However, areas of papillary growth may be seen as well as others with spindle cell proliferation. When the last of those components is extensive, such tumors are designated as "sclerosing" MECs.

Low-grade tumors characteristically lack necrosis and hemorrhage. As mentioned above, the cytologic features of these tumors are bland and mitotic activity is minimal or absent (Fig. 16.37). High-grade tumors share some of the architectural features seen in low-grade lesions but

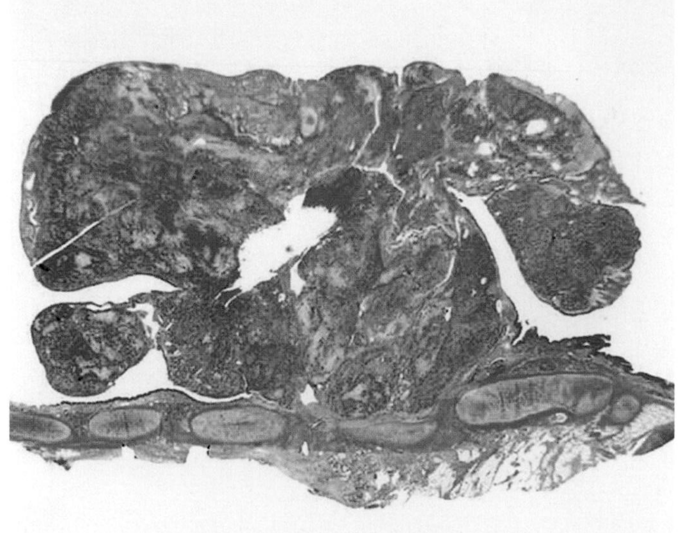

Fig. 16.36 Mucoepidermoid carcinoma is represented by a well-defined endobronchial mass in this photomicrograph.

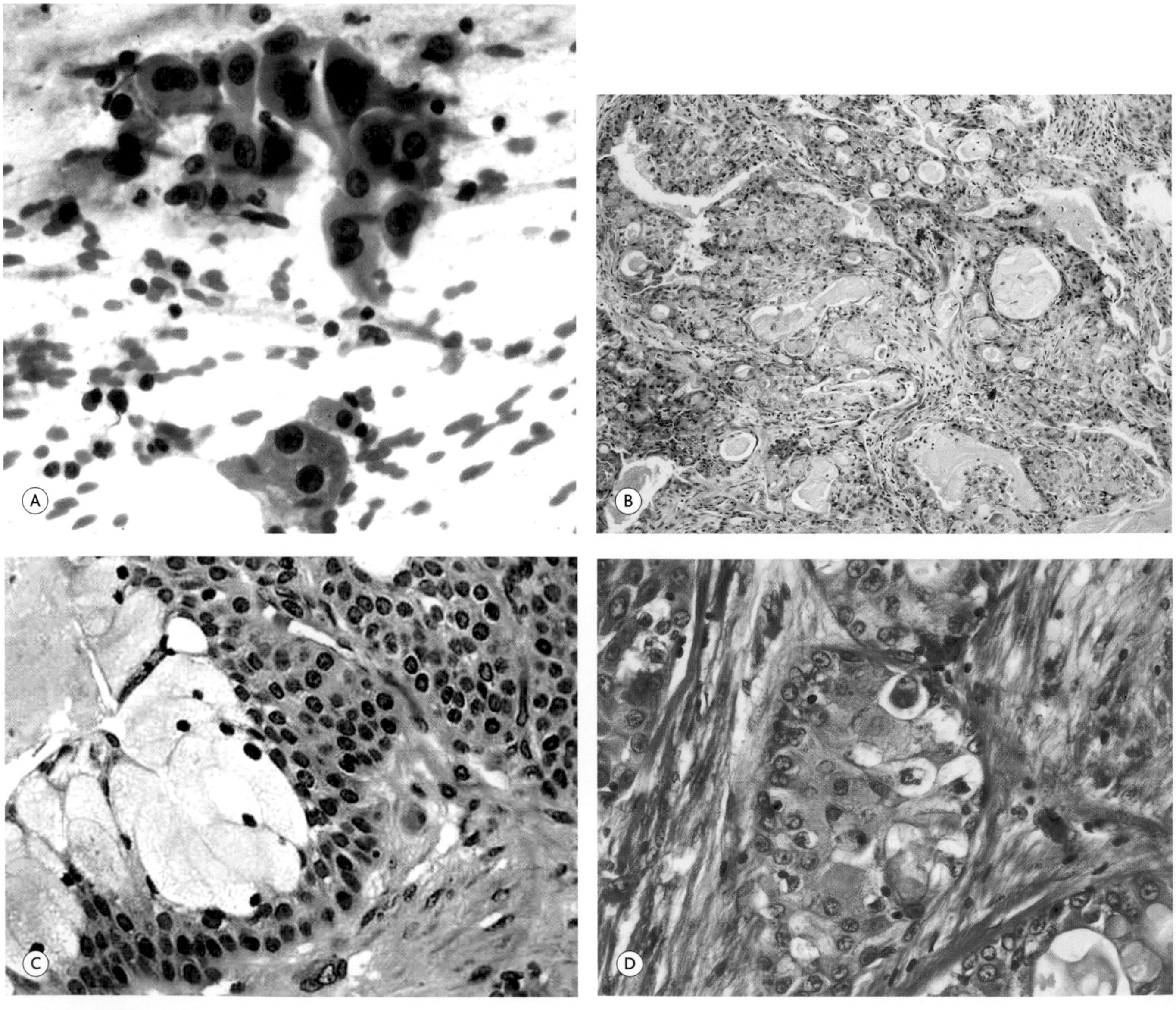

Fig. 16.37 (A) Fine-needle aspiration biopsy specimen from pulmonary mucoepidermoid carcinoma, showing aggregates of relatively bland squamoid cells in a mucoid background. (B–D) A juxtaposition of squamoid and mucinous glandular cells is apparent in this low-grade tumor.

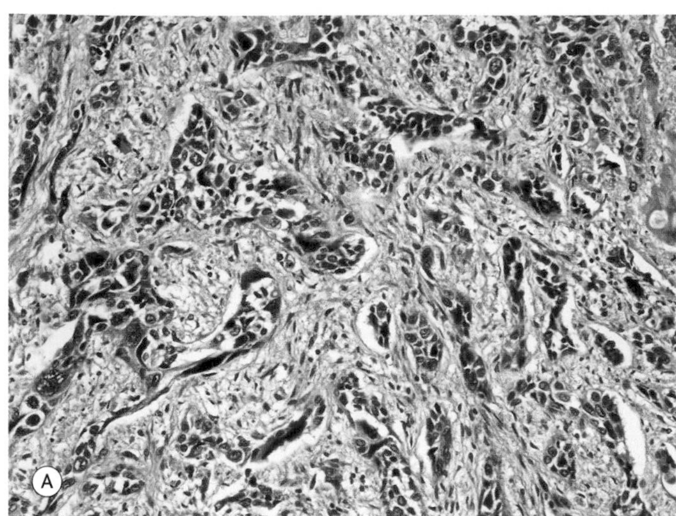
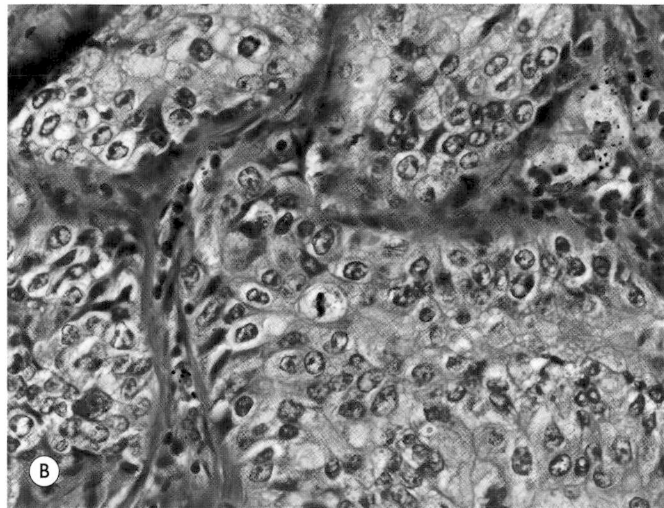

Fig. 16.38 (A,B) High-grade mucoepidermoid carcinoma demonstrates a greater degree of cytologic anaplasia in both its squamoid and glandular elements (compare with Fig. 16.37).

manifest a much higher degree of cytologic atypia and mitotic activity (Fig. 16.38). In some cases, necrosis and hemorrhage are also present.

In regard to low-grade MECs, especially in small biopsies, the most important tumor that poses a differential diagnostic problem is mucus gland adenoma. Unfortunately, a distinction between those two entities may not be possible until a complete resection of the tumor is performed. Mucus gland adenomas are generally confined to the internal aspect of bronchi in which they arise (luminal to the bronchial cartilage). In contrast, mucoepidermoid carcinomas commonly invade through the entirety of the bronchial wall. Another differential diagnostic problem is that of well-differentiated squamous cell carcinoma; in the context under discussion here, the presence of marked keratinization would favor an interpretation of a purely squamous tumor over one of MEC.

A separation of high-grade MEC from adenosquamous carcinoma may be largely academic, practically speaking, but it is usually based on the absence of foci of conventional-type adenocarcinoma in MEC and their presence in adenosquamous carcinoma. Other features that have been used in this separation include a central location for MEC, the absence of an in-situ carcinomatous component in mucoepidermoid tumors, and the presence of low-grade mucoepidermoid areas in some high-grade MECs.

The behavior of these neoplasms is best related to their stage and grade. Tumors in the low-grade MEC category can be managed by resection alone, and an indolent course is expected. However, in those that are categorized as high grade, surgical resection is usually followed by adjuvant radiation or chemotherapy and their behavior approximates that of more ordinary forms of lung cancer.

Adenoid cystic carcinoma

Adenoid cystic carcinoma (ACC) represents the second most common SGTTL,[94–101] and typically occurs in adults. In one large series on this tumor[94] patients ranged from 29 to 79 years in age (mean: 54 years), with a male-to-female ratio of 2:1. Clinically, because of their characteristic central location, pulmonary ACCs present with symptoms and signs of bronchial erosion or obstruction, including pneumonia, dyspnea, cough, wheezing, and hemoptysis. However, tumors arising in the peripheral lung have been reported as well, and these are usually asymptomatic. The average size of a pulmonary ACC is 4 cm, and the lesions are deceptively circumscribed on gross examination, with a soft yellow-white cut surface.

Adenoid cystic carcinoma is a prototypical tumor from a histologic perspective, being composed of monotonous arrays of compact polyhedral cells with uniformly round and hyperchromatic nucleoli and amphophilic cytoplasm.

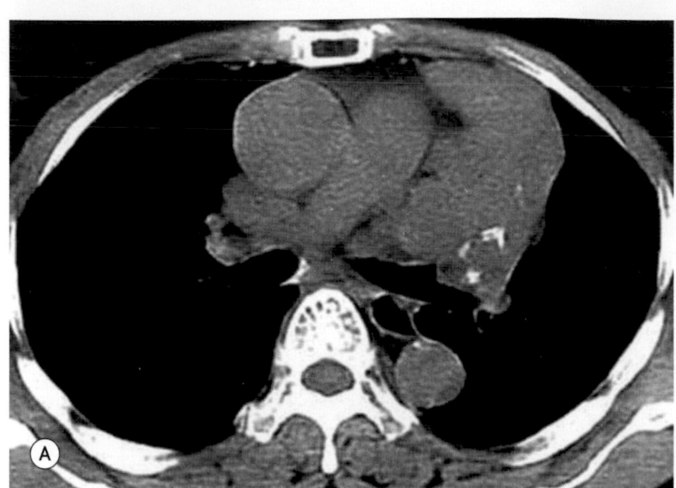

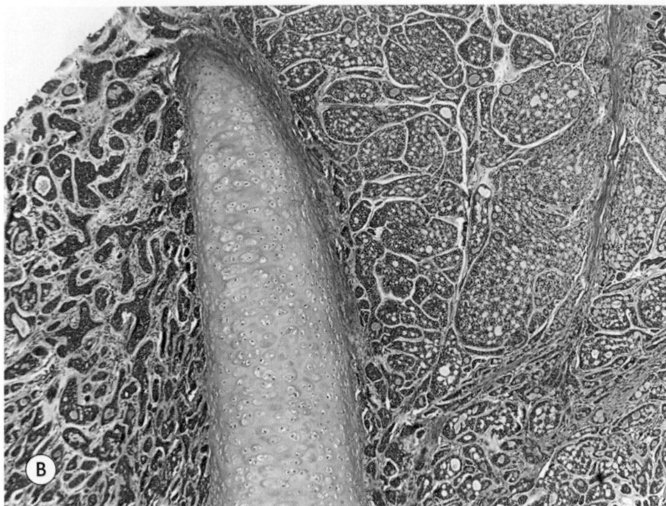

Fig. 16.39 (A) Computed tomogram of the thorax, showing infiltration and distortion of the left mainstem bronchus by adenoid cystic carcinoma of the lung. (B) The tumor is composed of monotonous small polygonal cells, which engulf plates of cartilage in the bronchial wall.

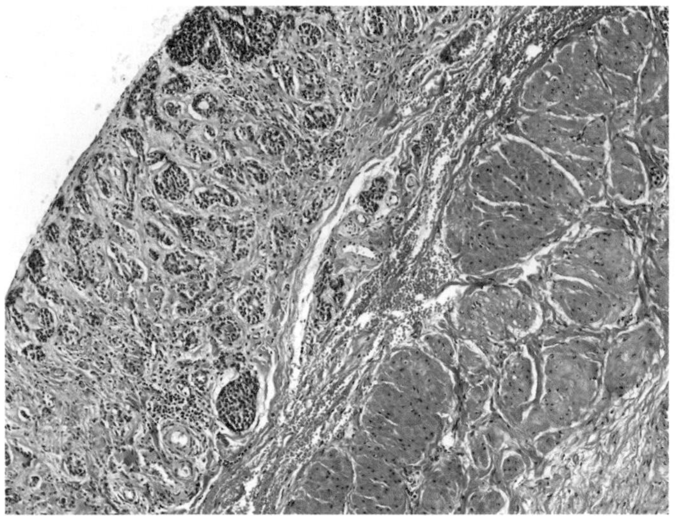

Fig. 16.40 Infiltration of the vascular adventitia of a pulmonary artery by adenoid cystic carcinoma of the lung.

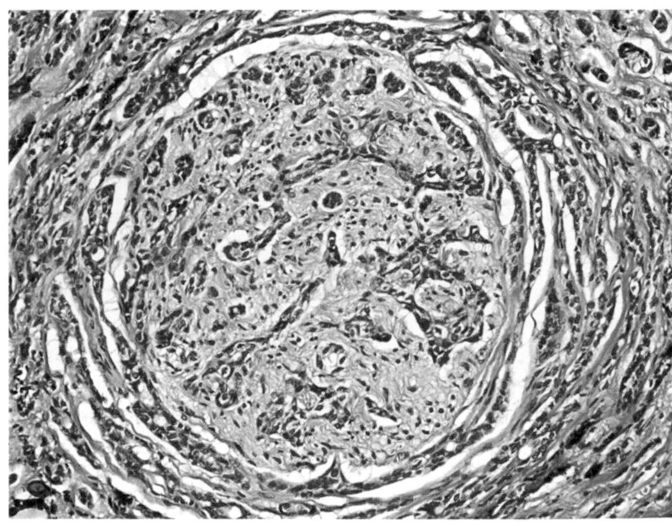

Fig. 16.41 Perineurial infiltration in the bronchial submucosa, by pulmonary adenoid cystic carcinoma.

Indeed, were it not for the obviously infiltrative growth that the neoplasms exhibit – with permeation of bronchial walls, blood vessels, and perineurial sheaths (Figs 16.39–16.41) – the cytologic features of ACC would not lead one to immediately interpret it as a malignant lesion. Fine-needle aspiration is effective in demonstrating the cytologic homogeneity of the tumor,[102] and it also shows interspersed cylinders or spheres of eosinophilic matrical material contained within the epithelial cell groups (Fig. 16.42). The most common histologic growth pattern is the "cylindromatous" one, reflected by islands and cords of tumor cells that are arranged in characteristic "jigsaw puzzle piece" pattern (Figs 16.43–16.45). Many cell groups encompass luminal or pseudoluminal spaces that may contain mucinous material – potentially yielding a cribriform image – and the nests are separated by bands of fibroconnective tissue with variable thickness. Cystic foci in ACC are lined by at least two layers of cells. Mitotic figures, nuclear pleomorphism, necrosis, and hemorrhage are almost always absent.

There are two additional growth patterns in pulmonary ACC which may pose a problem in regard to differential diagnosis. The "tubular" pattern characteristically shows arrangement of the neoplastic cells in small gland-like

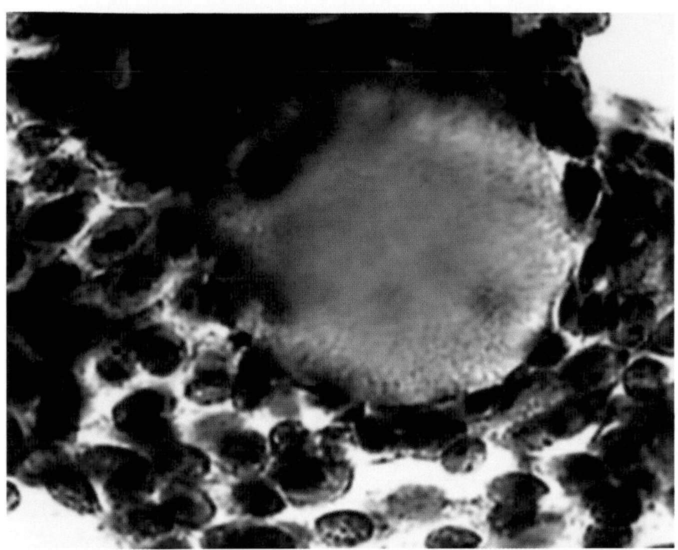

Fig. 16.42 Fine-needle aspiration biopsy specimen from bronchial adenoid cystic carcinoma, demonstrating monotonous small round tumor cells that encompass rounded profiles of eosinophilic basement membrane material.

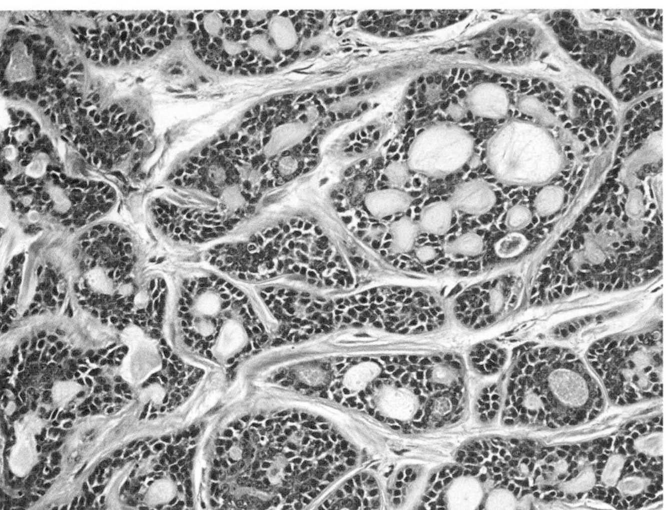

Fig. 16.44 The presence of a cribriform pattern of growth is well seen in the cell nests of this bronchial adenoid cystic carcinoma.

spaces or elongated cylinders (Fig. 16.46). Cytologically, the tumor cells in that variant are similar to those seen in cylindromatous ACC. The "solid" variant of ACC exhibits a medullary or insular proliferation of tumor cells with few if any intercellular spaces and only scant stromal matrix (Fig. 16.47). Mitotic activity is more brisk in that subtype as well. The diagnosis is suggested if abortive areas of cylindromatous differentiation can be identified; otherwise, several other tumor types with a basaloid cellular constituency enter diagnostic consideration. Purely tubular or solid adenoid cystic carcinomas are rare, with most cases demonstrating mixed histologic patterns from field to field in the lesion.

Adenoid cystic carcinoma of the lung may show ultrastructural or immunohistologic evidence of partial myoepithelial differentiation. Hence, potential reactivity for keratin, vimentin, actin, and S100 protein is observed. Labeling for CD117 (c-*kit* protein) has recently been described as well (Fig. 16.48).[103] Immunohistologic studies are usually not necessary for diagnosis, with the exception of some cases of "solid" ACC; in those lesions, stains for collagen type IV or laminin may be useful in highlighting small cylindrical stromal accumulations of basement membrane material. Tubular ACC may be confused with conventional well-differentiated adenocarcinoma of the lung; however, the latter tumor type typically contains larger cells with more discernible nucleoli.

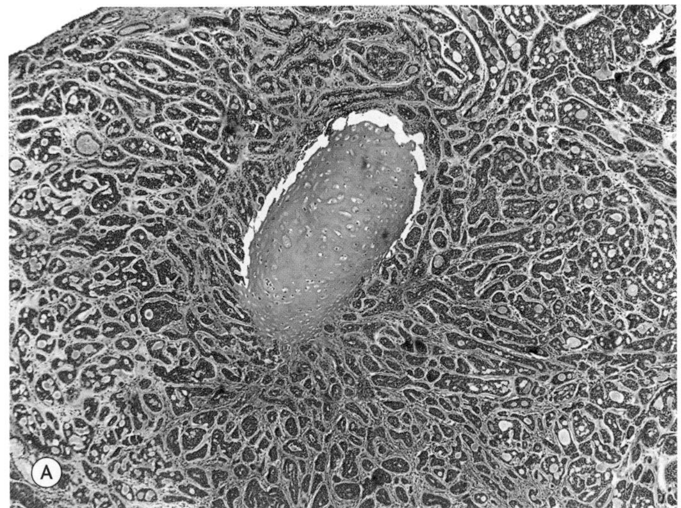

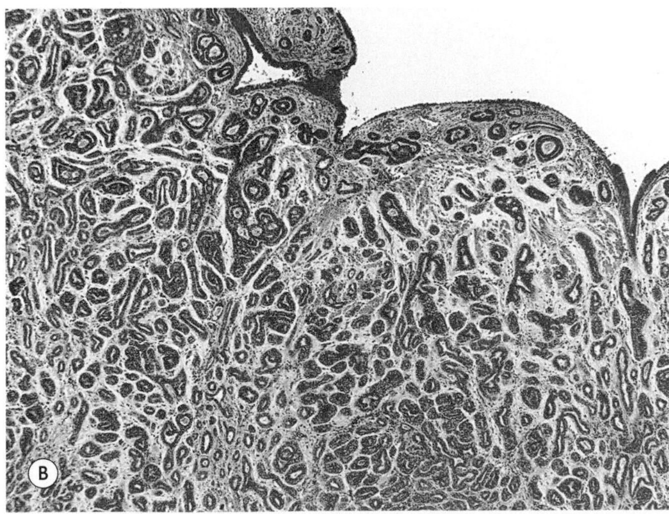

Fig. 16.43 (A,B) Bronchial adenoid cystic carcinoma, in which the nesting pattern of the tumor cells resembles pieces of a jigsaw puzzle.

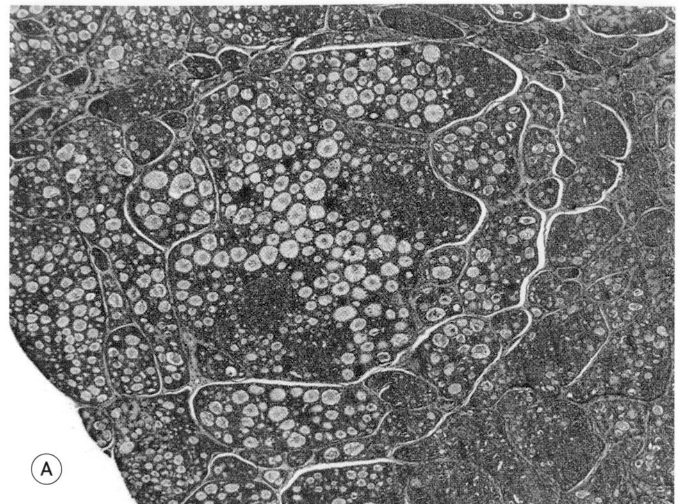

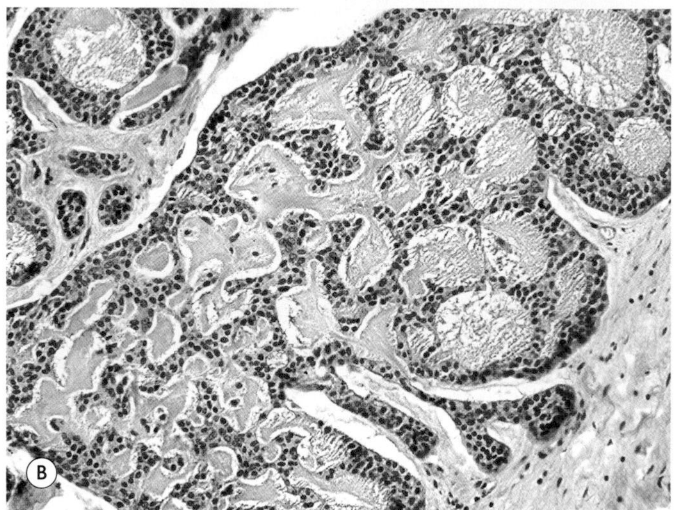

Fig. 16.45 (A,B) Many mucoid "cylinders" are contained within nests of monotonous small polygonal tumor cells in bronchial adenoid cystic carcinoma.

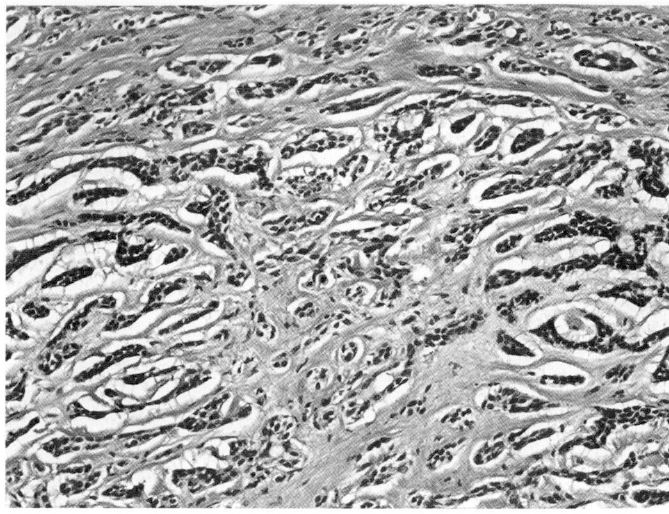

Fig. 16.46 Tubular profiles of tumor cells permeate a dense fibrohyaline stroma in this well-differentiated bronchial adenoid cystic carcinoma.

Adenoid cystic carcinomas are generally considered to be slowly growing tumors of low-grade malignancy. However, that view is deceptive in many cases. The lesions often pursue a tenaciously persistent course with recalcitrant intrathoracic recurrences over several years, culminating eventually with distant metastasis. Tumor stage at initial diagnosis is important in determining the clinical outcome, inasmuch as complete surgical excision offers the best chance of cure.

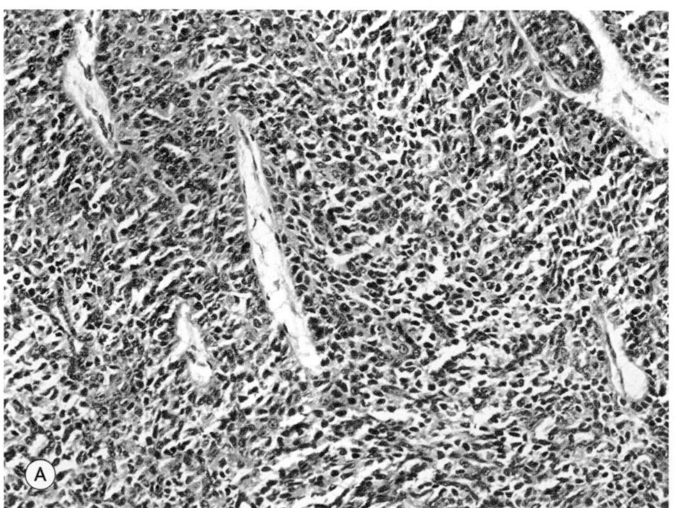

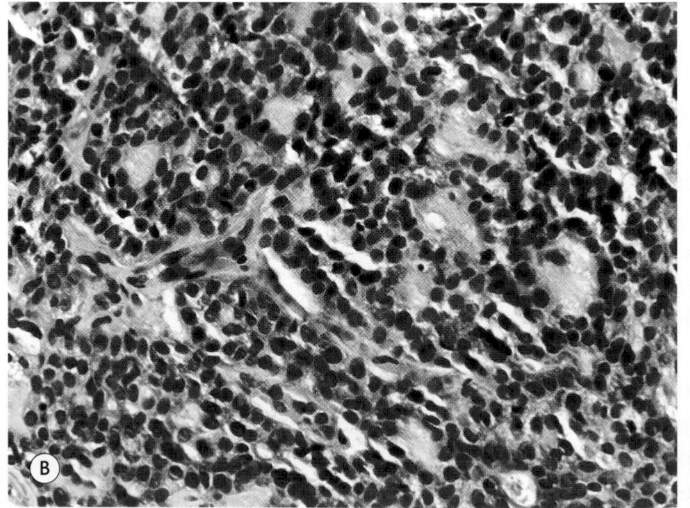

Fig. 16.47 (A,B) High-grade "solid" bronchial adenoid cystic carcinoma shows large nests of compact polygonal tumor cells in which only rare glandular foci are apparent.

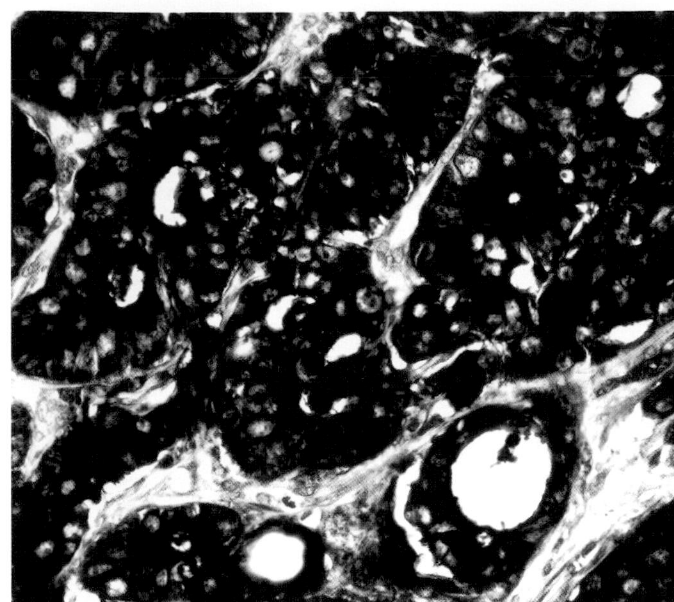

Fig. 16.48 Intense immunoreactivity is seen for CD117 (c-*kit* protein) in this bronchial adenoid cystic carcinoma.

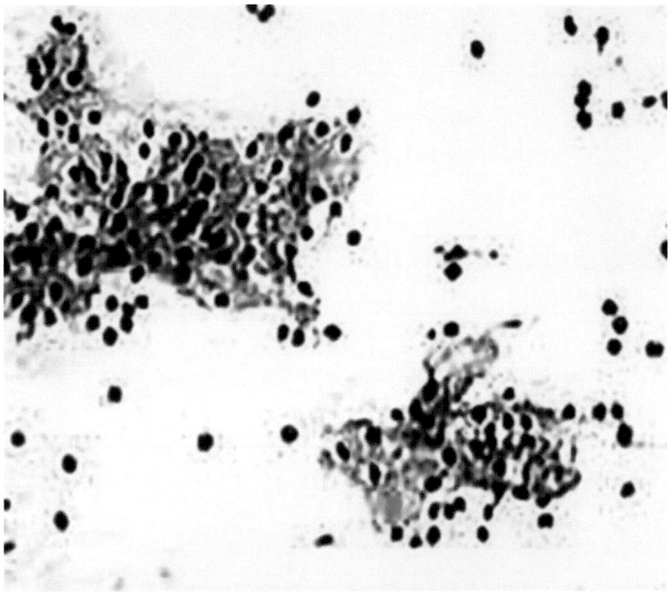

Fig. 16.49 Fine-needle aspiration biopsy specimen from acinic cell carcinoma, showing discrete nests of bland epithelial tumor cells with granulated cytoplasm.

Acinic cell carcinoma of the lung (Fechner's tumor)

Intrapulmonary acinic cell carcinoma has been designated as "Fechner's tumor" to honor the first description of this neoplasm by Dr. Robert Fechner.[104] It is an uncommon primary lesion in the lung but may be seen either as an endobronchial mass or a peripheral neoplasm that abuts a tubular airway.[105–107] Most descriptions of Fechner's tumors have been as isolated case reports. In the series that do exist on acinic cell carcinomas of the lung,[105] the authors noted that such tumors occur predominantly in adults, with an equal frequency in men and women. Because the majority of the lesions were peripherally located, most patients were asymptomatic and their tumors were discovered on screening chest radiographs. When Fechner's tumor assumes a central location, the patient is more likely to complain of dyspnea, cough, or hemoptysis.

These lesions are usually well circumscribed but not encapsulated, and they vary in size from 1 to 5 cm in greatest dimension. Their cut surfaces are tan-gray and homogeneous.

Scanning microscopy shows a circumscribed lesional image with internal effacement of the normal lung parenchyma. Solid growth is typical, with a composition of round-to-polygonal cells with prominently granular eosinophilic cytoplasm, round nuclei, and inconspicuous nucleoli. Mitotic activity and nuclear atypia are minimal, and areas of hemorrhage or necrosis are lacking (Figs 16.49–16.52). Occasionally, Fechner's tumor may comprise a proliferation of clear cells with granular cytoplasm and nuclei that are displaced towards the periphery of the cells, superficially simulating "signet ring" cells. The neoplastic cells also may be arranged in ill-defined nests separated by delicate fibroconnective tissue, with interspersed lymphocytes and plasma cells. Finally, as in the salivary glands, intrapulmonary acinic cell carcinoma may show acinar, oncocytic, cystic, and papillocystic growth patterns.

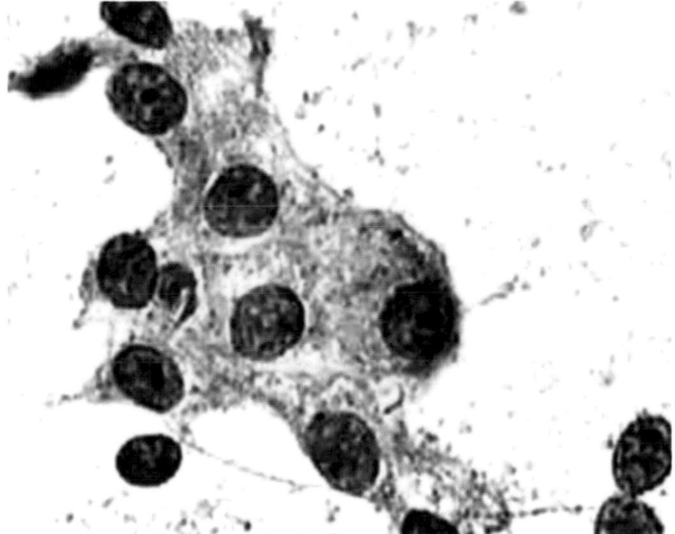

Fig. 16.50 The granular nature of the cytoplasm in acinic cell carcinoma is well seen in this fine-needle aspiration biopsy sample.

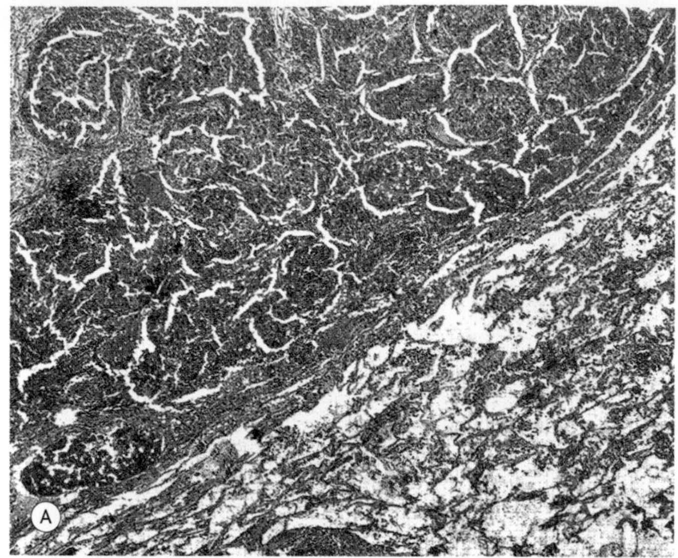

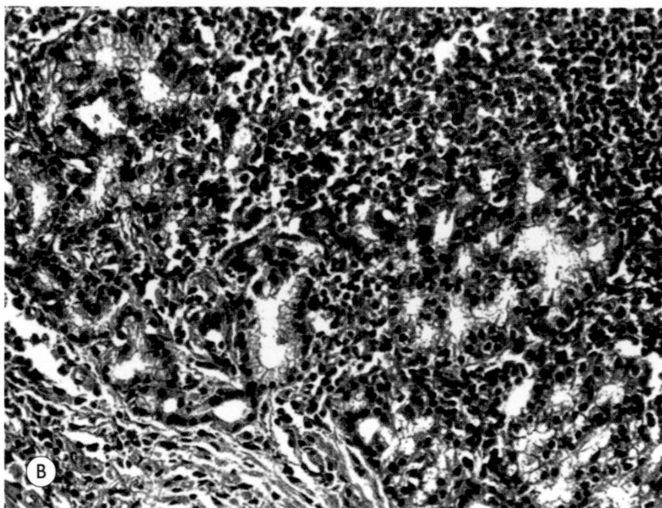

Fig. 16.51 (A) Acinic cell carcinoma of the lung (Fechner's tumor), demonstrating a circumscribed image with a relatively sharp interface with the surrounding lung parenchyma. (B) The tumor cells are bland, with granular to clear cytoplasm; they are arranged in small tubules, admixed with chronic inflammatory cells.

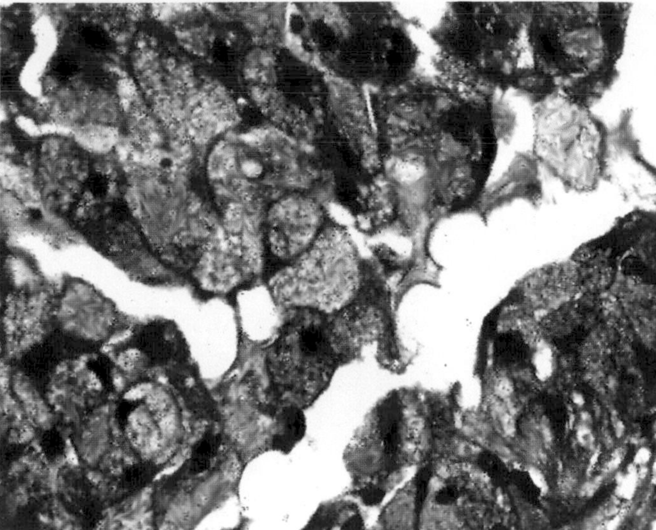

Fig. 16.52 In this example of pulmonary acinic cell carcinoma, the tumor cells have more amphophilic or lightly basophilic cytoplasm, which is granular in nature.

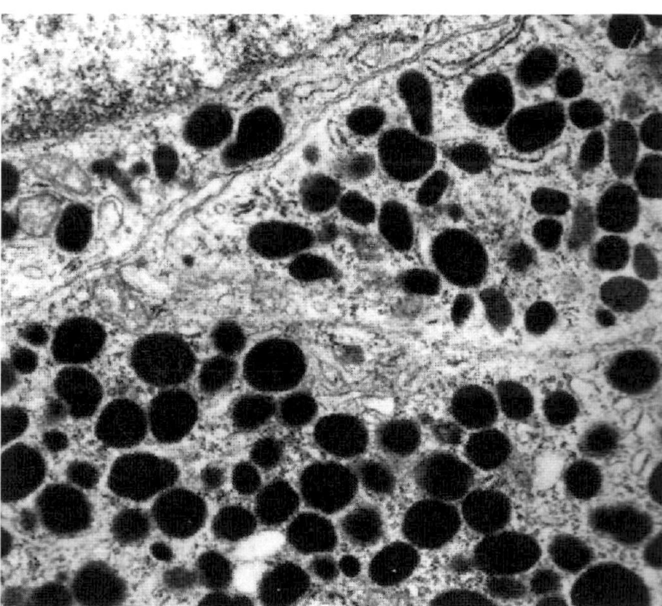

Fig. 16.53 Numerous zymogen-type granules are present in the cytoplasm of the tumor cells in acinic cell carcinoma, as seen in this electron photomicrograph.

One of the most useful histochemical stains in the evaluation of acinic cell carcinoma is the periodic acid–Schiff (PAS) method, used to demonstrate the presence of glycogen in the tumor cells. Mucicarmine stains may show foci of intracellular mucin production as well. Immunostains may demonstrate positivity for such lysosomal proteins as alpha-1-antitrypsin and amylase in the tumor cell granules.

Electron microscopy is still extremely helpful in the diagnosis of acinic cell carcinoma. The finding of large dark electron-dense or electron-lucent (immature) zymogen granules in the cytoplasm of the neoplastic cells is characteristic (Fig. 16.53).

The differential diagnosis of Fechner's tumor variants depends largely on the histologic growth pattern and cell type. When the lesion has prominently oncocytic features, the most important differential diagnosis is with oncocytoid carcinoid tumor (grade I neuroendocrine carcinoma). In this specific setting, immunohistochemical positivity for chromogranin-A, CD56, and synaptophysin is helpful in recognizing neuroendocrine tumors and excluding acinic cell carcinoma. On the other hand, when acinic cell tumors contain clear cells with "signet-ring-cell"-like features, the most important alternative diagnostic consideration is that of a conventional pulmonary adenocarcinoma with similar cytologic attributes. In that context, histochemical evaluations for intracellular mucin are helpful, because the intracytoplasmic vacuoles of true signet-ring-cell carcinomas should label with the mucicarmine or digested PAS methods. "Sugar tumor" (myomelanocytoma) of the lung is another possible differential diagnosis in cases of acinic cell carcinoma. The former of those entities may also show strong PAS-positivity, but, unlike acinic cell carcinoma, sugar tumors also display immunoreactivity with HMB-45 and MART-1.

Fechner's tumors are low-grade malignancies, and they have limited but definite potential to metastasize. Examples have been reported that involved regional lymph nodes in the thorax,[108,109] but the overall clinical evolution is usually favorable.

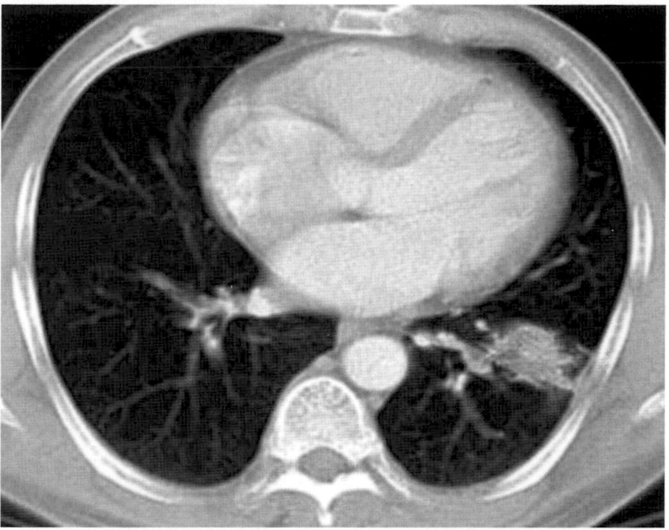

Fig. 16.54 Computed tomogram of the thorax, showing an irregularly shaped mass in the left lung field which represents an intrapulmonary mixed tumor.

Pleomorphic adenoma (mixed tumor)

Pleomorphic adenoma – also known as mixed tumor – is an uncommon primary tumor of the lung.[110–114] It occurs predominantly in adults with a slight predominance in women. The age range in which this tumor has been described is between 35 and 75 years. The lesion may present either as a central or a peripheral mass in any portion of either lung. Symptoms are again related to the location of the tumor, with those in the central bronchi manifesting with complaints relating to obstruction. Peripheral lesions sometimes present with chest pain but more frequently are discovered incidentally in screening chest radiographs (Fig. 16.54).

Macroscopically, endobronchial lesions are commonly polypoid tumors, whereas those in the periphery of the lung present as well-circumscribed tumors that are usually attached to bronchi (Fig. 16.55). The size of the neoplasms varies from 1 to 16 cm in greatest diameter. The cut surfaces of mixed tumors may be chondroid and firm, or they may have a soft consistency with only focal induration.

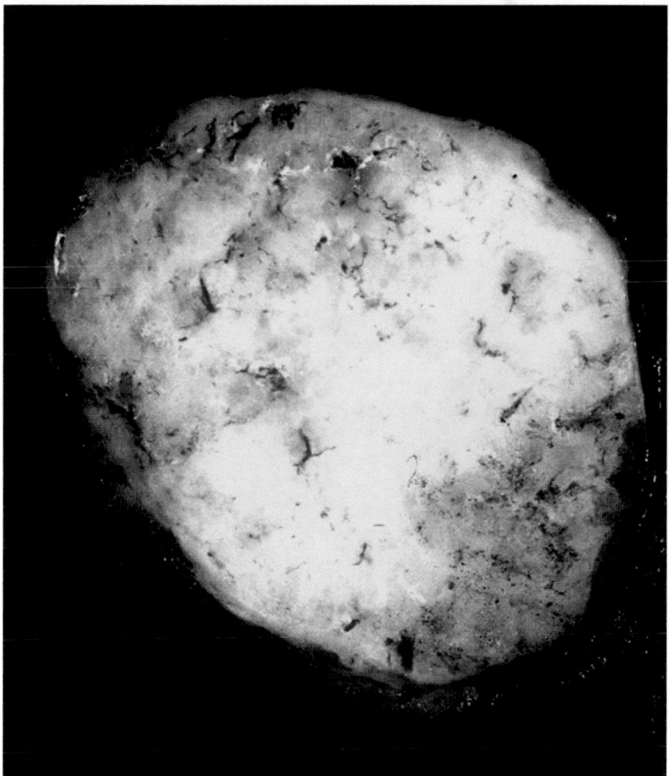

Fig. 16.55 Gross photograph of an excised pulmonary mixed tumor, demonstrating a blue-gray, translucent, "chondroid" cut surface.

By definition, pleomorphic adenomas of the lung tumors show at least a biphasic microscopic image; they are characteristically composed of epithelial tubules and nests that are embedded in a chondromyxoid stroma (Figs 16.56 and 16.57). Interestingly, however, intrapulmonary mixed tumors rarely show the amount of mature cartilaginous stroma that one observes in mixed tumors of the salivary glands. In some lesions, the predominant growth pattern may be that of a solid myoepithelial proliferation which approximates that of "cellular" mixed tumors in the head and neck. Those neoplasms comprise compact epithelioid cells with

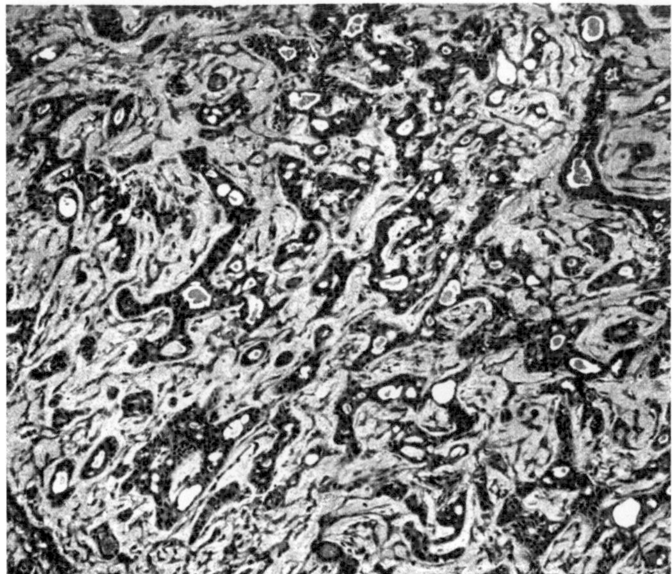

Fig. 16.56 Pulmonary mixed tumor, showing irregularly branching tubules of bland epithelial cells that are embedded in a myxochondroid stroma.

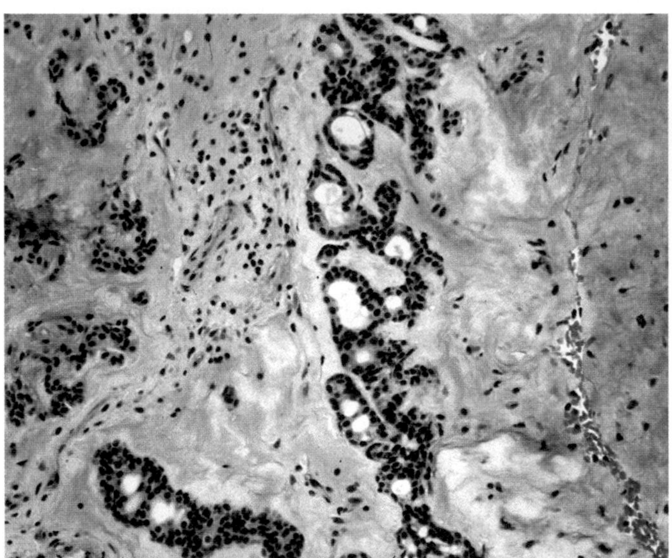

Fig. 16.57 The two components of pulmonary mixed tumor are well seen in this photomicrograph.

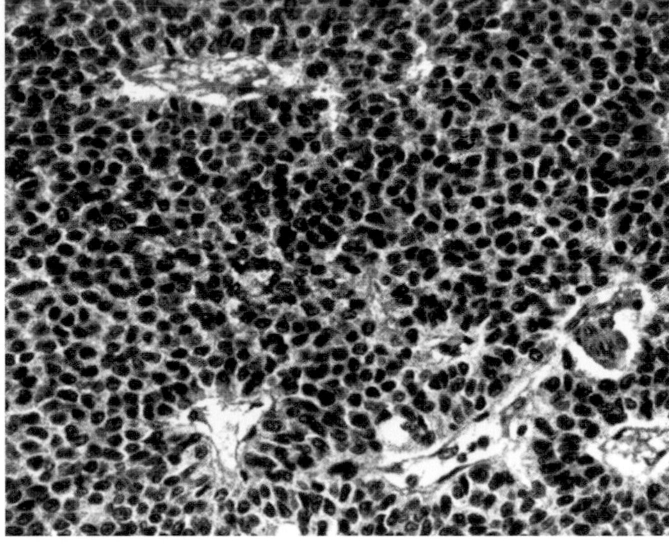

Fig. 16.58 "Cellular" mixed tumor lacks notable myxochondroid stroma throughout much of the mass, yielding an image which can be confused with that of other basaloid neoplasms.

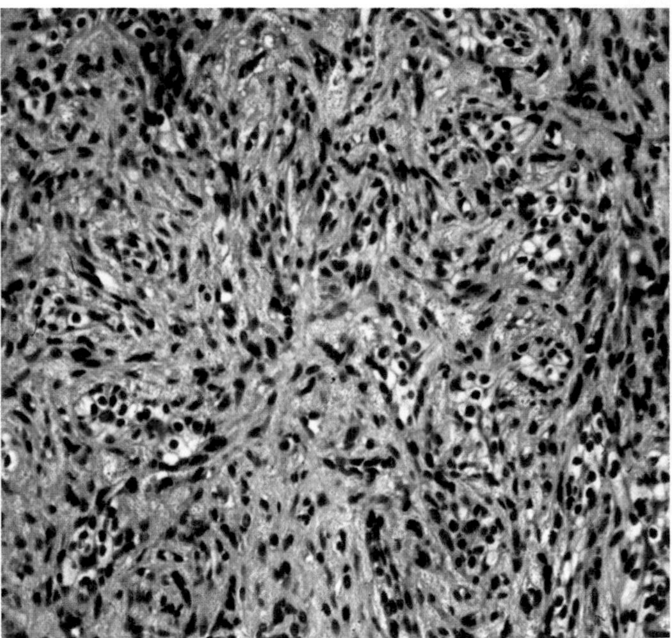

Fig. 16.59 The "myoepithelioma" variant of mixed tumor comprises fusiform tumor cells in a chondroid or hyalinized stroma, with little or no evidence of tubular epithelial differentiation.

round or oval nuclei, which generally lack nuclear atypia, necrosis, hemorrhage, and mitotic activity (Fig. 16.58). Notably, there have been no well-documented cases of carcinoma arising from pre-existing mixed tumors of the lung, as may rarely occur in salivary glandular sites. Other variants of mixed tumor include a "myoepitheliomatous" subtype that may manifest either a spindle cell composition (Fig. 16.59) or a plasmacytoid constituency; a form with extensive squamous metaplasia (Fig. 16.60); a subtype in which sizable zones of the lesion demonstrate an adenoid cystic carcinoma-like cribriform architecture; and a chondroid-rich form that simulates bronchial chondroma or chondromatous hamartoma.

Differential diagnosis depends on whether one is dealing with a biopsy specimen or a complete resection of the tumor. In the former instance, mixed tumors can be confused with other SGTTLs such as adenoid cystic carcinoma, as well as with hamartoma/chondroma, squamous cell carcinoma (when squamous metaplasia is

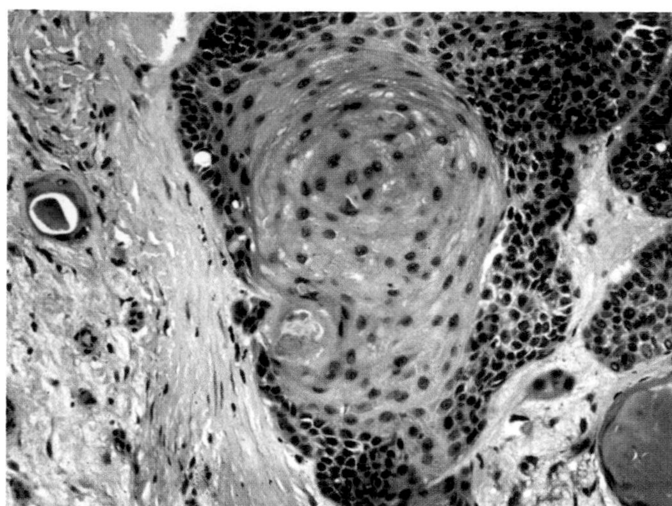

Fig. 16.60 Prominent squamous metaplasia is apparent in this bronchial mixed tumor.

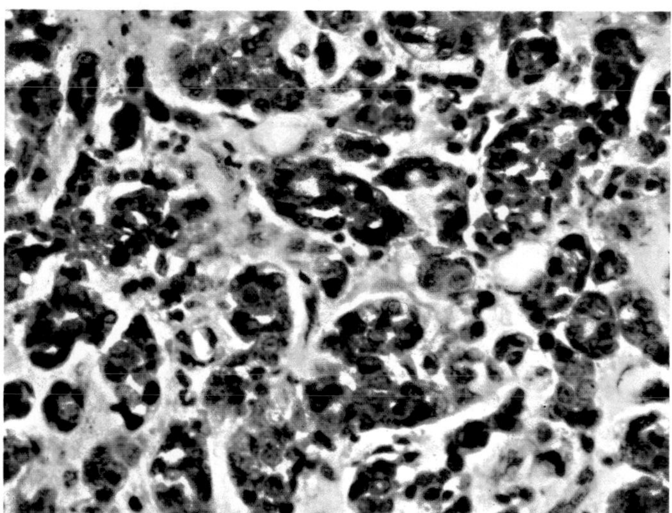

Fig. 16.61 Immunoreactivity for glial fibrillary acidic protein in mixed tumor, providing a helpful differential diagnostic marker for this lesion.

dominant), and biphasic malignancies such as sarcomatoid carcinoma. In resection specimens, the diagnosis is typically straightforward. However, if mixed tumors demonstrate an overwhelmingly prominent solid pattern with spindle cell ("myoepitheliomatous") differentiation, sarcomas may also enter into consideration. In this setting, concurrent immunoreactivity for keratin, S100 protein, actin, and glial fibrillary acidic protein (Fig. 16.61)[115] would provide the necessary evidence for the diagnosis of a mixed tumor variant.

Mixed tumors of the lung behave in an indolent fashion. There are only anecdotal reports of metastasizing lesions of this type,[116] in analogy to rare examples in the salivary glands. No particular pathologic features of such neoplasms can be utilized to predict this unusual adverse behavior. Complete but conservative excision is the treatment of choice.

Epithelial–myoepithelial carcinoma

Epithelial–myoepithelial carcinoma (EMC) is one of the most unusual primary tumors of the lung, and it belongs to the SGTTL group. Only a few cases of this lesion have been reported:[117–121] they have involved adults with endobronchial masses, and, because of their central location, the neoplasms were associated with obstructive symptoms and signs. Epithelial–myoepithelial carcinoma is considered a low-grade malignancy. It is reported to be well circumscribed but not encapsulated and may measure up to 4 cm in greatest dimension.

The scanning image of EMC is that of a predominantly glandular proliferation which is transected by thin fibroconnective stromal septa. It is centered in a large tubular airway but extends into and obliterates the adjacent lung parenchyma. On closer inspection, the glandular components of EMC show a characteristically biphasic cellular population, with inner ductal epithelial cells surrounded by an outer layer of myoepithelium (Figs 16.62 and 16.63).[13–15] This neoplasm does not have a high mitotic rate or notable nuclear atypia; similarly, necrosis and hemorrhage are absent. Hence, the diagnosis must be made on the basis of an infiltrative architecture, together with the aforementioned cytologic attributes. Immunohistochemically, the inner cell layer in tumoral glands shows strong reactivity for keratin, whereas the outer layer demonstrates positivity for alpha-isoform actin, p63 protein, and S-100 protein.[121]

Because of the prominently glandular appearance of EMC, it can be easily confused with a well-differentiated adenocarcinoma. Detailed morphologic examination, coupled with demonstration of a myoepithelial immunophenotype, are keys to the correct diagnostic interpretation. Mixed tumors also manifest a similar immunohistologic profile but differ substantially on morphologic grounds from EMC (see above).

In light of the rarity of this tumor in the lungs, it is difficult to draw meaningful conclusions regarding the behavior of pulmonary EMC. Pelosi et al.[121] have reviewed the pertinent literature and concluded that the term "pulmonary epithelial–myoepithelial tumor of unproven malignant potential" was preferable to EMC, because of a lack of metastasis in the reported cases to date. In any event, complete excision is recommended for this tumor.

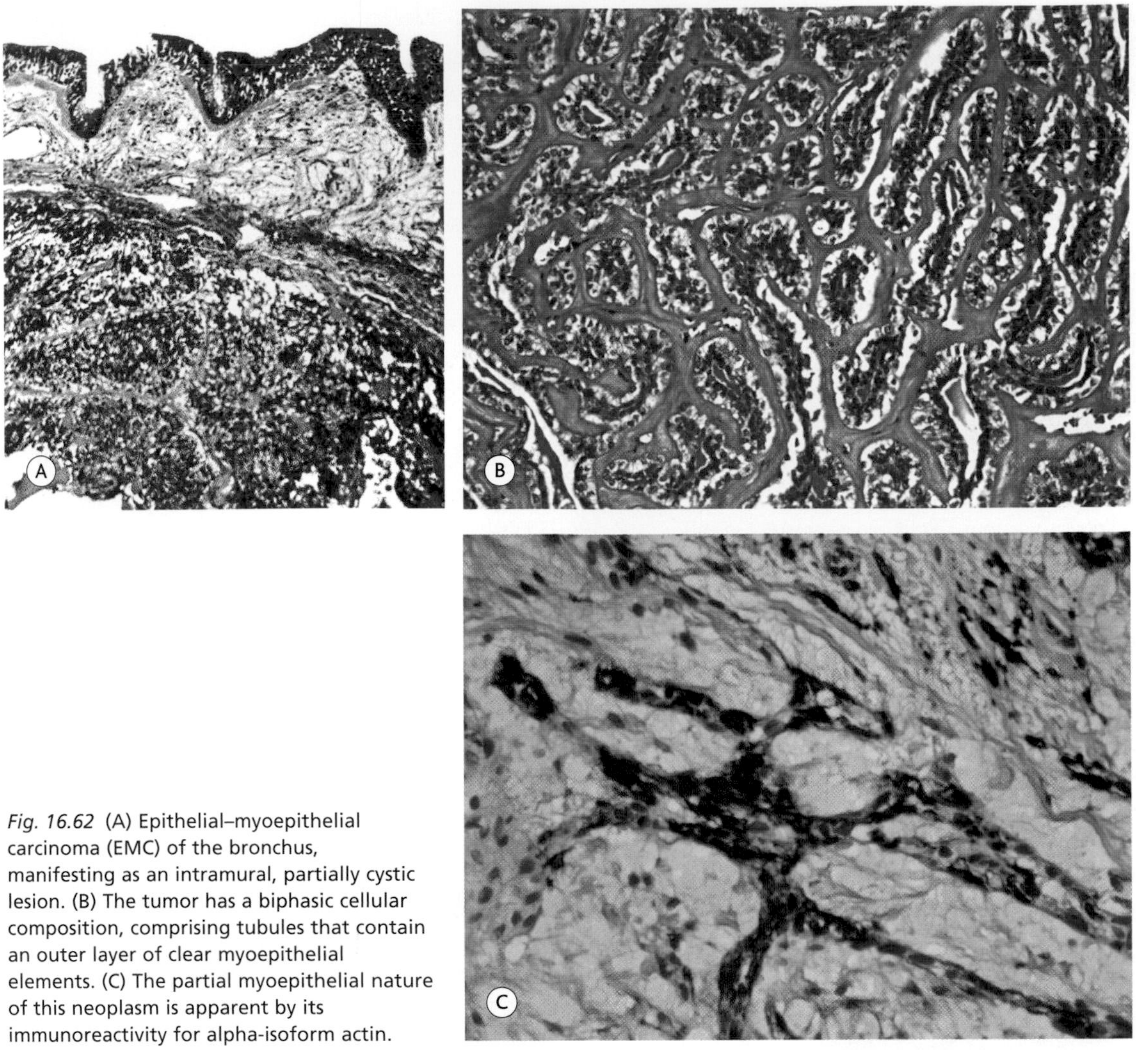

Fig. 16.62 (A) Epithelial–myoepithelial carcinoma (EMC) of the bronchus, manifesting as an intramural, partially cystic lesion. (B) The tumor has a biphasic cellular composition, comprising tubules that contain an outer layer of clear myoepithelial elements. (C) The partial myoepithelial nature of this neoplasm is apparent by its immunoreactivity for alpha-isoform actin.

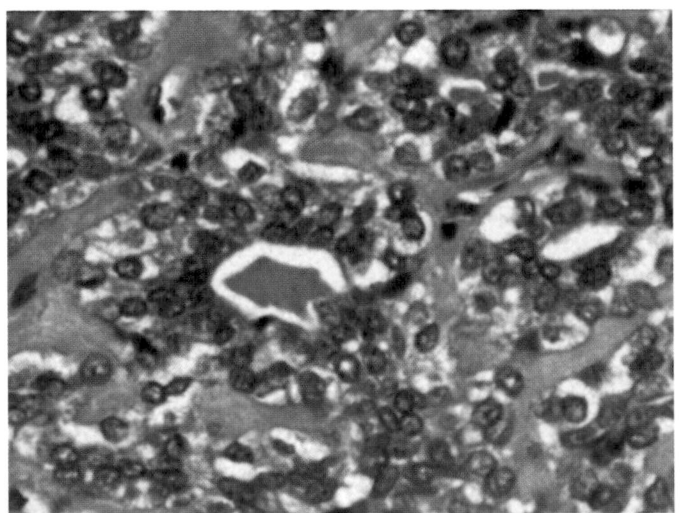

Fig. 16.63 This photograph shows the relationship between inner layers of epithelial cells and outer layers of myoepithelial elements in the tubules of epithelial–myoepithelial carcinoma.

Oncocytoma

Oncocytoma is a rare neoplasm in the lung, and there are only a few reported cases in the literature.[122–124] They exhibit similarities to comparable tumors in the salivary glands, showing a composition by nests of uniformly large polygonal cells with prominently eosinophilic granular cytoplasm and bland nuclei (Figs 16.64 and 16.65) . In view of the existence of other, more common pulmonary tumors that can show oncocytic changes, it is important to properly exclude those other possibilities by adjunctive studies. Primary pulmonary neuroendocrine tumors showing oncocytic features (oncocytic carcinoids; grade I neuroendocrine carcinomas) are by far more common than oncocytomas, and are recognizable by their

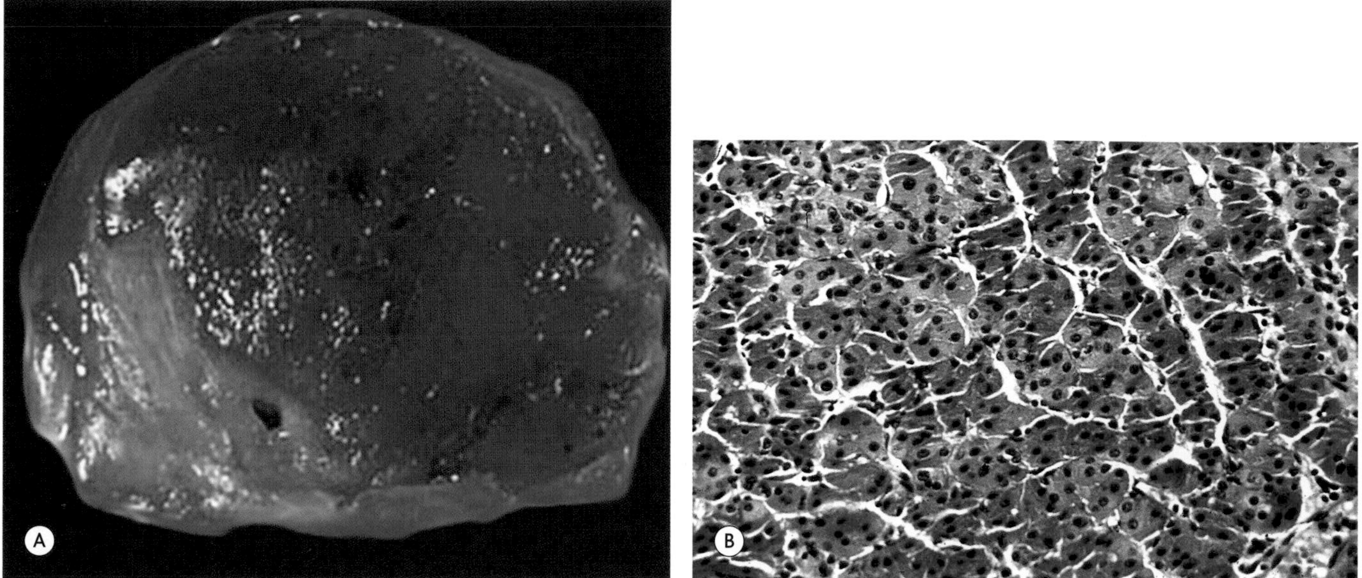

Fig. 16.64 (A) Endobronchial oncocytoma is represented by a homogeneous, soft, brownish mass, as seen in this gross photograph. (B) The tumor cells are arranged in compact nests.

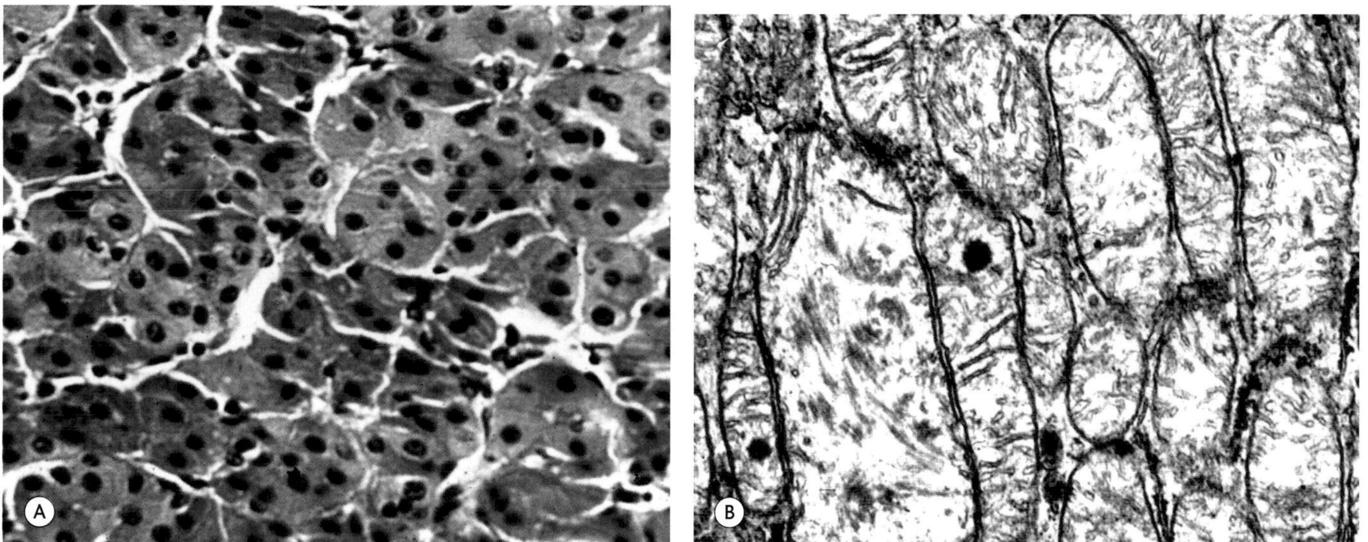

Fig. 16.65 (A) Bronchial oncocytoma shows granular eosinophilic cytoplasm and bland compact nuclei. (B) Electron microscopy demonstrates numerous mitochondria in the tumor cell cytoplasm.

immunoreactivity for chromogranin-A, synaptophysin, and CD56.[125] Metastatic tumors from extrathoracic sites such as the salivary glands and kidneys also need to be considered. Clinical information is important in this context, because electron microscopic and immunophenotypic properties of primary and metastatic oncocytic neoplasms may be very similar. Because of problems with the definition of pulmonary oncocytoma, as noted above, meaningful comments are precluded on its behavior.

Histopathologic and oncogenetic factors with putative prognostic significance for carcinomas of the lung

Several histologic factors that can be observed in conventionally stained microscopic sections have putative prognostic significance. Principal among these are, quite simply, the histologic type of the tumor, its level of

Table 16.2 TNM staging of lung carcinoma

T – Tumor size or extent of involvement	
TX	Tumor proven by the presence of malignant cells in bronchopulmonry secretions but not visualized roentgenographically or bronchoscopically, or any tumor that cannot be assessed as in treatment staging
T0	No evidence of primary tumor
Tis	Carcinoma in situ
T1	A tumor that is 3 cm or less in greatest dimension, surrounded by lung or visceral pleura, and without evidence of invasion proximal to a lobar bronchus at bronchoscopy. (Note: the uncommon superficial tumor of any size with its invasive component limited to the bronchial wall which may extend proximal to the main bronchus is also classified as T1.)
T2	A tumor more than 3.0 cm in greatest dimension or a tumor of any size that either invades the visceral pleura or has associated atelectasis or obstructive pneumonitis extending to the hilar region. At bronchoscopy, the proximal extent of demonstrable tumor must be within a lobar bronchus or at least 2.0 cm distal to the carcinoma. Any associated atelectasis or obstructive pneumonitis must involve less than an entire lung
T3	A tumor of any size with direct extension into the chest wall (including superior sulcus tumors), diaphragm, or the mediastinal pleura or pericardium without involving the heart, great vessels, trachea, esophagus, or vertebral body, or a tumor in the main bronchus within 2 cm of the carina without involving the carina
T4	A tumor of any size with invasion of the mediastinum or involving heart, great vessels, trachea, esophagus, vertebral body, or carina, or presence of malignant pleural effusion. (Note: most pleural effusions associated with lung cancer are due to tumor. There are, however, a few patients in whom cytopathologic examination of pleural fluid – on more than one specimen – is negative for tumor, the fluid is nonbloody, and is not an exudate. In such cases where these elements and clinical judgment dictate that the effusion is not related to the tumor, the patient should be staged TI, T2, or T3, excluding effusion as a staging element.) Also, the occurrence of separate tumor nodule(s) in the same lobe.
N – Nodal status	
NX	Regional lymph nodes cannot be assessed
N0	No demonstrable metastasis to regional lymph nodes
N1	Metastasis to lymph nodes in the peribronchial or the ipsilateral hilar region, or both, including direct extension
N2	Metastasis to ipsilateral mediastinal lymph nodes or subcarinal lymph nodes
N3	Metastasis to contralateral mediastinal lymph nodes, contralateral hilar nodes, ipsilateral or contralateral scalene, or supraclavicular lymph nodes
M – Distant metastases	
MX	Presence of distant metastases cannot be assessed
M0	No (known) distant metastasis
M1	Distant metastasis present – specify site(s). Also, separate tumor nodule(s) in a different lobe (ipsilateral or contralateral).

Table 16.3 Clinical stage groupings according to TNM subsets

Stage	Percent of cases	T factor	N factor	M factor	Surgical candidate
Occult	<1	TX	N0	M0	Yes
0	<1	Tis	N0	M0	Yes
I	13	T1 or T2	N0	M0	Yes
II	10	T1 or T2	N1	M0	Yes
IIIA	22	T3	N0 or N1	M0	Yes
		T1 through T3	N2	M0	Yes
IIIB	22	Any T	N3	M0	No
		T4	Any N	M0	No
IV	32	Any T	Any N	M1	No

For definitions of the T, N, and M factors see Table 16.2.

differentiation, and the status of the surgical margins and resected lymph nodes (if any) (Tables 16.2 and 16.3).[126–128] In addition, invasion of the visceral pleura by lung cancers increases their T substages and worsens survival, all other variables being equal.[129] Bunker et al. have shown that application of the Verhoeff–van Gieson elastic stain to paraffin sections enhances the pathologist's ability to recognize this feature.[130] A semiquantitative estimate of the degree of tumor necrosis was also reported to have predictive value by Elson et al.,[131] in a study of non-neuroendocrine carcinomas of the lung. Moreover, documentation of angiolymphatic vascular invasion by tumor was found to have similar importance by Haque and colleagues,[132] and, because it is more frequently observed in adenocarcinoma, may explain the worsened survival with which that tumor type is associated, vis-à-vis squamous cell carcinoma of the lung.

In other anatomic sites, particularly the head and neck and axillae, the presence of extranodal extension by tumor metastases of carcinomas has been associated with worsened prognosis. It is currently unknown as to whether this is also true of lung cancers that involve regional lymph nodes, and prospective analyses will be necessary to definitively address this point.

A number of investigators have examined the use of adjunctive techniques for the evaluation of proliferative activity in lung cancer. One may apply flow cytometry to measure the S-phase fraction of the tumor cell population,[126] or immunohistology to assess the expression of S-phase-related nuclear proteins such as Ki-67/MIB-1/PCNA.[133] To date, however, published work on such markers has not found them to offer a great deal more information than simple counting of mitotic figures. Similarly, measurement of DNA-ploidy in pulmonary carcinomas does not appear to provide prognostically valuable data.[126]

Over the past decade, a great deal of research has addressed the possible role of genetic alterations in predicting the clinical outcome of lung cancer cases. In particular, aberrations of the p53, c-*erb*B-2, K-*ras*, RB-1, *myc*, and *bcl*-2 genes have been evaluated in the greatest detail, but with conflicting and inconclusive results.[134–144] At present, therefore, the authors do not regard such assessments as clinically applicable or reliable in a prognostic context. Despite the work of Fontanini et al.,[145] purportedly demonstrating the predictive utility of microvessel counts in lung cancers, it is felt that, at present, a similar comment applies to that adjunctive area of analysis as well.[139]

Stylized surgical pathology reports on carcinoma of the lung

Obviously, not all pulmonary carcinomas are resectable. Colby and Deschamps[146] have nicely summarized the clinicopathologic features of these tumors, including that subset which is surgically approachable (Table 16.4). For those lesions that can be completely excised, pathology organizations such as the College of American Pathologists and the Association of Directors of Anatomic & Surgical Pathology (ADASP) have published guidelines for the current reporting of morphologic findings.[147,148] In the authors' opinion, the most tenable is that provided by the latter of those two organizations, which is reproduced in slightly modified form below.

Suggested ADASP reporting format for resected lung carcinomas[147]

A. Gross description

1. How the specimen was received – fresh, in formalin, opened, unopened, etc.
2. How the specimen was identified – labeled with (name, number) and designated as (e.g. right upper lobe).
3. Part(s) of lung included – including measurements in three dimensions and weights, and description of other attached structures (i.e. parietal pleura, hilar lymph nodes, etc.)
4. Tumor description:
   - Tumor location, including relationship to lobe(s), segment(s), and, if pertinent, major airway(s), and pleura. Involvement of lobar or mainstream bronchus should be specified.
   - Proximity to bronchial resection margin, and to other surgical margins (i.e. chest wall soft tissue, hilar vessels) as appropriate.

Table 16.4 Comparison of clinicopathologic features by histologic types of carcinoma of the lung

Tumor type	Percent of cases	Percent of smokers	Central lesions (%)	Localized (%)	5-year survival
Squamous cell	30	98	64	21.5	15.4%
Adenocarcinoma	31	82	5	22.2	16.6%[a]
Grade 3 NE, small-cell	19	99	74	8.2	4.6%
Other[b]	15	95	42	15	11.5%

Source: modified from Colby and Deschamps.[146]
NE = Neuroendocrine.
[a] Bronchioloalveolar carcinomas are associated with a 42% 5-year survival.
[b] Statistics in this group encompass large cell "undifferentiated," grade 3 neuroendocrine carcinoma, large cell type, and sarcomatoid carcinoma, but not salivary gland analogue tumors.

– Tumor size (three dimensions if possible).
– Presence or absence of satellite tumor nodules.

5. Description of non-tumorous lung – i.e. presence or absence of postobstructive changes or other abnormalities (e.g. bronchiectasis, mucus plugs, obstructive pneumonia, atelectasis).

B. Diagnostic information

1. Site of tumor (i.e. side, lobe, specific segment if appropriate) and surgical procedure (i.e. segmentectomy, lobectomy, pneumonectomy), including portion of lung resected.
2. Histologic type – i.e. a modified World Health Organization (WHO) classification[10] is recommended. Although the WHO classification is based on light microscopic criteria, the results of ancillary studies (i.e. histochemistry, immunohistochemistry, electron microscopy) should be reported when appropriate (e.g. large cell neuroendocrine carcinoma):
   - Squamous cell carcinoma (keratinization and/or intercellular bridges). Variant: spindle cell (squamous carcinoma).
   - Adenocarcinoma (tubular, acinar, or papillary growth pattern) and/or mucus production; acinar adenocarcinoma (i.e. adenocarcinoma, not otherwise specified); papillary adenocarcinoma; solid carcinoma with mucus formation; and variants including bronchioloalveolar adenocarcinoma and spindle cell adenocarcinoma.
   - Large cell carcinoma (large nuclei, prominent nucleoli, abundant cytoplasm, without characteristic features of squamous cell, small cell, or adenocarcinoma) including variants of giant cell carcinoma and clear cell carcinoma (large cell carcinomas composed extensively [>90%] of large cells with clear or foamy cytoplasm without mucin; clear cell features can also be prominent in squamous cell carcinomas and adenocarcinomas and in metastatic renal cell carcinoma).
   - Adenosquamous carcinoma.
   - Neuroendocrine carcinomas including carcinoid tumor; atypical carcinoid tumor (well-differentiated neuroendocrine carcinoma); large cell neuroendocrine carcinoma; and small cell neuroendocrine carcinoma. Variants can be mixed small cell/large cell carcinoma or composite small cell carcinoma (typical small cell carcinoma intimately admixed with areas of squamous cell carcinoma or adenocarcinoma).
   - Bronchial gland (salivary gland analogue) carcinomas (adenoid cystic carcinoma, mucoepidermoid carcinoma, acinic cell carcinoma)
   - Other specific carcinoma types
3. Histologic grade – WHO classification (i.e. well, moderately, and poorly differentiated) recommended for squamous cell carcinoma and adenocarcinomas of acinar (i.e. adenocarcinoma, not further specified) or papillary type.
4. Histologic assessment of surgical margins – includes comment regarding involvement of lobar or mainstem bronchi by invasive or in-situ carcinoma, and microscopic relationship of tumor to bronchial and/or vascular margin(s).
5. Pleural involvement – specify whether tumor invades into but not through visceral pleura without involving parietal pleura (T2), or into parietal pleura (T3) (elastic tissue stains can be helpful in defining the limiting elastic layer of visceral pleura).
6. Lymph node metastases – indicate the number of involved nodes and the total number of nodes received. (Precise node counts may be difficult for fragmented specimens such as those received from mediastinoscopy.) The nodal groups (N) should be specifically identified using the American Joint Committee on Cancer intraoperative staging system for regional lymph nodes.[149] N2 lymph nodes (with the exception of level 11 interlobar nodes) are generally received separately and must be appropriately identified by the submitting surgeon; these are to be reported separately. Pneumonectomies are usually accompanied by attached N2 lymph nodes, which should be specifically identified by location. If the nodal involvement is only by direct extension, this feature should be noted.
7. Non-neoplastic lung – any significant abnormalities (e.g. granulomas, pneumonia, etc.) should be recorded.

C. Optional features

The following features are considered optional in the final report because they represent specific institutional preferences or they are considered inconclusive vis-à-vis prognostic significance:

1. Stage – surgical pathology reports containing the previously listed information will contain all of the necessary data to establish the International TNM Staging System for lung carcinoma. It should be emphasized that pathologic tumor stage may be based on incomplete information and therefore may differ from clinical tumor stage.

2. Angiolymphatic invasion – whenever possible, it should be specified whether the structures involved are blood vessels or lymphatic vessels, and whether the involved blood vessels are muscular arteries, elastic arteries, or veins.
3. Perineural invasion.
4. Presence or absence of extranodal (extracapsular) tumor invasion.
5. Results of ancillary investigations (e.g. molecular pathology evaluations).

REFERENCES

1. Wingo PA, Tong T, Boldens S: Cancer statistics, 1995. *Ca* 1995; 45: 8–30.
2. Andre F, Jacot W, Pujol JL, Grunenwald D, LeChevalier T: Epidemiology, prognostic factors, staging, and treatment of non-small cell lung cancer. Bull Cancer 1999; 3(suppl): 17–41.
3. Fraire AE: Pathology of lung cancer. In: Comprehensive textbook of thoracic oncology, Aisner J, Arriagada R, Green MR, Martini N, Perry MC, Eds. 1996, Williams & Wilkins, Baltimore, pp 245–275.
4. Davila DG, Williams DE: The etiology of lung cancer. Mayo Clin Proc 1993; 68: 170–182.
5. Franceschi S, Bidoli E: The epidemiology of lung cancer. Ann Oncol 1999; 10(suppl): S3–S6.
6. Emmons KM: Smoking cessation and tobacco control: an overview. Chest 1999; 116(suppl3): 490S–492S.
7. Kubina M, Hedelin G, Charloux A, et al.: Do patients with squamous cell carcinoma or adenocarcinoma of the lung have different smoking histories? Rev Mal Respir 1999; 16: 539–549.
8. Boffetta P, Nyberg F, Agudo A, et al.: Risk of lung cancer from exposure to environmental tobacco smoke from cigars, cigarillos, and pipes. Int J Cancer 1999; 83: 805–806.
9. Lubin JH: Estimating lung cancer risk with exposure to environmental tobacco smoke. Environ Health Perspect 1999; 107(suppl 6): 879–883.
10. The World Health Organization histological typing of lung tumors, 2nd edn. Am J Clin Pathol 1982; 77: 123–136.
11. Yesner R, Seydel G, Asbell SO, et al.: Biopsies of non-small cell lung cancer: central review in cooperative studies of the radiation therapy oncology group. Mod Pathol 1991; 4: 432–440.
12. Olcott CT: Cell types and histologic patterns in carcinoma of the lung: observations on the significance of tumors containing more than one type of cell. Am J Pathol 1955; 31: 975–995.
13. Fraire AE, Cooper SP, Greenberg SD, Buffler PA: Carcinoma of the lung: changing cell distribution and histopathologic cell types. Prog Surg Pathol 1992; 12: 129–149.
14. Roggli VL, Vollmer RT, Greenberg SD, et al.: Lung cancer heterogeneity: a blinded and randomized study of 100 consecutive cases. Hum Pathol 1985; 16: 569–579.
15. Fraire AE, Roggli VL, Vollmer RT, et al.: Lung cancer heterogeneity: prognostic implications. Cancer 1987; 60: 370–379.
16. Vincent RG, Pickren JW, Lane NVW, et al.: The changing histopathology of lung cancer: a review of 1682 cases. Cancer 1977; 39: 1617–1655.
17. Fishback NF, Travis WD, Moran CA, et al.: Pleomorphic (spindle/giant-cell) carcinoma of the lung: a clinicopathologic correlation of 78 cases. Cancer 1994; 73: 2936–2945.
18. Nappi O, Swanson PE, Wick MR: Pseudovascular adenoid squamous cell carcinoma of the lung: clinicopathologic features of three cases and comparison with true pleuropulmonary angiosarcoma. Hum Pathol 1994; 25: 373–378.
19. Ritter JH, Mills SE, Nappi O, Wick MR: Angiosarcoma-like neoplasms of epithelial organs: true endothelial tumors or variants of carcinoma? Semin Diagn Pathol 1995; 12: 270–282.
20. Chang YL, Wu CT, Shih JY, Lee YC: New aspects in clinicopathologic and oncogene studies of 23 pulmonary lymphoepithelioma-like carcinomas. Am J Surg Pathol 2002; 26: 715–723.
21. Brambilla E, Moro D, Veale D, et al.: Basal cell (basaloid) carcinoma of the lung: a new morphologic and phenotypic entity with separate prognostic significance. Hum Pathol 1992; 23: 993–1003.
22. Koss MN, Travis WD, Moran CA, Hochholzer L: Pseudomesotheliomatous adenocarcinoma: a reappraisal. Semin Diagn Pathol 1992; 9: 117–123.
23. Dessy E, Pietra GG: Pseudomesotheliomatous adenocarcinoma of the lung: an immunohistochemical and ultrastructural study of three cases. Cancer 1991; 68: 1747–1753.
24. Lin JI, Tseng CH, Tsung SH: Pseudomesotheliomatous carcinoma of the lung. South Med J 1980; 73: 655–657.
25. DaCosta N, Sivararnan A, Kinare SG: Carcinoma of lung with special reference to adenocarcinoma: an autopsy study of 122 cases. Ind J Cancer 1993; 30: 42–47.
26. Weidner N: Pulmonary adenocarcinoma with intestinal-type differentiation. Ultrastruct Pathol 1992; 16: 7–10.
27. Hayashi H, Kitamura H, Nakatani Y, et al.: Primary signet-ring-cell carcinoma of the lung: histochemical and immunohistochemical characterization. Hum Pathol 1999; 30: 378–383.
28. Moran CA, Hochholzer L, Fishback N, Travis WD, Koss MN: Mucinous (so-called colloid) carcinomas of lung. Mod Pathol 1992; 5: 634–638.
29. Gaffey MJ, Mills SE, Ritter JH: Clear cell tumors of the lower respiratory tract. Semin Diagn Pathol 1997; 14: 222–232.
30. Nakatani Y, Kitamura H, Inayama Y, et al.: Pulmonary adenocarcinomas of the fetal lung type: a clinicopathologic study indicating differences in histology, epidemiology, and natural history of low-grade and high-grade forms. Am J Surg Pathol 1998; 22: 399–411.
31. Colby TV, Koss MN, Travis WD: Tumors of the lower respiratory tract. In: Atlas of tumor pathology, Series 3, Fascicle 13. 1995, Armed Forces Institute of Pathology, Washington, DC, pp 203–234.
32. Higashiyama M, Doi O, Kodama K, et al.: Extramammary Paget's disease of the bronchial epithelium. Arch Pathol Lab Med 1991; 115: 185–188.
33. Ordonez NG: Immunohistochemical diagnosis of epithelioid mesothelioma: a critical review of old markers and new markers. Hum Pathol 2002; 33: 953–967.
34. Liebow AA: Bronchioloalveolar carcinoma. Adv Intern Med 1960; 10: 329–358.
35. Clayton F: Bronchioloalveolar carcinomas: cell types, patterns of growth, and prognostic correlates. Cancer 1986; 57: 1555–1564.
36. Clayton F: The spectrum of significance of bronchioloalveolar carcinomas. Pathol Annu 1988; 23(2): 361–394.
37. Feldman ER, Eagan RT, Schaid J: Metastatic bronchioloalveolar carcinoma and metastatic adenocarcinoma of the lung: comparison of clinical manifestations, chemotherapeutic responses, and prognosis. Mayo Clin Proc 1992; 67: 27–32.
38. Grover FL, Piantadosi S: Recurrence and survival following resection of bronchioloalveolar carcinoma of the lung – the Lung Cancer Study Group experience. Ann Surg 1989; 209: 779–790.
39. Lozowski W, Hajdu SI: Cytology and immunocytochemistry of bronchioloalveolar carcinoma. Acta Cytol 1987; 31: 717–725.
40. Manning JT Jr, Spjut HJ, Tschen JA: Bronchioloalveolar carcinoma: the significance of two histopathologic types. Cancer 1984; 54: 525–534.
41. Marcq M, Galy P: Bronchioloalveolar carcinoma: clinicopathological relationships, natural history, and prognosis in 29 cases. Am Rev Resp Dis 1973; 107: 621–629.
42. Rosenblatt MB, Lisa JR, Collier F: Primary and metastatic bronchioloalveolar carcinoma. Chest 1967; 52: 147–152.
43. Schulze ES, Mattia AR, Chew FS: Bronchioloalveolar carcinoma. Am J Roentgenol 1994; 162: 1294.
44. Sutton LN, Morrison JF, Rees MR: Radiographic features and prognosis in bronchioloalveolar carcinoma: a local experience. Resp Med 1989; 83: 471–477.
45. Mizutani Y, Nakajima T, Morinaga S, et al.: Immunohistochemical localization of pulmonary surfactant apoproteins in various lung tumors, with special reference to lung adenocarcinoma subtypes. Cancer 1988; 61: 532–537.
46. Sorensen JB, Hirsch FR, Gazdar A, Olsen JE: Interobserver variability in histopathologic subtyping and grading of pulmonary adenocarcinoma. Cancer 1993; 71: 2971–2976.
47. Barsky SH, Grossman DA, Ho J, Holmes EC: The multifocality of bronchioloalveolar lung carcinoma: evidence and implications of a multiclonal origin. Mod Pathol 1994; 7: 633–640.
48. Grotte D, Stanley MW, Swanson PE, et al.: Reactive type II

pneumocytes in bronchoalveolar lavage fluid from acute respiratory syndrome can be mistaken for cells of adenocarcinoma. Diagn Cytopathol 1990; 6: 317–322.
49. Ritter JH, Wick MR, Reyes AR, Coffin CM, Dehner LP: False-positive interpretations of carcinoma in exfoliative respiratory cytology: report of two cases and a review of underlying disorders. Am J Clin Pathol 1995; 104: 133–140.
50. Mori M, Chiba R, Takahashi T: Atypical adenomatous hyperplasia of the lung and its differentiation from adenocarcinoma: characterization of atypical cells by morphometry and multivariate cluster analysis. Cancer 1993; 72: 2331–2340.
51. Hegg CA, Flint A, Singh G: Papillary adenoma of the lung. Am J Clin Pathol 1992; 97: 393–397.
52. Kitamura H, Kameda Y, Ito T, et al.: Atypical adenomatous hyperplasia of the lung: implications for the pathogenesis of peripheral lung adenocarcinoma. Am J Clin Pathol 1999; 111: 610–622.
53. Miller RR, Nelerris B, Evans KG, et al.: Glandular neoplasia of the lung: a proposed analogy to colonic tumors. Cancer 1988; 61: 1009–1014.
54. Huang MS, Colby TV, Goellner JR, et al.: Utility of bronchoalveolar lavage in the diagnosis of drug-induced pulmonary toxicity. Acta Cytol 1989; 33: 533–538.
55. Rao SK, Fraire AE: Alveolar cell hyperplasia in association with adenocarcinoma of the lung. Mod Pathol 1995; 8: 165–169.
56. Miller RR: Bronchioloalveolar cell adenomas. Am J Surg Pathol 1990; 14: 904–912.
57. Nakanishi K: Alveolar epithelial hyperplasia and adenocarcinoma of the lung. Arch Pathol Lab Med 1990; 114: 363–368.
58. Travis WD, Linnoila RI, Horowitz M, et al.: Pulmonary nodules resembling bronchioloalveolar carcinoma in adolescent cancer patients. Mod Pathol 1988; 1: 372–377.
59. Niho S, Yokose T, Suzuki K, et al.: Monoclonality of atypical adenomatous hyperplasia of the lung. Am J Pathol 1999; 154: 249–254.
60. Greenberg AK, Yee H, Rom WN: Preneoplastic lesions of the lung. Respir Res 2002; 3: 20.
61. Meyer EC, Leibow AA: Relationship of interstitial pneumonia honeycombing and atypical epithelial proliferation to cancer of the lung. Cancer 1965; 18: 322–351.
62. Shimosato Y, Noguchi M, Matsuno Y: Adenocarcinoma of the lung: its development and malignant progression. Lung Cancer 1993; 9: 99–108.
63. Cagle PT, Cohle SD, Greenberg SD: Natural history of pulmonary scar cancers: clinical and prognostic implications. Cancer 1985; 56: 2031–2035.
64. Barsky SH, Huang SJ, Bhuta S: The extracellular matrix of pulmonary scar carcinomas is suggestive of a desmoplastic origin. Am J Pathol 1986; 124: 412–419.
65. Takamori S, Noguchi M, Morinaga S, et al.: Clinical pathologic characteristics of adenosquamous carcinoma of the lung. Cancer 1991; 67: 649–654.
66. Sridhar KS, Bounassi MJ, Raub W, Richman SP: Clinical features of adenosquamous lung carcinoma in 127 patients. Am Rev Respir Dis 1990; 142: 19–23.
67. Ishida T, Kaneko S, Yokohama H, et al.: Adenosquamous carcinoma of the lung: clinicopathologic and immunohistochemical features. Am J Clin Pathol 1992; 97: 678–695.
68. Carter D, Patchefsky AS: Tumors & tumor-like conditions of the lung. 1998, WB Saunders, Philadelphia, pp 266–285.
69. Nash G, Stout AP: Giant cell carcinoma of the lung: report of 5 cases. Cancer 1958; 11: 369–376.
70. Ginsberg SS, Buzaid AC, Stern H, Carter D: Giant cell carcinoma of the lung. Cancer 1992; 70: 606–610.
71. Attanoos RL, Papagiannis A, Suttinont P, et al.: Pulmonary giant cell carcinoma: pathological entity or morphological phenotype? Histopathology 1998; 32: 225–231.
72. Sawyers CL, Golde DW, Quan S, Nimer SD: Production of granulocyte-macrophage colony stimulating factor in two patients with lung cancer, leukocytosis, and eosinophilia. Cancer 1992; 69: 1342–1346.
73. Shimosato Y: Lung tumors of uncertain histogenesis. Semin Diagn Pathol 1995; 12: 185–192.
74. Yoshida J, Nagai K, Hasebe T, et al.: Pulmonary metastasis of renal cell carcinoma resected sixteen years after nephrectomy. Jpn J Clin Oncol 1995; 25: 20–24.
75. Bonetti F, Pea M, Martignoni G, et al.: Clear cell ("sugar") tumor of the lung is a lesion strictly related to angiomyolipoma – the concept of a family of lesions characterized by the presence of the perivascular epithelioid cell (PEC). Pathology 1994; 26: 230–236.
76. Gaffey MJ, Mills SE, Frierson HF Jr, Askin FB, Maygarden SJ: Pulmonary clear cell carcinoid tumor: another entity in the differential diagnosis of pulmonary clear cell neoplasia. Am J Surg Pathol 1998; 22: 1020–1025.
77. Nowak MA, Fatteh SM, Campbell TE: Glycogen-rich malignant melanomas and glycogen-rich balloon cell malignant melanomas: frequency and pattern of PAS positivity in primary and metastatic melanomas. Arch Pathol Lab Med 1998; 122: 353–360.
78. MacDowell EM, Wilson TS, Trump BF: Atypical endocrine tumors of the lung. Arch Pathol Lab Med 1981; 105: 20–28.
79. Hammond ME, Sause WT: Large cell neuroendocrine tumors of the lung. Cancer 1985; 56: 1624–1629.
80. Piehl MR, Gould VE, Warren WH, et al.: Immunohistochemical identification of exocrine and neuroendocrine subsets of large cell lung carcinomas. Pathol Res Pract 1988; 183: 675–682.
81. Wick MR, Berg LC, Hertz M: Large cell carcinoma of the lung with neuroendocrine differentiation: a comparison with large cell "undifferentiated" pulmonary tumors. Am J Clin Pathol 1992; 97: 796–805.
82. Cavazza A, Colby TV, Tsokos M, Rush W, Travis WD: Lung tumors with a rhabdoid phenotype. Am J Clin Pathol 1996; 105: 182–188.
83. Wick MR, Ritter JH, Dehner LP: Malignant rhabdoid tumors: a clinicopathologic review and conceptual discussion. Semin Diagn Pathol 1995; 12: 233–248.
84. Moran CA. Primary salivary gland-type tumors of the lung. Semin Diagn Pathol 1995; 12:106–122.
85. Dowling EA, Miller RE, Johnson IM, et al.: Mucoepidermoid tumors of the bronchi. Surgery 1962; 52: 600–609.
86. Ozlu C, Christopherson WM, Allen JD: Mucoepidermoid tumors of the bronchi. J Thorac Cardiovasc Surg 1961; 42: 24–31.
87. Axelsson C, Burcharth F, Johansen A: Mucoepidermoid lung tumors. J Thorac Cardiovasc Surg 1973; 65: 902–908.
88. Turnbull AD, Huvos AG, Goodner JT, et al.: Mucoepidermoid tumors of bronchial glands. Cancer 1971; 28: 539–544.
89. Reichle FA, Rosemond GP: Mucoepidermoid tumors of the bronchus. J Thorac Cardiovasc Surg 1966; 51: 443–448.
90. Klacsmann PG, Olson JL, Eggleston JC: Mucoepidermoid carcinoma of the bronchus. Cancer 1979; 43: 1720–1733.
91. Barsky SH, Martin SE, Matthews M, et al.: "Low grade" mucoepidermoid carcinoma of the bronchus with "high grade" biologic behavior. Cancer 1983; 51: 1505–1509.
92. Seo IS, Warren J, Mirkin D, et al.: Mucoepidermoid carcinoma of the bronchus in a 4-year-old child. Cancer 1984; 53:1600–1604.
93. Yousem SA, Hochholzer L: Mucoepidermoid tumors of the lung. Cancer 1987; 60: 1346–1352.
94. Moran CA, Suster S, Koss MN: Primary adenoid cystic carcinoma of the lung: a clinicopathological and immunohistochemical study of 16 cases. Cancer 1994; 73: 1390–1397.
95. Ishida T, Nishino T, Oka T, et al.: Adenoid cystic carcinoma of the tracheobronchial tree: clinicopathology and immunohistochemistry. J Surg Oncol 1989; 41: 52–59.
96. Heilbrunn AA, Crosby IK: Adenoid cystic carcinoma and mucoepidermoid carcinoma of the tracheobronchial tree. Chest 1972; 61: 145–149.
97. Nomori H, Kaseda S, Kobayashi K, et al.: Adenoid cystic carcinoma of the trachea and main stem bronchus: a clinical, histopathologic, and immunohistochemical study. J Thorac Cardiovasc Surg 1988; 96: 271–277.
98. Inoue H, Iwashita A, Kanegae H, et al.: Peripheral pulmonary adenoid cystic carcinoma with substantial submucosal extension of the proximal bronchus. Thorax 1991; 46: 147–148.
99. Conlan AA, Payne WS, Woolner LB, et al.: Adenoid cystic carcinoma (Cylindroma) and mucoepidermoid carcinoma of the bronchus. J Cardiothorac Surg 1978; 76: 369–377.
100. Markel SF, Abell MR, Haight L, et al.: Neoplasms of the bronchus commonly designated as adenomas. Cancer 1964; 17: 590–604.
101. Payne WS, Ellis FH, Woolner LB, et al.: The surgical treatment of cylindroma (adenoid cystic carcinoma) and mucoepidermoid tumors of the bronchus. J Thorac Cardiovasc Surg 1959; 38: 709–726.
102. Sterman DH, Sztejman E, Rodriguez E, Friedberg J: Diagnosis and

staging of "other bronchial tumors." Chest Surg Clin N Am 2003; 13: 79–94.
103. Holst VA, Marshall CE, Moskaluk CA, Frierson HF Jr: KIT protein expression and analysis of *c-kit* gene mutation in adenoid cystic carcinoma. Mod Pathol 1999; 12: 956–960.
104. Fechner RE, Bentnick BR, Askew JB Jr: Acinic cell tumor of the lung: a histologic and ultrastructural study. Cancer 1972; 29:501–508.
105. Moran CA, Suster S, Koss MN: Acinic cell carcinoma of the lung ("Fechner Tumor"): a clinicopathologic, immunohistochemical, and ultrastructural study of five cases. Am J Surg Pathol 1992; 16: 1039–1050.
106. Latz DR, Bubis JJ: Acinic cell tumor of the bronchus. Cancer 1976; 38: 830–832.
107. Gharpure KJ, Desphande RK, Vishweshvara RN, et al.: Acinic cell tumor of the bronchus (a case report). Indian J Cancer 1985; 22: 152–156.
108. Lee HY, Mancer K, Koong HN: Primary acinic cell carcinoma of the lung with lymph node metastasis. Arch Pathol Lab Med 2003; 127: e216–e219.
109. Ukoha OO, Quartararo P, Carter D, Kashgarian M, Ponn RB: Acinic cell carcinoma of the lung with metastasis to lymph nodes. Chest 1999; 115: 591–595.
110. Davis PW, Briggs JC, Leal RME, et al.: Benign and malignant mixed tumors of the lung. Thorax 1972; 27: 657–673.
111. Hayes MM, Van der Westhuizen NG, Forgie R: Malignant mixed tumors of the bronchus: a biphasic neoplasm of epithelial and myoepithelial cells. Mod Pathol 1993; 6: 85–88.
112. Payne WS, Scier J, Woolner LB: Mixed tumors of the bronchus (salivary gland type). J Thorac Cardiovasc Surg 1965; 49: 663–668.
113. Sakamoto H, Uda H, Tanaka T, et al.: Pleomorphic adenoma in the periphery of the lung: report of a case and review of the literature. Arch Pathol Lab Med 1991; 115: 393–396.
114. Moran CA, Suster S, Askin FB, Koss MN: Benign and malignant salivary gland-type tumors of the lung: clinicopathologic and immunohistochemical study of eight cases. Cancer 1994; 73: 2481–2490.
115. Angelov A, Dikranian K, Trosheva M: Immunomorphological characteristics of pleomorphic adenoma of salivary glands. Bull Group Int Rech Sci Stomatol Odontol 1996; 39: 67–75.
116. Takeuchi E, Shimizu E, Sano N, et al.: A case of pleomorphic adenoma of the lung with multiple distant metastases – observations on its oncogene and tumor suppressor gene expression. Anticancer Res 1998; 18: 2015–2020.
117. Nistal M, Garcia-Viera M, Martinez-Garcia C, et al.: Epithelial-myoepithelial tumor of the bronchus. Am J Surg Pathol 1994; 18: 421–425.
118. Strickler JG, Hegstrom J, Thomas MJ, et al.: Myoepithelioma of the lung. Arch Pathol Lab Med 1987; 111: 1082–1086.
119. Tsuji N, Tateisha R, Ishiguro S, et al.: Adenomyoepithelioma of the lung. Am J Surg Pathol 1995; 19: 956–962.
120. Wilson RW, Moran CA: Epithelial-myoepithelial carcinoma of the lung: immunohistochemical and ultrastructural observations and review of the literature. Hum Pathol 1997; 28: 631–635.
121. Pelosi G, Fraggetta F, Maffini F, et al.: Pulmonary epithelial-myoepithelial tumor of unproven malignant potential: report of a case and review of the literature. Mod Pathol 2001; 14: 521–526.
122. Fechner RE, Bentnick BR: Ultrastructure of bronchial oncocytoma. Cancer 1973; 31: 1451–1457.
123. Nielsen AL. Malignant bronchial oncocytoma: a case report and review of the literature. Hum Pathol 1985; 16: 852–854.
124. Santos-Briz A, Jenron J, Sastre R, Romero L, Valle A: Oncocytoma of the lung. Cancer 1977; 40: 1330–1336.
125. Ritter JH, Nappi O: Oxyphilic proliferations of the respiratory tract and paranasal sinuses. Semin Diagn Pathol 1999; 16: 105–116.
126. Volm M, Hahn EW, Mattern J, et al.: Five year followup study of independent clinical and flow cytometric prognostic factors for the survival of patients with non-small cell carcinoma. Cancer Res 1988; 48: 2923–2928.
127. Mountain CF: Revisions in the International System for Staging Lung Cancer. Chest 1997; 111: 1710–1717.
128. Asamura H, Naruke T: Lung carcinoma. In: Prognostic factors in cancer, Hermanek P, Gospodarowicz MK, Henson DE, Hutter RVP, Sobin LH, Eds. 1995, Springer-Verlag, Berlin, pp 118–129.
129. Gallagher B, Urbanski SJ: The significance of pleural elastic invasion by lung carcinoma. Hum Pathol 1990; 21: 512–517.
130. Bunker ML, Raab SS, Landreneau RJ, Silverman JF: The diagnosis and significance of visceral pleural invasion in lung carcinoma: histologic predictors and the role of elastic stains. Am J Clin Pathol 1999; 112: 777–783.
131. Elson CE, Roggli VL, Vollmer RT, et al.: Prognostic indicators for survival in stage I carcinoma of the lung: a histologic study of 47 surgically resected cases. Mod Pathol 1988; 1: 288–291.
132. Haque AK, Adegboyega P, Sanchez RL: Vascular invasion in carcinoma of the lung. Mod Pathol 1993; 6: 131A.
133. Brown RNV, Fraire AE, Roggli V, Cagle PT: Assessment of proliferative fraction by PCNA in stage I non-small cell lung cancer. Mod Pathol 1993; 6: 129A.
134. Miyarnoto H, Flarada M, lsobe A, et al.: Prognostic value of nuclear DNA content and expression of the ras oncogene product in lung cancer. Cancer Res 1991; 51: 6346–6350.
135. Gazdar AF: Molecular markers for the diagnosis and prognosis of lung cancer. Cancer 1992; 69: 1592–1599.
136. Noguchi M, Hirohashi S, Hara F, et al.: Heterogeneous amplification of myc family oncogenes in small cell lung carcinomas. Cancer 1990; 66: 2053–2058.
137. Ritter JH, Dresler CM, Wick MR: Expression of bcl-2 protein in stage T1N0M0 non-small cell lung carcinoma. Hum Pathol 1995; 26: 1227–1232.
138. Ponder TB, Wick MR, Dresler CM, Ritter JH: Expression of ABH antigen, p53 protein, bcl-2 protein, and tumor grade as prognostic factors in T1N0M0 non-small cell lung carcinoma. Am J Clin Pathol 1996; 105: 493.
139. Ponder TB, Wick MR, Dresler CM, Ritter JH: Microvessel counts and lymphovascular invasion as prognostic indicators in T1N0M0 non-small cell lung carcinoma. Am J Clin Pathol 1996; 106: 402–403.
140. Haque AK, Abegboyega P, Al-Salalmeh A, Vrazel DP, Zwischenberger J: p53 and p-glycoprotein expression do not correlate with survival in non-small cell lung cancer: a long-term study and literature review. Mod Pathol 1999; 12: 1158–1166.
141. Hashimoto T, Tokuchi Y, Hayashi M, et al.: p53 null mutations undetected by immunohistochemical staining predict a poor outcome with early-stage non-small cell lung carcinomas. Cancer Res 1999; 59: 5572–5577.
142. Tomizawa Y, Kohno T, Fujita T, et al.: Correlation between the status of the p53 gene and survival in patients with stage I non-small cell lung carcinomas. Oncogene 1999; 18: 1007–1014.
143. Dosaka-Akita H, Hu SX, Fujino M,et al.: Altered retinoblastoma protein expression in non-small cell lung cancer: its synergistic effects with altered ras and p53 protein status on prognosis. Cancer 1997; 79: 1329–1337.
144. Maitra A, Amirkhan RH, Saboorian MH, Frawley WH, Ashfaq R: Survival in small cell lung carcinoma is independent of bcl-2 expression. Hum Pathol 1999; 30: 712–717.
145. Fontanini G, Vignati S, Bigini D, et al.: Recurrence and death in non-small cell lung carcinomas: a prognostic model using pathological parameters, microvessel count, and gene protein products. Clin Cancer Res 1996; 2: 1067–1075.
146. Colby TV, Deschamps C: The lung and pleura. In: Pathology for the surgeon, Banks PM, Kraybill WG, Eds. 1996, WB Saunders, Philadelphia, pp 155–168.
147. Nash G, Hutter RVP, Henson DE: Practice protocol for the examination of specimens from patients with lung cancer. Cancer Committee Task Force on the Examination of Specimens from Patients with Lung Cancer. Arch Pathol Lab Med 1995; 119: 695–700.
148. Association of Directors of Anatomic & Surgical Pathology: Recommendations for the reporting of resected primary lung carcinomas. Am J Clin Pathol 1995; 104: 371–374.
149. Fleming ID, Cooper JS, Henson DE, et al. (Eds): American Joint Committee on Cancer – Cancer staging manual, 5th edn. 1997, Lippincott-Raven, Philadelphia, pp 127–137.
150. Moran CA, Wick MR, Suster S: The role of immunohistochemistry in the diagnosis of malignant mesothelioma. Semin Diagn Pathol 2000; 17: 178–183.

17

Metastatic tumors in the lung: a practical approach to diagnosis

Stephen S Raab   Charles D Sturgis   Mark R Wick

The most common form of pulmonary neoplasm is a metastasis from outside the lungs. Based on autopsy data, the lungs are involved by metastatic lesions in 25% to 55% of malignant diseases,[1–5] and, in up to one-quarter of those cases, the pulmonary parenchyma and pleura are the *only* sites of distant spread.[4] On the other hand, the most common lung tumor encountered by a practicing surgical pathologist or cytopathologist is primary bronchogenic carcinoma; hence, the separation of primary from secondary pulmonary neoplasms is a major challenge. This chapter first provides a short background on the pathobiologic principles and clinico-radiologic findings attending metastases in the lungs, and then offers a framework for the practitioner to identify such lesions with an optimal level of certainty.

Routes of spread for intrapulmonary metastases

Extrapulmonary malignancies may spread to the lungs through the vascular system or the lymphatics, or by direct extension; technically, the last of those routes does not represent "metastasis" as it is usually defined. Primary lung cancers likewise may involve other pleuro-pulmonary zones by similar means or by aerogenous dissemination through the alveolar pores of Kohn. Clinical and radiologic features of a particular metastatic lesion depend on which of these avenues of spread applies.

Vascular metastases

The majority of metastatic tumors in the lungs have arrived at that destination hematogenously. There are two principal reasons for this: the lungs receive the entire cardiac output and they contain a rich vascular network, comprising a huge capillary bed. The detailed principles underlying vascular metastasis have been outlined elsewhere.[6–8] Malignant tumors may contain subclones[9] of cells with differing metastatic potential, and some of them acquire the ability to enter the bloodstream as microemboli. At selected distant sites, they adhere to endothelial basement membranes, and, through a process known as extravasation, the tumor cells move through the extracellular matrix to form metastatic deposits in various parenchymal structures. In this paradigm, the original micrometastasis then proliferates to yield a larger mass which, at a later time (often as long as several years), may become visible clinically or radiographically. Most pulmonary metastases show nests of neoplastic cells that are surrounded by, and intercalated with, a variable quantity of fibrous stroma. At this stage, no cells typically remain inside the pulmonary arterial, venous, or capillary system.

The rate at which potentially metastasizing cellular subclones develop (if they do at all) in primary tumors varies considerably; the probability that such lesions will spread hematogenously depends on both tumor-related factors and conditions in the milieu of the host tissues. For reasons that are largely unknown, some tumors – such as osteosarcoma- – often shed micrometastases at a time before the primary tumor is detected clinically, whereas other tumors may demonstrate metastasis only very late in their biologic evolution.[10]

The clinical presentation of patients with hematogenous pulmonary metastases is variable. The majority of individuals have no symptoms,[11] and their lesions are detected only through imaging studies that are under-taken for staging purposes or for surveillance during treatment. The radiographic appearance of metastatic pulmonary lesions may be that of a single central or peripheral mass, multiple central or peripheral masses, diffuse infiltrates, or a combination of the latter two possibilities. If a patient is symptomatic, the clinical findings reflect the location and extent of the metastatic deposits and commonly include chest pain, dyspnea, cough, hemoptysis, and wheezing, to name but a few.

In addition to the concept of microembolization as outlined above, tumors may also spread as macroscopic emboli that involve large- or medium-sized pulmonary arteries.[12] Large-vessel tumor emboli may cause acute heart failure, sudden death, rapidly evolving pulmonary hypertension, and pulmonary infarction, as also seen with banal intravascular thromboemboli that are associated with deep venous thrombosis.[13–15] The tumors that most commonly give rise to macroscopic emboli are those associated with major systemic veins (e.g. renal or hepatic carcinomas invading the renal and hepatic veins), and primary tumors of the heart (myxomas and sarcomas).

In rare instances, hematogenous metastasis principally manifests itself in the lung by the presence of occlusive luminal tumor plugs in small vessels (arterioles and capillaries) without interstitial involvement or formation of masses.[17] In a sense, those tumors have not gone through all of the biologic steps that are normally associated with the metastatic sequence, but are none-theless potentially lethal because they may cause severe pulmonary hypertension. Neoplasms that may demonstrate that pattern of spread (sometimes called tumor-related thrombotic pulmonary microangiopathy[17a]) include carcinomas of the breast, gastrointestinal tract, liver, pancreas, uterus, gallbladder, prostate, and ovary.[17]

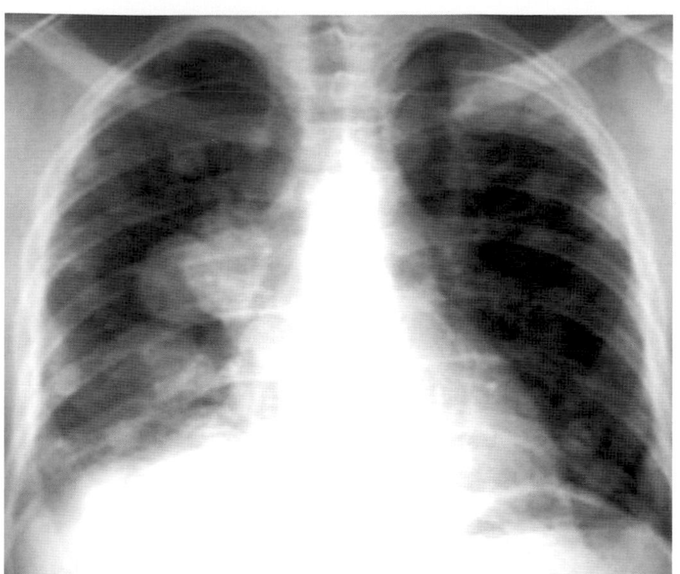
Fig. 17.1 Chest radiograph in a case of metastatic colorectal carcinoma involving the lungs. Tumor nodules are distributed throughout both lung fields; they are nodular and of variable sizes.

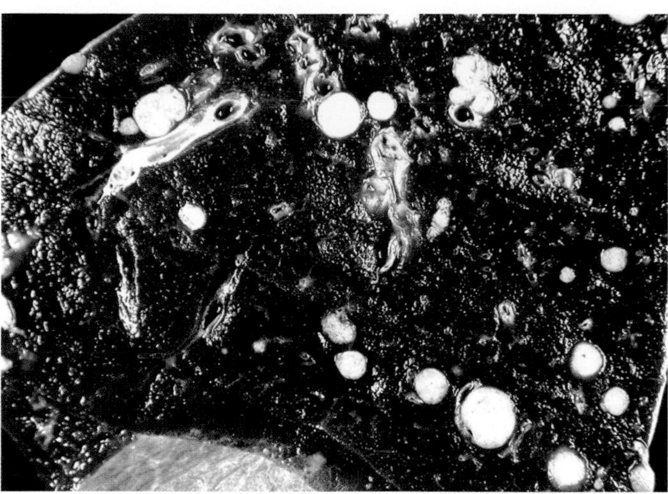
Fig. 17.3 Gross photograph from another case of metastatic carcinoma involving the lungs (from a primary tumor in the breast). Findings are similar to those described in reference to Fig. 17.2.

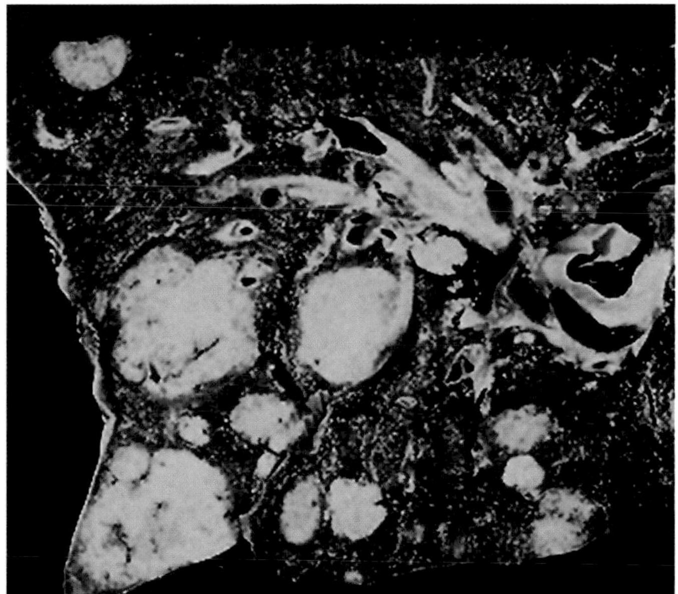
Fig. 17.2 Gross photograph of metastatic carcinoma in the lungs, demonstrating intraparenchymal and subpleural nodules of varying sizes.

Soares et al. reported that most malignant tumors that occlude small pulmonary vascular channels also can be seen simultaneously within larger vessels.[18] Patients with metastatic microvascular occlusion typically present with progressive dyspnea and cor pulmonale.[17,17a]

As a general rule of physiology, all caval venous blood flows through the lungs and portal venous return passes through the liver. Consequently, depending on the primary site of the tumor in question, metastases preferentially will be seen in one of those two organs. Malignant neoplasms that arise in sites with other pathways of vascular drainage (for example, prostatic tumors preferentially shed into the paravertebral venous plexus) only infrequently involve the lungs secondarily. Arterially-borne metastases to the lungs are relatively rare and are usually mediated by the bronchial arteries; the most common source of such lesions is a primary lung cancer that has gained access to the pulmonary venous system.

Hematogenous metastasis in the lung is associated with a spectrum of radiologic findings. The most common roentgenographic appearance is that of multiple, bilateral, variably sized masses (Figs 17.1–17.3); occasionally, a solitary intraparenchymal nodule is observed instead. The metastasic implants usually appear in the mid-to-lower lung fields, because that is where greatest parenchymal perfusion occurs. In up to 90% of patients with bilateral secondary disease, the lesions are peripheral and subpleural in location (Fig. 17.4).[1,19] Variability in the size of the metastatic nodules is related to different "ages" of the lesions, dissimilar growth rates, and other factors. Such lesions are usually smaller than primary pulmonary carcinomas, measuring <3–4 cm in maximum diameter. Metastases also enlarge more rapidly than bronchogenic carcinomas do.

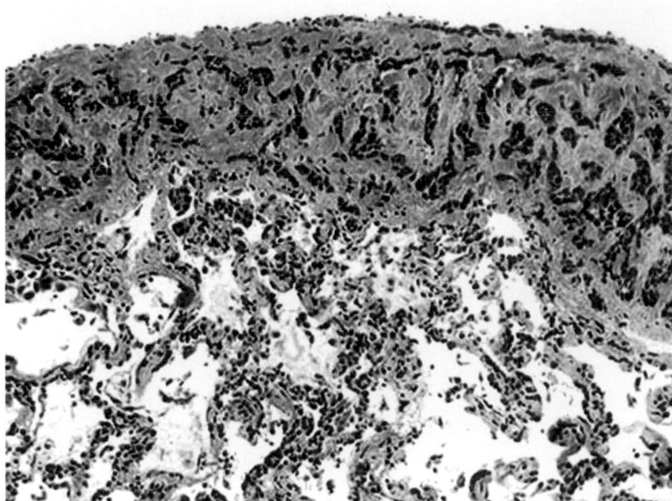

Fig. 17.4 Photomicrograph from a case of metastatic breast carcinoma in the lung, demonstrating a subpleural peripheral distribution of tumor within the pulmonary parenchyma.

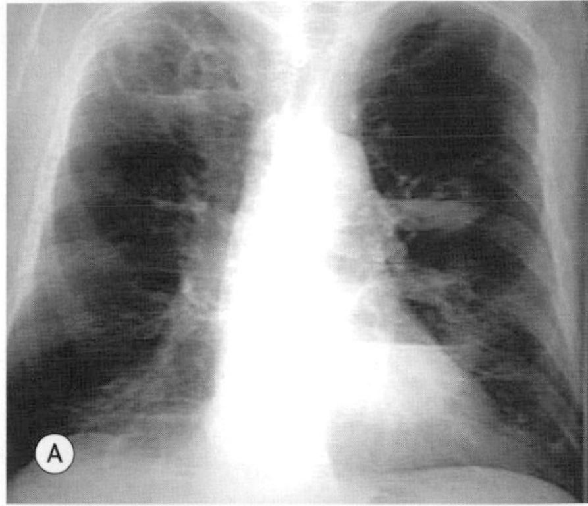

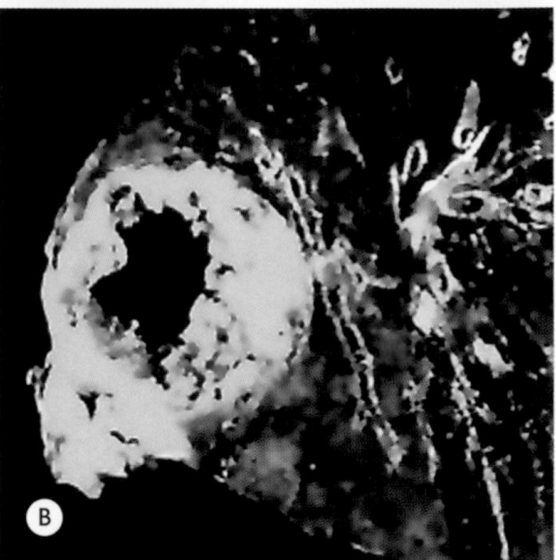

Fig. 17.5 (A) Chest radiograph from a case of metastatic oropharyngeal squamous cell carcinoma involving the lungs, demonstrating cavitating nodular lesions throughout both lung fields. (B) The cavitary nature of the lesions is well-shown in this gross photograph.

Tumors involving small vessels may produce linear parenchymal infiltrates, and patients who have both masses and metastases in small vessels or lymphatic spaces present with opacities and linear streaks. Embolic tumors in large pulmonary arteries may produce the radiographic appearance of an infarct, with a wedge-shaped peripheral zone of consolidation and possible pleural effusion.

Solitary metastases in the lungs are seen in up to 10% of all malignant tumors involving those organs.[20–22] Filderman et al. suggested that solitary lesions >5 cm in diameter most likely originate in the breast, kidney, or soft tissue.[6] It should be noted that metastasis taking the form of a solitary mass on plain films may in fact be represented by multiple contiguous or coalescent masses on computed tomograms. Quint and colleagues reported that, on statistical grounds, patients with carcinomas of the head and neck, bladder, breast, cervix, bile ducts, esophagus, ovary, prostate, or stomach were more likely to have a solitary metastasis to the lung than a new primary bronchogenic tumor, even when a significant period of time had elapsed after diagnosis of the extra-pulmonary neoplasms.[23] On the other hand, patients with prior malignant melanoma, sarcoma, or malignant germ cell tumor were more likely to have a second primary malignancy of the lung under the same circumstances.[23]

Large metastatic foci may undergo cavitation or result in pneumothorax or bronchopleural fistulization (Fig. 17.5). The most common secondary tumor that cavitates is squamous cell carcinoma, often originating in the head and neck.[24] Metastatic sarcoma and adenocarcinoma also may exhibit that feature on occasion.[24] Pneumothoraces and transpleural fistulae result from erosion by the metastatic tumor through the pleura, as seen most frequently with pediatric mesenchymal malignancies (e.g. osteosarcoma).[25]

Lymphogenous metastases

One study[26] reported that up to 56% of pulmonary metastases were lymphogenously mediated, although a more generally accepted figure is between 5% and 8%.[27,28] The majority of patients with lymphatic-borne lung metastases have a poor prognosis, with 90% dying in 6 months or less.[28]

The radiographic appearance of lymphangitic metastasis is variable; in 50% of cases plain chest films show no apparent abnormality.[29] Yang and Lin described four radiological patterns for this condition:

1. bilateral linear infiltrates without hilar enlargement or intrapulmonary masses
2. hilar masses with centripetal parenchymal extension (seen most commonly with cervical, gastric, and breast cancers) (Fig. 17.6)
3. focal linear infiltration of the parenchyma associated with a central primary tumor
4. parenchymal radiations from a peripheral primary tumor.[28]

With the first two patterns representing secondary tumors, pleural or less frequently hilar-lymph nodal involvement may be seen. Over 90% of these cases concern metastatic adenocarcinomas.[28] It is estimated that <1% of patients with pulmonary metastases from tumors arising outside the thorax also have hilar adenopathy.[30] Although this figure may appear low, hilar adenopathy in patients with secondary pulmonary malignancies is actually not uncommon in absolute terms because of the high prevalence of patients with metastatic disease.

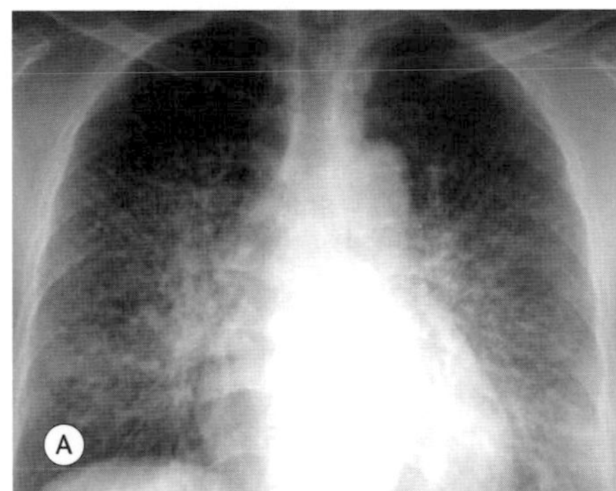

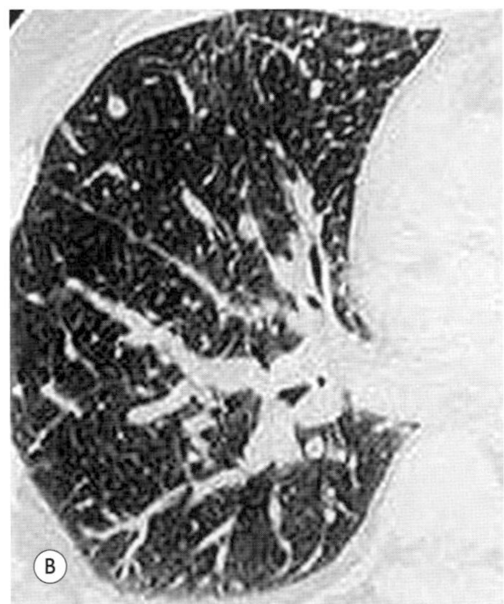

Fig. 17.6 (A,B) Chest radiograph and CT scan in a case of metastatic breast carcinoma in the lungs, assuming a centripetal lymphangitic pattern. Tumor is seen in lymph nodes in both hilar regions, and it also involves the lung fields in an arborizing pattern that follows the lymphatic channels.

Carcinomas may gain access to the pulmonary lymphatic system by retrograde spread; direct invasion of pulmonary lymphatics; and passage through adjacent blood vessels. The most common route of spread is the last of these three possibilities;[31] tumor first spreads hematogenously to the lung and results in small areas of interstitial growth. The neoplastic cells are then absorbed into lymphatics and permeate further throughout the lungs (Fig. 17.7). Tumor in alveolar spaces may likewise be absorbed through lymphatics adjacent to terminal bronchioles. Hence, patients who have lymphangitic intrapulmonary metastases generally also have had prior hematogenous spread.[31] Direct lymphatic invasion is most often associated with tumors arising in the breast or stomach;[28,32,33] in this mode, metastases may be seen exclusively in the pulmonary lymphatic spaces without the formation of mass lesions. Other metastatic carcinomas capable of showing the same pattern of spread are those arising in the ovary, thyroid, bladder, esophagus, and liver.[28,31]

Direct seeding

Metastatic disease arising through direct "seeding" occurs when a malignant tumor gains access to a serosally lined cavity such as the pleural space. Neoplasms that directly seed the pleura include primary lung cancers and malignancies of various lineages that originate in the chest wall or the mediastinum. In some cases, primary lung tumors such as peripheral pulmonary

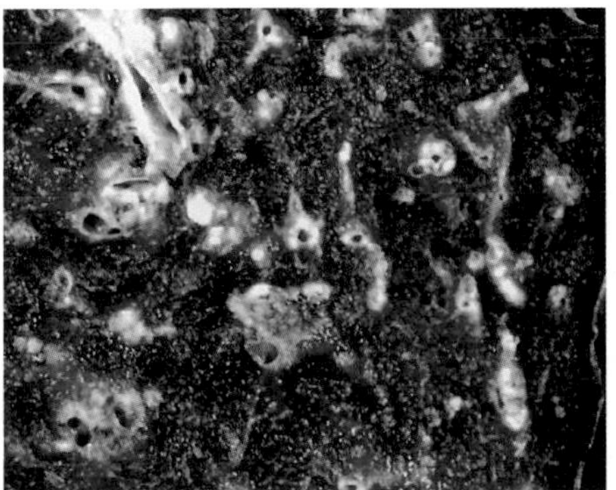

Fig. 17.7 A linear pattern of lymphangitic metastatic disease in the lung parenchyma is demonstrated in this gross photograph.

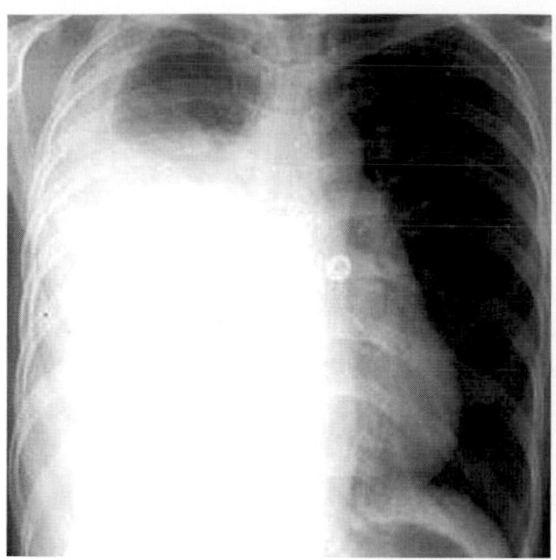

Fig. 17.8 Chest radiograph from a case of metastatic leiomyosarcoma massively involving the right pleura. The right hemithorax is largely obliterated by the tumor mass and an accompanying pleural effusion.

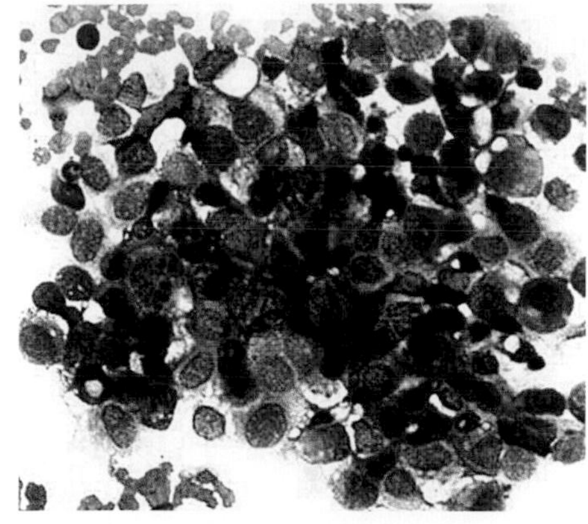

Fig. 17.9 Metastatic adenocarcinoma of pulmonary origin is seen in this preparation of a cytologic specimen of pleural fluid. The tumor cells are arranged in a vaguely three-dimensional configuration, and they demonstrate small nucleoli.

carcinoma grow through the visceral pleura; this phenomenon is less common in cases of chest wall sarcoma. The malignant cells attach themselves to multiple pleural sites and invade the subjacent tissues thereafter. Hence, multiple subpleural nodules may eventuate near a larger serosally-based secondary lesion.

Pleural metastases

Metastases are the commonest form of pleural malignancy. Most derive from primary neoplasms of the chest wall, mediastinum, or lungs,[6] although extrathoracic primary malignancies are also well-represented. The largest tumor nodules tend to be basally situated in the chest[34] (Fig. 17.8).

At least two-thirds of malignant pleural effusions can be diagnosed by cytologic sampling of the pleural fluid. More than 90% of cases are recognized on the first specimen,[35,36] but sensitivity predictably increases with successive sampling; three specimens are routinely recommended if the clinical suspicion of pleural metastasis is high.[37]

Malignancy is second only to congestive heart failure as a cause of pleural effusions.[38] Neoplastic effusions are typically described as "massive" or "copious," ranging up to 2500 ml in volume,[39] and they are often bloody. Nevertheless, malignant involvement of the pleura may also be associated with scant fluid production and a serous character.[34] Obviously, not all pleural effusions in patients with a history of malignancy contain tumor cells;[40] benign effusions in such cases may be secondary to lymphatic obstruction, altered lymphatic drainage caused by chemotherapy or radiation therapy,[41] heart failure, or other causes. It is interesting that because most sarcomas do not spread via lymphatic channels, their metastases in the lung and pleura are uncommonly accompanied by a tumorous effusion.[42] Up to 90% of malignant pleural effusions caused by metastatic lung or breast cancers are ipsilateral with regard to the site of the original tumor.[34] Patients with malignant pleural effusions typically have a dismal prognosis and most die within a few months of diagnosis.[43–45] Selected subgroups, such as those with lymphoma, breast cancer, or some pediatric malignancies, may fare somewhat better.

Chretien and Jaubert reported that 42% of cytologically sampled pleural effusions contained malignant cells.[46] The likely site of tumor origin in such cases appears to depend on patient demographics, although most series have reported that primary pulmonary carcinomas are the most common.[44,47] Squamous cell carcinomas of the lung only unusually involve the pleural fluid; adenocarcinomas most frequently do so (Fig. 17.9), followed by small cell neuroendocrine carcinoma.[48,49] Almost any other extrathoracic malignancy may metastasize to the pleural space, but the most common tumors that do so are carcinomas arising in the breasts, gastrointestinal tract, and ovary; non-Hodgkin's lymphoma is also well-represented.[44,47,50] Up to 7% of metastatic carcinomas in the pleura must be classified as originating in an unknown primary location.[47] In one analysis of malignant pleural effusions women predominated by a ratio of 2:1,[39] but no gender preferences have been seen in other series.[44]

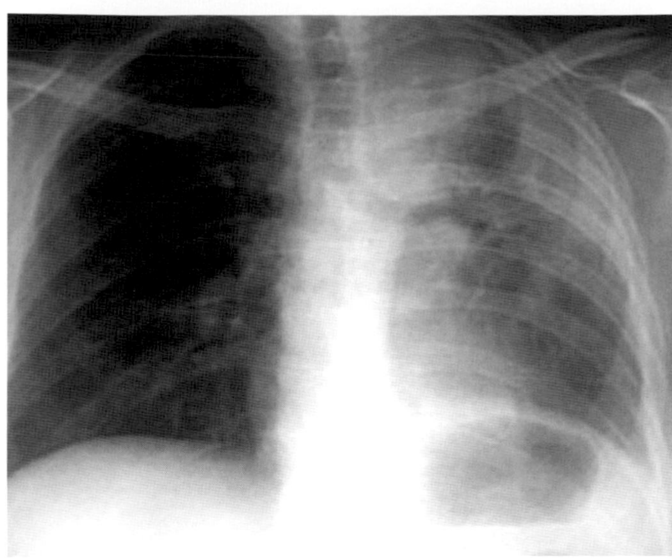

Fig. 17.10 Chest radiograph showing left upper lobar atelectasis, in a case of intrabronchial metastasis of renal cell carcinoma.

Endobronchial metastases

Endobronchial metastases are considered in a separate category because of the distinctive clinical findings that are associated with them, principally represented by the syndrome of "adult-onset asthma." The reported incidence of endobronchial and endotracheal metastatic disease ranges from 1% to 18% of patients who also have intrapulmonary metastases.[11,51,52] The most common sites of tumor origin in patients from North America and Western Europe are the breast, bone, soft tissue, large intestine, kidney, and skin (melanoma).[11,53–57] Over one-third of endobronchial metastases are sarcomatous in nature.[52,56] In populations with a high prevalence of acquired immunodeficiency syndrome, the most common secondary malignancies of the bronchi are Kaposi's sarcoma and malignant lymphoma.[58] Nasopharyngeal and laryngeal carcinomas are frequent sources of endobronchial metastasis in Asian countries.[59]

Endobronchial metastases may be either hematogenous or lymphogenous in nature.[11,52,56] Aerogenous spread of an upper airway malignancy has also been suggested as a possibility. Tumors that originate in the lung, hilar lymph nodes, or mediastinum may spread by direct extension into the bronchial system. Endobronchial lesions cause symptoms early in their course of growth: namely, cough with sputum production, dyspnea, wheezing, infection, and hemoptysis.[59,60] However, up to 25% of patients are asymptomatic.[57] Radiographically, an endobronchial mass is typically visible only on CT or MR scans; plain film studies commonly show only post-obstructive consolidation or atelectasis (Fig. 14.10). The mean interval between diagnosis of the original tumor and appearance of endobronchial metastasis is between 4 and 5 years.[60] Patients with this problem have a poor survival, with a median of 11 months;[60] patients with breast cancer may have a better prognosis.[53,56,57]

In histologic and cytologic specimens, endobronchial metastases may be confused with primary tumors. However, it should be remembered that primary endobronchial neoplasms are typically squamous cell carcinomas, neuroendocrine carcinomas, or salivary gland-type tumors. Endobronchial adenocarcinomas other than salivary morphotypes should therefore raise the suspicion of metastatic disease. An exuberant reactive stromal proliferation around such lesions may also be confused with metastatic spindle cell sarcoma.

Modalities for the diagnosis of pleuropulmonary metastases

The diagnostic tests that are typically used for any suspected pleuropulmonary tumor are also applicable to the study of metastatic disease. These include sputum cytology,[61,62] bronchoscopy with brushing, washing, alveolar lavage, transbronchial or transtracheal aspiration, and biopsy,[63–65] transthoracic fine-needle aspiration (FNA),[66,67] thoracoscopic biopsy (video-assisted thoracic surgery),[68–70] open thoracotomy and biopsy, and effusion cytology.[45] In some cases, expectant management is undertaken, following the lesions with sequential radiologic studies.[71,72] Computed tomography (CT) may be obtained to further delineate abnormalities and possibly to aid in the separation of primary from secondary malignancies; for example, the presence of mediastinal adenopathy would favor a primary lung tumor.[73] When multiple radiographic lesions of the lung or pleura are detected radiographically in some patients with well-documented histories of malignancy, further diagnostic evaluations may be eschewed.

For the most part, the diagnostic accuracy of tests that yield tissue for pathologic examination generally has not been determined in the specific context being discussed here. It is thought to depend principally on lesional size and location rather than the specific histologic nature of the tumor. For example, the sensitivity of FNA is 93% if the lesion is >2 cm in diameter and 60% for those <1 cm in size. Higher sensitivity is realized in the sampling of peripheral nodules as compared with central lesions, regardless of whether they are primary or secondary in character.[74] Pilotti et al. reported that the sensitivity of

FNA in the detection of metastatic pleuropulmonary disease was 89%, whereas it was 92% for primary malignancies.[75] Another inter-institutional study reported 96% specificity for transthoracic FNAs.[76] The sensitivity of bronchoscopy also depends on lesional location; as expected, that technique is particularly well-suited for the visualization and sampling of endobronchial metastases.[63–65] Thoracoscopy is a sensitive means of accessing peripheral lesions and has a high level of accuracy overall. It may be viewed as a treatment option as well as a diagnostic test in patients who have limited metastatic disease, especially if lung function is compromised.[68–70]

Kern and Schweizer concluded that the sensitivity of sputum cytology for the detection of intrapulmonary metastasis was similar to that associated with primary lung cancers.[77] That technique is more likely to be productive if the metastatic lesions are large and centrally located.[77]

Practical approach to differential diagnosis

A definite challenge in pulmonary pathology is represented by determining if a newly detected lung mass is primary or secondary in patients with or without a history of extrapulmonary malignancy. If no prior tumor has been seen and the lesion in question has the morphologic attributes of a non-pulmonary proliferation, one is faced with the need to search for a primary site. Malignancies that are clinically occult and which present with pulmonary metastases are not unusual, and they approximate 2–5% of all metastatic carcinomas of unknown origin (MCUOs).[78,79] Because of the treatment-related and prognostic issues pertaining to secondary malignancies of the lung, it may be decided that additional resources are not justified in order to determine the primary location of the tumor.[80]

In regard to the general distinction of primary and metastatic pulmonary tumors, one generally depends on radiographic findings, histologic features; microscopic comparison of the current lesion with any previous malignancies; and the use of ancillary pathologic studies such as immunohistochemistry, cytochemistry, molecular biologic techniques, cytogenetic methods,[81] and electron microscopy. If paraffin-embedded tissue from prior tumor material is available, immunopathologic studies of it and the current specimen can be obtained comparatively.

Useful information for the separation of primary and secondary neoplasms in the lung may be derived from details of the clinical evaluation and physical findings.[82,83] For example, the characteristically "spiculated" appearance of primary lung cancers (Fig. 17.11) on imaging studies of the chest separates them from the more rounded and well-delimited appearances of metastases. Unfortunately, such information is often not made available to pathologists despite the fact that it is well known to enhance diagnostic accuracy.[84] Open communication is

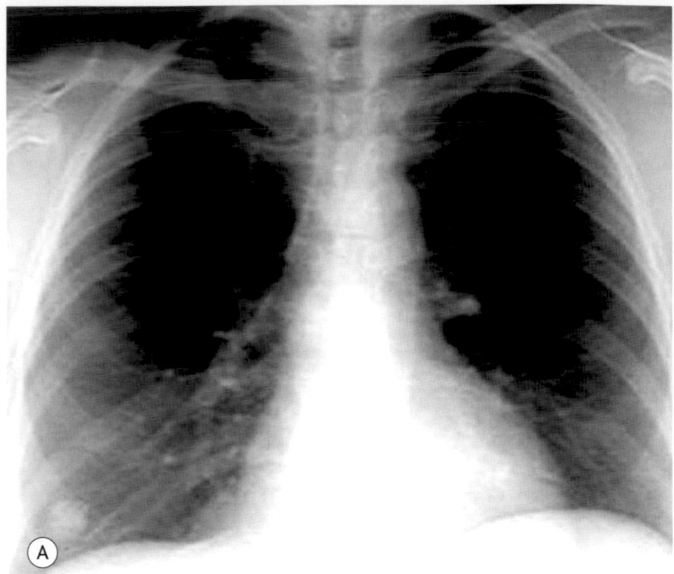

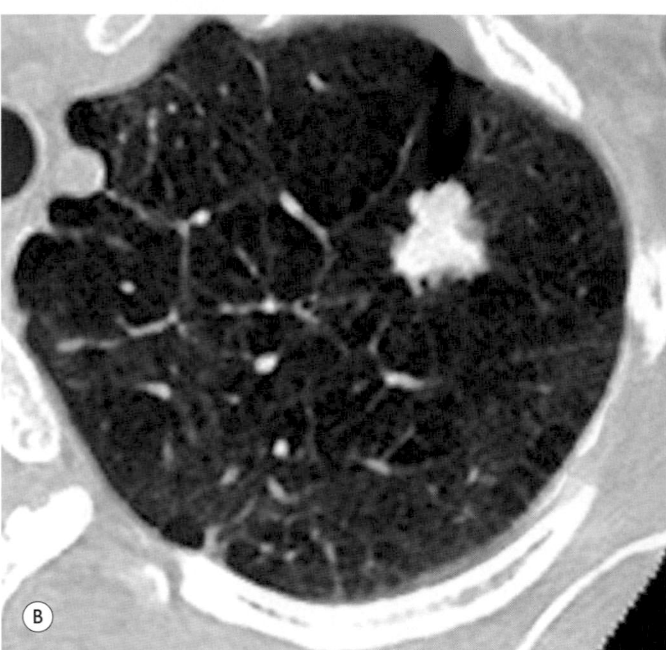

Fig. 17.11 (A) Chest radiograph from a case of primary adenocarcinoma of the lung, demonstrating a peripheral nodule in the lower right lung field. (B) A CT scan shows that the lesion has irregular "spiculated" margins, typical of a primary pulmonary neoplasm.

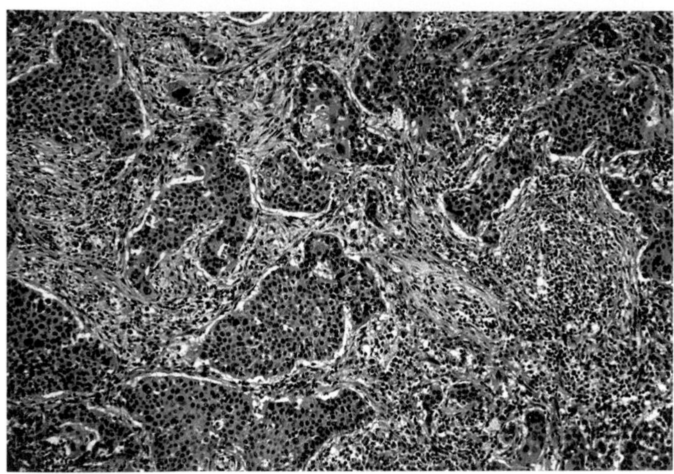

Fig. 17.12 Fibroinflammatory host reaction is seen in and around this primary squamous cell carcinoma of the lung, serving as a marker of its pulmonary origin.

essential if there has been a previous history of oncologic disease in any given case.

Light microscopic features of any given lesion are the cornerstone of pathologic diagnosis. Indeed, its appearance after hematoxylin and eosin (H&E) staining is often sufficient to answer the question of whether the tumor is primary or metastatic. In particular, carcinomas arising in the lung typically have evolved over several years before coming to clinical attention. As a consequence, the host responds to such lesions by surrounding them with an irregular cuff of fibroinflammatory tissue (Fig. 17.12). Moreover, the mixture of proliferation and degeneration that characterizes primary carcinomas commonly causes central zones of fibrosis as well, with entrapment of some residual native pulmonary structures. In contrast, metastases *to* the lung parenchyma have a "clean" interface with the surrounding tissue and are not associated with peripheral zones of fibroinflammatory response. Because they are rapidly growing vis-à-vis bronchogenic neoplasms, metastatic carcinomas also lack centrally sclerotic regions. These "rules" do not apply universally to all tumor types. Specifically, primary and metastatic sarcomas, adenocarcinomas with a "lepidic" growth pattern, and small cell neuroendocrine carcinomas are essentially superimposable morphologically.

The remainder of this section will consider five categories of tumors in patients with a known history of extrapulmonary malignant neoplasms:

1. adenocarcinoma variants
2. spindle cell and pleomorphic malignancies
3. small round cell neoplasms
4. squamous cell carcinomas and their simulants
5. undifferentiated large polygonal cell malignancies.

In each group, the differential diagnosis includes at least one primary pulmonary lesion. Although specific neoplastic entities are indeed discussed hereafter, our presentation of them is not all-inclusive. Rather, the approach summarized here is intended to serve as an exemplary differential diagnostic framework. Also, it should be recognized that there will inevitably be some overlap in the categories in which a particular tumor class may reside. For example, in selected cases hepatocellular carcinomas potentially may present the morphologic appearances of adenocarcinoma, not further specified; oncocytoid carcinoma; clear cell carcinoma; an undifferentiated large polygonal cell malignancy; and even sarcomatoid (spindle cell and pleomorphic) carcinoma. Accordingly, we have organized the presentation to reflect the most *common* morphologic groups in which specific neoplasms are usually placed.

The ensuing discussion also incorporates information on immunohistologic panels that can be used in the separation of nosologically different but structurally similar tumors. These panels have been presented in that manner because immunohistochemistry is today such an integral part of cytopathology and histopathology. However, we would certainly emphasize that differential diagnosis does not rest on adjuvant studies alone, but rather involves the melding of light microscopic observations, clinical information, and data derived from ancillary procedures. The availability of such techniques varies between medical institutions; therefore, the antibody profiles presented here again serve to illustrate our approach but should not be regarded as definitive or mandatory, especially in light of the rapid evolution of adjunctive technology in pathology.

Adenocarcinoma variants

Adenocarcinoma is the most common form of primary lung cancer, and, in patients who have a history of an extrapulmonary tumor of that type, the distinction between a primary and secondary lesion may be challenging. In some cases, morphologic appearances alone are sufficient to accomplish that task, as considered below. Immunopathology also is helpful in the recognition of some of these tumors. Table 17.1 shows the immunohistological profile of specific adenocarcinomas based on their sites of origin.[85]

Papillary adenocarcinomas

Silver and Askin reported that primary papillary pulmonary adenocarcinomas – defined as such if ≥75% of the neoplasm demonstrates a micropapillary architecture

Table 17.1 Immunophenotypes of carcinomas potentially seen in the lung

Origin	PK	CK7	CK20	EMA	THY	CEA	ER	HEP	GCDFP	S100	TTF1	PSA	INHB	CA125	CA19-9	CD10
Lung	P	P	N	P	N	P	N	N	N	N	P	N	N	N	PN	N
Breast	P	P	N	P	N	P	P	N	P	PN	N	N	N	PN	N	N
Thyroid gland	P	P	N	PN	P	PN	N	N	N	PN	P	N	N	N	N	N
Salivary duct	P	P	P	P	N	PN	N	N	PN	PN	N	PN	N	N	N	N
Ovary (serous)	P	P	N	P	N	N	P	N	N	PN	N	N	N	P	N	N
Kidney	P	PN	N	P	N	N	N	N	N	PN	N	N	N	N	N	P
Stomach	P	PN	PN	PN	N	PN	N	N	N	PN	N	PN	N	PN	PN	N
Pancreas	P	P	PN	P	N	P	N	N	N	N	N	N	N	PN	P	N
Colorectal	P	PN	P	P	N	P	N	N	N	PN	N	N	N	PN	PN	N
Prostate	P	PN	PN	PN	N	PN	N	N	PN	N	N	P	N	N	N	N
Adrenocortical	N	N	N	N	N	PN	N	N	N	N	N	N	P	N	N	N
Hepatocellular	P	PN	PN	PN	N	P	N	P	N	PN	N	N	N	N	N	PN

PK = pan-keratin; EMA = epithelial membrane antigen; THY = thyroglobulin; CEP P = carcinoembryonic antigen, polyclonal; ER = estrogen receptor; HEP = hepatocyte-related antigen in paraffin sections-1; GCDFP = gross cystic disease fluid protein; TTF1 = thyroid transcription factor-1; PSA = prostate specific antigen; INHB = inhibin; P = >75% of tumors; PN = between 10% and 75% of tumors; N = <10% of tumors.

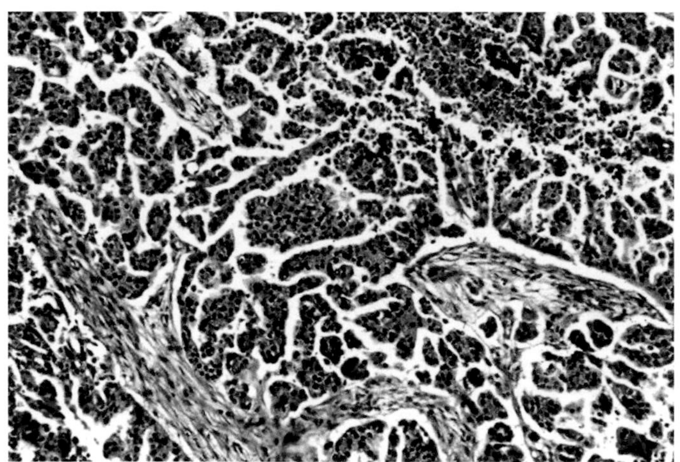

Fig. 17.13 Micropapillary architecture is apparent in this bronchioloalveolar carcinoma of the lung. This feature can be seen in both primary and secondary pulmonary epithelial tumors.

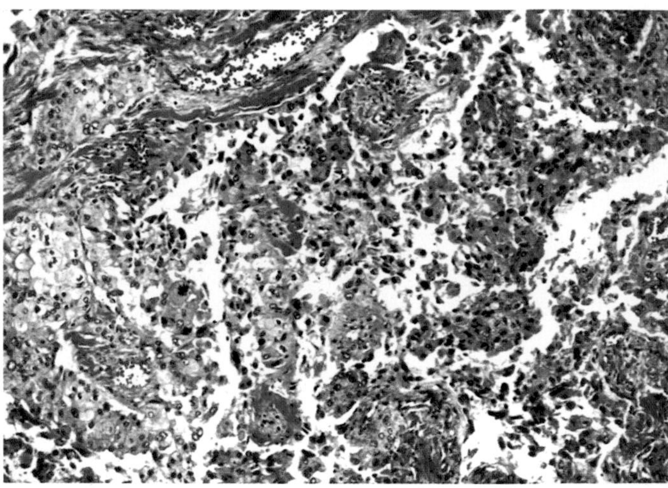

Fig. 17.14 Metastatic renal cell carcinoma with a micropapillary architecture.

– are not uncommon[86] moreover, micropapillae may be seen in conventional adenocarcinomas of the lung as well,[87,88] and bronchioloalveolar adenocarcinomas commonly have the potential for papillary growth (Fig. 17.13). Metastatic adenocarcinomas in the lung also may contain micropapillary structures. In FNA specimens, such tumors show fibrovascular fragments covered by cuboidal or low-columnar neoplastic cells.

Metastatic papillary adenocarcinomas may originate in the thyroid, breasts, ovaries, and kidneys (Fig. 17.14). Thyroid carcinomas of all histologic subtypes have the potential to metastasize to the lung. Indeed, of all thyroid carcinomas that spread to distant sites other than lymph nodes, up to 50% involve the pulmonary parenchyma.[89–91] Papillary thyroid carcinoma (PTC) almost always metastasizes to regional cervical lymph nodes beforehand;[89] in addition, that tumor type may directly invade the trachea and produce an endoluminal mass. Anaplastic thyroid carcinoma shares the latter potential. Hilar-intrathoracic and mediastinal lymph nodes are also involved by PTC in one-half of the cases with lung metastasis.[92] Secondary PTC is a tumor that may grow

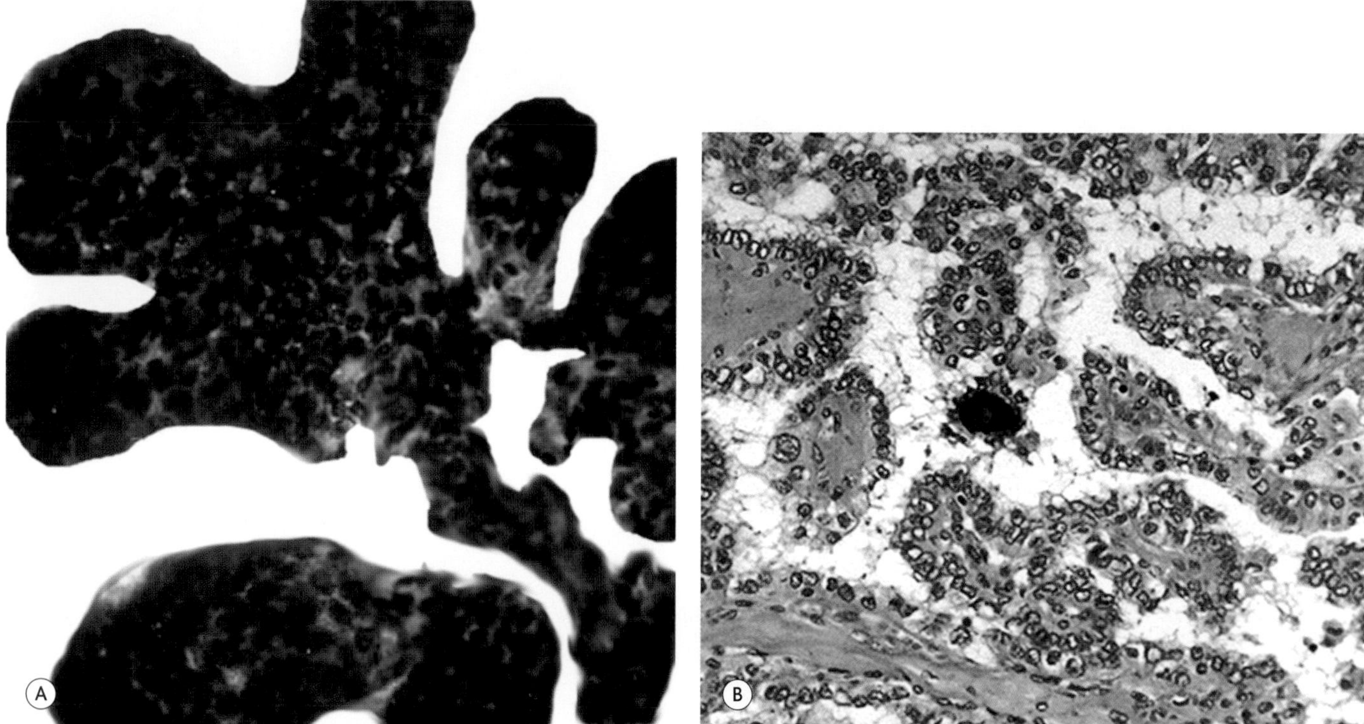

Fig. 17.15 (A) Fine-needle aspirate of metastatic papillary thyroid carcinoma in the lung, demonstrating an arborizing micropapillary image. (B) Nuclear overlap, intranuclear pseudoinclusions of cytoplasm, and psammomatous microcalcifications are observed in the cell block preparation from this case.

very slowly and remain solitary for extended periods of time, simulating the biologic characteristics of a primary pulmonary neoplasm.[89] In addition to its papillary substructure, other cytologic clues in cases of metastatic PTC include its characteristic nuclear features – including nuclear grooves, nuclear membrane irregularities, cytoplasmic invaginations (pseudoinclusions), and nuclear overlap – as well as the formation of colloid and psammoma bodies (Fig. 17.15). All types of ovarian carcinoma may metastasize to the lungs, and up to 50% of stage IV cases feature pulmonary involvement.[93] The papillary serous form of ovarian cancer is the most common subtype. The pleura is often involved early, by lymphatic spread through the diaphragm, and the peripheral lung parenchyma is then affected. Malignant pleural effusions caused by papillary serous carcinomas are seen in 40% of all cases with metastases,[93] and solitary pulmonary nodules are present in 7%.[94] Lymphangitic intrapulmonary growth of ovarian malignancies is associated with a rapid demise.[95,96]

Immunopathologic studies to determine the site of origin of a papillary carcinoma in the lung are outlined in Table 17.2.[85] We recommend using at least one marker (e.g. vimentin or pan-keratin) that should be positive in each of the differential diagnostic possibilities in order to establish the antigenic integrity of the tissue.[97] In this specific setting, the highest specificity of immunopathologic identification is associated with tumors of thyroid glandular, pulmonary, or mammary origin. Metastatic papillary tumors arising in the kidneys or ovaries are more difficult to segregate from others

Table 17.2 Immunohistologic differential diagnosis of papillary adenocarcinoma

	Antibody							
Origin	PK	TTF1	CK20	THY	ERP	GCDFP	CEA	S100
Lung	P	P	N	N	N	N	P	N
Thyroid gland	P	P	N	P	N	N	PN	PN
Breast	P	N	N	N	P	P	P	PN
Ovary (serous)	P	N	N	N	P	N	N	PN
Kidney	P	N	N	N	N	N	N	PN

P = positive (>80% of cases); PN = variably positive (between 10% and 80% of cases); N = negative (fewer than 10% of cases). PK = pan-keratin; TTF1 = thyroid transcription factor-1; CK20 = cytokeratin 20; THY = thyroglobulin; ERP = estrogen receptor protein; GCDFP = gross cystic disease fluid protein-15; CEA = carcinoembryonic antigen; S100 = S100 protein.

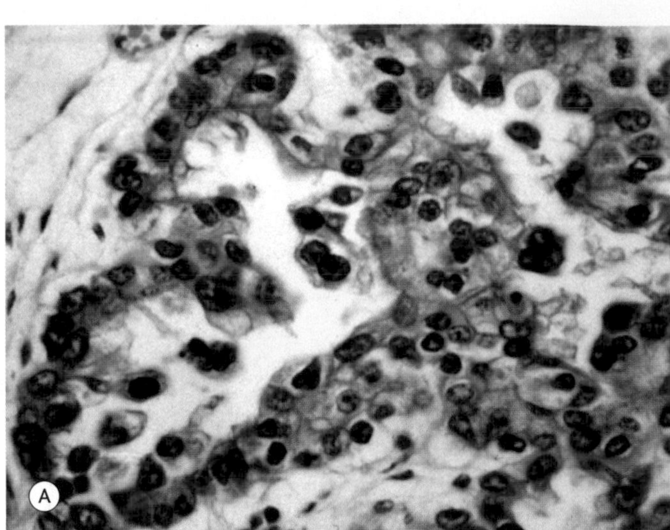

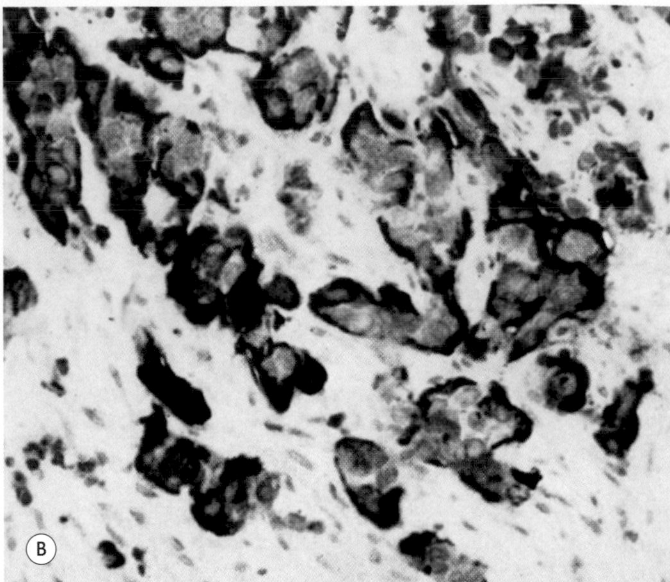

Fig. 17.16 (A) Metastatic clear-cell carcinoma of the ovary, showing glandular formations containing tumor cells with a "hobnail" appearance. (B) Immunostaining with CA-125 supports the müllerian origin of this tumor.

definitively using immunohistology, although CA-125 reactivity is a consistent feature of ovarian epithelial neoplasms (Fig. 17.16).

Another malignancy that often has a papillary "pseudocarcinomatous" appearance, especially in pleural fluid specimens, is the epithelioid variant of malignant mesothelioma (Fig. 17.17). Renshaw et al. estimated that the sensitivity of pleural fluid cytology for the diagnosis of mesothelioma was only 32%,[98] because epithelioid tumor cells often have a bland appearance and the sarcomatoid variant of mesothelioma rarely sheds into the pleural space. Many reports have considered the diagnostic separation of mesothelioma from metastatic adenocarcinoma, and this topic is discussed in detail in Chapter 20 (page 750).[99–101] Immunopathologic and electron microscopic studies generally represent the definitive methods that are used to make this distinction.[99,102] Table 17.3 shows a typical immunopathologic antibody panel that can be employed to separate mesothelial proliferations from epithelial tumors.[99,103,104] Imlay and Raab examined the utility of immunohistochemistry in this context in hospital practice.[44] They reported that immunopathologic techniques were applied to 2.6% of all cases concerning pleural fluid specimens. In 71.9% of those, a firm interpretation was facilitated by the results of such analyses.[44] However, none of the diagnoses in that series were based solely on immunopathology.[44] The low prevalence of mesothelioma in the general population explains the rarity of that interpretation in the experiences of most practicing pathologists.

Table 17.3 Immunohistologic differential diagnosis between malignant mesothelioma and metastatic adenocarcinoma

	Antibody						
Tumor	PK	CK5/6	CEA	CD15	Ber-EP4	B72.3	CALR
Malignant mesothelioma	P	P	N	N	N	N	P
Adenocarcinoma	P	N	P	P	P	P	N

CK = cytokeratin; VIM = vimentin; CEA P = carcinoembryonic antigen, polycolonal; CAL = calretinin; P = positive (>80% of cases); PN = variably positive (between 10% and 80%); N = negative (fewer than 10% of cases); PK = pan-keratin; CK 5/6 = cytokeratin 5/6; CEA = carcinoembryonic antigen; CALR = calretinin.

Clear cell adenocarcinomas

Clear cell features are best appreciated in histologic specimens, in which the cytoplasm of the neoplastic cells is lucent and only the cell borders are apparent. Clear cell change is often an artifact of formalin fixation, and, in cytologic specimens, the cytoplasm of the neoplastic cells has a more vacuolated appearance. Primary clear cell tumors of the lung are rare and are variable in cellular lineage; they are usually peripherally located[105] and are described in greater detail in Chapters 16 (page 571) and 19 (page 713). Clear cell change also may be seen focally in common tumor types. For example, biopsies of primary squamous cell carcinomas may show that alteration. Interestingly, that phenomenon is seen less frequently in cytologic specimens, in which the cytoplasm

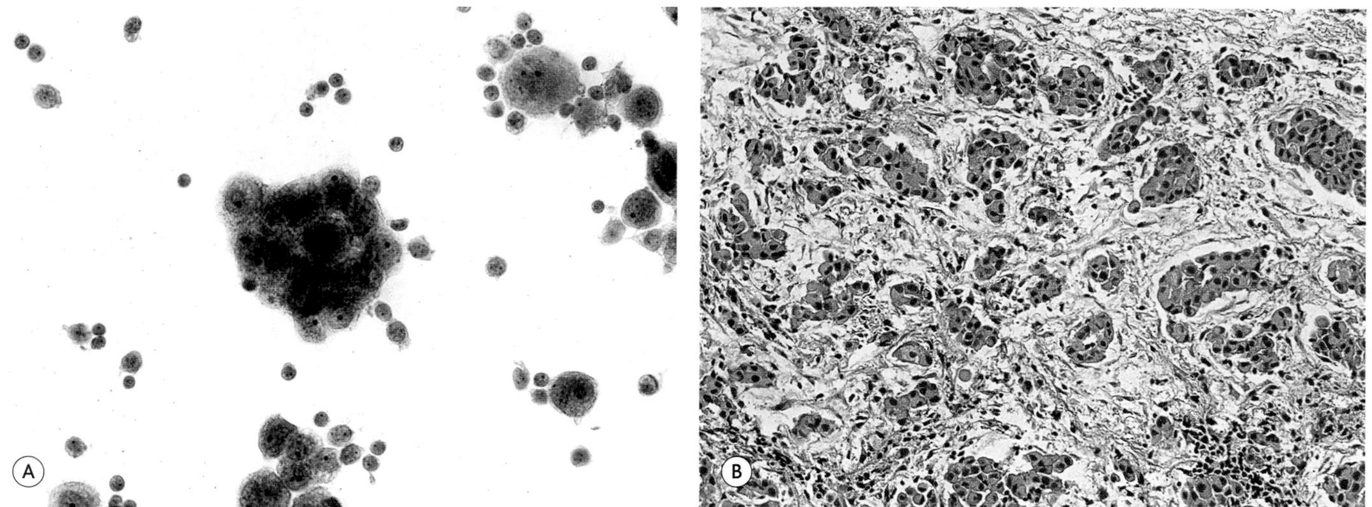

Fig. 17.17 (A) Cytologic preparation of pleural fluid in a case of malignant epithelioid mesothelioma shows a micropapillary array of atypical mesothelial cells. (B) A subsequent biopsy confirmed the micropapillary nature of the neoplasm, as shown here.

of the neoplastic cells maintains a classic "metaplastic" appearance.

Metastatic clear cell adenocarcinomas in the lungs may emanate from the kidneys, breasts, adrenal cortices, salivary glands, or other locations; indeed, primary clear cell malignancies have been described in practically every organ. The most common clear cell neoplasm in the lung is metastatic renal cell adenocarcinoma (Figs 17.18 and 17.19).[106] Hughes et al. reported that among 12 lung FNA specimens with clear cell features, 10 originated in the kidney, 1 in the cervix, and 1 in an undetermined site.[107] Clear cell carcinomas represent only a subset of renal tumors that may metastasize to the lungs; papillary, oncocytic, and sarcomatoid neoplasms may also do so. Because epithelial malignancies of the kidney have a proclivity to invade the renal veins and bypass the hepatic circulation, the first site of secondary disease may be in the lungs;[106,108] the pulmonary parenchyma is involved in up to 75% of cases of metastatic renal cell carcinoma.[108,109] Almost one-half of those patients have no symptoms suggesting the presence of extrathoracic disease[109] (Fig. 17.20). Metastatic disease in the lungs may take several radiographic forms, including a solitary mass, multiple nodules, miliary spread (innumerable small nodules), large- or small-vessel emboli, lymphatic space disease, hilar or mediastinal lymph nodal disease, and endobronchial tumor.[110–114] Metastatic renal cell carcinoma is an example of a neoplasm that may grow very slowly and become clinically evident only many years after the primary diagnosis was made.[115]

Like ovarian carcinomas, clear cell carcinomas of the kidney are difficult to identify definitively by immunohistologic studies. Nonetheless, the great majority of them are reactive for CD10 and cytokeratin 8 (Figs 17.21 and 17.22), which, in combination, are highly suggestive of the diagnosis in question.[114ab] Another monoclonal antibody to renal cell carcinoma, designated as "RCC," does show restricted reactivity with that tumor but is technically challenging to employ effectively.[114c]

Signet ring cell adenocarcinomas

A signet ring cell is relatively small and has an eccentrically placed nucleus indented by a large cytoplasmic vacuole or multiple vacuoles. Such cells generally are considered to be part of the spectrum of poorly differentiated mucin-forming adenocarcinoma, and some tumors of that type are composed almost entirely of signet ring cell forms. Signet ring cell differentiation is uncommon in most primary pulmonary adenocarcinomas, and if it is present a secondary malignancy should be favored (Fig. 17.23). Sources of metastases with that appearance include the stomach and other gastrointestinal sites, breasts, and pancreas. Metastatic signet ring cell carcinomas are usually associated with a dismal prognosis; they characteristically spread initially to regional lymph nodes before involving the lungs. Some esophageal signet ring cell tumors originating in foci of Barrett's esophagus may directly invade the lung or pleura. Metastatic pancreatic adenocarcinomas, including signet ring cell variants, often involve the liver in addition to the lungs.[116] In those cases, multiple pulmonary nodules are virtually always seen rather than a solitary secondary lesion.[116]

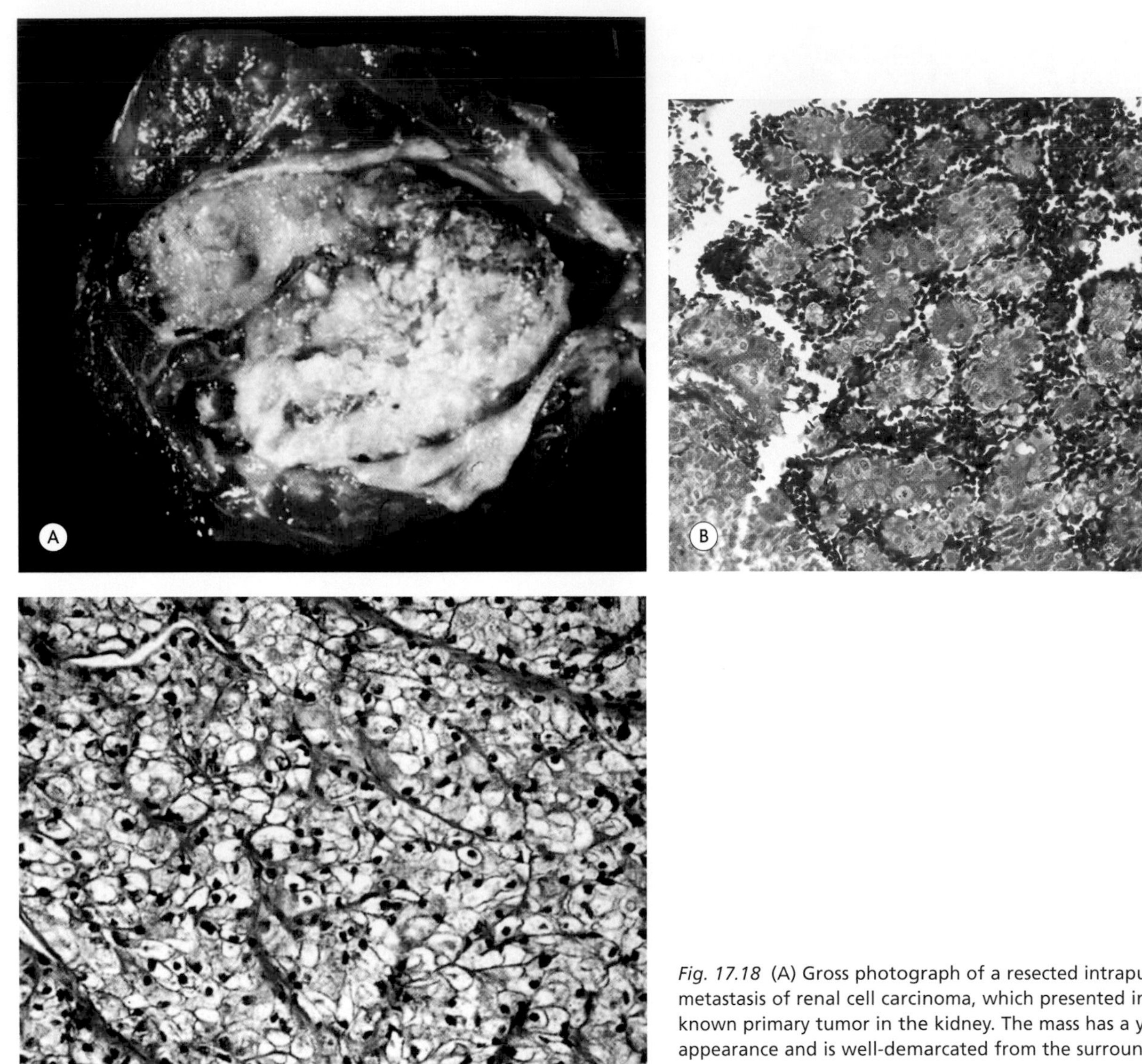

Fig. 17.18 (A) Gross photograph of a resected intrapulmonary metastasis of renal cell carcinoma, which presented in the absence of a known primary tumor in the kidney. The mass has a yellowish appearance and is well-demarcated from the surrounding lung parenchyma. (B) Typical blood "lakes" in the tumor serve as evidence of its renal origin. (C) The renal cell carcinoma in this case is otherwise composed of tubular arrays of clear cells.

Well-differentiated adenocarcinomas

The authors use the term "well-differentiated adenocarcinoma" in more than just a descriptive fashion to mean a malignant glandular proliferation that is morphologically difficult to separate from benign or reactive pulmonary proliferations. The recognition of these tumors is often extremely difficult in cytologic specimens because of the lack of contextual architecture. Well-differentiated primary adenocarcinomas of the lung include some "conventional" (acinar) adenocarcinomas, selected bronchioloalveolar adenocarcinomas, and salivary gland-type adenocarcinomas (see Chapter 17). These tumors show relatively low nuclear-to-cytoplasmic ratios and lack the degree of nuclear atypia seen in more overtly malignant lesions. Bronchioloalveolar adenocarcinomas, in particular, often pose a diagnostic conundrum, especially in cytologic preparations where one cannot see the malignant cells lining alveolar septa in a "lepidic" manner. Nevertheless, well-differentiated adenocarcinomas in the lung may also represent metastases, especially when they are sharply defined mass lesions macroscopically. Sites of origin for secondary adenocarcinomas with those attributes include the breasts, pancreas, kidneys, thyroid, and salivary glands.

Mammary carcinomas may metastasize to the lungs, the pleura, or both of those sites. In most instances the malignant cells are easily identified, but, in some FNA or

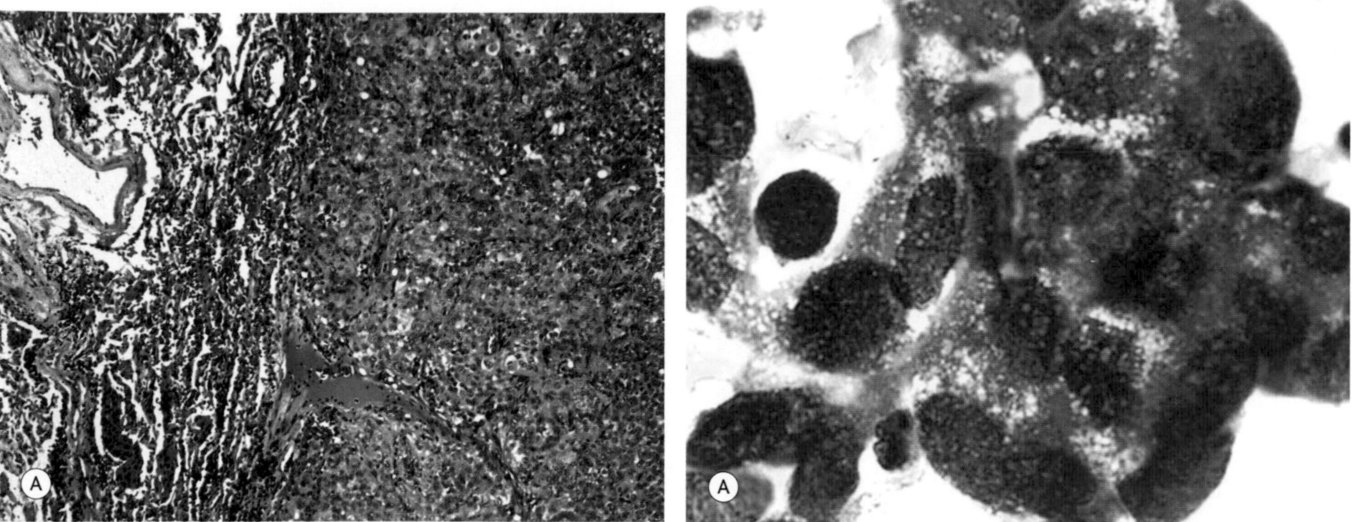

Fig. 17.19 (A) This example of resected metastatic renal cell carcinoma is more solid and comprises tumor cells with an oncocytoid appearance. (B) A prior fine-needle aspirate in the same case does show fine cytoplasmic vacuolization, serving as a clue to the renal nature of the lesion.

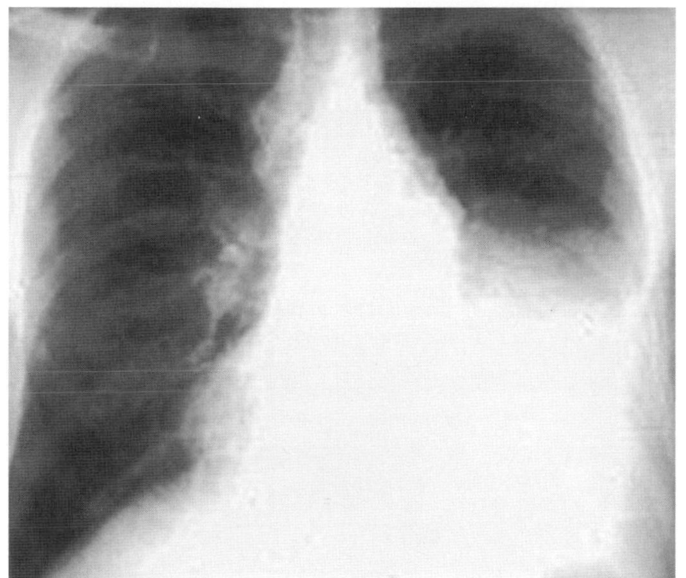

Fig. 17.20 This chest radiograph is from another patient with "occult" renal cell carcinoma, presenting with metastasis to the pleura and lungs. The left hemithorax is partially opacified by metastatic tumor and an accompanying pleural effusion.

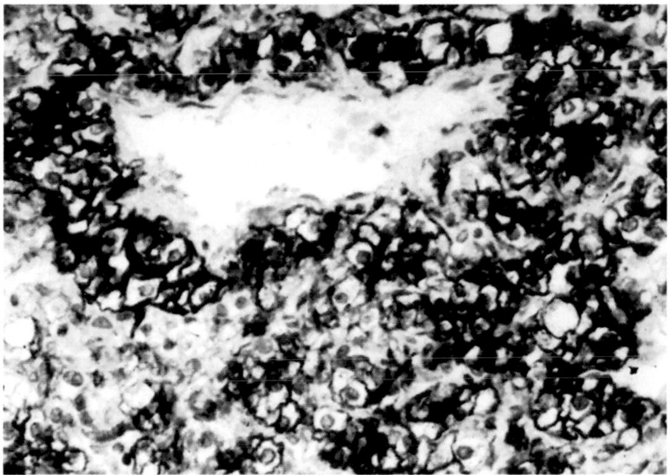

Fig. 17.21 Immunoreactivity for CD10 in metastatic renal cell carcinoma. This marker is found in the great majority of malignant renal epithelial tumors.

pleural fluid specimens, the malignant cells are very bland (Fig. 17.24). Intrapulmonary metastatic foci are often nodular, but other presentations such as endobronchial lesions, lymphangitic spread, and intravascular tumor emboli may be encountered as well.[117–120] Approximately 50% of metastatic breast cancers are associated with pleural effusions.[32,121] Casey et al. reported that 3% of primary mammary carcinomas were associated with a lung mass at the time of initial diagnosis; 43% of the pulmonary lesions represented metastases and 52% were concurrent primary lung cancers; the remainder were non-neoplastic.[120] The lungs and pleura are the first sites of tumor recurrence in 10% of cases of mammary carcinoma.[119] In patients who had a history of breast carcinoma and an adenocarcinoma in the lung, Raab et al. showed, with immunohistochemical studies (for estrogen receptor, gross cystic disease fluid protein-15, S-100 protein, and carcinoembryonic antigen) that 50% of the pulmonary lesions were metastatic mammary tumors, 37% were primary pulmonary carcinomas, and 13% were indeterminate (Figs 17.25 and 17.26).[122] Dabbs et al. found that some primary lung cancers may label for hormone receptor proteins, but not for the other specified markers.[123] Positivity for thyroid transcription factor-1 (Fig. 17.27) is compelling evidence in favor of pulmonary derivation in this particular context, as further discussed below.

Oncocytic and granular cell carcinomas

Neoplasms composed of cells containing granular cytoplasm may be oncocytic or non-oncocytic in nature. Both subtypes contain cells that have an eosinophilic appearance in conventional stains. In oncocytic cells, this reflects the presence of numerous cytoplasmic mitochondria. Non-oncocytic cells instead contain a preponderance of other cytoplasmic organelles, especially lysosomes. Primary pulmonary malignancies that may have a granular cell constituency include conventional adenocarcinomas and salivary gland-type adenocarcinomas. For the most part, however, this cytologic feature is rare in lung tumors.

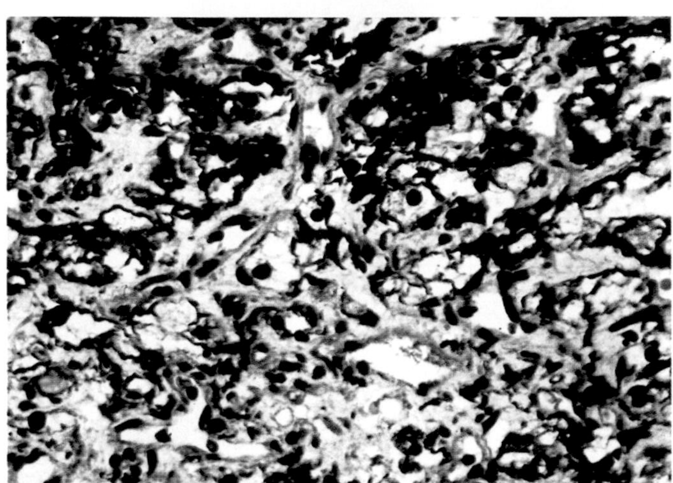

Fig. 17.22 Immunoreactivity for cytokeratin 8 in metastatic renal cell carcinoma. This keratin subtype is characteristic of non-oncocytic tumors of the kidney.

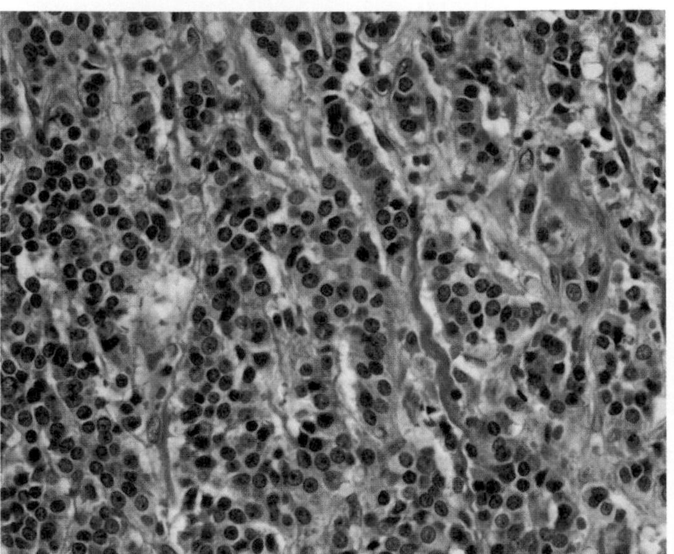

Fig. 17.24 Bland nuclear features are apparent in this metastatic lobular carcinoma of the breast involving the lung parenchyma.

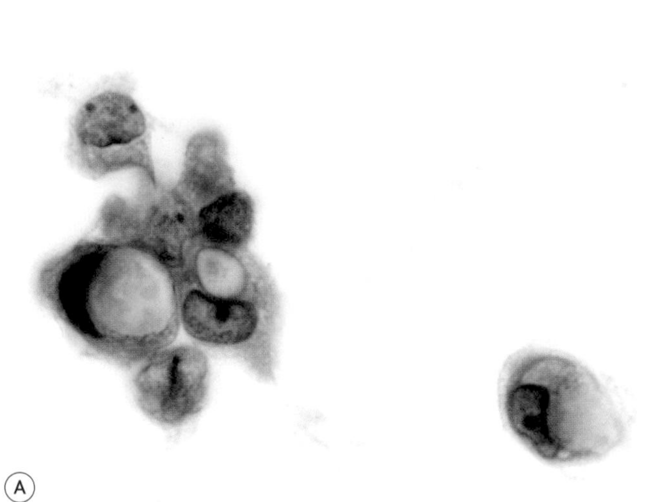

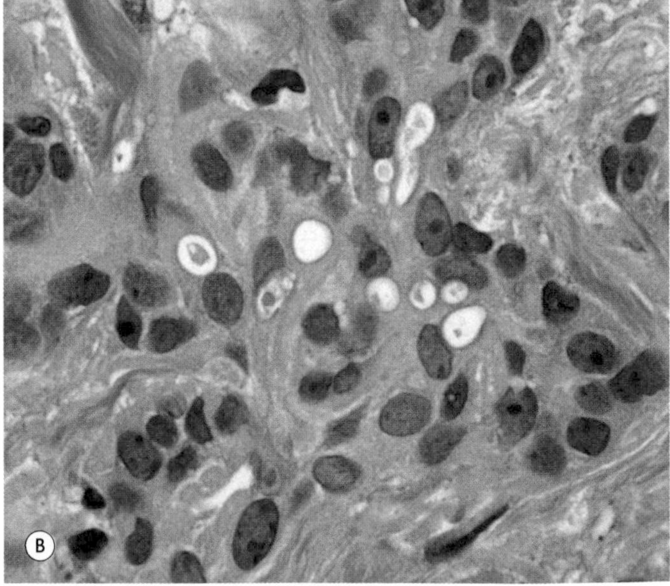

Fig. 17.23 (A) Metastatic adenocarcinoma in a fine-needle aspiration specimen, showing focal "signet ring cell" differentiation with formation of cytoplasmic vacuoles. (B) The same feature is seen in this cell block preparation. The primary tumor was lobular carcinoma of the breast.

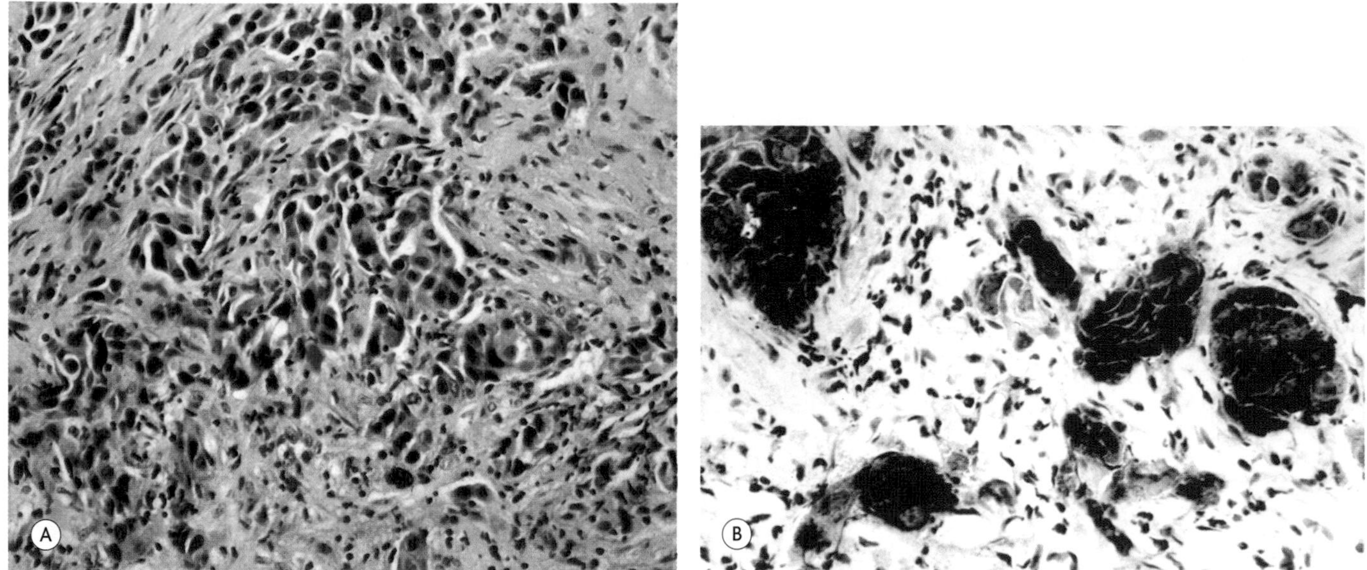

Fig. 17.25 (A) Adenocarcinoma in the lung with a histologically indeterminate appearance. It is unclear morphologically whether the tumor is primary or secondary. (B) Immunoreactivity for gross cystic disease fluid-protein-15, a breast marker, establishes the diagnosis of metastatic ductal mammary carcinoma.

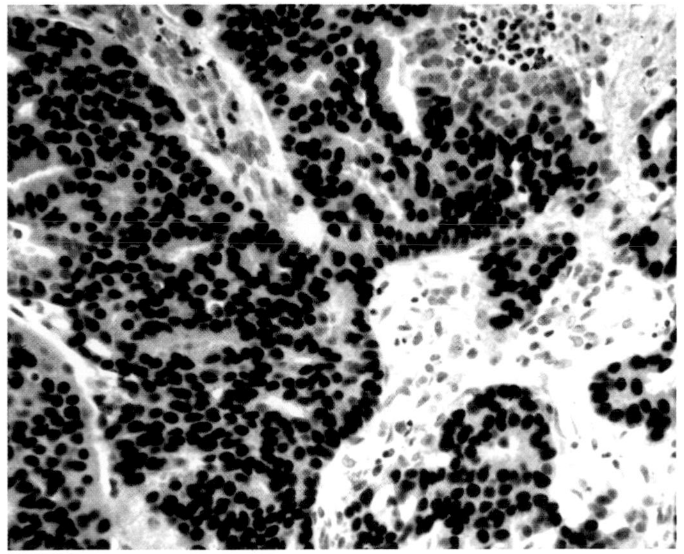

Fig. 17.26 Metastatic breast carcinoma in the lung, showing intense immunoreactivity for estrogen receptor protein.

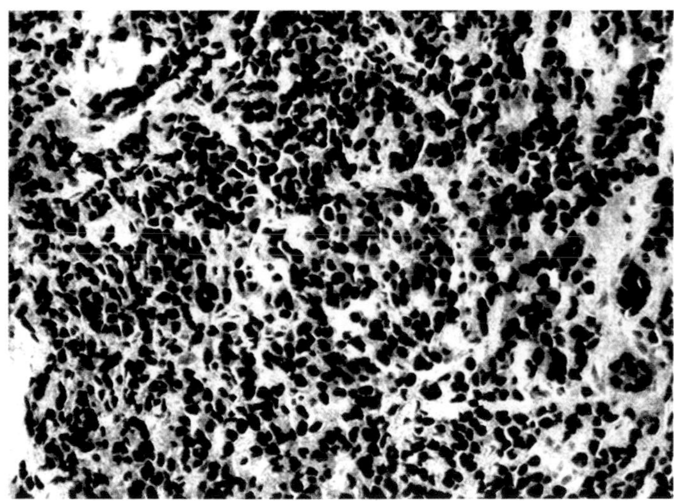

Fig. 17.27 Immunoreactivity for thyroid transcription factor-1 in primary adenocarcinoma of the lung. This marker is present only in thyroid and pulmonary proliferations.

Secondary neoplasms with granular cytoplasm include carcinomas of the kidney, thyroid, and liver (Fig. 17.28).

The lungs are involved in up to 70% of cases of metastatic hepatocellular carcinoma (HCC).[124–126] Several patterns of intrapulmonary spread have been reported; through transdiaphragmatic lymphatics, HCC may enter the right lower lobe; in this setting, several parenchymal mass lesions and pleural involvement are typically observed.[127,128] Alternatively, HCC may transit the venous system via the hepatic vein and inferior vena cava, presenting as a large intravascular mass or "showering" the lungs with small emboli that become manifest as miliary tumor.[127] Cytologically, the cells of this neoplasm often exhibit multinucleation; this feature is uncommon

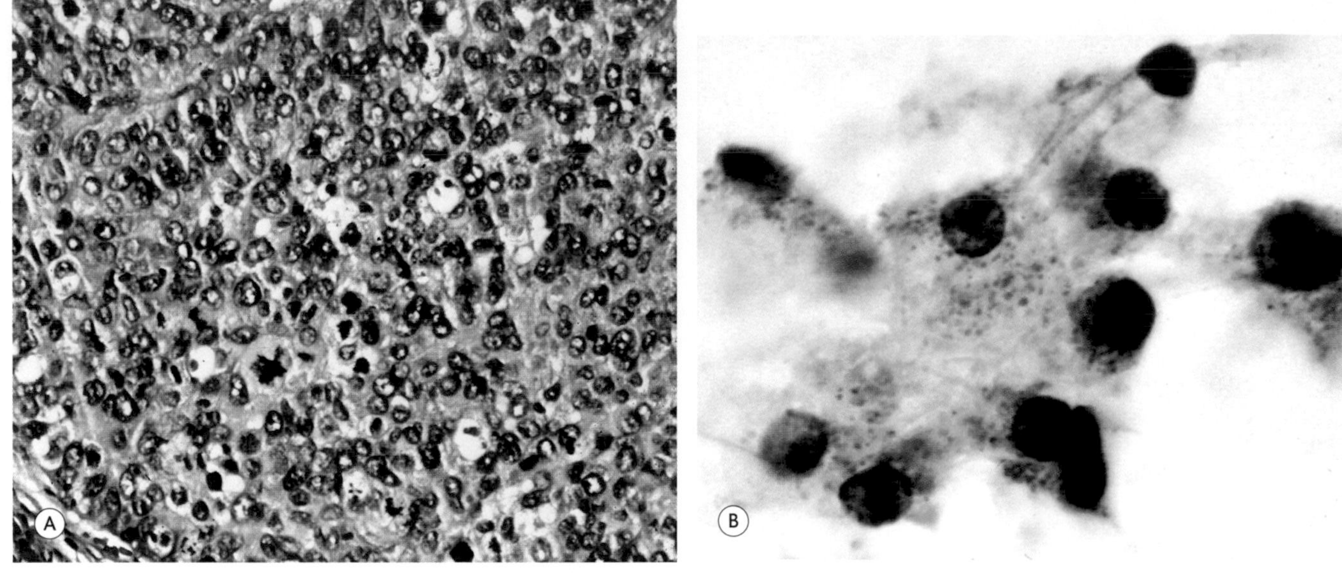

Fig. 17.28 (A) Metastatic large cell carcinoma in the lung with a granular cytoplasmic appearance. (B) Cytoplasmic granules are more evident in a fine-needle aspiration specimen. The primary tumor was in the liver.

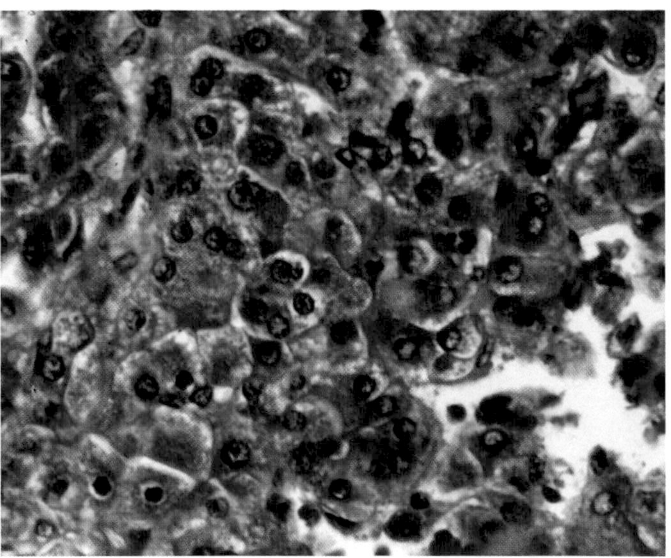

Fig. 17.29 Multifocal bile formation (right of figure) in metastatic hepatocellular carcinoma.

in most primary pulmonary malignancies. Moreover, bile formation may be present in metastatic HCC (Fig. 17.29). In addition, the tumor cells cluster around intralesional blood vessels, and "stripped" nuclei are seen as well.[129] Lastly, cytopathologists must guard against a misinterpretation of FNA specimens from the right lower pulmonary lobe as well-differentiated oncocytic or granular cell carcinomas; instead, such specimens may simply represent normal liver that has been mistakenly sampled instead of the lung. A monoclonal antibody raised against paraffin-embedded tissue from HCC, and designated "Hep-PAR1," has shown reasonably good discrimination in labeling that tumor.[129a]

Largely necrotic adenocarcinomas

The most commonly necrotic primary tumors of the lung are squamous cell carcinoma, small cell neuroendocrine carcinoma, and large cell undifferentiated or large cell neuroendocrine carcinoma. Primary pulmonary adenocarcinomas rarely demonstrate this alteration unless the tumors are very large or poorly differentiated. Thus, necrotic adenocarcinomas are more likely statistically to represent secondary malignancies in the lungs. Metastatic colorectal carcinomas characteristically show central necrosis cytologically, regardless of their degree of differentiation. FNA biopsy specimens of such lesions also show fusiform nuclei arranged in a "picket fence" pattern or in small glandular formations. Other extrapulmonary tumors that may yield the image of necrotic metastatic carcinoma include renal cell carcinoma, pancreatic carcinoma, esophageal squamous cell carcinoma or adenocarcinoma, breast cancer, and prostatic carcinoma.

In up to 50% of metastatic colorectal adenocarcinomas, the lungs are involved.[130] The majority of those cases show multiple pulmonary masses radiographically,[130] but roughly 40% of all solitary metastases in the lung are also derived from the large intestine.[20,21] Right-sided colonic tumors may produce lung metastases without

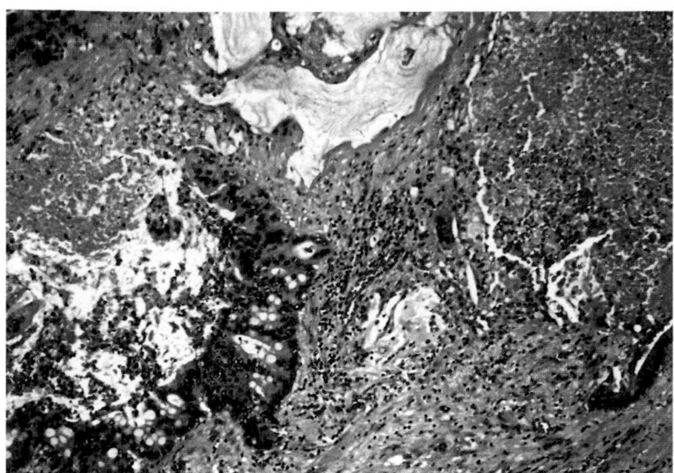

Fig. 17.30 Metastatic colonic adenocarcinoma in the lung, showing characteristically "incomplete" tumor glands and basally oriented tumor cell nuclei.

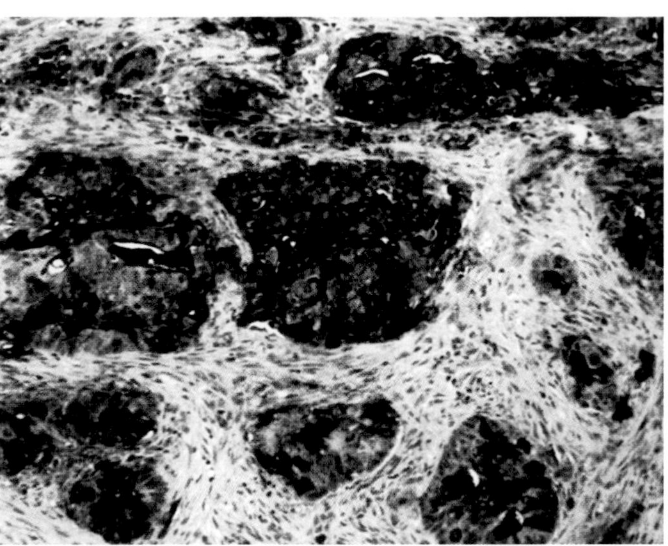

Fig. 17.32 Immunoreactivity for villin, a gut marker, in metastatic poorly differentiated colonic adenocarcinoma involving the lung.

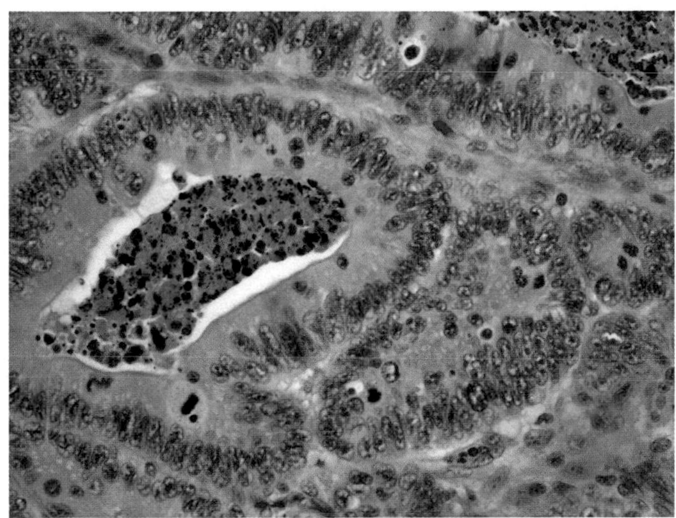

Fig. 17.31 "Dirty" necrosis is apparent in the centers of tumoral glands in metastatic colonic adenocarcinoma.

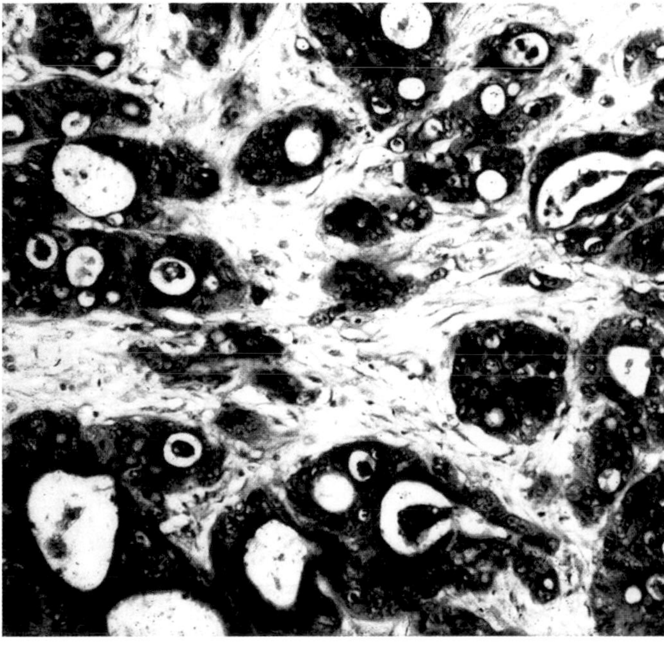

Fig. 17.33 Immunoreactivity for CA19.9, another gastrointestinal tract-related protein, in metastatic colonic adenocarcinoma.

liver metastases.[131–134] These lesions are often cystic and FNA specimens from them may be mistaken as showing cavitary squamous cell carcinoma. In histologic sections, zones of necrosis may be surrounded by only limited numbers of viable tumor cells; in cytologic preparations, rare viable cells may likewise be observed. Flint and Lloyd suggested that "dirty" (karyorrhectic) necrosis (Figs 17.30 and 17.31) was more often seen in metastatic colorectal tumors than in primary adenocarcinomas of the lung.[135] Immunopathologic studies are often helpful in separating secondary colonic malignancies from primary adenocarcinomas of the lung. Colorectal tumors generally are reactive for cytokeratin 20 but negative for cytokeratin 7 and thyroid transcription factor-1; the converse of that profile applies to primary pulmonary adenocarcinomas, even to those that have an "enteric" morphologic image on conventional microscopy.[136,141,141a] A cytoskeletal protein known as "villin" is also selectively seen in gastrointestinal malignancies, as is the plasmalemmal glycoprotein recognized by monoclonal antibody CA19-9 (Figs 17.32 and 17.33).[141bc]

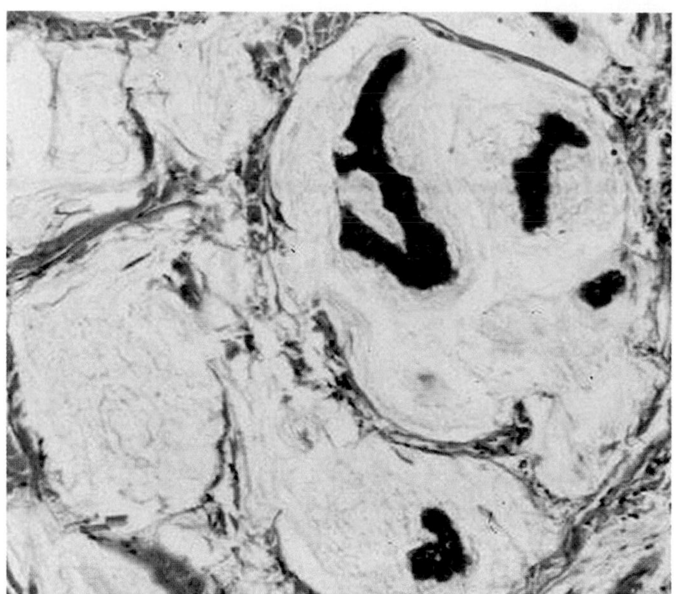

Fig. 17.34 Metastatic "colloid" carcinoma (mucinous adenocarcinoma) from the rectum, involving the lung. Narrowly branching profiles of tumor cells are suspended in pools of extracellular mucin. This image is highly suggestive of metastasis rather than a primary pulmonary tumor.

Mucinous adenocarcinomas

Primary mucin-producing carcinomas of the lung include some bronchioloalveolar carcinomas, selected muco-epidermoid carcinomas, and other rare primary mucinous tumors, some of which have the appearance of "colloid" carcinomas (Fig. 17.34).[141d] Most of these tumors have relatively specific radiologic attributes and when those images are absent and a mucinous carcinoma is present microscopically, metastasis may be suspected. However, it must be remembered that large amounts of post-obstructive mucin production by the lung may surround non-mucinous malignancies. Consequently, cyto-pathologists should be cautious in interpreting FNA specimens containing carcinoma cells and abundant mucin as bona fide mucinous carcinomas. The most common sites of origin for metastatic mucinous adeno-carcinomas are the intestine (including the vermiform appendix), ovaries, and breasts. Pathologic specimens of these secondary tumors in the lung may show only rare malignant cells and copious mucin pools. The neoplastic cells are often well differentiated and they are arranged in small clusters. The immunopathologic features of metastatic colorectal adenocarcinoma of the "colloid" type are essentially the same as those of ordinary colon cancers, and that statement also applies to secondary mucinous carcinoma of the breast. However, mucinous ovarian carcinomas differ from other epithelial malignancies of the ovary immunophenotypically; they typically lack CA-125 and instead exhibit an enteric antigenic profile like that of intestinal neoplasms.[141e]

Other metastatic malignancies that mimic adenocarcinomas of the lung

Other metastatic malignancies that may mimic a primary pulmonary adenocarcinoma include prostatic carcinoma, predominantly epithelioid synovial sarcoma, clear cell sarcoma, endometrial carcinoma, epithelioid sarcoma, malignant melanoma, adrenocortical carcinoma, and some germ cell malignancies such as metastatic embryonal carcinoma. Some of those lesions are discussed in later sections.

The immunopathologic profiles of prostatic, endometrial, and adrenocortical carcinomas are shown in Table 17.1. Prostatic and endometrial tumors rarely metastasize selectively to the lungs;[142,143] only 10% of all prostatic carcinomas yield lung metastases[144,145] and <3% of endometrial carcinomas do so.[143] Both of those malignancies usually first involve other sites, such as lymph nodes, bones, or liver.[142] When these lesions do spread to the lungs, multiple masses usually are apparent.[146] Metastatic prostatic carcinomas may produce endobronchial masses, lymphangitic carcinomatosis, or thoracic lymph nodal spread.[147–149] Antibodies to prostate-specific antigen (PSA), prostate-specific acid phosphatase (PSAP), and prostate-specific membrane antigen (PSMA) are highly specific for tumors of prostatic origin (Figs 17.35–17.37).[150] No such specific markers are currently available to identify endometrial neoplasms. Biopsies of metastatic adrenocortical carcinoma may show lipidized cytoplasm in the tumor cells and extensive cellular dyshesion; the immunoprofile of this neoplasm is unusual in that it features scant keratin production (if any); vimentin-reactivity, and labeling for inhibin, or MART-1/Melan-A (Figs 17.38 and 17.39), or both, despite S100 protein-negativity. Inhibin and MART-1 are typically associated with ovarian stromal tumors and melanocytic proliferations, respectively. Why they should be present in an epithelial tumor is an unanswered question, but their presence makes adrenocortical carcinoma a singularly identifiable form of metastasis in the lung.

Spindle cell and sarcomatoid tumors

The most common primary pulmonary malignancy with a spindle cell or pleomorphic growth pattern is sarcomatoid bronchogenic carcinoma. It must be separated from primary and metastatic sarcomas and other types of malignant spindle cell tumors (such as

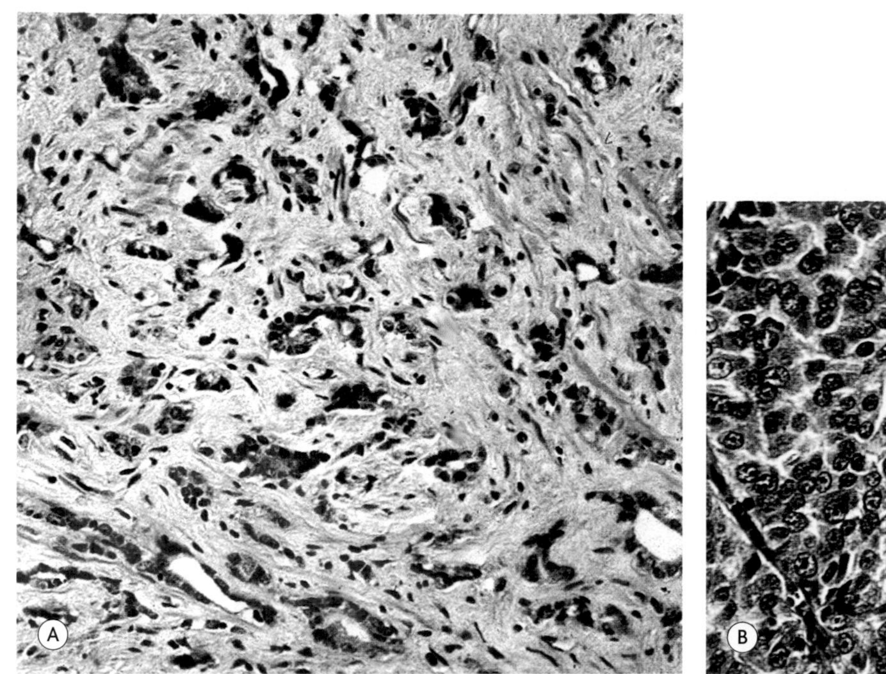

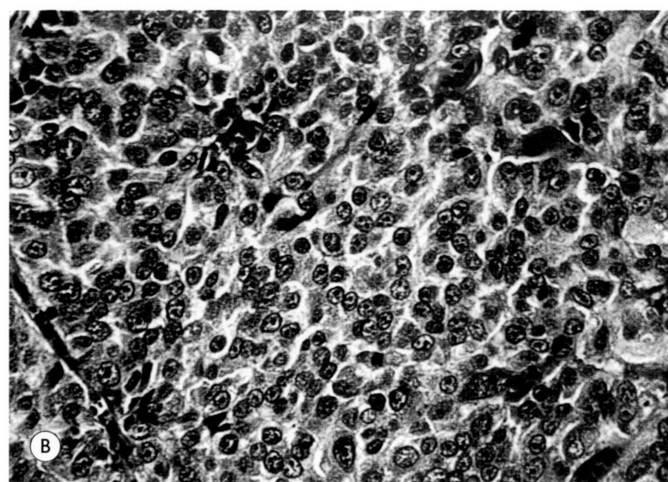

Fig. 17.35 Metastatic prostatic adenocarcinoma with intermediate (A) and high (B) Gleason scores, involving the lung parenchyma.

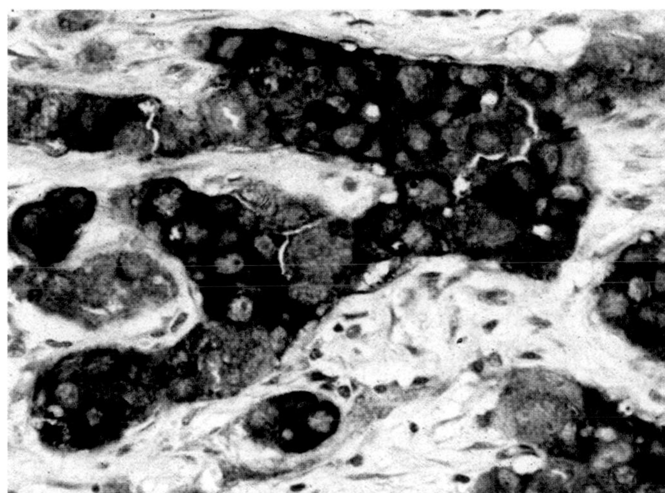

Fig. 17.36 Immunoreactivity for prostate-specific antigen in metastatic prostatic adenocarcinoma.

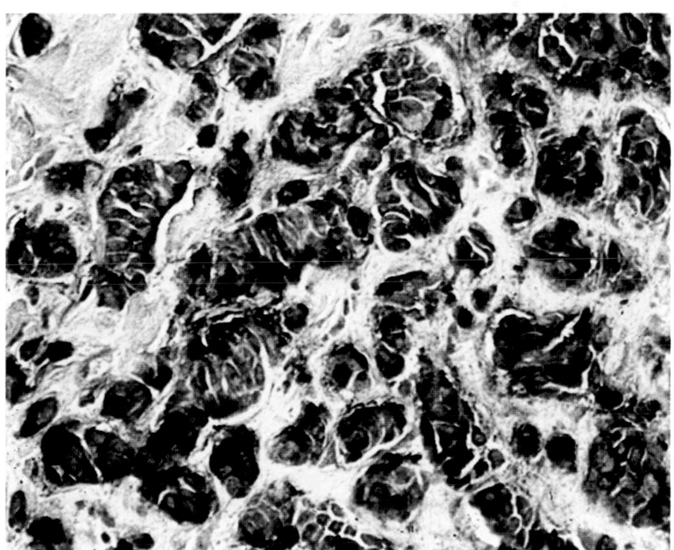

Fig. 17.37 Immunoreactivity for prostate-specific membrane antigen in metastatic prostatic adenocarcinoma.

sarcomatoid mesothelioma). Primary sarcomatoid carcinomas of the lung are extremely poorly differentiated, and many have been classified simply as "non-small cell carcinomas" in the past. Pathologic specimens of such tumors often show foci of spindle cell growth that are admixed with areas of more obvious epithelial differentiation (so-called "biphasic" sarcomatoid carcinoma) (Fig. 17.40), but monomorphic examples with no epithelioid components also exist ("monophasic" sarcomatoid carcinoma) (Fig. 17.41). Sarcomatoid carcinomas may contain homologous or heterologous foci of divergent mesenchymal-like differentiation, the latter of which resembles osteosarcoma, myogenous sarcomas, chondrosarcoma, and other forms of sarcoma (Fig. 17.42). This potentiality further confuses the diagnostic picture. Primary neuroendocrine carcinoma, especially "spindle cell carcinoid," may also enter the differential diagnosis, but sarcomatoid carcinomas do not exhibit the nuclear features that are seen in neuroendocrine lesions.

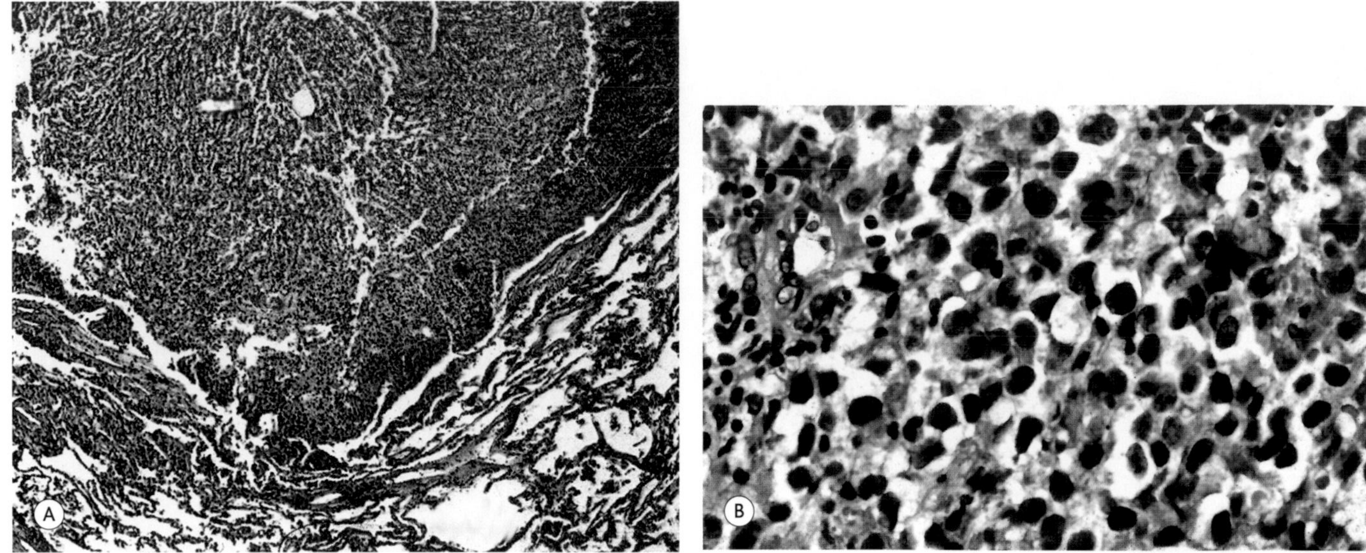

Fig. 17.38 (A,B) Metastatic adrenocortical carcinoma involving the lung, presenting as a solitary nodule composed of anaplastic large polygonal cells.

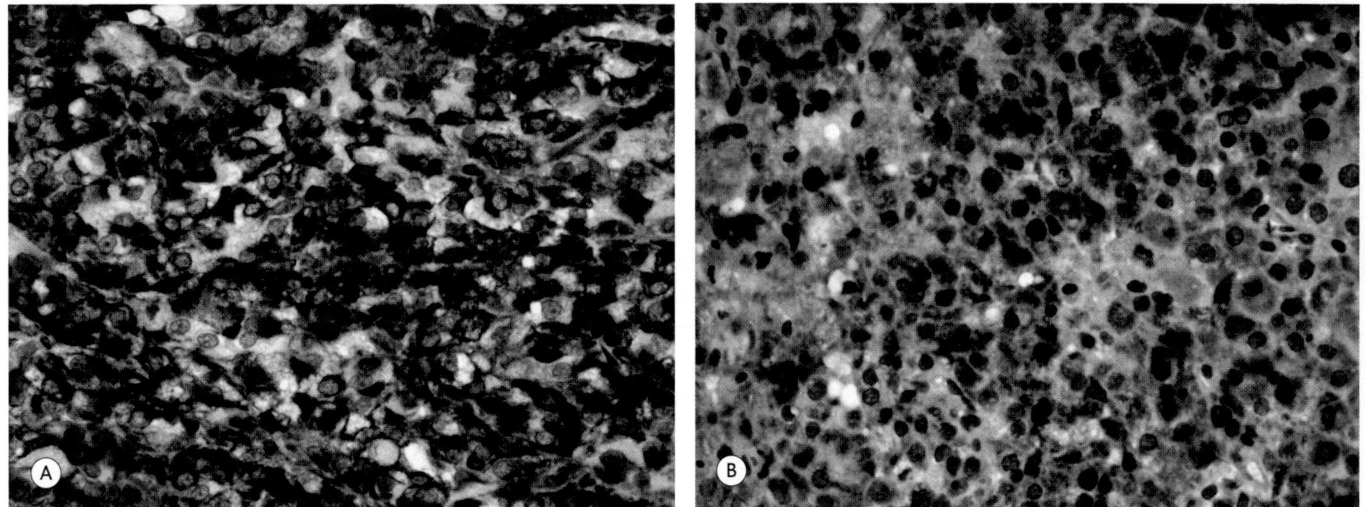

Fig. 17.39 Immunoreactivity was seen for (A) inhibin and (B) MART-1 in the tumor shown in Fig. 17.38, suggesting an adrenocortical origin.

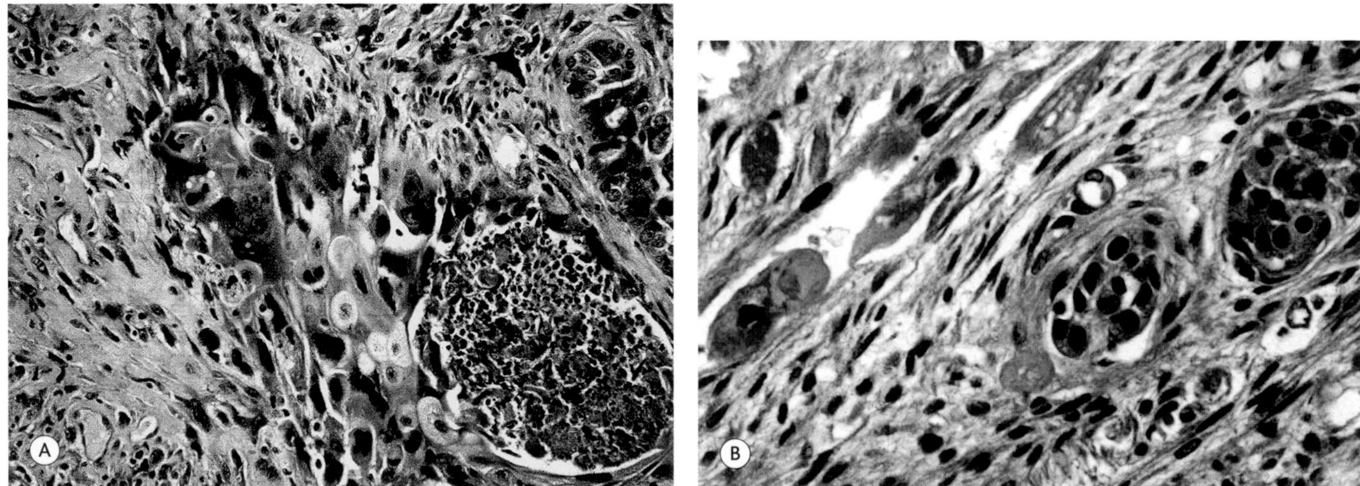

Fig. 17.40 (A) Metastatic biphasic sarcomatoid carcinoma of thyroidal origin, involving the lung. (B) Another view of the lesion shows the juxtaposition of sarcoma-like elements, including rhabdomyoblasts (top left) and obvious carcinoma (bottom right).

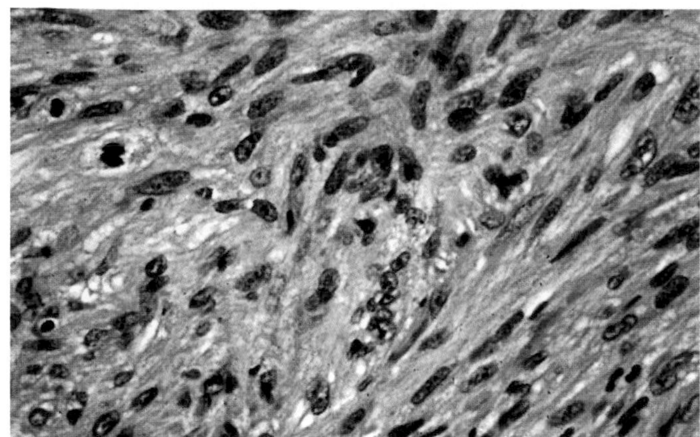

Fig. 17.41 Metastatic monophasic sarcomatoid carcinoma, comprising fusiform cells with no obvious sign of epithelial differentiation. Distinction from carcinoma is virtually impossible on conventional morphologic studies of such tumors.

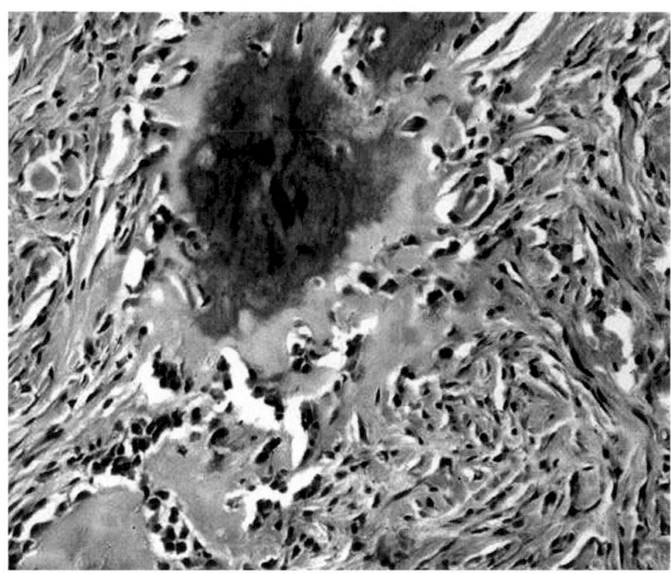

Fig. 17.42 Divergent osseous differentiation is present in this metastatic sarcomatoid carcinoma of uterine origin, involving the lung.

Table 17.4 Immunohistologic differential diagnosis of spindle cell malignancies in the lung

	Antibody										
Tumor	VIM	CEA	PK	ACT	CALR	CD31	CD34	S100	MART	CD99	EMA
Carcinoma	P	PN	PN	N	N	N	N	N	N	N	PN
Mesothelioma	P	N	PN	PN	PN	N	N	N	N	PN	PN
Melanoma	P	N	N	N	N	N	N	P	PN	PN	N
Synovial sarcoma	P	PN	PN	PN	PN	N	N	N	N	PN	PN
MPSNT	P	N	PN	PN	PN	N	PN	PN	N	N	PN
Leiomyosarcoma	P	N	PN	P	N	N	PN	N	N	N	N
Angiosarcoma	P	PN	PN	PN	N	PN	PN	N	N	N	N
Kaposi's sarcoma	P	N	N	PN	N	PN	P	N	N	N	N
MFH	P	N	PN	PN	N	N	PN	N	N	PN	PN

MPNST = malignant peripheral nerve sheath tumor; MFH = malignant fibrous histiocytoma; VIM = vimentin; PK = pan-keratin; ACT = actin; CALR = calretinin; MART = MART-1; S100 = S100 protein; EMA = epithelial membrane antigen; P = positive (>80% of cases); PN = variably positive (between 10% and 80% of cases); N = negative (<10% of cases).

Table 17.4 shows the immunophenotypes of specific spindle cell tumors in the lung.[151] In practice, the number of antibodies that are applied in immunohistologic studies varies according to the specific clinicopathologic setting. However, the ultimate diagnosis of sarcomatoid pulmonary lesions may require extensive use of adjunctive pathologic analyses.

Most patients with clinically apparent, metastatic, intrapulmonary spindle cell malignancies have metastatic sarcomas. Secondary spindle cell carcinoma is very unusual in the lungs; nevertheless, it should be remembered that sarcomas are uncommon as well; only 5000 to 6000 new cases of the latter tumors are seen each year in the United States.[152] In most cases of metastatic sarcoma in the lungs, a previous history of the tumor is well-known when pulmonary involvement becomes apparent. Thus, there is no need to institute a search for the primary lesion in that context. Solitary sarcomatous lesions of the lung and pleura are more difficult to recognize diagnostically, because the sarcoma morphotypes that occur primarily in those locations are also encountered in extrathoracic tissues and organs. That topic is considered in detail in Chapter 14.

Extrathoracic sarcomas are associated with a high

incidence of pulmonary metastasis overall. Autopsy series considering that point have found involvement of the lungs in up to 95% of cases.[153,154] Most metastatic sarcomas form multiple nodules in the pulmonary parenchymal or pleural surfaces, although solitary or multifocal endobronchial disease occasionally is seen as well.[155,156] Lymphatic spread of sarcomas is extremely unusual. Metastatic subpleural mesenchymal malignancies also may cavitate; this eventuality potentially causes pneumothorax formation or results in bronchopleural fistulae.[157–160] Foci of metastatic sarcoma may demonstrate a varied morphological appearance, even if the primary lesion did not; this phenomenon, termed "clonal evolution" is well-documented and may be an indicator of aggressive tumor growth.[160a] Irradiation and chemotherapy may facilitate its appearance.

Metastatic uterine smooth muscle tumors deserve special mention. Both high-grade leiomyosarcomas and low-grade myogenous tumors of the uterus (sometimes termed "metastasizing leiomyomas") may spread secondarily to the lungs.[161,162] In either instance, multiple and occasionally cystic nodular lesions are seen in the parenchyma and pleura; in rare cases, the metastatic tumor assumes a miliary pattern of spread.[163,164] Metastases of uterine smooth muscle neoplasms are usually seen in women of reproductive age or older,[165,166] but secondary intrapulmonary leiomyosarcoma has also been reported in men with primary soft tissue tumors.[165] Many of these patients have no symptoms at all, although dyspnea, cough, and cyanosis can be present. Indeed, some lesions may lead to respiratory failure.[165,167] Large smooth muscle tumors can yield neoplastic emboli and tumor-related pulmonary infarction.[168]

Grossly, metastatic smooth muscle tumors are white and well circumscribed with a "whorled" cut surface. Histologically, the constituent spindle cells may have a very bland appearance, especially in "metastasizing uterine leiomyomas." In those particular lesions, mitoses are rare or absent (Fig. 17.43).[165,166] Other examples of secondary leiomyosarcoma are easily recognized as malignant lesions because of the degree of nuclear atypia and mitotic activity that they demonstrate.

Some authors have suggested that "metastasizing leiomyomas" are actually multifocal pulmonary hamartomas, rather than metastatic tumors. That argument has focused on the bland appearance of the smooth muscle cells, the lack of mitoses, and the occasional presence of admixed glandular elements. Despite those points, we believe that "metastasizing leiomyomas" do indeed exist as a separate pathologic entity.[165] This opinion is based partly on aggregated clinicopathologic information. Most patients with such lesions have a history of surgical removal of uterine smooth muscle tumors (usually diagnosed as leiomyomas), or neoplasms of that type are found at autopsy. Synchronous metastatic implants have also been observed in abdominal, retroperitoneal, and pelvic soft tissue and lymph nodes in women who have "metastasizing leiomyomas" in the lungs.[169] In postmenopausal women, the metastatic lesions tend to be slowly growing or static, but they are associated with more rapid evolution and pulmonary morbidity in premenopausal patients. Some may even cause death. "Metastasizing leiomyomas" must be distinguished from lymphangioleiomyomatosis of the lungs, a condition that is discussed in detail in Chapter 7.

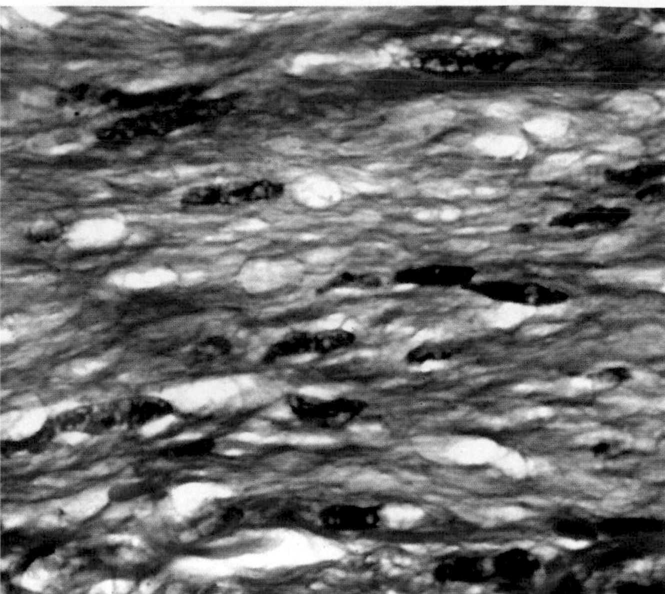

Fig. 17.43 "Metastasizing leiomyoma" of the uterus involving the lung. There is no appreciable nuclear atypia or mitotic activity in this bland spindle cell proliferation.

Malignant small round cell tumors

Malignant small round cell tumors prototypically are composed of cells with round-to-oval nuclei, scant cytoplasm, and extensive cellular dissociation. On scanning microscopy one often sees a "sheet" of nuclei; accordingly, these neoplasms are sometimes termed "small blue-cell" malignancies. An organoid growth pattern is also potentially apparent (Figs 17.44 and 17.45). The primary pleuropulmonary lesions in this category include neuroendocrine carcinomas, malignant lymphomas, and rare malignancies such as Askin's tumor or small cell mesothelioma. Metastatic small round cell tumors also include neuroendocrine carcinomas of extrapulmonary sites and malignant lymphomas, but additional sarcomas

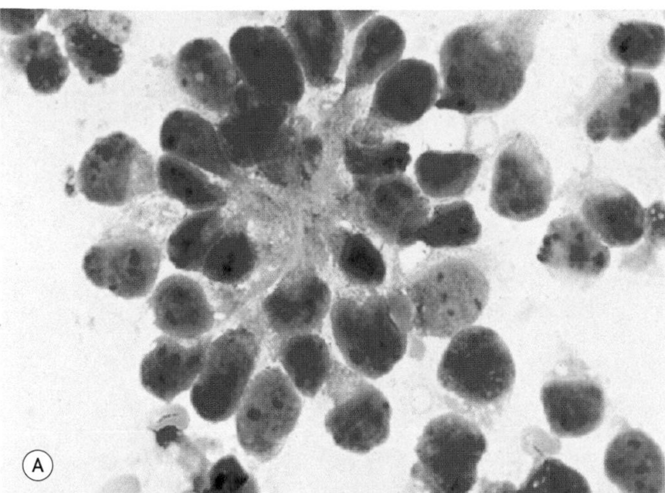

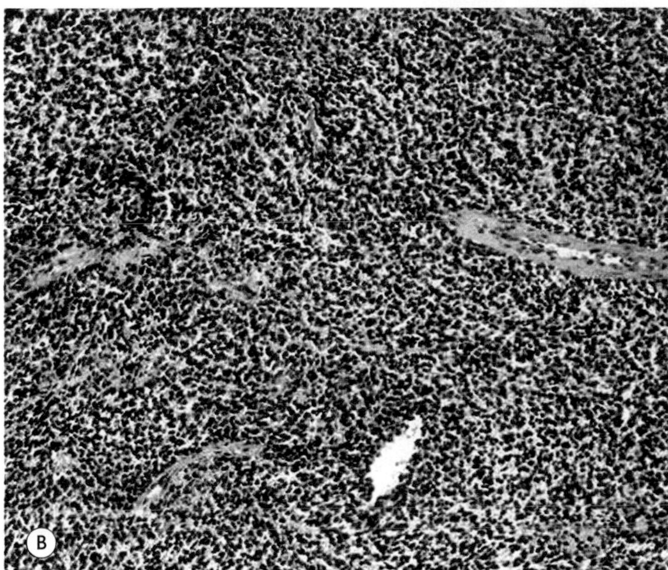

Fig. 17.44 (A) Fine-needle aspiration biopsy of primitive neuroectodermal tumor, metastatic to the lungs from a primary site in the chest wall. Relatively uniform small cells mold to one another and demonstrate only small nucleoli with dispersed chromatin. (B) The original biopsy specimen in this case shows sheets of small round cells that are transected by a delicate fibrovascular stroma.

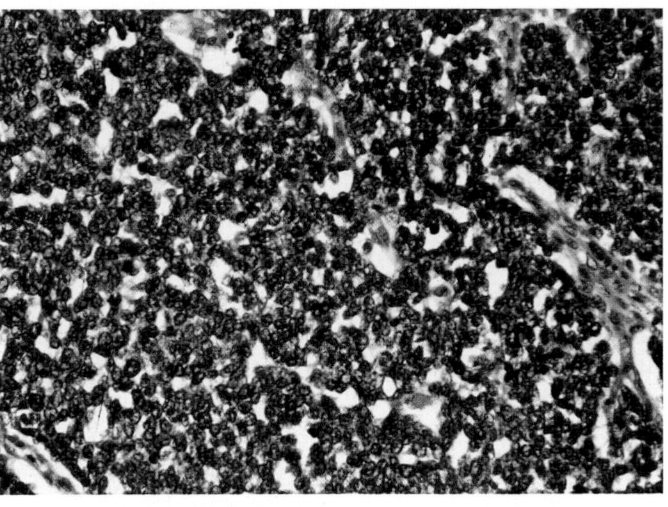

Fig. 17.45 Primitive rosette formation is apparent in primitive neuroectodermal tumor.

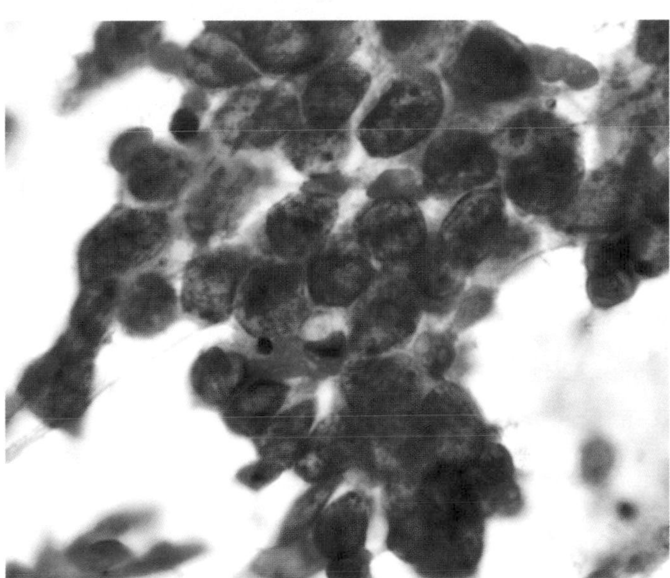

Fig. 17.46 Metastatic Merkel-cell carcinoma of the skin, involving the lung. This fine-needle aspirate shows tumor cells with scant cytoplasm and nuclear molding.

and other tumor types must also be considered (e.g. malignant melanoma, rhabdomyosarcoma, mesenchymal chondrosarcoma, small cell osteosarcoma, hepatoblastoma, neuroblastoma, and Wilms' tumor). Selected primary and secondary non-neuroendocrine carcinomas also may have a small cell composition.[170,171]

The most common primary intrathoracic small round cell malignancy is small cell neuroendocrine carcinoma of the lung (SCNCL).[171] That tumor is histologically and cytologically identical to small cell carcinomas originating in other sites (Figs 17.46 and 17.47). Clinically, most SCNCLs are centrally located and accompanied by enlarged mediastinal lymph nodes; they quickly metastasize and are usually advanced in stage at diagnosis. Regardless of their anatomic origins, metastatic foci of small cell neuroendocrine carcinoma (SCNC) are typically characterized radiographically by multiple intrapulmonaory masses; mediastinal involvement is often lacking when the tumor has arisen outside the lungs. The morphologic features of these lesions include granular dispersed nuclear chromatin, nuclear fragility, nuclear molding, and cellular clumping. Those attributes are generally associated with neuroendocrine differentiation. Immunopathologically, SCNCs often demonstrate a

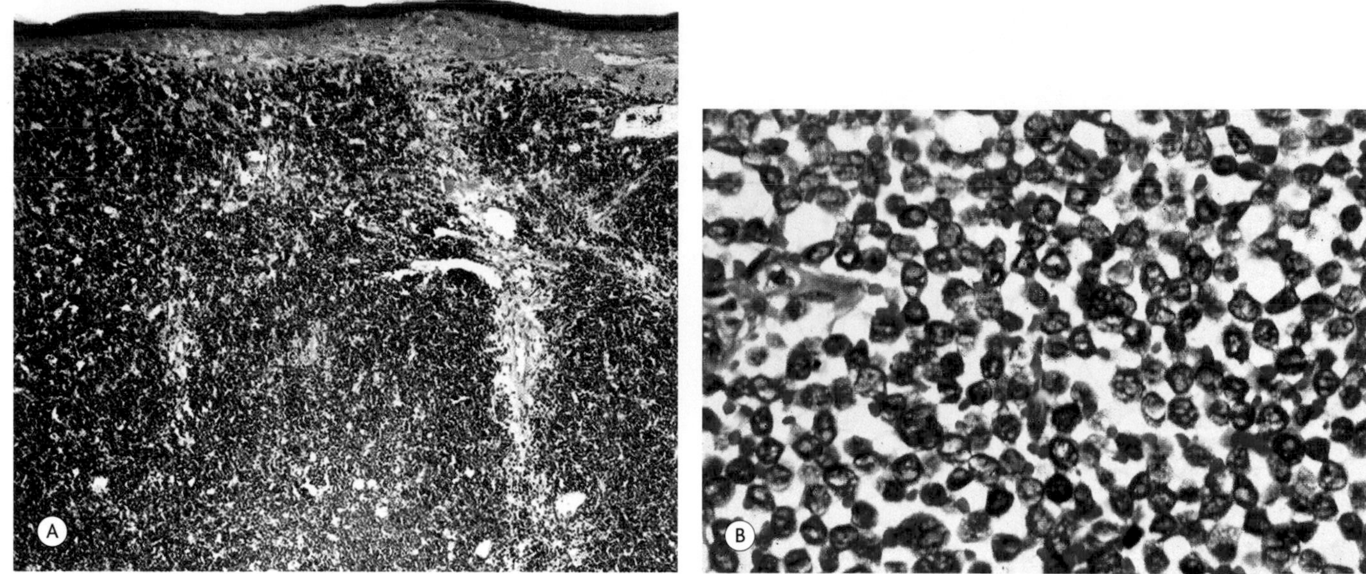

Fig. 17.47 (A,B) The primary tumor of the skin is shown here, corresponding to the lesion depicted in Fig. 17.46.

characteristic reactivity pattern for keratin, with dot-like perinuclear labeling. They may or may not show additional positivity for synaptophysin, chromogranin-A, CD56, CD57, and neuron-specific enolase. Byrd-Gloster et al. also reported that 97% of SCNCLs were reactive for thyroid transcription factor-1 (TTF1), whereas most (but not all) SCNCs of non-pulmonary derivation lacked that marker.[172] On the other hand, cytokeratin 20 positivity is potentially seen in primary extrathoracic SCNCs but it is uncommon in primary pulmonary small cell carcinoma.[173,174] SCNC of the lung and other sites may also contain a non-small cell component (so-called "composite" or "combined" SCNCL; see Chapter 13).

Metastatic well- or moderately-differentiated neuroendocrine carcinomas in the lung include "carcinoids" of gastrointestinal, uterine cervical, or other topographic derivations; neuroendocrine pancreatic tumors; and medullary thyroid carcinomas (Fig. 17.48).[175,176] Many of those tumors are associated with specific symptoms, owing to their production of various neuropeptides or amines. However, in histologic or cytologic specimens, such lesions are potentially identical to primary neuroendocrine neoplasms of the lung. Data on discriminating immunostains are still in evolution for this group of tumors, but TTF1-reactivity again may favor a pulmonary origin.[176a]

Primary pulmonary lymphomas are discussed in Chapter 15, but most malignant lymphoid tumors of the lung represent secondary lesions that occur in the context of systemic dissemination. Primary malignant lymphomas in this organ are typically low grade, whereas secondary hematolymphoid malignancies may represent any histologic subtype and grade. For example, 30% of patients with mediastinal Hodgkin's lymphoma will have lung involvement by direct extension.[177] It is felt that malignant lymphomas that secondarily affect the pulmonary parenchyma are not truly metastatic, because they populate lymphoid structures that are normally present in the lungs and pleura. One form of lymphomatous involvement is characterized by diffuse interstitial lymphocytic permeation, with focal formation of micronodules (Fig. 17.49).[178,179] When the constituent cells are relatively mature, the image of "lymphocytic interstitial pneumonia" may be obtained (see Chapters 7, 15). However, discrete nodules also may occur, especially with high-grade large cell neoplasms (Fig. 17.50), and these commonly simulate metastatic non-hematopoietic lesions on clinical and pathologic levels. Involvement of the pleura may be unilateral or bilateral in malignant lymphoma, but lymphoma and metastatic carcinoma are the two most common causes of malignant bilateral pleural effusion.[38] In cytological practice, it is difficult to be certain that effusion specimens containing atypical lymphoid cells are definitively positive for lymphoma; such cells may represent contamination of the sample by lymphocytes from the peripheral blood, and, especially when they are relatively mature, discrimination from

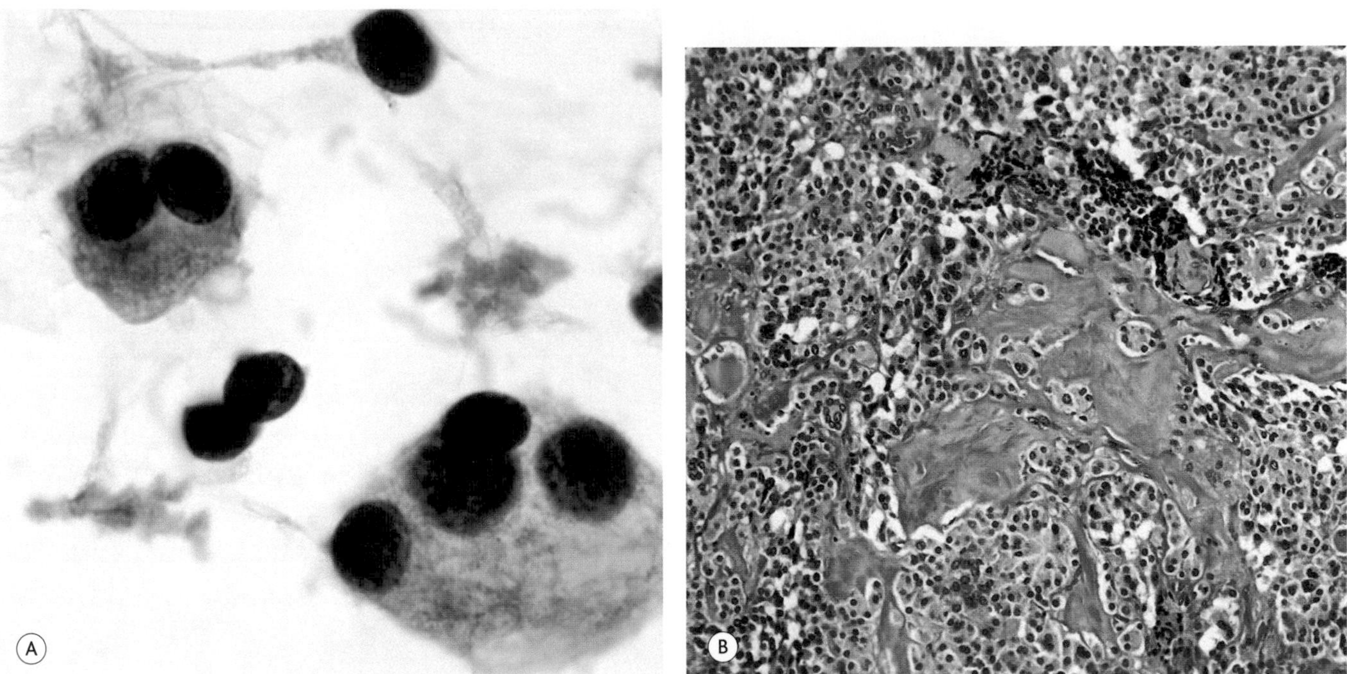

Fig. 17.48 (A) Multinucleated and plasmacytoid mononuclear tumor cells are present in this fine-needle aspirate of metastatic medullary thyroid carcinoma involving the lung. (B) The primary tumor is demonstrated here, showing an organoid growth pattern and production of stromal amyloid.

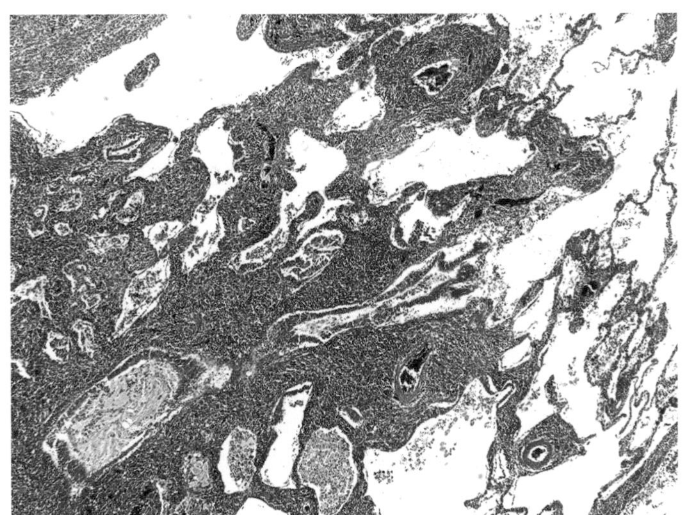

Fig. 17.49 Micronodular arrays of small lymphocytes are present in the pulmonary interstitium in this example of mucosal-type lymphoma involving the lungs.

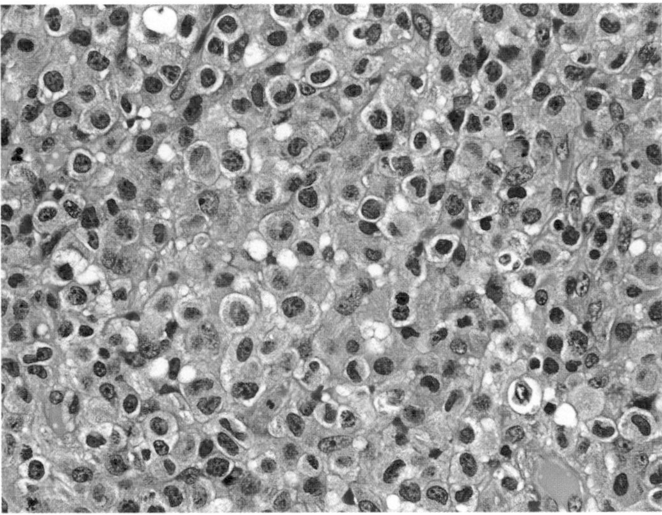

Fig. 17.50 Nodules of anaplastic polygonal cells are seen in this case of large cell non-Hodgkin's lymphoma involving the lungs.

other causes of lymphoid pleural effusion depends mainly on adjunctive studies.[180] Flow cytometry is probably optimally suited for this application.[181]

In the pediatric age group, a number of small round cell malignancies may metastasize to the lungs, as cited earlier (Fig. 17.51). Immunohistochemical studies and electron microscopy are helpful in separating among these lesions in difficult cases,[170] and cytogenetic analyses may also be valuable. Table 17.5 shows the immunopathological profile of several primary and secondary small round cell tumors.[170]

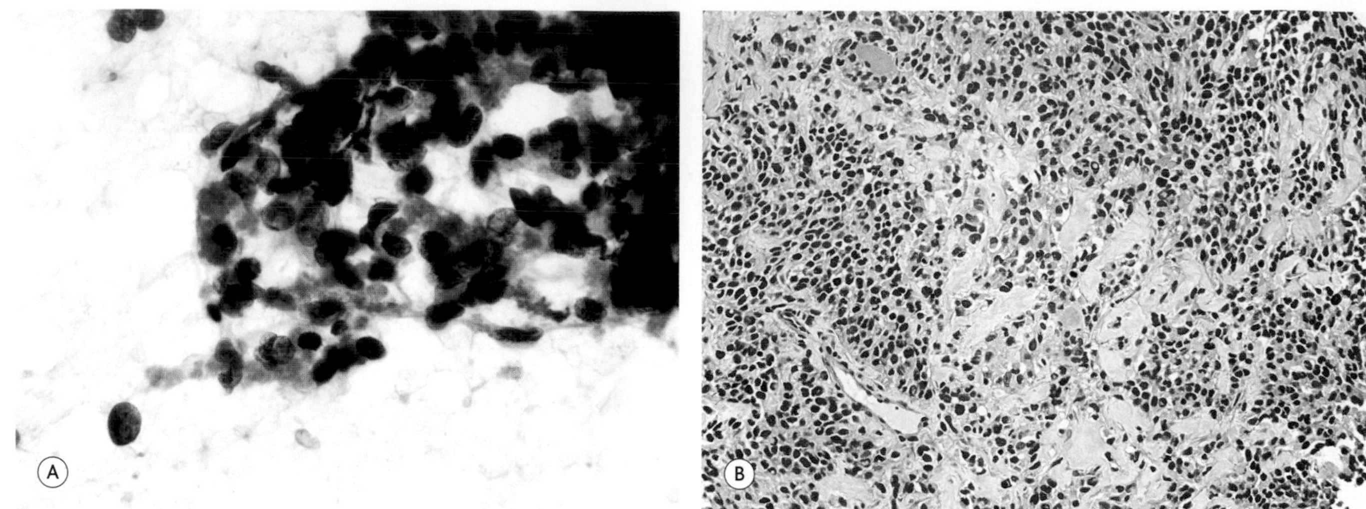

Fig. 17.51 (A,B) Metastatic alveolar rhabdomyosarcoma in the lung in a child. The tumor is composed of sheets of small round undifferentiated cells. (A = Fine needle aspirate)

Table 17.5 Immunohistological differential diagnosis of small round cell malignancies in the lung

	Antibodies								
Tumor	VIM	PK	S100	TTF1	CD45	CD56	DES	SYN	CD99
Small cell NE carcinoma	N	P	N	P	N	PN	N	PN	PN
Rhabdomyosarcoma	P	N	N	N	N	N	P	N	PN
Non-Hodgkin's lymphoma	P	N	N	N	P	N	N	N	N
Malignant melanoma	P	N	P	N	N	N	N	N	N
Ewing's sarcoma/PNET	PN	N	N	N	N	PN	N	PN	P
Metastatic NE carcinomas	N	P	N	PN	N	PN	N	PN	PN
Metastatic neuroblastoma	PN	N	N	N	N	P	N	P	N

NE = neuroendocrine; VIM = vimentin; PK = pan-keratin; S100 = S100 protein; TTF1 = thyroid transcription factor-1; DES = desmin; SYN = synaptophysin; P = positive (>80% of cases); PN = variably positive (between 10% and 80% of cases); N = negative (< 10% of cases).

Squamous cell carcinomas and morphologic simulants

The differential diagnosis of primary squamous cell carcinomas of the lung obviously includes secondary carcinomas with squamous differentiation, as well as other epithelioid malignancies that have "metaplastic" or "hard" eosinophilic cytoplasm. Some examples of such lesions are represented by transitional cell carcinoma and selected cases of malignant melanoma.

Based on morphology alone, the site of origin for squamous cell carcinoma (SCC) is impossible to determine (Figs 17.52 and 17.53). Most squamous carcinomas in the lung have arisen there, and, although the presence of multifocal SCCs suggests metastatic disease, that picture can also be observed with multiple primary synchronous bronchogenic carcinomas. The usual sources of metastastic SCC in the lung are mucosal sites of the head and neck, the esophagus, the uterine cervix, and the skin.

Squamous cell carcinomas from the head and neck that involve the lungs may originate in the larynx, nasopharynx, oropharynx, or hypopharynx, and lesions in the lungs may be single or multiple.[82,182,183] Because all of these tumors are associated with the use of alcohol and/or tobacco and/or infection with the human papillomavirus, patients with squamous carcinoma in one of the specified locations also commonly develop separate metachronous or synchronous primary squamous malignancies in other mucosal sites or in the lungs.[184] Among those patients with both pulmonary lesions and SCC in the head and/or neck, Malfetto et al. reported that 53% had separate primary bronchogenic carcinomas and

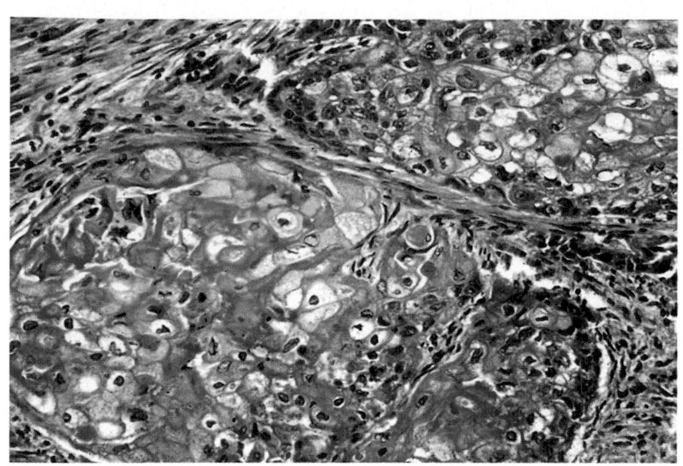

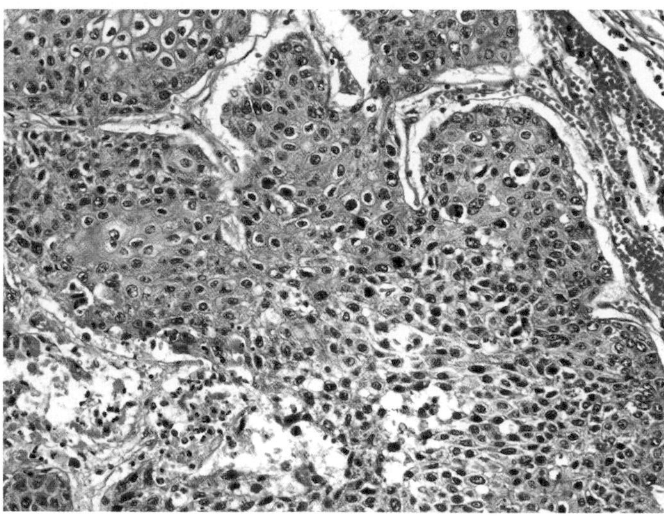

Fig. 17.52, 17.53 Metastatic well-differentiated (Fig. 17.52) and moderately differentiated (Fig. 17.53) squamous cell carcinoma of the head and neck, involving the lungs. Tumors such as these cannot be distinguished reliably from primary squamous pulmonary carcinomas.

19% had metastatic SCC in the lung.[184] Cervical lymph nodal involvement is also present in up to 80% of cases of metastatic intrapulmonary SCC.[82,83] The cumulative incidence of second malignancies in patients who have SCC of the head and neck is approximately 4% per year, and 30% of those tumors arise in the lungs.[185]

Sostman and Matthay reported that uterine cervical squamous cell carcinomas spread to the lungs less frequently (4%) than cervical adenocarcinomas do (20%).[186] In most instances, single or multiple lesions are present, and, as true of all squamous cell carcinomas, there is a tendency toward cavitation in the tumors.[187,188] Metastatic cervical SCC also may involve pulmonary hilar or mediastinal lymph nodes, endobronchial mucosal sites,[189,190] or the intrapulmonary lymphatics.[28,191]

Metastatic malignant melanoma has a myriad of histologic and cytologic appearances, and consequently, it may rightly be considered in the differential diagnosis with selected adenocarcinomas, malignant small round cell tumors, spindle cell neoplasms, large polygonal cell malignancies, and some squamous cell carcinomas. The appearance of single cells with "metaplastic" cytoplasm, large ovoid nuclei, and prominent nucleoli is common in the cytologic evaluation of malignant melanoma (Figs 17.54 and 17.55). Melanin production is a helpful clue to the identity of that tumor (Fig. 17.56), but it may be confused with other pigments such as hemosiderin, and requires histochemical verification. A history of prior ocular, cutaneous, or mucosal melanoma is often known when that neoplasm involves the lungs metastatically. However, some metastatic melanomas represent the initial signs of that tumor. Virtually all examples of melanoma in the lungs and pleura are metastatic; only anecdotal examples of putatively primary pulmonary malignancies with melanocytic differentiation have been documented.[191a] Metastatic melanomas usually involve multiple organs, but DasGupta and Brasfield found that the lungs were involved in 70% of such cases.[192] The secondary lesions are usually represented by multiple intrapulmonary nodules, but solitary lesions, lymphangitic or miliary disease, or endobronchial implants may also be seen.[193–196] Balch et al. reported that a solitary pulmonary mass was the first evidence of metastatic disease in 38% of cases.[197] Conversely, Pogrebniak and colleagues found that 33% of lung

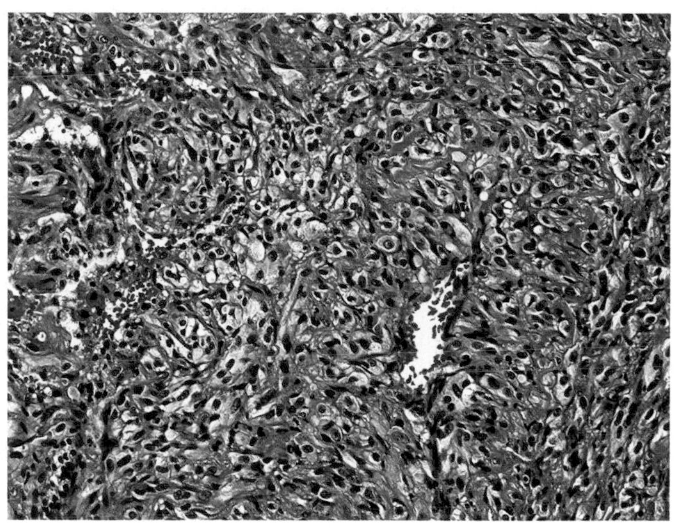

Fig. 17.54 Metastatic malignant melanoma in the lung parenchyma. The tumor is composed of large anaplastic polyhedral cells; melanin pigment is scarce.

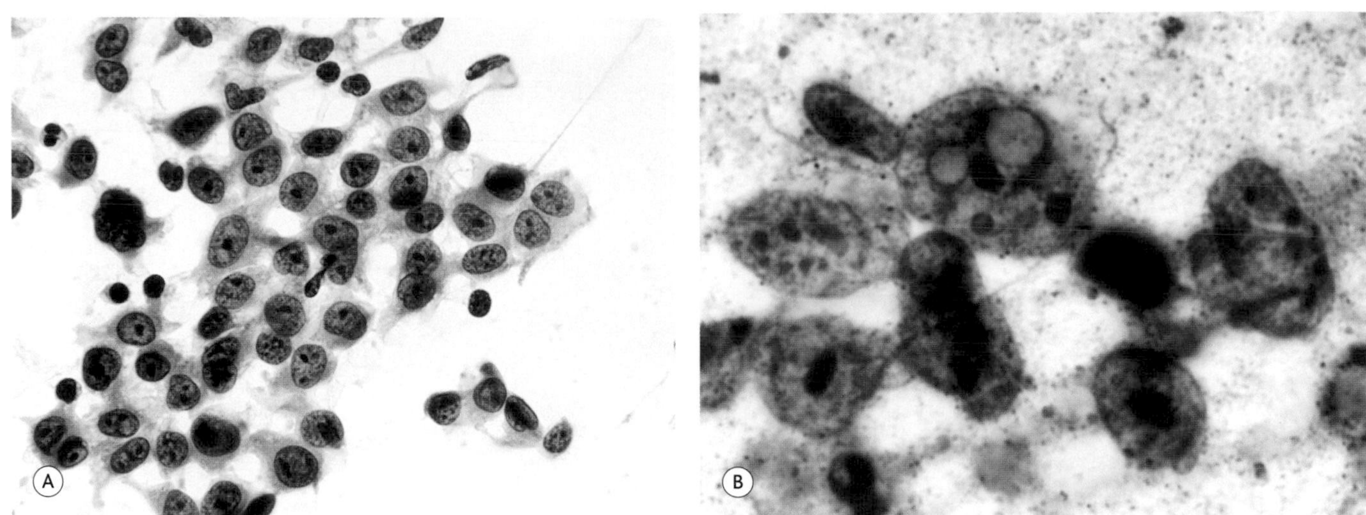

Fig. 17.55 (A) Fine-needle aspiration biopsy of metastatic melanoma, showing dyshesive tumor cells with high nucleocytoplasmic ratios. (B) Some of the neoplastic cells contain intranuclear invaginations of cytoplasm.

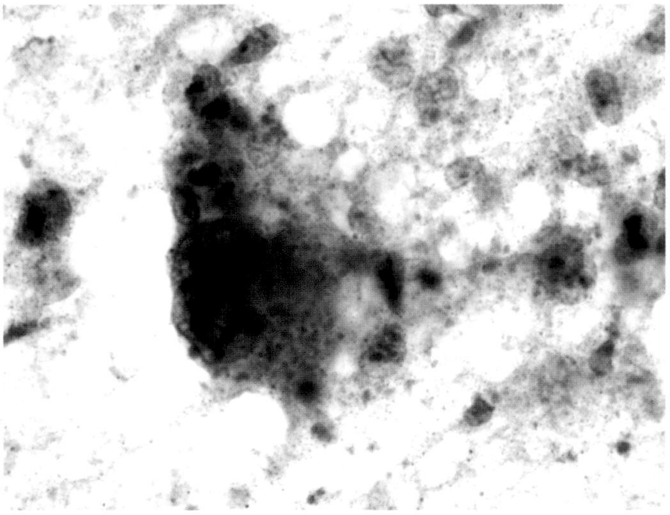

Fig. 17.56 Melanin pigment is seen in this fine-needle aspirate of metastatic melanoma.

Table 17.6 Immunohistologic differential diagnosis of squamous cell carcinomas and their potential simulators

	Antibody			
Tumor	**TBM**	**CK 5/6 or P63**	**S100**	**EMA**
Squamous cell carcinoma of lung	PN	P	N	PN
Squamous cell carcinoma of cervix	PN	P	N	PN
Squamous cell carcinoma of head and neck	PN	P	N	PN
Squamous cell carcinoma of esophagus	PN	P	N	PN
Melanoma	N	N	P	N
Transitional cell carcinoma	P	P	N	P
"Squamoid" hepatocellular carcinoma	N	N	N	N

TBM = thrombomodulin; CK 5/6 = cytokeratin 5/6; S100 = S100 protein; EMA = epithelial membrane antigen; P = positive (>80% of cases); PN = variably positive (between 10% and 80% of cases); N = negative (< 10% of cases).

nodules in patients with melanoma were unrelated and benign.[198]

Metastatic transitional cell carcinomas (TCCs) of the urinary tract often have a squamoid cytoplasmic appearance, and true squamous differentiation may be seen as well in those neoplasms. Cytologic specimens of such lesions show extensive cellular dyshesion and necrosis. Some authors have reported that cercariform cells – containing nucleated globular bodies and bulbous cytoplasmic processes – are suggestive of metastatic TCC.[98,199] These tumors often form mass lesions in the lungs and have also been known to spread lymphangitically.

Table 17.6 shows the immunopathologic profile of squamous cell carcinomas, based on their sites of origin; the immunophenotypes of their morphologic mimics are also included. If metastatic malignant melanoma is in the differential diagnosis, it can be easily characterized by its reactivity for S100 protein, HMB-45, MART-1, and tyrosinase.[200] Transitional cell carcinomas may label for cytokeratin 20 but are negative for cytokeratin 7 in most cases; this profile is the opposite of that seen in primary pulmonary adenocarcinoma.[138–141] Thrombomodulin (TBM; CD141) is potentially shared by both of the latter tumors, but it is more commonly present in TCC; similarly, p63 protein is present in TCC but not adenocarcinoma. Squamous carcinomas of all sites share with TCC the potential for TBM and p63 reactivity.

Undifferentiated large polygonal cell malignancies

Large polygonal cell undifferentiated tumors of the lung include primary large cell carcinomas, malignant lymphomas, metastatic malignant melanoma, metastatic germ cell tumors, metastatic "histiocytoid" malignant fibrous histiocytoma, metastatic epithelioid sarcoma, metastatic alveolar soft parts sarcoma, metastatic adrenocortical carcinoma, and other secondary carcinomas and sarcomas. The diagnostic difficulty attending this group lies in the fact that such tumors have an anaplastic appearance that often defies a determination of basic lineage.

Ultrastructural studies have shown that primary large cell carcinomas of the lung often exhibit squamous or glandular differentiation; indeed, these features may be demonstrated focally in histologic or cytologic preparations. As their name implies, the cells that comprise these tumors contain a relatively large amount of cytoplasm and correspondingly large nuclei. In cytologic specimens, some large cell carcinomas show significant cellular dyshesion (Fig. 17.57). Clinically, they are often bulky masses that are associated with mediastinal lymphadenopathy. Primary large cell carcinomas of the lung have an immunopathologic profile which is similar to that of other primary non-small cell carcinomas.

Many of the other neoplasms in the differential diagnosis have been discussed previously. Sarcomas that imitate primary large cell carcinomas have an epithelioid appearance, but, except for the pathologic *entities* known as epithelioid sarcoma and epithelioid synovial sarcoma, they are non-reactive for keratin immunohistochemically. Moreover, it is unusual for mesenchymal malignancies to *present* with pulmonary metastases, with the possible exceptions of alveolar soft parts sarcoma and selected examples of malignant fibrous histiocytoma. The primary foci of those tumors may indeed be occult and yet produce extensive distant disease in the lungs, brain, and other organs.[200ab]

Poorly differentiated adrenocortical carcinomas may show lipidized cytoplasm, which is an unusual feature in primary large cell carcinoma. The most common metastatic germ cell malignancies that simulate primary pulmonary large cell carcinoma are embryonal carcinoma (Fig. 17.58) and choriocarcinoma. When these neoplasms metastasize, they are often admixed with other germ cell components such as seminoma or teratoma, features that aid in their separation from other large polygonal cell tumors. The clinical history of patients with secondary germ cell lesions is often distinctive, vis-à-vis that which accompanies primary lung cancers. For example, metastatic choriocarcinomas are most commonly seen in young women,[201] whereas primary large cell carcinomas more often occur in older patients with a significant smoking history.[202] Furthermore, individuals with metastatic choriocarcinoma typically have multiple lung lesions[203] and an elevated level of beta-human chorionic gonadotropin in serum. Secondary embryonal carcinomas are

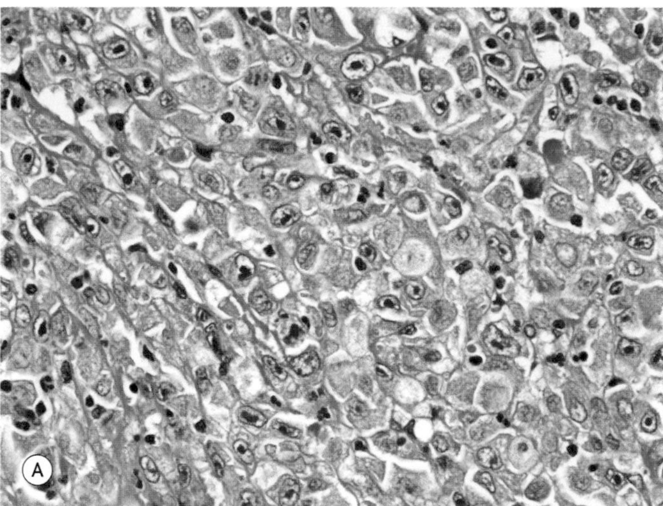

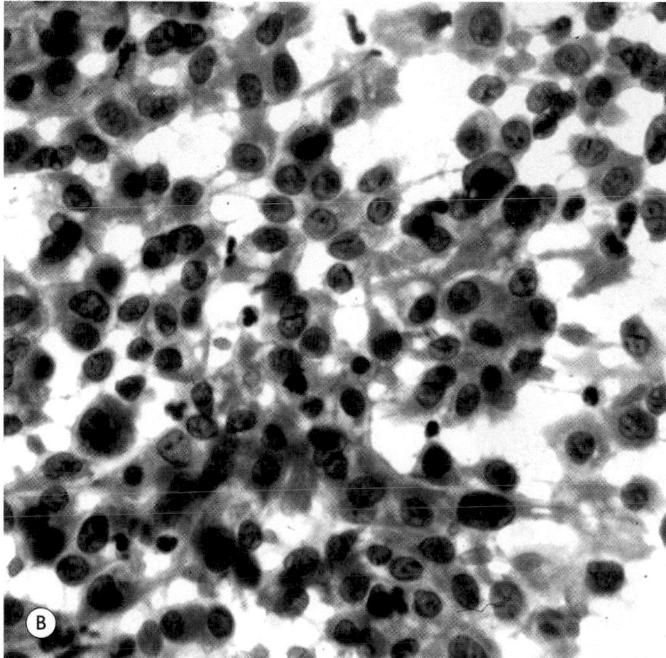

Fig. 17.57 Primary large cell undifferentiated carcinoma of the lung (A), showing sheets of anaplastic tumor cells with no distinguishing characteristics. (B) A fine-needle aspiration specimen in the same case shows no evidence of squamous or glandular differentiation.

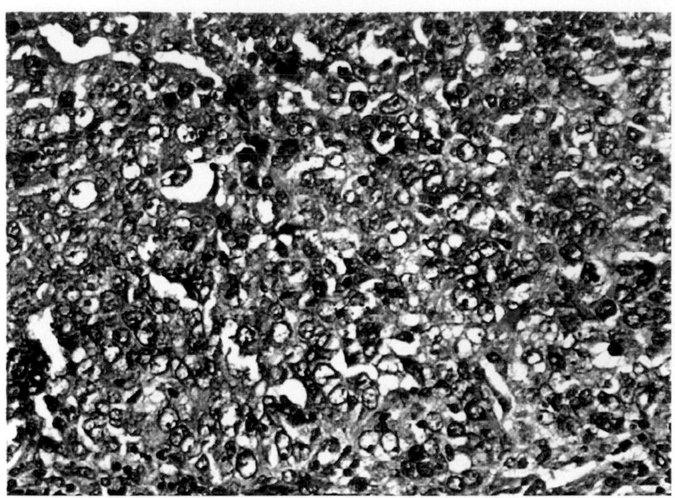

Fig. 17.58 Metastatic "solid" embryonal carcinoma of the testis, involving the lung. The tumor in this case is virtually indistinguishable from that shown in Fig. 17.57.

usually seen in men, who also have gonadal, intracranial, mediastinal, or retroperitoneal masses.

The histologic image of metastatic germ cell tumors is often sufficient for their definitive recognition, especially when it includes two or more morphologic subtypes of such lesions. Moreover, yolk sac tumor commonly demonstrates the presence of distinctive intercellular and intracytoplasmic eosinophilic globules, and choriocarcinoma is singular in its biphasic composition by cytotrophoblastic and syncytiotrophoblastic elements (Fig. 17.59). Nevertheless, the existence of primary somatic carcinomas of the lung with areas resembling germ cell tumor confounds the evaluation of these lesions.[203a]

Table 17.7 presents the immunopathologic profile of specific large polygonal cell tumors. The panel of antibody reagents listed there is particularly helpful in distinguishing primary large cell carcinoma from its diagnostic alternatives. Placental-like alkaline phosphatase is seen in most germ cell tumors, but occasionally is present in primary large cell carcinomas as well;[204] CD117 and CD30 are also selective markers for seminoma and embryonal carcinoma, respectively (Fig. 17.60). Those lesions may be separated from somatic tumors by their differential expression of epithelial membrane antigen (EMA); it is present in primary lung cancers but not in germ cell malignancies.[85,204] CD45 is restricted to large cell lymphoma (Fig. 17.61), MART-1 is limited to melanoma and adrenocortical carcinoma, and, except for epithelioid sarcoma and clear cell sarcoma, metastatic mesenchymal neoplasms are typified by positivity for vimentin but are devoid of keratin and melanocyte-related markers.

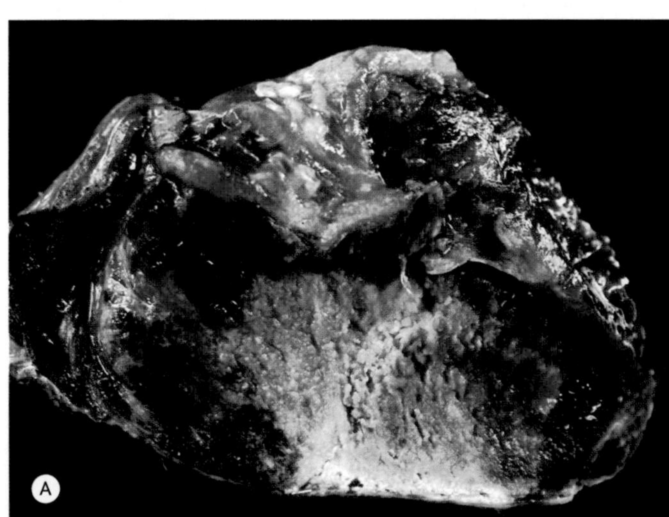

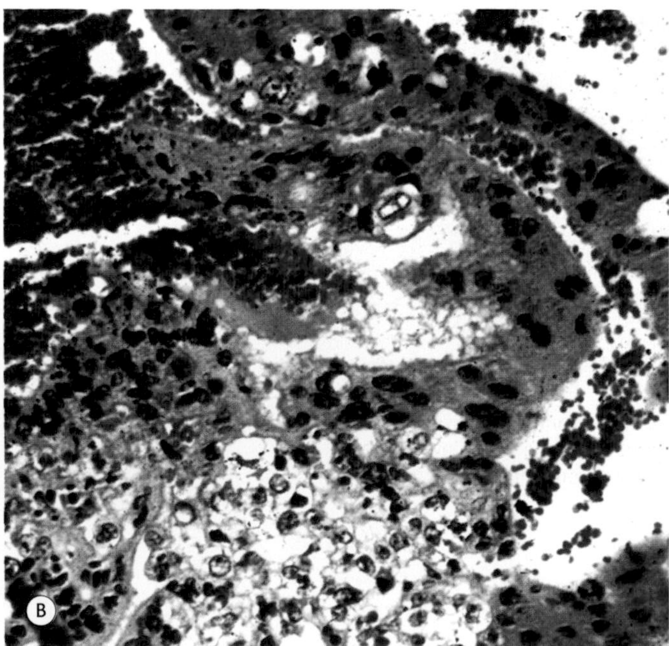

Fig. 17.59 (A) Gross photograph of metastatic choriocarcinoma of the ovary, involving the lung. The tumor nodule is internally hemorrhagic and necrotic. (B) Choriocarcinoma is typified by a juxtaposition of cytotrophoblastic and syncytiotrophoblastic elements.

Table 17.7 Immunohistologic differential diagnosis of large polygonal cell malignancies in the lung

	Antibody						
Tumor	**PK**	**VIM**	**CD45**	**EMA**	**MART**	**S100**	**PLAP**
Primary large-cell carcinoma of lung	P	PN	N	P	N	PN	PN
Met. epithelioid sarcoma	P	P	N	P	PN	N	N
Large-cell lymphoma	N	P	P	N	N	N	N
Met. malignant melanoma	N	P	N	N	P	P	N
Met. embryonal carcinoma	P	PN	N	N	N	N	P
Met. histiocytoid malignant fibrous histiocytoma	N	P	N	N	N	N	N
Met. adrenocortical carcinoma	N	PN	N	N	N	N	N
Met. hepatocellular carcinoma	P	N	N	N	N	N	N
Met. renal cell carcinoma	P	PN	N	P	N	N	N

Met. = metastatic; PK = pan-keratin; EMA = epithelial membrane antigen; MART = MART-1; VIM = vimentin; S100 = S100 protein; PLAP = placental-like alkaline phosphatase; P = positive (>80% of cases); PN = variably positive (between 10% and 80% of cases); N = negative (<10% of cases).

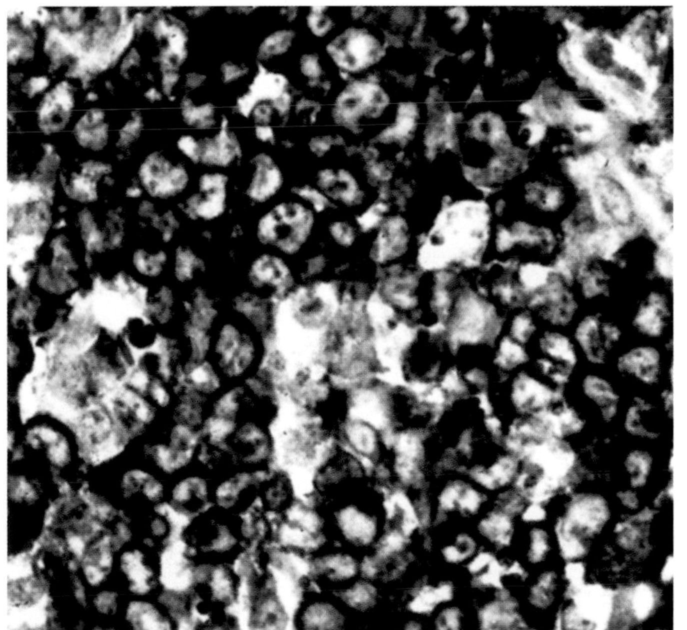

Fig. 17.60 Immunoreactivity for CD30 in metastatic embryonal carcinoma of the testis, involving the lung. This marker is not expected in primary pulmonary tumors.

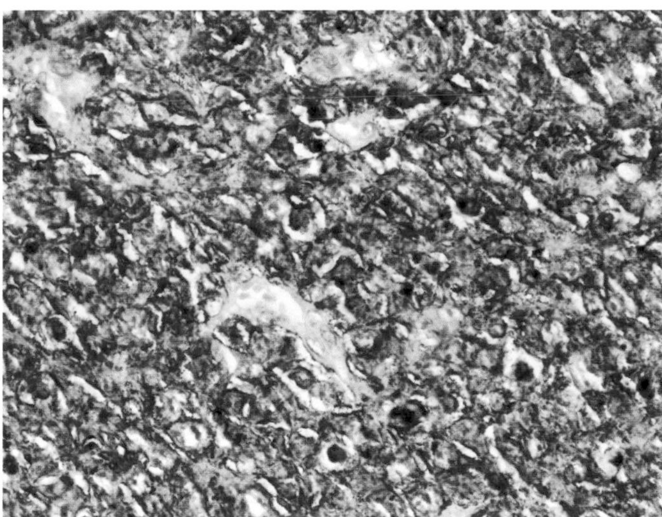

Fig. 17.61 Immunoreactivity for CD45 – a marker that is restricted to hematopoietic proliferations – in large cell non-Hodgkin's lymphoma involving the lung.

Other adjunctive pathologic techniques for the diagnosis of metastatic carcinoma

Although electron microscopy has been used progressively less in recent years in the diagnosis of tumors in surgical pathology, it still has considerable value in that context. In particular, there are several settings in the evaluation of possibly metastatic tumors in the lung where ultrastructural studies are useful.[205–215] Adenocarcinomas – including those arising in the pulmonary parenchyma – are characterized generically by the presence of short, non-branched plasmalemmal microvilli with a length-to-diameter ratio (LDR) of <10:1 (Figs 17.62 and 17.63).[216–218] Specialized features of specific lesions in that category include the presence of laminated cytoplasmic granules (primitive surfactant bodies) in some examples of primary adenocarcinoma of the lung (Fig. 17.64); cytoplasmic mucin granules and "terminal webs" of intermediate filaments that insert into the microvilli in adenocarcinomas with enteric differentiation (Fig. 17.65); glycogen pools and lipid droplets in metastatic renal cell carcinomas (Fig. 17.66); and tubular cristae in the mitochondria of steroid-producing tumors such as adrenocortical carcinoma (Fig. 17.67).[208,209,213,214] Malignant mesothelioma, a simulant of adenocarcinoma at a light microscopic level, is typified by elongated, bushy, branching microvilli with an LDR of >10:1, together with complex desmosomal complexes and cytoplasmic tonofilaments (Figs 17.68 and 17.69).[216–218] Mucin granules and surfactant bodies are absent in that tumor type.

Neuroendocrine carcinomas may be identified with certainty because of their synthesis of dense-core (neurosecretory) granules measuring 150–400 nm in diameter.

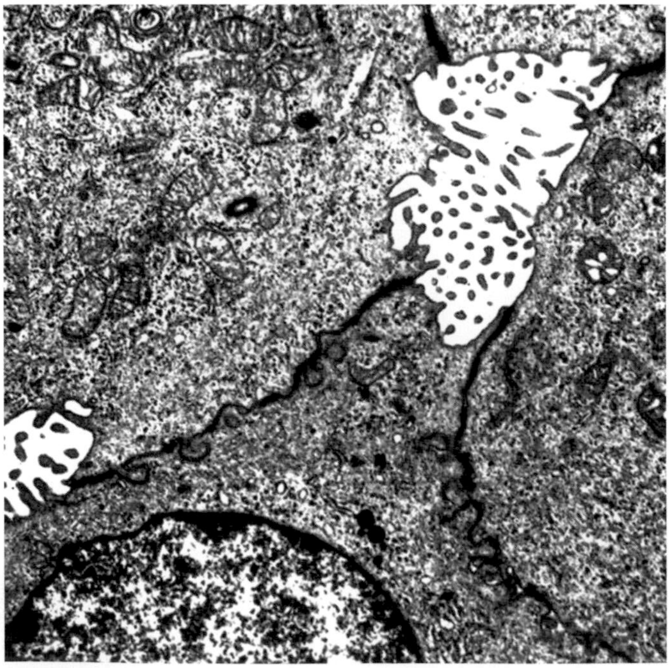

Fig. 17.62 Electron photomicrograph of primary pulmonary adenocarcinoma, showing prominent intercellular junctions bordering a tumor gland microlumen. Short non-branching plasmalemmal microvilli are also apparent.

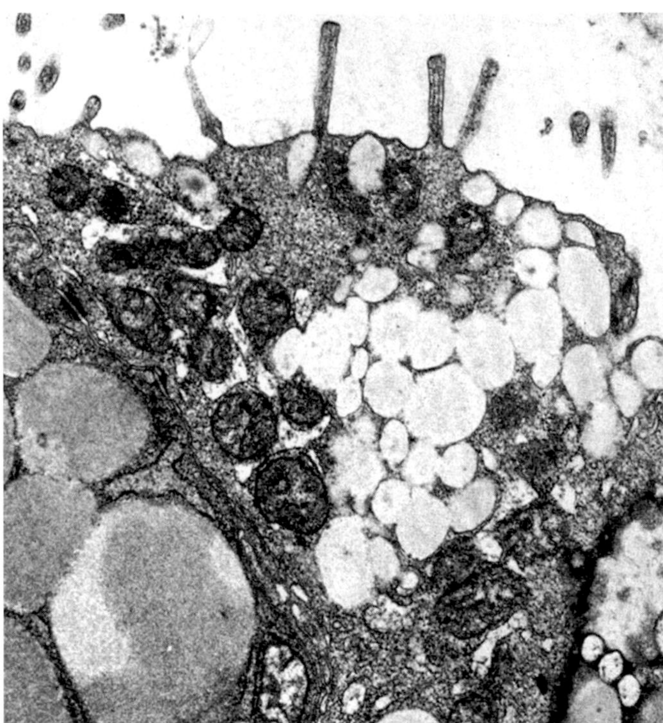

Fig. 17.63 Short cell surface microvilli and cytoplasmic mucin granules are apparent in this metastatic adenocarcinoma with mucinous features, arising in the breast.

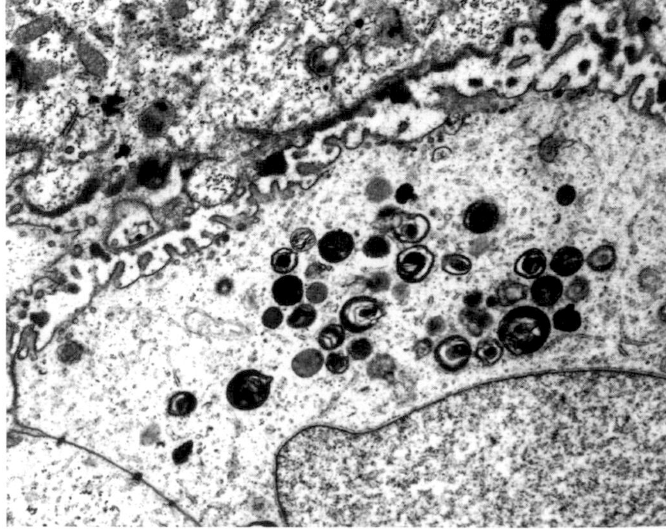

Fig. 17.64 Lamellated "myelinoid" figures are present in the cytoplasm of the tumor cells in this primary pulmonary adenocarcinoma. It is thought that such structures may represent primitive surfactant bodies.

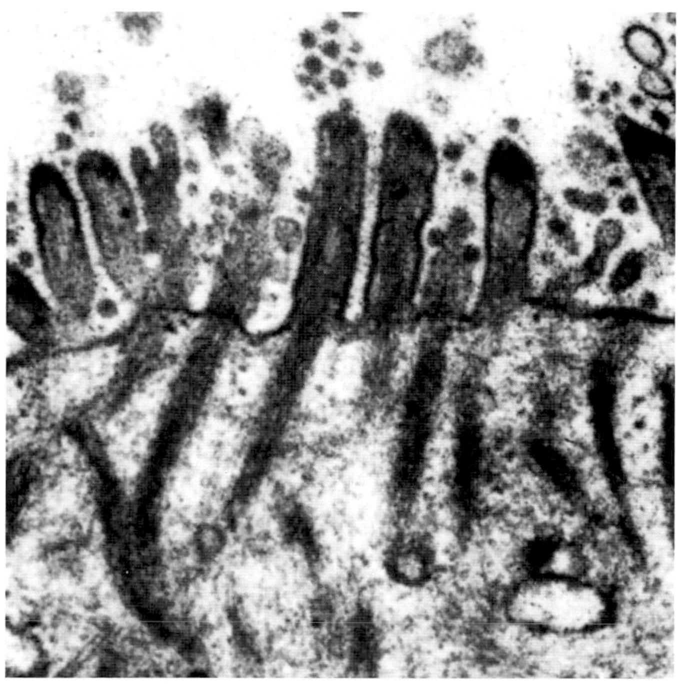

Fig. 17.65 A "terminal web" of thin filaments inserts into plasmalemmal microvilli in the tumor cells of this metastatic colonic adenocarcinoma. This structure is highly suggestive of an enteric anatomic origin.

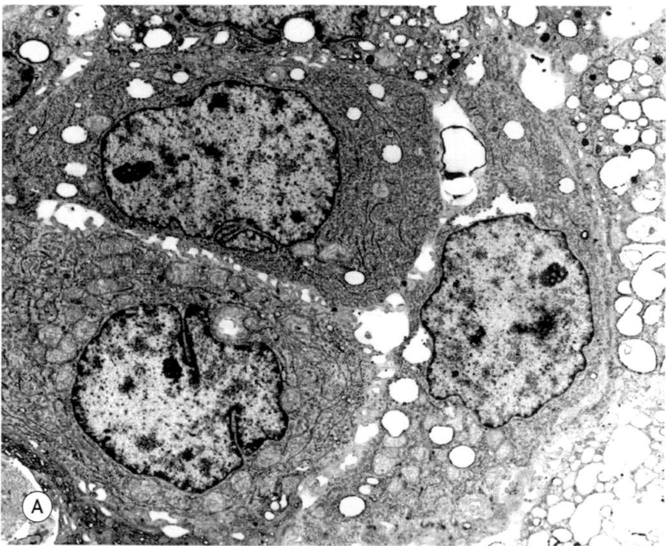

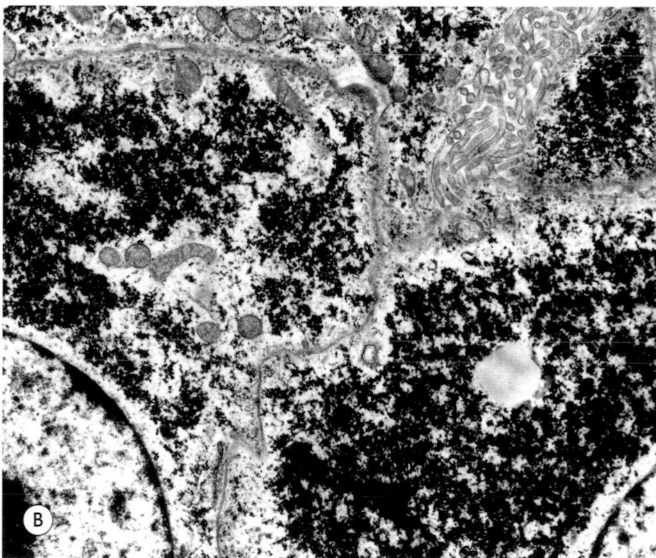

Fig. 17.66 (A) Numerous lipid droplets are present in the tumor cell cytoplasm in this metastatic renal cell carcinoma. (B) Another area of the same tumor demonstrates abundant cytoplasmic glycogen.

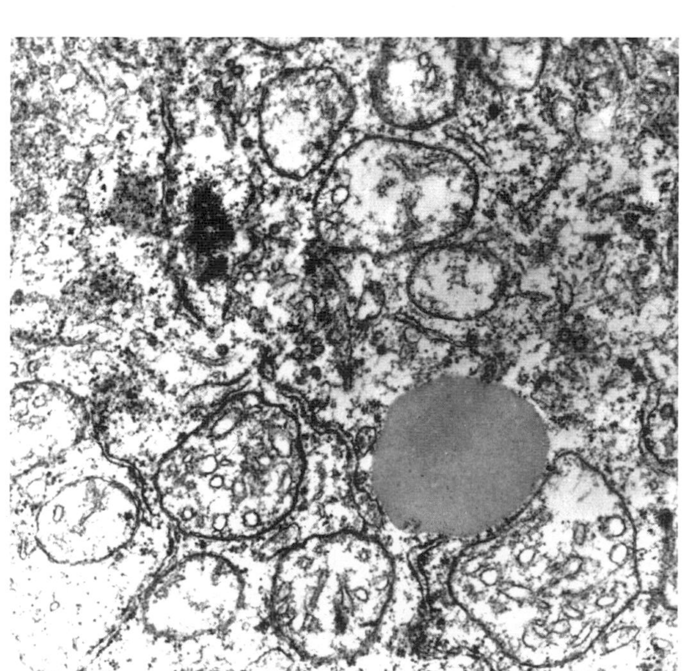

Fig. 17.67 Tubular mitochondrial cristae are seen in this metastatic adrenocortical carcinoma.

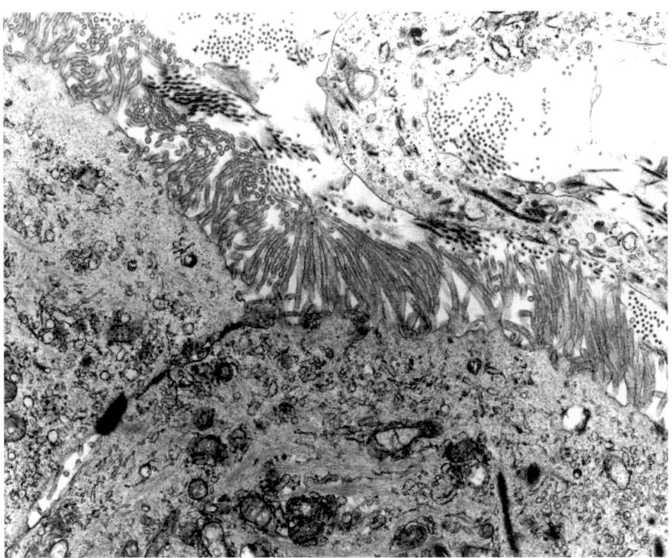

Fig. 17.68 Electron photomicrograph of malignant mesothelioma of the pleura, showing branching, "bushy" cell surface microvilli and elaborate, elongated intercellular junctional complexes.

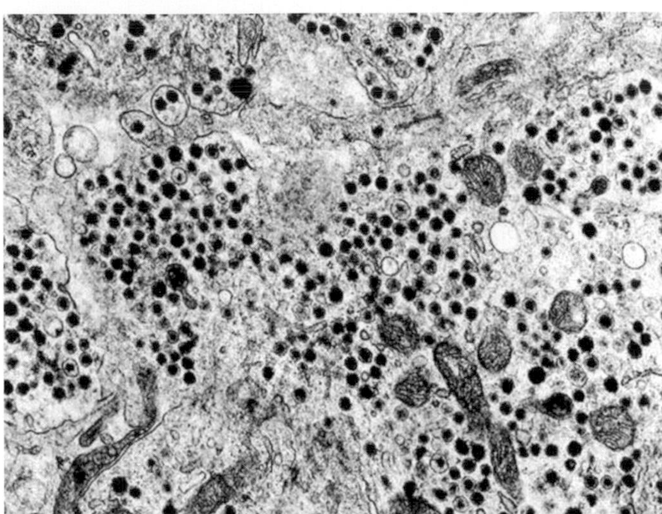

Fig. 17.70 Numerous dense-core neurosecretory granules are dispersed throughout the cytoplasm in this electron photomicrograph of metastatic well-differentiated neuroendocrine carcinoma ("carcinoid") from the ileum, involving the lungs.

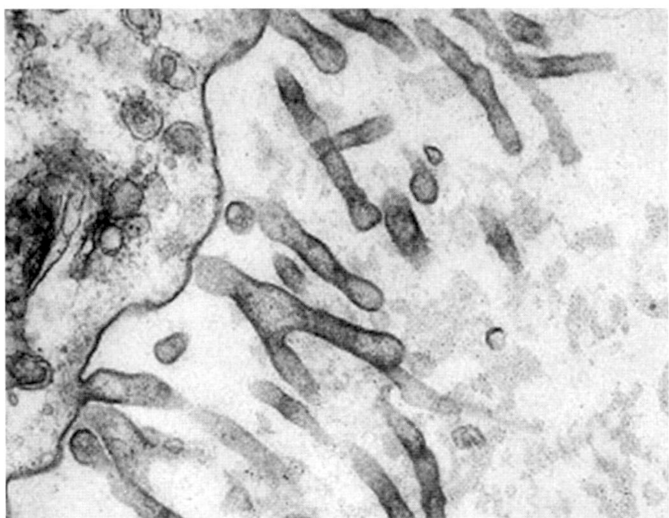

Fig. 17.69 The branching nature of plasmalemmal microvilli in mesothelioma is well-seen in this electron photomicrograph.

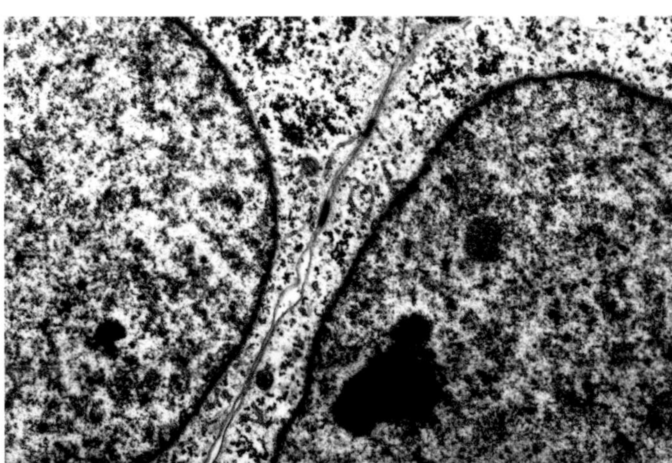

Fig. 17.71 This electron photomicrograph of metastatic seminoma shows complex nucleolar structure, abundant cytoplasmic glycogen, and macular-type intercellular junctions. Cytoplasmic organelles are otherwise rudimentary.

Those inclusions have peripheral zones of lucency and tend to be clustered together in the cytoplasm (Fig. 17.70), often near the Golgi apparatus.[205–208] Macular intercellular junctional complexes are also evident in such lesions, and small whorls of perinuclear intermediate filaments are common. These characteristics are the same regardless of the site of origin of neuroendocrine tumors; hence, electron microscopy cannot be used to distinguish primary pulmonary lesions from metastases.

Germ cell tumors exhibit electron microscopic characteristics that potentially simulate those of somatic carcinomas. Seminomas are undifferentiated at a fine structural level, showing only primitive appositional intercellular junctional complexes, prominent nucleoli, and the usual constituency of basic metabolic organelles (Fig. 17.71). One salient feature of those tumors is the presence of cytoplasmic glycogen pools, but those are shared by many non-germinal tumors as well.[208] Embryonal carcinomas largely resemble somatic adenocarcinomas – including the formation of plasmalemmal microvilli and intercellular gland-like spaces (Fig. 17.72) – and yolk sac tumors share the same potentialities. Choriocarcinomas are indeed relatively distinctive ultrastructurally, in that they demonstrate cytoplasmic

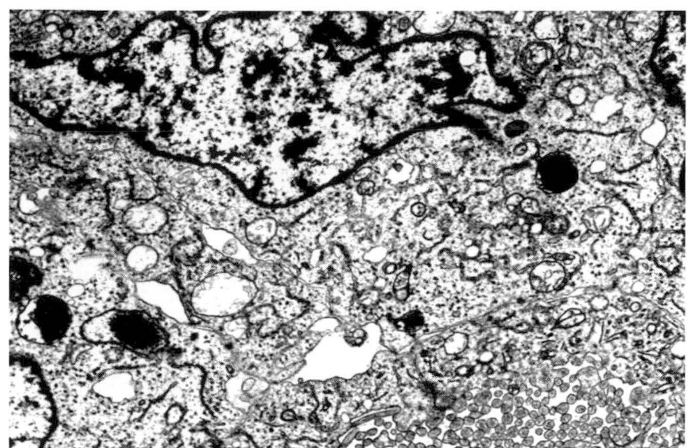

Fig. 17.72 Metastatic embryonal carcinoma of the testis shows the presence of cell surface microvilli (lower right of photograph), simulating the appearance of a somatic adenocarcinoma at a fine structural level.

tonofibrils that are reminiscent of those seen in squamous tumors.[212] The latter lesions are not part of the light microscopic differential diagnosis of choriocarcinomas, and that discrepancy may serve as a clue to the proper interpretation.

Non-epithelial malignancies with specific electron microscopic attributes are represented by rhabdomyosarcoma, leiomyosarcoma, alveolar soft part sarcoma, neuroblastoma, melanoma (and clear cell sarcoma), and endothelial sarcomas.[219] These neoplasms manifest primitive sarcomeric differentiation, with thick and thin cytoplasmic myofilaments (Fig. 17.73); cytoplasmic skeins of thin filaments punctuated by dense bodies; paracrystalline cytoplasmic inclusions (Fig. 17.74); complex interdigitating cytoplasmic extensions containing microtubules (Fig. 17.75); premelanosomes (Fig. 17.76); and Weibel–Palade bodies (Fig. 17.77), respectively. All of those structures are absent in primary pulmonary tumors, except for sarcomatoid carcinomas. Those lesions exhibit a mixture of cells with epithelial characteristics (e.g. intercellular junctions, tonofibrils, microvilli) and others with mesenchymal attributes.

The electron microscopic attributes of other mesenchymal neoplasms are nondescript or even misleading diagnostically. For example, primitive neuroectodermal tumors ([PNETs] and other blastomas such as hepatoblastoma or Wilms' tumor) are composed of primordial round cells joined by macular attachment plaques and often containing only basic organelles (Fig. 17.78).[210,219] In a minority of cases, glycogen deposits or nascent cytoplasmic extensions may be seen, the latter of

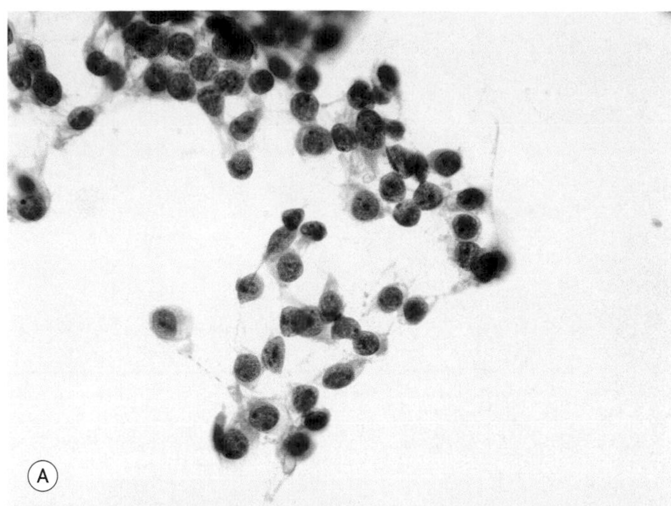

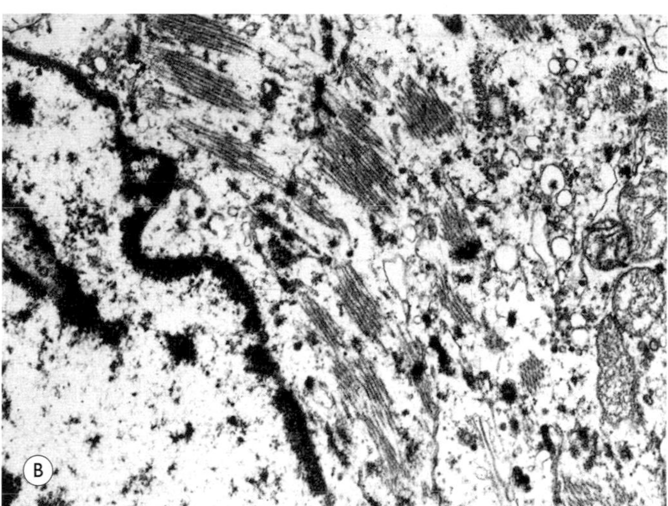

Fig. 17.73 (A) Metastatic embryonal rhabdomyosarcoma in a fine-needle aspirate, showing dyshesive cells with high nucleocytoplasmic ratios and naked nuclei. (B) An electron photomicrograph from a similar case demonstrates the presence of cytoplasmic thin and thick filaments, representing primitive sarcomeric differentiation.

which contain neurosecretory granules or synaptic-type vesicles. Despite the fact that they are soft tissue neoplasms, epithelioid sarcomas and synovial sarcomas mirror their immunohistologic features ultrastructurally, because they manifest the presence of polygonal cells joined by well-formed intercellular attachment plaques (Figs 17.79) and may even demonstrate microvillous differentiation.[219]

Hematopoietic proliferations are perhaps the most primitive at an electron microscopic level. They demonstrate only basic cytoplasmic constituents – often containing abundant dispersed ribosomes, with or without rough endoplasmic reticulum – but lacking other distinguishing features (Fig. 17.80).[214,220]

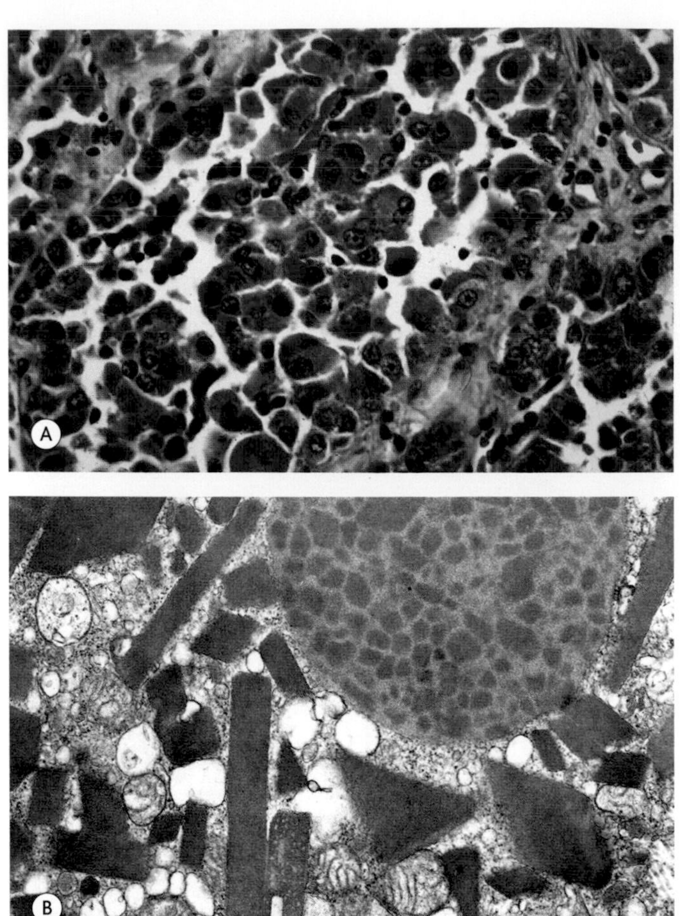

Fig. 17.74 (A) Metastatic alveolar soft part sarcoma, presenting in the lungs in an adolescent boy in the absence of a known soft tissue tumor. (B) An electron photomicrograph of the lesion shows characteristic paracrystalline cytoplasmic inclusions.

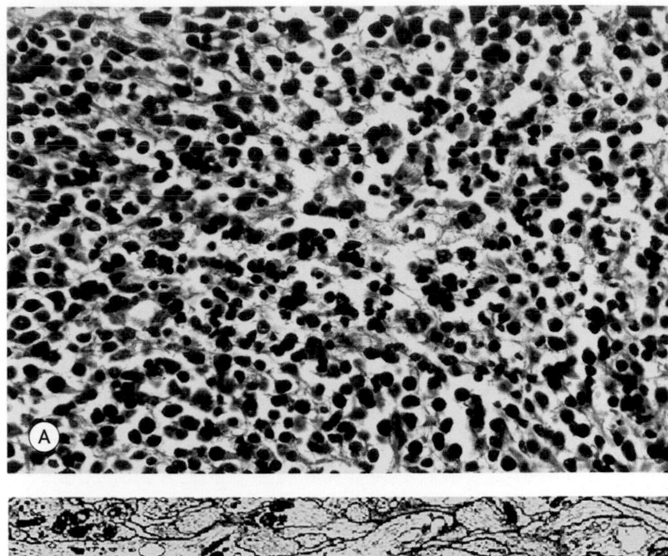

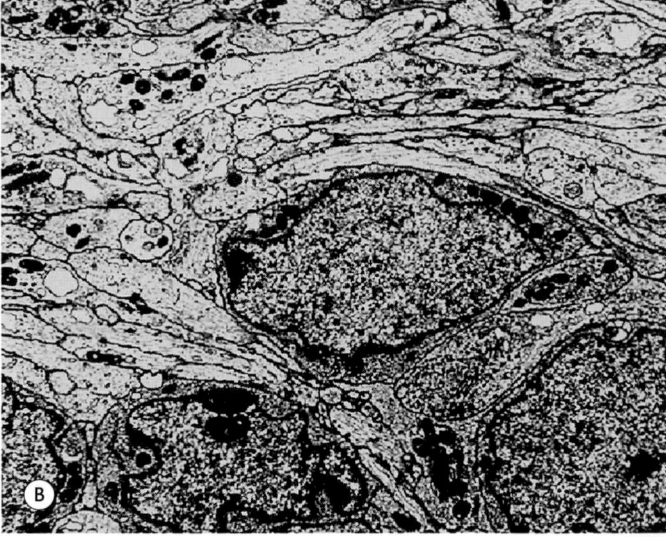

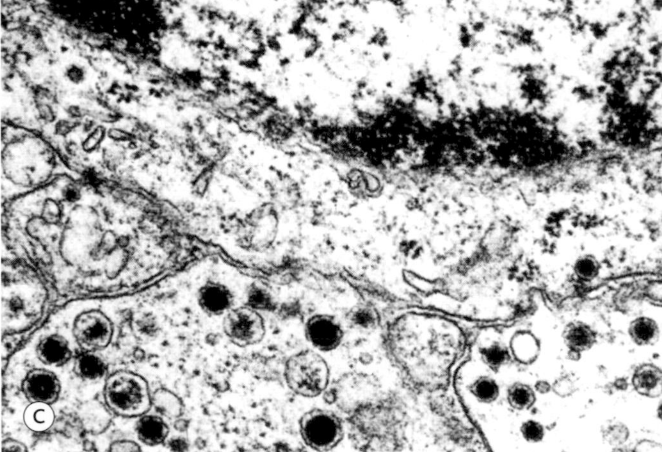

Fig. 17.75 (A) Metastatic neuroblastoma involving the lungs of a child, represented by sheets of small round undifferentiated tumor cells. (B,C) Electron microscopy of the lesion shows interdigitating cytoplasmic processes containing microtubules, as well as dense-core granules.

Cytogenetic information is rapidly accumulating on a variety of tumor types, and it holds the promise of serving as helpful differential diagnostic data in the context being discussed here. For example, several neoplasms have unique chromosomal abnormalities that serve to exclude other possibilities. These include deletions of the short arm of chromosome 3 in renal cell carcinoma; an unrelated deletion in the same chromosomal segment in primary SCNC of the lung; the t(11;22) translocation of PNET/Ewing's sarcoma; t(1;13) or t(2;13) translocations in alveolar rhabdomyosarcoma; the t(12;22) translocation of clear cell sarcoma; the der(17)t(X;17) translocation of alveolar soft part sarcoma; the t(X;18) translocation of synovial sarcoma; isochromosome 12p in germ cell malignancies; and a group of semispecific or specific karyotypic abnormalities in malignant lymphomas and

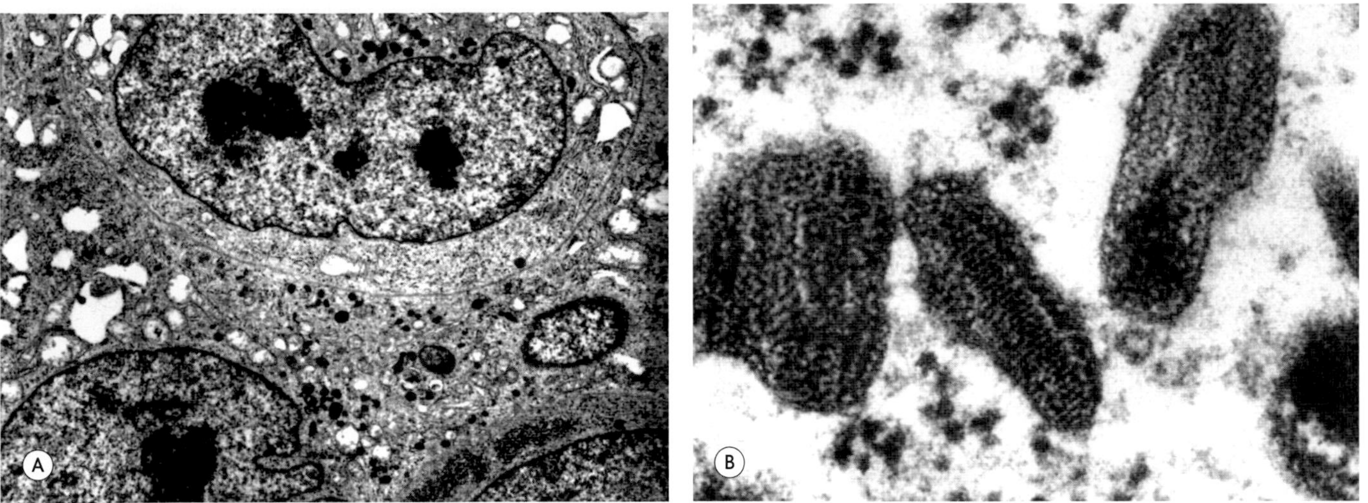

Fig. 17.76 (A) Electron photomicrograph of metastatic melanoma in the lung, showing epithelioid tumor cells joined by primitive appositional plaques. (B) Characteristic premelanosomes were present in the cytoplasm.

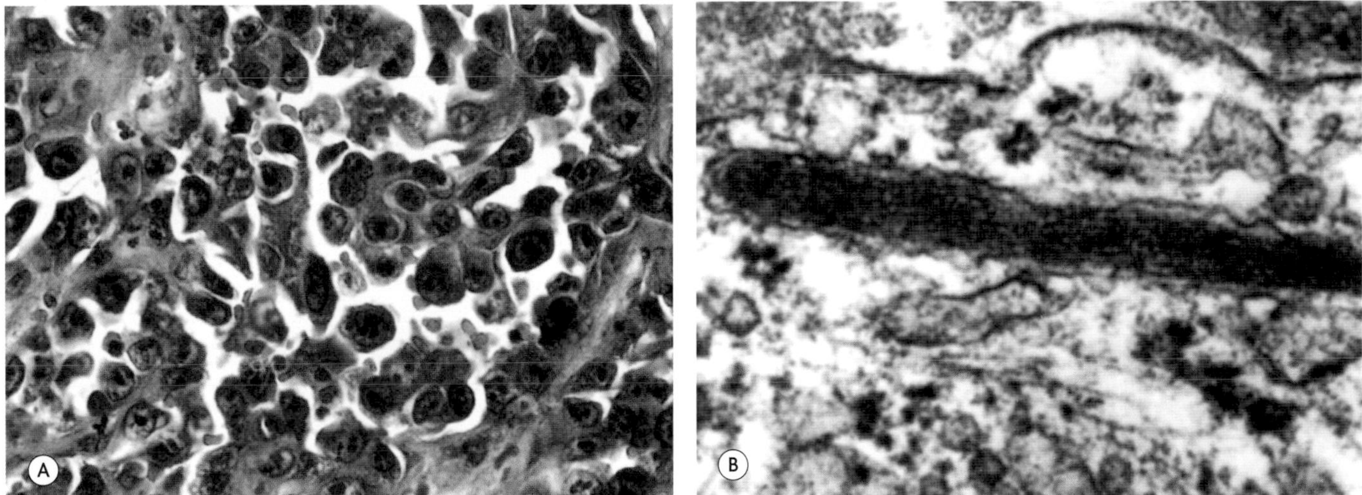

Fig. 17.77 (A) Metastatic epithelioid angiosarcoma in the lung, originating in the scalp in an elderly man. (B) A Weibel–Palade body is present in a tumor cell, marking the proliferation as endothelial in nature.

leukemias.[221–232] These markers are best assessed using fresh tissue, but assays for them that are based on the polymerase chain reaction or fluorescent in-situ hybridization studies are also becoming available for use in hospital practice.

Outcomes analysis

Optimal diagnostic testing strategies, principally pertaining to the *sequence* of tests, are controversial in regard to the assessment of patients with pulmonary lesions that are suspicious for metastases. In countries with available resources, a "definitive" diagnosis is usually based on the pathologic examination of tissue specimens. The methods used to obtain those have been previously discussed, but several factors affect the choice of a subsequent diagnostic testing approach. They include the preferences of patients and physicians; cost; testing characteristics such as sensitivity, specificity, rate, and complexity; and clinical attibutes (e.g. radiological findings, age, and general patient health).

Most decision-related analytic studies that have attempted to determine optimal testing strategies have focused on patients with solitary pulmonary nodules, and the authors generally have assumed that there was no known history of malignancy. In those publications the optimal testing paradigm was also equated with the most cost-effective strategy, meaning that it resulted in

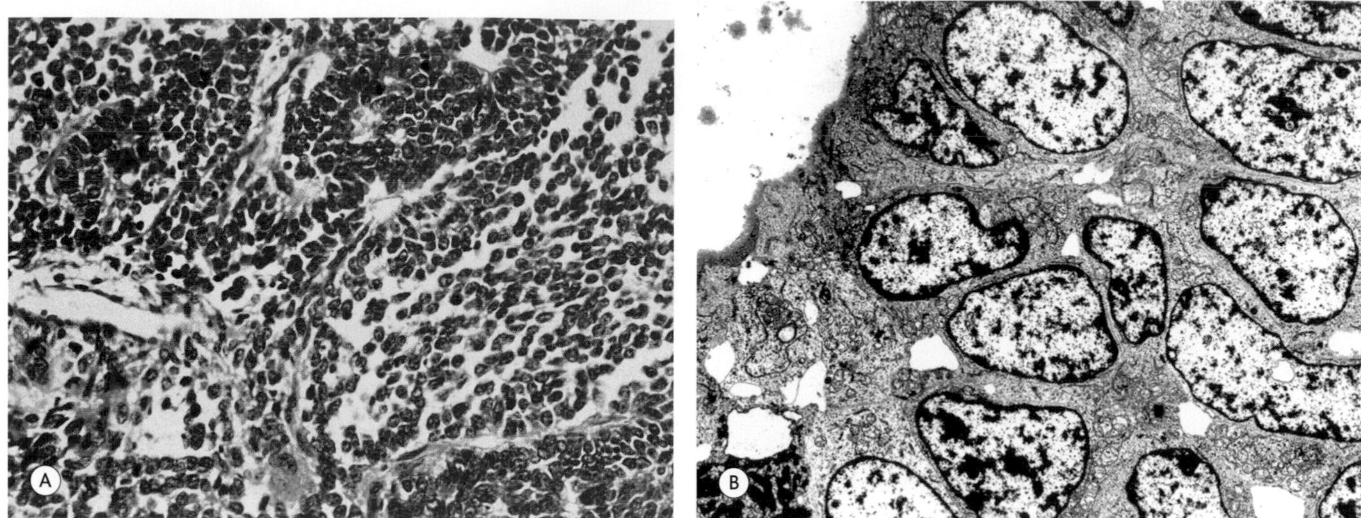

Fig. 17.78 (A) Metastatic Wilms' tumor, showing primitive tubules that punctuate a small round-cell (blastematous) background population of tumor cells. (B) Electron photomicrographs from the same case show a relatively nondescript population of cells that are joined by primitive appositional plaques and surrounded in part by basal lamina.

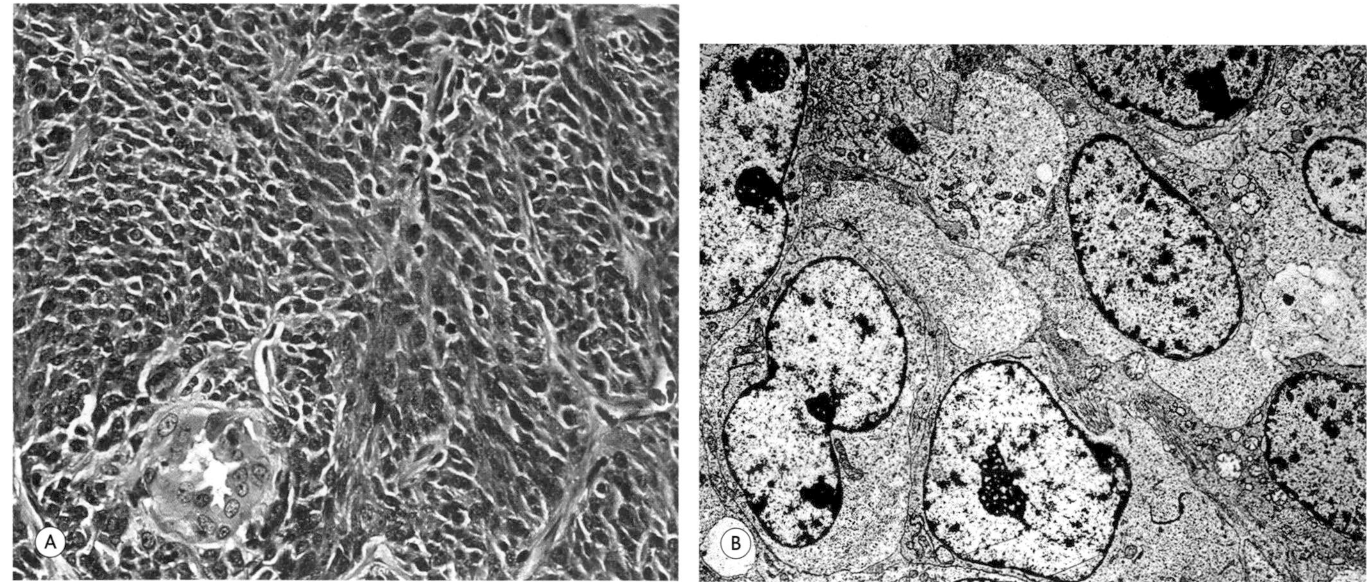

Fig. 17.79 (A) Metastatic synovial sarcoma originating in the soft tissue of the arm, involving the lungs. (B) Electron microscopy of the lesion shows investment of the tumor cells by basal lamina and the presence of intercellular junctions. These ultrastructural features may be misinterpreted as those of a carcinoma.

the greatest increase in population-related life expectancy for the lowest cost. Evaluations of this type have reached contradictory conclusions; some have stated that open biopsy or excision was the procedure of choice, whereas others suggested that sputum cytology should precede other testing methods in the specified context.[233–236] Potential reasons for these disagreements are several, including study bias, assumptions based on incomplete data, and the overall complexity of analytic modeling. One study that included theoretical patient preferences showed that the cost-effectiveness of testing strategies was variable, depending on patient values such as risk aversion (aversion to a false-negative diagnosis or a testing complication).[237] Although these factors have yet to be measured in actual practice, the specified results of the latter study indicate that a single testing strategy may not apply for all patient populations, including those with potential metastatic disease in the lungs.

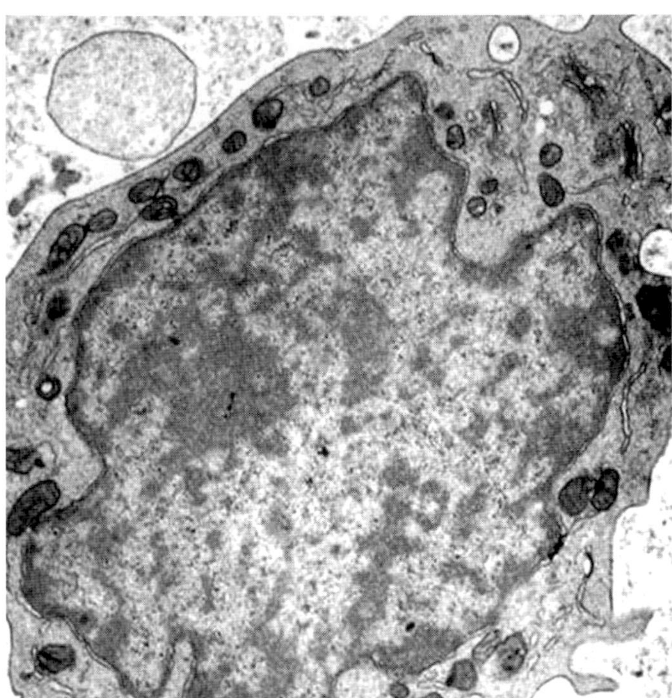

Fig. 17.80 Electron photomicrograph of granulocytic sarcoma (tumefactive acute myelogenous leukemia) involving the lungs. The tumor cells contain only primitive organelles and are not distinctive ultrastructurally.

Raab et al. assessed the sensitivity and cost-effectiveness of percutaneous FNA in a group of patients with known extrapulmonary malignancies and solitary lung masses.[238] Using data from two hospitals with active FNA programs, those authors showed that pathologists were able to correctly classify 87% of the pulmonary lesions as primary or secondary malignancies. Over 90% of them were metastases, indicating that the probability of a primary lung tumor is low in this particular clinical setting. As mentioned earlier, the separation of primary and secondary malignancies depended on light microscopic features; morphologic comparison with previous specimens, when available; and the judicious use of immunocytochemistry. Raab et al. found that the latter method was needed in only 20% of cases, but it yielded a definitive diagnosis in 78% of cases in which it was used.[238] The cost-effectiveness of percutaneous FNA – as compared with bronchoscopy and thoracoscopy – depends on several factors, such as test sensitivity and the pre-FNA probability of malignancy. An underlying assumption is that patients with metastatic disease do not need pulmonary resections, although those procedures may indeed be deemed appropriate in some patient populations by some physicians. At pre-FNA probabilities of malignancy of >50% and FNA sensitivities of >75%, FNA was more cost-effective than thoracoscopy in the cited series.[238] In most clinical scenarios, percutaneous FNA was also more cost-effective than bronchoscopy. Nonetheless, clinicians still tend to use a wide variety of testing strategies in the diagnostic evaluation of pulmonary masses.[239]

Another question of increasing importance is the utilitarian value of ancillary studies such as immunopathology in tumor subtyping. Raab showed that immunocytochemistry was cost-effective in three theoretical scenarios: increasing patient life expectancy, diagnostic certainty, and the ability to predict patient prognosis.[240] However, as Wick et al. have indicated, it has never been proven formally that the correct immunohistologic diagnosis of a specific tumor type, particularly concerning non-hematolymphoid malignancies, does, in fact, produce a benefit regarding patient outcome.[176] Accurate pathologic diagnosis is believed to be advantageous in some instances, such as those concerning small cell pediatric malignancies. Nonetheless, for the most part, patient survival in oncology cases generally depends more on non-pathologic variables such as tumor stage, patient age, and overall health.[241–245] The actual effect of accurate diagnoses was not reported in the latter study, which investigated cost-effectiveness of FNA in evaluation of lung masses, but Imlay and Raab separately showed that the use of immunopathology had no effect on patient survival in reference to pleural fluid evaluation.[44]

Some immunologic markers do have a potentially predictive role as applied to secondary pulmonary malignancies, such as estrogen receptor protein and progesterone receptor protein in cases of metastatic breast cancer. Those determinants may forecast the clinical response to appropriate treatment regimens, the response to which, in turn, may be prognostic (indicative of overall patient survival).[176] The actual benefit of most other markers of that type has not yet been thoroughly assessed with regard to cost-effectiveness.[176]

REFERENCES

1. Crow J, Slavin G, Kreel L: Pulmonary metastasis: a pathologic and radiologic study. Cancer 1981; 47: 2595–2603.
2. Johnson RM, Lindskog GE: 100 cases of tumor metastatic to the lung and mediastinum. JAMA 1967; 202: 94–98.
3. Abrams HJ, Spiro R, Goldstein N. Metastates in carcinoma, analysis of 1000 autopsied cases. Cancer 1950; 3: 74–75.
4. Farrell JT: Pulmonary metastasis: a pathologic, clinical, roentgenologic study based on 78 cases seen at necropsy. Radiology 1935; 24: 444–451.
5. Matthay R, Coppage L, Shaw C, Filderman A: Malignancies metastatic to the pleura. Invest Radiol 1990; 25: 601–619.
6. Filderman AE, Coppage L, Shaw C, Matthay RA: Pulmonary and pleural manifestations of extrathoracic malignancies. Clin Chest Med 1989; 10: 747–807.

7. Fidler IJ: Review: Biologic heterogeneity of cancer metastases. Breast Cancer Res Treat 1987; 17: 17.
8. Fidler IJ: The evolution of biologic heterogeneity in metastatic neoplasms. In: Cancer invasion and metastases: biologic and therapeutic aspects, Nicholson GL, Milas L, Eds. 1984, Raven Press, New York: p 5.
9. Liotta LA: Editorial. H-ras p21 and the metastatic phenotype. J Natl Cancer Inst 1988; 80: 468.
10. Cotran RS, Kumar V, Collins T, Robbins SL: Neoplasia. In: Robbins pathologic basis of disease. 1999, WB Saunders, Philadelphia, pp 241–304.
11. Braman SS, Whitcomb ME: Endobronchial metastasis. Arch Intern Med 1975; 135: 543–547.
12. Winterbauer RH, Elfenbein IB, Jr: WCB. Incidence and clinical significance of tumor embolization to the lungs. Am J Med 1968; 45: 271–290.
13. Goldhaber SZ, Dricker E, Buring JE: Clinical suspicion of autopsy-proven thrombotic and tumor pulmonary embolism in cancer patients. Am Heart J 1987; 114: 1432–1435.
14. Chan CK, Hutcheon MA, Hyland RH, et al.: Pulmonary tumor embolism: a critical review of clinical, imaging, and hemodynamic features. J Thorac Imaging 1987; 2: 4–14.
15. Gonzalez-Vitale JC, Garcia-Bunuel R: Pulmonary tumor emboli and cor pulmonale in primary carcinoma of the lung. Cancer 1976; 38: 2105–2110.
16. Abbondanzo SL, Klappenbach RS, Tsou E: Tumor cell embolism to pulmonary alveolar capillaries. Arch Pathol Lab Med 1986; 110: 1197–1198.
17. Kane RD, Hawkins HK, Miller JA: Microscopic pulmonary tumor emboli associated with dyspnea. Cancer 1975; 36: 1473–1482.
17a. Pinckard JK, Wick MR: Tumor-related thrombotic pulmonary microangiopathy: review of pathologic findings and pathophysiologic mechanisms. Ann Diagn Pathol 2000; 4: 154–157.
18. Soares FA, Landell GAM, deOliveira JAM: Pulmonary tumor embolism to alveolar septal capillaries: a prospective study of 12 cases. Arch Pathol Lab Med 1991; 115: 127–130.
19. Scholten ET, Kreel L: Distribution of lung metastases in the axial plane. Radiol Clin North Am 1977; 46: 248–265.
20. Steele JD: The solitary pulmonary nodule. J Thorac Cardiovasc Surg 1963; 46: 21–39.
21. Toomes H, Delphendahl A, Manke H, Vogt-Moykopf I: The coin lesion of the lung: a review of 955 resected coin lesions. Cancer 1983; 51: 534–537.
22. Viggiano RW, Swensen SJ, Rosenow EC: Evaluation and management of solitary and mulitple pulmonary nodules. Clin Chest Med 1992; 13: 83–95.
23. Quint LE, Park CH, Iannettoni MD: Solitary pulmonary nodules in patients with extrapulmonary neoplasms. Radiology 2000; 217: 257–261.
24. Dodd GD, Boyle JJ: Excavating pulmonary metastases. AJR 1961; 85: 277–293.
25. D'Angio GJ, Iannaccone G: Spontaneous pneumothorax as a complication of pulmonary metastases in malignant tumors of childhood. Am J Roentgenol 1961; 86: 1092–1102.
26. Fichera G, Hagerstrand I: The small lymph vessels of the lungs in lymphangiosis carcinomatosa. Acta Pathol Microbiol Scand 1965; 65: 505–513.
27. Harold JT: Lymphangitis carcinomatosa of the lungs. Q J Med 1952; 21: 353–360.
28. Yang SP, Lin CC: Lymphangitic carcinomatosis of the lungs: the clinical significance of its roentgenologic classification. Chest 1972; 62: 179–187.
29. Trapnell DH: The radiological appearance of lymphangitic carcinomatosa of the lung. Thorax 1964; 19: 251–260.
30. Winterbauer RH, Belic N, Moores KD: A clinical interpretation of bilateral hilar adenopathy. Ann Intern Med 1973; 78: 65–71.
31. Janower ML, Blennerhassett JB: Lymphangitic spread of metastatic cancer to the lung: a radiologic–pathologic classification. Radiology 1971; 101: 267–273.
32. Goldsmith HS, Bailey HD, Callahan EL, Beattie EJ: Pulmonary lymphangitic metastases from breast cancer. Arch Surg 1967; 94: 483–488.
33. Thurlbeck WM: Neoplasia of the pulmonary vascular bed. In: Pulmonary vascular disease, Moser KM, Ed. 1979, Marcel Dekker, New York, pp 629–649.
34. Canto-Armengod A: Macroscopic characteristics of pleural metastases arising from the breast and observed by diagnostic thorascopy. Am Rev Respir Dis 1990; 142: 616–618.
35. Hsu C: Cytologic detection of malignancy in pleural effusion: review of 5,255 samples from 3,811 patients. Diagn Cytopathol 1987; 3: 8–12.
36. Johnson WW: The malignant pleural effusion: a review of cytopathologic diagnoses of 584 specimens from 472 consecutive patients. Cancer 1985; 56: 905–909.
37. Venrick MG, Sidaway MK: Cytologic evaluation of serous effusions: processing techniques and optimal number of smears for routine preparation. Am J Clin Pathol 1993; 99: 182–186.
38. DeMay RM: Fluids. In: The art and science of cytopathology. 1996, ASCP Press, Chicago, pp 257–325.
39. Chernow B, Sahn SA: Carcinomatous involvement of the pleura: an analysis of 96 patients. Am J Med 1977; 63: 695–702.
40. Edoute Y, Kuten A, Ben-Haim SA: Symptomatic pericardial effusion in breast cancer patients: the role of fluid cytology. J Surg Oncol 1990; 45: 265–269.
41. Sahn SA: Malignant pleural effusions. Semin Respir Med 1987; 9: 43–53.
42. Canto A, Ferrer G, Romagosa V, Moya J, Bernat R: Lung cancer and pleural effusion. Clincal significance and study of pleural metastic locations. Chest 1985; 87: 649–852.
43. DiBonito L, Falconieri G, Colautti I: Cytopathology of malignant mesothelioma: a study of its patterns and histological bases. Diagn Cytopathol 1993; 9: 25–31.
44. Imlay SP, Raab SS: Pleural fluid cytology: immunocytochemistry usage patterns and significance of nondefinitive diagnosis. Diagn Cytopath 1999; 22: 281–285.
45. VandeMolengraft FJJM, Vooijs GP: Survival of patients with malignancy-associated effusions. Acta Cytol 1989; 33: 911–916.
46. Chretien J, Jaubert F: Pleural responses in malignant metastatic tumors. In: The pleura in health and disease, Chretien J, Bignon J, Hirsch A, Eds. 1985, Marcel Dekker, New York, pp 489–505.
47. Sahn SA: Malignant pleural effusion. In: Pulmonary diseases and disorders, 2nd edn, Fishman AP, Ed. 1988, McGraw-Hill, New York, pp 2159–2169.
48. Spriggs AI. Malignant cells in serous effusions complicating bronchial carcinoma. Thorax 1954; 9: 26–34.
49. Smith-Purslow MJ, Kini SR, Naylor B: Cells of squamous cell carcinoma in pleural, peritoneal and pericardial fluids: origina and morphology. Acta Cytol 1989; 84: 125–128.
50. Light RW: Tumors of the pleura. In: Textbook of respiratory medicine, Murray JF, Nadel JA, Eds. WB Saunders, Philadelphia, pp 1770–1780.
51. Bourke SA, Henderson AF, Stevenson RD, Banham SW: Endobronchial metastases simulating primary carcinoma of the lung. Respir Med 1989; 83: 151–152.
52. King DS, Castleman B: Bronchial involvement in metastatic pulmonary malignancy. J Thorac Surg 1943; 12: 305–315.
53. Katsimbri PP, Bamias AT, Froudarakis ME, et al.: Endobronchial metastases secondary to solid tumors: report of eight cases and review of the literature. Lung Cancer 2000; 28: 163–170.
54. Casino AR, Bellmunt J, Salud A, et al.: Endobronchial metastases in colorectal adenocarcinoma. Tumori 1992; 78: 270–273.
55. Schoenbaum S, Viamonte M: Subepithelial endobronchial metastases. Diagn Radiol 1971; 101: 63–69.
56. Fitzgerald RH: Endobronchial metastases. South Med J 1977; 79: 440–443.
57. Heitmiller R, Marasco W, Hruban R, Marsh B: Endobronchial metastasis. J Thorac Cardiovasc Surg 1993; 106: 537–542.
58. Argyros G, Torrington K: Fiberoptic bronchoscopy in the evaluation of carcinoma metastatic to the lung. Chest 1994; 105: 454–457.
59. Wang YH, Wong SL, Lai YF, Lin AS, Chang HW: Endobronchial metastatic disease. Chang Keng I Hsueh Tsa Chih 1999; 22: 240–245.
60. Salud A, Porcel JM, Rovirosa A, Bellmunt J: Endobronchial metastatic disease: analysis of 32 cases. J Surg Oncol 1996; 62: 249–252.
61. Mehta AC, Marty JJ, Lee FWY: Sputum cytology. Lung Cancer 1993; 14: 36–85.

62. Koss L, Melamed M, Goodner J: Pulmonary cytology: a brief survey of diagnostic results from July 1st, 1952 until December 31st, 1960. Acta Cytol 1964; 8: 104–113.
63. Arroliga A, Matthay R: The role of bronchoscopy in lung cancer. Lung Cancer 1993; 14: 87–98.
64. Harrow EM, Wang KP: The staging of lung cancer by bronchoscopic transbronchial needle aspiration. Chest Surg Clin North Am 1996; 6: 223–235.
65. Wang KP: Transbronchial needle aspiration and percutaneous needle aspiration for staging and diagnosis of lung cancer. Clin Chest Med 1995; 16: 535–552.
66. Salazar A, Westcott J: The role of thoracic needle biopsy for the diagnosis and staging of lung cancer. Lung Cancer 1993; 14: 99–110.
67. Garcia RF, Lobato SD, Pino JM: Value of CT-guided fine needle aspiration in solitary pulmonary nodules with negative fiberoptic bronchoscopy. Acta Radiol 1994; 35: 478–480.
68. Sonett J: Pulmonary metastases: biologic and historical justification for VATS. Video assisted thoracic surgery. Eur J Cardiothorac Surg 1999; 16(suppl): S13–15.
69. Coosemans W, Lerut T, Raemdonck DV: Thoracoscopic surgery: the Belgian experience. Ann Thorac Surg 1993; 56: 621–660.
70. Miller J: The present role and future considerations of video-assisted thorascopy in general thoracic surgery. Ann Thorac Surg 1993; 56: 804–806.
71. Nathan M, Colloing V, Adams R: Differentation of benign and malignant pulmonary nodules by growth rate. Radiology 1962; 79: 221–232.
72. Nathan M: Management of solitary pulmonary nodules: an organized approach based on growth rate and statistics. JAMA 1974; 227: 1141–1144.
73. Godwin JP, Speckman JM, Fram EK: Distinguishing benign from malignant pulmonary nodules by computed tomography. Radiology 1982; 144: 349–352.
74. Layfield LJ, Coogan A, Johnston WW, Patz EF: Transthoracic fine needle aspiration biopsy. Sensitivity in relation to guidance technique and lesion size and location. Acta Cytol 1996; 40: 687–690.
75. Pilotti S, Rilke F, Gribaudi G, Damascelli B: Fine needle aspiration biopsy cytology of primary and metastatic pulmonary tumors. Acta Cytol 1982; 26: 661–666.
76. Zarbo R, Fenoglio-Preiser C: Interinstitutional database for comparison of performance in lung fine-needle aspiration cytology. A College of American Pathologists Q-Probe Study of 5264 cases with histologic correlation. Arch Pathol Lab Med 1992; 116: 463–470.
77. Kern WH, Schweizer CW: Sputum cytology of metastatic carcinoma of the lung. Acta Cytol 1976; 20: 514–520.
78. Perchalski JE, Hall KL, Dewar MA: Metastasis of unknown orgin. Prim Care 1992; 19: 747–757.
79. Fizazi K, Culine S: Metastatic carcinoma of unknown orgin. Bull Cancer 1998; 85: 609–617.
80. Schapira DV, Jerrett AR: The need to consider survival, outcome, and expense when evaluating and treating patients with unknown primary carcinoma. Arch Intern Med 1995; 155: 2050–2054.
81. Heim S, Mitleman F: Solid tumors. In: Cancer cytogenetics. 1987, Alan R Liss, New York, pp 227–261.
82. Papec R: Distant metastases from head and neck. Cancer 1984; 53: 342–345.
83. Probert J, Thompson R, Bagshaw M: Patterns of spread of distant metastases in head and neck cancer. Cancer 1974; 33: 127–133.
84. Raab SS, Oweity T, Hughes JH, et al.: The effect of patient history on diagnostic accuracy in the interpretation of bronchial brush specimens. Am J Clin Pathol 2000; 114: 78–83.
85. DeYoung BR, Wick MR: Immunohistologic evaluation of metastatic carcinomas by unknown origin: an algorithmic approach. Semin Diagn Pathol 2000; 17: 184–193.
86. Silver SS, Askin FB: True papillary carcinoma of the lung. A distinct clinicopathologic entity. Am J Surg Pathol 1997; 21: 43–51.
87. Nakamura S, Koshikawa T, Sato T, Hayashi K, Suchi T: Extremely well differentiated papillary adenocarcinoma of the lung with prominent cilia formation. Acta Pathol Jpn 1992; 42: 745–750.
88. Salisbury JR, Darby AJ, Whimster WF: Papillary adenocarcinoma of lung with psammoma bodies: report of a case derived from type II pneumocytes. Histopathology 1986; 10: 877–884.
89. Massin J-P, Savoie J-C, Garnier H, et al.: Pulmonary metastases in differentiated thyroid carcinoma. Study of 58 cases with implications for the primary tumor treatment. Cancer 1984; 53: 982–992.
90. Samaan NA, Schultz PN, Haynie TP, Ordonez NG: Pulmonary metastasis of differential thyroid carcinoma: treatment results in 101 patients. J Clin Endocrinol Metab 1985; 60: 376–380.
91. Venkatesh YSS, Ordonez NG, Schultz PN, et al.: Anaplastic carcinoma of the thyroid: a clinicopathologic study of 121 cases. Cancer 1990; 66: 321–330.
92. Shepherd MP: Endobronchial metastatic disease. Thorax 1982; 37: 362–365.
93. Kerr VE, Cadman E: Pulmonary metastases in ovarian cancer. Cancer 1985; 56: 1209–1213.
94. Dvoretsky PM, Richards KA, Angel C: Distribution of disease at autopsy in 100 women with ovarian cancer. Hum Pathol 1988; 19: 57–63.
95. Oosterlee J: Peritoneovenous shunting for ascites in cancer patients. Br J Surg 1980; 67: 663–666.
96. Fildes J, Narvarez GP, Baig KA, Pai N, Gerst PH: Pulmonary tumor embolization after peritoneovenous shunting for malignant ascites. Cancer 1988; 61: 1973–1976.
97. Werner M, Chott A, Fabiano A, Battifora H: Effect of formalin tissue fixation and processing on immunohistochemistry. Am J Surg Pathol 2000; 24: 1016–1019.
98. Renshaw AA, Dean BR, Antman KH, Sugarbaker DJ, Cibas ES: The role of cytologic evaluation of pleural fluid in the diagnosis of malignant mesothelioma. Chest 1997; 111: 106–109.
99. Moran CA, Wick MR, Suster S: The role of immunohistochemistry in the diagnosis of malignant mesothelioma. Semin Diagn Pathol 2000; 17: 178–183.
100. Moch H, Oberholzer M, Dalquen P: Diagnostic tools for differentiating between pleural mesothelioma and lung adenocarcinoma in paraffin embedded tissue. Virch Arch A 1993; 423: 19–27.
101. Moch H, Oberholzer M, Christen H: Diagnostic tools for differentiating plural mesothelioma from lung adenocarcinoma in paraffin embedded tissue. Part II. Virch Arch A 1993; 423: 493–496.
102. Wang N-S: Electron microscopy in the diagnosis of pleural mesotheloma. Cancer 1973; 31: 1046–1054.
103. Batiffora H, Kopinski MI: Distinction of mesothelioma from adenocarcinoma. An immunohistochemical approach. Cancer 1985; 55: 655–662.
104. Strickler JG, Hemdier BG, Rouse RV: Immunohistochemical staining in malignant mesotheliomas. Am J Clin Pathol 1987; 88: 610–614.
105. Gaffey M, Mills S, Askin F, et al.: Clear cell tumor of the lung. A clinicopathologic, immunohistochemical, and ultrastructural study of eight cases. Am J Surg Pathol 1990; 14: 248–259.
106. Greenberg BE, Young JM: Pulmonary metastasis from occult primary sites resembling bronchogenic carcinoma. Dis Chest 1958; 33: 496–505.
107. Hughes JH, Jensen CS, Donnelly AD, et al.: The role of fine-needle aspiration cytology in the evaluation of metastatic clear cell tumors. Cancer 1999; 87: 380–389.
108. Saitoh H: Distant metastasis of renal adenocarcinoma in patients with a tumor thrombus in the renal vein and/or vena cava. J Urol 1982; 127: 652–653.
109. Latour A, Shulman HS: Thoracic manifestations of renal cell carcinoma. Radiology 1976; 121: 43–48.
110. Coppage L, Shaw C, Curtis AM: Metastatic disease to the chest in patients with extrathoracic malignancy. J Thoracic Imag 1987; 2: 24–37.
111. Gerle R, Felson B: Metastatic endobronchial hypernephroma. Dis Chest 1963; 44: 225–233.
112. Noy S, Michowitz M, Lazebnik N, Baratz M: Endobronchial metastasis of renal cell carcinoma. J Surg Oncol 1986; 31: 268–270.
113. Amer E, Guy J, Vaze B: Endobronchial metastasis from renal adenocarcinoma simulating a foreign body. Thorax 1981; 36: 183–184.
114. King TE, Fisher J, Schwarz MI, Patzelt LH: Bilateral hilar adenopathy: an unusual presentation of renal cell carcinoma. Thorax 1982; 37: 317–318.
114a. Chu P, Arber DA: Paraffin section detection of CD10 in 505 nonhematopoietic neoplasms: frequent expression in renal cell carcinoma and endometrial stromal sarcoma. Am J Clin Pathol 2000; 113: 374–382.
114b. Scarpatetti M, Tsybrovskyy O, Popper HH: Cytokeratin typing as an aid in the differential diagnosis of primary versus metastatic lung

carcinoma, and comparison with normal lung. Virchows Arch 2002; 440: 70–76.
114c. Avery AK, Beckstead J, Renshaw AA, Corless CL: Use of antibodies to RCC and CD10 in the differential diagnosis of renal neoplasms. Am J Surg Pathol 2000; 24: 203–210.
115. Katzenstein A-LA, Purvis RW, Gmelich JT, Askin FB: Pulmonary resection for metastatic renal adenocarcinoma. Cancer 1978; 41: 712–723.
116. Lisa JR, Trinidad S, Rosenblatt MB: Pulmonary manifestations of carcinoma of the pancreas. Cancer 1964; 17: 395–401.
117. Cutler SJ, Asire AJ, Taylor SG: Classification of patients with disseminated cancer of the breast. Cancer 1969; 24: 861–869.
118. DeBeer RA, Garcia RL, Alexander SC: Endobronchial metastasis from cancer of the breast. Chest 1978; 73: 94–96.
119. Winchester DP, Sener SF, Khandekar JD: Symptomatology as an indicator of recurrent or metastatic breast cancer. Cancer 1979; 43.
120. Casey JJ, Stempel BG, Scanlon EF, Fry WA: The solitary pulmonary nodule in the patient with breast cancer. Surgery 1984; 96: 801–805.
121. Fracchia AA, Knapper WH, Carey JT: Intrapleural chemotherapy for effusion from metastatic breast carcinoma. Cancer 1970; 26: 626–629.
122. Raab SS, Berg LC, Swanson PE, Wick MR: Adenocarcinoma in the lung in patients with breast cancer. A prospective analysis of the discriminatory value of immunohistology. Am J Clin Pathol 1993; 100: 27–35.
123. Dabbs DJ, Liu Y, Tung M, Raab SS, Silverman JF: Immunohistochemical detection of estrogen receptor in pulmonary adenocarcinomas is dependent upon the antibody used. Mod Pathol 2000; 13: 208A.
124. MacDonald RA: Primary carcioma of the liver. A clinicopathologic study of one hundred eight cases. Arch Intern Med 1957; 99: 266–279.
125. Katyal S, Oliver JH, Peterson MS, et al.: Extrahepatic metastases of hepatocellular carcinoma. Radiology 2000; 216: 698–703.
126. Patton RB, Horn RC: Primary liver carcinoma. Autopsy study of 60 cases. Cancer 1964; 17: 757–768.
127. Tsai GL, Liu JD, Siauw CP, Chen PA: Thoracic roentgenologic manifestations in primary carcinoma of the liver. Chest 1984; 86: 430–434.
128. Levy JI, Geddes EW, Kew MC: The chest radiograph in primary liver cancer. An analysis of 449 cases. S Afr Med J 1976; 50: 1323–1326.
129. Cohen MB, Haber MM, Holly EA, et al.: Cytologic criteria to distinguish hepatocellular carcinoma from nonneoplastic liver. Am J Clin Pathol 1991; 95: 125–130.
129a. Wieczorek TJ, Pinkus JL, Glickman JN, Pinkus GS: Comparison of thyroid transcription factor-1 and hepatocyte antigen immunohistochemical analysis in the differential diagnosis of hepatocellular carcinoma, metastatic adenocarcinoma, renal cell carcinoma, and adrenal cortical carcinoma. Am J Clin Pathol 2002; 118: 911–921.
130. August DA, Ottow RT, Sugarbaker PH: Clinical perspective of human colorectal cancer metastasis. Cancer Metastasis Rev 1984; 5: 303–324.
131. Dionne L: The pattern of blood-borne metastasis from carcinoma of rectum. Cancer 1965; 18: 775–781.
132. Taylor FW: Cancer of the colon and rectum: a study of routes of metastases and death. Surgery 1962; 52: 302–308.
133. Langer B: Managing distant metastases. Can J Surg 1985; 28: 419–421.
134. McCormack PM, Attiyeh FF: Resected pulmonary metastases from colorectal cancer. Dis Colon Rectum 1979; 22: 553–556.
135. Flint A, Lloyd RV: Colon carcinoma metastatic to the lung. Cytologic manifestations and distinction from primary pulmonary adenocarcinoma. Acta Cytol 1992; 36: 230–235.
136. Harlamert HA, Mira J, Bejarano PA: Thyroid transcription factor-1 and cytokeratins 7 and 20 in pulmonary and breast carcinoma. Acta Cytol 1998; 42: 1382–1388.
137. Bohinski RJ, Bejarano PA, Balko G: Determination of lung as the primary site of cerebral metastatic adenocarcinomas using monoclonal antibody to thyroid transcription factor-1. J Neurooncol 1998; 40: 227–231.
138. Wang NP, Zee S, Zarbo RJ, Bacchi CE, Gown AM: Coordinate expression of cytokeratins 7 and 20 defines unique subsets of carcinomas. Appl Immunohistochem 1995; 3: 99–107.
139. Baars JH, DeRuijter JL, Smedts F, et al.: The applicability of a keratin 7 monoclonal antibody in routinely Papanicolaou-stained cytologic specimens for the differential diagnosis of carcinomas. Am J Clin Pathol 1994; 101: 257–261.
140. Sack MJ, Roberts SA: Cytokeratins 20 and 7 in the differential diagnosis of metastatic carcinoma in cytologic specimens. Diagn Cytopathol 1997; 16: 132–136.
141. Wauters CC, Smedts F, Gerrits LG, Bosman FT, Ramakers FC: Keratins 7 and 20 as diagnositc markers of carcinomas metastatic to the ovary. Hum Pathol 1995; 26: 852–855.
141a. Tsao MS, Fraser RS: Primary pulmonary adenocarcinoma with enteric differentiation. Cancer 1991; 68: 1754–1757.
141b. Bacchi CE, Gown AM: Distribution and pattern of expression of villin, a gastrointestinal-associated cytoskeletal protein, in human carcinomas: a study employing paraffin-embedded tissue. Lab Invest 1991; 64: 418–424.
141c. Gatalica Z, Miettinen M: Distribution of carcinoma antigens CA19-9 and CA15-3: an immunohistochemical study of 400 tumors. Appl Immunohistochem 1994; 2: 205–211.
141d. Moran CA, Hocchholzer L, Fishback N, Travis WD, Koss MN: Mucinous (so-called colloid) carcinomas of lung. Mod Pathol 1992; 5: 634–638.
141e. Cathro HP, Stoler MH: Expression of cytokeratins 7 and 20 in ovarian neoplasia. Am J Clin Pathol 2002; 117: 944–951.
142. Ware JL: Prostate tumor progression and metastasis. Biochim Biophys Acta 1987; 907: 279–298.
143. Ballon SC, Donaldson RC, Growdon WA: Pulmonary metastases in endometrial carcinoma. In: Pulmonary metastasis, Weiss L, Gilbert HW, Eds. 1978, GK Hall, Boston.
144. Mintz ER, Smith GG: Autopsy finding in 100 cases of prostatic cancer. N Engl J Med 1934; 211: 479–487.
145. Elkin M, Mueller HP: Metastasis from cancer of the prostate: autopsy and roentgenological findings. Cancer 1954; 7: 1246–1248.
146. Kume H, Takai K, Kameyama S, Kawabe K: Multiple pulmonary metastasis of prostatic carcinoma with little or no bone or lymph node metastasis. Report of two cases and review of the literature. Urol Int 1999; 62: 44–47.
147. Scherz H, Schmidt JD: Endobronchial metastasis from prostate carcinoma. Prostate 1986; 8: 319–324.
148. Legge DA, Good CA, Ludwig J: Roentgenologic features of pulmonary carcinomatosis from carcinoma of the prostate. AJR 1971; 11: 360–364.
149. Apple JS, Paulson DF, Baber C, Putman CE: Advanced prostatic carcinoma: pulmonary manifestations. Radiology 1985; 54: 601–604.
150. Miller GJ: The use of histochemistry and immunohistochemistry in evaluating prostatic neoplasia. Prog Surg Pathol 1982; 5: 115–126.
151. Suster S: Recent advances in the application of immunohistochemical markers for the diagnosis of soft tissue tumors. Semin Diagn Pathol 2000; 17: 225–235.
152. Lewis J, Brennan M: Soft tissue sarcomas. Curr Probl Surg 1996; 33:817–872.
153. Scranton PE, DeCicco FA, Totten RS: Prognostic factors in osteosarcoma. A review of 20 year's experience at the University of Pittsburgh Health Center Hospitals. Cancer 1975; 36: 2179–2191.
154. Vezeridis MP, Moore R, Karakousis CP: Metastatic patterns in soft-tissue sarcomas. Arch Surg 1983; 118: 915–918.
155. Flynn KJ, Kim HS: Endobronchial metastasis of uterine leiomyosarcoma. JAMA 1978; 1978.
156. Aronchick JM, Palevsky HI, Miller WT: Cavitary pulmonary metastases in angiosarcoma. Diagnosis by trans-thoracic needle aspiration. Am Rev Respir Dis 1989; 139: 252–253.
157. Shaw AB: Spontaneous pneumothorax from secondary sarcoma of lung. Br Med J 1951; 1: 278–280.
158. Spittle MF, Heal J, Harmer C, White WF: The association of spontaneous pneumothorax with pulmonary metastases in bone tumours of children. Clin Radiol 1968; 19: 400–403.
159. Lodmell EA, Capps SC: Spontaneous pneumothorax associated with metastatic sarcoma. Radiology 1949; 52: 88–93.
160. Dines DE, Cortese DA, Brennan MD, Hahn RG, Payne WS: Malignant pulmonary neoplasms predisposing to spontaneous pneumothorax. Mayo Clin Proc 1973; 48: 541–544.
160a. Brooks JJ: The significance of double phenotypic patterns and markers in human sarcomas: a new model of mesenchymal differentiation. Am J Pathol 1986; 125: 113–123.
161. Gal AA, Brooks JSJ, Pietra GG: Leiomyomatous neoplasms of the lung: a clinical, histologic and immunohistochemical study. Mod Pathol 1989; 2: 209–216.

162. Cho KR, Woodrumm JD, Epstein JI: Leiomyoma of the uterus with multiple extrauterine smooth muscle tumors: a case report suggesting multifocal orgin. Hum Pathol 1989; 20: 80–83.
163. Sherman RS, Brant EE: An x-ray of spontaneous pneumothorax due to cancer metastases to the lungs. Chest 1954; 26: 328–337.
164. Lipton JH, Fong TC, Burgess KR: Miliary pattern as presentation of leiomyomatosis of the lung. Chest 1987; 91: 781–782.
165. Wolff M, Kaye G, Silva F: Pulmonary metastases (with admixed epithelial elements) from smooth muscle neoplasms. Report of nine cases, including three males. Am J Surg Pathol 1979; 3: 325.
166. Horstmann JP, Pietra GG, Harman JA: Spontaneous regression of pulmonary leiomyomas during pregnancy. Cancer 1977; 39: 314.
167. Kaplan C, Katoh A, Shamoto M: Multiple leiomyomas of the lung: benign or malignant. Am Rev Respir Dis 1973; 108: 656–659.
168. Norris HJ, Parmley T: Mesenchymal tumors of the uterus.V: Intravenous leiomyomatosis. A clinical and pathologic study of 14 cases. Cancer 1975; 36: 2164–2178.
169. Bachman D, Wolff M: Pulmonary metastases from benign smooth muscle tumors of the uterus. AJR. 1976; 127: 441.
170. Devoe K, Widner N: Immunohistochemistry of small round-cell tumors. Semin Diagn Pathol 2000; 17: 216–224.
171. Meis-Kindblom JM, Stenman G, Kindblom LG: Differential diagnosis of small round cell tumors. Semin Diagn Pathol 1996; 13: 213–241.
172. Byrd-Gloster AL, Khoor A, Glass LF, et al.: Differential expression for thyroid transcription factor 1 in small cell lung carcinoma and Merkel cell tumor. Hum Pathol 2000; 31: 58–62.
173. Moll R, Lower A, Laufer J: Cytokeratin 20 in human carcinomas. A new histodiagnostic marker detected by monoclonal antibodies. Am J Pathol 1992; 140: 427–447.
174. Schmidt U, Muller U, Metz KA: Cytokeratin and neurofilament protein staining in Merkel cell carcinoma and of the small cell type and small cell carcinoma of the lung. Am J Dermatopathol 1998; 20: 346–351.
175. Wick MR: Immunohistology of neuroendocrine and neuroectodermal tumors. Semin Diagn Pathol 2000; 17: 194–203.
176. Wick MR, Ritter JH, Swanson PE: The impact of diagnostic immunohistochemistry on patient outcomes. Clin Lab Med 1999; 19: 797–814.
176a. Oliveira AM, Tazelaar HD, Myers JL, Erickson LA, Lloyd RV: Thyroid transcription factor-1 distinguishes metastatic pulmonary from well-differentiated neuroendocrine tumors of other sites. Am J Surg Pathol 2001; 25: 815–819.
177. Juhl J: Tumors of the lungs and bronch. In: Essentials of radiologic imaging. 1998, Lippincott-Raven, Philadelphia.
178. Colby TV, Carrington CB: Malignant lymphoma simulating lymphomatoid granulomatosis. Am J Surg Pathol 1982; 6: 19–32.
179. Colby TV, Carrington CB: Lymphoreticular tumors and infiltrates of the lung. Pathol Annu 1983; 18: 27–70.
180. Melamed MR: The cytological presentation of malignant lymphomas and related diseases in effusions. Cancer 1963; 16: 413–431.
181. Meda BA, Buss DH, Woodruff RD, et al.: Diagnosis and subclassification of primary and recurrent lymphoma. The usefulness and limitations of combined fine-needle aspiration cytomorphology and flow cytometry. Am J Clin Pathol 2000; 113: 688–689.
182. Demington M, Carter D, Meyers A: Distant metastases in head and neck epidermoid carcinoma. Laryngoscope 1980; 90: 196–201.
183. O'Brien PH, Carlson R, Steubner EA: Distant metastases in epidermoid cell carcinoma of the head and neck. Cancer 1971; 27: 204–307.
184. Malefetto JP, Kasimis BS, Moran EM, Wuerker RB, Stein JJ: The clinical significance of radiographically detected pulmonary neoplastic lesions in patients with head and neck cancer. J Clin Oncol 1984; 2: 625–630.
185. Leon X, Quer M, Diez S, et al.: Second neoplasm in patients with head and neck cancer. Head Neck 1999; 21: 204–210.
186. Sostman HD, Matthay RA: Thoracic metastases from cervical carcinoma: current status. Invest Radiol 1980; 15: 113–119.
187. D'Orsi CJ, Bruckman J, Mauch P, Smith EH: Lung metastases in cervical and endometrial carcinoma. AJR 1979; 133: 719–722.
188. Kirubakaran MG, Pulimood BM, Ray D: Excavating pulmonary metastases in carcinoma of the cervix. Postgrad Med J 1975; 51: 243–245.
189. Scott I, Bergin CJ, Muller NL: Mediastinal and hilar lymphadenopathy as the only manifestation of metastatic carcinoma of the cervix. J Can Assoc Radiol 1986; 37: 52–53.
190. King TE, Neff TA, Ziporin P: Endobronchial metastasis from the uterine cervix: presentation as primary lung abscess. JAMA 1979; 242: 1651–1652.
191. Buchsbaum HJ: Lymphangitis carcinomatosis secondary to carcinoma of cervix. Obstet Gynecol 1970; 36: 850–860.
191a. Wilson RW, Moran CA: Primary melanoma of the lung: a clinicopathologic and immunohistochemical study of eight cases. Am J Surg Pathol 1997; 21: 1196–1202.
192. DasGupta T, Brasfield R: Metastic melanoma: a clinopathological study. Cancer 1964; 17: 1323–1339.
193. Harpole DH, Johnson CM, Wolfe WG, George SL, Seigler HF: Analysis of 945 cases of pulmonary metastatic melanoma. J Thorac Cardiovasc Surg 1992; 103: 743–750.
194. Chen JTT, Dahmash NS, Ravin CE: Metastatic melanoma to the thorax: report of 130 patients. AJR 1981; 137: 293–298.
195. Dwyer AJ, Reichert CM, Woltering EA, Flye MW: Diffuse pulmonary metastasis in melanoma: radiographic–pathologic correlation. AJR 1984; 143: 983–984.
196. Webb WR, Gamsu G: Thoracic metastasis in malignant melanoma. Chest 1977; 71: 176–181.
197. Balch CM, Soong SJ, Murad TM, et al.: A multifactorial analysis of melanoma: prognostic factors in 200 melanoma patients with distant metastases. J Clin Oncol 1983; 1: 126–134.
198. Pogrebniak HW, Stovroff M, Roth JA, Pass HI: Resection of pulmonary metastases from malignant melanoma: results of a 16-year experience. Ann Thorac Surg 1988; 46: 20–23.
199. Renshaw A, Madge R: Cercariform cells for helping distinguish transitional cell carcinoma from non-small cell lung carcinoma in fine needle aspirates. Acta Cytol 1997; 41: 999–1007.
200. Gown AM, Vogel AM, Hoak D, Gough F, McNutt MA: Monoclonal antibodies specific for melanocytic tumors distinguish subpopulations of melanocytes. Am J Pathol 1986; 123: 195–203.
200a. Munk PL, Connell DG, Muller NL, Lentle BC: Alveolar soft parts sarcoma with pulmonary metastases. Skeletal Radiol 1988; 17: 454–457.
200b. Weiss SW, Enzinger FM: Malignant fibrous histiocytoma: an analysis of 200 cases. Cancer 1978; 41: 2250–2266.
201. Hendin AS: Gestational trophoblastic tumors metastatic to the lungs. Cancer 1984; 53: 58–61.
202. Hatch KD, Shingleton HM, Gore H, Younger B, Boots LR: Human chorionic gonadotropin-secreting large cell carcinoma of the lung detected during follow-up of a patient previously treated for gestational trophoblastic disease. Gynecol Oncol 1980; 10: 98–104.
203. Kumar J, Ilancheran A, Ratnam SS: Pulmonary metastases in gestational trophoblastic disease: a review of 97 cases. Br J Obstet Gynecol 1988; 95: 70–74.
203a. Siegel RJ, Bueso-Ramos C, Cohen C, Koss M: Pulmonary blastoma with germ cell (yolk sac) differentiation: report of two cases. Mod Pathol 1991; 4: 566–570.
204. Wick MR, Swanson PE, Manivel JC: Placenta-like alkaline phosphatase reactivity in human tumors: an immunohistochemical study of 520 cases. Hum Pathol 1987; 18: 946–954.
205. Hammar S: The use of electron microscopy and immunohistochemistry in the diagnosis and understanding of lung neoplasms. Clin Lab Med 1987; 7: 1–30.
206. Hammar SP, Bolen JW, Bockus D, Remington F, Friedman S: Ultrastructural and immunohistochemical features of common lung tumors: an overview. Ultrastruct Pathol 1985; 9: 283–318.
207. Mennemeyer R, Hammar SP, Bauermeister DE, et al.: Cytologic, histologic, and electron microscopic correlations in poorly-differentiated primary lung carcinoma: a study of 43 cases. Acta Cytol 1979; 23: 297–302.
208. Mackay B, Silva EG: Diagnostic electron microscopy in oncology. Pathol Annu 1980; 15(part II): 241–270.
209. Tucker JA: The continuing value of electron microscopy in surgical pathology. Ultrastruct Pathol 2000; 24: 383–389.
210. Mierau GW, Berry PJ, Malott RL, Weeks DA: Appraisal of the comparative utility of immunohistochemistry and electron microscopy in the diagnosis of childhood round cell tumors. Ultrastruct Pathol 1996; 20: 507–517.
211. Erlandson RA, Rosai J: A realistic approach to the use of electron microscopy and other ancillary diagnostic techniques in surgical pathology. Am J Surg Pathol 1995; 19: 247–250.

212. Lombardi L, Orazi A: Electron microscopy in an oncologic institution: diagnostic usefulness in surgical pathology. Tumori 1988; 74: 531–535.
213. Williams MJ, Uzman BG: Uses and contributions of diagnostic electron microscopy in surgical pathology: a study of 20 Veterans Administration hospitals. Hum Pathol 1984; 15: 738–745.
214. Azar HA, Espinoza CG, Richman AV, Saba SR, Wang T: "Undifferentiated" large cell malignancies: an ultrastructural and immunocytochemical study. Hum Pathol 1982; 13: 323–333.
215. Seymour AE, Henderson DW: Electron microscopy in surgical pathology: a selective review. Pathology 1981; 13: 111–135.
216. Warhol MJ, Corson JM: An ultrastructural comparison of mesotheliomas with adenocarcinomas of the lung and breast. Hum Pathol 1985; 16: 50–55.
217. Warhol MJ, Hickey WF, Corson JM: Malignant mesothelioma: ultrastructural distinction from adenocarcinoma. Am J Surg Pathol 1982; 6: 307–314.
218. Warhol MJ, Hunter NJ, Corson JM: An ultrastructural comparison of mesotheliomas and adenocarcinoma of the ovary and endometrium. Int J Gynecol Pathol 1982; 1: 125–134.
219. Wick MR, Swanson PE, Manivel JC: Immunohistochemical analysis of soft tissue sarcomas. Comparisons with electron microscopy. Appl Pathol 1988; 6: 169–196.
220. Gonzalez-Crussi F, Mangkornkanok M, Hsueh W: Large-cell lymphoma: diagnostic difficulties and case study. Am J Surg Pathol 1987; 11: 59–65.
221. Weinstein MH, Dal Cin P: Genetics of epithelial tumors of the renal parenchyma in adults and renal cell carcinoma in children. Anal Quant Cytol Histol 2001; 23: 362–372.
222. Argani P, Antonescu CR, Illei PB, et al.: Primary renal neoplasms with the ASPL-TFE3 gene fusion of alveolar soft parts sarcoma: a distinctive tumor entity previously included among renal cell carcinomas of children and adolescents. Am J Pathol 2001; 159: 179–192.
223. Cerasoli S, Spada F, Buda R, Turci A, Giangaspero F: Cytogenetic analysis of 19 renal cell tumors. Pathologica 2001; 93: 118–123.
224. Dennis TR, Stock AD: A molecular cytogenetic study of chromosome 3 rearrangements in small cell lung cancer: consistent involvement of chromosome band 3q13.2. Cancer Genet Cytogenet 1999; 113: 134–140.
225. Onuki N, Wistuba II, Travis WD, et al.: Genetic changes in the spectrum of neuroendocrine lung tumors. Cancer 1999; 85: 600–607.
226. Kovatich A, Friedland DM, Druck T, et al.: Molecular alterations to human chromosome 3p loci in neuroendocrine lung tumors. Cancer 1998; 83: 1109–1117.
227. Sandberg AA: Cytogenetics and molecular genetics of bone and soft-tissue tumors. Am J Med Genet 2002; 115: 189–193.
228. Parham DM: Neuroectodermal and neuroendocrine tumors principally seen in children. Am J Clin Pathol 2001; 115(suppl): S113–S128.
229. Summersgill B, Goker H, Osin P, et al.: Establishing germ cell origin of undifferentiated tumors by identifying gains of 12p material using comparative genomic hybridization analysis of paraffin-embedded samples. Diagn Mol Pathol 1998; 7: 260–266.
230. Ahmed S, Siddiqui AK, Rai KR: Low-grade B-cell bronchial associated lymphoid tissue (BALT) lymphoma. Cancer Invest 2002; 20: 1059–1068.
231. Hedvat CV, Hegde A, Chaganti RS, et al.: Application of tissue microarray technology to the study of non-Hodgkin's and Hodgkin's lymphoma. Hum Pathol 2002; 33: 968–974.
232. Mehra S, Messner H, Minden M, Chaganti RS: Molecular cytogenetic characterization of non-Hodgkin lymphoma cell lines. Genes Chromosomes Cancer 2002; 33: 225–234.
233. Minna JD: Neoplasms of the lung. In: Harrison's principles of internal medicine, Favei AS, Braunwald E, Isselbacher KJ, Eds. 1998, McGraw-Hill, New York, pp 552–562.
234. Snyder CL, Saltzman DA, Ferrell KL, Thompson RC, Leonard AS: A new approach to the resection of pulmonary osteosarcoma metastases. Results of aggressive metastasectomy. Clin Orthop 1991; 270: 247–253.
235. Todd TR: The surgical treatment of pulmonary metastases. Chest 1997; 112: 287S–290S.
236. Downey RJ: Surgical treatment of pulmonary metastases. Surg Oncol Clin N Am 1999; 8: 341.
237. Raab SS, Hornberger J, Raffin T: The importance of sputum cytology in the diagnosis of lung cancer. A cost-effectiveness analysis. Chest 1997; 112: 937–945.
238. Barlow PB, Beck JR: The solitary pulmonary nodule: a decision analysis [Abstract]. Chest 1985; 88: 45S.
239. Cummings SR, Lillington GA, Richards RJ: Managing solitary pulmonary nodules: the choice of strategy is a "close call". Am Rev Respir Dis 1986; 134: 453–460.
240. Kunstaetter R, Wolkove N, Kreisman H: The solitary pulmonary nodule: decision analysis. Med Decis Making 1985; 5: 61–75.
241. Raab SS, Hornberger J: The effect of a patient's risk-taking attitude on the cost effectiveness of testing strategies in the evaluation of pulmonary lesions. Chest 1997; 111: 1583–1590.
242. Raab SS, Slagel DD, Hughes JH, Thomas PA, Silverman JF: Sensitivity and cost-effectiveness of fine needle aspiration with immunocytochemistry in the evaluation of patients with a pulmonary malignancy and a history of cancer. Arch Pathol Lab Med 1997; 121: 695–700.
243. Raab S, Gross T, Grzybicki D, Silverman J: Clinical perception of the utility of sputa and other tests in patients with lung masses. Mod Pathol 1999; 12: 188A.
244. Raab SS: The cost-effectiveness of immunohistochemistry. Arch Pathol Lab Med 2000; 124: 1185–1191.
245. Alberts AS, Falkson G, Falkson HC, Merwe MPvd: Treatment and prognosis of metastatic carcinoma of unknown primary: analysis of 100 patients. Med Pediatr Oncol 1989; 17: 188–192.

18

Pseudoneoplastic lesions of the lungs and pleural surfaces

Mark R Wick Jon H Ritter Osamu Matsubara

There is a limited group of pulmonary lesions that one can classify as pseudoneoplastic, but those conditions comprise a significant aggregation in absolute numbers. Some are categorized as malformative or reactive in nature, including pulmonary hamartomas; selected inflammatory pseudotumors ("plasma cell granulomas"); tumefactive lymphoid hyperplasias; inflammatory or reparative conditions simulating carcinomas; unusual granulomatous reactions; tumefactive pleural plaques; and florid examples of pleural mesothelial hyperplasia. Other clinical "pseudotumors" such as amyloidoma and rounded atelectasis[1] are confused with neoplasms only by non-pathologists and are not included for discussion here. On the other hand, the variant of inflammatory pseudotumor now known as "inflammatory myofibroblastic tumor" demonstrates clonal characteristics and can rightly be regarded as a true neoplasm.[2,3] Accordingly, it likewise has been omitted from this chapter.

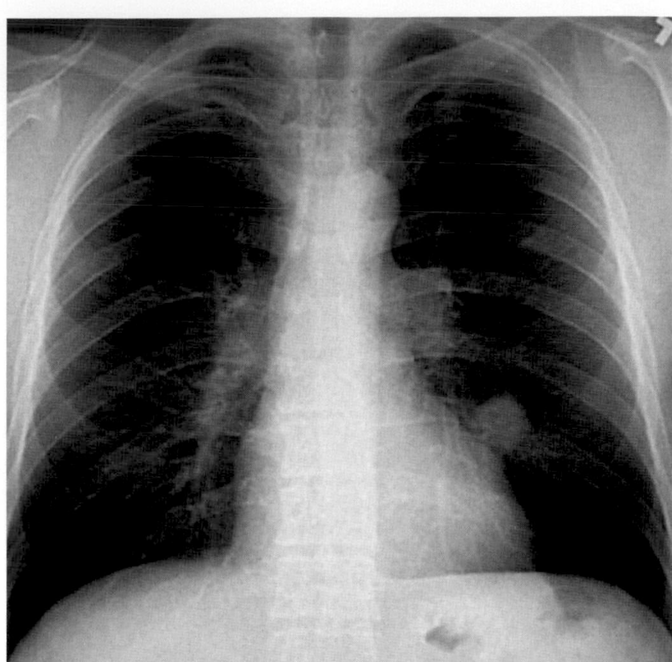

Fig. 18.1 Chest radiograph of pulmonary hamartoma, showing a well-circumscribed peripheral mass abutting the left cardiac border in this posteroanterior view.

Pulmonary hamartomas

The term "hamartoma" is intended to denote tumefactive malformations that exhibit an architecturally abnormal constituency by tissue components that are appropriate to the organ site in which they arise.[4] Other terms for these lesions in the lung include "benign mesenchymoma," "fibroma," "chondroma," "fibrochondrolipoma," "fibrolipomyochondroma," "hamartoma-chondroma," "cartilage-containing tumor of the lung," "adenochondroma," "lipochondroadenoma," "adenofibrolipochondromyxoma," and "mixed tumor."[5]

In autopsy studies, pulmonary hamartomas have been encountered in approximately 0.25% of all cases.[6] They have two forms – central and peripheral – and the second is more common in men than in women.[7–10] Radiographically, hamartomas of the lung are nodules that are found incidentally, usually in patients between 40 and 60 years of age; nevertheless, pediatric cases are also represented in the literature.[10] Uncommonly, these lesions may be multiple or syndromic. In particular, Carney et al. have documented a constellation of masses in young women wherein bronchial cartilaginous hamartomas are part of a lesional triad that includes extra-adrenal paragangliomas and gastric epithelioid stromal tumors.[11,12] Another practical clinical problem is that hamartomas may coexist with primary or secondary malignancies of the lung.[13,14]

Macroscopically, most pulmonary hamartomas are peripherally located, and they sometimes show a topographical relationship to small bronchi or bronchioles.[15–18] Tomiyasu and colleagues documented an unusual example that penetrated the visceral pleura.[19] These lesions are well-demarcated, (Figs 18.1 and 18.2) and they range from several millimeters to 20 cm in diameter. The central form of hamartoma is encountered in association with large bronchi, as an endoluminal polypoid protuberance covered by intact mucosa.[10] All hamartomas of the lung are lobulated, and their cut surfaces reflect their microscopic constituency (Figs 18.3 and 18.4). Most of

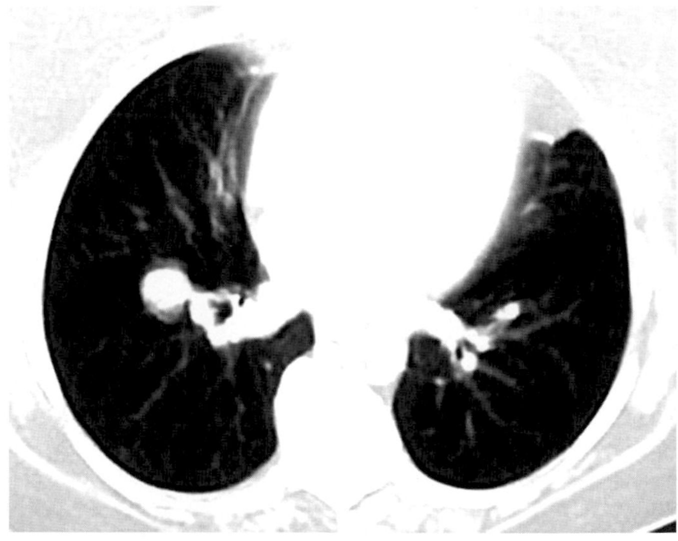

Fig. 18.2 CT of the thorax showing pulmonary hamartoma as a sharply demarcated nodular lesion near the right hilum.

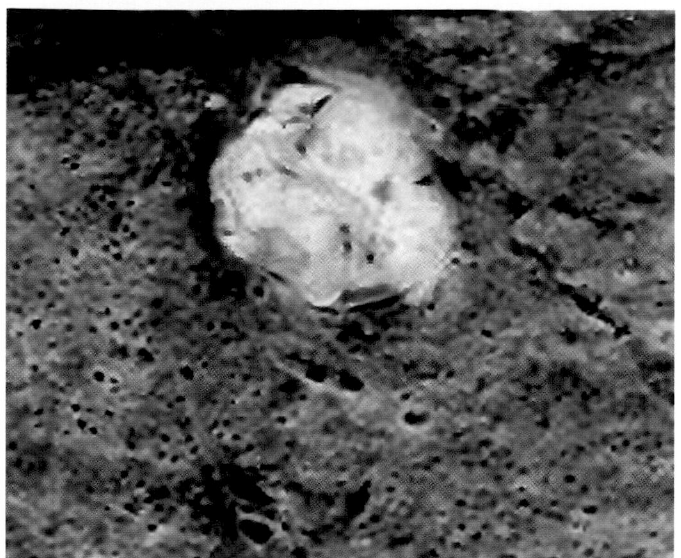

Fig. 18.3 Gross photograph of pulmonary hamartoma, showing a firm homogeneous yellow-tan nodule that stands away from the cut surface of the lung.

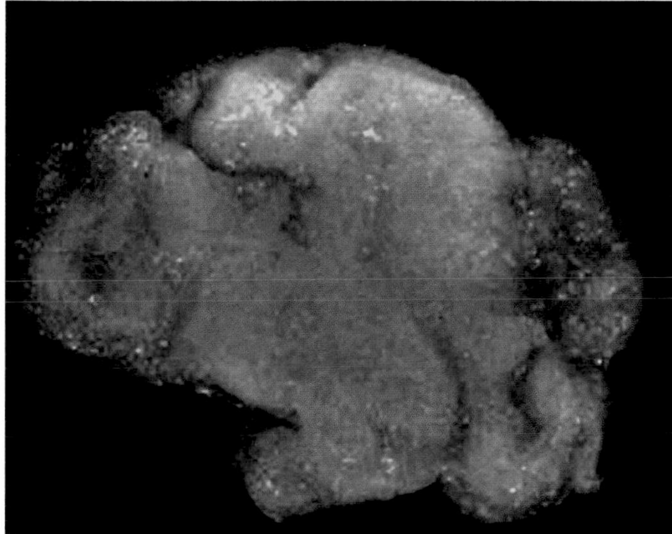

Fig. 18.4 Another macroscopic image of pulmonary hamartoma, demonstrating internal lobulation and a glistening translucent cut surface.

these lesions contain predominantly cartilaginous tissue and are therefore firm to hard, relatively homogeneous, and translucent when transected.

On histologic examination, pulmonary hamartomas (PHs) manifest the presence of mature mesenchymal tissues, but with abnormal configurations. These elements are usually represented by hyaline cartilage, but fibrous tissue, smooth muscle, or adipocytic components also may be seen relatively frequently. Those masses lacking chondroid elements have been termed "intrabronchial lipoma," "myxoma," "leiomyoma," or "fibroadenoma."[15–18]

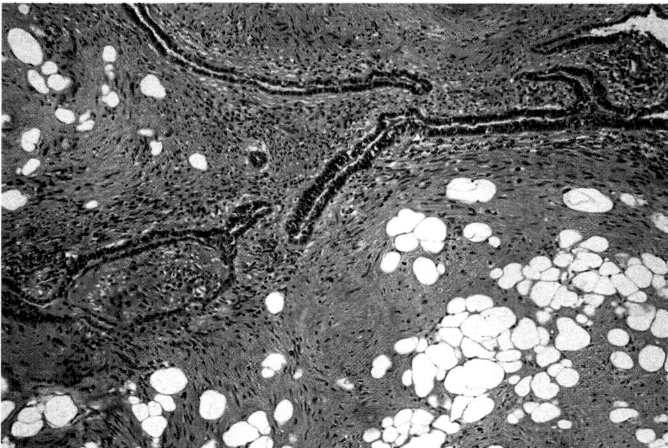

Fig. 18.5 Bronchiolar epithelium is entrapped by relatively mature chondroid and adipocytic tissues in this pulmonary hamartoma.

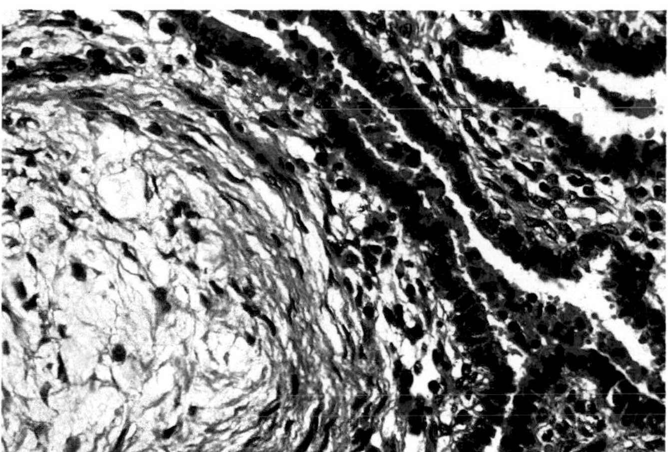

Fig. 18.6 The juxtaposition of lesional mesenchyme (left) and trapped epithelium (right) is seen in this photomicrograph of pulmonary hamartoma.

During the growth of PH, the mesenchymal portions of the lesion engulf and trap small tubular airways and the latter structures thus spuriously appear to represent an integral part of the lesion (Figs 18.5 and 18.6). The incorporated epithelium is cuboidal or low-columnar. Metaplasia, hyperplasia, and papillary proliferation may be present as well in the entrapped airways (Fig. 18.7). Indeed, the last of those changes can be prominent, and Xu et al. have noted that it may produce a morphologic likeness to placental tissue;[20] they termed this feature "placental transmogrification," and regarded it as an inductive phenomenon. Transthoracic fine-needle aspiration biopsy is a common method for the initial pathologic sampling of mass lesions in the lung. In fact, if PH is the favored diagnosis of the radiologist, fine-needle aspiration biopsy is usually done with the anticipation

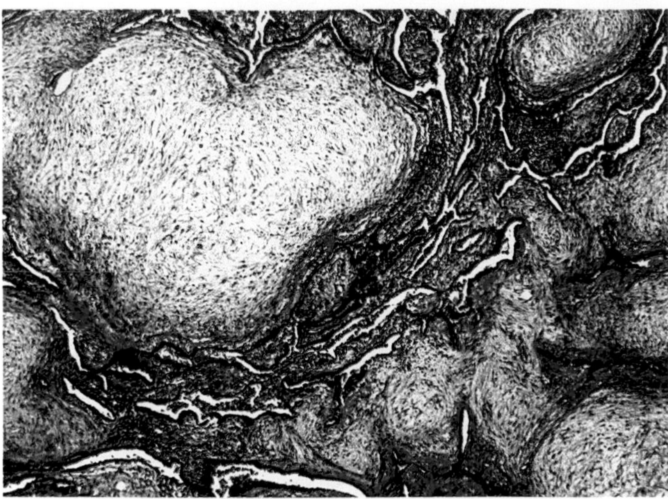

Fig. 18.7 Nodules of cellular mesenchymal tissue with a chondroid "aura" alternate with trapped and proliferating epithelial profiles in another example of pulmonary hamartoma.

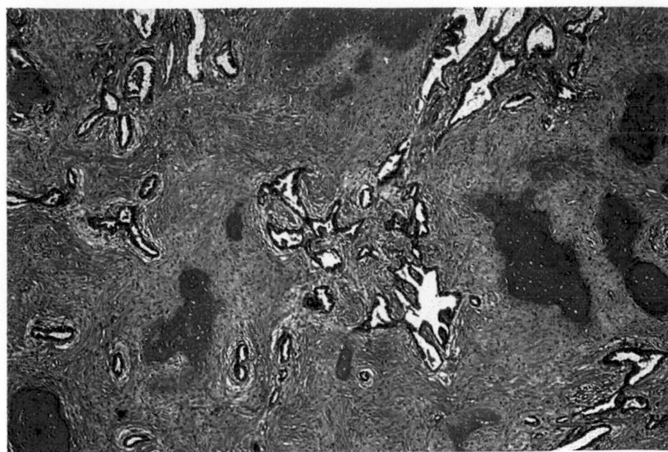

Fig. 18.8 Differential diagnosis in cases of pulmonary hamartoma includes "metaplastic" (sarcomatoid) carcinoma with a biphasic configuration, as shown here.

that a thoracotomy can be avoided if that interpretation is correct. The cytological features of that lesion include the presence of dispersed bland fusiform and stellate cells in a myxoid background, as seen histologically.[21,22]

Surfactant-containing intranuclear inclusions can be seen in the trapped epithelium of PH,[23] like those observed in bronchioloalveolar carcinomas composed of neoplastic type II pneumocytes. Electron microscopic studies show primitive stellate mesenchymal tissue in PH that demonstrates a transition to cartilaginous foci.[24,25] Cytogenetic evaluations have demonstrated an abnormal karyotype in several instances, principally represented by an exchange of material between various chromosomes.[26–29] Those data beg the question of whether PH might actually be neoplastic after all, but the clinical evolution of this lesion (see below) speaks strongly against such a possibility, in our opinion.

PH must be distinguished from primary or metastatic mesenchymal malignancies in the lungs, as well as primary or secondary biphasic sarcomatoid carcinomas.[30–33] The presence of multinucleated cells, nuclear pleomorphism, necrosis, and mitotic activity is rare in PH, in contrast to those diagnostic alternatives. In histologically similar biphasic carcinomas (Fig. 18.8), keratin immunoreactivity is present both in the mesenchymal-like and the overtly epithelial components, whereas PH shows positivity for epithelial markers only in trapped epithelial elements.

PH will continue to enlarge slowly if left in place after diagnosis, but it rarely causes significant clinical difficulty. Simple excision of the lesion is typically performed today, especially with the availability of thoracoscopic video-assisted surgical techniques.[34] Laser treatment has also been offered for patients with central PH.[35] The clinical result of these treatments is excellent.

Inflammatory pseudotumor – plasma cell granuloma of the lung

The most common form of the proliferative spindle cell lesion known as "inflammatory pseudotumor" of the lung has undergone scrutiny in the recent past, and is generally regarded currently as a true neoplasm composed of myofibroblasts.[2,3] That particular entity has been called the "fibrohistiocytic" subtype of pulmonary pseudotumor in the past,[36–38] but has now been renamed "inflammatory myofibroblastic tumor (IMT)".[3] The lesion known as "calcifying fibrous pseudotumor"[39–42] probably represents a closely related entity, bound to IMT by its common manifestation of a t(2;17) chromosomal translocation and potential expression of the *ALK*-1 protein.[43–45] With that having been said, other lesions of the lung that also have been included in the category of inflammatory pseudotumor (IPT) – namely, "plasma cell granuloma" and "hyalinizing granuloma" (HG)[44–51] – probably *do* represent *non*-neoplastic masses with variable etiologies. Both of them are composed of inflammatory and mesenchymal cells, potentially including mature lymphocytes, plasma cells, mast cells, macrophages, eosinophils, fibroblasts, and myofibroblasts.

As just defined, the true incidence of pulmonary IPT is uncertain. It is not commonly encountered in general surgical pathology practice, but its frequency is somewhat dependent upon definitions. Some observers have used "inflammatory pseudotumor" broadly, to describe both circumscribed nodules and irregular inflammatory masses or segmental or lobar consolidations.[52]

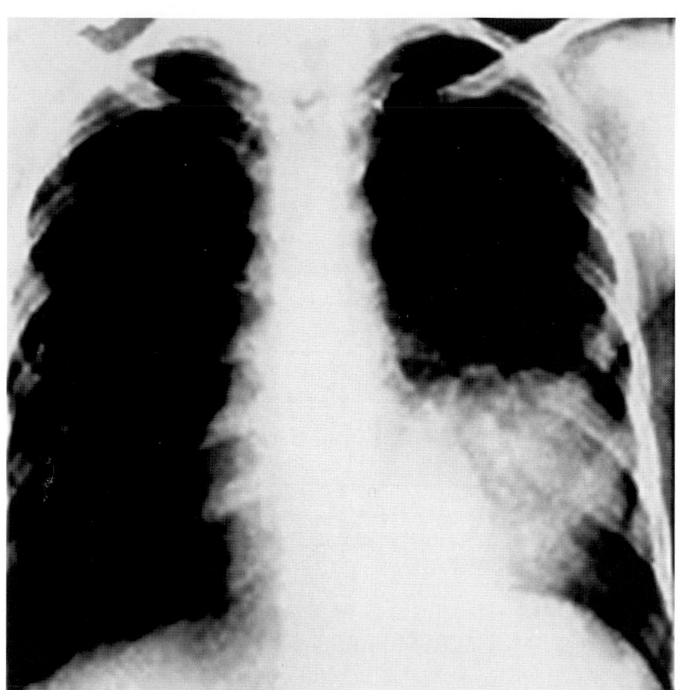

Fig. 18.9 Plasma cell granuloma-type pulmonary inflammatory pseudotumor, seen in this chest radiograph as a large nodular mass in the right lower lung field.

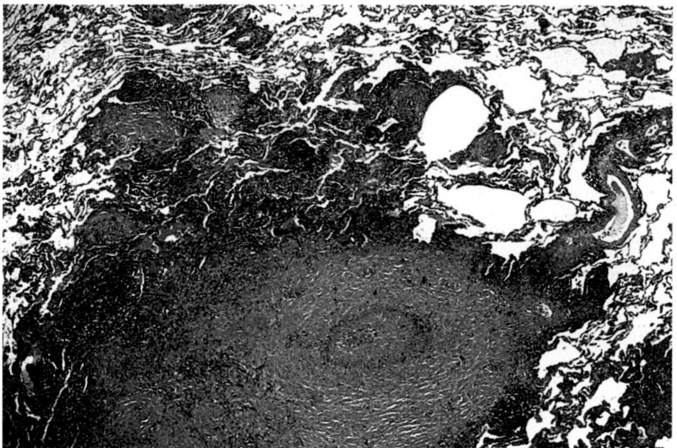

Fig. 18.10 This photomicrograph of inflammatory pseudotumor of the lung shows an irregular interface with the surrounding parenchyma, multiple foci of chronic inflammation, and central sclerosis.

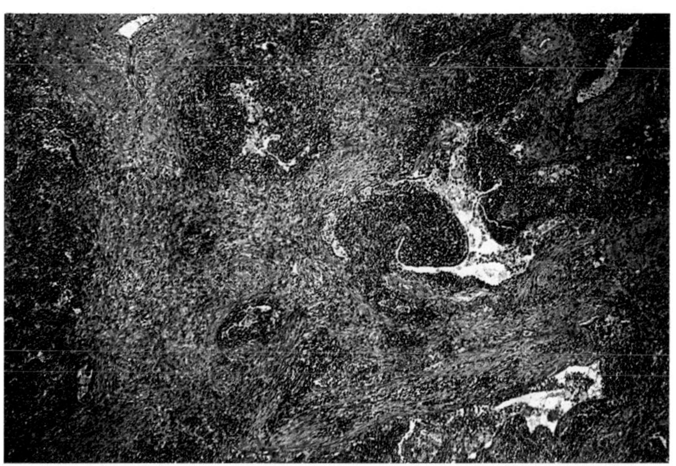

Fig. 18.11 Marked chronic inflammation and peripheral sclerosis in pulmonary inflammatory pseudotumor.

This lesion shows no sex predilection and occurs over a broad range of ages. Patients have ranged in age from 1 to 77 years at diagnosis, with a mean between 27 and 50 years.[38] Approximately 50% complained of cough, hemoptysis, shortness of breath, or chest pain, or combinations thereof. Chest radiographs usually show a single, sharply marginated, round or oval mass (Fig. 18.9), but the edges of large lesions may be more ill-defined.[53,54] Some IPTs involve the pleural surface and retract it as seen on computed tomography (CT) of the thorax;[54] as expected, those findings may falsely suggest the possibility of malignancy. Calcification and cavitation also are potentially present in IPTs of the lung as seen in imaging studies.

Pulmonary IPTs range in size from 0.5 to >30 cm.[37,38] Most have well-defined margins macroscopically but do not show true fibrous capsules; the color and texture of such lesions on cut section is variable. Those that contain numerous inflammatory cells are tan-white and fleshy, and those with a predominance of mesenchymal tissue are gray and firm. IPTs with secondary xanthomatization may be bright yellow and can be friable as well. A few of these masses also exhibit areas of hemorrhage, necrosis, or calcification. Occasionally, IPTs may be sessile intrabronchial lesions, and they also can be attached to the pleura. In typical pulmonary IPT, the microscopic architecture of the lung is replaced by the lesional fibroinflammatory proliferation. Depending on their dominant cellular elements and major growth patterns, they may be subclassified into two types: namely, "tumefactive organizing pneumonia-like" and "lymphoplasmacytic" variants.[37] These may simply represent different stages in the evolution of IPT, and have no special clinicopathologic significance other than potentially invoking different histopathologic diagnostic considerations. The "organizing pneumonia-like" form of IPT shows intra-alveolar lymphohistiocytic inflammation and peripheral as well as central fibrosis (Figs 18.10 and 18.11). Fibroblastic proliferation is admixed with fibrinoinflammatory exudate in alveoli, alveolar ducts, and bronchioles. The alveolar architecture is preserved in early lesions and the peripheral portions of "mature" IPT,

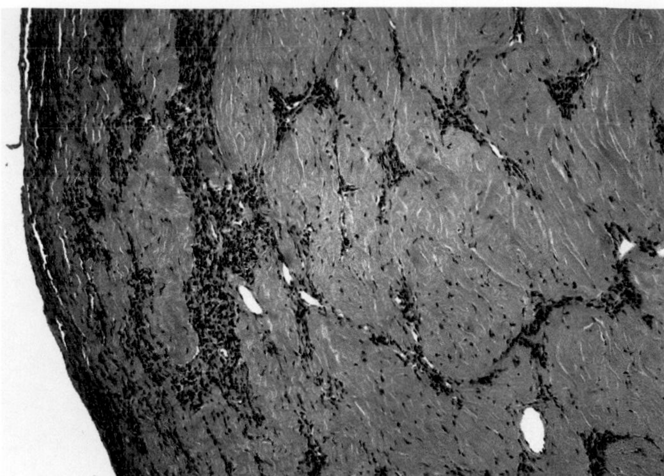

Fig. 18.12 "Mature" plasma cell granuloma-type pulmonary inflammatory pseudotumor demonstrates filling of the distal airspaces by densely collagenized stroma, with residual foci of lymphoplasmacytic inflammation.

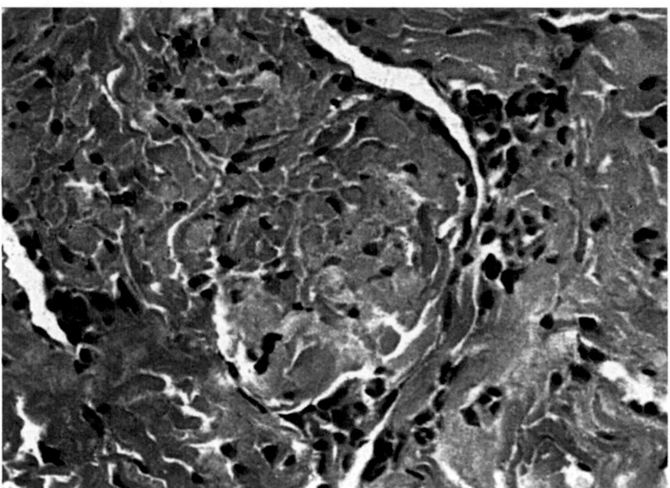

Fig. 18.13 Sclerotic collagenous profiles fill alveolar spaces in this late-stage plasma cell granuloma-type pulmonary inflammatory pseudotumor.

but it is obscured by superimposed fibrous tissue which tends to assume a whorled configuration (Figs 18.12 and 18.13). Neutrophils are sometimes interspersed with the lymphocytes and plasma cells, and they may form intralesional microabscesses that result in small areas of cavitation. Alveoli bordering IPTs are often filled with foamy macrophages and mantled by hyperplastic pneumocytes. Multinucleated cells of the Touton type are sometimes apparent within the masses, sometimes with foci of dystrophic calcification, osseous metaplasia, or myxomatous change. Lipoid pneumonia may develop adjacent to areas where IPT has caused bronchial obstruction by intraluminal proliferation or impingement on the airway. Late in the evolution of IPTs and in their central aspects, the lung parenchyma is replaced by deposition of mature collagen in broad bundles that transect the lesion; it may sometimes assume a keloidal appearance.

In the "lymphoplasmacytic" IPT variant, plasma cells and lymphocytes comprise the bulk of the lesion and germinal centers may be prominent. Fibroblasts and xanthoma cells are usually relatively scant. The two histologic subtypes of IPT overlap one another morphologically, and it is relatively uncommon to find "pure" examples of either one. Neither of them is composed of solid sheets of lymphocytes or plasma cells, tending to prevent diagnostic confusion with lymphoma or plasmacytoma. Matsubara et al.[37] found lymphocytic infiltration and scarring of vascular walls in several examples of IPT, often in association with organizing thrombi. These changes were thought to be secondary rather than a reflection of a primary vasculitic process. Both kappa and lambda light chain immunoglobulins are detectable immunohistologically in the lesional plasma cells, indicating a polytypic population;[49] lymphocyte subset markers similarly show an admixture of B cells and T cells.[3]

The specific etiologic factors underlying the development of pulmonary IPT are unknown. The premise that it represents a peculiar form of localized pneumonia has support from a history of a previous febrile illness with respiratory complaints in up to 40% of cases. Some case reports have suggested that there is an overlap in appearance between IPT and tumefactive pulmonary infections with aspergillus, rickettsiae, mycoplasma, various viruses, mycobacteria, *Cryptococcus*, corynebacteria, and other microorganisms.[52–61] Rare examples have also been documented after trauma to the lung.[62]

The differential diagnosis of pulmonary IPT has been partially cited above. It includes plasmacytoma,[63] malignant lymphoma,[64,65] and lymphoid hyperplasia,[66] selected examples of "sclerosing hemangioma" of the lung (called "epithelial plasma cell granuloma-like tumors" by Michal and Mukensnabl[67]), and the peculiar variant of lung cancer known as "inflammatory sarcomatoid carcinoma"[68] (ISC; see Ch. 14). Among those conditions, plasmacytomas are recognized by their monotypism for cytoplasmic immunoglobulin, and selected lymphomas may also demonstrate that characteristic. Furthermore, malignant lymphomas are generally less well-circumscribed than IPTs, and exhibit more cytologically monotonous infiltrates of atypical lymphoid cells. Localized and diffuse forms of pulmonary lymphoid hyperplasia are composed predominantly of mature lymphocytes, in contrast to the heterogeneous cellular composition of IPT. ISC can be separated from inflammatory simulators by its diffuse immunoreactivity for keratin. There is some minor difference of opinion as to whether or not "pulmonary hyalinizing granuloma"[69] is a part of the spectrum of IPT in the lung. Pulmonary hyalinizing granuloma shows more lamellar hyalinized collagen than is seen in classical IPT. Hyalinizing granulomas of the lung are commonly multiple, whereas "usual" IPT is not.[69] Sclerosing hemangiomas[70] were once considered to be related to IPTs, but they are now appreciated as epithelial neoplasms with pneumocytic differentiation.[71] The latter lesions may exhibit sclerosis, but they also contain aggregates of bland cuboidal cells together with micropapillary and angiomatoid areas. Inflammation is absent or scanty in sclerosing hemangiomas, and their constituent cells express thyroid transcription factor-1;[71] those of IPT do not. Ledet et al[72] have examined the utility of immunostains for mutant p53 protein in the diagnostic separation of IPTs from low-grade intrapulmonary sarcomas. In their hands, p53 was restricted to malignant lesions, albeit with less than absolute sensitivity for such tumors.

Some examples of pulmonary IPT have been monitored for extended periods of time before excision or autopsy examination.[73–75] Information from these cases indicates that the lesions tend to remain stable or grow very slowly. Spontaneous complete resolution has also been documented, and a few lesions have shrunken after small biopsies were taken of them or systemic corticosteroids or irradiation were administered.[73,75] Surgical removal is usually necessary to establish a definitive diagnosis of IPT, and, if the lesion has been completely excised, no further therapy is needed.[53] Long-term follow-up of patients with pulmonary IPTs has revealed no untoward clinical events in such cases.

Mycobacterial spindle cell pseudotumor

Spindle cell pseudotumors that are reactions to mycobacterial infection have been documented in several organ sites in immunosuppressed patients.[76–78] These proliferations show a close histologic resemblance to "histoid" leprosy,[79,80] and most reports on them have documented numerous intralesional mycobacteria (see Chapter 6). Only one case of mycobacterial pseudotumor (MP) has been reported in the lung,[81] and we have encountered another example in a 41-year-old male patient with acquired immunodeficiency syndrome (AIDS). The patient documented by Sekosan et al.[81] was a 32-year-old male with diabetes; he had undergone kidney and pancreatic transplantation with multiple subsequent episodes of acute rejection, treated with aggressive immunomodulation. Respiratory failure then ensued, and disseminated alveolar infiltrates were seen on chest films. Sputum cultures were positive for *Mycobacterium tuberculosis*, and although multi-drug therapy was given to treat that organism, the patient died. Autopsy examination showed that the lungs contained many yellow-gray nodules, with partial bronchocentricity. Microscopic sections of those lesions demonstrated aggregates of spindle cells with a fascicular growth pattern, and without significant atypia or mitoses. Scattered lymphocytes and plasma cells were apparent throughout, but overt granulomas were lacking. The cytoplasm of the spindle cells was described as "foamy," with focal hemosiderosis as well. The lesional cells were immunoreactive for lysozyme, with no labeling for S100 protein, keratin, actin, desmin, or von Willebrand factor. Ziehl–Neelsen staining showed innumerable acid-fast bacilli in the fusiform elements. Our patient had had cutaneous Kaposi's sarcoma and pneumocystis pneumonia in the past, and presented with a radiographically detected nodule in the upper lobe of the right lung. Histologic attributes of the lesion were as described above (Figs 18.14 and 18.15). Although mycobacterial organisms were obvious histologically (Fig. 18.16), cultures had not been obtained of the lesion. Most examples of MP in other anatomic locations have been related to *Mycobacterium avium-intracellulare* or *M. kansasii*.

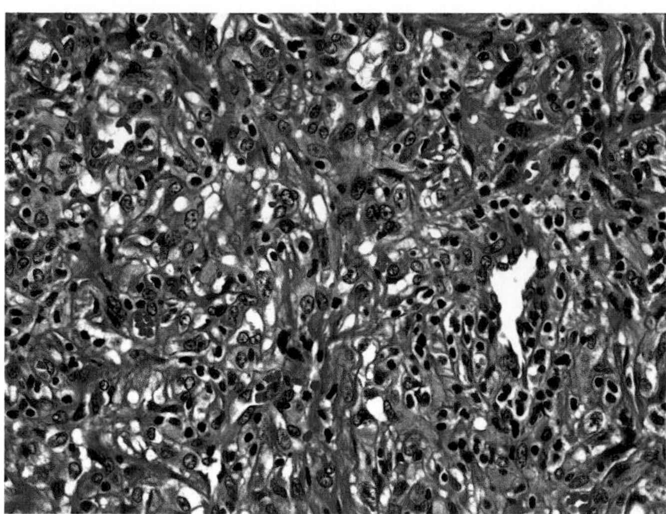

Fig. 18.14 Mycobacterial pseudotumor of the lung in a patient with acquired immunodeficiency syndrome, represented by a disorganized proliferation of spindle cells admixed with lymphocytes and histiocytes.

Another reported feature of MPs in other sites is a possible source of diagnostic error. That is, a reproducible cross-reaction has been seen with mycobacterial antigens using certain desmin antibodies,[82] spuriously suggesting the presence of a myogenous proliferation. This observation is especially troublesome in the setting being

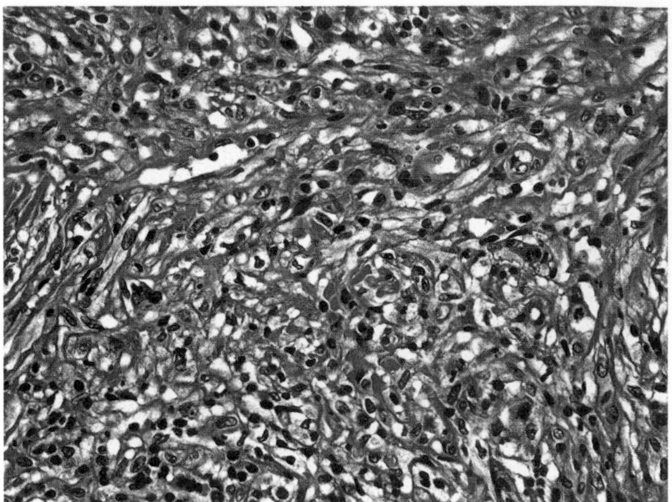

Fig. 18.15 This image of pulmonary mycobacterial pseudotumor is reminiscent of the "myofibroblastic tumor" form of inflammatory pseudotumor of the lung.

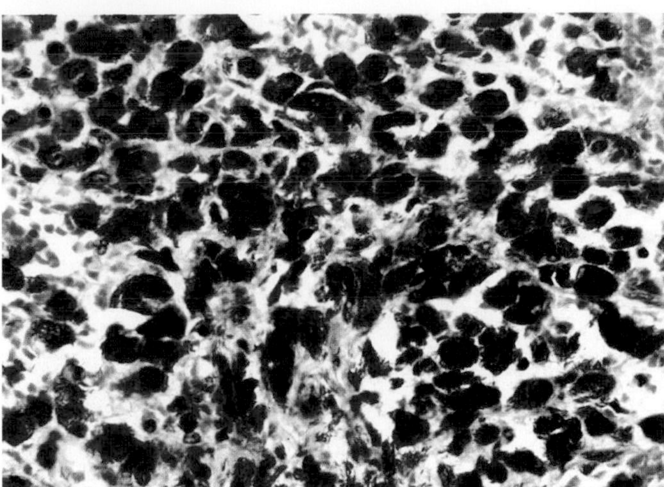

Fig. 18.16 Innumerable intralesional mycobacteria are present in the proliferating cells of pulmonary mycobacterial pseudotumor, as seen in this Ziehl–Neelsen stain.

discussed here, because smooth muscle or myofibroblastic tumors enter prominently into the differential diagnosis of MPs. However, a documented lack of immunoreactivity for actin and electron microscopic attributes that support histiocytic differentiation in MP argue against those alternative interpretations. Other lesions that must be separated from pulmonary MP include Kaposi's sarcoma, malignant fibrous histiocytoma (MFH), spindle cell melanoma, and neural proliferations.[81] Obviously, acid-fast stains should be done in all cases concerning immunocompromised individuals, and these consistently confirm mycobacterial causation. In some instances, the nature of MP is more obvious because of overtly granulomatous foci in the lung tissue around the spindle cell lesion. Characteristics of malignancy such as necrosis, nuclear atypia, and pathologic mitoses are absent in MP.[76–78] Thus, diagnoses of pulmonary sarcomatoid carcinoma, MFH, or other sarcomas would be unlikely.

Pulmonary lymphoid hyperplasia (see also Chapter 15)

Controversy surrounds the nature of selected pulmonary lymphoid infiltrates, relating to the diagnostic terms "lymphoid interstitial pneumonia (LIP)," "lymphoplasmacytic pneumonia," "plasmacytic interstitial pneumonia," and "pseudolymphoma."[83] We believe that some of those entities – in particular, selected examples of LIP and most "pseudolymphomas" – are, in fact, low-grade malignant lymphomas of the bronchus-associated lymphoid tissue.[84,85] However, in this section, we concentrate on those forms of LIP that seem to lack molecular evidence of clonality, and therefore have the features of peculiar tumefactive hyperplasias. In line with that approach, we concur with Koss in his opinion that LIP (and, perhaps, other forms of pulmonary lymphoid hyperplasia) " … is not a single etiological or pathogenetic entity, but rather a morphological expression in the lung of a variety of diseases."[86]

The clinical manifestations of LIP are variable, potentially including cough, dyspnea, weight loss, fever, hemoptysis, chest pain, and joint pain.[86,87] The last of these complaints may be associated with laboratory findings suggesting an autoimmune disorder or collagen vascular disease, such as rheumatoid arthritis and its variants, lupus erythematosus, or myasthenia gravis.[86–89] Other conditions in which immune function is altered – such as primary biliary cirrhosis, Blackfan–Diamond syndrome, lupoid chronic hepatitis, and AIDS – have also been linked to pulmonary lymphoid hyperplasia in some cases.[86,87] Paraproteinemias are common in patients with LIP, especially polyclonal hypergammaglobulinemia.[90] In a minority of cases, *hypo*gammaglobulinemia may be seen. Results of spirometric testing are usually unremarkable.

Radiologic findings on chest roentgenograms are also inconstant, potentially including interstitial densities throughout one or both lungs; randomly situated nodular lesions of variable sizes; or a combination of those abnormalities[66,86,87,91] (Figs 18.17 and 18.18). Approximately one-half of patients present with a localized single mass, raising the suspicion of a non-lymphoid neoplasm or an infectious lesion.[86] As summarized by Liebow and Carrington,[90] mediastinal lymphadenopathy and pleural

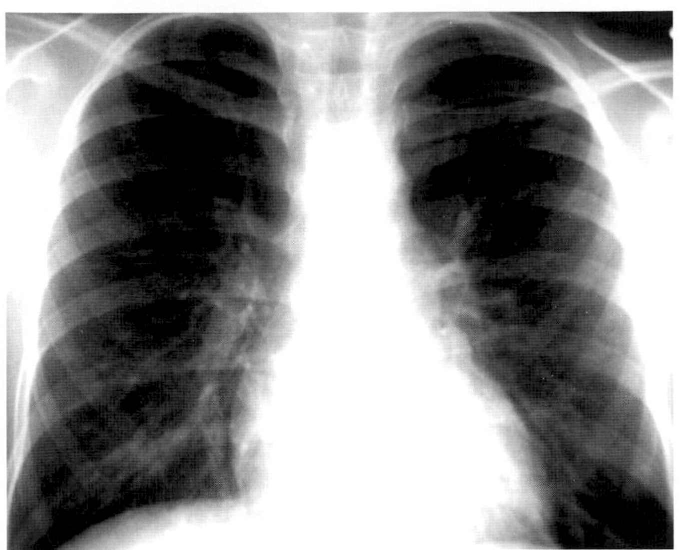

Fig. 18.17 Modestly increased interstitial markings are seen bilaterally in this chest film from a patient with lymphoid interstitial pneumonia.

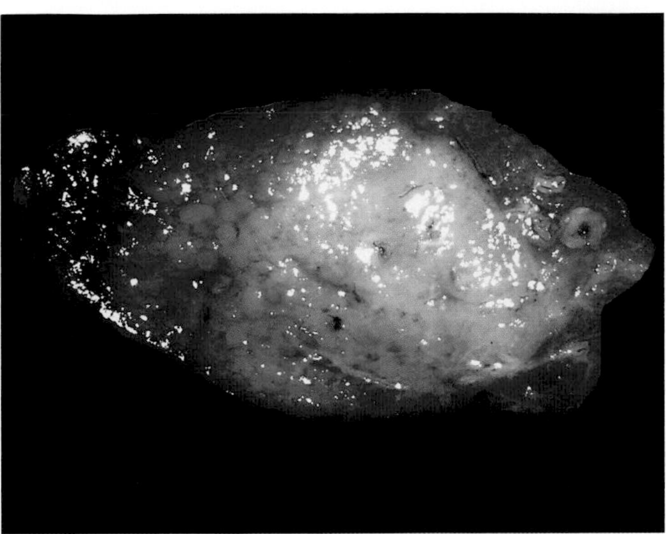

Fig. 18.19 Gross photograph of lymphoid interstitial pneumonia, showing similar macroscopic features to those portrayed in Fig. 18.18.

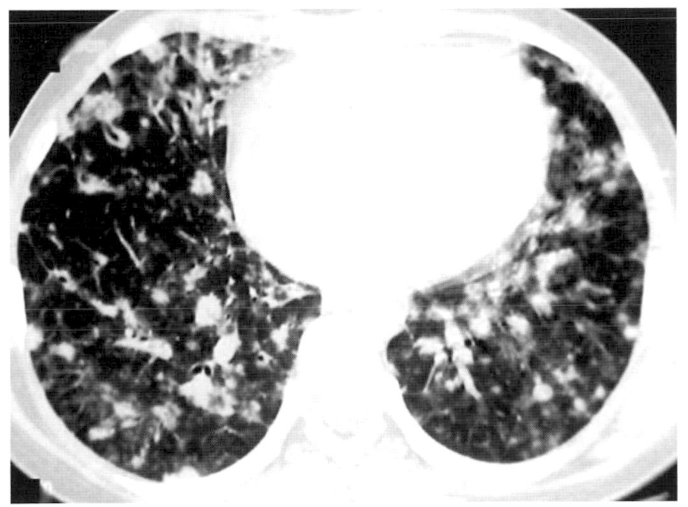

Fig. 18.18 This thoracic CT from another case of lymphoid interstitial pneumonia demonstrates more florid reticulonodular interstitial infiltrates throughout both lungs, with zones of confluence.

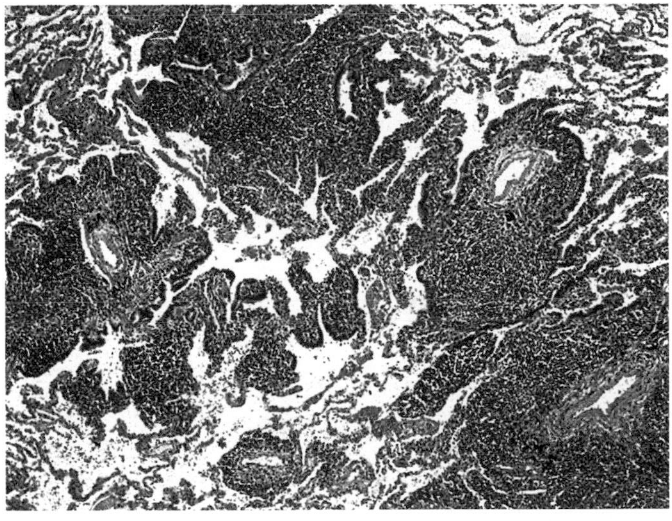

Fig. 18.20 Dense "coat-sleeve" lymphocytic infiltrates are seen around blood vessels in the interstitium in lymphoid interstitial pneumonia.

effusions are uncommon in LIP and their presence suggests another diagnosis.

The biologic evolution of pulmonary lymphoid hyperplasias is difficult to predict. Most observers have found that as many patients die with this condition as those who improve or have stable disease. Overall mortality is roughly 50% at 5 years after diagnosis.[86,87,91] Treatment with corticosteroids or antineoplastic drugs has been employed for LIP with random success. Using modern technologies, it should be possible to define lymphoid infiltrates of the lung that are monotypic and have the characteristics of malignant lymphomas.[92] However, it remains to be seen whether prospective culling of such cases from series of "LIP" will narrow the behavioral spectrum of that disorder. In the past, approximately 5–10% of patients with "LIP" have developed systemic lymphoma with long-term follow-up.[93]

Lymphoid infiltrates in LIP tend to follow the routes of pulmonary lymphatic drainage. Hence, they are centered around blood vessels and tubular airways in a "coat-sleeve" distribution or as nodular groupings[86,94] (Figs 18.19–18.21). In most instances, permeation outward into the alveolar septa is also present. Constituent cells are polymorphous, but they are principally represented by

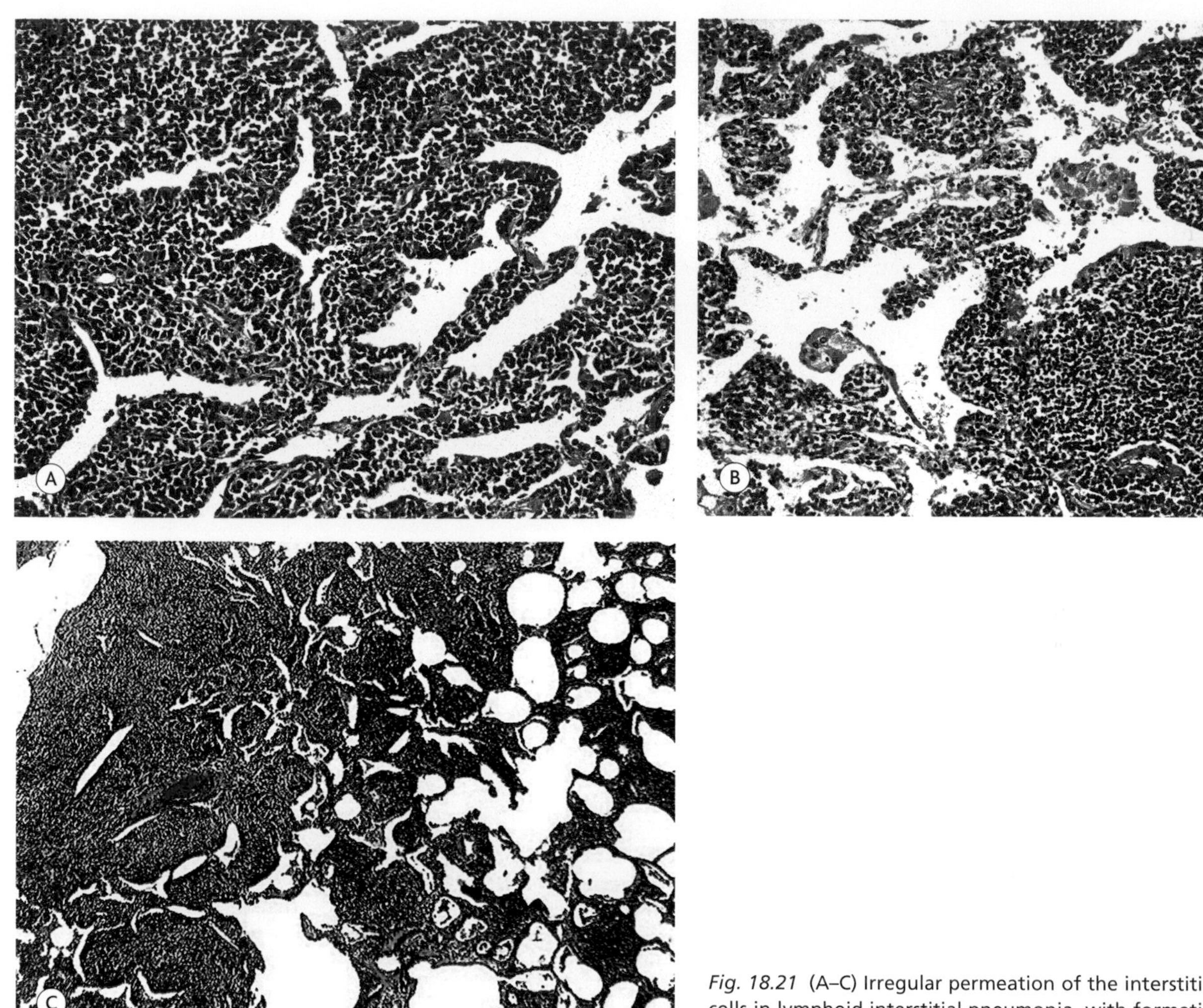

Fig. 18.21 (A–C) Irregular permeation of the interstitium by lymphoid cells in lymphoid interstitial pneumonia, with formation of lymphocytic micronodules. (see Chapter 7 for additional discussion)

Fig. 18.22 The constituent cells of lymphoid interstitial pneumonia are small lymphocytes.

small mature lymphocytes (Fig. 18.22). Transformed cells with larger, more irregular nuclear contours, and immunoblasts are consistently seen as well, together with scattered plasma cells, macrophages, and neutrophils. Germinal centers are apparent in 20–30% of cases, and they are most prominent in those cases where the lymphoid infiltrate is nodular. Unlike neoplastic lymphoid follicles, the germinal centers show a heterogeneous population of immunoblasts and phagocytic "tingible body" macrophages. Their central portions may contain amorphous hyalinized material surrounding blood vessels, analogous to the core structures of hyaline-vascular-type Castleman's disease. Stromal amyloid may also be observed in lymphoid hyperplasia of the lung, as well as epithelioid granulomas. Nevertheless, neither of those features is a reliable discriminator from low-grade lymphoid neoplasia. On the other hand, cellular monomorphism, subendothelial intravascular aggregates of lymphocytes, apoptosis, mitotic activity, and nuclear irregularity indicate the diagnostic likelihood of lymphoma.

As referenced earlier, malignant lymphoproliferative diseases are also characterized by their aberrant immunophenotypes – with monotypism for light-chain immunoglobulins or deletion of pan-B-cell or pan-T-cell cell antigens – or rearrangement of immunoglobulin heavy-chain genes or T-cell receptor genes in molecular studies.[95,96] Frozen tissue is the most suitable substrate for immunohistology or genotypic evaluations. It is best to cryopreserve a representative portion of any pulmonary wedge biopsy if lymphoproliferative disease is considered in the clinical differential diagnosis. If only paraffin-embedded specimens are available, a dominance ($\geq$75%) of $CD20^+$ lymphocytes or coexpression of CD20 and CD43 in the same cells argues in favor of a neoplastic B-cell infiltrate in immunohistochemical analyses.[95,97] Studies for gene rearrangement also may be attempted using paraffin sections and the polymerase chain reaction,[98] but these are substantially less sensitive in detecting monoclonality than comparable evaluations done on fresh tissue (also see Chapter 15 for further discussion).

Several theories have addressed potential causes for pulmonary lymphoid hyperplasia.[66,85,87–90] These have centered on two principal pathogenetic mechanisms – dysregulation of immunity and virally-mediated lymphoproliferation – which are not necessarily mutually exclusive. Many patients with LIP have clinical and serologic evidence of an autoimmune disease.[87] It is similarly notable that genomic segments of the Epstein–Barr virus have been identified in some examples of LIP;[99–101] furthermore, that agent may exert a mitogenic effect together with the human immunodeficiency virus in the setting of AIDS-related LIP.[99] Regardless of whether or not those constructs are valid, they unfortunately have no role in separating LIP from malignant lymphoma because that disease likewise may have an association with autoimmunity or viral infection.[102]

It has been stated repeatedly in the foregoing discussion that the major differential diagnosis for LIP is that of low-grade malignant lymphoma of the bronchus-associated lymphoid tissue (BALT).[82,92] At the risk of reiteration, the immunohistochemical demonstration of lymphoid monotypism or genotypic analysis are the best methods for separation of these disorders with certainty. There are no conventional morphologic features of either disease that allow for definitive identification by themselves.

In selected instances, Castleman's disease (angiofollicular lymph node hyperplasia; ALNH),[103] involves the lungs and could be confused with multinodular LIP histologically. Careful inspection of such cases reveals the prototypical "onion-skinning" of lymphocytes around distorted germinal centers in "hyaline-vascular" ALNH, or sheets of plasma cells in its plasmacellular subtype. Neither of those architectural findings is seen in LIP. Pulmonary Castleman's disease may also be separated from LIP by the integration of Kaposi's sarcoma-associated herpesvirus (human herpesvirus-8) nuclei acid sequences in the former, but not the latter, of those entities, as detected by polymerase chain reaction studies.[104]

Isolated examples of acute viral pneumonia may demonstrate exuberant interstitial lymphoid infiltration. Nevertheless, the clinical context of that disorder – featuring a rapidly evolving course and other symptoms of acute infectious disease – usually facilitates its accurate recognition. It is somewhat more difficult to distinguish LIP from extrinsic allergic alveolitis (hypersensitivity pneumonitis; HP) pathologically, because both of those disorders potentially feature the presence of lymphoid infiltrates and epithelioid granulomas.[105] Typically, clinical data on hypersensitivity to certain fungi and other organic antigens are necessary to identify HP definitively. On the other hand, the presence of histologic bronchiolitis obliterans would indicate a diagnostic likelihood of LIP.

Rosai–Dorfman disease (Sinus histiocytosis with massive lymphadenopathy)

Another form of pseudoneoplastic hematopoietic proliferation may involve the lung: namely, sinus histiocytosis with massive lymphadenopathy (SHML; Rosai–Dorfman disease).[106] It can be seen in either sex and over a wide range of patient ages. Despite the name of this condition, lymphadenopathy does not always coexist with extranodal disease. When it affects the pulmonary parenchyma, this condition appears to have its epicenter in the hilar tissue and follows lymphatics peripherally into both lungs.[106,107] Accordingly, chest radiographs show an accentuation of central bronchovascular markings and bilateral interstitial prominence CT scans (Fig. 18.23) may show areas of pleural-based consolidation. Confluence of the infiltrates may yield mass-like densities in the lung fields as well (Fig. 18.24). In likeness to LIP, clinical evidence of associated immune dysfunction may be apparent in SHML, including autoantibody formation, polyarthritis, immune-complex glomerulonephritis, asthma, and juvenile diabetes mellitus. Fever, night sweats, and weight loss can be seen as well.[106] Justification for the classification of Rosai–Dorfman

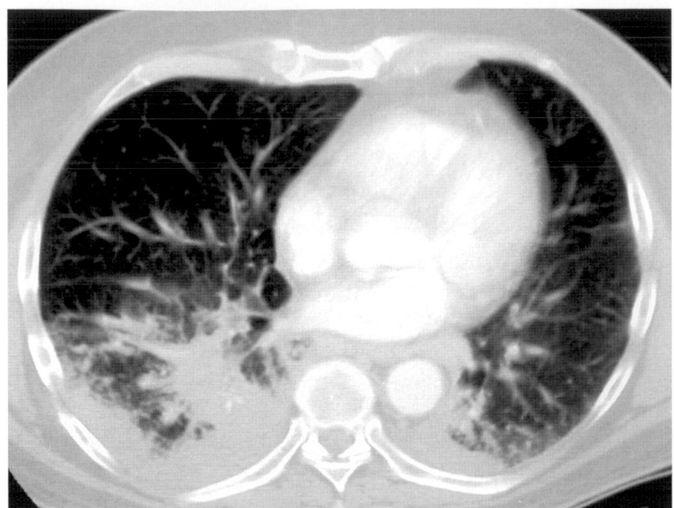

Fig. 18.23 CT scan from a patient with Rosai–Dorfman disease. Note the accentuation of the bronchovascular bundles and pleural-based consolidation.

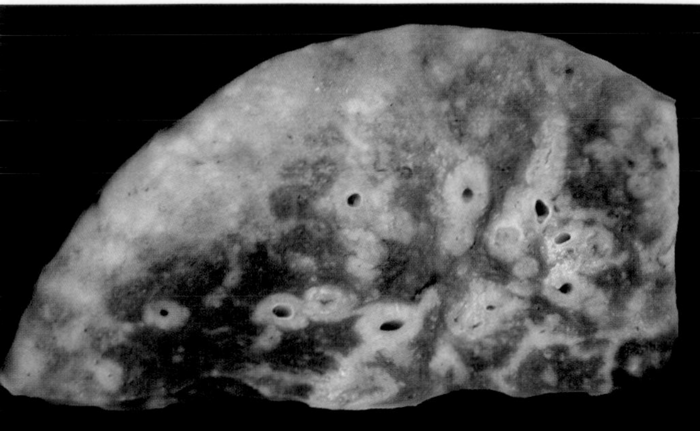

Fig. 18.24 Gross photograph of Rosai–Dorfman disease involving lung (from the patient illustrated in Fig. 18.23).

disease as non-neoplastic comes from molecular data indicating its polyclonal nature.[108]

Pathologic specimens of the lung or lymph nodes in SHML demonstrate comparable morphologic findings. Dilated lymphatic spaces in the pulmonary parenchyma contain large pale histiocytes with abundant amphophilic cytoplasm, surrounded by lymphoid infiltrates that are punctuated by germinal centers and fibrous septa (Figs 18.25 and 18.26). The large histiocytes demonstrate a peculiar tendency to engulf intact, mature lymphocytes, representing a phenomenon known as "lymphemperipolesis" (Fig. 18.27). The overall image of foci of SHML in extranodal sites is therefore reminiscent of abnormal lymph nodes.[106] The immunophenotype of the lesional histiocytes is singular in that it features prominent reactivity for S100 protein (Fig. 18.28) and CD45 in the absence of CD1a. Labeling for CD68, lysozyme, MAC387, and alpha-1-antichymotrypsin may also be observed.

Differential diagnoses in cases of SHML potentially include metastatic carcinoma, metastatic melanoma, large cell non-Hodgkin's lymphoma, and Hodgkin's disease.[106] The large tumor cells in these conditions differ from Rosai–Dorfman disease immunohistologically, in their respective reactivity for keratin, MART-1/melan-A, CD3 or CD20, and CD30. Practically speaking, all of them show a much higher degree of cytologic atypicality than that seen in SHML, and special diagnostic studies are usually not required to make the cited distinctions.

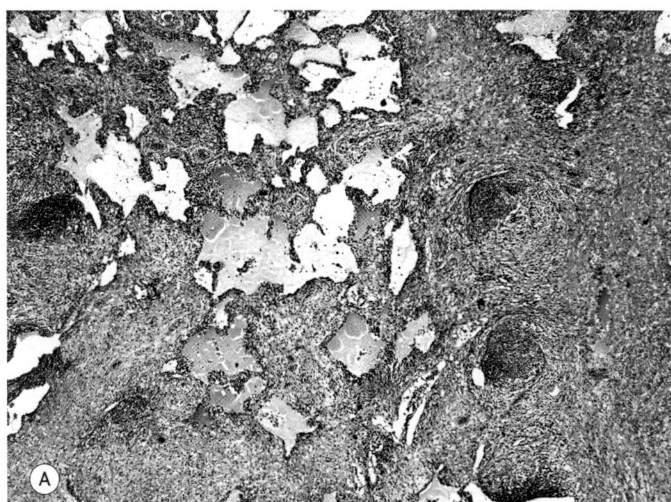

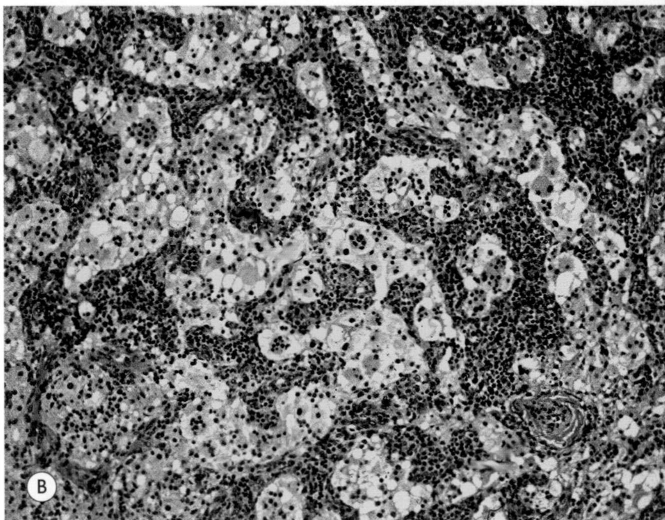

Fig. 18.25 (A) Rosai–Dorfman disease involving the lung showing dense but heterogeneous lymphoid infiltrates with discrete lymphoid aggregates visible. (B) Large pale histiocytes are visible at higher magnification.

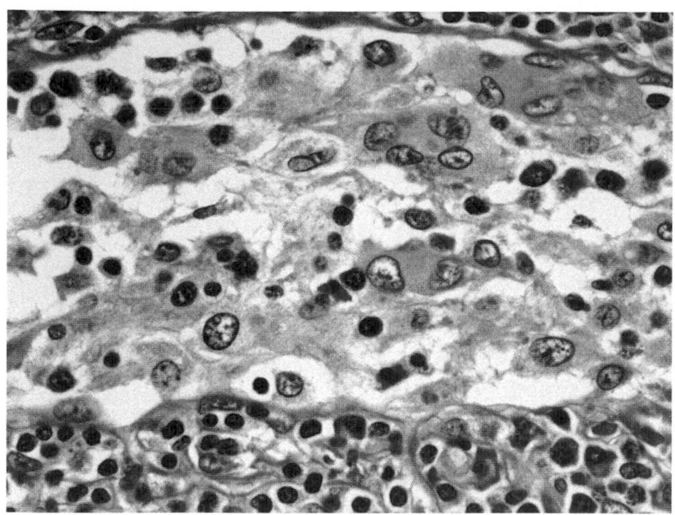

Fig. 18.26 Rosai–Dorfman disease, demonstrating the presence of large pale histiocytic elements amongst a background of small lymphocytes and plasma cells.

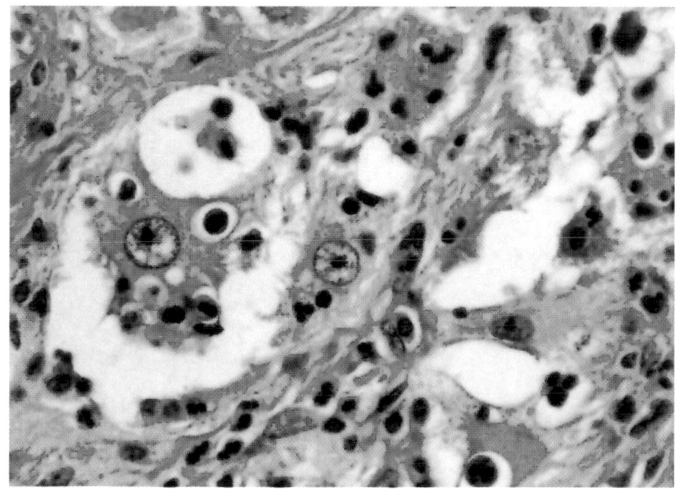

Fig. 18.27 The large cells in Rosai–Dorfman disease contain numerous engulfed lymphocytes ("lymphemperipolesis"); this feature is characteristic of that condition, but may be difficult to identify in the pulmonary manifestation.

The clinical course of Rosai–Dorfman disease is unpredictable. In a comprehensive summary by Foucar et al.,[106] it was noted that patients with more than one site of extranodal disease and obvious immune dysfunction more often suffered significant morbidity and possible mortality from this condition. Spontaneous remissions have been seen as well. Treatment is individualized, with antineoplastic therapy being reserved for those patients with serious organ dysfunction.

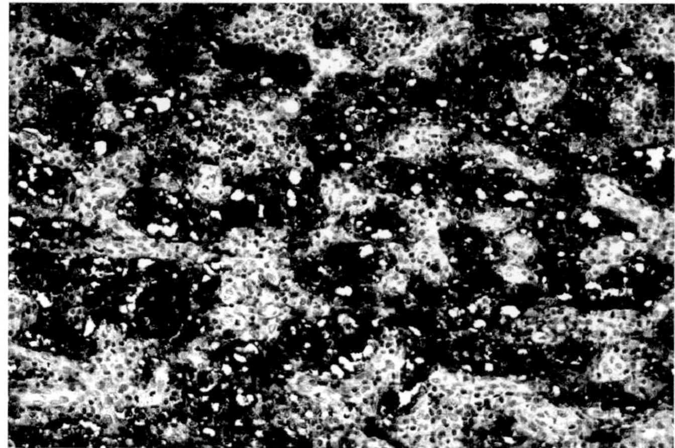

Fig. 18.28 Intense immunoreactivity for S100 protein is seen in the lesional histiocytes of Rosai–Dorfman disease.

Pseudoneoplastic changes as a consequence of lung injury

Exfoliative cytology of the respiratory tract has been used effectively for several decades in the diagnosis of pulmonary disorders.[110] Nonetheless, inherent shortcomings in this method have been well-documented, and some of them relate to the potential for the over-diagnosis of benign reparative or inflammatory conditions in the lungs as neoplastic. The incidence of this eventuality should be $\leq$ 0.25% of all cytologic specimens according to accepted standards.[111] Generally speaking, similar pitfalls accompany the interpretation of small transbronchial biopsy specimens in surgical pathology.

There are several possible reasons for mistakes in the cytologic diagnosis of malignancy in the lung. One may simply misinterpret reparative conditions or inflammatory epithelial atypia as carcinoma, but this should be rare.[112,113] Another potential source of confusion is the shedding or artifactual introduction of malignant cells from the mouth or upper airway into a sputum or bronchial washing specimen.[114,115] Both of these scenarios are troublesome *only* if there are accompanying abnormalities on chest films that might cause clinicians to consider a neoplasm diagnostically. Thus, it is obvious that radiologic data are essential to optimal cytopathologic interpretation.

With that having been said, however, there are some mass lesions that may, under selected circumstances, incite benign but atypical epithelial proliferations in the surrounding lung. Exfoliated cells in those cases may thus be mistaken as carcinomatous. The underlying conditions associated with this trap include symptomatically "occult" pulmonary infarcts, granulomas, and

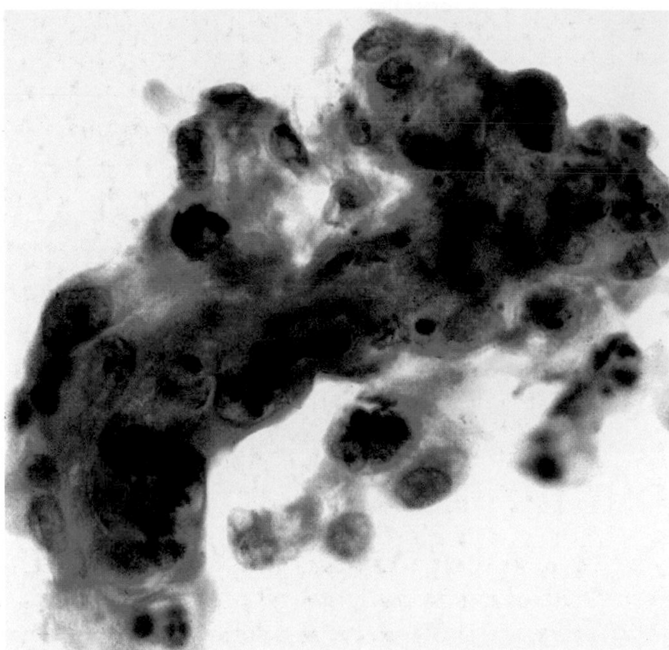

Fig. 18.29 Cytologic specimen from a bronchial brushing biopsy in a case of isolated granuloma of the lung, demonstrating a markedly atypical squamoid cell group with irregular nuclear chromatin and high nuclear-to-cytoplasmic ratios. Although cellular aggregates such as this were ultimately proven to be reactive in nature, they caused marked diagnostic consternation over the possibility of squamous carcinoma.

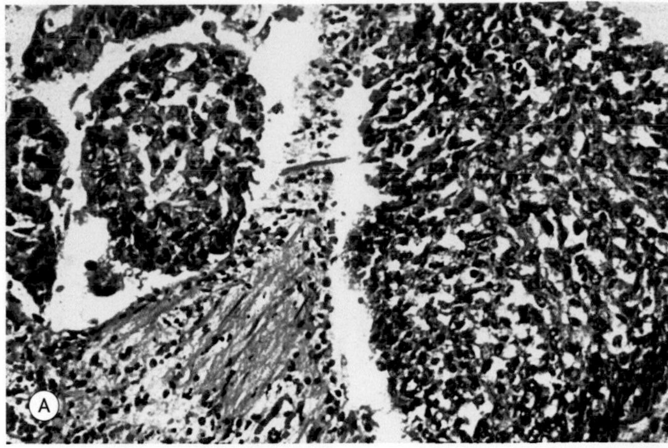

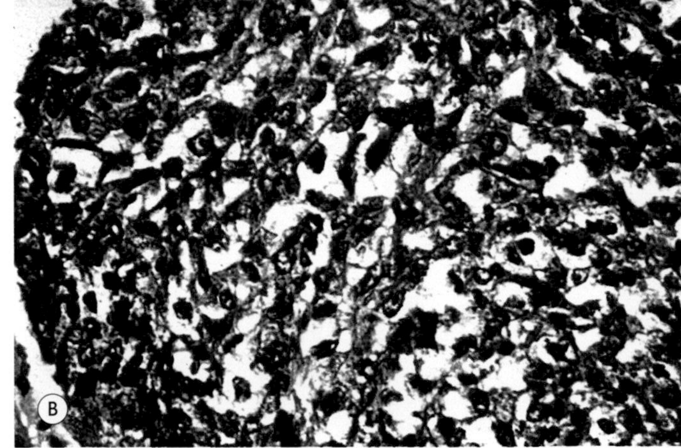

Fig. 18.30 (A,B) Atypical squamous metaplasia adjacent to an intrapulmonary granuloma. Changes such as these account for cytologic findings like those shown in Fig. 18.29.

bronchiectasis with surrounding pneumonia, typically associated with atypical squamous metaplasia in adjacent bronchi[116–122] (Figs 18.29 and 18.30). As expected, a misdiagnosis of squamous carcinoma is the usual error in such instances.

Another more heterogeneous collection of diseases that may imitate *adeno*carcinoma in cytologic samples or small biopsies includes radiation pneumonitis, post-chemotherapy atypia in alveolar lining cells, bronchiectasis, pulmonary infarcts, viral pneumonias of various types, pulmonary vasculitides, lung injury caused by toxic chemicals, non-infectious interstitial pneumonitides, and diffuse alveolar damage[123–130] (Figs 18.31 and 18.32). These conditions are again most misleading in the context of localized radiographic abnormalities in the lungs. Moreover, because of the broad roentgenographic spectrum of such tumors as bronchioloalveolar adenocarcinoma – including an imitation of uncomplicated pneumonia[131] – the study of chest films is, unfortunately, an imperfect safeguard in this specific setting. Stanley et al.[132] have suggested that pseudomalignant glandular pulmonary metaplasias show greater cellular heterogeneity than that seen in true adenocarcinomas. Lower nuclear-to-cytoplasmic ratios, "scalloping" of cell borders, and focal intercellular "windows" in pseudoneoplastic gland-

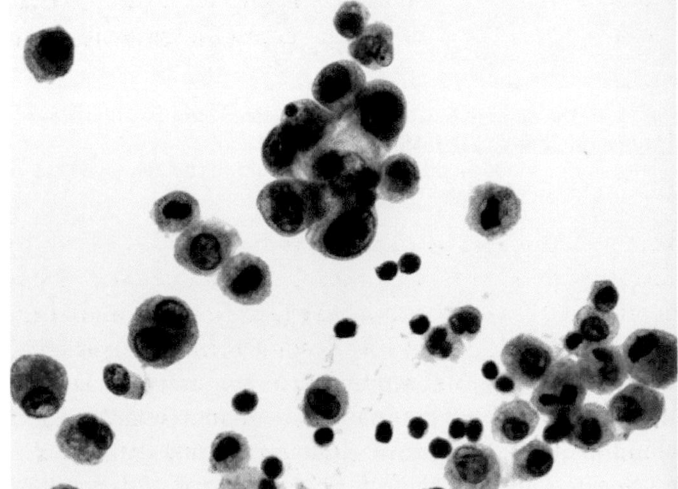

Fig. 18.31 Atypical groups of glandular cells are present in this bronchial washing specimen from a patient who had received chemotherapy for metastatic adenocarcinoma of the pancreas. They were thought to represent secondary involvement of the lung by tumor, ultimately proven to be post-chemotherapy atypia.

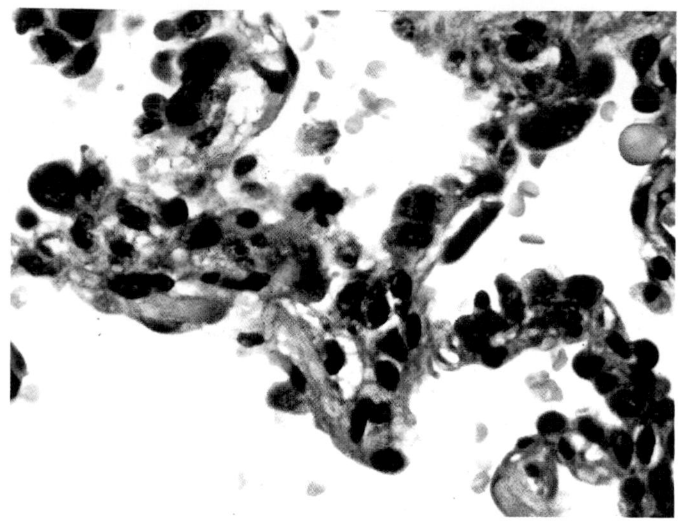

Fig. 18.32 An open biopsy of lung tissue in the case referenced in Fig. 18.31 showed only atypical pneumocytic proliferation, thought to reflect the effects of chemotherapy. This change probably accounted for the abnormal cytologic findings that were observed.

like profiles also typify atypical metaplasias. It is also important to realize that special techniques – such as immunostains for tumor-associated glycoprotein-72 (with the antibody B72.3) – are *not* able to make the distinction in question and may even contribute further to misdiagnosis.[133] Indeed, there are no universally effective methods to avoid mistakes in the cytologic or biopsy diagnosis of pulmonary malignancy. Patients and clinicians should probably be apprised of that reality.

Pseudoneoplastic lesions of the pleural surfaces

Pseudoneoplastic lesions of the pleura comprise a relatively small group. Perhaps the most common of them is principally seen by cytopathologists: namely, mesothelial hyperplasia in pleural effusion specimens. Indeed, cytologic simulators of malignancy encompass such a wide variety of entities that they cannot be addressed completely in this text. We will consider selected aspects of this topic, but for a more complete discussion the reader should consult comprehensive treatises on cytopathology.[134–136]

The microscopic classification of mesothelial lesions can be challenging, both in cytology and surgical pathology. Pertinent problems in this area include the distinction of reactive proliferations from mesothelioma or metastatic carcinoma, and the separation of benign and malignant lymphocytic effusions. Approaches to the last of these topics are identical to techniques discussed above in reference to pulmonary lymphoid lesions, and will not be recounted here.

Reactive mesothelial proliferations

Reactive mesothelial lesions have often been given the descriptive but nebulous label of "atypical mesothelial cell proliferation" in cytologic practice.[137] However, because that terminology implies a possible connection to malignancy, or, at least, premalignancy, we do not advocate its use. Rather, one should simply state that mesothelial cells are hyperplastic or reactive if their morphologic features are clearly benign.[138] Such proliferations are associated with a number of underlying pathologic conditions, including cirrhosis, anemia, viral infections, collagen vascular diseases, radiation-induced pleuritis, reactions to bronchogenic carcinomas or pleural metastases, and a variety of chronic pleural infections.[139] An adequate clinical history is obviously necessary to the accurate interpretation of pleural tissue samples. Cytologic features that favor malignancy include the presence of papillae or other architectural complexities, obvious nuclear atypia, necrosis, and pathologic mitotic figures.[134,140] As outlined by Bedrossian et al.,[141] there are contrasting criteria for the recognition of reactive or hyperplastic mesothelial lesions. They are characterized only by superficial entrapment of mesothelial cell nests in the pleural stroma; an intense inflammatory infiltrate that is densest near the pleural surface; vascular proliferation with few associated spindle cells; an absence of overt nuclear atypia; and a lack of atypical mitoses (Figs 18.33 and 18.34).

Despite an almost-universal reference to cytologic atypia in the literature on mesothelioma, our experience with that tumor type suggests that nuclear aberrations are often unimpressive in it. Conversely, they may be striking in reactive mesothelium.[142] In general, the cytologic criteria associated with malignant mesothelioma include an elevated nucleocytoplasmic ratio, irregularity of the nuclear membranes, and coarsely clumped chromatin.[140] However, even by morphometric evaluation, conflicting results regarding such features have been obtained. Studies by Marchevsky et al.,[143] Kwee and colleagues,[144] and Oberholzer and coworkers[145] all suggested that nuclear morphometry was capable of discriminating between benign and malignant mesothelial

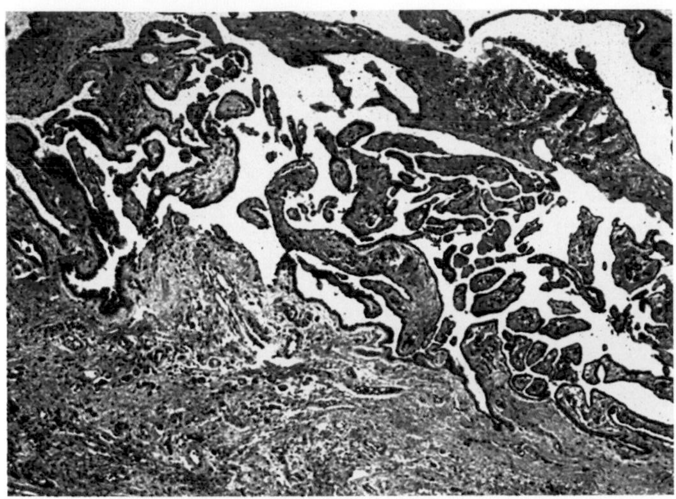

Fig. 18.33 Markedly papillary profiles of proliferative mesothelium are seen on the pleural surface in this patient with lupus erythematosus, who had recurrent pleural effusions. Although this image is worrisome, the lesion was ultimately felt to be reactive in nature.

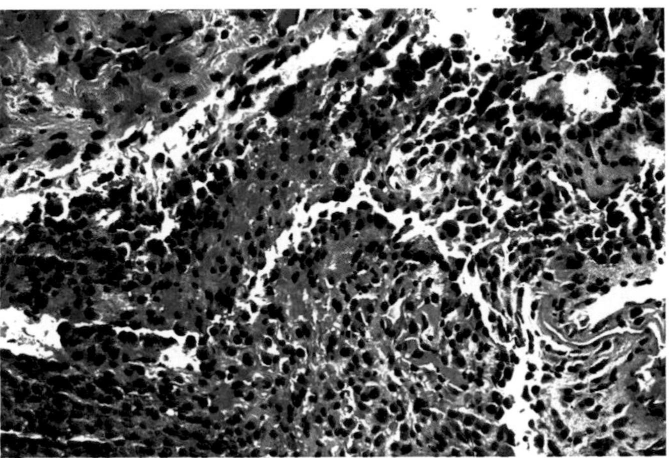

Fig. 18.34 Solid sheets of reactive benign mesothelial cells are admixed with fibrin and inflammation in the case shown in Fig. 18.33. The cytologic features of the mesothelium caused concern over the diagnostic possibility of malignant mesothelioma.

cells. Nonetheless, other evaluations have concluded that the latter technique was *not* useful in that context.[146]

Several attributes of mesothelial cells are potentially shared by both benign and malignant proliferations in cytologic samples. They include cytoplasmic vacuolization, binucleation or multinucleation, and a brush-border pattern that extends over the entire free surface of the cells, correlating with the ultrastructural finding of elongated microvilli.[134,140] Reactive cells generally tend to exfoliate singly or in small groups; on the other hand, large formations, including morular structures with "knobby" cellular outlines or papillary structures, raise the likelihood of mesothelioma.[140,147] A similar comment applies to uniformly dense mesothelial hypercellularity in an effusion specimen. It should also be understood that the comments just offered apply only to epithelial or biphasic subtypes of malignant mesothelioma, because sarcomatoid variants rarely shed into body cavities. If effusions are present in the latter cases, they usually contain only inflammatory cells and reactive but cytologically benign mesothelial cells.[148] The large hypothetical concept of "mesothelioma in situ" has been introduced for putatively malignant but microscopic lesions that are limited to the pleural surface,[149,150] but we regard the distinction of that condition from reactive mesothelial proliferations to be an unsettled area diagnostically.

Immunohistochemistry has limited value in the separation of reactive and malignant mesothelial cells.[151] Some analyses have suggested that purely epithelioid mesotheliomas show dense plasmalemmal labeling for epithelial membrane antigen (EMA) and vimentin,[152] whereas benign mesothelial cells lack both markers. Nevertheless, those determinants have been shared by both pathologic entities in our experience. Both cell types are consistently negative for carcinoembryonic antigen (CEA), tumor-associated glycoprotein-72, and CD15 (all of which are expected in carcinomas), and positive for HBME-1, calretinin, WT-1, and keratin 5/6.[140,153] Although that panel of reactants is useful in distinguishing adenocarcinoma from mesothelioma, it cannot separate benign and malignant mesothelial lesions.

Interest has also arisen regarding the immunostaining of mesothelial lesions for selected gene products that might be correlated with malignancy. In particular, mutant p53 proteins have been assessed in that context, with the expectation that they would be present in malignant mesothelioma but not in benign pleural proliferations.[154,155] In fact, when they are immunoreactive for p53 protein, reactive mesothelia usually shows weak nuclear labeling or both cytoplasmic and nuclear staining that should raise suspicion of a spurious result.[155] In contrast, mesotheliomas can exhibit convincing and intense nuclear positivity, but up to 40% are completely nonreactive for p53.[154] Although it may provide adjunctive diagnostic information, we believe that p53 protein immunotyping should not be used in isolation. It must be integrated with morphologic findings as well as radiographic details.

In view of the poor outcome of most mesothelioma cases and the limited therapy for that tumor type, diagnostic circumspection is appropriate in this specific context. It would be very undesirable to label a patient with a reactive proliferation as having a mesothelioma, and, with the passage of time, true examples of that tumor will declare themselves clinicopathologically.

Regarding the distinction of reactive mesothelium from metastatic carcinoma, one has the advantage of much more clear-cut criteria.[141] Carcinomatous effusions often feature a distinctly dimorphic cellular population, although this may be subtle in cases of mammary or gastric cancers.[134] Immunohistologic differences have been outlined above. Periodic acid–Schiff stains, performed with and without diastase digestion, will label neutral mucins in at least 50% of metastatic adenocarcinomas but not in mesothelial proliferations. Some intracytoplasmic vacuoles in mesothelial cells also contain hyaluronic acid that may stain with the Alcian blue method at pH 2.5; it is digestible with hyaluronidase. Such inclusions may show weak cross-reactivity with mucicarmine stains, potentially causing a mistaken diagnosis of carcinoma; however, spurious mucicarmine staining again disappears after hyaluronidase treatment, unlike the pattern of adenocarcinoma.

Hyaline pleural plaques

Hyaline pleural plaques (HPP) are important because of their value as markers of occupational-level dust exposure (Fig. 18.35). Moreover, they occasionally may simulate the radiographic and pathologic appearances of selected mesothelial neoplasms or metastases of malignant tumors in the pleural space.

Many studies have linked asbestos exposure to the emergence of fibrohyaline plaques (Fig. 18.36).[156–162] There is also a variable but generally low incidence of these lesions in routine necropsies. Asbestos fibers are absent in the plaques themselves, and, if present, are seen only in the subjacent pulmonary parenchyma. Publications by Churg[156] and others[157-162] have found that there is an increase in commercial-type amphibole asbestos content in the lungs in most patients with HPPs. The number of fibers is above that seen in the "background" population, but less than the number found in individuals with asbestosis. The foregoing comments best apply to those individuals with *bilateral* pleural plaques. Unilateral plaques may develop as a consequence of chronic pleural irritation of any type; they are commonly associated with infections such as tuberculosis or empyema, chronic or recurrent pleural hemorrhage, and chest wall trauma.[161]

HPPs are most often detected after the age of 50 years, and males predominate. Those lesions associated with occupational asbestos exposure show an average latency of ≥20 years from the time of initial dust inhalation.[161,162] HPPs characteristically arise in the lower thorax (especially the diaphragm) and preferentially involve the parietal pleura, often with a parallel orientation to the ribs. Much less commonly, they may affect the pericardial surfaces as well.[157] Individuals with HPPs lack symptoms

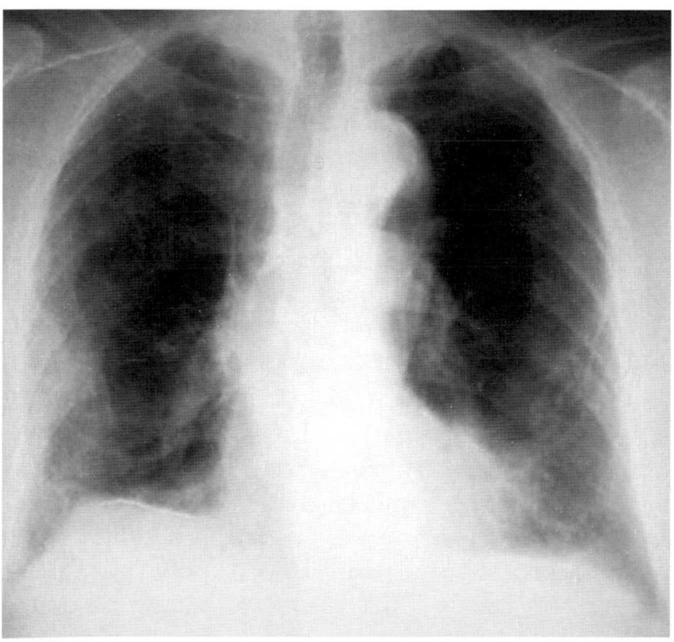

Fig. 18.35 This posteroanterior chest film demonstrates a large nodular mass in the right basal pleura, with linear internal calcification. It represents a pseudotumoral fibrohyaline pleural plaque in a patient with occupational-level asbestos exposure.

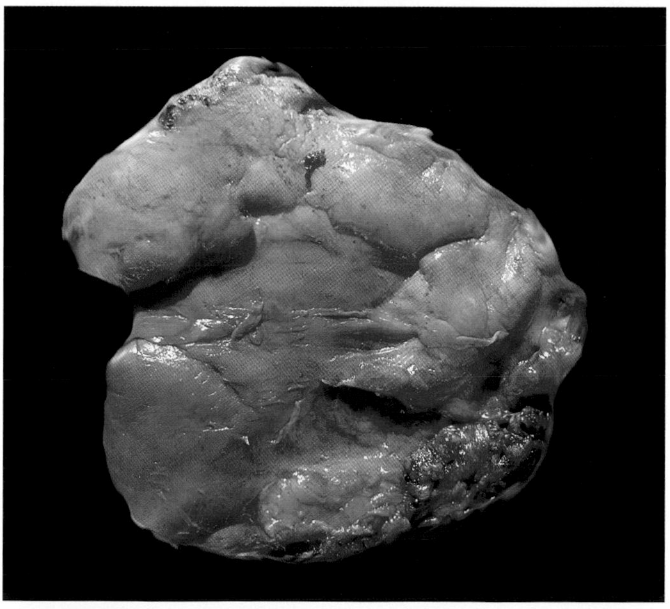

Fig. 18.36 Gross image of fibrohyaline pleural plaques, represented by well-demarcated sessile white-yellow excrescences.

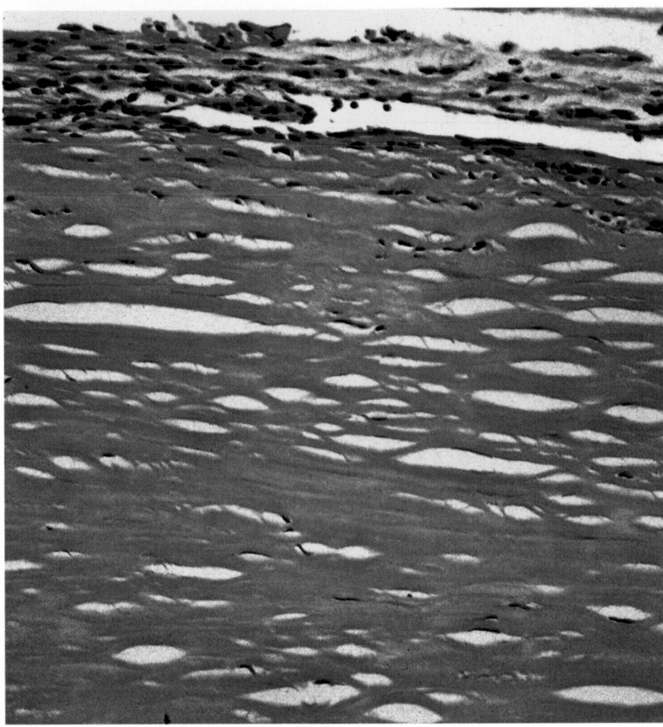

Fig. 18.37 Photomicrograph of fibrohyaline pleural plaque, showing a "basket-weave" configuration of laminated, markedly hypocellular, mature collagen. The surface of the plaque contains chronic inflammatory cells.

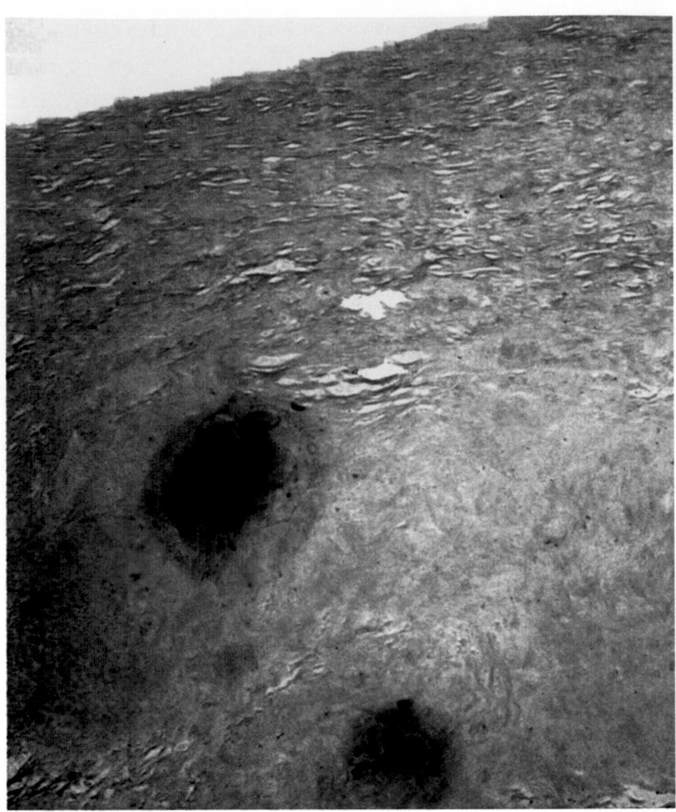

Fig. 18.38 Another example of fibrohyaline pleural plaque, containing internal foci of dystrophic calcification.

that are directly related to the plaques themselves, and they are regarded as tissue reactions rather than a true disease process. Most associated pulmonary function abnormalities are due to accompanying emphysema or interstitial lung disease.[156] Plain films have limited sensitivity for the detection of uncomplicated HPPs, but that statistic increases markedly if the plaques are calcified. The use of CT has greatly improved the ease with which these lesions are recognized.[163]

The typical pattern of HPP features hypocellular, dense bundles of hyalinized collagen, often with a "basket-weave" arrangement[161] (Fig. 18.37). Chronic inflammation may be present in and around the lesion and, in some cases, acute inflammation or fibrin deposition may be seen on the pleural surface. Those changes likely reflect the proposed mechanism of formation of the lesion: namely, that of recurrent and organizing pleuritis. Dystrophic calcification is often evident pathologically (Fig. 18.38).

The main pathologic diagnostic alternative in cases of HPP is that of desmoplastic mesothelioma (DM). That tumor shares many of the microscopic characteristics of HPP; both are composed of relatively bland cells that are separated by dense bands of collagen. Nonetheless, there is greater cellularity in DM, at least focally, with areas of storiform growth and a greater degree of nuclear pleomorphism.[164] Necrosis is also possible in mesothelioma but does not occur in HPP. Involvement of the visceral pleura or diffuse effacement of the pleural space are features usually associated with DM, and they argue against an interpretation of HPP. Adjunctive studies are of very little use in this context. Immunoreactivity for mutant p53 protein does show a preference to occur in DM, but is not restricted to that lesion.[165] Furthermore, a substantial portion of DM cases are completely p53-negative, mirroring the expected immunophenotype of HPP.

Although some solitary fibrous tumors of the pleura (SFTs) may contain keloidal collagen like that seen in HPPs,[166] they show much greater cellularity and a dissimilar histologic pattern overall. Furthermore, SFT typically presents as a localized, polypoid intrapleural mass, rather than a sessile plaque, and it has no causal relationship to asbestos exposure.

There is no indication for surgical removal of HPPs, except in those rare cases where their radiologic images cause clinical concern over a possible diagnosis of

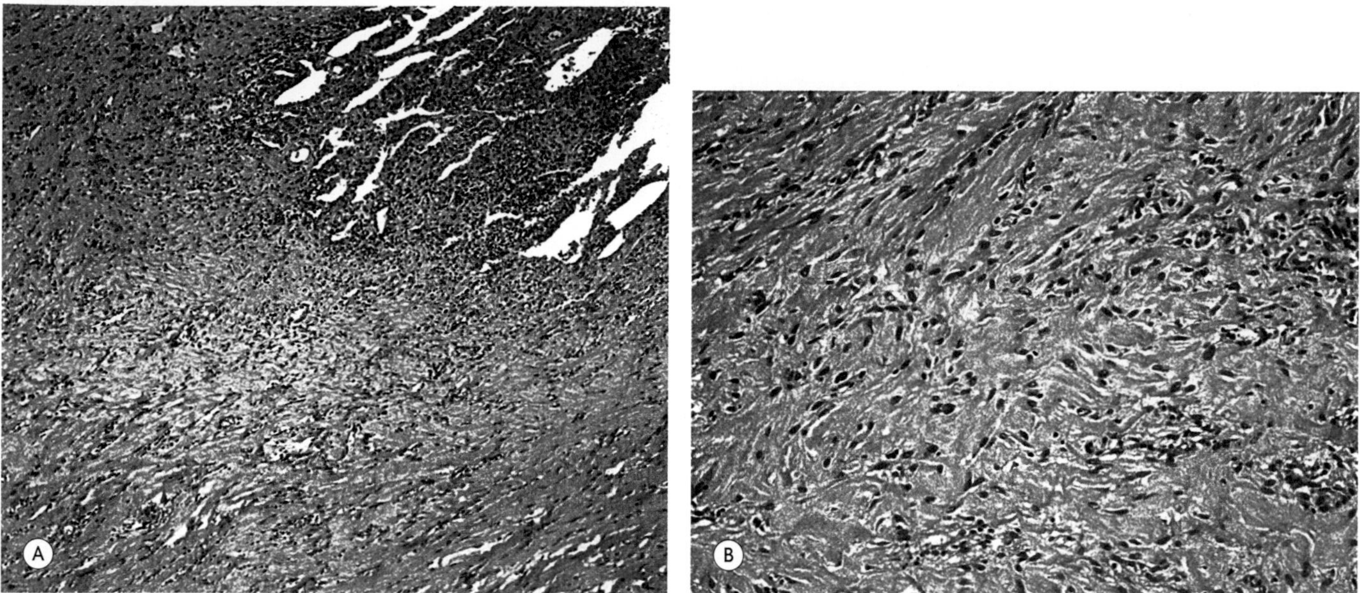

Fig. 18.39 (A,B) Diffuse pleural fibrosis, showing a disorganized deposition of hypocellular, fully mature collagen in the visceral pleura.

malignancy. Their possible relationship to bronchogenic carcinoma or mesothelioma has been examined, as reviewed elsewhere.[167] The plaques themselves appear not to be precursor lesions for malignancies, but are simple markers of dust exposure.

Diffuse pleural fibrosis

A related pathologic process is that of diffuse pleural fibrosis (DPF). It may be associated with connective tissue disorders such as lupus erythematosus or rheumatoid arthritis, as well as chronic infections; however, as true of HPPs, there is a link to occupational asbestos exposure in some cases.[168–170] DPF often involves the visceral pleura and there may be apical fibrous "capping" analogous to that seen in association with bullous emphysema. In extreme cases, obliteration of the pleural space may eventuate.

Microscopically, DPF is characterized by the deposition of bland, hypocellular fibrous tissue in the pleura, without the basket-weave pattern of hyaline plaques (Fig. 18.39). The subjacent tissue may demonstrate hypervascularity and scattered foci of chronic inflammation containing plasma cells, lymphocytes, and histiocytes (Fig. 18.40). Associated exudate may be apparent on the luminal pleural surface. Differential diagnosis again centers on the exclusion of a DM. The clinicopathologic similarities of that tumor and DPF are even closer than the likenesses between DM and HPP, because both DM and DPF have the ability to encase the lung in a "rind" of tissue.[165] Once more, however, DPF lacks the level of cellularity, nuclear atypia, potential necrosis, and invasive growth of mesothelioma. Special studies are generally noncontributory to this diagnostic separation.

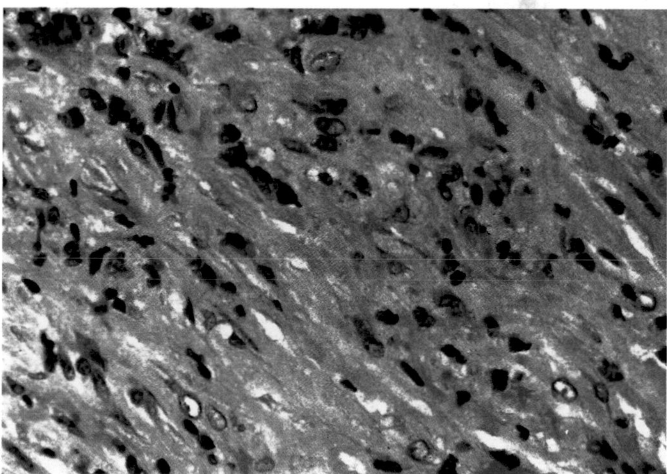

Fig. 18.40 Diffuse pleural fibrosis, demonstrating a scant admixture of lymphocytes and plasma cells in the mature collagen.

REFERENCES

1. Koss MN: Unusual tumor-like conditions of the lung. Adv Pathol Lab Med 1994; 7: 123–150.
2. Su LD, Atayde-Perez A, Sheldon S, Fletcher JA, Weiss SW: Inflammatory myofibroblastic tumor: cytogenetic evidence supporting clonal origin. Mod Pathol 1998; 11: 364–368.
3. Coffin CM, Dehner LP, Meis-Kindblom JM: Inflammatory myofibroblastic tumor, inflammatory fibrosarcoma, and related

lesions: an historical review with differential diagnostic considerations. Semin Diagn Pathol 1998; 15: 102–110.
4. Albrecht E: Uber Harmartome. Verh Dtsch Ges Pathol 1904; 7: 153–157.
5. Takeshima Y, Furukawa K, Inai K: Adenomyomatous hamartoma of the lung. Pathol Int 2000; 50: 984–986.
6. McDonald JR, Harrington SW, Clagett OT: Hamartoma (often called chondroma) of the lung. J Thorac Cardiovasc Surg 1945; 14: 128–143.
7. Tomashefski JF Jr: Benign endobronchial mesenchymal tumors: their relationship to parenchymal pulmonary hamartomas. Am J Surg Pathol 1982; 6: 531–540.
8. Koutras P, Urschel HC, Paulson DL: Hamartoma of the lung. J Thorac Cardiovasc Surg 1971; 61: 768–776.
9. Cosio BG, Villena V, Echave-Sustaeta J, et al.: Endobronchial hamartoma. Chest 2002; 122: 202–205.
10. Ge F, Tong F, Li Z: Diagnosis and treatment of pulmonary hamartoma. Chin Med J 1998; 13: 61–62.
11. Carney JA: The triad of gastric epithelioid leiomyosarcoma, functioning extra-adrenal paraganglioma, and pulmonary chondroma. Cancer 1979; 43: 374–382.
12. Wick MR, Ruebner BH, Carney JA: Gastric tumors in patients with pulmonary chondroma or extra-adrenal paraganglioma: an ultrastructural study. Arch Pathol Lab Med 1981; 105: 527–531.
13. Higashita R, Ichikawa S, Ban T, et al.: Coexistence of lung cancer and hamartoma. Jpn J Thorac Cardiovasc Surg 2001; 49: 258–260.
14. Aggarwal P, Handa R, Wali JP, Wig N, Biswas A: Pulmonary hamartoma in a patient with testicular seminoma. J Assoc Physicians India 1999; 47: 552–553.
15. Van Den Bosch JMM, Wagenaar SS, Corrin B, et al.: Mesenchymoma of the lung (so called hamartoma): a review of 154 parenchymal and endobronchial cases. Thorax 1987; 42: 790–793.
16. Salminen US: Pulmonary hamartoma: a clinical study of 77 cases in a 21 year period and review of the literature. Eur J Cardiothorac Surg 1990; 4: 15–18.
17. Hansen CP, Holtveg H, Francis D, Raasch L, Bertelsen S: Pulmonary hamartoma. J Thorac Cardiovasc Surg 1992; 104: 674–678.
18. Wang SC: Lung hamartoma: a report of 30 cases and review of 477 cases. Chung Hua Wai Ko Tsa Chih 1992; 30: 540–542.
19. Tomiyasu M, Yoshino I, Suemitsu R, Shoji F, Sugimachi K: An intrapulmonary chondromatous hamartoma penetrating the visceral pleura: report of a case. Ann Thorac Cardiovasc Surg 2002; 8: 42–44.
20. Xu R, Murray M, Jagirdar J, Delgado Y, Melamed J: Placental transmogrification of the lung is a histologic pattern frequently associated with pulmonary fibrochondromatous hamartoma. Arch Pathol Lab Med 2002; 126: 562–566.
21. Azua-Blanco J, Azua-Romeo J, Ortego J, Perez-Cacho MJ: Cytologic features of pulmonary hamartoma: report of a case diagnosed by fine needle aspiration cytology. Acta Cytol 2001; 45: 267–270.
22. Hamper UM, Khouri NF, Stitik FP, Siegelman SS: Pulmonary hamartoma: diagnosis by transthoracic needle aspiration biopsy. Radiology 1985; 155: 15–18.
23. Incze JS, Lui PS: Morphology of the epithelial component of human lung hamartomas. Hum Pathol 1977; 8: 411–419.
24. Stone FJ, Churg AM: The ultrastructure of pulmonary hamartoma. Cancer 1977; 39: 1064–1070.
25. Perez-Atayde AR, Seiler MW: Pulmonary hamartoma: an ultrastructural study. Cancer 1984; 53: 485–492.
26. Johansson M, Dietrich C, Mandahl N, et al.: Recombinations of chromosomal bands 6p21 and 14q24 characterize pulmonary hamartomas. Br J Cancer 1993; 67: 1236–1241.
27. Fletcher JA, Pinkus GS, Donovan K, et al.: Clonal rearrangement of chromosome band 6p21 in the mesenchymal component of pulmonary chondroid hamartoma. Cancer Res 1992; 52: 6224–6228.
28. Rogalla P, Lemke I, Kazmierczak B, Bullerdiek J: An identical HMGIC-LPP fusion transcript is consistently expressed in pulmonary chondroid hamartomas with t(3;12)(q27-28;q14-15). Genes Chromosomes Cancer 2000; 29: 363–366.
29. Kazmierczak B, Meyer-Bolte K, Tran KH, et al.: A high frequency of tumors with rearrangements of genes and the HMGI(Y) family in a series of 191 pulmonary chondroid hamartomas. Genes Chromosomes Cancer 1999; 26: 125–133.
30. Yilmaz A, Rush DS, Soslow RA: Endometrial stromal sarcomas with unusual histologic features: a report of 24 primary and metastatic tumors emphasizing fibroblastic and smooth muscle differentiation. Am J Surg Pathol 2002; 26: 1142–1150.
31. Erasmus JJ, Connolly JE, McAdams HP, Roggli VL: Solitary pulmonary nodules: Part I. Morphologic evaluation for differentiation of benign and malignant lesions. Radiographics 2000; 20: 43–58.
32. Chell SE, Nayar R, De Frias DV, Bedrossian CW: Metaplastic breast carcinoma metastatic to lung mimicking a primary chondroid lesion: report of a case with cytohistologic correlation. Ann Diagn Pathol 1998; 2: 173–180.
33. Nappi O, Glasner SD, Swanson PE, Wick MR: Biphasic and monophasic sarcomatoid carcinomas of the lung. Am J Clin Pathol 1994; 102: 331–340.
34. Landreneau RJ, Hazelrigg SR, Ferson PF, et al.: Thoracoscopic resection of 85 pulmonary lesions. Ann Thorac Surg 1992; 54: 415–420.
35. Nakano M, Fukuda M, Sasayama K, et al.: Nd–YAG laser treatment for central airway lesions. Nippon Kyoubu Shikkan Gakkai Zasshi 1992; 30: 1007–1015.
36. Spencer H: The pulmonary plasma cell/histiocytoma complex. Histopathology 1984; 8: 903–916.
37. Matsubara O, Tan-Liu NS, Kenney RM, Mark EJ: Inflammatory pseudotumors of the lung: progression from organizing pneumonia to fibrous histiocytoma or to plasma cell granuloma in 32 cases. Hum Pathol 1988; 19: 807–814.
38. Pettinato G, Manivel JC, Rosa ND, Dehner LP: Inflammatory myofibroblastic tumor (plasma cell granuloma): clinicopathologic study of 20 cases with immunohistochemical and ultrastructural observations. Am J Clin Pathol 1990; 94: 538–546.
39. Cavazza Gelli MC, Agostini L, et al.: Calcified pseudotumor of the pleura: description of a case. Pathologica 2002; 94: 201–205.
40. Fetsch JF, Montgomery EA, Meis JM: Calcifying fibrous pseudotumor. Am J Surg Pathol 1993; 17: 502–508.
41. Pinkard NB, Wilson RW, Lawless N, et al.: Calcifying fibrous pseudotumor of the pleura: a report of three cases of a newly described entity involving the pleura. Am J Clin Pathol 1996; 105: 189–194.
42. Pomplun S, Goldstraw P, Davies SE, Burke MM, Nicholson AG: Calcifying fibrous pseudotumor arising within an inflammatory pseudotumor: evidence of progression from one lesion to the other? Histopathology 2000; 37: 380–382.
43. Nascimento AF, Ruiz R, Hornick JL, Fletcher CDM: Calcifying fibrous "pseudotumor:" clinicopathologic study of 15 cases and analysis of its relationship to inflammatory myofibroblastic tumor. Int J Surg Pathol 2002; 10: 189–196.
44. Bahadori M, Liebow AA: Plasma cell granulomas of the lung. Cancer 1973; 31: 191–208.
45. Anthony PP: Inflammatory pseudotumor (plasma cell granuloma) of lung, liver, and other organs. Histopathology 1993; 23: 501–503.
46. Ahn JM, Kim WS, Yeon KM, et al.: Plasma cell granuloma involving the tracheobronchial angle in a child: a case report. Pediatr Radiol 1995; 25: 204–205.
47. Copin MC, Gosselin BH, Ribet ME: Plasma cell granuloma of the lung: difficulties in diagnosis and prognosis. Ann Thorac Surg 1996; 61: 1477–1482.
48. Mas Estelles F, Andres V, Vallcanera A, Muro D, Cortina H: Plasma cell granuloma of the lung in childhood: atypical radiologic findings and association with hypertrophic osteoarthropathy. Pediatr Radiol 1995; 25: 369–372.
49. Monzon CM, Gilchrist GS, Burgert EO, et al.: Plasma cell granuloma of the lung in children. Pediatrics 1982; 70: 268–274.
50. Tomita T, Dixon A, Watanabe I, Mantz F, Richany S: Sclerosing vascular variant of plasma cell granuloma. Hum Pathol 1980; 11: 197–202.
51. Toccanier MF, Exquis B, Groebli Y: Granulome plasmocytaire du poumon. Neuf observations avec etude immunohistochemique. Ann Pathol 1982; 2: 21–28.
52. Mohsenifar Z, Bein ME, Mott LJM, Tashkin DP: Cystic organizing pneumonia with elements of plasma cell granuloma. Arch Pathol Lab Med 1979; 103; 600–601.
53. Cerfolio RJ, Allen MS, Nascimento AG, et al.: Inflammatory pseudotumors of the lung. Ann Thorac Surg 1999; 67: 933–936.
54. Agrons GA, Rosado-de-Christenson ML, Kirejczyk WM, Conran RM, Stocker JT: Pulmonary inflammatory pseudotumor: radiologic features. Radiology 1998; 206: 511–518.
55. Park SH, Choe GY, Kim CW, Chi JG, Sung SH: Inflammatory pseudotumor of the lung in a child with *Mycoplasma* pneumonia. J Korean Med Sci 1990; 5: 213–223.

56. Harjula A, Mattila S, Kyoesola K, Heikkilae L, Maekinen J: Plasma cell granuloma of lung and pleura. Scand J Thorac Cardiovasc Surg 1986; 20: 119–121.
57. Loo KT, Seneviratne S, Chan JKC: Mycobacterial infection mimicking inflammatory pseudotumor of the lung. Histopathology 1989; 14: 217–219.
58. Kim I, Kim WS, Yeon KM, Chi JG: Inflammatory pseudotumor of the lung manifesting as a posterior mediastinal mass. Ped Radiol 1992; 22: 467–468.
59. Kuhr H, Svane S: Pulmonary pseudotumor caused by *Cryptococcus neoformans*. Tidsskr Norweg Laegeforen 1991; 111: 3288–3290.
60. Bishopric GA, D'Agay MF, Schlemmer B, Sarfati E, Brocheriou C: Pulmonary pseudotumor due to *Corynebacterium equi* in a patient with the acquired immunodeficiency syndrome. Thorax 1988; 43: 486–487.
61. Yanagisawa K, Traquina DN: Inflammatory pseudotumor: an unusual case of recurrent pneumonia in childhood. Int J Ped Otorhinolaryngol 1993; 25: 261–268.
62. Freschi P, Pocecco M, Carini C, Silvestri F, Alcaro P: Pseudotumor inflammatorio polmonare post-traumatico: descrizione di un caso. Ped Med e Chir 1989; 11: 93–96.
63. Roikjaer O, Thomsen JK: Plasmacytoma of the lung. Cancer 1986; 58: 2671–2674.
64. Weiss LM, Yousem SA, Warnke RA: Non-Hodgkin's lymphomas of the lung. Am J Surg Pathol 1985; 9: 480–490.
65. Toh HC, Ang PT: Primary pulmonary lymphoma – clinical review from a single institution in Singapore. Leuk Lymphoma 1997; 27: 153–163.
66. Kradin RL, Mark EJ: Benign lymphoid disorders of the lung with a theory regarding their development. Hum Pathol 1983; 14: 857–867.
67. Michal M, Mukensnabl P: Epithelial plasma cell granuloma-like tumors of the lungs: a hitherto-unrecognized tumor. Pathol Res Pract 2002; 198: 311–316.
68. Wick MR, Ritter JH, Nappi O: Inflammatory sarcomatoid carcinoma of the lung: report of three cases and comparison with inflammatory pseudotumors in adult patients. Hum Pathol 1995; 26: 1014–1021.
69. Yousem SA, Hochholzer L: Pulmonary hyalinizing granuloma. Am J Clin Pathol 1987; 87: 1–6.
70. Alvarez-Fernandez E, Carretero-Albinana L, Menarguez-Palance J: Sclerosing hemangioma of the lung: an immunohistochemical study of intermediate filaments and endothelial markers. Arch Pathol Lab Med 1989; 113: 121–124.
71. Illei PB, Rosai J, Klimstra DS: Expression of thyroid transcription factor-1 and other markers in sclerosing hemangioma of the lung. Arch Pathol Lab Med 2001; 125: 1335–1339.
72. Ledet SC, Brown RW, Cagle PT: p53 immunoreactivity in the differentiation of inflammatory pseudotumor from sarcoma involving the lung. Mod Pathol 1995; 8: 282–286.
73. Doski JJ, Priebe CJ Jr, Driessnack M, et al.: Corticosteroids in the management of unresected plasma cell granuloma (inflammatory pseudotumor) of the lung. J Ped Surg 1991; 26: 1064–1066.
74. Umeki S: A case of plasma cell granuloma which resolved after steroid therapy. Nippon Kyoubu Shikkan Gakkai Zasshi 1993; 31: 123–126.
75. Imperato JP, Folkman J, Sagerman RH, Cassady JR: Treatment of plasma cell granuloma of the lung with radiation therapy: a report of two cases and a review of the literature. Cancer 1986; 57: 2127–2129.
76. Wood C, Nickoloff BJ, Todes-Taylor NR: Pseudotumor resulting from atypical mycobacterial infection: a "histoid" variety of *Mycobacterium avium-intracellulare* complex infection. Am J Clin Pathol 1985; 83: 524–527.
77. Brandwein M, Choid HSH, Strauchen J, Stoler M, Jagirdar J: Spindle cell reaction to nontuberculous mycobacteriosis in AIDS mimicking a spindle cell neoplasm: evidence for dual histiocytic and fibroblast-like characteristics of the cells. Virchows Arch Pathol Anat 1990; 416: 281–286.
78. Chen KTK: Mycobacterial spindle cell pseudotumor of lymph nodes. Am J Surg Pathol 1992; 16: 276–281.
79. Wade HW: The histoid variety of lepromatous leprosy. Int Lepr 1963; 31: 129–142.
80. Triscott JA, Nappi O, Ferrara G, Wick MR: "Pseudoneoplastic" leprosy. Histoid leprosy revisited. Am J Dermatopathol 1995; 17: 297–302.
81. Sekosan M, Cleto M, Senseng C, Farolan M, Sekosan J: Spindle cell pseudotumors in the lungs due to *Mycobacterium tuberculosis* in a transplant patient. Am J Surg Pathol 1992; 18: 1065–1068.
82. Umlas J, Federman M, Crawford C, O'Hara BAC, Fitzgibbons JF, Modeste A: Spindle cell pseudotumor due to *Mycobacterium avium-intracellulare* in patients with acquired immunodeficiency syndrome (AIDS): positive staining of mycobacteria for cytoskeletal filaments. Am J Surg Pathol 1991; 15: 1181–1187.
83. Poletti V, Kitaichi M: Facts and controversies in the classification of idiopathic interstitial pneumonias. Sarcoidosis Vasc Diffuse Lung Dis 2000; 17; 229–238.
84. Isaacson PG, Spencer J: Malignant lymphoma of mucosa-associated lymphoid tissue. Histopathology 1987; 11: 445–462.
85. Addis BJ, Hyjek E, Isaacson PG: Primary pulmonary lymphoma: a reappraisal of its histogenesis and its relationship to pseudolymphoma and lymphoid interstitial pneumonia. Histopathology 1988; 13; 1–7.
86. Koss MN: Lymphoproliferative disorders of the lung. In: Surgical pathology of lung neoplasms, Marchevsky AM, Ed. 1990, Marcel Dekker, New York, pp. 433–486.
87. Koss MN, Hochholzer L, Langloss JM, Wehunt WD, Lazarus AA: Lymphoid interstitial pneumonia: clinicopathological and immunopathological findings in 18 cases. Pathology 1987; 19: 178–185.
88. Morris JC, Rosen MJ, Marchevsky AM, Teirstein AS: Lymphocytic interstitial pneumonia in patients at risk for the acquired immune deficiency syndrome. Chest 1987; 91: 63–67.
89. Strimlan CV, Rosenow EC III, Divertie MB, Harrison EG Jr: Pulmonary manifestations of Sjogren's syndrome. Chest 1976; 70: 354–361.
90. Liebow AA, Carrington CB: Diffuse pulmonary lymphoreticular infiltrations association with dysproteinemia. Med Clin North Am 1973; 57: 809–843.
91. Vath RR, Alexander CB, Fulmer JD: The lymphocytic infiltrative lung diseases. Clin Chest Med 1982; 3: 619–634.
92. Salhany KE, Pietra GG: Extranodal lymphoid disorders. Am J Clin Pathol 1993; 99: 472–485.
93. Banerjee D, Dildar A: Malignant lymphomas complicating lymphoid interstitial pneumonia. Hum Pathol 1982; 13: 780–782.
94. Koss MN, Hochholzer L, Nichols PW, Wehunt WD, Lazarus AA: Primary non-Hodgkin's lymphomas and pseudolymphomas of the lung: a study of 161 patients. Hum Pathol 1983; 14: 1024–1038.
95. Begueret H, Vergier B, Parrens M, et al.: Primary lung small B-cell lymphoma versus lymphoid hyperplasia: evaluation of diagnostic criteria in 26 cases. Am J Surg Pathol 2002; 26: 76–81.
96. Philippe B, Delfau-Larue MH, Epardeau B, et al.: B-cell pulmonary lymphoma: gene rearrangement analysis of bronchoalveolar lymphocytes by polymerase chain reaction. Chest 1999; 115: 1242–1247.
97. Ritter JH, Adesokan PN, Fitzgibbon JF, Wick MR: Paraffin section immunohistochemistry as an adjunct to morphologic analysis in the diagnosis of cutaneous lymphoid infiltrates. J Cutan Pathol 1994; 21: 481–493.
98. Bagg A, Braziel RM, Arber DA, Bijwaard KE, Chu AY: Immunoglobulin heavy chain gene analysis in lymphomas: a multicenter study demonstrating the heterogeneity of performance of polymerase chain reaction assays. J Molec Diagn 2002; 4: 81–89.
99. Andiman WA, Eastman R, Martin K, et al.: Opportunistic lymphoproliferations associated with Epstein–Barr viral DNA in infants and children with AIDS. Lancet 1985; 2: 1390–1393.
100. Schooley RT, Carey RW, Miller G, et al.: Chronic Epstein–Barr virus infection associated with fever and interstitial pneumonitis. Ann Intern Med 1986; 104: 636–646.
101. Resnick L, Pitchenik AE, Fisher E, Croney R: Detection of HTLV-III/LAV-specific IgG and antigen in bronchoalveolar lavage fluid from two patients with lymphocytic interstitial pneumonia associated with AIDS-related complex. Am J Med 1987; 82: 553–556.
102. Kim EA, Lee KS, Johkoh T, et al.: Interstitial lung diseases associated with collagen vascular diseases: radiologic and histopathologic findings. Radiographics 2002; 22 (suppl): S151–65.
103. Keller AR, Hochholzer L, Castleman B: Hyaline-vascular and plasma cell types of giant lymph node hyperplasia of the mediastinum and other locations. Cancer 1972; 29: 670–676.
104. Hayashi M, Aoshiba K, Shimada M, et al.: Kaposi's sarcoma-associated herpesvirus infection in the lung in multicentric Castleman's disease. Intern Med 1999; 38: 279–282.
105. Nicholson AG: Classification of idiopathic interstitial pneumonias: making sense of the alphabet soup. Histopathology 2002; 41: 381–391.
106. Foucar E, Rosai J, Dorfman R: Sinus histiocytosis with massive lymphadenopathy (Rosai–Dorfman disease): review of the entity. Semin Diagn Pathol 1990; 7: 19–73.

107. Wright DH, Richards DB: Sinus histiocytosis with massive lymphadenopathy (Rosai–Dorfman disease): report of a case with widespread nodal and extranodal dissemination. Histopathology 1981; 5: 697–709.
108. Paulli M, Bergamaschi G, Tonon L, et al.: Evidence for a polyclonal nature of the cell infiltrate in sinus histiocytosis with massive lymphadenopathy (Rosai–Dorfman disease). Br J Haematol 1995; 91: 415–418.
109. Eisen RN, Buckley PJ, Rosai J: Immunophenotypic characterization of sinus histiocytosis with massive lymphadenopathy (Rosai–Dorfman disease). Semin Diagn Pathol 1990; 7: 74–82.
110. Wandall HH: A study on neoplastic cells in sputum as a contribution to the diagnosis of primary lung cancer. Acta Chir Scand 1944; 91 (suppl 93): 1–143.
111. Koss LG: Diagnostic cytology & its histologic basis, 4th edn. 1992, JB Lippincott, Philadelphia, pp 849–864.
112. Erozan YS: Cytopathologic diagnosis of pulmonary neoplasms in sputum and bronchoscopic specimens. Semin Diagn Pathol 1986; 3: 188–195.
113. Jay SJ, Wehr K, Nicholson DP, Smith AL: Diagnostic sensitivity and specificity of pulmonary cytology. Acta Cytol 1980; 24: 304–312.
114. Pearson FG, Thompson DW, Delarue NC: Experience with the cytologic detection, localization, and treatment of radiographically undemonstrable bronchial carcinoma. J Thorac Cardiovasc Surg 1967; 54: 371–382.
115. Zavala DC: Diagnostic fiberoptic bronchoscopy: techniques and results of biopsy in 600 patients. Chest 1975; 68: 12–19.
116. Truong LD, Underwood RD, Greenberg SD, McLarty JW: Diagnosis and typing of lung carcinomas by cytopathologic methods: a review of 108 cases. Acta Cytol 1985; 29: 379–384.
117. Berkheiser JW: Bronchiolar proliferation and metaplasia associated with bronchiectasis, pulmonary infarct, and anthracosis. Cancer 1959; 12: 499–508.
118. Berkheiser JW: Bronchiolar proliferation and metaplasia associated with thromboembolism: a pathological and experimental study. Cancer 1963; 16: 205–211.
119. Kawecka M: Cytological evaluation of the sputum in patients with bronchiectasis and the possibility of erroneous diagnosis of carcinoma. Acta Union Int Cancer 1959; 15: 469–473.
120. Marchevsky AM, Nieburgs HE, Olenko F, et al.: Pulmonary tumorlets in cases of "tuberculoma" of the lung with malignant cells in brush biopsy. Acta Cytol 1982; 26: 491–494.
121. Johnston WW, Frable WJ: Cytopathology of the respiratory tract: a review. Am J Pathol 1976; 84: 371–424.
122. Ritter JH, Wick MR, Reyes A, Coffin CM, Dehner LP: False-positive interpretations of carcinoma in exfoliative respiratory cytology. Am J Clin Pathol 1995; 104: 133–140.
123. Saccomanno G, Archer VE, Saunders RD, et al.: Development of carcinoma of the lung as reflected in exfoliated cells. Cancer 1974; 33: 256–270.
124. Koss LG, Richardson HI: Some pitfalls of cytological diagnosis of lung cancer. Cancer 1955; 8: 937–947.
125. Plamenac P, Nikulin A, Pikula B: Cytologic changes of the respiratory tract in young adults as a consequence of high levels of air pollution exposure. Acta Cytol 1973; 17: 241–244.
126. Kern WH: Cytology of hyperplastic and neoplastic lesions of terminal bronchioles and alveoli. Acta Cytol 1965; 9: 372–379.
127. McKee G, Parums DV: False positive cytodiagnosis in fibrosing alveolitis. Acta Cytol 1990; 34: 105–107.
128. Meyer EC, Liebow AA: Relationship of interstitial pneumonia and honey-combing and typical epithelial proliferation to cancer of the lung. Cancer 1965; 18: 322–351.
129. Williams JW: Alveolar metaplasia: its relationship to pulmonary fibrosis in industry and development of lung cancer. Br J Cancer 1957: 11: 30–42.
130. Johnston WW: Type II pneumocytes in cytologic specimens: a diagnostic dilemma. Am J Clin Pathol 1992; 97: 608–609.
131. Clayton F: The spectrum and significance of bronchioloalveolar carcinoma. Pathol Annu 1988; 23(part 2): 361–394.
132. Stanley MW, Henry-Stanley MJ, Gajl-Peczakska KJ, Bitterman PB: Hyperplasia of type II pneumocytes in acute lung injury. Am J Clin Pathol 1992; 97: 669–677.
133. Grotte D, Stanley MW, Swanson PE, Henry-Stanley MJ, Davies S: Reactive type II pneumocytes in bronchoalveolar lavage fluid from acute respiratory distress syndrome can be mistaken for cells of adenocarcinoma. Diagn Cytopathol 1990; 6: 317–322.
134. Cibas ES: Effusions (pleural, pericardial, & peritoneal) and peritoneal washings. In: Atlas of diagnostic cytopathology, Atkinson B, Ed. WB Saunders, Philadelphia.
135. Bibbo M: Comprehensive cytopathology. 1991, WB Saunders, Philadelphia.
136. DeMay RM: The art & science of cytopathology. 1996, ASCP Press, Chicago.
137. Kobayashi TK, Gotoh T, Nakano K, et al.: Atypical mesothelial cells associated with eosinophilic pleural effusions: nuclear DNA content and immunocytochemical staining reaction with epithelial markers. Cytopathology 1993; 4: 37–46.
138. Chen CJ, Chang SC, Tseng HH: Assessment of immunocytochemical and histochemical staining in the distinction between reactive mesothelial cells and adenocarcinoma in body effusions. Chinese Med J 1994; 54: 149–155.
139. Schultenover SJ: Body cavity fluids. In: Clinical cytopathology & aspiration biopsy, Ramzi I, Ed. 1990, Appleton-Lange, East Norwalk, CT, pp 165–180.
140. Leong AS-Y, Stevens MW, Mukherjee TM: Malignant mesothelioma: cytologic diagnosis with histologic, immunohistochemical, and ultrastructural correlation. Semin Diagn Pathol 1992; 9: 141–150.
141. Bedrossian CWM, Bonsib S, Moran C: Differential diagnosis between mesothelioma and adenocarcinoma: a multimodal approach based on ultrastructure and immunocytochemistry. Semin Diagn Pathol 1992; 9: 91–96.
142. Kutty CPK, Remeniuk E, Varkey B: Malignant-appearing cells in pleural effusion due to pancreatitis. Acta Cytol 1981; 25: 412–416.
143. Marchevsky AM, Hauptman E, Gil J, Watson C: Computerized interactive morphometry as an aid in the diagnosis of pleural effusions. Acta Cytol 1987; 31: 131–136.
144. Kwee WS, Veldhuizen RW, Alons CA, et al.: Quantitative and qualitative differences between benign and malignant mesothelial cells in pleural fluid. Acta Cytol 1982; 26: 401–406.
145. Oberholzer M, Ettlin R, Christen H, et al.: The significance of morphometric methods in cytologic diagnostics: differentiation between mesothelial cells, mesothelioma cells, and metastatic adenocarcinoma cells in pleural effusions with special emphasis on chromatin texture. Analyt Cell Pathol 1991; 3: 25–42.
146. Ranaldi R, Marinelli F, Barbatelli G, et al.: Benign and malignant mesothelial lesions of the pleura: quantitative study. Appl Pathol 1986; 4: 55–64.
147. Roberts GH, Campbell GH: Exfoliative cytology of diffuse mesothelioma. J Clin Pathol 1972; 25: 557–582.
148. Bolen JW: Tumors of serosal tissue origin. Clin Lab Med 1987; 7: 31–50.
149. Whitaker D, Henderson DW, Shilkin KB: The concept of mesothelioma *in situ*: implications for diagnosis and histogenesis. Semin Diagn Pathol 1992; 9: 151–161.
150. Henderson DW, Shilkin KB, Whitaker D: Reactive mesothelial hyperplasia vs. mesothelioma, including mesothelioma in-situ: a brief review. Am J Clin Pathol 1998; 110: 397–404.
151. Lee A, Baloch ZW, Yu G, Gupta PK: Mesothelial hyperplasia with reactive atypia: diagnostic pitfalls and role of immunohistochemical studies: a case report. Diagn Cytopathol 2000; 22: 113–116.
152. Singh HK, Silverman JF, Berns L, Haddad MG, Park HK: Significance of epithelial membrane antigen in the workup of problematic serous effusions. Diagn Cytopathol 1995; 13: 3–7.
153. Ferrandez-Izquierdo A, Navarro-Fos S, Gonzalez-Devesa M, Gil-Benso R, Llombart-Bosch A: Immunocytochemical typification of mesothelial cells in effusions: in vivo and in vitro models. Diagn Cytopathol 1994; 10: 256–262.
154. Cagle PT, Brown RW, Lebovitz RM: p53 immunostaining in the differentiation of reactive processes from malignancy in pleural biopsy specimens. Hum Pathol 1994; 25: 443–448.
155. Walts AE, Said JW, Koeffler HP: Is immunoreactivity for p53 useful in distinguishing benign from malignant effusions? Localization of p53 gene product in benign mesothelial and adenocarcinoma cells. Mod Pathol 1994; 7: 462–468.
156. Churg A. Asbestos fibers and pleural plaques in a general autopsy population. Am J Pathol 1982; 109: 88–96.
157. Fondimare A, Duwoos H, Desbordes J, et al.: Plaques fibroyalines calcifiees du foie dans l'asbestose. Nouv Presse Med 1973; 3: 893.
158. Hourihane DO, Lessof L, Richardson PC. Hyaline and calcified

pleural plaques as an index of exposure to asbestos: a study of radiological and pathological features of 100 cases with a consideration of epidemiology. Br Med J 1966; 1: 1069–1074.
159. Kishimoto T, Ono T, Okada K, Ito H: Relationship between numbers of asbestos bodies in autopsy lung and pleural plaques on chest x-ray film. Chest 1989; 95: 549–552.
160. Mattson S, Ringqvist T: Pleural plaques and exposure to asbestos. Scand J Respir Dis 1970; 75: 1–41.
161. Roberts GH: The pathology of parietal pleural plaques. J Clin Pathol 1961: 348–353.
162. Warnock Ml, Prescott BT, Kuwahara TJ: Numbers and types of asbestos fibers in subjects with pleural plaques. Am J Pathol 1982; 109: 37–46.
163. Kuhlman JE, Singha NK: Complex disease of the pleural space: radiographic and CT evaluation. Radiographics 1997; 17: 63–79.
164. Wilson GE, Hasleton PS, Chatterjee AK: Desmoplastic malignant mesothelioma: a review of 17 cases. J Clin Pathol 1992; 45: 295–298.
165. Mangano EW, Cagle PT, Churg A, Voller RT, Roggli VL: The diagnosis of desmoplastic malignant mesothelioma and its distinction from fibrous pleurisy: a histologic and immunohistochemical analysis of 31 cases including p53 immunostaining. Am J Clin Pathol 1998; 110: 191–199.
166. Moran CA, Suster S, Koss MN: The spectrum of histologic growth patterns in benign and malignant fibrous tumors of the pleura. Semin Diagn Pathol 1992; 9: 169–180.
167. Wain SL, Roggli VL, Foster WL Jr: Parietal pleural plaques, asbestos bodies and neoplasia: a clinical, pathologic and roentgenographic correlation of 25 consecutive cases. Chest 1985; 86: 707–713.
168. Epler GR, McCloud TC, Gaensler EA: Prevalence and incidence of benign asbestos pleural effusion in a working population. JAMA 1982; 247: 617–622.
169. Gibbs AR, Stephens M, Griffiths DM, Blight BJN, Pooley FD: Fiber distribution in the lungs and pleura of subjects with asbestos-related diffuse pleural fibrosis. Br J Industr Med 1991; 48: 762–770.
170. Stephens M, Gibbs AR, Pooley FD, Wagner JC: Asbestos-induced diffuse pleural fibrosis: pathology and mineralogy. Thorax 1987; 42: 583–588.

19

Benign and borderline tumors of the lungs and pleura

Mark R Wick   *Stacey E Mills*

Malignant neoplasms are more common, by far, than benign tumors in the lower respiratory tract. In the United States, lung carcinoma is the leading cause of cancer-related death in both sexes, and it accounts for >0.7% of new malignancies each year in men.[1] In Europe, the situation is even worse; for example, >3% of newly diagnosed malignant neoplasms in Germany are lung cancers.[2] These data reflect the continuing use of cigarettes worldwide, and the relative potency which tobacco smoke has as a carcinogenic agent.

Because of the prognostic gravity attending the diagnosis of lung cancers and their frequency, lesser literary attention has been given to benign pulmonary neoplasms and those that have "borderline" malignant potential. Nonetheless, they comprise an interesting array of lesions with diverse lineages, the causes of which are known only in a minority of cases. This chapter will provide an overview of such tumors, with an emphasis on differential diagnosis.

Bronchoscopic examination and endobronchial biopsy will be productive diagnostically if the tumor in question protrudes significantly into the lumen of the airway. However, brushing cytology is only variably effective in sampling such growths, depending on whether the mucosa over them is intact, and the level of intercellular cohesion in the tumor itself. With respect to deeply seated masses in the parenchyma, transthoracic or transbronchial aspirates or needle biopsies are usually necessary for adequate sampling. In that setting, it should be remembered that those procedures are most effective in the diagnosis of *malignant* neoplasms; if the pathologist sees only histologically banal tissue elements in the latter specimens, it is often impossible to discern whether they truly represent the lesion or are simply part of the adjacent lung. Moreover, in small biopsies, the morphologic attributes of some cytologically low-grade malignancies may be virtually identical to those of benign tumors belonging to the same general cellular lineage.

Benign pleuropulmonary neoplasms

Clinical features

The clinical characteristics of benign tumors in the lower respiratory tract can be considered in an overview, because they are generally not specific to any particular diagnosis. Most benign intrapulmonary lesions are associated with no symptoms or signs whatsoever, and are found incidentally with screening radiographic studies. As discussed elsewhere in this book, hamartomas are often separable from other benign but truly neoplastic masses of the lung on imaging studies, because of their common content of distinctive calcifications, or fat densities, or both[3] (Fig. 19.1). Otherwise, the radiologist is not typically able to distinguish between specific histologic entities in this context. Endotracheal and endobronchial tumors are more often related to clinical complaints such as wheezing, hemoptysis, obstructive pneumonia, and postobstructive pulmonary hyperinflation, depending on their anatomic localization.

In the past, radiologists felt more comfortable in simply observing a pulmonary mass over time, if it had reassuring morphologic characteristics. In fact, statistical paradigms have been constructed to aid them in this process.[4] However, because of the unfortunate pressure of litigation involving putative "delays in diagnosis" of malignant neoplasms in various sites[5] – together with the modern availability of techniques such as video-assisted thoracoscopic surgery[6] – many more benign lesions of the lungs are excised today than in previous years.

Benign tumors that are principally tracheal and endobronchial

Solitary tracheobronchial papilloma

Solitary papillomas of the tracheobronchial tree (SPTT) are uncommon. They are most often seen in adults – who are typically middle-aged – with a slight male predominance.[7–21] Occasionally, even though only one papillomatous lesion of the lower respiratory tract may be present, it may coexist with papillary squamous proliferations of the larynx or oropharynx. If located near a bronchial orifice, an SPTT may cause obstructive

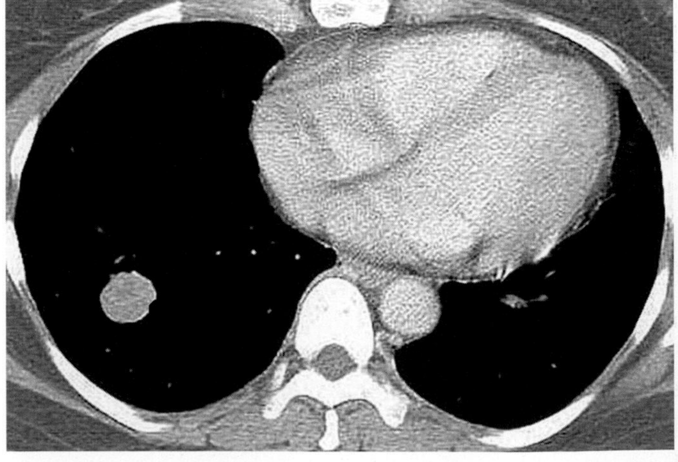

Fig. 19.1 This computed tomogram of the lung shows a well-demarcated peripheral nodule with internal calcification, typical of pulmonary hamartoma.

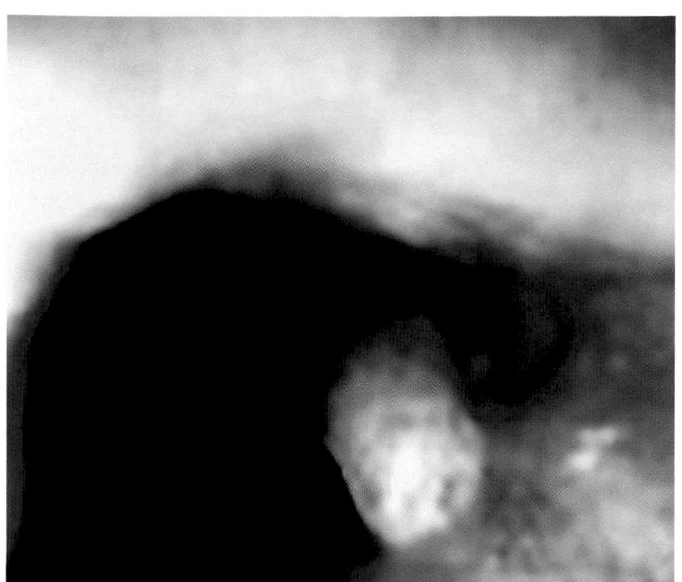

Fig. 19.2 Bronchoscopic image of solitary bronchial papilloma, showing a smooth-surfaced lesion protruding into the bronchial lumen.

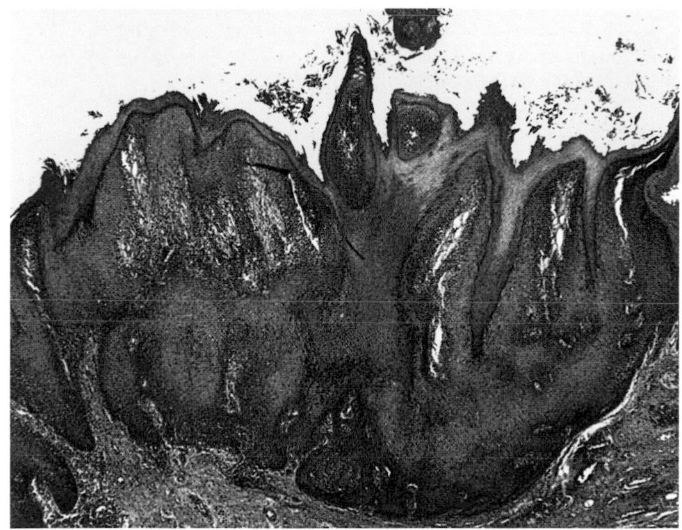

Fig. 19.3 Solitary papilloma of the bronchus, represented by a papillary proliferation of bland squamous epithelium supported by well-formed fibrovascular stroma.

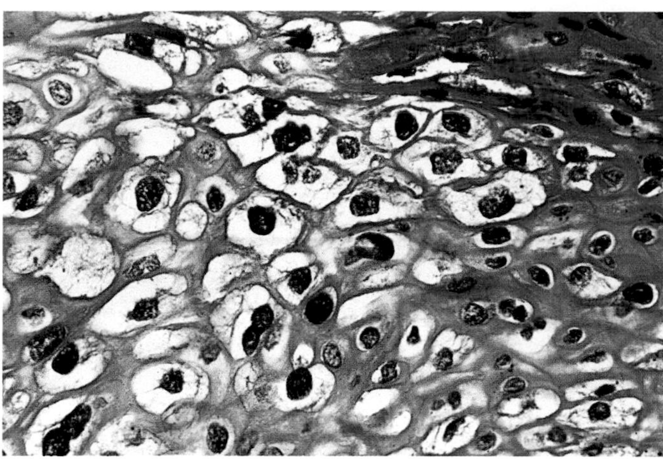

Fig. 19.4 Koilocytotic change in the squamous cells of a solitary bronchial papilloma, represented by nuclear hyperchromasia and crenation, and perinuclear clearing of the cytoplasm.

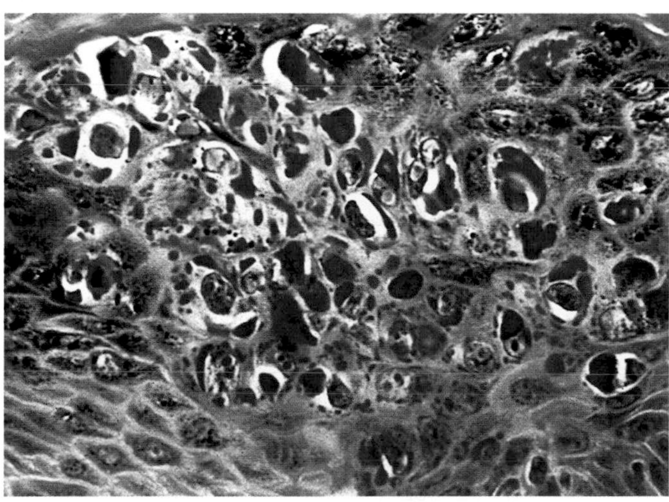

Fig. 19.5 Clumped keratohyaline and eosinophilic cytoplasmic inclusions are seen in the lesional cells of this solitary squamous papilloma of the bronchus with a viral causation.

pneumonia;[19] otherwise, the patient may be entirely asymptomatic.

Macroscopically, one sees a pedunculated tan-white polypoid excrescence in the mucosa of the airway, with variable compromise of its lumen (Fig. 19.2). The surface may either be smooth or slightly verrucoid.

The microscopic image of SPTTs is almost always similar to that of viral papillomas elsewhere in the body, particularly in the genitoperineal region. They are constituted by arborizing fronds with fibrovascular cores, mantled by relatively bland squamous epithelial cells (Fig. 19.3). These often exhibit nuclear hyperchromasia and crenation, but the nuclear chromatin may instead be homogenized and glassy. The cytoplasm is commonly unremarkable; alternatively, it shows perinuclear clearing, eosinophilic globular inclusions, or hypergranulation with clumping of keratohyaline granules (Figs 19.4 and 19.5). Nuclear atypia has been observed in squamous SPTT, and Popper et al. reported several cases in which overt squamous cell carcinoma developed.[22,23]

Another even rarer variant of SPTT is the columnar papilloma, showing a constituency by columnar epithelial cells rather than squamous elements.[14] Putatively, it has no potential at all for malignant change.

Interestingly, the biologic associations between squamous SPTT and human papillomavirus (HPV) types

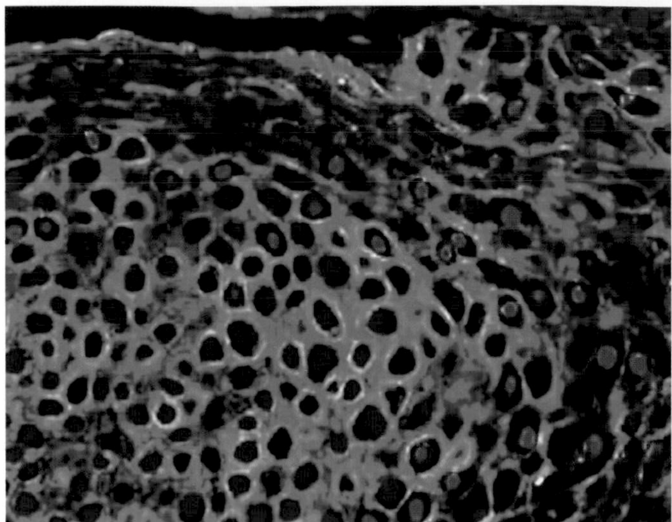

Fig. 19.6 The presence of human papillomavirus type 11 is apparent in this in-situ hybridization preparation, as evidenced by nuclei that show a red-pink fluorescence signal.

are comparable to those which apply in the genital tract. Specifically, HPV types 7 and 11 are most commonly seen in uncomplicated SPTT; in contrast, HPV types 16 and 18 are associated with dysplastic nuclear features and a higher risk of carcinomatous transformation.[22,23] The presence of those viral agents can be evaluated using in-situ hybridization (ISH) (Fig. 19.6), hybrid capture methodology (HCM), or the polymerase chain reaction (PCR).[22–26]

In light of the usual behavior of SPTT, conservative therapeutic approaches such as endoscopic removal, cryotherapy, or fulguration are typically applied. Those lesions in which malignancy appears must be treated in a manner appropriate for "ordinary" lung cancers.[27–30]

Multifocal respiratory tract papillomatosis

Respiratory tract papillomatosis (RTP) is the multifocal form of viral papillomagenesis, as described above. Its onset is early in life, owing to the fact that the mode of transmission is natal inhalation of virally infected genital tract secretions during vaginal delivery.[31–40] Children with RTP typically develop oropharyngeal or laryngeal disease initially; it may remain localized there or spread with time to involve the lower airways as well, as seen in 5% of cases.[39] In the latter instance, growth into the lung parenchyma may supervene, with the eventual appearance of cavitary lesions that can simulate carcinomas radiographically.[31,40] Obstruction of the tracheal or bronchial lumina is associated with recurrent pneumonia, hemoptysis, and asthma-like symptoms. Even though RTP is often said to be "recurring," the entire respiratory tract is at risk for infection by HPV in this disorder. Thus, it is more apropos to consider separate lesions as metachronously or synchronously independent of one another pathogenetically.

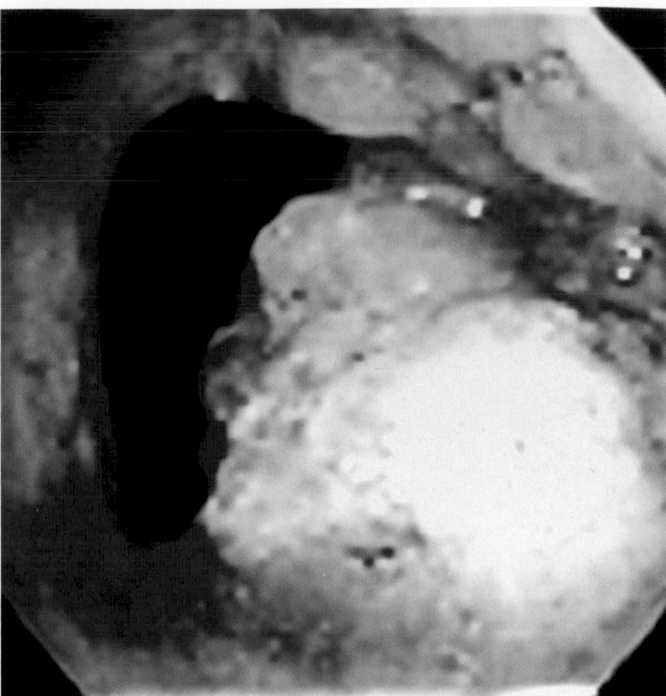

Fig. 19.7 Bronchoscopic appearance of multifocal respiratory papillomatosis, showing a multiplicity of smooth-domed and confluent lesions in the bronchial mucosa.

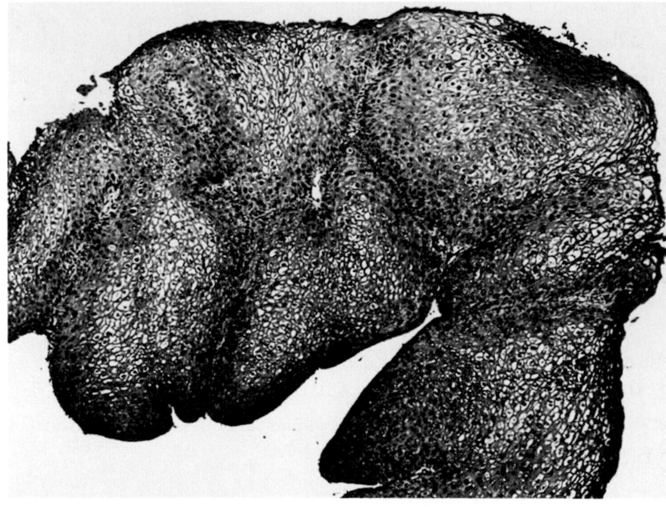

Fig. 19.8 An individual lesion of multifocal respiratory papillomatosis, demonstrating comparable features to those depicted in Fig. 19.3.

Gross and histologic features of RTP are largely the same as those of SSTP. Exceptions to that statement concern the multiplicity of lesions in the first of those diseases (Fig. 19.7), and the greater tendency for "inverting" or tissue-destructive growth of the papillomatous lesions in RTP (Figs 19.8 and 19.9). The HPV profiles of RTP and

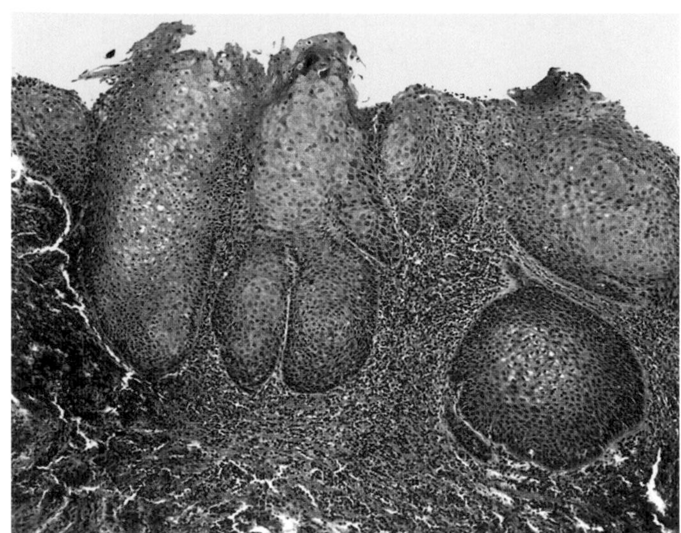

Fig. 19.9 Inverting growth into the bronchial submucosa by an individual lesion of multifocal respiratory papillomatosis.

SSTP are also comparable, with the notable proviso that HPV-11 is overwhelmingly the most common viral type that is seen in RTP. Mutations of the p53 gene have been linked to malignant transformation of individual lesions in both conditions.[22,23,26,40–45]

The incidence of preceding HPV integration was assessed by Clavel et al.[24] using HCM in a series of bronchopulmonary carcinomas. They found evidence of oncogenic HPV integration in only 2.7% of those tumors. On the other hand, Yousem and colleagues[46] demonstrated similar positivity by ISH in 30% of squamous carcinomas and 17% of large cell undifferentiated carcinomas of the lung; Syrjanen[27] likewise observed histologic viral changes in adjacent metaplastic bronchial mucosa in 26/104 squamous carcinomas (25%). Based on these data, it must be acknowledged that HPV may play a greater role in the etiology of lung carcinomas (particularly of the squamous type) than previously thought.

Bronchial mucus gland adenoma

The term "bronchial adenoma" has been plagued by many misconceptions and misapplications since its introduction by Liebow in 1952.[47] That is because tumors with well-documented malignant potential were initially included under that rubric; these included both neuroendocrine carcinomas and salivary gland-type carcinomas. With that having been said, two benign neoplastic entities remain in reference to the tracheobronchial tree – mucus gland adenoma (MGA) and mixed tumor (pleomorphic adenoma). The second of those is discussed in Chapter 16, (page 591).

MGA is an extraordinarily rare lesion. As support for that statement, England and Hochholzer[48] noted that one series of >3000 pulmonary tumors included no examples of MGA,[49] and only one was represented in another report of 130 benign neoplasms of the lung that were seen at a large referral center.[50] In the vast experience of the US Armed Forces Institute of Pathology (AFIP), only 10 examples of MGA were found; men and women were equally affected, and the patients ranged in age from 25 to 67 years.[48] Some of these tumors are asymptomatic, whereas others produce symptoms and signs relating to airway obstruction. There is no particular predilection for anatomic localization; MGAs may arise in any of the major lobar or segmental bronchi. Radiographs either show changes of post-obstructive pneumonia or hyperinflation, or they may demonstrate a discrete nodule or coin lesion that is centered on a bronchus[51–63] (Fig. 19.10).

Grossly, MGAs measure between 0.5 and 7 cm in maximal dimension. They often demonstrate encapsulation, with slimy mucoid cut surfaces; internal fibrous septations may yield a loculated appearance as well.

Histologic descriptions of MGA have varied from series to series, and, in our opinion, some reports of these lesions have been contaminated with epithelial-predominant mixed tumors or predominantly-cystic mucoepidermoid carcinomas. As succinctly stated by England and Hochholzer,[48] "cystic change [is] the cardinal feature of MGA of the bronchus" at a microscopic level. One observes microcystic arrays of cuboidal or columnar tumor cells that may permeate the bronchial wall to the level of the cartilaginous plates; however, growth beyond that point is absent (Fig. 19.11). Cystic contents are either overtly mucinous or more serous in nature. Secondary formation of cholesterol clefts and dystrophic calcifications may also be seen, and squamous metaplasia in the most luminal aspect of the lesion is another possibility. Nuclei are generally bland with small nucleoli, and cytoplasm may be amphophilic, oxyphilic, clear, or foamy. Mitotic figures are scarce.

The internal substructure of MGA has been divided into two morphologic patterns: glandular-tubulocystic (Fig. 19.12) and papillocystic (Fig. 19.13). Within each of these categories, England and Hochholzer described a spectrum of appearances, ranging from a monotonous tubular pattern to a complex arborizing aggregation of papillary structures.[48] Stromal sclerosis is potentially present in MGA, but mesenchymal cellularity may be notable as well. Intralesional inflammation is chronic in nature and tends to be concentrated towards the luminal surface.

Immunohistologic features of MGA are comparable to those of non-neoplastic bronchial glands. The constituent

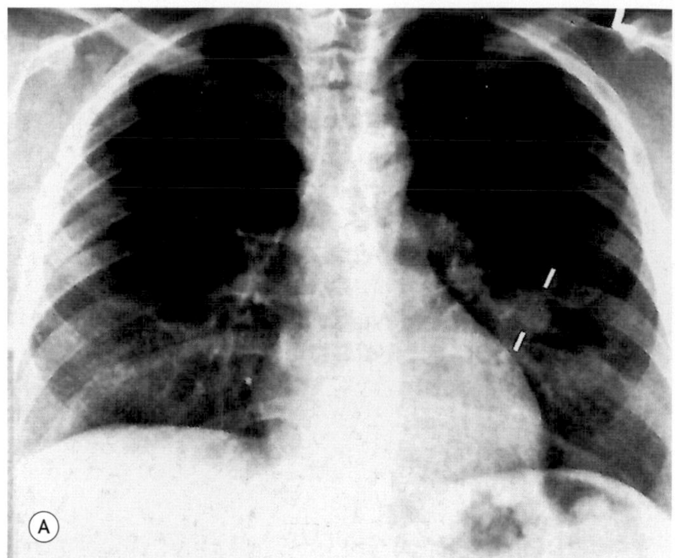

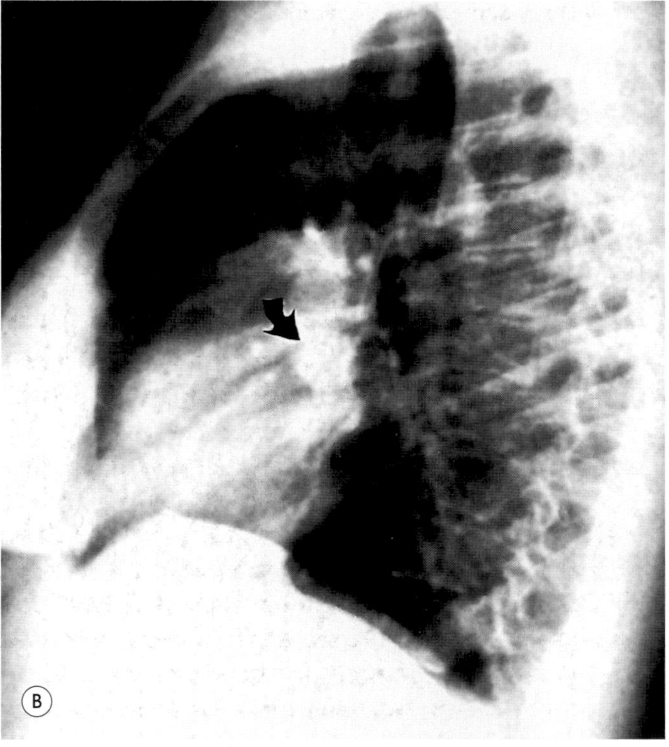

Fig. 19.10 Posteroanterior (A) and lateral (B) chest radiographs, showing a nodular lesion that is centered on a bronchus (arrow) and which proved to be a mucus gland adenoma. (Reproduced with permission from England and Hochholzer[48] and by courtesy of Dr. Douglas England.)

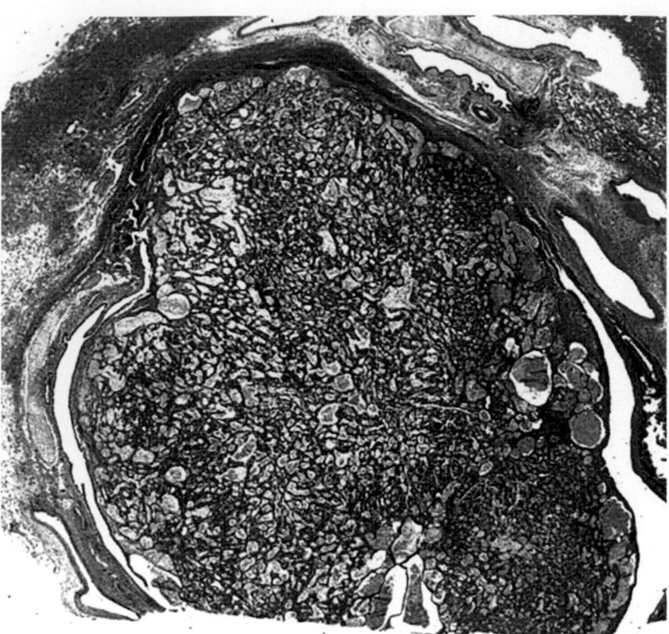

Fig. 19.11 Scanning microscopic view of a mucus gland adenoma of the bronchus, demonstrating an epithelial lesion that fills the bronchial lumen and shows internal gland formation. (Courtesy of Dr. Douglas England.)

cells are consistently labeled for cytokeratin, epithelial membrane antigen, and blood group isoantigens, with less uniform reactivity for carcinoembryonic antigen. Stromal cells have been found to show myoepithelial features, with concurrent staining for keratin, actin, and S100 protein.[48]

Differential diagnosis includes predominantly-cystic mucoepidermoid carcinoma (MEC), mixed tumor (MT), "sclerosing hemangioma" (pneumocytoma), and primary or metastatic mucinous ("colloid") adenocarcinoma. Of those possibilities, the first two are the most problematic, necessitating adequate biopsies for visualization of tumor architecture.

An admixture of squamous elements throughout the mass, or infiltrative growth through the bronchial wall, or both, would tend to argue for a diagnosis of MEC. Although MGA does not manifest the presence of chondromyxoid stroma or immunoreactivity for glial fibrillary acidic protein (GFAP), as seen in a proportion of MTs,[64] the possibility that MGA is related nosologically to monomorphic adenoma – a variant of MT – cannot be dismissed entirely. In any event, it represents a distinctive clinicopathologic entity that is felt to deserve its own diagnostic designation.

Treatment of MGA can be conservative, with sleeve resection of the bronchus and reconstruction whenever that is clinically feasible.[48,54] It is admittedly difficult to be definitively diagnostic when given a small biopsy of a lesion that may be a MGA. Thus, the surgeon may sometimes need to perform a second procedure to adequately treat tumors that are originally interpreted as adenomas, but which are found to actually represent MECs after an initial excision has been done.

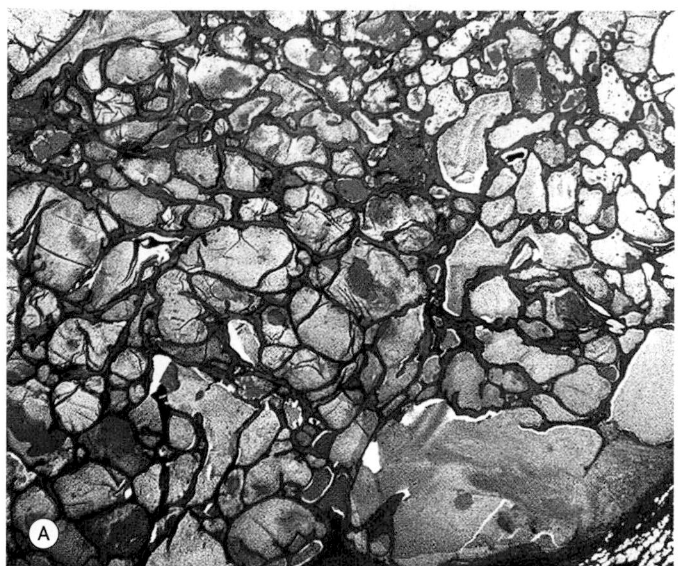

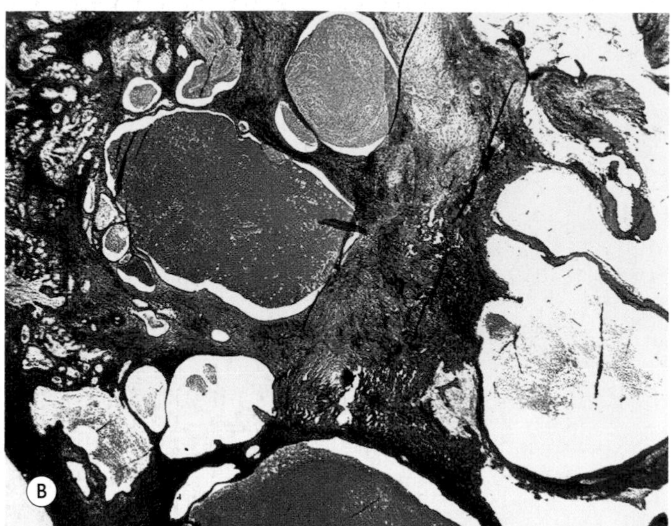

Fig. 19.12 (A, B) A glandular-tubulocystic growth pattern is present in this mucus gland adenoma of the bronchus. (Courtesy of Dr. Douglas England.)

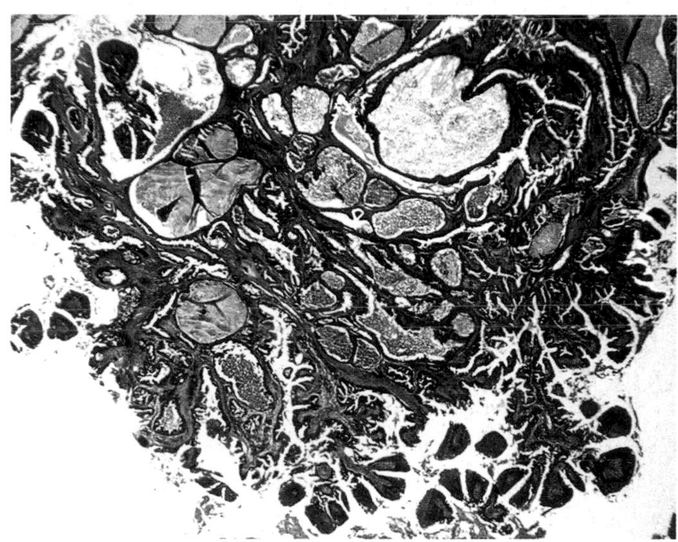

Fig. 19.13 This mucus gland bronchial adenoma shows a papillocystic configuration. (Courtesy of Dr. Douglas England.)

Peripheral nerve sheath tumors of the respiratory tract

Primary neoplasms of the lung that demonstrate schwannian or perineurial differentiation are rare. They are more often located in the walls of major bronchi than in the peripheral lung parenchyma, although the latter possibility does indeed exist. Patients with these lesions are asymptomatic, or they manifest nonspecific complaints such as cough or vague chest pain.[65–78] Chest radiographs show nodular or irregular masses that are associated with bronchi; secondary atelectasis is sometimes noted as well[65] (Fig. 19.15). Some patients with primary neurogenic pulmonary tumors have neurofibromatosis type 1 (NF1; von Recklinghausen's disease), and that is true regardless of whether the lung lesion in question is a neurofibroma or a neurilemmoma.[79] Neurogenic sarcomas do arise in the lungs as well,[80–82] but it is unclear from a review of the pertinent literature as to how many have occurred in the context of NF1 in association with pre-existing pulmonary neurofibromas.

Macroscopically, peripheral nerve sheath tumors (PNSTs) of the bronchus are well-demarcated yellow-white masses that are centered on the bronchial wall and often protrude into the bronchial lumen (Figs 19.16 and 19.17). Gross foci of hemorrhage, necrosis, or cystification are absent in benign lesions of this type.

The histologic images associated with benign PNSTs are varied. Prototypical neurofibromas are "plexiform" in NF1 (Fig. 19.18), putatively reflecting a neoplastic attempt to recapitulate a neural plexus. Constituent cells are serpiginous in contour, with attenuated fusiform nuclei and delicately fibrillar cytoplasm (Fig. 19.19). The supporting matrix is myxedematous or collagenized, and may contain scattered foam cells, mast cells, and lymphocytes. Mitotic activity is typically absent. Neurilemmomas – also termed "schwannomas" – are biphasic in classical form, with compactly cellular ("Antoni A") areas alternating with zones of loose cellularity and myxoid change ("Antoni B" foci) (Figs 19.20 and 19.21). Nuclei may be aligned in register in Antoni A areas, representing so-called Verocay bodies (Fig. 19.22). Intralesional blood vessels have thick walls

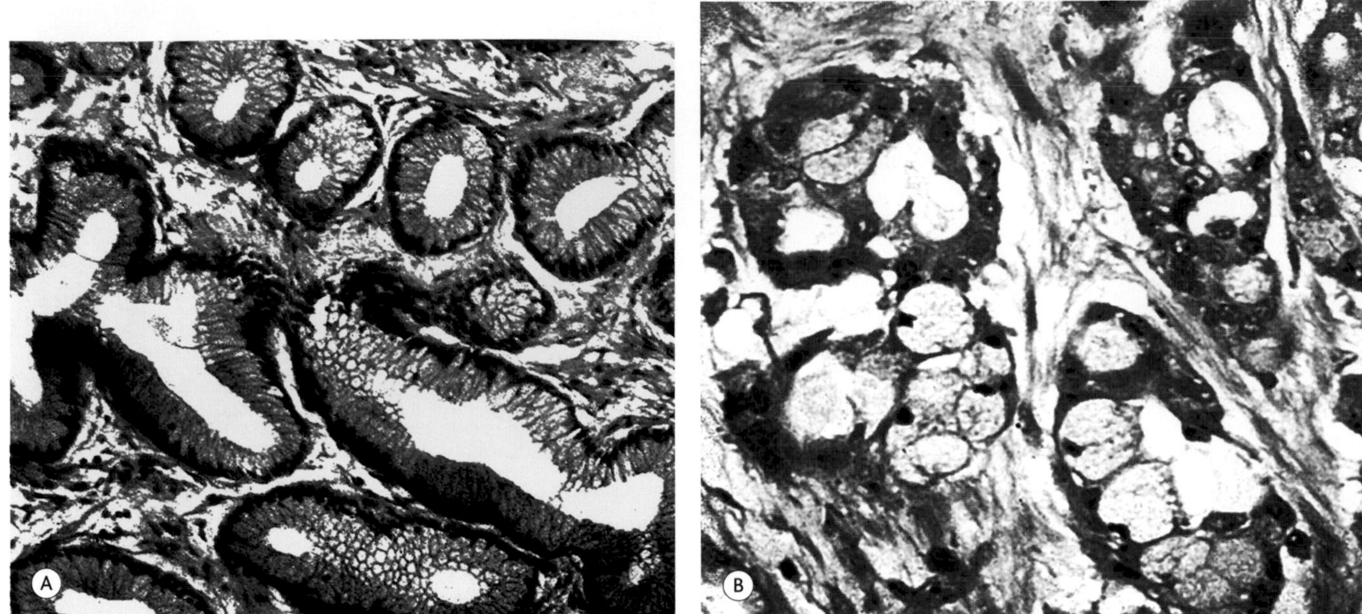

Fig. 19.14 (A, B) Lesional tubules are composed of bland mucinous epithelium in this glandular-tubulocystic mucus gland bronchial adenoma. (Courtesy of Dr. Douglas England.)

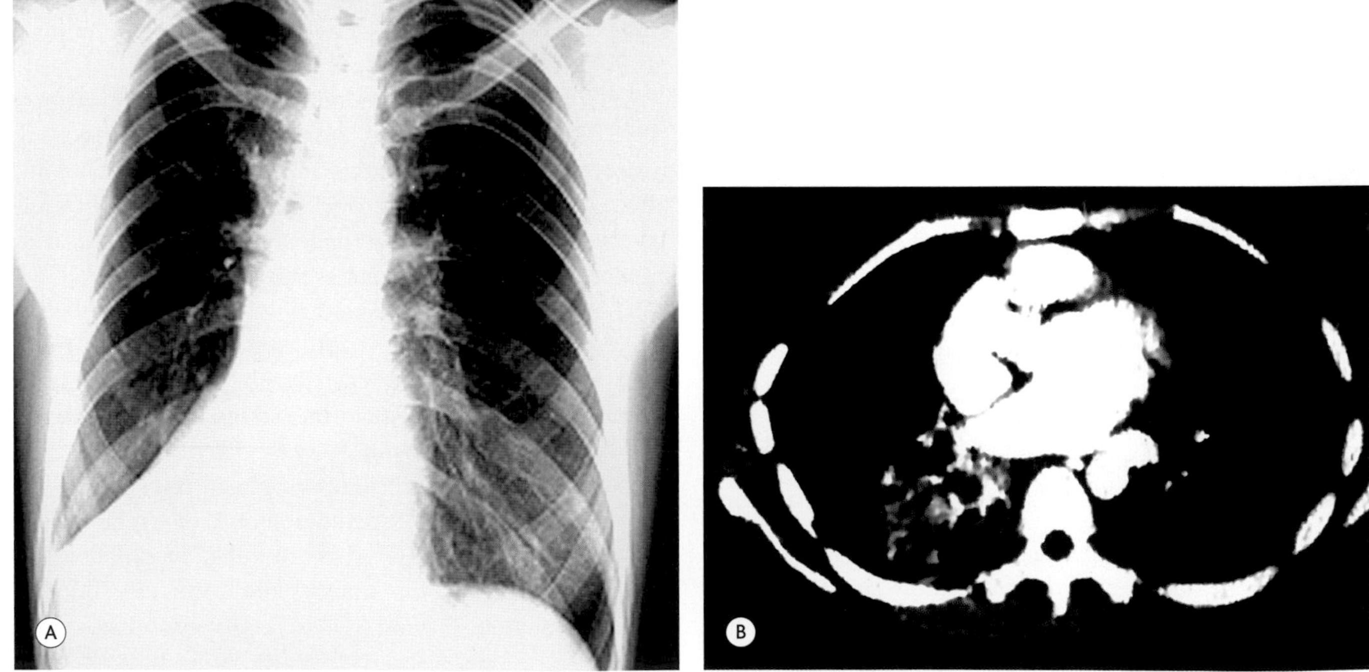

Fig. 19.15 This chest radiograph in a case of intrabronchial neurilemmoma demonstrates atelectasis of the right lower lobe, owing to obstruction of the corresponding bronchus by the tumor. (A) A CT image (B) demonstrates segmental opacification.

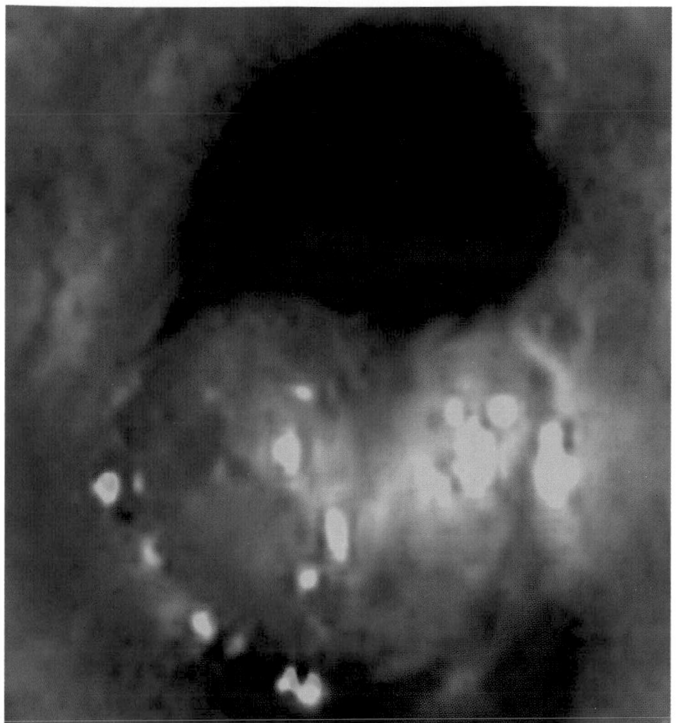

Fig. 19.16 This bronchoscopic image of a bronchial neurilemmoma shows a sessile polypoid lesion that is covered by intact mucosa.

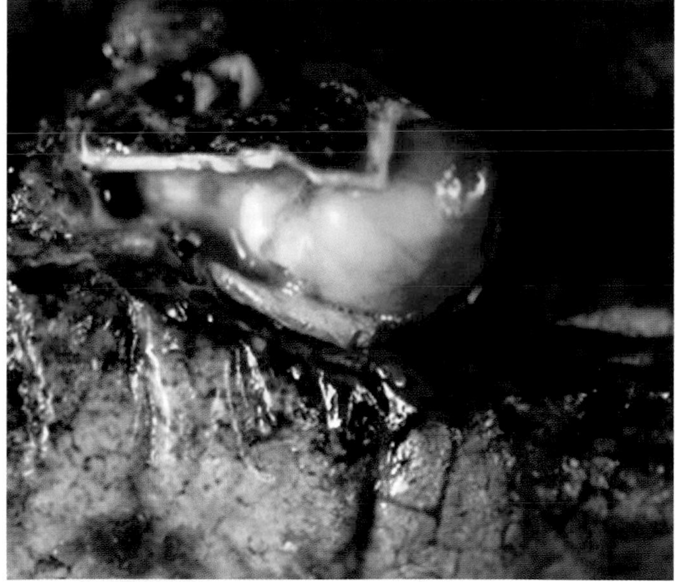

Fig. 19.17 The resected lung in a case of bronchial neurilemmoma demonstrates occlusion of the bronchial lumen by a uniform, yellow, solid tumor.

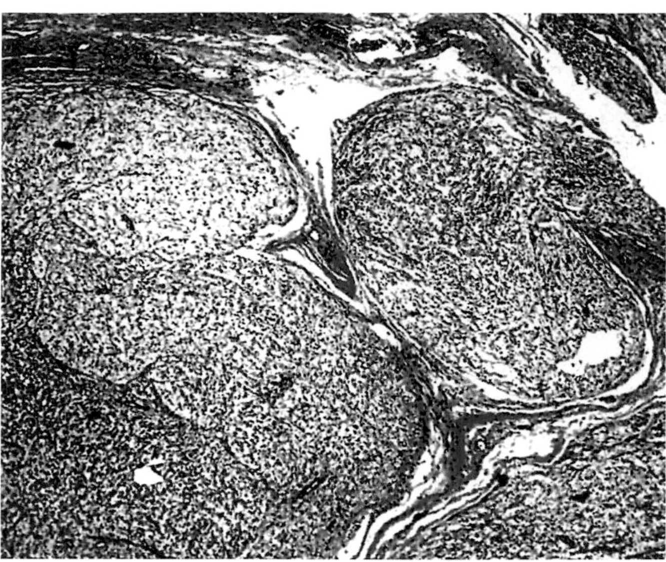

Fig. 19.18 Plexiform neurofibroma, showing internal compartmentalization of the tumor into neoplastic cell fascicles that simulate a developing nerve plexus.

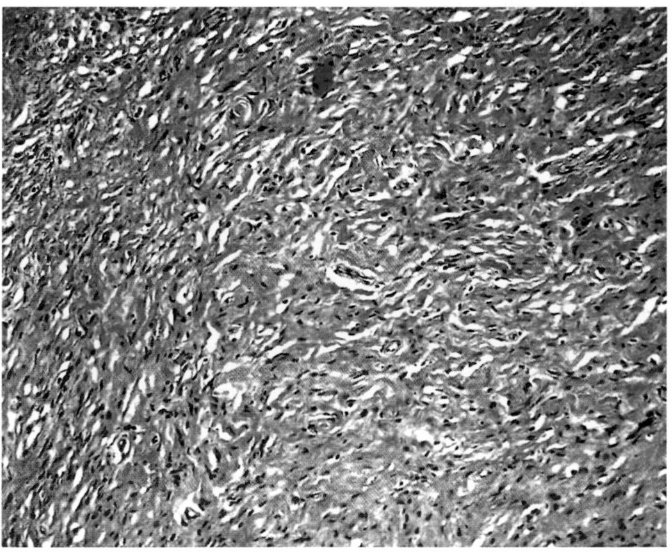

Fig. 19.19 The tumor cells in neurofibroma show serpiginous nuclear profiles and eosinophilic cytoplasm. They are bland, with no nuclear atypia or mitotic activity.

in many neurilemmomas, and a well-defined peripheral tumor capsule may be identified in some instances. Variants of neurilemmoma include "cellular" schwannoma, which manifests intersecting bundles of densely apposed, focally mitotic spindle cells in the context of an encapsulated mass[78] (Fig. 19.23); "glandular" schwannoma, in which scattered foci of divergent benign glandular differentiation are seen; "ancient" schwannoma, showing scattered pleomorphic hyperchromatic nuclei in degenerative cells (Fig. 19.24); plexiform schwannoma, in which broad plexiform fascicles of tumor cells show the substructure of neurilemmoma; and melanotic psammomatous schwannoma, exhibiting concentric microcalcifications

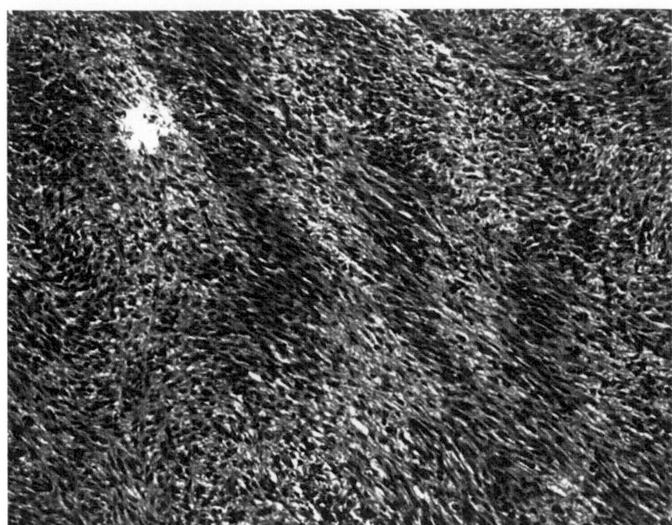

Fig. 19.20 An "Antoni A" area of growth is shown in a bronchial neurilemmoma, represented by compact cellular apposition and a tendency for nuclei to be aligned in register.

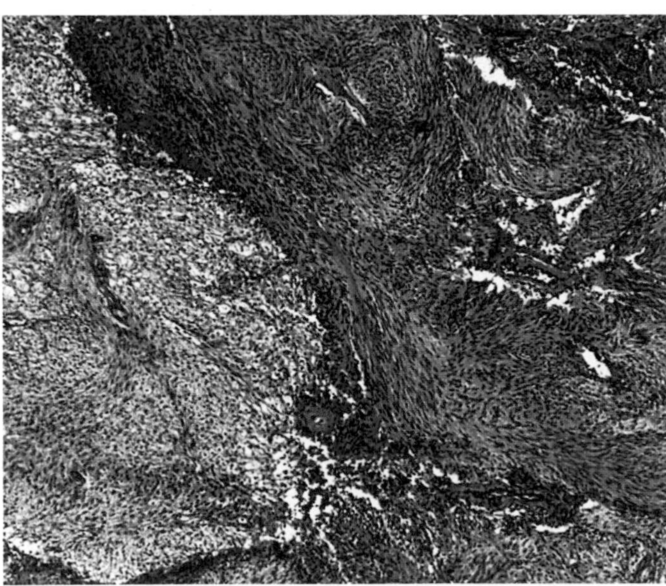

Fig. 19.21 An "Antoni B" focus in bronchial neurilemmoma shows the presence of intercellular myxoid matrix (lower left portion of figure).

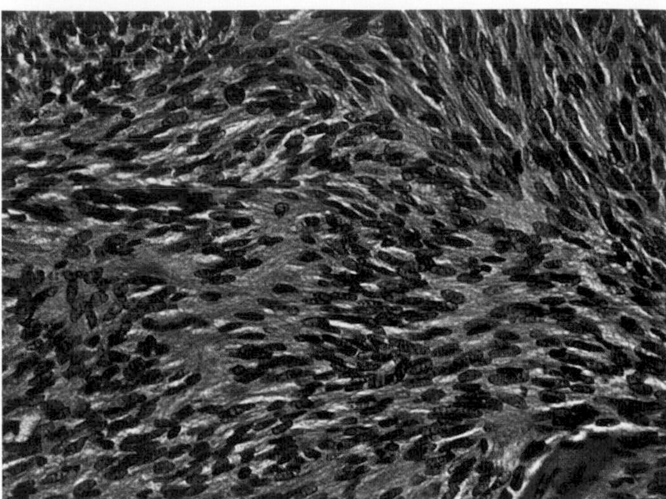

Fig. 19.22 "Verocay bodies" are zones in Antoni A areas of neurilemmoma in which nuclei form linear "stacks."

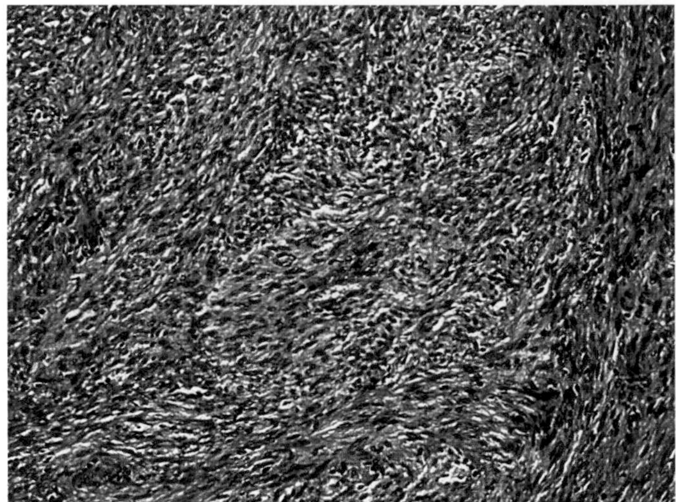

Fig. 19.23 Cellular schwannoma (neurilemmoma), demonstrating densely agglomerated spindle cells with focal mitotic activity.

and melanin pigmentation[83] (Fig. 19.25). The last of those subtypes may be associated with myxomas of the skin, heart, and breast; the presence of cutaneous ephelides; and overactivity of endocrine glands.

Benign PNSTs of the bronchus respect the cartilaginous plates and therefore do not permeate more deeply into the bronchial wall. In keeping with their gross characteristics, necrosis is not expected in these lesions, but areas of degenerative change, with edema and sclerosis, are relatively common.

The immunophenotype of PNSTs features reactivity for vimentin, and variable labeling for S100 protein, CD56, CD57, GFAP, and epithelial membrane antigen (Fig. 19.26). The last of those markers is felt to represent perineurial differentiation in this context. Keratin positivity is absent, except in the glands of glandular schwannoma, and myogenous markers are similarly lacking in benign nerve sheath neoplasms.

As true of all spindle cell lesions of the lung, it is necessary to exclude the possibility of sarcomatoid carcinoma before making a final diagnosis of PNST; immunohistologic evaluation is the most expeditious means of doing so. In addition, other mesenchymal lesions of the lung – especially leiomyoma and leiomyomatous

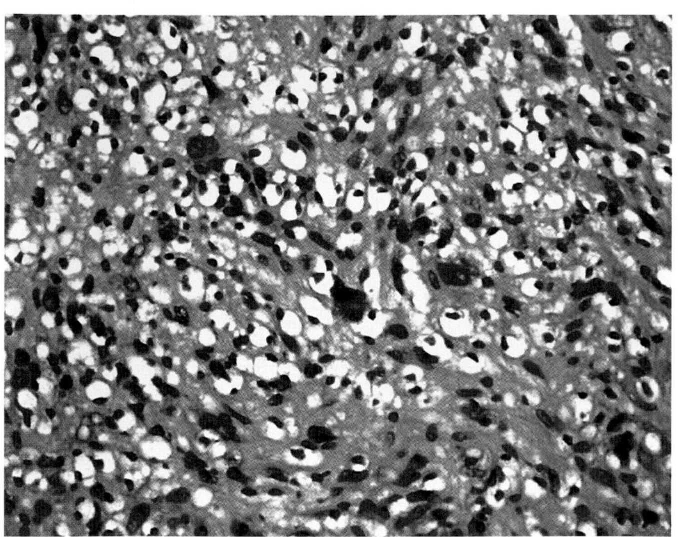

Fig. 19.24 "Ancient" neurilemmoma, showing degenerative atypia of tumor cell nuclei with mild pleomorphism and hyperchromasia.

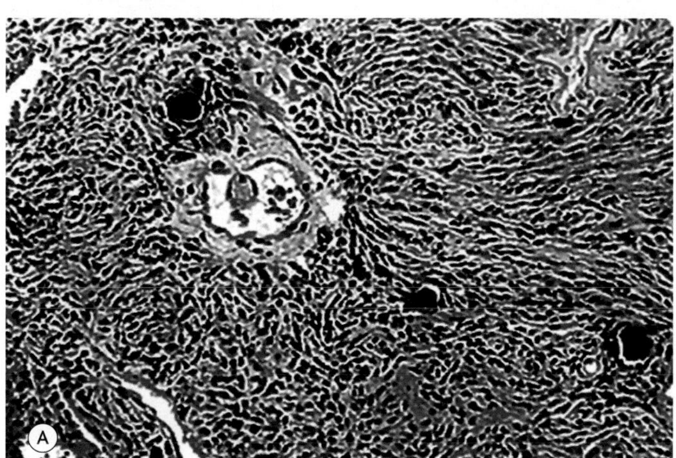

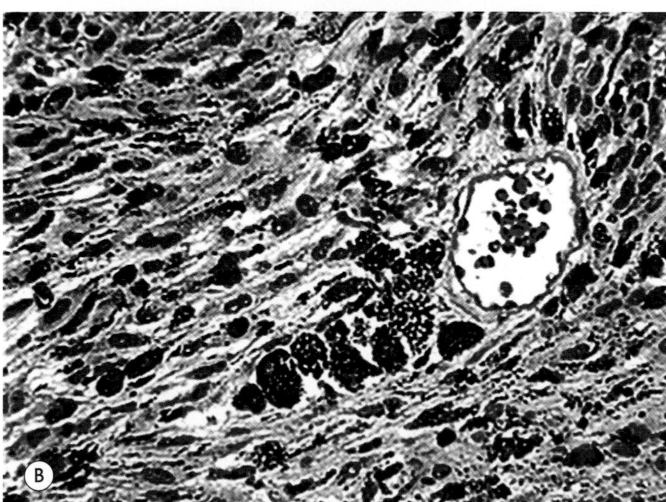

Fig. 19.25 Melanotic psammomatous schwannoma (neurilemmoma), exhibiting (A) microcalcifications and (B) cytoplasmic melanin pigment.

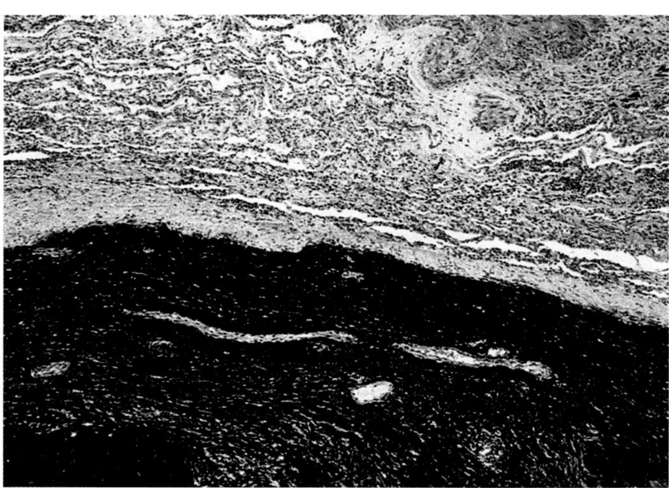

Fig. 19.26 Intense immunoreactivity for S100 protein is seen in this bronchial neurilemmoma.

hamartoma – must be considered as alternatives to an interpretation of neurofibroma or neurilemmoma. The immunoprofiles of those lesions are dissimilar as well.

If the identification of PNST can be established in evaluations of bronchial biopsy specimens, and radiographic findings support a benign diagnosis, the surgeon can undertake a conservative approach to the removal of such lesions.[69,72] However, small samples of neurogenic neoplasms are notoriously unreliable in predicting the biologic potential of PNSTs, and should not be used in isolation to govern decisions on therapy.

Granular cell tumors of the lung

Granular cell tumor (GCT; also known as Abrikossoff's tumor[84]) may be seen in many anatomic locations, including the skin, oral cavity, breast, larynx, esophagus, biliary tree, vulva, penis, soft tissue, and lower respiratory tract.[85] Among those sites, it is relatively rare in the trachea and lungs, with less than 200 cases having been reported therein.[86–104] Patients of any age may develop such lesions, and multiple tumors in the same individual have been reported.[100]

With respect to tracheobronchial GCTs, some are asymptomatic and are found incidentally,[103] whereas others present with obstructive signs and symptoms; hemoptysis; or cough.[97,100] Endoscopic examination often reveals a sessile polypoid endoluminal component, with intact overlying mucosa[96] (Fig. 19.27). Radiographic studies confirm that characteristic, but also demonstrate an infiltrative aspect to many GCTs that may lead to a mistaken preoperative diagnosis of malignancy.[95–101] GCTs in the peripheral lung parenchyma are unusual,[103] but these likewise assume a spiculated appearance which

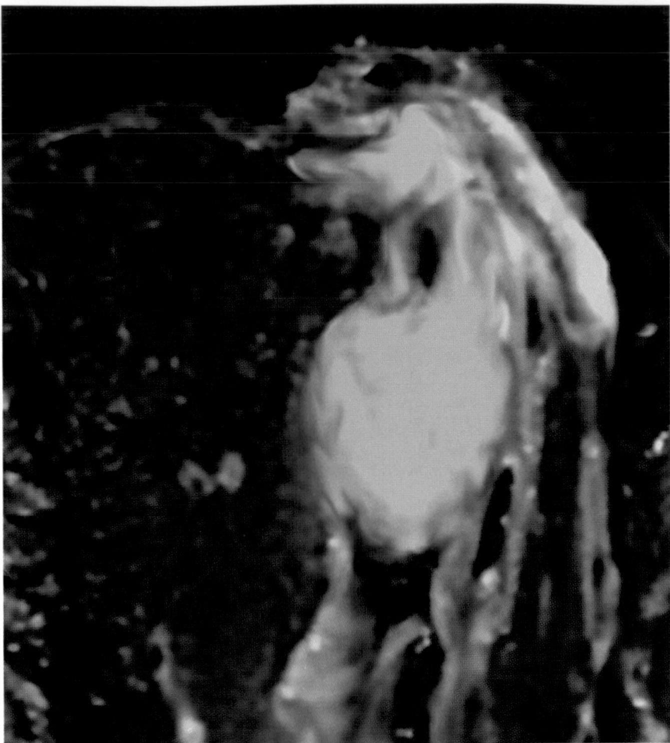

Fig. 19.27 A small polypoid intrabronchial lesion (arrow) is apparent in this photograph, representing a granular cell tumor.

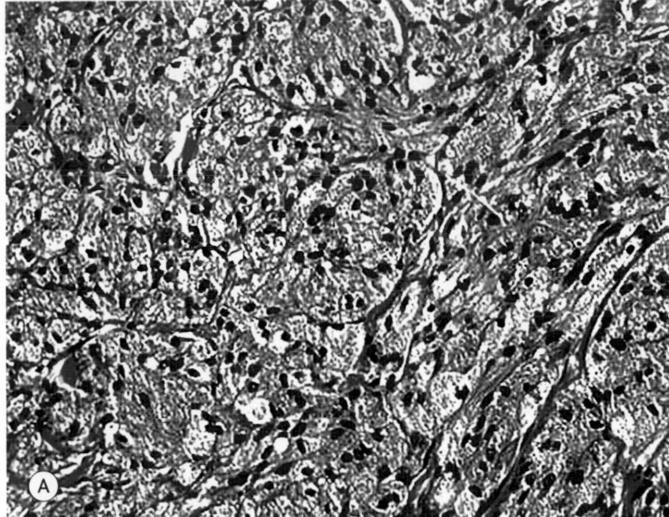

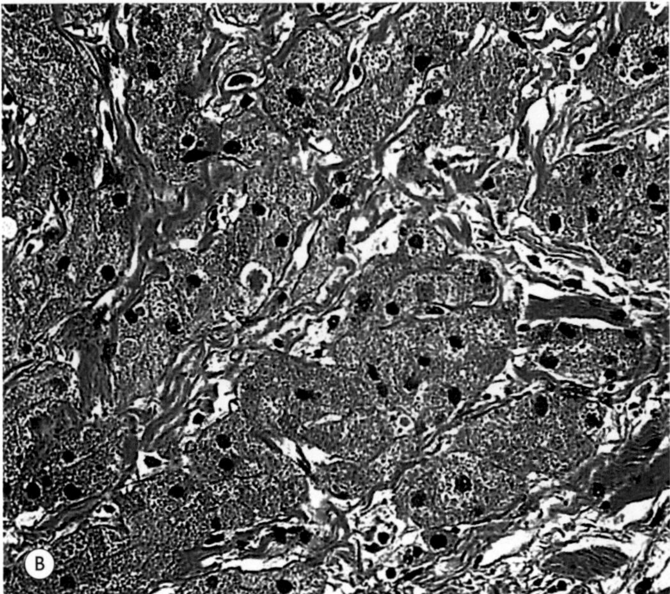

Fig. 19.28 Sheets of polygonal eosinophilic cells (A) with bland nuclei and prominently granular cytoplasm (B) are seen in this pulmonary granular cell tumor.

closely simulates that of adenocarcinoma. This situation is further complicated by occasional case reports of GCTs that coexisted with malignant neoplasms.[105,106]

Grossly, GCT is a white-tan, ill-defined mass with a gritty cut surface, again simulating the features of an infiltrating carcinoma at that level of observation. However, necrosis and hemorrhage are distinctly unusual. Maximum tumor size approximates 5 cm.

Microscopically, one sees a uniform population of polygonal or fusiform cells that contain small ovoid hyperchromatic nuclei with indistinct nucleoli (Fig. 19.28). The cytoplasm is abundant, eosinophilic or amphophilic, and coarsely granulated, often with the additional presence of rounded inclusions that superficially resemble Michaelis–Gutman bodies (Fig. 19.29). The latter structures may also have a targetoid configuration. Mitotic figures are typically scarce and physiologic in shape; necrosis and vascular invasion are absent. The advancing border of granular cell tumors may be "pushing" or irregular and permeative. Indeed, a proportion of these lesions infiltrate deeply into the bronchial wall or even through it into the adjacent parenchyma. In non-pulmonary sites, such a growth pattern has been linked to a greater risk of recurrence,[107] but that correlation does not seem to apply to GCTs in the airways or lungs. Indeed, the existence of primary *malignant* granular cell tumor of the respiratory tract has never been convincingly documented, and recurrent neoplasms are typically those that have never been completely excised in the first place.

Electron microscopy of GCTs shows a distinctive multiplicity of secondary and tertiary lysosomes in the cytoplasm of the tumor cells, virtually to the exclusion of other organelles[108,109] (Fig. 19.30). Immunohistologic evaluation most often reveals evidence of schwannian differentiation, with reactivity for S100 protein, CD56, CD57, myelin basic protein, and combinations thereof, in 80–85% of cases.[109–112] The abundance of lysosomes in such lesions is reflected by their CD68 reactivity.

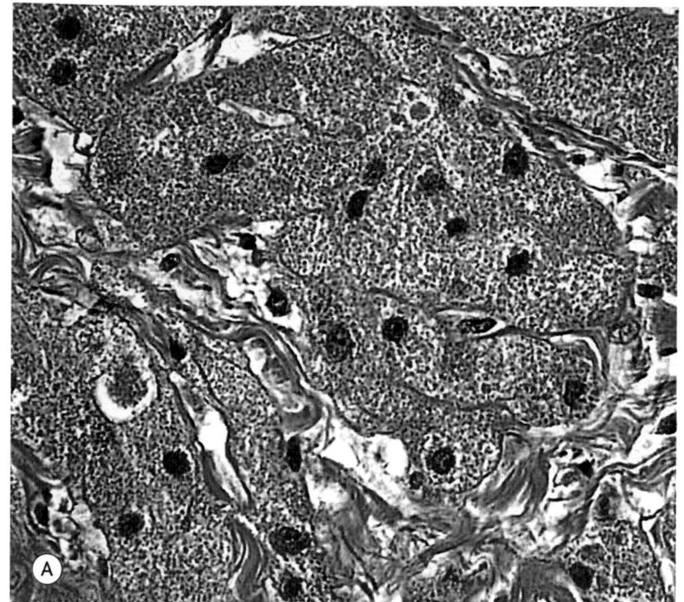

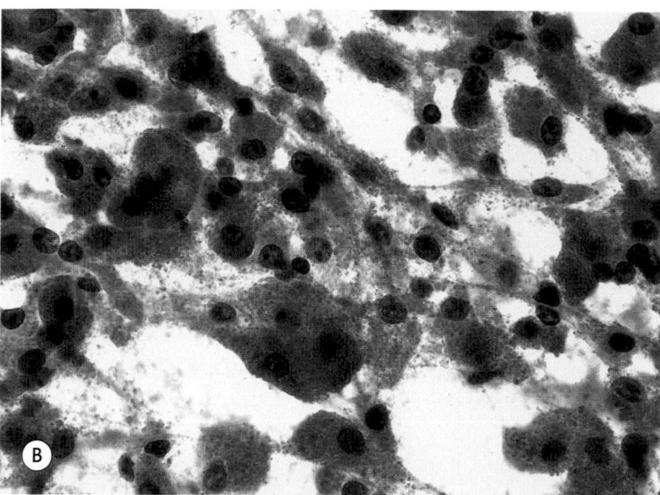

Fig. 19.29 Granular cytoplasm and the presence of targetoid intracytoplasmic inclusions resembling Michaelis–Gutman bodies (top center and left of figure) are seen in this bronchial granular cell tumor (A). A fine-needle aspiration biopsy specimen (B) in the same case demonstrates the numerous cytoplasmic granules in the lesion and its tendency towards cellular dyshesion in this type of sample.

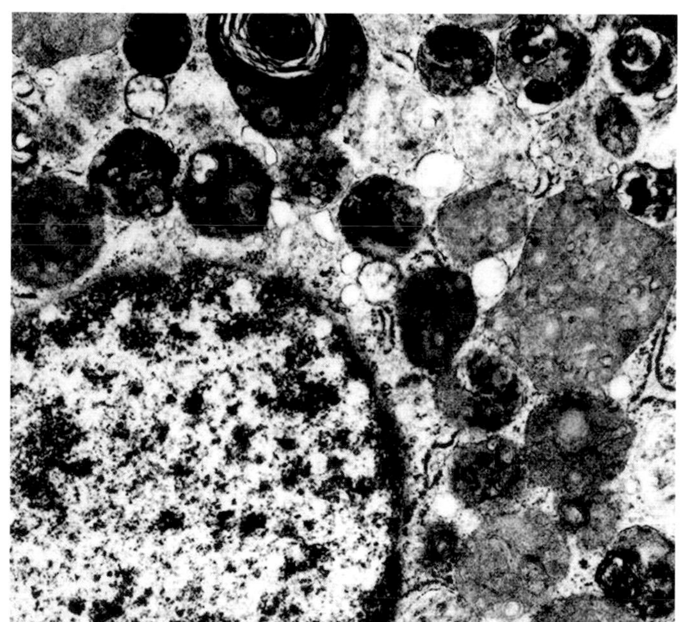

Fig. 19.30 This electron photomicrograph of granular cell tumor demonstrates innumerable secondary and tertiary cytoplasmic lysosomes.

Recently, the presence of calretinin and alpha-inhibin has also been reported in GCT.[113]

An important caveat regarding the immunophenotype of this tumor type is that *non*-schwannian lesions containing granular cells comprise a heterogenous group.[114] Carcinomas (both neuroendocrine and non-endocrine,[115,116] smooth muscle tumors, endothelial proliferations, and neoplasms of uncommitted lineage have all been described with a granular cell phenotype. Therefore, it is important to include immunohistologic evaluations to address those possibilities in differential diagnosis, with or without ultrastructural studies as well. Oncocytoid granular cell grade 1 neuroendocrine carcinoma ("carcinoid") of the lung is the most common simulator of GCT,[117,118] making chromogranin-A and synaptophysin (both of which are absent in GCT) important markers in this context. Neurosecretory granules are also apparent in ultrastructural studies of neuroendocrine lesions, but not in GCTs.

As mentioned above, aggressive behavior by bronchopulmonary GCT has not been observed. Therefore, conservative therapy for this neoplasm is warranted.

Benign lesions affecting either large airways or the parenchyma

Leiomyoma/leiomyomatous hamartoma and "benign metastasizing leiomyoma"

Solitary leiomyoma of the respiratory tract has been reported as an independent entity, by several authors. They may be located in the trachea, bronchial walls, or pulmonary parenchyma.[119–124] Because of the relatively common content of smooth muscle in hamartomas of the lung (see Ch. 18), we believe that it is difficult – if not

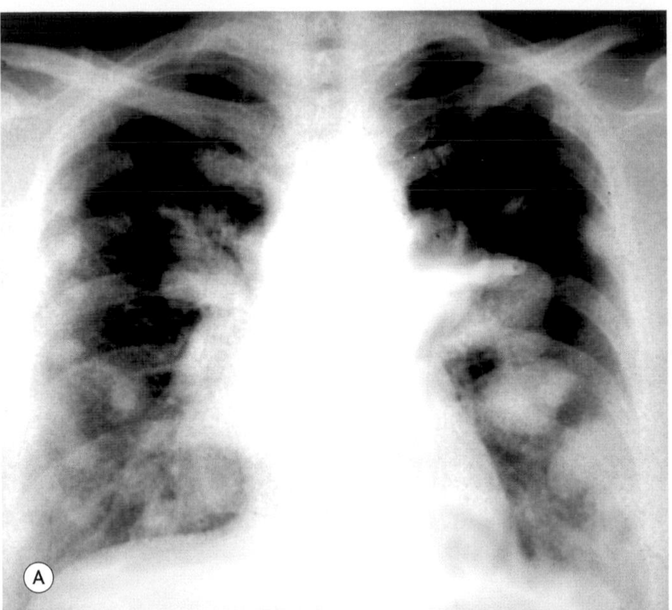

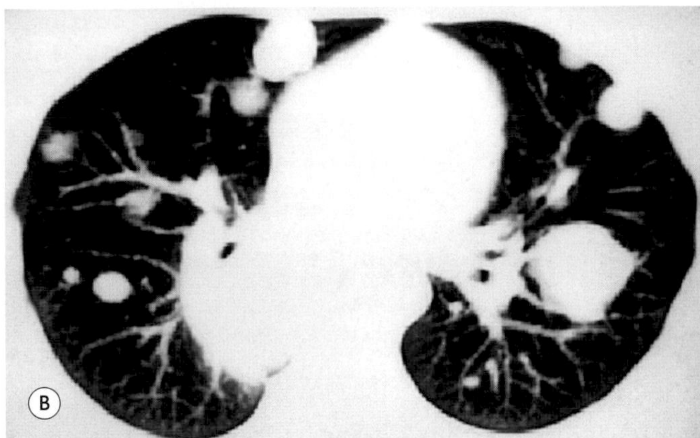

Fig. 19.31 (A) "Benign metastasizing leiomyoma" takes the form of multiple bilateral intrapulmonary nodules of variable size in a plain-film chest radiograph. A computed tomogram (B) from another case of "benign metastasizing leiomyoma" of the lung demonstrates comparable findings.

impossible – to separate them definitively from pulmonary "leiomyomas;" indeed, because hamartomas are comparatively common, it is also statistically likely that at least some "leiomyomas" actually represented variants thereof.

In any event, patients with bronchopulmonary leiomyomas (BPLs) have typically been adults, with women substantially outnumbering men. Most of these tumors are discovered because of cough, asthma-like symptoms and signs, hemoptysis, or obstructive pneumonia.[122–124] Bronchoscopic evaluation in those instances shows a dome-shaped endoluminal mass, usually with a smooth mucosal surface. In contrast, parenchymal leiomyomas are oval or round coin lesions in the peripheral lung fields, and these are discovered incidentally on chest radiographs in asymptomatic individuals.[120,122]

A most peculiar variant of smooth muscle proliferation in the lung is represented by the tumor variously known as "benign metastasizing leiomyoma"[125–135] or "(adeno)fibroleiomyomatous hamartoma."[136–138] It is a multifocal multinodular proliferation in the lung parenchyma, typically assuming the radiographic appearance of metastatic lesions (Fig. 19.31), and is confined to women. Most of those patients have undergone previous hysterectomies for uterine smooth muscle tumors, or are found to have such neoplasms concurrently with their pulmonary tumors.

The macroscopic image of smooth muscle tumors in the lung is comparable to the same lesions in other locations, being represented by sharply circumscribed firm tan-gray masses with a "whorled" internal fascicular pattern. Solitary pulmonary lesions may be several centimeters in greatest dimension, whereas those in the large airways are small.[124] "Benign metastasizing leiomyomas" (BMLs) likewise vary considerably in size, but some cases feature the presence of innumerable small nodules that reproduce the appearance of miliary granulomatous disease.[134]

The histologic appearance of these tumors features a uniform population of fusiform cells with blunt-ended nuclei, dispersed chromatin, fibrillary eosinophilic cytoplasm, few if any mitotic figures, and an absence of necrosis (Figs 19.32–19.34). Some also contain zones of stromal fibrosis, with or without entrapment of bronchiolar epithelium. It is the latter lesions which, in multifocal form, are either termed BMLs or adeno-fibroleiomyomatous hamartomas. These proliferations beg the question of whether they are multifocal (but primary) malformations in the lung in patients with extrapulmonary smooth muscle tumors, or, alternatively, intrathoracic metastases of such neoplasms. Recent molecular–genetic analysis has argued in favor of the latter interpretation, indicating that BMLs have a clonal (neoplastic) nature.[131]

The fine structural features of smooth muscle tumors in the lung include the presence of pericellular basal

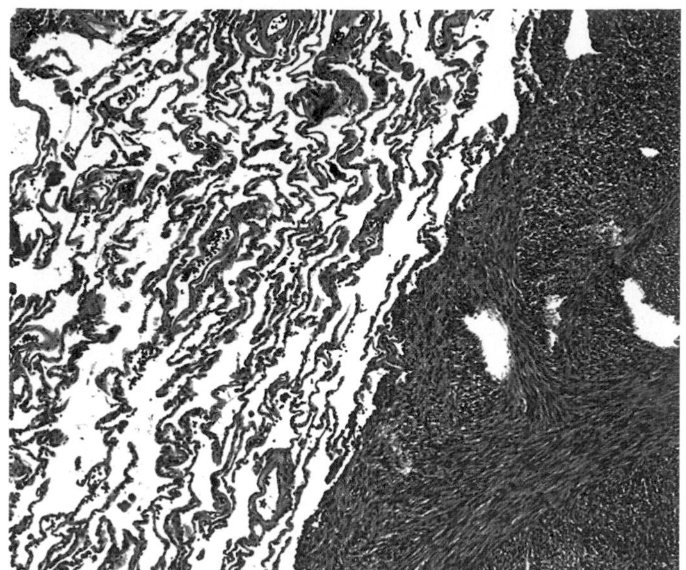

Fig. 19.32 This low-power microscopic image of a pulmonary "benign metastasizing leiomyoma" shows sharp circumscription of a cellular spindle cell tumor, with no associated fibrosis or inflammation.

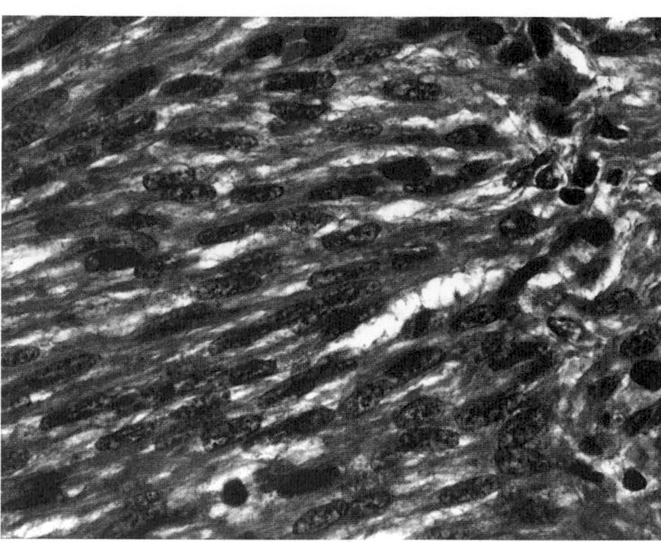

Fig. 19.34 Fibrillar eosinophilic cytoplasm and blunt-ended nuclear profiles are evident in this pulmonary "benign metastasizing leiomyoma."

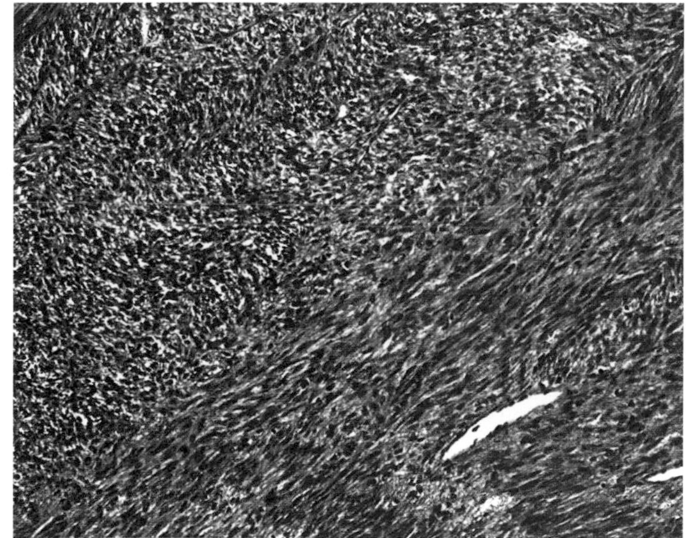

Fig. 19.33 Internal fascicles of fusiform tumor cells are apparent in this "benign metastasizing leiomyoma" of the lung.

lamina; plasmalemmal hemidesmosomes and micropinocytotic vesicles; skeins of cytoplasmic thin filaments; and intrafilamentous dense bodies.[126,136] Immunohistologically, one typically sees reactivity for muscle-specific actin, alpha-isoform ("smooth-muscle") actin, desmin, calponin, and caldesmon, with an absence of S100 protein, CD56, CD57, and keratin.[124,130,132] Several reports have also documented the presence of receptor proteins in the tumor cells for estrogen and progesterone[126,133] (Fig. 19.35).

Differential diagnosis of primary smooth muscle tumors of the respiratory tract includes hamartomas (see above), as well as peripheral nerve sheath tumors and sarcomatoid carcinomas. Although conventional histologic analysis is usually sufficient to distinguish between those possibilities, the special studies just cited may be necessary as well.

Solitary smooth muscle tumors are treated with simple but complete excision, if thorough clinical evaluation has excluded an extrapulmonary lesion of the same type. The latter proviso relates to the fact that some leiomyosarcomas (particularly in the retroperitoneum) are extremely low-grade proliferations that may still produce metastases which simulate leiomyomas histologically.[139] Despite the likelihood that they are also secondary in nature, BMLs may nonetheless regress spontaneously or in response to pharmacologic hormonal modulation.[125] Women with those neoplasms have a favorable prognosis despite the alarming appearances of their chest radiographs, and growth of such lesions typically stops with the onset of the menopause.

Glomus tumor and glomangioma

Glomus tumor/glomangioma (GTG) is an uncommon pulmonary lesion, with less than 15 cases having been reported to date.[140–145] It is most often seen in the skin and superficial soft tissue,[146] but also occurs with relative frequency in the alimentary tract.[147] The clinicopathologic characteristics of this lesion in the trachea, lungs, and

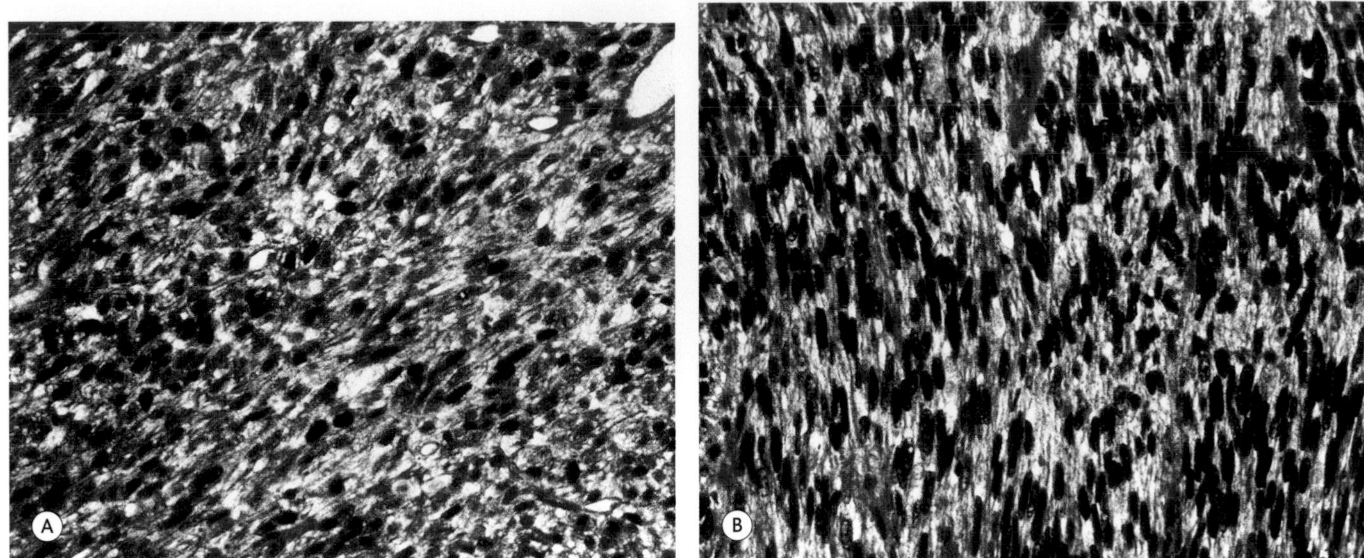

Fig. 19.35 Nuclear immunoreactivity for estrogen receptor protein (A) and progesterone receptor protein (B) in "benign metastasizing leiomyoma" of the lung.

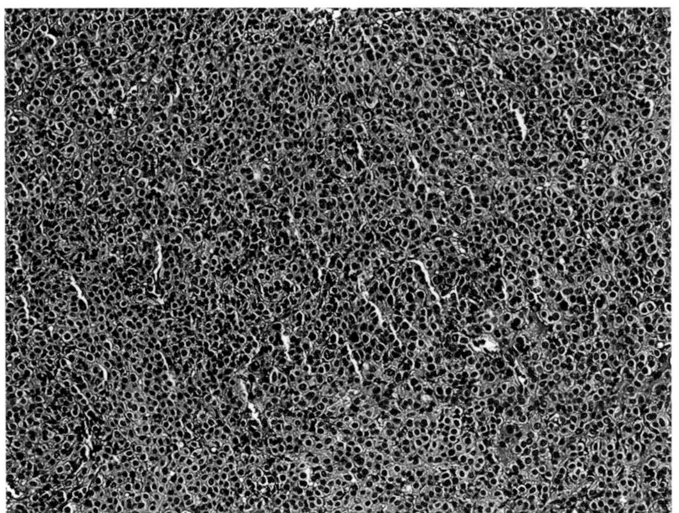

Fig. 19.36 Sheets of monotonous, bland epithelioid cells are seen in this glomus tumor.

mediastinum have been summarized recently by Gaertner et al.[144]

Pulmonary GTG has affected adults, with the youngest patient being 20 years of age and the oldest being 69 at diagnosis. The majority of the lesions were found incidentally on chest radiographs in asymptomatic individuals, but some were associated with hemoptysis, upper abdominal pain, and pneumothorax. One tumor arose in the left mainstem bronchus, whereas the others were peripheral neoplasms that affected each of the major pulmonary compartments except for the right middle lobe.[144] They were treated variably with lobectomy, sleeve resection of the bronchus, or wedge resection of the subpleural lung parenchyma, and all except one patient (see below) were alive without recurrence at last follow-up.

The macroscopic features of GTG include a nodular configuration, with uniform gray-white or yellow cut surfaces and a maximum dimension of 6.5 cm. These attributes have led to erroneous gross diagnoses of "carcinoid" in some cases.[145]

Microscopically, the lesions are constituted by compact polygonal or round cells, which are closely apposed (Fig. 19.36). Nuclei are round or oval with dispersed chromatin, scarce mitotic activity, and little if any pleomorphism. Cytoplasm is modest in amount and amphophilic or eosinophilic (Fig. 19.37). Supporting stroma consists of delicate fibrovascular septations. In those lesions that lie toward the "glomangioma" pole of the spectrum, dilated vascular spaces also punctuate the lesions (Fig. 19.38), and some of these may assume a "moose-antler" shape like the vessels seen in hemangiopericytomas. A proportion of pulmonary GTGs are infiltrative; accordingly, they may permeate through the bronchial wall into the adjacent parenchyma, or grow irregularly in the peripheral lung tissue. Nevertheless, the usual image has been that of a circumscribed lesion on low-power examination, having a distinct interface with the surrounding parenchyma.

One exception to the foregoing description (mentioned above) was represented by a tumor in the series of

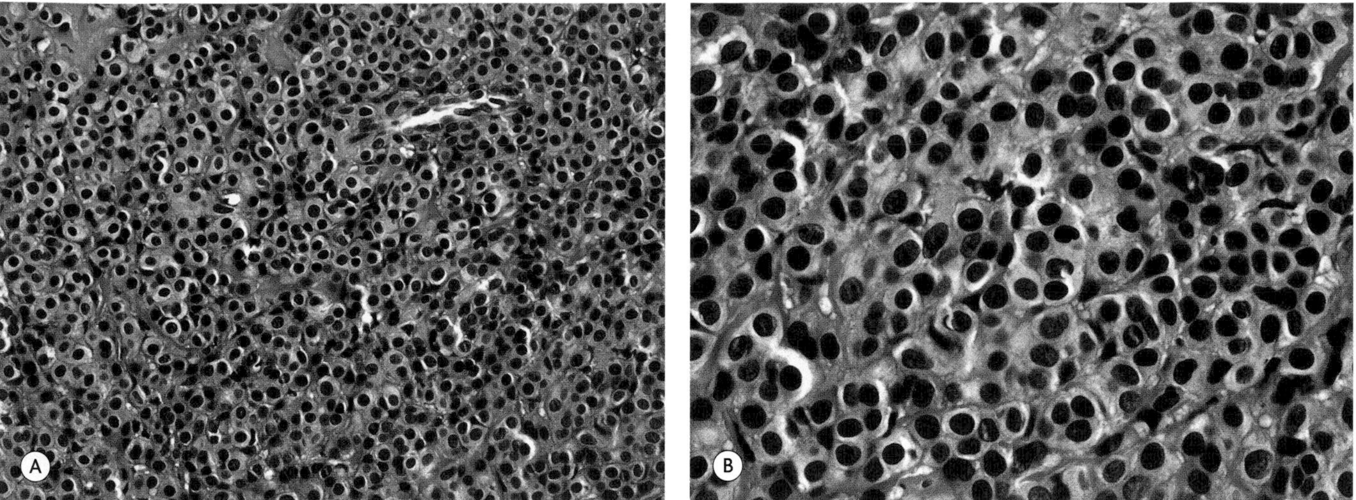

Fig. 19.37 (A, B) Cytoplasm is eosinophilic and modest in quantity in glomus tumor cells. Nuclei in glomus tumor are regular, round, and bland, with no nucleoli and only very rare mitotic figures.

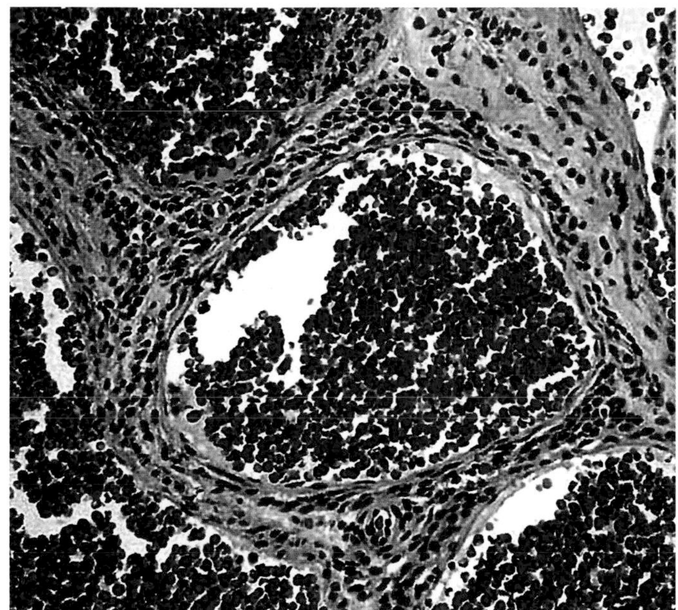

Fig. 19.38 This example of glomangioma demonstrates dilated vascular structures.

Gaertner et al., which demonstrated infiltrative growth, obvious nuclear atypia with prominent nucleoli, necrosis, and brisk mitotic activity.[144] That neoplasm metastasized to several visceral sites and soft tissue, causing death in 1.3 years. Thus, it was classified as a "glomangiosarcoma."

Electron microscopic examination of GTGs shows evidence of specialized smooth muscle differentiation (see above section on leiomyoma), as expected in pericytic perivascular cells.[143,144] The immunophenotype of GTG includes reactivity for vimentin, actin, laminin, and collagen type IV, with an absence of keratin, neuroendocrine markers, CD31, and CD34.[144]

The differential diagnosis of GTG centers on the alternatives of grade 1 neuroendocrine carcinoma ("carcinoid"), primitive neuroectodermal tumor (PNET) of the lung, intrapulmonary paraganglioma, and hemangiopericytoma. The first three of those lesions reproducibly demonstrate neuroendocrine or neuroectodermal markers such as chromogranin-A, synaptophysin, CD56, and CD99 – all of which are absent in GTG – and hemangiopericytomas consistently lack the actin positivity that is expected in glomus tumors.

Chondroma, myxoma, and fibromyxoma

Although some authors have posited that true chondromas and (fibro)myxomas of the lung[148,149] exist apart from hamartomas[150–153] (see Ch. 18), we believe that conclusion to be debatable. At the present time, we are unconvinced that examples of pulmonary chondroma or myxoma can be found in the literature which differ significantly enough from hamartomatous myxochondroid lesions to stand alone as definable entities.

Hemangioma and "hemangiomatosis"

True hemangiomas of the tracheobronchial tree and lung are vanishingly rare. They are usually detected in childhood, sometimes with hemoptysis and in other cases with indirect signs of intrathoracic disease such as digital clubbing.[154] Discrete, variably-dense and sometimes-cystic masses are present on chest radiographs in examples of parenchymal hemangioma, and they may be multiple. The maximum size of individual lesions can be several

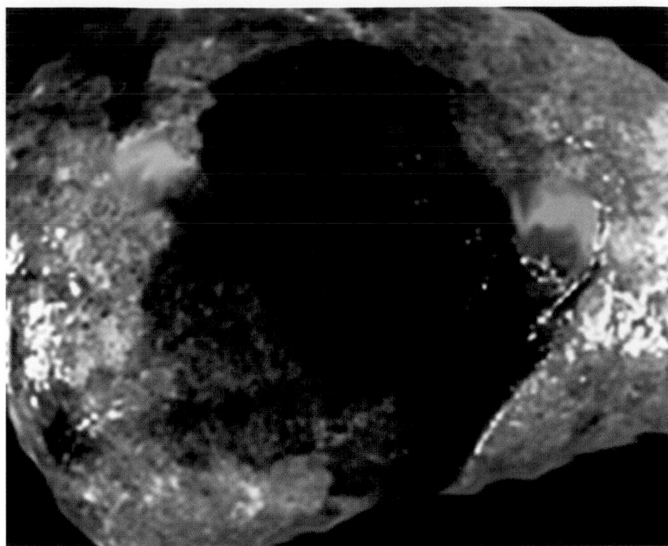

Fig. 19.39 This gross photograph of an intrapulmonary hemangioma shows a well-defined, dark, blood-filled lesion measuring several centimeters in diameter.

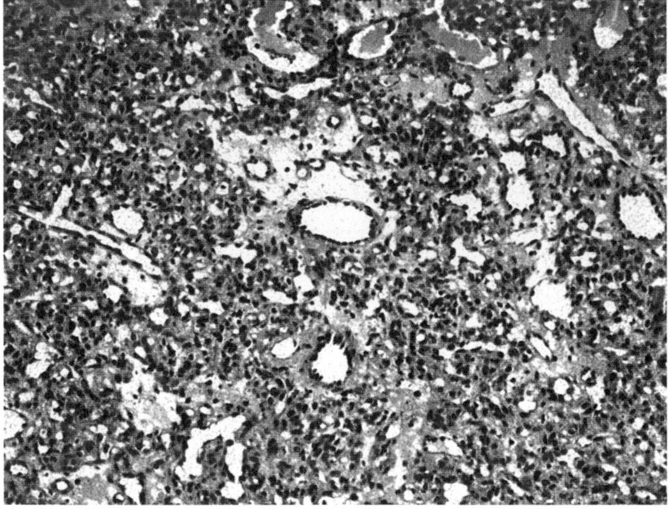

Fig. 19.40 Numerous, closely set, small tubular vascular lumina are apparent in this capillary hemangioma.

centimeters (Fig. 19.39). In at least one case, an intrapulmonary hemangioma was interpreted radiographically as an intrapulmonary bronchogenic cyst.[154] Simple excision has been curative.

Microscopically, true hemangiomas of the airways and lungs completely replace a portion of the native tissue with a proliferation of tubular vascular spaces that are lined by bland endothelial cells. A "capillary hemangioma" pattern appears to be most common, in which the caliber of the neoplastic vessels approximates that of normal small venules or capillaries (Fig. 19.40). It is of course implicit in this diagnosis that no other tumoral elements are identified; this is an important caveat because several other neoplasms in the lung – including some carcinomas – may contain blood lakes or pseudovascular foci that resemble the image of vascular proliferations.[155]

Another salient differential diagnostic consideration is that of "pulmonary hemangiomatosis" (see Chapter 11, page 396). That is a condition in which capillary-sized blood vessels proliferate throughout the pre-existing pulmonary parenchyma and stroma, including the alveolar septa, interlobular and interlobar septa, bronchial and bronchiolar walls, intrapulmonary vasa vasorum, and pleural surfaces.[156,157] In reality, it may not be a neoplastic process at all, but rather a malformative or reactive proliferation. For example, some cases of pulmonary hemangiomatosis have been associated with long-standing passive congestion of the lungs, as seen in left-sided heart failure.[157]

Lipoma and lipoblastoma

Lipoma of the major bronchi (LMB) is an uncommon lesion, with <150 cases in the literature;[158–163] however, once again, it is difficult to separate examples of LMB from lipocytic hamartomas of the lung with certainty, and pathologic criteria for doing so are arbitrary.[164] Patients with LMB are adults, usually in the fifth or sixth decades of life, who present with symptoms and signs of airway obstruction, cough, shortness of breath, or secondary pneumonia.[161] Endoscopic examination shows a variably-polypoid submucosal nodule in one of the first three subdivisions of the tracheobronchial tree; radiographs demonstrate secondary atelectasis, obstructive pneumonia, or a mass in 80% of cases, but the remainder have no radiologic abnormalities on plain films.[159] Computed tomograms (CTs) are more sensitive in revealing the presence of an endobronchial lesion.[163] Current treatment recommendations are for conservative endoscopic resection after a transbronchial biopsy has established the adipocytic nature of the lesion (Fig. 19.41).

Lipomas are also rarely seen in the peripheral lung fields, again with <125 reported cases.[159,163,164–168] Demographic data on affected patients are similar to those associated with LMB. Intrapulmonary lipomas are often subpleural and may even protrude into the pleural space, but are associated with few if any symptoms. Accordingly, these nodular lesions are typically detected incidentally on chest radiographs. Computed tomography shows that lipomas of the lung have a density approximating that of pleural adipose tissue.[163] Occasional

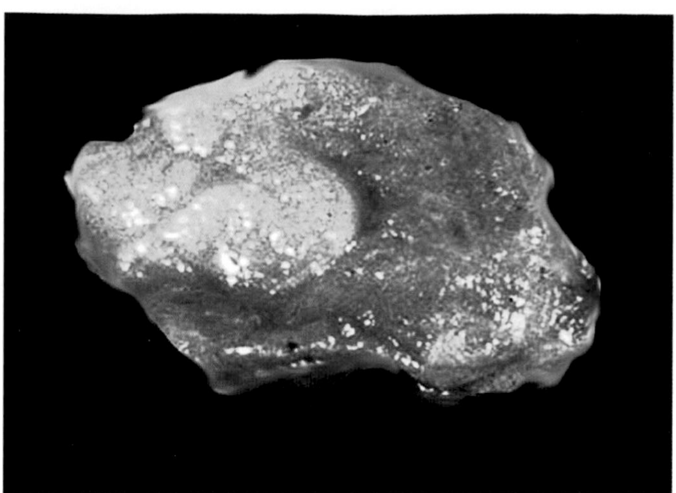

Fig. 19.41 This bronchoscopically resected endobronchial lipoma shows internal lobulation and uniformly yellow tissue.

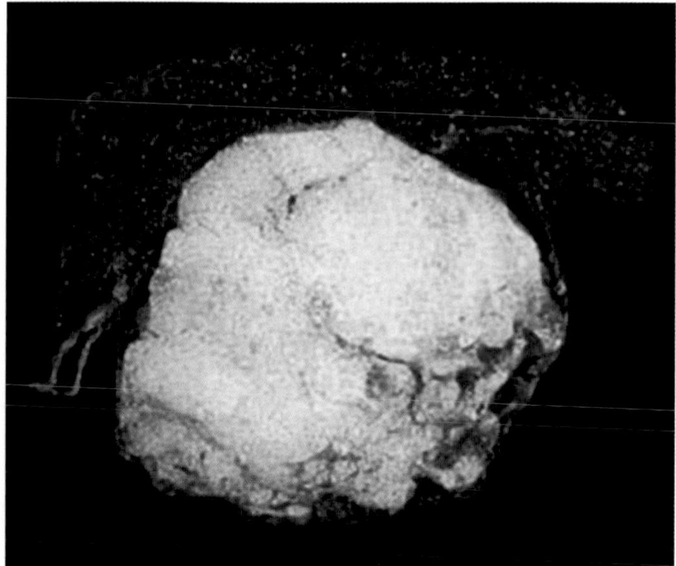

Fig. 19.42 Peripheral intrapulmonary lipoma, represented by a large globular tan-yellow lesion beneath the pleural surface.

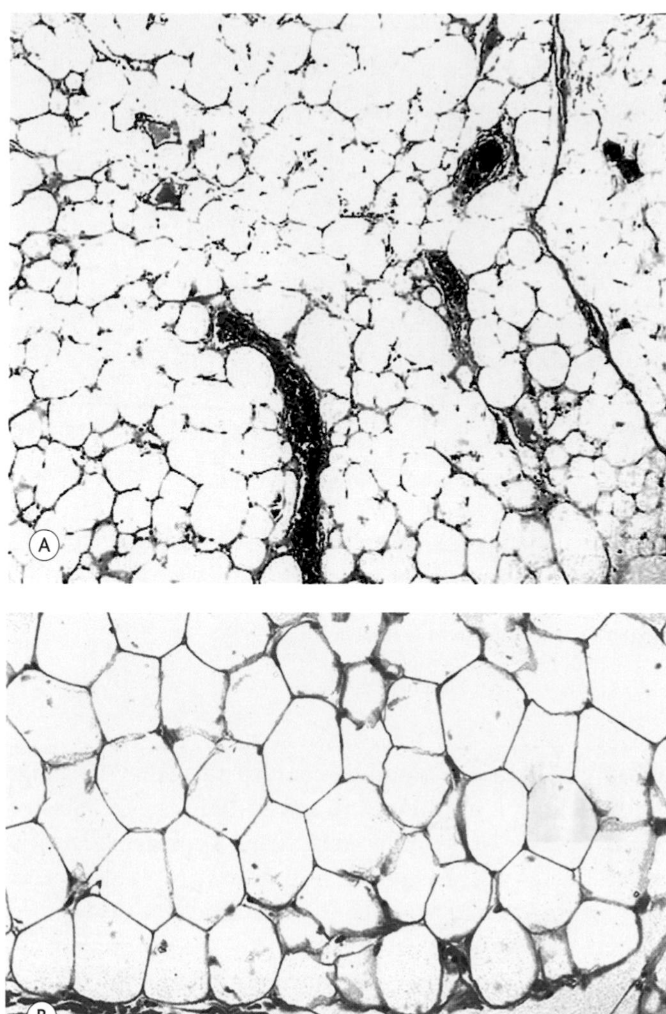

Fig. 19.43 (A) Lobulated arrays of mature adipocytes with (B) compact eccentric nuclei and abundant lipid-filled cytoplasm are evident in this pulmonary lipoma.

lesions of this type have been found coincidentally in patients with pulmonary carcinomas.[160]

The remaining fatty tumor that may arise very rarely within the respiratory tract is the lipoblastoma. These neoplasms are seen in young children, usually in the soft tissue of the trunk, extremities, head and neck, or retroperitoneum.[169] Some have affected the pleura and chest wall as well, but only anecdotal reports exist of intrapulmonary lipoblastomas (ILBs).[170,171] At least one of these neoplasms was extremely large and occupied almost one entire hemithorax.[170] Excision was curative in the few cases with meaningful follow-up.

The principal macroscopic feature of intrapulmonary adipocytic tumors is that of a yellow, globular, relatively soft mass in the parenchyma (Fig. 19.42). Internal fibrous septation may be apparent, as may a circumferential capsule or small foci of intralesional sclerosis. There is no necrosis or hemorrhage.

Microscopically, one sees sheets of fully mature adipocytes in ordinary lipomas, supported by delicate fibrovascular stroma (Fig. 19.43). Matsuba et al. have described a single example of atypical intrapulmonary lipoma, showing scattered multinucleated “floret” cells.[166] However, that finding did not influence behavior unfavorably. Lipoblastomas have a more lobulated substructure, with an admixture of uncommitted

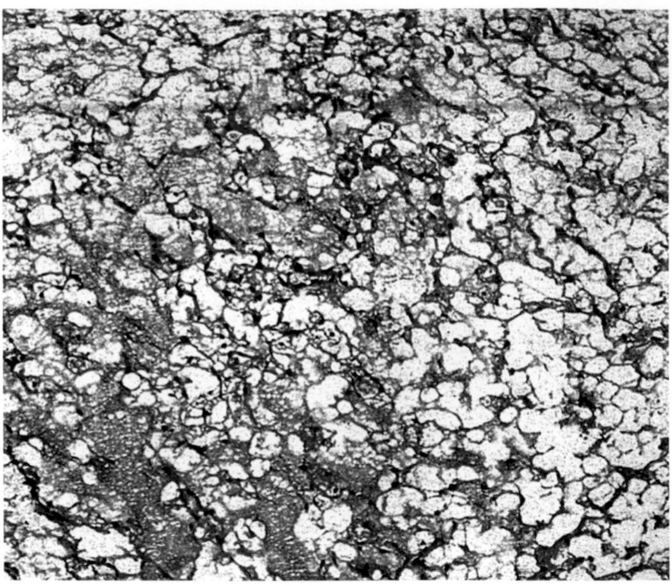

Fig. 19.44 A lobulated admixture of mature lipocytes, stellate cells, and myxoid stroma is apparent in lipoblastoma.

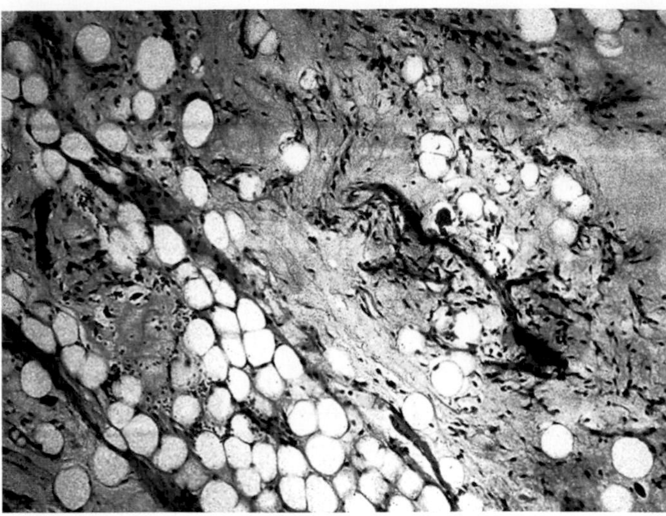

Fig. 19.45 Internal vascular stroma is evident in this lipoblastoma, superficially simulating the appearance of myxoid liposarcoma.

fibromyxoid tissue amongst mature fat cells[169,172] (Fig. 19.44). The first of those elements contains aggregates of bland stellate or spindle cells. True lipoblasts may be apparent as well, rare mitotic figures may be evident, and supporting stromal tissue contains a delicately arborizing capillary network (Fig. 19.45). The overall image of lipoblastoma therefore may be quite similar to that of myxoid liposarcoma, and the mutually exclusive occurrence of those tumors in different age groups – with liposarcomas being seen in adults – is important to their proper identification.

If the latter point is in doubt, karyotypic analysis may be useful, using fluorescent in-situ hybridization (FISH). Abnormalities in chromosome 8q are most common in lipoblastomas,[172] whereas myxoid liposarcoma demonstrates a reproducible t(12;16) chromosomal translocation.[173] Parenthetically, cytogenetic profiles are somewhat less helpful in the distinction between lipomas of the lung and lipomatous hamartomas, both of which may show abnormalities in chromosome 12.[167,174] However, exchanges of material between chromosomes 6 and 14 are also potentially observed in hamartomas but not lipomas.[175]

Immunohistology of fatty tumors of the lungs shows consistent reactivity for S100 protein in the adipocytic elements, as well as "high-mobility-group" (HMG) proteins.[174] Lipoblastoma may also show positivity for factor XIIIa in its stellate and fusiform cells.[172]

The differential diagnosis of lipoma and lipoblastoma in the lung has been mentioned above. However, to reiterate, it centers on lipomatous hamartoma and metastatic lipoma-like liposarcoma in respect to primary pulmonary lipoma, and metastatic or primary myxoid liposarcoma in regard to primary lipoblastoma of the lung. Again, cytogenetic studies are probably the most productive in discriminating between primary fatty tumors of various types; historic information is typically sufficient to address the possibility of metastatic sarcoma.

Angiomyolipoma

In recent years, it has become apparent that a family of neoplasms – which may arise in the kidney, pancreas, alimentary system, liver, soft tissue, and respiratory tract – demonstrates differentiation towards a unique cell type that has both myogenous and melanocytic features.[176–178] These tumors have been variously called "angiomyolipomas," "perivascular epithelioid cell neoplasms" (PEComas), and "myomelanocytomas."[176–179] If a typical morphologic image including smooth muscle, fat, and vascular proliferation is observed, the first of those terms is still preferred; a few lesions with such characteristics have been reported in the lung.[180–184] Another member of this nosologic group – the pulmonary "sugar tumor" – will be discussed later in this chapter. All of these proliferations potentially share immunoreactivity with the melanocyte-related antibody human melanin black (HMB)-45, as well as anti-actins.[177] Other immunohistochemical markers of melanocytic and smooth muscle differentiation – e.g. antibodies to S100 protein, tyrosinase, HMB-50, melanoma antigen related to T-cells-1 (MART-1), caldesmon, calponin, and desmin – may also label them.[178]

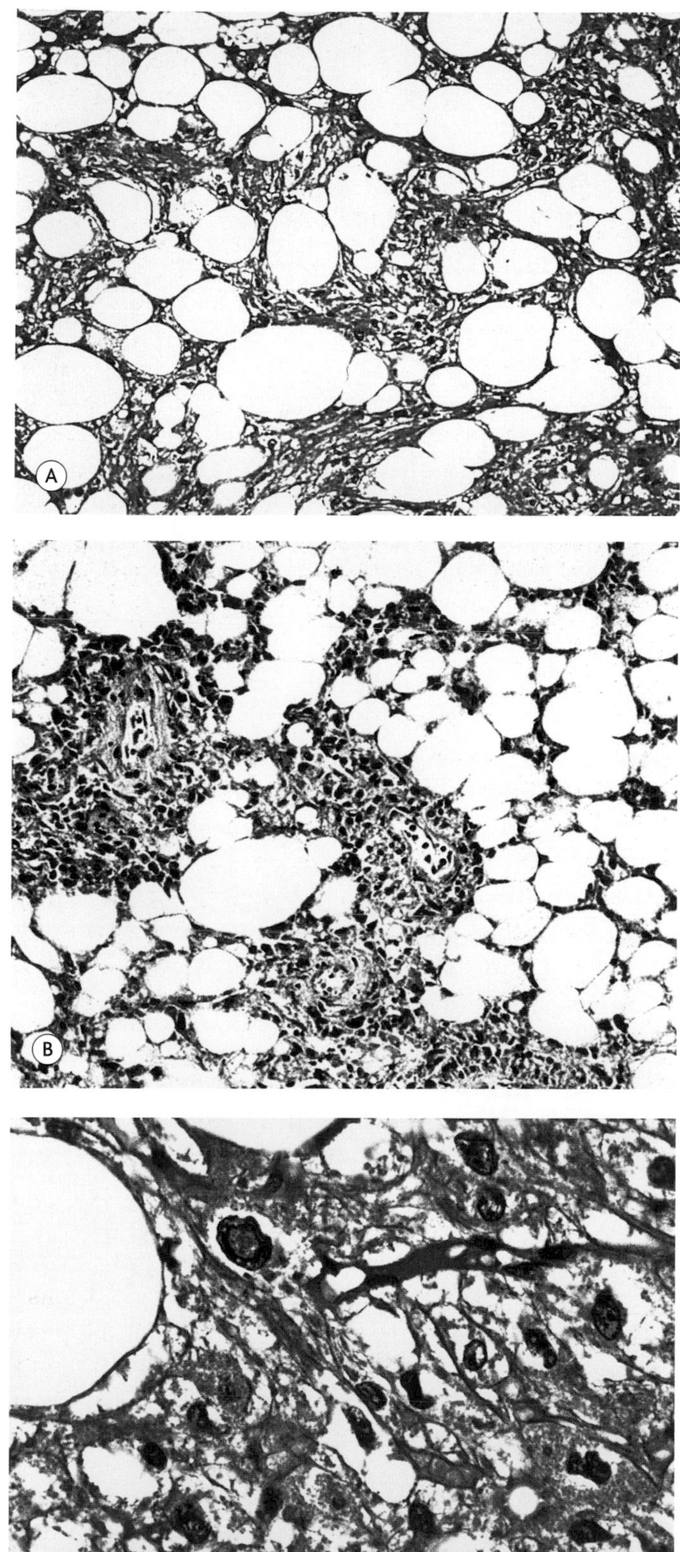

Fig. 19.46 (A–C) These angiomyolipomas show a tripartite constituency by mature adipocytes, large blood vessels, and epithelioid and fusiform myogenous cells, with variable prominence of each component.

A proportion of patients with angiomyolipomas, regardless of their anatomic locations, will have the phakomatosis known as tuberous sclerosis (Bourneville's syndrome). It classically includes nodular periventricular glial proliferations and subependymal giant cell astrocytomas in the brain; cutaneous connective tissue nevi; often-multifocal renal angiomyolipomas; and pulmonary lymphangioleiomyomatosis (LAM), with or without multifocal micronodular pneumocytic hyperplasia (MMPH) (discussed further in Chapter 7).[181,185–187]

Pulmonary angiomyolipoma is extremely rare, with less than 10 documented cases in the literature.[180–184] It has been discovered as an incidental finding on chest radiographs, in one case occasioned by the presence of hemothorax.[183] In another instance, there were several angiomyolipomas in both lung fields, simulating the macroscopic image of metastatic disease.[180] Wu and Tazelaar[181] were the first to report angiomyolipoma of the lung in a patient with other morphologic lesions of tuberous sclerosis, including renal angiomyolipoma and MMPH.

The lung tumors in these cases have individually been <2 cm in maximal dimension. They showed sharp interfaces with the surrounding lung tissue and uniform yellow-tan cut surfaces.

Microscopically, pulmonary angiomyolipoma is essentially identical to its better-known renal counterpart. Prototypically, it manifests a concatenation of mature fat, variably sized and haphazardly arranged blood vessels with muscular walls, and nests or skeins of fusiform or epithelioid smooth muscle elements (Fig. 19.46) The first or last of those components may dominate the histologic picture and cause diagnostic confusion with either pure adipocytic neoplasms or sarcomas, respectively. Nuclear atypia has been seen in the smooth muscle elements of angiomyolipomas in extrapulmonary sites, and rare cases outside the lung have even shown overtly malignant transformation with necrosis and atypical mitotic activity.[188] Those attributes have not been seen in pulmonary lesions of this type.

Electron microscopic analysis of angiomyolipoma demonstrates findings that recall the characteristics of smooth muscle cells, including pericellular basal lamina and plasmalemma-associated pinocytotic vesicles.[180] Cytoplasmic bundles of thin filaments have not been found. Approximately 50% of such neoplasms do show the presence of cytoplasmic premelanosomes.[178]

The principal immunohistologic findings in angiomyolipomas have been listed above (Fig. 19.47). Additional features of note include negativity for keratin, desmoplakin, epithelial membrane antigen, carcino-embryonic antigen, and Ber-EP4 antigen.

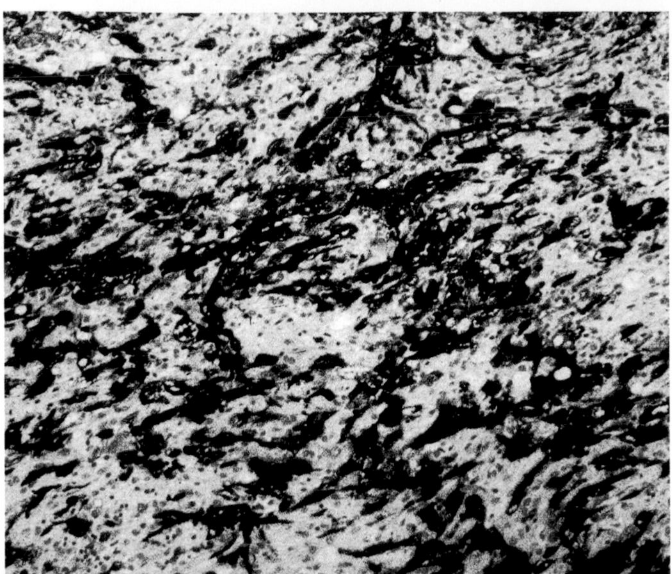

Fig. 19.47 HMB-45 immunoreactivity in angiomyolipoma.

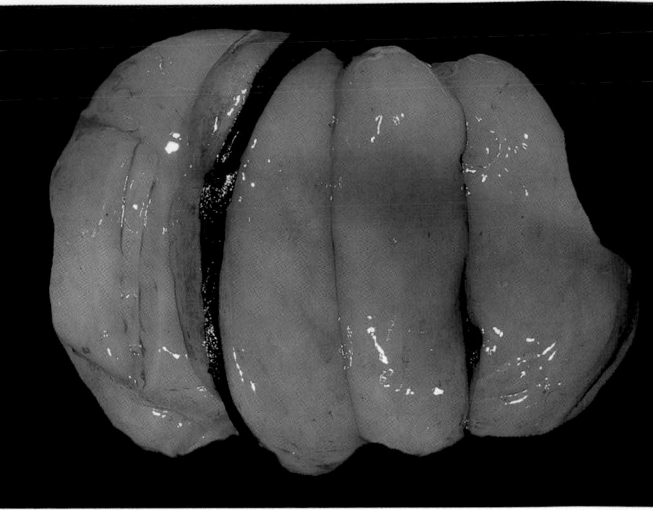

Fig. 19.48 This gross photograph of myelolipoma shows a lobulated circumscribed yellow lesion, resembling a lipoma.

In its usual form, angiomyolipoma has no realistic differential diagnostic alternatives. Nevertheless, as mentioned above, its morphologic variants may be difficult to distinguish from metastastic melanomas, carcinomas, or sarcomas in the lung. Before an unqualified diagnosis of a pure pulmonary smooth muscle tumor or melanoma is made, additional immunocytochemical evaluation with HMB-45 and anti-actins is probably a prudent step.

Myelolipoma

Myelolipoma is a peculiar lesion that is typically located in the adrenal glands or the retroperitoneum.[189,190] As its name suggests, it comprises a tumefactive admixture of mature adipose tissue and hematopoietic precursor cells, including megakaryocytes (Figs 19.48 and 19.49). It is still unclear whether myelolipoma represents a true neoplasm or a peculiar form of extramedullary hematopoiesis; indeed, the difference between those entities may be only a semantic one. Alternatively, myelolipoma could be regarded as a lipoma that is secondarily populated by bone marrow elements.

In any event, anecdotal reports have been made of primary pulmonary myelolipoma, all of which occurred in adult patients.[191–194] Hunter et al. described a case in which multiple lesions of this type were seen in the lungs, simulating the radiographic appearance of metastatic malignancy.[191] In contrast, Sabate and Shahian documented a pulmonary myelolipoma that had been present in chest

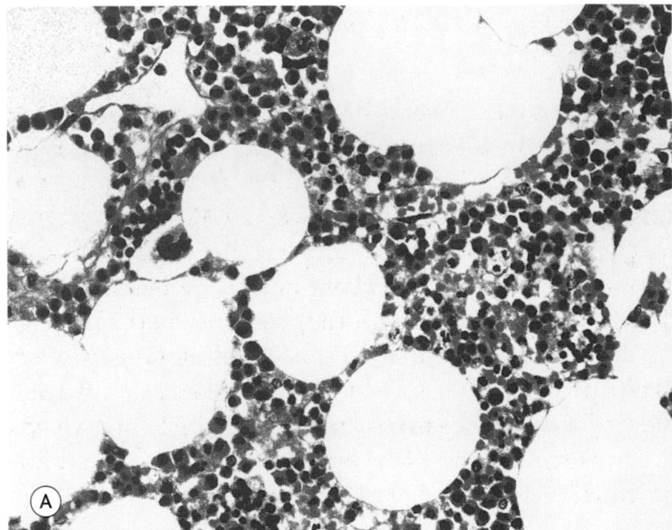

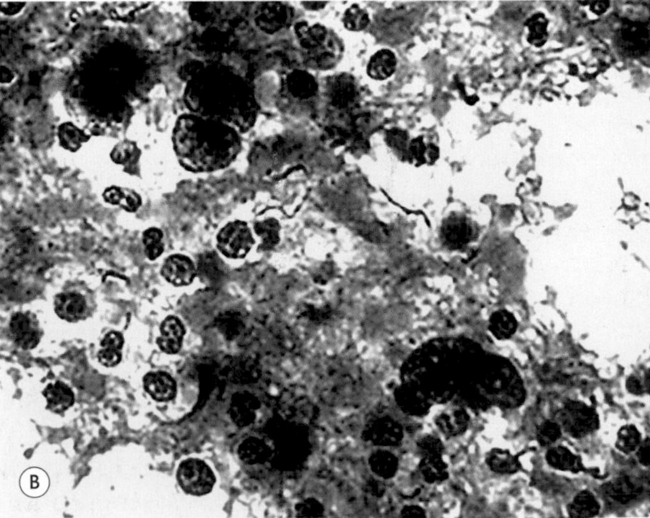

Fig. 19.49 (A,B) Photomicrograph of myelolipoma, showing an admixture of mature adipocytes and hematopoietic precursors.

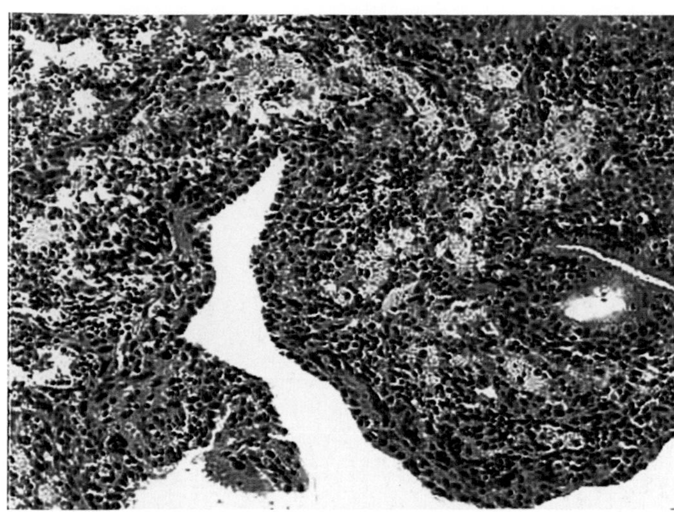

Fig. 19.50 Cystic fibrohistiocytic tumor of the lung, showing a central lesional space mantled by a proliferation of spindled and xanthomatous cells.

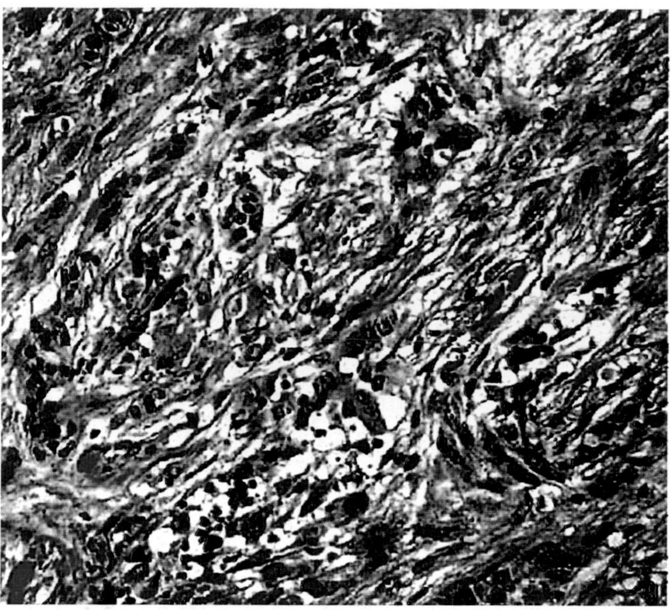

Fig. 19.51 The neoplastic elements in a cystic fibrohistiocytic tumor are represented by relatively bland fusiform elements arranged in a vaguely storiform pattern.

radiographs taken over a 20-year period, and which was eventually excised from a 54-year-old man.[192] Another patient studied by Zunarelli and colleagues had a concurrent myelolipoma and carcinoid tumor of the lung.[193] Two final cases documented by Ziolkowski and coworkers presented as solitary peripheral lung nodules, one of which was found for the first time at autopsy.[194]

The pathologic features of myelolipoma are so distinctive that it has no viable differential diagnosis. Nevertheless, it is again probably worthwhile to evaluate the peripheral blood picture to exclude the possibility of functional extramedullary hematopoiesis.

Cystic fibrohistiocytic tumor of the lung

Joseph and colleagues have described two adult patients who were found to have variably cystic lung lesions, represented by multiple parenchymal abnormalities on chest radiographs.[195] One patient had pneumothorax and shortness of breath, and lesions in the other case were asymptomatic. Open lung biopsies showed a proliferation of relatively bland spindle cells and histiocyte-like elements, mantling cystic spaces that were lined by metaplastic bronchiolar epithelium, squamous cells, or type II pneumocytes (Figs 19.50 and 19.51). Some of the cysts contained erythrocytes and hemosiderin deposits. Another case has been illustrated anecdotally by Han.[196]

Although the lesions in the report by Joseph et al.[195] enlarged very slowly over time, the biologic potential and recommended treatment of pulmonary cystic fibrohistiocytic tumors is unclear. For now, we have arbitrarily included them in this section on benign lesions.

Differential diagnosis centers primarily on metastases of low-grade malignant fibrous histiocytoma or "borderline" fibrohistiocytic tumors. However, those lesions have typically been well documented historically before they involve the lungs. In particular, Colome-Grimmer and Evans have described cystic change in pulmonary metastases of low-grade cutaneous fibrohistiocytic tumors.[197]

Benign tumors of the pleura

Adenomatoid tumor of the pleura

It is an unfortunate truism that completely benign neoplasms of the pleura are a distinct rarity. Indeed, the only representative of that diagnostic category is the adenomatoid tumor. That neoplasm is a lesion with mesothelial differentiation, which is most often encountered in the adnexal soft tissue surrounding the uterus and testes.[198,199] Only four cases have been described in the pleura, by Kaplan et al.,[200] Handra-Luca et al.,[201] and Umezu et al.[202] These lesions occurred in a middle-aged man, a middle-aged woman, an elderly woman, and an elderly man, and all were asymptomatic. They were incidental findings in lung resections that were done for other unrelated lesions (squamous cell carcinoma,

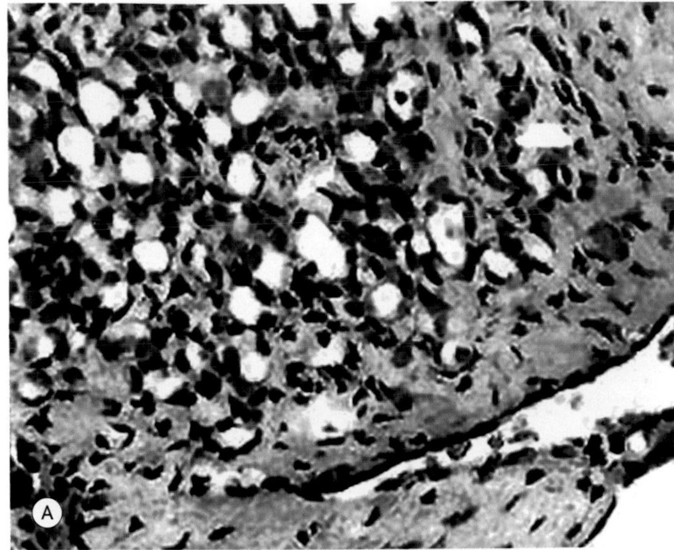

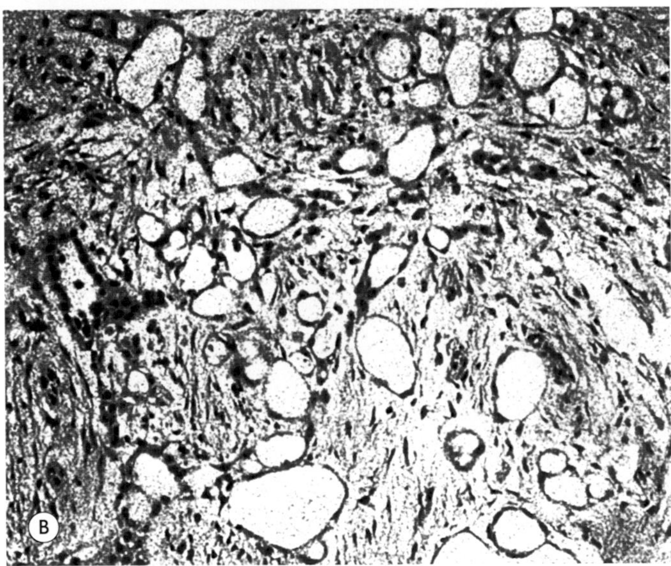

Fig. 19.52 (A, B) Adenomatoid tumor of the pleura, comprising microcystic arrays of bland epithelioid cells.

mesothelioma, adenosquamous carcinoma, and histoplasmoma), and they showed no subsequent evidence of aggressive behavior. We have seen one similar case (unreported) in a 55-year-old man with an adenocarcinoma of the lung.

All reported pleural adenomatoid tumors were unencapsulated, and they measured 0.5–2.5 cm in greatest dimension. Microscopically, the lesions were composed of epithelioid cells that were organized into compact gland-like profiles (Fig. 19.52). They had vesicular nuclear chromatin, inconspicuous nucleoli, and relatively abundant eosinophilic or vacuolated cytoplasm. No areas of nuclear pleomorphism were noted and no mitoses

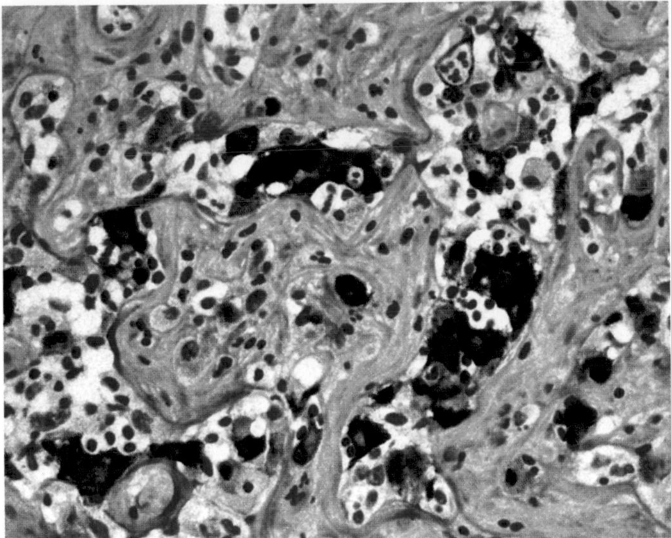

Fig. 19.53 Immunoreactivity for calretinin in pleural adenomatoid tumor.

were apparent. The lesions did not invade the subjacent lung parenchyma. The case in our files was essentially identical.

Electron microscopy in the cases of Kaplan and colleagues[200] showed branching plasmalemmal microvilli and prominent intercellular attachment complexes, typical of mesothelial lesions. Immunohistologically, the tumor cells labeled for keratin, but were negative for carcinoembryonic antigen, CD15, CD34, Ber-EP4 antigen, and tumor-associated glycoprotein-72. Our case manifested comparable characteristics, and was also reactive for calretinin (Fig. 19.53).

The principal differential diagnostic alternatives to pleural adenomatoid tumor (PAT) are metastatic adenocarcinoma and malignant mesothelioma. Both of those possibilities are rendered unlikely by the bland histologic images of PAT, with no evidence of infiltrative growth. That is an important point, inasmuch as the immunohistologic and ultrastructural attributes of PAT and mesothelioma are identical (see Ch. 20).

Calcifying fibrous pseudotumor of the pleura

A unique entity known as calcifying fibrous "pseudotumor" (CFPT) has been described in the pleura.[203–206] This lesion is histologically similar, if not identical, to calcifying fibrous "pseudotumors" of the soft tissue, as originally described by Rosenthal and Abdul-Karim.[207]

The five described cases of pleural CFPT have all occurred in adults (age range 23–46 years); four were women. Two patients manifested with chest pain, and the

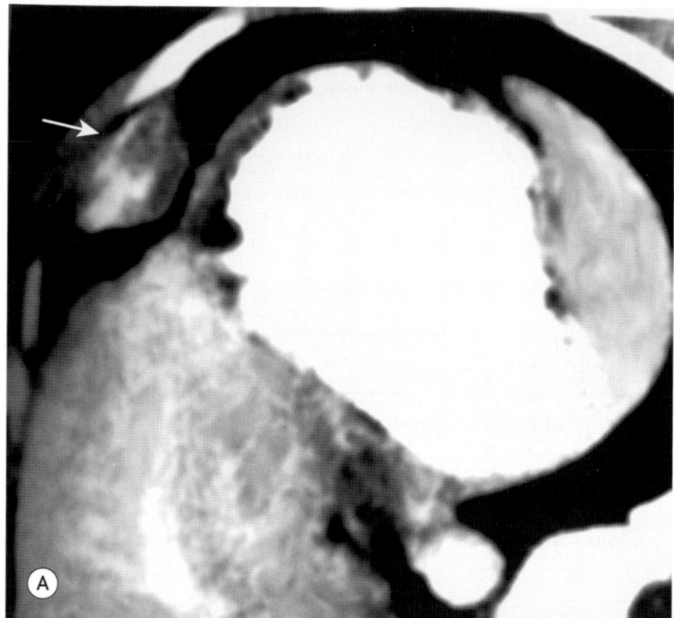

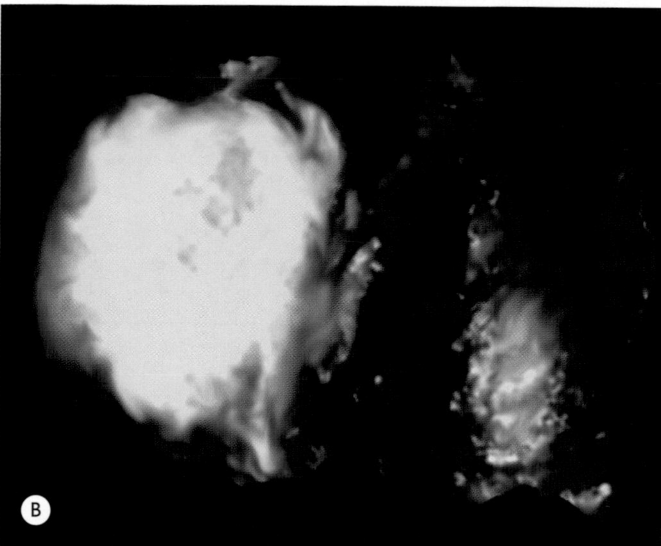

Fig. 19.54 This computed tomogram (A; arrow) and gross photograph (B) of a calcifying fibrous pseudotumor of the pleura show a well-demarcated nodular lesion. (Reproduced from Pinkard et al.[203] with permission.)

remainder were asymptomatic. Pleural-based masses were seen by chest radiographs in all cases and CT scans also demonstrated well-demarcated, partially calcified nodular lesions, measuring up to 12 cm in diameter (Fig. 19.54). Two individuals had multiple masses.

Histologically, all patients had circumscribed but non-encapsulated fibrous lesions that were composed of dense, hyalinized, collagenous tissue, with interspersed bland spindle cells (Fig. 19.55). The masses were generally hypocellular, particularly at their peripheries, and no nuclear atypia of the fusiform cells was present. A scant chronic inflammatory infiltrate was seen, without lymphoid aggregates, giant cells, or necrosis. All lesions also featured calcifications of the psammomatous (Fig. 19.56) as well as dystrophic types. These histologic features are identical to those of calcifying fibrous pseudotumors of soft tissue.[208–210]

Nascimento et al.[210] studied 15 examples of CFPT in non-pleural locations, and compared them with published examples of inflammatory myofibroblastic tumor (IMT; see below). The immunohistologic profile of CFPT featured reactivity for vimentin and scattered cells that labeled for actin, desmin, and CD34 in most instances. In contrast, there was no reactivity for *ALK*-1 or p80 proteins. That constellation of findings differed from the immunophenotype of IMT, and it was concluded that CFPT is distinct from the latter neoplasm. Accordingly,

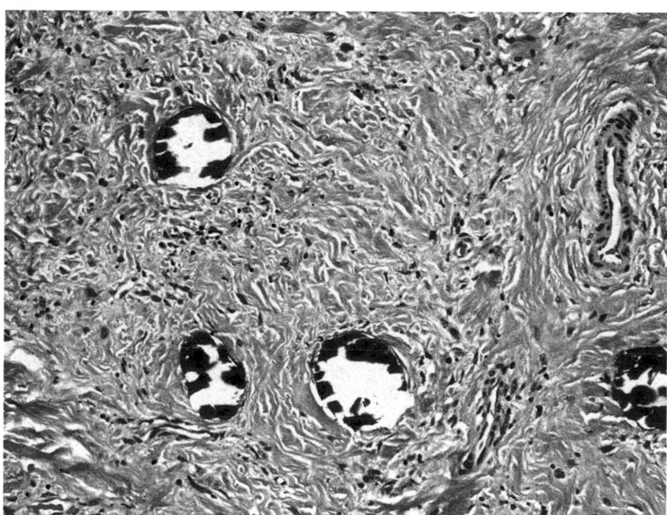

Fig. 19.55 Calcifying pseudotumor of the pleura, represented by a hypocellular proliferation of bland spindle cells that are set in a dense and hyalinized collagenous stroma.

Nascimento and colleagues recommended using the term "calcifying fibrous tumor" in reference to CFPT.[210]

Other differential diagnostic considerations include hyaline pleural plaques, tumefactive pleural fibrosis, calcified or hyalinizing granulomas, and amyloidosis. The clinical presentation, gross features, and microscopic

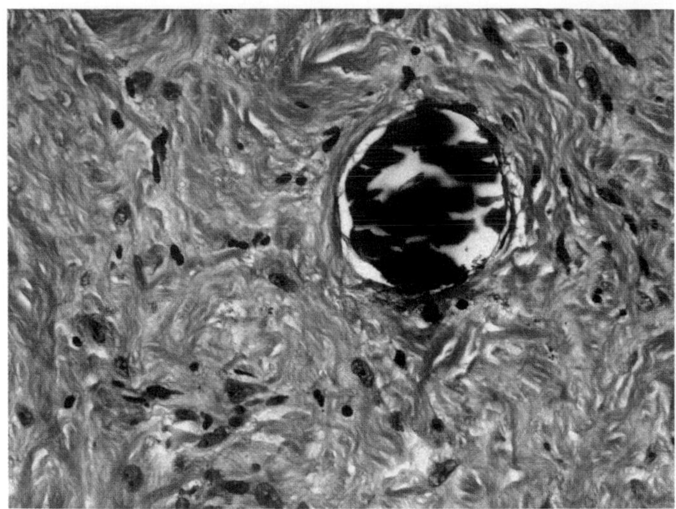

Fig. 19.56 Psammomatous calcification in calcifying fibrous pseudotumor of the pleura.

features of CFPT argue against any of those considerations, as does its regular content of psammomatous calcifications. Follow-up has shown no examples of untoward behavior.

Biologically borderline tumors of the lung and pleura

The biologic difference between "benign" and "borderline" (very low-grade malignant) tumors is a subtle one, inasmuch as very few of the latter neoplasms cause significant mortality. For purposes of this discussion, we have defined "borderline" lesions of the lung and pleura as those that have shown a potential for local recurrence after apparently adequate excision, or for rare embolic metastasis, or both. It is readily acknowledged that other observers may regard the same tumors as either benign or overtly malignant.

Inflammatory myofibroblastic tumor ("inflammatory pseudotumor") of the lung

In 1939, Brunn described two pulmonary lesions that were composed of spindle cells admixed with inflammatory elements, in patients with fever and weight loss.[211] The systemic complaints disappeared after surgical removal of the lung tumors. Although they were felt to be true neoplasms of probable smooth muscle lineage, subsequent authors espoused the theory that masses with the same attributes were inflammatory and reparative lesions.[212,213] Hence, the term "inflammatory pseudotumor" gained favor for diagnostic use. However, Spencer noted that a proportion of such proliferations behaved in a biologically malignant fashion,[214] and other reports also documented the presence of vascular invasion and recurrence in some cases.[215–217] Molecular analyses in the 1990s revealed a clonal character for "inflammatory pseudotumors" in the lungs and other anatomic sites,[218–220] and, together with aggregated clinicopathologic information on them, those data resulted in amendment of their name to "inflammatory myofibroblastic tumors" (IMTs).[221] It is now accepted that IMTs form a conceptual continuum with "inflammatory fibrosarcoma," as described by Meis and Enzinger.[222,223] Because they may recur and occasionally metastasize as well, IMTs are best considered as biologically "borderline" neoplasms.

The lung is most frequently affected by IMT, among all potential topographic locations.[223] Although the majority of pulmonary lesions of this type are seen in children and young adults, they may in fact be encountered in patients of all ages with no gender predilection.[217] Some IMTs are situated in the large airways with no parenchymal involvement, but they are exceptional; most arise in the peripheral lung fields. Systemic complaints of a paraneoplastic nature have been reported in up to 50% of cases, including such findings as anemia, fever, weight loss, hyperglobulinemia, leukothrombocytosis, and elevations in erythrocyte sedimentation rate.[223] As referenced above, those abnormalities typically remit when the IMT is removed. The remaining cases present with cough, vague chest discomfort, or hemoptysis, or are asymptomatic, with the lesions being found incidentally on chest radiographs.[221] On imaging studies, IMT is typically a lobulated or globoid mass (Fig. 19.57), usually measuring <5 cm in maximum dimension. Occasionally, it may attain a size of >10 cm; internal calcifications are commonly seen in this lesion as well. Infiltration of great vessels, mediastinal soft tissue, or chest wall is apparent radiographically in a minority of cases.

Macroscopic examination of IMTs shows a deceptively circumscribed appearance, with a gray-tan or yellow cut surface (Fig. 19.58). Grittiness may be encountered during sectioning with the knife blade because of aforementioned microcalcification. Foci of gross necrosis and hemorrhage are exceptional. When the tumor is in proximity to large airways or blood vessels, growth into those structures can sometimes be seen with compromise of their lumina by tumor tissue.

The histologic profile of IMT features a proliferation of relatively bland spindle cells, which are arranged haphazardly or in vague fascicles[221,223,224] (Figs 19.59 and 19.60). In contrast to the gross appearance referenced

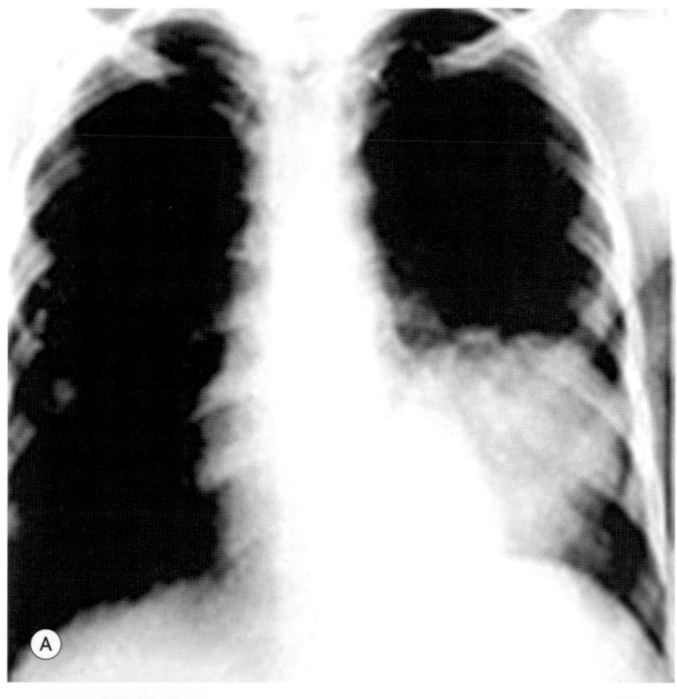

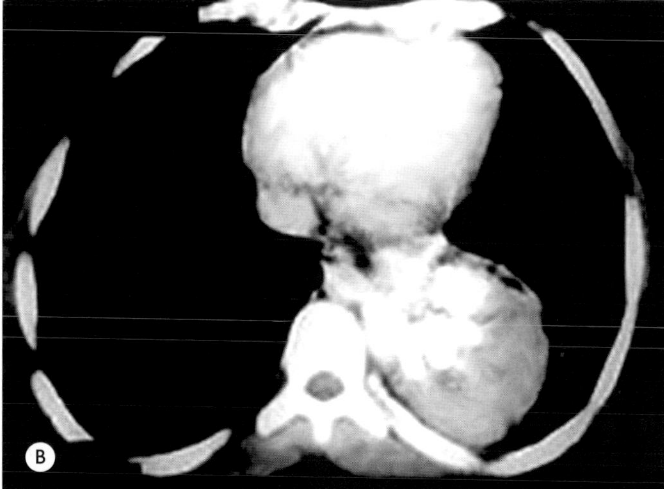

Fig. 19.57 Inflammatory myofibroblastic tumor of the lung, manifest in a plain-film chest radiograph (A) and a computed tomogram (B) as an irregularly lobulated mass with internal heterogeneity.

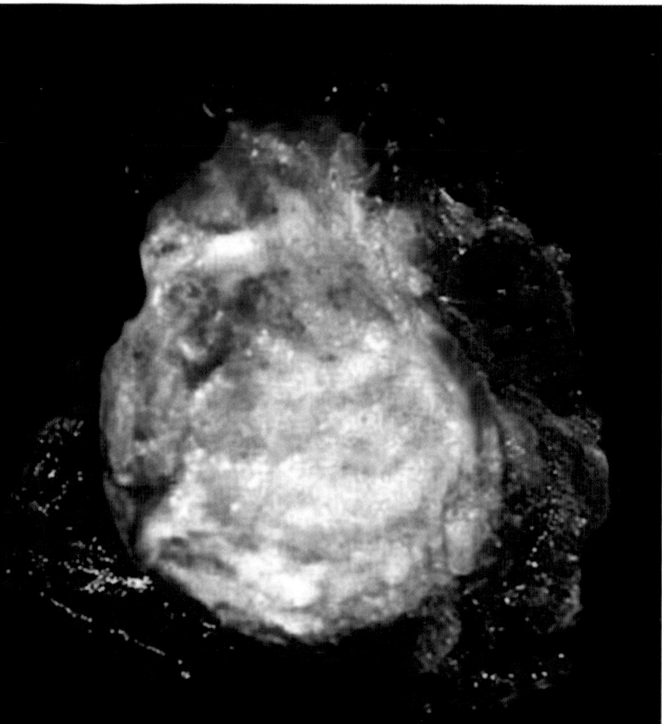

Fig. 19.58 This gross photograph of a pulmonary inflammatory myofibroblastic tumor demonstrates a relatively circumscribed lesion with a slightly fasciculated white-yellow cut surface.

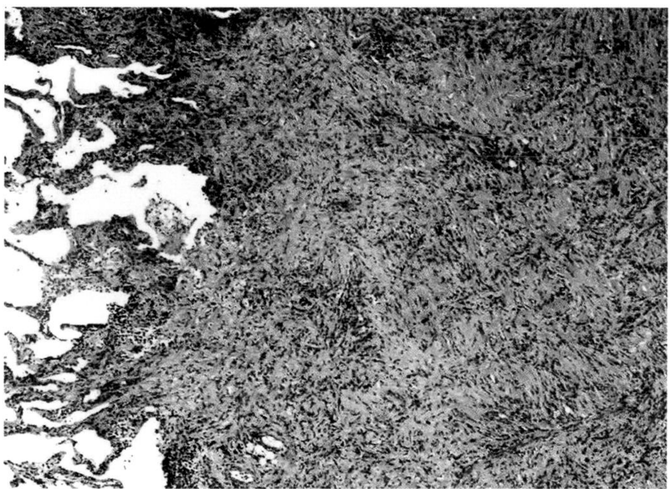

Fig. 19.59 Inflammatory myofibroblastic tumor of the lung showing a spindle cell proliferation demonstrating an irregular interface with the surrounding lung parenchyma.

previously, this lesion has an irregular peripheral zone of growth microscopically, with tongues of tumor that comingle with adjacent normal tissues. Not surprisingly, infiltration of blood vessels, bronchi, and pleura may be evident. Nuclei in the neoplastic fusiform elements usually contain dispersed or vesicular chromatin with compact nucleoli (Fig. 19.61). Mitotic activity is typically easily found, but without pathologic division figures. Cytoplasm is amphophilic or lightly eosinophilic and may show a faintly fibrillar character. Admixed inflammatory cells are greatly variable in density and type, and some cases of IMT show virtually none. Lymphocytes, plasma cells, macrophages, eosinophils, and neutrophils are also potentially represented (Fig. 19.62), and intralesional aggregates of xanthomatized foam cells are sometimes apparent as well. Some cases demonstrate rather striking zones of sclerosis, and these may even be

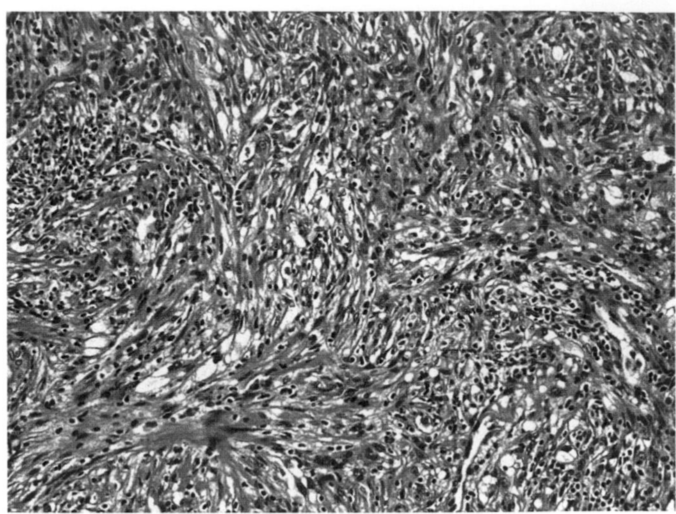

Fig. 19.60 The spindle cells in this pulmonary inflammatory myofibroblastic tumor are arranged in vague fascicles.

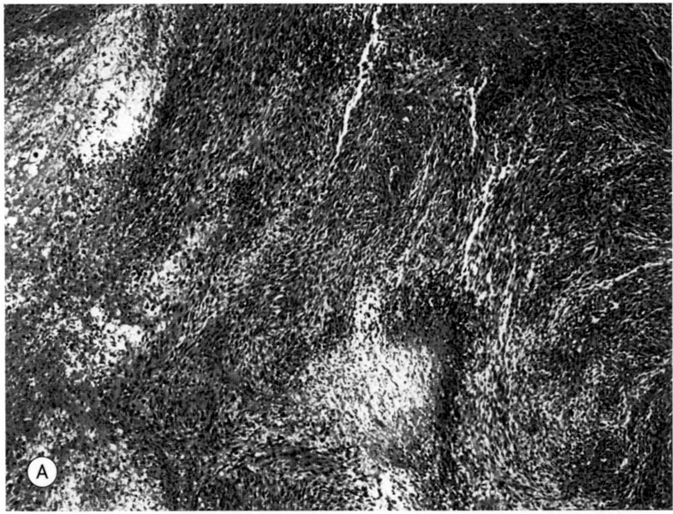

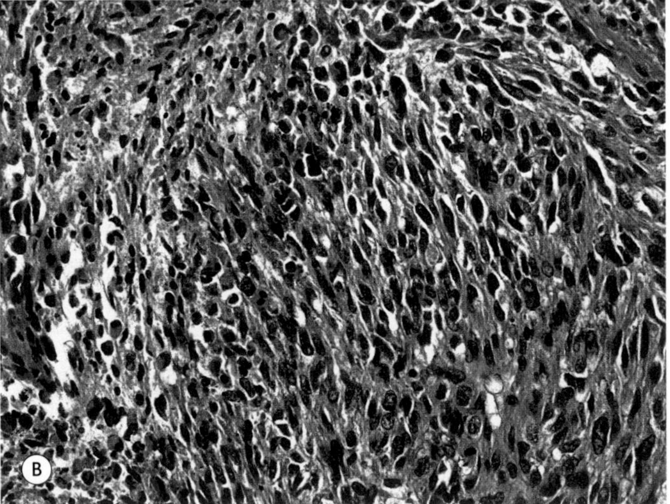

Fig. 19.61 (A; top of figure) A zone of spontaneous necrosis is present in this inflammatory myofibroblastic tumor of the lung, and (B) fusiform tumor cell nuclei show the presence of slightly clumped chromatin and small nucleoli.

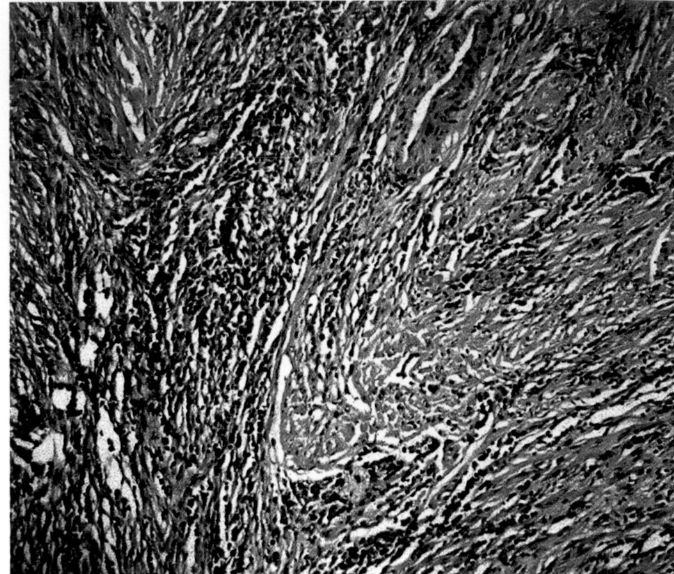

Fig. 19.62 Intralesional lymphocytes and plasma cells are numerous (left of figure) in this pulmonary inflammatory myofibroblastic tumor.

hyalinized. On the other hand, 20–30% of these lesions show dense cellularity with focal or global nuclear atypia, relatively high nuclear-to-cytoplasmic ratios, nuclear hyperchromasia, mild nuclear pleomorphism, and zones of necrosis.[217]

Electron microscopic evaluation of IMTs shows that the tumor cells possess some features which are associated with smooth muscle: namely, plasmalemmal dense patches, pinocytotic vesicles, and cytoplasmic bundles of thin (actin-type) filaments. Pericellular basal lamina is variably present, but there are no intercellular attachment complexes.[221]

By immunohistochemical assessment, one finds reactivity for vimentin, alpha-isoform and muscle-specific actins, and calponin, but usually not for desmin, caldesmon, CD34, or keratin.[223] Mutant p53 protein is detectable immunohistologically in <10% of cases.[220] On the other hand, two proteins that relate to reproducible cytogenetic abnormalities in chromosome 2p23 in IMTs are detectable in approximately 40% of these lesions. These are known as "*ALK*-1 (anaplastic lymphoma kinase-1)" (Fig. 19.63) and "p80," and were originally studied in anaplastic large-cell ("Ki-1") lymphomas.[225]

The differential diagnosis of pulmonary IMT includes tumefactive organizing pneumonia[224] (also termed "true inflammatory pseudotumor" or "plasma cell granuloma" in Ch. 18), smooth muscle proliferations in the lung, inflammatory sarcomatoid carcinoma (ISC)[217] (Fig. 19.64), and inflammatory malignant fibrous histiocytoma (IMFH). *ALK*-1/p80 reactivity is diagnostic of IMT in this

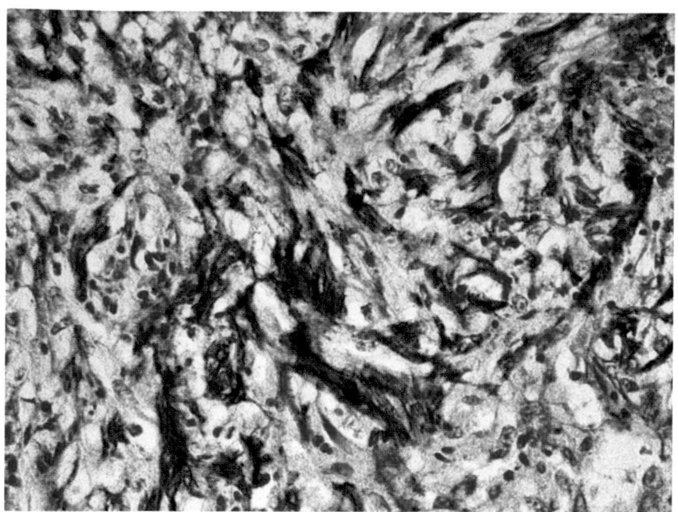

Fig. 19.63 Diffuse immunoreactivity is present for *ALK-1* protein in this inflammatory myofibroblastic tumor of the lung.

setting, but, as mentioned, is seen in only a minority of cases. The spindle cells of ISC can be labeled for keratin and epithelial membrane antigen, in contrast to those of IMT[217] conversely, IMFH is typically not reactive for actins or calponin. Spindle cells in organizing pneumonia usually comprise foci of repair in organizing bronchiolitis or alveolitis, and, as such, are much more organized than the neoplastic elements of IMT.[224]

There are few if any pathologic variables that can be used successfully in any given individual case of IMT to predict its biologic behavior with certainty.[226] Some examples of pulmonary IMT that have been observed for extended periods of time before surgical excision or autopsy examination have shown that the lesions often remain stable or increase in size very slowly. Spontaneous complete resolution has also been recorded, and a few lesions have diminished in size after non-surgical

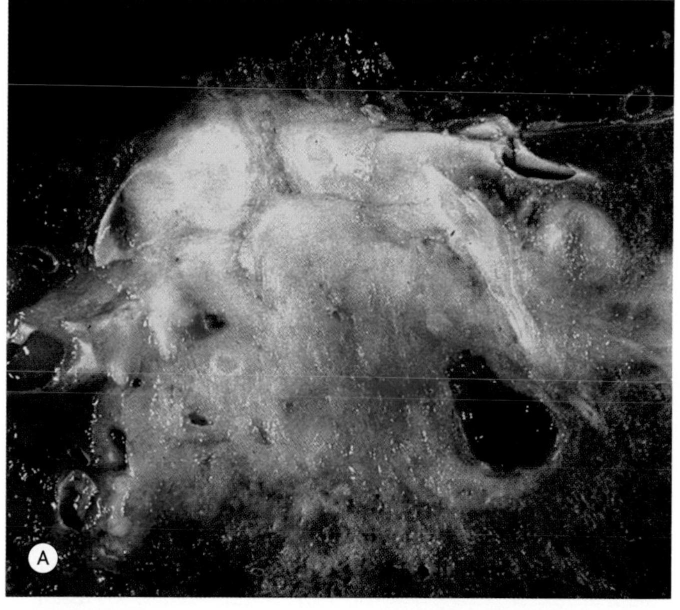

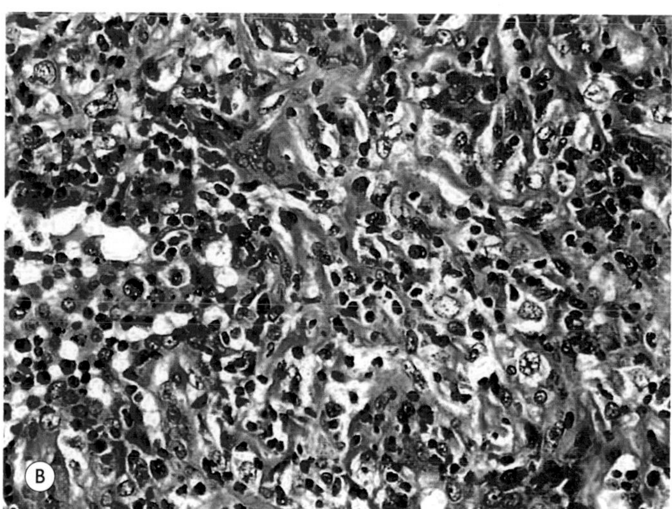

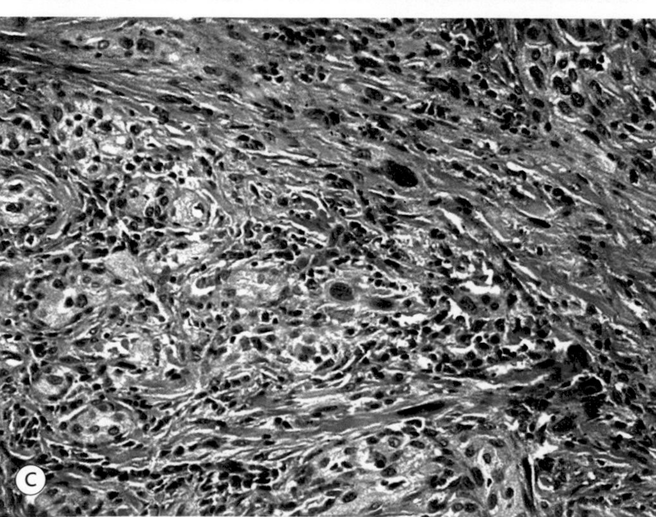

Fig. 19.64 Inflammatory sarcomatoid carcinoma (ISC) represents an important differential diagnostic alternative to inflammatory myofibroblastic tumor (IMT). The gross appearance of such a carcinoma is shown in (A), and is quite similar to that of many IMTs. Similarly, admixed chronic inflammatory cells are seen in both IMT and ISC (B). These may obscure the tumor cells, which are better seen in (C). Immunostains for keratin and epithelial membrane antigen are positive in ISC but negative in IMT.

therapy.[223] Operative removal is usually necessary to establish a firm diagnosis of IMT, and, if the lesion has been completely excised, no further intervention is required or advised at the present time. On the other hand, it is logical to expect that incomplete removal – particularly if invasion of adjacent extrapulmonary tissues is present – might, in some instances, be followed by continued growth.[227] In particular, involvement of the pleura, pulmonary hilum, diaphragm, or mediastinum is associated with morbidity from IMTs of the lung. They may even, exceptionally, prove fatal if they are massive and infiltrate the mediastinum extensively, or if distant spread occurs. Overall, recurrence of IMT is seen in approximately 25% of cases, but <1% metastasize.[223]

Pneumocytoma

Almost 50 years ago, Liebow and Hubbell described a peculiar tumor of the peripheral lung parenchyma with a sclerosing, angiomatoid, and papillary architecture.[228] They gave it the name "sclerosing hemangioma," but this designation was chosen in unfortunate mimicry of a convention then extant in dermatopathology. In the 1950s, the lesion now known as "dermatofibroma" or "cutaneous fibrous histiocytoma" was likewise commonly called "sclerosing hemangioma,"[229] because it sometimes showed internal blood lakes and hemosiderosis. In their seminal description of "sclerosing hemangioma" of the lung, Liebow and Hubbell disavowed an endothelial derivation for the tumor and appended the alternative appellations of "histiocytoma" and "xanthoma," perhaps in deference to the true identity of its alleged dermal analogue. This enigmatic series of nosologic and terminological choices set the stage for confusion in the succeeding decades. Indeed, various studies on the cellular nature of pulmonary "sclerosing hemangioma" have suggested vascular, fibrohistiocytic, mesothelial, and epithelial lineages for it,[230–234] and controversies over such proposals still persist today to some extent.

Based on the aggregated data on this tumor entity – to be reviewed below – we believe that it is best considered as a neoplasm showing differentiation which is most like that of embryonic (uncommitted) respiratory epithelium. Moreover, we also feel that it encompasses a spectrum of pulmonary lesions that have been given separate names in their own rights: namely, "papillary adenoma,"[235–238] "alveolar adenoma,"[239] and "Clara cell adenoma."[240] Therefore, the entity in question is best designated as "pneumocytoma," as suggested by Shimosato.[241] Up until the current century, the literature contained reports of <200 such lesions.[242–261] Devouassoux-Shisheboran et al.[262] then published a comprehensive review of 100

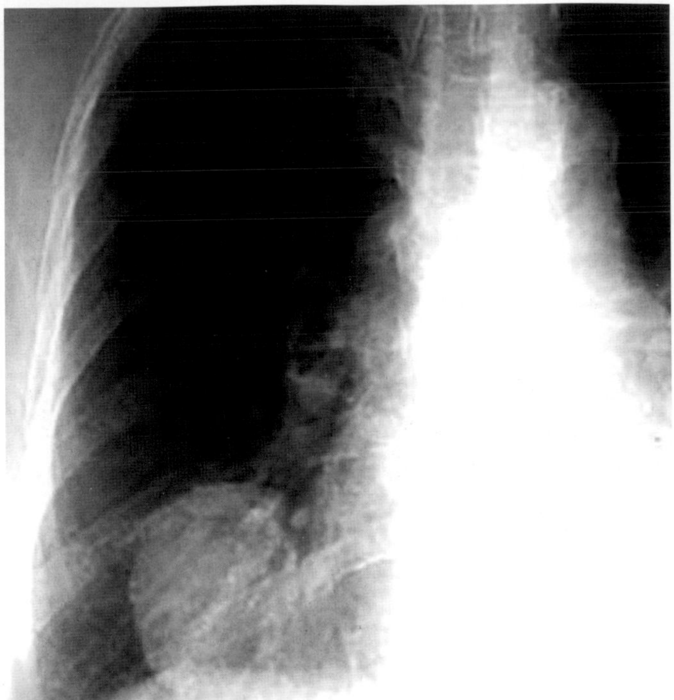

Fig. 19.65 This plain-film chest radiograph demonstrates a well-delineated nodular lesion in the basal right lung field, representing a pneumocytoma ("sclerosing hemangioma").

additional cases, providing valuable insights on their clinicopathologic attributes, and others have followed.[263–273]

Pneumocytomas can affect patients of almost any age, from early childhood[267] through the end of life. Females predominate by a factor of 5:1.[262] Only roughly 20% of patients have any respiratory complaints at the time their tumors are found, including cough, hemoptysis, or chest pain. In some cases, chest radiographs that are done in the evaluation of previous or concurrent neoplasms – such as germ cell tumors, lymphomas, melanomas, or extrapulmonary carcinomas – show the presence of a peripheral lung lesion that ultimately proves to be a pneumocytoma. It may arise in any of the pulmonary lobes; a localization in the large airways, pleura, and mediastinum is also rarely possible.[262]

Radiographically, most patients with pneumocytomas have solitary peripheral masses with well-defined homogeneous round or oval profiles on chest roentgenograms (Fig. 19.65). Computed tomography of the thorax shows a homogeneity and high density to the lesions in the great majority of cases; low-density areas may be apparent in some tumors because of cystic changes in pneumocytomas (Fig. 19.66). In addition, the "air meniscus sign" (also known as the "air trapping" or "air crescent" sign)[257,268,269] – a rim of air that partially or circumferentially surrounds

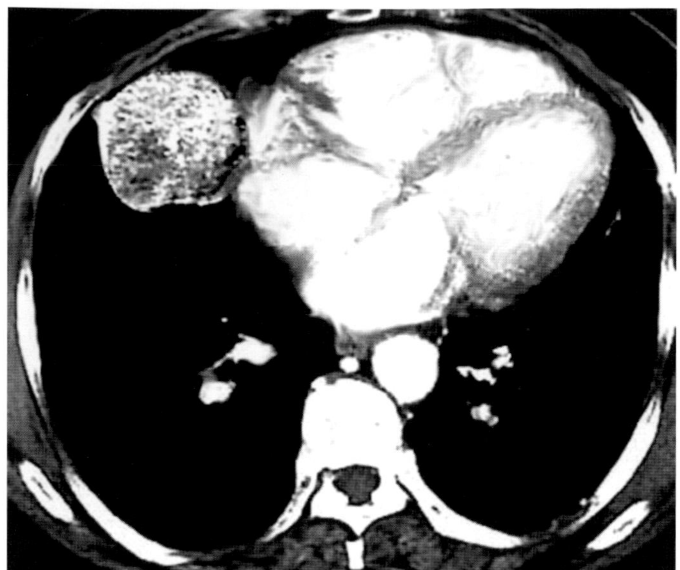

Fig. 19.66 Internal variegation in density is seen in this computed tomogram of the lesion shown in Fig. 19.65, owing to partial cystification.

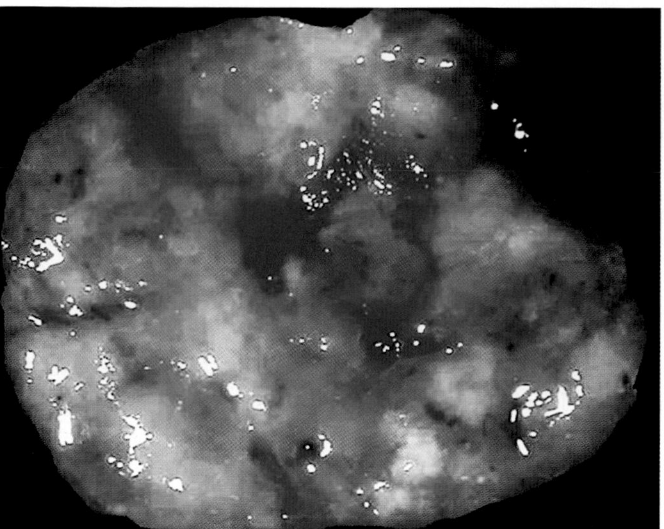

Fig. 19.68 This pneumocytoma ("sclerosing hemangioma") was "shelled out" by the surgeon and demonstrates little if any adherent peripheral alveolated pulmonary tissue.

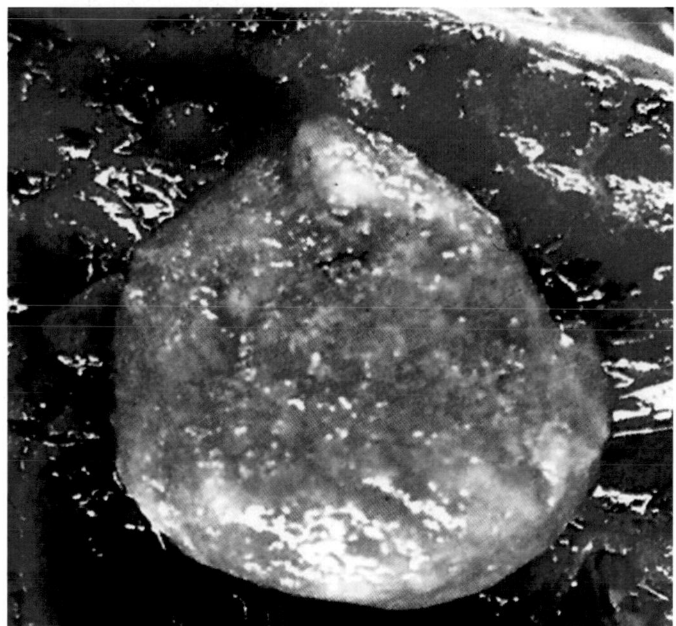

Fig. 19.67 Gross photograph of pneumocytoma ("sclerosing hemangioma"), showing a sharply circumscribed and internally homogeneous tan-pink nodule in the peripheral lung parenchyma.

a mass – is evident in the lung parenchyma adjacent to occasional lesions of this type.

Grossly, most pneumocytomas are <3 cm in maximum dimension (Fig. 19.67), but sometimes they may attain a size of up to 10 cm. Multifocality,[245,254,262,265] sometimes featuring a satellitotic configuration of small nodules around a dominant central one,[262] is apparent in approximately 4% of cases. Roughly the same proportion are pleural-based and may be polypoid, potentially simulating the appearance of solitary fibrous tumors[262] (see below). Sharp circumscription from the surrounding lung parenchyma is the rule, so much so that pneumocytomas are sometimes "shelled out" by the surgeon with little if any attached alveolated tissue (Fig. 19.68). Their cut surfaces are tan-gray, yellow, or mottled. Cystic areas are evident in roughly 3% of cases; 20% show areas of intralesional hemorrhage, which may be extensive.

The histologic images of pneumocytoma include varying admixtures of four basic growth patterns, i.e. sclerotic (Fig. 19.69), papillary (Fig. 19.70), solid (Fig. 19.71), and hemorrhagic/angiomatoid (Fig. 19.72) configurations; only approximately 15% of cases are monomorphic (including papillary, alveolar, papillary-cystic, and Clara cell adenomas), and roughly 20% contain areas representing all of the patterns in the same lesion. Two basic cell types comprise the neoplastic elements in pneumocytomas – "surface" cells, which mantle papillary projections, and "round" cells, seen in the cores of papillary structures and in solid sheets within the lesions. Surface cells often show the presence of intranuclear invaginations of cytoplasm, yielding "pseudoinclusions" like those seen in type II pneumocytes and Clara cells. They also may be multinucleated. Round cells are actually polygonal, with oval nuclei, dispersed chromatin, indiscernible nucleoli, and extremely rare mitotic figures. They may focally exhibit cytoplasmic vacuolation (Fig. 19.73) and even assume a

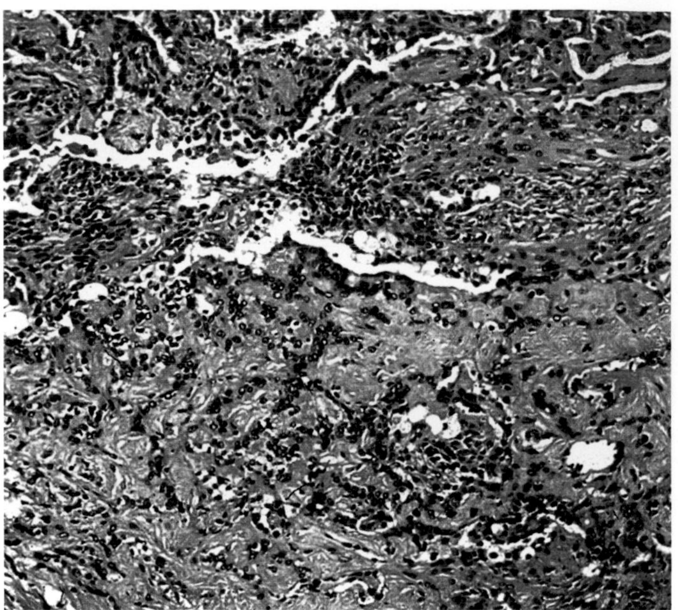

Fig. 19.69 Stromal sclerosis is prominent in this pneumocytoma ("sclerosing hemangioma"), with only a minor component of papillary epithelial growth.

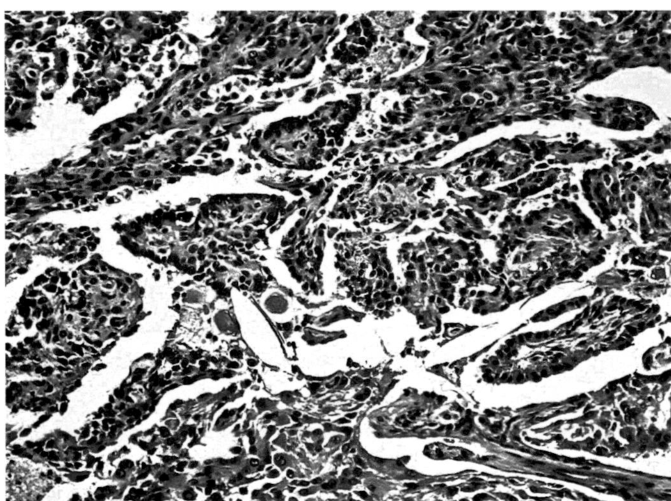

Fig. 19.70 Papillary epithelial groups are numerous in this pneumocytoma ("sclerosing hemangioma"), yielding a configuration that has also been termed "papillary adenoma."

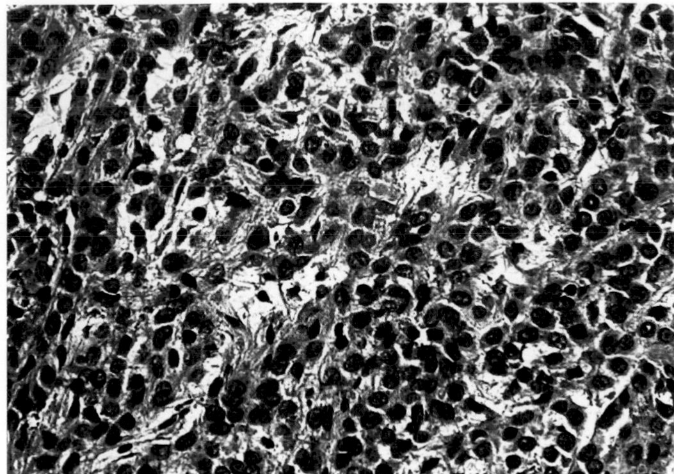

Fig. 19.71 Solid growth of polygonal cells is apparent in this pneumocytoma ("sclerosing hemangioma").

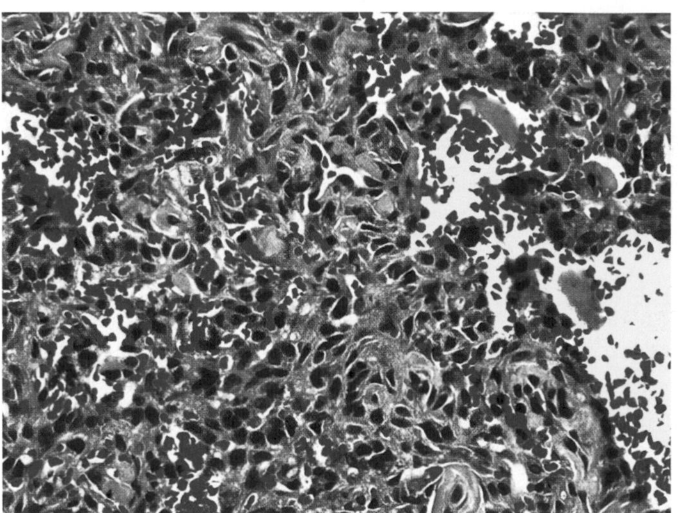

Fig. 19.72 An angiomatoid focus is evident in pneumocytoma ("sclerosing hemangioma").

signet-ring-cell image. Rarely, nuclear hyperchromasia and moderate pleomorphism is appreciated in the round cell element.[242,262]

Secondary features of pneumocytoma include blood lakes in angiomatoid foci; limited areas of necrosis; stromal hemosiderosis, calcification, cholesterolosis, or combinations thereof; internal cystification, with mucinous contents; granulomatous inflammation; and a potential association with foci of neuroendocrine hyperplasia ("tumorlets") in the surrounding lung parenchyma.[242,248,262,263]

Several publications have addressed fine-needle aspiration (FNA) biopsy findings in pneumocytomas, and most have noted substantial morphologic overlap between those lesions and well-differentiated adenocarcinomas (particularly of the bronchioloalveolar type).[244,260,261,266,270,271] Indeed, a shared potential for nuclear atypia, intranuclear pseudoinclusions, and micropapillary growth in both of those tumor entities makes the definitive cytologic recognition of pneumocytoma very difficult. In fact, despite assertions that it can indeed be accomplished, we believe that an unqualified interpretation of pneumocytoma by FNA biopsy is unwise. In

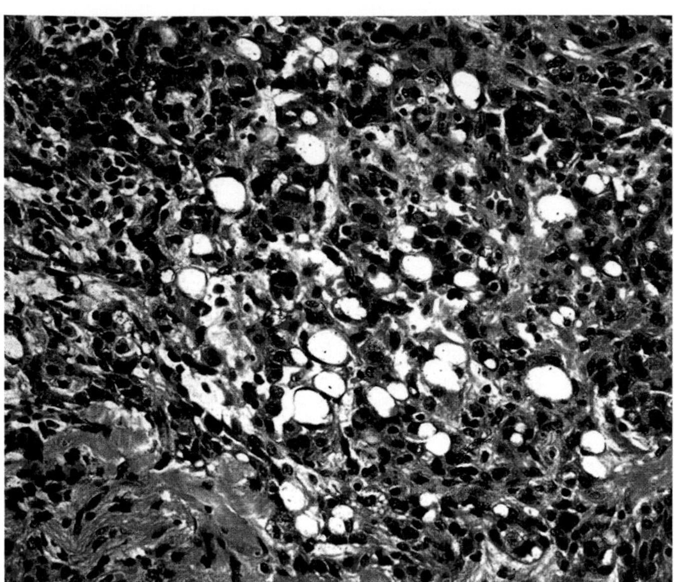

Fig. 19.73 Cytoplasmic vacuolization is apparent in the tumor cells of pneumocytoma ("sclerosing hemangioma"), probably representing accumulation of surfactant proteins.

appropriate cases that possibility can be included in the diagnostic report, hopefully prompting an intraoperative frozen section examination to further guide the surgeon's choice of procedure thereafter. This proviso relates to the *very* close similarity we have noted between pneumocytoma and selected adenocarcinomas at a cytologic level.

Electron microscopy of pneumocytomas has shown that both the surface cell and round cell components of those lesions demonstrate type II pneumocytic features, containing cytoplasmic lamellar bodies with variable levels of maturation.[232,236,262] Other organelles are nonspecific.

Immunohistologically, variable reactivity has been seen for keratin, EMA, surfactant-related proteins, Clara cell antigen, and thyroid transcription factor-1 in both cellular components of pneumocytomas[240,243,244,249–253,255,262,272,273] (Fig. 19.74). Receptors for estrogen and progesterone are also demonstrable in a minority of cases.[262] On the other hand, mesothelial markers such as calretinin, HBME-1, cytokeratin 5/6, and WT-1 protein are absent in these lesions, as are neuroendocrine, neural, and myogenous determinants.

Justification for our inclusion of pneumocytoma as a "borderline" lesion stems from reports of lymph nodal metastases of this tumor in 8 patients to date.[246,262,264,269] In the series from the AFIP, this behavior was observed in 1% of cases.[262] Despite that observation, no patient with metastatic pneumocytoma has died of the tumor, and Miyagawa-Hayashino et al.[264] found that lymph node involvement did not affect survival at all. In that regard, this neoplasm is very roughly analogous biologically to such very low-grade epithelial malignancies as "borderline" ovarian serous tumors or classical papillary thyroid carcinoma.

As mentioned above, the principal differential diagnostic alternative to pneumocytoma is that of low-grade adenocarcinoma of bronchioloalveolar or conventional types.[260,261,271] An adequate tissue sample – allowing for evaluation of the architecture of the entire mass – is essential to making that distinction. Another diagnostic possibility is the papillary variant of low-grade mucoepidermoid carcinoma,[274] but its particular histologic pattern, with an intimate admixture of mucinous and squamous epithelium, should allow for a distinction from pneumocytoma.

Pulmonary mucinous cystadenoma and borderline mucinous tumor

Mucinous cystadenomas and cystic mucinous tumors of low malignant potential – "borderline" mucinous neoplasms (BMTs) – are well-known to gynecologic and gastrointestinal pathologists, because they rather commonly arise in the ovaries, gut, and pancreas.[275,276] However, a primary origin in the lung for such lesions is distinctly unusual, and less than 15 cases have been reported in that organ.[277–286] These have affected adult patients as solitary lesions in the peripheral parenchyma, and were associated with no symptoms. Both plain films and CTs of the thorax clearly showed the cystic nature of the tumors, which generally measured several centimeters in diameter.

Grossly, mucinous cystadenomas and BMTs are sharply demarcated from the surrounding lung parenchyma and may even "shell out" for the surgeon. Their walls are relatively thick and fibrous, enclosing locules that contain thick viscous mucoid material. Foci of granular tissue are present on the internal aspects of the cysts, representing epithelial projections.

Histologically, the latter structures are constituted by cytologically bland mucin-containing tumor cells that are cuboidal or low-columnar (Fig. 19.75). Nuclei are generally basally located and relatively banal, with no pleomorphism or mitotic activity (Fig. 19.76). Neither cystadenomas nor BMTs demonstrate invasive growth into the fibrous walls of the lesions, but borderline tumors do manifest a "piling up" of lesional epithelium that yields complex micropapillary structures (Fig. 19.77). Davison et al. and Butnor & colleagues also reported cases in which adenocarcinoma evolved from pre-existing pulmonary mucinous cystadenoma.[278,284]

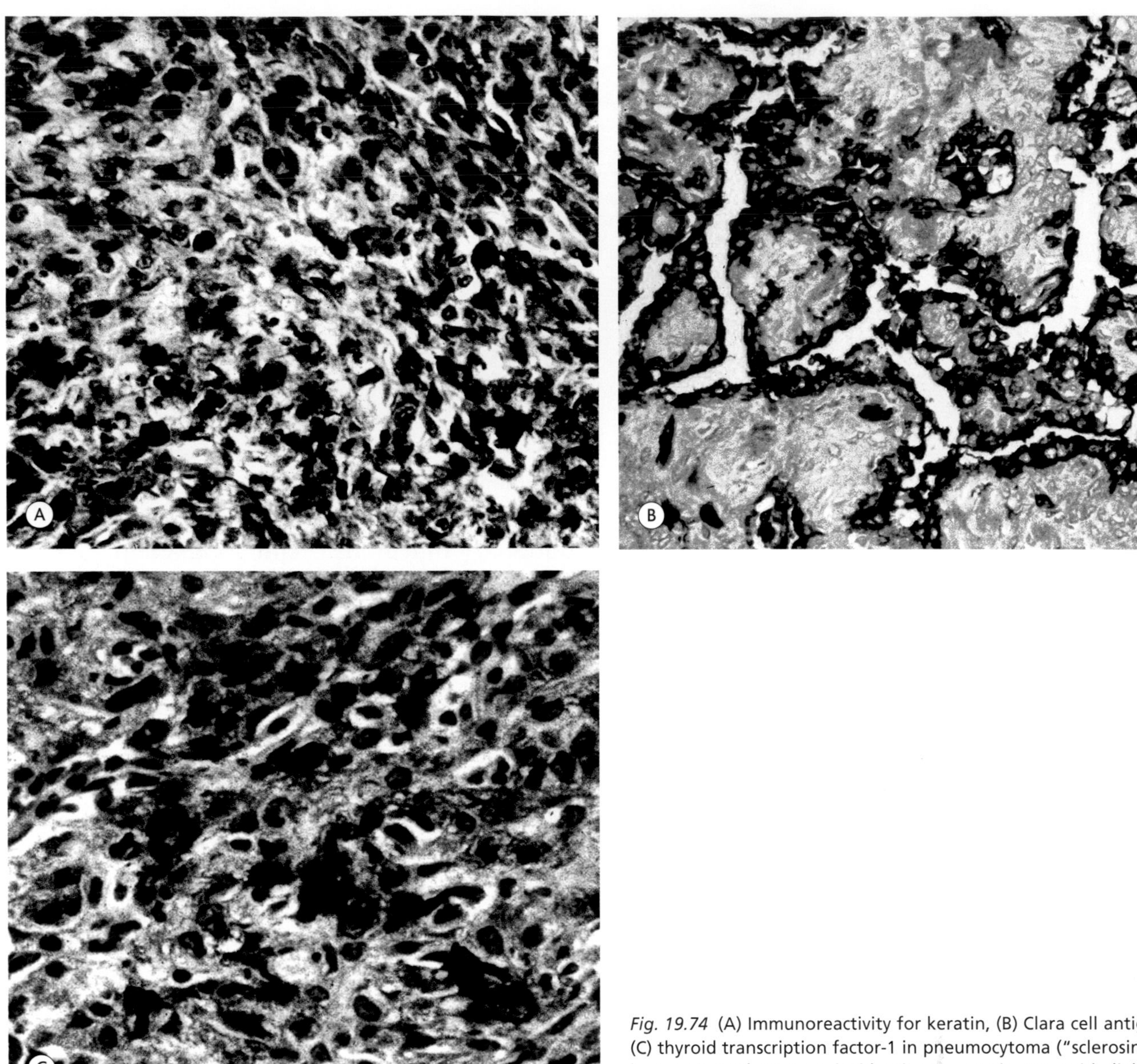

Fig. 19.74 (A) Immunoreactivity for keratin, (B) Clara cell antigen, and (C) thyroid transcription factor-1 in pneumocytoma ("sclerosing hemangioma") supports its identity as a respiratory epithelial neoplasm.

Differential diagnosis for these lesions is largely academic, because mucinous cystadenomas and BMTs in extrapulmonary locations do not metastasize to the lungs. Moreover, the clinical and histologic features of such tumors are quite different from those of other respiratory tract lesions that may contain mucin. The latter include mucoepidermoid carcinoma, mucus gland adenoma, and bronchioloalveolar carcinoma.

The classification of pulmonary BMT as a neoplasm with low malignant potential is inferential, based solely on its morphologic homology with lesions in other organs. In fact, none of the pulmonary tumors has recurred locally, as those arising in the pancreas, gut, or ovaries may do.

Solitary fibrous tumor

Solitary fibrous tumor (SFT; also called "fibroma" [287,288]) of the lung and pleura is still confused by some clinicians with mesothelial neoplasms. That is because of a nosologic scheme advanced by Klemperer and Rabin in 1931,[289] which was used for many years thereafter and gave SFT the designation of "localized fibrous mesothelioma." Particularly in the past two decades, much work has been done which unequivocally shows that SFT *lacks* mesothelial differentiation;[290] instead, it is composed of facultative fibroblastic elements like those seen in the submesothelial zone of the normal lung. Even though it may occasionally recur and sometimes

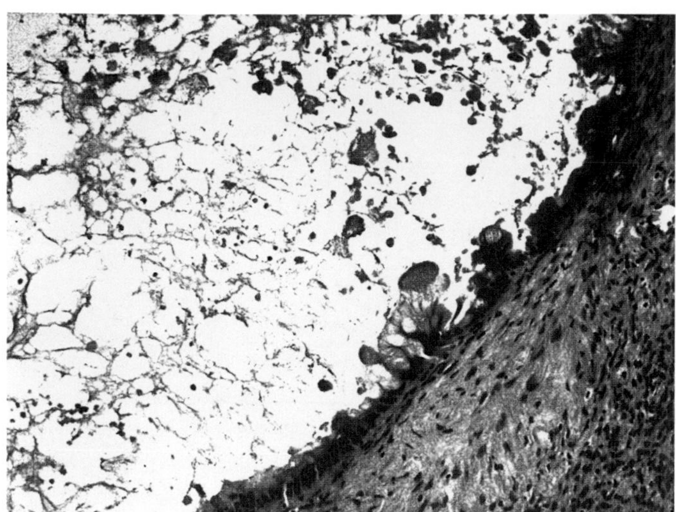

Fig. 19.75 Mucinous cystadenoma of the lung, showing a fibrous cyst wall that is mantled by bland mucinous epithelial cells. The cavity of the lesion contains abundant and inspissated mucinous material.

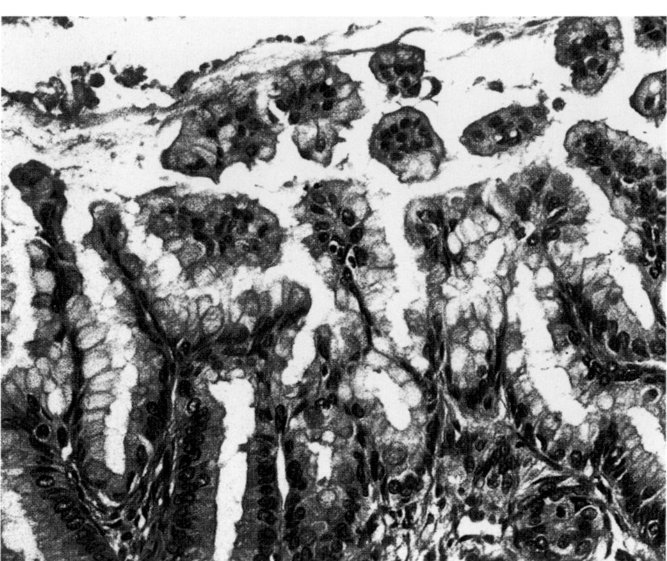

Fig. 19.77 Micropapillary growth is evident in some cystic mucinous tumors of the lung, justifying use of the term "borderline" in reference to them.

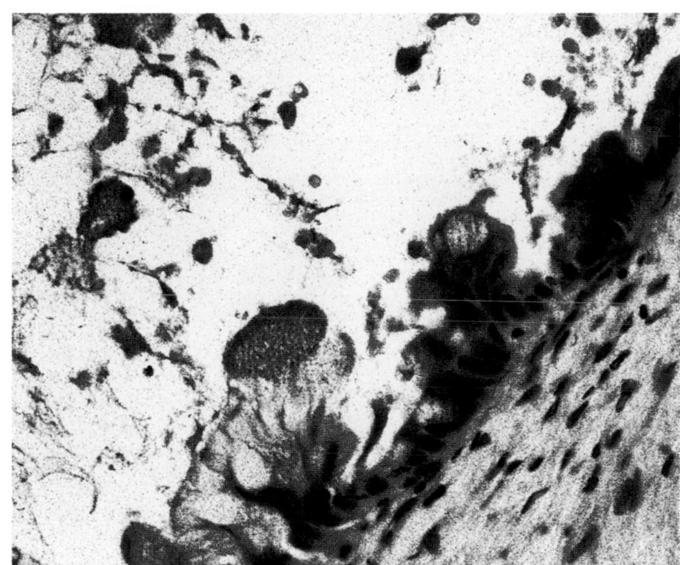

Fig. 19.76 The neoplastic epithelial cells of pulmonary mucinous cystadenoma are banal, with no significant nuclear atypia. Cytoplasmic mucin is apparent.

demonstrates locally aggressive growth – justifying its classification as a "borderline" mesenchymal tumor – SFT generally has a favorable prognosis that differs markedly from that of mesothelioma.[290–300] Likewise, pleural fibrous tumors have no etiologic relationship whatsoever to occupational-level asbestos exposure, in contrast to a proportion of mesotheliomas.[298]

Approximately two mesotheliomas are encountered for every SFT in general thoracic surgical practice.[290] Outside of infancy, patients of any age may develop an SFT, but it is most often seen in individuals over 40 years old, with no gender predilection. The great majority of cases present with an asymptomatic pleuropulmonary mass that is seen on screening radiographs. Other patients may complain of chest pain, shortness of breath, fever, general malaise, night sweats, hemoptysis, weight loss, backache, and syncope. Rarely, one of two paraneoplastic complexes accompanies SFT; those are represented by hypertrophic osteoarthropathy and tumor-associated hypoglycemia (Doege–Potter syndrome)[298] The cause of the first condition is still unknown; the second is related to an insulin-like growth factor that is produced directly by the neoplastic cells.

Radiographically, SFT may be as small as 1 cm in maximal dimension or as large as 36 cm. Indeed, occasional lesions of this type have occupied virtually an entire hemithorax and weighed in excess of 5 kg.[297] They are usually globoid neoplasms with a relatively homogeneous internal density, but cystic change, calcification, or foci of necrosis are sometimes apparent (Fig. 19.78). A minority of cases demonstrate a pedicle that attaches an SFT in the pleural space to the pleura itself. Conversely, other lesions "invert" into the lung parenchyma or may arise from interlobar pleural reflections, producing the appearance of a peripheral intrapulmonary mass;[287,288,301] large tumors may displace the trachea or intramediastinal structures as well.[290] Rarely, overt invasion of the chest wall, vertebral bodies, or adjacent lung tissue is apparent on imaging studies.[301,302]

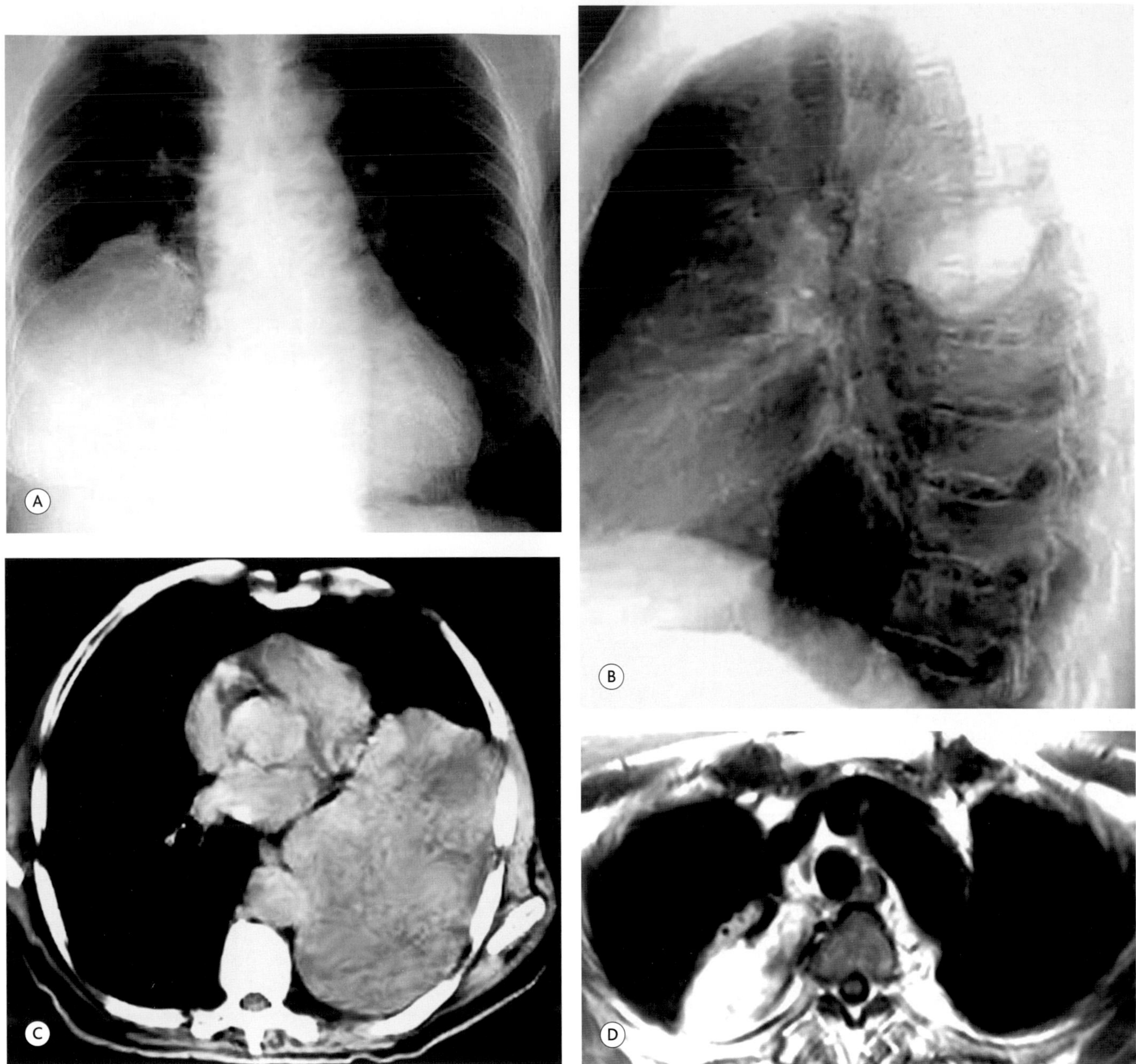

Fig. 19.78 Solitary fibrous tumors of the pleura, appearing as globoid sessile neoplasms in two chest radiographs (A, B). Internal homogeneity is apparent by computed tomography. (D) Another lesion seen in a magnetic resonance image has a slightly infiltrative peripheral aspect.

Macroscopic examination of resected SFTs shows a lobulated mass that is invested by pleural tissue (Fig. 19.79). Their cut surfaces can be homogeneous, tan-gray, and vaguely "whorled," or they may show distinct internal septa and foci of degeneration, mucoid change, hemorrhage, calcification, or necrosis[300,301] (Fig. 19.80). Intralesional cysts can also be appreciated in some instances.

The microscopic spectrum of pleuropulmonary SFT has been reviewed by Moran et al.[300] In their review of 50 cases and a redaction of the literature, it was found that solid spindle cell growth and a diffuse sclerosing pattern were most frequently encountered. In the first of those configurations, fusiform cells were arranged in random arrays (a "patternless pattern") (Fig. 19.81), fascicular groupings, storiform or herringbone patterns, regimented arrays with nuclear palisading, or a pattern featuring the presence of epithelioid cells and branched intralesional blood vessels resembling "moose antlers," as seen in hemangiopericytoma or synovial sarcoma (Fig. 19.82). Zones of fibrosis were interspersed with cellular zones and dominated those lesions classified as "diffuse sclerosing" SFT (Fig. 19.83). Focal collagenous degeneration was occasionally apparent, simulating true necrosis. Less frequent patterns included the presence of multinucleated tumor giant cells, "amianthoid" arrays of collagen fibers, and metaplastic ossification. Mitotic activity in most SFTs is present but not prominent, and division figures are physiological in shape. Myxoid stromal changes, limited areas of spontaneous necrosis, and hemorrhage are potentially seen as well.

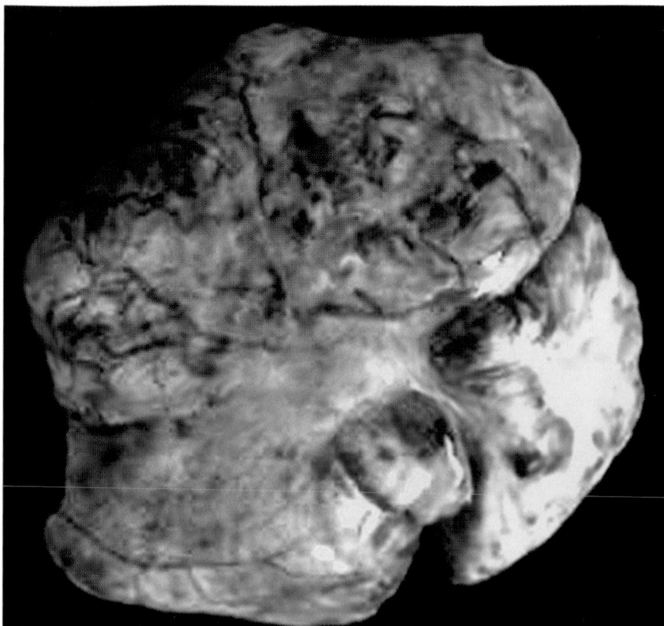

Fig. 19.79 The external surface of this solitary fibrous tumor of the pleura is covered by serosal membrane.

England et al.[301] attempted a codification of criteria for malignancy in SFT, in a study of archival cases at the AFIP. These included dense cellularity with overlapping nuclei; nuclear hyperchromasia and pleomorphism (Fig. 19.84); mitotic activity above 4 division figures per 10 ×400 microscopic fields, coupled with necrosis and hemorrhage. However, only 55% of the lesions with such features actually pursued an aggressive course in the AFIP series, with recurrence, or metastasis, or both. Vallat-Decouvelaere et al.[292] also emphasized that histologic findings in SFTs may not be accurate predictors of their behavior. In line with that admonition, a small proportion of histologically banal tumors of this type also manifest untoward behavior, typically with invasion of the bony structures and soft tissues of the thorax, or recurrence.[290,298] Because of these attributes, it is best to consider SFT as a borderline neoplasm. As Vallat-Decouvelaere and colleagues stated, "it is probably unwise to regard any such lesion as definitely benign."[292]

Ali et al.[302] and others[303,304] have addressed the cytologic features of SFT as seen in FNA biopsy specimens. In typical examples of this neoplasm, one observes variably cohesive and pleomorphic spindle cells in a bloody background (Fig. 19.85), representing an image that corresponds to a sizable differential diagnosis. Preparation

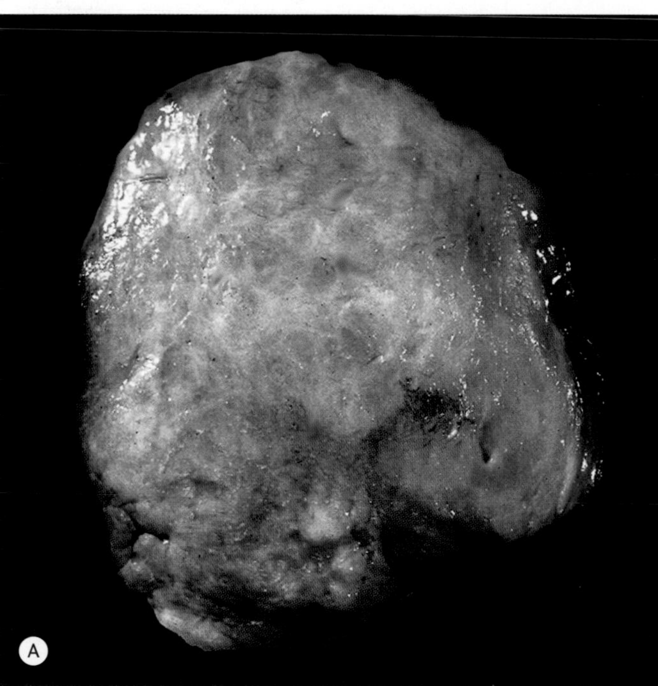

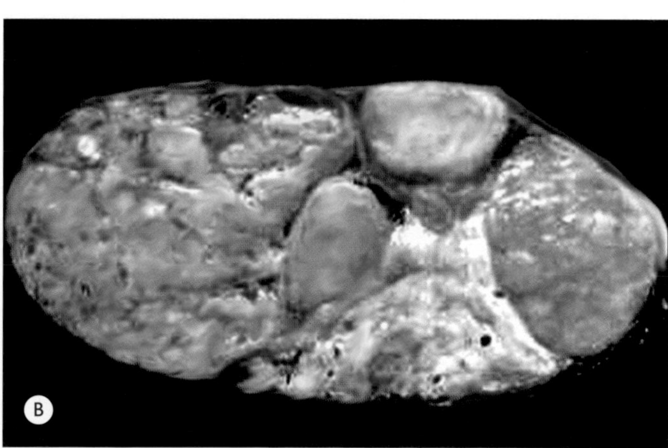

Fig. 19.80 The cut surfaces of solitary fibrous pleural tumors may be either homogeneous and tan-pink (A), or septated, with or without foci of degeneration or necrosis (B).

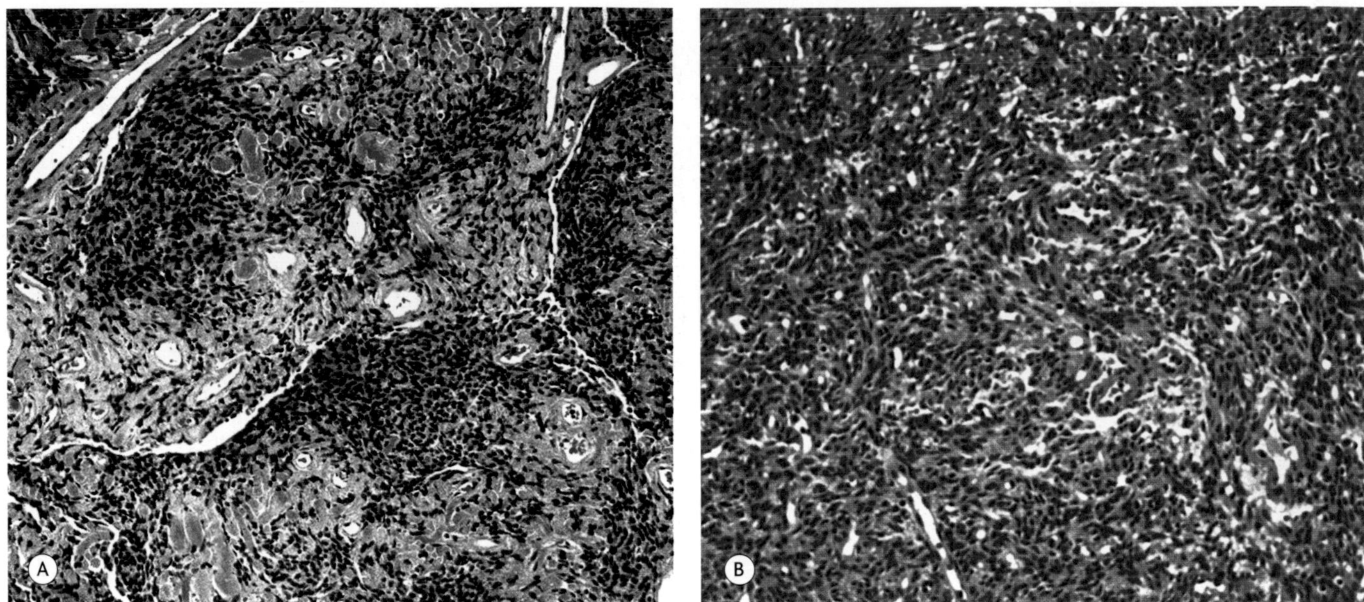

Fig. 19.81 (A,B) A "patternless pattern" is apparent in this solitary fibrous pleural tumor, wherein spindle cells are randomly arranged with some variation in cellularity from region to region within the neoplasm.

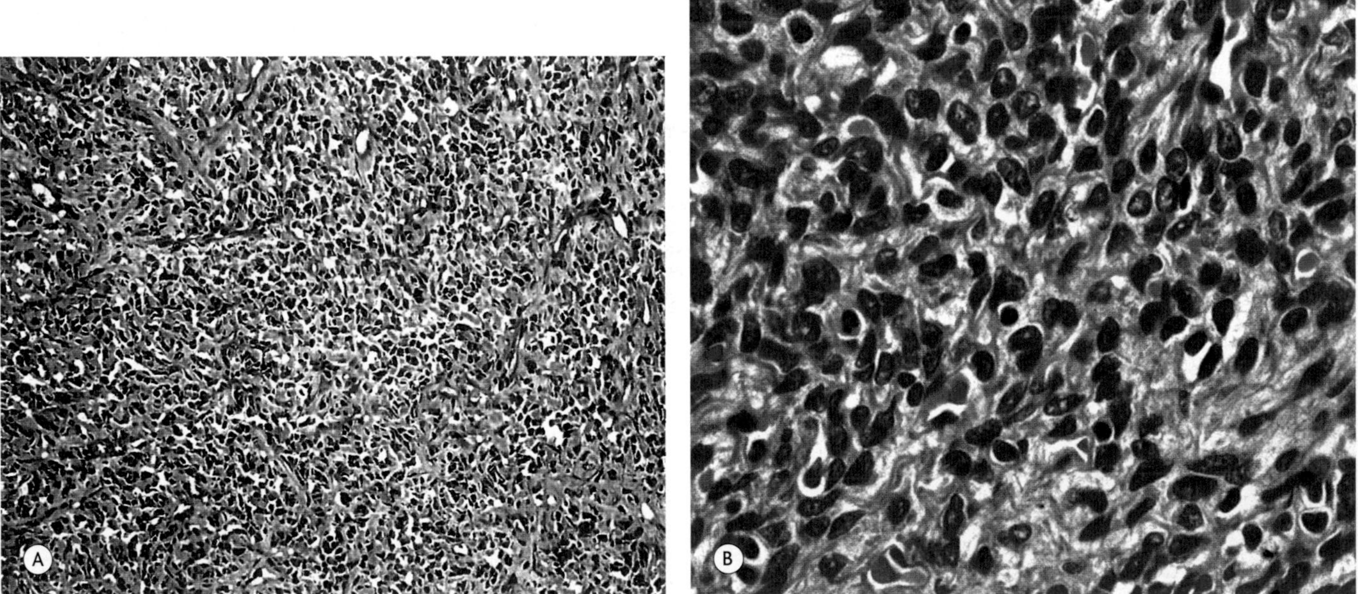

Fig. 19.82 (A,B) An epithelioid cytologic composition is seen in this solitary fibrous tumor of the pleura, potentially simulating the appearance of synovial sarcoma or hemangiopericytoma.

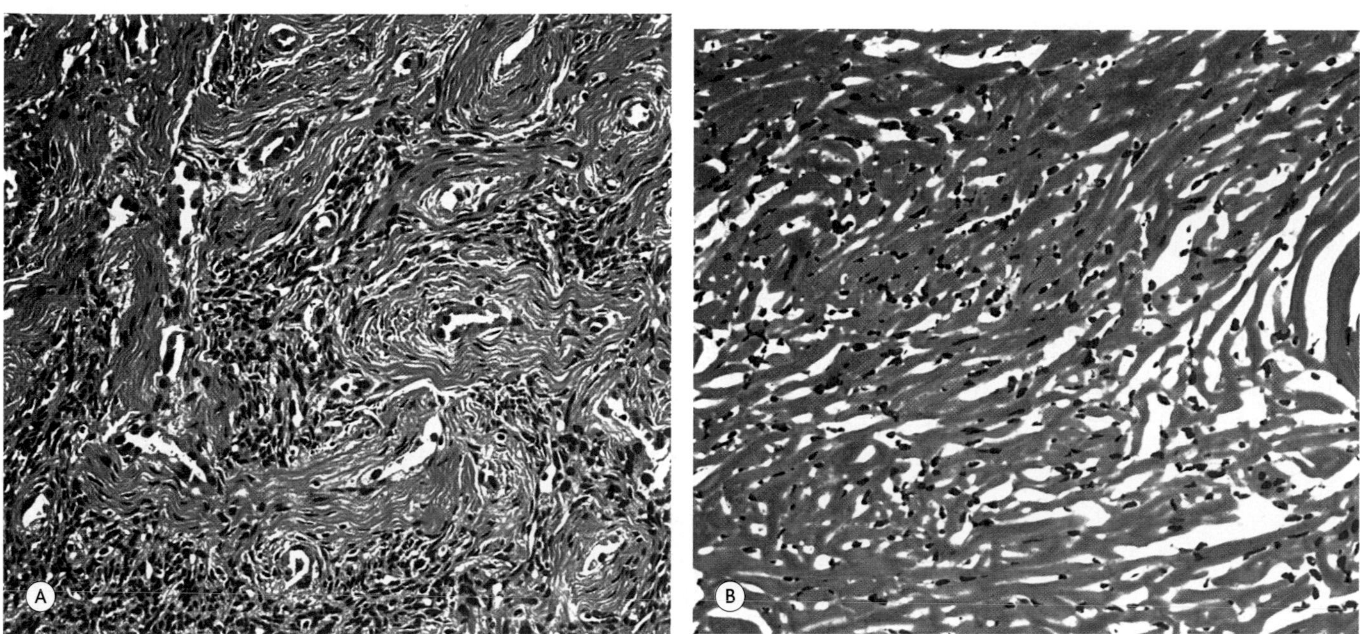

Fig. 19.83 (A,B) Hyalinizing collagenous stroma is prominent in this solitary fibrous pleural tumor.

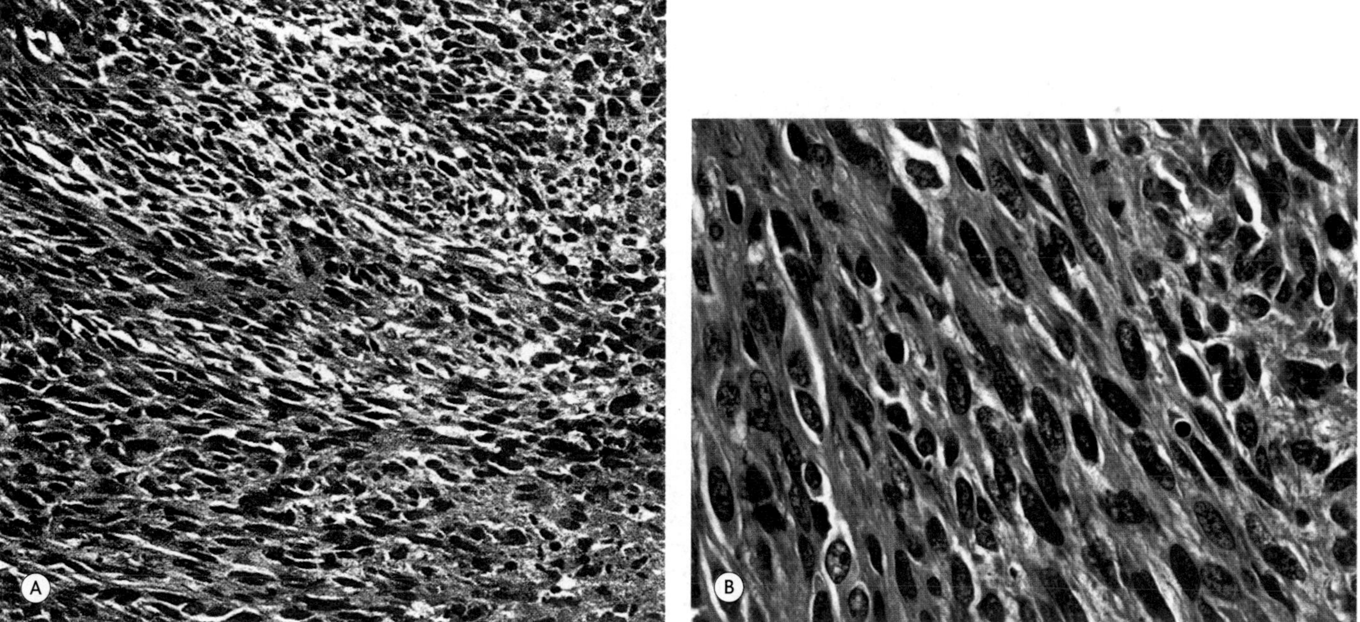

Fig. 19.84 Atypical features in solitary fibrous pleural tumor, which raise the possibility of malignancy, include uniformly dense cellularity (A) and nuclear overlapping with vesicular change in chromatin (B).

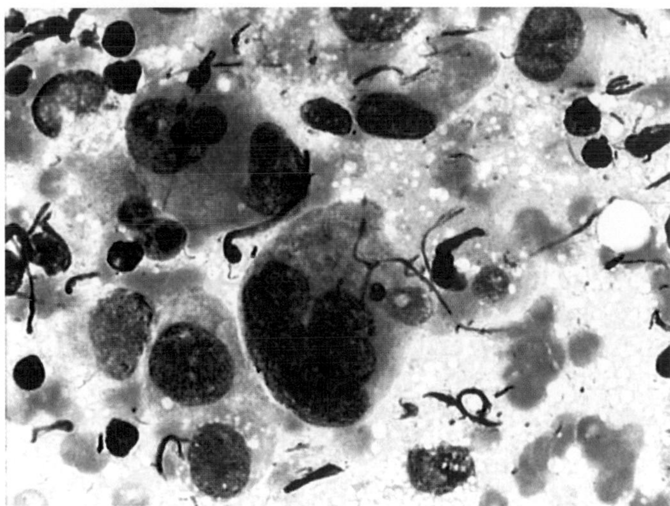

Fig. 19.85 This fine-needle aspiration biopsy specimen of a pleural solitary fibrous tumor shows dyshesive pleomorphic mesenchymal cells in a bloody background.

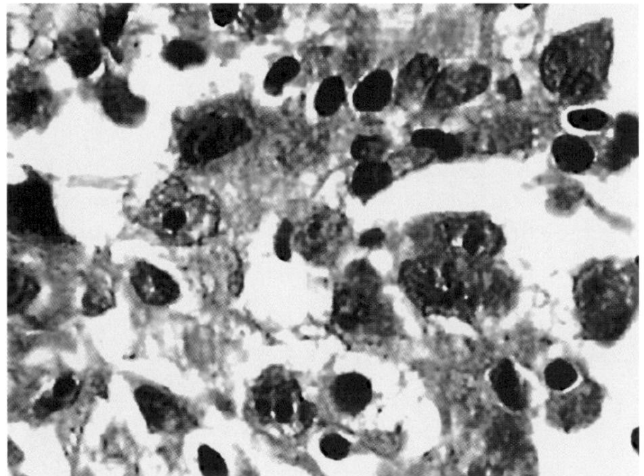

Fig. 19.86 A cell block preparation from the case shown in Fig. 19.85, demonstrating typical histologic features of solitary fibrous tumor.

of cell block sections (Fig. 19.86) and the procurement of adjunctive pathologic studies is essential to a specific diagnosis.

Electron microscopic analysis of SFT has shown that the tumor cells are fibroblast-like. They lack basal lamina, intercellular junctions, and plasmalemmal microvilli, as expected in epithelial or mesothelial cells, and instead contain only basic intracellular organelles.[298] Occasionally, intrareticular collagen fibrils are apparent within profiles of endoplasmic reticulum.

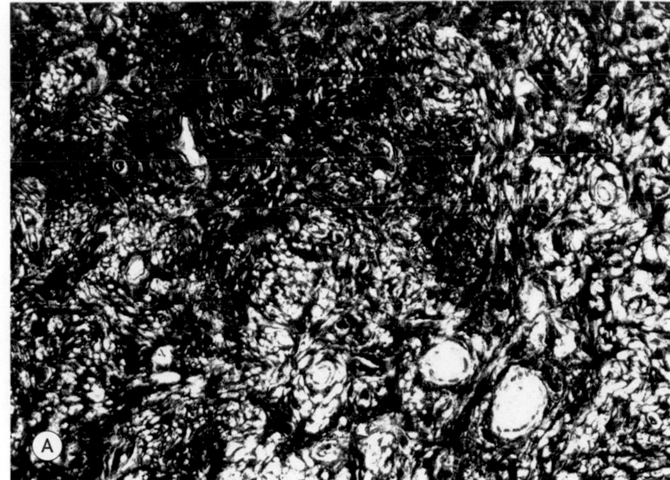

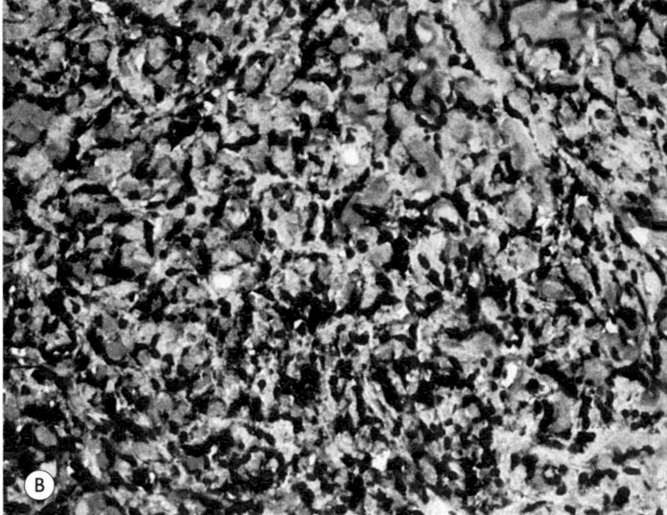

Fig. 19.87 Diffuse immunoreactivity for CD34 (A) and CD99 (B) is characteristic of solitary fibrous tumor.

Immunophenotypically, SFT demonstrates reactivity for vimentin, CD34, CD99, and *bcl*-2 protein in >85% of cases[292,299,301,302,304–308] (Fig. 19.87). There is typically no labeling for keratin, EMA, desmin, actins, S100 protein, collagen type IV, CD31, or CD57. Anecdotally, it may be true that those lesions with malignant histologic features are prone to exhibit mutant p53 protein immunoreactivity[309] (Fig. 19.88), but that relationship has not been subjected to rigorous evaluation.

Cytogenetic assessment of SFT is still in its infancy. However, the most frequent defects reported in this tumor type have involved chromosomes 4q, 8, 13q, 15q, and 21q.[310,311] One case reported by Dal Cin et al. showed a balanced t(4;15)(q13;q26) translocation.[311]

The differential diagnosis of pleuropulmonary SFT includes primary and secondary sarcomatoid carcinoma; sarcomatoid or desmoplastic mesothelioma; fibrosarcoma;

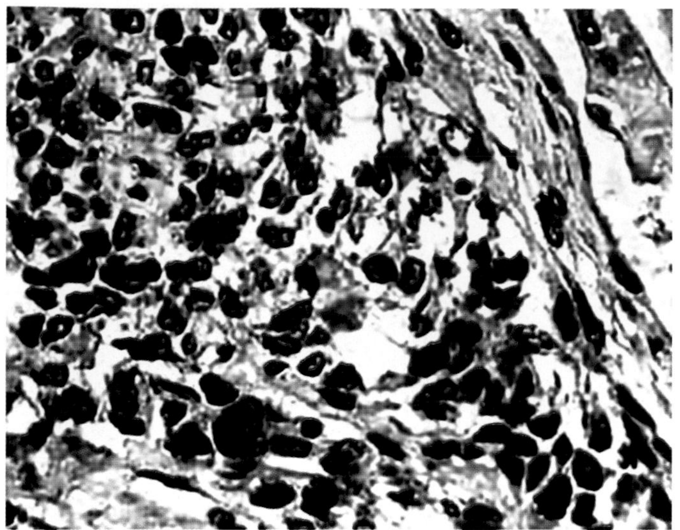

Fig. 19.88 Immunoreactivity for mutant p53 protein, shown here, has been anecdotally linked to malignancy in solitary fibrous tumor.

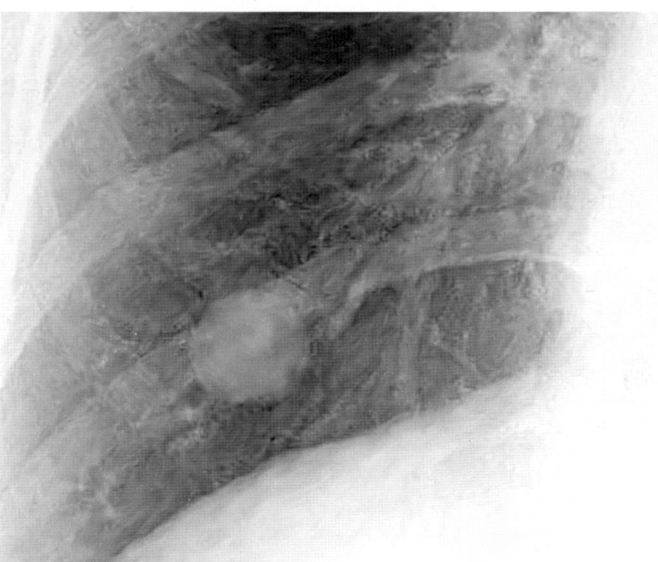

Fig. 19.89 This highlighted plain-film chest radiograph of a clear cell pulmonary "sugar tumor" demonstrates a nondescript well-defined nodule in the right lung field.

storiform malignant fibrous histiocytoma (MFH); synovial sarcoma; hemangiopericytoma; and metastatic endometrial stromal sarcoma.[300] Among these possibilities, carcinomas, mesotheliomas, and synovial sarcomas may be excluded because of their immunoreactivity for keratin, or EMA, or both. In addition, synovial sarcoma reproducibly shows a t(X;18) translocation,[312] which is absent in SFT. Even though hemangiopericytomas share CD34-positivity with SFTs, the former tumors are also reactive for CD57 but lack CD99;[313] that immunoprofile separates them from SFT. Likewise, consistent CD10 reactivity in endometrial stromal sarcoma differs from the properties of SFT.[314] Fibrosarcoma and MFH lack CD34, CD99, and *bcl*-2 protein, all of which are typically manifest in SFT.

The biologic attributes of SFT have been largely covered by previous comments. However, some of its characteristics merit reiteration. Approximately 10% of "ordinary" intrathoracic SFTs (lacking histologic indicators of possible malignancy) will recur, sometimes massively.[290] This behavior has most often been linked with incomplete lesional excision at initial surgery, and salvage of the patient is still a distinct possibility if total removal of the tumor can still be accomplished.[293,295] Metastastic disease is very unusual, but it tends to be refractory to oncological intervention.

Pulmonary "sugar tumor" (epithelioid myomelanocytoma)

The general premises underlying the nosologic family of "myomelanocytomas" (MMCs) have been described previously in reference to angiomyolipomas. Another member of that conceptual group – the clear cell "sugar" tumor of the lung (STL) – may be viewed as a purely epithelioid MMC,[178] which, for reasons to be discussed, is probably best regarded as biologically "borderline."

Pulmonary "sugar tumor" was first described noncommittally as "clear cell tumor of the lung" by Liebow and Castleman 40 years ago,[315] and <100 additional examples of that entity in the respiratory tract have been documented in the interim.[316–333] It has usually been observed in patients over 40 years old, typically as an asymptomatic peripheral lung nodule that is found incidentally by screening radiography. However, occasional examples have been reported in the trachea or large bronchi,[319,330] and these have presented with dyspnea, cough, or hemoptysis. Like angiomyolipoma, STL has also been found concurrently with lymphangioleiomyomatosis and multifocal micronodular pneumocyte hyperplasia in some patients with tuberous sclerosis.[327] Tumors in such patients demonstrate a loss of heterozygosity in the TSC2 region of chromosome 16p13.[334,335]

The radiographic attributes of STL are nondescript.[318,323] It is a homogeneously dense, round to ovoid, peripheral lung mass that may be seen in any region of the lung (Fig. 19.89). Computed tomography has typically shown sharp circumscription.

These same features are reflected in gross examination of pulmonary sugar tumors. Their cut surfaces are pink to brown and uniform, although necrotic foci may sometimes be present. Maximum diameter is generally <5 cm.

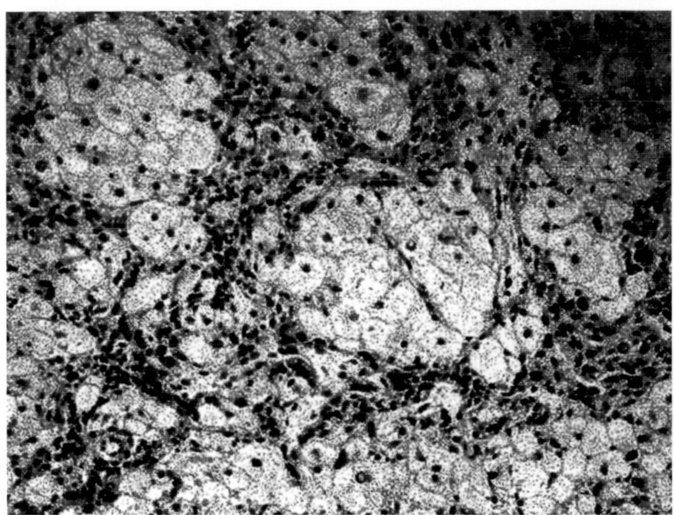

Fig. 19.90 One potential histologic configuration of pulmonary clear cell sugar tumor is shown in this photograph, wherein vague nests of clear, cytologically bland epithelioid cells are separated by fibrous stroma.

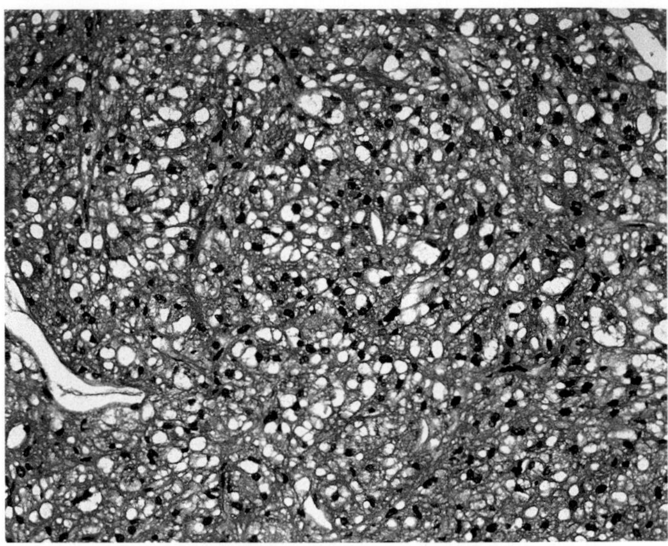

Fig. 19.91 Another growth pattern in pulmonary sugar tumor is medullary in nature, comprising sheets of clear neoplastic cells with indistinct internal fibrovascular septations.

Histologic examination shows one of two general growth patterns in STLs. The first is organoid, with broad cords and rounded nests of cells being separated by a variably prominent fibrovascular stroma (Fig. 19.90). The second configuration is a medullary image, showing sheets of epithelioid cells with little internal clustering (Fig. 19.91). Pre-existing small bronchi and bronchioles are often entrapped by the neoplastic cells. Nuclei are round to ovoid with small nucleoli; intranuclear invaginations of cytoplasm also may be apparent, but mitotic figures are usually difficult to find. Cytoplasm is clear or lightly eosinophilic, and may be finely granular. Intralesional blood vessels can be markedly sclerotic in some cases; spontaneous necrosis is occasionally seen; and sparse intratumoral chronic inflammatory cells may be identified.

Ultrastructural studies of STL have shown attributes suggesting a "hybrid" cell type that incorporates elements of modified perivascular smooth muscle and melanocytes. These include interdigitating cellular processes, pericellular basal lamina, primitive intercellular attachment complexes, plasmalemmal pinocytosis, membrane-bound and free cytoplasmic glycogen granules, and variant-form premelanosomes.[317,320,321,324,326,329]

Immunohistologically, one sees a uniform lack of reactivity for epithelial markers in STL, but consistent positivity for vimentin, CD117, collagen type IV, HMB-45, MART-1, and microophthalmia transcription factor-1 (with the last three determinants all being related to melanocytes)[177,321,322,326,328] (Fig. 19.92). Inconsistent but generally positive results are obtained for muscle-specific actin, S100 protein, and neuron-specific enolase. Recently, Panizo-Santos et al. have described aberrant but virtually exclusive cytoplasmic immunoreactivity for Myo-D1 in members of the MMC family of tumors.[336] That marker is a *nuclear* transcription factor that is related to striated muscle development, and bona fide labeling for it would not be expected in the cytoplasm. Hence, it appears that the cited pattern of staining probably represents a reproducible artifact, but it is one which, if corroborated, could prove to be useful diagnostically.

The differential diagnosis for STL is a lengthy one, including primary carcinomas of the lung with clear cell features; metastatic clear cell carcinomas from the kidney, urogenital tract, breast, and other locations; metastatic clear cell sarcoma (CCS); and metastatic "balloon cell" melanoma.[337] The generic possibility of carcinoma can be relatively quickly excluded by the lack of keratin and EMA in STL (Fig. 19.93), but CCS and melanoma are not as easily dismissed because they potentially share the entire complement of immunohistologic melanocyte markers with MMCs. Reactivity for actin, CD117, or Myo-D1 would strongly argue in favor of STL in this setting, because those determinants have not been reported in metastatic malignant melanocytic neoplasms.

Returning to the biologic nature of STL, it has traditionally been considered as a benign pulmonary tumor. Nonetheless, at least two examples of that lesion – reported by Gaffey et al.[329] and Sale and Kulander[331] – metastasized to other visceral sites, and one proved fatal.

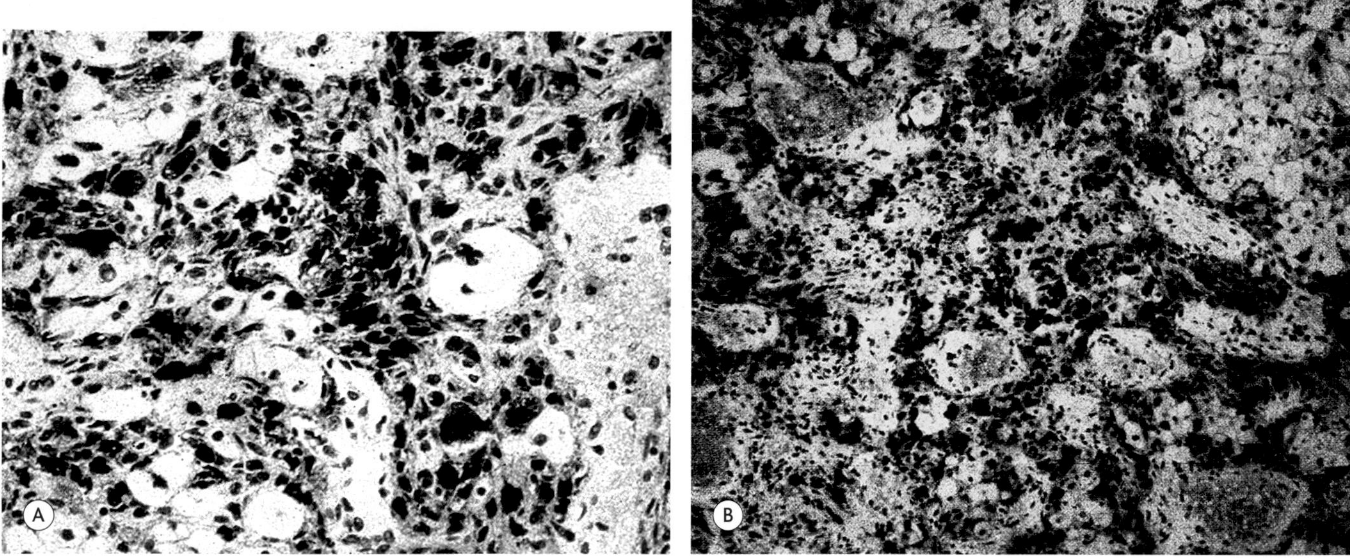

Fig. 19.92 (A) Immunoreactivity with HMB-45 and (B) for melan-A/MART-1 is typical of clear cell pulmonary sugar tumor.

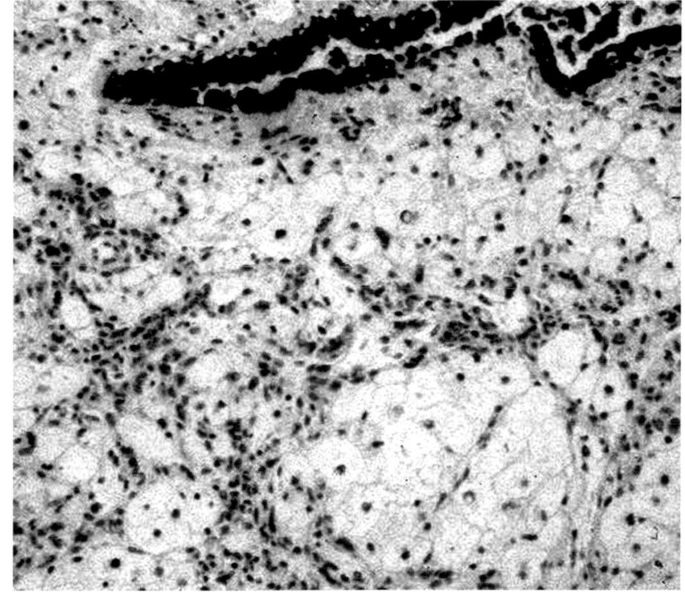

Fig. 19.93 Sugar tumors of the lung are consistently nonreactive for keratin, as shown in this figure (note positive staining of the epithelium of a small airway at the top of the figure).

That behavior parallels the biologic potential of MMCs in other organs, notably the kidney. Thus, it would seem appropriate to regard STL as another borderline neoplasm of the lung. With that having been said, however, simple surgical removal of the lesion – with wedge excision of the peripheral lung parenchyma, if possible – is felt to represent adequate therapy.

Primary pleuropulmonary thymoma

Even though thymomas typically arise in the anterosuperior mediastinum, the literature contains ample evidence of their ability to develop in ectopic sites as well. These tumors have been described in the soft tissue of the lower neck, as well as the thyroid, pericardium, lungs, and pleura.[338–341] Because of their ability to show a relatively wide morphologic spectrum, heterotopic thymic tumors may be quite difficult to recognize diagnostically.

Intrapulmonary thymoma is seen in adults between the ages of 20 and 80 years. In the minority of cases where the lesion is linked to one of several distinctive thymoma-related paraneoplastic syndromes – principally including myasthenia gravis, pure red cell aplasia, and acquired hypogammaglobulinemia – its identity may be suspected clinically.[342] However, the majority of these tumors present as asymptomatic masses that are found radiographically. They can be situated centrally, close to the hilum, and even endobronchially in rare instances, as well as in the mid-lung fields or beneath the pleural surfaces[343–353] (Fig. 19.94). Occasionally, two or more intrapulmonary masses are seen concurrently. In analogy to mediastinal thymomas, those arising in the lungs may either be circumscribed or infiltrative, and some demonstrate prominent intralesional cystification.

Pleural thymomas may simulate the appearance of any other solitary serosal neoplasm. In rare examples, they have diffusely effaced the pleural space in one or both hemithoraces, reproducing the radiographic and gross pathologic image of diffuse pleural mesothelioma or metastatic serosal carcinoma.[351–353]

All of the scenarios just listed include an absence of any abnormalities in the anterior mediastinum. With that in mind, it is easy to understand that a definitive radiographic interpretation of ectopic thymoma is virtually impossible.

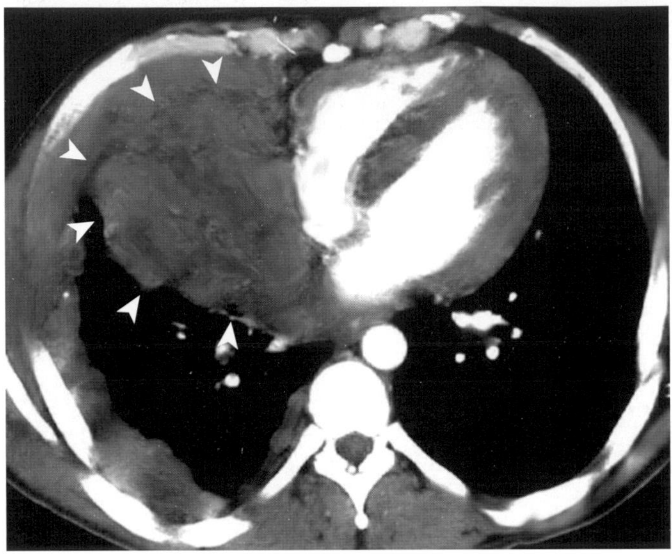

Fig. 19.94 This computed tomogram of the thorax shows a lobulated mass in the anterior right lung field (arrowheads), representing a primary intrapulmonary thymoma.

Many of the gross features of pulmonary and pleural thymomas have been mentioned above. However, others that merit mention include the tendency for such lesions to show internal fibrous septations, subdividing the masses into angulated tissue compartments. They have a fleshy pink-tan cut surface that closely resembles that of lymphoreticular neoplasms (Fig. 19.95), but areas of necrosis, hemorrhage, or cyst formation are much more common than they are in lymphomas. Dystrophic calcification also may be present.

Microscopically, circumferential fibrous encapsulation of pulmonary or pleural thymomas is unusual, in contrast to their intrathymic counterparts. As a result, ectopic lesions in the hemithoraces must commonly be classified as "invasive," almost by definition (Fig. 19.96). As stated previously, intralesional fibrous septa intersect one another at acute angles (Fig. 19.97), differing from the obtuse connections that are seen in nodular sclerosing Hodgkin's lymphoma or sclerosing non-Hodgkin's lymphomas in the chest. We utilize the classical Bernatz system of histologic classification for thymic epithelial tumors, which has five subdivisions:

- lymphocyte-predominant thymoma (≥66% lymphocytes)
- mixed thymoma (34–65% lymphocytes)
- epithelial-predominant thymoma (≤33% lymphocytes)
- spindle cell thymoma (a variant of epithelial-predominant thymoma in which the majority of the neoplastic cells are fusiform) (Fig. 19.98)

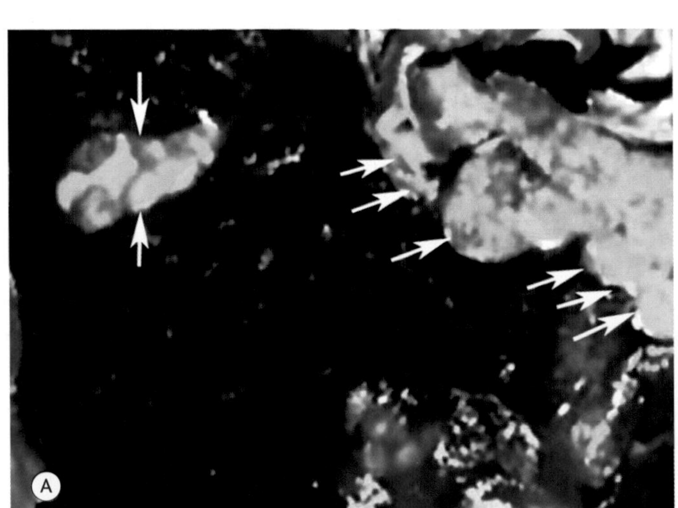

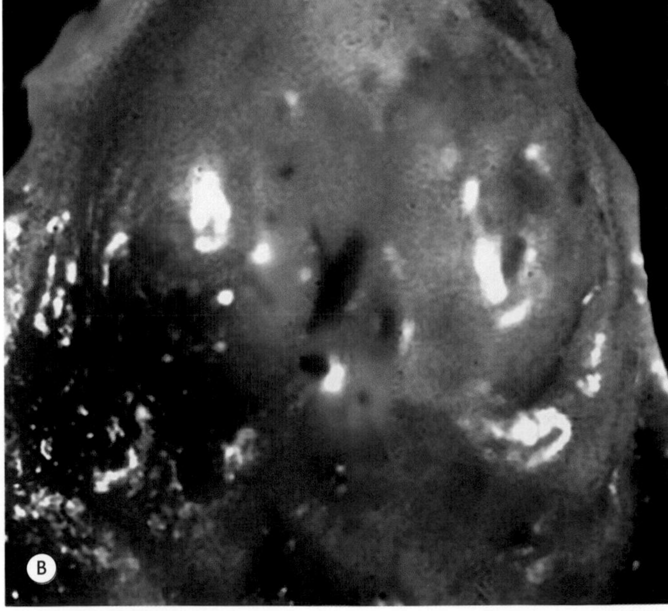

Fig. 19.95 (A; arrows) These gross photographs of intrapulmonary thymomas show that such lesions are often centered on interlobar septa and (B) invested by the serosal membrane. They otherwise resemble lymphoreticular neoplasms.

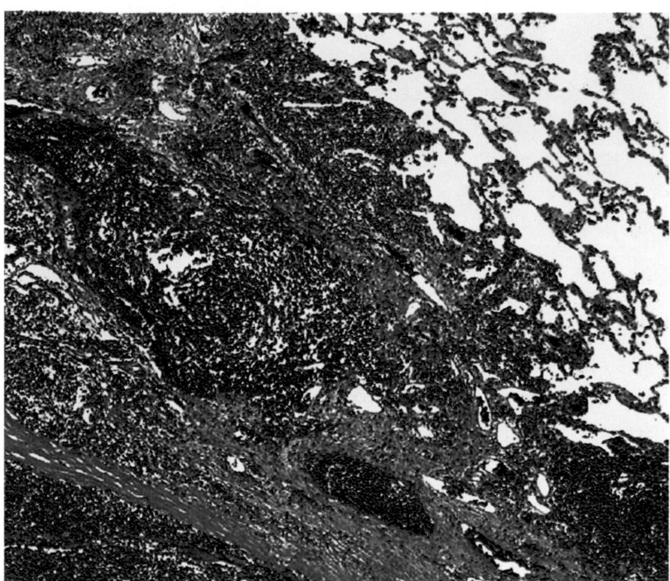

Fig. 19.96 Invasion of the lung parenchyma is seen in this case of intrapulmonary thymoma.

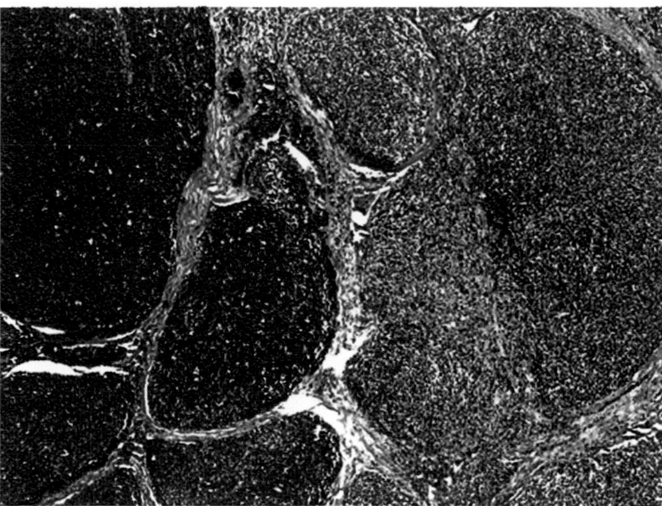

Fig. 19.97 Internal fibrous septa in thymomas intersect one another at acute angles, yielding a distinctive image.

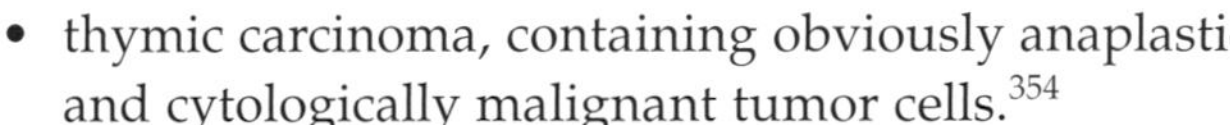

- thymic carcinoma, containing obviously anaplastic and cytologically malignant tumor cells.[354]

Each of the five lesional categories may also be either circumscribed or invasive, based on gross findings at surgery. Other alternative nosologic constructions for thymic tumors have entered common use as well, including the Marino–Muller-Hermelink scheme,[355] the World Health Organization system,[356] and the Suster–Moran codification.[357] The last one can be linked with the Bernatz system to specifically address those tumors that demonstrate a notable degree of nuclear atypia, yet whose features are insufficient for an outright diagnosis of carcinoma; such neoplasms are termed "atypical" thymomas.

The epithelial cells of thymomas – not the lymphoid cells – are the neoplastic elements therein, and they are characterized by a range of cytologic images. Some have vague cellular borders, oval nuclear contours, dispersed chromatin, and indistinct nucleoli. At the other end of the spectrum, one sees rather clear-cut plasmalemmal interfaces, moderate nuclear irregularity and hyperchromasia, and the presence of distinct nucleoli (Fig. 19.99). As mentioned earlier, spindle cell change is another potential image in thymomas, and the nuclei in such lesions tend to have bland and uniform morphologic characteristics. Mitotic activity in thymic tumors is greatly variable as well, and it achieves importance as a possible marker of thymic carcinoma only in those neoplasms that also show nuclear abnormalities.

Secondary architectural changes in thymomas include the formation of perivascular "lakes" of serum, in which lymphoid cells are suspended; pseudoglandular arrays or pseudorosettes of epithelial cells; microcysts or areas of macroscopic cystic change, with or without necrosis; stromal blood lakes and vascular dilatation; and "medullary differentiation," in which loose and vaguely nodular aggregates of stromal lymphocytes are present.[354] Hassall's corpuscles are seen in only a small minority of cases. Some spindle cell thymomas contain a vascular network comprising numerous vessels with a "moose-antler" configuration, yielding a pattern which virtually perfectly imitates that of hemangiopericytomas.

Epithelial-predominant thymomas with nuclear atypia, an organoid growth pattern, and distinct cellular borders have been called "well-differentiated thymic carcinomas" by Kirchner et al.[358] However, their generic clinicopathologic characteristics are clearly dissimilar to those of outright thymic carcinomas, and most observers believe they are more properly termed "atypical thymomas," as referenced above.[357]

The cytologic attributes of thymic epithelial neoplasms have been adeptly summarized by Wakely[359] and others,[360,361] as seen in FNA specimens. Thymomas are morphologically heterogeneous in that context, paralleling their histologic appearances. Mature lymphocytes are admixed with thymic epithelial cells, which show a tendency to cohesion. However, scattered single epithelial cells may also be evident. As in tissue sections, epithelial cell nuclei are generally monomorphic, with dispersed chromatin and small chromocenters. Cytoplasm is amphophilic, with indistinct cell borders. A fusiform

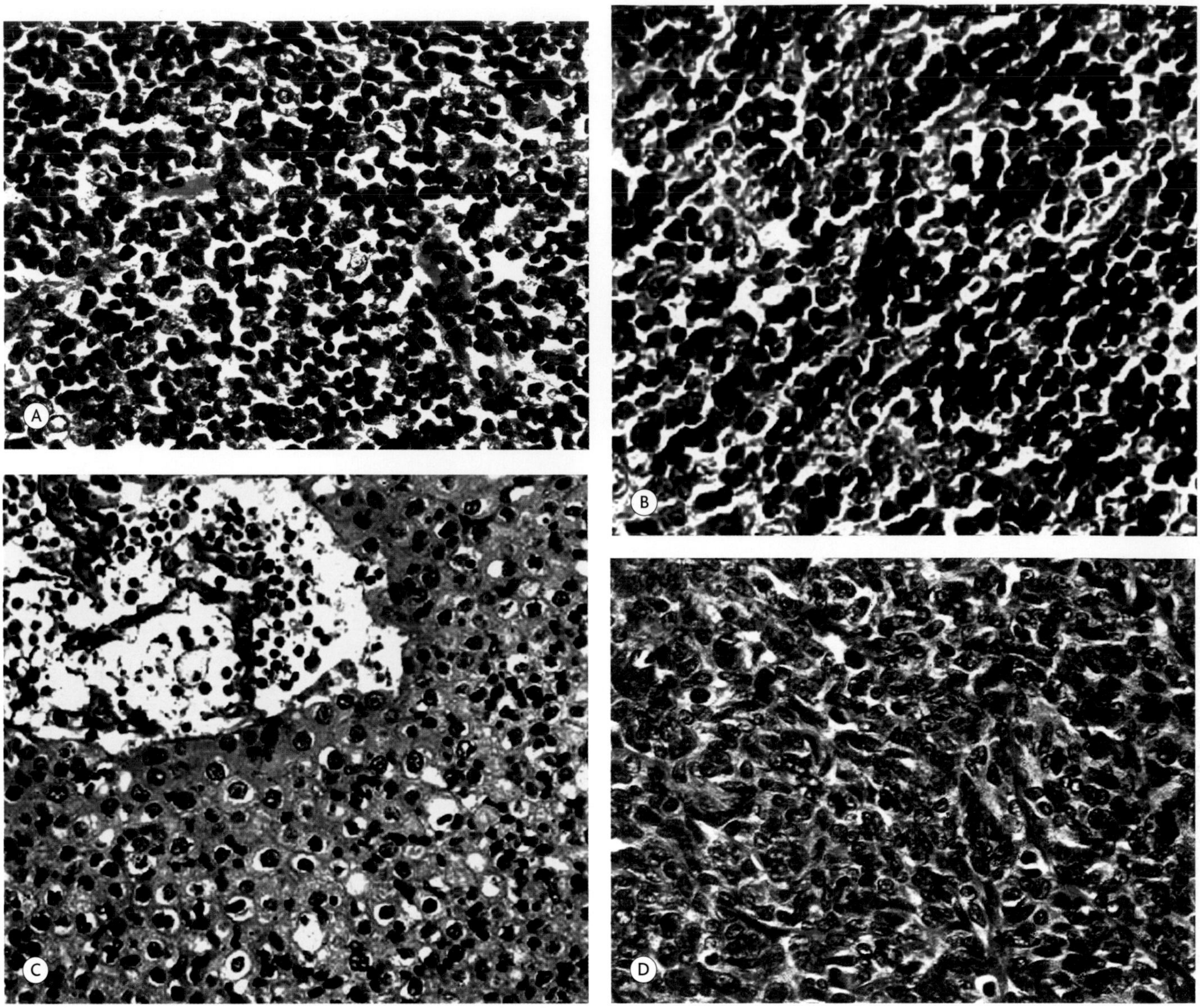

Fig. 19.98 (A) Lymphocyte-predominant thymoma. (B) Mixed lymphoepithelial thymoma. (C) Predominantly epithelial and polygonal cell thymoma. Note the presence of an intratumoral perivascular zone of serous fluid in which blood cells are suspended; this secondary feature is characteristic of thymomas in general. (D) Predominantly epithelial and spindle cell thymoma.

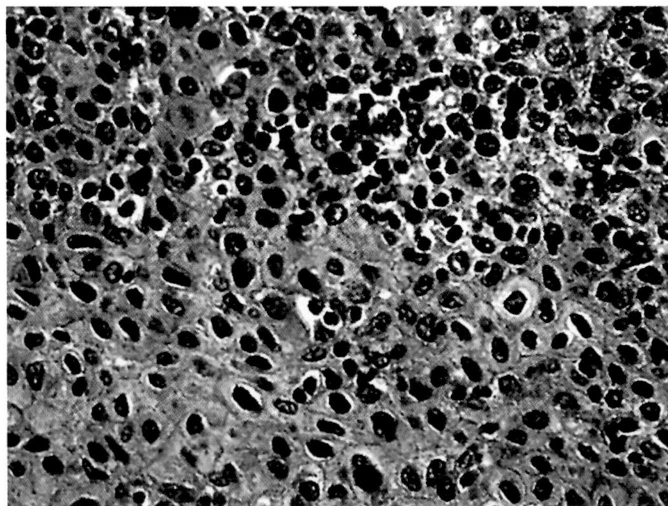

Fig. 19.99 "Atypical" epithelial-predominant thymoma shows increased nucleocytoplasmic ratios, the presence of nucleoli, nuclear hyperchromasia, and distinct intercellular membranes. However, these changes fall short of the cytomorphologic threshold for thymic carcinoma.

cellular shape may be encountered in spindle cell tumors, but the grouping of such cells into small clusters helps to distinguish them from mesenchymal proliferations. The lymphoid elements in thymoma are a potential diagnostic pitfall, in that nuclear "activation" may be seen with increases in the nuclear-to-cytoplasmic ratios. Convolution of the nuclear borders can also be present, as may mitotic figures. The overall image of "activated" intratumoral lymphocytes is quite similar to that of lymphoblastic lymphoma, and a misdiagnosis may ensue unless adjunctive studies are performed to detect the epithelial elements of thymoma.[346,359] Predictably, invasive thymomas cannot be distinguished from encapsulated tumors using the FNA technique.

Electron microscopy of thymomas shows the presence of elongated and interdigitating cytoplasmic processes emanating from constituent epithelial cells, and these are joined to one another by well-formed desmosomes into which broad tonofibrils insert. Plasmalemmal microvilli are absent, and intralesional lymphoid cells are usually intercalated between the epithelial elements.[362]

Cytogenetic analysis has shown no consistent karyotypic aberrations in thymomas. Several different abnormalities have been documented, including deletions of chromosome 6p; t(1;8) and t(15;22) chromosomal translocations; pseudodicentric (16;12)(q11;p11.2); and ring chromosome 6.[363–365] However, none of these findings is typically associated with other primary pleuropulmonary tumors.

Immunohistologic studies are paramount in confirming the cellular nature of ectopic thymomas. Keratin immunostains show a characteristically arborizing network of reactivity, reflecting the presence of interconnecting cytoplasmic processes[366] (Fig. 19.100). The keratin subtype 5/6 is also characteristic of thymic epithelium.[367] p63 protein, a member of the p53 protein "family," is likewise consistently present in thymoma, as it is in squamous neoplasms.[368] Finally, the lymphoid cells in thymomas are true thymocytes; as such, they express CD1a, nuclear terminal deoxynucleotidyl transferase (TdT) and CD99[346] (Fig. 19.101). The latter phenotype is shared only by the tumor cells of lymphoblastic lymphomas, but those hematopoietic neoplasms are uniformly nonreactive for p63 and keratin. Thus, a truly diagnostic immunoprofile exists in reference to thymoma. Parenthetically, it should be noted that "pseudomesotheliomatous" pleural thymomas may be

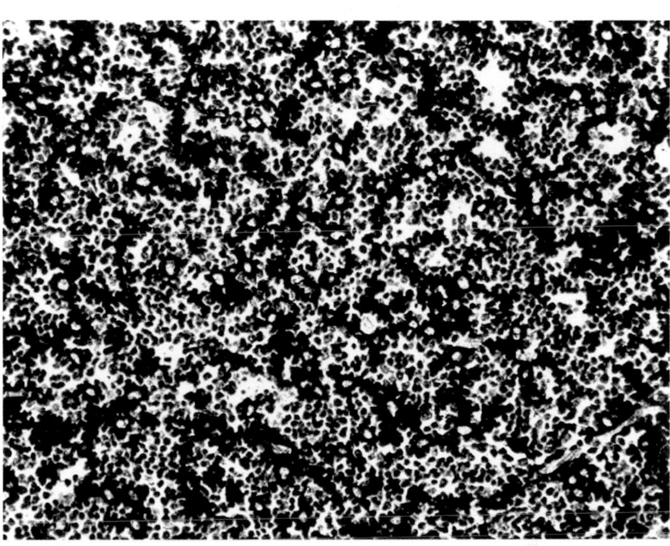

Fig. 19.100 Delicately interconnecting cell processes in thymoma are labeled for keratin, yielding a "lacy" staining pattern.

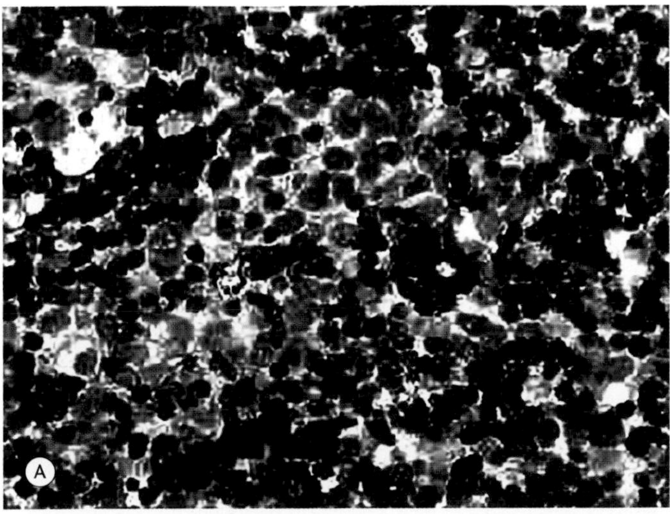

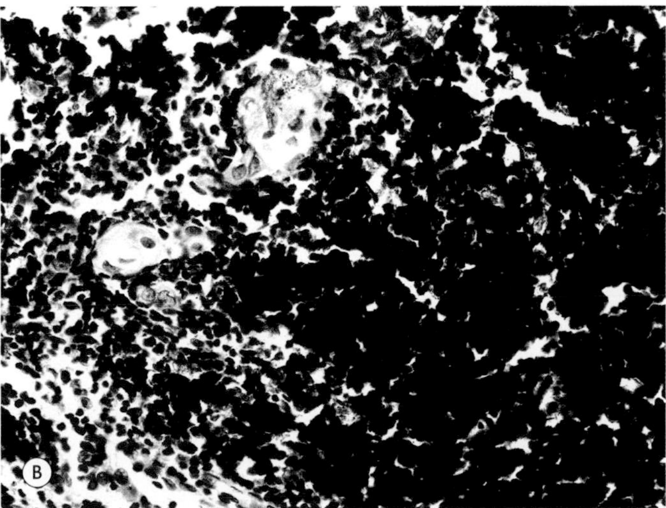

Fig. 19.101 (A) Lymphoid cells in thymomas are true thymocytes which label for CD99 and (B) nuclear terminal deoxynucleotidyl transferase.

reactive for calretinin, keratin 5/6, and thrombomodulin, all of which are commonly associated with mesothelial cells.[353] That concatenation of results may easily lead to misdiagnosis if studies for p63, CD1a, TdT, and CD99 are omitted.

Differential diagnostic considerations in cases of pleuropulmonary thymoma include lymphoma, metastatic somatic carcinoma, metastatic seminoma, mesothelioma, and pleural sarcomas (especially synovial sarcoma and hemangiopericytoma), depending on the microscopic nuances of the lesion being studied. The immunophenotype of thymoma presented above is unique among all those possibilities.

Behaviorally, ectopic thymomas in the lung and pleura are typically indolent lesions and can usually be cured by complete surgical resection. However, several examples have been reported in which recurrence, or distant metastasis, or both, was observed.[343–350] Moreover, lesions that simulate mesothelioma because of their encasement of the lungs or heart are associated with a greater risk of adverse behavior.[351–353] Because a minority of all pleuropulmonary thymomas are fatal, they are justifiably considered borderline in nature.

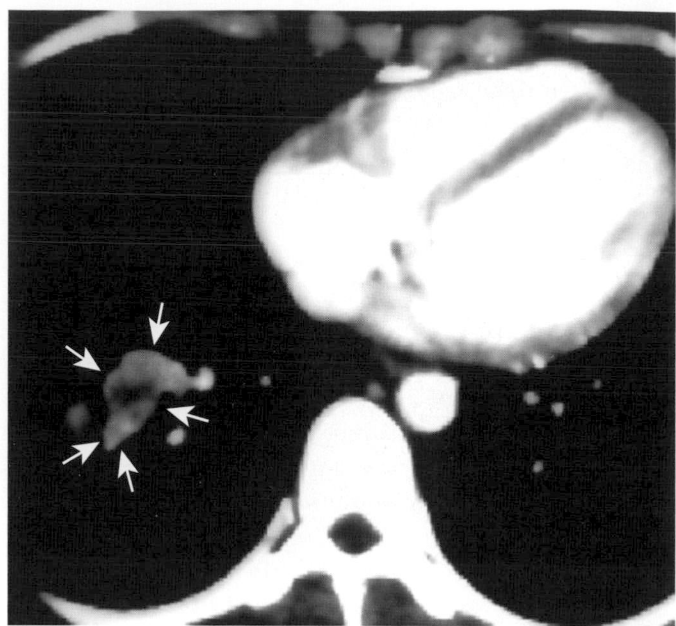

Fig. 19.102 This computed tomogram of the thorax shows a slightly spiculated nodular mass in the mid right lung field (arrows), which proved to be a primary pulmonary meningioma.

Heterotopic meningeal proliferations

Meningiomas are typically regarded as neoplasms of the main neural axis, but they are, perhaps, the most widely distributed of any tumor in that group. Tumefactive proliferations with meningothelial features have been reported in the skull and other bones, sinonasal tract, orbits, oropharynx, skin, middle ear, salivary glands, mediastinum, retroperitoneum, peripheral soft tissue, and lungs, in the absence of involvement of the coverings of the brain and spinal cord.[369] Patients with such lesions seem to be somewhat younger on average than those with intracranial meningiomas, most of whom are adults in middle age or older. Because these neoplasms are clearly not expected outside of their usual confines, their clinical presentation in heterotopic locations is typically undiagnosed at a clinical level.[370] For example, those in the lung are usually felt to represent granulomas or adenocarcinomas radiographically (Fig. 19.102). Ectopic meningiomas generally pursue a relatively favorable clinical course; although local recurrence is a possibility, these lesions are uncommonly associated with distant metastasis.[371]

At a gross level, meningioma of the lung is usually sharply marginated and easily dissected from the surrounding parenchyma (Fig. 19.103). It measures between 1 and 5 cm in diameter, and has a globoid configuration and a uniformly white-gray cut surface.

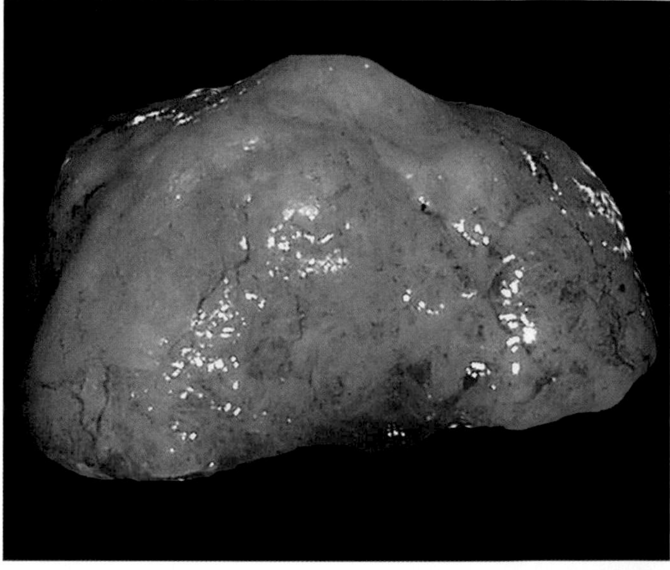

Fig. 19.103 This gross photograph of a primary intrapulmonary meningioma shows a globose mass that was "shelled out" by the surgeon from the surrounding parenchyma.

Those rare lesions that are malignant may show areas of necrosis and hemorrhage, as well as infiltration of the adjacent lung.[371,372]

Histologically, our experience with heterotopic meningiomas and that in reported cases has shown a preferential expression of meningothelial, fibroblastic, or "transitional" growth patterns in such tumors.[373–383]

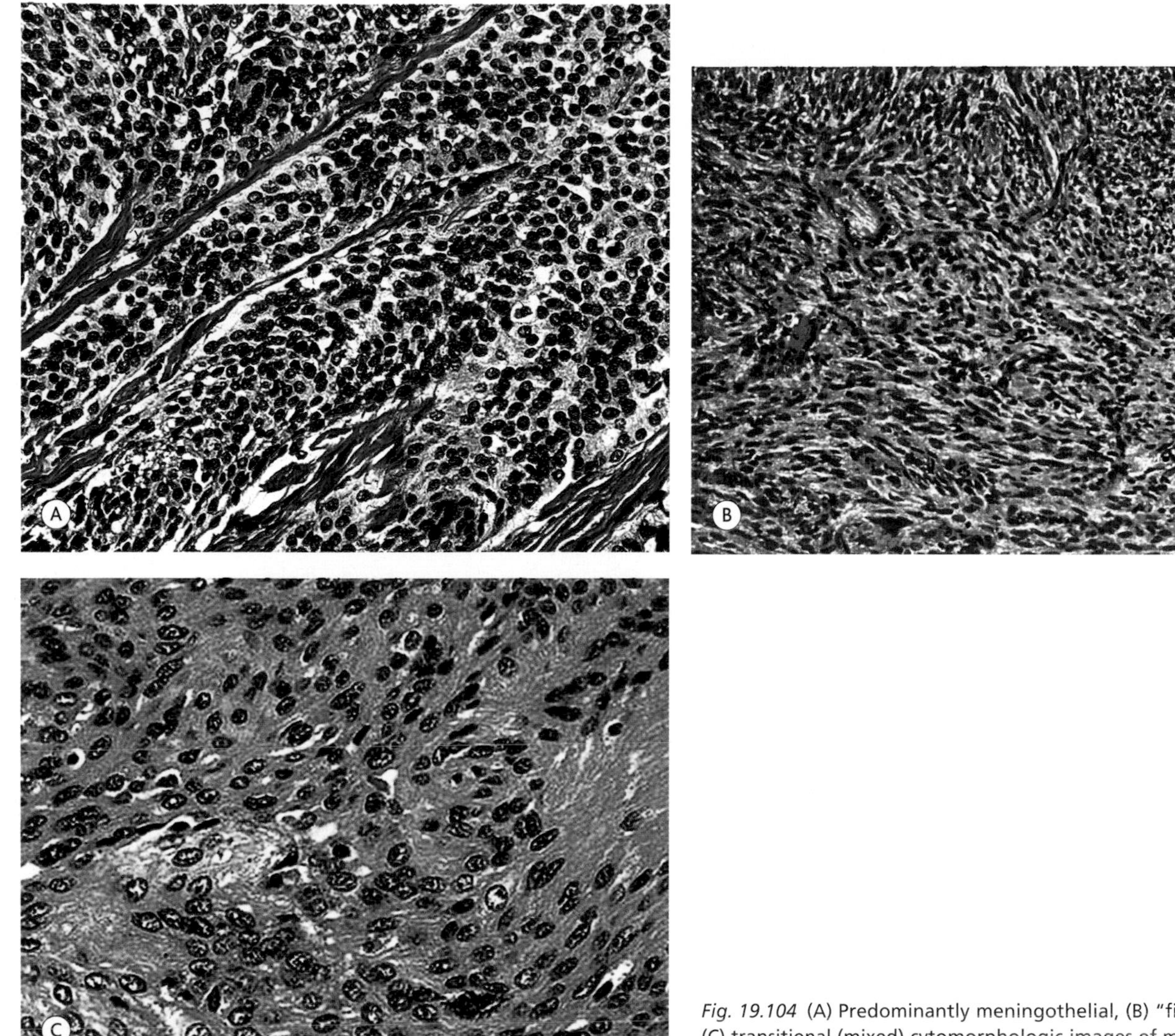

Fig. 19.104 (A) Predominantly meningothelial, (B) "fibrous", and (C) transitional (mixed) cytomorphologic images of meningioma are shown in this figure.

Although other microscopic variants such as papillary, chordoid, secretory, microcystic, anaplastic, lipomatous, rhabdoid, and "meshy" meningioma have been described in reference to lesions of the neuraxis, those forms appear to be absent in the lung. As such, meningiomas of the lung are composed of polygonal or fusiform cells with monomorphic oval nuclei and dispersed chromatin (Fig. 19.104). Whorled aggregates of tumor cells may be observed multifocally, with or without secondary psammomatous microcalcifications (Fig. 19.105). In some cases, the latter structures are numerous. Purely meningotheliomatous lesions – comprising a pure population of polygonal cells – may simulate the appearance of a carcinoma; at the other pole of the spectrum, "fibroblastic" or solely spindle cell meningiomas can imitate the configuration of solitary fibrous tumor, hemangiopericytoma, or other primary soft tissue neoplasms[369,372] (Fig. 19.106). Mitotic activity is limited, nuclear atypia is only modest, and necrosis is usually absent in benign pulmonary meningiomas, and the presence of those findings should raise concern over the rare possibility of malignancy.

The premise has been advanced by some authors that primary pulmonary meningioma may arise from so-called meningothelial-like micronodules (MLMs) in the lung[373,375] (formerly and erroneously called "minute pulmonary chemodectomas"), which are related to parenchymal damage from cardiac failure, chronic obstructive pulmonary disease, and thromboemboli[384] (Fig. 19.107). The conclusion that they are the precursors of meningioma has derived from the fact that both lesions have been seen together in the same case; however, no molecular analyses have been done to date to further address that possibility. In our opinion,

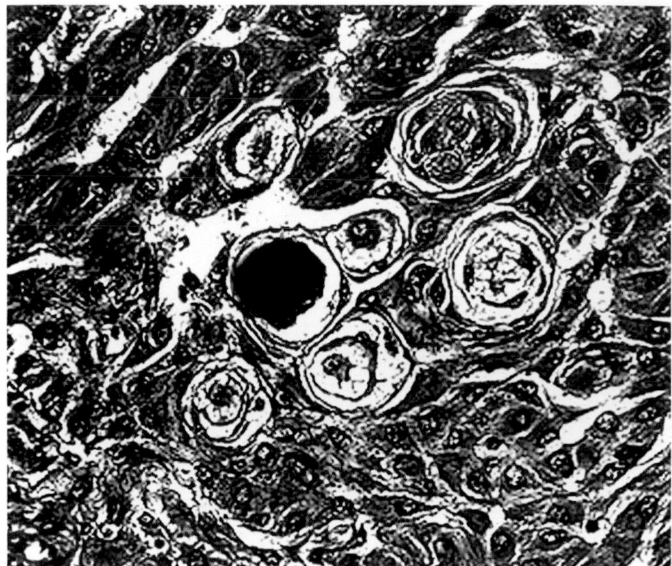

Fig. 19.105 Vaguely whorled microaggregates of tumor cells are often seen in meningioma, with focal psammomatous calcification, as shown here.

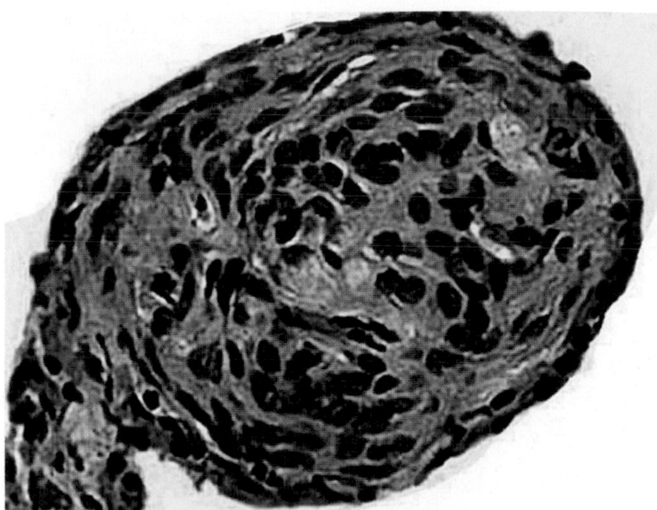

Fig. 19.107 Microscopic nodules of meningothelial-like cells, as shown in this figure, may be associated with heart failure or chronic non-neoplastic pulmonary diseases of various types. They have been proposed as possible precursors for intrapulmonary meningiomas.

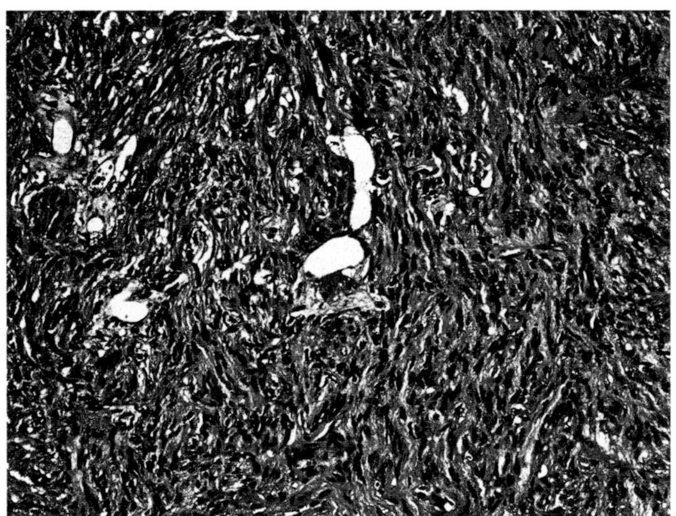

Fig. 19.106 Blunt spindle cells are arranged around a central vascular structure resembling a "staghorn" in meningioma, potentially simulating the appearance of hemangiopericytoma.

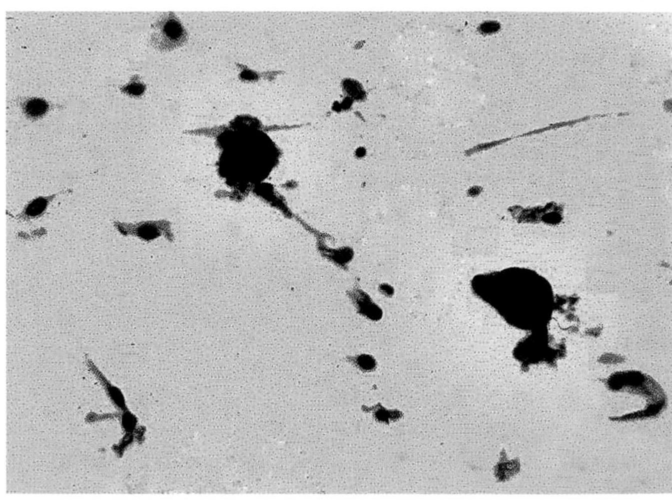

Fig. 19.108 This fine-needle aspiration biopsy specimen of a primary pulmonary meningioma shows microcalcifications and scant, dyshesive, nondescript tumor cells.

however, this is unlikely; recent studies have shown that MLMs are polyclonal and probably reactive in nature.[385]

Fine-needle aspiration biopsies of pulmonary meningioma have been obtained in a few cases.[373,377] These specimens have shown scanty material, represented by whorls of cells with a concentric internal configuration, as well as isolated individual cells (Fig. 19.108). Intranuclear inclusions may be apparent, and psammomatous calcifications can be observed as well in rare instances.

Electron microscopy is still an extremely useful tool for the resolution of differential diagnostic questions surrounding these tumors.[386] Meningioma has a singular ultrastructural appearance that features numerous interdigitating cell processes, which are attached by prominent desmosomes (Fig. 19.109). Skeins of well-formed tonofibrils insert into those attachment complexes. To our knowledge, this particular constellation of findings is not recapitulated by any other tumor type.

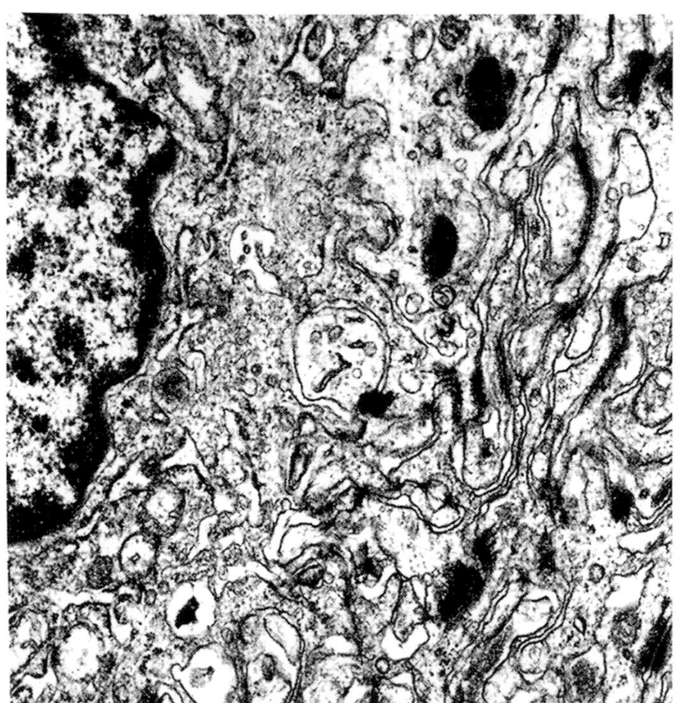

Fig. 19.109 Electron microscopy of meningiomas shows complexly interdigitating cytoplasmic processes, as well as prominent desmosomes and cytoplasmic tonofibrils.

Prototypically, meningiomas are reactive for vimentin to the exclusion of other intermediate filament proteins; EMA is also present universally, as is immunoreactivity for desmoplakin, a desmosomal constituent.[369,372–374,386] Immunophenotypic characteristics of ectopic meningiomas differ from those of their neuraxis analogues, in that the former lesions appear to more often express keratin. Admittedly, that attribute is probably influenced by sites of origin. Additional markers that are germane to differential diagnosis, such as CD34 and S100 protein, have also been reported sporadically in heterotopic meningiomas in some sites.

Other pertinent diagnostic considerations for primary pulmonary meningiomas include carcinomas with or without spindle cell features; solitary fibrous tumors; hemangiopericytomas; schwannomas; and amelanotic malignant melanomas.[372] To reiterate, electron microscopy is still very effective in resolving such uncertainties, because of the distinctive profile of meningioma. Immunohistochemical analyses require the application of antibodies to Ber-EP4, MOC-31, carcinoembryonic antigen, CD56, CD57, CD99, melan-A/Mart-1, and tyrosinase. Another useful modality of investigation is that of FISH, which demonstrates monosomy of chromosome 22 in a majority of meningiomas,[387] a cytogenetic abnormality that is not shared by other differential diagnostic possibilities. None of these studies is effective in separating primary ectopic from *metastatic* neuraxis-based meningiomas.[382,388] However, it is an exceedingly rare situation for the latter neoplasms to present in distant sites with no prior knowledge of a primary tumor within the cranial vault or spine.[388]

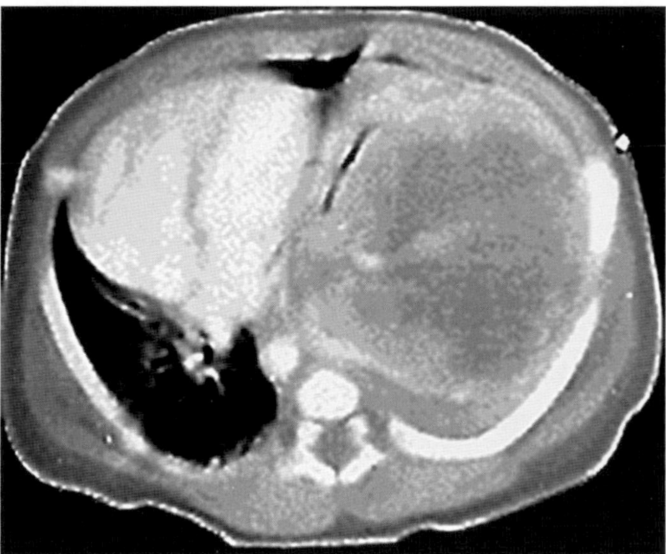

Fig. 19.110 This computed tomogram of the chest in a young adult man shows a solid mass that occupies virtually the entire left hemithorax. It proved to be an immature teratoma, apparently arising in the lung.

Intrapulmonary teratomas

Examples of primary intrapulmonary teratoma have been reported only with extraordinary rarity[389–392] (Fig. 19.110). Indeed, the overwhelming majority of teratoid tumors in the lungs and pleura represent altered metastases of gonadal germ cell tumors, in which malignant histologic components were formerly present but have been extirpated by chemotherapy. Another small group of cases comprises primary teratoid tumors of the lung which contain seminoma, embryonal carcinoma, yolk sac carcinoma, or choriocarcinoma.[394–396] Primary pulmonary teratomas that *lack* such cytologically malignant components are so uncommon as to be anecdotal. However, they have principally been seen as variably cystic masses in young adults, and at least one such lesion was associated with pyothorax.[389]

Grossly, the most obvious constituents of such neoplasms are squamous epithelium with associated keratinous debris, and cartilage (Fig. 19.111). Mucoid contents may sometimes be seen in cystic areas and nondescript solid foci may also be present.

Microscopically, teratomas of the lung can be divided into mature and immature varieties, as true elsewhere in the body. The first of those subtypes is self-explanatory (Fig. 19.112), but the term "immature" refers specifically in this context to the presence of primitive neurectodermal tissue that resembles the developing neural tube (Fig. 19.113). Otherwise, virtually any tissue in the body can be reflected in the constituents of teratoid lesions, including such unexpected elements as retina (Fig. 19.114). In order to qualify as teratomatous, the tumor must demonstrate the presence of derivatives from at least two of the three germinal lines (ectoderm, endoderm, and mesoderm).

Special pathologic studies are generally unnecessary diagnostically in reference to teratoid neoplasms. However, immunostains may sometimes be undertaken to search for possible production of such oncofetal proteins as alpha-fetoprotein by endodermally derived elements, including intestinal and hepatic tissue.

Too few cases of mature or immature primary intrapulmonary teratoma have been studied to determine

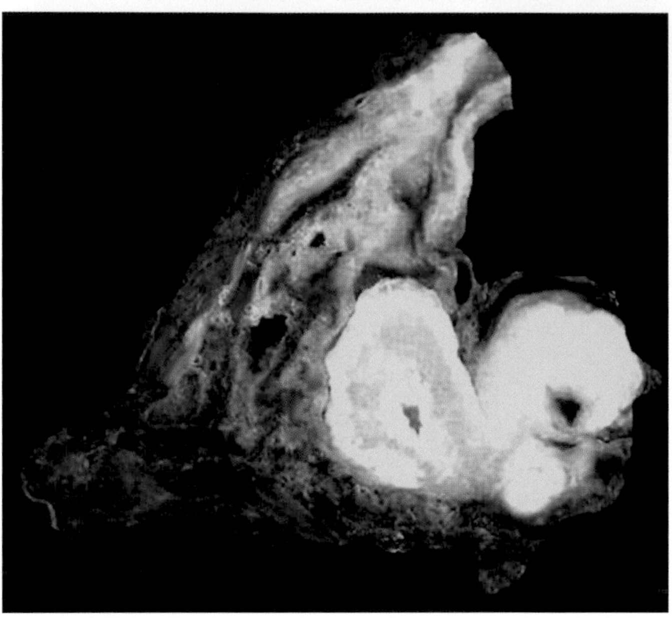

Fig. 19.111 This gross photograph of an intrapulmonary teratoma shows a largely-solid white-gray mass in the parenchyma with some central cystification.

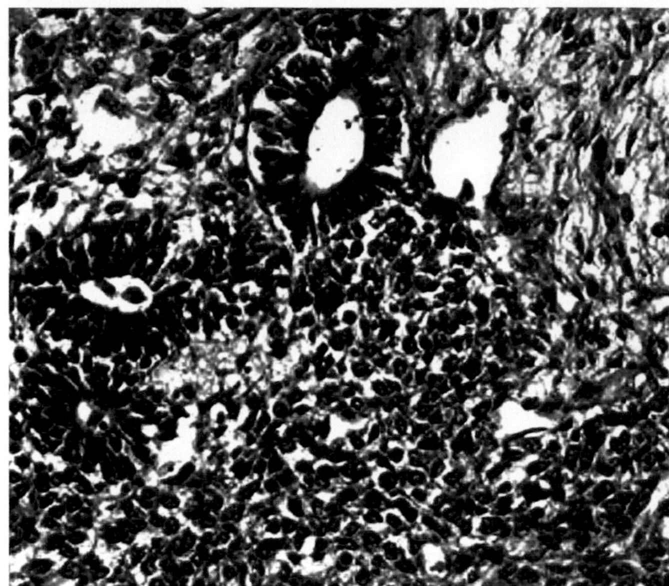

Fig. 19.113 Immature teratoma, as shown in this figure, contains foci of primitive neuroepithelial differentiation, simulating the developing neural tube.

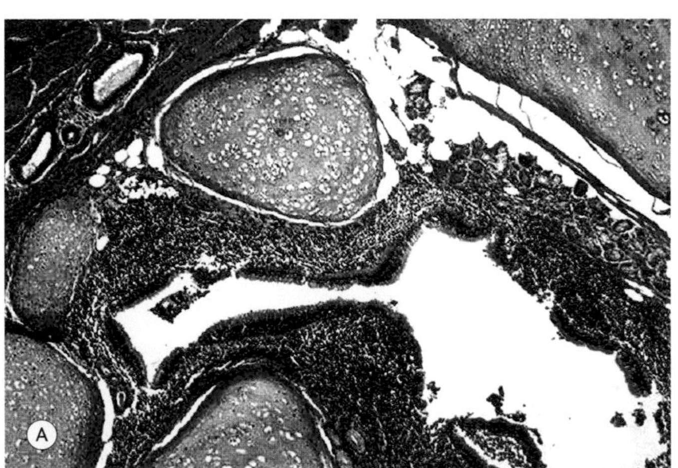

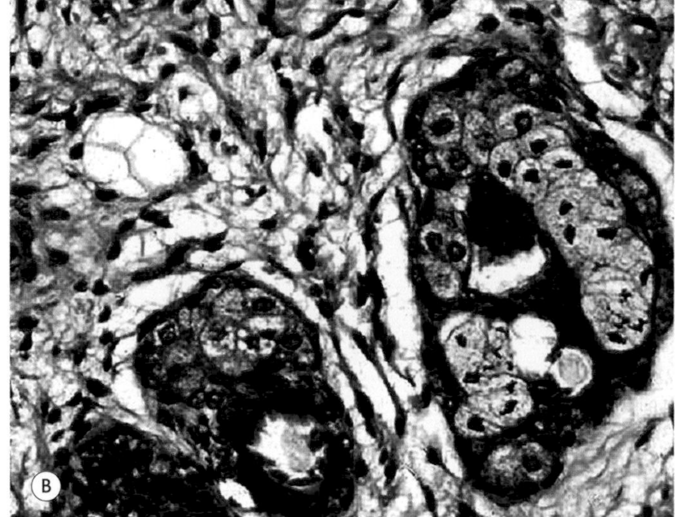

Fig. 19.112 (A) Mature teratoma contains fully-developed tissues from at least two of the three germ cell lines, potentially including cartilage and respiratory epithelium or (B) cutaneous tissue complete with appendages.

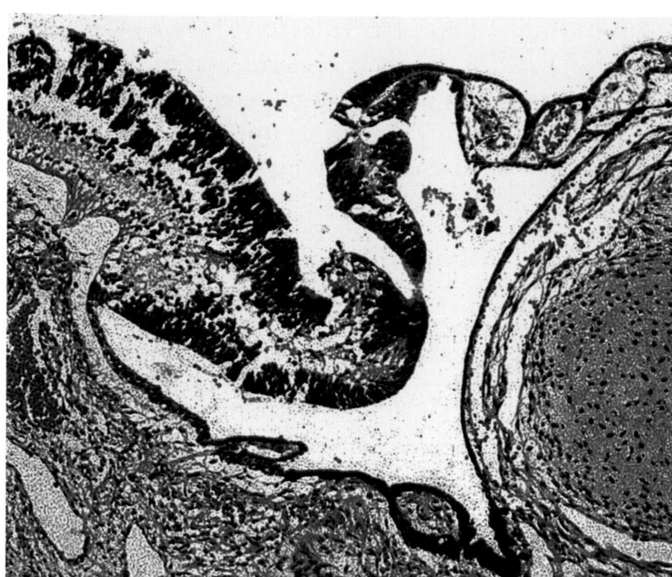

Fig. 19.114 Retinal pigment epithelium is apparent in this teratoma.

their biologic potential with certainty. However, by extrapolation from other anatomic locations, immature teratomas are known to have a potential for recurrence or metastasis. Thus, as a group, we have tentatively classified these lesions as borderline neoplasms.

Other lesions

Well-differentiated papillary mesothelioma (WDPM) of the pleura, and intrapulmonary paraganglioma represent other borderline lesions that are properly mentioned here. Because of its specialized nature and possible relationship to malignant mesotheliomas, WDPM will be discussed in Chapter 20 of this book. In like manner, intrapulmonary paraganglionic tumors have been included in Chapter 13, dealing with neuroendocrine neoplasms. Because its biologic characteristics are more aggressive than those of most other "borderline lesions," we have elected to include epithelioid hemangio-endothelioma in Chapter 14, on malignant mesenchymal tumors of the lung and pleura.

REFERENCES

1. Wingo PA, Cardinez CJ, Landis SH, et al.: Long-term trends in cancer mortality in the United States, 1930–1998. Cancer 2003; 97(12 suppl): 3133–3275.
2. Lutz JM, Francisci S, Mugno E, et al.: Cancer prevalence in Central Europe: the EUROPREVAL study. Ann Oncol 2003; 14: 313–322.
3. Oei TK, Wouters EF, Visser R, VanEngelshoven JM, Greve LH: The value of conventional radiography and computed tomography (CT) in diagnosis of pulmonary hamartoma. Rontgenblatter 1983; 36: 324–327.
4. Erasmus JJ, Connolly JE, McAdams HP, Roggli VL: Solitary pulmonary nodules: Part I. Morphologic evaluation for differentiation of benign and malignant lesions. Radiographics 2000; 20: 43–58.
5. Petticrew MP, Sowden AJ, Lister-Sharp D, Wright K: False-negative results in screening programs: systematic review of impact and implications. Health Technol Assess 2000; 4: 1–120.
6. Cardillo G, Regal M, Sera F, et al.: Videothoracoscopic management of the solitary pulmonary nodule: a single-institution study on 429 cases. Ann Thorac Surg 2003; 75: 1607–1611.
7. Barzo P, Molnar L, Minik K: Bronchial papilloma of various origins. Chest 1987; 92: 132–136.
8. Spencer H, Dail DH, Arneaud J: Noninvasive bronchial epithelial papillary tumors. Cancer 1980; 45: 1486–1497.
9. Zimmerman A, Lang HR, Muhlberger F, Bachman M: Papilloma of the bronchus. Respiration 1980; 39: 286–290.
10. Maxwell RJ, Gibbons JR, O'Hara MD: Solitary squamous papilloma of the bronchus. Thorax 1985; 40: 68–71.
11. Laubscher FA: Solitary squamous cell papilloma of bronchial origin. Am J Clin Pathol 1969; 52: 599–603.
12. Greene JG, Tassin L, Saberi A: Endobronchial epithelial papilloma associated with a foreign body. Chest 1990; 97: 229–230.
13. Miura H, Tsuchida T, Kawate N, et al.: Asymptomatic solitary papilloma of the bronchus: review of occurrence in Japan. Eur Respir J 1993; 6: 1070–1073.
14. Basheda S, Gephardt GN, Stoller JK: Columnar papilloma of the bronchus: case report and literature review. Am Rev Resp Dis 1991; 144: 1400–1402.
15. Trillo A, Guha A: Solitary condylomatous papilloma of the bronchus. Arch Pathol Lab Med 1988; 112: 731–733.
16. Desai AV, Scolyer RA, McCaughan B, Torzillo PJ: Middle lobe syndrome due to obstructing solitary bronchial papilloma. Aust N Z J Med 1999; 29: 745–747.
17. Hurt R: Benign tumors of the bronchus and trachea, 1951–1981. Ann Roy Coll Surg Engl 1984; 66: 22–26.
18. Roviaro GC, Varoli F, Pagnini CA: Is the solitary papilloma of the bronchus always a benign tumor? J Otorhinolaryngol Relat Spec 1981; 43: 301–308.
19. Katial RK, Ranlett R, Whitlock WL: Human papillomavirus associated with solitary squamous papilloma complicated by bronchiectasis and bronchial stenosis. Chest 1994; 106: 1887–1889.
20. Roglic M, Jukic S, Damjanov I: Cytology of the solitary papilloma of the bronchus. Acta Cytol 1975; 19: 11–13.
21. Flieder DB, Koss MN, Nicholson A, et al.: Solitary pulmonary papillomas in adults: a clinicopathologic and in-situ hybridization study of 14 cases combined with 27 cases in the literature. Am J Surg Pathol 1998; 22: 1328–1342.
22. Popper HH, El-Shabrawi Y, Wockel W, et al.: Prognostic importance of human papillomavirus typing in squamous cell papilloma of the bronchus: comparison of in-situ hybridization and the polymerase chain reaction. Hum Pathol 1994; 25: 1191–1197.
23. Popper HH, Wirnsberger G, Juttner-Smolle FM, Pongratz MG, Sommersgutter M: The predictive value of human papillomavirus (HPV) typing in the prognosis of bronchial squamous cell papillomas. Histopathology 1992; 21: 323–330.
24. Clavel CE, Nawrocki B, Bosseaux B, et al.: Detection of human papillomavirus DNA in bronchopulmonary carcinomas by hybrid capture. II. A study of 185 tumors. Cancer 2000; 88: 1347–1352.
25. Smith E, Pignatari S, Gray S, Haugen T, Turak L: Human papillomavirus infection in papillomas and nondiseased respiratory sites of patients with recurrent respiratory papillomatosis, using the polymerase chain reaction. Arch Otolaryngol Head Neck Surg 1993; 119: 554–557.
26. Rady PL, Schnadig VJ, Weiss RL, Hughes TK, Tyring SK: Malignant transformation of recurrent respiratory papillomatosis associated with integrated human papillomavirus type 11 DNA and mutation of p53. Laryngoscope 1998; 108: 735–740.
27. Syrjanen RJ: Epithelial lesions suggestive of a condylomatous origin found closely associated with invasive bronchial squamous cell carcinomas. Respiration 1980; 40: 150–160.
28. DiMarco AF, Montenegro H, Payne CB Jr, Kwon KH: Papillomas of the tracheobronchial tree with malignant degeneration. Chest 1978; 74: 464–465.
29. Bejui-Thivolet F, Chardonnet Y, Patricot LM: Human papillomavirus type 11 DNA in papillary squamous cell lung carcinoma. Virchows Arch A 1990; 417: 457–461.
30. Inoue Y, Oka M, Ishii H, et al.: A solitary bronchial papilloma with malignant changes. Intern Med 2001; 40: 56–60.

31. Kramer S, Wehunt W, Stocker J, Kashima H: Pulmonary manifestations of juvenile laryngotracheal papillomatosis. Am J Roentgenol 1985; 144: 687–694.
32. Fechner RE, Fitz-Hugh G: Invasive tracheal papillomatosis. Am J Surg Pathol 1980; 4: 79–86.
33. Peterson BL, Buchwald C, Gerstoft J, Bretlau P, Lindeberg H: An aggressive and invasive growth of juvenile papillomas involving the total respiratory tract. J Laryngol Otol 1998; 112: 1101–1104.
34. Franzmann MB, Buchwald C, Larsen P, Balle V: Tracheobronchial involvement of laryngeal papillomatosis at onset. J Laryngol Otol 1994; 108: 164–165.
35. Shykhon M, Kuo M, Pearman R: Recurrent respiratory papillomatosis. Clin Otolaryngol 2002; 27: 237–243.
36. Blackledge RA, Anandi VK: Tracheobronchial extension of recurrent respiratory papillomatosis. Ann Otol Rhinol Laryngol 2000; 109: 812–818.
37. Harada H, Miura K, Tsutsui Y, et al.: Solitary squamous cell papilloma of the lung in a 40 year old woman with recurrent laryngeal papillomatosis. Pathol Int 2000; 50: 431–439.
38. Weingarten J: Cytologic and histologic findings in a case of tracheobronchial papillomatosis. Acta Cytol 1981; 25: 167–170.
39. Kashima H, Mounts P, Leventhal B, Hruban RH: Sites of predilection in recurrent respiratory papillomatosis. Ann Otol Rhinol Laryngol 1993; 102: 580–583.
40. Al-Saleem T, Peale AR, Norris CM: Multiple papillomatosis of the lower respiratory tract: clinical and pathologic study of eleven cases. Cancer 1968; 22: 1173–1184.
41. Rahman A, Ziment I: Tracheobronchial papillomatosis with malignant transformation. Arch Intern Med 1983; 143: 577–578.
42. Batsakis JG, Raymond AK, Rice DH: The pathology of head and neck tumors: papillomas of the upper aerodigestive tracts, Part 18. Head Neck Surg 1983; 5: 332–344.
43. Zarod A, Rutherford J, Corbitt G: Malignant progression of laryngeal papilloma associated with human papillomavirus type 6 (HPV-6). J Clin Pathol 1988; 41: 280–283.
44. Byrne J, Tsao MS, Fraser R, Howley P: Human papillomavirus-11 DNA in a patient with chronic laryngotracheobronchial papillomatosis and metastatic squamous cell carcinoma of the lung. N Engl J Med 1987; 317: 873–878.
45. Wilde E, Duggan M, Field S: Bronchogenic squamous cell carcinoma complicating localized recurrent respiratory papillomatosis. Chest 1994; 105: 1887–1888.
46. Yousem SA, Ohori NP, Sonmez-Alpan E: Occurrence of human papillomavirus DNA in primary lung neoplasms. Cancer 1992; 69: 693–697.
47. Liebow AA: Tumors of the lower respiratory tract. In: Atlas of tumor pathology, Series 1, Fascicle 17. 1952, Armed Forces Institute of Pathology, Washington, DC, p 22.
48. England DM, Hochholzer L: Truly benign "bronchial adenoma:" report of 10 cases of mucous gland adenoma with immunohistochemical and ultrastructural findings. Am J Surg Pathol 1995; 19: 887–899.
49. Markel SF, Abell MR, Haight C, French AJ: Neoplasms of the bronchus commonly designated as adenomas. Cancer 1964; 17: 590–608.
50. Payne WS, Fontana RS, Woolner LB: Bronchial tumors originating from mucous glands: current classification and unusual manifestations. Med Clin North Am Dis Respir 1964; 48: 945–960.
51. Spencer H: Bronchial mucous gland tumors. Virchows Arch Pathol Anat 1979; 383: 101–115.
52. Allen MS Jr, Marsh WL Jr, Greissinger WT: Mucous gland adenoma of the bronchus. J Thorac Cardiovasc Surg 1974; 67: 966–968.
53. Emory WB, Mitchel WT Jr, Hatch HG Jr: Mucous gland adenoma of the bronchus. Am Rev Respir Dis 1973; 108: 1407–1410.
54. Edwards CW, Matthews HR: Mucous gland adenoma of the bronchus. Thorax 1981; 36: 147–148.
55. Kroe DJ, Pitcock JA: Benign mucous gland adenoma of the bronchus. Arch Pathol 1967; 84: 539–540.
56. Heard BE, Corrin B, Dewar A: Pathology of seven mucous cell adenomas of the bronchial glands with particular reference to ultrastructure. Histopathology 1985; 9: 687–701.
57. Akhtar M, Young I, Reyes F: Bronchial adenoma with polymorphous features. Cancer 1974; 33: 1572–1576.
58. Rosenblum P, Klein RI: Adenomatous polyp of the right main bronchus producing atelectasis. Pediatrics 1936; 78: 791–796.
59. Smith AG: Benign epithelial tumors of the bronchus. South Med J 1965; 58: 1535–1541.
60. Courtin P, Janin A, Sault MC, et al.: Pure bronchial adenoma. Anatomic, clinical, and ultrastructural study of a case. Ann Pathol 1987; 7: 315–319.
61. Weinberger MA, Katz S, Davis EW: Peripheral bronchial adenoma of mucous gland type: clinical and pathological aspects. J Thorac Surg 1955; 29: 626–635.
62. Key BM, Pritchett PS: Mucous gland adenoma of the bronchus. South Med J 1979; 72: 83–85.
63. Arrigoni MG, Woolner LB, Bernatz PE, Miller WE, Fontana RS: Benign tumors of the lung: a ten-year experience. J Thorac Cardiovasc Surg 1970; 60: 589–599.
64. Moran CA, Suster S, Askin FB, Koss MN: Benign and malignant salivary gland-type mixed tumors of the lung: clinicopathologic and immunohistochemical study of eight cases. Cancer 1994; 73: 2481–2490.
65. Bartley TD, Arean VM: Intrapulmonary neurogenic tumors. J Thorac Cardiovasc Surg 1965; 50: 114–123.
66. Roviaro G, Montorsi M, Varoli F, Binda R, Cecchetto A: Primary pulmonary tumors of neurogenic origin. Thorax 1983; 38: 942–945.
67. Silverman JF, Leffers BR, Kay S: Primary pulmonary neurilemmoma: report of a case with ultrastructural examination. Arch Pathol Lab Med 1976; 100: 644–648.
68. Yamakawa H: Intrapulmonary schwannoma: a case report. J Jpn Assoc Chest Surg 1993; 7: 165–169.
69. Sugita M, Fujimura S, Hasumi T, Kondo T, Sagawa M: Sleeve superior segmentectomy of the right lower lobe for endobronchial neurinoma: report of a case. Respiration 1996; 63: 191–194.
70. McCluggage WG, Bharucha H: Primary pulmonary tumors of nerve sheath origin. Histopathology 1995; 26: 247–254.
71. Lin YC, Lin MC, Chen TC, Huang CC, Lee CH: Tracheal neurilemmoma mimicking bronchial asthma – a dilemma of difficult diagnosis: case report. Chang Yi Xue Za Zhi 1999; 22: 525–529.
72. Tsukada H, Hsada H, Kojima K, Yamata N: Bronchial wall schwannoma removed by sleeve resection of the right mainstem bronchus without lung resection. J Cardiovasc Surg 1998; 39: 511–513.
73. Ashkan K, Casey AT: Pulmonary apex schwannoma. J Neurol Neurosurg Psych 1997; 63: 719.
74. Bosch X, Ramirez J, Font J, et al.: Primary intrapulmonary benign schwannoma: a case with ultrastructural and immunohistochemical confirmation. Eur Respir J 1990; 3: 234–237.
75. Muhrer KH, Fischer HP: Primary pulmonary neurilemmoma. Thorac Cardiovasc Surg 1983; 31: 313–316.
76. Imaizumi M, Takahashi T, Niimi T, et al.: A case of primary intrapulmonary neurilemmoma and review of the literature. Jpn J Surg 1989; 19: 740–746.
77. Feldhaus RJ, Anene C, Bogard P: A rare endobronchial neurilemmoma (schwannoma). Chest 1989; 95: 461–462.
78. Nesbitt JC, Vega DM, Burke T, Mackay B: Cellular schwannoma of the bronchus. Ultrastruct Pathol 1996; 20: 349–354.
79. Unger PD, Geller SA, Anderson PJ: Pulmonary lesions in a patient with neurofibromatosis. Arch Pathol Lab Med 1984; 108: 654–657.
80. Bacha EA, Wright CD, Grillo HC, et al.: Surgical treatment of primary pulmonary sarcomas. Eur J Cardiothorac Surg 1999; 15: 456–460.
81. Moran CA, Suster S, Koss MN: Primary malignant "triton" tumor of the lung. Histopathology 1997; 30: 140–144.
82. Attanoos RL, Appleton MA, Gibbs AR: Primary sarcomas of the lung: a clinicopathological and immunohistochemical study of 14 cases. Histopathology 1996; 29: 29–36.
83. Simansky DA, Aviel-Ronen S, Reder I, et al.: Psammomatous melanotic schwannoma: presentation of a rare primary lung tumor. Ann Thorac Surg 2000; 70: 671–672.
84. Abrikossoff A: Uber Myome ausgehend von der quergestreiften willkurlichen Muskulatur. Virchows Arch Pathol Anat Physiol Klin Med 1926; 260: 215–233.
85. Lack EE, Worsham GF, Callihan MD, et al.: Granular cell tumor: a clinicopathologic study of 110 patients. J Surg Oncol 1980; 13: 301–316.
86. Alvarez-Fernandez E, Carretero-Albinana L: Bronchial granular cell tumor: presentation of three cases with tissue culture and ultrastructural study. Arch Pathol Lab Med 1987; 111: 1065–1069.
87. DeClerq D, Van der Straten M, Roels H: Granular cell myoblastoma of the bronchus. Eur J Respir Dis 1983; 64: 72–76.
88. Hurwitz SS, Conlan AA, Gritzman MC, Krut LH: Granular cell myoblastoma. Thorax 1982; 37: 392–393.

89. Hosaka T, Suzuki S, Niikawa H, et al.: A rare case of a pulmonary granular cell tumor presenting as a coin lesion. Jpn J Thorac Cardiovasc Surg 2003; 51: 107–109.
90. Abdulhamid I, Rabah R: Granular cell tumor of the bronchus. Pediatr Pulmonol 2000; 30: 425–428.
91. Husain M, Nguyen GK: Cytopathology of granular cell tumor of the lung. Diagn Cytopathol 2000; 23: 294–295.
92. Al-Ghamdi AM, Flint JD, Muller NL, Stewart KC: Hilar pulmonary granular cell tumor: a case report and review of the literature. Ann Diagn Pathol 2002; 4: 245–251.
93. Scala R, Naldi M, Fabianelli F, et al.: Endobronchial granular cell tumor. Monaldi Arch Chest Dis 1999; 54: 404–406.
94. Thomas de Montpreville V, Dulmet EM: Granular cell tumors of the lower respiratory tract. Histopathology 1995; 27: 257–262.
95. Deavers M, Guinee D, Koss MN, Travis WD: Granular cell tumors of the lung: clinicopathologic study of 20 cases. Am J Surg Pathol 1995; 19: 627–635.
96. Hernandez OG, Haponik EF, Summer WR: Granular cell tumor of the bronchus: bronchoscopic and clinical features. Thorax 1986; 41: 927–931.
97. Mullen CV Jr, Hewan-Lowe K, Gilman MJ: Massive hemoptysis associated with granular cell tumor of the bronchus. South Med J 1983; 76: 1452.
98. Lack EE, Harris GB, Eraklis AJ, Vawter GF: Primary bronchial tumors in childhood: a clinicopathologic study of six cases. Cancer 1983; 51: 492–497.
99. Guillou L, Gloor E, Anani PA, Kaelin R: Bronchial granular cell tumor: report of a case with preoperative cytologic diagnosis on bronchial brushings and immunohistochemical studies. Acta Cytol 1991; 35: 375–380.
100. Majmudar B, Thomas J, Gorelkin L, Symbas PN: Respiratory obstruction caused by a multicentric granular cell tumor of the laryngotracheobronchial tree. Hum Pathol 1981; 12: 283–286.
101. Oparah SS, Subramanian VA: Granular cell myoblastoma of the bronchus: report of 2 cases and review of the literature. Ann Thorac Surg 1976; 22: 199–202.
102. Robinson JM, Knoll R, Henry DA: Intrathoracic giant cell myoblastoma. South Med J 1988; 81: 1453–1457.
103. Schulster PL, Khan FA, Azueta V: Asymptomatic pulmonary granular cell tumor presenting as a coin lesion. Chest 1975; 68: 256–258.
104. Chen KTK: Cytology of bronchial benign granular cell tumor. Acta Cytol 1991; 35: 381–384.
105. Muhammed AA, Sikka P, Dhillon RS, Gibbons WJ, Ahmed A: Coexisting granular cell tumor and adenocarcinoma of the lung: a case report and review of the literature. Respir Care 2001; 46: 702–704.
106. Cutlan RT, Eltorky M: Pulmonary granular cell tumor coexisting with bronchogenic carcinoma. Ann Diagn Pathol 2001; 5: 74–79.
107. Althausen AM, Kowalski DP, Ludwig ME, Curry SL, Greene JF: Granular cell tumors: a new clinically important histologic finding. Gynecol Oncol 2000; 77: 310–313.
108. Sobel HJ, Marquet E, Avrin E, Schwarz R: Granular cell myoblastoma: an electron microscopic and cytochemical study illustrating the genesis of granules and aging of myoblastoma cells. Am J Pathol 1971; 65: 59–78.
109. Miettinen M, Lehtonen E, Lehtola H, et al.: Histogenesis of granular cell tumor: an immunohistochemical and ultrastructural study. J Pathol 1984; 142: 221–229.
110. Mazur M, Shultz JJ, Myers JL: Granular cell tumor: immunohistochemical analysis of 21 benign tumors and one malignant tumor. Arch Pathol Lab Med 1990; 114: 692–696.
111. Liu Z, Mira JL, Vu H: Diagnosis of malignant granular cell tumor by fine needle aspiration cytology. Acta Cytol 2001; 45: 1011–1021.
112. Ordonez NG, Mackay B: Granular cell tumor: a review of the pathology and histogenesis. Ultrastruct Pathol 1999; 23: 207–222.
113. Fine SW, Li M: Expression of calretinin and the alpha-subunit of inhibin in granular cell tumors. Am J Clin Pathol 2003; 119: 259–264.
114. Nappi O, Ferrara G, Wick MR: Neoplasms composed of eosinophilic polygonal cells: an overview with consideration of different cytomorphologic patterns. Semin Diagn Pathol 1999; 16: 82–90.
115. Franzblau MJ, Manwaring M, Plumhof C, Listrom JB, Burgdorf WHC: Metastatic breast carcinoma mimicking granular cell tumor. J Cutan Pathol 1989; 16: 218–221.
116. Reuter VE: Renal tumors exhibiting granular cytoplasm. Semin Diagn Pathol 1999; 16: 135–145.
117. Ogino S, Al-Kaisi N, Abdul-Karim FW: Cytopathology of oncocytic carcinoid tumor of the lung mimicking granular cell tumor: a case report. Acta Cytol 2000; 44: 247–250.
118. Ritter JH, Nappi O: Oxyphilic proliferations of the respiratory tract and paranasal sinuses. Semin Diagn Pathol 1999; 16: 105–116.
119. Tomashefski JF: Benign endobronchial mesenchymal tumors: their relationship to parenchymal pulmonary hamartomas. Am J Surg Pathol 1982; 6: 531–540.
120. Yellin A, Roserman Y, Lieberman Y: Review of smooth muscle tumors of the lower respiratory tract. Br J Dis Chest 1984; 78: 337–351.
121. White SH, Ibrahim NBN, Forrester-Wood CP, Jeyasingham R: Leiomyomas of the lower respiratory tract. Thorax 1985; 40: 306–311.
122. Orlowski TM, Stasiak K, Kolodziej J: Leiomyoma of the lung. J Thorac Cardiovasc Surg 1978; 76: 257–261.
123. Van den Bosch JM, Wagenaar SS, Corrin B, et al.: Mesenchymoma of the lung (so-called hamartoma): a review of 154 parenchymal and endobronchial cases. Thorax 1987; 42: 790–793.
124. Gal AA, Brooks JJ, Pietra GG: Leiomyomatous lung neoplasms: a clinical, histologic, and immunohistochemical study. Mod Pathol 1989; 2: 209–216.
125. Horstman JP, Pietra GG, Harman JA, et al.: Spontaneous regression of pulmonary leiomyomas during pregnancy. Cancer 1977; 39: 314–321.
126. Cramer SF, Meyer JC, Kraner JF, et al.: Metastasizing leiomyoma of the uterus: S-phase fraction, estrogen receptor, and ultrastructure. Cancer 1980; 45: 932–937.
127. Wolff M, Kaye G, Silva F: Pulmonary metastases (with admixed epithelial elements) from smooth muscle neoplasms: report of nine cases, including three males. Am J Surg Pathol 1979; 3: 325–342.
128. Sentinelli S, Covello R, Venevolo M, Licci S, Perrone-Donnorso R: Benign metastasizing pulmonary leiomyoma: description of a case and review of the literature. Pathologica 2002; 94: 253–256.
129. Abramson S, Gilkeson RC, Goldstein JD, et al.: Benign metastasizing leiomyoma: clinical, imaging, and pathologic correlation. Am J Roentgenol 2001; 176: 1409–1413.
130. Kayser K, Zink S, Schneider T, et al.: Benign metastasizing leiomyoma of the uterus: documentation of clinical, immunohistochemical, and lectin-histochemical data of ten cases. Virchows Arch A 2000; 437: 284–292.
131. Tietze L, Gunther K, Horbe A, et al.: Benign metastasizing leiomyoma: a cytogenetically balanced but clonal disease. Hum Pathol 2000; 31: 126–128.
132. Esteban JM, Allen WM, Schaerf RH: Benign metastasizing leiomyoma of the uterus: histologic and immunohistochemical characterization of primary and metastatic lesions. Arch Pathol Lab Med 1999; 123: 960–962.
133. Jautzke G, Muller-Ruchholtz E, Thalmann U: Immunohistological detection of estrogen and progesterone receptors in multiple and well-differentiated leiomyomatous lung tumors in women with uterine leiomyomas (so-called benign metastasizing leiomyomas): a report on 5 cases. Pathol Res Pract 1996; 192: 215–223.
134. Lipton JH, Fong TC, Burgess KR: Miliary pattern as presentation of leiomyomatosis of the lung. Chest 1987; 91: 781–782.
135. Sabatini R, Ferreri R, Distante G, Loizzi V, Loizzi P: Benign metastasizing leiomyoma in the lung: a case report. Eur J Gynecol Oncol 2002; 23: 445–446.
136. Silverman JF, Kay S: Multiple pulmonary leiomyomatous hamartomas: report of case with ultrastructural examination. Cancer 1976; 38: 1199–1204.
137. Hull MT, Gonzalez-Crussi F, Grosfeld JL: Multiple pulmonary fibroleiomyomatous hamartomata in childhood. J Pediatr Surg 1979; 14: 428–431.
138. Itoh H, Yanagi M, Setoyama T, et al.: Solitary fibroleiomyomatous hamartoma of the lung in a patient without a preexisting smooth muscle tumor. Pathol Int 2001; 51: 661–665.
139. Shmookler BM, Lauer DH: Retroperitoneal leiomyosarcoma: a clinicopathologic analysis of 36 cases. Am J Surg Pathol 1983; 7: 269–280.
140. Mackay B, Legha SS: Coin lesion of the lung in a 19 year old male. Ultrastruct Pathol 1981; 2: 289–294.
141. Alt B, Huffer WE, Belchis DA: A vascular lesion with smooth muscle differentiation presenting as a coin lesion in the lung: glomus tumor versus hemangiopericytoma. Am J Clin Pathol 1983; 80: 765–771.
142. Fabich DR, Hafez GR: Glomangioma of the trachea. Cancer 1980; 45: 2337–2341.

143. Tang C, Toker CK, Foris NP, Trump BF: Glomangioma of the lung. Am J Surg Pathol 1978; 2: 103–109.
144. Gaertner EM, Steinberg DM, Huber M, et al.: Pulmonary and mediastinal glomus tumors: report of five cases including a pulmonary glomangiosarcoma. A clinicopathologic study with literature review. Am J Surg Pathol 2000; 24: 1105–1114.
145. Yilmaz A, Bayramgurler B, Aksoy F, et al.: Pulmonary glomus tumor: a case initially diagnosed as carcinoid tumor. Respirology 2002; 7: 369–371.
146. Shugart RR, Soule EH, Johnson EW: Glomus tumors. Surg Gynecol Obstet 1963; 117: 334–340.
147. Miettinen M, Paal E, Lasota J, Sobin LH: Gastrointestinal glomus tumors: a clinicopathologic, immunohistochemical, and molecular genetic study of 32 cases. Am J Surg Pathol 2002; 26: 301–311.
148. Littlefield JB, Drash EC: Myxoma of the lung. J Thorac Surg 1959; 37: 745–749.
149. Pollak ER, Naunheim KS, Little AG: Fibromyxoma of the trachea. Arch Pathol Lab Med 1985; 109: 926–929.
150. Butler C, Kleinerman J: Pulmonary hamartoma. Arch Pathol 1969; 88: 584–592.
151. Gjevre JA, Myers JL, Prakash UBS: Pulmonary hamartomas. Mayo Clin Proc 1996; 71; 14–20.
152. Hamper UM, Khouri NF, Stitik FP, et al.: Pulmonary hamartoma: diagnosis by transthoracic needle-aspiration biopsy. Radiology 1985; 155: 15–18.
153. Wiatrowska BA, Yazdi HM, Matzinger FR, MacDonald LL: Fine needle aspiration biopsy of pulmonary hamartomas: radiologic, cytologic, and immunocytochemical study of 15 cases. Acta Cytol 1995; 39: 1167–1174.
154. Abrahams NA, Colby TV, Pearl RH, et al.: Pulmonary hemangiomas of infancy and childhood: report of two cases and review of the literature. Pediatr Dev Pathol 2002; 5: 283–292.
155. Ritter JH, Mills SE, Nappi O, Wick MR: Angiosarcoma-like neoplasms of epithelial organs: true endothelial tumors or variants of carcinoma? Semin Diagn Pathol 1995; 12: 270–282.
156. Almagro P, Julia J, Sanjaume M, et al.: Pulmonary capillary hemangiomatosis associated with primary pulmonary hypertension: report of 2 new cases and review of 35 cases from the literature. Medicine 2002; 81: 417–424.
157. Havlik DM, Massie LW, Williams WL, Crooks LA: Pulmonary capillary hemangiomatosis-like foci: an autopsy study of 8 cases. Am J Clin Pathol 2000; 113: 655–662.
158. Eastridge CF, Young JM, Steplock AL: Endobronchial lipoma. South Med J 1984; 77: 759–761.
159. Politis J, Funahashi A, Gehlsen JA, et al.: Intrathoracic lipomas: report of three cases and review of the literature with emphasis on endobronchial lipoma. J Thorac Cardiovasc Surg 1979; 77: 550–556.
160. Kamiyoshihara M, Sakata K, Ohtani Y, et al.: Endobronchial lipoma accompanied with primary lung cancer: report of a case. Surg Today 2002; 32: 402–405.
161. Moran CA, Suster S, Koss MN: Endobronchial lipomas: a clinicopathologic study of four cases. Mod Pathol 1994; 7: 212–214.
162. Muraoka M, Oka T, Akamine S, et al.: Endobronchial lipoma: review of 64 cases reported in Japan. Chest 2003; 123: 293–296.
163. Gaerte SC, Meyer CA, Winer-Muram HT, Tarver RD, Conces DJ Jr: Fat-containing lesions of the chest. Radiographics 2002; 22 (suppl): S61–S78.
164. Solli P, Rossi G, Carbagnani P, et al.: Pulmonary abnormalities in Cowden's disease. J Cardiovasc Surg 1998; 40: 753–755.
165. Sekine I, Kodama T, Yokose T, et al.: Rare pulmonary tumors – a review of 32 cases. Oncology 1998; 55: 431–434.
166. Matsuba K, Saito T, Ando K, Shirakusa T: Atypical lipoma of the lung. Thorax 1991; 46: 685.
167. Bridge JA, Roberts CA, Degenhardt J, et al.: Low-level chromosome 12 amplification in a primary lipoma of the lung: evidence for a pathogenetic relationship with common adipose tissue tumors. Arch Pathol Lab Med 1998; 122: 187–190.
168. Hirata J, Reshad K, Itoi K, Muro K, Akiyama J: Lipomas of the peripheral lung – a case report and review of the literature. Thorac Cardiovasc Surg 1989; 37: 385–387.
169. Coffin CM: Lipoblastoma: an embryonal tumor of soft tissue related to organogenesis. Semin Diagn Pathol 1994; 11: 98–103.
170. Kanu A, Oermann CM, Malicki D, Wagner M, Langston C: Pulmonary lipoblastoma in an 18-month-old child: a unique tumor in children. Pediatr Pulmonol 2002; 34: 150–154.
171. Mathew J, Sen S, Chandi SM, et al.: Pulmonary lipoblastoma: a case report. Pediatr Surg Int 2001; 17: 543–544.
172. Hicks J, Dilley A, Patel D, et al.: Lipoblastoma and lipoblastomatosis in infancy and childhood: histopathologic, ultrastructural, and cytogenetic features. Ultrastruct Pathol 2001; 25: 321–333.
173. Meis-Kindblom JM, Sjogren H, Kindblom LG, et al.: Cytogenetic and molecular genetic analyses of liposarcoma and its soft tissue simulators: recognition of new variants and differential diagnosis. Virchows Arch 2001; 439: 141–151.
174. Tallini G, Vanni R, Manfioletti G, et al.: HMGI-C and HMGI(Y) immunoreactivity correlates with cytogenetic abnormalities in lipomas, pulmonary chondroid hamartomas, endometrial polyps, and uterine leiomyomas and is compatible with rearrangement of the HMGI-C and HMGI(Y) genes. Lab Invest 2000; 80: 359–369.
175. Johansson M, Dietrich C, Mandahl N, et al.: Recombinations of chromosomal bands 6p21 and 14q24 characterize pulmonary hamartomas. Br J Cancer 1993; 67: 1236–1241.
176. Pea M, Bonetti F, Zamboni G, et al.: Clear cell tumor and angiomyolipoma. Am J Surg Pathol 1991; 15: 199–202.
177. Bacchi CE, Bonetti F, Pea M, Martignoni G, Gown AM: HMB-45: a review. Appl Immunohistochem Molec Morphol 1996; 4: 73–85.
178. Bonetti F, Pea M, Martignoni G, et al.: Clear cell ("sugar") tumor of the lung is a lesion strictly related to angiomyolipoma – the concept of a family of lesions characterized by the presence of the perivascular epithelioid cell (PEC). Pathology 1994; 26: 230–236.
179. Folpe AL, McKenney JK, Li Z, Smith SJ, Weiss SW: Clear cell myomelanocytic tumor of the thigh: report of a unique case. Am J Surg Pathol 2002; 26: 809–812.
180. Garcia TR, Mestre-de-Juan MJ: Angiomyolipoma of the liver and lung: a case explained by the presence of perivascular epithelioid cells. Pathol Res Pract 2002; 198: 363–367.
181. Wu K, Tazelaar HD: Pulmonary angiomyolipoma and multifocal micronodular pneumocyte hyperplasia associated with tuberous sclerosis. Hum Pathol 1999; 30: 1266–1268.
182. Papla B, Malinowski E: Angiomyolipoma of the lung. Pol J Pathol 1999; 50: 47–50.
183. Ito M, Sugamura Y, Ikari H, Sekine I: Angiomyolipoma of the lung. Arch Pathol Lab Med 1998; 122: 1023–1025.
184. Guinee DG Jr, Thornberry DS, Azumi N, et al.: Unique pulmonary presentation of an angiomyolipoma: analysis of clinical, radiographic, and histopathologic features. Am J Surg Pathol 1995; 19: 476–480.
185. Chu SC, Horiba K, Usuki J, et al.: Comprehensive evaluation of 35 patients with lymphangioleiomyomatosis. Chest 1999; 115: 1041–1052.
186. Kitaichi M, Nishimura K, Itoh H, Izumi T: Pulmonary lymphangioleiomyomatosis: a report of 46 patients including a clinicopathologic study of prognostic factors. Am J Respir Crit Care Med 1995; 151: 527–533.
187. Matsumoto S, Nishioka T, Akiyama T: Renal angiomyolipoma associated with micronodular pneumocyte hyperplasia of the lung with tuberous sclerosis. Int J Urol 2001; 8: 242–244.
188. Takahashi N, Kitihara R, Hishimoto Y, et al.: Malignant transformation of renal angiomyolipoma. Int J Urol 2003; 10: 271–273.
189. Gee WF, Chikos PM, Greaves JP, Ikemoto N, Tremann JA: Adrenal myelolipoma. Urology 1975; 5: 562–566.
190. Singla AK, Kechejian G, Lopez MJ: Giant presacral myelolipoma. Am Surg 2003; 69: 334–338.
191. Hunter SB, Schemankewitz EH, Patterson C, Varma VA: Extraadrenal myelolipoma: a report of two cases. Am J Clin Pathol 1992; 97: 402–404.
192. Sabate CJ, Shahian DM: Pulmonary myelolipoma. Ann Thorac Surg 2002; 74: 573–575.
193. Piccinini L, Barbolini G: A case of lung myelolipomatosis in a patient with bronchial carcinoid. Panminerva Med 1999; 41: 175–178.
194. Ziolkowski P, Muszczynska-Bernhard B, Dziegiel P: Myelolipoma: the report of two cases in a pulmonary location. Pol J Pathol 1996; 47: 141–142.
195. Joseph MB, Colby TV, Swensen SJ, Mikus JP, Gaensler EA: Multiple cystic fibrohistiocytic tumors of the lung: report of two cases. Mayo Clin Proc 1990; 65: 192–197.
196. Han JH: Uncommon tumors of the lung (Internet presentation). www.pathology.or.kr/studygroup/cardiopulmonary/lecture/lenote/hjh.htm.

197. Colome-Grimmer MI, Evans HL: Metastasizing cellular dermatofibroma: a report of two cases. Am J Surg Pathol 1996; 20: 1361–1367.
198. Quigley JC, Hart WR: Adenomatoid tumors of the uterus. Am J Clin Pathol 1981; 76: 627–635.
199. Srigley JR, Hartwick RW: Tumors and cysts of the paratesticular region. Pathol Annu 1990; 25: 51–108.
200. Kaplan MA, Tazelaar HD, Hayashi T, Schroer KR, Travis WD: Adenomatoid tumors of the pleura. Am J Surg Pathol 1996; 20: 1219–1223.
201. Handra-Luca A, Couvelard A, Abd-Alsamad I, et al.: Adenomatoid tumor of the pleura: case report. Ann Pathol 2000; 20: 369–372.
202. Umezu H, Kuwata K, Ebe Y, et al.: Microcystic variant of localized malignant mesothelioma accompanying an adenomatoid tumor-like lesion. Pathol Int 2002; 52: 416–422.
203. Pinkard NB, Wilson RW, Lawless N, et al.: Calcifying fibrous pseudotumor of the pleura: a report of three cases of a newly described entity involving the pleura. Am J Clin Pathol 1996; 105: 189–194.
204. Murray JG, Pinkard NB: Calcifying fibrous pseudotumor of the pleura: radiologic features in three cases. J Comput Assist Tomogr 1996; 20: 763–765.
205. Hainaut P, Lesage V, Weynand B, Coche E, Noirhomme P: Calcifying fibrous pseudotumor (CFPT): a patient presenting with multiple pleural lesions. Acta Clin Belg 1999; 54: 162–164.
206. Cavazza A, Gelli MC, Agostini L, et al.: Calcified pseudotumor of the pleura: description of a case. Pathologica 2002; 94: 201–205.
207. Rosenthal NS, Abdul-Karim FW: Childhood fibrous tumor with psammoma bodies: clinicopathologic features in two cases. Arch Pathol Lab Med 1988; 112: 798–800.
208. Maeda T, Hirose T, Furuya K, Kameoka K: Calcifying fibrous pseudotumor: an ultrastructural study. Ultrastruct Pathol 1999; 23: 189–192.
209. Hill KA, Gonzalez-Crussi F, Chou PM: Calcifying fibrous pseudotumor versus inflammatory myofibroblastic tumor: a histological and immunohistochemical comparison. Mod Pathol 2001; 14: 784–790.
210. Nascimento AF, Ruiz R, Hornick JL, Fletcher CDM: Calcifying fibrous "pseudotumor": clinicopathologic study of 15 cases and analysis of its relationship to inflammatory myofibroblastic tumor. Int J Surg Pathol 2002; 10: 189–196.
211. Brunn H: Two interesting benign lung tumors of contradictory histopathology. J Thorac Cardiovasc Surg 1939; 9: 119–131.
212. Umiker WO, Iverson L: Postinflammatory "tumors" of the lung: report of four cases simulating xanthoma, fibroma, or plasma cell tumor. J Thorac Cardiovasc Surg 1954; 28: 55–63.
213. Bahadori M, Liebow AA: Plasma cell granulomas of the lung. Cancer 1973; 31: 191–208.
214. Spencer H: The pulmonary plasma cell/histiocytoma complex. Histopathology 1984; 8: 903–916.
215. Berardi RS, Lee SS, Chen HP, et al.: Inflammatory pseudotumors of the lung. Surg Gynecol Obstet 1983; 156: 89–96.
216. Souid AK, Ziemba MC, Dubansky AS, et al.: Inflammatory myofibroblastic tumor in children. Cancer 1993; 72: 2042–2048.
217. Wick MR, Ritter JH, Nappi O: Inflammatory sarcomatoid carcinoma of the lung: report of three cases with comparison with inflammatory pseudotumors in adult patients. Hum Pathol 1995; 26: 1014–1021.
218. Su LD, Atayde-Perez A, Sheldon S, Fletcher JA, Weiss SW: Inflammatory myofibroblastic tumor: cytogenetic evidence supporting a clonal origin. Mod Pathol 1998; 11: 364–368.
219. Snyder CS, Dell'Aquila M, Haghighi P, et al.: Clonal changes in inflammatory pseudotumor of the lung: a case report. Cancer 1995; 76: 1545–1549.
220. Yamamoto H, Oda Y, Saito T, et al.: p53 mutation and MDM2 amplification in inflammatory myofibroblastic tumors. Histopathology 2003; 42: 431–439.
221. Pettinato G, Manivel JC, DeRosa N, et al.: Inflammatory myofibroblastic tumor (plasma cell granuloma): a clinicopathologic study of 20 cases with immunohistochemical and ultrastructural observations. Am J Clin Pathol 1990; 94: 538–546.
222. Meis JM, Enzinger FM: Inflammatory fibrosarcoma of the mesentery and retroperitoneum: a tumor closely simulating inflammatory pseudotumor. Am J Surg Pathol 1991; 15: 1146–1156.
223. Coffin CM, Dehner LP, Meis-Kindblom JM: Inflammatory myofibroblastic tumor, inflammatory fibrosarcoma, and related lesions: an historical review with differential diagnostic considerations. Semin Diagn Pathol 1998; 15: 102–110.
224. Matsubara O, Tan-Liu NS, Kenney RM, et al.: Inflammatory pseudotumors of the lung: progression from organizing pneumonia to fibrous histiocytoma or to plasma cell granuloma in 32 cases. Hum Pathol 1988; 19: 807–814.
225. Cessna MH, Zhou H, Sanger WG, et al.: Expression of *ALK1* and p80 in inflammatory myofibroblastic tumor and its mesenchymal mimics: a study of 135 cases. Mod Pathol 2002; 15: 931–938.
226. Hussong JW, Brown M, Perkins SL, Dehner LP, Coffin CM: Comparison of DNA ploidy, histologic, and immunohistochemical findings with clinical outcome in inflammatory myofibroblastic tumors. Mod Pathol 1999; 12: 279–286.
227. Messineo A, Mognato G, D'Amore ES, et al.: Inflammatory pseudotumors of the lung in children: conservative or aggressive approach? Med Pediatr Oncol 1998; 31: 100–104.
228. Liebow AA, Hubbell DS: Sclerosing hemangioma (histiocytoma, xanthoma) of the lung. Cancer 1956; 9: 53–75.
229. Gross RE, Wolbach SB: Sclerosing hemangiomas: their relationship to dermatofibroma, histiocytoma, xanthoma, and to certain pigmented lesions of the skin. Am J Pathol 1943; 19: 533–546.
230. Katzenstein AL, Weise D, Fuilling K, Battifora H: So-called sclerosing hemangioma of the lung: evidence for mesothelial origin. Am J Surg Pathol 1983; 7: 3–14.
231. Kennedy A: "Sclerosing hemangioma" of the lung: an alternative view of its development. J Clin Pathol 1973; 26: 792–799.
232. Hill GS, Eggleston JC: Electron microscopic study of so-called pulmonary "sclerosing hemangioma": report of a case suggesting an epithelial origin. Cancer 1972; 30: 1092–1106.
233. Kay S, Still WJ, Borochovitz D: Sclerosing hemangioma of the lung: an endothelial or epithelial neoplasm? Hum Pathol 1977; 8: 468–474.
234. Spencer H, Nambu S: Sclerosing hemangiomas of the lung. Histopathology 1986; 10: 477–487.
235. Hegg CA, Flint A, Singh G: Papillary adenoma of the lung. Am J Clin Pathol 1992; 97: 393–397.
236. Fantone JC, Geisinger KR, Appelman HD: Papillary adenoma of the lung with lamellar and electron-dense granules. Cancer 1982; 50: 2839–2844.
237. Noguchi M, Kodama T, Shimosato Y, et al.: Papillary adenoma of type II pneumocytes. Am J Surg Pathol 1986; 10: 134–139.
238. Sanchez-Jimenez J, Ballester-Martinez A, Lodo-Besse J, et al.: Papillary adenoma of type II pneumocytes. Pediatr Pulmonol 1994; 17: 396–400.
239. Yousem SA, Hochholzer L: Alveolar adenoma. Hum Pathol 1986; 17: 1066–1071.
240. Nagata N, Dairaku M, Ishida T, Sueishi K, Tanaka K: Sclerosing hemangioma of the lung: immunohistochemical characterization of its origin as related to surfactant protein. Cancer 1985; 55: 116–123.
241. Shimosato Y: Lung tumors of uncertain histogenesis. Semin Diagn Pathol 1995; 12: 185–192.
242. Katzenstein AL, Gmelich J, Carrington C: Sclerosing hemangioma of the lung: a clinicopathologic study of 51 cases. Am J Surg Pathol 1980; 4: 343–356.
243. Yousem SA, Wick MR, Singh G, et al.: So-called sclerosing hemangiomas of lung: an immunohistochemical study supporting a respiratory epithelial origin. Am J Surg Pathol 1988; 12: 582–590.
244. Wojcik E, Sneige N, Lawrence D, Ordonez NG: Fine needle aspiration cytology of sclerosing hemangioma of the lung: case report with immunohistochemical study. Diagn Cytopathol 1993; 9: 304–309.
245. Noguchi M, Kodama T, Morinaga S, et al.: Multiple sclerosing hemangiomas of the lung. Am J Surg Pathol 1986; 10: 429–435.
246. Tanaka I, Inoue M, Matsui Y, et al.: A case of pneumocytoma (so-called sclerosing hemangioma) with lymph node metastasis. Jpn J Clin Oncol 1986; 16: 77–86.
247. Barbareschi M, Colombetti V, Ferrero S, Yousem SA, Singh G: Sclerosing hemangioma of the lung. Histo Histopathol 1992; 7: 209–212.
248. Moran CA, Zeren H, Koss MN: Sclerosing hemangioma of the lung: granulomatous variant. Arch Pathol Lab Med 1994; 118: 1028–1030.
249. Satoh Y, Tsuchiya E, Weng SY, et al.: Pulmonary sclerosing hemangioma of the lung: type II pneumocytoma by immunohistochemistry and immunoelectron microscopic studies. Cancer 1989; 64: 1310–1317.
250. Alvarez-Fernandez B, Carretero-Albinana L, Menarquez-Palanca J: Sclerosing hemangioma of the lung: an immunohistochemical study of intermediate filaments and endothelial markers. Arch Pathol Lab Med 1989; 113: 121–124.

251. Fukayama M, Mikoike M: So-called sclerosing hemangioma of the lung: an immunohistochemical, histochemical, and ultrastructural study. Acta Pathol Jpn 1988; 38: 627–642.
252. Leong ASY, Chan KW, Seneviratne HS: A morphological and immunohistochemical study of 25 cases of so-called sclerosing hemangioma of the lung. Histopathology 1995; 27: 121–128.
253. Nagata N, Dairaku M, Sueishi K, Tanaka K: Sclerosing hemangioma of the lung: an epithelial tumor composed of immunohistochemically heterogeneous cells. Am J Clin Pathol 1987; 88: 552–559.
254. Nicholson AG, Magkou C, Snead D, et al.: Unusual sclerosing haemangiomas and sclerosing haemangioma-like lesions, and the value of TTF-1 in making the diagnosis. Histopathology 2002; 41: 404–413.
255. Xu HM, Li WH, Hou N, et al.: Neuroendocrine differentiation in 32 cases of so-called sclerosing hemangioma of the lung, identified by immunohistochemistry and ultrastructural study. Am J Surg Pathol 1997; 21: 1013–1022.
256. Papla B: Sclerosing hemangioma of the lung – benign sclerosing pneumocytoma. Pol J Pathol 1999; 50: 99–106.
257. Guibaud L, Pracros JP, Rode V, et al.: Sclerosing hemangioma of the lung: radiological findings and pathological diagnosis. Pediatr Radiol 1995; 25(suppl 1): S207–S208.
258. Mori M, Chiba R, Tezuka F, et al.: Papillary adenoma of type II pneumocytes might have malignant potential. Virchows Arch A 1996; 428: 195–200.
259. Yamamoto T, Horiguchi H, Shibagaki J, et al.: Encapsulated type II pneumocyte adenoma: a case report and review of the literature. Respiration 1993; 60: 373–377.
260. Gottschalk-Sabag S, Hadas-Halpern I, Glick T: Sclerosing hemangioma of lung mimicking carcinoma, diagnosed by fine needle aspiration (FNA) cytology. Cytopathology 1995; 6: 115–120.
261. Krishnamurthy SC, Naresh KN, Soni M, Bhasin SD: Sclerosing hemangioma of the lung: a potential source of error in fine needle aspiration cytology. Acta Cytol 1995; 38: 111–112.
262. Devouassoux-Shisheboran M, Hayashi T, Linnoila R, Koss MN, Travis WD: A clinicopathologic study of 100 cases of pulmonary sclerosing hemangiooma with immunohistochemical studies: TTF-1 is expressed in both round and surface cells, suggesting an origin from primitive respiratory epithelium. Am J Surg Pathol 2000; 24: 906–916.
263. Kuo KT, Hsu WH, Wu YC, Huang MH, Li WY: Sclerosing hemangioma of the lung: an analysis of 44 cases. J Chin Med Assoc 2003; 66: 33–38.
264. Miyagawa-Hayashino A, Tazelaar HD, Langel DJ, Colby TV: Pulmonary sclerosing hemangioma with lymph node metastases: report of 4 cases. Arch Pathol Lab Med 2003; 127: 321–325.
265. Hayashi A, Takamori S, Mitsuoka M, et al.: Unilateral progressive multiple sclerosing hemangioma in a young female successfully treated by pneumonectomy: report of a case. Int Surg 2002; 87: 69–72.
266. Iyoda A, Baba M, Saitoh H, et al.: Imprint cytologic features of pulmonary sclerosing hemangioma: comparison with well-differentiated papillary adenocarcinoma. Cancer 2002; 96: 146–149.
267. Batinica S, Gunek G, Raos M, Jelasic D, Bogovic M: Sclerosing hemangioma of the lung in a 4-year-old child. Eur J Pediatr Surg 2002; 12: 192–194.
268. Nam JE, Ryu YH, Cho SH, et al.: Air-trapping zone surrounding sclerosing hemangioma of the lung. J Comput Assist Tomogr 2002; 26: 358–361.
269. Yano M, Yamakawa Y, Kiriyama M, Hara M, Murase T: Sclerosing hemangioma with metastases to multiple nodal stations. Ann Thorac Surg 2002; 73: 981–983.
270. Gal AA, Nassar VH, Miller JI: Cytopathologic diagnosis of pulmonary sclerosing hemangioma. Diagn Cytopathol 2002; 26: 163–166.
271. Ng WK, Fu KH, Wang E, Tang V: Sclerosing hemangioma of lung: a close cytologic mimicker of pulmonary adenocarcinoma. Diagn Cytopathol 2001; 25: 316–320.
272. Illei PB, Rosai J, Klimstra DS: Expression of thyroid transcription factor-1 and other markers in sclerosing hemangioma of the lung. Arch Pathol Lab Med 2001; 125: 1335–1339.
273. Chan AC, Chan JKC: Pulmonary sclerosing hemangioma consistently expresses thyroid transcription factor-1 (TTF-1): a new clue to its histogenesis. Am J Surg Pathol 2000; 24: 1531–1536.
274. Guillou L, DeLuze P, Zysset F, Costa J: Papillary variant of low-grade mucoepidermoid carcinoma – an unusual bronchial neoplasm: a light microscopic, ultrastructural, and immunohistochemical study. Am J Clin Pathol 1994; 101: 269–274.
275. Rodriguez IM, Prat J: Mucinous tumors of the ovary: a clinicopathologic analysis of 75 borderline tumors (of intestinal type) and carcinomas. Am J Surg Pathol 2002; 26: 139–152.
276. Izumo A, Yamaguchi K, Eguchi T, et al.: Mucinous cystic tumor of the pancreas. Oncol Rep 2003; 10: 515–525.
277. Sambrook-Gowar FJ: An unusual mucous cyst of the lung. Thorax 1978; 33: 796–799.
278. Butnor KJ, Sporn TA, Dodd LG: Fine needle aspiration cytology of mucinous cystadenocarcinoma of the lung: report of a case with radiographic and histologic correlation. Acta Cytol 2001; 45: 779–783.
279. Monaghan H, Salter DM, Ferguson T: Pulmonary mucinous cystic tumor of borderline malignancy: a rare variant of adenocarcinoma. J Clin Pathol 2002; 55: 156.
280. Divisi D, Battaglia C, Giusti L, et al.: Mucinous cystadenoma of the lung. Acta Biomed Ateneo Parmense 1997; 68: 115–118.
281. Papla B, Malinowski E, Harazda M: Pulmonary mucinous cystadenoma of borderline malignancy: a report of two cases. Pol J Pathol 1996; 47: 87–90.
282. Roux FJ, Lantuejoul S, Brambilla E, Brambilla C: Mucinous cystadenoma of the lung. Cancer 1995; 76: 1540–1544.
283. Pelletier B, Dubigeon P, Despins P, Dehajartre AY: Cystic mucinous pulmonary tumor of borderline malignancy: report of a case. Ann Pathol 1993; 13: 405–408.
284. Davison AM, Lowe JW, DaCosta P: Adenocarcinoma arising in a mucinous cystadenoma of the lung. Thorax 1992; 47: 129–130.
285. Traub B: Mucinous cystadenoma of the lung. Arch Pathol Lab Med 1991; 115: 740–741.
286. Kragel PJ, Devaney KO, Meth BM, et al.: Mucinous cystadenoma of the lung: a report of two cases with immunohistochemical and ultrastructural analysis. Arch Pathol Lab Med 1990; 114: 1053–1056.
287. Kleinert R, Popper H: Giant fibroma of the lung: a morphologic study. Virchows Arch A 1987; 410: 363–367.
288. Sauk JJ, Pliego M, Anderson WR: Primary pulmonary fibroma. Minn Med 1972; 55: 220–223.
289. Klemperer P, Rabin CB: Primary neoplasms of the pleura. Arch Pathol 1931; 11: 385–412.
290. Briselli MF, Mark EJ: Solitary fibrous tumors of the pleura and benign extrapleural tumors of mesothelial origin. In: Asbestos-related malignancy, Antman K, Aisner J, Eds. 1986, Grune & Stratton, Philadelphia, pp 165–178.
291. Dalton W, Zollike A, McCaughey WT, Jacques J, Kannerstein M: Localized primary tumors of the pleura. Cancer 1979; 44: 1465–1475.
292. Vallat-Decouvelaere AV, Dry SM, Fletcher CDM: Atypical and malignant solitary fibrous tumors in extrathoracic locations: evidence of their comparability to intrathoracic tumors. Am J Surg Pathol 1998; 22: 1501–1511.
293. Magdeleinat P, Alifano M, Petino A, et al.: Solitary fibrous tumors of the pleura: clinical characteristics, surgical treatment, and outcome. Eur J Cardiothorac Surg 2002; 21: 1087–1093.
294. Cardillo G, Facciolo F, Cavazzana AO, et al.: Localized (solitary) fibrous tumors of the pleura: an analysis of 55 patients. Ann Thorac Surg 2000; 70: 1808–1812.
295. Duster P, Mayer E, Kramm T, et al.: Solitary fibrous pleural tumors – rare tumors with unpredictable clinical behavior. Pneumologie 2000; 54: 16–19.
296. Meyer M, Krause U: Solitary fibrous tumors of the pleura. Chirurgie 1999; 70: 949–952.
297. Khan JH, Rahman SB, Clary-Macy C, et al.: Giant solitary fibrous tumor of the pleura. Ann Thorac Surg 1998; 65: 1461–1464.
298. Briselli MF, Mark EJ, Dickersin GR: Solitary fibrous tumors of the pleura: eight new cases and review of 360 cases in the literature. Cancer 1981; 47: 2678–2689.
299. Hanau CA, Miettinen M: Solitary fibrous tumor: histological and immunohistochemical spectrum of benign and malignant variants presenting at different sites. Hum Pathol 1995; 26: 440–449.
300. Moran CA, Suster S, Koss MN: The spectrum of histologic growth patterns in benign and malignant fibrous tumors of the pleura. Semin Diagn Pathol 1992; 9: 169–180.
301. England DM, Hochholzer L, McCarthy MJ: Localized benign and malignant fibrous tumors of the pleura. Am J Surg Pathol 1989; 13: 640–658.

302. Ali SZ, Hoon V, Hoda S, Heelan R, Zakowski MF: Solitary fibrous tumor: a cytologic–histologic study with clinical, radiologic, and immunohistochemical correlations. Cancer 1997; 81: 116–121.
303. Weynand B, Collard P, Galant C: Cytopathological features of solitary fibrous tumor of the pleura: a study of 5 cases. Diagn Cytopathol 1998; 18: 118–124.
304. Caruso RA, LaSpada F, Gaeta M, Minutoli I, Inferrera C: Report of an intrapulmonary solitary fibrous tumor: fine needle aspiration cytologic findings, clinicopathological, and immunohistochemical features. Diagn Cytopathol 1996; 14: 64–67.
305. Khalifa MA, Montgomery EA, Azumi N, et al.: Solitary fibrous tumors: a series of lesions, some in unusual sites. South Med J 1997; 90: 793–799.
306. Van de Rijn M, Lombard CM, Rouse RV: Expression of CD34 by solitary fibrous tumors of the pleura, mediastinum, and lung. Am J Surg Pathol 1994; 18: 814–820.
307. Suster S, Fisher C, Moran CA: Expression of *bcl-2* oncoprotein in benign and malignant spindle cell tumors of soft tissue, skin, serosal surfaces, and gastrointestinal tract. Am J Surg Pathol 1998; 22: 863–872.
308. Flint A, Weiss SW: CD34 and keratin expression distinguishes solitary fibrous tumor (fibrous mesothelioma) of pleura from desmoplastic mesothelioma. Hum Pathol 1995; 26: 428–431.
309. Ledet SC, Brown RW, Cagle PT: p53 immunostaining in the differentiation of inflammatory pseudotumor from sarcoma involving the lung. Mod Pathol 1995; 8: 282–286.
310. Krismann M, Adams H, Jaworska M, Muller KM, Johnen G: Patterns of chromosomal imbalances in benign solitary fibrous tumors of the pleura. Virchows Arch A 2000; 70: 1808–1812.
311. Dal Cin P, Pauwels P, Van den Berghe H: Solitary fibrous tumor of the pleura with t(4;15)(q13;q26). Histopathology 1999; 35: 94–95.
312. Carbone M, Rizzo P, Powers A, et al.: Molecular analyses, morphology, and immunohistochemistry together differentiate pleural synovial sarcomas from mesotheliomas: clinical implications. Anticancer Res 2002; 22: 3443–3448.
313. Nappi O, Ritter JH, Pettinato G, Wick MR: Hemangiopericytoma: histopathological pattern or clinicopathologic entity? Semin Diagn Pathol 1995; 12: 221–232.
314. Sumathi VP, McCluggage WG: CD10 is useful in demonstrating endometrial stroma at ectopic sites and in confirming a diagnosis of endometriosis. J Clin Pathol 2002; 55: 391–392.
315. Liebow AA, Castleman B: Benign "clear cell tumors" of the lung. Am J Pathol 1963; 43: 13–14.
316. Liebow AA, Castleman B: Benign clear cell ("sugar") tumors of the lung. Yale J Biol Med 1971; 43: 213–222.
317. Hoch WS, Patchefsky AS, Takeda M, Gordon G: Benign clear-cell tumor of the lung: an ultrastructural study. Cancer 1974; 33: 1328–1336.
318. Ozdemir IA, Zaman NU, Rullis I, Webb WR: Benign clear cell tumor of lung. J Thorac Cardiovasc Surg 1974; 68: 131–133.
319. Kung M, Landa JF, Lubin J: Benign clear cell tumor ("sugar tumor") of the trachea. Cancer 1984; 54: 517–519.
320. Hashimoto T, Oka K, Hakozaki H, et al.: Benign clear cell tumor of the lung. Ultrastruct Pathol 2001; 25: 479–483.
321. Slodkowska J, Suilkowska-Rowinska A, Dorosz P, Radomski P, Wasiutynski A: Benign clear cell tumor of the lung ("sugar tumor"): morphologic, immunohistochemical, and ultrastructural evaluation. Pneumonol Allergol Pol 2000; 68: 60–64.
322. Gaffey MJ, Mills SE, Ritter JH: Clear cell tumors of the lower respiratory tract. Semin Diagn Pathol 1997; 14: 222–232.
323. Jeanfaivre T, Savary L, Richard C: Benign clear cell tumor ("sugar tumor"): an unusual cause of intrapulmonary coin lesion. Rev Mal Respir 1997; 14: 223–224.
324. Andrion A, Mazzucco G, Gugliotta P, Monga G: Benign clear-cell ("sugar") tumor of the lung: a light microscopic, histochemical, and ultrastructural study with a review of the literature. Cancer 1985; 56: 2657–2663.
325. Sale GE, Kulander BG: Benign clear-cell tumor of lung with necrosis. Cancer 1976; 37: 2355–2358.
326. Lantuejoul S, Isaac S, Pinel N, et al.: Clear cell tumor of the lung: an immunohistochemical and ultrastructural study supporting a pericytic differentiation. Mod Pathol 1997; 10: 1001–1008.
327. Flieder DB, Travis WD: Clear cell "sugar" tumor of the lung associated with lymphangioleiomyomatosis and multifocal micronodular pneumocyte hyperplasia in a patient with tuberous sclerosis. Am J Surg Pathol 1997; 21: 1242–1247.
328. Gal AA, Koss MN, Hochholzer L, Chejfec G: An immunohistochemical study of benign clear-cell ("sugar") tumor of the lung. Arch Pathol Lab Med 1991; 115: 1034–1038.
329. Gaffey MJ, Mills SE, Askin FB, et al.: Clear cell tumor of the lung: a clinicopathologic, immunohistochemical, and ultrastructural study of eight cases. Am J Surg Pathol 1991; 15: 199–202.
330. Stolz AJ, Schutzner J, Lischke R, et al.: Benign clear cell tumors of the lung – sugar tumors. Rozhl Chir 2003; 82: 149–151.
331. Sale GE, Kulander BG: "Benign" clear-cell tumor (sugar tumor) of the lung with hepatic metastases ten years after resection of pulmonary primary tumor. Arch Pathol Lab Med 1988; 112: 1177–1178.
332. Cavazza A, Sgarbi G, Ferrari G, Putrino I, Gardini G: Clear cell tumor of the lung: description of a case 1 mm. in diameter ("micro-sugar tumor"). Pathologica 2001; 93: 556–560.
333. Justrabo E, Mergey E, Piard F, Michiels R, Viard H: Benign clear cell tumour of the lung. Sem Hop 1982; 58: 673–677.
334. Urban T: Clinical and molecular epidemiology of lymphangioleiomyomatosis and pulmonary pathology in tuberous sclerosis. Rev Mal Respir 2000; 17: 597–603.
335. Knowles MA, Hornigold N, Pitt E: Tuberous sclerosis complex (TSC) gene involvement in sporadic tumors. Biochem Soc Trans 2003; 31: 597–602.
336. Panizo-Santos A, Sola I, DeAlava E, et al.: Angiomyolipoma and PEComa are immunoreactive for Myo-D1 in a cell cytoplasmic staining pattern. Appl Immunohistochem Molec Morphol 2003; 11: 156–160.
337. Nappi O, Mills SE, Swanson PE, Wick MR: Clear-cell tumors of unknown nature and origin: a systematic approach to diagnosis. Semin Diagn Pathol 1997; 14: 164–174.
338. Rosai J, Limas C, Husband EM: Ectopic hamartomatous thymoma. A distinctive benign lesion of lower neck. Am J Surg Pathol 1984; 8: 501–513.
339. Cohen JB, Troxell M, Kong CS, McDougall JR: Ectopic intrathyroidal thymoma: a case report and review. Thyroid 2003; 13: 305–308.
340. Ben-Hami B, Caulet-Maugendre S, Valla J, et al.: Primary pericardial thymoma: an unusual etiology of neoplastic pericarditis. Ann Pathol 1996; 16: 445–448.
341. Marchevsky AM: Lung tumors derived from ectopic tissues. Semin Diagn Pathol 1995; 12: 172–184.
342. Velojic D, Marsenic B, Nikolic D, Bosnic M, Djordjevic A: Ectopic thymoma with myasthenic and cardiac symptomatology. Plucne Bolesti Tuberk 1972; 24: 199–204.
343. Veynovich B, Masetti P, Kaplan PD, et al.: Primary pulmonary thymoma. Ann Thorac Surg 1997; 64: 1471–1473.
344. Moran CA, Suster S, Fishback NF, Koss MN: Primary intrapulmonary thymoma: a clinicopathologic and immunohistochemical study of eight cases. Am J Surg Pathol 1995; 19: 304–312.
345. James CL, Iyer PV, Leong ASY: Intrapulmonary thymoma. Histopathology 1992; 21: 175–177.
346. Fukayama M, Maeda Y, Funata N, et al.: Pulmonary and pleural thymoma: diagnostic application of lymphocyte markers to the thymoma of unusual site. Am J Clin Pathol 1988; 89: 617–621.
347. Green WR, Pressoir R, Gumbs RV, et al.: Intrapulmonary thymoma. Arch Pathol Lab Med 1987; 111: 1074–1076.
348. Kung IT, Loke SL, So SY, et al.: Intrapulmonary thymoma: report of two cases. Thorax 1985; 40: 471–474.
349. Yeoh CB, Ford JM, Lattes R, Wylie RH: Intrapulmonary thymoma. J Thorac Cardiovasc Surg 1966; 51: 131–136.
350. Shih DF, Wang JS, Tseng HH, Tiao WM: Primary pleural thymoma. Arch Pathol Lab Med 1997; 121: 79–82.
351. Honma K, Shimada K: Metastasizing ectopic thymoma arising in the right thoracic cavity and mimicking diffuse pleural mesothelioma – an autopsy study of a case with review of literature. Wien Klin Wochenschr 1986; 98: 14–20.
352. Fushimi H, Tanio Y, Kotoh K: Ectopic thymoma mimicking diffuse pleural mesothelioma: a case report. Hum Pathol 1998; 29: 409–410.
353. Attanoos RL, Galateau-Salle F, Gibbs AR, et al.: Primary thymic epithelial tumors of the pleura mimicking malignant mesothelioma. Histopathology 2002; 41: 42–49.
354. Bernatz PE, Harrison EG, Clagett OT: Thymoma: a clinicopathologic study. J Thorac Cardiovasc Surg 1961; 42: 424–444.
355. Muller-Hermelink HK, Marino M, Palestro G: Pathology of thymic epithelial tumors. Curr Top Pathol 1986; 75: 207–268.

356. Dadmanesh F, Sekihara T, Rosai J: Histologic typing of thymoma according to the new World Health Organization classification. Chest Surg Clin N Am 2001; 11: 407–420.
357. Suster S, Moran CA: Thymoma, atypical thymoma, and thymic carcinoma: a novel conceptual approach to the classification of thymic epithelial neoplasms. Am J Clin Pathol 1999; 111: 826–833.
358. Kirchner T, Schalke B, Buchwald J, et al.: Well-differentiated thymic carcinoma: an organotypical low-grade carcinoma with relationship to cortical thymoma. Am J Surg Pathol 1992; 16: 1153–1169.
359. Wakely PE Jr: Cytopathology–histopathology of the mediastinum: epithelial, lymphoproliferative, and germ cell neoplasms. Ann Diagn Pathol 2002; 6: 30–43.
360. Chhieng DC, Rose D, Ludwig ME, Zukowski MF: Cytology of thymomas: emphasis on morphology and correlation with histologic subtypes. Cancer 2000; 90: 24–32.
361. Shabb NS, Fahl M, Shabb B, Haswani P, Zaatari G: Fine needle aspiration of the mediastinum: a clinical, radiologic, cytologic, and histologic study of 42 cases. Diagn Cytopathol 1998; 19: 428–436.
362. Levine GD, Rosai J: Thymic hyperplasia and neoplasia: a review of current concepts. Hum Pathol 1978; 9: 495–515.
363. Mirza I, Kazimi SN, Ligi R, Burns J, Braza F: Cytogenetic profile of a thymoma: a case report and review of the literature. Arch Pathol Lab Med 2000; 124: 1714–1716.
364. Goh SG, Lau LC, Sivaswaren C, et al.: Pseudodicentric (16;12)(q11;p11.2) in a type AB (mixed) thymoma. Cancer Genet Cytogenet 2001; 131: 42–47.
365. Van den Berghe I, Debiec-Rychter M, Proot L, Hagemeijer A, Michielssen P: Ring chromosome 6 may represent a cytogenetic subgroup in benign thymoma. Cancer Genet Cytogenet 2002; 137: 75–77.
366. Kuo TT: Cytokeratin profiles of the thymus and thymomas: histogenetic correlations and proposal for a histological classification of thymomas. Histopathology 2000; 36: 403–414.
367. Chu PG, Weiss LM: Expression of cytokeratin 5/6 in epithelial neoplasms: an immunohistochemical study of 509 cases. Mod Pathol 2002; 15: 6–10.
368. DiComo CJ, Urist MJ, Babayan I, et al.: p63 expression profiles in human normal and tumor tissues. Clin Cancer Res 2002; 8: 494–501.
369. Wick MR, Nappi O: Ectopic neural and neuroendocrine neoplasms. Semin Diagn Pathol, in press.
370. Cesario A, Galetta D, Margaritora S, Granone P: Unsuspected primary pulmonary meningioma. Eur J Cardiothorac Surg 2002; 21: 553–555.
371. Prayson RA, Farver CF: Primary pulmonary malignant meningioma. Am J Surg Pathol 1999; 23: 722–726.
372. Moran CA, Hochholzer L, Rush W, Koss MN: Primary intrapulmonary meningiomas: a clinicopathologic and immunohistochemical study of ten cases. Cancer 1996; 78: 2328–2333.
373. Gomez-Aracil V, Mayayo E, Alvira R, Arraiza A, Ramon y Cajal S: Fine needle aspiration cytology of primary pulmonary meningioma associated with minute meningothelial-like nodules. Report of a case with histologic, immunohistochemical, and ultrastructural studies. Acta Cytol 2002; 46: 899–903.
374. Falleni M, Roz E, Dessy E, et al.: Primary intrathoracic meningioma: histopathological, immunohistochemical, and ultrastructural study of two cases. Virchows Arch A 2001; 439: 196–200.
375. Spinelli M, Claren R, Colombi R, Sironi M: Primary pulmonary meningioma may arise from meningothelial-like nodules. Adv Clin Pathol 2000; 4: 35–39.
376. DePerrot M, Kurt AM, Robert J, Spiliopoulos A: Primary pulmonary meningioma presenting as lung metastasis. Scand Cardiovasc J 1999; 33: 121–123.
377. Ueno M, Fujiyama J, Yamazaki I, et al.: Cytology of primary pulmonary meningioma: report of the first multiple case. Acta Cytol 1998; 42: 1424–1430.
378. Kaleem Z, Fitzpatrick MM, Ritter JH: Primary pulmonary meningioma: report of a case and review of the literature. Arch Pathol Lab Med 1997; 121: 631–636.
379. Lockett L, Chiang V, Scully N: Primary pulmonary meningioma: report of a case and review of the literature. Am J Surg Pathol 1997; 21: 453–460.
380. Maiorana A, Ficarra G, Fano RA, Spagna G: Primary solitary meningioma of the lung. Pathologica 1996; 88: 457–462.
381. Flynn SD, Yousem SA: Pulmonary meningiomas: report of two cases. Hum Pathol 1991; 22: 469–474.
382. Kodama K, Doi O, Higashiyama M, et al.: Primary and metastatic pulmonary meningioma. Cancer 1991; 67: 1412–1417.
383. Strimlan CV, Golembiewski RS, Celko DA, Fino GJ: Primary pulmonary meningioma. Surg Neurol 1988; 29: 410–413.
384. Churg AM, Warnock ML: So-called "minute pulmonary chemodectoma:" a tumor not related to paragangliomas. Cancer 1976; 37: 1759–1769.
385. Ionescu DN, Sasatomi E, Aldeeb D, Omalu BI, Finkelstein SD, Swalsky PA, Yousem SA: Pulmonary meningothelial-like nodules: a genotypic comparison with meningiomas.
386. Drlicek M, Grisold W, Lorber J, et al.: Pulmonary meningioma: immunohistochemical and ultrastructural features. Am J Surg Pathol 1991; 15: 455–459.
387. Ishino S, Hashimoto N, Fushiki S, et al.: Loss of material from chromosome arm 1p during malignant progression of meningioma revealed by fluorescent in-situ hybridization. Cancer 1998; 83: 360–366.
388. Adlakha A, Rao K, Adlakha H, et al.: Meningioma metastatic to the lung. Mayo Clin Proc 1999; 74: 1129–1133.
389. Tandon S, Kant S, Singh AK, et al.: Primary intrapulmonary teratoma presenting as pyothorax. Indian J Chest Dis Allied Sci 1999; 41: 51–55.
390. Kayser K, Gabius HJ, Hagemeyer O: Malignant teratoma of the lung with lymph node metastasis of the ectodermal compartment: a case report. Ann Cell Pathol 1993; 5: 31–37.
391. Eggerath A, Ammon J, Karstens JH, Rubben H, Morales MR: Extragonadal germ cell tumors – diagnostic and therapeutic aspects. Strahlentherapie 1984; 160: 1–7.
392. Hartman GE, Shochat SJ: Primary pulmonary neoplasms of childhood: a review. Ann Thorac Surg 1983; 36: 108–119.
393. Moran CA, Travis WD, Carter D, Koss MN: Metastatic mature teratoma in lung following testicular embryonal carcinoma and teratocarcinoma. Arch Pathol Lab Med 1993; 117: 641–644.
394. Kakkar N, Vashishta RK, Banerjee AK, et al.: Primary pulmonary malignant teratoma with yolk sac elements associated with hematologic neoplasia. Respiration 1996; 63: 52–54.
395. Stair JM, Stevenson DR, Schaefer RF, Fullenwider JP, Campbell GS: Primary teratocarcinoma of the lung. J Surg Oncol 1986; 33: 262–267.
396. Berghout A, Mallens WM, TeVelde J, Haak HL: Teratoma of the lung in a hemophilic patient. Acta Hematol 1983; 70: 330–334.

Malignant and borderline mesothelial tumors of the pleura

20

Mark R Wick   Cesar A Moran   Jon H Ritter   Stacey E Mills

The number of publications on the pathologic features of primary pleural mesothelial tumors has gone from meager to innumerable in a little over 40 years. As late as the 1960s, a strong opinion in the medical community suggested that a diagnosis of malignant mesothelioma (MM) could not be established with certainty during life, and that neoplasms effacing the serosal lining of the chest cavity were probably metastatic from other sites.[1] Accordingly, a diagnostic interpretation of MM was largely consigned to autopsy pathologists.

Another problem, which persists to some extent even today, relates to the widely-cited paradigm for classification of mesothelial tumors that was first advanced by Klemperer and Rabin in 1931.[2] Those authors divided such lesions into four broad categories, depending on whether they were benign or malignant, and localized or diffuse. However, using that model, such neoplasms as solitary fibrous tumors and pleural sarcomas – which are not mesothelial at all – are still confused by some clinicians with true MM.

Developments in the sphere of technology have shed a great deal of light on these subjects in the recent past. Accurate classification of mesothelial neoplasms can now be accomplished, and their differential diagnosis from morphologically similar lesions is facilitated by the use of several adjunctive study modalities.

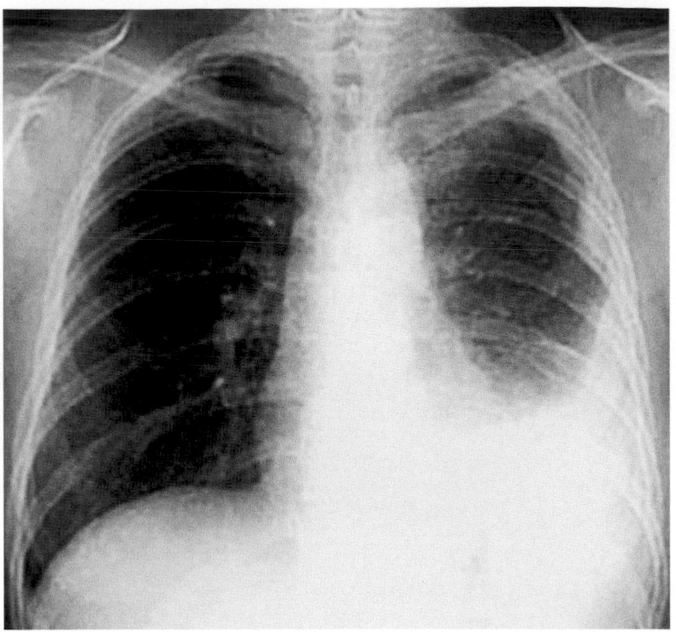

Fig. 20.1 Chest radiograph from a patient with malignant pleural mesothelioma, demonstrating a large left pleural effusion.

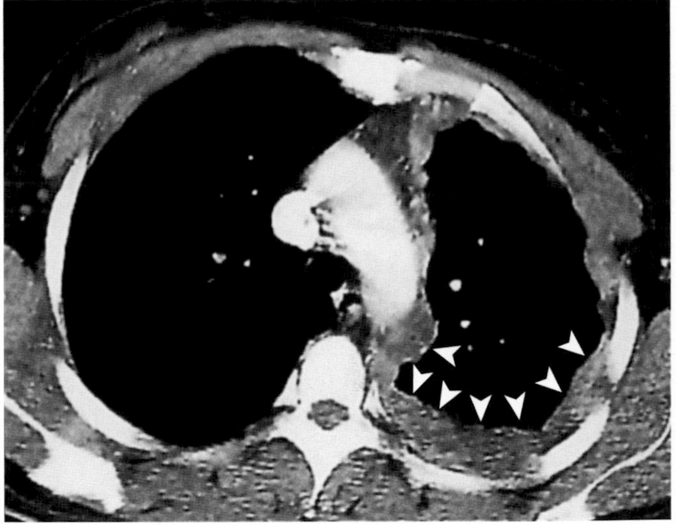

Fig. 20.2 Computed tomographic scan of the chest from a patient with pleural mesothelioma. A multinodular and confluent tumor of the left chest is apparent (arrowheads).

Malignant mesothelioma

Clinical findings in cases of pleural mesothelioma

Patients with malignant pleural mesothelioma are typically adults over the age of 50 years,[3–6] but there have also been several well-documented examples of this tumor in children.[7–9] Very rarely, familial clustering of MM has been reported, with parent–child or sibling–sibling combinations being represented.[10–13] To date, there have been no reports of spouse–spouse concurrences.

The most common presentation of MM is with progressive shortness of breath.[4,5,14,15] Unilateral chest pain is also relatively frequent, and this may or may not have pleuritic characteristics. Another possible but rarer manifestation is that of flu-like illness, with malaise, anorexia, low-grade fever, myalgias, and weight loss.[16–19] Distant metastasis of MM to lymph nodes or other anatomic sites at presentation is extraordinarily uncommon.[20,21]

Plain-film chest radiographs typically show a unilateral pleural effusion, which may be massive in volume despite relatively minor symptoms (Fig. 20.1). Re-imaging after thoracentesis often reveals diffuse pleural thickening; more rarely, a single discrete pleural mass may be observed.[22–25] Computed tomographic (CT) and magnetic resonance imaging (MRI) scans of the thorax are more sensitive than plain films for demonstrating tumor invasion of contiguous anatomic structures[25–27] (Fig. 20.2). They are also superior in showing the presence of pleural plaques and pleural calcifications, which are sensitive markers of asbestos exposure; one or both of them are

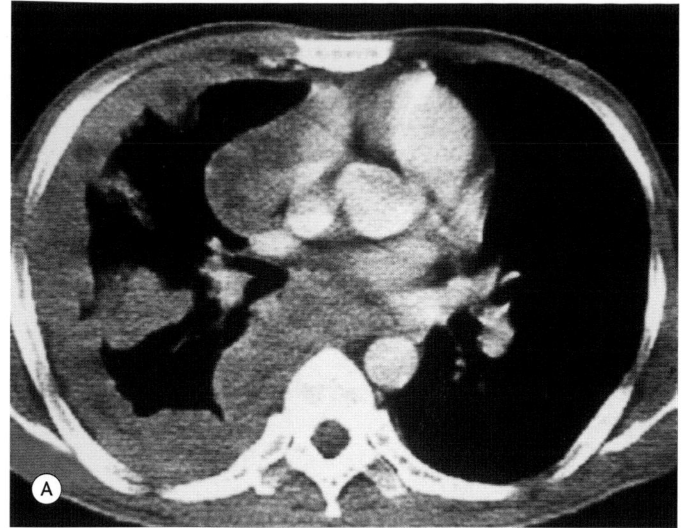

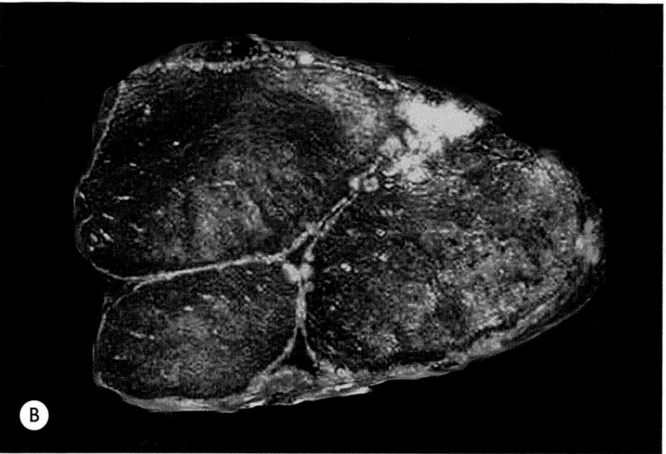

Fig. 20.3 (A) Computed tomographic scan of the chest and (B) autopsy specimen from a patient with pseudomesotheliomatous adenocarcinoma of the right lung. The tumor encases the right lung both radiographically and grossly, recapitulating the features of mesothelioma.

seen in 85% or more of all individuals who are exposed to that mineral group at an above-background level.[28,29]

Other laboratory abnormalities in MM cases are relatively few and nondescript. However, a substantial proportion of patients have tumor-related thrombocytosis, with platelet counts >400,000 mm^3.[30–30c] That finding may relate to the elaboration of interleukin-6 by the tumor cells, inasmuch as that cytokine is known to stimulate thrombopoiesis and is often elevated in both pleural fluid and serum in individuals with MM.[33] As expected, an excess of thrombotic events is associated with MM-related thrombocythemia.[30]

It must be emphasized that none of the clinical findings just mentioned is specific for MM, and they may also be encountered in connection with other primary pleural neoplasms or metastases to the pleura. In particular, the peculiar form of lung cancer known as "pseudomesotheliomatous" (pleurotropic) adenocarcinoma (see Ch. 16) is capable of reproducing the symptomatic and radiographic constellation of abnormalities associated with mesothelioma[31–33] (Fig. 20.3).

Regarding the procurement of diagnostic biopsy specimens in MM cases, video-assisted thoracoscopic surgery (VATS) is now the preferred method for obtaining such tissue.[34,35] Video-assisted thoracoscopic surgery is superior to cytologic sampling of pleural fluid and closed-needle biopsies because of its much greater yield. It also produces a specimen of sufficient size for visualization of microarchitectural landmarks. Finally, the morbidity associated with VATS is very low. In particular, cytologic examination of pleural fluid produces positive results in only a minority of cases. That is probably because the free surfaces of MMs are often coated with layers of fibrinoinflammatory exudates, with or without a benign mesothelial reaction. This process "walls off" the tumor cells and prevents them from shedding freely into the pleural fluid.[36,37]

One unwanted but common complication of thoracic biopsies in MM cases is the growth of tumor along needle or instrumentation tracks in the chest wall.[38,39] The reason for this peculiar behavior is currently unknown.

In general, once the clinical presence of diffuse pleural MM has been established, ensuing survival is limited. Most patients live roughly 1 year after diagnosis, regardless of the type of therapeutic intervention that is used.[40–43] However, a small minority of individuals with good overall performance status and limited intrathoracic disease may be candidates for extrapleural pneumonectomy (EPP).[41,44] That procedure has resulted in lengthened median survivals in some published series;[44] however, a significant proportion of patients go on to demonstrate the presence of distant metastases of MM under such circumstances, perhaps because of this shift in the natural history of the tumor. Radiotherapy has also been given after EPP, especially for the attempted salvage of patients with recurrent tumor.[43] Nevertheless, along with most chemotherapeutic approaches and immunomodulation,[45] that treatment modality has not produced uniformly encouraging results. Pisani et al.[18] assessed the outcome of patients with MM who were seen at one large tertiary care facility. They concluded that an epithelial histologic subtype, a favorable overall performance score, relatively young age, and the absence of chest pain were all correlated with better survival.

A more favorable prognosis is associated with *localized* malignant pleural mesothelioma, a rare lesion.[46–48] It often grows preferentially into the soft tissue of the chest wall rather than along the pleural surface, and thus presents itself as a discrete mass. Radical surgery removal of localized mesothelioma results in long-term survival in up to 50% of cases.[48]

Etiologic considerations regarding malignant pleural mesothelioma

The potential causal association between pleural mesotheliomas and occupational-level asbestos exposure is well known. Practically speaking, however, physicians rarely concern themselves with the etiology of these tumors at a clinical level, because diagnosis and therapy are the principal focuses of their attention. In that context, pathologic findings are, by far, the most important consideration.

However, the nearly-ubiquitous involvement of attorneys in mesothelioma cases, as part of the burgeoning field known as "toxic tort" law,[49] has compelled physicians to acquire a working familiarity with the pathogenetic underpinnings of MM. Because of this reality, a brief review of that subject will be provided here; additional information is housed in Chapter 9, which deals specifically with pneumoconioses.

In the early-to-mid 1960s, a causal connection between high-level inhalation of amphibole-class asbestos fibers and mesothelioma was first established to the satisfaction of the medical community at large, through the efforts of Wagner et al. and others.[50–53] At first, epidemiologic study was the principal tool whereby this association was identified. However, that avenue of investigation – in which exposures are determined primarily by word-of-mouth information – is applicable to patient *groups* rather than individuals. In the current social environment of the 21st century, epidemiologic questioning and medical history taking are plagued by significant problems in trying to determine the causation of any given single case of MM. This is true because media-related exposure of the potential linkage between mesothelioma and asbestos has been robust. Therefore, patients with that tumor are inculcated with the belief that they *must* have been exposed to asbestos somewhere and somehow in the past. Moreover, another very real issue concerning the pathogenesis of MM is whether chrysotile-type asbestos – the most commonly used representative of that mineral group in the past several decades – is effective as a carcinogen in this specific context. Current data suggest that chrysotile has very weak activity in regard to mesotheliomagenesis.[54–57] Hence, "asbestos exposure" as a generic term has an indefinite and imprecise meaning for individual patients in the absence of other data.[58]

Fortunately, objective information is available to address this area of causation; this is important not only for the courts – where it can be used to provide concrete fact instead of hearsay – and also for physicians who are committed to the principles of evidence-based medicine. Examination of pathologic specimens continues to be a lynchpin in this setting. If conventional light microscopic scrutiny of sections of lung parenchyma demonstrates asbestos bodies at an above-background density, or those structures are seen in intrathoracic lymph nodes, it may be concluded that a mesothelioma in the same case is indeed asbestos-related. Similarly, the radiographic or pathologic presence of pleural plaques or pleural calcifications serves a comparable purpose.[59] Ultimately, the most direct and best approach to evaluating the presence of asbestos in lung tissue is to perform a digestion analysis of representative parenchymal samples (Fig. 20.4), comparing the density of asbestos fibers found by such methods to that which is present in a carefully assembled age- and sex-matched control population, acquired from the same geographic region as that in which the patient lived.[60]

Using the last of these techniques, Roggli et al. have shown that a bimodal distribution of pulmonary asbestos burdens is associated with pleural MMs.[61] The majority of patients (group I) have a density of asbestos bodies above 20 per gram of wet lung tissue using the methods

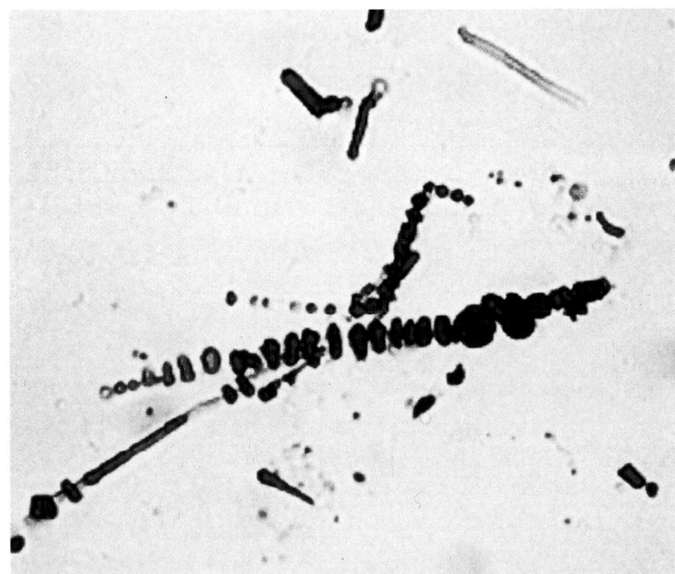

Fig. 20.4 Multiple asbestos bodies are present in this lung tissue digest preparation, taken from a patient with above-background asbestos exposure.

of those authors. The remaining population of cases (group II) manifests an asbestos burden identical to that seen in appropriate reference cohorts. These data strongly support the conclusion that group II MMs are *not* etiologically related to asbestos, and, in the absence of other potential causes (see below), those cases are properly termed "idiopathic" or "spontaneous" mesotheliomas. Practically speaking, one can employ the latter designation if no objective support for asbestos causation is apparent in a case in question, based on a review of thoracic imaging studies, pleuropulmonary tissue biopsies, or autopsy specimens of lung and pleura.[62] The proportion of MMs that is idiopathic in nature has varied from study to study in the published literature, probably as a function of geographic and chronological bias.[63] Cited percentages for this group have generally been between 25% and 40% of all pleural mesotheliomas.[64] In the authors' experience, using the objective approach just outlined, 40– 50% of MMs are spontaneous neoplasms with no definable etiologic linkage to asbestos.

Pleural mesotheliomas that are caused by asbestos develop after a long latency period, typically >20 years in duration.[65] The reason for this hiatus is not clear, but it appears that the carcinogenic effect of this mineral group requires a prolonged time – and probably a complicated set of intermediate cellular events[66–68] – to become manifest.

Other documented etiologies for pleural MM besides asbestos undeniably exist.[62,63,69] These include prior therapeutic irradiation to the anatomic region in which the mesothelioma develops;[70–75] chronic serosal inflammation, such as that associated with tuberculosis, pleural empyema, familial Mediterranean fever, or chronic collagen vascular diseases (e.g. rheumatoid arthritis or lupus erythematosus);[76–79] membership in familial "cancer kindreds" ("Lynch families");[12,13,80] prior administration of Thorotrast, a radiological imaging agent;[81,82] and inhalational exposure to erionite, a mineral group that is largely restricted geographically to Turkey.[83,84] Infection with Simian virus-40 has recently been examined as another possible cause of human mesothelioma, with contradictory conclusions.[85–89] For now, it would be premature to make a definite determination on a potential etiologic role for that agent, singly or in combination with other factors. Interestingly, mesothelioma is a well-documented malignancy of cattle and other animals (both wild and domesticated) in veterinary practice, and the clinicopathologic attributes of such animal tumors are comparable in every way to those of spontaneous human MMs.[90–96] Further attention to the potential pathogeneses of veterinary mesotheliomas could possibly be illuminating in a mechanistic sense.

Pathological features of pleural mesothelioma

The pathologic attributes of mesotheliomas can be considered at several levels of examination, beginning with their macroscopic features and extending through their molecular–biological characteristics. This information is summarized in the following sections.

Gross attributes of mesothelioma of the pleura

Pleural mesothelioma may occasionally produce striking clinical symptoms, including large pleural effusions, while the tumor is still invisible radiographically. Moreover, direct examination of the pleural surfaces in such cases – via such techniques as VATS – likewise may be relatively unrevealing, and a pathologic diagnosis of MM in biopsies done in such circumstances is often met with disbelief. Only the passage of time, with progressive development of the characteristic phenotype of mesothelioma, may suffice to convince all concerned that the tumor is actually present.

More typically, however, clinical abnormalities are accompanied by multifocal "studding" of the visceral or parietal pleural surfaces – or both –by firm white-gray nodules that individually measure up to several centimeters in diameter. With time, these become innumerable and confluent, obliterating the pleural cavity and often forming a thick layer of constricting neoplastic tissue (Figs 20.5 and 20.6). Invasion of contiguous structures, including the peripheral lung parenchyma, pericardium

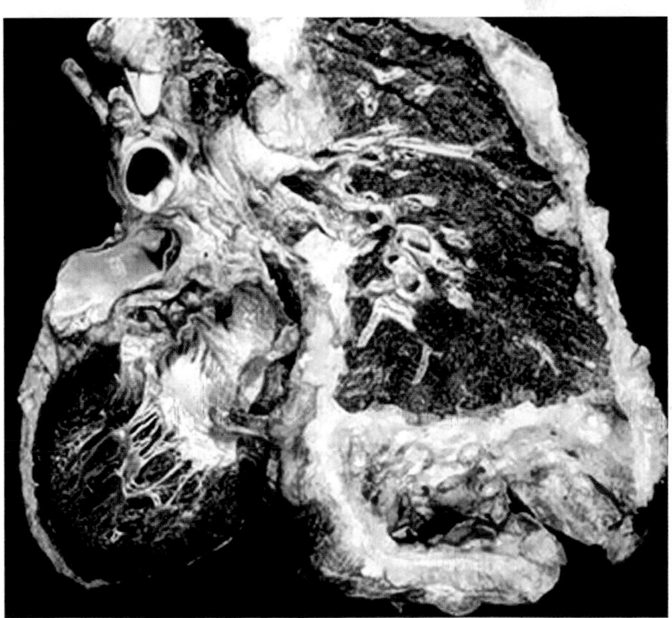

Fig. 20.5 Gross photograph of malignant pleural mesothelioma, taken at autopsy. The tumor envelops one lung and is adherent to mediastinal structures as well.

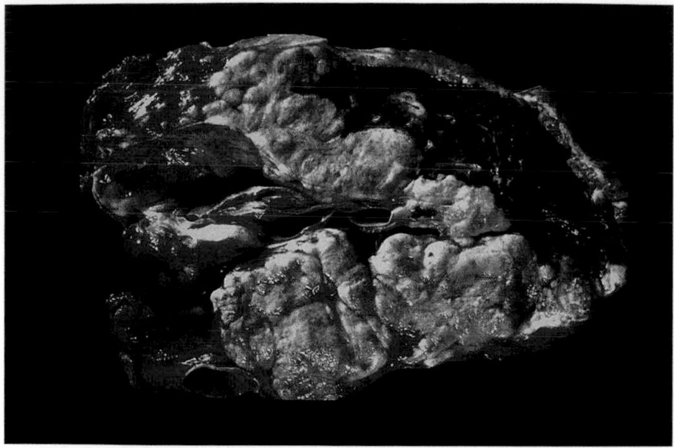

Fig. 20.6 Gross photograph of malignant pleural mesothelioma, showing a bulky mass that effaces the pleural space and compresses the lung.

and myocardium, adventitia of the great thoracic blood vessels, and soft tissue of the chest wall, is common as tumor growth advances. In addition, mesotheliomas of the pleura may cross the central apertures of the diaphragm to secondarily involve the peritoneal cavity,[97] and they are also capable of crossing the mediastinum to involve the contralateral hemithorax. If the patient survives long enough, the terminal image of the tumor may be that of a dense rind of tissue that encases the viscera of the chest.[98] Grossly visible metastases in regional lymph nodes and distant sites may also be appreciated, but they generally appear only late in the clinical course. It should be noted that there is nothing specific about the macroscopic characteristics just outlined. They are potentially common to MM, metastatic carcinoma in the pleural spaces, pleural lymphoma, and primary pleural sarcomas.[31–33,99,100]

Solitary (localized) MMs of the pleura most often grow exophytically into the soft tissue of the chest or, alternatively, into the subjacent lung parenchyma, rather than spreading along the serosal surfaces.[48] As such, they can macroscopically simulate peripheral carcinomas of the lung.

The cut surfaces of mesotheliomas are nondescript. Most often these neoplasms are white-gray with a relatively firm consistency on sectioning, because of the stromal fibrosis they incite. Desmoplastic MMs are particularly dense when they are incised in the operating room or the gross pathology laboratory.

Cytopathologic features of malignant pleural mesothelioma

Mesothelial proliferations in the pleura have a wide spectrum of potential cytomorphologic appearances, and can rightfully be included in several generic cytologic categories that encompass small round cell tumors,

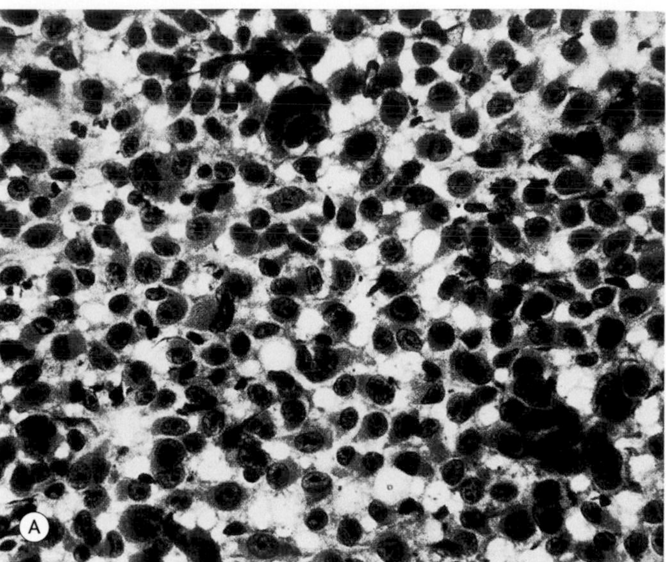

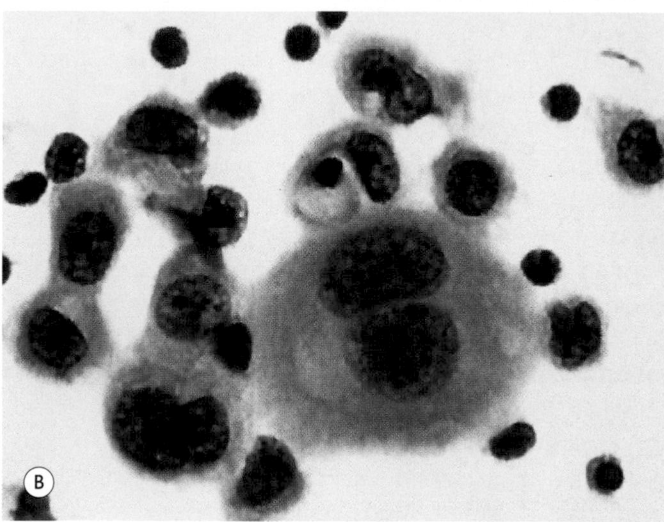

Fig. 20.7 (A) Dense cellularity is evident in this cytologic preparation of pleural fluid from a patient with pleural mesothelioma. (B) The tumor cells show substantial nuclear pleomorphism, with coarse chromatin.

polygonal cell malignancies, spindle cell and pleomorphic lesions, and neoplasms with mixed cellular features.[101] Traditionally, however, three broad histopathologic patterns of mesothelioma have been considered: epithelial (including tubulopapillary, oncocytoid/deciduoid, clear cell, and small cell subtypes), sarcomatoid (including desmoplastic and "lymphohistiocytoid" variants), and biphasic. These lesions may, on occasion, show other unusual histopathologic features, such as the presence of extensive myxoid change, adenomatoid tumor-like images, "rhabdoid" features, and metaplastic formation of bone and cartilage.

Epithelial mesothelioma is composed of sheets and clusters of variably atypical epithelioid cells in effusion cytology specimens. Such samples are typically densely cellular (Fig. 20.7). Mitotic figures and background necrosis are uncommon, but those two features may certainly be apparent in high-grade lesions. Epithelial MMs may also show papillary or tubulopapillary cell groups (Fig. 20.8), and, in thoracentesis specimens, the malignant cells may be surprisingly bland cytologically.[102–107] Conversely, benign reactive mesothelia can show an alarming degree of nuclear atypia, compounding their diagnostic separation from malignancies.[104,108] Groups of both reactive and neoplastic mesothelial cells may demonstrate intercellular spaces or "windows," and sufficient dispersion of such elements shows the presence of fuzzy cell membranes owing to the presence of elongated plasmalemmal microvilli (Fig. 20.9). Nuclear-to-cytoplasmic ratios are high in obviously anaplastic MMs, but many tumors lack this feature. Small cell epithelial mesothelioma demonstrates tightly clustered cell groups with scant cytoplasm and no obvious microvilli; it may be exceedingly similar cytomorphologically to other small cell malignant neoplasms, particularly small cell neuroendocrine carcinoma[109] (Fig. 20.10). *Sarcomatoid mesothelioma* comprises cytologically malignant dyshesive

Fig. 20.8 A tubular profile of tumor cells is apparent in this pleural fluid cytology preparation of malignant mesothelioma.

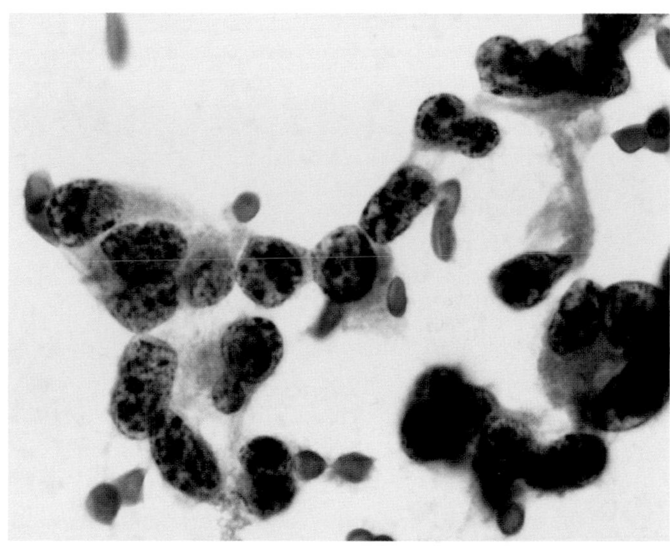

Fig. 20.10 Cytologic specimen from a case of small cell malignant mesothelioma of the pleura. A morphological similarity to small cell lung carcinoma is readily evident.

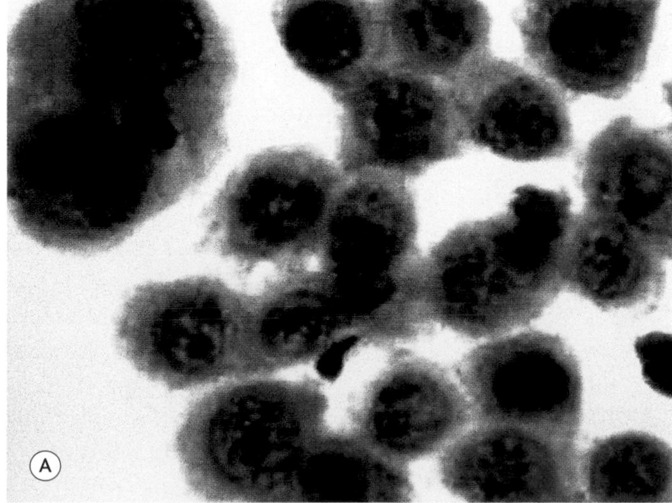

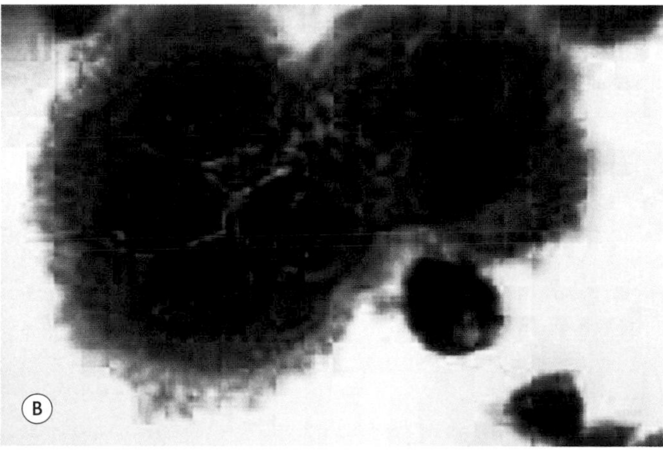

Fig. 20.9 (A,B) "Fuzzy" cell membranes are apparent in this example of malignant mesothelioma in a pleural fluid cytology specimen. That finding relates to the presence of elaborate plasmalemmal microvilli.

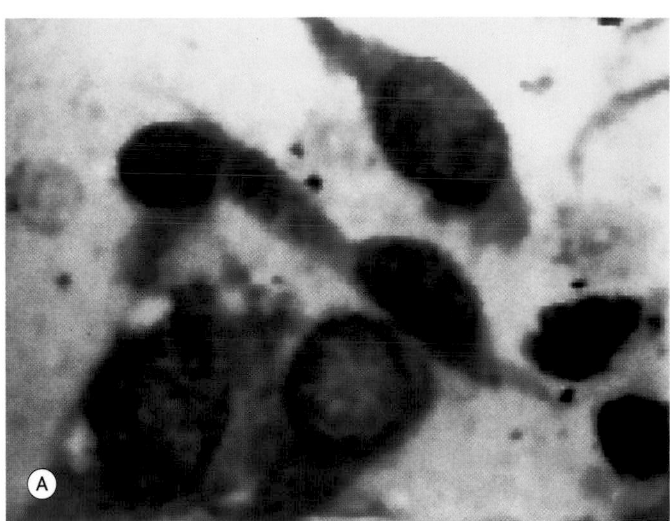

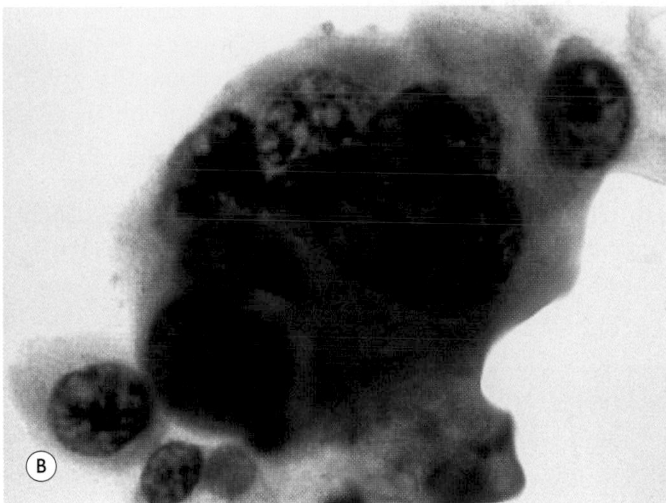

Fig. 20.11 (A,B) Cytologic specimen of sarcomatoid malignant pleural mesothelioma, showing dyshesive and pleomorphic tumor cells.

fusiform cell proliferations that cytologically imitate other tumors of mesenchymal origin, i.e. sarcomas[110] (Fig. 20.11). In pleural effusions, the tumor cells of sarcomatoid MM are few in number if they are present at all, with scant cytoplasm, elongated nuclei, and rare mitotic figures. A subtype of this variant is the *desmoplastic mesothelioma*, which is characterized histologically by a bland appearance of the spindle cells that are embedded in a hypocellular, abundantly collagenized stroma.[111] As one might expect, diagnostic tumor cells from desmoplastic tumors rarely, if ever, are shed into effusions. *"Lymphohistiocytoid"* mesothelioma has also been regarded as a sarcomatoid MM variant,[112] but it actually bears more resemblance to "lymphoepithelioma-like" carcinomas of various organs than to true sarcomas. In that lesion, one sees syncytia of polyhedral cells with prominent nucleoli, admixed with numerous mature lymphocytes. *Biphasic mesotheliomas* manifest a combination of the cytomorphologic patterns that are expected in epithelial and sarcomatoid tumors.[103]

In the past, many pathologists have been reluctant to make a definitive diagnosis of mesothelioma based only on effusion cytology specimens, in light of the pitfalls mentioned above. However, the authors' experience in recent years has been that this hesitancy is often unnecessary. If several pleural fluid samples in a given case consistently show dense cellularity, an overwhelming dominance of cells with clearly mesothelial morphologic features, three-dimensional cellular aggregates, and at least some nuclear atypia, a diagnosis of MM is likely. This interpretation can be solidified by preparation of cell block sections (Fig. 20.12) and application of adjunctive studies.[113,114] Therefore, a conclusive opinion can indeed be rendered by the cytopathologist in a sizable proportion of mesothelioma cases.

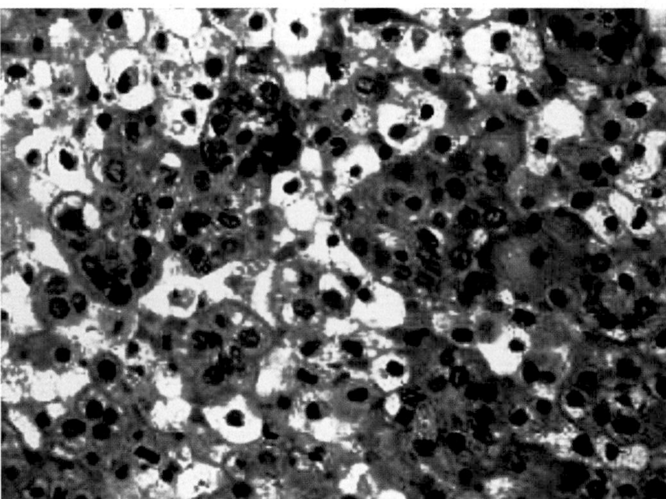

Fig. 20.12 Cell block preparation of pleural fluid in a case of malignant mesothelioma, demonstrating a solid sheet of epithelioid tumor cells with atypical nuclear profiles.

Histopathologic attributes of pleural mesotheliomas

Mesothelioma generally – but not always – spreads multifocally throughout the pleural soft tissues, demonstrating invasion of the peripheral-most subpleural lung tissue in many cases. Other uncommon histologic patterns of growth have been noted by Nind et al.,[115] including lymphangitic spread in the lung; pulmonary alveolar permeation through the pores of Kohn; and lepidic intra-

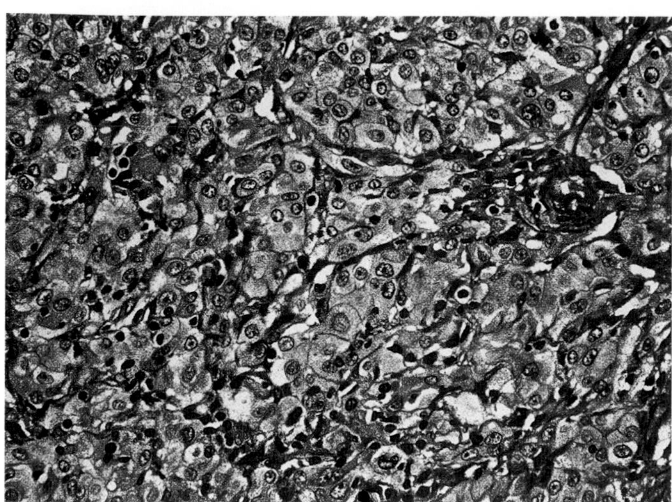

Fig. 20.13 "Solid" malignant mesothelioma of the pleura, comprising confluent sheets and nests of polygonal tumor cells.

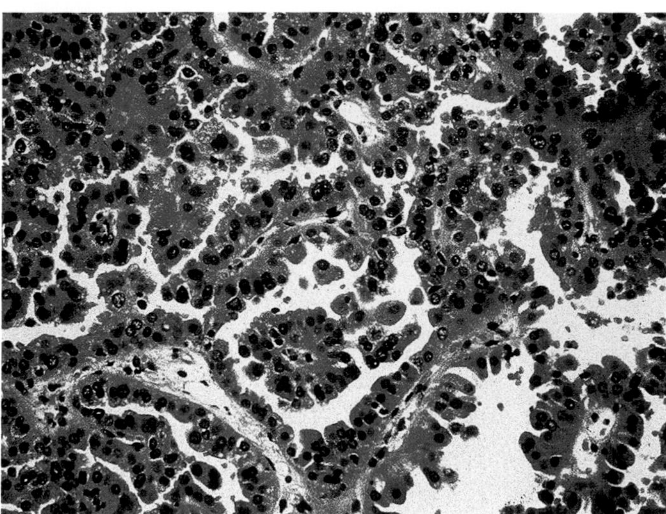

Fig. 20.14 Tubulopapillary malignant pleural mesothelioma, demonstrating micropapillary profiles of polyhedral cells.

pulmonary growth, mantling alveolar septa. The general histologic categorization of MMs has been outlined above. However, additional details will be provided in the following sections.

Epithelioid mesothelioma

Epithelioid MM (EMM) is the most commonly encountered microscopic subtype of mesothelioma.[116] In the majority of cases, one sees a lesion composed of sheets and nests of polyhedral cells with moderately atypical nuclear features, and clear infiltration of the pleural soft tissue, or subjacent lung, or both. Lesions comprising uniform expanses of densely apposed polygonal cells are known as *"solid"* epithelioid MMs (Fig. 20.13). In other tumors, gland-like profiles are common; indeed, some cases demonstrate a predominance of such structures, prompting use of the terms "tubular" or "pseudoglandular" EMM. Micropapillary cell groups are also frequent, and, when they uniformly characterize the lesion, the term *"tubulopapillary" MM* is rightly applied (Fig. 20.14). Although psammomatous microcalcifications are associated with other epithelial malignancies having a papillary configuration, they are only very rarely seen in pleural mesotheliomas.[117]

A useful diagnostic finding in EMM concerns the tinctorial properties of the tumoral stroma. Lightly hematoxylinophilic and myxoid material may be seen between epithelioid cell groups in this lesion, representing the presence of stromal mucin.[118] Although it is not absolutely specific, this observation does favor an interpretation of MM over one of carcinoma. An extension of the same property is reflected by the cytoplasmic characteristics of some tumor cells in EMM, which demonstrate macrovacuoles having a bluish cast (Fig. 20.15). These probably represent intracellular inclusions of the same stromal material.

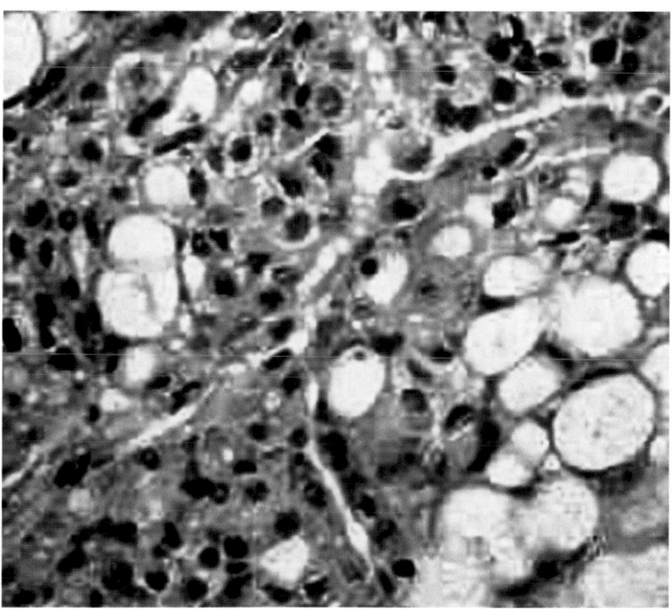

Fig. 20.15 Large cytoplasmic vacuoles are apparent in this example of malignant epithelioid pleural mesothelioma. These probably contain stromal-type mucin that is produced by the tumor cells.

One subtype of EMM has been called *"deciduoid" mesothelioma*, because of the impression that its constituent cells resemble those of decidua in the female genital tract.[119–121] As such, they assume a large polygonal cell image with relatively abundant eosinophilic cytoplasm

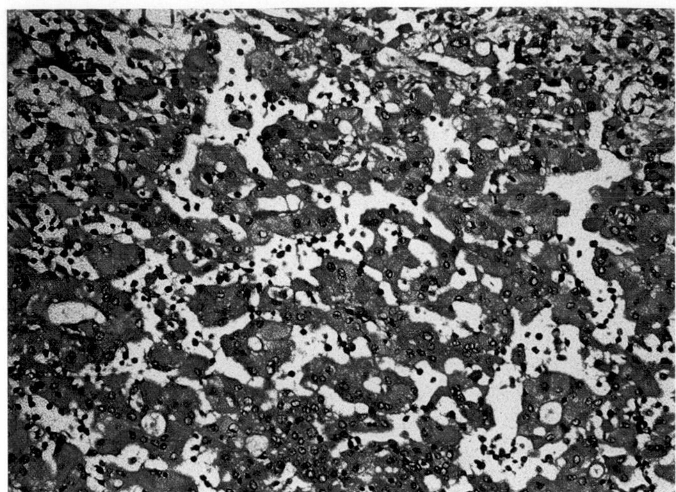

Fig. 20.16 "Deciduoid" malignant pleural mesothelioma is composed of large epithelioid cells with lightly eosinophilic cytoplasm, simulating the image of true decidua.

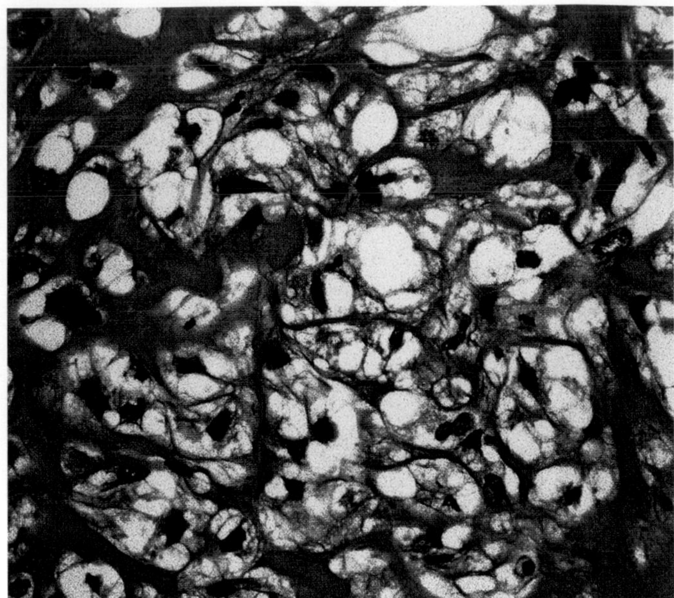

Fig. 20.17 Clear cell malignant pleural mesothelioma, demonstrating uniform cytoplasmic lucency. This change may be caused by accumulation of glycogen or lipid in the neoplastic cells.

and oval vesicular nuclei (Fig. 20.16). This relatively bland appearance belies the invasive nature of deciduoid MM, the biologic features of which are fully comparable to other forms of mesothelioma. Synonyms for this variant are "oxyphilic" or "oncocytoid" MM.[101]

Another form of EMM comprises polyhedral cells with strikingly lucent cytoplasm, and is accordingly known as *"clear cell" mesothelioma*[122–124] (Fig. 20.17). This variant is extremely uncommon, at least in pure form, and is also related to *"foam cell"* or *"lipid-rich"* MM.[125]

Rarely, foci in EMM may simulate the microscopic appearance of pleural adenomatoid tumors (see Ch. 19), with bland microcystic gland-like profiles comprising compact epithelioid cells.[126] However, other areas in those lesions typically have the conventional image of ordinary mesothelioma.

Mention must also be made here of the concept of "mesothelioma in-situ." That term has been applied to cytologically atypical proliferations of epithelioid mesothelial cells that are confined to the pleural surface, with no evidence of invasion across its basement membrane[127,128] (Fig. 20.18). Reports on that finding have been limited to cases where other areas of the pleura *did* demonstrate infiltrative MM. Hence, it is still not clear as to whether pleural mesothelioma can truly exist in an exclusively in-situ form. In fact, the authors have never seen an autopsy case which included that finding.

Sarcomatoid (spindle cell) mesothelioma

Sarcomatoid mesothelioma (SMM) comprises fusiform cells with variable degrees of atypia and pleomorphism.[110,116,129–131] These may be arranged in fascicles, storiform arrays, or random configurations (Figs 20.19 and 20.20). Tumoral collagenogenesis is likewise heterogeneous. The prevalence of mitotic activity and necrosis in such lesions generally parallels their histologic grade. A special variant of SMM is that which shows divergent differentiation into "heterologous" mesenchymal tissues such as osteoid, cartilage, and striated muscle (Fig. 20.21). It could rightly be called *"metaplastic" sarcomatoid mesothelioma*. Tumors with angiosarcoma-like foci in this category have also been termed *"pseudovascular"* or *"angiomatoid"* mesotheliomas. Myxoid stroma may also dominate the microscopic picture in occasional examples of SMM. When cellular atypia in sarcomatoid mesothelioma is extreme, the designations of "anaplastic" or *"pleomorphic"* MM are appropriate.[135]

Desmoplastic mesothelioma

As mentioned above, desmoplastic MM (DMM) is a special subtype of SMM in which spindle-shaped or stellate neoplastic cells are quite bland cytologically.[111,136–138] They are set in a markedly collagenized and hyalinized stromal matrix, often with a "basket-weave" configuration like that of pleural plaques or fibrohyaline pleuritis ("fibrous pleurisy")[111] (Fig. 20.22). Mitoses are sparse and necrosis is limited if it is present at all in desmoplastic mesothelioma. That diagnosis should be used in reference to lesions which are *entirely* composed of tissue with the

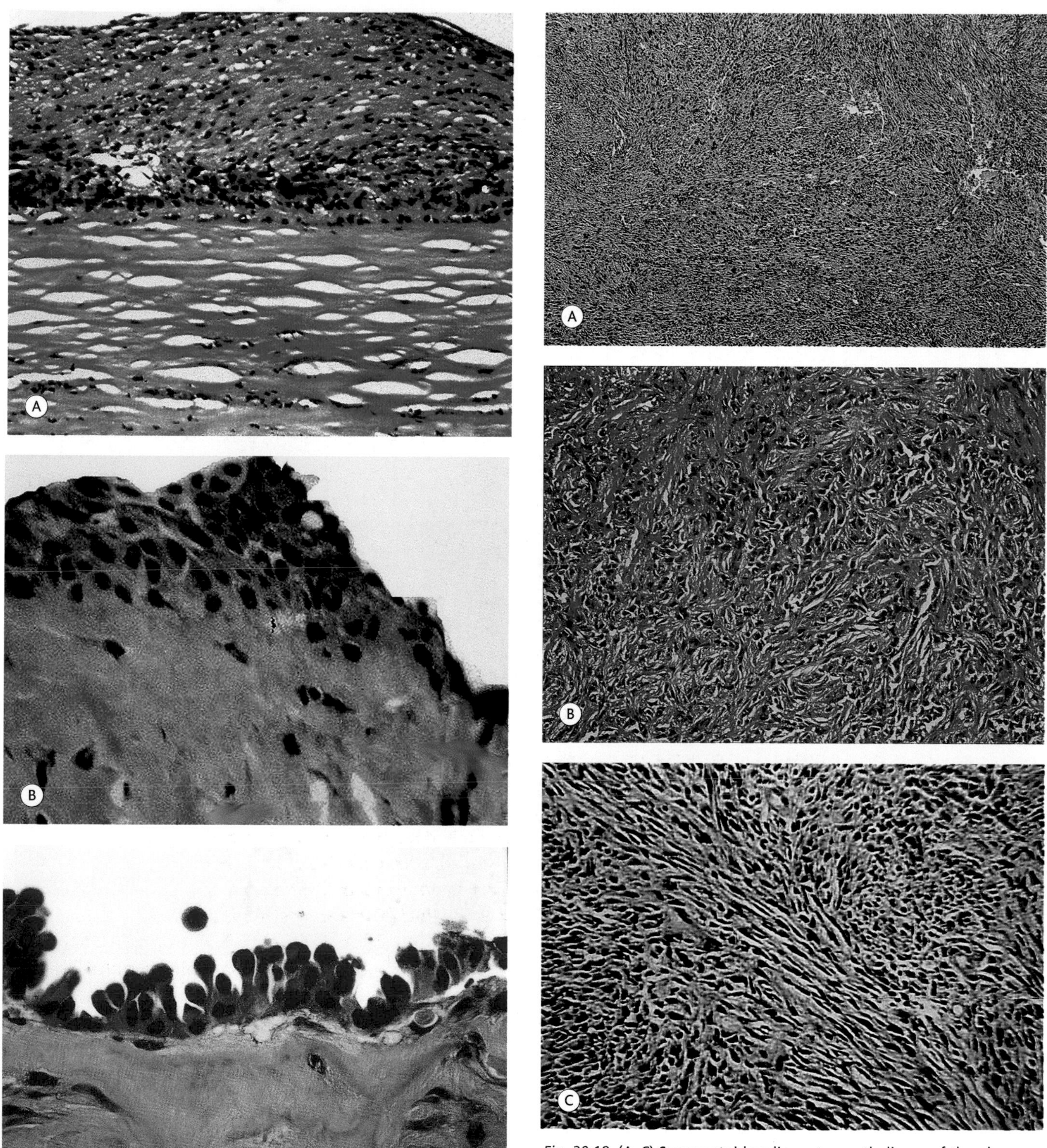

Fig. 20.18 (A–C) So-called in-situ mesothelioma, showing non-invasive foci of atypical mesothelial cells. The tumor in (A) is colonizing a pre-existing pleural plaque.

Fig. 20.19 (A–C) Sarcomatoid malignant mesothelioma of the pleura, showing a disorganized proliferation of highly atypical spindle cells.

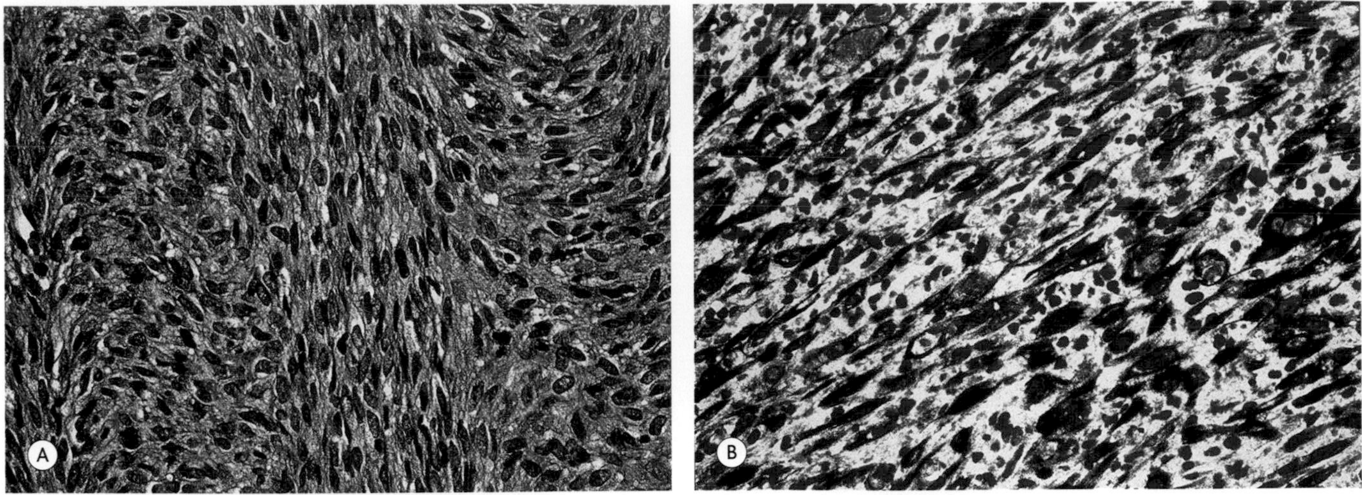

Fig. 20.20 (A) Atypical spindle cells are arranged in fascicles in another example of sarcomatoid mesothelioma. (B) A keratin immunostain demonstrates strong reactivity in the neoplastic cells.

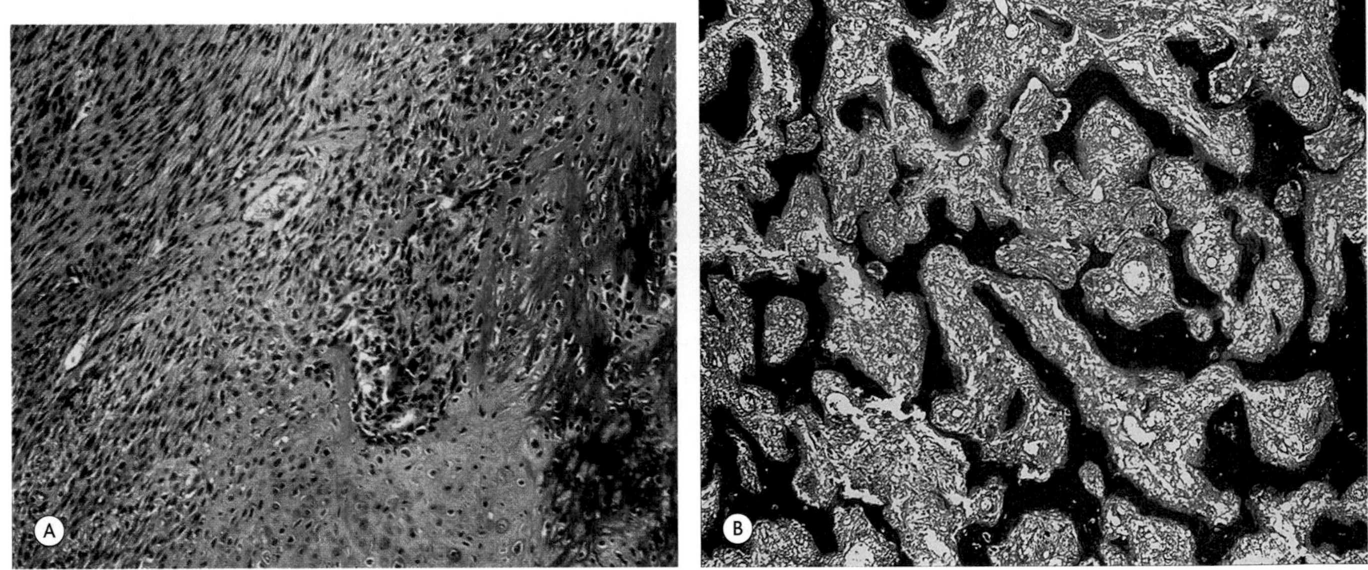

Fig. 20.21 (A,B) Divergent osteochondroid differentiation in sarcomatoid malignant pleural mesothelioma.

aforementioned characteristics. Many sarcomatoid MMs also contain small foci in which a desmoplastic image is seen.

The malignant nature of DMM is manifest by its invasion of underlying lung or adjacent soft tissues (Fig. 20.23). In addition, careful scrutiny of the tumor usually (but not always) reveals a level of cellular atypism and a degree of cellular density which exceed that of benign pleural lesions (Fig. 20.24). Moreover, there is no microscopic "zonation" in DMM. That phenomenon is best represented in fibrohyaline pleuritis, in which lesional cellularity decreases as one moves spatially from the pleural space into the subjacent tissues.[139]

Biphasic mesothelioma

As their name suggests, biphasic mesotheliomas (BMMs) are typified by admixtures of two morphologic configurations – usually at least one variant of EMM and at least one in the spectrum of SMM. Those components may be abruptly juxtaposed to one another or blend imperceptibly[116] (Fig. 20.25).

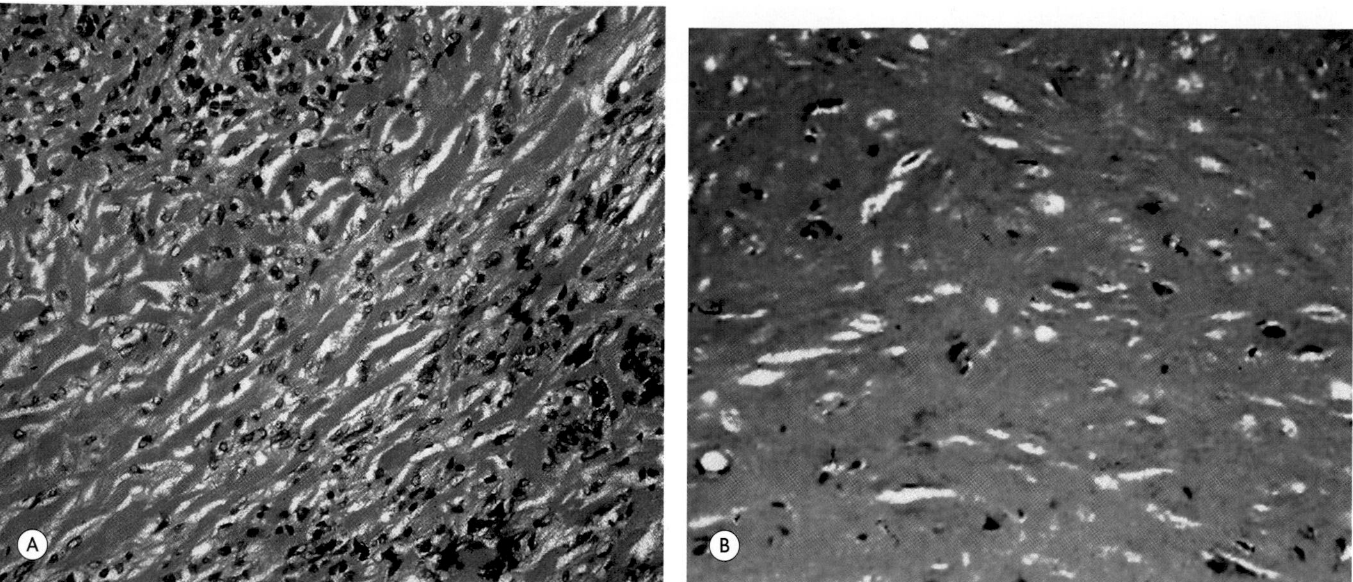

Fig. 20.22 (A,B) This example of desmoplastic pleural mesothelioma shows a relatively bland, pleural plaque-like morphologic appearance.

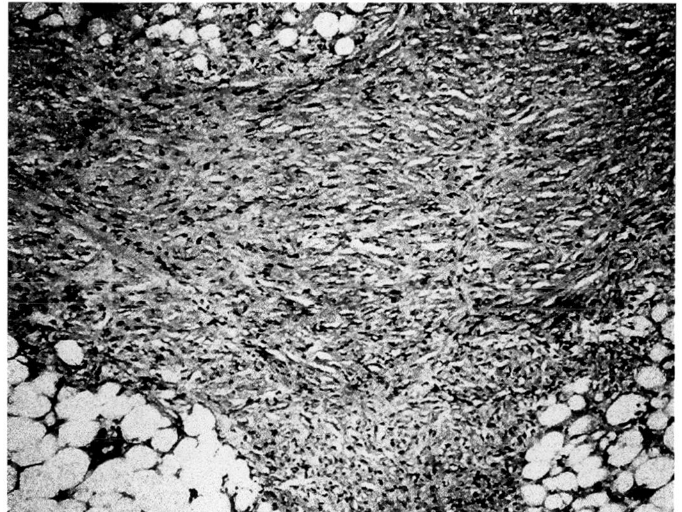

Fig. 20.23 Invasion of pleural soft tissue is apparent in this example of desmoplastic mesothelioma. Confirmation with immunohistologic stain for cytokeratin are often helpful.

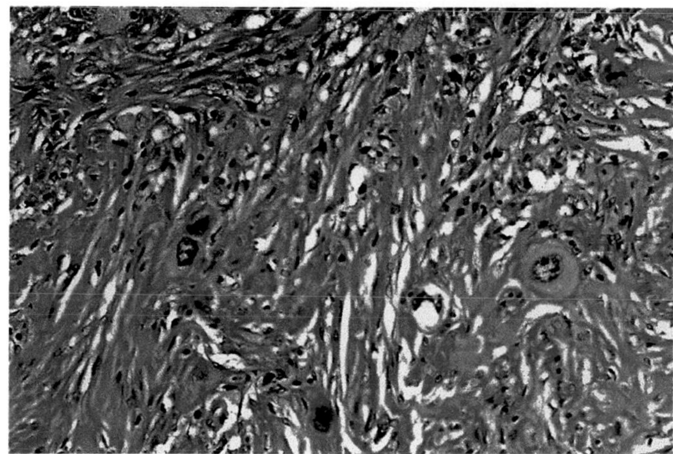

Fig. 20.24 At least focally, most examples of desmoplastic mesothelioma show significant nuclear atypia, as shown here. However, that finding is dependent on sampling.

Small cell mesothelioma

Another uncommon form of MM is that represented by small cell mesothelioma, which is technically a subtype of EMM.[109,140] It is only rarely seen in "pure" form, and usually comprises a portion of tumors with other histologic patterns. This lesion is composed of compact round cells with high nuclear-to-cytoplasmic ratios, oval nuclei with dispersed chromatin, variably discernible nucleoli, and scant amphophilic cytoplasm (Figs 20.26 and 20.27). As such, it is morphologically similar to several other malignant small cell/basaloid neoplasms, including basaloid carcinoma, high-grade neuroendocrine carcinoma, small cell melanoma, small round cell sarcomas, and non-Hodgkin lymphomas.

Rhabdoid mesothelioma

Over the past decade, it has become apparent that a relatively broad spectrum of malignant tumors may exhibit a "rhabdoid" phenotype, akin to that seen in high-grade pediatric renal neoplasms. *Extrarenal rhabdoid tumors* (ERTs) may be "pure" histologically, or they may represent a new clonal element that has arisen from another recognizable tumor type.[141] Hence, one may see ERT in combination with a definable carcinoma, melanoma,

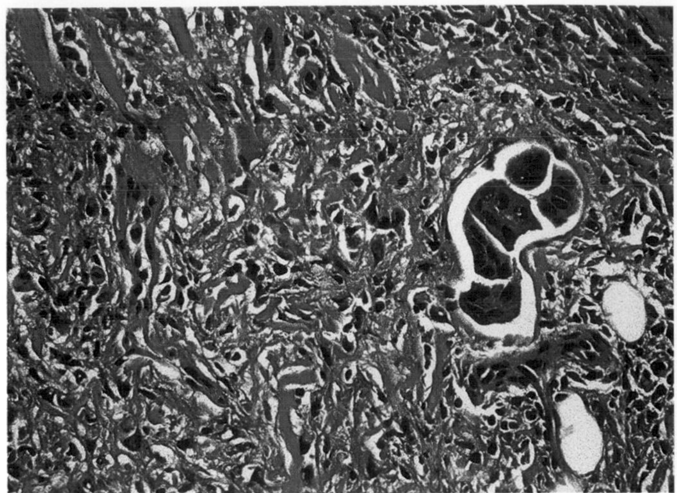

Fig. 20.25 Biphasic malignant pleural mesothelioma, showing a focus of overtly epithelioid tumor cells (right) in the midst of fusiform and pleomorphic (sarcomatoid) elements.

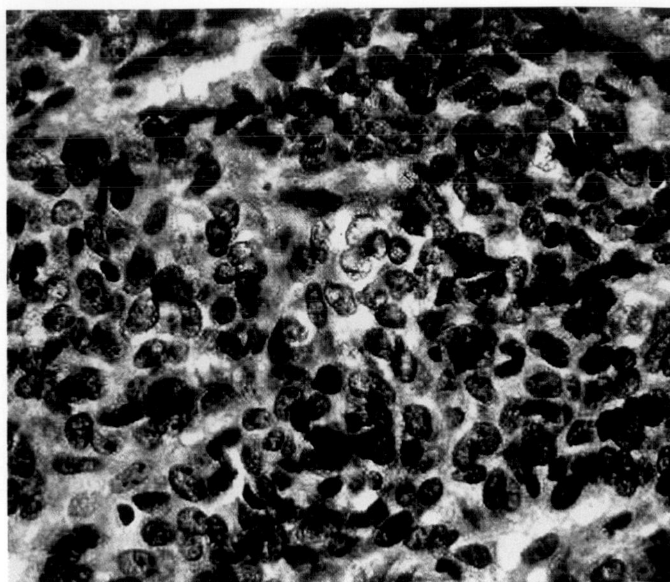

Fig. 20.27 The uniformity of tumor cells in small cell mesothelioma is well-shown in this photograph.

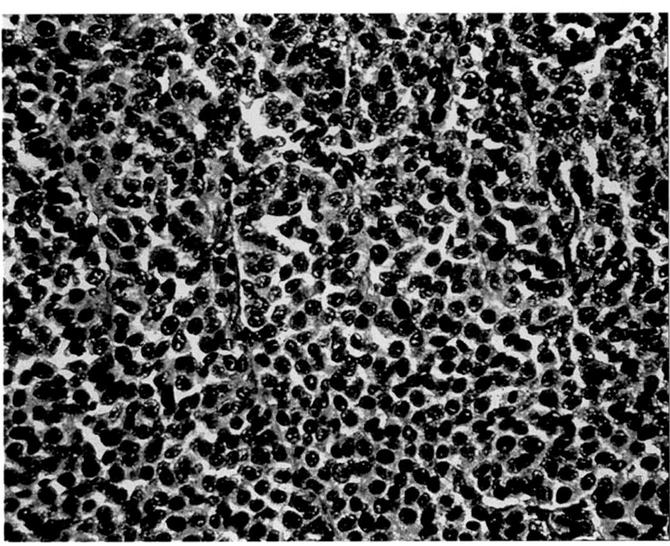

Fig. 20.26 Small cell malignant pleural mesothelioma, represented by a sheet of relatively monomorphic and compact tumor cells.

or sarcoma. In the latter instance, the term "composite" ERT is *apropos*. Malignant mesothelial tumors are no exception to these precepts. Thus, wholly rhabdoid MMs may be encountered in some cases, whereas other pleural mesotheliomas may show an "ordinary" morphotype that is admixed with ERT.[142]

Rhabdoid cells are characterized by a moderately pleomorphic epithelioid shape, eccentric nuclei with vesicular chromatin and prominent nucleoli, and distinctive eosinophilic cytoplasm having a "hard" globular quality (Fig. 20.28). They are relatively dyshesive; occasional spindle cell change and multinucleation may be seen as well.

The principal significance of a rhabdoid phenotype is the biologic aggressiveness with which it is associated, regardless of other clinicopathologic details of that individual tumor.[141] Nonetheless, because mesotheliomas as a group have such an adverse outcome, the behavioral impact of rhabdoid change is not as great in this particular context.

Histochemical features of malignant mesotheliomas of the pleura

Up until 20 years ago, the separation of MM from other histologically similar neoplasms was based largely on histochemical results. The capacity for adenocarcinomas to synthesize epithelial mucin had been recognized quickly after the application of specialized biochemical methods in surgical pathology, and it was also known that mesotheliomas did not possess that ability[143–150] (Figs 20.29 and 20.30). Conversely, MMs were found to manufacture *stromal* mucin – which was labeled by the colloidal iron (CI) or alcian blue (AB) methods at pH 2.5 – and prior treatment of tissue sections with hyaluronidase removed that substance[143,146,149,151] (Fig. 20.31). Thus, these observations set the stage for the use of the periodic acid–Schiff (PAS) technique, with and without diastase predigestion (to remove glycogen, which, like epithelial mucin, is PAS-positive); the mucicarmine method (to label epithelial mucin); and the CI or AB procedures,

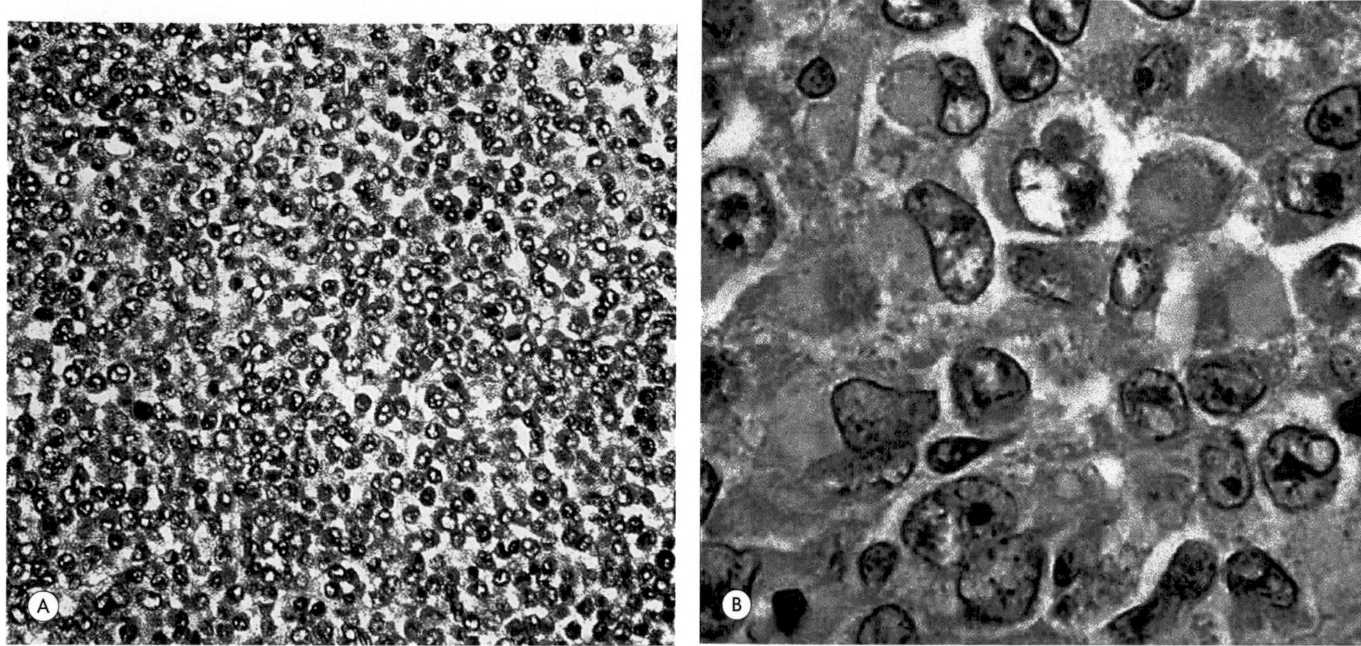

Fig. 20.28 (A) Rhabdoid malignant mesothelioma, showing a sheet of large ovoid cells which contain (B) "hard" eosinophilic paranuclear inclusions.

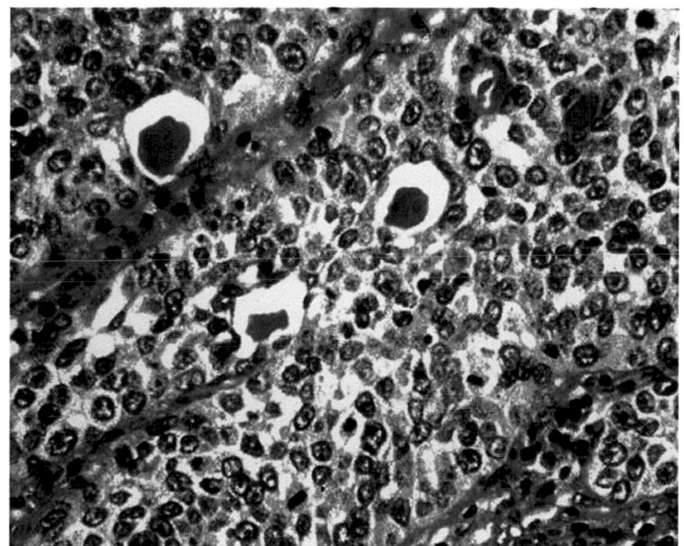

Fig. 20.29 Histochemical reactivity with the digested periodic acid–Schiff (D-PAS) method in pseudomesotheliomatous adenocarcinoma of the pleura.

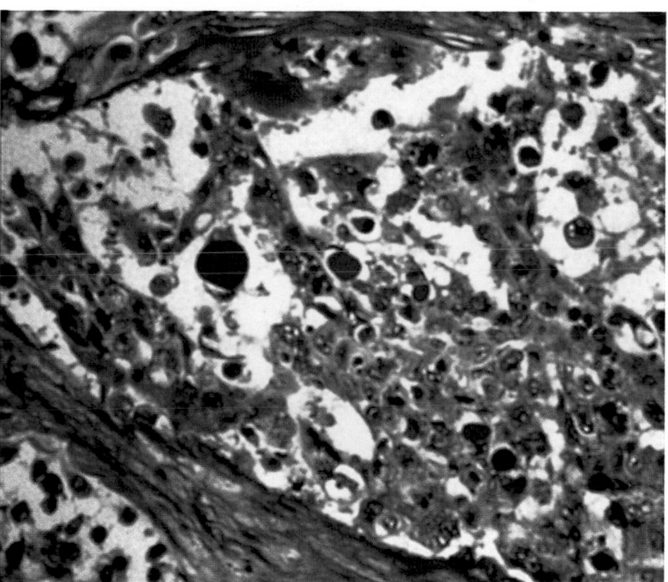

Fig. 20.30 Mucicarmine positivity is seen in this pseudomesotheliomatous adenocarcinoma.

with and without hyaluronidase pretreatment, for the histochemical delineation of adenocarcinomas and mesotheliomas.

Such an approach is still useful, but there are several caveats that must be borne in mind in this context. First, histochemical studies are most useful in the distinction of *epithelioid* mesothelioma variants from other tumors, and they lose much of their value if the differential diagnosis is that of *sarcomatoid* MM versus spindle cell carcinoma or true sarcoma. Those statements derive from the reality that carcinomas which are not overtly gland-forming lack epithelial mucin; on the other hand, sarcomatoid carcinomas and various sarcomas do have the ability to produce stromal mucin.

Providing that one observes the cautions just cited, epithelioid mesotheliomas can be distinguished from carcinomas histochemically in approximately 50% of cases.[150] The PAS-diastase technique is the most useful for

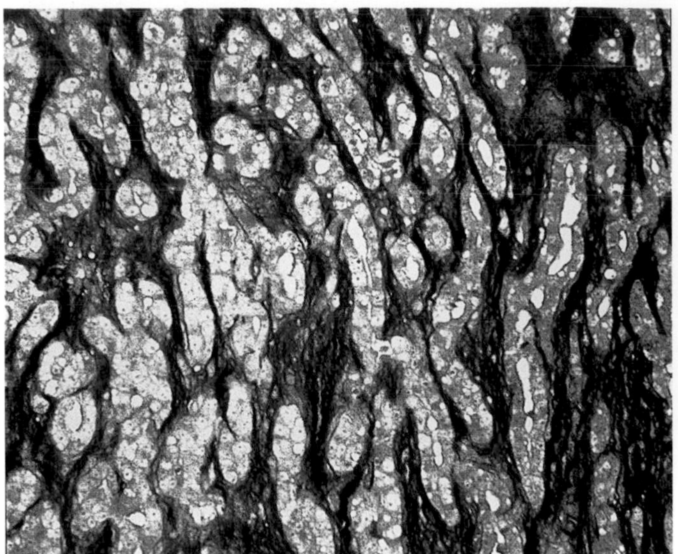

Fig. 20.31 Colloidal iron (CI) staining of malignant epithelioid pleural mesothelioma, showing the presence of intercellular stromal mucin. It is represented by blue matrix in this photomicrograph. Pretreatment of histologic sections from this case with hyaluronidase abolished the CI positivity.

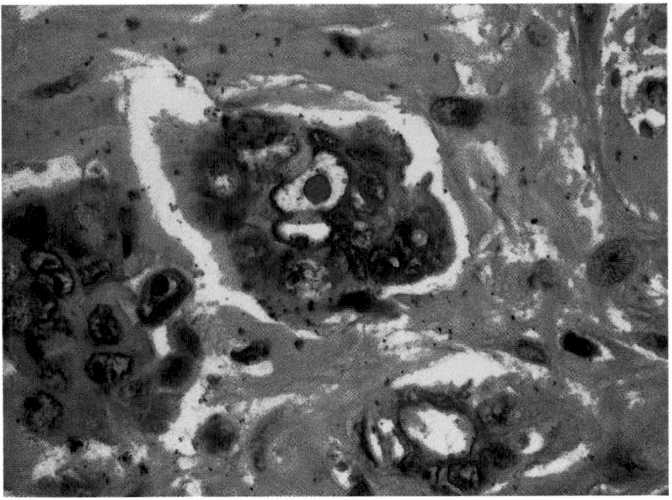

Fig. 20.32 Aberrant mucicarmine positivity in malignant epithelioid mesothelioma, which was abrogated by pretreatment of tissue sections with hyaluronidase.

that purpose, because, at least, in the authors' experience, it is more sensitive than the mucicarmine stain. Moreover, there have been sporadic reports of MMs that were spuriously labeled with the mucicarmine procedure, apparently because it unexpectedly recognized a form of stromal mucin[152] (Fig. 20.32). Pretreatment with hyaluronidase is successful in abrogating that aberrant reactivity, and therefore it should be employed routinely if mucicarmine is utilized in differential diagnoses that include epithelioid MM.

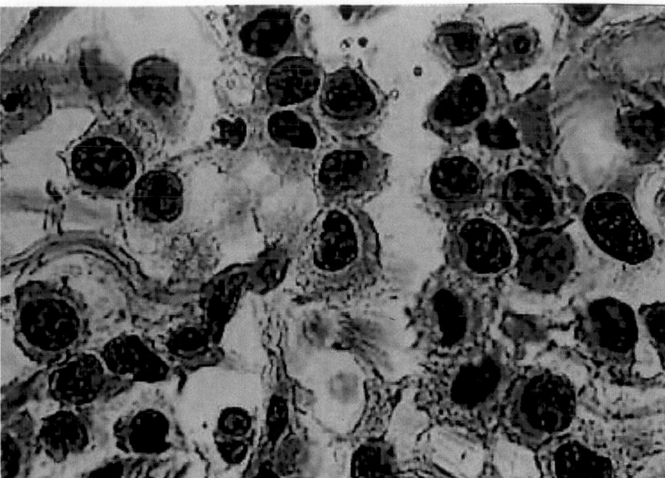

Fig. 20.33 Argyrophilic nucleolar organizer regions (AgNORs) in this malignant mesothelioma are visible as black intranuclear deposits.

In the same vein, CI and AB methods will commonly label epithelial mucin. Hence, only those epithelioid lesions that lose their CI/AB positivity after hyaluronidase predigestion are consistent with mesothelial neoplasms.[143,145–147] Again, roughly 50% of polygonal cell MMs manifest this pattern of reactivity.

During the 1980s, it was recognized that silver impregnation methods were able to label accumulations of intranuclear proteins that are associated with active transcription of nucleic acid. Known as "silver-stained nucleolar organizing regions" (argyrophilic nucleolar organizer regions or AgNORs), these silver-positive areas are now known to be related to double chromosomal "satellites," chromosome polymorphisms, and structural abnormalities involving chromosomal satellite regions.[153–155] Silver nitrate (in colloidal suspension) has an affinity for them, yielding a black precipitate, and discrete globular deposits of it are then visible in positive nuclei on conventional microscopy (Fig. 20.33). Several authors have confirmed the fact that MMs and carcinomas both have higher AgNOR counts per nucleus than do reactive mesothelial proliferations.[156–158] Therefore, the usual application of this method is not to separate mesothelioma from adenocarcinoma, but to distinguish MM from an atypical but benign mesothelial proliferation.[156,157] AgNOR values in those two groups have ranged from slightly >1 in minimally atypical benign mesothelial cells to >7.5 in highly anaplastic mesothelioma cells, usually showing a bimodal distribution in mesotheliosis and MM.[159] Despite the hopeful nature of those results, it is also unfortunately true that substantial numerical overlap exists between the two lesional groups in question. Recently, Pomjanski et al. have shown that further assessment with image

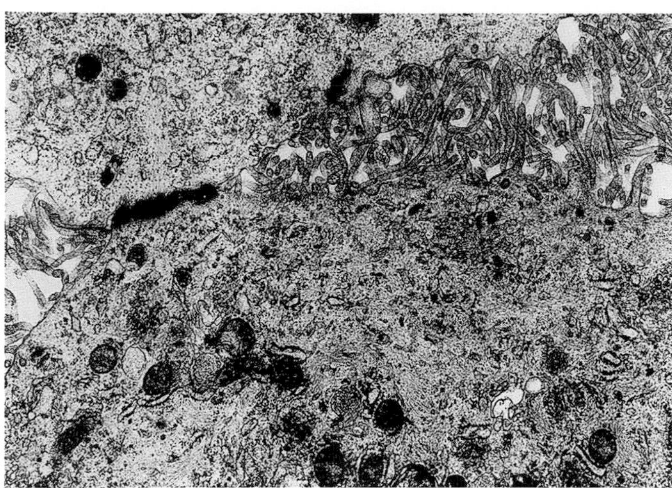

Fig. 20.34 Prominent, elongated desmosomes (left center) join the tumor cells of a malignant mesothelioma in this electron photomicrograph.

cytometry may improve the situation, and, in their hands, >95% of malignant pleural effusions were successfully separated diagnostically from benign mesothelial diatheses.[160] It remains to be seen whether or not these techniques will enter the sphere of practical surgical pathology.

Electron microscopic features of malignant mesothelioma

In the early 1970s, several investigators began to catalogue the ultrastructural characteristics of MM and compare them with those of histologically similar neoplasms.[161–163] Through the ensuing years, it has become apparent that transmission electron microscopy is an extremely effective tool in the delineation of mesothelial differentiation, and it provides valuable information in differential diagnosis with other malignancies.[164,165]

In epithelioid mesotheliomas, a constellation of findings that includes abundant tangles of cytoplasmic intermediate filaments – with focal formation of perinuclear tonofibrils – elongated and complex desmosomes (Fig. 20.34), an absence of mucin droplets, and the presence of long, branching, plasmalemmal microvilli (with a length-to-diameter ratio (LDR) of 10:1 or more)[164,167,168] (Fig. 20.35) is typical. Other common findings include cytoplasmic glycogen deposits, dilated intercellular spaces, and intracellular lumina, which are also often lined by microvilli. External microvillous projections are sometimes difficult to evaluate with regard to their dimensions, because they can be compressed and distorted when caught between adjacent tumor cells. Basal lamina is also

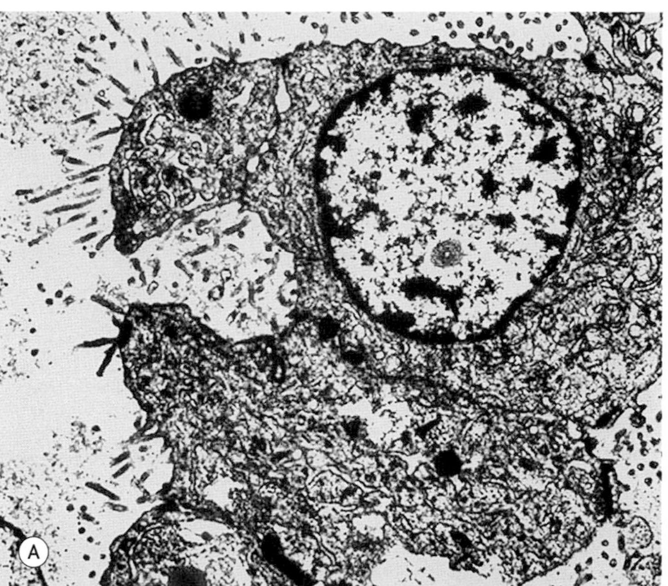

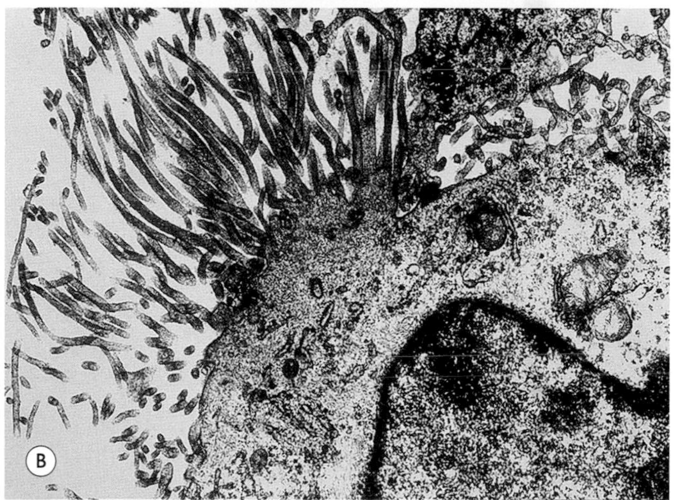

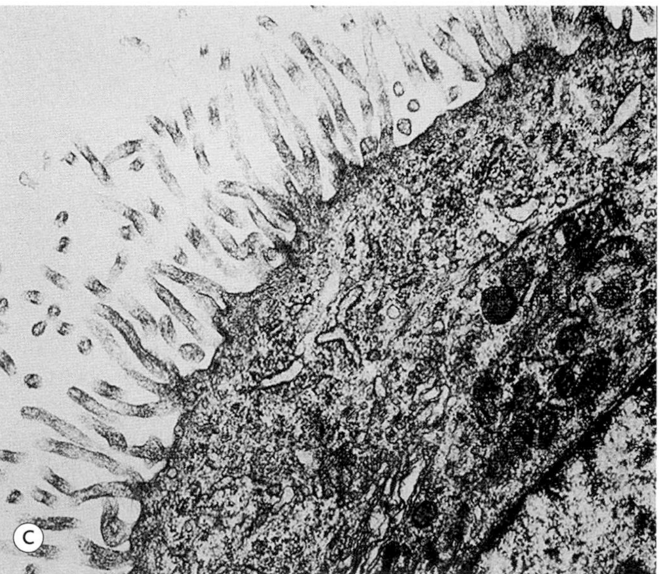

Fig. 20.35 (A–C) Elongated and "bushy" plasmalemmal microvilli are seen in these epithelioid mesotheliomas ultrastructurally.

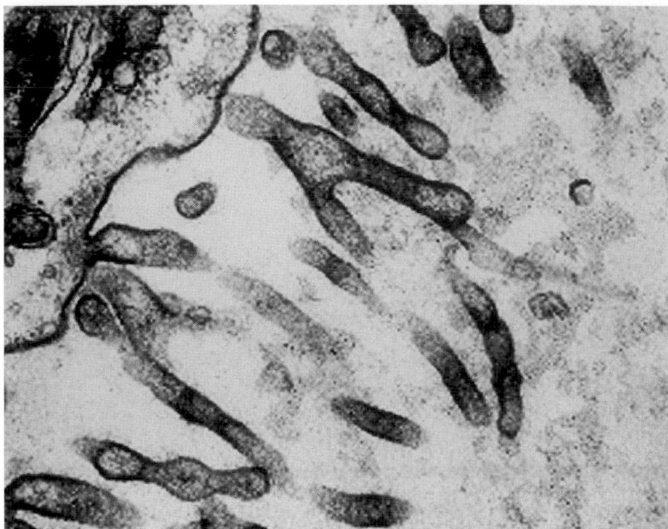

Fig. 20.36 A delicate granular coating of electron-dense material is seen on the surfaces of microvilli in this epithelioid mesothelioma.

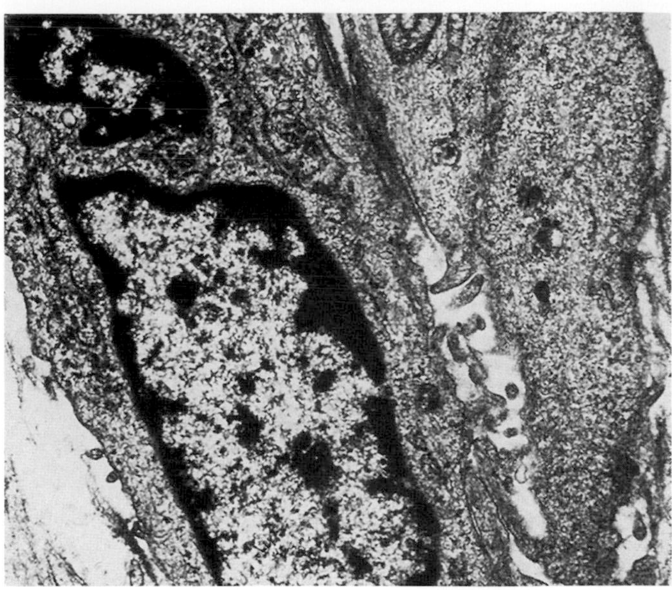

Fig. 20.37 Sarcomatoid mesothelioma differs substantialliy from epithelioid tumors by electron microscopy; this example resembles fibrosarcoma ultrastructurally.

present around many of the neoplastic cells in mesotheliomas, and the microvilli are often coated by an amorphous granular material[169,170] (Fig. 20.36).

Unfortunately, relatively few neoplasms show all of the "classical" characteristics of MM,[169] but most mesothelial tumors manifest enough of them to make their identification straightforward. In contrast, metastatic adenocarcinomas (MACs) of various anatomic origins – which represent the principal diagnostic alternative to malignant mesothelioma – exhibit short truncated microvilli and an absence of tonofibrils, and may contain intracytoplasmic mucin granules as well.[164,171–173] Wick et al.[150] performed a comparative study of electron microscopy and immunohistology in the distinction between epithelioid MM and MACs, and those two techniques were found to be comparable in diagnostic efficacy.

The polygonal cells in biphasic mesotheliomas exhibit ultrastructural features that are comparable to those of purely epithelioid MM. Thus, electron microscopy is similarly helpful in separating such tumors from biphasic sarcomatoid carcinomas involving the pleura.

On the other hand, sarcomatoid MMs lose the distinctive plasmalemmal modifications that characterize their epithelioid counterparts. Spindle cell and pleomorphic mesotheliomas most closely resemble true sarcomas at an ultrastructural level (Fig. 20.37), except for the presence of rare intercellular junctional complexes and intermediate filament bundles.[110,167,174,175] In this specific context, electron microscopic assessment is not often definitive diagnostically.

Immunohistochemical findings in malignant mesothelioma

Mesothelioma has been vigorously studied immunohistochemically over the past decade. From a histopathologic point of view, there are basically four settings in which immunophenotyping plays an important role in its diagnosis:

1. epithelioid MM versus adenocarcinoma
2. sarcomatoid mesothelioma versus primary or metastatic pleural sarcoma versus metastatic sarcomatoid carcinoma
3. epithelioid mesothelioma versus reactive mesothelial hyperplasia
4. desmoplastic sarcomatoid mesothelioma versus fibrohyaline pleuritis.

Among these problems, the one that is most commonly encountered is that of mesothelioma versus metastatic carcinoma. Despite the more uncommon nature of sarcomatoid MM, immunohistochemistry is nonetheless equally useful in its distinction from true sarcomas affecting the pleural space. However, in the remaining settings, in which differential diagnosis involves a benign or reactive condition, the practical contribution of immunophenotyping is much more limited. With specific reference to desmoplastic mesothelioma, it has been properly suggested that because of its poor prognosis and the lack of effective treatment, underdiagnosis of that tumor is preferable to overdiagnosis.[136] It may well take several biopsies to establish a definitive interpretation in such cases.

Each of the previously cited diagnostic questions is associated with differing panels of immunohistochemical reagents. For instance, in cases of possible spindle cell or desmoplastic mesothelioma, the antibodies used should principally include those to keratin, calretinin, and WT1 gene product, and other markers are necessary only to subtype a mesenchymal neoplasm if and when the keratin reaction is negative. In this context, the application of antibodies that are used to recognize overtly epithelial tumors – e.g. Ber-Ep4, CD15, CA72-4, and carcinoembryonic antigen (CEA) – is illogical. That is true because neither sarcomas nor sarcomatoid carcinomas generally synthesize the targets of those reagents.[176] In the following sections, we will review the different analytes that have been tested clinically in the study of MM, in order to provide a guide for a practical approach to immunohistochemical analysis.

Antibodies often used in the analysis of possible mesotheliomas

General and "exclusionary" markers

Keratins. Keratin antibodies have been extensively applied to MMs and their simulators, with the principal goal of distinguishing mesothelioma from adenocarcinomas[177–182] and true sarcomas. Some authors have concluded that particular staining patterns for specific keratins may allow for the separation of those tumor types, and differing degrees of contextual specificity and sensitivity have been ascribed to various keratin subsets. Most recently, antibodies to keratin 5/6 have been promoted as helpful immunohistochemical markers for MM[182] (Fig. 20.38). In one assessment, Ordoñez found that 40 examples of mesothelioma were positive for keratin 5/6, whereas 30 pulmonary adenocarcinomas were negative. However, he also observed focal reactivity in 14 of 93 cases of nonpulmonary adenocarcinoma, to some extent limiting the utility of keratin 5/6 in the exclusion of metastases to the pleura.[182] Another study reported 92% keratin 5/6 positivity in MM, and 14% labeling in cases of MAC.[183] Despite these drawbacks, keratin 5/6 does appear to be a helpful presumptive marker for mesothelioma when used in the proper fashion and the appropriate morphologic setting.

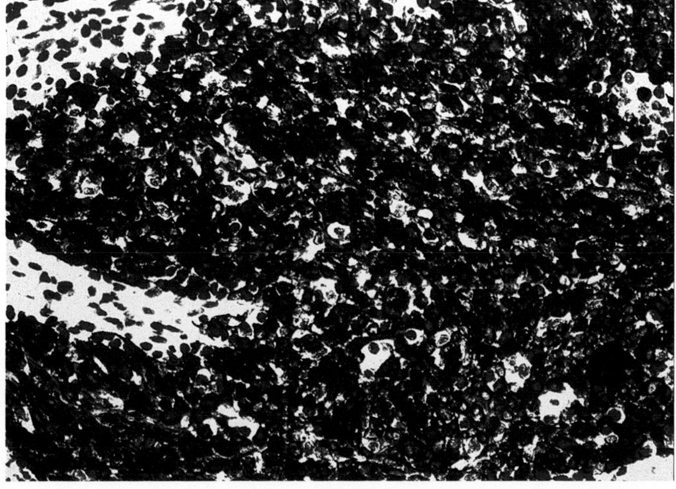

Fig. 20.38 Immunoreactivity for keratin 5 in small cell mesothelioma.

In general, it has been noted that reagents against high-molecular-weight keratins will label most mesotheliomas and relatively few adenocarcinomas, whereas antibodies to low-molecular-weight keratins recognize both of those tumor groups.[184] Keratins 7, 8, 18, and 19 are present in all MMs and adenocarcinomas, whereas cytokeratins 5, 6, 14, and 17 are found in some types of mesothelioma but are lacking in MACs.[184] Unfortunately, the latter four proteins are absent in cases of sarcomatoid mesothelioma.

Epithelial membrane antigen (EMA). Studies dealing with anti-EMA have shown that it commonly yields positive results in both MACs and MMs.[185–187] Antibodies to EMA potentially label mesotheliomas of all histologic subtypes. It has been claimed that this protein generally shows a double-density ("tram track") cell-membranous pattern of staining in MMs, whereas MAC cells demonstrate more delicate membrane labeling.[188] It also has been contended that *reactive* mesothelial hyperplasia is EMA-negative, in contrast with primary malignancies of the serosal surfaces.[189] However, in our experience, both of those claims are open to question; in practical usage, we have found that the reactivity patterns in question are not universally present as depicted in the literature.

Carcinoembryonic antigen (CEA). Carcinoembryonic antigen has been considered by most observers to be one of the most reliable markers for distinguishing MM from adenocarcinoma.[150,190–192] The vast majority of mesotheliomas lack CEA. Positivity for that determinant has been reported in up to 5% of cases of MMs, but studies describing that phenomenon have generally used unabsorbed heteroantisera to CEA that undoubtedly recognized unrelated molecules. Monoclonal antibodies to specific CEA epitopes are more reliable in this context. However, the use of anti-CEA reagents has no role in the diagnosis of sarcomatoid mesotheliomas, as mentioned earlier.

Thyroid transcription factor-1 (TTF1). Thyroid transcription factor-1 is a 38 kDa intranuclear polypeptide that is synthesized by a gene located on chromosome 14q13; it is also known as "NKX2A protein." [193,194] Among epithelial elements, this homeodomain-containing nuclear transcription factor is restricted to follicular and parafollicular thyroid cells, glandular and alveolar-lining cells of the lung, and anterior pituicytes. TTF1-positive neoplasms are largely encompassed by those same tissues, with the addition of moderately and poorly differentiated neuroendocrine carcinomas of various organs and the unexpected omission of parathyroid and pituitary tumors.[193] Approximately 75–85% of pulmonary adenocarcinomas and adenosquamous carcinomas are labeled for TTF1.[195,196] In contrast, mesotheliomas of all histologic types have been consistently nonreactive for that marker.[197] It is important to require that *nuclear* labeling be regarded as the only true pattern of positivity for TTF1.[198]

CD15. CD15 has a high level of specificity for MACs,[150,191,192,199–201] but some examples of MM have also shown focal labeling for this marker: that finding appears to be more common in peritoneal tumors than in pleural lesions.[202] Like CEA, the use of CD15 is most appropriate in the evaluation of biphasic or epithelial mesotheliomas, because sarcomatoid tumors consistently lack it.

CA72-4 (recognized by monoclonal antibody B72.3). CA72-4, which is also known as tumor-associated glycoprotein-72, is a generic epithelial determinant that is a high-molecular-weight cell-membranous glycoprotein.[202–207] Regardless of their sites of origin, the majority of MACs show strong reactivity for this marker. Rare examples of MM may also show focal labeling.[208]

Ber-Ep4. Ber-Ep4 is another epithelial marker that was initially thought to be specific for adenocarcinomas,[209,210] and it does indeed demonstrate a high level of sensitivity for those neoplasms as a generic group. Nevertheless, it is now known that approximately 15% of mesotheliomas can show focal staining with this antibody,[211,212] and it has no value in the evaluation of purely sarcomatoid tumors.

MOC-31. MOC-31 is a monoclonal antibody that labels a 35–4 kDa transmembrane glycoprotein in the plasmalemma of most glandular cells.[213,214] That molecule is closely related to lung cancer-associated antigen-2,[215] but, in addition to pulmonary adenocarcinomas, MOC-31 is reactive with glandular malignancies arising in most other organ sites as well.[216,217] Mesotheliomas are reproducibly negative for this marker.[212,217]

BG8. "BG8" is a synonym for Lewis blood group antigen Y (Le^y; CD174), a glycoprotein that is overrepresented in malignant epithelium and is again widely distributed in glandular cells throughout the body.[218–220] Accordingly, its immunohistochemical characteristics in neoplasia generally parallel those of the MOC-31 antigen.[197,221]

p53. The p53 gene is a nuclear phosphoprotein that regulates DNA replication, cell proliferation, and apoptosis.[222] In cases featuring atypical spindle cell proliferations that are morphologically suspicious for desmoplastic MM, p53 immunolabeling of >10% of the lesional cells favors a diagnosis of mesothelioma over one of a cellular pleural plaque or fibrohyaline pleuritis.[223] Nevertheless, that characteristic is not observed in all desmoplastic MMs, nor are all cases of pleuritis necessarily p53-negative.

Another salient observation is that mutant p53 proteins – which are generally recognized by immunohistologic studies – are relatively restricted to MMs and are not typically seen in resting or reactive mesothelial cells.[224–227] On the face of things, mutant p53 therefore would seem to have potential value in the distinction of cytologically bland malignant mesothelioma from mesothelial hyperplasia. Nevertheless, based on our clinical experience with that problem, we would suggest avoiding exclusive reliance on that marker under such circumstances. We have seen several examples of benign mesothelial proliferations that were unexpectedly immunoreactive for p53.

Inclusionary markers for mesothelioma

The aforementioned antibodies are those which have been recommended by the US & Canadian Mesothelioma Panel,[149] and they are probably still the most commonly used markers in surgical pathology laboratories for the evaluation of malignant pleural neoplasms. However, except for p53, all of the markers presented thus far assist in the diagnosis of MM *by exclusion*. Over the past several years, efforts have been directed at identifying "proactive" markers of mesothelioma; i.e. those that would be *present* in the majority of MMs. Some such antibodies have been used diagnostically, whereas others have been analyzed as prognostic indicators. A brief discussion of those reagents follows.

Calretinin. Calretinin is a member of a large family of cytoplasmic calcium-binding proteins.[228] This marker is seen in >95% of mesothelioma cases of the epithelioid and biphasic types[212,229–231] (Fig. 20.39). Antibodies to other related polypeptides are also available, including anti-parvalbumin and anti-calbindin, but they fail to recognize mesotheliomas and non-neoplastic mesothelium.[232] Interestingly, there are conflicting reports regarding the expression of calretinin in sarcomatoid mesothelioma; some observers have seen universal staining of such neoplasms, but others have claimed that they are negative.[233–235] The authors' experience is that approximately 50% of sarcomatoid lesions do, in fact, label for calretinin, albeit in a multifocal fashion. Recent studies have shown that this antibody may also stain selected adenocarcinomas,[230] but, if one requires *nuclear* labeling for calretinin as a truly positive result, these are few in number.

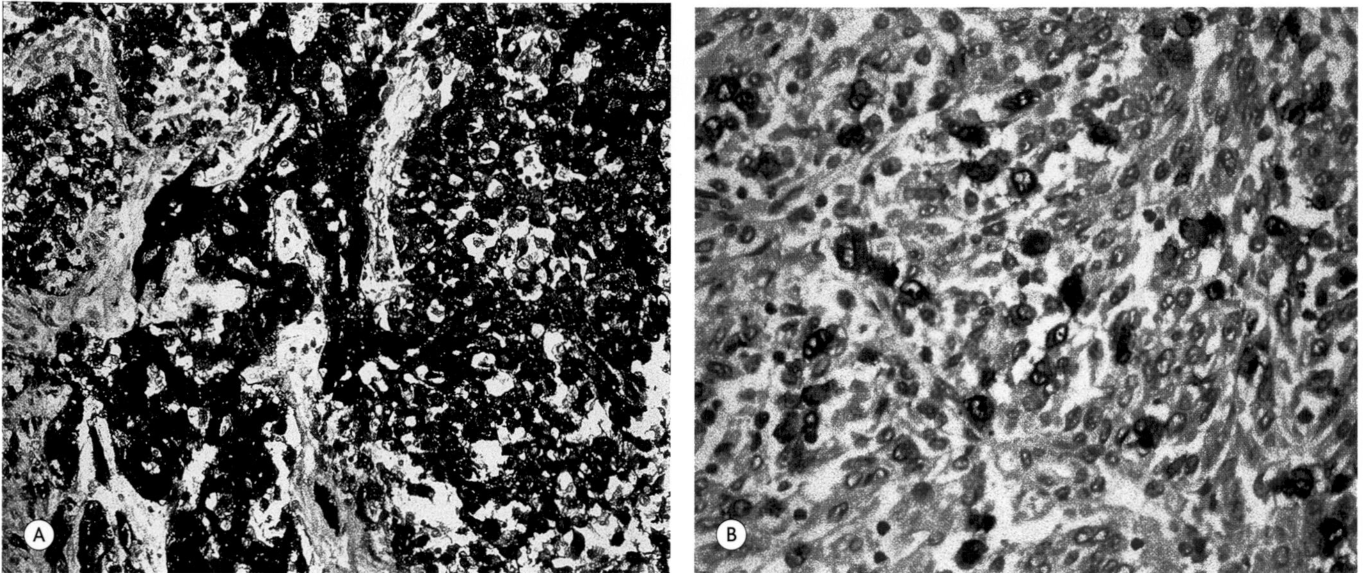

Fig. 20.39 (A) Diffuse nucleocytoplasmic labeling for calretinin is apparent in epithelioid mesothelioma, whereas (B) sarcomatoid mesothelioma demonstrates more focal reactivity.

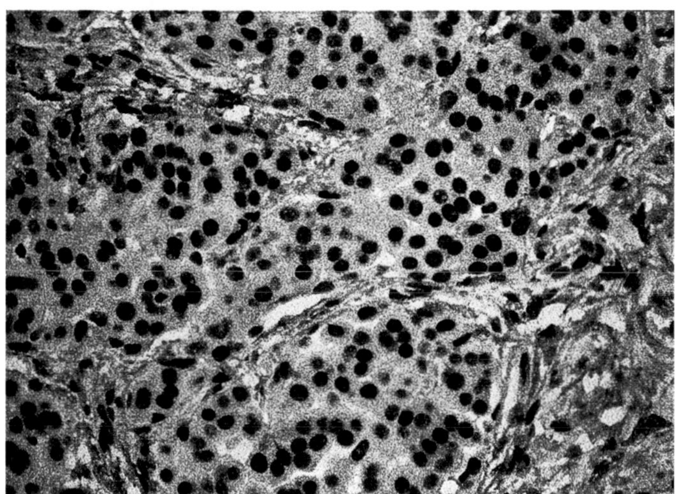

Fig. 20.40 Crisp nuclear staining for WT1 protein is apparent in this malignant mesothelioma.

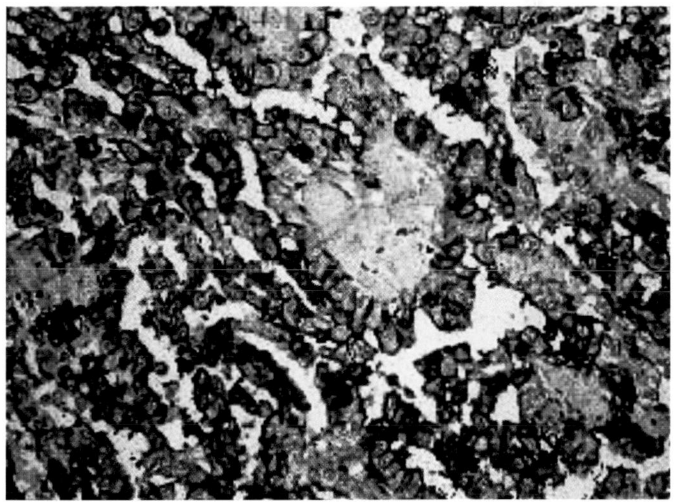

Fig. 20.41 Cell-membranous labeling for thrombomodulin in epithelioid pleural mesothelioma.

WT1 gene product. The WT1 gene resides on the short arm of chromosome 11; when it is deleted constitutively, patients have a tendency to develop nephroblastoma, an embryonic renal tumor.[236] Because of that association, WT1 has generally been regarded as a tumor-suppressor gene, but it is conversely *over*-expressed in other malignancies, including mesothelioma, and therefore also may function as an oncogene.[237] Nuclear immunolabeling for WT1 gene product is apparent in >80% of epithelioid and biphasic MMs (Fig. 20.40), but sarcomatoid tumors again demonstrate lesser positivity, in approximately 30% of cases.[197,212,234,235,238–240] WT1 is not restricted to mesothelial proliferations, and is also present in carcinomas of the thyroid, kidney, ovaries, and endometrium, some of which enter into differential diagnosis with MM.[241,242] Because it is typically absent in adenocarcinoma of the lung, WT1 has greatest applicability when that tumor is the principal diagnostic alternative to epithelioid mesothelioma.[197] Its use in the analysis of sarcomatoid tumors is complicated by the fact that true sarcomas can also be WT1-positive.[243]

Thrombomodulin (CD141). Thrombomodulin, or CD141, converts thrombin from a procoagulant protease to an anticoagulant.[244] It is found in endothelial cells, syncytiotrophoblast, mesothelium, and various epithelia, principally including squamous and transitional cells.[245,246] The majority of MMs (approximately 65%) will label for CD141[183,191,212,221,231,247] (Fig. 20.41), as well as squamous cell carcinomas and transitional cell carcinomas.[230,248] Glandular malignancies of various origins (including the lung) have also demonstrated unexpected reactivity in some series, and as many as 13% of adenocarcinomas have been positive.[230] Hemangioendotheliomas and angiosarcomas, which may occasionally enter differential diagnosis with mesothelioma, are also potentially immunoreactive for CD141.[249]

Other markers

Oncofetal proteins. The use of antibodies to oncofetal proteins is most commonly undertaken in the study of germ cell tumors. However, their role in the differential diagnosis of mesothelioma has been assessed in a few studies. Beta-human chorionic gonadotropin (HCG), pregnancy-specific glycoprotein (PSG), human placental lactogen (HPL), and placental-like alkaline phosphatase (PLAP) have been principally found in adenocarcinomas of various sites.[250] However, the sensitivity of these determinants is relatively low, and some examples of HCG production by pleural mesotheliomas have indeed been described.[251]

Blood group isoantigens. In addition to Lewis blood group antigens – as typified by BG8 (see above) – some studies have compared the relative reactivities of MM and adenocarcinomas for blood group isoantigens A, B, and H.[150,218,252] Their staining patterns generally mirror those of BG8, being restricted to carcinomas, but with lesser sensitivity.

Mesothelin. Mesothelin is a 40 kDa plasmalemmal protein that may function in intercellular adhesion. It is seen in roughly 70% of epithelioid and biphasic MMs, but sarcomatoid mesothelial tumors are negative.[253] Controversy has surrounded the differential diagnostic specificity of this marker vis-à-vis mesothelioma, and recent studies have reported mesothelin reactivity in a broad range of carcinomas as well.[254]

HBME-1 and CA-125. HBME-1 is a monoclonal antibody that was raised against mesothelial cells, and it recognizes a membranous glycoprotein. Although it demonstrates a high degree of sensitivity for MM[217,240,247] (Fig. 20.42), several studies over the past decade have shown that it clearly is not a mesothelium-specific reagent. Adenocarcinomas of several sites, including the lung, kidney, thyroid, and female genital tract, are also potentially HBME-1-reactive.[212,255–257] Similar comments apply to another mesothelium-related marker, OC125 (recognized by the monoclonal antibody CA-125);[257] in fact, that determinant is widely used to label müllerian carcinomas.[258]

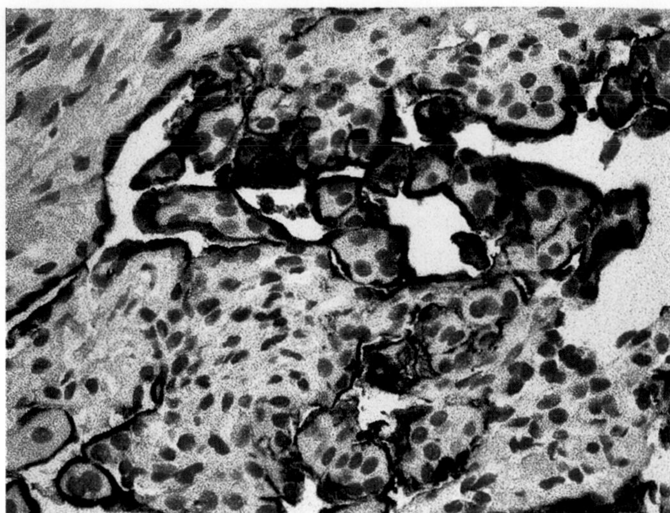

Fig. 20.42 Membrane-based positivity with HBME-1 in tubulopapillary mesothelioma.

Neuroendocrine determinants. Small cell MM may be confused with metastatic neuroendocrine carcinoma in the pleura. With that in mind, it is noteworthy that small cell mesotheliomas commonly manifest immunoreactivity for determinants that are generally regarded as "neuroendocrine" markers: namely, neuron-specific (gamma-dimer) enolase and CD57.[259] However, more specific indicators of a neuroendocrine lineage, such as chromogranin-A, CD56, and synaptophysin, are absent in MMs.

Additional hematopoietic markers. CD15 and CD141 have already been discussed with reference to their relative presence in mesothelial tumors. Other hematopoietic markers of interest in this setting include CD10 (neutral endopeptidase; common acute lymphoblastic leukemia antigen) and CD138 (syndecan-1). Among epithelial malignancies, CD10 is most commonly used as a potential indicator for renal cell carcinoma and hepatocellular carcinoma,[260,261] and pleural metastases of those tumors can certainly imitate MM morphologically. Unfortunately, mesotheliomas may also express CD10,[262] making it necessary to rely on additional discriminants in this context. On the other hand, CD138 is seen in a variety of carcinomas (e.g. pulmonary, colonic, pancreaticobiliary, hepatocellular, prostatic, renal, transitional cell, mammary, ovarian, endometrial, cutaneous, thyroid, adrenal, and salivary glandular) in differing percentages. MM is consistently CD138-negative.[263]

Additional supplementary reagents. Several other antibodies have been applied to the identification of epithelioid MM in the past, and more are likely to appear in the future. For the most part, those which have not been mentioned specifically in this review are not considered to be standard diagnostic markers. However, for purposes of completeness, their relative reactivity patterns in epithelioid mesotheliomas and MACs are provided in Table 20.1 (see also Table 16.1).

In a critical review of the numerous publications on the immunohistochemistry of malignant mesothelioma, one sees graphic proof of the tenet that single immunostains cannot be used to establish that diagnosis. It is therefore mandatory that a panel of reagents must be used which includes at least four discriminatory antibodies. Similar conclusions have been drawn by other authors, who have noted that the proportion of mesotheliomas lending themselves to confident diagnosis increases in direct proportion to the number of antibodies employed.[212,221,264] In particular, Ordonez has recommended that:

> the best discriminators among the antibodies considered to be negative markers for [epithelioid] mesothelioma are CEA, MOC-31, Ber-EP4, BG8, and B72.3. A panel of four markers (two positive and two negative) selected based upon availability and which ones yield good staining results in a given laboratory is recommended. Because of their specificity and sensitivity for mesotheliomas, the best combination appears to be calretinin and cytokeratin 5/6 (or WT1) for the positive markers and CEA and MOC-31 (or B72.3, Ber-EP4, or BG-8) for the negative markers.[212]

Table 20.1 Supplementary immunohistochemical reagents (see text) used to distinguish epithelioid mesothelioma from adenocarcinoma[a]

Marker	Mesothelioma[b]	Adenocarcinomas
Desmin	± 37%	–
Human milk fat globule protein-2	± 15%	± 75%
N-cadherin	+ 73%	± 30%
CD44S	+ 73%	± 48%
LN1	± 48%	+ 86%
CD56	–	± 16%
CD138	± 4%	± 51%
LN2	± 5%	+ 91%
p21 *ras* oncoproteins	± 13%	± 16%

[a]See also Table 16.1.
[b]Percentages are derived from a synthesis of the pertinent literature.

Independent of current advances in methodology and the availability of new markers, it is also important to recognize that, unfortunately, infallible reliability can still not be expected of immunohistochemistry. In occasional instances, electron microscopy may still be the best way to resolve diagnostic dilemmas in this area of tumor pathology.

Cytogenetic and molecular features of pleural mesothelioma

Cytogenetic studies on human MMs have shown no consistent chromosomal abnormalities. Of those which have been reported, monosomy 6, assorted trisomies and polysomies, allelic losses of 4p and 4q, deletions of 1p22, 3p, 7q, and 14q, and complete loss of chromosomes 21, 22, and Y appear to be relatively random events.[265–271] On the other hand, a relatively consistent deletion of 9p21-22, involving the CDKN2A/INK4A gene, has been seen in up to 60% of cases in some studies.[272–274]

Mutations in the p53 gene have received substantial attention as possible differential diagnostic tools in mesothelial proliferations.[224–227,275–279] However, MM does not inevitably manifest such abnormalities and they have been reported in 33–70% of cases in various series.[227,277,279] Point mutations also may occur in the INK4A gene.[280]

On the other hand, several genes and their protein products may be overexpressed in mesothelioma. They include those coding for platelet-derived growth factors, hepatocyte growth factor, c-*met*, insulin-like growth factor-1, transforming growth factor-beta, and *bcl*-2.[281–284] HER-2/c-*erb*B-2, the target of a commercially available immunotherapy, conversely is *not* amplified in MM.[285] Interestingly, Ramos-Nino et al. have found that the activator protein-1 gene complex, encoding transcription factors that include c-*fos*, *Fos*-B, *Fra*-1, *Fra*-2, c-*jun*, *Jun*-B, and *Jun*-D, is activated in those mesotheliomas which are etiologically related to asbestos.[286] That observation could potentially have important epidemiologic and medicolegal implications.

Differential diagnosis of pleural mesothelioma: special considerations

Several differential diagnostic alternatives to the various morphologic forms of MM have already been mentioned through the course of this discussion. Some of these will be addressed in greater detail, and others merit special consideration, as outlined below.

Differential diagnosis of benign versus malignant mesothelial proliferations

Florid mesothelial hyperplasia versus epithelioid mesothelioma

Mesothelial hyperplasia that is seen in the context of infectious or inflammatory pleural effusions can be exuberant and moderately atypical cytologically (Fig. 20.43). Especially when the mesothelium becomes entrapped in organizing fibrinous exudates, histologic images in pleural biopsies may engender serious concern over the possibility of epithelioid MM.

Differential diagnosis centers on the presence of actual invasion by the proliferation in question, and this can only be identified in an adequate tissue sample. If a deep enough portion of pleura is obtained, one can usually see a zonal phenomenon in mesothelial hyperplasia, wherein the cellularity of the tissue decreases with increasing distance from the pleural surface, and no mesothelial aggregates are visualized in the pleural fibroadipose tissue.[139] Otherwise, the superficial portions of such specimens may be markedly cellular, even with formation of micropapillary structures that are mantled by atypical mesothelial cells.

As stated above, we are not strong proponents of adjunctive immunohistochemical studies in this setting. It has been suggested by others that strong labeling for EMA and p53 protein in the proliferating mesothelium is an indicator of malignancy.[185,188,189,226] However, we have observed several cases in which both of those markers were unequivocally present in mesothelial proliferations that proved to be benign.

Another intriguing recent publication concerns the use of cyclin-dependent kinase inhibitor-2A (CDKN2A; INK4A; p16) in this setting. That moiety inhibits cyclin-dependent kinase-4 and is encoded by a gene on chromosome 9p21. Using fluorescence in-situ hybridization and ThinPrep^R cytologic preparations of pleural effusion specimens, Illei et al. found that mesotheliomas exhibited homozygous deletion for CDKN2A, whereas reactive benign mesothelium showed retention of at least one copy of the gene.[287] The number of cases in that series was modest, and additional work will be required on this marker before it can be used clinically.

Fibrohyaline pleuritis versus desmoplastic mesothelioma

One of the most difficult problems confronting thoracic surgeons and surgical pathologists is the patient who has had a long-standing or recurrent pleural effusion, culminating in a "rind" of organized and densely collagenized tissue that obliterates the pleural space and encompasses the lung. Under those circumstances, the diagnostic alternatives are those of fibrohyaline pleuritis ("fibrous pleurisy") and DMM. The distinction between those conditions can be challenging even with a complete pleurectomy specimen in hand, but sufficient sampling is

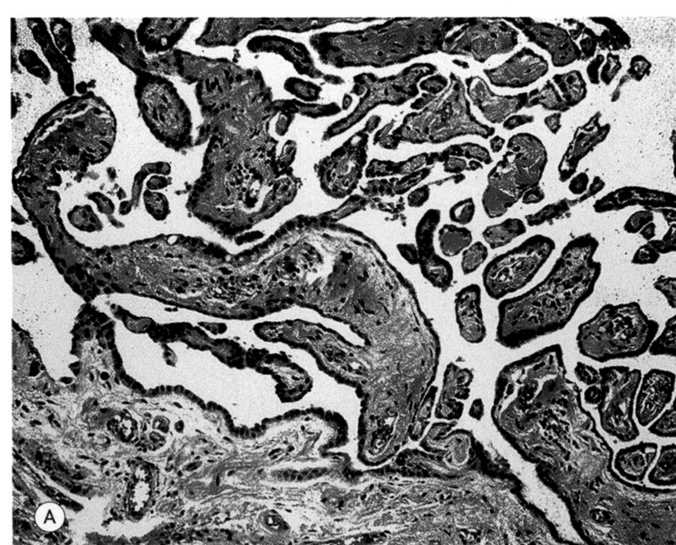

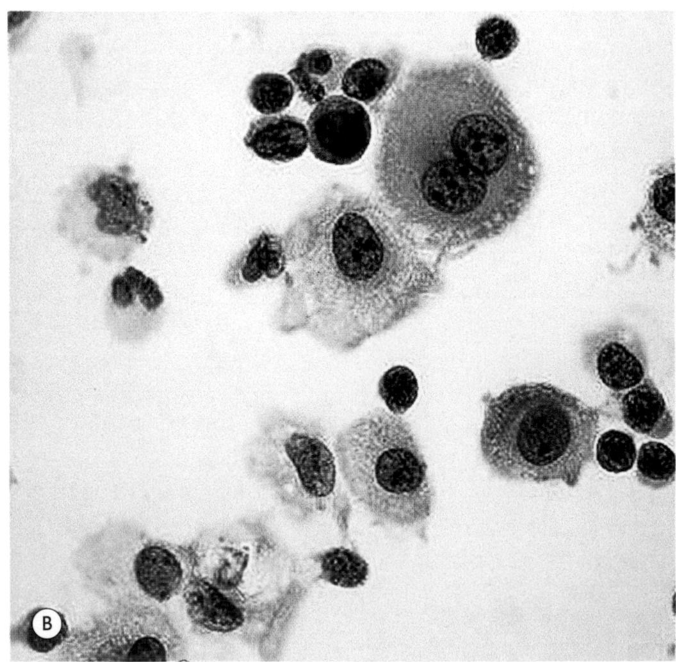

Fig. 20.43 (A) Mesothelial hyperplasia, as seen in a biopsy specimen and (B) cytologically. This condition may closely simulate the morphologic images of mesothelioma.

again the key to proper diagnosis. Criteria that are used for recognition of DMM include foci of necrosis, obvious invasion of pleural adipose tissue or subjacent lung, and the presence of obvious focal cellular anaplasia.[136,137] p53 immunostaining has again been used by some authors in this context,[223] but results of that analysis are similar conceptually to those attending the evaluation of mesothelial hyperplasia, as discussed above.

Differential diagnosis of cytologically malignant pleural neoplasms

Epithelioid mesothelioma versus hematopoietic malignancies

Uncommonly, hematopoietic malignancies such as large cell non-Hodgkin lymphoma, syncytial or "sarcomatoid" Hodgkin lymphoma, and granulocytic sarcoma (tumefactive acute myelogenous leukemia) may be primary neoplasms of the pleura and simulate MM, both clinically and morphologically.[288–291] The former three tumors are constituted by large polygonal or round cells, like epithelioid MM, and their histologic images are accordingly very similar to that of the solid-anaplastic variety of mesothelioma. Hematopoietic malignancies demonstrate a much more notable degree of apoptosis than that seen in MM, with greater irregularity in the nuclear contours of the tumor cells and more numerous mitoses. Electron microscopic analysis fails to show any intercellular attachment complexes in such lesions, in contrast to their prominence in MMs; similarly, plasmalemmal microvilli are absent in lymphoma and leukemia. (Parenthetically, there is a form of large cell non-Hodgkin lymphoma, known as "anemone cell lymphoma," in which numerous cell-surface projections are evident,[292] but those structures are not true microvilli.) Immunohistologic studies reveal a lack of keratin and calretinin in hematopoietic tumors, which instead exhibit variable positivity for CD15, CD20, CD43, and CD45.[293] Those phenotypes are mutually exclusive with regard to respective diagnoses of MM and lymphoma/leukemia. However, a pitfall in this area is the potential reactivity for CD30 and the WT1 gene product in mesothelioma as well as in hematopoietic malignancies.[294,295] The latter marker is particularly prevalent in granulocytic sarcoma.

Epithelioid mesothelioma versus epithelioid endothelial neoplasms

The capacity of epithelioid mesothelioma to exhibit cytoplasmic macrovacuolation has been noted earlier. That particular feature likens some lesions of this type to epithelioid vascular tumors such as epithelioid hemangio-

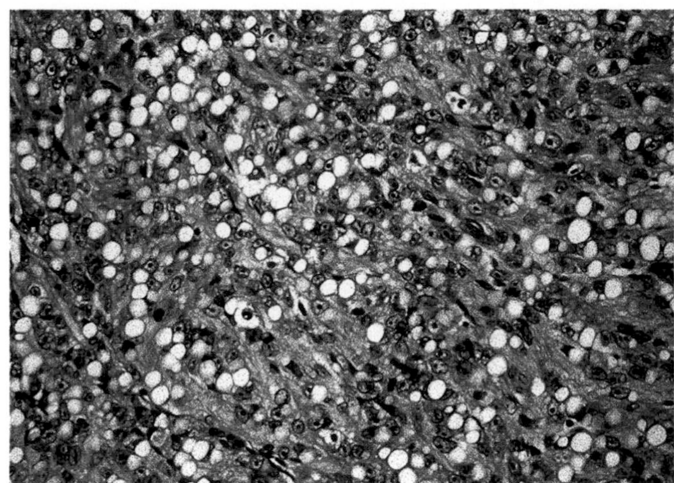

Fig. 20.44 Pleural epithelioid hemangioendothelioma, comprising densely apposed and vacuolated polygonal cells. This lesion can imitate the gross and microscopic appearance of mesothelioma.

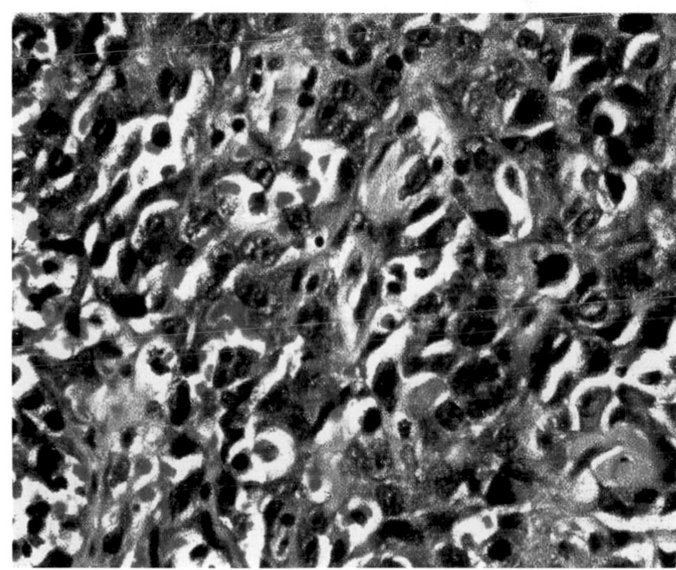

Fig. 20.45 Epithelioid angiosarcoma of the pleura, as shown here, may also be confused diagnostically with epithelioid mesothelioma.

endothelioma (EHE) and epithelioid angiosarcoma (EAS), both of which can represent primary pleural neoplasms[100,296–300] (Figs 20.44 and 20.45).

Ultrastructural studies are usually definitive in separating epithelioid MM from EHE and EAS. The first of those three tumor types shows elaborate microvillous differentiation, complex desmosomes, and cytoplasmic tonofibrils, none of which is apparent in vascular lesions. On the other hand, the cells of EHE and EAS contain variable numbers of Weibel–Palade bodies, which are elongated, tubular, electron-dense cytoplasmic structures

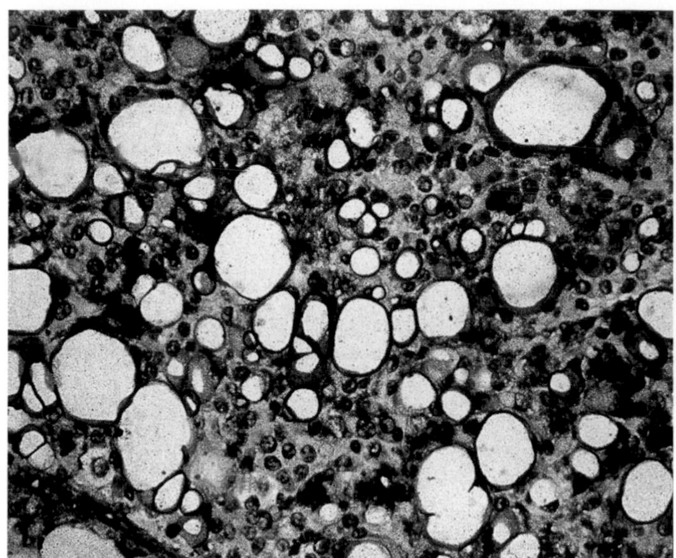

Fig. 20.46 Immunoreactivity for CD34 in pleural epithelioid hemangioendothelioma. That marker is not seen in mesotheliomas.

with internal striations,[301,302] and mesotheliomas lack such inclusions.

Immunohistologically, epithelioid vascular tumors are unusual mesenchymal neoplasms because they quite commonly exhibit "aberrant" expression of keratin.[303] They are also reactive for CD141,[249] as are mesothelial proliferations. However, EHE and EAS lack calretinin, WT1 protein, and keratin 5/6, and instead are consistently positive for CD31 and CD34[304] (Fig. 20.46). Both of the last two markers are absent in mesotheliomas.

Primary pleural myxoid chondrosarcoma versus mesothelioma

Extraskeletal myxoid chondrosarcoma (EMC) is a soft tissue tumor that is cytogenetically characterized by two chromosomal translocations –t(9;22)(q22;q11-12) or t(9;17)(q22;q11) – which yield the EWS/CHN or RBP56/CHN fusion genes, respectively.[305] It has rarely been reported as a primary pleural malignancy,[306] and its histologic image may simulate that of epithelioid mesothelioma. However, EMC lacks the microvillous plasmalemmal differentiation of MM on electron microscopy. It is also consistently non-reactive for keratin and calretinin, instead labeling for vimentin and variably for S100 protein, neuron-specific enolase, and protein gene product 9.5,[307,308] none of which is seen in mesotheliomas. The characteristic fusion-gene proteins of EMC can also be demonstrated rapidly using the polymerase chain reaction,[305] and they are consistently lacking in mesothelial tumors.

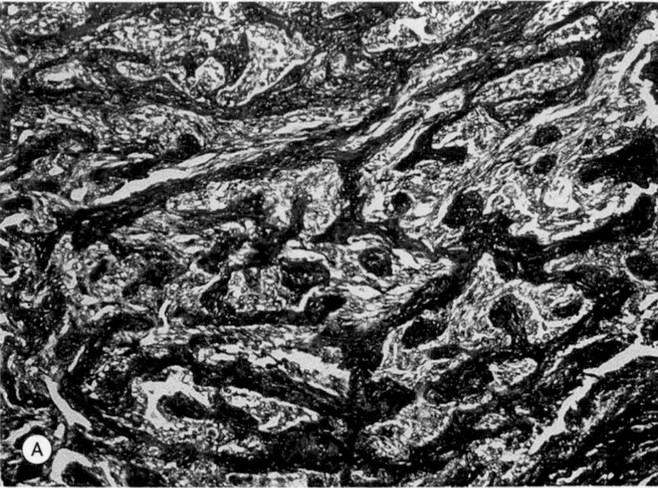

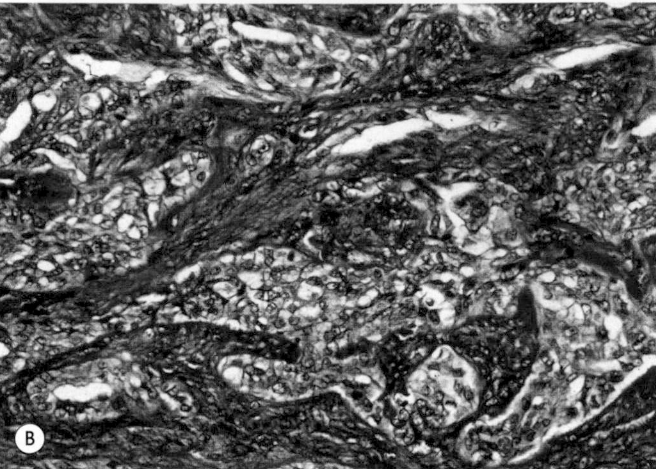

Fig. 20.47 (A,B) Biphasic synovial sarcoma of the pleura, demonstrating tubular arrays of epithelioid cells set in a neoplastic spindle cell background. A likeness to biphasic mesothelioma is apparent.

Synovial sarcoma versus mesothelioma

The clinicopathologic characteristics of pleuropulmonary synovial sarcoma have been provided in Chapter 14, including the potential for that tumor to mimic biphasic or sarcomatoid mesotheliomas (Figs 20.47 and 20.48). Specialized pathologic studies are most productive in biphasic tumors, where the microvillous ultrastructural nature of epithelioid cells in MM is not reproduced in synovial sarcoma.[309] Miettinen et al. have examined this specific differential diagnosis by immunohistochemical means,[310] showing that biphasic synovial sarcoma often manifests Ber-Ep4 positivity, a rarity of CD141, and a lack of WT1 in its epithelioid elements. Mesotheliomas usually demonstrated the converse of that profile. Diffuse expression of keratin 7 and keratin 19 in mesotheliomas was also contrasted with focal labeling for those proteins

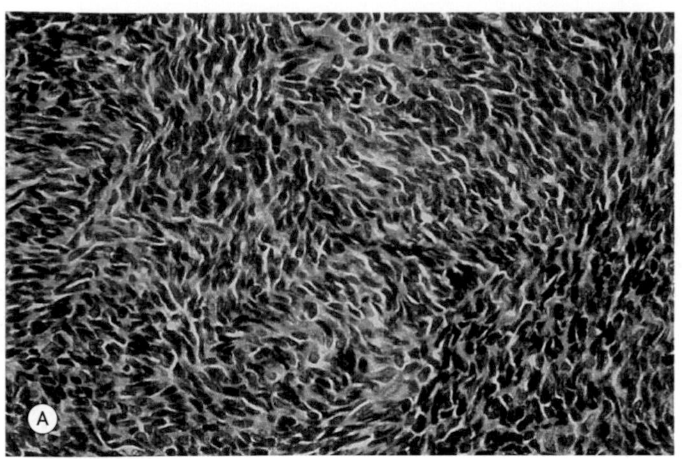

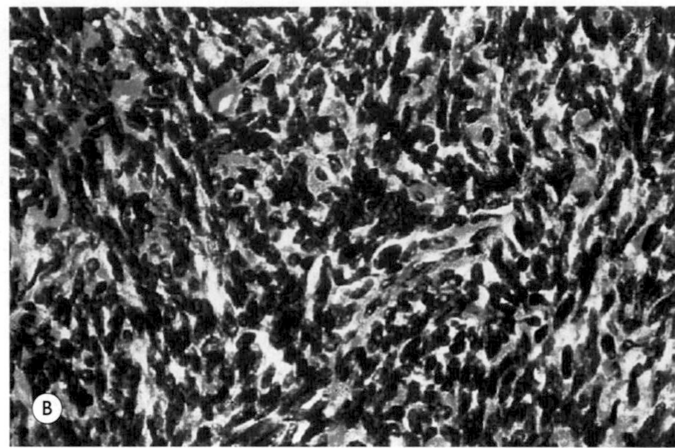

Fig. 20.48 (A,B) Monophasic pleural synovial sarcoma, demonstrating fascicular growth by nondescript fusiform tumor cells. This neoplasm may imitate either sarcomatoid mesothelioma or malignant solitary fibrous tumor of the pleura.

in synovial sarcoma, whereas keratin 14 was seen in the latter lesion but not most mesotheliomas. Calretinin was potentially common to both monophasic spindle cell synovial sarcoma and purely sarcomatoid mesothelioma, but WT1 protein was only encountered in MMs. Other markers were not discriminatory between those particular tumor variants.[310]

Ultimately, molecular analysis may be necessary to establish a definitive interpretation in this setting. Virtually all synovial sarcomas show a reproducible t(X;18) chromosomal translocation, which is not seen in MMs. Its presence can be assessed indirectly by using the polymerase chain reaction with primers designed to identify the *SYT–SSX1* and *SYT–SSX2* fusion proteins that are produced by the translocation in question.[311]

Pseudomesotheliomatous sarcomatoid carcinoma versus mesothelioma

A related morphologic problem is represented by sarcomatoid carcinomas that extensively involve the pleura and simulate mesothelioma; these likewise may show biphasic or spindle cell/pleormorphic images.[33] As true in biphasic synovial sarcomas, the ultrastructural and immunophenotypic attributes of epithelioid components in biphasic carcinomas are distinct from those of biphasic MMs.[311a] Purely non-epithelioid lesions in both categories are more difficult to separate from one another; however, the presence of immunoreactivity for calretinin and WT1 strongly favors mesothelioma, in our experience.

From the perspective of patient management, this diagnostic distinction is not crucial, because pseudomesotheliomatous carcinomas and mesotheliomas generally manifest the same limited response to therapy and a comparably adverse prognosis.[31–33] However, medicolegal issues attending the two neoplasms are potentially quite different.

Small cell mesothelioma versus other small cell malignancies

In limited biopsy specimens, small cell mesothelioma may be difficult to distinguish from metastatic small cell neuroendocrine carcinoma (SCNC) involving the pleura,[312] or from Askin's tumor (primary thoracopulmonary primitive neuroectodermal tumor, PNET). The latter two lesions have been considered in greater detail in Chapters 13 and 14. To date, ultrastructural studies on small cell MM have not been performed; hence, it is not known whether it shares the microvillous electron microscopic attributes of conventional epithelioid mesotheliomas, or, alternatively, manifests the formation of blunt neuritic-type cytoplasmic extensions as seen in PNET. Immunohistologically, all three lesions in this differential diagnostic cluster may exhibit positivity for pan-keratin; however, SCNC tends to show a distinctive globule of paranuclear keratin reactivity that is not shared by MM or PNET[313] (Fig. 20.49). Moreover, keratin 5/6 and calretinin are more often observed in small cell MM than in SCNC,[230] and they have not been reported in Askin's tumor. Other helpful determinants for the separation of such lesions are hematopoietic in nature. CD99 is unique to PNET in this group; CD56 and CD57 are seen in SCNC and PNET but not small cell MM; and CD141 is seen in mesothelioma but tends to be absent in the other neoplasms.[230,313] Finally, MOC-31 and anti-TTF1 characteristically label metastatic small cell carcinoma of the

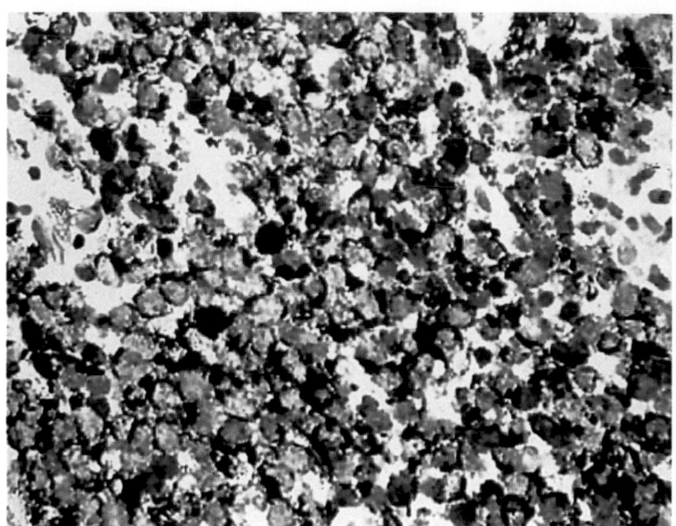

Fig. 20.49 Globular perinuclear immunoreactivity for keratin, as seen in this metastatic small cell neuroendocrine carcinoma, distinguishes that tumor from small cell mesothelioma.

lung,[314,315] whereas MM and Askin's tumor are negative for those markers.

Primary pleural thymomatosis versus mesothelioma

The capability for thymomas to arise and spread in the pleura, simulating mesothelioma clinicopathologically,[316] has been discussed in Chapter 19. To reiterate, although both of those tumor types share potential immunoreactivity for keratin 5/6, thrombomodulin, and calretinin, only thymomas contain lymphoid cells that express CD1a and CD99. Similarly, the p63 positivity of thymomas[317] is not seen in MMs. Lastly, microvilli are not evident in thymic epithelial neoplasms ultrastructurally.[318]

Solitary fibrous tumor of the pleura versus sarcomatoid mesothelioma

When provided only with small biopsy specimens and given no clinical information, pathologists may conceivably confuse atypical variants of solitary fibrous tumor (SFT) of the pleura with sarcomatoid MM on morphologic grounds. Nevertheless, the immunophenotypes of those neoplasms are mutually exclusive. Solitary fibrous tumor is reactive for CD34, with or without CD99, but it lacks keratin. Mesothelioma shows the opposite of those results.[319]

Clear cell mesothelioma versus metastatic renal cell carcinoma

Clear cell mesotheliomas are rare, but they may be closely simulated by metastases of "conventional" renal cell carcinoma (RCC)[320] (Fig. 20.50). The latter of those neoplasms lacks unique and easily detected markers, and, particularly because it also shares potential positivity for several proteins with mesothelioma (including keratin, vimentin, CD10, WT1, and thrombomodulin),[260,321] a tailored immunohistologic approach to differential diagnosis is necessary in this specific instance. Those markers which are most discriminatory between RCC and clear cell MM include keratin 5/6, calretinin, CD15, Ber-Ep4, and BG8. The presence of the first two determinants strongly favors an interpretation of mesothelioma, whereas positivity for CD15, Ber-Ep4, and BG8 is representative of RCC.[322]

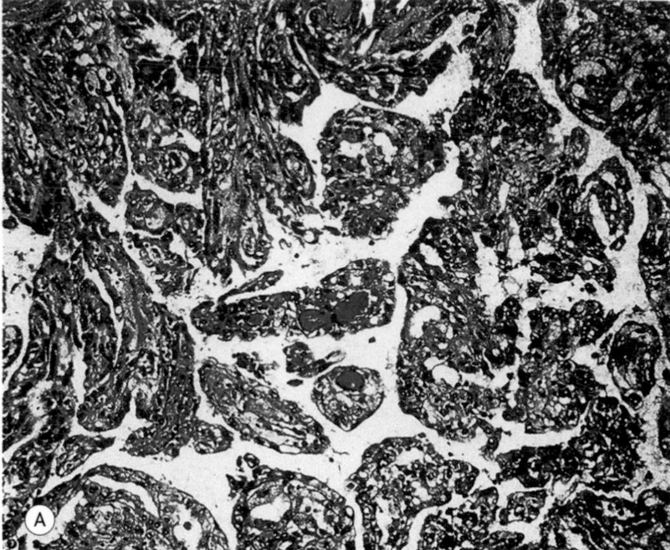

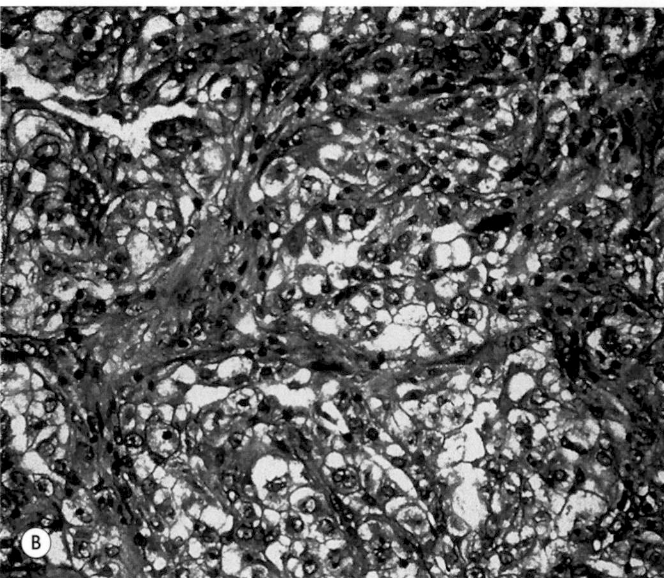

Fig. 20.50 (A,B) Metastatic renal cell carcinoma in the pleura, showing papillary and solid growth patterns. This tumor was felt to represent a clear cell mesothelioma on initial clinicopathologic evaluation.

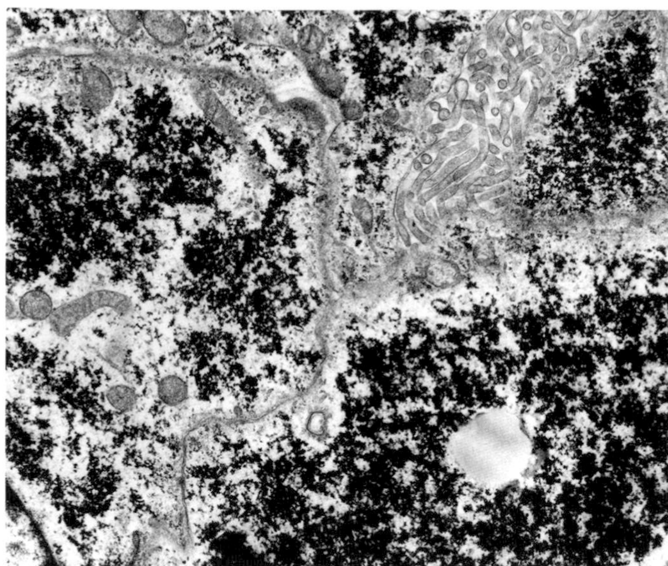

Fig. 20.51 Electron photomicrograph of renal cell carcinoma, showing abundant cytoplasmic glycogen and only rudimentary plasmalemmal microvilli. These features contrast with those of epithelioid clear cell mesothelioma.

This is a circumstance where electron microscopic study is probably superior in specificity to immunohistochemical analysis. Renal cell carcinomas have poorly formed plasmalemmal microvilli and no cytoplasmic tonofibrils, and, instead, they contain prominent cytoplasmic collections of glycogen, or lipid, or both[323] (Fig. 20.51). Clear cell mesothelioma does not share those ultrastructural characteristics.

Oncocytoid/deciduoid mesothelioma versus other "pink cell" malignancies

Deciduoid/oncocytoid mesothelioma can be simulated by pleural metastases of carcinomas that are constituted by large "pink" cells. These principally include hepatocellular carcinoma (HCC), adrenocortical carcinoma (ACC), and RCC.[324] Electron microscopy provides valuable information in this particular context, because none of the cited tumors, except for deciduoid MM, contains elongated plasmalemmal microvilli, complex desmosomes, or tonofilaments. Moreover, ACC (and sometimes RCC) may also manifest the presence of tubulovesicular mitochondrial cristae[325] (Fig. 20.52), which are absent in mesotheliomas. Immunohistologic separation of such tumors centers on a few key determinants. Epithelial membrane antigen is consistently present in oncocytoid MM and RCC but is absent in HCC and ACC.[326] On the other hand, keratin is paradoxically absent in paraffin sections of ACC, even though it is undeniably epithelial.[327] Those two markers are particularly important in regard to the separation of MM and adrenocortical neoplasms, because both of them are commonly positive for calretinin.[328] However, ACC also shows reactivity for inhibin (Fig. 20.53) and CD56, both of which are not seen in mesotheliomas.[263] The distinction of oncocytoid RCC and MM is basically comparable to that attending their clear cell variants, as discussed above. Lastly, an antibody known as HEP-Par1 is selective for HCC, and reproducibly allows for a distinction of that tumor type from mesotheliomas.[261]

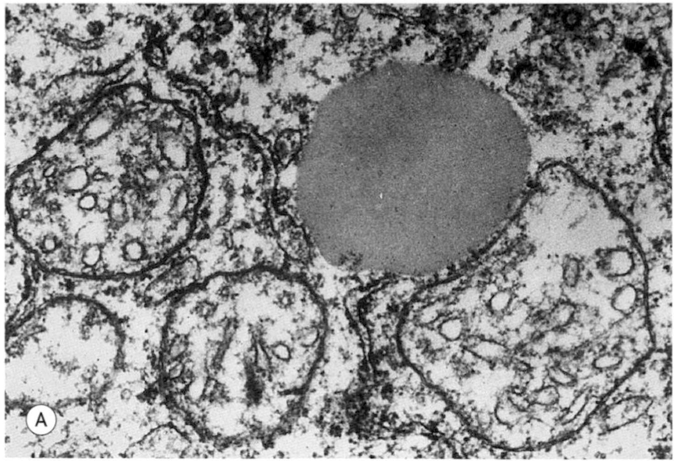

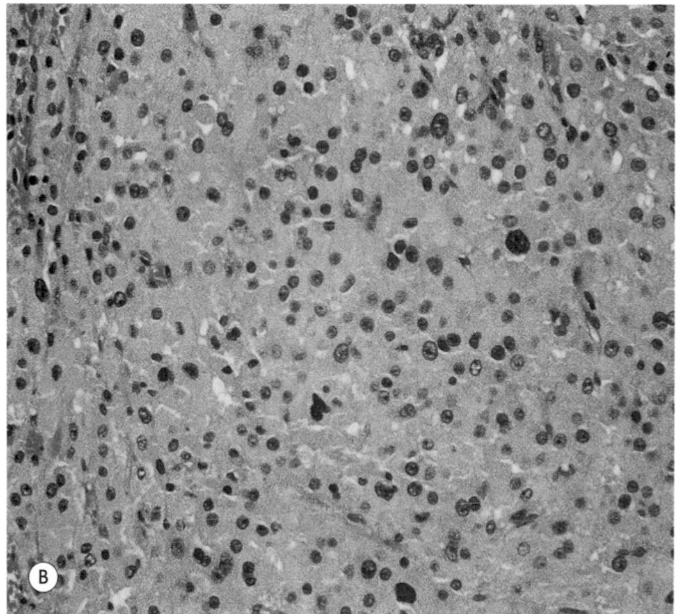

Fig. 20.52 (A) Tubular mitochondrial cristae are apparent in the tumor cells of (B) adrenocortical carcinoma, which might be confused with deciduoid mesothelioma if it involves the pleura.

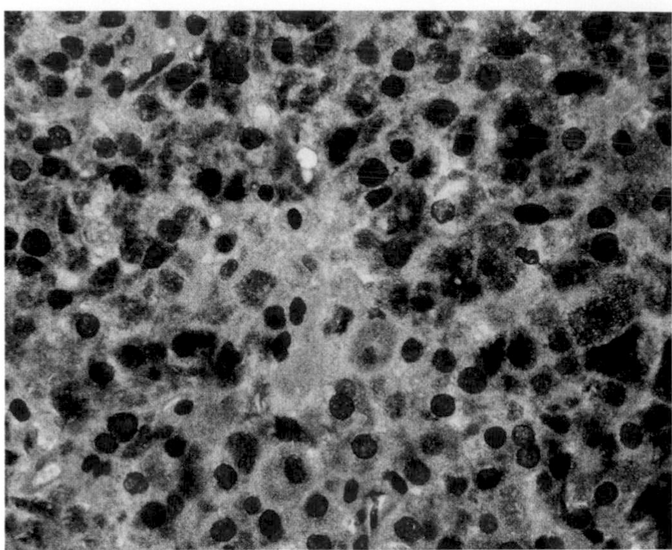

Fig. 20.53 Inhibin immunoreactivity, as shown here, is typical of adrenocortical carcinoma but is not seen in mesothelioma.

Rhabdoid mesothelioma versus metastases of extrarenal malignant rhabdoid tumors

As mentioned earlier, "extrarenal malignant rhabdoid tumor" (EMRT) is probably a phenotype as well as a neoplastic entity. In other words, a spectrum of tumor types – including mesothelioma – may demonstrate clonal evolution and assume a rhabdoid image.[141,142] When that occurs, ultrastructural and immunophenotypic characteristics of the original lesion are usually lost in the rhabdoid component. Regardless of its derivation, EMRT has the ability to show paranuclear whorls of intermediate filaments by electron microscopy, as well as potential immunoreactivity for keratin, vimentin, desmin, EMA, actins, CD99, and WT1 protein.[142] Other markers of potential mesothelial differentiation (e.g. calretinin, CD141, keratin 5/6, etc.) are absent.[141] Hence, a rhabdoid mesothelioma will not be identifiable as such unless it also has a minor "conventional" MM component that is concurrently sampled.

Epithelioid mesothelioma versus primary or metastatic germ cell malignancies

Very uncommonly, malignant germ cell tumors – principally represented by embryonal carcinoma and yolk sac carcinoma, or combinations thereof – may arise primarily in the pleuropulmonary compartment.[329] In addition, metastases from occult neoplasms of those types in other anatomic sites rarely can secondarily involve the pleura. The histologic image of such tumors may imitate that of solid "anaplastic" MM. Electron microscopy is an effective means of separating germ cell neoplasms from mesotheliomas, because plasmalemmal microvilli are absent in the former of those tumor groups.[330]

Immunohistologic studies will show positivity for placental alkaline phosphatase in germ cell tumors, with or without CD117,[326,331] but they lack calretinin and WT1 protein. Once again, those results are incompatible with the phenotype of MM.[332]

Metastatic intranodal mesothelioma versus lymph nodal mesothelial rests

Several reports have been made on the presence of mesothelial inclusions (rests) in the sinusoids of intrathoracic lymph nodes[333–335] (Figs 20.54 and 20.55). They may be found incidentally and unexpectedly in nodes that are removed in the treatment of other clinical conditions. Under such circumstances, specialized pathologic evaluations are incapable of distinguishing such benign and probably developmental abnormalities from metastatic intranodal mesothelioma. However, in all cases documented to date, the affected patients had absolutely no evidence of pleural disease and therefore a diagnosis of MM would have been untenable. Metastatic adenocarcinoma is another consideration under these circumstances, but that possibility can be dismissed by appropriate immunohistochemical studies.[333]

Borderline (low-grade malignant) mesothelial tumors

Even though Chapter 19 was devoted to both benign and borderline neoplasms of the thorax, only pleural adenomatoid tumors were included there. That decision was made to allow for a more unified discussion at this point of mesothelial proliferations with either low-grade malignant or obviously aggressive features. Two additional lesions with mesothelial differentiation are considered in the following sections, both of which have a limited potential for local recurrence or distant spread. These are represented by well-differentiated papillary mesothelioma (WDPM) and multicystic mesothelial tumor of borderline biologic potential (MMTBBP; formerly called "multicystic mesothelioma").

Etiologic considerations

Both WDPM and MMTBBP were initially described as abdominal lesions in young individuals who were typically female.[336,337] They were thought to be unassociated

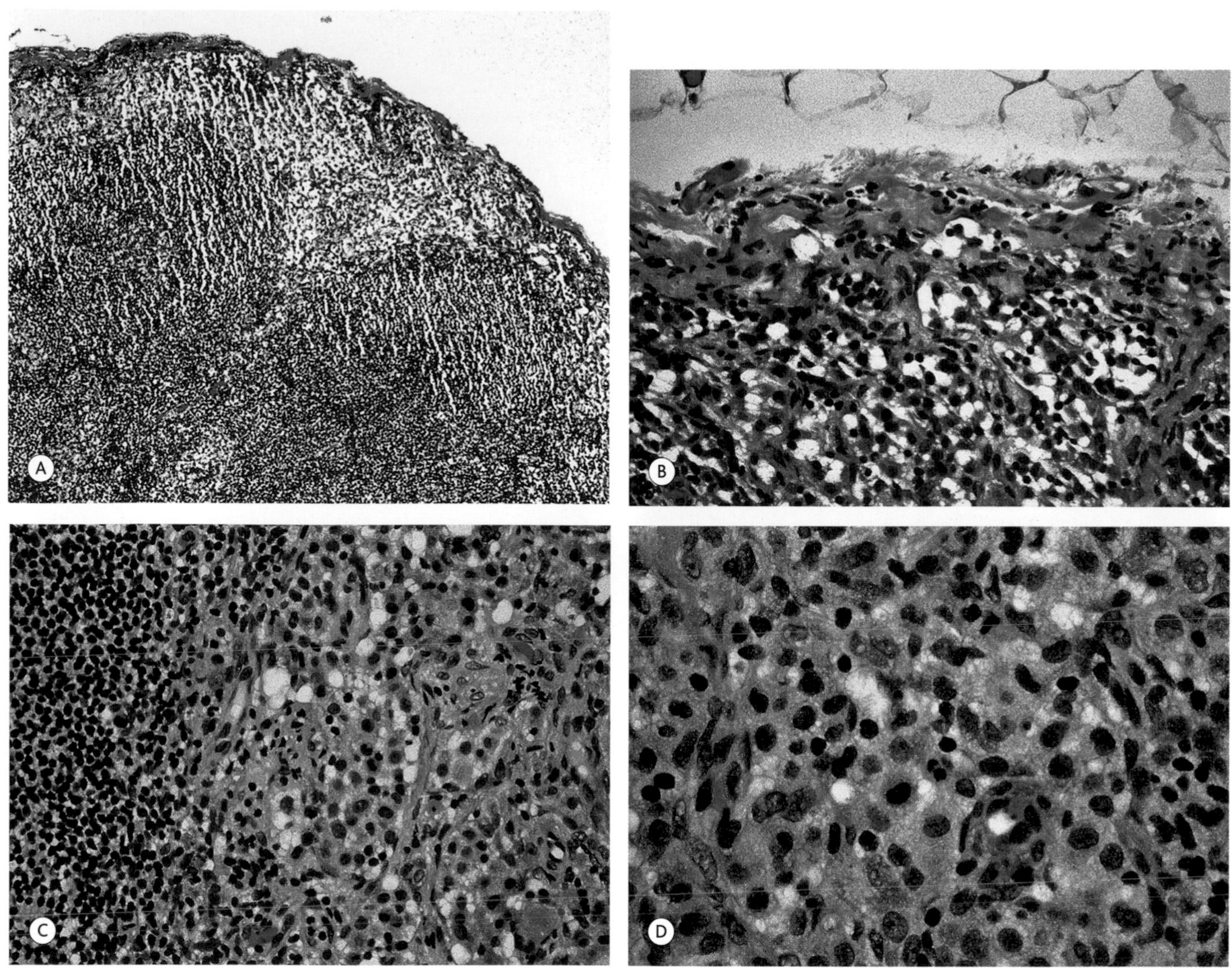

Fig. 20.54 (A–D) Mesothelial rests in a mediastinal lymph node, seen principally in the nodal sinusoids. The node was removed incidentally during cardiac surgery.

causally with asbestos exposure, representing idiopathic proliferations. That precept is still accepted in reference to peritoneal tumors of these types.

Very few examples of *pleural* WDPM and MMTBBP have been described, and it would therefore be premature to draw definite conclusions on their pathogeneses. Multicystic mesothelial tumor of borderline biologic potential of the thorax has yet to be linked with any definable etiologic agent. However, Butnor et al. recently described seven examples of pleural WDPM, two of which occurred in patients with objective radiographic or pathologic evidence of above-background asbestos exposure.[338] Such evidence was reflected by the presence of fibrohyaline pleural plaques.

As the authors of the latter report suggested, those data raise the prospect that asbestos may indeed cause some examples of pleural WDPM. However, it should also be noted that all cases in the series by Butnor et al. were taken from the consultation files of two other coauthors who are well-known in the area of asbestos-related litigation. Therefore, the possibility of etiologic bias is very real in that publication. Many more additional cases of intrathoracic WDPM will need to be evaluated – with close attention to objectifiable markers of asbestos exposure – before this issue can be resolved conclusively.

Clinical findings

Well-differentiated papillary mesothelioma of the pleura has presented similarly to conventional forms of epithelioid mesothelioma, with dyspnea and a serosal effusion.[338,339] To date, no other clinical complaints have been documented

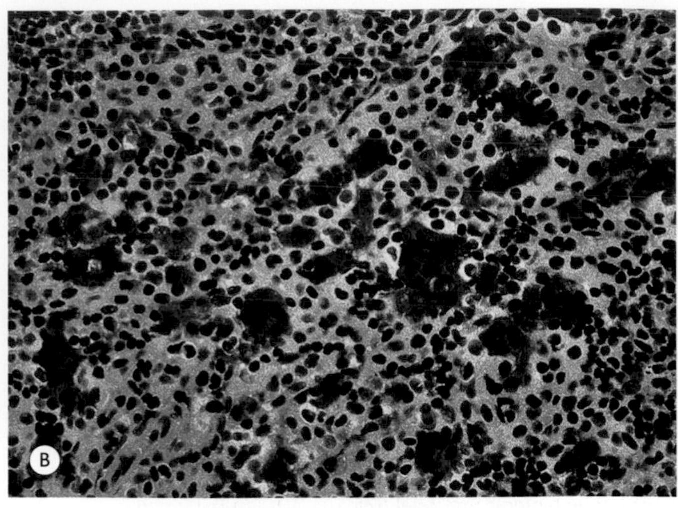

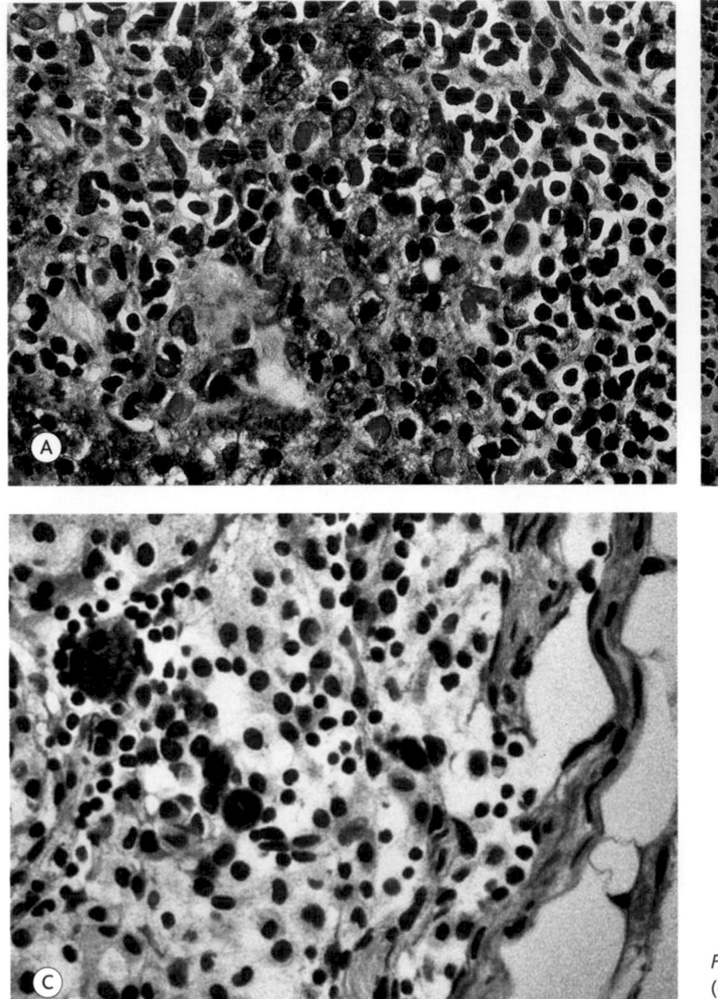

Fig. 20.55 (A) Reactivity with HBME-1 and (B) for calretinin and (C) keratin 5 in the lesion shown in the Fig. 20.54. Other immunostains for glandular epithelial markers were negative.

in association with those lesions. Radiographic assessment has shown pleural nodularity in association with an effusion.[338]

Multicystic mesothelial tumor of borderline biologic potential of the pleura is extraordinarily rare, with only one published example. That patient was a 37-year-old woman who presented with a localized, multiloculated intrapleural mass that was found on imaging studies. No pleural effusion was apparent.[340] We have recently seen one other lesion of this type in a 34-year-old woman with a unilateral pleural mass.

The evolution of pleural WDPM has been variable; however, of four cases in the report by Butnor and colleagues in which follow-up was available, all of the patients were alive with persistent tumor at least 6 months after diagnosis.[338] None of the lesions metastasized outside the thorax or crossed the anatomic midline. The single reported MMTBBP of the pleura was cured by excision.[340]

Pathologic observations

Pleural WDPM has manifested itself either as a multifocal nodular proliferation, with firm white-tan lesions on the serosal surface, or as a single exophytic growth that projected into the pleural space. The size of individual nodules in such cases has ranged from <1 cm to 5 cm in greatest dimension.[338] Those descriptions obviously overlap with the macroscopic features of conventional mesotheliomas. On the other hand, MMTBBP has a distinctive image, represented by a well-circumscribed agglomeration of thin-walled cysts filled with serous fluid (Fig. 20.56). No internal nodularity is apparent when the cystic cavities are opened.

Microscopically, WDPM is typified by arborescent fibrovascular papillary projections of variable width and length, which are covered by one or two layers of relatively bland cuboidal mesothelium (Fig. 20.57). Nuclei

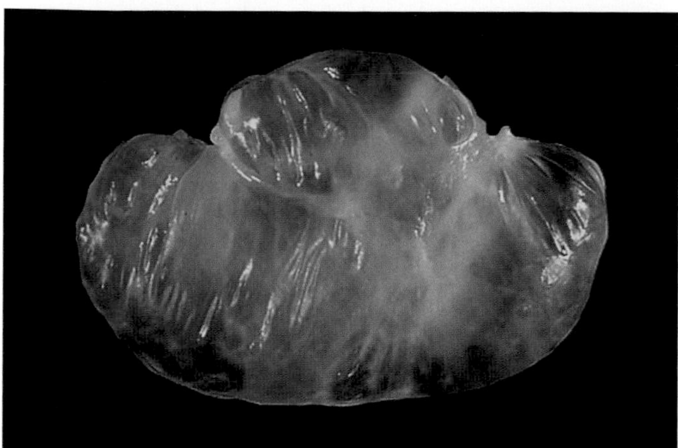

Fig. 20.56 Gross photograph of pleural multicystic mesothelial tumor of borderline biologic potential (MMTBBP). It is a thin-walled, internally loculated cyst that was easily dissected from surrounding tissues.

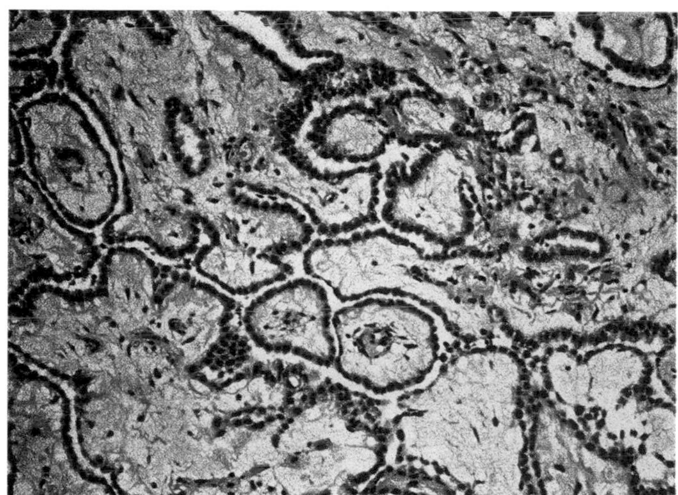

Fig. 20.57 Well-differentiated papillary mesothelioma (WDPM) of the pleura, showing broad fronds of tumor tissue that are mantled by uniform cuboidal cells.

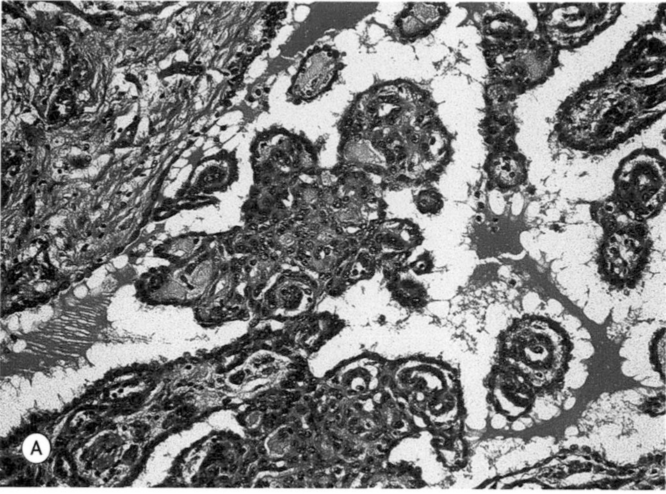

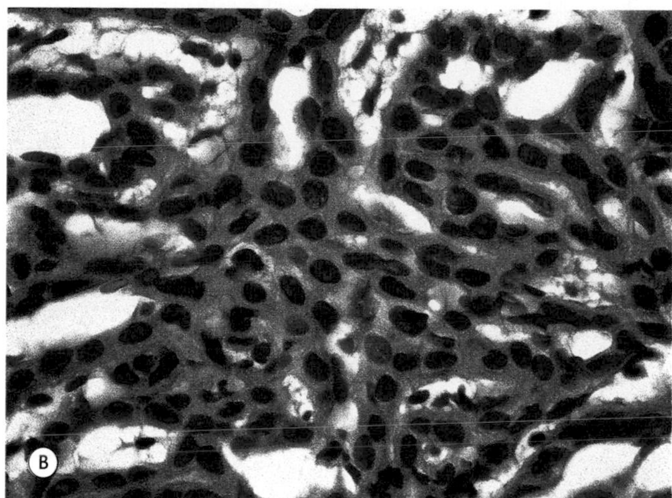

Fig. 20.58 Smaller papillae are evident in this (A) pleural well-differentiated papillary mesothelioma (WDPM), as are (B) areas of tubule formation. Note the cytologic blandness of the tumor cells.

are round to oval, with vesicular or dispersed chromatin and focally prominent nucleoli; mitotic figures are sparse (Fig. 20.58). Some examples show hyalinization of the papillary cores, or psammoma bodies, or both. Limited infiltration of the subjacent pleural soft tissue by tubular cell profiles is seen in a minority of cases. Histochemical, ultrastructural, and immunohistochemical attributes of WDPM are comparable to those that are associated with conventional mesothelioma morphotypes.

The multicystic mesothelial tumor histologically comprises relatively large macrocystic spaces that are bounded by hypocellular collagenized stroma and filled with lightly eosinophilic serous fluid (Fig. 20.59). The cysts are mantled by a single layer of bland cuboidal mesothelial cells with "hobnail" nuclear profiles (Fig. 20.60). No nucleoli or mitotic activity are apparent, and, although tubular profiles may surround the cystic spaces, there is no infiltration of the surrounding tissue by the lesional cells.

Results of adjunctive studies in MMTBBP again mirror those obtained in mesothelial proliferations in general. However, the morphologic image of that lesion is so singular that specialized evaluations are not necessary.

Staging and prognosis of malignant mesothelioma

In general, tumor stage is the most powerful predictor of biologic behavior for any given malignancy. Several

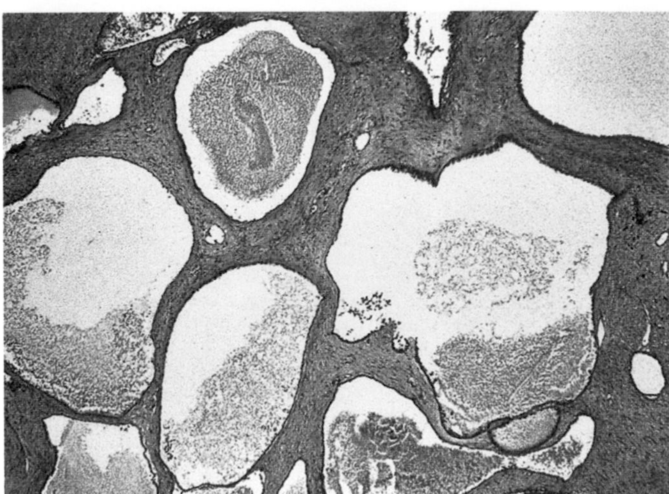

Fig. 20.59 Multicystic mesothelial tumor of borderline biologic potential (MMTBBP) is a multilocular lesion on scanning microscopy, with proteinaceous contents.

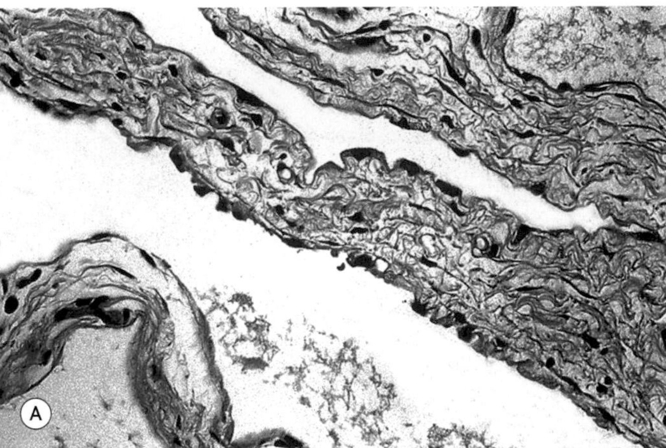

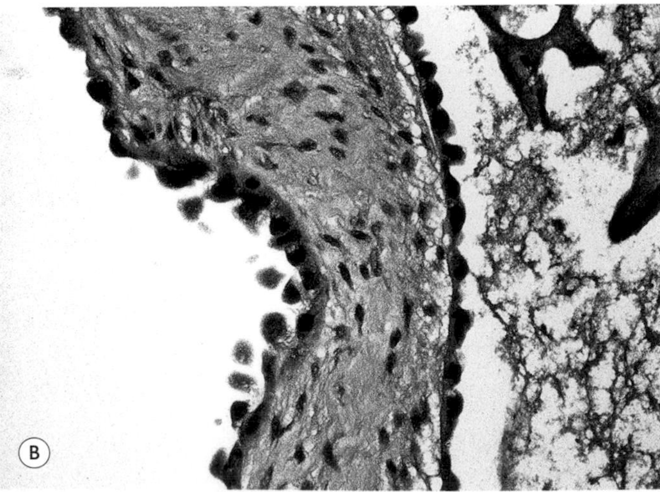

Fig. 20.60 Internal fibrous septa (A) are lined by plump epithelioid cells with a "hobnail" configuration (B) in multicystic mesothelial tumor of borderline biologic potential (MMTBBP).

staging systems have been used to document the locoregional and distant growth of MM. The first of these was the Butchart (English) scheme, proposed in 1976.[341] It dealt descriptively with the general growth characteristics of individual tumors. That same principle was later expanded by the International Mesothelima Interest Group[342] and codified by the American Joint Committee on Cancer, in a formal tumor–node–metastasis (TNM) format.[343] The Thoracic Oncology Group at the Brigham & Women's Hospital has also advanced a pragmatic surgery-oriented staging system which has entered clinical use.[344] These three schemes are summarized in Table 20.2.

Some of the other clinicopathologic factors affecting prognosis have been mentioned earlier in this discussion. In multivariate statistical analyses, those that have been associated with longer survivals include an epithelial histologic subtype, stage I disease, a good clinical performance (Karnofsky) score, female gender, patient age of <65 years old at diagnosis, tumor-related symptoms for >6 months before diagnosis, weight loss of <5%, negative tissue margins in surgically resected cases, serum levels of lactate dehydrogenase <500 IU/L, and the absence of chest pain.[345–348] Conversely, asbestos causation, cigarette smoking, and thrombocytosis have *not* held up as independent negative prognosticators.[345]

Table 20.2A Butchart (British) staging system for malignant pleural mesothelioma

Stage	Location
I	Tumor confined to the ipsilateral pleura, lung, or pericardium
II	Tumor invading the chest wall or mediastinal structures or metastases to thoracic lymph nodes
III	Tumor penetrating the diaphragm to involve the peritoneum or metastases to extrathoracic lymph nodes
IV	Distant blood-borne metastases

Table 20.2B Brigham & Women's Hospital staging system for pleural mesothelioma

Stage	Description
I	Can be extirpated surgically; no involvement of regional lymph nodes by tumor
II	Can be removed surgically but regional lymph nodes are involved by tumor
III	Inoperable; tumor involves chest wall, pericardium, or diaphragm/peritoneum. Regional lymph nodes may or may not contain metastases
IV	Inoperable; distant (extrathoracic) metastases are present

Table 20.2C TNM staging system for malignant pleural mesothelioma

Stage	Description of tumor
T1a	Limited to ipsilateral parietal pleura (including mediastinal and diaphragmatic pleura), with no involvement of visceral pleura
T1b	Ipsilateral parietal pleural involvement (including mediastinal and diaphragmatic pleura), with scattered foci of visceral pleural involvement
T2	Ipsilateral pleural involvement, with at least 1 of the following: Diaphragmatic muscle involvement Confluent visceral pleural tumor involvement (including fissures) Extension from visceral pleura into pulmonary parenchyma
T3	Locally advanced but resectable tumor; each ipsilateral pleural surface shows at least 1 of the following: Involvement of the endothoracic fascia Extension into the mediastinal fat Solitary, completely resectable tumor focus in chest wall soft tissues Nontransmural involvement of the pericardium
T4	Locally advanced, technically unresectable tumor; each ipsilateral pleural surface shows at least 1 of the following: Diffuse extension or multifocal chest wall masses with or without rib destruction Direct transdiaphragmatic extension into the peritoneum Direct extension to contralateral pleura Direct extension to 1 or more mediastinal organs Direct extension into spine Extension through to internal surface of pericardium, with or without pericardial effusion or myocardial involvement
NX	Regional lymph nodes are not evaluable
N0	No regional lymph nodes metastases are present
N1	Metastases in ipsilateral bronchopulmonary or hilar lymph nodes
N2	Metastases in subcarinal or ipsilateral mediastinal lymph nodes, including ipsilateral internal mammary nodes
N3	Metastases in contralateral mediastinal, contralateral internal mammary, and ipsilateral or contralateral supraclavicular lymph nodes
MX	Presence of distant metastases is not evaluable
M0	No distant metastases are present
M1	Distant (extrathoracic) metastases are present

Stage grouping: Stage IA – T1a/N0/M0; Stage IB – T1b/N0/M0; Stage II – T2/N0/M0; Stage III – T3/Any N/M0 *or* T1 or T2/N1 or N2/M0; Stage IV – T4/Any N/M0 *or* Any T/N3/M0 *or* Any T/Any N/M1.

Recent analyses have also examined the prognostic influence of cell-cycle-related proteins in the tumor cells: p27 (*kip1*) is a cell-cycle inhibitor that is downregulated in rapidly replicating tissues; accordingly, it is not surprising that several studies have concluded that its level correlates directly with prognosis in MM cases.[349–351] On the other hand, the Ki-67 protein, an S-phase-related nuclear moiety, is preferentially *expressed* in actively dividing cells. Thus, one would expect that high Ki-67 indices (>30%) would be seen in aggressive MMs, and based on the results of pertinent publications,[351,352] that supposition appears to be valid.

REFERENCES

1. Millard M: Lung, pleura, and mediastinum. In: Pathology, Anderson WAD, Ed., 6th edn. 1971, CV Mosby, St. Louis, pp 875–997.
2. Klemperer P, Rabin CB: Primary neoplasms of the pleura. Arch Pathol 1931; 11: 385–401.
3. DeLajarte M, deLaJarte AY: Mesothelioma on the coast of Brittany, France. Ann NY Acad Sci 1979; 330: 323–332.
4. Legha SS, Muggia FM: Pleural mesotheliomas: clinical features and therapeutic implications. Ann Intern Med 1977; 87: 613–620.
5. Elmes PC, Simpson MJC: The clinical aspects of mesothelioma. Q J Med 1976; 45: 427–441.
6. Aziz T, Jilaihawi A, Prakash D: The management of malignant pleural mesothelioma: single center experience in 10 years. Eur J Cardiothorac Surg 2002; 22: 298–305.
7. Grundy GW, Miller RW: Malignant mesothelioma in childhood. Cancer 1972; 30: 1216–1218.
8. Coffin CM, Dehner LP: Mesothelial and related neoplasms in children and adolescents: a clinicopathologic and immunohistochemical analysis of eight cases. Pediatr Pathol 1992; 12: 333–347.
9. Fraire AE, Cooper S, Greenberg SD, Buffler P, Langston C: Mesothelioma of childhood. Cancer 1988; 62: 838–847.
10. Ascoli V, Scalzo CC, Bruno C, et al.: Familial pleural malignant mesothelioma: clustering in three sisters and one cousin. Cancer Lett 1998; 130: 203–207.
11. Dawson A, Gibbs A, Browne K, Pooley F, Griffiths M: Familial mesothelioma: details of 17 cases with histopathologic findings and mineral analysis. Cancer 1992; 70: 1183–1187.
12. Krousel T, Garcas N, Rothschild H: Familial clustering of mesothelioma: a report on three affected persons in one family. Am J Prev Med 1986; 2: 186–188.

13. Lynch HT, Katz D, Markvicka SE: Familial mesothelioma: review and family study. Cancer Genet Cytogenet 1985; 15: 25–35.
14. Law MR, Hodson ME, Turner-Warwick M: Malignant mesothelioma of the pleura: clinical aspects and symptomatic treatment. Eur J Respir Dis 1984; 65: 162–168.
15. Bonomo L, Feragalli B, Sacco R, et al.: Malignant pleural disease. Eur J Radiol 2000; 34: 98–118.
16. Bueno R: Mesothelioma – clinical presentation. Chest 1999; 116 (Suppl 6): 444S–445S.
17. Neumeister W, Gillisseu A, Rasche K, et al.: Pleural mesothelioma. I. Historical, epidemiological, and clinical aspects (symptoms and diagnosis). Med Klin 2001; 96: 722–729.
18. Pisani RJ, Colby TV, Williams DE: Malignant mesothelioma of the pleura. Mayo Clin Proc 1988; 63: 1234–1244.
19. Ruffie PA: Pleural mesothelioma. Curr Opin Oncol 1991; 3: 328–334.
20. Dutt PL, Baxter JW, O'Malley FP, Glick AD, Page DL: Distant cutaneous metastasis of pleural mesothelioma. J Cutan Pathol 1992; 19: 490–495.
21. Sussman J, Rosai J: Lymph node metastasis as the initial manifestation of malignant mesothelioma: report of six cases. Am J Surg Pathol 1990; 14: 819–828.
22. Achatzy R, Beba W, Ritschler R, et al.: The diagnosis, therapy, and prognosis of diffuse malignant mesothelioma. Eur J Cardiothorac Surg 1989; 3: 445–448.
23. Mischler NE, Chuprevich T, Johnson RO, Tormey DC: Malignant mesothelioma presenting in the pleura and peritoneum. J Surg Oncol 1979; 11: 185–191.
24. Metintas M, Icgun I, Elbek O, et al.: Computed tomographic features in malignant pleural mesothelioma and other commonly seen pleural diseases. Eur J Radiol 2002; 41: 1–9.
25. Marom EM, Erasmus JJ, Pass HI, Patz EF Jr: The role of imaging in malignant pleural mesothelioma. Semin Oncol 2002; 29: 26–35.
26. Eibel K, Tuengerthal S, Schoenberg SO: The role of new imaging techniques in diagnosis and staging of malignant pleural mesothelioma. Curr Opin Oncol 2003; 15: 131–138.
27. Knuuttila A, Kivisaari L, Kivisaari A, et al.: Evaluation of pleural disease using MR and CT, with special reference to malignant pleural mesothelioma. Acta Radiol 2001; 42: 502–507.
28. Hammar SP: The pathology of benign and malignant pleural disease. Chest Surg Clin N Am 1994; 4: 405–430.
29. Hillerdal G: The human evidence: parenchymal and pleural changes. Ann Occup Hyg 1994; 38: 561–567.
30. Chahinian AP, Pajak TF, Holland JF, et al.: Diffuse malignant mesothelioma: prospective evaluation of 69 patients. Ann Intern Med 1982; 96: 746–755.
30a. DePangher-Manzini V, Brollo A, Bianchi C: Thrombocytosis in malignant pleural mesothelioma. Tumori 1990; 76: 576–578.
30b. Nakano T, Fujii J, Tamura S, Hada T, Higashino K: Thrombocytosis in patients with malignant pleural mesothelioma. Cancer 1986; 58: 1699–1701.
30c. Nakano T, Chahinian AP, Shinjo M, et al.: Interleukin-6 and its relationship to clinical parameters in patients with malignant pleural mesothelioma. Br J Cancer 1998; 77: 907–912.
31. Shah I, Salvatore JR, Kummet T, Gani OS, Wheeler LA: Pseudomesotheliomatous carcinoma involving pleura and peritoneum: a clinicopathologic and immunohistochemical study of three cases. Ann Diagn Pathol 1999; 3: 148–159.
32. Koss MN, Fleming M, Przygodski RM, et al.: Adenocarcinoma simulating mesothelioma: a clinicopathologic and immunohistochemical study of 29 cases. Ann Diagn Pathol 1998; 2: 93–102.
33. Hartmann CA, Schutze H: Mesothelioma-like tumors of the pleura: a review of 72 autopsy cases. Cancer Res Clin Oncol 1994; 120: 331–347.
34. Jaklitsch MT, Grondin SC, Sugarbaker DJ: Treatment of malignant mesothelioma. World J Surg 2001; 25: 210–217.
35. Grossebner MW, Arifi AA, Goddard M, Ritchie AJ: Mesothelioma – VATS biopsy and lung mobilization improves diagnosis and palliation. Eur J Cardiothorac Surg 1999; 16: 619–623.
36. Roberts GH, Campbell GH: Exfoliative cytology of diffuse mesothelioma. J Clin Pathol 1972; 25: 557–582.
37. Nguyen GK, Akin MR, Villanueva RR, Slatnik J: Cytopathology of malignant mesothelioma of the pleura in fine needle aspiration biopsies. Diagn Cytopathol 1999; 21: 253–259.
38. Antman KH: Clinical presentation and natural history of benign and malignant mesothelioma. Semin Oncol 1981; 8: 313–320.
39. Lee YC, Light RW, Musk AW: Management of malignant pleural mesothelioma: a critical review. Curr Opin Pulm Med 2000; 6: 267–274.
40. Butchart EG: Contemporary management of malignant pleural mesothelioma. Oncologist 1999; 4; 488–500.
41. Zellos LS, Sugarbaker DJ: Diffuse malignant mesothelioma of the pleural space and its management. Oncology 2002; 16: 916–925.
42. Kindler HL: Malignant pleural mesothelioma. Curr Treat Options Oncol 2000; 1: 313–326.
43. Senan S: Indications and limitations of radiotherapy in malignant pleural mesothelioma. Curr Opin Oncol 2003; 15: 144–147.
44. Grondin SC, Sugarbaker DJ: Pleuropneumonectomy in the treatment of malignant pleural mesothelioma. Chest 1999; 116 (Suppl 6): 450S–454S.
45. Kaiser LR: New therapies in the treatment of malignant pleural mesothelioma. Semin Thorac Cardiovasc Surg 1997; 9: 383–390.
46. Erkilic S, Sari I, Tuncozgur B: Localized pleural malignant mesothelioma. Pathol Int 2001; 51: 812–815.
47. Okamura H, Kamai T, Mitsuno A, et al.: Localized malignant mesothelioma of the pleura. Pathol Int 2001; 51: 654–660.
48. Crotty TB, Myers JL, Katzenstein AL, et al.: Localized malignant mesothelioma: a clinicopathologic and flow cytometric study. Am J Surg Pathol 1994; 18: 357–363.
49. Christoffel T, Teret SP: Epidemiology and the law: courts and confidence intervals. Am J Public Health 1991; 81: 1661–1666.
50. Wagner JC, Sleggs CA, Marchand P: Diffuse pleural mesothelioma and asbestos exposure in North-Western Cape Province. Br J Ind Med 1960; 17: 260–271.
51. Smither WJ: Asbestos, asbestosis, and mesothelioma of the pleura. Proc R Soc Med 1966; 59: 57–59.
52. Hill ID, Doll R, Knox JF: Mortality among asbestos workers. Proc R Soc Med 1966; 59: 59–60.
53. Mann RH, Grosh JL, O'Donnell WM: Mesothelioma associated with asbestosis: a report of 3 cases. Cancer 1966; 19: 521–526.
54. Butnor KJ, Sporn TA, Roggli VL: Exposure to brake dust and malignant mesothelioma: a study of 10 cases with mineral fiber analyses. Ann Occup Hyg 2003; 47: 325–330.
55. Valic F: The asbestos dilemma. I. Assessment of risk. Arh Hig Rada Toksikol 2002; 53: 153–167.
56. Roggli VL, Sharma A, Butnor KJ, Sporn TA, Vollmer RT: Malignant mesothelioma and occupational exposure to asbestos: a clinicopathological correlation of 1445 cases. Ultrastruct Pathol 2002; 26: 55–65.
57. McDonald JC, Armstrong BG, Edwards CW, et al.: Case-referent study of young adults with mesothelioma. I. Lung fiber analyses. Ann Occup Hyg 2001; 45: 513–518.
58. Britton M: The epidemiology of mesothelioma. Semin Oncol 2002; 29: 18–25.
59. Marchevsky AM, Wick MR: Current controversies regarding the role of asbestos exposure in the causation of malignant mesothelioma: the need for an evidence-based approach to develop medicolegal guidelines. Ann Diagn Pathol, in press.
60. Roggli VL, Pratt PC, Brody AR: Asbestos content of lung tissue in asbestos-associated diseases: a study of 110 cases. Br J Ind Med 1986; 43: 18–28.
61. Roggli VL, Pratt PC, Brody AR: Analysis of tissue mineral fiber content. In: Pathology of asbestos-associated diseases, Roggli VL, Greenberg SD, Pratt PC, Eds. 1992, Little Brown, Boston, pp 299–345.
62. Ilgren EB, Wagner JC: Background incidence of mesothelioma: animal and human evidence. Regul Toxicol Pharmacol 1991; 13: 133–149.
63. Peterson JT Jr, Greenberg SD, Buffler PA: Non-asbestos-related malignant mesothelioma: a review. Cancer 1984; 54: 951–960.
64. Craighead JE, Mossman BT: Pathogenesis of mesothelioma. In: Asbestos-related malignancy, Antman KH, Aisner J, Eds. 1987, Grune & Stratton, New York, pp 151–162.
65. Lanphear BP, Buncher CR: Latent period for malignant mesothelioma of occupational origin. J Occup Med 1992; 34: 718–721.
66. Pass HI, Mew DJ: In-vitro and in-vivo studies of mesothelioma. J Cell Biochem 1996; 24 (Suppl): 142–151.
67. Manning CB, Vallyathan V, Mossman BT: Diseases caused by asbestos: mechanisms of injury and disease development. Int Immunopharmacol 2002; 2: 191–200.

68. Fitzpatrick DR, Peroni DJ, Bielefeldt-Ohmann H: The role of growth factors and cytokines in the tumorigenesis and immunobiology of malignant mesothelioma. Am J Resp Cell Mol Biol 1995; 12: 455–460.
69. Huncharek M: Non-asbestos-related diffuse malignant mesothelioma. Tumori 2002; 88: 1–9.
70. Falchero L, Coiffier B, Guibert B, et al.: Malignant mesothelioma of the pleura following radiotherapy of Hodgkin's disease. Bull Cancer 1996; 83: 964–968.
71. Mizuki M, Yukishige K, Abe Y, Tsuda T: A case of malignant pleural mesothelioma following exposure to atomic radiation in Nagasaki. Respirology 1997; 2: 201–205.
72. Antman KH, Ruxer RL Jr, Aisner J, Vawter G: Mesothelioma following Wilms' tumor in childhood. Cancer 1984; 54: 367–369.
73. Neugut AI, Ahsen H, Antman KH: Incidence of malignant pleural mesothelioma after thoracic radiotherapy. Cancer 1997; 80: 948–950.
74. Weissmann LB, Corson JM, Neugut AI, Antman KH: Malignant mesothelioma following treatment for Hodgkin's disease. J Clin Oncol 1996; 14: 2098–2100.
75. Cavazza A, Travis LB, Travis WD, et al.: Post-irradiation malignant mesothelioma. Cancer 1996; 77: 1379–1385.
76. Hillerdal G, Berg J: Malignant mesothelioma secondary to chronic inflammation and old scars. Cancer 1985; 55: 1968–1972.
77. Vertun-Baranowska B, Szymanska D, Szturmowicz M: Malignant mesothelioma. I. Evaluation of autopsy specimens. Pneumonol Pol 1988; 56: 47–54.
78. Livneh A, Langevitz P, Pras M: Pulmonary associations in familial Mediterranean fever. Curr Opin Pulm Med 1999; 5; 326–331.
79. Lidar M, Pras M, Langevitz P, Livneh A: Thoracic and lung involvement in familial Mediterranean fever. Clin Chest Med 2002; 23: 505–511.
80. Huncharek M, Kelsey K, Muscat J, Christiani D: Parental cancer and genetic predisposition in malignant pleural mesothelioma: a case-control study. Cancer Lett 1996; 102: 205–208.
81. Van Kaick G, Dalheimer A, Hornick S, et al.: The German Thorotrast Study: recent results and assessment of risks. Radiat Res 1999; 152 (Suppl 6): S64–S71.
82. Andersson M, Wallin H, Jonsson M, et al.: Lung carcinoma and malignant mesothelioma in patients exposed to Thorotrast: incidence, histology, and p53 status. Int J Cancer 1995; 63: 330–336.
83. Emri S, Demir A, Dogan M, et al.: Lung diseases due to environmental exposures to erionite and asbestos in Turkey. Toxicol Lett 2002; 127: 251–257.
84. Dumortier P, Gocmen A, Laurent K, Manco A, DeVuyst P: The role of environmental and occupational exposures in Turkish immigrants with fiber-related disease. Eur Respir J 2001; 17: 922–927.
85. Strickler HD, Goedert JJ, Fleming M, et al.: Simian virus 40 and pleural mesothelioma in humans. Cancer Epidemiol Biomarkers Prev 1996; 5; 473–475.
86. Dopp E, Poser I, Papp T: Interphase FISH analysis of cell cycle genes in asbestos-treated human mesothelial cells (HMC), SV40-transformed HMB, and mesothelioma cells. Cell Mol Biol 2002; 48: OL271–OL277 (online publication).
87. Mutti L, Carbone M, Giordano GG, Giordano A: Simian virus-40 and human cancer. Monaldi Arch Chest Dis 1998; 53: 198–201.
88. Simsir A, Fetsch P, Bedrossian CW, Ioffe OB, Abati A: Absence of SV-40 large-T antigen (Tag) in malignant mesothelioma effusions: an immunocytochemical study. Diagn Cytopathol 2001; 25: 203–207.
89. Foddis R, DeRienzo A, Broccoli D, et al.: SV40 infection induces telomerase activity in human mesothelial cells. Oncogene 2002; 21: 1434–1442.
90. Hashimoto N, Oda T, Kadota K: An ultrastructural study of malignant mesotheliomas in two cows. Jpn J Vet Sci 1989; 51: 327–336.
91. Colbourne CM, Bolton JR, Mills JN, et al.: Mesothelioma in horses. Aust Vet J 1992; 69: 275–278.
92. Misdorp W: Tumors in calves: comparative aspects. J Comp Pathol 2002; 127: 96–105.
93. Cunningham AA, Dhillon AP: Pleural malignant mesothelioma in a captive clouded leopard (*Neofelis nebulosa nebulosa*). Vet Rec 1998; 143: 22–24.
94. Baskerville A: Mesothelioma in the calf. Pathol Vet 1967; 4: 149–156.
95. Shibuya K, Tajima M, Yamate J: Histological classification of 62 spontaneous mesotheliomas in F344 rats. Jpn J Vet Sci 1990; 52: 1313–1317.
96. Rostami M, Tateyama S, Uchida K, et al.: Tumors in domestic animals examined during a ten-year period (1980–1989) at Miyazaki University. J Vet Med Sci 1994; 56: 403–405.
97. Rusch VW, Godwin JD, Shuman WP: The role of computed tomography scanning in the initial assessment and the followup of malignant pleural mesothelioma. J Thorac Cardiovasc Surg 1988; 96: 171–177.
98. Golla B, Singh SP, Pinkard NB, Klemm KM, Nath H: Rapidly fatal bilateral malignant mesothelioma. Semin Roentgenol 1998; 33: 306–308.
99. Nakatsuka S, Yao M, Hoshida Y, et al.: Pyothorax-associated lymphoma: a review of 106 cases. J Clin Oncol 2002; 20: 4255–4260.
100. Falconieri G, Bussani R, Mirra M, Zanella M: Pseudomesotheliomatous angiosarcoma: a pleuropulmonary lesion simulating pleural mesothelioma. Histopathology 1997; 30: 419–424.
101. Wick MR: Pleural cytology, tumor markers, and immunohistochemistry. In: Textbook of pleural diseases, Light RW, Lee YCG, Eds. 2003, Arnold, Publishers, London, pp 256–281.
102. DiBonito L, Falconieri G, Colautti I, et al.: Cytopathology of malignant mesothelioma: a study of its patterns and histological bases. Diagn Cytopathol 1993; 9: 25–31.
103. Sherman ME, Mark EJ: Effusion cytology in the diagnosis of malignant epithelioid and biphasic pleural mesothelioma. Arch Pathol Lab Med 1990; 114: 845–851.
104. Johnston WW: The malignant pleural effusion: a review of cytopathologic diagnoses of 584 specimens from 472 consecutive patients. Cancer 1985; 56: 905–909.
105. Matzel W: Biochemical and cytological features of diffuse mesothelioma of the pleura. Arch Geschwulstforsch 1985; 55: 259–264.
106. Castelain G, Castelain C, Pretet S, Kreis B: Cytodiagnosis of pleural mesotheliomas. Presse Med 1969; 77: 197–199.
107. Castelain G, Ioannou J, Castelain C, Pretet S: Cytodiagnosis in lung diseases: its importance and its value. A study of 945 cases. Presse Med 1968; 76: 2219–2221.
108. Yokoi T, Mark EJ: Atypical mesothelial hyperplasia associated with bronchogenic carcinoma. Hum Pathol 1991; 22: 695–699.
109. Cavazza A, Rossi G, Agostini L, et al.: Small-cell mesothelioma of the pleura: description of a case. Pathologica 2002; 94: 247–252.
110. Hammar SP, Bolen JW: Sarcomatoid pleural mesothelioma. Ultrastruct Pathol 1985; 9: 337–343.
111. Colby TV: Malignancies in the lung and pleura mimicking benign processes. Semin Diagn Pathol 1995; 12: 30–44.
112. Khalidi HS, Medeiros LJ, Battifora H: Lymphohistiocytoid mesothelioma: an often-misdiagnosed variant of sarcomatoid malignant mesothelioma. Am J Clin Pathol 2000; 113: 649–654.
113. Cibas ES, Corson JM, Pinkus GS: The distinction of adenocarcinoma from malignant mesothelioma in cell blocks of effusions. Hum Pathol 1987; 18: 67–74.
114. Renshaw AA, Dean BR, Antman KH, Sugarbaker DJ, Cibas ES: The role of cytologic evaluation of pleural fluid in the diagnosis of malignant mesothelioma. Chest 1997; 111: 106–109.
115. Nind AR, Attanoos RL, Gibbs AR: Unusual intraparenchymal growth patterns of malignant pleural mesothelioma. Histopathology 2003; 42: 150–155.
116. Corson JM: Pathology of diffuse malignant pleural mesothelioma. Semin Thorac Cardiovasc Surg 1997; 9: 347–355.
117. Donaldson JC, Elliott RC, Kaminsky DB, Walsh TE, Newby JG: Psammoma bodies in pleural fluid associated with a mesothelioma: case report. Mil Med 1979; 144: 476–479.
118. Suzuki Y: Diagnostic criteria for human diffuse malignant mesothelioma. Acta Pathol Jpn 1992; 42: 767–786.
119. Shia J, Erlandson RA, Klimstra DS: Deciduoid mesothelioma: a report of 5 cases and literature review. Ultrastruct Pathol 2002; 26: 355–363.
120. Monaghan H, Al-Nafussi A: Deciduoid pleural mesothelioma. Histopathology 2001; 39: 104–106.
121. Ordonez NG: Epithelial mesothelioma with deciduoid features: report of four cases. Am J Surg Pathol 2000; 24: 816–823.
122. Ordonez NG, Mackay B: Glycogen-rich mesothelioma. Ultrastruct Pathol 1999; 23: 401–406.
123. Dessy E, Falleni M, Braidotti P, et al.: Unusual clear-cell variant of epithelioid mesothelioma. Arch Pathol Lab Med 2001; 125: 1588–1590.
124. Ordonez NG, Myhre M, Mackay B: Clear cell mesothelioma. Ultrastruct Pathol 1996; 20: 331–336.

125. Chang HT, Yantiss RK, Nielsen GP, McKee GT, Mark EJ: Lipid-rich diffuse malignant mesothelioma: a case report. Hum Pathol 2000; 31: 876–879.
126. Umezu H, Kuwata K, Ebe Y, et al.: Microcystic variant of localized malignant mesothelioma accompanying an adenomatoid tumor-like lesion. Pathol Int 2002; 52: 416–422.
127. Henderson DW, Shilkin KB, Whitaker D: Reactive mesothelial hyperplasia versus mesothelioma, including mesothelioma in-situ: a brief review. Am J Clin Pathol 1998; 110: 397–404.
128. Whitaker D, Henderson DW, Shilkin KB: The concept of mesothelioma in-situ: implications for diagnosis and histogenesis. Semin Diagn Pathol 1992; 9: 151–161.
129. Bolen JW: Tumors of serosal tissue origin. Clin Lab Med 1987; 7: 31–50.
130. Carter D, Otis CN: Three types of spindle cell tumors of the pleura: fibroma, sarcoma, and sarcomatoid mesothelioma. Am J Surg Pathol 1988; 12: 747–753.
131. Avellini C, Alampi G, Cocchi V, et al.: Malignant sarcomatoid mesothelioma of the pleura. Pathologica 1991; 83: 335–340.
132. Andrion A, Mazzucco G, Bernardi P, Mollo F: Sarcomatous tumor of the chest wall with osteochondroid differentiation: evidence of mesothelial origin. Am J Surg Pathol 1989; 13: 707–712.
133. Okamoto T, Yokota S, Shinkawa K, et al.: Pleural malignant mesothelioma with osseous, cartilaginous, and rhabdomyoblastic differentiation. J Jpn Resp Soc 1998; 36: 696–701.
134. Yousem SA, Hochholzer L: Malignant mesotheliomas with osseous and cartilaginous differentiation. Arch Pathol Lab Med 1987; 111: 62–66.
135. Sterrett GF, Whitaker D, Shilkin KB, Walters MN: Fine needle aspiration cytology of malignant mesothelioma. Acta Cytol 1987; 31: 185–193.
136. Colby TV: The diagnosis of desmoplastic malignant mesothelioma. Am J Clin Pathol 1998; 110: 135–136.
137. Wilson GE, Hasleton PS, Chatterjee AK: Desmoplastic malignant mesothelioma: a review of 17 cases. J Clin Pathol 1992; 45: 295–298.
138. Cantin R, Al-Jabi M, McCaughey WTE: Desmoplastic diffuse mesothelioma. Am J Surg Pathol 1982; 6: 215–222.
139. Churg A, Colby TV, Cagle PT, et al.: The separation of benign and malignant mesothelial proliferations. Am J Surg Pathol 2000; 24: 1183–2000.
140. Mayall FG, Gibbs AR: The histology and immunohistochemistry of small cell mesothelioma. Histopathology 1992; 20: 47–51.
141. Wick MR, Ritter JH, Dehner LP: Malignant rhabdoid tumors: a clinicopathologic review and conceptual discussion. Semin Diagn Pathol 1995; 12: 233–248.
142. Puttagunta L, Vriend RA, Nguyen GK: Deciduoid epithelial mesothelioma of the pleura with focal rhabdoid change. Am J Surg Pathol 2000; 24: 1440–1443.
143. Kannerstein M, Churg J, Magner D: Histochemistry in the diagnosis of malignant mesothelioma. Ann Clin Lab Sci 1973; 3: 207–211.
144. Cook HC: A histochemical characterization of malignant tumor mucins as a possible aid in the identification of metastatic deposits. Med Lab Technol 1973; 30: 217–224.
145. Griffiths MH, Riddell RJ, Xipell JM: Malignant mesothelioma: a review of 35 cases with diagnosis and prognosis. Pathology 1980; 12: 591–603.
146. Kwee WS, Veldhuizen RW, Golding RP, et al.: Histologic distinction between malignant mesothelioma, benign pleural lesions, and carcinoma metastasis. Virchows Arch Pathol Anat 1982; 397: 287–299.
147. Bertoldo E, Bernardi P, Gugliotta P: Histochemical and immunohistochemical methods in the diagnosis of mesothelioma. Pathologica 1987; 79: 447–455.
148. Lucas JG, Tuttle SE: Diagnostic histochemical and immunohistochemical studies in malignant mesothelioma. J Surg Oncol 1987; 35: 30–34.
149. McCaughey WTE, Colby TV, Battifora H, et al.: Diagnosis of diffuse malignant mesothelioma: experience of a US/Canadian Mesothelioma Panel. Mod Pathol 1991; 4: 342–353.
150. Wick MR, Loy T, Mills SE, Legier JF, Manivel JC: Malignant epithelioid pleural mesothelioma versus peripheral pulmonary adenocarcinoma: a histochemical, ultrastructural, and immunohistologic study of 103 cases. Hum Pathol 1990; 21: 759–766.
151. Arai H, Endo M, Sasai Y, et al.: Histochemical demonstration of hyaluronic acid in a case of pleural mesothelioma. Am Rev Respir Dis 1975; 111: 699–702.
152. Hammar SP, Bockus DE, Remington FL, Rohrbach KA: Mucin-positive epithelial mesotheliomas: a histochemical, immunohistochemical, and ultrastructural comparison with mucin-producing pulmonary adenocarcinomas. Ultrastruct Pathol 1996; 20: 293–325.
153. McMeekin W, Kennedy A, McNicol AM: Combined immunocytochemical and nucleolar organizer region staining: some technical aspects. Med Lab Sci 1989; 46: 11–15.
154. Smith PJ, Skilbeck NQ, Harrison A, Crocker J: The effect of a series of fixatives on the AgNOR technique. J Pathol 1988; 155: 109–112.
155. Leong ASY, Raymond WA: Demonstration of AgNOR-related proteins in microwave-fixed tissues. J Pathol 1988; 156: 352.
156. Ayres JG, Crocker JG, Skilbeck NQ: Differentiation of malignant from normal and reactive mesothelial cells by the argyrophil technique for nucleolar organizer region-asssociated proteins. Thorax 1988; 43: 366–370.
157. Bethwaite PB, Delahunt B, Holloway LJ, Thornton A: Comparison of silver-staining nucleolar organizer region (AgNOR) counts and proliferating cell nuclear antigen (PCNA) expression in reactive mesothelial hyperplasia and malignant mesothelioma. Pathology 1995; 27: 1–4.
158. Ramesh K, Gahukamble L, Al-Fituri O: Utility of AgNOR technique in distinguishing reactive mesothelial hyperplasia, malignant mesothelioma, and pulmonary adenocarcinoma. Cent Afr J Med 1994; 40: 265.
159. Wolanski KD, Whitaker D, Shilkin KB, Henderson DW: The use of epithelial membrane antigen and silver-stained nucleolar organizer region testing in the differential diagnosis of mesothelioma from benign reactive mesothelioses. Cancer 1998; 82: 583–590.
160. Pomjanski N, Motherby H, Buckstegge B, et al.: Early diagnosis of mesothelioma in serous effusions using AgNOR analysis. Anal Quant Cytol Histol 2001; 23: 151–160.
161. Wang NS: Electron microscopy in the diagnosis of pleural mesotheliomas. Cancer 1973; 31: 1046–1054.
162. McDonald AD, Magner D, Eyssen G: Primary malignant mesothelial tumors in Canada, 1960–1968: a pathologic review by the Mesothelioma Panel of the Canadian Tumor Reference Center. Cancer 1973; 31: 869–876.
163. David JM: Ultrastructure of human mesotheliomas. J Natl Cancer Inst USA 1974; 52: 1715–1725.
164. Warhol MJ, Hickey WF, Corson JM: Malignant mesothelioma: ultrastructural distinction from adenocarcinoma. Am J Surg Pathol 1982; 6: 307–314.
165. Kobzik L, Antman KH, Warhol MJ: The distinction of mesothelioma from adenocarcinoma in malignant effusions by electron microscopy. Acta Cytol 1985; 29: 219–225.
166. Suzuki Y, Kannerstein M: Ultrastructure of human malignant diffuse mesothelioma. Am J Pathol 1976; 85: 241–262.
167. Stoebner P, Brambilla E: Ultrastructure of pleural tumors. Pathol Res Pract 1982; 173: 402–416.
168. Leong ASY, Stevens MW, Mukherjee TM: Malignant mesothelioma: cytologic diagnosis with histologic, immunohistochemical, and ultrastructural correlation. Semin Diagn Pathol 1992; 9; 141–150.
169. Dardick I, Jabi M, McCaughey WTE, et al.: Diffuse epithelial mesothelioma: a review of the ultrastructural spectrum. Ultrastruct Pathol 1987; 11: 503–533.
170. Oury TD, Hammar SP, Roggli VL: Ultrastructural features of diffuse malignant mesotheliomas. Hum Pathol 1998; 29: 1382–1392.
171. Ferenczy A: Diagnostic electron microscopy in gynecologic pathology. Pathol Annu 1979; 14 (part I): 353–381.
172. Chen HP, Berardi RS: A light and electron microscopic study of lung cancers: clinical implications. Int Surg 1993; 78: 124–126.
173. McGregor DH, Dixon AY, McGregor DK: Adenocarcinoma of the lung: a comparative diagnostic study using light and electron microscopy. Hum Pathol 1988; 19: 910–913.
174. Klima M, Bossart MI: Sarcomatous type of malignant mesothelioma. Ultrastruct Pathol 1983; 4: 349–358.
175. Dardick I, Srigley JR, McCaughey WTE, van Nostrand AW, Ritchie AC: Ultrastructural aspects of the histogenesis of diffuse and localized mesothelioma. Virchows Arch Pathol Anat 1984; 402: 373–388.
176. Leong ASY, Wick MR, Swanson PE: Immunohistology & electron microscopy of anaplastic & pleomorphic tumors. 1997, Cambridge University Press, Cambridge, UK, pp 59–108.

177. Corson JM, Pinkus GS: Mesothelioma: profile of keratin proteins and carcinoembryonic antigen. Am J Pathol 1982; 108: 80–87.
178. Bejui-Thivolet F, Patricot LM, Vauzelle JL: Keratins in malignant mesothelioma and pleural adenocarcinomas. Pathol Res Pract 1984; 179: 67–73.
179. Churg A: Immunohistochemical staining for vimentin and keratin in malignant mesothelioma. Am J Surg Pathol 1985; 9: 360–365.
180. Moll R, Dhouailly D, Sun TT: Expression of keratin 5 as a diagnostic feature of epithelial and biphasic mesotheliomas. Virchows Arch B 1989; 58: 129–145.
181. Kahn HJ, Thorner PS, Yeger H, Bailey D, Baumal R: Distinct keratin patterns demonstrated by immunoperoxidase staining of adenocarcinoma, carcinoids, and mesotheliomas using polyclonal and monoclonal antikeratin antibodies. Am J Clin Pathol 1986; 86: 566–574.
182. Ordonez NG: Value of cytokeratin 5/6 immunostaining in distinguishing epithelial mesothelioma of the pleura from lung adenocarcinoma. Am J Surg Pathol 1998; 22: 1215–1221.
183. Cury PM, Butcher DN, Fisher C, Corrin B, Nicholson DM: Value of the mesothelium-associated antibodies thrombomodulin, cytokeratin 5/6, calretinin, and CD44H in distinguishing epithelioid pleural mesothelioma from adenocarcinoma metastatic to the pleura. Mod Pathol 2000; 13: 107–112.
184. Blobel GA, Moll R, Franke WW, Kayser KW, Gould VE: The intermediate filament cytoskeleton of malignant mesothelioma and its diagnostic significance. Am J Pathol 1985; 121: 235–247.
185. Van Der Kwast TH, Versnel MA, Delahaye M, et al.: Expression of epithelial membrane antigen on malignant mesothelioma cells: an immunocytochemical and immunoelectron microscopic study. Acta Cytol 1988; 32: 169–174.
186. Kawai T, Greenberg SD, Truong LD, et al.: Differences in lectin binding of malignant pleural mesothelioma and adenocarcinoma of the lung. Am J Pathol 1988; 130: 401–410.
187. Pfaltz M, Odermatt B, Christen B, Ruttner JR: Immunohistochemistry in the diagnosis of malignant mesothelioma. Virchows Arch Pathol Anat 1987; 411: 387–393.
188. Leong ASY, Parkinson R, Milios J: "Thick" cell membranes revealed by immunocytochemical staining: a clue to the diagnosis of mesothelioma. Diagn Cytopathol 1990; 6: 9–13.
189. Dejmek A, Hjerpe A: Reactivity of six antibodies in effusions of mesothelioma, adenocarcinoma, and mesotheliosis: stepwise logistic regression analysis. Cytopathology 2000; 11: 8–17.
190. Villena V, Lopez-Encuentra A, Echave-Sustaeta J, et al.: Diagnostic value of CA-549 in pleural fluid: comparison with CEA, CA15-3, and CA72-4. Lung Cancer 2003; 40: 289–294.
191. Comin CE, Novelli L, Boddi V, Paglierami M, Dini S: Calretinin, thrombomodulin, CEA, and CD15: a useful combination of immunohistochemical markers for differentiating pleural epithelioid mesothelioma from peripheral pulmonary adenocarcinoma. Hum Pathol 2001; 32: 529–536.
192. Carella R, Deleonardi G, D'Errico A, et al.: Immunohistochemical panels for differentiating epithelial malignant mesothelioma from lung adenocarcinoma: a study with logistic regression analysis. Am J Surg Pathol 2001; 25: 43–50.
193. Lau SK, Luthringer DJ, Eisen RN: Thyroid transcription factor-1: a review. Appl Immunohistochem Molec Morphol 2002; 10: 97–102.
194. Hecht JL, Pinkus JL, Weinstein LJ, Pinkus GS: The value of thyroid transcription factor-1 in cytologic preparations as a marker for metastatic adenocarcinoma of lung origin. Am J Clin Pathol 2001; 116: 483–488.
195. Yatabe Y, Mitsudomi T, Takahashi T: Thyroid transcription factor-1 expression in pulmonary adenocarcinomas. Am J Surg Pathol 2002; 26: 767–773.
196. Zamecnik J, Kodet R: Value of thyroid transcription factor-1 and surfactant apoprotein-A in the differential diagnosis of pulmonary carcinomas: a study of 109 cases. Virchows Arch A 2002; 440: 353–361.
197. Ordonez NG: Value of thyroid transcription factor-1, E-cadherin, BG8, WT1, and CD44S immunostaining in distinguishing epithelial pleural mesothelioma from pulmonary and non-pulmonary adenocarcinoma. Am J Surg Pathol 2000; 24: 598–606.
198. Bejarano PA, Mousavi F: Incidence and significance of cytoplasmic thyroid transcription factor-1 immunoreactivity. Arch Pathol Lab Med 2003; 127: 193–195.
199. Ordonez NG: The immunohistochemical diagnosis of epithelial mesothelioma. Hum Pathol 1999; 30: 313–323.
200. Dejmek A, Brockstedt U, Hjerpe A: Optimization of a battery using nine immunocytochemical variables for distinguishing between epithelial mesothelioma and adenocarcinoma. APMIS 1997; 105: 889–894.
201. Sheibani K, Battifora H, Burke JS: Antigenic phenotype of malignant mesotheliomas and pulmonary adenocarcinomas: an immunohistologic analysis demonstrating the value of Leu-M1 antigen. Am J Pathol 1986; 123: 212–219.
202. Roberts F, Harper CM, Downie I, Burnett RA: Immunohistochemical analysis still has a limited role in the diagnosis of malignant mesothelioma: a study of thirteen antibodies. Am J Clin Pathol 2001; 116: 253–262.
203. Shield PW, Callan JJ, Devine PL: Markers for metastatic adenocarcinoma in serous effusion specimens. Diagn Cytopathol 1994; 11: 237–245.
204. Moch H, Oberholzer M, Dalquen P, Wegmann W, Gudat F: Diagnostic tools for differentiating between pleural mesothelioma and lung adenocarcinoma in paraffin embedded tissue. Part I: Immunohistochemical findings. Virchows Arch Pathol Anat 1993; 423: 19–27.
205. Bedrossian CW, Bonsib S, Moran C: Differential diagnosis between mesothelioma and adenocarcinoma: a multimodal approach based on ultrastructure and immunocytochemistry. Semin Diagn Pathol 1992; 9: 124–140.
206. Thor A, Ohuchi N, Szpak CA, Johnston WW, Schlom J: Distribution of oncogetal antigen tumor-associated glycoprotein-72, defined by monoclonal antibody B72.3. Cancer Res 1986; 46: 3118–3124.
207. Szpak CA, Johnston WW, Roggli VL, et al.: The diagnostic distinction between malignant mesothelioma of the pleura and adenocarcinoma of the lung as defined by a monoclonal antibody (B72.3). Am J Pathol 1986; 122: 252–260.
208. Wirth PR, Legier JF, Wright GL Jr: Immunohistochemical evaluation of seven monoclonal antibodies for differentiation of pleural mesothelioma from lung adenocarcinoma. Cancer 1991; 67: 655–662.
209. Latza U, Niedobitek G, Schwarting R, Nekarda H, Stein H: Ber-EP4: new monoclonal antibody which distinguishes epithelia from mesothelia. J Clin Pathol 1990; 43: 213–219.
210. Sheibani K, Shin SS, Kezirian J, Weiss LM: Ber-EP4 antibody as a discriminant in the differential diagnosis of malignant mesothelioma versus adenocarcinoma. Am J Surg Pathol 1991; 15: 779–784.
211. Gaffey MJ, Mills SE, Swanson PE, et al.: Immunoreactivity for Ber-EP4 in adenocarcinomas, adenomatoid tumors, and malignant mesotheliomas. Am J Surg Pathol 1992; 16: 593–599.
212. Ordonez NG: The immunohistochemical diagnosis of mesothelioma: a comparative study of epithelioid mesothelioma and lung adenocarcinoma. Am J Surg Pathol 2003; 27: 1031–1051.
213. Ruitenbeek T, Gouw AS, Poppema S: Immunocytology of body cavity fluids: MOC-31, a monoclonal antibody discriminating between mesothelial and epithelial cells. Arch Pathol Lab Med 1994; 118: 265–269.
214. Niemann TH, Hughes JH, DeYoung BR: MOC-31 aids in the differentiation of metastatic adenocarcinoma from hepatocellular carcinoma. Cancer 1999; 87: 295–298.
215. Kempner DH, Jay MR, Stevens RH: Human lung tumor-associated antigens of 32,000 daltons molecular weight. J Natl Cancer Inst USA 1979; 63: 1121–1129.
216. Lau SK, Prakash S, Geller SA, Alsabeh R: Comparative immunohistochemical profile of hepatocellular carcinoma, cholangiocarcinoma, and metastatic adenocarcinoma. Hum Pathol 2002; 33: 1175–1181.
217. Gonzalez-Lois C, Ballestin C, Sotelo MT, et al.: Combined use of novel epithelial (MOC-31) and mesothelial (HBME-1) immunohistochemical markers for optimal first-line diagnostic distinction between mesothelioma and metastatic carcinoma in pleura. Histopathology 2001; 38: 528–534.
218. LePender J, Marionneau S, Cailleau-Thomas A, et al.: ABH and Lewis histo-blood group antigens in cancer. APMIS 2001; 109: 9–31.
219. Steplewska-Mazur K, Gabriel A, Zajecki W, Wylezol M, Gluek M: Breast cancer progression and expression of blood group-related tumor-associated antigens. Hybridoma 2000; 19: 129–133.

220. Jordon D, Jagirdar J, Kaneko M: Blood group antigens Lewis X and Lewis Y in the diagnostic determination of malignant mesothelioma versus adenocarcinoma. Am J Pathol 1989; 135: 931–937.
221. Riera JR, Astengo-Osuna C, Longmate JA, Battifora H: The immunohistochemical diagnostic panel for epithelial mesothelioma: a reevaluation after heat-induced epitope retrieval. Am J Surg Pathol 1997; 21: 1409–1419.
222. Humphrey PA: p53: mutations and immunohistochemical detection, with a focus on alterations in urologic malignancies. Adv Pathol Lab Med 1994; 7: 579–596.
223. Mangano WE, Cagle PT, Churg A, Vollmer RT, Roggli VL: The diagnosis of desmoplastic malignant mesothelioma and its distinction from fibrous pleurisy: a histologic and immunohistochemical analysis of 31 cases including p53 immunostaining. Am J Clin Pathol 1998; 110: 191–199.
224. Attanoos RL, Griffin A, Gibbs AR: The use of immunohistochemistry in distinguishing reactive from neoplastic mesothelium: a novel use for desmin and comparative evaluation with epithelial membrane antigen, p53, platelet-derived growth factor receptor, P-glycoprotein, and *bcl*-2. Histopathology 2003; 43: 231–238.
225. Esposito V, Baldi A, DeLuca A, et al.: p53 immunostaining in differential diagnosis of pleural mesothelial proliferations. Anticancer Res 1997; 17: 733–736.
226. Cagle PT, Brown RW, Lebovitz RM: p53 immunostaining in the differentiation of reactive processes from malignancy in pleural biopsy specimens. Hum Pathol 1994; 25: 443–448.
227. Kafiri G, Thomas DM, Shepherd NA, et al.: p53 expression is common in malignant mesothelioma. Histopathology 1992; 21: 331–332.
228. Dei Tos AP, Doglioni C: Calretinin: a novel tool for diagnostic immunohistochemistry. Adv Anat Pathol 1998; 5: 61–66.
229. Ordonez NG: In search of a positive immunohistochemical marker for mesothelioma: an update. Adv Anat Pathol 1998; 5: 53–60.
230. Miettinen M, Sarlomo-Rikala M: Expression of calretinin, thrombomodulin, keratin 5, and mesothelin in lung carcinomas of different types: an immunohistochemical analysis of 596 tumors in comparison with epithelioid mesotheliomas of the pleura. Am J Surg Pathol 2003; 27: 150–158.
231. Abutaily AS, Addis BJ, Roche WR: Immunohistochemistry in the distinction between malignant mesothelioma and pulmonary adenocarcinoma: a critical evaluation of new antibodies. J Clin Pathol 2002; 55: 662–668.
232. Gotzos V, Vogt P, Celio MR: The calcium binding protein calretinin is a selective marker for malignant pleural mesotheliomas of the epithelial type. Pathol Res Pract 192; 137–147.
233. Doglioni C, Dei Tos AP, Laurino L, et al.: Calretinin: a novel immunocytochemical marker for mesothelioma. Am J Surg Pathol 1996; 20: 1037–1046.
234. Attanoos RL, Dojcinov SD, Webb R, Gibbs AR: Anti-mesothelial markers in sarcomatoid mesothelioma and other spindle-cell neoplasms. Histopathology 2000; 37: 224–231.
235. Lucas DR, Pass HI, Madan SK, et al.: Sarcomatoid mesothelioma and its histological mimics: a comparative immunohistochemical study. Histopathology 2003; 42: 270–279.
236. Haber DA, Buckler AJ, Glaser T, et al.: An internal deletion within an 11p13 zinc finger gene contributes to the development of Wilms' tumor. Cell 1990; 61: 1257–1269.
237. Loeb DM, Sukumar S: The role of WT1 in oncogenesis: tumor suppressor or oncogene? Int J Hematol 2002; 76: 117–126.
238. Gulyas M, Hjerpe A: Proteoglycans and WT1 as markers for distinguishing adenocarcinoma, epithelioid mesothelioma, and benign mesothelium. J Pathol 2003; 199: 479–487.
239. Foster MR, Johnson JE, Olson SJ, Allred DC: Immunohistochemical analysis of nuclear versus cytoplasmic staining of WT1 in malignant mesotheliomas and primary pulmonary adenocarcinomas. Arch Pathol Lab Med 2001; 125: 1316–1320.
240. Oates J, Edwards C: HBME-1, MOC-31, WT1, and calretinin: an assessment of recently-described markers for mesothelioma and adenocarcinoma. Histopathology 2000; 36: 341–347.
241. Campbell CE, Kuriyan NP, Rackley RR, et al.: Constitutive expression of the Wilms tumor suppressor gene (WT1) in renal cell carcinoma. Int J Cancer 1998; 78: 182–188.
242. Goldstein NS, Bassi D, Uzieblo A: WT1 is an integral component of an antibody panel to distinguish pancreaticobiliary and some ovarian epithelial neoplasms. Am J Clin Pathol 2001; 116: 246–252.
243. Ueda T, Oji Y, Naka N, et al.: Overexpression of the Wilms tumor gene WT1 in human bone and soft tissue sarcomas. Cancer Sci 2003; 94: 271–276.
244. Esmon CT: The protein C pathway. Chest 2003; 124 (Suppl 3): 26S–32S.
245. Ishii H, Nakano M, Tsubouchi J, Kazama M, Majerus PW: Distribution of thrombomodulin in human tissues and characterization of thrombomodulin in plasma. Acta Hematol Jpn 1988; 51: 1228–1233.
246. Boffa MC, Burke B, Haudenschild C: Different localization of thrombomodulin. Ann Biol Clin 1987; 45: 191–197.
247. Attanoos RL, Goddard H, Gibbs AR: Mesothelioma-binding antibodies: thrombomodulin, OV632, and HBME-1 and their use in the diagnosis of malignant mesothelioma. Histopathology 1996; 29: 209–215.
248. Ordonez NG: Thrombomodulin expression in transitional cell carcinoma. Am J Clin Pathol 1998; 110: 385–390.
249. Appleton MA, Attanoos RL, Jasani B: Thrombomodulin as a marker of vascular and lymphatic tumors. Histopathology 1996; 29: 153–157.
250. Ordonez NG: The immunohistochemical diagnosis of mesothelioma: differentiation of mesothelioma and lung adenocarcinoma. Am J Surg Pathol 1989; 13: 276–291.
251. Gibbs AR, Harach R, Wagner JC, Jasani B: Comparison of tumor markers in malignant mesothelioma and pulmonary adenocarcinoma. Thorax 1985; 40: 91–95.
252. Kawai T, Suzuki M, Torikata C, Suzuki Y: Expression of blood group-related antigens and *Helix pomatia* agglutinin in malignant pleural mesothelioma and pulmonary adenocarcinoma. Hum Pathol 1991; 22: 118–124.
253. Ordonez NG: Value of mesothelin immunostaining in the diagnosis of mesothelioma. Mod Pathol 2003; 16: 192–197.
254. Frierson HF Jr, Moskaluk CA, Powell SM, et al.: Large-scale molecular and tissue microarray analysis of mesothelin expression in common human carcinomas. Hum Pathol 2003; 34: 605–609.
255. Cheung CC, Ezzat S, Freeman JL, Rosen IB, Asa SL: Immunohistochemical diagnosis of papillary thyroid carcinoma. Mod Pathol 2001; 14: 338–342.
256. Fetsch PA, Abati A, Higazi YM: Utility of the antibodies CA19-9, HBME-1, and thrombomodulin in the diagnosis of malignant mesothelioma and adenocarcinoma in cytology. Cancer 1998; 84: 101–108.
257. Bateman AC, Al-Talib RK, Newman T, Williams JH, Herbert A: Immunohistochemical phenotype of malignant mesothelioma: predictive value of CA125 and HBME-1 expression. Histopathology 1997; 30: 49–56.
258. Loy TS, Quesenberry JT, Sharp SC: Distribution of CA-125 in adenocarcinomas: an immunohistochemical study of 481 cases. Am J Clin Pathol 1992; 98: 175–179.
259. Mayall FG, Jasani B, Gibbs AR: Immunohistochemical positivity for neuron-specific enolase and Leu-7 in malignant mesotheliomas. J Pathol 1991; 165: 325–328.
260. Kim MK, Kim S: Immunohistochemical profile of common epithelial neoplasms arising in the kidney. Appl Immunohistochem Molec Morphol 2002; 10: 332–338.
261. Fan Z, van de Rijn M, Montgomery K, Rouse RV: Hep-Par1 antibody staining for the differential diagnosis of hepatocellular carcinoma: 676 tumors tested using tissue microarrays and conventional tissue sections. Mod Pathol 2003; 16: 137–144.
262. Cohen AJ, Bunn PA, Franklin W, et al.: Neutral endopeptidase: variable expression in human lung, inactivation in lung cancer, and modulation of peptide-induced calcium flux. Cancer Res 1996; 56: 831–839.
263. Chu PG, Arber DA, Weiss LM: Expression of T/NK-cell and plasma cell antigens in nonhematopoietic epithelioid neoplasms. Am J Clin Pathol 2003; 120: 64–70.
264. Brown RW, Clark GM, Tandon AK, Allred DC: Multiple-marker immunohistochemical phenotypes distinguishing malignant pleural mesothelioma from pulmonary adenocarcinoma. Hum Pathol 1993; 24: 347–354.
265. Segers K, Ramael M, Singh S, et al.: Detection of numerical chromosomal aberrations in paraffin-embedded malignant pleural mesothelioma by non-isotopic in-situ hybridization. J Pathol 1995; 175: 219–226.

266. Shivapurkar N, Virmani AK, Wistuba I, et al.: Deletions of chromosome 4 at multiple sites are frequent in malignant mesothelioma and small-cell lung carcinoma. Clin Cancer Res 1999; 5: 17–23.
267. Bjorkqvist AM, Wolf M, Nordling S, et al.: Deletions at 14q in malignant mesothelioma detected by microsatellite marker analysis. Br J Cancer 1999; 81: 1111–1115.
268. Lee WC, Balsara B, Liu Z, Jhanwar SC, Testa JR: Loss of heterozygosity analysis defines a critical region in chromosome 1p22 commonly deleted in human malignant mesothelioma. Cancer Res 1996; 56: 4297–4301.
269. Huncharek M: Genetic factors in the etiology of malignant mesothelioma. Eur J Cancer 1995; 31A: 1741–1747.
270. Garlepp MJ, Leong CC: Biological and immunological aspects of malignant mesothelioma. Eur Respir J 1995; 8: 643–650.
271. Popescu NC, Chahinian AP, DiPaolo JA: Nonrandom chromosome alterations in human malignant mesothelioma. Cancer Res 1988; 48: 142–147.
272. Illei PB, Rusch VW, Zakowski MF, Ladanyi M: Homozygous deletion of CDKN2A and codeletion of the methylthioadenosine phosphorylase gene in the majority of pleural mesotheliomas. Clin Cancer Res 2003; 9: 2108–2113.
273. Dreyling MH, Bohlander SK, Adeyanju MO, Olopade OI: Detection of CDKN2 deletions in tumor cell lines and primary glioma by interphase fluorescence in-situ hybridization. Cancer Res 1995; 55: 984–988.
274. Cheng JQ, Jhanwar SC, Lu YY, Testa JR: Homozygous deletions within 9p21-p22 identify a small critical region of chromosomal loss in human malignant mesotheliomas. Cancer Res 1993; 53: 4761–4763.
275. Kitamura F, Araki S, Suzuki Y, et al.: Assessment of the mutations of the p53 suppressor gene and Ha- and Ki-*ras* oncogenes in malignant mesothelioma in relation to asbestos exposure: a study of 12 American patients. Ind Health 2002; 40: 175–181.
276. Roberts F, McCall AE, Burnett RA: Malignant mesothelioma: a comparison of biopsy and postmortem material by light microscopy and immunohistochemistry. J Clin Pathol 2001; 54: 766–770.
277. Mayall FG, Jacobson G, Wilkins R: Mutations of the p53 gene and SV40 sequences in asbestos-associated and non-asbestos-associated mesotheliomas. J Clin Pathol 1999; 52: 291–293.
278. Murthy SS, Testa JR: Asbestos, chromosomal deletions, and tumor suppressor gene alterations in human malignant mesothelioma. J Cell Physiol 1999; 180: 150–157.
279. Liu BC, Fu DC, Miao Q, Wang HH, You BR: p53 gene mutations in asbestos-associated cancers. Biomed Environ Sci 1998; 11: 226–232.
280. Kirao T, Bueno R, Chen CJ, et al.: Alterations of the p16 (INK4) locus in human malignant mesothelial tumors. Carcinogenesis 2002; 23: 1127–1130.
281. Van der Meerden A, Seddon MB, Betscholtz CA, Lechner JF, Gerwin BI: Tumorigenic conversion of human mesothelial cells as a consequence of platelet-derived growth factor-A chain overexpression. Am J Respir Cell Molec Biol 1993; 8: 214–221.
281a. Tolnay E, Kuhnen C, Wiethage T, et al.: Hepatocyte growth factor/scatter factor and its receptor c-*met* are overexpressed and associated with an increased microvessel density in malignant pleural mesothelioma. J Cancer Res Clin Oncol 1998; 124: 291–296.
282. Hodzic D, Delacroix L, Willemsen P, et al.: Characterization of the IGF system and analysis of the possible molecular mechanisms leading to IGF-II overexpression in mesothelioma. Horm Metab Res 1997; 29: 549–555.
283. Kumar-Singh S, Weyler J, Martin MJ, Vermeulen PB, Van Marck E: Angiogenic cytokines in mesothelioma: a study of VEGF, FGF-1 and 2, and TGF-beta expression. J Pathol 1999; 189: 72–78.
284. Segers K, Ramael M, Singh SK, et al.: Immunoreactivity for *bcl*-2 protein in malignant mesothelioma and non-neoplastic mesothelium. Virchows Arch A 1994; 424: 631–634.
285. Horvai AE, Li L, Xu Z, et al.: Malignant mesothelioma does not demonstrate overexpression or gene amplification despite cytoplasmic immunohistochemical staining for c-*erb*B-2. Arch Pathol Lab Med 2003; 127: 465–469.
286. Ramos-Nino ME, Timblin CR, Mossman BT: Mesothelial cell transformation requires AP-1 binding activity and ERK-dependent Fra-1 expression. Cancer Res 2002; 62: 6065–6069.
287. Illei PB, Ladanyi M, Rusch VW, Zakowski MF: The use of CDKN2A deletion as a diagnostic marker for malignant mesothelioma in body cavity effusions. Cancer 2003; 99: 51–56.
288. Nakatsuka S, Yao M, Hoshida Y, et al.: Pyothorax-associated lymphoma: a review of 106 cases. J Clin Oncol 2002; 20: 4255–4260.
289. Wakely PE Jr, Menezes G, Nuovo G: Primary effusion lymphoma: cytopathologic diagnosis using in-situ molecular genetic analysis for human herpesvirus 8. Mod Pathol 2002; 15: 944–950.
290. Aquino SL, Chen MY, Kuo WT, Chiles C: The CT appearance of pleural and extrapleural disease in lymphoma. Clin Radiol 1999; 54: 647–650.
291. Lee MJ, Grogan L, Meehan S, Breatnach E: Pleural granulocytic sarcoma: CT characteristics. Clin Radiol 1991; 43: 57–59.
292. Blakolmer K, Essop MF, Close PM: Diagnosis of an anemone cell tumor as a B-cell lymphoma by molecular analysis. Ultrastruct Pathol 1996; 20: 189–193.
293. Nappi O, Boscaino A, Wick MR: Extramedullary hematopoietic proliferations, extraosseous plasmacytomas, and ectopic splenic implants (splenosis). Semin Diagn Pathol, in press.
294. Inoue K, Ogawa H, Sonoda Y, et al.: Aberrant overexpression of the Wilms tumor gene (WT1) in human leukemia. Blood 1997; 89: 1405–1412.
295. Hirose M, Kuroda Y: p53 may mediate mdr-1 expression via the WT1 gene in human vincristine-resistant leukemia/lymphoma cell lines. Cancer Lett 1998; 129: 165–171.
296. Lin BT, Colby TV, Gown AM, et al.: Malignant vascular tumors of the serous membranes mimicking mesothelioma. A report of 14 cases. Am J Surg Pathol 1996; 20: 1431–1439.
297. Zhang PJ, LiVolsi VA, Brooks JJ: Malignant epithelioid vascular tumors of the pleura: report of a series and literature review. Hum Pathol 2000; 31: 29–34.
298. Ximenes M III, Miziara HL: Hemangioendothelioma of the lung and pleura: report of three cases. Int Surg 1981; 55: 67–70.
299. Battifora H: Epithelioid hemangioendothelioma imitating mesothelioma. Appl Immunohistochem 1993; 1: 220–222.
300. Del Frate C, Mortele K, Zanardi R, et al.: Pseudomesotheliomatous angiosarcoma of the chest wall and pleura. J Thorac Imaging 2003; 18: 200–203.
301. McKay B, Ordonez NG, Huang WL: Ultrastructural and immunocytochemical observations on angiosarcomas. Ultrastruct Pathol 1989; 13: 97–110.
302. Weiss SW, Enzinger FM: Epithelioid hemangioendothelioma: a vascular tumor often mistaken for a carcinoma. Cancer 1982; 50: 970–981.
303. Miettinen M, Fetsch JF: Distribution of keratins in normal endothelial cells and a spectrum of vascular tumors: implications in tumor diagnosis. Hum Pathol 2000; 31: 1062–1067.
304. Miettinen M, Lindenmayer AE, Chaubal A: Endothelial cell markers CD31, CD34, and BNH9 antibody to H- and Y- antigens: evaluation of their specificity and sensitivity in the diagnosis of vascular tumors and comparison with von Willebrand factor. Mod Pathol 1994; 7: 82–90.
305. Panagopoulos I, Mertens F, Isaksson M, et al.: Molecular genetic characterization of the EWS/CHN and RBP56/CHN fusion genes in extraskeletal myxoid chondrosarcoma. Genes Chromosomes Cancer 2002; 35: 340–352.
306. Goetz SP, Robinson RA, Landas SK: Extraskeletal myxoid chondrosarcoma of the pleura: report of a case clinically simulating mesothelioma. Am J Clin Pathol 1992; 97: 498–502.
307. Okamoto S, Hisaoka M, Ishida T, et al.: Extraskeletal myxoid chondrosarcoma: a clinicopathologic, immunohistochemical, and molecular analysis of 18 cases. Hum Pathol 2001; 32: 1116–1124.
308. Dei Tos AP, Wadden C, Fletcher CDM: Extraskeletal myxoid chondrosarcoma: an immunohistochemical reappraisal of 39 cases. Appl Immunohistochem 1997; 5: 73–77.
309. Fisher C: Synovial sarcoma. Ann Diagn Pathol 1998; 2: 401–421.
310. Miettinen M, Limon J, Niezabitowski A, Lasota J: Calretinin and other mesothelial markers in synovial sarcoma: analysis of antigenic similarities and differences with malignant mesothelioma. Am J Surg Pathol 2001; 25: 610–617.
311. Carbone M, Rizzo P, Powers A, et al.: Molecular analyses, morphology, and immunohistochemistry together differentiate pleural synovial sarcoma from mesotheliomas: clinical implications. Anticancer Res 2002; 22: 3443–3448.
311a. Nappi O, Glasner SD, Swanson PE, Wick MR: Biphasic and monophasic sarcomatoid carcinomas of the lung. Am J Clin Pathol 1994; 102: 331–340.

312. Falconieri G, Zanconati F, Bussani R, DiBonito L: Small cell carcinoma of the lung simulating pleural mesothelioma: report of 4 cases with autopsy confirmation. Pathol Res Pract 1995; 191: 1147–1152.
313. Wick MR: Immunohistology of neuroendocrine and neuroectodermal tumors. Semin Diagn Pathol 2000; 17: 194–203.
314. Beiske K, Myklebust AT, Aamdal S, et al.: Detection of bone marrow metastases in small cell lung carcinoma patients: comparison of immunologic and morphologic methods. Am J Pathol 1992; 141: 531–538.
315. Chhieng DC, Ko EC, Yee HT, et al.: Malignant pleural effusions due to small cell lung carcinoma: a cytologic and immunocytochemical study. Diagn Cytopathol 2001; 25: 356–360.
316. Attanoos RL, Galateau-Salle F, Gibbs AR, et al.: Primary thymic epithelial tumors of the pleura mimicking malignant mesothelioma. Histopathology 2002; 41: 42–49.
317. DiComo CJ, Urist MJ, Babayan I, et al.: p63 expression profiles in human normal and tumor tissues. Clin Cancer Res 2002; 8: 494–501.
318. Hammond EH, Flinner RL: The diagnosis of thymoma: a review. Ultrastruct Pathol 1991; 15: 419–438.
319. Flint A, Weiss SW: CD34 and keratin expression distinguishes solitary fibrous tumor (fibrous mesothelioma) of pleura from desmoplastic mesothelioma. Hum Pathol 1995; 26: 428–431.
320. Gaffey MJ, Mills SE, Ritter JH: Clear cell tumors of the lower respiratory tract. Semin Diagn Pathol 1997; 14: 222–232.
321. Fleming S: Genetics of renal tumours. Cancer Metastasis Rev 1997;16: 127–140.
322. Osborn M, Pelling N, Walker MM, Fisher C, Nicholson AG: The value of "mesothelium-associated" antibodies in distinguishing between metastatic renal cell carcinomas and mesotheliomas. Histopathology 2002; 41: 301–307.
323. Herrera GA, Turbat-Herrera EA: The role of ultrastructural pathology in the diagnosis of epithelial and unusual renal tumors. Ultrastruct Pathol 1996; 20: 7–26.
324. Nappi O, Ferrara G, Wick MR: Neoplasms composed of eosinophilic polygonal cells: an overview with consideration of different cytomorphologic patterns. Semin Diagn Pathol 1999; 16: 82–90.
325. Mackay B, El-Naggar A, Ordonez NG: Ultrastructure of adrenal cortical carcinoma. Ultrastruct Pathol 1994; 18: 181–190.
326. DeYoung BR, Wick MR: Immunohistologic analysis of metastatic carcinomas of unknown origin: an algorithmic approach. Semin Diagn Pathol 2000; 17; 184–193.
327. Gaffey MJ, Traweek ST, Mills SE, et al.: Cytokeratin expression in adrenocortical neoplasia. Hum Pathol 1992; 23: 144–153.
328. Zhang PJ, Genega EM, Tomaszewski JE, Pasha TL, LiVolsi VA: The role of calretinin, inhibin, melan-A, *bcl*-2, and c-*kit* in differentiating adrenal cortical and medullary tumors: an immunohistochemical study. Mod Pathol 2003; 16: 591–597.
329. Vaideeswar P, Deshpande JR, Jambhekar NA: Primary pleuropulmonary malignant germ cell tumors. J Postgrad Med 2002; 48: 29–31.
330. Srigley JR, Mackay B, Toth P, Ayala A: The ultrastructure and histogenesis of male germ cell neoplasia with emphasis on seminoma with early carcinomatous features. Ultrastruct Pathol 1988; 12: 67–86.
331. Devouassoux-Shisheboran M, Manduit C, Tabone E, Droz JP, Benahmed M: Growth regulating factors and signalling proteins in testicular germ cell tumors. APMIS 2003; 111: 212–224.
332. Horvai AE, Li L, Xu Z, et al.: c-*kit* is not expressed in malignant mesothelioma. Mod Pathol 2003; 16: 818–822.
333. Brooks JJ, LiVolsi VA, Pietra GG: Mesothelial cell inclusions in mediastinal lymph nodes, mimicking metastatic carcinoma. Am J Clin Pathol 1990; 93: 741–748.
334. Parkash V, Vidwans M, Carter D: Benign mesothelial cells in mediastinal lymph nodes. Am J Surg Pathol 1999; 23: 1264–1269.
335. Isotalo PA, Veinot JP, Jabi M: Hyperplastic mesothelial cells in mediastinal lymph node sinuses with extranodal lymphatic involvement. Arch Pathol Lab Med 2000; 124: 609–613.
336. Hoekman K, Tognon G, Risse EK, Bloesma CA, Vermorken JB: Well-differentiated papillary mesothelioma of the peritoneum: a separate entity. Eur J Cancer 1996; 32A: 255–258.
337. Weiss SW, Tavassoli FA: Multicystic mesothelioma: an analysis of pathologic findings and biologic behavior in 37 cases. Am J Surg Pathol 1988; 12: 737–746.
338. Butnor KJ, Sporn TA, Hammar SP, Roggli VL: Well-differentiated papillary mesothelioma. Am J Surg Pathol 2001; 25: 1304–1309.
339. Yesner R, Hurwitz A: Localized pleural mesothelioma of epithelial type. J Thorac Surg 1953; 26: 325–329.
340. Ball NJ, Urbanski SJ, Green FH, Kieser T: Pleural multicystic mesothelial proliferation: the so-called "multicystic mesothelioma." Am J Surg Pathol 1990; 14: 375–378.
341. Butchart EG, Ashcroft T, Barnsley WC, Holden MP: Pleuropneumonectomy in the management of diffuse malignant mesothelioma of the pleura: experience with 29 patients. Thorax 1976; 31: 15–24.
342. Rusch VW: A proposed new international TNM staging system for malignant pleural mesothelioma from the International Mesothelioma Interest Group. Lung Cancer 1996; 14: 1–12.
343. Greene FL, Ed.: American Joint Committee on Cancer (AJCC) Cancer Staging Manual, 6th edn. 2002, Springer-Verlag, New York, pp 139–141.
344. Sugarbaker DJ, Strauss GM, Lynch TJ, et al.: Node status has prognostic significance in the multimodality therapy of diffuse malignant mesothelioma. J Clin Oncol 1993; 11: 1172–1178.
345. Koong HN, Battafarano RJ, Ginsberg RJ: Malignant pleural mesothelioma. In: Prognostic factors in cancer, 2nd edn, Gospodarowicz MK, Henson DE, Hutter RVP, et al., Eds. 2001, Wiley-Liss, New York, pp 371–385.
346. Johansson L, Linden CJ: Aspects of histopathologic subtype as a prognostic factor in 85 pleural mesotheliomas. Chest 1996; 109: 109–114.
347. Rusch VW, Venkatraman ES: Important prognostic factors in patients with malignant pleural mesothelioma, managed surgically. Ann Thorac Surg 1999; 68: 1799–1804.
348. Metintas M, Metintas S, Ucgun I, et al.: Prognostic factors in diffuse malignant pleural mesothelioma: effects of pretreatment clinical and laboratory characteristics. Respir Med 2001; 95: 829–835.
349. Beer TW, Shepherd P, Pullinger NC: p27 immunostaining is related to prognosis in malignant mesothelioma. Histopathology 2001; 38: 535–541.
350. Bongiovanni M, Cassoni P, DeGiuli P, et al.: p27 (kip1) immunoreactivity correlates with long-term survival in pleural malignant mesothelioma. Cancer 2001; 92; 1245–1250.
351. Leonardo E, Zanconati F, Bonifacio D, Bonito LD: Immunohistochemistry for MIB-1 and p27/kip1 as a prognostic factor for pleural mesothelioma. Pathol Res Pract 2001; 197: 253–256.
352. Comin CE, Anichini C, Boddi V, Novelli L, Dini S: MIB-1 proliferation index correlates with survival in pleural malignant mesothelioma. Histopathology 2000; 36: 26–31.

APPENDIX Miscellaneous distinctive histopathologic findings

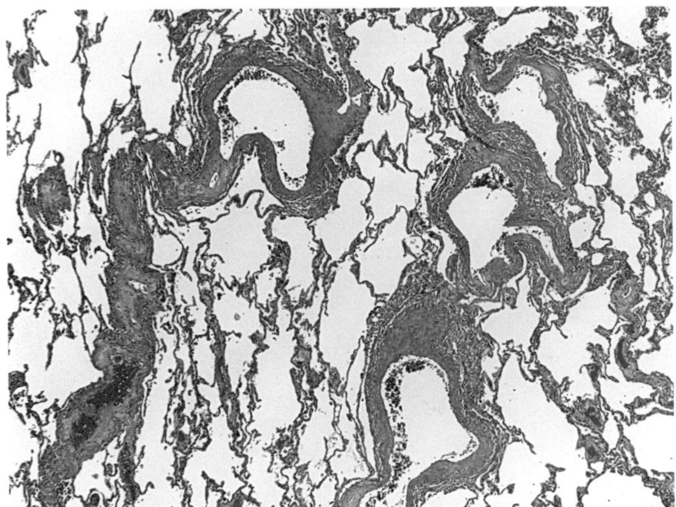

Fig. A1 **Aging changes in arteries.** Abnormalities in pulmonary arteries can be observed in many surgical lung biopsies, unrelated to clinical evidence of pulmonary hypertension. This phenomenon is seen most commonly in aging smokers and in the vicinity of localized scars. Vessel tortuosity is the common denominator, and if medial thickening is present, it tends to be patchy and somewhat eccentric (possibly representing tangent sectioning).

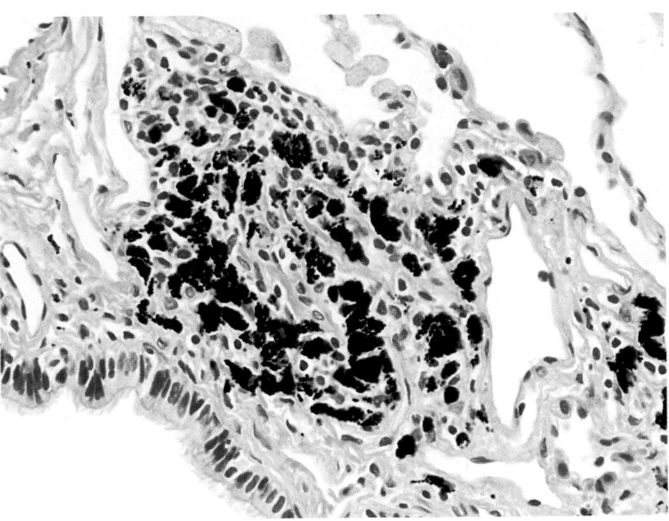

Fig. A2 **Anthracosis (focal) parenchymal.** Anthracotic pigment is a common incidental finding in surgical lung biopsies and transbronchial biopsies. A characteristic distribution is often discernible, with dust being deposited along lymphatic routes in the pleura and bronchovascular sheaths. It is always prudent to seek clinical and radiologic correlation before ascribing such changes to a pneumoconiosis.

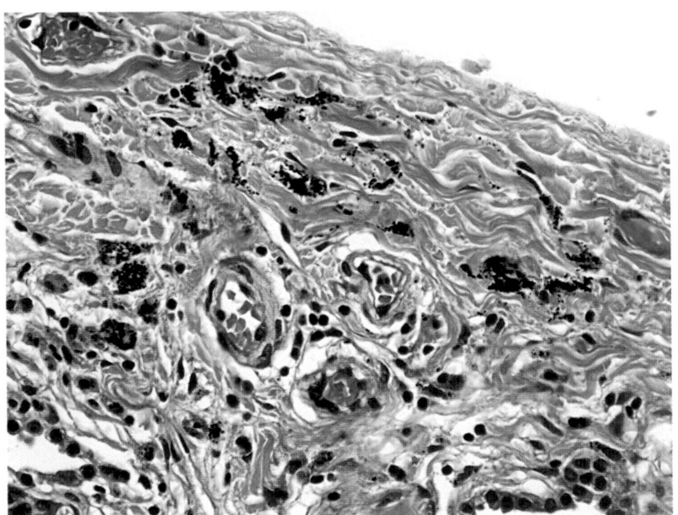

Fig. A3 **Anthracosis (focal) in pleura.** Small foci of dust accumulation along pleural lymphatic routes are an expected finding in smokers and city dwellers.

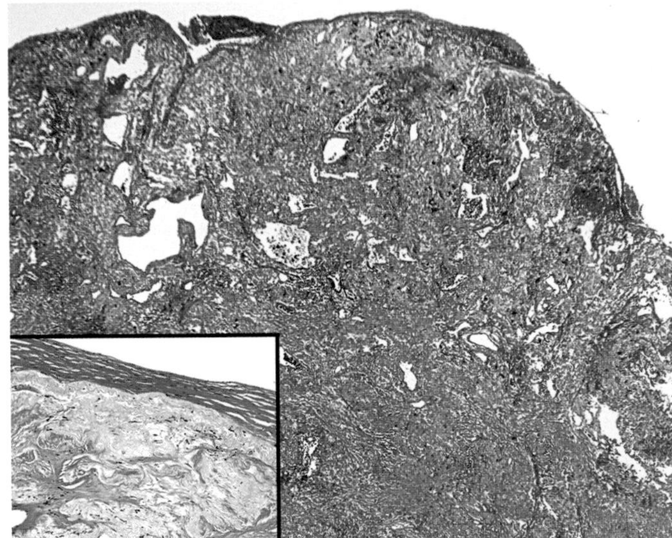

Fig. A4 **Apical cap fibrosis.** Subpleural zones of elastofibrotic scar occur as an incidental finding in the upper lung zones. The phenomenon is easy to recognize and is important because such incidental scars may be mistaken surgically for tumor. If apical cap is identified by frozen section analysis, the pathologist can encourage additional biopsies in search of more specific findings. (Inset: higher magnification view of the distinctive elastotic collagen of the apical cap.)

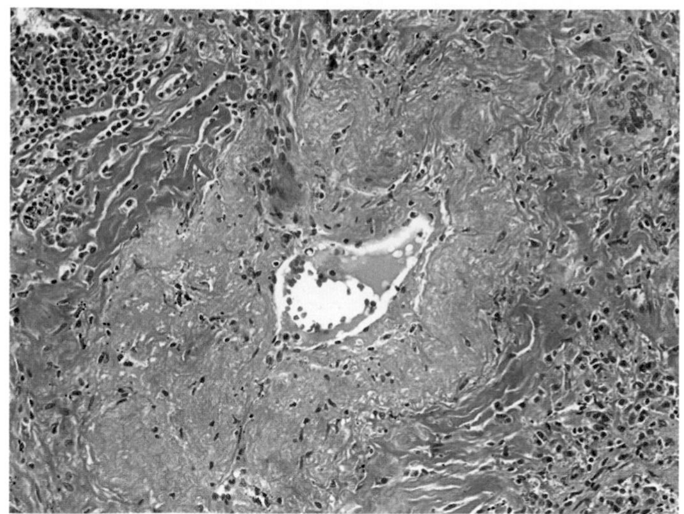

Fig. A5 **Arterial medial hyaline sclerosis.** Hyaline sclerosis of the pulmonary arterial media can occur as a consequence of fibrosis and other lung injury (here in a case of sarcoidosis, note multinucleated giant cell in upper right).

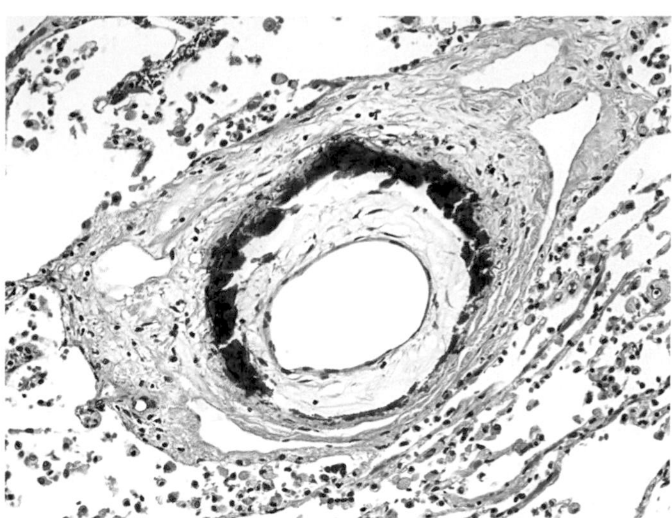

Fig. A6 **Arterial medial calcification.** Calcification may occur in the media of large pulmonary arteries as an incidental finding. This small artery has dramatic medial calcification in the setting of chronic mitral stenosis.

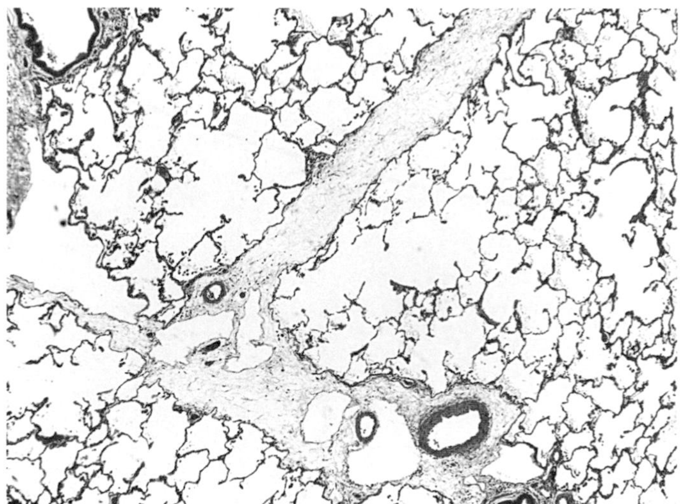

Fig. A7 **Artifactual lymphatic dilation from injection fixation.** The optimal method for achieving fixation of the surgical wedge biopsy can be achieved using injection of fixative with a small gauge (22–25) needle and 5 ml syringe. Overzealous injection can produce distinctive artifacts, such as the septal lymphatic dilatation seen in this photomicrograph (see Chapter 2 for a discussion of fixation methods).

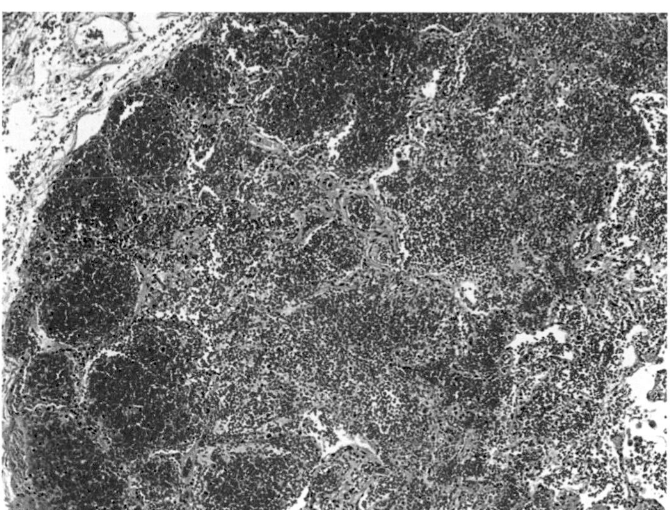

Fig. A8 **Artifactual hemorrhage.** Fresh blood in alveolar spaces may occur as a consequence of operative manipulation. To distinguish such artifactual hemorrhage from pathologic alveolar hemorrhage, a search for hemosiderin-laden macrophages and abnormal cellularity of the alveolar interstitium is often helpful (see Chapter 10 – diffuse alveolar hemorrhage – for further discussion).

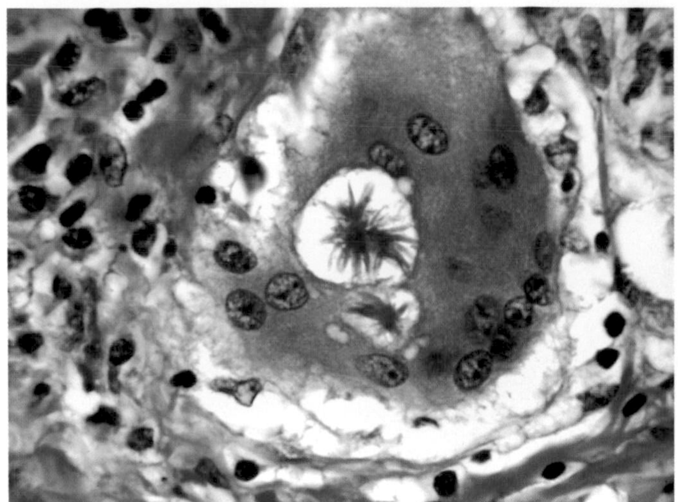

Fig. A9 **Asteroid body in a multinucleated giant cell.** Asteroid bodies are distinctive eosinophilic inclusions composed of cytoskeletal components and collagen. Asteroid bodies are not specific for sarcoidosis and are actually seen in a minority of patients with this disease.

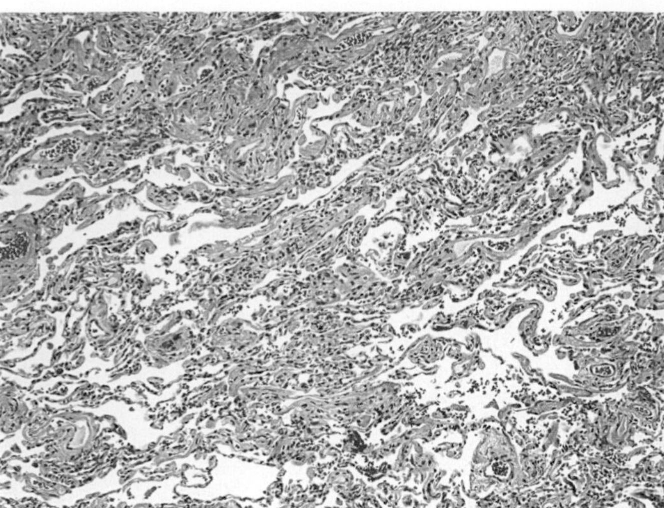

Fig. A10 **Atelectasis.** The lung must be collapsed as part of the video-assisted thoracoscopic surgical (VATS) procedure. For this reason, biopsies allowed to fix by immersion, without removal of staples, may be difficult to interpret, given the dense approximation of alveolar walls. Agitation fixation or inflation is a preferable technique (see Chapter 2 for a discussion of fixation methods).

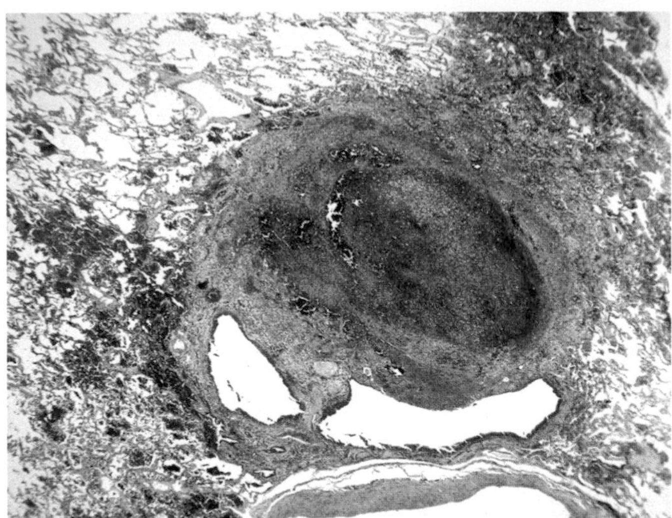

Fig. A11 **Biopsy site.** On rare occasions, a prior biopsy procedure may result in a reparative reaction that can be seen in subsequent wedge biopsy or lobectomy specimens.

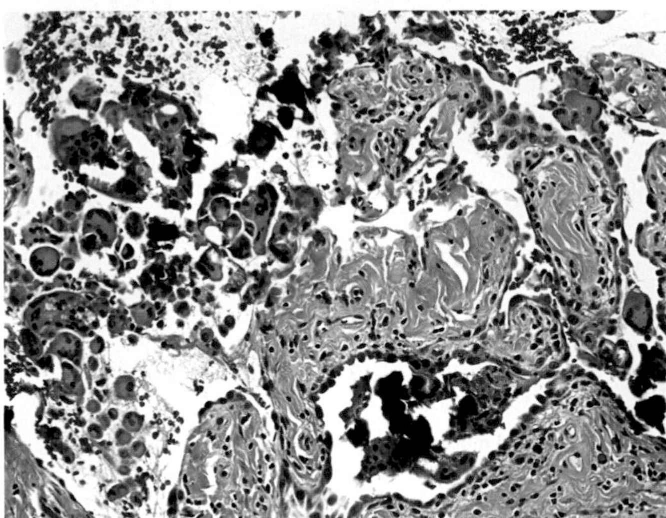

Fig. A12 **Blue bodies.** These distinctive laminated and calcified hematoxyphilic bodies are a nonspecific finding. They may be seen in the alveolar spaces focally in a number of interstitial lung diseases where alveolar macrophages accumulate.

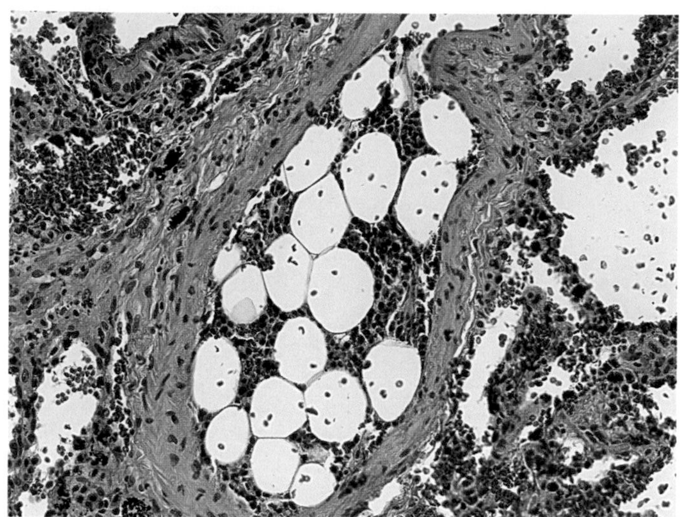

Fig. A13 **Bone marrow embolus.** Embolized fragments of bone marrow are incidental findings in resected lung tissue.

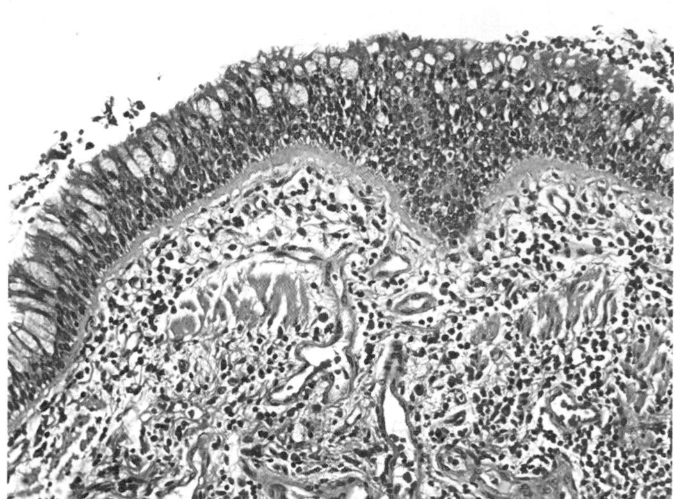

Fig. A14 **Bronchial mucosa basement membrane thickening.** This classic finding in asthma can also be seen as a nonspecific finding in smokers.

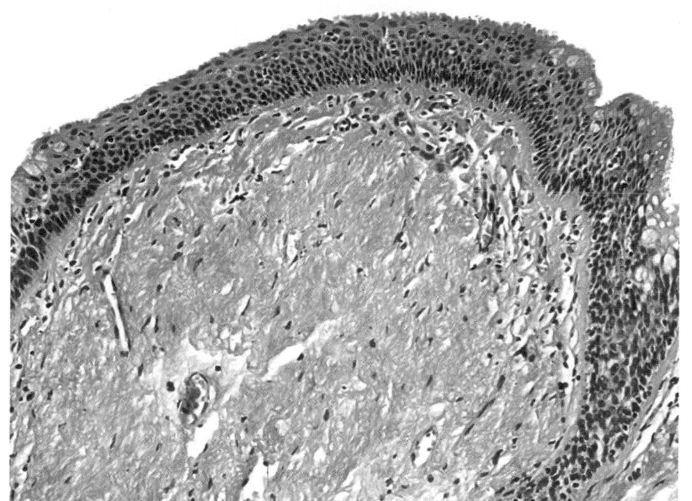

Fig. A15 **Bronchial mucosa subepithelial elastosis.** This change is a nonspecific finding seen on occasion in lung biopsies from older patients.

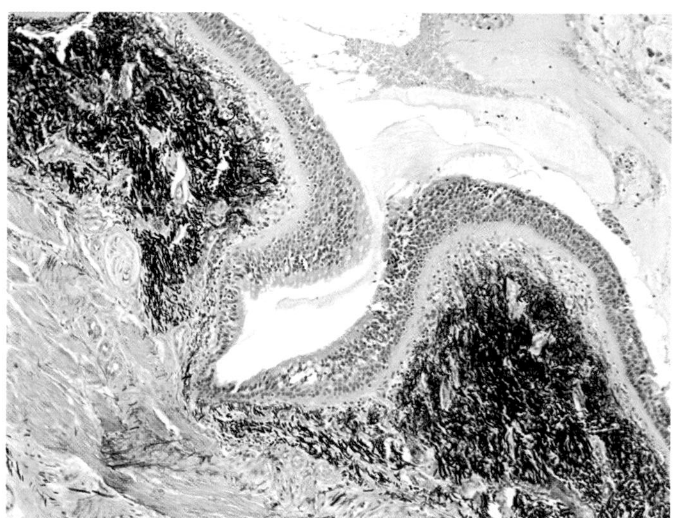

Fig. A16 **Bronchial mucosa subepithelial elastosis.** Elastic tissue stains, such as this Verhoeff's stain, nicely highlight in black the abnormal accumulation of elastic fibers.

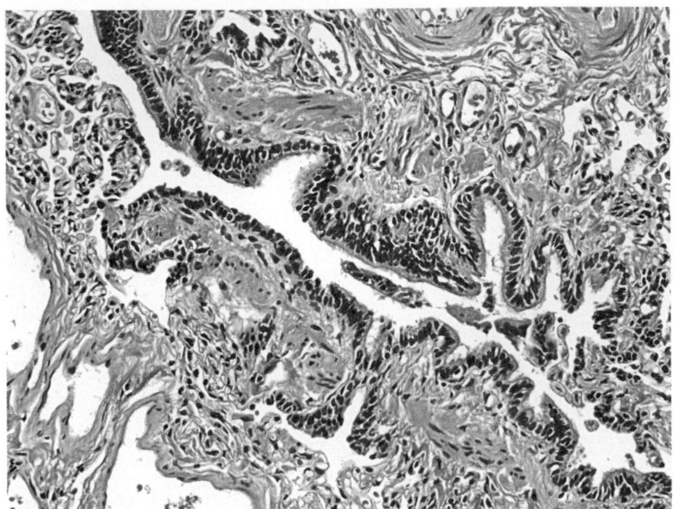

Fig. A17 **Bronchiolar tortuosity.** This clearly abnormal finding is commonly observed in the lungs of chronic smokers with degrees of chronic obstructive pulmonary disease (COPD), and in the vicinity of parenchymal scars or bulla. When this process is widespread in the biopsy material, consideration of small airways disease with constrictive bronchiolitis is always worthwhile (see Chapter 8).

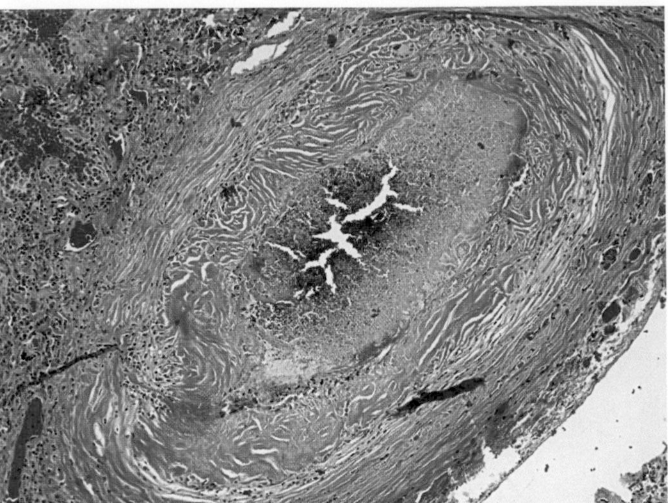

Fig. A18 **Calcified granuloma in pleura.** The presence of rare fibrotic and calcified granulomas varies in accordance with the distribution of regional endemic infections such as histoplasmosis (Mississippi and Ohio River valleys) and coccidioidomycosis (desert Southwest and California) (see Chapter 6).

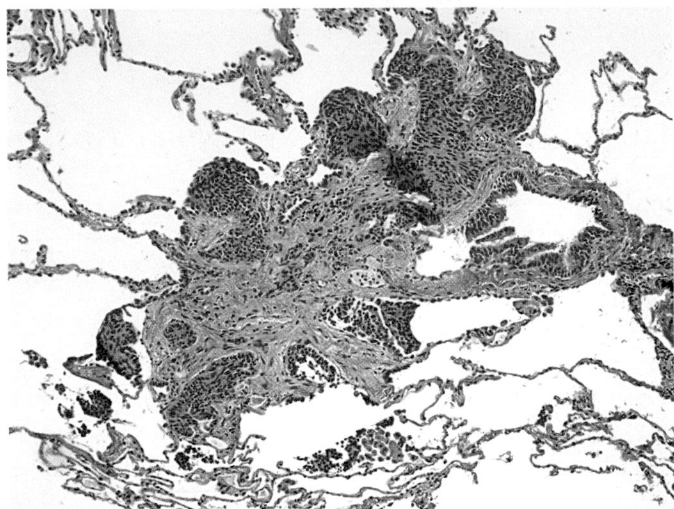

Fig. A19 **Carcinoid tumorlet.** These benign neuroendocrine cellular proliferations resemble their carcinoid tumor counterparts in peripheral lung, with a tendency toward spindled cellular profiles. They always occur within and around the bronchovascular sheaths. By definition, carcinoid tumorlets must not exceed 4 mm in maximal radial dimension. They may be longer than this on occasion, as they follow the terminal airways. They may occur with or without associated lung disease (see Chapter 13).

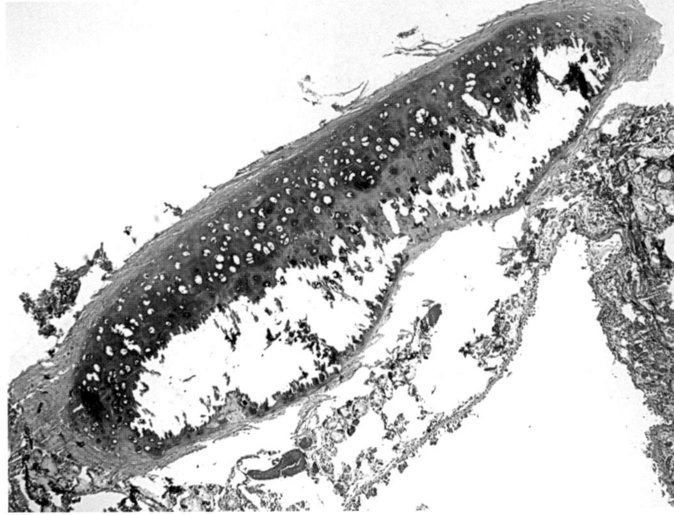

Fig. A20 **Cartilage ossification.** This phenomenon is a consequence of aging and has no clinical relevance.

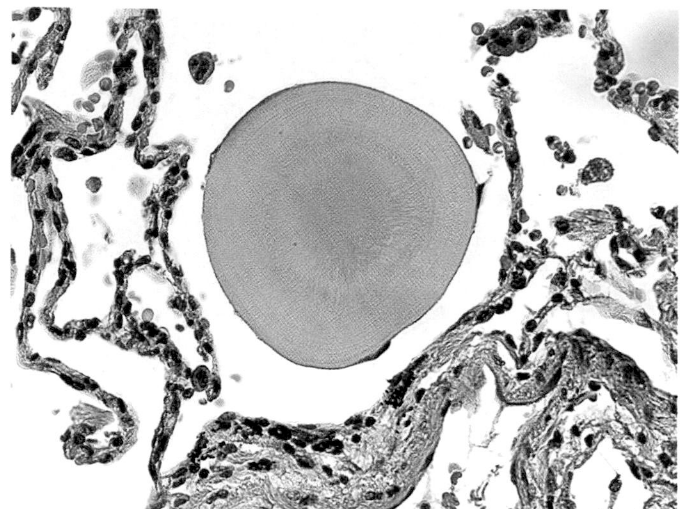

Fig. A21 **Corpora Amylacea.** These eosinophilic spherical structures are found sporadically within the airspaces. They are entirely nonspecific findings and they rotate plane-polarized light, weakly.

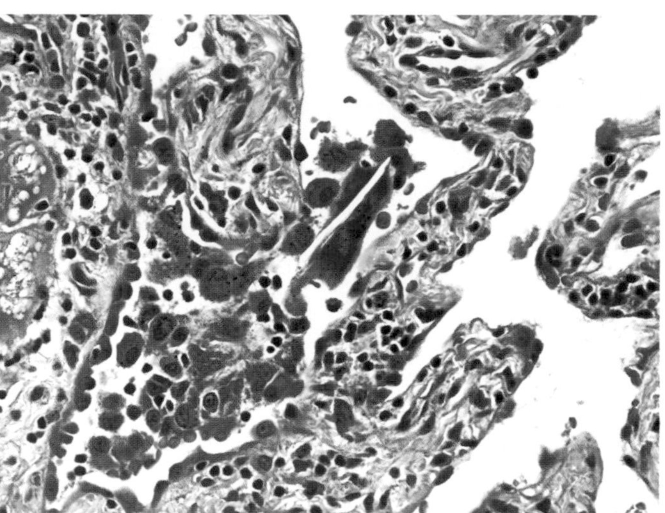

Fig. A22 **Cholesterol cleft in giant cell.** A common finding seen in association with granulomatous inflammation, cholesterol clefts in giant cells are more a manifestation of chronic airway obstruction than hypersensitivity pneumonitis (which is typically the first response from clinicians when they see these in biopsies).

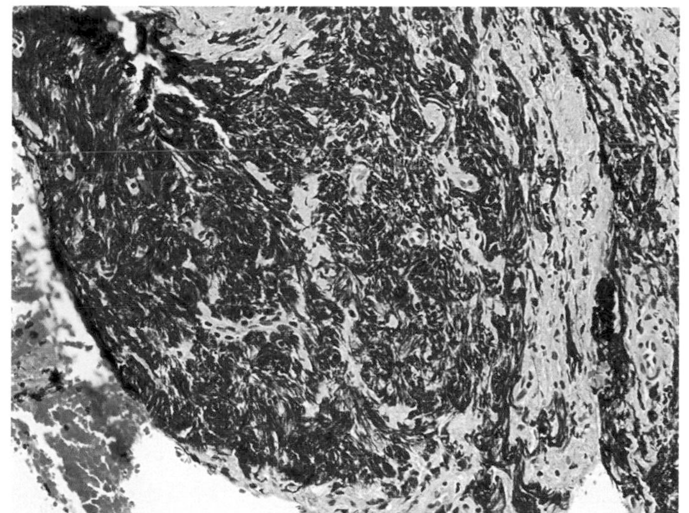

Fig. A23 **Crush artifact.** Acquisition and processing of lung samples may result in irrevocable tissue damage by crushing, especially so when the involved tissue is composed of fragile cells (typically lymphocytes or undifferentiated tumor cells). This example proved to be small cell undifferentiated carcinoma.

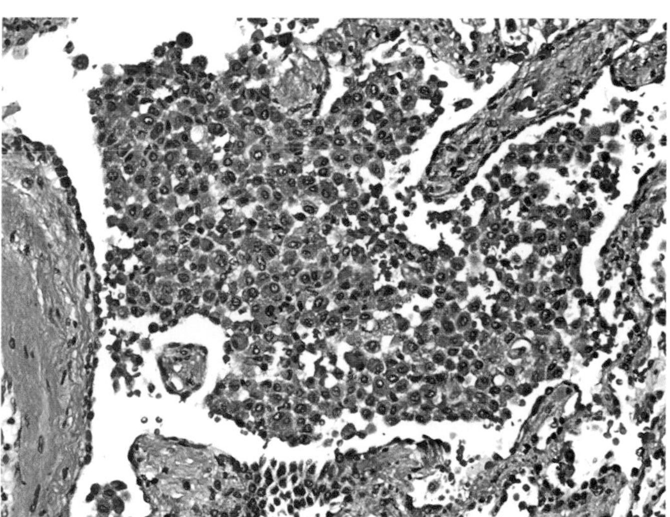

Fig. A24 **Desquamative interstitial pneumonia reaction (DIP-like).** Accumulation of macrophages in the alveolar spaces is the hallmark of the smoking-related diffuse lung disease known as "desquamative interstitial pneumonia." Unfortunately, a wide spectrum of diseases with increased alveolar macrophages occur and the simple presence of dense alveolar macrophages is insufficient for a diagnosis of DIP (see Chapter 7). The term DIP-like reaction may be useful in situations where this finding is focal in the biopsy.

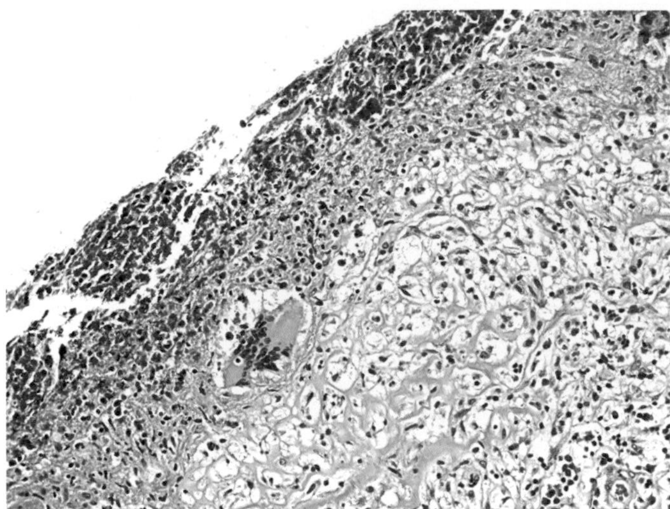

Fig. A25 **Eosinophilic pleuritis following pneumothorax.** Some occurrences of spontaneous pneumothorax may result in surgical intervention for repair of a persistent air leak. When this occurs, a portion of lung in the vicinity of the perforation may be sent to pathology. Dramatic inflammatory changes and peculiar parenchymal fibrosis may be seen, often accompanied by tissue eosinophilia.

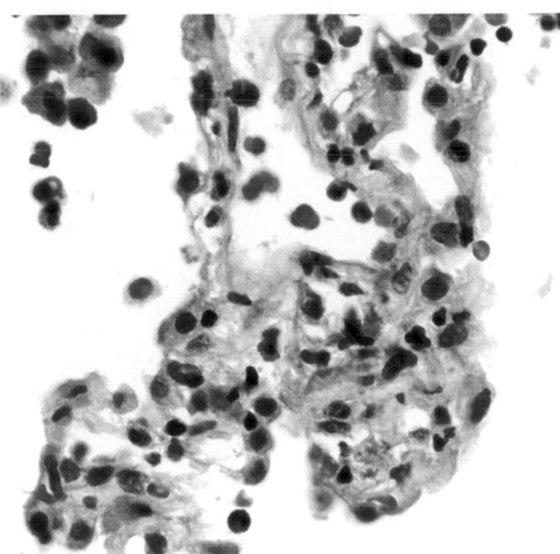

Fig. A26 **Eosinophils in a smoker.** As a general rule, extravascular eosinophils are a significant finding in lung biopsies. It is essential to remember that smokers typically have increased tissue eosinophils, but never accompanied by evidence of acute lung injury, unless significant.

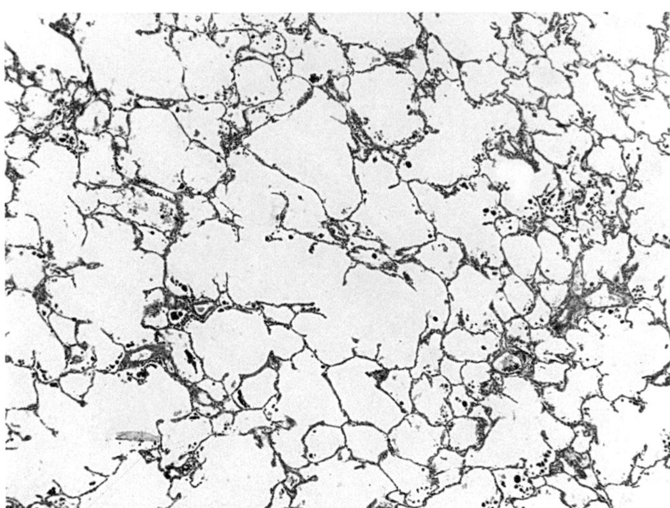

Fig. A27 **Emphysema centriacinar, mild.** As a general rule, mild emphysema is not graded microscopically, although its presence is clearly evident.

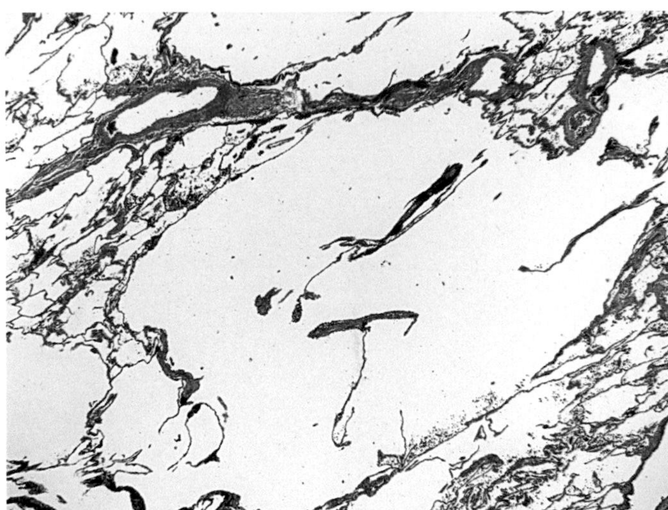

Fig. A28 **Emphysema centriacinar, severe.** When this degree of emphysema is observed throughout the biopsy specimen, the patient typically has well-recognized chronic obstructive pulmonary disease (COPD) clinically.

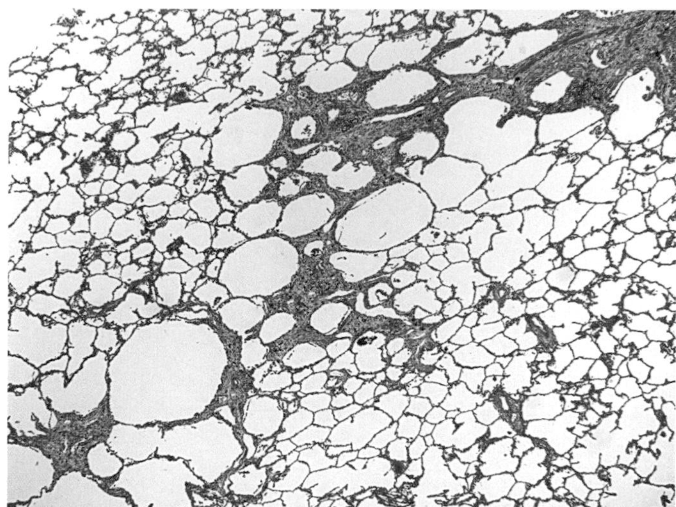

Fig. A29 **Emphysema, paraseptal.** This form of airspace dilatation presumably occurs as a result of traction accentuated at the periphery of the lobule. This phenomenon occurs more commonly in the upper lobes and probably plays a role in the formation of apical bulla and the occurrence of pneumothorax.

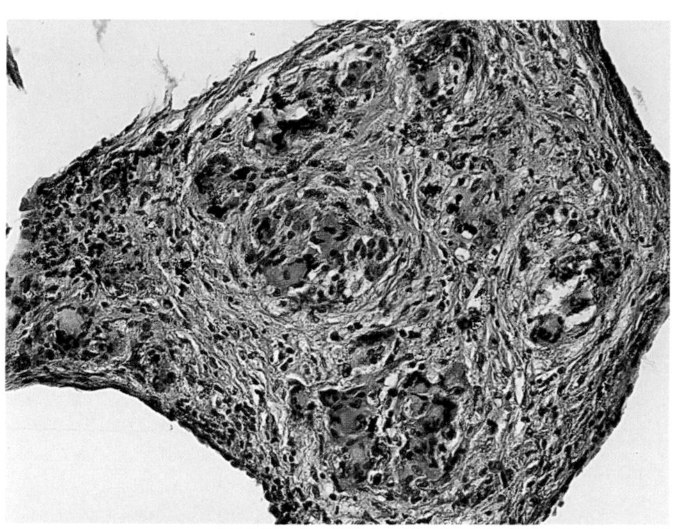

Fig. A30 **Vascular elastic tissue encrustation ("endogenous pneumoconiosis").** Elastic fibers of pulmonary veins may become encrusted with iron in situations where chronic passive congestion or other forms of chronic hemorrhage supervene. The encrusted fibers may appear brown, gray or black, and stain with the Prussian blue histochemical method for iron. A giant cell reaction, with engulfed fiber fragments, often occurs in the immediate vicinity of the affected vessel.

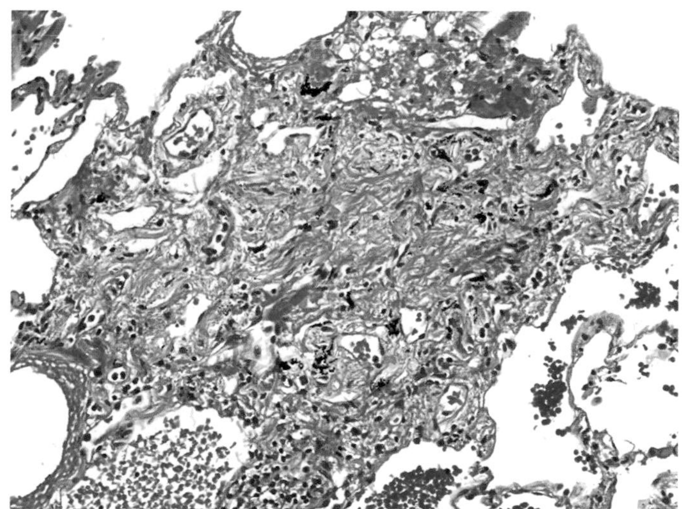

Fig. A31 **Focal parenchymal scar.** Focal scars, such as that illustrated here, are entirely nonspecific, especially when they occur singly.

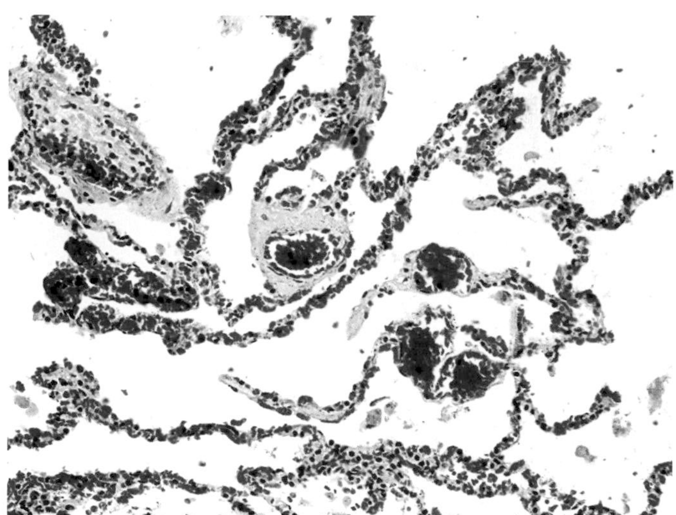

Fig. A32 **Formalin (artifactual) pigmentation.** Inadequately buffered formalin interacts with blood to produce a brown crystalline precipitate.

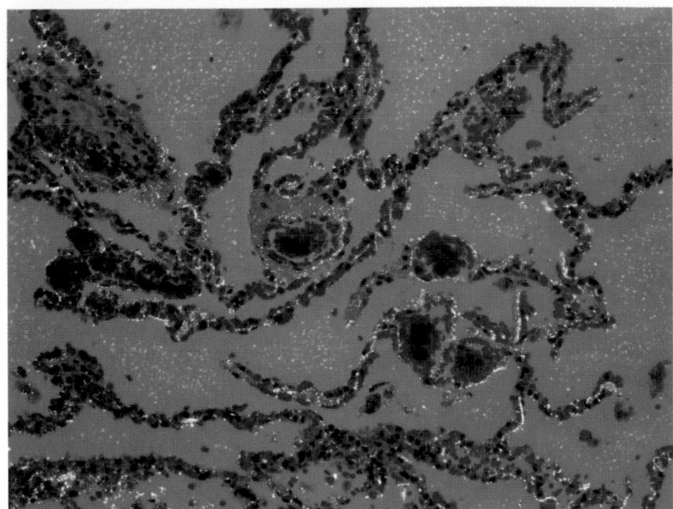

Fig. A33 **Formalin pigmentation under polarized light.** A simple method to verify the presence of formalin pigment is the use of plane-polarized light. Formalin pigment is birefringent.

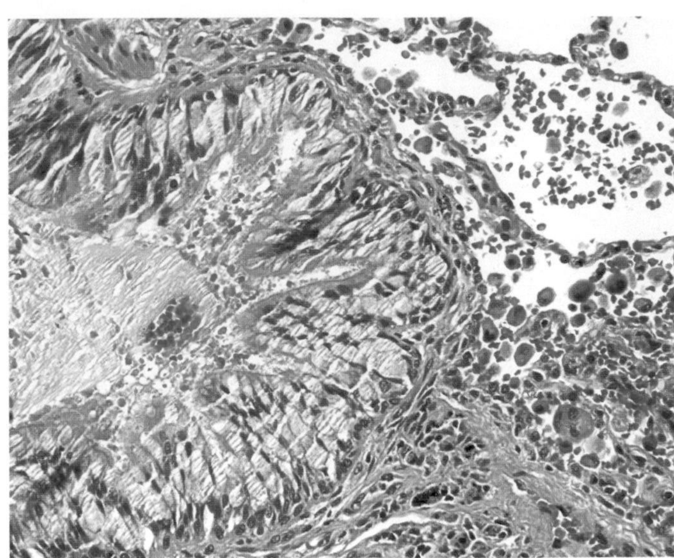

Fig. A34 **Goblet cell hyperplasia in a smoker.** Chronic irritation caused by cigarette smoke induces hyperplasia of mucus-secreting goblet cells in bronchial epithelium.

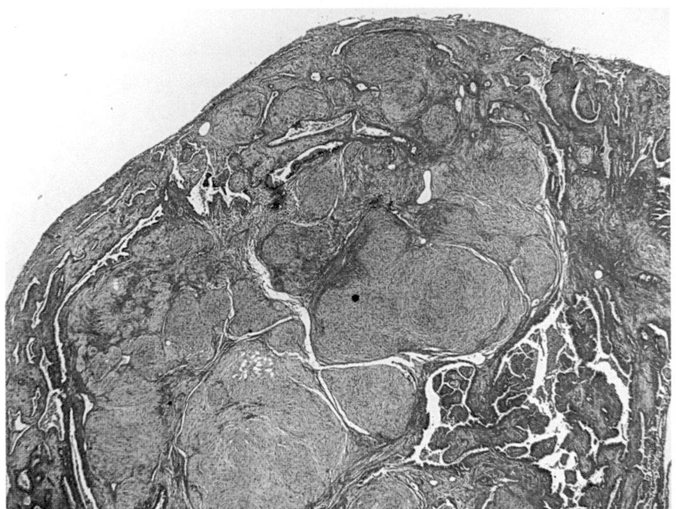

Fig. A35 **Hamartoma.** These distinctive benign lung lesions are so well circumscribed that they tend to "shell out" of the lung parenchyma on gross examination. They are composed of an admixture of mesenchymal cells, mature cartilage, fat, and epithelium. Calcification may be present.

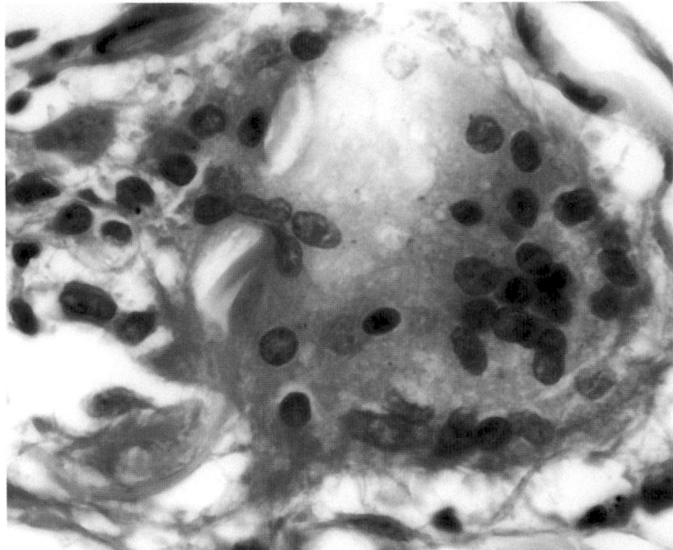

Fig. A36 **Iatrogenic foreign material in giant cell.** Patients who undergo extensive surgical procedures, or require recurrent venous access for therapy, may have isolated giant cells containing foreign material.

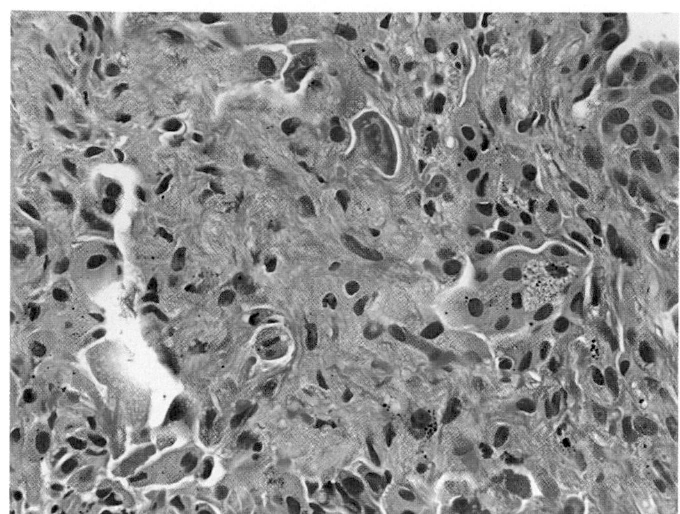

Fig. A37 **Kuhn's hyaline.** Eosinophilic material resembling Mallory's hyaline, may be observed in type II epithelial cells as a nonspecific finding in a number of lung diseases and disorders. The material is composed of condensed intermediate filaments.

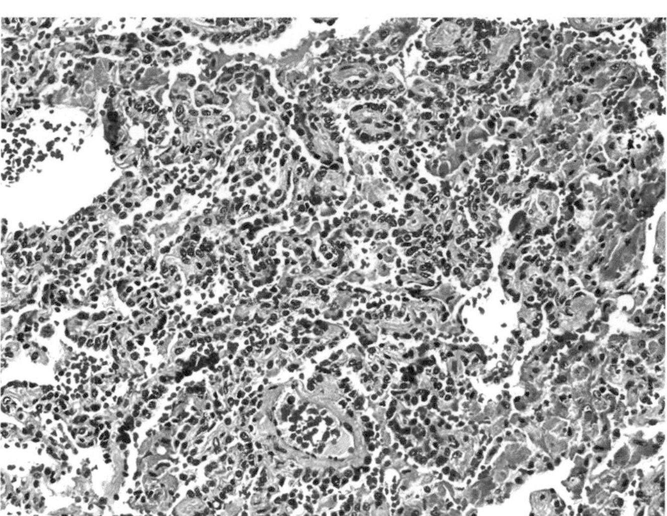

Fig. A38 **Lambertosis (bronchiolar metaplasia).** Bronchiolar epithelial metaplasia may occur as a consequence of chronic irritation and other injury to the terminal airways. Because the canals of Lambert (direct communication channels that exist between terminal airways and laterally adjacent alveoli) are often involved, the term *lambertosis* has been coined. A better term is *bronchiolar* or *peribronchiolar metaplasia*.

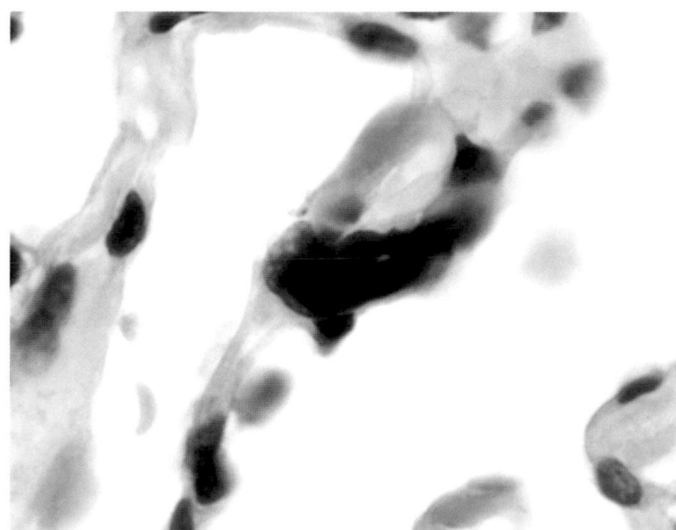

Fig. A39 **Megakaryocyte in alveolar septum.** Megakaryocytes may be seen frequently in surgical lung biopsy specimens as an incidental finding.

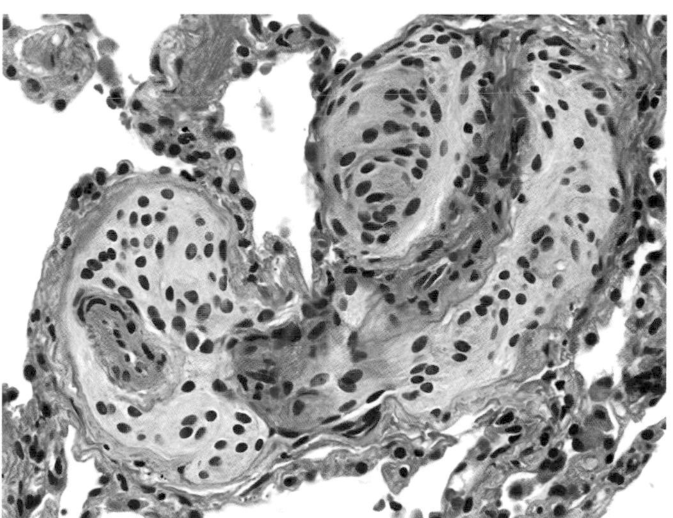

Fig. A40 **Meningothelial-like nodule.** Previously referred to as "minute pulmonary chemodectomas," these perivenular lesions seem to be associated with chronic hypoxia, although no specific etiology or normal cellular progenitor for them has yet been identified.

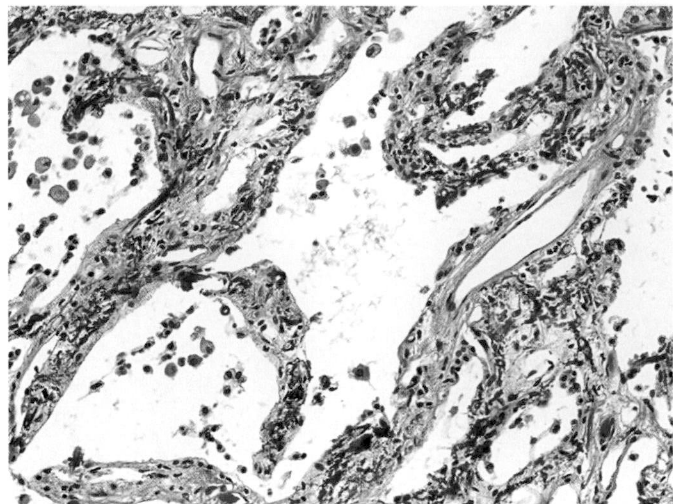

Fig. A41 **Metastatic alveolar calcification.** Chronic hemodialysis and disorders that result in hypercalcemia may lead to extensive pulmonary calcification. The finding is often asymptomatic clinically and differs from dystrophic calcification by the lack of osseous metaplasia (see Chapter 7 –Dendriform calcification).

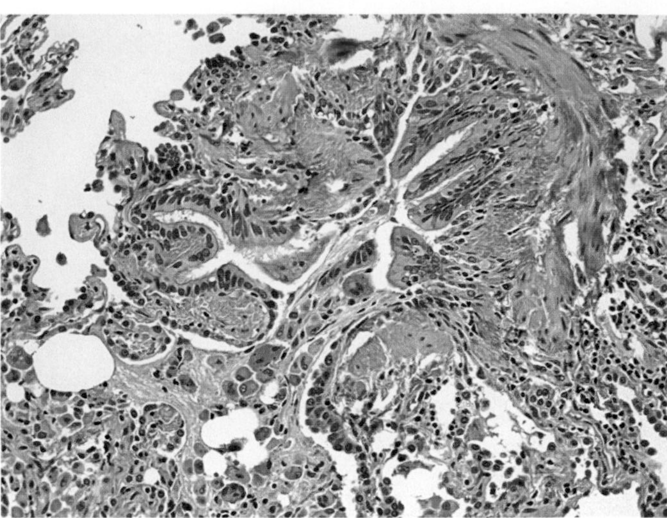

Fig. A42 **Mucostasis, early.** The early manifestation of goblet cell hyperplasia and excess mucus production may be seen as extrusion of mucus into alveolar ducts from terminal airways.

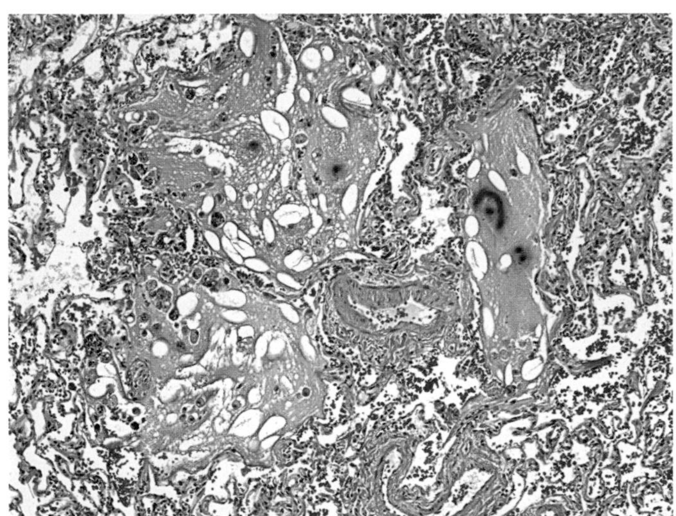

Fig. A43 **Mucostasis, advanced.** Alveolar spaces may become filled with mucin in settings of advanced mucus obstruction of the airways. When more than a few airspaces are involved, a careful search for neoplastic epithelium is in order, as mucinous infiltrates may be a manifestation of mucinous bronchioloalveolar carcinoma.

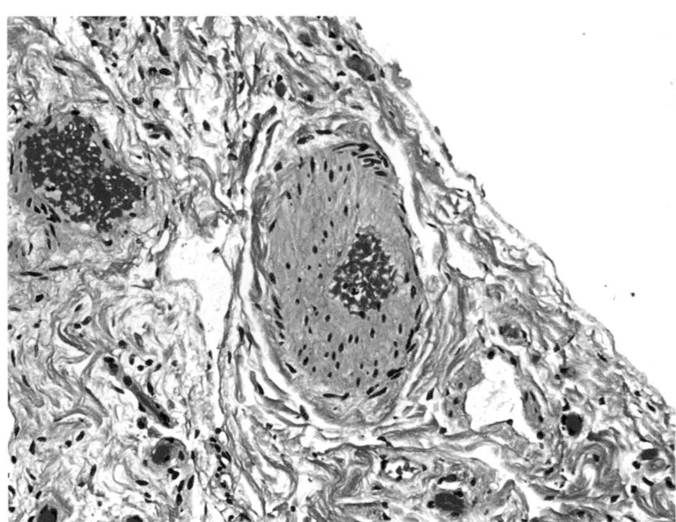

Fig. A44 **Muscular hyperplasia in pleural vein.** This incidental finding can be quite dramatic. Such focal nonspecific muscular hyperplasia in veins traversing the pleura is probably an age-related phenomenon.

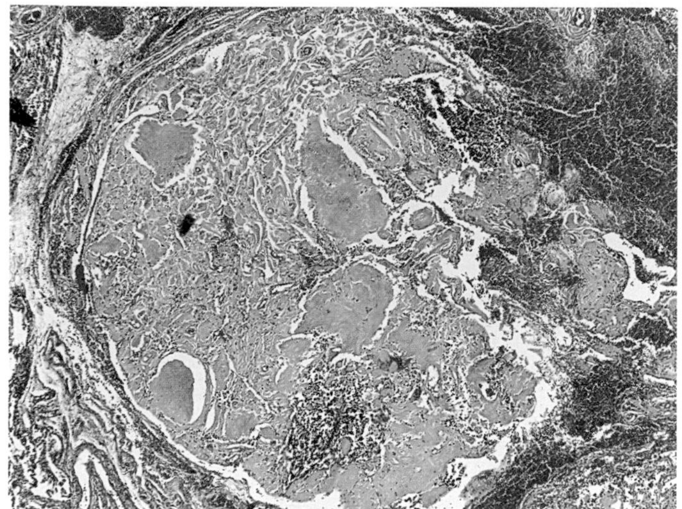

Fig. A45 **Nodular amyloid.** A specific manifestation of amyloid, nodular amyloid produces mass lesions, but most often has no relation to systemic amyloidosis.

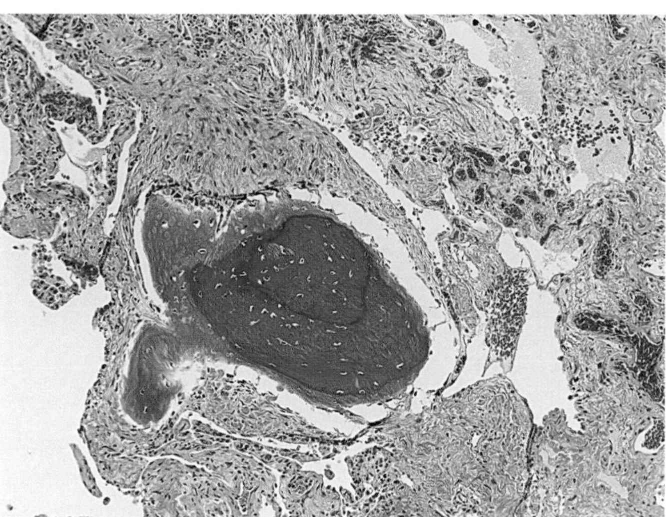

Fig. A46 **Osseous metaplasia in fibrosis.** Small nodules of bone may be seen in lung processes that produce fibrosis.

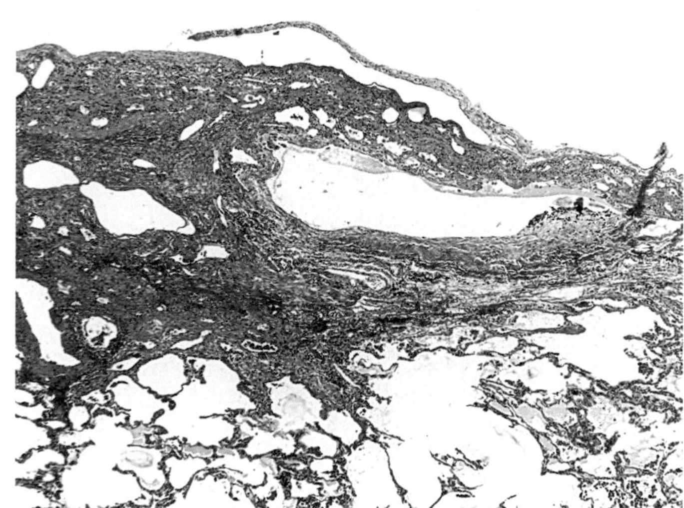

Fig. A47 **Pleural bleb.** In contrast to *bulla,* blebs are entirely intrapleural.

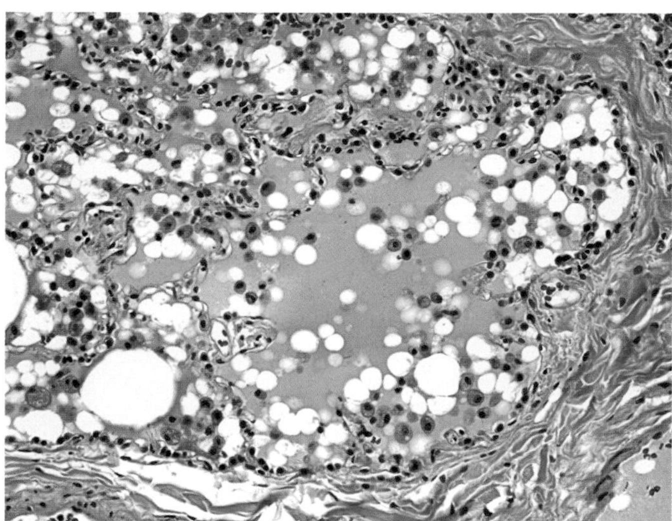

Fig. A48 **"Pseudo" lipid.** Distinctive artifactual gas vacuoles may occur in areas of hemorrhage or inflammation.

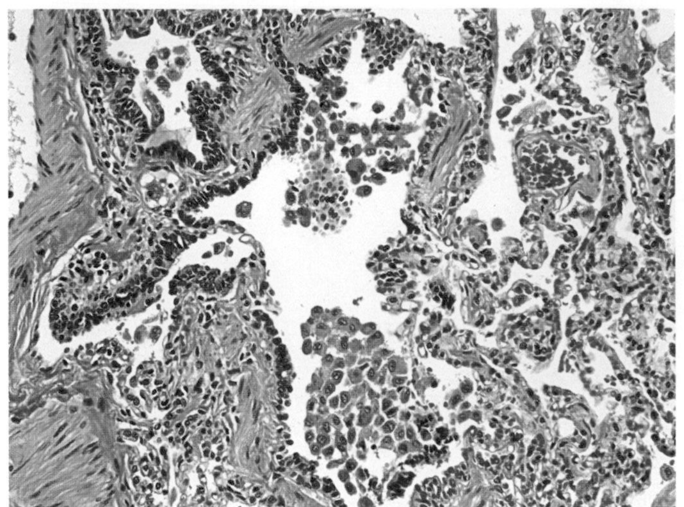

Fig. A49 **Respiratory bronchiolitis.** This very common smoking-related airway injury is often not the principal pathology of the biopsy sample. Rarely, respiratory bronchiolitis may occur as the primary pathologic process in a relatively specific clinical–radiologic context, and absent findings to suggest another disease (see Chapters 7 and 8 for further discussion of respiratory bronchiolitis).

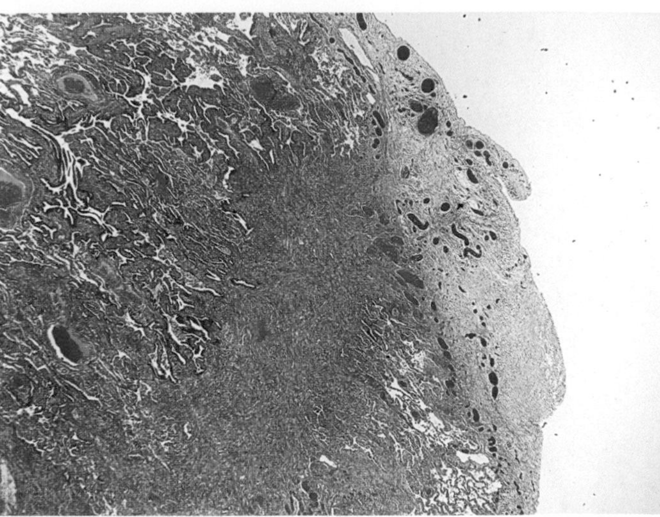

Fig. A50 **Scar at the tip of a lobe.** Nonspecific scarring may occur in peripheral lung, often in characteristic locations (such as the tip of the middle lobe or lingula).

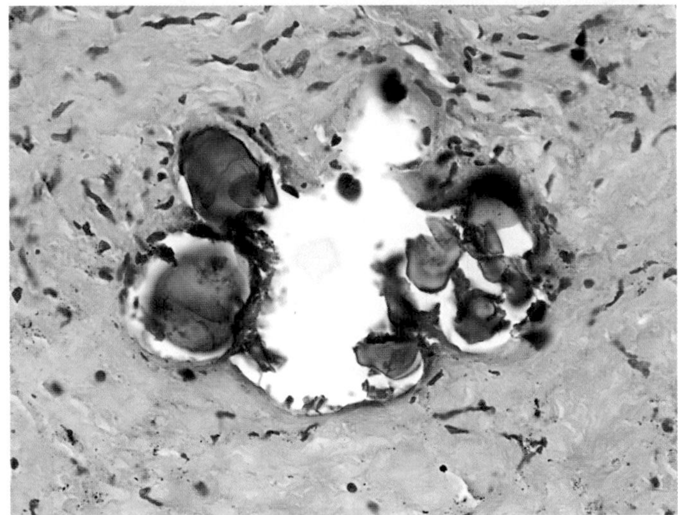

Fig. A51 **Schaumann bodies in fibrosis.** These irregular calcified lamellar bodies (also known as conchoidal bodies) are an indicator of granulomatous inflammation, whether current or resolved. They are commonly observed in the granulomas of patients with sarcoidosis, but are not specific for this disease.

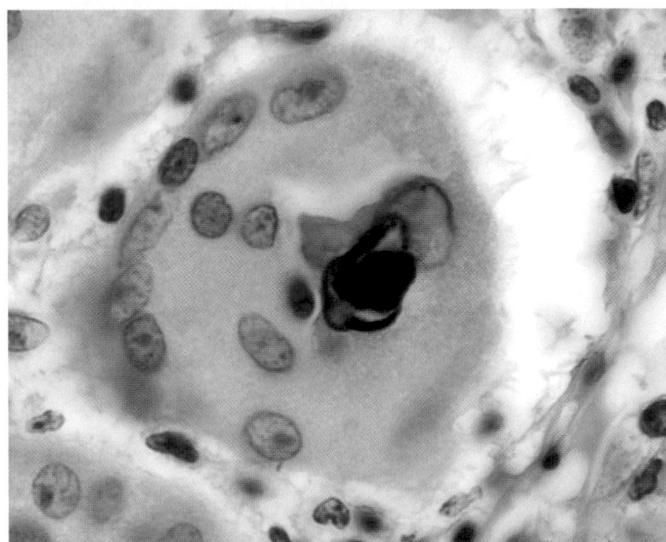

Fig. A52 **Schaumann bodies in a giant cell.** Schaumann bodies in giant cells are a nonspecific finding in granulomatous inflammation and alone do not constitute evidence for sarcoidosis.

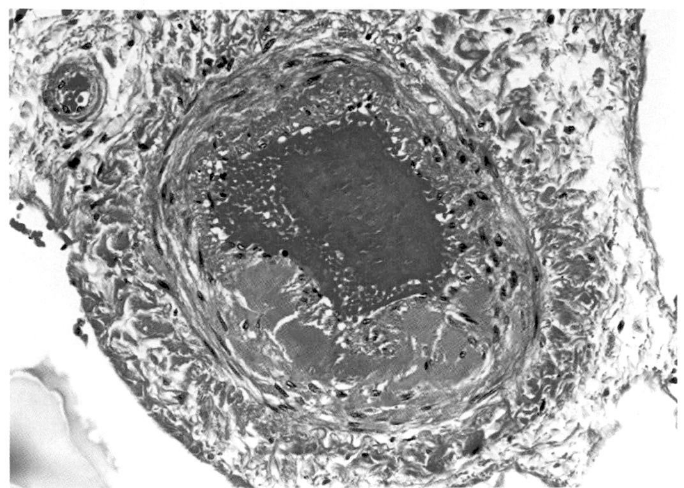

Fig. A53 **Senile amyloid in pulmonary arteries.** Generalized senile amyloidosis is an incidental finding, and may be widespread at autopsy. The biochemical type is ATTR (transthyretin).

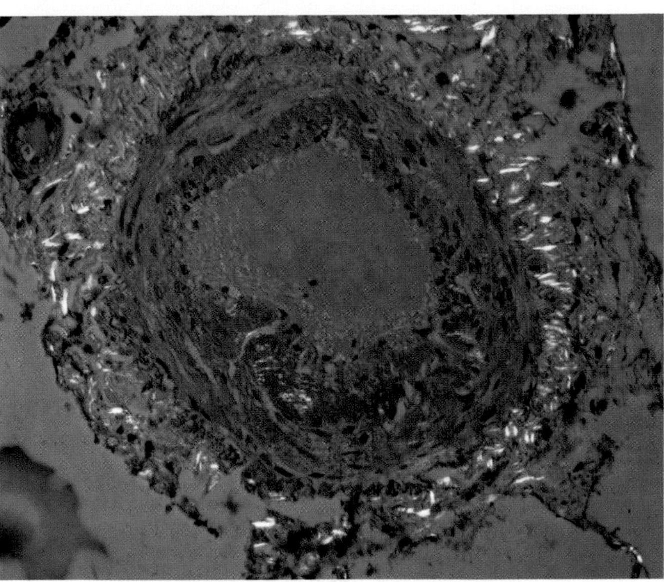

Fig. A54 **Senile amyloid (Congo red–polarized light).** Apple green birefringence is evident in a Congo red stain.

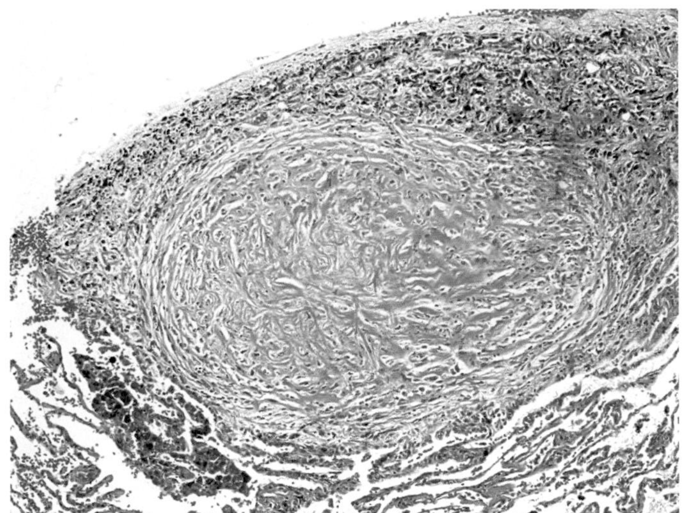

Fig. A55 **Silicate nodule in pleura.** Rare small silicate nodules may be seen in patients following inhalational exposure. The mere presence of a silicate nodule is not sufficient evidence for the pneumoconiosis (see Ch. 9 for further discussion).

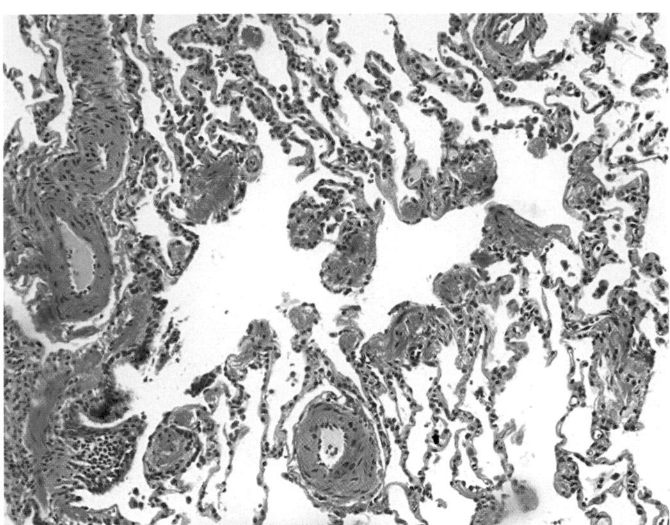

Fig. A56 **Smooth muscle hyperplasia of alveolar ducts in a smoker.** Prominence of the smooth muscle bundles, present at the tips of alveoli opening onto alveolar ducts, may be seen as a consequence of smoking and other airway irritation.

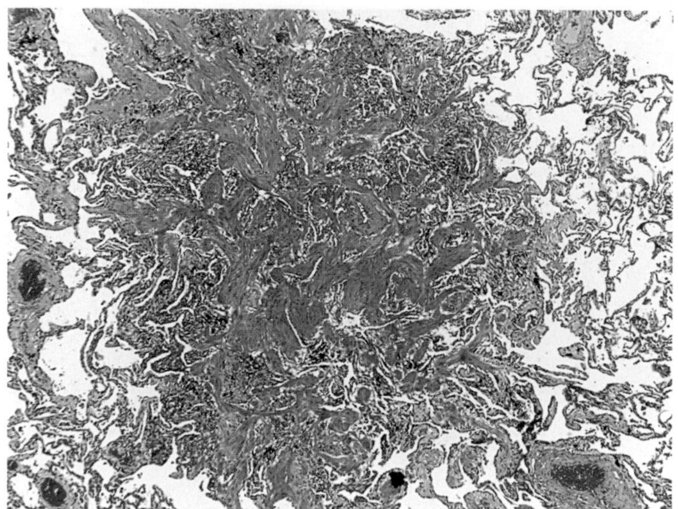

Fig. A57 **Smooth muscle nodule.** Peculiar nodules of smooth muscle fascicles arranged in a stellate shape (sometimes with admixed fibrosis) are frequently seen in the lungs of smokers. They differ from the stellate scars of resolved (inactive) pulmonary Langerhans cell histiocytosis by the presence of excess smooth muscle. They probably represent obliterated terminal airways with associated smooth muscle proliferation.

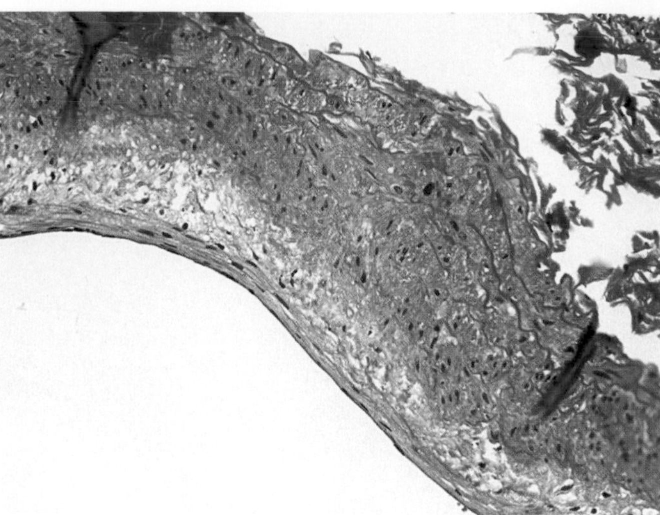

Fig. A58 **Subendothelial fibrosis in pulmonary arteries.** This finding is often more evident in larger pulmonary arteries. The significance is unknown in the absence of other vasculopathic changes to suggest hypertension, or thrombosis/embolization with recanalization.

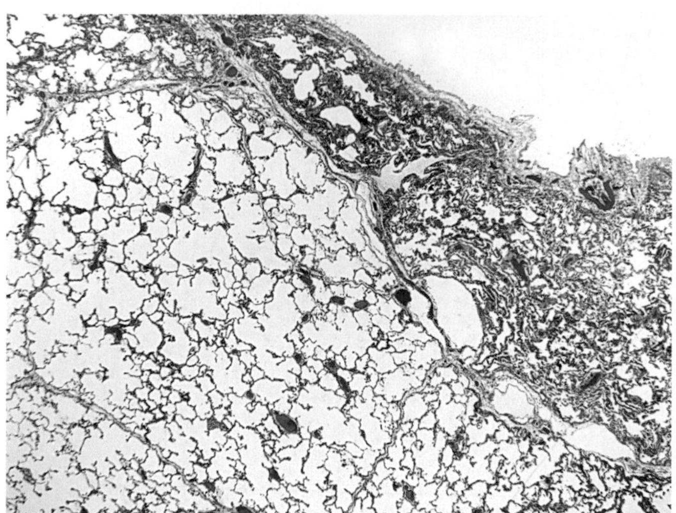

Fig. A59 **Technical artifact from inflation fixation.** Although uncommon, aggressive fixation by syringe and needle may result in distinctive artifacts. Fortunately, the benefits outweigh the risks, as it is often easier to ignore prominent septal and lymphatic dilatation than to diagnose disease accurately in a poorly fixed, atelectatic lung biopsy.

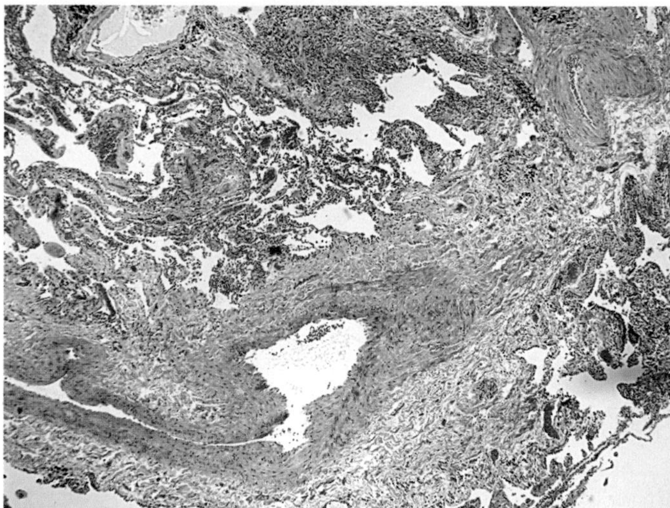

Fig. A60 **Tortuous arteries near scar.** Scar tissue in the lung may produce peculiar vascular tortuosity. If the presence of such change causes concern, a search for other vessels away from scar may be helpful in excluding true vasculopathic disease.

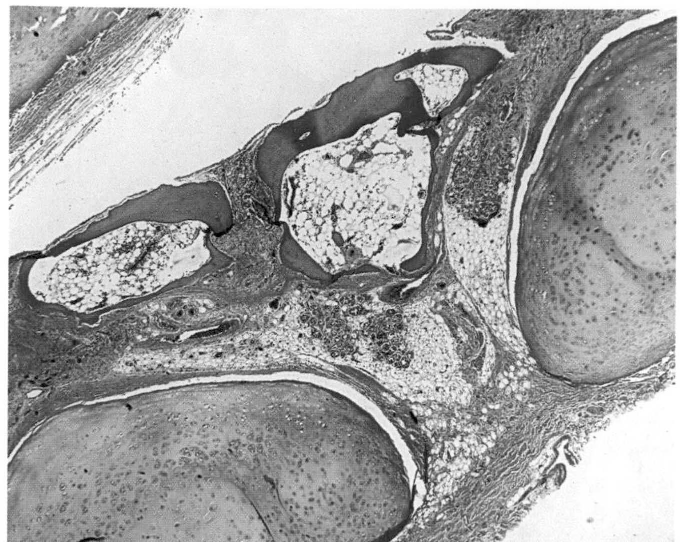

Fig. A61 **Tracheobronchopathia osteochondroplastica.** This rare condition is characterized by the presence of submucosal nodules of metaplastic bone and cartilage typically identified endoscopically in the trachea and major bronchi. In this photomicrograph, nodules of mature bone can be seen between the tracheal cartilage rings, on the mucosal side.

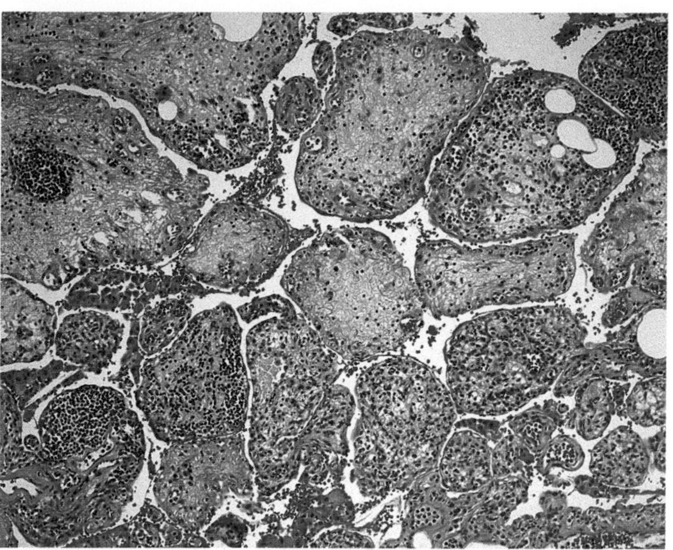

Fig. A61a **Transmogrification.** Bullous placental transmogrification (also known as localized giant bullous emphysema) is a rare but distinctive localized cystic lesion that occurs in young to middle aged adults. This lesion has been traditionally regarded as a form of emphysema, but recent studies suggest an abnormality of interstitial cells with secondary formation of cysts (Cavazza A, Lantuejoul S, Sartori G, Bigiani N, Maiorana A, Pasquinelli G, Paci M, Rossi G.: Placental transmogrification of the lung: clinicopathologic, immunohistochemical and molecular study of two cases, with particular emphasis on the interstitial clear cells. Hum Pathol. 2004 Apr;35(4):517-21.) The etiology is unknown and local resection is curative.

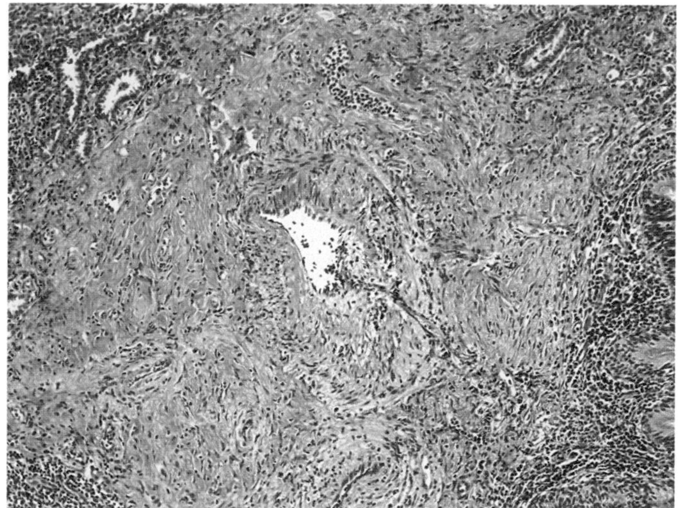

Fig. A62 **Vascular sclerosis in scar tissue.** Arteries entrapped in dense scar may develop medial fibroelastosis.

Index

B

D

E

F

G

H

I

J

K

L

M

N

Q

R

S

T

U

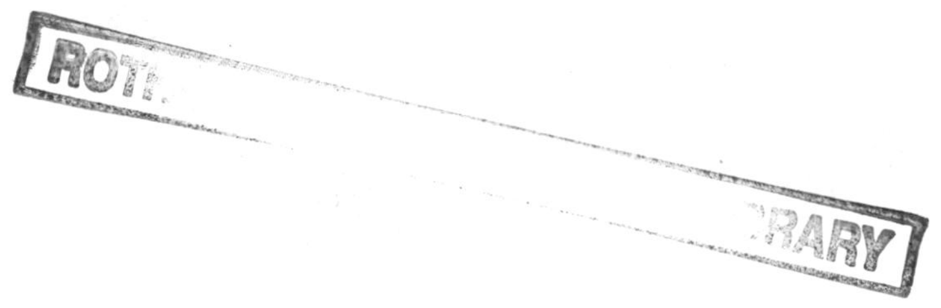